# CURRENT PRACTICE OF RADIOLOGY

# CURRENT THERAPY/CURRENT PRACTICE SERIES

***Bardin***
Current Therapy in Endocrinology and Metabolism
***Bayless***
Current Therapy in Gastroenterology and Liver Disease
***Brain, Carbone***
Current Therapy in Hematology-Oncology
***Callaham***
Current Practice of Emergency Medicine
***Cameron***
Current Surgical Therapy
***Cherniack***
Current Therapy in Respiratory Disease
***Cooke, Frohlich***
Current Management of Hypertensive and Vascular Diseases
***Ernst, Stanley***
Current Therapy in Vascular Surgery
***Fazio***
Current Therapy in Colon and Rectal Surgery
***Foley, Payne***
Current Therapy of Pain
***Garcia, Mastroianni, Amelar, Dubin***
Current Therapy of Infertility
***Gates***
Current Therapy in Otolaryngology—Head and Neck Surgery
***Glassock***
Current Therapy in Nephrology and Hypertension
***Grillo, Austen, Wilkins, Mathisen, Vlahakes***
Current Therapy in Cardiothoracic Surgery
***Horowitz***
Current Management of Arrhythmias
***Hurst***
Current Therapy in Cardiovascular Disease
***Jeejeebhoy***
Current Therapy in Nutrition
***Johnson, Griffin***
Current Therapy in Neurologic Disease
***Kadir***
Current Practice of Interventional Radiology
***Kaplan***
Current Therapy in Pediatric Infectious Disease
***Kass, Platt***
Current Therapy in Infectious Disease
***Kassirer***
Current Therapy in Internal Medicine
***Lichtenstein, Fauci***
Current Therapy in Allergy, Immunology, and Rheumatology
***Long***
Current Therapy in Neurological Surgery
***Marsh***
Current Therapy in Plastic and Reconstructive Surgery
***Myerson***
Current Therapy in Foot and Ankle Surgery
***Nelson***
Current Therapy in Neonatal-Perinatal Medicine
***Niederhuber***
Current Therapy in Oncology
***Parrillo***
Current Therapy in Critical Care Medicine
***Resnick, Kursh***
Current Therapy in Genitourinary Surgery
***Rogers***
Current Practice in Anesthesiology
***Spaeth, Katz***
Current Therapy in Ophthalmic Surgery
***Thrall***
Current Practice of Radiology
***Torg, Welsh, Shephard***
Current Therapy in Sports Medicine
***Trunkey, Lewis***
Current Therapy of Trauma

# CURRENT PRACTICE OF RADIOLOGY

JAMES H. THRALL, M.D.

*Juan M. Taveras Professor of Radiology*
*Harvard Medical School*
*Radiologist-in-Chief*
*Massachusetts General Hospital*
*Boston, Massachusetts*

*with* 1851 *illustrations*

B.C. Decker
An Imprint of Mosby–Year Book, Inc.

Mosby

B.C. Decker

Executive Editor: Susan M. Gay
Senior Managing Editor: Lynne Gery
Project Supervisor: Allan S. Kleinberg
Manufacturing Supervisor: Betty Richmond



Printed in the United States of America.

Mosby–Year Book, Inc.
11830 Westline Industrial Drive
St. Louis, Missouri 63146

**NOTICE:** The authors and publisher have made every effort to ensure that the patient care recommended herein, including choice of drugs and drug dosages, is in accord with the accepted standards and practice at the time of publication. However, since research and regulation constantly change clinical standards, the reader is urged to check the product information sheet included in the package of each drug, which includes recommended doses, warnings, and contraindications. This is particularly important with new or infrequently used drugs.

**Library of Congress Cataloging-in-Publication Data**

Current practice of radiology / [edited by] James H. Thrall.
p. cm. – (Current therapy series)
Includes bibliographical references and index.
ISBN 1-55664-385-3
1. Radiography, Medical. I. Thrall, James H. II. Series.
[DNLM: 1. Technology, Radiologic. 2. Radiography. WN 160 C976 1993]
RC78.C86 1993
616.07′57–dc20
DNLM/DLC
for Library of Congress

93-10273
CIP

93 94 95 96 97 GW/MY 9 8 7 6 5 4 3 2 1

# CONTRIBUTORS

RONALD S. ADLER, Ph.D., M.D.
Assistant Professor of Radiology, University of Michigan Medical School; Director, Musculoskeletal Division, University of Michigan Medical Center, Ann Arbor, Michigan

BENNETT A. ALFORD, M.D.
Associate Professor of Radiology and Pediatrics, University of Virginia Hospital and Children's Medical Center, Charlottesville, Virginia

PIRAN ALIABADI, M.D.
Visiting Associate Professor of Radiology, Harvard Medical School; Radiologist, Director of Emergency Radiology Service, and Director, Division of Quality Assurance, Brigham and Women's Hospital, Boston, Massachusetts

HANNU J. ARONEN, M.D., Ph.D.
Assistant Professor of Radiology, University of Helsinki, Helsinki, Finland; Postdoctoral Research Fellow, Nuclear Magnetic Resonance Center, Massachusetts General Hospital, Boston, Massachusetts

JUDITH M. ASH, M.D., FRCPC, ABNM
Associate Professor of Radiology, University of Toronto Faculty of Medicine; Senior Staff Radiologist, Department of Diagnostic Imaging, The Hospital for Sick Children, Toronto, Ontario, Canada

GREGORY V. BABIGIAN, M.D.
Assistant Professor of Radiology, Sections of Neuroradiology and Vascular Interventional Radiology, State University of New York at Stony Brook Health Sciences Center, Stony Brook, New York

DEMETRIUS H. BAGLEY, M.D.
Professor of Urology and Radiology, Jefferson Medical College of Thomas Jefferson University, Philadelphia, Pennsylvania

STEPHEN R. BAKER, M.D.
Professor and Chairman, Department of Radiology, University of Medicine and Dentistry of New Jersey/New Jersey Medical School; Director of Radiology, University Hospital, Newark, New Jersey

WILLIAM S. BALL, Jr., M.D.
Associate Professor of Radiology and Pediatrics, University of Cincinnati College of Medicine and Children's Hospital Medical Center; Chief, Section of Pediatric Neuroradiology, Children's Hospital Medical Center, Cincinnati, Ohio

EMIL J. BALTHAZAR, M.D.
Professor of Radiology and Chief of Gastrointestinal Radiology, New York University–Tisch–Bellevue Medical Center, New York, New York

MICHAEL A. BETTMANN, M.D.

Professor of Radiology, Boston University School of Medicine; Interim Director of Radiology, University Hospital, and Chief, Cardiovascular Radiology, Boston University Medical Center, Boston, Massachusetts

EDWARD I. BLUTH, M.D., FACR

Clinical Professor of Radiology, Tulane University School of Medicine; Associate Head, Section of Ultrasound, Ochsner Clinic, New Orleans, Louisiana

ROBERT L. BREE, M.D.

Associate Professor of Radiology, University of Michigan Medical Center; Chief, Radiology Services, Veterans Affairs Medical Center, Ann Arbor, Michigan

R. JAMES BRENNER, M.D., J.D.

Associate Clinical Professor of Radiology, University of California, Los Angeles, School of Medicine; Director, Tower Breast Imaging Center, Los Angeles, California

BRADLEY R. BUCHBINDER, M.D.

Instructor in Radiology, Harvard Medical School; Staff Neuroradiologist, Massachusetts General Hospital, Boston, Massachusetts

WILLIAM H. BUSH, Jr., M.D., FACR

Professor of Radiology, and Director of Genitourinary Radiology, Department of Radiology, University of Washington School of Medicine, Seattle, Washington

BARBARA L. CARTER, M.D.

Professor of Radiology and Otolaryngology, Tufts University School of Medicine; Chief, ENT Radiology, New England Medical Center, Boston, Massachusetts

MAURICIO CASTILLO, M.D.

Associate Professor of Radiology and Chief of Neuroradiology, University of North Carolina at Chapel Hill School of Medicine, Chapel Hill, North Carolina

STANLEY M. CHERNISH, M.D.

Associate Professor of Medicine, Indiana University School of Medicine; Consultant in Research, Methodist Hospital of Indiana, Indianapolis, Indiana

ROBERT H. CLEVELAND, M.D.

Associate Professor of Radiology, Harvard Medical School; Radiologist, The Children's Hospital, Boston, Massachusetts

R. EDWARD COLEMAN, M.D.

Professor of Radiology and Director of Nuclear Medicine, Duke University Medical Center, Durham, North Carolina

B. DAVID COLLIER, Jr., M.D.

Professor of Radiology and Director of Nuclear Medicine, Medical College of Wisconsin; Chief, Nuclear Medicine Service, Clement J. Zablocki Veterans Affairs Medical Center, and Director of Nuclear Medicine, Milwaukee County Medical Complex and Froedtert Memorial Hospital, Milwaukee, Wisconsin

HUGH D. CURTIN, M.D.

Professor of Radiology and Otolaryngology, University of Pittsburgh School of Medicine; Director of Radiology, Eye and Ear Institute, Pittsburgh, Pennsylvania

DAVID J. CURTIS, M.D., FACR

Professor of Radiology, George Washington University School of Medicine and Health Sciences, Washington, D.C.; Clinical Professor of Radiology and Nuclear Medicine, Uniformed Services University of the Health Sciences, Bethesda, Maryland

THOMAS R. DAMIANO, M.D.

Assistant Clinical Professor of Radiology, University of Colorado Health Sciences Center, Denver; Neuroradiologist, Fitzsimons Army Medical Center, Aurora, Colorado

KENNETH R. DAVIS, M.D.

Professor of Radiology, Harvard Medical School; Staff Neuroradiologist, Massachusetts General Hospital, Boston, Massachusetts

SHEILA D. DAVIS, M.D.

Associate Professor of Radiology, Cornell University Medical College; Associate Attending Radiologist, The New York Hospital, New York, New York

GERALD D. DODD III, M.D.

Assistant Professor of Radiology, University of Pittsburgh School of Medicine; Director of Sonography, Presbyterian-University Hospital, Pittsburgh, Pennsylvania

ANDRÉ J. DUERINCKX, M.D., Ph.D.

Assistant Professor, University of California, Los Angeles, School of Medicine, Los Angeles, and Veterans Administration Medical Center, West Los Angeles, California

ROBERT R. EDELMAN, M.D.

Associate Professor of Radiology, Harvard Medical School; Director of Magnetic Resonance Imaging, Beth Israel Hospital, Boston, Massachusetts

ALLEN D. ELSTER, M.D.

Professor of Radiology and Director of Magnetic Resonance Imaging, Bowman Gray School of Medicine of Wake Forest University; Staff Neuroradiologist, North Carolina Baptist Hospital, Winston-Salem, North Carolina

PETER J. FECZKO, M.D.

Staff Radiologist, William Beaumont Hospital, Royal Oak, Michigan

MICHAEL P. FEDERLE, M.D.

Professor of Radiology, University of Pittsburgh School of Medicine, Pittsburgh, Pennsylvania

ARTHUR C. FLEISCHER, M.D.

Professor of Radiology and of Obstetrics and Gynecology, and Chief, Diagnostic Sonography, Vanderbilt University Medical Center, Nashville, Tennessee

BARRY D. FLETCHER, M.D.

Chairman, Department of Diagnostic Imaging, St. Jude Children's Research Hospital; Professor of Radiology and Pediatrics, University of Tennessee College of Medicine, Memphis, Tennessee

CALVIN H. FLOWERS, M.D.

Staff, Department of Radiology, Cook County Hospital, Chicago, Illinois

EDMUND A. FRANKEN, Jr., M.D.

Professor and Head, Department of Radiology, The University of Iowa College of Medicine; Director, Department of Radiology, The University of Iowa Hospitals and Clinics, Iowa City, Iowa

MARY F. GASKILL-SHIPLEY, M.D.

Assistant Professor of Radiology, University Hospital, Cincinnati, Ohio

G. SCOTT GAZELLE, M.D.

Instructor in Radiology, Harvard Medical School; Assistant Radiologist, Division of Gastrointestinal/Interventional Radiology, Massachusetts General Hospital, Boston, Massachusetts

WARREN B. GEFTER, M.D.

Professor of Radiology, University of Pennsylvania School of Medicine, Philadelphia, Pennsylvania

DAVID W. GELFAND, M.D.

Professor of Radiology, Bowman Gray School of Medicine of Wake Forest University; Attending Radiologist, North Carolina Baptist Hospital, Winston-Salem, North Carolina

HARRY K. GENANT, M.D.

Professor of Radiology, Medicine, and Orthopaedic Surgery; Chief, Skeletal Section, and Director, Osteoporosis Research Group, Department of Radiology, University of California, San Francisco, School of Medicine, San Francisco, California

MARYELLEN L. GIGER, Ph.D.

Associate Professor of Radiology, University of Chicago Pritzker School of Medicine, Chicago, Illinois

BARRY B. GOLDBERG, M.D.

Professor of Radiology, and Director, Division of Diagnostic Ultrasound, Department of Radiology, Jefferson Medical College of Thomas Jefferson University, Philadelphia, Pennsylvania

LUÍS FLÁVIO GONÇALVES, M.D.

Research Fellow in Ultrasound, Department of Radiology, Vanderbilt University Medical Center, Nashville, Tennessee

R. GILBERTO GONZÁLEZ, M.D., Ph.D.

Assistant Professor of Radiology, Harvard Medical School; Assistant Radiologist, Massachusetts General Hospital, Boston, Massachusetts

PHILIP C. GOODMAN, M.D.

Clinical Professor of Radiology, Duke University Medical Center, Durham, North Carolina

EDWARD G. GRANT, M.D.

Professor of Radiological Sciences, University of California, Los Angeles, School of Medicine; Chief, Radiology Services, Veterans Affairs Medical Center–West Los Angeles, Los Angeles, California

BARRY H. GROSS, M.D.

Professor of Radiology, University of Michigan Medical Center, Ann Arbor, Michigan

PETER F. HAHN, M.D., Ph.D.

Assistant Professor of Radiology, Harvard Medical School; Assistant Radiologist, Massachusetts General Hospital, Boston, Massachusetts

JACK O. HALLER, M.D.

Professor and Vice Chairman, Department of Radiology, State University of New York Downstate Medical Center; Director of Pediatric Radiology, King County Hospital, Brooklyn, New York

MARGARET E. HANSEN, M.D.

Assistant Professor of Radiology, University of Texas Southwestern School of Medicine; Attending Radiologist, Special Procedures Section, Parkland Memorial Hospital, Veterans Affairs Medical Center, and Zale-Lipshy University Hospital, Dallas, Texas

MICHAEL W. HANSON, M.D.

Assistant Professor of Radiology, Associate in Internal Medicine, and Chief of Nuclear Cardiology, Duke University Medical Center, Durham, North Carolina

JOHN H. HARRIS, Jr., M.D., D.Sc., FACR

John S. Dunn Chair in Radiology, and Professor and Chief of Emergency Radiology, University of Texas Medical School at Houston; Chief of Emergency Radiology, Hermann Hospital, Houston, Texas

MICHAEL F. HARTSHORNE, M.D.

Vice Chairman and Associate Professor of Radiology, University of New Mexico School of Medicine, Albuquerque, New Mexico

VICTOR M. HAUGHTON, M.D.

Professor of Radiology and Biophysics, and Director of Magnetic Resonance Imaging Research, Medical College of Wisconsin, Milwaukee, Wisconsin

ROBERT S. HELLMAN, M.D.

Associate Professor of Radiology, Medical College of Wisconsin; Staff Physician, Milwaukee County Medical Complex and Clement J. Zablocki Veterans Affairs Medical Center, Milwaukee, Wisconsin

CHARLES B. HIGGINS, M.D.

Professor of Radiology, University of California, San Francisco, School of Medicine; Chief, Magnetic Resonance Imaging, The Medical Center at University of California, San Francisco, California

NANCY YANES HOFFMAN, M.Sc.

Writer-in-Residence, Elizabeth Wende Breast Clinic, Rochester, New York

HEDVIG HRICAK, M.D., Ph.D.

Professor of Radiology, Urology, and Radiation Oncology, and Chief, Uroradiology Section, University of California, San Francisco, School of Medicine, San Francisco, California

CONRADE CARL JAFFE, M.D.

Professor of Diagnostic Radiology and Internal Medicine, Yale University School of Medicine; Attending Radiologist, Yale-New Haven Hospital, New Haven, Connecticut

DIEGO JARAMILLO, M.D.

Instructor in Radiology, Harvard Medical School; Radiologist, The Children's Hospital, Boston, Massachusetts

PHILIPPE JEANTY, M.D., Ph.D.

Associate Professor of Radiology, and Assistant Professor of Obstetrics and Gynecology, Vanderbilt University School of Medicine, Nashville, Tennessee

J. RANDY JINKINS, M.D.

Associate Professor and Director of Neuroradiology, Department of Radiology, The University of Texas Health Science Center at San Antonio, San Antonio, Texas

SIMON CHING-SHUN KAO, M.D.

Associate Professor of Radiology, The University of Iowa College of Medicine, Iowa City, Iowa

COLIN KARMODY, M.D., FRCSE, FACS

Professor of Otolaryngology, Tufts University School of Medicine; Senior Surgeon, New England Medical Center, Boston, Massachusetts

DAVID J. KASTAN, M.D.

Senior Staff, Henry Ford Hospital, Detroit, Michigan

SUSAN V. KATTAPURAM, M.D.

Assistant Professor of Radiology, Harvard Medical School; Associate Radiologist, Massachusetts General Hospital, Boston, Massachusetts

ROBERT A. KAUFMAN, S.B., M.D.

Professor of Radiology and Pediatrics, University of Tennessee, Memphis, College of Medicine; Former Director of Radiology, Le Bonheur Children's Medical Center; Consultant in Radiology, St. Jude Children's Hospital, Memphis, Tennessee

JOYCE KELLY, R.D.M.S.

Staff Sonographer, Department of Radiology, Vanderbilt University Medical Center, Nashville, Tennessee

PHILIP J. KENNEY, M.D.

Associate Professor of Radiology, University of Alabama School of Medicine, Birmingham, Alabama

ARFA KHAN, M.D.

Associate Professor of Radiology, Albert Einstein College of Medicine of Yeshiva University, Bronx; Chief, Division of Thoracic Radiology, and Director, Computed Body Tomography, Long Island Jewish Medical Center, New Hyde Park, New York

WILLIAM C. KLINGENSMITH III, M.D.

Associate Clinical Professor, University of Colorado School of Medicine, Denver; Radiologist, Radiology Imaging Associates, Englewood, Colorado

SPYROS S. KOLLIAS, M.D.

Neuroradiology Research Fellow, Children's Hospital Medical Center, Cincinnati, Ohio

DANIEL B. KOPANS, M.D.

Associate Professor of Radiology, Harvard Medical School; Assistant Director, Ambulatory Care Radiology, and Director, Breast Imaging, Massachusetts General Hospital, Boston, Massachusetts

JONATHAN KRAMER, M.D.

Instructor in Radiology, Harvard Medical School; Neuroradiologist, Beth Israel Hospital, Boston, Massachusetts

JANET E. KUHLMAN, M.D.

Assistant Professor and Director, Chest Radiology Section, The Johns Hopkins Hospital, Baltimore, Maryland

FRED J. LAINE, M.D.

Assistant Professor of Radiology, and Clinical Director of Magnetic Resonance, Medical College of Virginia, Richmond, Virginia

TAL LAOR, M.D.

Fellow in Pediatric Radiology, Harvard Medical School; Assistant in Radiology, The Children's Hospital, Boston, Massachusetts

ROBERT L. LAPIDUS, M.D.

Resident Physician, Department of Radiology, Vanderbilt University Medical Center, Nashville, Tennessee

RICHARD E. LATCHAW, M.D.

Professor of Radiology and Neurosurgery, Margaret and H. O. Peterson Chair of Neuroradiology, University of Minnesota Medical School; Chief of Neuroradiology, University of Minnesota Hospital and Clinic, Minneapolis, Minnesota

IGOR LAUFER, M.D.

Professor of Radiology, University of Pennsylvania School of Medicine; Chief, Gastrointestinal Radiology, Hospital of the University of Pennsylvania, Philadelphia, Pennsylvania

EVERETT MARC LAUTIN, M.D.

Associate Professor of Diagnostic Radiology, Albert Einstein College of Medicine of Yeshiva University; Attending Radiologist, Montefiore Medical Center, Bronx, New York

JEFFREY LEWIS LAUTIN, M.D.

Resident in Radiology, Mt. Sinai Hospital, New York, New York

J. NASH LAWRASON, M.D.

Clinical Instructor in Radiology, Harvard Medical School; Assistant Radiologist, Massachusetts General Hospital, Boston, Massachusetts

THOMAS L. LAWSON, M.D.

Professor and Chairman, Department of Radiology, Loyola University of Chicago Stritch School of Medicine, Maywood, Illinois

ROBERT L. LEBOWITZ, M.D.

Professor of Radiology, Harvard Medical School; Associate Radiologist-in-Chief, The Children's Hospital, Boston, Massachusetts

MICHAEL J. LEE, M.Sc., MRCPI, FRCR, FFR (RCSI)

Clinical Instructor of Radiology, Harvard Medical School; Assistant Radiologist, and Assistant Director of Ultrasound, Massachusetts General Hospital, Boston, Massachusetts

VICTOR W. LEE, M.D.

Professor of Radiology, Boston University School of Medicine; Chief of Nuclear Medicine, Boston City Hospital, Boston, Massachusetts

LEE R. LISKEY, M.D.

Private Practice, Clearwater Imaging Associates, Clearwater, Florida

JI-BIN LIU, M.D.

Research Assistant Professor, Division of Diagnostic Ultrasound, Department of Radiology, Jefferson Medical College of Thomas Jefferson University, Philadelphia, Pennsylvania

YU LIU, M.D.

Research Associate, Nuclear Medicine Division, Department of Radiology, Medical College of Wisconsin, Milwaukee, Wisconsin

WENDE WESTINGHOUSE LOGAN-YOUNG, M.D.

Director, The Elizabeth Wende Breast Clinic, Rochester, New York

VINCENT H. S. LOW, M.B.B.S., FRACR

Fellow in Gastrointestinal Radiology, Hospital of the University of Pennsylvania, Philadelphia, Pennsylvania

ROBERT R. LUKIN, M.D., FACR

Professor of Radiology, Director of Neuroradiology, and Adjunct Professor of Neurosurgery, University Hospital, Cincinnati, Ohio

HEBER MacMAHON, M.D.

Associate Professor of Radiology, The University of Chicago Hospitals, Chicago, Illinois

DEAN D. T. MAGLINTE, M.D., FACR

Clinical Professor of Radiology, Indiana University School of Medicine; Chief, Gastrointestinal Section, Department of Radiology, Methodist Hospital of Indiana, Indianapolis, Indiana

JOHN F. MATHEWS, M.B., Ch.B., FRACR

Lecturer in Radiology, The University of Michigan Hospitals, Ann Arbor, Michigan; Consultant Radiologist, Diagnostic Imaging, Campbelltown, New South Wales, Australia

JAMES J. McCORT, M.D.

Emeritus Clinical Professor of Radiology, Stanford University School of Medicine, Stanford; Radiologist, Santa Clara Valley Medical Center, San Jose, California

I. ROSS McDOUGALL, M.B., Ch.B., Ph.D.

Division of Nuclear Medicine, Stanford University Medical Center, Stanford, California

FRANK P. McGRATH, M.B., M.Sc., FFR (RCSI), FRCR, FRCPC

Assistant Professor of Diagnostic Radiology, and Active Staff, McMaster University Medical Center, Hamilton, Ontario, Canada

JOAN McILHENNY, M.D.

Assistant Professor of Radiology and Pediatrics, University of Virginia Hospital and Children's Medical Center, Charlottesville, Virginia

THERESA C. McLOUD, M.D.

Associate Professor of Radiology, Harvard Medical School; Chief, Thoracic Radiology Division, and Radiologist, Department of Radiology, Massachusetts General Hospital, Boston, Massachusetts

ELLEN B. MENDELSON, M.D.

Clinical Associate Professor of Diagnostic Radiology, University of Pittsburgh School of Medicine; Director, Breast Diagnostic Imaging Center, The Western Pennsylvania Hospital, Pittsburgh, Pennsylvania

ROBERT E. MINDELZUN, M.D.

Associate Professor of Radiology, Stanford University School of Medicine, Stanford, California

STUART E. MIRVIS, M.D.

Associate Professor of Radiology, University of Maryland School of Medicine; Director, Trauma Radiology, Maryland Institute for Emergency Medical Services Systems, Baltimore, Maryland

SHEILA G. MOORE, M.D.

Assistant Professor of Radiology, Stanford University School of Medicine, Stanford, California

CONRAD E. NAGLE, M.D., FACNP, FACSM

Chief, Nuclear Medicine Services, William Beaumont Hospital, Troy, Michigan; President, American College of Nuclear Physicians

JEFFREY H. NEWHOUSE, M.D.

Professor of Radiology, Columbia University College of Physicians and Surgeons; Attending Radiologist, Presbyterian Hospital, New York, New York

ROBERT A. NOVELLINE, M.D.

Associate Professor of Radiology, Harvard Medical School; Director, Emergency Radiology, Massachusetts General Hospital, Boston, Massachusetts

JOHN F. O'CONNOR, M.D.

Professor of Radiology, Pediatrics, and Anatomy, Boston University School of Medicine; Director, Pediatric Radiology, Boston University Medical Center and Boston City Hospital, Boston; Chief Radiologist, Franciscan Children's Hospital, Brighton; and Director of Radiology, North Shore Children's Hospital, Salem, Massachusetts

JAMES OSKIN, D.O.

Fellow, Neuroradiology, Northwestern University Medical School and Northwestern Memorial Hospital, Chicago, Illinois

CHRISTOPHER J. PALESTRO, M.D.

Associate Professor of Nuclear Medicine and Radiology, Albert Einstein College of Medicine of Yeshiva University, Bronx; Attending Physician and Chief, Division of Nuclear Medicine, Long Island Jewish Medical Center, New Hyde Park, New York

EDWIN L. PALMER, M.D.

Instructor in Radiology, Harvard Medical School; Associate Radiologist, Massachusetts General Hospital, Boston, Massachusetts

WILLIAM E. PALMER, M.D.

Instructor in Radiology, Harvard Medical School; Radiologist, Massachusetts General Hospital, Boston, Massachusetts

ELLEN PANAGEAS, M.D.

Assistant Professor of Radiology, Westchester County Medical Center, Valhalla, New York

NICHOLAS PAPANICOLAOU, M.D.
Associate Professor of Radiology, Harvard Medical School; Head, Division of Genitourinary Radiology, Massachusetts General Hospital, Boston, Massachusetts

STEVE H. PARKER, M.D
Staff Radiologist, Radiology Imaging Associates, Englewood, Colorado

ROBERT S. PERRET, M.D.
Assistant Professor of Radiology, Section of Digital Imaging, Medical College of Wisconsin; Co-Director, Abdominal Imaging, Veterans Affairs Medical Center, Milwaukee, Wisconsin

ANN C. PRICE, M.D.
Associate Professor of Radiology, Harvard Medical School, Boston, Massachusetts

ROBERT M. QUENCER, M.D.
Professor and Chairman, Department of Radiology, University of Miami School of Medicine; Chief, Radiological Services, Jackson Memorial Hospital, Miami, Florida

LESLIE E. QUINT, M.D.
Associate Professor of Radiology, University of Michigan Hospitals, Ann Arbor, Michigan

HELEN C. REDMAN, M.D.
Professor of Radiology, University of Texas Southwestern Medical Center, Dallas, Texas

JAMES C. REED, M.D.
Professor of Radiology, Bowman Gray School of Medicine of Wake Forest University, Winston-Salem, North Carolina

CHARLES L. ROBERTSON, M.D.
Clinical Associate, Department of Radiology, Massachusetts General Hospital, Boston, Massachusetts; Director, Breast Imaging, St. Luke's Regional Medical Center, Boise, Idaho

BRUCE R. ROSEN, M.D., Ph.D.
Associate Professor of Radiology, Harvard Medical School; Co-Director, Nuclear Magnetic Resonance Center, Massachusetts General Hospital, Boston, Massachusetts

EVA RUBIN, M.D.
Associate Professor of Radiology, and Chief, Mammography Section, University of Alabama at Birmingham Medical Center, Birmingham, Alabama

VAL M. RUNGE, M.D.
Rosenbaum Professor of Diagnostic Radiology, and Director, Magnetic Resonance Imaging and Spectroscopy Center, University of Kentucky College of Medicine, Lexington, Kentucky

ERIC J. RUSSELL, M.D.
Associate Professor of Radiology, Northwestern University Medical School; Director of Neuroradiology, Northwestern Memorial Hospital, Chicago, Illinois

RICHARD SACKNOFF, M.D.
Instructor in Radiology, Harvard Medical School; Associate Radiologist, Massachusetts General Hospital, Boston, Massachusetts

SANJAY SAINI, M.D.
Associate Professor of Radiology, Harvard Medical School; Assistant Radiologist, and Director, Computed Tomography, Massachusetts General Hospital, Boston, Massachusetts

YUTAKA SATO, M.D.
Professor of Radiology (Pediatric Radiology and Neuroradiology), The University of Iowa Hospitals and Clinics, Iowa City, Iowa

DONALD S. SCHAUWECKER, Ph.D., M.D.
Professor of Radiology, Indiana University School of Medicine; Chief of Nuclear Medicine, Wishard Memorial Hospital, Indianapolis, Indiana

JAMES A. SCOTT, M.D.
Assistant Professor of Radiology, Harvard Medical School; Associate Radiologist, Massachusetts General Hospital, Boston, Massachusetts

JANE CHRESTMAN SHARE, M.D.
Instructor in Radiology, Harvard Medical School; Radiologist, The Children's Hospital, Boston, Massachusetts

FRANK G. SHELLOCK, Ph.D., FACSM, FACC
Assistant Professor of Radiological Sciences, University of California, Los Angeles, School of Medicine; Director of Research, Development, and Advanced Applications, Tower Imaging, Los Angeles, California

JO-ANNE O. SHEPARD, M.D.
Assistant Professor of Radiology, Harvard Medical School; Associate Radiologist, Massachusetts General Hospital, Boston, Massachusetts

P. C. SHETTY, M.D.
Vice Chairman, Department of Diagnostic Radiology, and Division Head, Special Procedures and Interventional Radiology, Henry Ford Hospital, Detroit, Michigan

EDWARD A. SICKLES, M.D.
Professor of Radiology, University of California, San Francisco, School of Medicine; Chief, Breast Imaging Section, Department of Radiology, The Medical Center at the University of California, San Francisco, California

JOSEPH F. SIMEONE, M.D.
Professor of Radiology, Harvard Medical School; Head of Ultrasound, Department of Radiology, and Radiologist, Massachusetts General Hospital, Boston, Massachusetts

CARLOS J. SIVIT, M.D.
Assistant Professor of Radiology and Pediatrics, George Washington University School of Medicine; Staff Radiologist, Children's National Medical Center, Washington, D.C.

M. LEON SKOLNICK, M.D.
Professor of Radiology, University of Pittsburgh School of Medicine; Attending Radiologist, Presbyterian-University Hospital, Pittsburgh, Pennsylvania

JAMES G. SMIRNIOTOPOULOS, M.D.
Associate Professor of Radiology and Nuclear Medicine, Uniformed Services University of the Health Sciences, Bethesda, Maryland; Associate Clinical Professor of Radiology, Georgetown University, and Associate Professorial Lecturer in Radiology, George Washington University School of Medicine and Health Sciences, Washington, D.C.

WENDY R. K. SMOKER, M.D.
Professor of Radiology and Director of Neuroradiology, Medical College of Virginia, Richmond, Virginia

DAVID L. SPIZARNY, M.D.
Director, Division of Body Computed Tomography, Department of Radiology, Henry Ford Hospital, Detroit, Michigan

PAUL STARK, M.D.
Associate Professor of Radiology, Harvard Medical School, Boston, Massachusetts, and Professor of Radiology, Loma Linda University School of Medicine, Loma Linda, California; Co-Director, Division of Thoracic Radiology, Brigham and Women's Hospital, Boston, Massachusetts

FRED STEINBERG, M.D.
President, Steinberg Medical Imaging, Sherman Oaks, California

GILES W. STEVENSON, B.M., FRCP, FRCR, FRCPC
Professor and Chairman, Department of Radiology, McMaster University School of Medicine; Head of Section, Department of Radiology, Chedoke-McMaster Hospitals, Hamilton, Ontario, Canada

JOHN R. STY, M.D.
Clinical Professor of Radiology, Medical College of Wisconsin, Milwaukee, and University of Wisconsin Medical School, Madison; Chief of Radiology, Children's Hospital of Wisconsin, Milwaukee, Wisconsin

DENNIS P. SWANSON, R.Ph., M.S.
Associate Professor and Assistant Dean, University of Pittsburgh School of Pharmacy, and Adjunct Associate Professor, University of Pittsburgh School of Medicine; Manager, Radiology Pharmacy Services, University of Pittsburgh Medical Center, Pittsburgh, Pennsylvania

E. TURGUT TALI, M.D.

Chairman, Department of Radiology, Betemar CT and MRI Health Services Company, Ankara, Turkey

RITA LITTLEWOOD TEELE, M.D.

Radiologist and Ultrasonologist, The Children's Hospital, and Consultant in Neonatal Radiology, Brigham and Women's Hospital, Boston, Massachusetts

SHEKHAR C. THAKUR, M.D.

Resident, Nuclear Medicine, Medical College of Wisconsin, Milwaukee, Wisconsin

M. KRISTIN THORSEN, M.D.

Associate Professor of Radiology, Medical College of Wisconsin; Staff Radiologist, Milwaukee County Medical Complex, and Froedtert Memorial Lutheran Hospital, Milwaukee, Wisconsin

JAMES H. THRALL, M.D.

Juan M. Taveras Professor of Radiology, Harvard Medical School; Radiologist-in-Chief, Massachusetts General Hospital, Boston, Massachusetts

RONALD S. TIKOFSKY, Ph.D.

Research Assistant Professor, Department of Radiology, Section of Nuclear Medicine, Medical College of Wisconsin; Director, Brain Imaging Research, Clement J. Zablocki Veterans Affairs Medical Center, Milwaukee, Wisconsin

CHARLES L. TRUWIT, M.D.

Chief, Neuroradiology and Magnetic Resonance Imaging, Fitzsimons Army Medical Center, Aurora, Colorado

BARRY A. TURNBULL, Ph.D.

Associate Director of Biostatistics, Parexel International Corporation, Waltham, Massachusetts

CORNELIS VAN KUIJK, M.D., Ph.D.

Visiting Assistant Research Radiologist, Osteoporosis Research Group, Department of Radiology, The Medical Center at the University of California, San Francisco, California; Department of Radiology, Erasmus University, Rotterdam, The Netherlands

A. CHRISTINE WATT, M.B., Ch.B.

Department of Radiology, St. John Hospital and Medical Center, Detroit, Michigan

RALPH WEISSLEDER, M.D., Ph.D.

Director, Magnetic Resonance Pharmaceutical Program, Massachusetts General Hospital Nuclear Magnetic Resonance Center, Charlestown, Massachusetts

BARBARA N. WEISSMAN, M.D.

Associate Professor of Radiology, Harvard Medical School; Assistant Chairman, Radiology and Ambulatory Services, and Director, Musculoskeletal Radiology, Brigham and Women's Hospital, Boston, Massachusetts

ROBERT G. WELLS, M.D.

Associate Clinical Professor of Radiology, Medical College of Wisconsin; Staff Radiologist, Children's Hospital of Wisconsin, Milwaukee, Wisconsin

JACK WITTENBERG, M.D.

Professor of Radiology, Harvard Medical School; Radiologist, Massachusetts General Hospital, Boston, Massachusetts

AIZIK L. WOLF, M.D.

Assistant Professor of Neurosurgery and Neurology, University of Maryland Medical System, Veterans Hospital, and Mercy Medical Center, Baltimore, Maryland

NANCY WOLF, M.S., R.Ph., B.C.N.P.

Clinical Nuclear Pharmacist, Veterans Affairs Medical Center, Albuquerque, New Mexico

BEVERLY P. WOOD, M.D.

Professor of Radiology and Pediatrics, University of Southern California School of Medicine; Radiologist-in-Chief, Children's Hospital of Los Angeles, Los Angeles, California

TINA I. YOUNG, M.D.

Instructor in Radiology, Harvard Medical School; Assistant Radiologist, Massachusetts General Hospital, Boston, Massachusetts

E. KENT YUCEL, M.D.

Instructor in Radiology, Harvard Medical School; Assistant Radiologist, Massachusetts General Hospital, Boston, Massachusetts

WILLIAM T. C. YUH, M.D., M.S.E.E.

Director of Magnetic Resonance Imaging, The University of Iowa College of Medicine, Iowa City, Iowa

ROBERT A. ZIMMERMAN, M.D.

Professor of Radiology, University of Pennsylvania School of Medicine; Chief, Pediatric Neuroradiology and Pediatric Magnetic Resonance Imaging, Children's Hospital of Philadelphia, Philadelphia, Pennsylvania

# PREFACE

*Current Practice of Radiology* is a departure from the style of both textbooks and review articles. The intention of the book is to provide an opportunity for recognized experts in radiology to share their current approaches to common and important diagnostic problems. It is a logical extension of the *Current Therapy* series, which has been very successful using the same philosophy of asking experts to describe their own approaches to practice.

Each author was charged with presenting his or her viewpoint rather than presenting a comprehensive spectrum of opinion from the literature or the point and counterpoint of controversies. It is the goal of this book to give the reader a clear statement from an authoritative figure, recognizing that many background details are not included. The authors also have kept the suggested readings to a minimum, emphasizing only the more important articles that can serve as an entry point to a wider pursuit of the literature.

It was not possible or practical to be encyclopedic or exhaustive in selecting material for this book. Rather, emphasis has been placed on topics that reflect the forefront of current practice. Other chapters are contemporary presentations of areas of longstanding interest in radiology.

The intended audience for this work is primarily the practicing radiologist who needs to stay abreast of contemporary thinking in the specialty. The book should also be of interest to radiologists in training who have mastered the fundamentals and are ready for more advanced material in which the fundamentals are put into practice.

A unique feature of this work is the "book-within-the-book" concept. One of the problems with radiology is the taxonomy of our specialty. The academic framework for radiology has increasingly become organ-system specialization. However, many individual radiologists also have an interest in the technical modalities that cross organ-system boundaries. The basic organization of the book into sections follows an organ-system outline. The table of contents is then restated so that all chapters dealing with nuclear medicine, ultrasonography, computed tomography, or magnetic resonance imaging can be readily accessed.

It is hoped that *Current Practice of Radiology* will become an enduring part of the educational resource in radiology. Contributors to this first edition have done a marvelous job in capturing the spirit of presenting a personal statement of their practice. Feedback and critique will guide topical selections for future editions.

I would like to thank the many authors for their excellent contributions to the book. Lynne Gery provided excellent editorial support, and Doreen Flynn did yeoman work in keeping the many correspondences going to the right people.

*James H. Thrall, M.D.*

# CONTENTS

## THORACIC RADIOLOGY



## GASTROINTESTINAL RADIOLOGY

# GENITOURINARY RADIOLOGY

## NEURORADIOLOGY AND HEAD AND NECK RADIOLOGY

## PEDIATRIC RADIOLOGY



## CARDIOVASCULAR RADIOLOGY

# CONTENTS BY IMAGING MODALITY

## NUCLEAR MEDICINE



## ULTRASONOGRAPHY

## COMPUTED TOMOGRAPHY

## MAGNETIC RESONANCE IMAGING

# THORACIC RADIOLOGY

## The Chest Radiograph in AIDS: Infections and Neoplasms

*PHILIP C. GOODMAN, M.D.*

The variety of opportunistic infections and lung neoplasms observed in patients with acquired immunodeficiency syndrome (AIDS) has changed little since the earliest manifestations of the epidemic in 1981. The clinical and imaging modalities used to diagnose these diseases have included blood gas measurements, pulmonary function tests, bronchoscopy with lavage and biopsy, gallium lung scans, computed tomography (CT), and magnetic resonance imaging. Each has had its advocates; nevertheless, chest radiography remains the primary imaging technique and in most patients provides not only evidence of pathology but also offers clues to specific diagnoses. This chapter reviews the radiographic findings of the most common pulmonary abnormalities observed in patients with AIDS. Special emphasis is placed on features helpful in differentiating between illnesses.

### Infections

#### Pneumocystis carinii *Pneumonia*

The most common pulmonary infection in patients with AIDS is *Pneumocystis carinii* pneumonia (PCP). This illness establishes an AIDS diagnosis or is ultimately discovered in 60 to 80 percent of individuals infected with the human immunodeficiency virus (HIV). Chest radiographs invariably demonstrate an abnormality; only 5 to 10 percent of patients with PCP have normal chest films. The primary radiographic feature and clue to diagnosis is a fine-to-medium reticulonodular opacity. This is usually distributed diffusely and symmetrically in both lungs (Fig. 1), but unusual patterns of involvement as discussed later may appear. In its mildest form, the chest film may be so subtle that inter- and intraobserver discrepancies in interpretation are common. Ultimately, the workup of a patient depends on more than the chest film, so that differences in opinion or misinterpretations seldom result in mistakes in patient therapy. Thus an individual at risk for HIV infection who presents with cough, fever, low diffusing capacity, or low $Po_2$ should proceed to further diagnostic steps irregardless of the chest film findings. In this circumstance other imaging tests such as gallium scanning or CT may be performed, but generally direct sampling procedures such as induced sputum, bronchoalveolar lavage, or transbronchial biopsy are indicated to obtain specimens for staining, culture, or cytologic evaluation. Patients who present with a "classic" chest radiograph for PCP may proceed to a sampling procedure or in some centers might be treated without further tests.

Occasionally chest film abnormalities seen with PCP are distributed in an unusual fashion. They may be bilateral but asymmetric, unilateral, or primarily involve the upper lobes (Fig. 2). This may initially be confusing, but the pattern of fine-to-medium reticulonodular opacities is generally unchanged and provides the strongest evidence for the underlying condition. Diagnostic considerations other than PCP for reticulonodular opacification include lymphocytic interstitial pneumonitis (LIP) and cytomegalovirus (CMV) pneumonia. LIP is chiefly seen in children with AIDS, is not as rapidly debilitating as PCP, and is usually suggested after PCP has been excluded. Hilar or mediastinal lymphadenopathy is sometimes seen with LIP, but is not observed with PCP. CMV is seldom cytopathologic in the lungs, so that consideration of CMV as the cause of pneumonia in this setting has low priority.

PCP on occasion produces unusual radiographic appear-

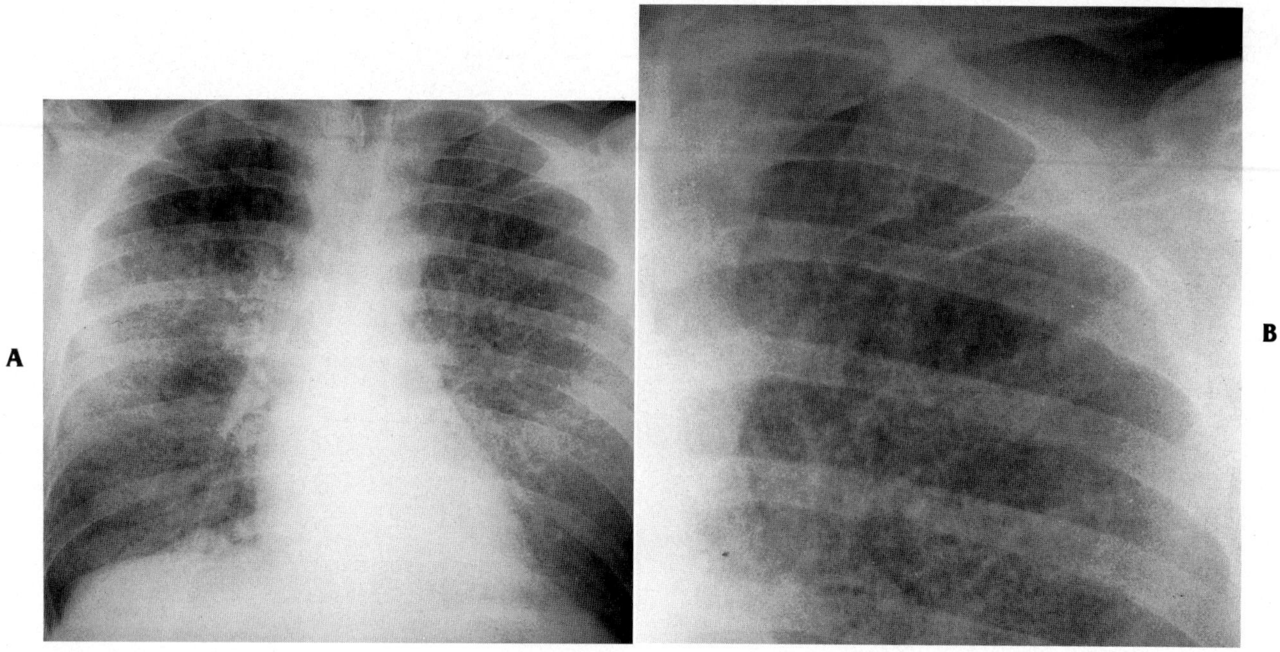

**FIGURE 1** PCP. *A,* An AP chest film demonstrates the characteristic diffuse and symmetric distribution of fine-to-medium reticulonodular opacities seen in patients with PCP. *B,* A close-up of the left upper lobe demonstrates in better detail the fine-to-medium reticulonodular pattern most typically observed in patients with PCP.

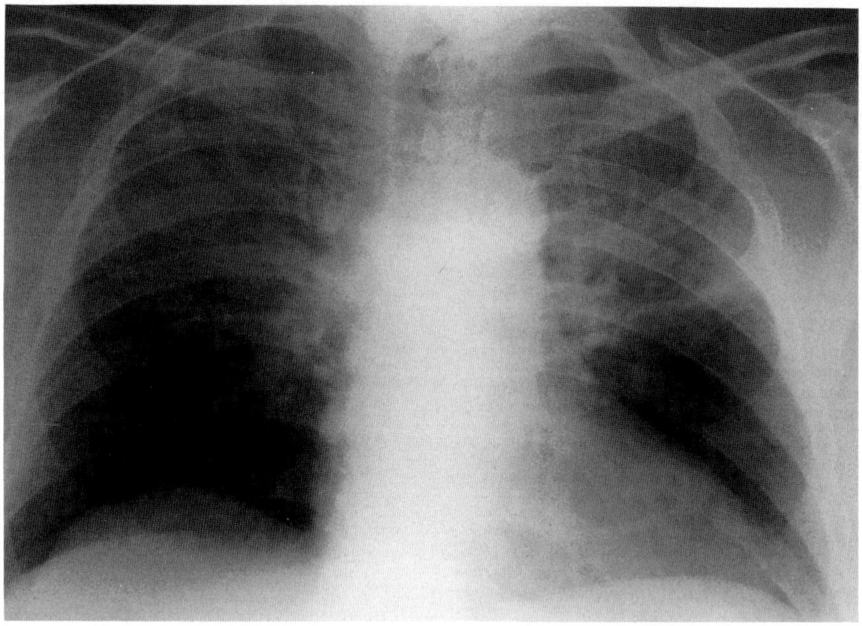

**FIGURE 2** PCP. A PA chest film reveals bilateral upper lobe fine-to-medium reticular opacities. This distribution may simulate reactivation tuberculosis, but in AIDS patients is most commonly associated with PCP developing in a patient who has undergone prophylactic aerosolized pentamidine therapy.

ances aside from those of atypical distribution. Rarely segmental or lobar homogeneous consolidation may be observed. *Pneumocystis carinii* infection may also take the form of poorly defined 1 to 2 cm nodules (Fig. 3). Cavitation may occur resulting in a medium- to thick-walled lesion. Diagnostic considerations other than PCP for a homogeneous area of opacification include bacterial pneumonias (e.g., caused by *Streptococcus pneumoniae, Haemophilus influenzae, Staphylococcus*), unusual infections (e.g., caused by *Legionella, Nocardia*), and focal hemorrhage secondary to pulmonary Kaposi's

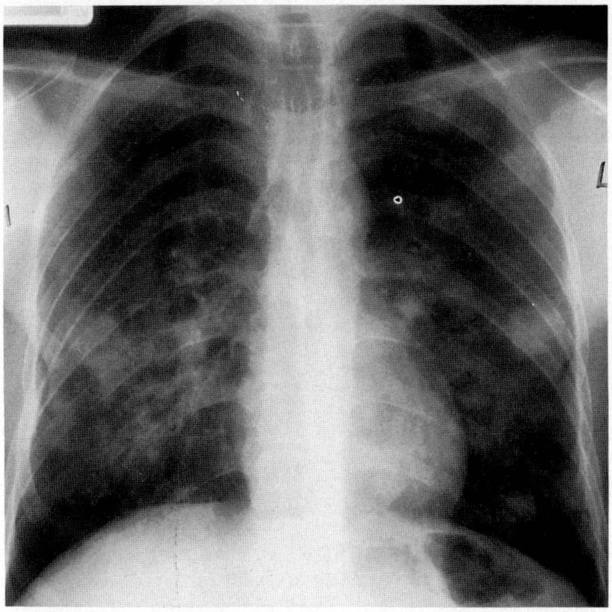

**FIGURE 3** PCP. A PA chest film reveals multiple, poorly defined, and fairly large nodules throughout both lungs. This is a most unusual appearance of PCP. Occasionally the nodules cavitate.

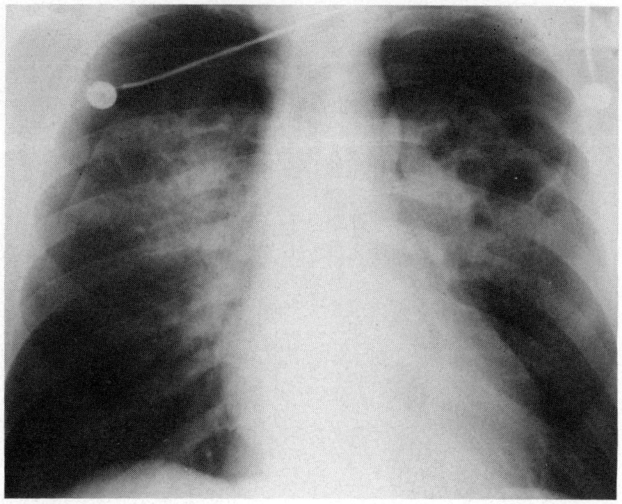

**FIGURE 5** PCP. A PA chest film demonstrates bilateral large pneumothoraces. In the underlying lungs, multiple thin-walled pneumatoceles can be identified adjacent to the visceral pleura.

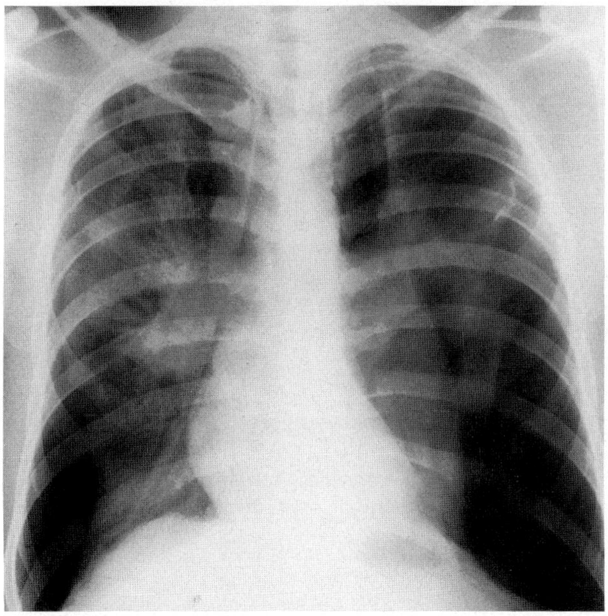

**FIGURE 4** PCP. A PA chest film demonstrates bilateral moderate-to-large pneumothoraces. Underlying fine reticulonodular opacification is best seen in the partially inflated right lung.

sarcoma (KS). The differential diagnosis for nodular or cavitary lesions in patients with AIDS includes fungal infections (cryptococcosis, aspergillosis), pulmonary KS, and septic emboli. Pulmonary non-Hodgkin's lymphoma tends to produce better-defined nodules than those caused by *P. carinii,* but differentiation can be difficult. Ancillary findings of hilar or mediastinal lymph node enlargement or pleural fluid favor a diagnosis other than PCP.

Spontaneous pneumothorax (Fig. 4) and pneumatocele formation are complications almost exclusively seen with PCP. The pneumatoceles, thin-walled air-containing structures, typically appear 5 to 6 days into the pneumonia, range from 0.5 to 6 cm in diameter, and persist after the pneumonia has resolved. Over 6 months they gradually resolve. They are frequently multiple, and this contributes to the difficulty in treating pneumothoraces resulting from their rupture into the pleural space (Fig. 5).

Radiographically demonstrable lymphadenopathy and pleural fluid are so uncommon with PCP that their appearance virtually excludes *P. carinii* as the sole disease-causing agent.

The course of treated PCP is one of steady, and at times rapid, improvement. Partial radiographic clearing should be seen within 3 to 4 days, and complete resolution can be noted within 2 weeks. With intravenous trimethoprimsulfamethoxazole therapy, a large fluid load may lead to an appearance of pulmonary edema within 4 days of institution of treatment. This may cause an erroneous impression of drug or treatment failure if not recognized.

When untreated, PCP worsens and the chest radiograph worsens in a linear fashion. The initial fine reticulonodular opacities spread to involve previously unaffected lung. Coalescence of opacities eventually leads to homogeneous opacification throughout the pulmonary parenchyma (Fig. 6). In its most fulminant case, this degree of deterioration may occur within 24 hours. With increasing physician and patient awareness of PCP, this severe type of lung involvement is not as frequently observed as it was in the early days of the AIDS epidemic.

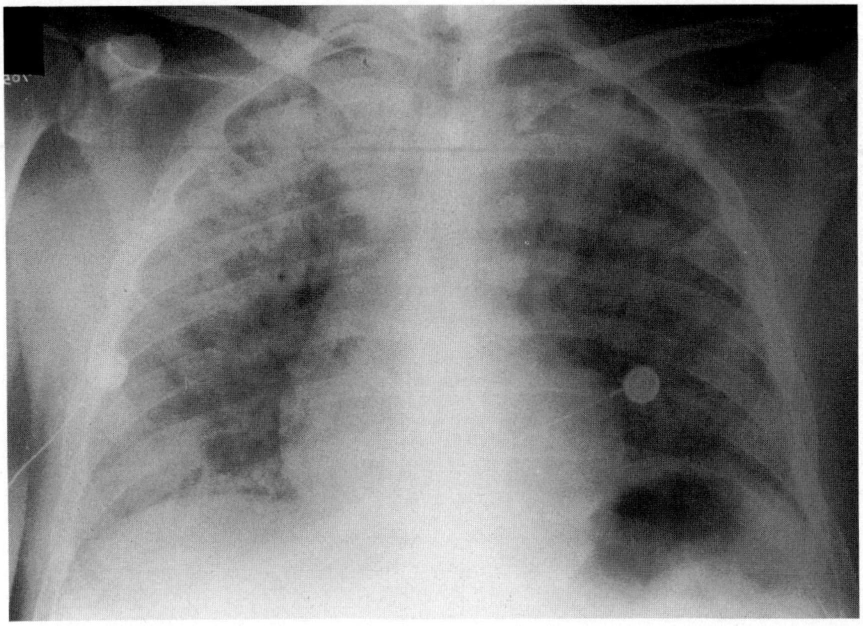

**FIGURE 6** PCP. An AP chest film demonstrates diffuse, bilateral, homogeneous opacification representing severe PCP.

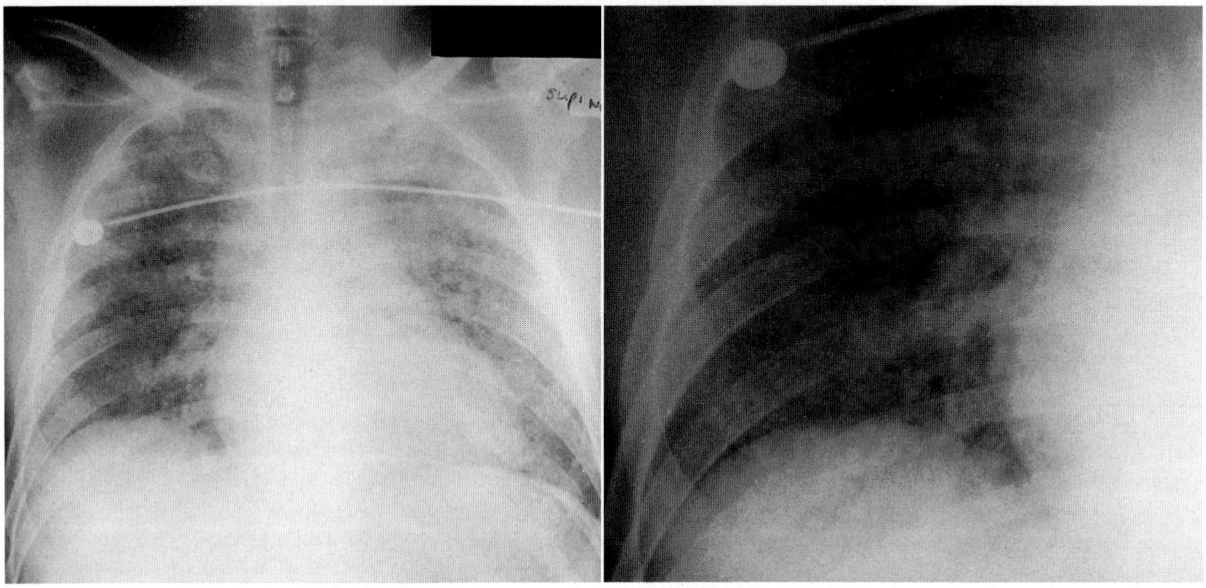

A B

**FIGURE 7** Histoplasmosis. *A,* An AP chest film demonstrates symmetric, bilateral, coarse, nodular opacities in a patient with histoplasmosis. *B,* A close-up of the right lower lobe demonstrates in better detail the nodular appearance typical of disseminated histoplasmosis or coccidioidomycosis.

## *Fungal Infections*

Several fungi have been identified as pulmonary pathogens in patients with AIDS. Among these are *Histoplasma capsulatum* and *Coccidioides immitis* seen endemically in the eastern and southwestern United States, respectively, and *Cryptococcus neoformans* and *Aspergillus* species seen with slowly increasing frequency throughout the country. Coccidioidomycosis and histoplasmosis have similar chest radiographic appearances. The chest films demonstrate bilateral, diffuse, symmetric, coarse, nodular opacities (Fig. 7). The nodules are poorly defined and generally measure approximately 3 to 5 mm in diameter. Although distribution of this abnormality is similar to that seen with PCP, the quality of the opacities is coarser and more nodular; thus a preliminary differentiation between these diseases is often possible. A more problematic situation arises when trying to distinguish these fungi from disseminated tuberculosis or pulmonary toxoplasmosis, which may both present with similar coarse nodular opacities. Hilar and mediastinal adenopathy have been reported as has homogeneous opacification simulating airspace pneumonia. Pleural fluid and cavitation are infrequent.

The appearance of cryptococcal pulmonary disease differs from that of the previously discussed fungi. The distinctive finding with this infection is a well-defined nodule with or without cavitation. Associated lymphadenopathy may be observed. Occasionally lymph node enlargement is observed without lung abnormalities (Fig. 8). Pleural fluid is also reported. Invasive pulmonary aspergillosis has been reported

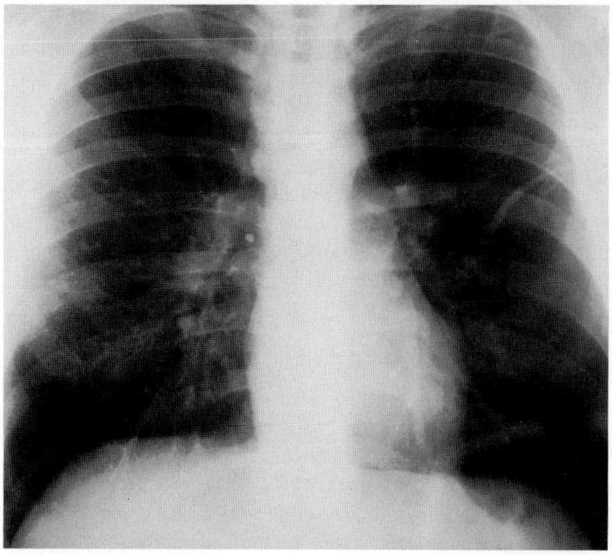

**FIGURE 8** Cryptococcosis. A PA chest film demonstrates right hilar and right paratracheal adenopathy. Although lung disease such as well-defined nodules or cavities is typically observed with cryptococcal pulmonary disease, occasionally, as in this case, isolated lymph node enlargement is the sole finding.

as a late complication in patients with AIDS. Some of these individuals were being treated with corticosteroid adjunctive therapy for PCP at the time that aspergillosis was diagnosed. The chest radiographs demonstrate focal areas of consolidation or nodules with or without cavitation. The differential diagnosis list for focal opacities with cavitation would thus include cryptococcosis, aspergillosis, PCP, and septic emboli. The nodules of KS and non-Hodgkin's lymphoma do not tend to cavitate.

## *Mycobacterial Disease*

The incidence of pulmonary tuberculosis has increased over the last several years in part related to the AIDS epidemic. The radiographic appearance of tuberculosis depends on the stage of HIV infection. Early in this disease, when the patient's immune status is mildly diminished, the pattern of tuberculosis is similar to that seen in the general population. Thus the chest radiograph demonstrates coarse linear and nodular opacities with or without cavitation in the apical and posterior segments of the upper lobes and superior segments of the lower lobes. In later stages of HIV infection, or following an AIDS diagnosis, the chest film demonstrates diffuse, symmetric, bilateral, coarse, reticulonodular opacities with a tendency toward nodularity (Fig. 9). In some AIDS populations (e.g., Haitians, intravenous drug abusers), an extremely high incidence of hilar and/or mediastinal adenopathy has been reported. Pleural fluid may also be observed in these patients. Although the diffuse nodular pattern at times simulates miliary disease (i.e., 1 to 2 mm in diameter), more frequently the opacities are larger and coarser (i.e., 3 to 5 mm in diameter). In this latter form, there is little to distinguish AIDS-associated

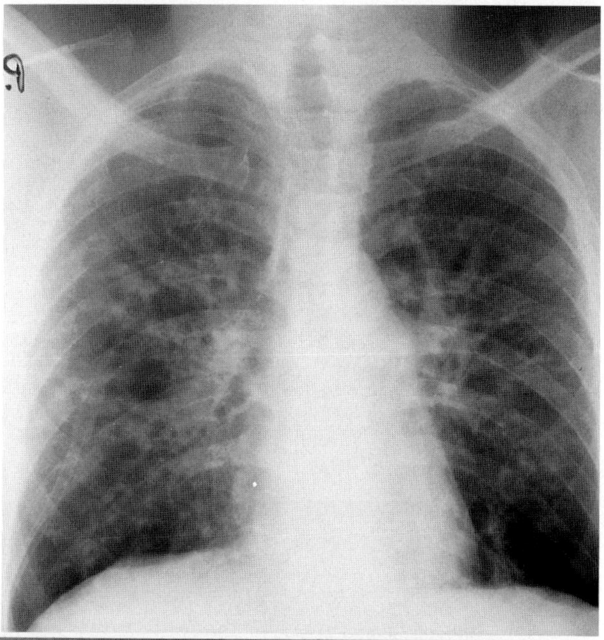

A

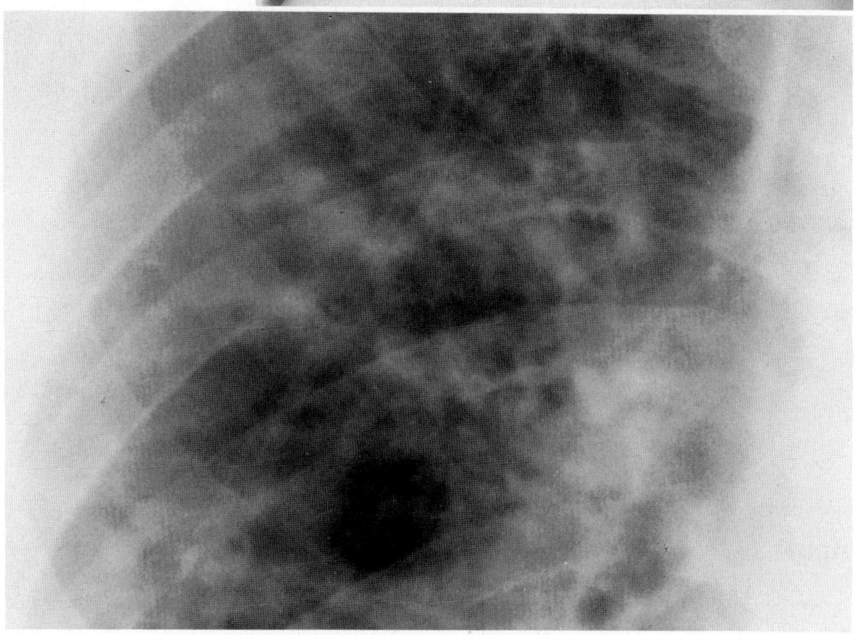

B

**FIGURE 9** Tuberculosis. *A,* A PA chest film demonstrates symmetric, bilateral, coarse, reticulonodular opacities. The distribution and quality of infiltrate are typical of that observed in patients with tuberculosis and late HIV infection. *B,* A close-up of the right midlung demonstrates in better detail the coarse quality of this reticulonodular pattern. (From Goodman PC, Microbacterial disease in AIDS. J Thoracic Imaging 1991; 6(4): 22–27, with permission of Aspen Publishers, Inc., © 1991.)

disseminated tuberculosis from disseminated fungal disease. There is, however, a greater tendency for lymph node enlargement and possibly pleural fluid accumulation in patients with tuberculosis. Differentiating PCP from tuberculosis is usually possible, since the parenchymal disease of PCP is rarely as coarse as that of tuberculosis, and lymphadenopathy and pleural fluid are not expected with PCP. Patients who are treated with antituberculosis medications show steady improvement on their chest radiographs. Worsening of the chest film should suggest the presence of a secondary infection rather than tuberculosis treatment failure.

Disseminated infections with *Mycobacterium avium*-complex (MAC) are generally observed in extrapulmonary sites; however, several reports of lung disease with this agent have been published. The chest radiograph has a nonspecific appearance and most commonly demonstrates diffuse reticulonodular opacities. Lymphadenopathy may be seen in up to 20 percent of individuals. Pleural fluid and parenchymal cavitation are rare.

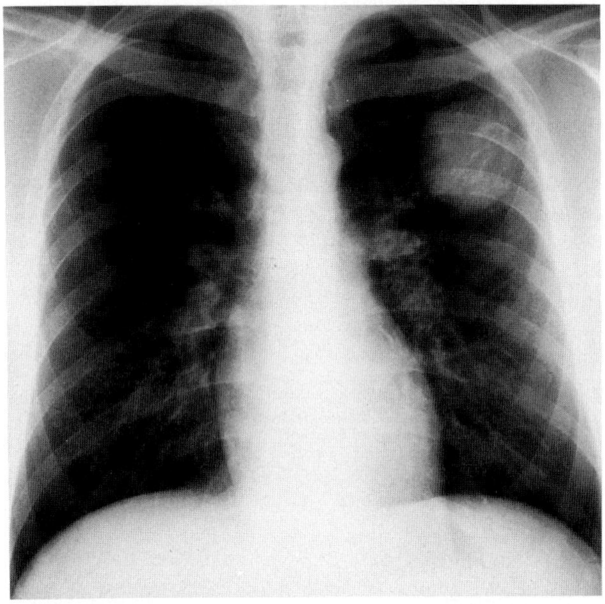

**FIGURE 10** Non-Hodgkin's lymphoma. A large, well-defined, homogeneous nodule is seen in the left upper lobe. Five weeks earlier this nodule representing non-Hodgkin's lymphoma had measured 1 cm in diameter. This rapid growth is characteristic of this form of neoplasm in patients with AIDS.

## Other Infections

Pyogenic pneumonias such as those caused by *S. pneumoniae, H. influenzae,* and staphylococcal species are commonly encountered in patients with AIDS. The chest radiograph demonstrates homogeneous segmental or lobar opacification no different than expected in the general population.

Parapneumonic effusions may accompany the pulmonary abnormalities. This type of homogeneous consolidation is rarely observed with PCP and fungal infections, and although typical of the pulmonary illnesses caused by *Nocardia* and *Legionella,* these latter diseases are so uncommon that pyogenic pneumonia should be suggested when this presentation is seen. Appropriate antibiotic therapy results in rapid radiographic and clinical improvement.

CMV was initially considered a common cause of pneumonia in patients with AIDS. However, investigators have noted little cytopathologic evidence of pneumonia caused by this agent. When CMV is thought to be the cause of pneumonia, the chest radiograph demonstrates diffuse, bilateral, symmetric, fine, reticular opacities indistinguishable from PCP. I generally do not include CMV on my differential list because current studies fail to demonstrate that it has significant clinical importance. CMV as a cause of pneumonia should be

A

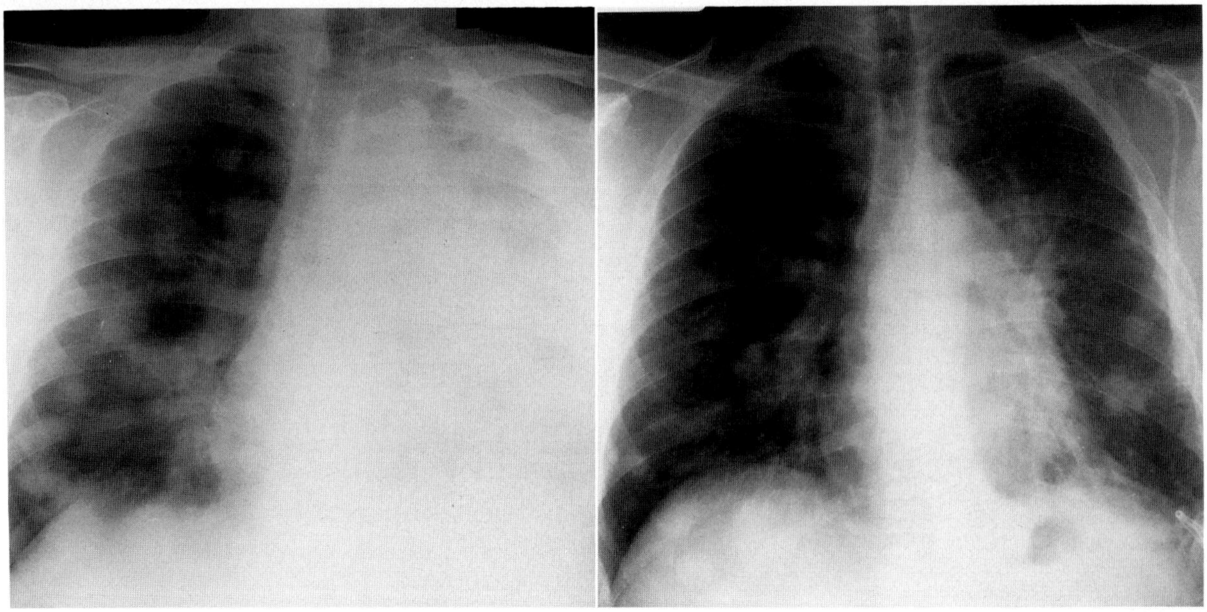

B

**FIGURE 11** Non-Hodgkin's lymphoma. *A,* A PA chest film demonstrates a large left pleural fluid collection and multiple well-defined nodules in the right lung. *B,* Two weeks later a PA chest film of the same patient demonstrates significant improvement in left pleural fluid and reduction in size of pulmonary nodules. Underlying left hilar adenopathy is now revealed. This rapid improvement is not uncommon in patients with non-Hodgkin's lymphoma and AIDS following appropriate chemotherapy.

considered only after more readily treatable diseases such as PCP or tuberculosis are excluded.

*Toxoplasma gondii,* while principally a disease of the central nervous system, has been identified as a cause of pneumonia in some patients with AIDS. The radiographic abnormality is a diffuse, bilateral, symmetric, coarse, nodular opacity similar in appearance to disseminated tuberculosis, coccidioidomycosis, or histoplasmosis. Pleural fluid has occasionally been identified in these patients. No definite mediastinal or hilar adenopathy has been observed.

## Neoplasms

### *Non-Hodgkin's Lymphoma*

Non-Hodgkin's lymphoma of AIDS patients is more aggressive and detected at more advanced stages of disease than in the general population. Involvement is most frequent in the central nervous system, intra-abdominal organs, and bone marrow. In a combined series, intrathoracic involvement was clinically identified in only 10 percent of patients, whereas in another study, it was observed in approximately 30 percent of individuals at autopsy. The common chest film abnormalities are hilar and/or mediastinal adenopathy, pleural fluid, and diffuse medium-to-coarse bilateral, reticular, and linear opacities. Well-defined parenchymal nodules are interesting and somewhat unique radiographic findings (Fig. 10). These nodules may be solitary or multiple, may or may not be associated with the other more common findings of pulmonary lymphoma, and demonstrate a propensity for rapid growth. This latter tendency, which may see nodule diameters increase three- to fourfold over 1 to 2 months, may erroneously suggest an infectious etiology. One must be alert to the possibility of neoplasm. Non-Hodgkin's lymphomas are generally extremely anaplastic, which probably accounts for their rapid growth but also can lead to equally rapid temporary improvement with radiation or chemotherapy (Fig. 11). The nodules may rarely cavitate following treatment. Other AIDS-related diseases to consider in the differential diagnosis include tuberculosis for lymphadenopathy, tuberculosis and KS for pleural fluid, KS, fungi, PCP for nodules, and perhaps KS and pulmonary edema from AIDS-related cardiomyopathy for the diffuse linear interstitial opacities.

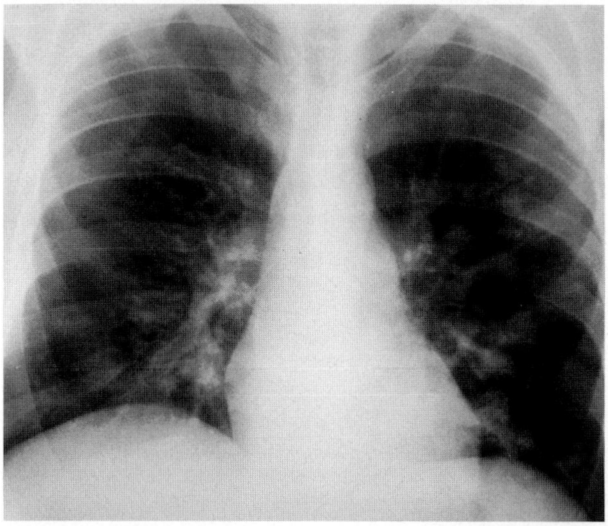

**FIGURE 12** Kaposi's sarcoma. An AP chest film demonstrates bilateral, poorly defined, oval and rounded nodular opacities. They measure approximately 1 to 2 cm in diameter and are typical of pulmonary KS.

### *Kaposi's Sarcoma*

KS is generally a disease of mucocutaneous surfaces of the body. The lungs are involved in approximately 8 percent of AIDS patients. The chest radiograph typically reveals 1 to 2 cm in diameter, poorly defined nodules, and/or coarse linear opacities with a variety of distributions (Fig. 12). Asymmetric, unilateral, or bilateral disease has been reported, whereas with extensive involvement a more symmetric diffuse appearance is commonly observed (Fig. 13). Intrathoracic lymphadenopathy is seen in less than 10 percent of patients with KS. Pleural fluid is extremely common and has been reported in 35 to 50 percent of individuals with this disease (Fig. 14). The radiographic appearance of KS is one of the most distinctive seen in patients

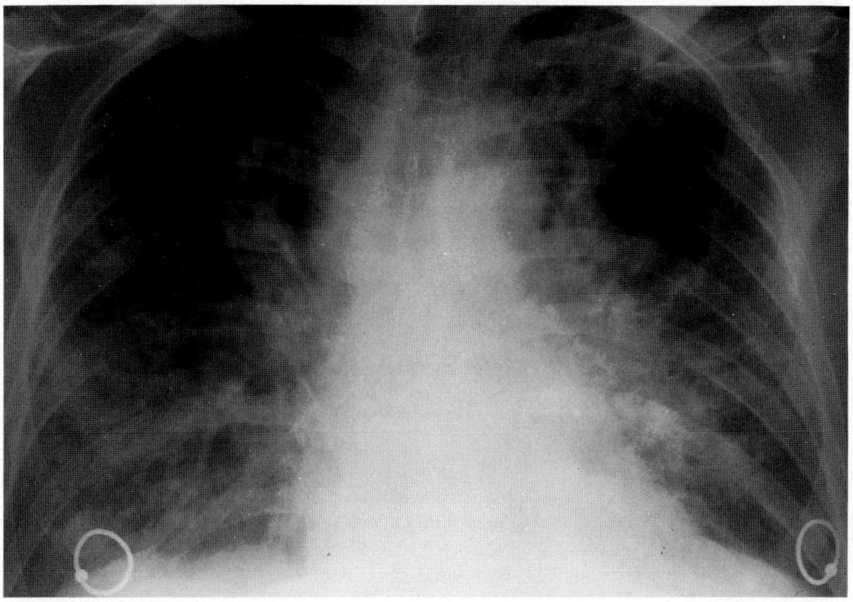

**FIGURE 13** Kaposi's sarcoma. An AP chest film demonstrates bilateral, coarse, linear densities distributed in a parahilar fashion. This type of abnormality may be combined with poorly defined nodules to give a nearly pathognomonic picture of pulmonary KS.

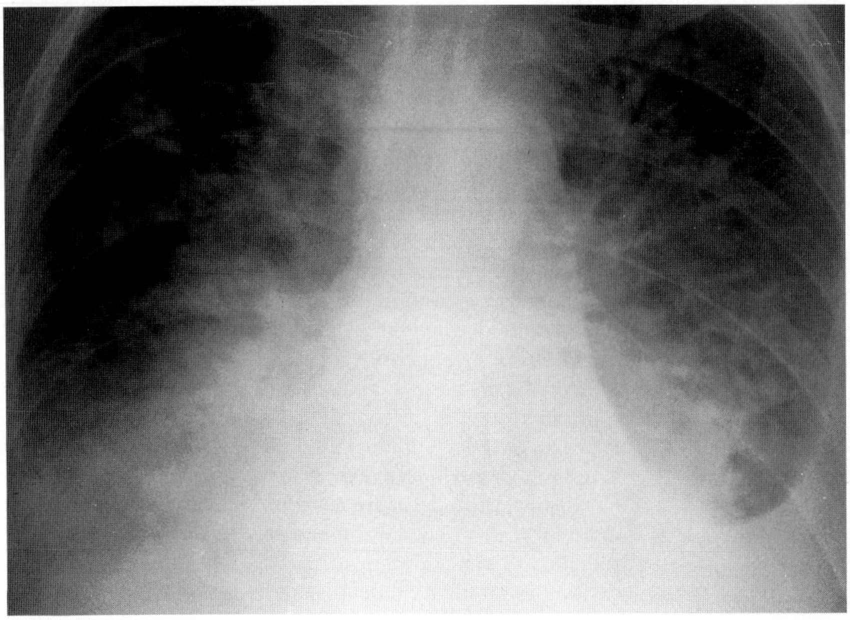

**FIGURE 14** Kaposi's sarcoma. A PA chest film demonstrates coarse, parahilar, linear, opacities characteristic of pulmonary KS. Pleural fluid is also demonstrated and is seen in up to 50 percent of patients with intrathoracic KS.

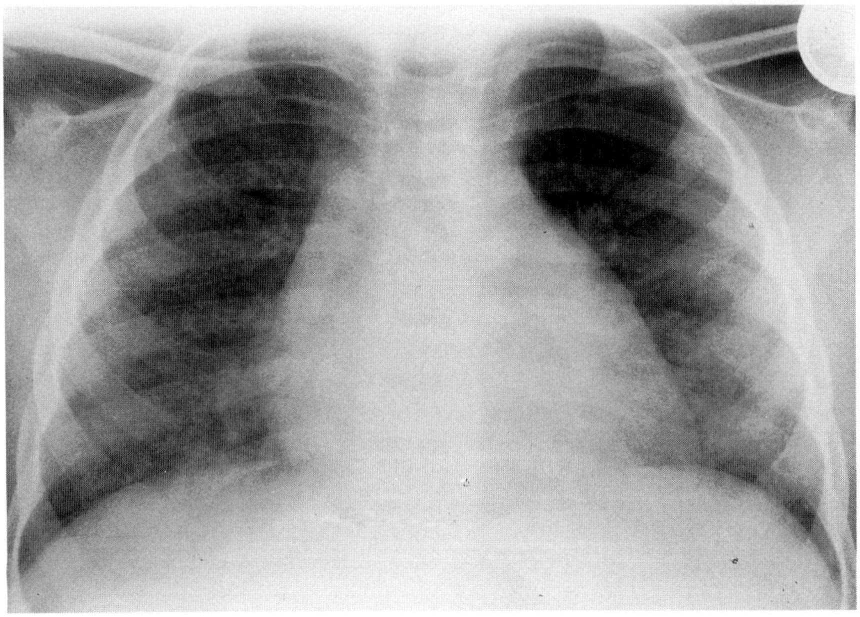

**FIGURE 15** Lymphocytic interstitial pneumonitis. An AP chest film of a child with AIDS demonstrates bilateral, symmetric, fine-to-medium nodular opacities. The nodularity would favor LIP, although PCP could not definitely be excluded.

with AIDS; nevertheless, the diagnosis is unlikely unless there is evidence of cutaneous involvement. Other differential considerations include septic emboli, the rare case of multinodular PCP, fungi (in particular, cryptococcosis and aspergillosis), and occasionally non-Hodgkin's lymphoma.

## Miscellaneous

### *Lymphocytic Interstitial Pneumonitis*

LIP is more common in children with AIDS than in adults and is characterized by interstitial accumulation of lymphocytes and plasma cells. The lymphocytes are typically evenly distributed in the alveolar and interlobular septae but occasionally form nodules. Chest radiographs reflect this pathology and reveal diffuse or focal fine-to-medium reticulonodular opacities. At times a predominantly nodular pattern is noted (Fig. 15). The disease slowly progresses over weeks to months. In later stages lymphadenopathy may be observed. Except for this latter finding and a tendency toward nodular opacities, LIP is indistinguishable from PCP.

## Suggested Reading

Goodman PC, ed. Thoracic manifestations of AIDS. J Thorac Imaging 1991; 6(4).

McLoud TC, Naidich DP. Thoracic disease in the immunocompromised patient. Radiol Clin North Am 1992; 30:525–554.

Sande MA, Volberding PA, eds. The Medical Management of AIDS. 3rd ed. Philadelphia: WB Saunders, 1992.

White DA, Stover DE, eds. Pulmonary effects of AIDS. Clin Chest Medicine 1988; 9:363–533.

# CT Evaluation of the Chest in AIDS

*JANET E. KUHLMAN, M.D.*

It is estimated that there are currently between 1.5 and 2 million individuals in the United States infected with the human immunodeficiency virus (HIV). The number of patients developing the acquired immunodeficiency syndrome (AIDS) continues to increase annually, and there are currently about 270,000 patients with AIDS in the United States. The epidemic has become nationwide and global and is no longer limited only to inner cities or high-risk patients. No matter where one practices radiology, one is called on increasingly to examine and evaluate patients with HIV disease. Thus a familiarity with the radiographic appearances and common presentations of chest diseases in AIDS is a timely topic.

AIDS is caused by HIV. Groups at high risk for exposure to the virus include homosexual males, intravenous drug users, Haitians, and patients transfused with HIV-contaminated blood products. AIDS is not, however, limited to these groups. Heterosexual transmission to female sexual partners of infected carriers of the virus has increased the number of women with HIV disease. Maternal-fetal transmission has spread the infection to newborns.

This chapter discusses the role of chest computed tomography (CT) in the evaluation of the patient with HIV disease. I prefer to use the term *HIV disease* rather than AIDS to emphasize that not all HIV-positive patients are alike. Some patients do not have known HIV disease at the time of their first presentation, and radiologic findings may be the first indication of HIV disease. Other patients are blood test positive for HIV, but they may not have yet manifested an AIDS-defining illness, and the extent of their immunosuppression may be relatively less severe. Other patients have "full-blown" AIDS with one or more manifestations of the disease and immunosuppression of varying severity. Chest disease in each of these HIV populations can be different in presentation and appearance.

Thoracic manifestations of HIV disease encompass a spectrum of chest disorders. This chapter concentrates on (1) CT manifestations of AIDS-related adenopathy in the chest, (2) CT patterns of lung involvement in opportunistic infection in AIDS, and (3) thoracic manifestations of AIDS-related neoplasms. I emphasize how and when to use chest CT scanning in the HIV-positive patient, with specific examples illustrating useful indications and applications of CT.

## Technique

One of the most common requests I receive for chest CT evaluation of a HIV-positive patient is to evaluate fever of unknown origin or unexplained respiratory symptoms. Indications for chest CT evaluation that I have found helpful in the HIV-positive patient include (1) searching for occult pulmonary infection in the setting of unexplained fever or respiratory symptoms, (2) characterizing the nature and extent of lung disease initially identified on chest radiographs, (3) evaluating the extent and distribution of adenopathy and staging known malignancies, and (4) planning biopsy procedures.

When examining the patient with known or suspected HIV disease and pulmonary symptoms, I use a modified high-resolution CT technique (HRCT). I find HRCT technique helpful in these patients for identifying subtle pulmonary infiltrates and ground glass opacities that may indicate occult lung infection. My technique employs thin sections (2 to 4 mm) obtained at 1 cm intervals using a high spatial frequency algorithm (a bone algorithm on most scanners). Typical exposure factors are 4 seconds, 310 mA, 125 kVp (Siemens Somatom DRH model scanner). I survey the entire chest from lung apices to diaphragm. In acutely ill patients who are unable to hold their breath, I find it useful to employ 1 second or subsecond scan times available on most state-of-the-art scanners. These fast scan times significantly diminish the amount of degradation from respiratory motion, while still maintaining sufficient diagnostic information in the images. Typical exposure parameters on the Siemens Somatom Plus scanner are 1 second, 260 mA, 137 kVp.

If, on the other hand, I am examining the HIV-positive patient specifically for adenopathy or to stage a known malignancy such as Kaposi's sarcoma (KS) or lymphoma, I prefer to use conventional CT scanning protocols consisting of 8 mm thick sections obtained at 1 cm intervals, from the lung apex to the diaphragm. Typical exposure parameters are 3 seconds, 230 mA, 125 kVp.

## HIV-related Adenopathy

Lymphadenopathy is extremely common in the patient with AIDS, as well as the HIV-positive patient who has yet to manifest an AIDS-defining illness. Many of these latter patients have the progressive generalized lymphadenopathy syndrome or the AIDS-related complex. The most common causes of nodal enlargement in HIV disease include reactive lymphoid hyperplasia (50 percent), AIDS-related lymphoma (20 percent), disseminated mycobacterial infection (17 percent), the lymphadenopathic form of KS (10 percent), and miscellaneous causes such as metastatic tumor, multiorganism infection, and drug reactions.

When performing chest CT on HIV-positive patients, I appreciate more extensive adenopathy than is identified on physical examination or by conventional radiography. Bilateral axillary adenopathy is a common chest CT finding (Fig. 1). It may be accompanied by bilateral inguinal adenopathy and is observed in patients with AIDS and the prodromal illness, progressive generalized lymphadenopathy syndrome. Progressive generalized lymphadenopathy is defined as chronic adenopathy involving two or more sites other than the inguinal regions that persists for 3 months, without evidence of an AIDS-defining illness as determined by the Centers for Disease Control. Biopsy of such nodes usually reveals reactive hyperplasia. Some of these patients also have bilateral cystic enlargement of the parotid glands known as benign lymphoepithelial cystic disease, another manifestation of reactive lymphoid hyperplasia, in this case surrounding the ductal system of the parotid gland causing duct obstruction and cyst formation (Fig. 2).

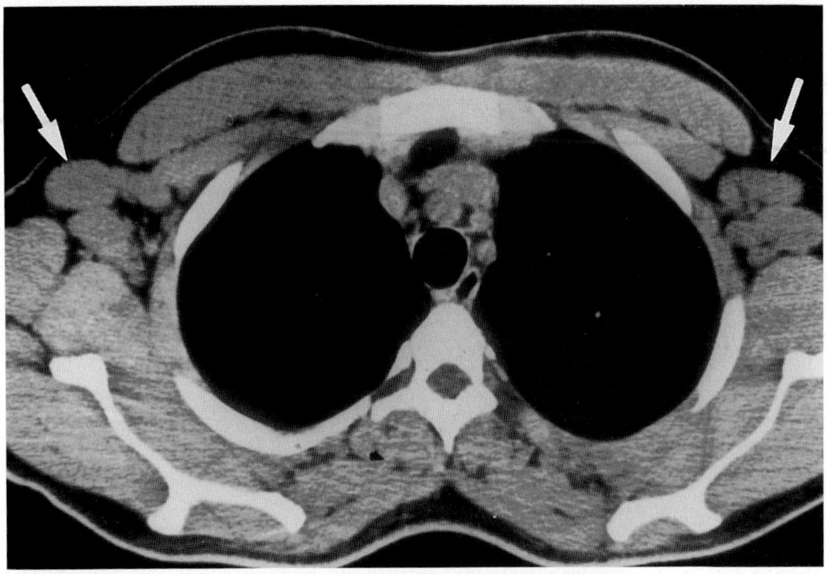

**FIGURE 1** AIDS-related lymphadenopathy. Bilateral axillary adenopathy *(arrows)* from reactive lymphoid hyperplasia. (From Kuhlman JE, Fishman EK, Hruban RH, et al. Diseases of the chest in AIDS: CT diagnosis. Radiographics 1989; 9:827; with permission.)

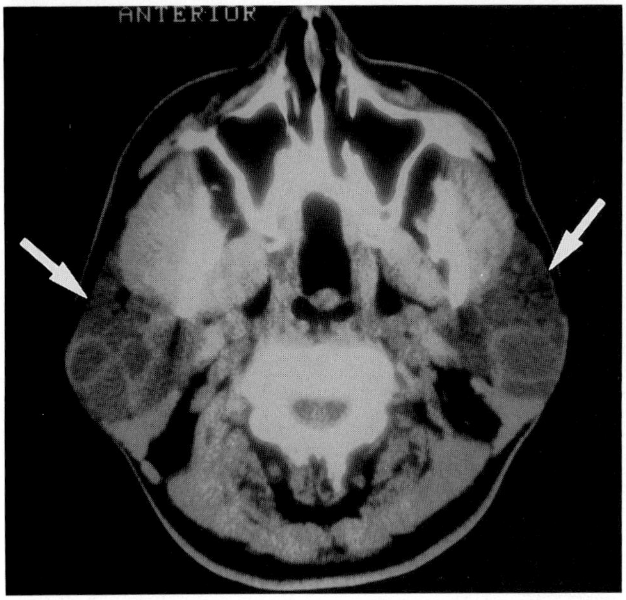

**FIGURE 2** Lymphoepithelial cystic disease of the parotid glands. Lymphoid hyperplasia in and around the parotid ductal system results in cystic obstruction of the ducts and bilateral parotid gland enlargement *(arrows)*.

When extensive mediastinal or hilar adenopathy is identified by chest CT (Fig. 3), usually one of three diseases is present: (1) an AIDS-related lymphoma, (2) disseminated mycobacterial infection either caused by *Mycobacterium avium-intracellulare* (MAI) or tuberculosis (TB), or (3) the lymphadenopathic form of KS.

There is one situation in the setting of enlarged mediastinal and hilar adenopathy in which a specific diagnosis can be made, that is, when calcification is identified within the enlarged lymph nodes (Fig. 4). This has recently been recognized in AIDS patients with the disseminated form of *Pneumocystis* infection. Patients with disseminated *Pneumocystis* infection present with calcifications in enlarged lymph nodes, calcifications in their spleen, and calcifications in other organs such as the liver and kidneys. At least some of these patients are being treated with aerosolized pentamidine, and it has been postulated that disseminated infection may occur because blood levels of pentamidine with aerosolized treatments are not high enough to clear the bloodstream of the infection. What causes calcification within the affected lymphatic tissues in this setting is not known, but appears to be a dystrophic response to the disseminated infection.

## CT Patterns of Lung Involvement Caused by Opportunistic Infections in HIV Disease

Opportunistic infections are common in patients with AIDS and account for significant morbidity and mortality. A pulmonary infection, in fact, is often the first AIDS-defining illness. The patient with HIV disease is susceptible to multiorganism infection and a variety of pulmonary infections caused by common bacterial organisms and unusual opportunistic pathogens. Although CT findings of lung infection in HIV disease are often nonspecific, certain characteristic CT patterns are more suggestive of certain infections than others. CT is also helpful in confirming the presence of occult lung infection in subtle or equivocal cases.

### Pneumocystis *Pneumonia*

*Pneumocystis carinii* pneumonia (PCP) is the most common life-threatening lung infection in patients with AIDS. It is estimated that over 60 percent of AIDS patients experience at least one episode of PCP during the course of their illness. Unlike its presentation in other immunocompromised hosts, PCP in AIDS can have an atypical course with insidious onset of malaise, fever, and nonproductive cough. Early in the course of infection, the chest radiograph may appear normal or show only minimal increased lung markings. It is in this setting that chest CT scanning can be helpful, primarily to confirm or exclude the presence of subtle lung infection.

Three CT patterns of pulmonary involvement are commonly observed in PCP: a ground glass pattern, a patchwork pattern, and an interstitial pattern.

The ground glass pattern of PCP is characterized on CT by

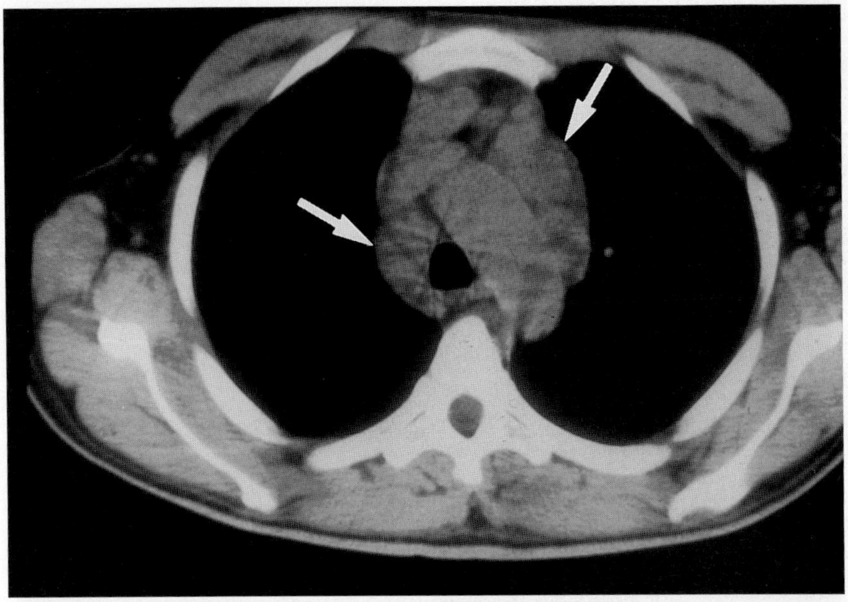

**FIGURE 3** Extensive mediastinal adenopathy *(arrows)* caused by an AIDS-related lymphoma.

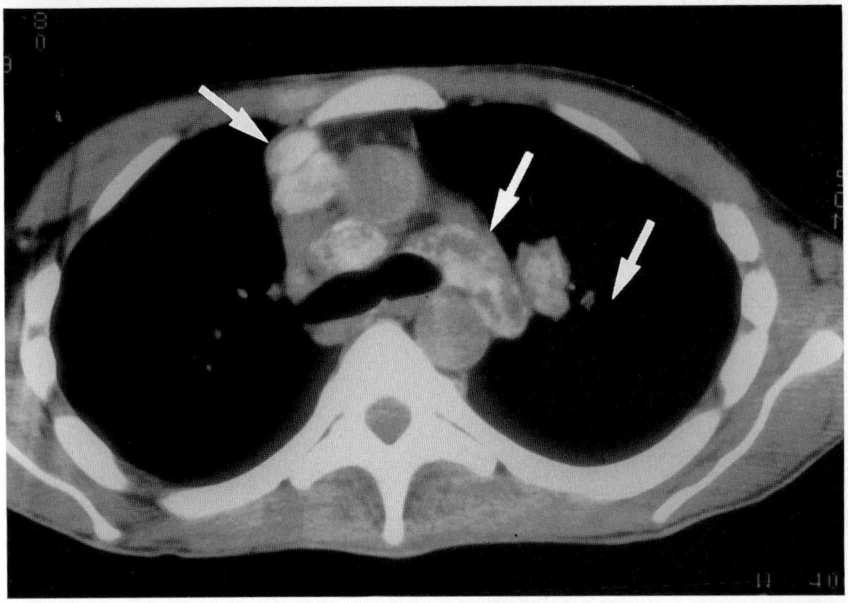

**FIGURE 4** Calcified enlarged mediastinal lymph nodes *(arrows)* caused by disseminated *Pneumocystis* infection. Calcifications have been reported in abdominal lymph nodes, the liver, spleen, and kidneys in disseminated pneumocystis infection.

diffuse, bilateral airspace disease that affects the lungs symmetrically. The patchwork pattern of PCP is characterized on CT by asymmetric involvement of both lungs that is distinctly patchy in its distribution, with sparing of segmental and subsegmental areas of the lung. The resultant CT pattern has a geographic or mosaic appearance. In my experience this is the most characteristic CT pattern suggesting PCP infection (Fig. 5). It typically consists of ground glass airspace opacities with or without a component of interstitial disease. An interstitial pattern may also be seen on CT in PCP, particularly in patients who have had recurrent infection. Up to 20 percent of AIDS patients have relapse of their PCP infection, and PCP heals with lung fibrosis. The interstitial pattern is characterized by increased interstitial markings that are primarily linear.

Other less common manifestations of PCP on chest radiographs and CT include focal infiltrates, cavities, and nodules. A solitary nodule identified on CT may be caused by PCP infection in those few HIV-positive patients who are still able to mount a granulomatous response to the infection.

One form of PCP that appears to be increasing in frequency is what I like to call "cavitary or cystic PCP" (Fig. 6). In this form of the infection, the lungs are replaced by a multitude of thin-walled cysts or cavities. The etiology of this form of cystic PCP is not known. It may or may not be related to the use of aerosolized pentamidine or zidovudine (AZT). This form of the infection is often associated with the disseminated form of the disease, which was discussed earlier.

CT findings that often accompany PCP infection in HIV disease include the presence of apical and paraseptal bullae (Fig. 7) and spontaneous pneumothoraces. Pleural effusions are uncommon in isolated PCP infection. Development of bullae and cystic spaces is important clinically because it predisposes AIDS patients to pneumothoraces, both spontaneous ones and those that result from diagnostic and therapeutic procedures. These pneumothoraces are often difficult to treat with persistent air leaks requiring surgical intervention with pleurectomy, pleurodesis, or lung-stapling procedures.

A

B

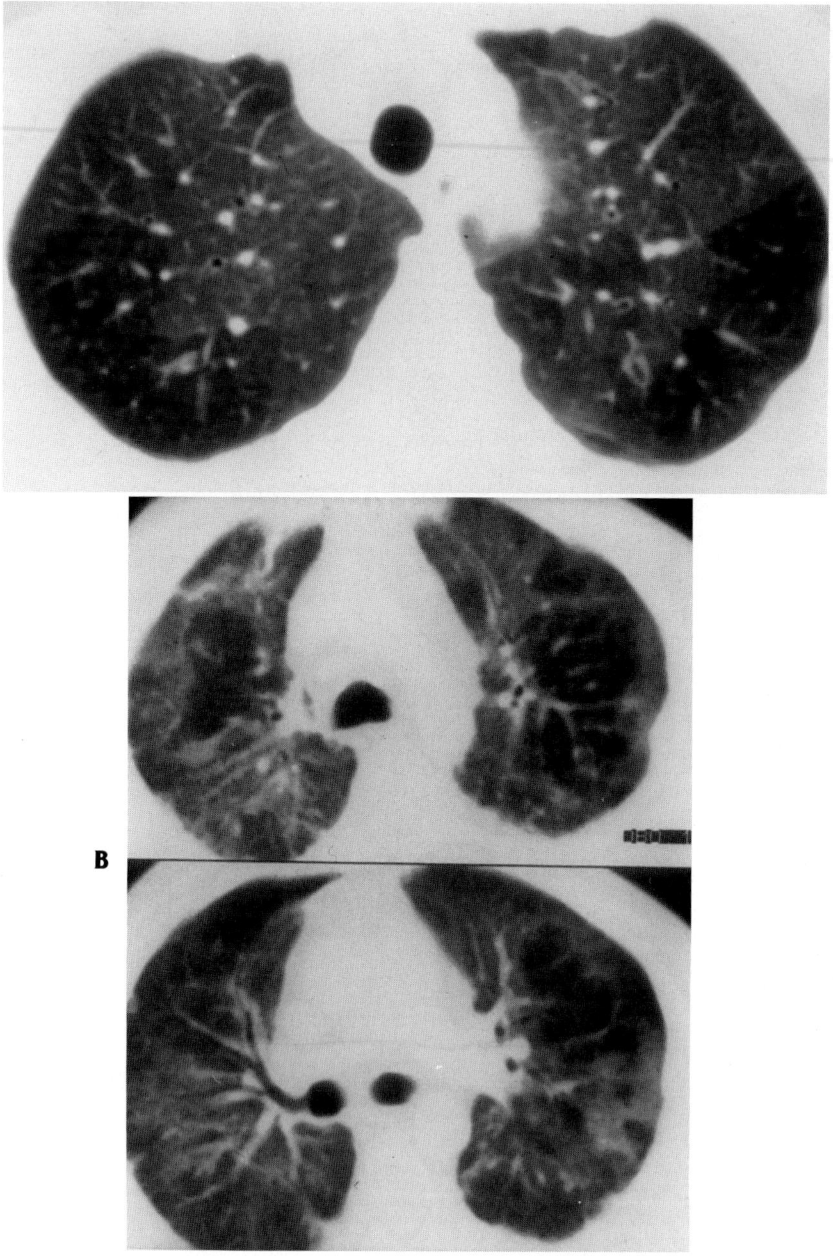

**FIGURE 5** *A* and *B*, CT patterns of *Pneumocystis* pneumonia: patchwork pattern. Both cases show patchy ground glass infiltrates in a geographic or mosaic distribution. (From Kuhlman JE, Kavuru M, Fishman EK, Siegelman SS. *Pneumocystis carinii* pneumonia: Spectrum of parenchymal CT findings. Radiology 1990; 175:711–714; with permission.)

## Nocardia, *Cytomegalovirus, Fungal, and Mycobacterial Disease*

*Nocardia* is an opportunistic lung pathogen that is seen in HIV disease. *Nocardia* infection usually presents as a necrotizing pneumonia with lobar, multilobar, or multisegmental cavitary disease. Nocardiosis in AIDS is shown in Figure 8. This segmental or lobar configuration of a cavitating pneumonia, particularly if it involves more than one area of the lung, should suggest *Nocardia* as a possible etiology. The cavitary disease also tends to be slowly progressive.

Cytomegalovirus (CMV) is almost ubiquitous in AIDS patients, and it is frequently cultured out of the blood, urine, and organs at autopsy. How much clinically significant lung disease CMV causes is controversial. It can produce diffuse infiltrates indistinguishable from PCP, and frequently both organisms are cultured out of lung specimens. CMV can cause serositis with pleural effusions and pericardial effusions. It also can produce severe disabling esophagitis (Fig. 9). Although CT is not used to diagnose esophagitis in AIDS patients, one can identify findings of severe esophagitis on CT including diffuse circumferential esophageal wall thickening. Such esophageal findings can be caused by CMV, *Candida,* or herpes simplex infection of the esophagus.

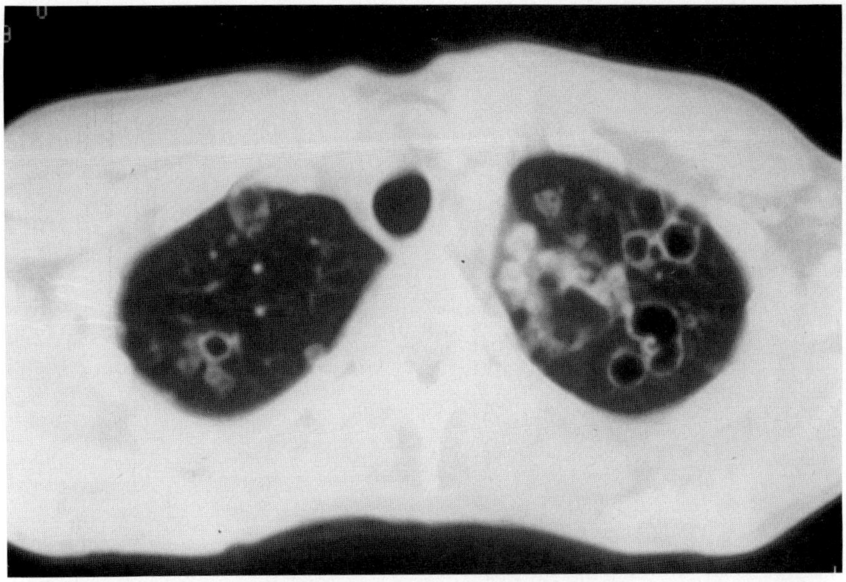

**FIGURE 6** CT patterns of *Pneumocystis* pneumonia: cystic or cavitary disease. Multiple thin-walled cysts or cavities characterize this form of the infection, which may be associated with CT findings of dissemination such as calcifications in lymph nodes and abdominal organs.

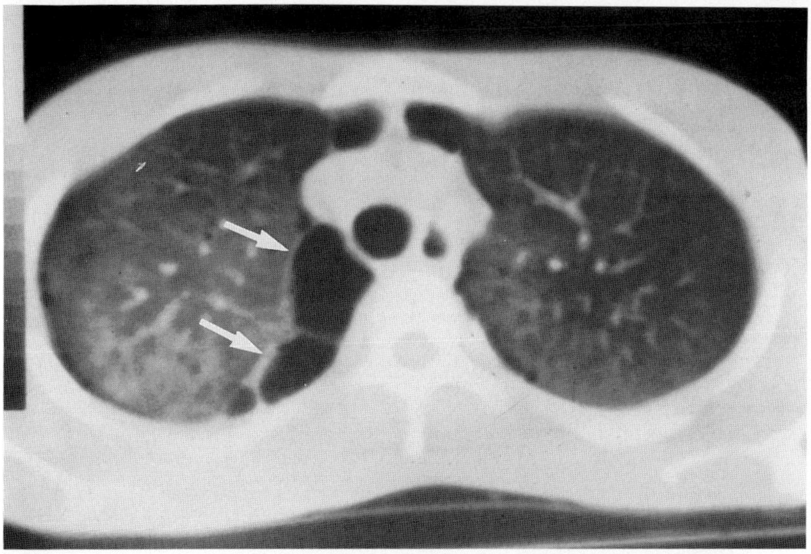

**FIGURE 7** Paraseptal and apical bullae *(arrows)* in AIDS. Notice ground glass infiltrates caused by PCP. (From Kuhlman JE, Knowles MC, Fishman EK, Siegelman SS. Premature bullous damage in AIDS: CT diagnosis. Radiology 1989; 173:23; with permission.)

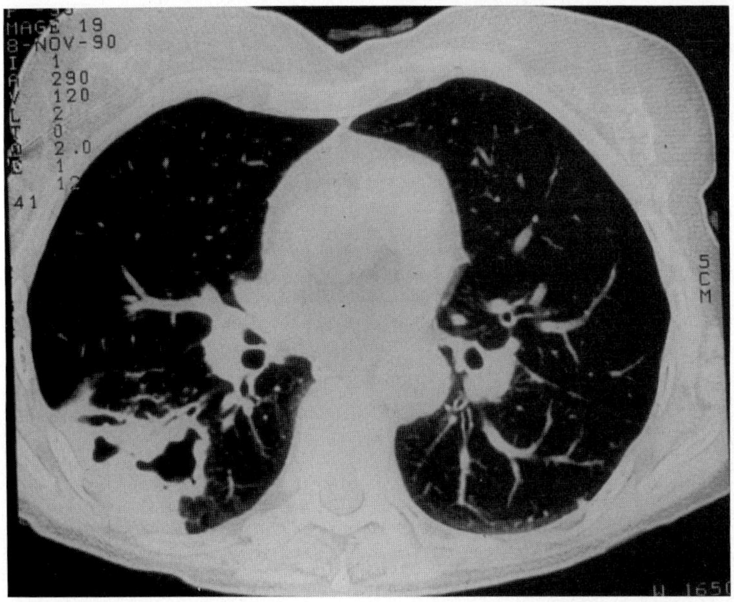


**FIGURE 8** Nocardiosis in AIDS. Progressive cavitary pneumonia characterizes this infection.

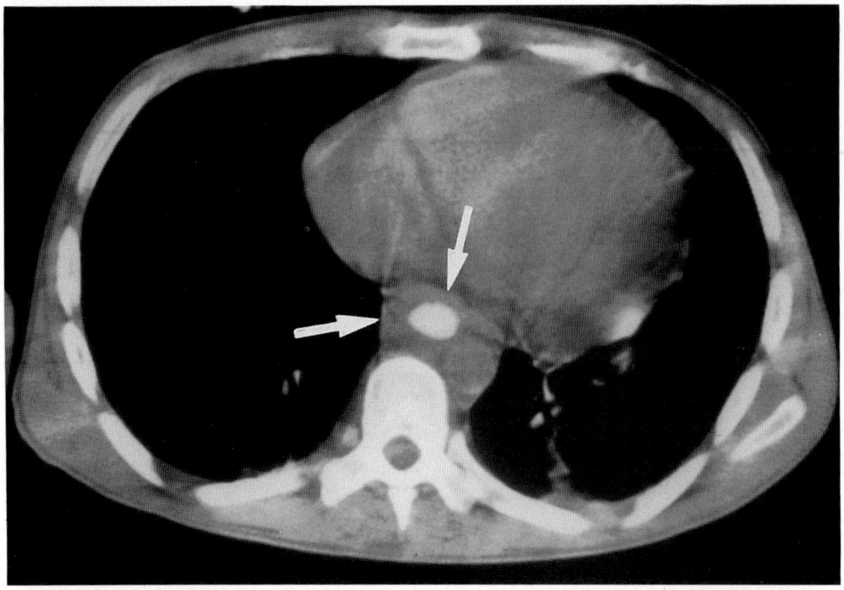

**FIGURE 9** CMV esophagitis. CT shows marked esophageal wall thickening *(arrows)*.

A

B

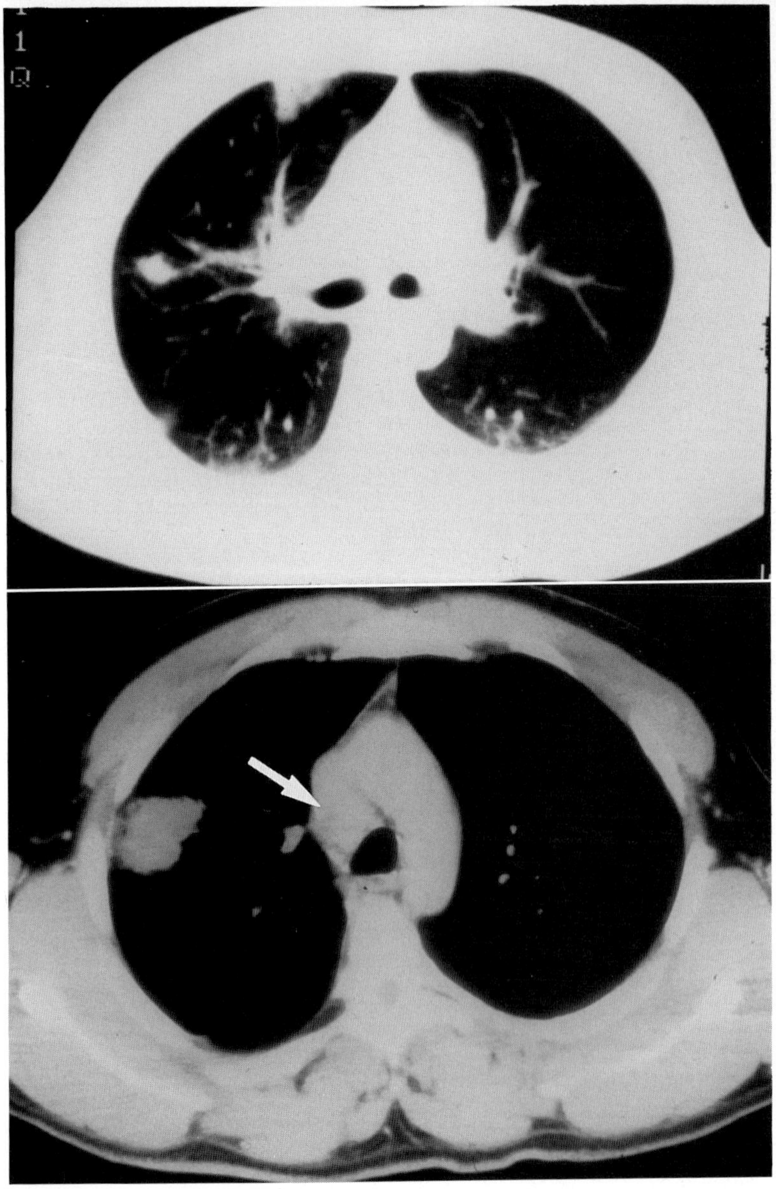

**FIGURE 10** *A* and *B,* Tuberculosis in AIDS. CT shows multiple lung masses *(arrow)* and mediastinal adenopathy. Adenopathy is the rule rather than the exception in HIV-positive adults with TB.

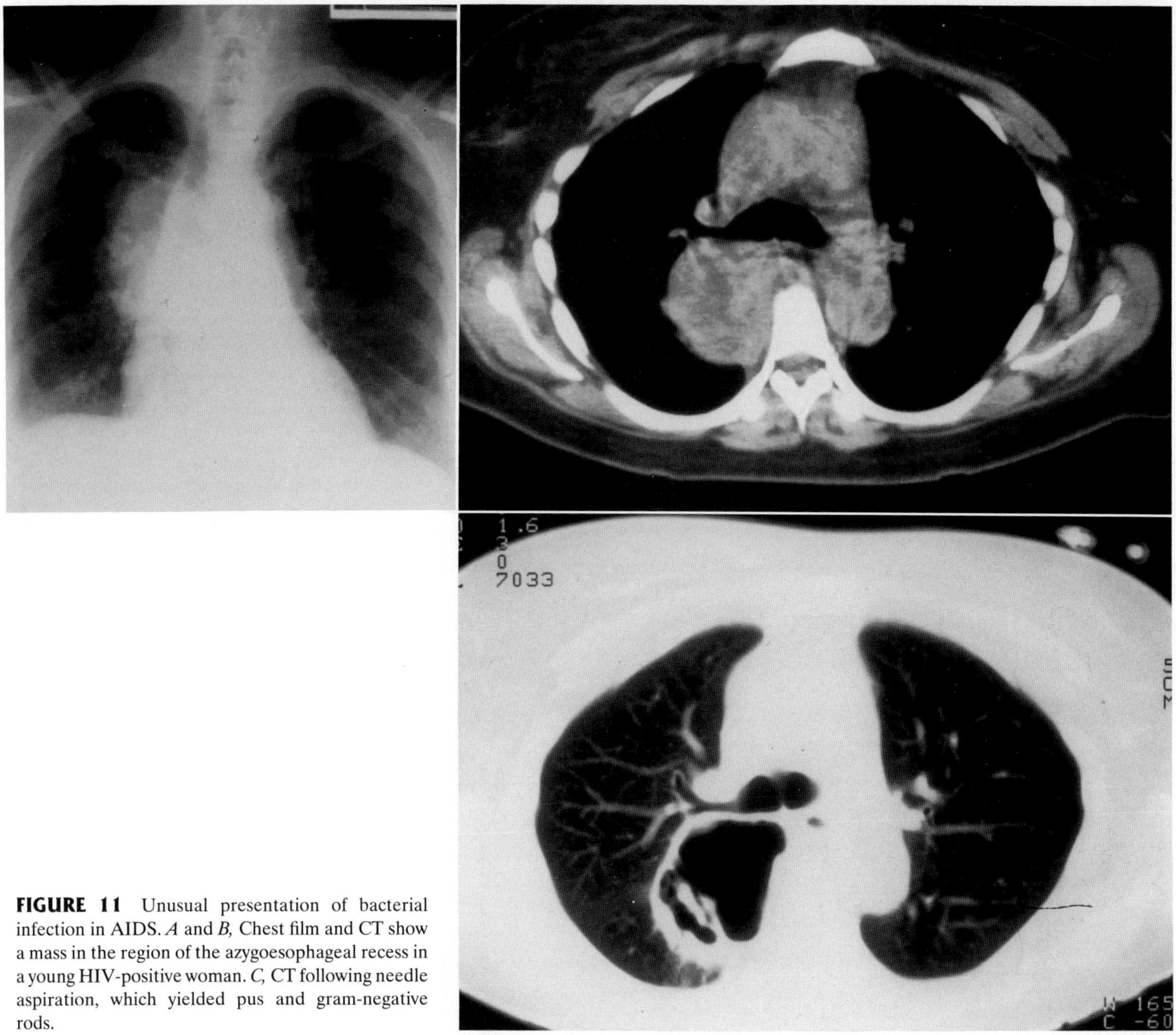

A B C

**FIGURE 11** Unusual presentation of bacterial infection in AIDS. *A* and *B,* Chest film and CT show a mass in the region of the azygoesophageal recess in a young HIV-positive woman. *C,* CT following needle aspiration, which yielded pus and gram-negative rods.

Fungal infections in the lung in HIV disease usually present as multiple inflammatory nodules or as cavities. Fungal pathogens include *Candida, Aspergillus,* and *Cryptococcus,* among other species. Definitive diagnosis of pulmonary fungal infection usually requires biopsy and cultures of lung tissue, and CT can be useful in localizing the most accessible site of lung infection for sampling.

Lung infection in HIV disease caused by mycobacterial disease may be from TB or atypical mycobacterium such as MAI. MAI most commonly manifests itself as adenopathy without pulmonary infiltrates, but it can cause cavities, nodules, or reticulonodular infiltrates on CT. Pulmonary disease caused by TB is increasing in this country as a result of the AIDS epidemic. For many years the incidence of TB was on the decline in the United States, but because of the AIDS epidemic the incidence of TB is now on the rise. The CT manifestations of TB in the chest vary in HIV disease and depend on how advanced the immunosuppression is. In early HIV disease, TB presents in a more "classic" fashion with cavitary disease and bronchogenic spread. In more advanced HIV disease, when immunosuppression is severe, TB presents in unusual forms. It tends to be widely disseminated and aggressive. Multiple pulmonary masses with significant adenopathy is another presentation of TB in the AIDS patient (Fig. 10). Adenopathy as a manifestation of TB in AIDS is the rule rather than the exception, unlike TB in the non-HIV adult patient with TB in which adenopathy is uncommon. TB is also a recognized cause of tracheoesophageal fistulas in AIDS patients.

### *Bacterial Infections*

Although one tends to concentrate on the unusual opportunistic infections in HIV disease, common bacterial pathogens also cause significant pulmonary disease in these patients (Fig. 11). In addition to T-cell deficiencies, these patients also have deficiencies in the humoral antibody system, making them prone to recurrent and more severe bacterial infections.

Intravenous drug users are one of the fastest-growing subpopulations of HIV-infected patients. Increasingly one observes manifestations of chest disease in these patients that

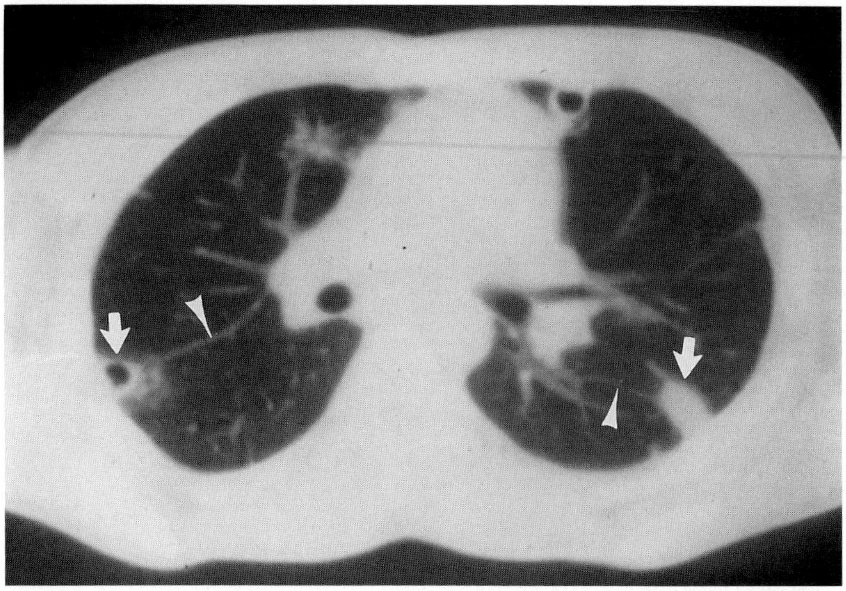

**FIGURE 12** Septic emboli are readily diagnosed with CT in the HIV-positive drug user. CT shows multiple peripheral nodules in varying stages of cavitation *(arrows)* and feeding vessels *(arrowheads)*.

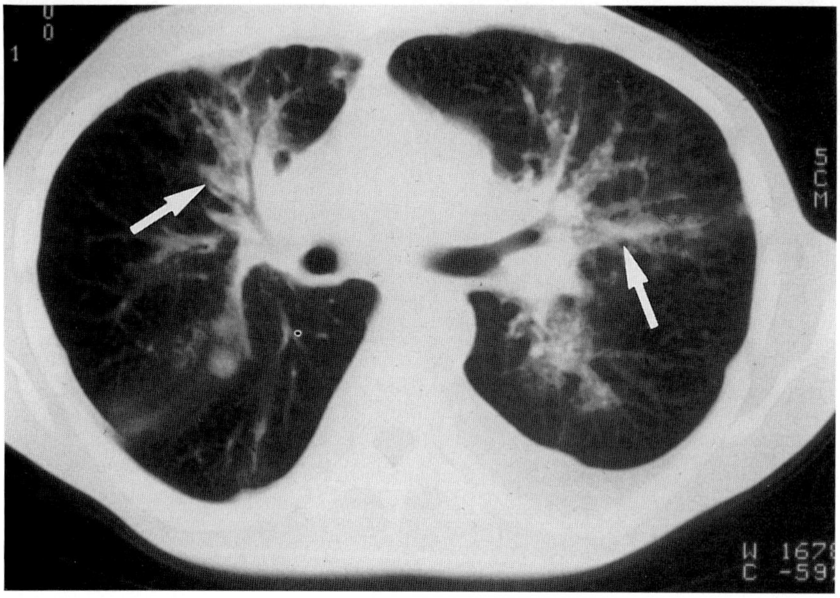

**FIGURE 13** CT features of parenchymal lung involvement in Kaposi's sarcoma. Lung disease as a result of Kaposi's sarcoma appears to radiate out from both pulmonary hilum along the bronchovascular bundles *(arrows)*.

reflect not only their HIV status, but also the fact that they use intravenous drugs. For example, septic pulmonary emboli are observed not uncommonly in the intravenous drug user with HIV disease (Fig. 12). In addition, as with other pulmonary infections in HIV disease, septic emboli in these patients tend to be more severe, more extensive, and more often complicated by abscess and empyema formation.

CT findings of septic pulmonary emboli include the presence of multiple peripheral nodules often demonstrating various stages of cavitation. A distinct feeding vessel leading to each nodule can often be identified by CT, indicating the hematogenous origin of the lesion. CT findings of septic emboli may be the first indication of endocarditis or intravascular infection in unsuspected cases. CT can be used to quickly confirm chest film findings that may be subtle or equivocal for septic emboli. CT documents the extent of disseminated infection and identifies complicating empyemas. Management of loculated empyemas is aided by CT examination and can be used to direct chest tube placement.

## Clinical Applications

The AIDS patient with unexplained fever or respiratory symptoms represents a difficult clinical problem. When routine radiographic evaluation fails to provide an answer in this setting, CT plays an important diagnostic and management role as follows:

1. CT helps detect early infection when the chest films remain negative or equivocal.
2. CT characterizes the type and extent of pulmonary disease, and in certain instances, CT patterns of parenchymal involvement may suggest the most likely diagnosis.
3. In the patient with a complex or difficult to interpret chest radiograph, CT clarifies radiographic abnormalities.

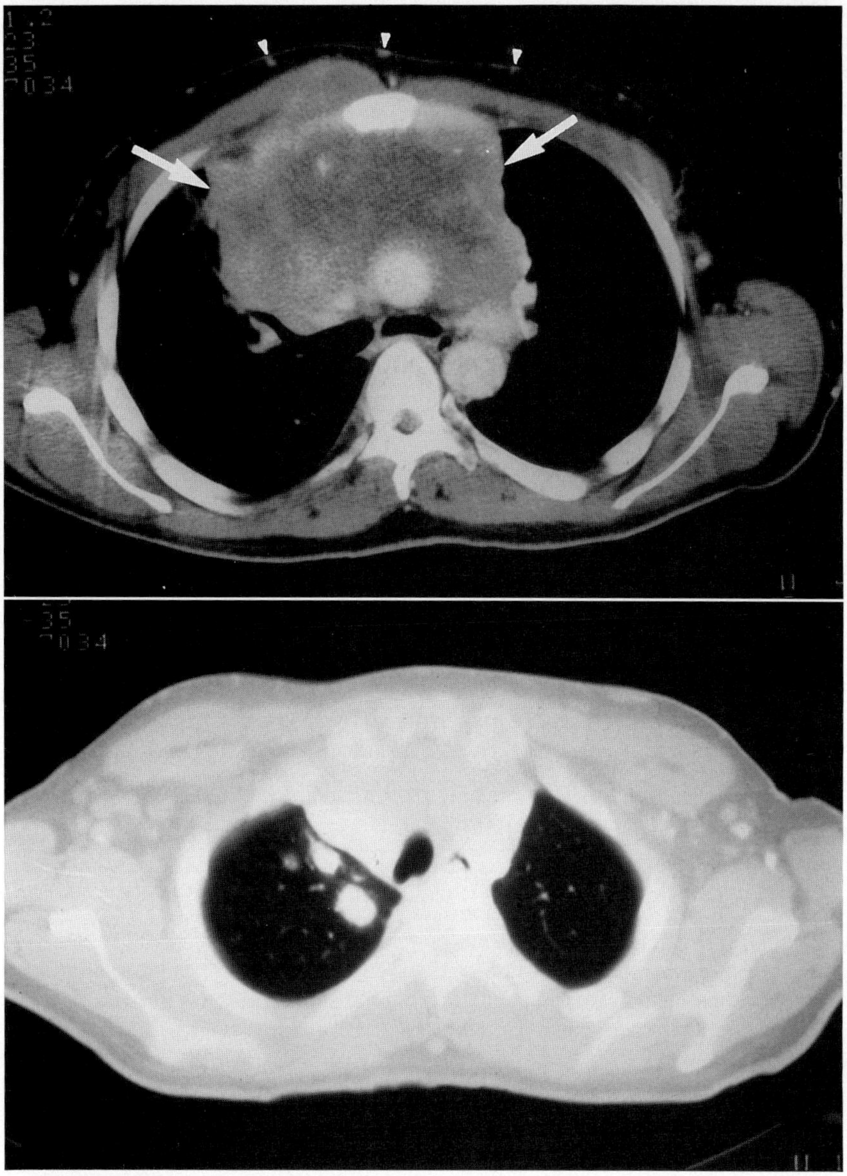

A

B

**FIGURE 14** AIDS-related lymphoma. *A,* A large anterior mediastinal mass is aggressively invading the chest wall *(arrows)* and causing superior vena cava obstruction. See chest wall collaterals *(arrowheads)*. *B,* At presentation, the patient also had multiple lung masses.

4. CT can direct invasive biopsy procedures, especially when there is CT evidence of multiorganism infection.

## AIDS-related Neoplasms

Neoplastic disorders in HIV disease that may affect the chest include AIDS-related lymphomas, lymphocytic interstitial pneumonitis (LIP), and KS. There are also anecdotal reports of other solid tumors that may or may not have an increased incidence in AIDS.

KS occurs in approximately 25 percent of patients with AIDS. Of those, an estimated 20 percent experience pulmonary involvement. Almost invariably these patients have extensive skin and other organ involvement at the time they present with pulmonary disease. CT findings of KS in the lung include the presence of poorly marginated nodular infiltrates that radiate out from the pulmonary hila along the bronchovascular bundles (Fig. 13). Disease appears to encase or coat the bronchi. Pleural disease can also be seen. KS causes pleural thickening and loculated bloody pleural effusions. In KS patients with pulmonary involvement, one can frequently identify on CT skin nodules and sometimes bone lesions caused by KS.

A spectrum of lymphoproliferative disorders affects the lung in AIDS including lymphoma and LIP. All types of lymphoma appear to have an increased incidence in AIDS, but the most common AIDS-related lymphoma is non-Hodgkin's lymphoma. Typically AIDS-related lymphomas are aggressive and show a predilection for extranodal sites of involvement such as the central nervous system, the gastrointestinal tract, the pulmonary parenchyma, and bone marrow. Thoracic involvement has been reported to occur in 9 to 31 percent of patients with AIDS-related lymphomas. Lymphoma may be the first AIDS-defining illness in some HIV-positive individuals. Only about 25 percent of patients with AIDS-related lymphomas present in a typical fashion for lymphoma, with mediastinal or hilar adenopathy. Unusual presentations of lymphoma seem to be the norm in HIV disease including CT findings such as pleural effusions, parenchymal nodules, alveolar and interstitial infiltrates, and paraspinal and chest wall masses. These may occur with or without associated adenopathy (Fig. 14).

## Suggested Reading

Barrio JL, Suarez M, Rodriguez JL, et al. *Pneumocystis carinii* pneumonia presenting as cavitating and noncavitating solitary pulmonary nodules in patients with the acquired immunodeficiency syndrome. Am Rev Respir Dis 1986; 134:1094.

Bottles K, McPhaul LW, Volberding P. Fine-needle aspiration biopsy of patients with acquired immunodeficiency syndrome (AIDS): Experience in an outpatient clinic. Ann Intern Med 1988; 108:42.

Kovacs JA, Hiemenz JW, Macher AM, et al. *Pneumocystis carinii* pneumonia: A comparison between patients with acquired immunodeficiency syndrome and patients with other immunodeficiencies. Ann Intern Med 1984; 100:633.

Kuhlman JE, Fishman EK, Hruban RH, et al. Diseases of the chest in AIDS: CT diagnosis. Radiographics 1989; 9:827.

Kuhlman JE, Fishman EK, Teigen C. Pulmonary septic emboli: Diagnosis with CT. Radiology 1990; 174:211.

Kuhlman JE, Kavuru M, Fishman EK, Siegelman SS. *Pneumocystis carinii* pneumonia: Spectrum of parenchymal CT findings. Radiology 1990; 175:711–714.

Kuhlman JE, Knowles MC, Fishman EK, Siegelman SS. Premature bullous damage in AIDS: CT diagnosis. Radiology 1989; 173:23.

Naidich DP, Garay SM, Goodman PC. Pulmonary manifestations of AIDS. In: Federle MD, Megibow AJ, Naidich DP, eds. Radiology of AIDS. New York: Raven, 1988:47.

Radin DR, Baker EL, Klatt EC, et al. Visceral and nodal calcification in patients with AIDS-related *Pneumocystis carinii* infection. AJR 1990; 154:27.

Sider L, Weiss AJ, Smith MD, et al. Varied appearance of AIDS-related lymphoma in the chest. Radiology 1989; 171:629.

# Radionuclide Evaluation of the Chest in AIDS

*VICTOR W. LEE, M.D. · ELLEN PANAGEAS, M.D.*
*BARRY A. TURNBULL, Ph.D.*

Since currently there is no effective cure for human immunodeficiency virus (HIV) infection, the management of patients with acquired immunodeficiency syndrome (AIDS) is limited to management of its complications including opportunistic infections and neoplasia. The common chest complications include *Pneumocystis carinii* pneumonia (PCP), bacterial pneumonia, tuberculous infections, Kaposi's sarcoma, non-Hodgkin's lymphoma, and other fungal infections. Chest complications are not only the most common, but also the leading causes of death among these patients. Chest radiography and computed tomography (CT) have been useful for evaluation of patients suspected of these complications, but their major limitation is their nonspecificity. For example, Kaposi's sarcoma cannot be reliably differentiated from lymphoma. The details of chest CT and radiography of these conditions are discussed in the two preceding chapters and thus are not covered here. Radionuclide scans have been used frequently to complement these anatomic imaging techniques.

## Gallium and Thallium Scintigraphy

Gallium scintigraphy has been the most commonly performed radionuclide study for patients with AIDS since the beginning of the epidemic. Earlier reports raised doubt about the clinical usefulness of gallium scans, because the sensitivity and specificity were highly variable. According to our own experience, as well as more recent reports in the literature, we find the following measures are crucial to obtain optimal, reproducible, and specific results from gallium scintigraphy (gallium scan technique is described in standard nuclear medicine textbooks and is not repeated here).

### *Grading the Intensity of Gallium Uptake in the Lung*

The "darkness" of the lungs in the gallium scan depends not only on the presence of pathology, but also on other technical factors such as the type of films used and the "gain" control of the cathode-ray tube. This variable often results in significant interobserver differences and subjectivity of interpretation. The grading system using a relative scale, comparing the intensity of gallium uptakes of the lung and the adjacent normal organs, has been found useful. *Grade 0:* lung uptake same as soft tissue, e.g., axilla; *grade 1:* lung uptake above soft tissue, but below that of bone (ribs); *grade 2:* lung uptake same as ribs, but below sternum or liver; *grade 3:* lung uptake same as sternum, but below liver (a negative cardiac shadow is also apparent); *grade 4:* lung uptake equal or above liver. Grades 0 and 1 are considered normal, grade 2 is borderline, and grades 3 and 4 are definitely abnormal. This grading system gives us more confidence in reading gallium scans, and it minimizes subjectivity.

When the interpretation is equivocal (grade 2), other patient information also should be used such as clinical presentations, radiologic findings, and prior gallium scans.

### *Pattern Approach of Gallium Scans*

The interpretation of gallium scans is more than just the recognition of presence or absence of chest pathology. The distribution pattern of abnormal gallium uptake is highly useful in helping the radiologist to identify or at least suggest the specific complicating pathologies. This approach is based on knowledge of the common complications in AIDS, as well as empiric knowledge in recent reports. Correlation with the

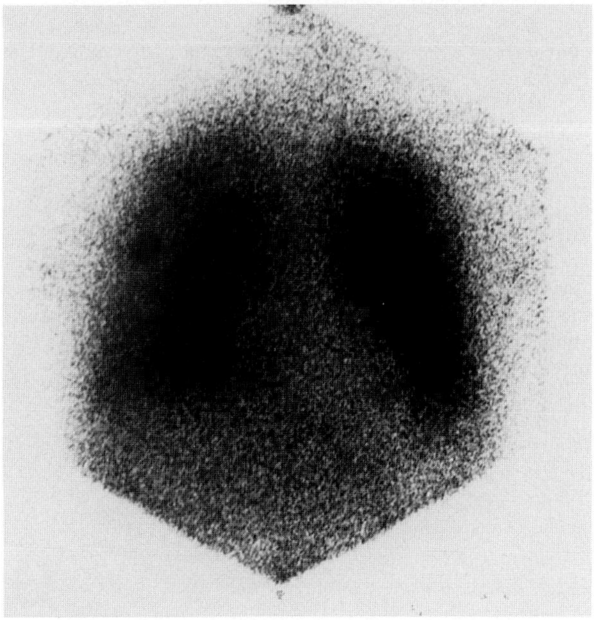

**FIGURE 1** A 37-year-old immunodeficient patient who complained of cough, fever, and shortness of breath. His chest radiographs showed only slight increase of reticulonodular density at the bases of lung. The gallium scan demonstrated diffuse, homogeneous, and markedly increased uptake of both lungs. The intensity of gallium uptake was above that of the sternum and liver (grade 4). The diagnosis of PCP was confirmed by bronchoscopy.

patient's clinical information and radiographs is indispensable for optimal results. This pattern approach should be combined with the grading system discussed previously.

### Diffuse Increase of Uptake of Gallium in Both Lungs

When the intensity of gallium lung uptake is grade 3 or 4 and the distribution is diffuse (homogeneous or patchy), the most common cause among patients with AIDS is PCP. The uptake in the lung is obviously above that of the mediastinum and heart, resulting in an appearance of a "negative cardiac shadow" (Fig. 1). Although the corresponding radiographs may show variable patterns in PCP, ranging from normal to interstitial reticulonodular appearance, they should always be compared with the gallium scans side by side before the diagnosis of PCP is made. Other common pathologies among patients with AIDS, such as adult respiratory distress syndrome (ARDS) and pulmonary edema caused by overhydration, may be the causes of marked and diffuse gallium uptake in the lungs. These causes can be seen in chest radiographs showing a diffuse alveolar pattern, which is different from PCP. Other causes of diffuse pulmonary infections, such as miliary tuberculosis and disseminated histoplasmosis, are also known to show similar pattern in gallium scans, but they are much less common among patients with AIDS. They need to be excluded on clinical grounds.

Lymphocytic interstitial pneumonia (LIP) should also be included in the differential diagnosis. Its diagnosis is usually made by exclusion or biopsy. Fortunately for the radiologist, it is rare among adult patients with AIDS. The abnormal lung gallium uptake is diffuse, but usually the intensity of uptake is only moderate (grade 2) in contrast to PCP. Among children with HIV infections, the disease should be considered or excluded, either on clinical grounds or by biopsy, whenever a diffuse pattern of grade 2 gallium uptake is present.

### Segmental or Lobar Uptake of Gallium in the Lung

This pattern is usually associated with common bacterial pneumonia caused by pneumococci, *Haemophilus influenzae,* staphylococci, *Legionella,* and so forth. The radiographs usually demonstrate consolidation in the same locations.

For patients who are on prophylactic inhalation therapy with pentamidine aerosol, PCP sometimes may show an unusual pattern, resulting in bilateral apical uptake of gallium. This is because pentamidine aerosol is usually given with the patient in the upright position, resulting in insufficient deposition of pentamidine in the apical regions. This characteristic pattern, together with the history of prophylactic inhalation therapy should point to the correct diagnosis. It is distinct from the segmental distribution of gallium uptake in bacterial pneumonia.

### Focal Uptake of Gallium in the Mediastinum and Hila

The common etiologies of this abnormal pattern are *Mycobacterium tuberculosis* infection (MTB), *Mycobacterium avium-intracellulare* (MAI), lymphoma, and less frequently, cytomegalovirus infection (CMV) (Fig. 2).

Especially among patients with advanced immunodeficiency, MTB infection often manifests differently from the "adult" type or reactivation of tuberculosis. It resembles more the primary type of infection, with hilar and mediastinal lymphadenopathy, which is gallium avid. MAI shows exactly the same pattern in chest radiographs and gallium scans. It can only be distinguished from MTB by bacterial culture results. MAI is not a pathogen among immunocompetent hosts. The treatment of MAI is difficult and controversial.

Non-Hodgkin's lymphoma is a fatal complication among patients with AIDS. It frequently causes lymphadenopathy and extranodal involvement. Gallium scan alone cannot differentiate lymphoma from tuberculosis or MAI. However, it may sometimes indicate an easy site for biopsy, e.g., positive supraclavicular nodes in addition to mediastinal adenopathy. Together with thallium scans, a more specific diagnosis can be made (Table 1; Fig. 3).

Although CMV has been isolated frequently in bronchoalveolar washing among patients with AIDS and among patients showing focal gallium uptake in the mediastinum and hila, its pathologic effects in the lung are considered only trivial. Probably it does not have any significant impact on the clinical course in most patients.

### Opacities in Radiographic and Negative Gallium Studies

This pattern is suggestive of pulmonary Kaposi's sarcoma, which can be confirmed with thallium scintigraphy (Table 1). Of the common chest complications of AIDS mentioned above, Kaposi's sarcoma is the only one that is consistently gallium negative. Although its appearance is variable in radiographs, it is commonly associated with pleural effusion. Cutaneous lesions are usually present, but pulmonary Kaposi's sarcoma may sometimes precede cutaneous manifestation. Clinically it is important to differentiate pulmonary Kaposi's sarcoma from other pulmonary complications such as PCP, since it is frequently the cause of major respiratory symptoms or even

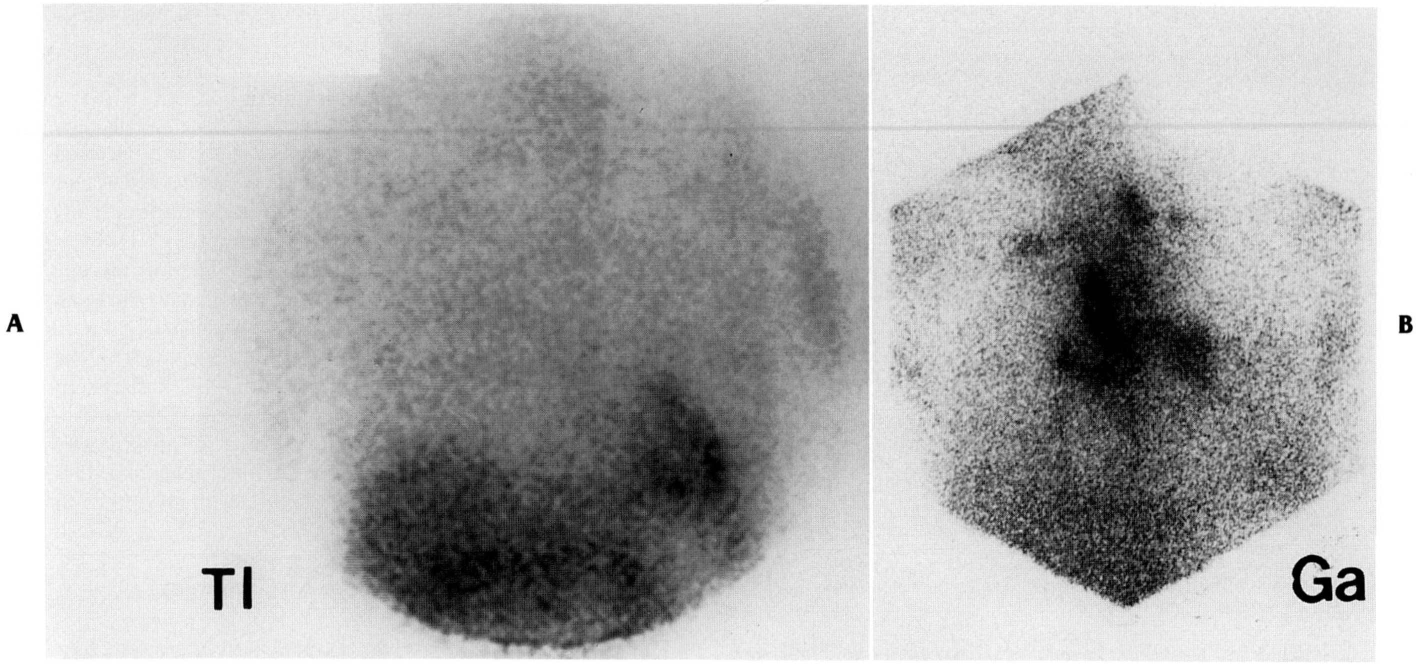


**FIGURE 2** A 39-year-old male with a known history of AIDS. He was readmitted to the hospital because of persistent fever, chills, and cough. The admission chest radiographs (not shown) demonstrated newly developed mediastinal and hilar adenopathy. *A,* The 3 hour thallium scans were negative. *B,* The gallium scans showed multiple, partly confluent foci of abnormal gallium uptake in the hilar, mediastinal, and supra-clavicular regions. The findings were consistent with infectious lymphadenitis. Biopsy and culture confirmed that it was *Mycobacterium tuberculosis.*

**TABLE 1** Findings of Gallium and Thallium Scintigraphy in Patients with Chest Complications of AIDS

| | Gallium | Thallium |
|---|---|---|
| PCP | Positive, diffuse | Negative |
| TB, MAI | Positive, focal | Negative |
| Lymphoma | Positive | Positive |
| Kaposi's sarcoma | Negative | Positive |

death. Even limited chemotherapy or radiation treatment may provide significant symptomatic relief. Its diagnosis by bronchoscopy or biopsy is difficult because of the high incidence of false negatives and potential complications such as bleeding.

### *Thallium Scintigraphy*

Thallium-201 in the form of thallous ion is a biochemical analog of potassium cation. It is an intracellular ion found in high concentration in normal myocardium, skeletal muscles, and many neoplastic cells such as observed in Kaposi's sarcoma and lymphoma. Thallium scintigraphy can be used to differentiate these tumors from infections, because cell culture experiments show infected or inflammatory cells exhibit only relatively low concentration of thallium.

In clinical settings it is crucial to perform delayed (3 hours after injection) scans of the chest, because pulmonary edema or congestion associated with infections is known to show relatively high early uptake of thallium. Although tumor uptake is persistent, the thallium uptake caused by congestion or edema decreases rapidly. Persistent thallium uptake in the lung is characteristic of both Kaposi's sarcoma and lymphoma. Since lymphoma is both gallium and thallium avid, and infections are gallium avid but thallium negative, these lesions can be differentiated from pulmonary Kaposi's sarcoma when combined thallium and gallium scans are used (Table 1; Fig. 4).

Technically a thallium scan should be performed first, before a gallium scan, because of its lower energy peaks (69 to 93 keV). Other technical details are described in standard textbooks and are not repeated here.

The patient's current chest radiographs should always be available for side-by-side comparison with the thallium and gallium scans. For patients in the advanced stage of AIDS, it is not rare to have more than one disease in the lungs simultaneously, e.g., Kaposi's sarcoma and PCP. Therefore it is not enough just to say that the gallium scan is positive. It is extremely important to locate the presence or absence, as well as the locations, of abnormal thallium and gallium uptake relative to the opacities seen on the current chest radiographs. This side-by-side comparison enables us to diagnose the presence of multiple chest pathologies.

## Tc-DTPA Aerosol Lung Scan and Clearance Test for Lung Infections

### *Rationale*

In most nuclear medicine departments, technetium diethylenetriaminepenta-acetic acid (Tc-DTPA) aerosol lung scans usually are performed together with perfusion lung scans for detection of pulmonary embolism. Tc-DTPA aerosol is administered to the patient by inhalation through a nebulizer. After administration, most of the small droplets of aerosol are deposited in the alveolar walls and terminal bronchiole. They are absorbed through the alveolar walls, passing through the pulmonary interstitium into the capillaries. The tracer is then transported through the bloodstream and excreted by the kidneys. The major barrier and limiting factor of clearance is the alveolar wall. The mucociliary and lymphatic pathways of

A

B

C

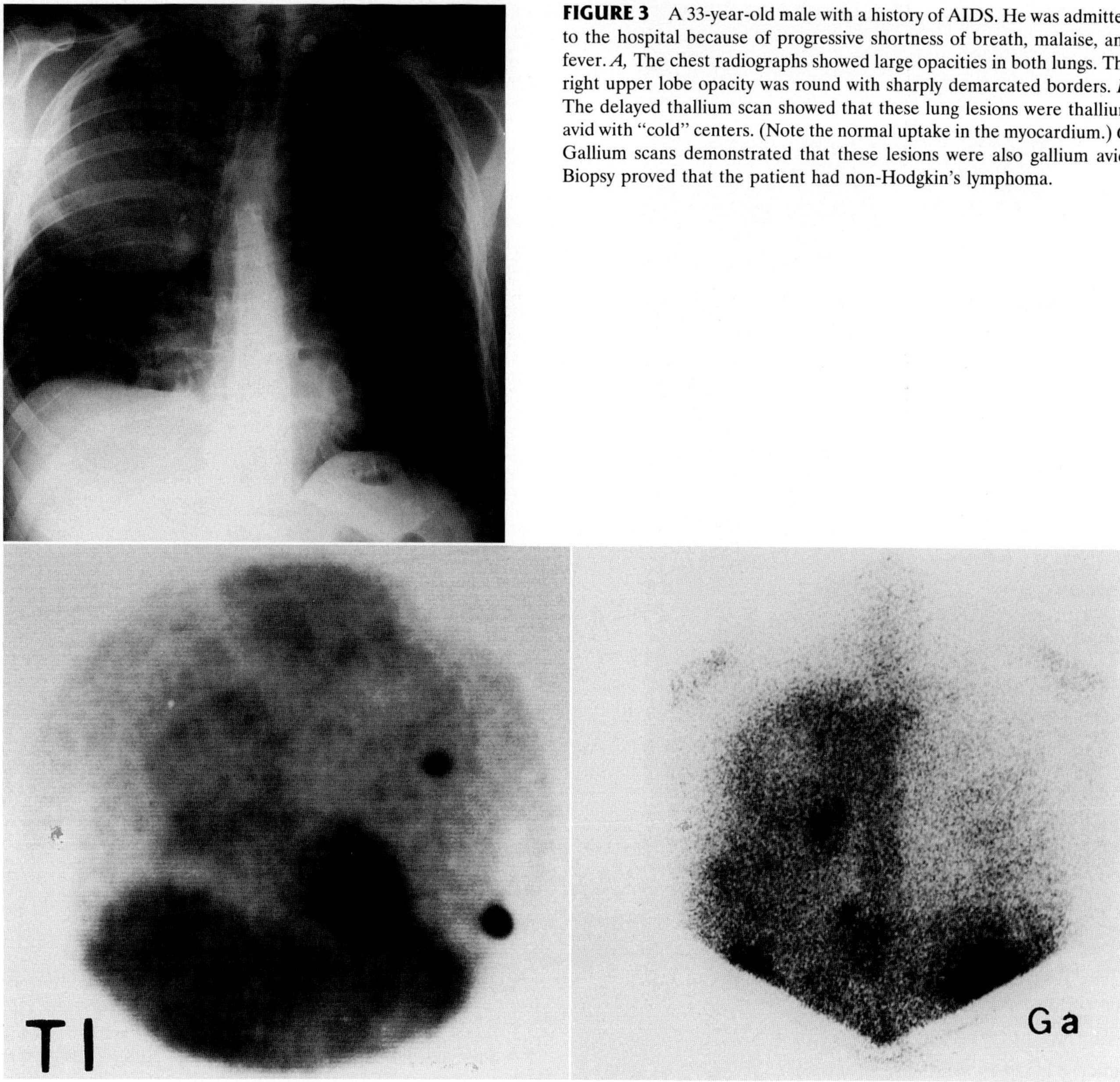


**FIGURE 3** A 33-year-old male with a history of AIDS. He was admitted to the hospital because of progressive shortness of breath, malaise, and fever. *A,* The chest radiographs showed large opacities in both lungs. The right upper lobe opacity was round with sharply demarcated borders. *B,* The delayed thallium scan showed that these lung lesions were thallium avid with "cold" centers. (Note the normal uptake in the myocardium.) *C,* Gallium scans demonstrated that these lesions were also gallium avid. Biopsy proved that the patient had non-Hodgkin's lymphoma.

clearance are insignificant. In disease states the alveolar wall is damaged and the major barrier is broken down. The clearance rate is markedly accelerated.

In the past this technique has been used for evaluation of patients suffering from many different pulmonary conditions such as sarcoidosis, ARDS, effects of cigarette smoking, and recently, AIDS-related infections. The pulmonary clearance rate of Tc-DTPA aerosol is accelerated among these patients.

Since our purpose is just to detect the presence or absence of accelerated aerosol clearance, imaging is not necessary, although we have included in the following paragraphs both the imaging (visual inspection) method and a quantitative measurement of Tc-DTPA pulmonary clearance.

### *Technique*

Tc-DTPA aerosols are inhaled through a nebulizer for 5 minutes with the patient lying supine so that 3 mCi of aerosol is delivered to the patient's lungs. An Anger camera is placed underneath the patient. Digital scintigrams are taken at one frame per minute for 7 minutes, using a 64 $\times$ 64 matrix. Analog scintigrams (optional) are taken at the rate of one frame every 5 minutes for 60 minutes, using a preset time format of 1 minute for each frame.

#### Computer Data Analysis

Regions of interest (ROIs) are marked to include both lungs to obtain a time-activity curve. Special attention is paid not to include in the ROI any gastric activity caused by the patient's inadvertent swallowing of aerosol. From the time-activity curve, the clearance half-time is calculated using standard computer programs, assuming the clearance rate curve is a simple monoexponential function. (The reason for using only the first 7 minutes of data for quantitative analysis is to minimize the effects of recirculation, which produces a complex exponential function.)

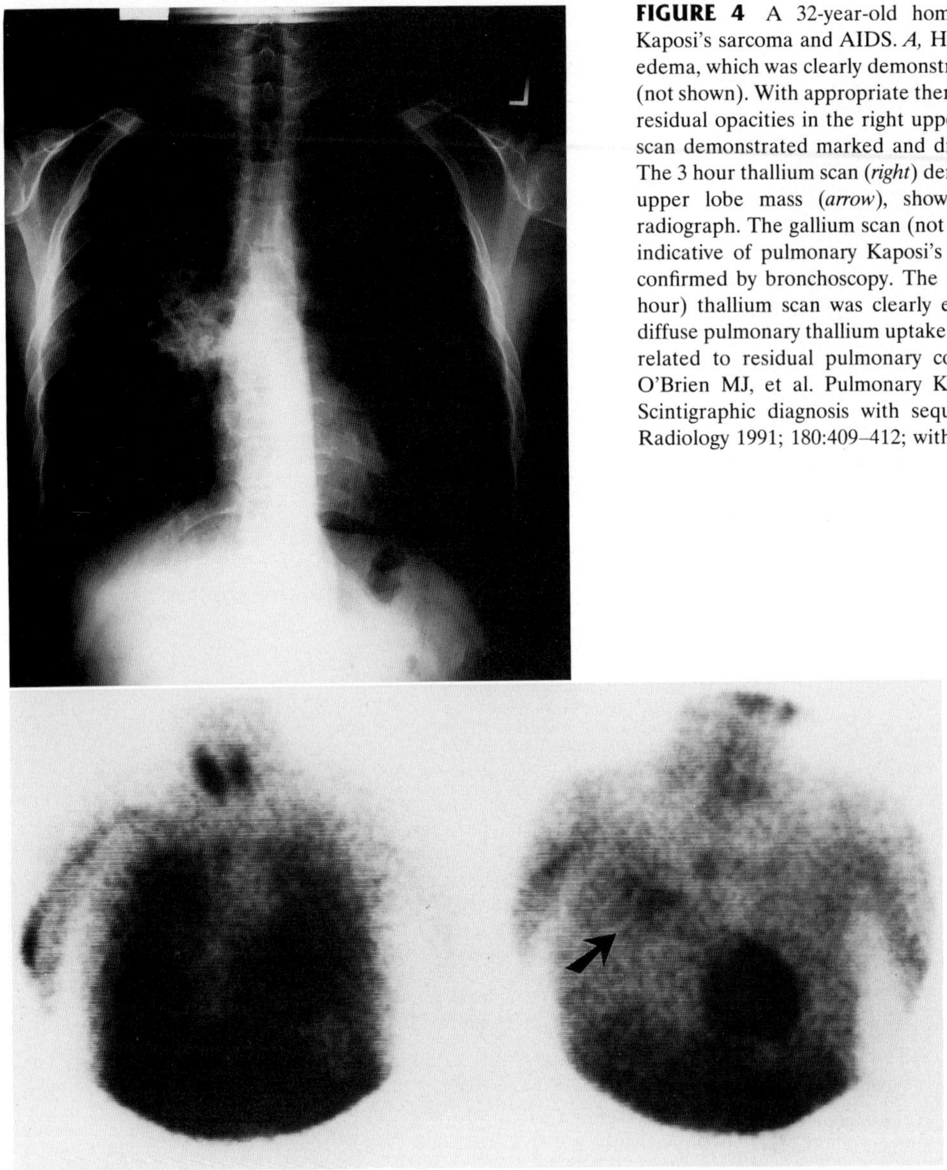

A

B

**FIGURE 4** A 32-year-old homosexual male with known cutaneous Kaposi's sarcoma and AIDS. *A,* He was readmitted because of pulmonary edema, which was clearly demonstrated in the admission chest radiographs (not shown). With appropriate therapy, the pulmonary edema subsided, but residual opacities in the right upper lobe remained. *B,* The early thallium scan demonstrated marked and diffuse pulmonary thallium uptake (*left*). The 3 hour thallium scan (*right*) demonstrated increased uptake in the right upper lobe mass (*arrow*), showing good correlation with the chest radiograph. The gallium scan (not shown) was negative. The findings were indicative of pulmonary Kaposi's sarcoma (Table 1). The diagnosis was confirmed by bronchoscopy. The importance of performing a delayed (3 hour) thallium scan was clearly exemplified in this case. The early and diffuse pulmonary thallium uptake was highly nonspecific and was probably related to residual pulmonary congestion. (From Lee VW, Fuller JD, O'Brien MJ, et al. Pulmonary Kaposi sarcoma in patients with AIDS: Scintigraphic diagnosis with sequential thallium and gallium scanning. Radiology 1991; 180:409–412; with permission.)

### Analog Images (Visual Inspection)

Assuming the patient's renal function is not significantly compromised, we assess the pulmonary clearance rate by comparing the intensity of lung and renal uptake in 1 hour by a grading system as follows:

*Grade 1:* No significant change in lung activity in 1 hour; renal uptake negligible in 1 hour

*Grade 2:* Visible decrease of lung activity in 1 hour; renal activity visible but less than lung activity in 1 hour

*Grade 3:* Moderate decrease of lung activity in 1 hour; renal activity equal to lung activity in 1 hour

*Grade 4:* Marked decrease of lung activity in 1 hour; renal activity higher than lung activity in 1 hour

## *Results and Interpretation*

The results of our experience in Boston City Hospital showed that among nonsmoking patients ($N = 14$) and healthy volunteers, there is significant augmentation of lung clearance with presence of lung infections (PCP, tuberculosis, bacterial). Normal clearance half-times are between 30 and 120 minutes (mean 55.3 minutes), whereas the half-times among patients with proven lung infections ranged from 11 to 29 minutes (mean 17.7 minutes). The separation between normal and infected groups is clear-cut. If 36 minutes is used as the cut point, the sensitivity and specificity of lung infection are 100 and 80 percent, respectively. Our results among nonsmoking patients are in general agreement with other recent reports in the literature.

Among smoking patients ($N = 34$), there are significant overlapping values between the infected and noninfected groups: noninfected group: 12 to 68 minutes (mean 29.2 minutes); lung infection group: 11 to 29 minutes (mean 17.0 minutes). If 23 minutes is used as the cut point, the sensitivity and specificity are only 86.7 and 56.0 percent, respectively.

Among nonsmokers the visual scores of analog imaging show good correlation with the clearance rate and presence or absence of lung infections. Grades 3 and 4 indicate the presence of infections with sensitivity and specificity of 100 and 86.7 percent. Among smokers the scores overlap too much to be of any clinical use.

### Clinical Uses of Tc-DTPA Pulmonary Clearance Test

The advantages of the clearance test are easy availability of Tc-DTPA, lower radiation exposure (compared to gallium), and rapid results (within minutes). Since imaging is not necessary, simple detection probes can be used instead of the more expensive Anger camera. It is also easily portable and can be used in remote geographic areas where gallium or an Anger camera is not available. A sophisticated computer is not necessary for calculation of the clearance half-time from the time-activity curves. Simple semilogarithmic paper and pencil are entirely adequate for the job. It is also a convenient screening test and can be used to monitor patients under treatment for lung infections. The major limitation of this test is the low sensitivity and specificity among smoking patients. Potentially this method may be useful as a screening test for nonsmokers or smokers who have quit smoking and for pediatric patients with AIDS.

The recent report by Russo and co-workers reconfirms that the Tc-DTPA aerosol clearance test is a highly sensitive test among symptomatic patients with AIDS for detection of chest complications. It is even more sensitive than gallium scans and radiographs. However, infectious and noninfectious causes (e.g., Kaposi's sarcoma and smoking) all result in accelerated aerosol clearance. It can be used clinically as a screening test.

## Discussion

Gallium scintigraphy is the most commonly used radionuclide screening test for chest complications among patients with AIDS. The diagnostic accuracy of gallium scans can be significantly improved if we use the grading scale, pattern approach, and correlate with thallium scans and current chest radiographs. Tc-DTPA clearance measurement may occasionally be useful.

## Suggested Reading

Bekerman, Bitran J. Gallium-67 in the clinical evaluation of human immunodeficiency virus infection: Indications and limitations. Semin Nucl Med 1988; 18:273–286.

Federle MP. A radiologist looks at AIDS imaging evaluation based on symptom complexes. Radiology 1988; 166:553–562.

Ganz WI, Serafini AD. The diagnostic role of nuclear medicine in AIDS. J Nucl Med 1989; 30:1935–1945.

Golden JA, Sollito RA. The radiology of pulmonary disease: Chest radiography, computed tomography, and gallium scanning. Clin Chest Med 1988; 9:481–495.

Kramer EL, Sanger JJ, Garay S, et al. Gallium scans of the chest in patients with acquired immunodeficiency syndrome. J Nucl Med 1987; 28:1107–1114.

Lee VW. The importance of performing a delayed thallium scan. (Letter.) J Nucl Med 1992; 33:463–464.

Lee VW, Fuller JD, O'Brien MJ, et al. Pulmonary Kaposi sarcoma in patients with AIDS: Scintigraphic diagnosis with sequential thallium and gallium scanning. Radiology 1991; 180:409–412.

Lee VW, Rosen MP, Baum A, et al. AIDS-related Kaposi sarcoma: Findings on thallium-201 scintigraphy. AJR 1988; 151:1233–1235.

Murray JF, Mills J. Pulmonary complications of human immunodeficiency virus infection. Part 1. Am Rev Respir Dis 1990; 141:1356–1372.

Murray JF, Mills J. Pulmonary complications of human immunodeficiency virus infection. Part 2. Am Rev Respir Dis 1990; 141:1582–1598.

Rosso J, Guillon JM, Parrot A, et al. Tc99m DTPA aerosol and gallium scanning in pulmonary complications of HIV infection. J Nucl Med 1992; 33:81–87.

Weissler JC, Mootz AR. Southwestern Internal Medicine Conference: Pulmonary disease in AIDS patients. Am J Med Sci 1990; 300:330–343.

# CT Evaluation of Interstitial Lung Disease

*THERESA C. McLOUD, M.D.*

A large number of chronic diseases may cause diffuse infiltration of the lungs. Many of these diseases involve both the interstitium and the airspaces, and I prefer the term *chronic infiltrative lung disease* (CILD). Over 100 such diseases have been described, and patterns identified on the chest radiograph are seldom specific. In addition, approximately 10 percent of patients with CILD have normal chest radiographs, even when symptoms and functional impairment are present. Computed tomography (CT), in particular, high-resolution CT (HRCT), has been shown over the past several years to play a major role in the assessment of patients with CILD. CT allows a better assessment of the type, distribution, and severity of parenchymal abnormalities.

## Indications and Clinical Utility

Several chronic diffuse lung diseases have been shown to have a characteristic appearance on CT. CT therefore can be helpful in the evaluation of patients suspected of having CILD with either nonspecific findings on the chest radiograph or a normal chest radiograph. CT can also serve as a useful guide to the choice of an optimal biopsy site, particularly when the disease process is uneven in distribution with patchy involvement in the lungs. In addition, because of its diagnostic value, CT may provide helpful information in regard to the type of biopsy that is most likely to produce diagnostic tissue. CT is also recommended in the follow-up of patients with CILD with clinical deterioration or failure to respond to treatment and for the assessment of progression, activity, and possible complications.

## Technical Approach

Technical factors used in HRCT include (1) thin collimation; (2) reconstruction using a high spatial frequency algorithm; (3) targeting of image reconstruction; and (4) increased kilovoltage and milliampere scan parameters. Scanning with thin collimation of 1 to 1.5 mm reduces volume averaging within the plane of section and optimizes spatial resolution. However, to avoid errors in interpretation, corresponding fixed, standard, thick-section 1 cm scans should be obtained for comparison. With conventional body CT, scan data are usually reconstructed with a relatively low spatial frequency algorithm that smooths the image, reduces visible image noise, and improves contrast resolution. Reconstruction of the image using a high spatial frequency algorithm reduces image smoothing and increases spatial resolution, making structures sharper. Retrospectively targeting image reconstruction to a single lung, instead of the entire thorax, significantly reduces image pixel size and thus increases the spatial resolution. However, image targeting is not always necessary, provided the other two parameters of thin collimation and reconstruction with a bone algorithm are employed. A number of protocols can be used to carry out HRCT of the lungs. I prefer to perform standard thick-section CT throughout the lungs followed by HRCT scans at five or six levels evenly spaced from the lung apices to the bases. Scans should be obtained at full inspiration in the supine position. If the lung disease is basilar, prone scans are recommended to differentiate dependent lung density from true interstitial pathology. When HRCT is employed primarily for the detection of early disease, particularly basilar interstitial lung disease such as asbestosis, it is preferable to perform three to five scans only through the lung bases in both the prone and supine positions.

## Diagnostic Approach

### *Normal Anatomy*

On HRCT the secondary pulmonary lobule, the basic unit of lung structure, can be visualized. The interlobular septa can be observed as thin straight lines of uniform thickness that are 1 to 2 cm in length and usually contact the pleural surface. These are better identified in the peripheral rather than the central lung. A linear, branching, or dotlike density seen within the lobule within a centimeter of the pleural surface represents the intralobular branch of the pulmonary artery. Usually, small bronchioles cannot be identified within the secondary pulmonary lobule.

### *Diagnostic Aspects*

A number of signs of infiltrative lung disease have been described on HRCT. These include thickening of the interlobular septa, intralobular lines or bands, irregular pleural surfaces, nodules, ground glass density, and alveolar disease. Müller and colleagues have provided a classification of HRCT findings in CILD that is based on the recognition of four types of patterns: the irregular linear pattern, the cystic pattern, the nodular pattern, and the ground glass pattern (Table 1).

Diseases that produce an irregular linear pattern include idiopathic pulmonary fibrosis, pulmonary lymphangitic carcinomatosis, and asbestosis. In idiopathic pulmonary fibrosis with honeycombing, the HRCT appearance is characteristic (Fig. 1). A linear pattern can be identified at the bases of the lungs, with associated cystic spaces several millimeters to several centimeters in diameter that are often peripheral and subpleural. Such honeycombing is associated with septal thickening and intralobular bands. Bronchioles within the center of the secondary pulmonary lobule can be identified in patients with fibrosis, because of a combination of bronchiolectasis and thickening of the peribronchiolar interstitium. In patients with lymphangitic spread of carcinoma, septal thickening is characteristic. It may be the predominant finding. In addition, the septum may have a beaded appearance indicating nodularity. A network of thickened interlobular septa creates a pattern of multiple polygonal structures that represent the secondary pulmonary lobules distributed throughout the lung. The lobules may contain a central dot. The dot is produced by the lobular artery and associated connective tissue and possibly tumor infiltration around the artery. A number of findings have been described in asbestosis. CT may detect early cases when the chest radiograph is normal. HRCT findings characteristic of asbestosis include (1) subpleural curvilinear lines; (2) parenchymal bands, which are linear densities 2 to 5 cm in length running through the lung, usually extending to the pleural surface; (3) thickened septal lines and thickening of structures within the secondary pulmonary lobule; and (4) honeycombing (Fig. 2). These findings are relatively nonspecific, and occasionally some of these can be identified in control

**TABLE 1** CT Patterns of Chronic Infiltrative Lung Disease

| |
|---|
| *Irregular Linear Pattern* |
| Idiopathic pulmonary fibrosis |
| Lymphatic spread to tumor |
| Asbestosis |
| *Cystic Pattern* |
| Lymphangioleiomyomatosis |
| Histiocytosis X |
| *Nodular Pattern* |
| Silicosis and coal worker's pneumoconiosis |
| Sarcoidosis |
| Hypersensitivity pneumonitis |
| *"Ground Glass" and Alveolar Pattern* |
| Alveolar proteinosis |
| Chronic eosinophilic pneumonia |
| Bronchiolitis obliterans organizing pneumonia |

Modified from Müller NL, Miller R. Computed tomography of chronic diffuse infiltrative lung disease. Am Rev Respir Dis 1990; 142:1206–1215; with permission.

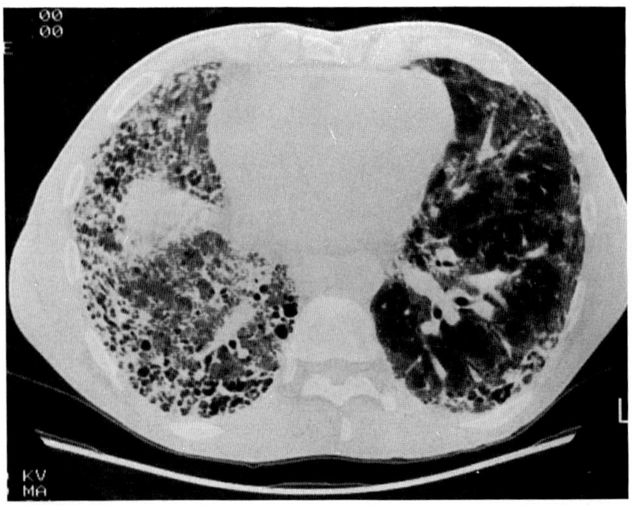


**FIGURE 1** Idiopathic pulmonary fibrosis. Peripheral subpleural honeycomb spaces are identified in both lung bases associated with coarse linear opacities.

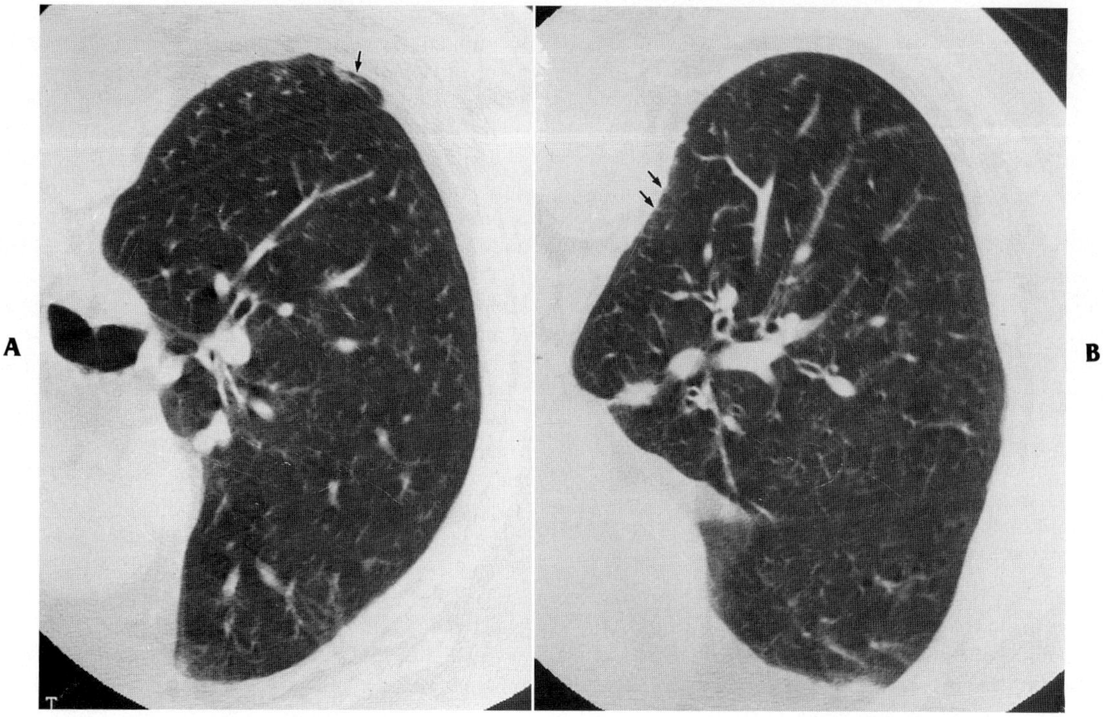

**FIGURE 2** Early asbestosis. *A* and *B*, Prone scans demonstrate a subpleural line *(arrow)* and thickened interlobular septa *(arrows)*.

populations without any history of exposure to asbestos. A combination of two or more of these findings is more indicative of asbestosis than a single finding alone.

The cystic pattern can be identified in lymphangioleiomyomatosis (LAM) and histiocytosis X. Histiocytosis X in addition may show nodular opacities. Characteristic HRCT findings have been described in LAM. These include thin-walled cystic airspaces of varying size distributed diffusely throughout the lungs (Fig. 3). In the early phases of the disease, the lung parenchyma surrounding the cystic spaces is normal. These spaces can be differentiated from honeycombing, because of the absence of a predominant basilar and subpleural distribution. The walls of the cysts in LAM are also extremely thin and surrounded by normal lung. In histiocytosis X a variety of patterns including cysts up to 4 cm in size with thin or indiscernible walls, a reticular nodular infiltrate, and nodules 2 mm to 2 cm in size have been described. Some of these nodules appear cavitated and are located along the terminal bronchioles in the secondary pulmonary lobules. The predominant cystic abnormality with lack of peripheral concentration and the thickness of the cyst walls help to distinguish histiocytosis X from idiopathic pulmonary fibrosis.

The nodular pattern can be identified in a number of diseases including the pneumoconioses, silicosis and coal worker's pneumoconiosis, sarcoidosis, and hypersensitivity pneumonitis. In regard to silicosis, the most characteristic finding on CT is the presence of nodules, which are usually localized in the posterior portions of the upper lobes. CT is particularly useful in determining the stage of disease, because it may detect coalescence of nodules that may not be apparent on the radiograph, indicating the presence of complicated silicosis. CT also has been shown to be more sensitive in the detection of early emphysema in patients with both silicosis

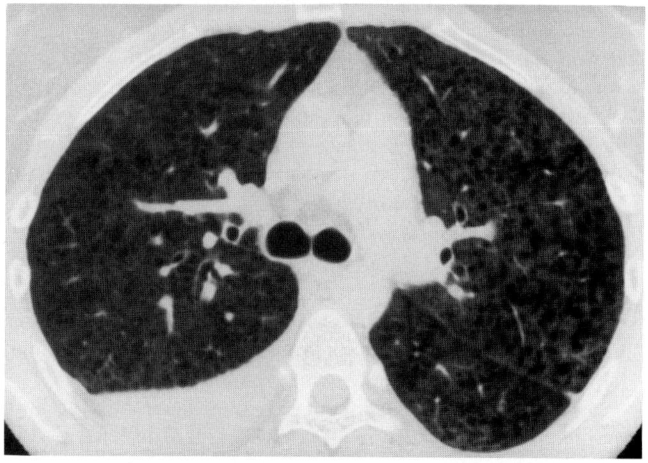

**FIGURE 3** Lymphangioleiomyomatosis in a 37-year-old woman. There is a right chylous pleural effusion. Thin-walled cystic spaces are distributed uniformly throughout the lungs.

and coal worker's pneumoconiosis. However, nodules may occasionally be missed when narrow collimation alone is used. Particularly in the assessment of patients with coal worker's pneumoconiosis and silicosis, we recommend the performance of standard 10 mm thick slices followed by HRCT scans through the area of interest.

In sarcoidosis the characteristic parenchymal abnormalities are nodular opacities along the bronchovascular bundles, interlobular septa, and subpleural regions including the fissures (Fig. 4). The nodules frequently have irregular margins. Occasionally these nodules may be confluent, and air bronchograms with alveolar consolidation may occur. As fibrosis develops, irregular linear opacities become a prominent feature and are accompanied by parenchymal distortion.

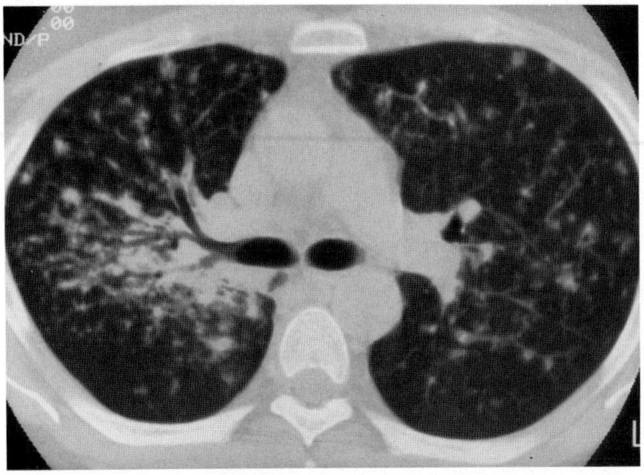

**FIGURE 4** Sarcoidosis. Multiple subpleural and central nodules are identified. Nodules radiate out centrally from the hilum along the bronchovascular bundles on the right side.

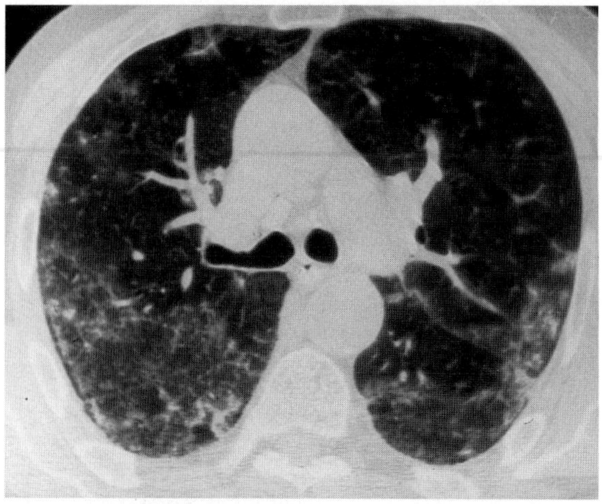

**FIGURE 5** Desquamative interstitial pneumonitis. Predominantly "ground glass" opacity can be observed in this stage of disease, which is characterized by active alveolitis.

Volume loss occurs in the upper lobes with posterior displacement of the main and upper lobe bronchi. CT may also be helpful in assessing the presence and extent of complications associated with sarcoidosis such as bullae, bronchiectasis, and mycetoma formation.

In hypersensitivity pneumonitis the CT appearance varies with the stage of the disease. With acute exposure diffuse airspace consolidation may be observed that resolves within a matter of days. In the subacute phase, a fine nodular or reticulonodular pattern is apparent. The chronic stage of hypersensitivity pneumonitis is characterized by the presence of fibrosis, which may occur months to years after initial exposure. HRCT scans in these patients often show irregular linear opacities presumably representing fibrosis. In the subacute stage, small rounded opacities less than 5 mm in diameter amid patchy areas of airspace opacification appear to be characteristic.

The "ground glass" pattern can be identified in diseases such as alveolar proteinosis, chronic eosinophilic pneumonia, and bronchiolitis obliterans with organizing pneumonia. The ground glass pattern consists of hazy opacification in the lung parenchyma observed on CT, in which the outlines of the pulmonary vessels are preserved. As ground glass density progresses, true alveolar consolidation may be identified with air bronchograms. However, ground glass opacification may be produced by interstitial as well as alveolar disease. Thickening of alveolar walls results in decreased air content of the alveoli and hazy ground glass opacification. Thus patchy areas of ground glass density may be seen occasionally in some of the interstitial lung diseases such as idiopathic pulmonary fibrosis.

In regard to the alveolar diseases mentioned earlier, the patterns are not particularly characteristic. However, in chronic eosinophilic pneumonia the distribution is classically in the peripheral portions of the lungs and is frequently seen in the upper lobes. In bronchiolitis obliterans with organizing pneumonia, a similar peripheral pattern may be identified in approximately half of the patients.

It appears that HRCT can sometimes allow a specific diagnosis of some types of infiltrative lung disease such as idiopathic pulmonary fibrosis, lymphangitic spread of carcinoma, or LAM. Several studies have compared the accuracy of chest radiographs to CT findings in predicting specific diagnoses in diffuse CILDs. These studies have consistently shown a higher accuracy for HRCT as compared with standard chest radiographs. In addition, HRCT leads to a higher level of confidence in making correct diagnoses.

HRCT may also be useful in accurately localizing areas of abnormal lung for lung biopsy. Biopsies may be obtained from areas most likely to yield a diagnosis. In addition, HRCT may be useful in helping to determine the correct biopsy approach. Transbronchial biopsy is appropriate in diseases involving the peribronchovascular spaces, such as sarcoidosis and lymphangitic spread of tumor. In other disorders an open-lung biopsy is usually more appropriate.

### *Correlation with Function and Activity of Disease*

Some preliminary work has been done correlating CT findings in interstitial lung disease with functional abnormalities. Data suggest that in idiopathic pulmonary fibrosis correlation of extent of disease with lung function studies is better than with standard radiographs. Staples and colleagues studied 23 patients with idiopathic pulmonary fibrosis with CT and standard radiography. The severity of disease on the CT scan was determined by extent rather than by profusion. Significant correlation was found between the extent of disease assessed with CT and the severity of dyspnea, as well as between CT and the impairment of gas exchange as measured by diffusing capacity. It has been suggested that the appearance of consolidation or ground glass density on HRCT correlates with disease activity in patients with fibrosing alveolitis (Fig. 5). More investigation needs to be carried out in these areas. It is possible that CT may provide a means of monitoring disease activity over time and determining which patients are likely to benefit from therapy.

## Suggested Reading

Aberle DR, Gamsu G, Ray CS, Feuerstein IM. Asbestos-related pleural and parenchymal fibrosis: Detection with high resolution CT. Radiology 1988; 166:729–734.

Brauner MW, Grenier P, Mompoint D, et al. Pulmonary sarcoidosis: Evaluation with high resolution CT. Radiology 1989; 172:467–471.

Lenoir S, Grenier P, Braunner MW, et al. Pulmonary lymphangiomyomatosis and tuberous sclerosis: Comparison of radiographic and thin section CT findings. Radiology 1990; 175:329–334.

Mathieson JR, Mayo JR, Staples CA, Müller NL. Chronic diffuse infiltrative lung disease: Comparison of diagnostic accuracy of CT and chest radiography. Radiology 1989; 171:111–116.

Moore ADA, Godwin JD, Müller NL, et al. Pulmonary histiocytosis X: Comparison of radiographic and CT findings. Radiology 1989; 172:249–254.

Müller NL, Miller RR. Computed tomography of chronic diffuse infiltrative lung disease. Part I. Am Rev Respir Dis 1990; 142:1206–1215.

Müller NL, Miller RR. Computed tomography of chronic diffuse infiltrative lung disease. Part II. Am Rev Respir Dis 1990; 142:1440–1448.

Müller NL, Miller RR, Webb WR, et al. Fibrosing alveolitis: CT-pathologic correlation. Radiology 1986; 160:585–588.

Stein MG, Mayo J, Müller N, et al. Pulmonary lymphangitic spread of carcinoma: Appearance on CT scans. Radiology 1987; 162:371–375.

# Imaging the Airways

*JO-ANNE O. SHEPARD, M.D.*

Computed tomography (CT) has gained wide acceptance as the imaging modality of choice for most airway lesions, because it is a noninvasive procedure and has high inherent spatial and contrast resolution. CT may provide valuable diagnostic information in a number of disease entities and clinical situations. The role of other preferred or complementary imaging studies, including magnetic resonance imaging (MRI), is discussed in the course of this chapter.

## Conventional Radiographic Studies

The plain chest radiograph in the posteroanterior (PA) and lateral projections is recommended as a screening evaluation in any patient with a suspected tracheal or bronchial abnormality. A high-kilovoltage technique (140 kVp) is preferred, because the visibility of the bony thorax is reduced and mediastinal interfaces are enhanced. Bilateral oblique chest radiographs are a useful adjunct to PA and lateral chest radiographs, because the trachea and carina are rotated away from the spine. However, it is often the case that tracheobronchial lesions are not detected on chest radiographs, because of the small size of the lesion or because of superimposition of mediastinal or bony structures.

The role of conventional tomography in detecting tracheobronchial lesions has been largely replaced by CT, because of the clarity of anatomic detail and the superior contrast resolution of CT. However, there are a few remaining indications for the use of conventional tomography. Because the trachea and bronchi are seen in the long axis on conventional tomograms, the length of a lesion is often better demonstrated on conventional tomograms than on axial CT images. Conventional tomograms are recommended before bronchoplastic surgery to obtain an accurate assessment of the length of a tracheal tumor and its distance from the larynx and carina. Conventional tomography can sufficiently evaluate the degree and extent of postintubation strictures in which mediastinal abnormalities are not expected to be present. CT is recommended to evaluate almost all other airway lesions.

Chest fluoroscopy is the preferred technique for evaluation of tracheobronchial malacia. Fluoroscopy provides a real-time assessment of airway dynamics during inspiration, expiration, coughing, and quiet breathing. Although the trachea, carina, and main bronchi are usually visible in multiple projections, the lobar and smaller airways are not adequately evaluated by this technique. Ultrafast CT scanning can provide information about the collapsibility of the airways, but unfortunately this technique has not been widely available.

Before the development of CT, bronchography was considered the definitive procedure for establishing the diagnosis and determining the extent of bronchiectasis. Bronchography is an invasive procedure with inherent risks including temporary impairment of ventilation and diffusion, allergic reactions, and alveolitis. Performance of an adequate study requires an experienced radiologist. In addition, underfilling of the bronchi can result in a false-negative evaluation. Recently, high-resolution CT techniques (HRCTs) have replaced bronchography in clinical practice and are discussed in further detail in the next section.

## CT Evaluation of the Airways

The routine protocol for screening CT evaluations includes a standard reconstruction algorithm, 10 mm contiguous scans from the thoracic inlet to the hila, 5 mm contiguous scans through the hilar regions, and 10 mm contiguous scans from the inferior portion of the hila through the diaphragm. Scanning is performed during suspended inspiration, with the patient in the supine position with the arms extended above the head. The use of 5 mm scans through the hila permits reliable visualization of all the lobar and segmental bronchi.

The HRCT technique includes 1.5 mm scan collimation, a high-resolution reconstruction algorithm (i.e., a bone algorithm), and targeted reconstruction. HRCT is the preferred technique for the diagnosis and evaluation of the extent of bronchiectasis.

CT scanning offers several advantages in evaluating the airways. An understanding of normal tracheobronchial anatomy can help to localize airway lesions, detect hilar disease, and serve as a road map to parenchymal lesions. The high-contrast resolution capability of CT is useful in determining mediastinal invasion by airway tumors and detecting extrinsic compression of the airways by vascular aneurysms or rings and mediastinal masses such as goiters. Similarly CT can detect the presence of fat within airway tumors, such as hamartomas and lipomas, and calcification within broncholiths, chondromas, and carcinoid tumors (Fig. 1). Small

A 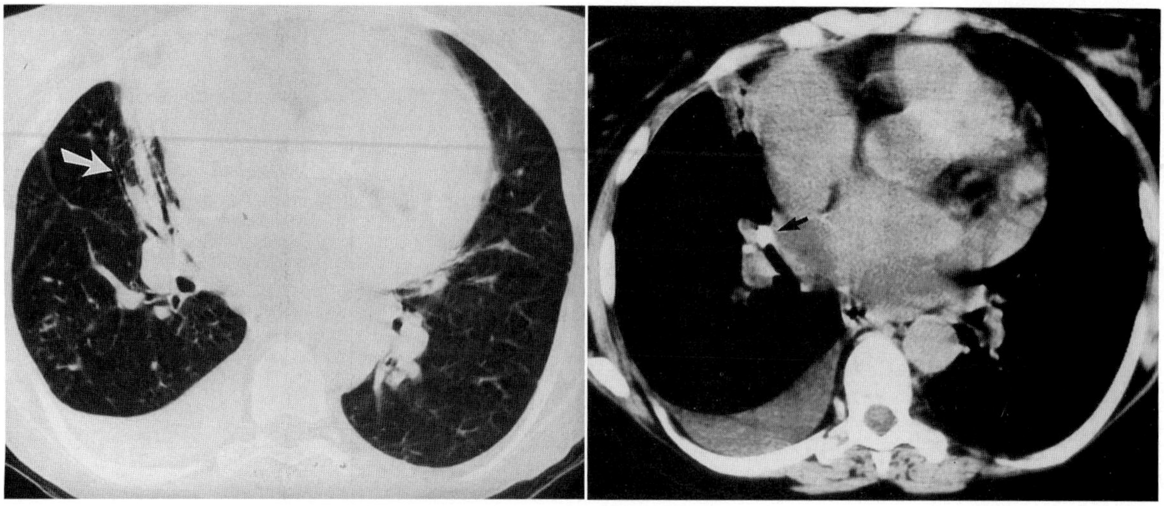 B

**FIGURE 1** Broncholith. *A,* CT scan demonstrates partial collapse of the right middle lobe (RML) adjacent to the right heart border *(arrow)*. *B,* CT scan shows a calcified broncholith obstructing the RML bronchus *(arrow)*.

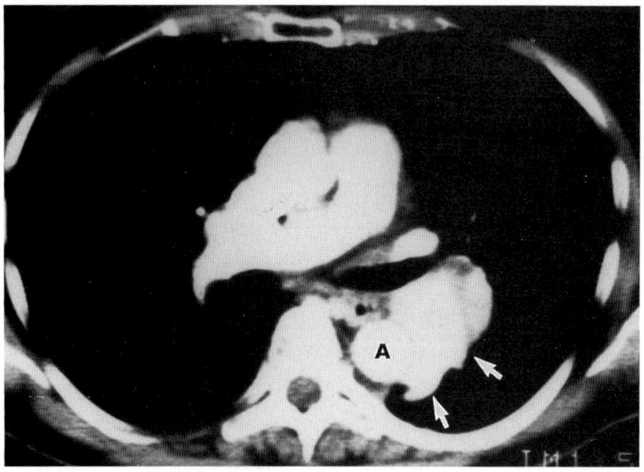


**FIGURE 2** Carcinoid tumor. CT scan during an intravenous contrast bolus demonstrates dense enhancement of a carcinoid tumor in the left hilum *(arrows),* abutting the aorta (A), and obstructing the superior segment bronchus of the left lower lobe.

peribronchial air collections can be visualized by CT in cases of tracheobronchial rupture or dehiscence of a bronchial anastomosis. The administration of a bolus of iodinated contrast material can provide information regarding the vascularity of tumors such as carcinoid tumors (Fig. 2). The principal disadvantage of CT lies in its inability to image the trachea and bronchi in the long axis.

The role of CT in detecting and determining the extent of bronchial tumors has been addressed by several studies that have compared the results of CT and bronchoscopy. Fiberoptic bronchoscopy (FOB) and CT of the bronchi are considered complementary procedures. CT is capable of detecting approximately 90 percent of airway tumors and correctly excluding lesions in 92 percent of cases. The findings of intraluminal nodularity or irregularity are considered the only specific signs of endobronchial disease on CT. However, in the absence of these specific signs, CT is inaccurate in predicting whether a given abnormality is endobronchial, submucosal, or peribronchial. Diffuse mucosal involvement is rarely identified by CT and is best evaluated by FOB. It is not

A 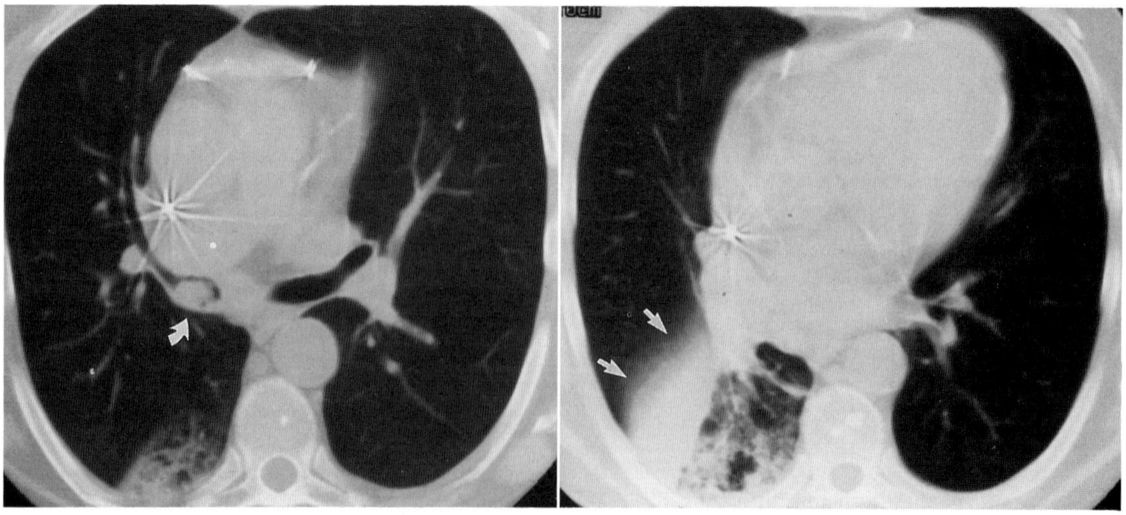 B

**FIGURE 3** Bronchogenic carcinoma. *A,* CT scan shows a nodular intraluminal mass nearly obstructing the distal right main bronchus *(arrow)*. *B,* CT scan demonstrates collapse of the right middle lobe and partial collapse and postobstructive pneumonia in the right lower lobe *(arrows)*.

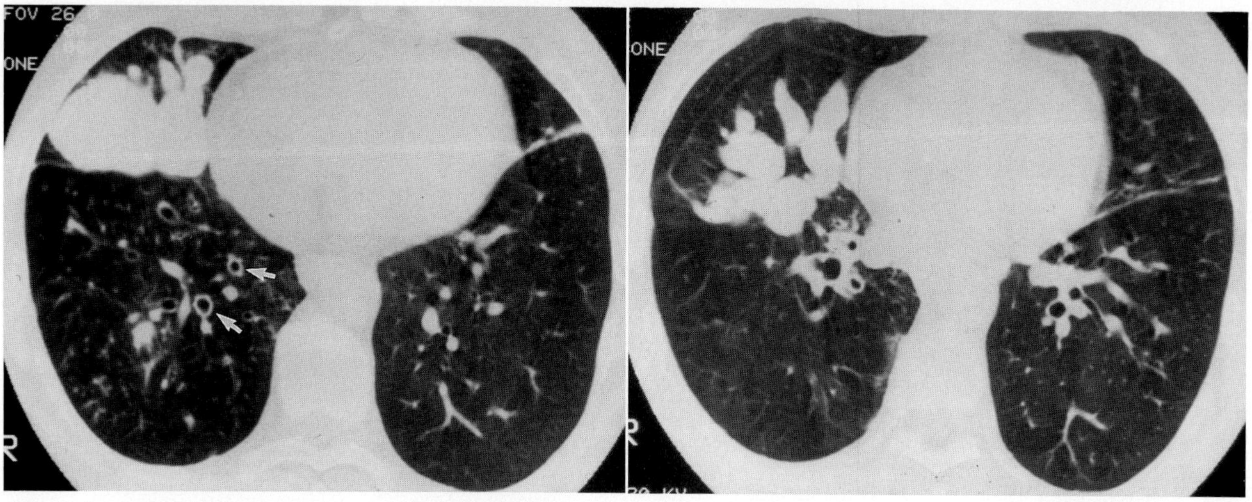

**FIGURE 4** Bronchiectasis and mucoid impaction. *A,* CT scan shows dilated bronchi with thickened walls in the right lower lobe *(arrows),* in contrast to the normal left lower lobe bronchi. *B,* CT scan through the right middle lobe demonstrates branching tubular opacities representing mucoid impaction.

possible to see bronchi distal to a tight stenosis by bronchoscopy, whereas distal bronchi and lung are well demonstrated by CT. The extraluminal portion of a tumor is well demonstrated by CT, but cannot be assessed by FOB. CT is also useful in guiding a transtracheal or transbronchial biopsy and is helpful in predicting the success of a transbronchial biopsy or needle aspiration biopsy. CT should not be considered a substitute for FOB.

CT has a highly important role in the evaluation of patients with atelectasis. CT has proven accurate in defining the site of bronchial obstruction in collapse secondary to endobronchial occlusion (Fig. 3). However, there is little specificity in the CT appearance of endobronchial lesions. Nonobstructive atelectasis can be identified when lobar bronchi are patent and air bronchograms are present within the collapsed lobe. In such cases tumor is considered unlikely. CT can reliably distinguish passive atelectasis secondary to large pleural effusions or pneumothorax or atelectasis related to scarring or radiation from collapse as a result of obstruction.

Recently CT has replaced bronchography as the preferred evaluation of bronchiectasis. Recent reports of the relative diagnostic accuracy of CT and bronchography have shown that CT is highly accurate in the diagnosis of bronchiectasis. When HRCT techniques are employed, using 1.5 mm collimation at 10 mm intervals, a specificity of 93 percent and sensitivity of 90 percent can be achieved. Several CT criteria for the diagnosis of bronchiectasis have been described. In cylindric bronchiectasis smooth dilatation and bronchial wall thickening are seen as "tram lines" or ring opacities, depending on the plane of imaging (Fig. 4). In varicose bronchiectasis the bronchi have a beaded appearance. In cystic bronchiectasis a cluster or string of cysts may be identified, some of which may contain air-fluid interfaces. In normal lung, bronchi can be identified only within the inner one-third of the lung on 10 mm images and within the inner two-thirds of the lung on 1.5 mm images. The presence of dilated bronchi with thickened walls in the periphery of the lung is a more subtle sign of bronchiectasis. These signs of bronchiectasis become unreliable in the setting of acute pneumonia when reversible bronchiectasis is sometimes found.

Inspissated secretions may accumulate distal to a bronchial obstruction forming a mucoid impaction. Mucoid impactions may also accumulate in the absence of obstruction in patients with disorders such as cystic fibrosis and bronchopulmonary aspergillosis. The CT findings of mucoid impaction include tubular opacities that usually emanate from larger central opacities, or branching tubular opacities with a V- or Y-shaped configuration (see Fig. 4). When an unusually shaped pulmonary mass is identified on a chest radiograph, or when mucoid impaction is suspected, CT is the procedure of choice to confirm or further define the abnormality.

In the evaluation of diffuse tracheobronchial narrowing, CT can determine the presence and extent of airway wall thickening and assess the degree of airway narrowing. CT evaluations can distinguish primary mediastinal abnormalities that may secondarily affect the tracheobronchial tree, such as fibrosing mediastinitis from diseases that primarily affect the airways. Diffuse tracheobronchial narrowing is observed in a number of situations including postintubation injuries, tuberculosis, fungal infections, and noninfectious conditions such as sarcoidosis, Wegener's granulomatosis, relapsing polychondritis, amyloidosis, tracheobronchopathia osteochondroplastica (Fig. 5), and idiopathic cases. There have been reports of CT findings in many of these entities. Unfortunately the CT findings are often not specific and require a biopsy for a specific diagnosis.

The diagnosis of tracheobronchomegaly (Mounier-Kuhn syndrome) can be overlooked on chest radiographs and is easily made by CT. A tracheal diameter greater than 3 cm, a right main bronchial diameter greater than 2.4 cm, and a left main bronchial diameter greater than 2.3 cm in an adult are considered abnormal. Redundant musculomembranous tissue protrudes between cartilaginous rings and creates a corrugated or scalloped appearance on CT (Fig. 6).

## MRI of the Airways

MRI represents a significant advance in diagnostic imaging and is particularly well suited to imaging the trachea and potentially the bronchi. One of the major advantages of MRI in

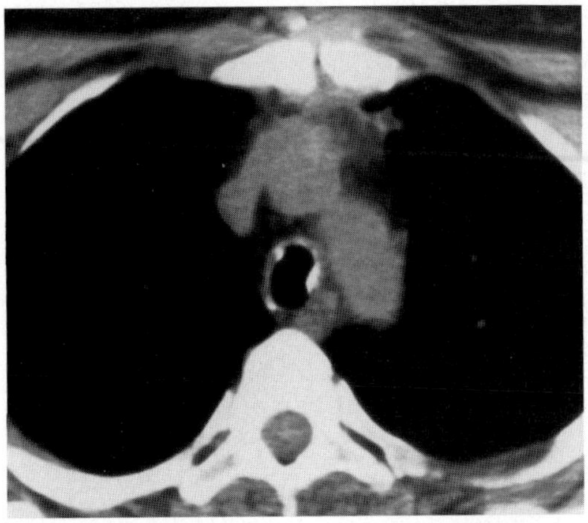

**FIGURE 5** Tracheobronchopathia osteochondroplastica. CT scan through the superior mediastinum demonstrates nodular thickening of the tracheal wall containing calcification.

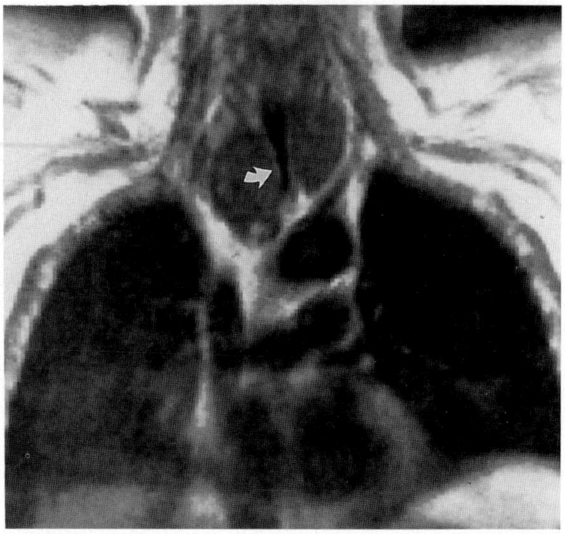

**FIGURE 7** Mediastinal goiter. Coronal T1-weighted MRI demonstrates a diffusely enlarged thyroid gland extending into the superior mediastinum, causing compression and narrowing of the trachea *(arrow)*.

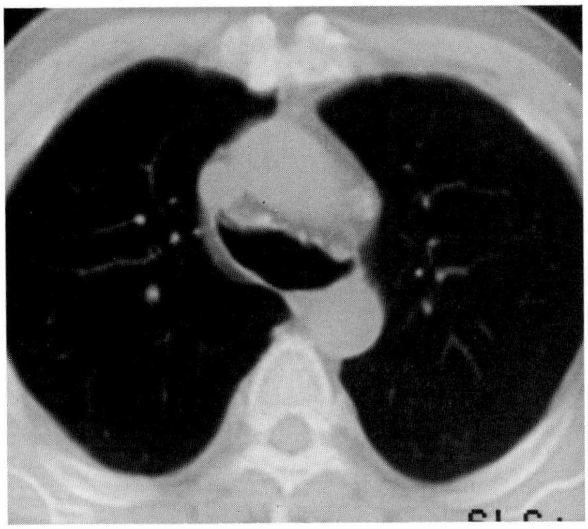

**FIGURE 6** Mounier-Kuhn syndrome. CT scan through the trachea shows a markedly dilated trachea with an abnormal "smile" shape. The anterior wall has a scalloped appearance.

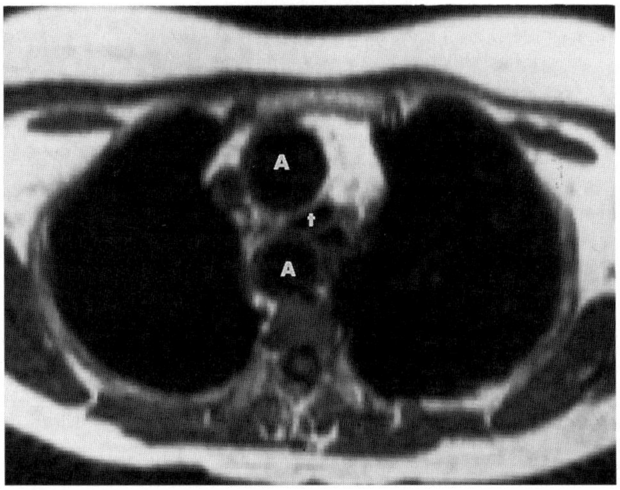


**FIGURE 8** Right aortic arch. Axial T1-weighted MRI through the ascending and descending portions of the aorta (A) demonstrates compression and narrowing of the trachea (t) by the aorta.

imaging the airways is the multiplanar capability of MRI. Imaging in the sagittal and coronal planes allows the trachea and bronchi to be imaged in the long axis, in contrast to the axial plane of CT images (Fig. 7). The use of "off-axis" coronal images can display the entire trachea and carina on a single image. MRI has been shown to be accurate in determining both the length and degree of occlusion within the trachea using spin-echo technique with short TR and TE pulsing sequences. MRI has also proven useful in infants and children in imaging vascular rings or compression of the trachea by the innominate artery or aorta without the hazards of intravenous contrast material and ionizing radiation (Fig. 8). In addition, MRI may be superior to CT in evaluating mediastinal invasion by tracheal tumors, because of better contrast resolution between fat and soft tissues on MRI compared with CT (Fig. 9).

At the present time, the major disadvantage to MRI appears to be decreased spatial resolution, particularly of the lobar and segmental bronchi largely because of respiratory artifact. The number of normal and abnormal bronchi demonstrated on CT has been shown to exceed the number seen on MRI. With faster scanning capabilities employing breath-holding techniques, the spatial resolution should improve. Ultrafast scanning techniques combined with multiplanar imaging may potentially allow real-time imaging of the tracheobronchial tree in the long axis. Presently the indications for MRI of the tracheobronchial tree are limited.

A

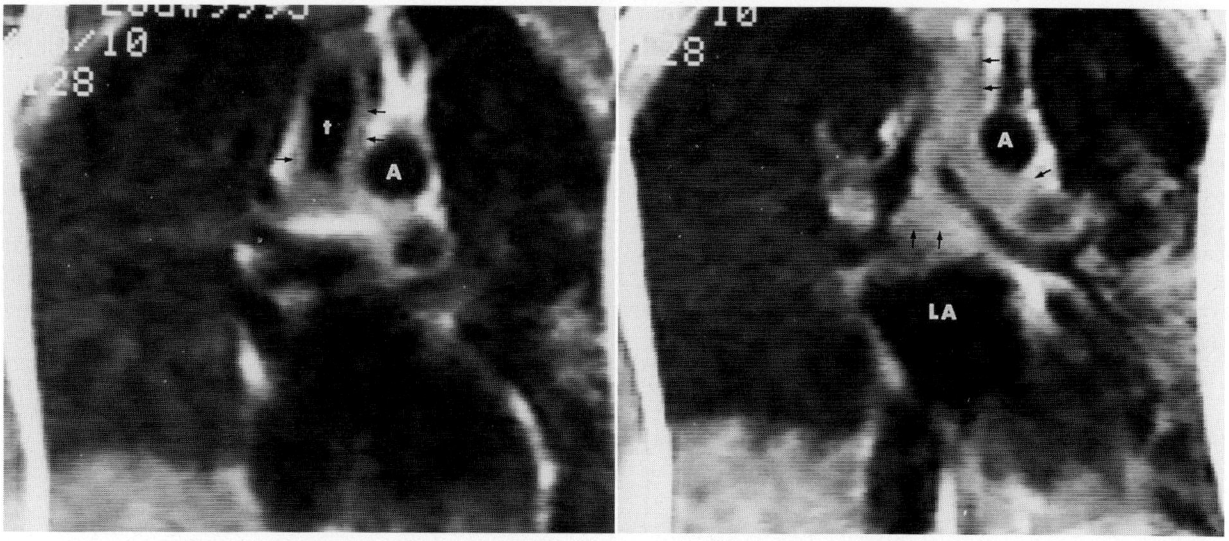


B

**FIGURE 9** Adenoidcystic carcinoma of the trachea. *A,* Coronal T1-weighted MRI through the trachea demonstrates diffuse tracheal wall thickening of intermediate signal intensity *(arrows)*. *B,* Coronal T1-weighted MRI through the trachea and main bronchi shows extensive mediastinal invasion by the tumor into the left paratracheal region, aortopulmonic window, and subcarinal region *(arrows)*. (t = trachea; A = aorta; LA = left atrium)

## Suggested Reading

Fletcher BD, Dearborn DG, Mulopulos GP. MR imaging in infants with airway obstruction: Preliminary observations. Radiology 1986; 160:245.

Gamsu G, Webb R. Computed tomography of the trachea and mainstem bronchi. Semin Roentgenol 1983; 18:51.

Grenier P, Frantz M, Musset D. Bronchiectasis: Assessment by thin-section CT. Radiology 1986; 161:95.

Mayo JR, Webb WR, Gould R, et al. High resolution CT of the lungs: An optimal approach. Radiology 1987; 163:507.

Mayr B, Heywang SH, Ingrisch H, et al. Comparison of CT with MR imaging of endobronchial tumors. J Comput Assist Tomogr 1987; 11:43.

McLoud TC, Ragozzino MW. MR imaging of the thorax. In: Edelman RR, ed. Clinical MR imaging: A Practical Text. Philadelphia: WB Saunders, 1989:731.

Naidich DP, Lee J-J, Garay SM. Comparison of CT and fiberoptic bronchoscopy in the evaluation of bronchial disease. AJR 1987; 148:1.

Naidich DP, McCauley DI, Khouri NF. Computed tomography of lobar collapse. 1. Endobronchial obstruction. J Comput Assist Tomogr 1983; 7:745.

Naidich DP, McCauley DI, Khouri NF. Computed tomography of lobar collapse. 2. Collapse in the absence of endobronchial obstruction. J Comput Assist Tomogr 1983; 7:758.

Shin MS, Jackson RM, Ho K-J. Tracheobronchomegaly (Mounier-Kuhn syndrome): CT diagnosis. AJR 1988; 50:777.

# CT Detection of Pulmonary Metastatic Disease

*SHEILA D. DAVIS, M.D.*

Pulmonary metastases are found in 20 to 54 percent of patients dying with malignancy. For certain patients with known extrathoracic malignancies (ETMs), the early diagnosis of pulmonary metastases may be critical for the institution of therapy and improvement in long-term survival. There is no question that computed tomography (CT) is much more sensitive than conventional radiography in detecting pulmonary metastases. Nevertheless, from the standpoint of cost-effectiveness and concerns about radiation exposure, one must define the clinical circumstances under which routine CT scanning of the chest is most appropriate.

In particular, the following questions should be considered:

1. For what ETMs would screening chest CT have the highest yield in diagnosing occult pulmonary metastases?
2. What are the key image signs for pulmonary metastases, and what factors influence the accuracy of CT?
3. What is the role of CT in patient management?
4. What is the optimal technical approach in performing CT for detection of pulmonary metastases?

## CT Screening for Pulmonary Metastases

Statistical analysis of autopsy data has suggested that certain malignancies have a high propensity for metastasizing initially to the lungs (group 1). These include the bone and soft-tissue sarcomas, testicular carcinoma, choriocarcinoma, most pediatric tumors (with the exception of neuroblastoma), head and neck carcinomas, and endocrine tumors. For patients with these ETMs, pulmonary metastases may be the major cause of death if left untreated.

Other malignancies tend to metastasize to the lungs sequentially, only after first disseminating to other sites (group

2). Tumors of the gastrointestinal tract (stomach, pancreas, colon) or ovary tend to metastasize first to the liver. Carcinoma of the prostate tends to metastasize initially to the bones.

Finally, there are certain malignancies that disseminate simultaneously to a number of sites, in addition to the lungs (group 3). Tumors of the bladder, cervix, and uterus may metastasize to both the liver and the lungs. Carcinoma of the breast may involve the lungs, vertebrae, or liver. Renal cell carcinoma frequently disseminates to the lungs, but may also involve the bones through connections between the renal veins and Batson's plexus. Melanoma has a high propensity for early metastases to the lungs, but also disseminates to multiple visceral sites. For ETMs in group 3, the patient's ultimate demise is not infrequently a result of advanced extrapulmonary disease.

This overall scheme, known as the "cascade theory," provides a useful guide for screening, although there are exceptions in individual cases. The yield of detecting occult lung metastases early in the clinical course should be highest for ETMs in group 1. For group 2, the yield of screening is expected to be relatively low if there is no radiologic evidence of metastases to the liver or bones. For group 3 there should be a concerted effort to exclude metastatic disease at multiple visceral sites.

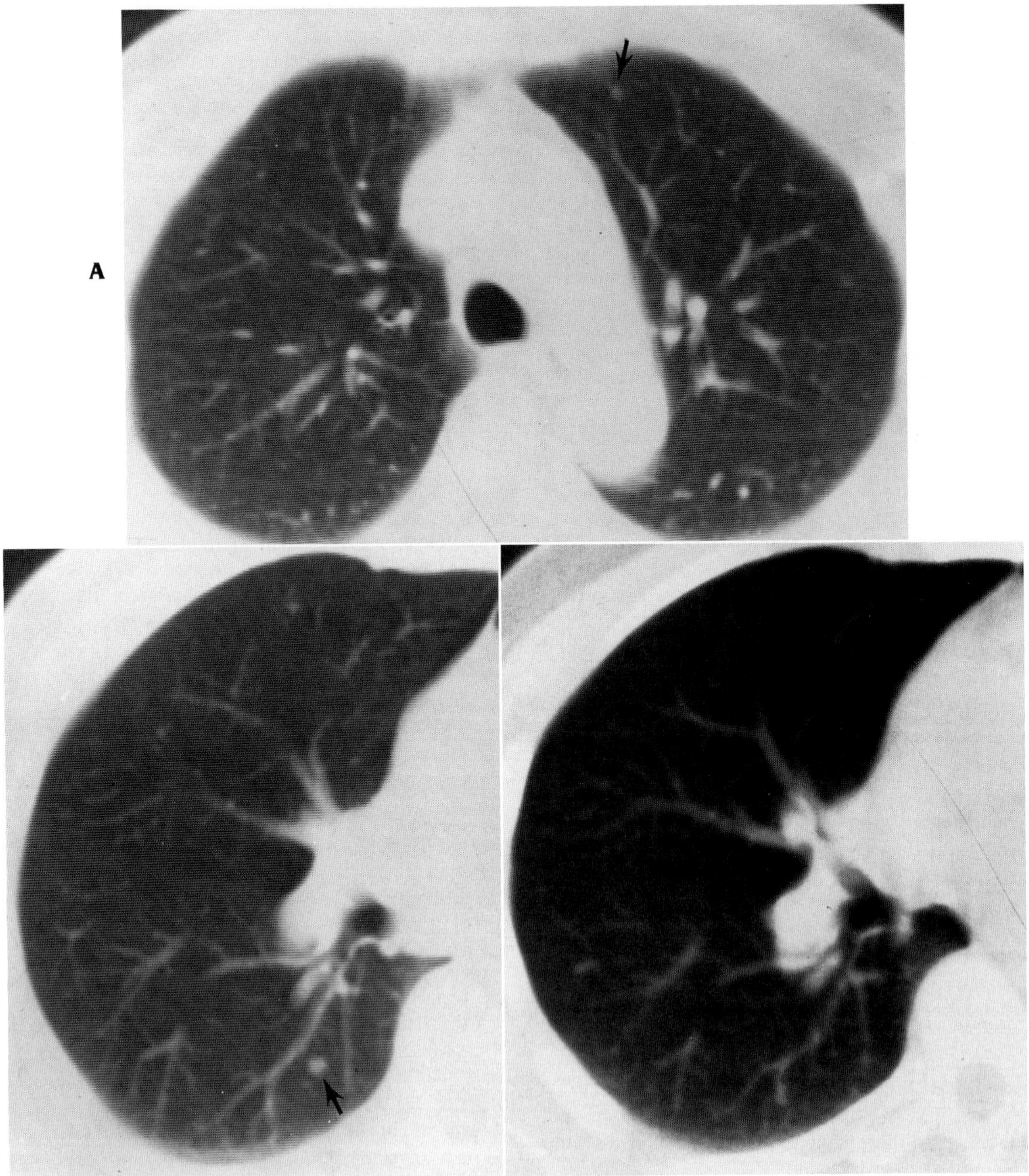


**FIGURE 1** A 57-year-old man with renal cell carcinoma. Chest radiograph appeared normal, but CT revealed small peripheral lesions, larger than adjacent vessels on end. *A,* A 2 mm nodule *(arrow)* in the left upper lobe. *B,* A 4 mm nodule *(arrow)* in the right lower lobe. *C,* As represented by this section at the same level as *(B),* lesions were not apparent on a scan 2 months earlier, suggesting that the nodules represent metastases.

## Diagnostic Approach

### *Morphology and Key Image Signs of Pulmonary Metastases*

Pulmonary nodules are the most common form of pulmonary metastases. These are generally spherical, well defined, multiple, and vary in size. Nodules are usually peripherally distributed, in the outer third or subpleural regions of the lungs, and tend to be more predominant in the mid and lower zones.

The greatest challenge in identifying nodules on CT is distinguishing the lesions from vessels on end. When nodules are 2 to 3 mm in diameter, they are usually easy to detect at the periphery, where they tend to be of larger caliber than adjacent vessels (Fig. 1). More centrally, lesions as large as 5 to 6 mm may be confused with the larger pulmonary vessels. Small nodules ( < 2 mm) are difficult to detect when they are isolated or few. However, if they are also numerous it becomes obvious that nodules must be present, since not all of the small densities seen in the plane of section can be accounted for by vessels alone (Fig. 2).

In searching for nodules of any size, one should evaluate contiguous sections for possible branching of structures to identify vessels. It is also important to remember that more vessels are observed on end with scans of narrow collimation. Thus, except for subpleural lesions, it is often more difficult to identify nodules on thin-section than on standard 10 mm collimation scans (Fig. 3).

Nodular pulmonary metastases are occasionally atypical in appearance. Ill-defined margins have been observed with metastases from choriocarcinoma, or even from other malignancies following chemotherapy, probably caused by some associated hemorrhage. At times nodular metastases contain calcification; this phenomenon occurs most frequently with metastases from sarcomas or mucinous or papillary adenocarcinomas (Fig. 4). Cavitation may also be present and is generally seen within metastases from sarcomas, squamous cell carcinomas, or other malignancies following treatment.

Although metastases are often multiple, they may be few or even solitary. For solitary lesions one must consider the additional diagnostic possibility of a primary lung carcinoma. A widely quoted rule of thumb states that a solitary pulmonary nodule in a patient with known ETM is (1) more likely to represent lung carcinoma if the underlying ETM is a carcinoma of the head and neck or breast; (2) more likely to represent a metastasis if the ETM is a sarcoma or melanoma; (3) equally likely to be lung carcinoma or a metastasis in cases of other ETMs.

Less common forms of pulmonary metastases include lymphangitic carcinomatosis, endobronchial lesions, and tumor embolization. In contrast with the nodular form, which tends to be asymptomatic, these entities are often clinically suspected because of respiratory symptoms. Lymphangitic carcinomatosis is usually seen with carcinomas of the breast, lung, stomach, pancreas, cervix, or thyroid. It is now well recognized that this pattern is better appreciated on CT than on chest radiographs, and better on high-resolution CT (HRCT) than on routine CT. HRCT findings include nodular thickening of septal lines, prominence of a reticular pattern or polygonal lines, and nodular thickening along bronchovascular bundles. Endobronchial metastases (Fig. 5) are most commonly seen with carcinomas of the breast, colon, or kidney. Tumor embolization is usually associated with renal cell carcinoma, choriocarcinoma, hepatoma, or hepatic metastases.

### *Accuracy of CT Imaging of Pulmonary Metastases*

Formal studies evaluating the sensitivity and specificity of CT in diagnosing pulmonary metastases have focused mainly on the nodular form of disease. The superior sensitivity of CT over conventional radiography is attributable to the lack of superimposition and the inherent high-contrast resolution of nodules against air-containing lung. It is well known that CT frequently demonstrates occult, multiple, or bilateral nodules when the plain radiographic studies are "negative" or show solitary or unilateral lesions. Nevertheless, an overall sensitivity of 51 to 73 percent reported in the literature indicates that generally more lesions are found at thoracotomy than are detected at CT. False-negative results (Table 1) are attributable to the limits of spatial resolution and other technical factors, as well as to problems of interpretation.

Limitations in specificity have been a more perplexing problem. Unlike sensitivity, which is technology and observer dependent, the specificity of CT is determined mainly by clinical factors. Nodules are more likely to be metastases if the underlying ETM is one at high risk for dissemination to the lungs or if there is locally advanced disease (e.g., Clark level IV

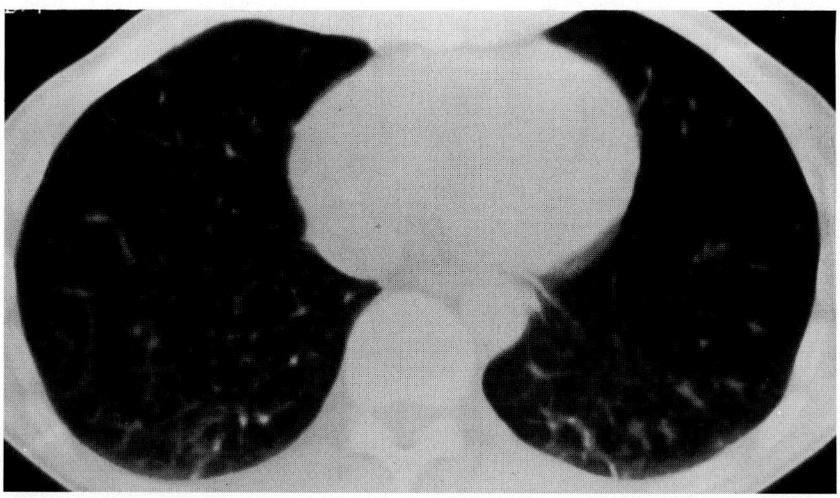

**FIGURE 2** A 53-year-old man with renal cell carcinoma. Chest radiograph appeared normal, but CT revealed innumerable tiny nodules (1 to 2 mm in diameter), more prominent in the right than in the left lung. Not all of these small densities can be accounted for by vessels on end. Subsequent growth of lesions on a follow-up scan confirmed that these represent metastases.

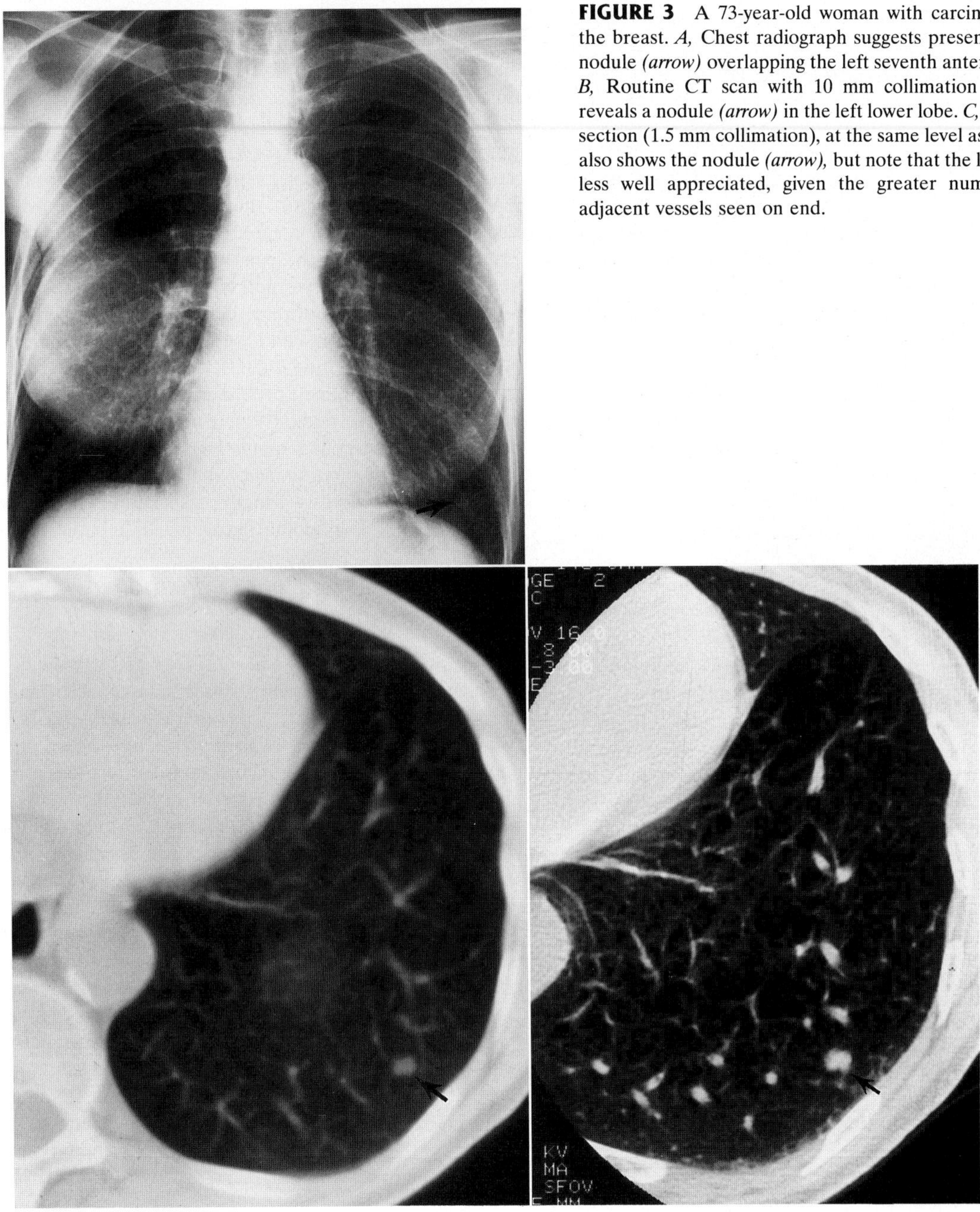


A

B

C

**FIGURE 3** A 73-year-old woman with carcinoma of the breast. *A,* Chest radiograph suggests presence of a nodule *(arrow)* overlapping the left seventh anterior rib. *B,* Routine CT scan with 10 mm collimation clearly reveals a nodule *(arrow)* in the left lower lobe. *C,* HRCT section (1.5 mm collimation), at the same level as in *(B),* also shows the nodule *(arrow),* but note that the lesion is less well appreciated, given the greater number of adjacent vessels seen on end.

or V melanoma). The frequency of false-positive results also influences specificity. As shown in Table 2, nodules are more likely to be metastases if (1) the patient is not from a region where granulomatous disease is endemic, (2) the patient is young (lower incidence of granulomatous disease, fibrosis, or intrapulmonary lymph nodes), or (3) the patient has not previously been treated.

## Impact of CT on Management

### *Tissue Diagnosis*

In view of the limited specificity of CT findings, tissue diagnosis is frequently necessary. For pulmonary nodules the diagnostic yield of percutaneous needle aspiration biopsy (PNAB) is generally higher than that of fiber-optic bronchoscopy (FOB), since nodular metastases tend to be peripheral in their distribution. PNAB can be accomplished under either fluoroscopic or CT guidance (see Fig. 4). Even if PNAB is performed under fluoroscopic guidance, preliminary CT is still helpful in selecting the optimal approach and ascertaining the distance to the lesion. On the other hand, if CT should reveal the presence of a central mass, lymphangitic carcinomatosis or an endobronchial lesion (see Fig. 5), tissue sampling should be accomplished through FOB.

### *Surgical Resection*

There has been increasing success with the surgical resection of pulmonary metastases, or "metastasectomy," in selected cases. Overall 5 year survival rates of 20 to 50 percent have been reported, and operative mortality now approaches zero.

A

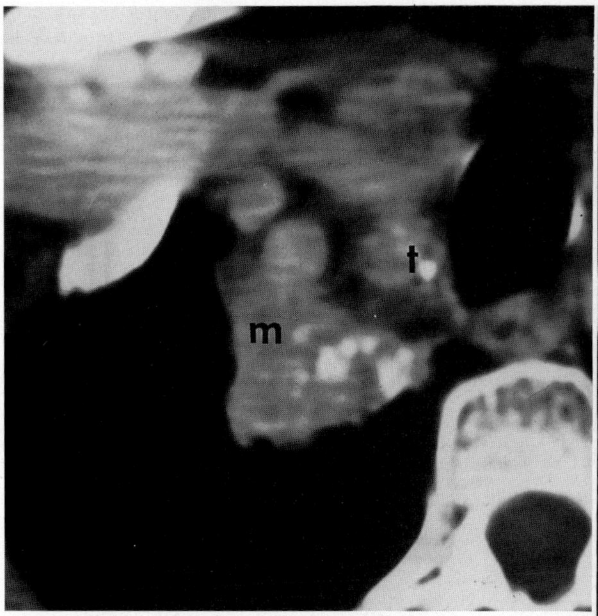


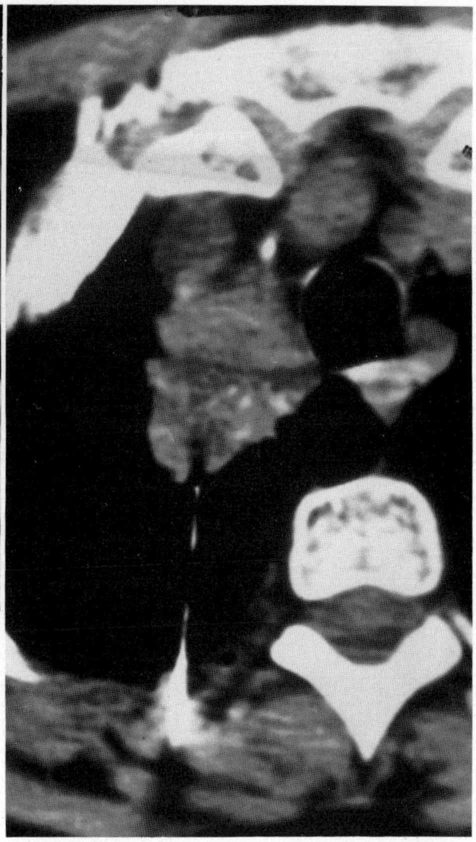

B

**FIGURE 4** A 65-year-old woman with carcinoma of the colon. *A,* CT scan reveals presence of a mass (m) with focal areas of calcification, posterior to and distinct from the right lobe of thyroid (t), which also contains some calcification. *B,* CT-guided needle aspiration biopsy, as well as subsequent surgical resection, revealed that this mass was a metastasis from the known carcinoma of the colon.

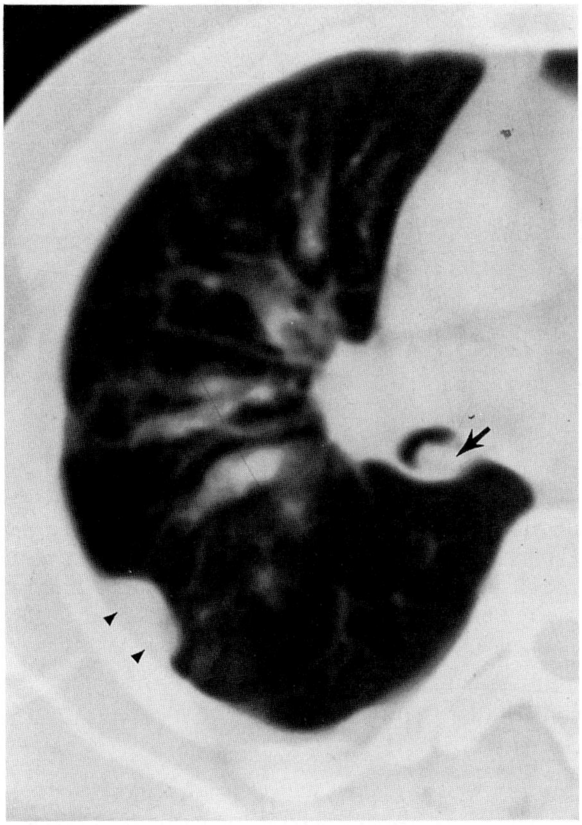

**FIGURE 5** A 54-year-old man with renal cell carcinoma. CT reveals an endobronchial metastasis *(arrow)* within the bronchus intermedius. Note also the presence of small lung parenchymal nodules and a larger pleural-based lesion *(arrowheads).*

Favorable results can be obtained with resection of multiple and bilateral lesions, or even repeated resections in the same patient.

The highest postresection 5 year survival rates are seen with the bone and soft-tissue sarcomas, choriocarcinoma, nonsem-

**TABLE 1** False-negative CT Results

| |
|---|
| Limits of spatial resolution |
| Technical factors: |
| Partial volume averaging |
| Respiratory motion artifact |
| Variability in degree of inspiration |
| Electronic window settings |
| Problems of interpretation: |
| Vessels on end |
| Parenchymal infiltration or atelectasis |
| Misdiagnosis |

**TABLE 2** False-positive CT Results

| |
|---|
| Benign neoplasms |
| Granulomatous diseases |
| Intrapulmonary lymph nodes |
| Inflammatory pseudotumor |
| Focal fibrosis |
| Pulmonary infarcts |
| Intrafissural pleural plaques |
| Post-treatment effects: |
| Postoperative scarring |
| Suture granulomas |
| Organized pneumonia |
| Chemotherapy-induced pulmonary toxicity |
| Sterilized metastases |
| Benign transformation of metastases |

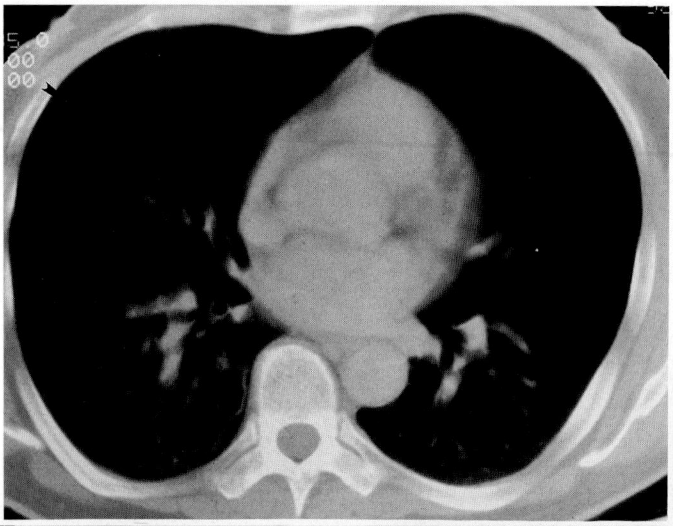

A

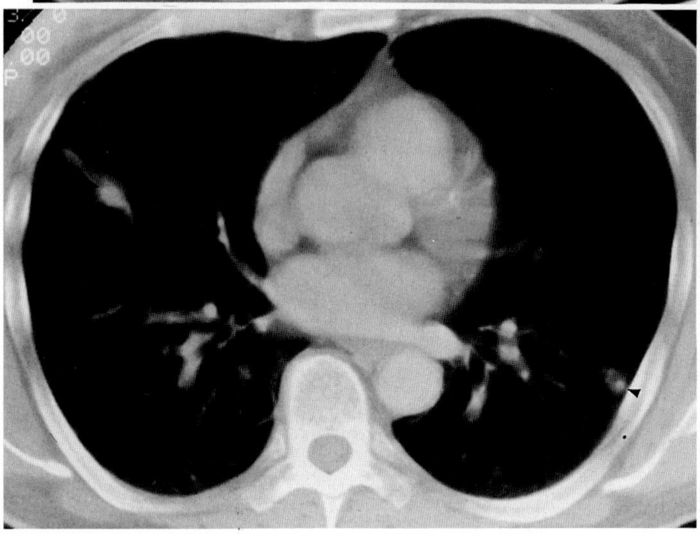

B

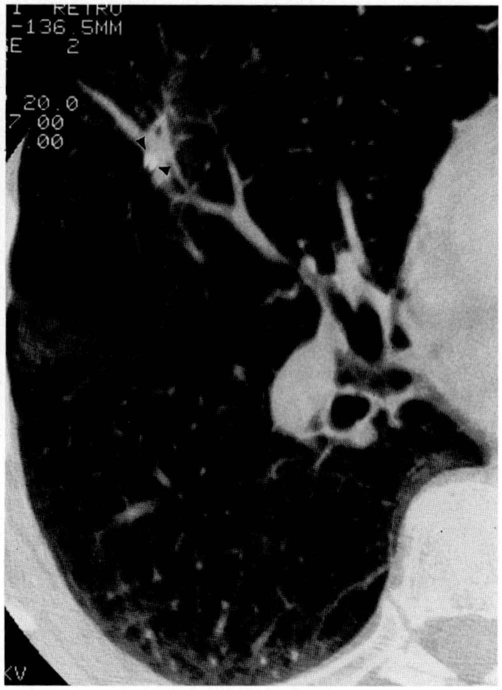

C

**FIGURE 6** A 69-year-old man with renal cell carcinoma. *A,* CT scan reveals an 8 mm nodule *(arrow)* in the right middle lobe. As confirmed by subsequent metastasectomy, this was a metastasis. *B,* Follow-up scan 8 months later reveals an apparent nodular density in the region of the wedge resection *(arrow)* and a new subpleural nodule *(arrowhead)* in the left lower lobe. The new left lower lobe nodule was proven to represent a second pulmonary metastasis, upon a repeat wedge resection procedure. *C,* The right-sided nodular density, investigated further by HRCT, most likely represents postoperative scarring around sutures *(arrowheads).*

inomatous testicular carcinoma, and Wilms' tumor. As mentioned previously, these tumors are among those at high risk for early dissemination to the lungs. Screening by chest CT is thus expected to be most valuable for these types of ETMs. Preoperative CT is essential for defining the size, number, and location of lesions, as well as for excluding unsuspected extrapulmonary disease affecting the mediastinum, pleura, chest wall, or upper abdomen. Follow-up CT scans are helpful in detecting recurrent metastases (Fig. 6).

### *Systemic Therapy*

Systemic therapy with combination chemotherapy, hormonal agents, or immunotherapy is frequently employed, either alone or in conjunction with metastasectomy. Pulmonary metastases that are most responsive to chemotherapeutic regimens originate from the bone and soft-tissue sarcomas, choriocarcinoma, nonseminomatous testicular carcinoma, and Wilms' tumor, i.e., the same types of malignancy associated with the highest postresection five-year survival rates. Again, it is expected that screening by chest CT should be particularly valuable in patients with these types of ETMs. Once systemic therapy is contemplated, a baseline CT scan is indicated to document the initial presence and extent of lesions; follow-up scans should then be obtained to quantify the response, progression, or recurrence of disease (Fig. 7).

### *"Unverifiable" CT-detected Lesions*

In clinical practice I often encounter small CT-detected nodules that are too small for biopsy and for which surgical resection is not feasible or immediately desired. Serial CT scans, with or without empiric treatment, are often helpful in evaluating these "unverifiable" lesions (Figs. 1, 7, 8). Nodules that are enlarging or newly appearing or that decrease in size on antineoplastic therapy are likely to be metastases; nodules that are initially present, remain stable for at least 12 months, or decrease in size without antineoplastic therapy are likely to be benign.

## Technical Approach

CT scanning for possible pulmonary metastases is usually performed without intravenous contrast medium, unless examination of the abdomen and pelvis is also required. In the exceptional case, when tumor embolus is suspected, contrast should be administered by bolus technique to opacify the central pulmonary vessels.

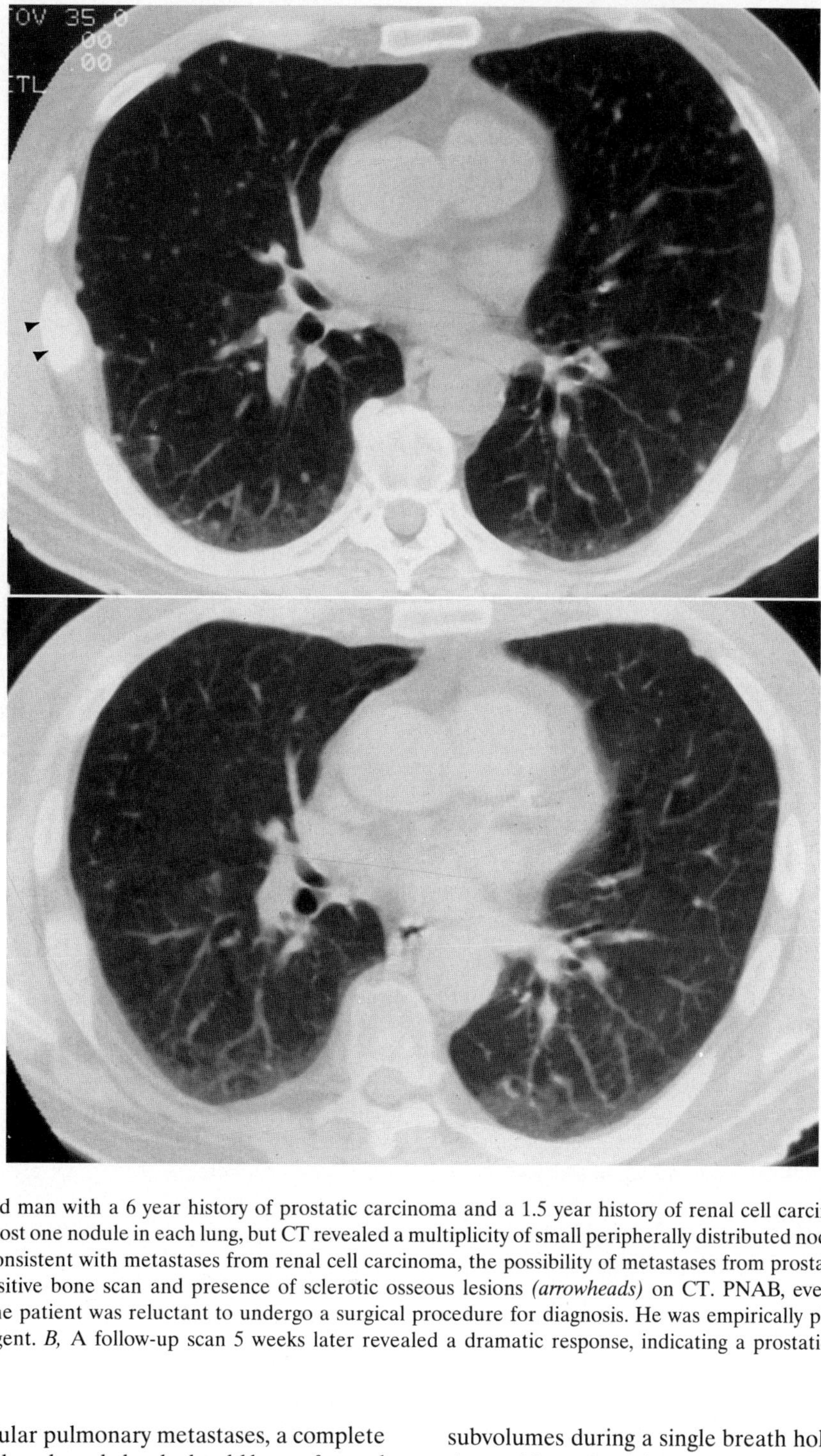

A

B

**FIGURE 7** A 67-year-old man with a 6 year history of prostatic carcinoma and a 1.5 year history of renal cell carcinoma. *A,* Chest radiograph suggested presence of at most one nodule in each lung, but CT revealed a multiplicity of small peripherally distributed nodules. Although this pattern was thought to be more consistent with metastases from renal cell carcinoma, the possibility of metastases from prostatic carcinoma could not be excluded, in view of a positive bone scan and presence of sclerotic osseous lesions *(arrowheads)* on CT. PNAB, even under CT guidance, was considered difficult and the patient was reluctant to undergo a surgical procedure for diagnosis. He was empirically placed on hormonal therapy with an antiandrogenic agent. *B,* A follow-up scan 5 weeks later revealed a dramatic response, indicating a prostatic origin for the pulmonary metastases.

In searching for nodular pulmonary metastases, a complete scan from the apices to the adrenal glands should be performed with 10 mm sections; contiguous 5 mm sections can be obtained in young children. As discussed earlier, isolated nodules may be more difficult to detect on thin-section scans, given the greater number of vessels seen on end. Nevertheless, even with contiguous 10 mm sections, small nodules can still be missed because of respiration-induced variability between sections. Such variability may also cause considerable frustration in comparing serial CT examinations for change in the size or number of lesions. If scans are obtained at suspended resting lung volumes, variability may be diminished. However, it is now clear that spiral volumetric CT, with scanning of large lung subvolumes during a single breath hold, does much to obviate the problem of respiratory-induced misregistration of nodules.

In addition to the complete routine scan, selected thin-section scans can be performed to evaluate the morphology of individual nodules in greater detail (see Fig. 6) and to ascertain the precise location of lesions (e.g., relationship to fissures) before surgical resection. CT densitometry, for identification of high-attenuation benign lesions, is often useful in the general population. However, this technique is not recommended for patients with ETMs known to be associated with occasional calcification within pulmonary metastases.

For patients who have ETMs that may give rise to lymphangitic carcinomatosis and/or who have clinical symp-

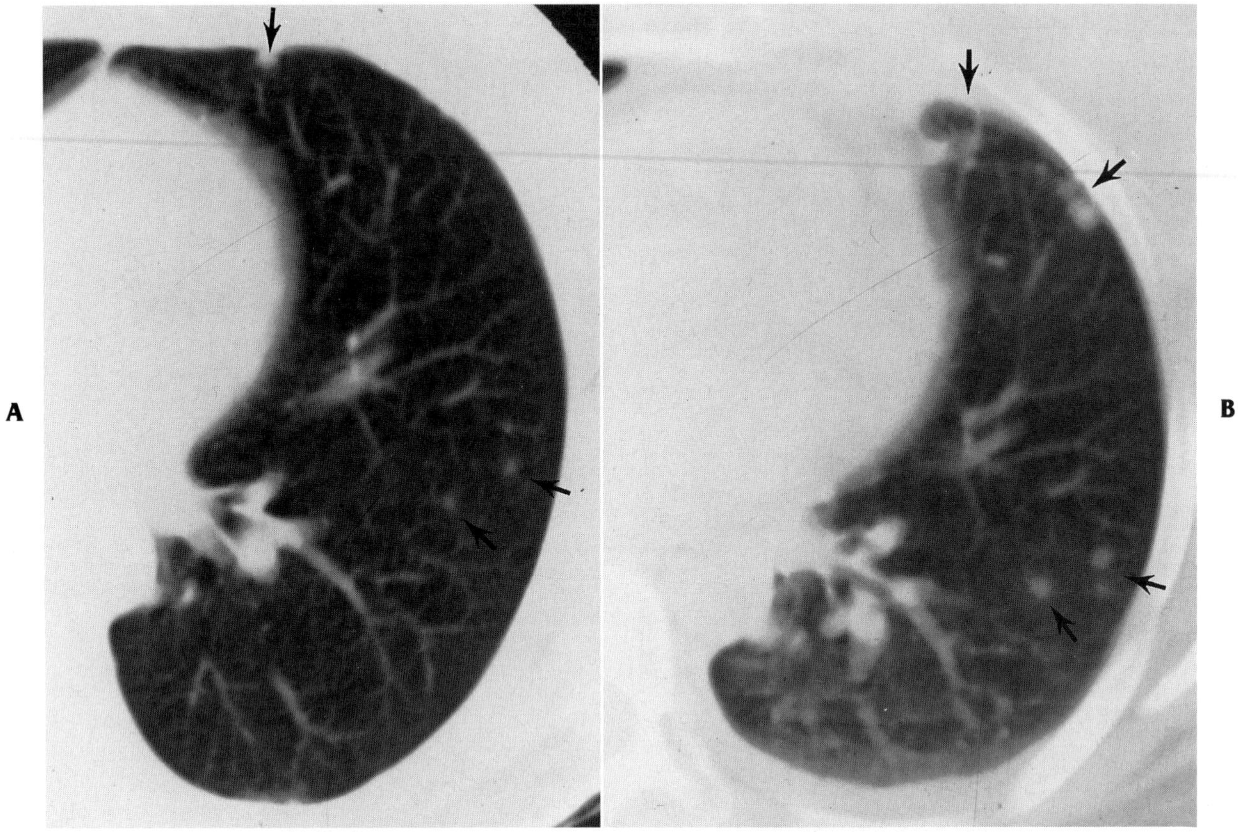


**FIGURE 8** A 44-year-old woman with carcinoma of the breast. *A,* CT scan reveals small subpleural nodules *(arrows)* in the left lung, two in the region of the major fissure and one anteriorly in the lingula. *B,* Ten months later a follow-up study revealed an increase in the size and number of lesions *(arrows),* evaluated at multiple levels; the scan shown here is at a level comparable to that in *(A),* although it was obtained with a greater degree of expiration.

toms suggestive of this pattern, three to six HRCT scans (through the apices, hila, and bases) should be performed in addition to the routine scan. If endobronchial metastases are suspected, contiguous 5 mm scans through the hila can be obtained.

There is appropriate concern regarding cumulative radiation dose, particularly in children and young adults who have tumors with a favorable prognosis and who require multiple follow-up CT examinations. Use of low-dose CT technique may be useful in this setting. Recent encouraging preliminary results suggest that magnetic resonance imaging (MRI) may be at least as sensitive as CT in detecting nodules larger than 5 mm. MRI would of course offer the advantage of avoiding ionizing radiation.

## Recommendations

Further prospective studies comparing MRI and CT in the diagnosis of pulmonary metastases would be of considerable interest, but presently CT remains the gold standard. CT is clearly more sensitive than conventional radiography in detecting nodular lesions. CT is also better able to reveal lymphangitic, endobronchial, or embolic manifestations of disease. The specificity of CT remains a problem, but attention to relevant clinical factors should be of assistance.

Evaluation of a patient with known ETM should always begin with a posteroanterior (PA) and lateral chest radiograph, and comparison with any prior studies is essential. If the chest radiograph is negative, screening by chest CT to detect occult metastases is recommended only for patients with those ETMs that are at high risk for early dissemination to the lungs and for which metastasectomy and/or systemic therapy is associated with prolonged survival, i.e., the bone and soft-tissue sarcomas, choriocarcinoma, nonseminomatous testicular carcinoma, and most pediatric tumors. Screening might also be performed for advanced melanoma, for which there is a high incidence of occult pulmonary metastases; however, there must also be an extensive search for concomitant extrapulmonary disease. For patients with high-risk ETMs, screening chest CT should perhaps be performed at 3 to 6 month intervals, for at least 2 years from the time of initial diagnosis.

If the chest radiograph reveals an apparent solitary nodule or an equivocal finding, not clarified by additional radiographic views or fluoroscopy, CT is indicated. If the chest radiograph demonstrates multiple nodules, CT is not required, unless tissue biopsy or definitive treatment is contemplated.

CT is frequently of great assistance in establishing a tissue diagnosis for a pulmonary abnormality; based on CT findings, one can decide whether PNAB or FOB should be performed. Serial CT scans are often helpful in determining the benign or malignant nature of "unverifiable" lesions that are too small for biopsy. Once surgical or systemic treatment has been selected, baseline and subsequent follow-up CT scans are essential. Finally, large prospective studies examining individual ETMs are needed to assess the impact of early CT detection of pulmonary metastases on long-term survival.

## Suggested Reading

Costello P, Anderson W, Blume D. Pulmonary nodule: Evaluation with spiral volumetric CT. Radiology 1991; 179:875–876.

Davis, Sheila D. Evaluation for pulmonary metastases in patients with known extrathoracic malignancy. Radiology 1991; 180:1–12.

Feuerstein IM, Jicha DL, Pass HI, et al. Pulmonary metastases: MR imaging with surgical correlation – a prospective study. Radiology 1992; 182:123–129.

Heaston DK, Putnam CE, Rodan BA, et al. Solitary pulmonary metastases in high-risk melanoma patients: A prospective comparison of conventional and computed tomography. AJR 1983; 141:169–174.

Marincola FM, Mark JBD. Selection factors resulting in improved survival after surgical resection of tumors metastatic to the lungs. Arch Surg 1990; 125:1387–1393.

Panicek DM. MR imaging for pulmonary metastases? Radiology 1992; 182:10–11.

Pass HI, Dwyer A, Makuch R, Roth JA. Detection of pulmonary metastases in patients with osteogenic and soft-tissue sarcomas: The superiority of CT scans compared with conventional linear tomograms using dynamic analysis. J Clin Oncol 1985; 3:1261–1265.

Peuchot M, Libshitz HI. Pulmonary metastatic disease: Radiologic-surgical correlation. Radiology 1987; 164:719–722.

Venn GE, Sarin S, Goldstraw P. Survival following pulmonary metastasectomy. Eur J Cardiothorac Surg 1989; 3:105–110.

Viadana E, Bross IDJ, Pickren JW. Cascade spread of blood-borne metastases in solid and nonsolid cancers of humans. In: Weiss L, Gilbert HA, eds. Pulmonary metastasis. Boston: GK Hall, 1978: 142.

# CT Evaluation of Solitary Pulmonary Nodules

*ARFA KHAN, M.D.*

A solitary pulmonary nodule (SPN) is described as a focal lung density, measuring less than 6 cm in diameter and not associated with atelectasis, adenopathy, or pleural effusion. The finding of a SPN in an asymptomatic patient is a common diagnostic problem in radiology occurring in about 1 to 2 per 1,000 chest radiographs. SPN is the most common presentation for asymptomatic bronchogenic carcinoma, as well as for benign pulmonary masses. In most reported series, the majority of resected SPNs are benign. To avoid unnecessary thoracotomies for benign disease, preoperative differentiation of a benign from a malignant nodule is a main goal of the radiologist.

In addition to history – age, history of smoking, pre-existing malignancy, and infection – helpful criteria to differentiate benign from malignant SPNs are the following:

1. Size – SPNs greater than 3 cm are usually malignant.
2. Edge – spiculated margins are suggestive of malignancy.
3. Lack of growth – lack of growth for 2 or more years is the most reliable criterion for benignancy.
4. Calcification – presence of calcification in a benign pattern is the second most reliable criterion for benignancy; benign patterns of calcification are central nidus, laminated, popcorn-like, and diffuse.

Radiographic methods for detection of calcium are as follows:

1. Chest radiograph
2. Low-kilovolt spot radiograph
3. Conventional tomogram
4. Computed tomogram
5. Dual-energy digital radiography
6. Digitized chest radiograph

Computed tomography (CT) owing to its superior contrast resolution is more accurate than traditional radiographic techniques in evaluating nodules for presence of calcifications. As a result of advances in CT densitometry and the availability of a reference phantom, CT has been increasingly used for characterization of SPNs. Not every pulmonary nodule can be differentiated as benign or malignant by CT evaluation.

An algorithm for the workup of SPN is proposed in Figure 1.

## Thin-section CT

CT evaluation of SPNs is performed by obtaining 1.5 mm thin sections through the nodule. Thin-section CT is more sensitive than standard 10 mm section CT in detecting calcifications. Thin-section CT detects calcifications in 36 percent of benign nodules, whereas standard CT detects calcifications in only 12 percent.

The pulmonary nodule is characterized as benign or indeterminate on the basis of size and edge characteristics and presence of calcification and fat on thin-section CT. Any SPN larger than 3 cm in diameter is considered indeterminate, even if it exhibits benign patterns of calcification (Fig. 2). The edge of the nodule is classified as spiculated, irregular, lobulated, or smooth. Spiculated margins are differentiated from irregular margins by the presence of sharp needle-like projections. A spiculated nodule larger than 1.5 cm is considered to be indeterminate, even if it fulfills other criteria of benignancy. CT is of greater value in evaluating smooth and lobulated nodules. The likelihood of benignity is decreased in spiculated lesions; even when benign, such lesions are less likely to be calcified. The presence of calcification on thin-section CT is determined by gross observation of all the sections through the nodule at narrow window width (0 to 400 H). The area of calcification is calculated on one or more sections with the use of a pixel ruler (Computed Imaging Reference System). Presence of calcification in a benign pattern (i.e., diffuse, central, laminated, or popcorn) and representing more than 10 percent of the cross-sectional area of the nodule is suggestive of a benign nodule (Fig. 3).

Presence of fat attenuation on thin-section CT is considered diagnostic for a hamartoma (Fig. 4). Areas of low density secondary to necrosis should not be mistaken for the presence of fat. Presence of fat attenuation is confirmed by comparing the CT numbers in the low-attenuation areas of the nodule with the CT numbers of subcutaneous fat. Fat is present in over

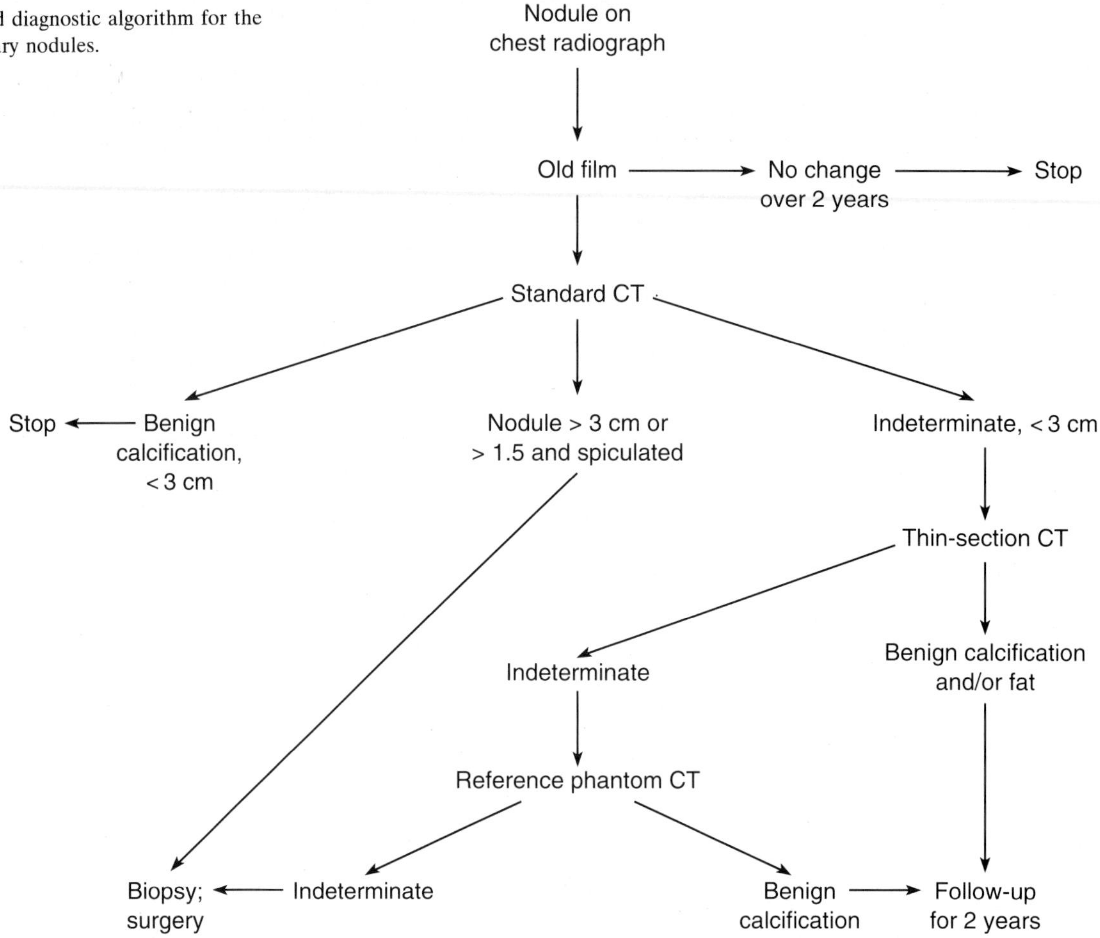


**FIGURE 1** Proposed diagnostic algorithm for the evaluation of pulmonary nodules.

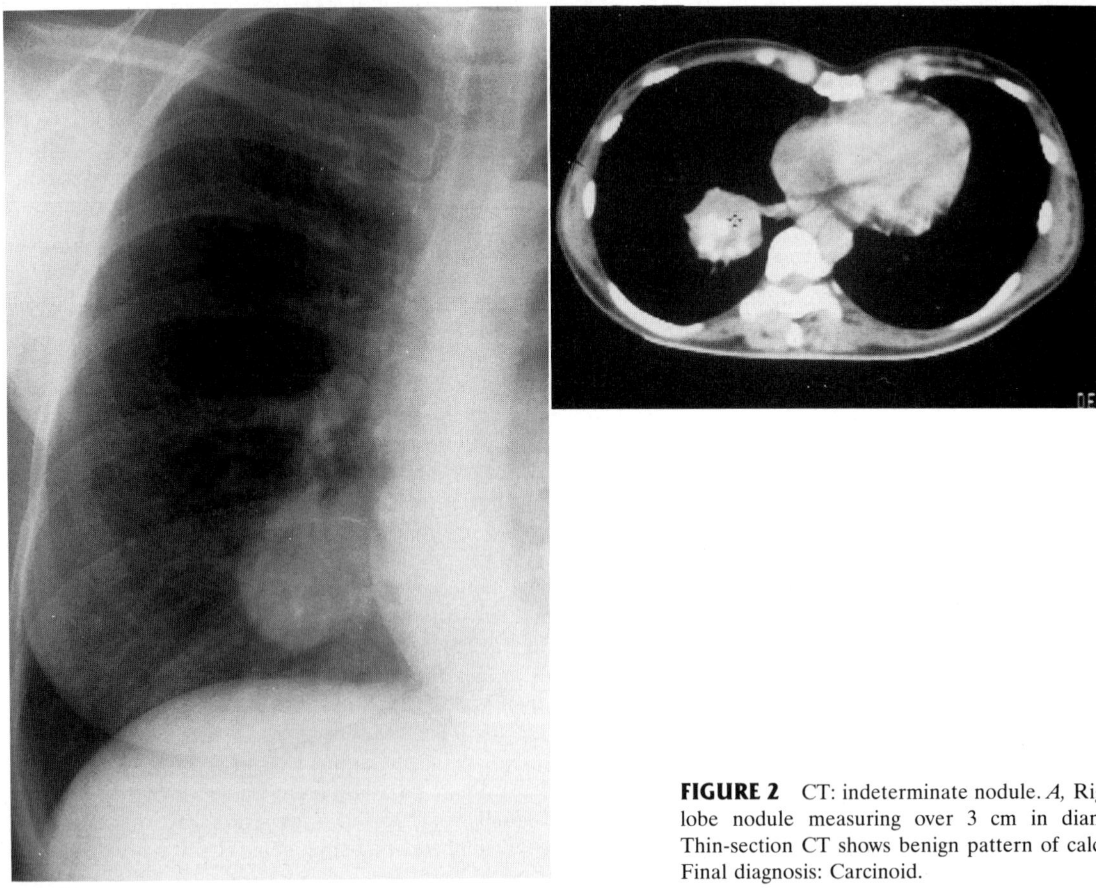

A

B

**FIGURE 2** CT: indeterminate nodule. *A*, Right lower lobe nodule measuring over 3 cm in diameter. *B*, Thin-section CT shows benign pattern of calcification. Final diagnosis: Carcinoid.

A

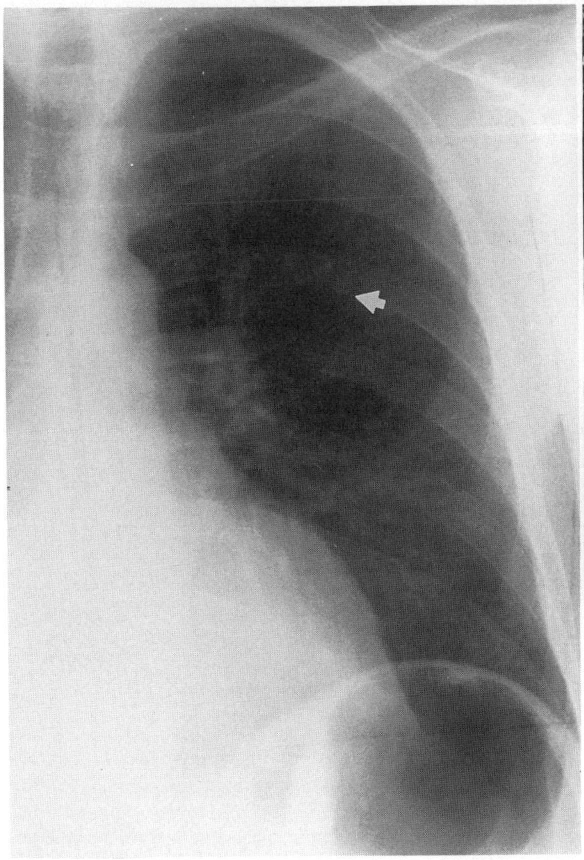

B

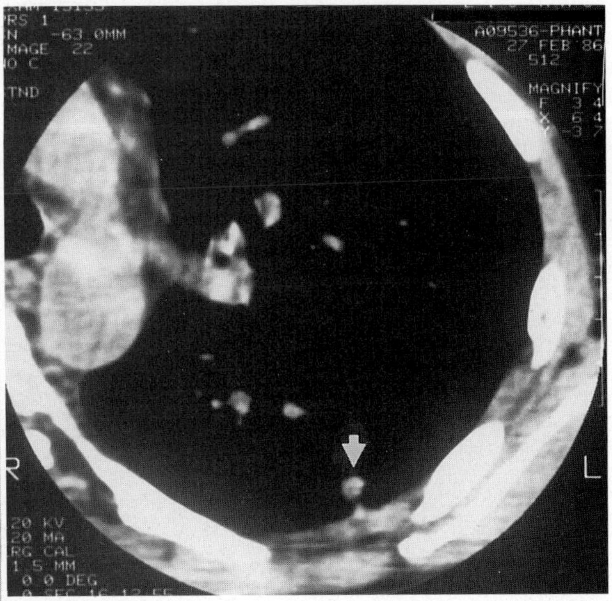


**FIGURE 3** CT: benign nodule. *A,* Chest radiograph shows a noncalcified 10 mm nodule *(arrow)* in the left upper lobe. *B,* Thin-section CT shows contiguous calcification of more than 10 percent of the surface area of the nodule *(arrow).* Final diagnosis: granuloma.

50 percent of hamartomas. Calcification with or without fat is present in 30 percent of hamartomas. One-third of hamartomas contain neither fat nor calcium and are assessed as indeterminate. Hamartoma is the third most common SPN after granuloma and carcinoma. It is the only benign nodule that may show growth over time. A smooth nodule less than 3 cm in diameter, with presence of fat and calcium, is characteristic of a hamartoma and does not require histologic confirmation (Fig. 5). The only other fat-containing lesion of lung is lipoid pneumonia, also a benign condition.

If the nodule is assessed as benign on thin-section CT, two follow-up chest radiographs at 3 month intervals, followed by three radiographs at 6 month intervals are recommended. If there is lack of growth for 2 years, the nodule is considered to be benign.

## Reference Phantom CT

If the SPN is characterized as indeterminate on thin-section CT, comparison with the reference phantom should be performed.

The reference phantom was first introduced by Zerhouni and co-workers in 1983. The reference phantom allows a standardized method of CT densitometric measurement of a pulmonary nodule. A large number of factors can affect the CT numbers of a pulmonary nodule (e.g., section thickness, partial volume effect, reconstruction algorithm, type of scanner, technique, nodule size and location, and electronic drift). The technique of reference phantom CT is simple, uniform, scanner independent, and reproducible.

Reference phantom CT is more sensitive than thin-section CT for identification of calcification in benign nodules. In our study of 75 consecutive patients, reference phantom CT increased the sensitivity for identification of calcification in benign nodules by 22 percent as compared with thin-section CT. Reference phantom CT also helps to increase the level of confidence of identification of calcifications at thin-section CT.

The reference phantom (Fig. 6) consists of three transaxial sections that simulate the anatomy of the thorax above the level of aortic arch, at the level of aortic arch, and at the level of left atrium. The phantom reproduces transverse sections of the thorax using epoxy resin plastics of various compositions that duplicate the shape and CT density of the structures within each section. Rings of "fat-equivalent" plastic of various widths are positioned around the phantom to duplicate the chest wall thickness of individual patients. Reference nodules are cylinders varying from 0.4 to 6 cm in diameter, made of epoxy resin mixed with calcium carbonate powder. The sections of the phantom can be mounted on a support board using Velcro surfaces. The reference nodule is positioned within the lung cavities of the phantom to simulate the clinical situation. At our institution, using a GE 9800 scanner, the reference phantom CT images are obtained with the use of the following technical factors: soft-tissue algorithm, 120 kVp, 170 mA, and 48 cm field of view.

The patient is examined at resting volume. The patient is instructed: "Breathe in, breathe out, relax and hold your breath." Several thin contiguous sections through the nodule are obtained, and the average diameter of the nodule is measured. The nodule diameter is defined as half the sum of the maximal and minimal diameters on the scan on which the nodule appears the largest at a window level of 500 HU and

A

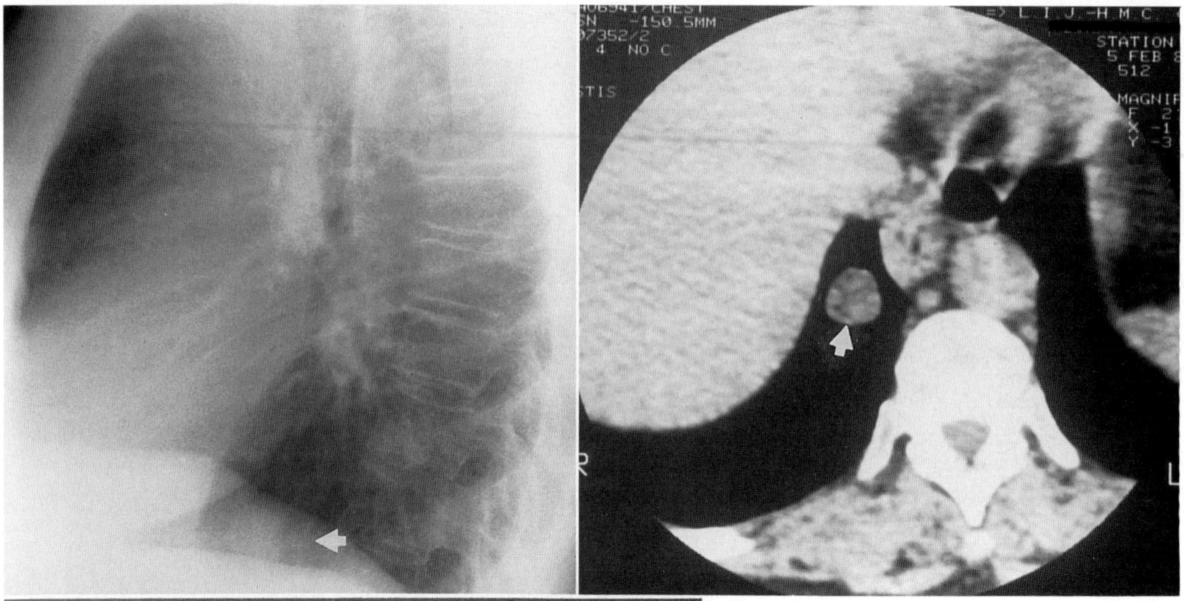


B

C

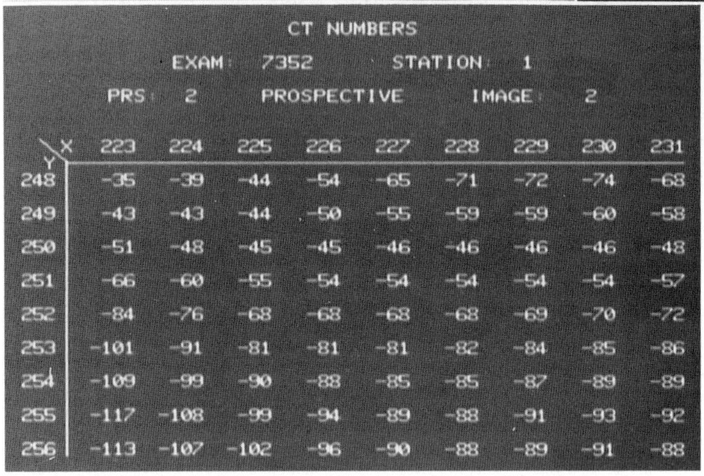

CT NUMBERS

EXAM: 7352 STATION: 1

PRS: 2 PROSPECTIVE IMAGE: 2

| Y \ X | 223 | 224 | 225 | 226 | 227 | 228 | 229 | 230 | 231 |
|---|---|---|---|---|---|---|---|---|---|
| 248 | -35 | -39 | -44 | -54 | -65 | -71 | -72 | -74 | -68 |
| 249 | -43 | -43 | -44 | -50 | -55 | -59 | -59 | -60 | -58 |
| 250 | -51 | -48 | -45 | -45 | -46 | -46 | -46 | -46 | -48 |
| 251 | -66 | -60 | -55 | -54 | -54 | -54 | -54 | -54 | -57 |
| 252 | -84 | -76 | -68 | -68 | -68 | -68 | -69 | -70 | -72 |
| 253 | -101 | -91 | -81 | -81 | -81 | -82 | -84 | -85 | -86 |
| 254 | -109 | -99 | -90 | -88 | -85 | -85 | -87 | -89 | -89 |
| 255 | -117 | -108 | -99 | -94 | -89 | -88 | -91 | -93 | -92 |
| 256 | -113 | -107 | -102 | -96 | -90 | -88 | -89 | -91 | -88 |

**FIGURE 4** Hamartoma containing fat. *A,* Lateral chest radiograph shows a 1.8 cm sharply marginated nodule in the right lower lobe *(arrow). B,* Thin-section CT scan shows low-attenuation areas within the nodule *(arrow). C,* Computer printout of CT numbers for the low-attenuation area show negative CT numbers in the range of fat. The presence of fat was confirmed at surgery and pathologic evaluation. (From Khan A, Herman PG, Vorwerk P, et al. Solitary pulmonary nodules: Comparison of classification with standard, thin-section, and reference phantom CT. Radiology 1991; 179:477–481, with permission.)

window width of 1,500 to 2,000 HU. The phantom section most resembling the actual anatomy at the level of the nodule is then selected, placing a "fat ring" around it if necessary so as to match the thickness of the chest wall. The phantom is mounted on its support in the same position as the patient. A phantom nodule equal in dimension to the average diameter of the patient's nodule is placed in the lung cavity in the same position as the nodule in the patient's chest. If the phantom nodule of same size as the patient's nodule is not available, the next larger phantom nodule should be selected. The phantom is scanned immediately after the patient, using the same technical factors to minimize temporal and technical variations. At least two scans are obtained. The scan showing the highest CT numbers for the phantom nodule is chosen for comparison with the patient's nodule.

The density of the patient's nodule is then compared with the reference phantom nodule using the following method (Fig. 7). The phantom scan is first viewed using a window width of 1 to 2 H, after which the window level is raised until the "nodule" disappears. The patient's scans are then viewed successively using the same window level and width.

Alternatively, the density of phantom nodule and patient's nodule can be compared by displaying the two images simultaneously on the screen on top of each other. Using the fixed window width of 1 to 2 H, the window level is raised until one of the nodules disappears. The nodule that disappears first is less dense than the other.

If the phantom nodule is denser than the patient's nodule, the latter is considered noncalcified and therefore indeterminate (Fig. 8). The nodule is considered calcified and benign only if a group of contiguous pixels representing at least 10 percent of the cross-sectional area of the nodule is of higher attenuation value than the highest pixel of the phantom nodule (see Fig. 7).

Cytologic or histologic confirmation is suggested in every case interpreted as indeterminate on CT scans. For cases interpreted as benign on CT scans, two follow-up chest radiographs at 3 month intervals, followed by three radiographs at 6 month intervals, are recommended. If there is no growth of the nodule over 2 years, the nodule is presumed to be benign.

## Pitfalls

CT densitometry is not suitable for all pulmonary nodules. Strict selection of criteria for CT densitometry of SPNs is

A

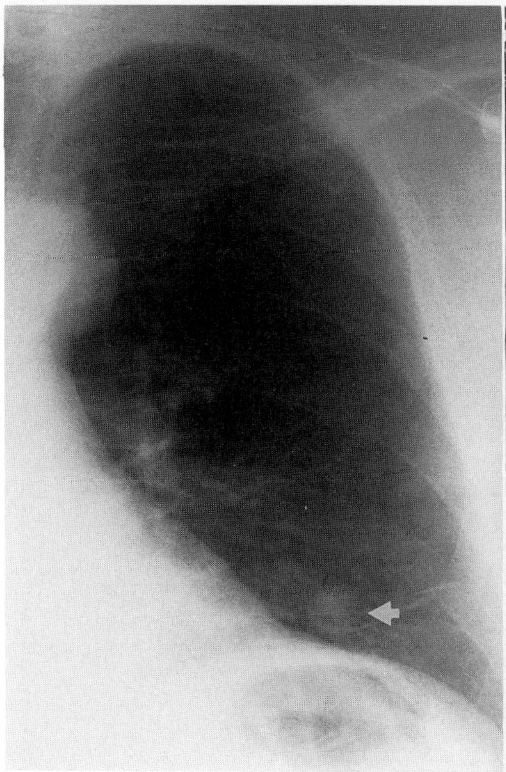

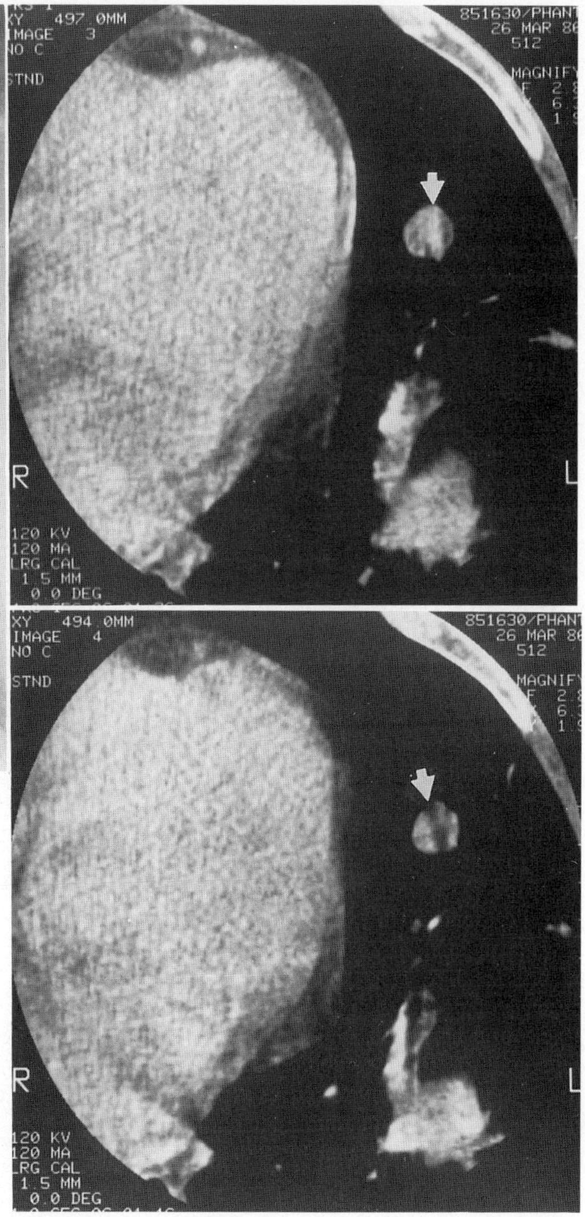


C

**FIGURE 5** Hamartoma containing fat and calcification. *A,* Chest radiograph shows a 1.5 cm left lower lobe nodule *(arrow). B,* Thin-section CT scan shows central calcification *(arrow). C,* Thin-section CT scan caudad to *(B)* shows the central low-attenuation area *(arrow),* which displayed CT numbers similar to the subcutaneous fat.

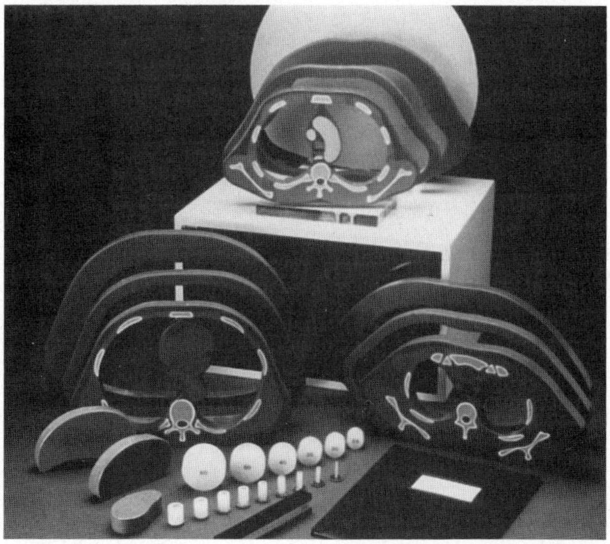

**FIGURE 6** Reference phantom (CIRS).

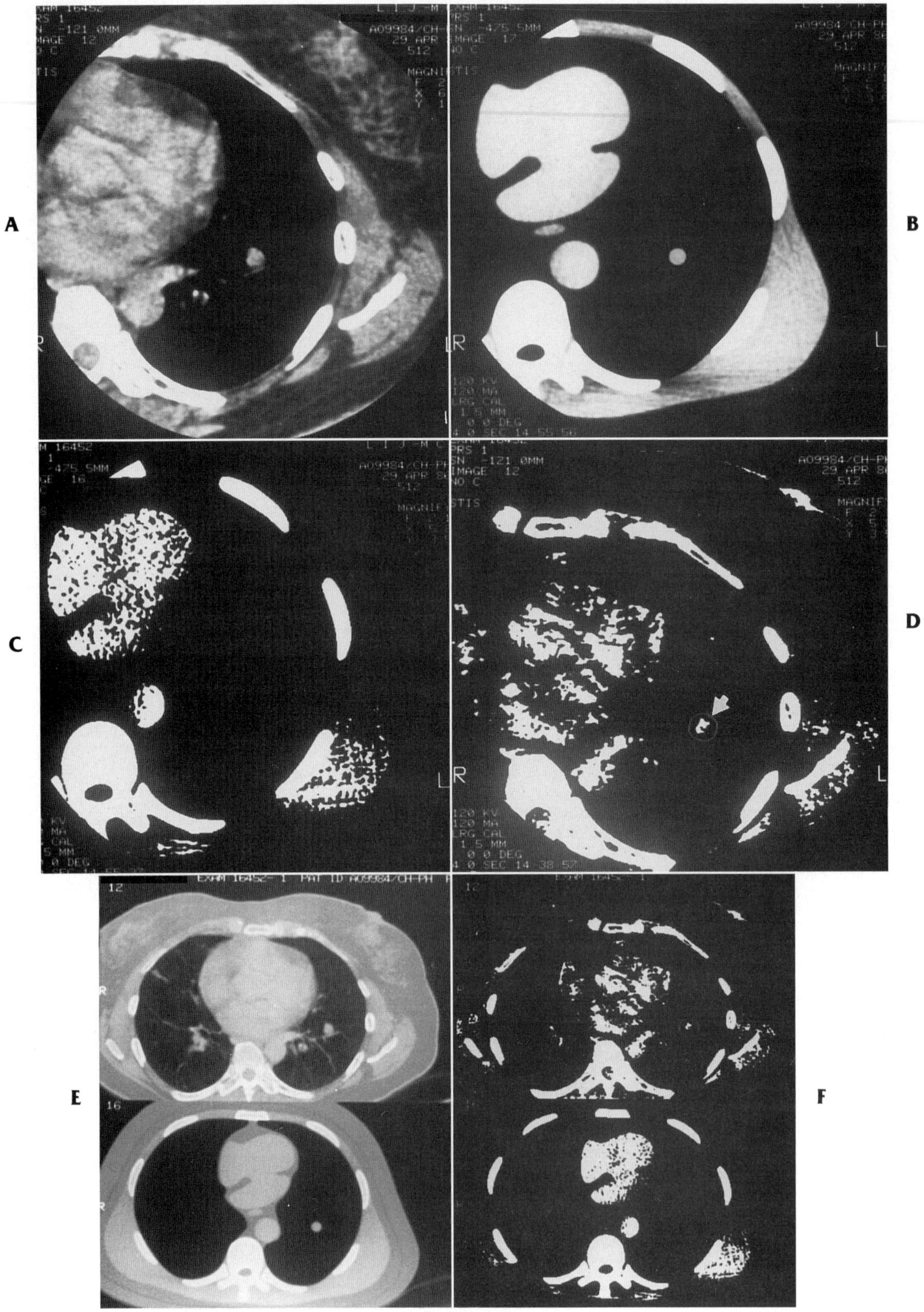

**FIGURE 7** Example of analysis of a solitary pulmonary nodule with a reference phantom (phantom: benign nodule). *A,* Thin-section CT scan of the patient's nodule. No visible calcification is observed. *B,* Phantom scan with the reference nodule. *C,* Phantom scan viewed at a window width of 2 HU and a window level at which the nodule disappears (38 HU in this case). *D,* Patient's scan viewed at the same window width and window length as *(C)*. A group of contiguous pixels *(arrow)* representing more than 10 percent of the cross-sectional area of the nodule is of higher attenuation value than the phantom nodule. The nodule is evaluated as calcified and benign. *E,* and *F,* Example of analysis of a solitary pulmonary nodule with side-by-side comparison. Patient *(top)*, phantom *(bottom)*. At a window level of 38 HU and a window width of 2 HU *(F),* the patient's nodule is still seen, whereas the phantom nodule is no longer visible indicating significant calcification in the patient's nodule.

A

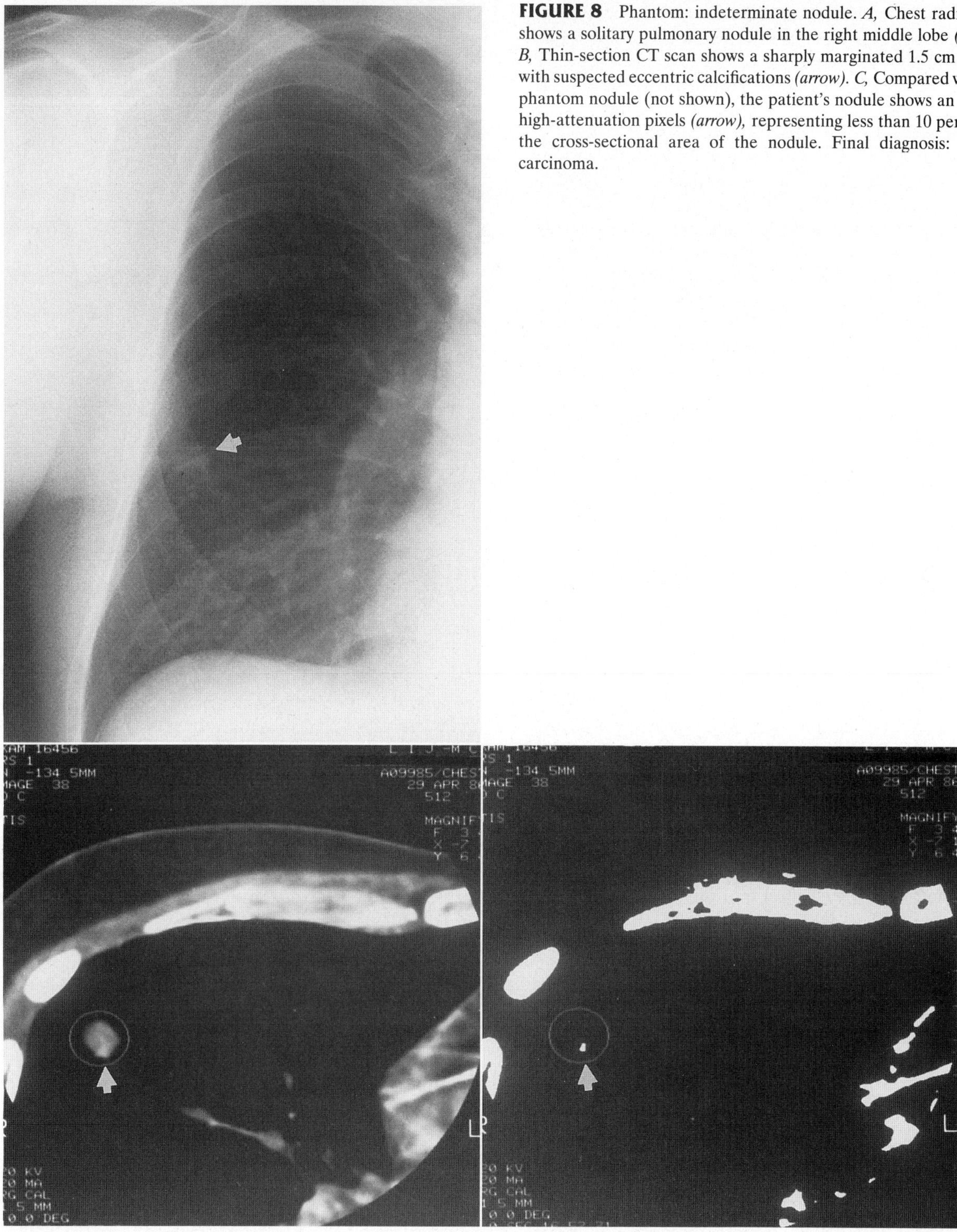

B

C

**FIGURE 8** Phantom: indeterminate nodule. *A,* Chest radiograph shows a solitary pulmonary nodule in the right middle lobe *(arrow). B,* Thin-section CT scan shows a sharply marginated 1.5 cm nodule with suspected eccentric calcifications *(arrow). C,* Compared with the phantom nodule (not shown), the patient's nodule shows an area of high-attenuation pixels *(arrow),* representing less than 10 percent of the cross-sectional area of the nodule. Final diagnosis: adenocarcinoma.

recommended to avoid errors in diagnosis. CT densitometry of SPNs should not be performed for the following:

1. Any nodule greater than 3 cm in diameter
2. Spiculated nodule greater than 1.5 cm in diameter
3. Cavitating nodule
4. Metastatic osteosarcoma
5. Uncooperative patient

All scans with motion artifacts should be excluded from consideration. Great care should be exercised for simulating the phantom as close as possible to patient's anatomy. The size of phantom nodule should never be smaller than patient's nodule.

To my knowledge no direct radiologic-pathologic correlative studies show that calcifications in a nodule are related to the high-attenuation pixels at reference phantom CT. In my experience foci of calcification observed at thin-section CT correlate exactly with high-attenuation pixels at reference phantom CT; this correlation offers indirect evidence that high-attenuation pixels on reference phantom CT represent foci of calcifications.

Mere presence of calcification is not a specific sign of benignancy, since malignant tumors may show calcification in rare instances. Calcification is found in 14 percent of cancers at histologic evaluation and in 7 percent at CT.

The pattern of calcification in a malignant tumor is usually eccentric or finely stippled. Metastatic pulmonary lesions in patients with mucinous carcinoma may contain diffuse fine calcifications that can render CT densitometry unreliable.

Ossified carcinoids (see Fig. 2) may be confused with calcified granuloma. A carcinoid is usually a central lesion with a proximal bronchus forming a margin or a portion of the lesion. Granulomas are peripheral lesions that do not have contact with a defined bronchus. Occasionally it is difficult to differentiate the two.

## Suggested Reading

Khan A, Herman PG, Vorwerk P, et al. Solitary pulmonary nodules: Comparison of classification with standard, thin-section, and reference phantom CT. Radiology 1991; 179:477–481.

Mahoney MC, Shipley RT, Corcoran HL, Dickson BA. CT demonstrations of calcification in carcinoma of lung. AJR 1990; 154:255–258.

Siegelman SS, Khouri NF, Leo FP, et al. Solitary pulmonary nodules: CT assessment. Radiology 1986; 160:307–312.

Siegelman SS, Khouri NF, Scott WW, et al. Pulmonary hamartoma: CT findings. Radiology 1986; 160:313–317.

Webb RW. Radiologic evaluation of the solitary pulmonary nodule. AJR 1990; 154:701–708.

Zerhouni EA, Boukadoum M, Siddiky MA, et al. Standard phantom for quantitative analysis of pulmonary nodules by computed tomography. Radiology 1983; 149:767–773.

Zerhouni EA, Spivey JF, Morgan RH, et al. Factors influencing quantitative CT measurements of solitary pulmonary nodules. J Comput Assist Tomogr 1982; 6:1075–1087.

# CT and MRI Evaluation of Mediastinal Masses

*BARRY H. GROSS, M.D. · DAVID L. SPIZARNY, M.D.*

I had the good fortune to do my diagnostic radiology residency at the University of Cincinnati at a time when both Felson and Proto were there. They were interested in the role that the emerging technology of chest computed tomography (CT) should play. Felson in particular viewed late 1970s chest CT with a somewhat jaundiced eye. This seemed to me to be a result of the not yet perfected technology, as well as his considerable skills in analysis of conventional radiographs. Cross-sectional chest imaging in 1992 bears little resemblance to the images of the 1970s, just as the interpretive skills that most of us bring to conventional chest radiography bear little resemblance to those of Felson and Proto. Presently we do not screen patients carefully to ensure that chest CT is indicated; the only significant requirement for chest CT is that the patient have a chest. However, one connecting thread from then to now is the primacy of chest CT in the evaluation of mediastinal masses. In this chapter we discuss the application of CT and magnetic resonance imaging (MRI) to the evaluation of mediastinal masses.

## Indications

First, a word about MRI. We don't use it to evaluate mediastinal masses. That isn't to say that there aren't patients in whom it can be helpful as a problem solver. For example, patients allergic to iodinated contrast media who have suspected vascular mediastinal masses (such as aneurysms) could benefit from MRI instead of CT. Nevertheless, we seldom use MRI (in fact, we seldom use MRI for any chest abnormalities).

The mediastinum is difficult to evaluate using conventional radiographs and easy to assess with CT. Among the advantages of CT over conventional radiographs are improved contrast resolution, mass characterization by attenuation measurements, cross-sectional anatomic display, evaluation of enhancement characteristics, and detection of associated neck, chest wall, and upper abdominal abnormalities. As the technology has evolved, so have the indications for chest CT. With regard to mediastinal masses, I used to recommend CT for patients with chest radiographic evidence of anterior or posterior mediastinal masses; for middle mediastinal masses I suggested barium swallow as the next diagnostic tool. Although I still teach this approach to medical students and radiology residents, in reality we do CT for any patient with a mediastinal mass at chest radiography. CT has also proven its value for mediastinal masses in high-risk patients with normal chest radiographs. Patients with myasthenia gravis undergo CT no matter what the chest radiograph shows, as do patients being staged for lymphoma. Patients with esophageal carcinoma typically undergo chest CT, even though CT is not an especially effective tool for detection or local staging of esophageal carcinoma. CT has been considered a sensitive tool for detecting mediastinal spread of lung cancer, even in patients with conventional radiographic T1N0M0 disease, although a recent report published in *Radiology* raises questions about just how sensitive CT really is for detecting mediastinal lymph node metastases in lung cancer.

When chest radiographic follow-up as a tool for evaluating questionable conventional radiographic abnormality is deemed clinically inappropriate, CT usually confirms or excludes a significant abnormality. Pathologic mediastinal widening and possible aortopulmonary window lymph node enlargement are examples of questionable abnormality frequently referred to CT.

In summary, CT is now used for patients with chest radiographic evidence, chest radiographic suspicion, or clinical suspicion of a mediastinal mass. There is no acceptable alternative technology.

## Technical Approach

CT technique is somewhat dependent on patient body habitus. In the average patient we scan at 120 kV, 140 mA, and 2 second scan time. We have one helical scanner, but pending a tube upgrade we have not used helical scanning to any significant extent.

The critical technical issue in CT of mediastinal masses is bolus infusion of intravenous contrast material. There are institutions and radiologists performing routine noncontrast chest CT, and with an exceptionally talented chest radiologist this may work out well. As for the rest of us, bolus infusion of intravenous contrast material makes detection of abnormality much easier. With vascular structures opacified by contrast material, mediastinal masses (even enhancing masses) stand out in sharp contrast as lower-attenuation lesions.

For the usual patient, we power inject 150 ml of 30 percent iodinated contrast medium (45 g of iodine) at 2 ml per second, preferably through an 18 gauge Angiocath. If nonionic contrast material is indicated, we use 125 ml of 35 percent contrast medium (43.75 g of iodine). Scanning is initiated 20 to 25 seconds into the bolus, beginning at the caudal hila and proceeding to the lung apices. Scans are routinely 1 cm in thickness and are obtained at 1 cm intervals. We only rarely use thin sections to decrease partial volume averaging (i.e., aortopulmonary window evaluation). Once the lung apices have been scanned, scanning resumes from the caudal hila into the abdomen, and is generally carried through the adrenal glands. Images are reviewed at the console before the patient leaves the department to ensure high quality. Interpretation is subsequently performed using images photographed at lung, soft-tissue, and liver windows (and selected bone window images, if necessary).

## Diagnostic Approach

Mediastinal mass is diagnosed when a mediastinal structure that does not correspond to normal mediastinal anatomy exceeds 1 cm in short-axis dimension. Smaller structures are considered normal mediastinal lymph nodes, although normal-size nodes may harbor tumor. Mediastinal parathyroid adenomas can also be small, making diagnosis difficult. Lymph nodes that are larger than 1 cm in short axis may not contain tumor, especially if there is preserved central nodal fat or extensive nodal calcification. However, the larger the lymph node, the more likely it represents a significant abnormality.

We have already extolled the virtues of CT in detecting mediastinal masses, but now comes a surprise: CT is not especially good at diagnosing the etiology of a mediastinal mass. Although attenuation features and enhancement characteristics may allow specific diagnoses, most masses are of soft-tissue attenuation. It is generally not possible to distinguish lymphoma from metastatic disease from benign entities (especially sarcoidosis) using CT; it is generally not possible to separate Hodgkin's lymphoma from non-Hodgkin's lymphoma, nor to separate metastatic lung carcinoma from metastatic extrapulmonary malignancy. In a study of 132 mediastinal masses, we arrived at a specific diagnosis in only 16.

Given that specific diagnosis is not the forte of CT, why use it at all? Justifications include mediastinal mass detection, confirmation of questionable abnormalities, delineation of disease extent, reduction in size of the differential diagnostic list, and facilitation of optimal diagnostic and therapeutic strategies. The advantages of disease detection and confirmation of questionable abnormalities are obvious. Accurate delineation of disease extent narrows the differential diagnosis in several ways. First, confirmation of mass location in a specific mediastinal compartment (anterior, middle, or posterior) is the cornerstone of differential diagnosis. Subcompartmentalization gives clues to etiology, because a mass centered on the location of normal thymus is more likely a thymoma than a mass centered near the location of normal thyroid. CT also distinguishes single mediastinal masses from multifocal masses. A single mass virtually excludes lymphoma; multifocal masses are unlikely to be thymoma or teratoma and usually indicate lymphoma, metastatic disease, or sarcoidosis. Finally, associated abnormalities such as focal pulmonary mass(es), focal liver lesions, or bone lesions suggest metastatic disease, whereas axillary lymph node enlargement favors lymphoma.

CT facilitates optimal diagnostic strategies by determining the available routes to obtain tissue. CT can show whether a lesion is accessible to mediastinoscopy and can guide bronchoscopic Wang needle aspiration. CT is also used for radiation therapy treatment planning.

The preceding paragraphs apply to the vast majority of cases—routine mediastinal CT. In a distinct minority of patients, mediastinal CT is interesting precisely because it makes specific diagnoses. Specific diagnoses rely on intrinsic attenuation features and enhancement characteristics of masses. An anterior mediastinal mass containing fat, water, calcium, and/or teeth is a teratoma. Thymoma may have a rim of calcification, whereas thymic cyst is a water-attenuation lesion. Pericardial fat pads and mediastinal lipomatosis are proven by their characteristic homogeneous fat attenuation, whereas thyroid enlargement and mediastinal hematoma demonstrate intrinsic high attenuation. In the middle mediastinum, bronchogenic cyst is usually a water-attenuation

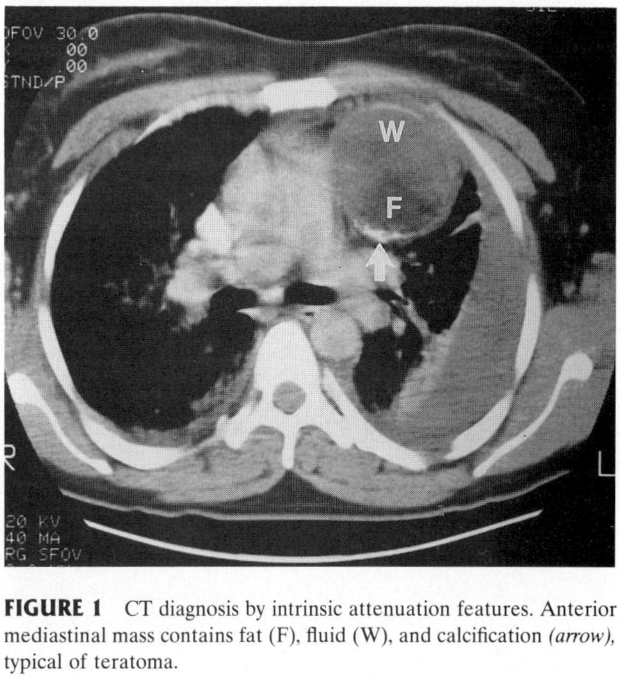


**FIGURE 1** CT diagnosis by intrinsic attenuation features. Anterior mediastinal mass contains fat (F), fluid (W), and calcification *(arrow)*, typical of teratoma.

A

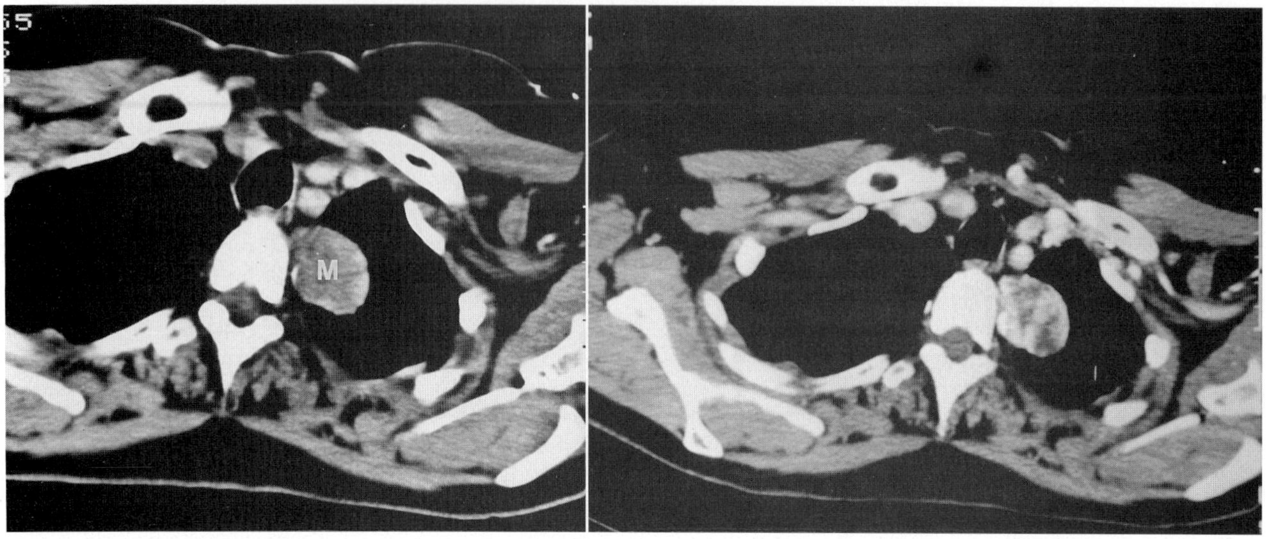


B

**FIGURE 2** CT diagnosis by enhancement characteristics. *A,* Noncontrast CT of posterior mediastinal mass (M). *B,* After bolus injection of intravenous contrast medium, there is peripheral puddling of contrast in this hemangioma.

**FIGURE 3** What is this rapidly disappearing mass? *A,* Chest radiograph reveals an anterior mediastinal mass (M) in a patient with treated lymphoma. *B,* Chest radiograph 5 days later is normal. *C,* CT 1 day after *(A)* displays high-attenuation anterior mediastinal mass (H) representing spontaneous mediastinal hematoma.

A

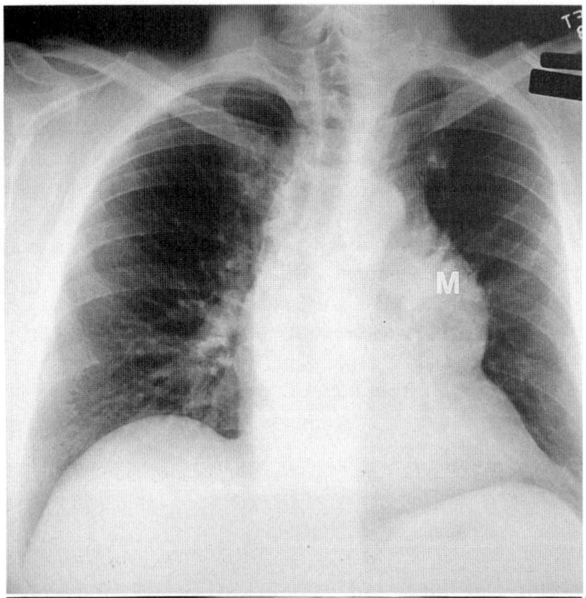


B

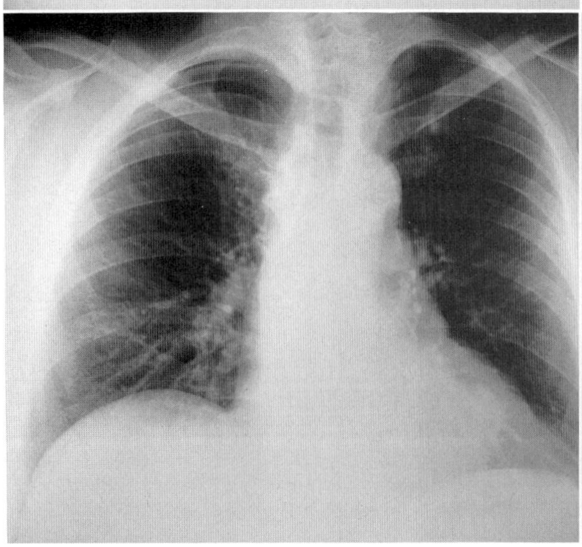

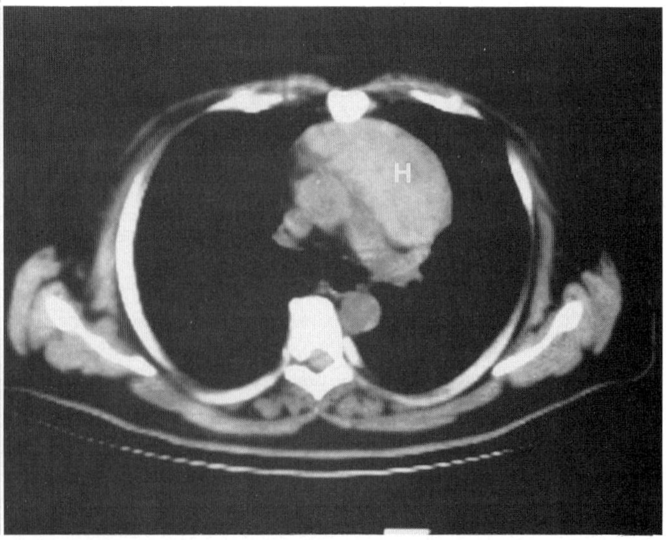


C

**TABLE 1** Differential Diagnosis of Mediastinal Masses

| Location | Entities | Clinical Clues | Special Features |
|---|---|---|---|
| *Anterior* | 4 T's: | | |
| | Thymoma | Older patient (>40) Myasthenia gravis | Single mass; ± calcification |
| | Teratoma | Younger patient (<20) | Single mass; fat, water, calcium, and/or teeth |
| | Thyroid | | Contiguity with thyroid in the neck; calcium, intrinsic high attenuation, enhancement |
| | Terrible lymphoma | Bimodal (any age) | Multiple masses; no de novo calcium, no enhancement |
| | And others: | | |
| | Metastases | Primaries – lung, breast, melanoma, genitourinary (renal or testicular), head and neck, gastric | |
| | Hematoma | ± Trauma | Intrinsic high attenuation, rapid resolution |
| | Parathyroid adenoma | Hyperparathyroid | ± Enhancement |
| | Vascular (aneurysm) | | Enhancement |
| *Middle* | Esophageal disease | Dysphagia | |
| | Bronchogenic cyst | | Water attenuation (or uniformly higher) |
| | Lymph node disease (sarcoidosis, lymphoma, metastases) | | |
| | Tuberculosis | | Low-attenuation nodes with enhancing rims |
| | Vascular | | Enhancement |
| | Castleman's disease | | Enhancement |
| *Posterior* | Neurogenic tumor | | |
| | Lateral meningocele | Neurofibromatosis | Water attenuation |
| | Disk space infection | | |
| | Vascular | | Enhancement |
| | Extramedullary hematopoiesis | Hereditary spherocytosis or thalassemia | Bilateral; lobulated |

lesion, although uniform higher attenuation of a bronchogenic cyst is a well-known phenomenon. Low-attenuation peripherally enhancing lymph nodes are typical of tuberculous lymphadenitis. As for posterior mediastinal lesions, calcification may be observed with certain neurogenic tumors, particularly those containing elements of neuroblastoma, whereas lateral meningoceles present as water-attenuation paravertebral masses.

Demonstration of mediastinal mass enhancement also results in a more specific differential diagnosis. Mediastinal thyroid is the most common enhancing mass. Extra-adrenal pheochromocytomas and other tumors derived from paraganglion cells such as aortic and carotid body tumors, chemodectomas, and glomus tumors often enhance. Other enhancing mediastinal masses include Castleman's disease, carcinoid tumor, and rare sarcomas. Contrast enhancement virtually eliminates lymphoma and metastatic disease.

Table 1 presents a differential diagnostic scheme for CT of mediastinal masses. Selected illustrative examples follow (Figs. 1 to 3).

## Suggested Reading


Aronberg DJ, Glazer HS, Sagel SS. MRI and CT of the mediastinum: Comparisons, controversies, and pitfalls. Radiol Clin North Am 1985; 23:439–448.

Batra P, Herrman C Jr, Mulder D. Mediastinal imaging in myasthenia gravis: Correlation of chest radiography, CT, MR, and surgical findings. AJR 1987; 148:515–519.

Feigin DS, Padua EM. Mediastinal masses: A system for diagnosis based on computed tomography. J Comput Tomogr 1986; 10:11–22.

Glazer GM, Orringer MB, Gross BH, Quint LE. The mediastinum in non-small cell lung cancer: CT-surgical correlation. AJR 1984; 142:1101–1105.

McLoud TC, Bourgouin PM, Greenberg RW, et al. Bronchogenic carcinoma: Analysis of staging in the mediastinum with CT by correlative lymph node mapping and sampling. Radiology 1992; 182:319–323.

Rebner M, Gross BH, Robertson JM, et al. CT evaluation of mediastinal masses. Comput Radiol 1987; 11:103–110.

Spizarny DL, Rebner M, Gross BH. Enhancing mediastinal masses: CT evaluation. J Comput Assist Tomogr 1987; 11:990–993.

# Pulmonary Vascular MRI

*WARREN B. GEFTER, M.D.*

Magnetic resonance imaging (MRI) has opened up new avenues for anatomic as well as quantitative physiologic imaging of the pulmonary vasculature. The technology is in evolution, and the methods will undoubtedly continue to be refined and advanced. The major advantage of the modality for conventional anatomic imaging is the ability to obtain superb images of the vessels in any desired plane without the requirement for intravenous contrast agents. In addition, the field of view can be varied as needed. The principal advantage of the quantitative techniques is the ability to calculate volume flow within the larger vessels completely noninvasively. This chapter reviews the major indications, strengths, and limitations of these MRI studies, technical approaches, and new investigational methods likely to have significant clinical impact in the near future (Tables 1 and 2).

## Indications, Strengths, and Limitations

The primary indications for conventional MRI of the pulmonary arteries include congenital abnormalities, involvement by extrinsic or intrinsic masses, and the identification of central thromboemboli. MRI is a particularly useful modality for evaluating pulmonary artery size and morphology including pulmonary artery stenosis and atresia, and congenital right ventricular outflow obstructive disorders. The presence of central pulmonary arteries of sufficient size to allow surgical shunt procedures may be difficult to ascertain by conventional angiography. Relative to echocardiography, MRI offers the advantages of a large field of view and the ability to fully image the proximal pulmonary arteries. The left pulmonary artery can be particularly difficult to image by echocardiography in older children and adults. Because the technique is completely noninvasive, it can readily be applied to serial studies demonstrating the development of the pulmonary arteries before and after the placement of surgical shunts, as well as in the evaluation of the size and patency of these shunts and conduits. Other congenital vascular abnormalities, including anomalous pulmonary artery/aortic relationships (e.g., truncus arteriosus [Fig. 1], transpositions, and more complex malpositions), pulmonary artery sling, and anomalies of the central pulmonary veins, are equally well studied.

The major drawback of MRI in these situations relates to image degradation by motion. Sources of this motion are primarily cardiac, respiratory, and vascular (blood flow and vessel pulsatility). Motion suppression techniques are therefore essential for such imaging, and include electrocardiographic (ECG) gating, respiratory motion compensation software (respiratory reordering of the phase-encoding steps) to suppress ghost artifacts caused by breathing, and the use of spatial presaturation pulses to suppress any flow-related signals within the vessels. For morphologic images of the central pulmonary vessels, conventional T1-weighted scans (short repetition time [TR] on the order of 400 to 600 msec together with short echo time [TE] in the range of 10 to 20 msec) are used. Axial images are supplemented by coronal, sagittal, and oblique views as indicated by the vascular anatomy of interest.

The demonstration of involvement of the central pulmonary arteries and/or veins by hilar, mediastinal, or juxtamediastinal masses has been particularly valuable in the staging of lung cancer (Fig. 2). A number of recent studies have demonstrated increased accuracy of MRI relative to computed tomographic (CT) scanning in identifying encasement or invasion of mediastinal vessels. This is of particular importance with regard to the recently revised staging classification for lung cancer, in which minimal invasion of the mediastinum (no involvement of major mediastinal structures) is regarded as stage IIIA and potentially resectable, as opposed to unresectable stage IIIB disease, in which there is significant involvement of vascular structures, heart, tracheobronchial tree, or esophagus. We have found MRI to be valuable in identifying such involvement of the central pulmonary arteries and veins in cases with indeterminate CT scans. This is particularly true

**TABLE 1** Pulmonary Vascular MRI: Current Clinical Applications

| |
|---|
| Congenital abnormalities: |
| Pulmonary artery stenosis, atresia |
| Right ventricular outflow tract obstruction |
| Surgical systemic-to-pulmonary shunts—preoperative and post-operative evaluation |
| Anomalous pulmonary artery/aortic relationships |
| Truncus arteriosus |
| Transpositions |
| Pulmonary artery sling |
| Pulmonary venous anomalies |
| Scimitar syndrome |
| Pulmonary sequestration |
| Staging of lung cancer (vascular involvement) |
| Chronic central thomboemboli |
| Vascular lesions in the lung: |
| Pulmonary arteriovenous malformations (AVMs) |
| Nodule vs. blood vessel (inconclusive CT scan) |
| Small ACTH-producing carcinoid tumors of lung |
| Pulmonary artery primary and metastatic tumors: |
| Intravascular tumor vs. bland thrombus |

**TABLE 2** Pulmonary Vascular MRI: Potential Applications

| |
|---|
| Pulmonary artery flow quantitation: |
| Pulmonary hypertension |
| Intracardiac shunts |
| Lung transplantation |
| Congenital, acquired pulmonary artery stenosis |
| Pulmonary angiography: |
| Acute, chronic pulmonary emboli |
| Pulmonary capillary permeability: |
| Characterization of pulmonary edema |
| Characterization of stages of lung injury (alveolitis vs. fibrosis) |
| Measurement of capillary blood flow and volume: |
| Evaluation of pulmonary tissue perfusion |

A

B

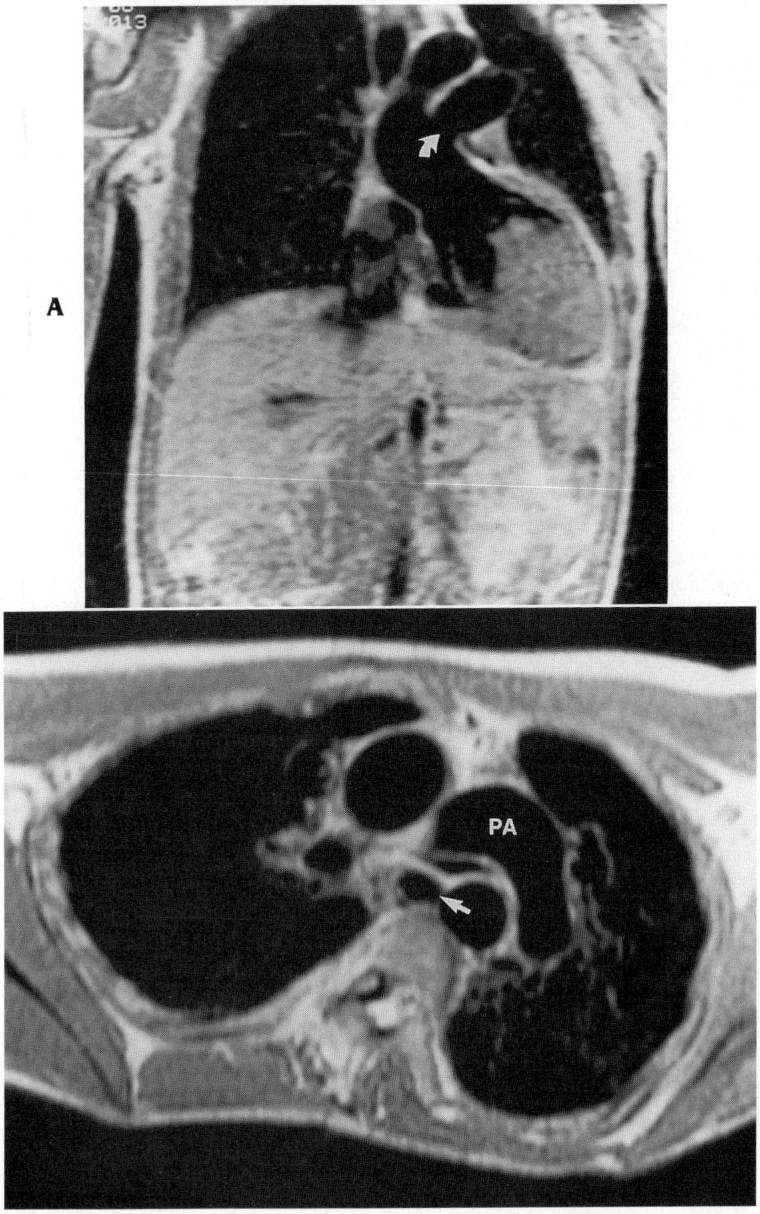


**FIGURE 1** Truncus arteriosus with aplasia of the right pulmonary artery. *A,* Coronal T1-weighted MR image shows origin of left pulmonary artery *(arrow)* from the truncus. *B,* Axial scan shows dilated left pulmonary artery (PA). No right pulmonary artery is present. The right lung is fed by a hypertrophic bronchial artery *(arrow)* originating from the descending thoracic aorta.

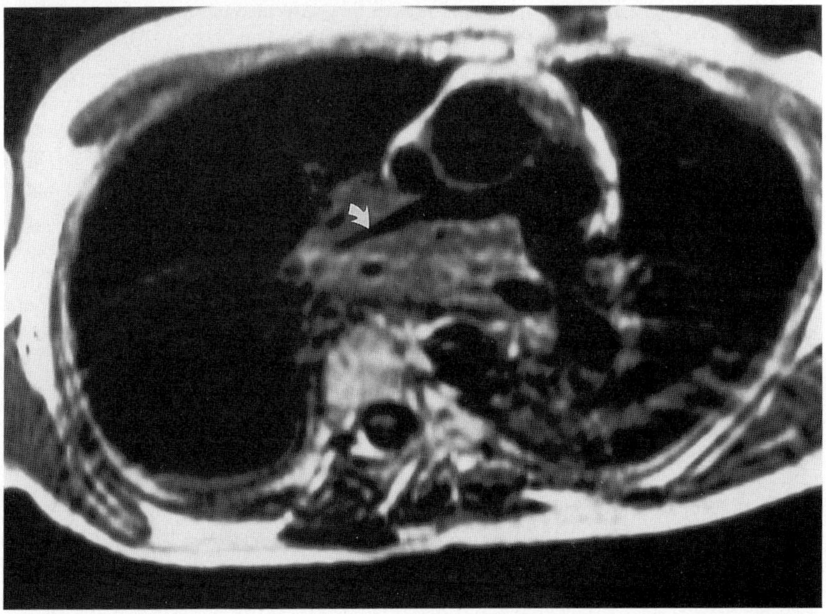

**FIGURE 2** Encasement of the right pulmonary artery by carcinoma of the lung. This anaplastic carcinoma with mediastinal invasion completely encases the right pulmonary artery *(arrow),* indicative of a stage IIIB unresectable tumor. Radionuclide $\dot{V}/\dot{Q}$ scan and conventional pulmonary angiogram both suggested a diagnosis of pulmonary embolism based on lack of perfusion to the right upper lobe.

A

B

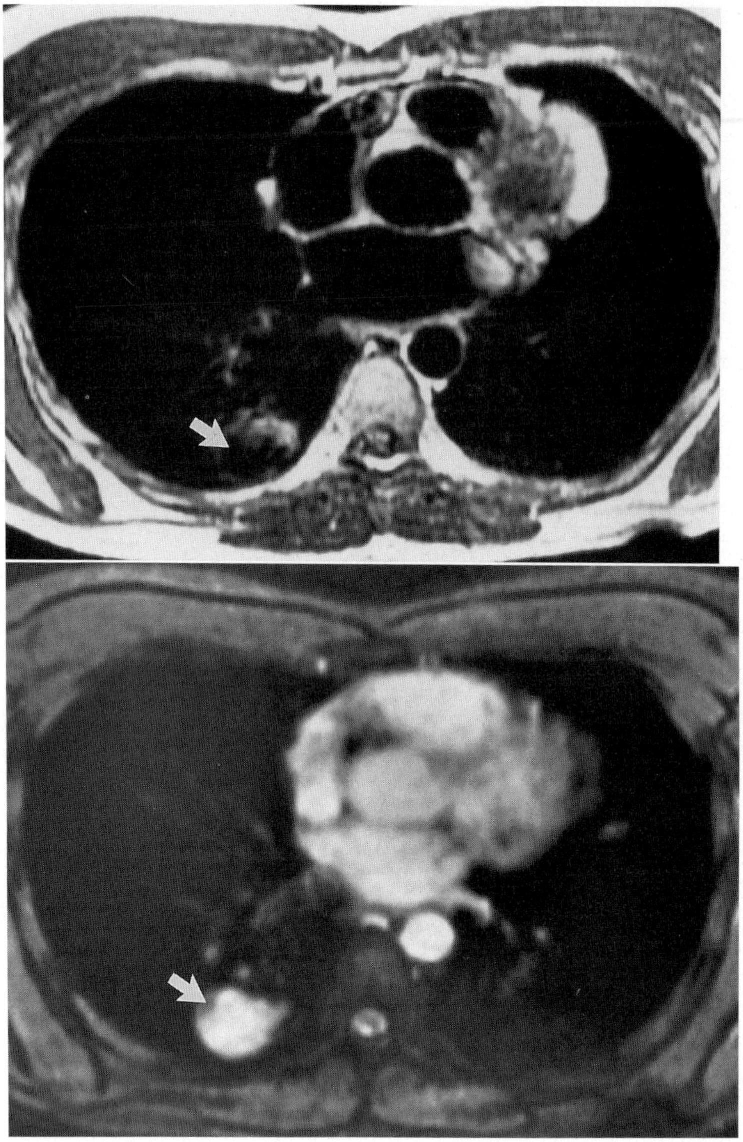

**FIGURE 3** Pulmonary arteriovenous malformation. *A,* The AVM *(arrow)* is difficult to visualize on the T1-weighted spin-echo image because of flow void within the lesion. *B,* Flow-sensitive gradient-echo image clearly shows high signal indicative of flow with the nodule *(arrow),* confirming the diagnosis of AVM.

when contrast enhancement on the CT evaluation is suboptimal or contraindicated.

One of the major problems with conventional spin-echo imaging by MRI is the differentiation of slow flow–related intravascular signal from that of intravascular tumor or bland thrombus. Fortunately the great versatility of MRI allows for a number of supplementary techniques that can assist in this differentiation. We have found that rapid gradient-echo images during suspended respiration provide the most rapid and accurate solution to this problem. Flowing blood appears bright on these flow-sensitive images, whereas intravascular tumor or thrombus appears as a low signal filling defect comparable to that of conventional angiography. A full, dynamic cine gradient-echo series can be obtained, if available, for difficult cases. Here, the ability to image the vessel throughout the cardiac cycle is advantageous, since true clot remains stationary throughout the varying cardiac phases as opposed to dynamic flow abnormalities. The dynamic motion of the central pulmonary arteries on cine gradient-echo MRI studies can also be helpful in suggesting whether extrinsic masses are fixed to the vessel wall.

MRI techniques have also proven to be efficacious for the noninvasive diagnosis of pulmonary sequestration, pulmonary arteriovenous malformations (AVMs), scimitar syndrome, etc. Lung nodules suspected of being pulmonary AVMs can be readily differentiated from nodules of other etiologies with MRI. A series of rapid gradient-echo images through the nodule during breath holding can quickly demonstrate the presence of high signal flow, which would indicate an AVM (Fig. 3). We always include conventional spin-echo images as well to be certain we are not dealing with high signal fat or blood clot (methemoglobin) within a solid nodule. Other MRI approaches to diagnosing flow within a pulmonary AVM include cine gradient-echo scans, and phase images (static or dynamic) in which the phase, rather than the magnitude of the signals, is displayed. These techniques are particularly useful in differentiating an AVM from lung nodules with rich capillary vascularity, such as carcinoid tumors, which can also show contrast enhancement on CT scans and thereby be misinterpreted as AVMs. MRI can also be used as a supplementary study to differentiate a small lung nodule from a pulmonary vessel, which may be problematic on CT scans. Likewise, MRI has been shown to be more sensitive than CT in the detection of small ACTH-producing carcinoid tumors in the lung, since these are frequently located adjacent to vessels.

Another important, although less common, clinical application for which we have found MRI of the pulmonary arteries especially useful is in the identification of chronic central clot in patients with chronic thromboembolic pulmonary hypertension. In this uncommon sequela of acute pulmonary emboli, organized clot becomes incorporated into the vessel wall, leading to the progressive development of pulmonary arterial hypertension. The distinction between this form of pulmonary hypertension and that of primary (idiopathic) pulmonary hypertension can be difficult clinically. Moreover, patients with thromboembolic pulmonary hypertension can show significant improvement with reduction in pulmonary artery pressures following surgical thromboendarterectomy for central clots. On the other hand, patients with clots limited to the smaller peripheral vessels are not considered candidates for this kind of surgery. The findings of central mural thrombi on pulmonary angiography can be subtle and are often overlooked. The ability of MRI to visualize both the vessel wall as well as the lumen provides an advantage over conventional angiography for identifying mural thrombus. Our experience has indicated significant utility and accuracy of MRI in evaluating patients with this disorder.

Again, studies to evaluate thromboemboli include T1-weighted images employing ECG gating, respiratory compensation, and spatial presaturation pulses (Fig. 4, *A*). Unfortunately, because the pulmonary artery flow is relatively slow in patients with more severe degrees of pulmonary hypertension, slow flow–related signal is often present in the pulmonary arteries despite the application of presaturation pulses, which are designed to suppress such signal. In these situations other supplementary techniques must be used to identify true clot. As described earlier, gradient-echo images, particularly cine images, have been particularly useful in this regard (Fig. 4, *B*). In addition, we have employed another technique known as spatial modulation of magnetization (SPAMM) to differentiate clot from slow flow. This technique, which has found principal application in heart wall motion studies, consists of magnetically tagging the tissues with a cross-hatched grid of low signal saturation stripes. The stripes can be incorporated into conventional spin-echo sequences, multiphase spin-echo scans displaying multiple phases of the cardiac cycle, or cine gradient-echo scans. The stripes are maintained in areas of stationary tissue, including that of clot, whereas the stripes become distorted and dispersed in areas of blood flow (Fig. 4, *C*). We have found accuracies of 90 to 95 percent in identifying central thromboemboli using cine gradient-echo scans and SPAMM, as opposed to an accuracy of only approximately 40 percent without these supplemental pulse sequences. In light of the high accuracy in identification of surgically resectable central clots, but limited visualization of distal vessels, MRI serves as a useful complementary study to conventional angiography in the evaluation of these patients. MRI is likely to further improve with the development of high-resolution MRI pulmonary angiography (described in the following section), as well as faster versions of cine MRI and SPAMM, which can be obtained within a single breath-hold. It should be noted that such clots have also been recently demonstrated with high spatial resolution using ultrafast and spiral CT scanning, which will likely prove to be competitive with MRI in this regard. MRI does have the advantage of not requiring any intravenous contrast agents, however.

Not all intravascular lesions in the pulmonary arteries are a result of thromboemboli or contiguous extension of adjacent neoplasms. Rarely primary and metastatic neoplasms may result in an intravascular soft-tissue mass. When there is no gross extension of these lesions outside the vessel lumen, such tumors must be differentiated from bland thromboemboli. In this situation MRI techniques can be helpful. We and others have encountered primary pulmonary artery sarcomas that demonstrate increased signal on T2-weighted (long TR, long TE) images relative to T1-weighted scans. This long T2 would not be expected in fibrotic, chronic clot, although it may be possible with acute emboli. However, differentiation is possible on postcontrast images following intravenous administration of gadolinium, since primary sarcomas have shown contrast enhancement to a significantly greater degree than bland thrombus (Fig. 5).

## Future Directions

The MRI techniques described thus far are capable of imaging only the proximal portions of the pulmonary arteries. Recently, however, techniques have been developed that enable imaging of more peripheral branches of the pulmonary arterial tree. These employ modifications of methods being used more generally in the head and body to create projection vascular images referred to as MR angiography (MRA). Several different approaches have been described for acquiring pulmonary MRAs, including two-dimensional (2D) and three-dimensional (3D) time-of-flight gradient-echo acquisitions, the use of the body coil versus surface coils, breath holding versus breathing, cardiac gating, the use of paramagnetic contrast agents, techniques to suppress signal in the pulmonary veins, and various postprocessing algorithms to create projection images analogous to those of conventional angiograms. The potential advantage of MRI, aside from not requiring a right ventricular catheterization procedure and traditional iodinated contrast agents, is the ability to acquire both tomographic and 3D volumetric displays of the pulmonary vessels which can be viewed from any desired angle. Along with several other groups, we have developed a pulmonary MRA technique that employs phased array surface coils to increase the signal-to-noise ratio relative to the standard body coil, ultrafast image acquisition ($<1$ second) using a gradient-echo pulse sequence with a short TR (8 to 12 msec) and TE (2 to 3 msec), and ECG triggering (Fig. 6). A series of approximately 15 sagittal images encompassing one entire lung can be obtained within one breath hold. To date we have not found significant additional benefit in using contrast enhancement with intravenous gadolinium. It is likely that in the future, however, intravascular contrast agents such as macromolecular forms of gadolinium may increase the visibility of smaller vessels. In addition to acquiring and evaluating the individual images, the data sets

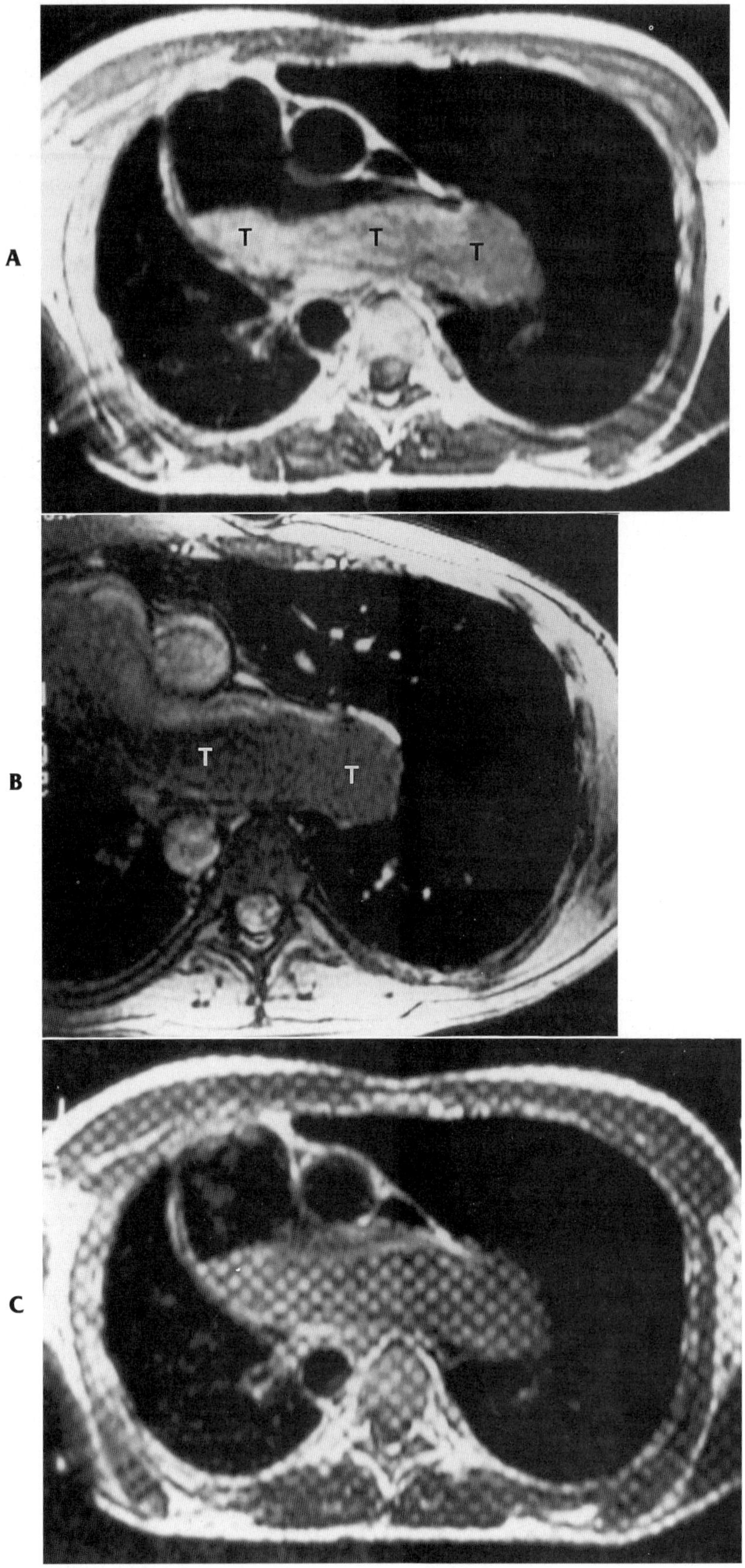


**FIGURE 4** Thromboembolic pulmonary hypertension with large central pulmonary artery clot. *A,* Spin-echo image. Prominent signal in the main and right pulmonary arteries (T) assumed to be thrombus, but requiring differentiation from slow flow–related signal. *B,* Breath-hold gradient-echo image demonstrates corresponding low signal consistent with thrombus (T). *C,* SPAMM image shows persistence of magnetic tagging stripes, confirming stationary clot.

A 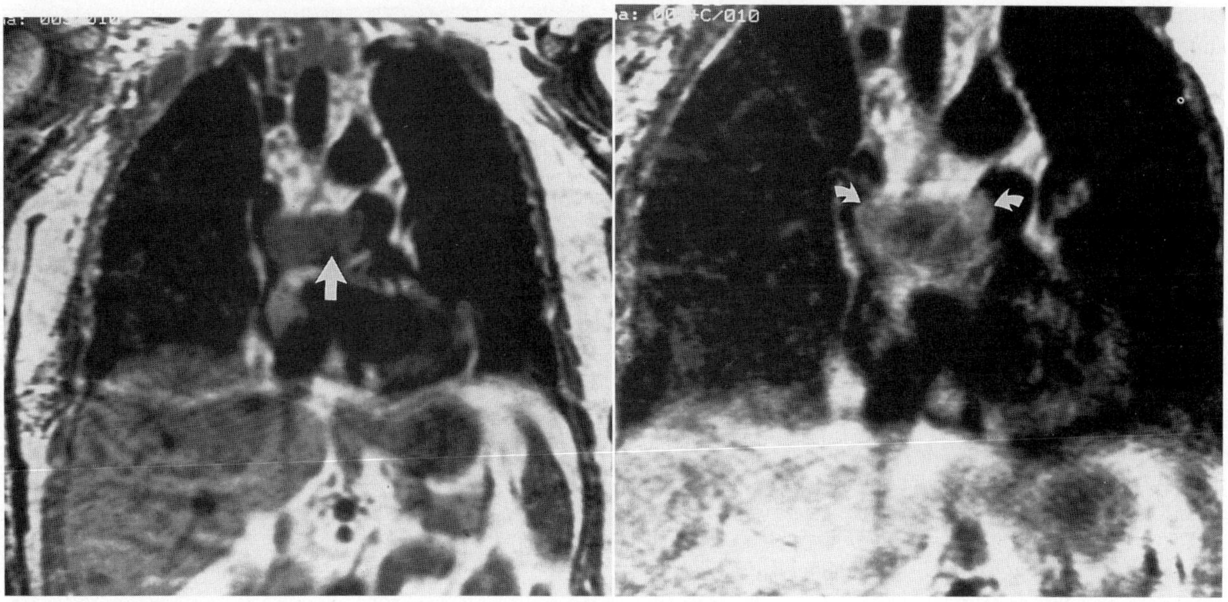 B

**FIGURE 5** Primary pulmonary artery leiomyosarcoma. *A,* Coronal T1-weighted image shows intravascular mass *(arrow)* in the right pulmonary artery. There is suggestion of extension to the superior vena cava, but otherwise mass cannot be differentiated from bland thrombus. *B,* Postcontrast scan following administration of Gd-DTPA demonstrates enhancement indicative of tumor *(arrows).*

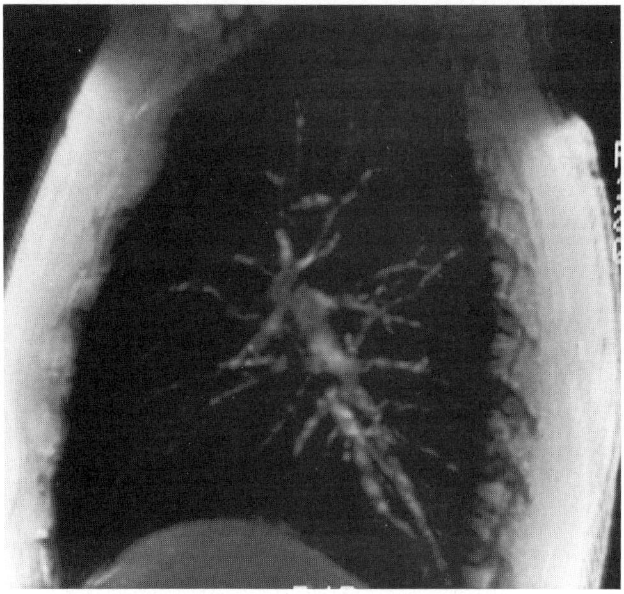

**FIGURE 6** Pulmonary MRA. Sagittal image of right lung was acquired using phased array multiple surface coils on anterior and posterior chest walls. An ECG-triggered ultrafast gradient-echo sequence was used to obtain approximately 15 images during a single breath hold.

are reconstructed using various modifications of a maximum intensity projection algorithm to yield a 3D display of the pulmonary vascular tree that can be rotated through multiple viewing angles and directions (Fig. 7). Early experience with such pulmonary MRAs has indicated that vessels on the order of sixth- and seventh-generation branches can be obtained, at least in normal subjects. Although some preliminary data indicate that the technique enables identification of smaller

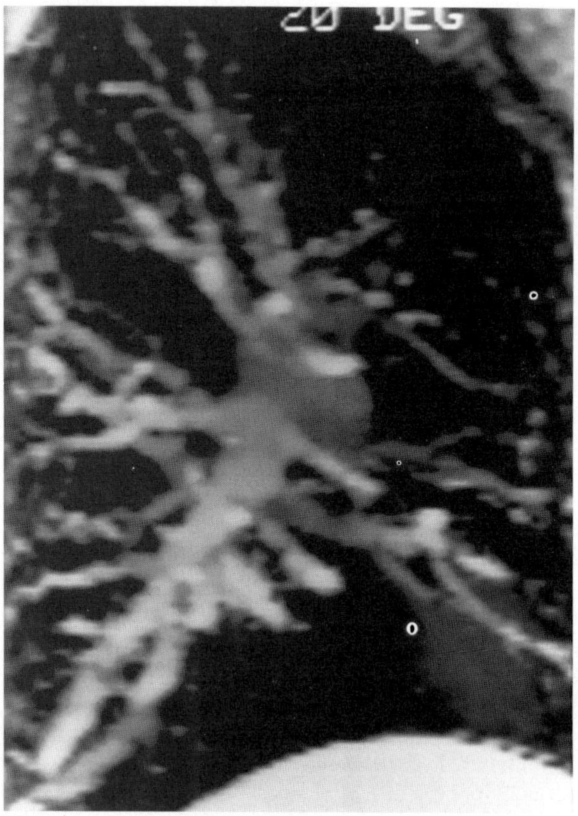


**FIGURE 7** Projection pulmonary MRA obtained using sequence described in text and using a modification of a maximum intensity projection algorithm (TRAP), which incorporates depth cues to enhance 3D relationships.

emboli, problems related to respiratory motion have been encountered in dyspneic patients. (This can be partially overcome with increased signal averaging.) Moreover, the spatial resolution is not consistently sufficient to visualize the smaller peripheral vessels in all patients. Further developments in image acquisition and in appropriate reconstruction algorithms designed to optimize clot detection are required. For these reasons, the technique cannot yet be adopted for routine clinical evaluation of acute pulmonary emboli. It is anticipated that with such refinements in the methodology, pulmonary MRA may be useful in patients with indeterminate radionuclide ventilation-perfusion ($\dot{V}/\dot{Q}$) scans, especially when there are contraindications to conventional pulmonary angiography. This noninvasive technique may also have value in the serial follow-up of patients being treated for large pulmonary emboli. It may well be feasible and cost-effective in the near future to combine pulmonary MRA with recently developed MR venography (MRV) of the lower extremities and pelvis for the simultaneous evaluation of deep venous thrombosis and pulmonary embolism. Pulmonary MRA will also be useful as a noninvasive modality for the diagnosis of other peripheral pulmonary vascular abnormalities including anomalous venous return (scimitar syndrome), AVMs, sequestration, and other conditions.

It is likely that MRI contrast agents currently under active investigation will be used in connection with MRI studies of pulmonary perfusion. The feasibility of obtaining perfusion images using a polymeric form of Gd-DTPA linked to polylysine, which remains in the intravascular space for prolonged periods, has recently been demonstrated in rats; in addition, ventilation images could be obtained using aerosolized Gd-DTPA in intubated rats. With the combination of these two agents, MRI-$\dot{V}/\dot{Q}$ scans were successfully obtained in rat models of pulmonary perfusion and airway obstruction. Such a $\dot{V}/\dot{Q}$ scan, which would have the advantages of high resolution and tomographic or 3D display, in conjunction with pulmonary MRA and possibly MRV for deep vein thrombosis (DVT) as indicated earlier, could provide a powerful, comprehensive, noninvasive evaluation of pulmonary thromboembolic disease, particularly since it may be possible to perform these evaluations sequentially in one session. Other applications of an intravascular contrast agent include imaging and quantitation of pulmonary capillary permeability and potentially the measurement of tissue capillary blood flow and blood volume.

One of the major strengths of MRI is the ability to obtain not only anatomic images, but also physiologic information with regard to blood flow. Initially this was accomplished using multiphase spin-echo imaging, in which a series of images was obtained throughout the cardiac cycle. Using such a technique, abnormally slow flow in cases of pulmonary hypertension was reflected in persistence of intravascular signal in the pulmonary arteries during systole. Cine gradient-echo images improved temporal resolution and provided the ability to image blood flow patterns and to assess vascular distensibility; abnormalities in these features were again identified in cases of pulmonary hypertension, thromboemboli, stenoses, and other conditions.

A major advance, however, occurred with the development of truly quantitative methods to measure flow velocities and volume flow in the pulmonary arteries (and central veins). Such techniques are based on the principle that spins moving along a magnetic gradient experience a phase change that is proportional to velocity. The subtraction of two phase-sensitive images with differing amounts of flow encoding can yield phase maps in which each pixel intensity corresponds to flow velocity and direction (Fig. 8). By multiplying these flow velocities by the cross-sectional area of the vessel lumen, flow volume can be derived. The incorporation of such a velocity-encoding technique into the dynamic cine pulse sequence yields velocity

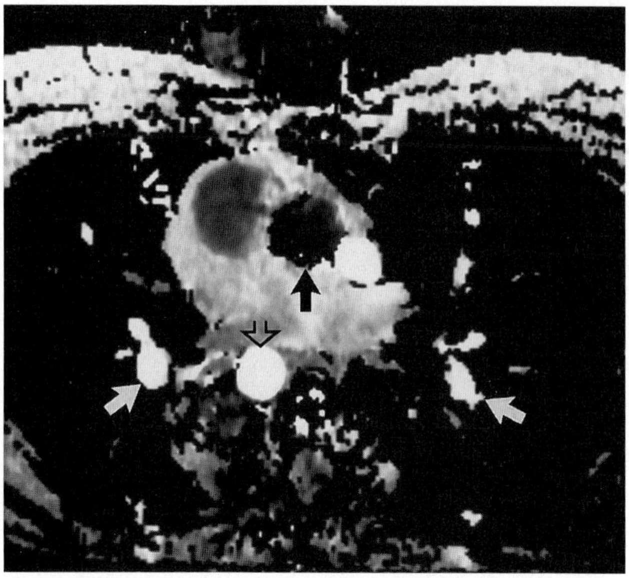

**FIGURE 8** Velocity-encoded MR image from a cine sequence (VINNIE). Pixel intensities are proportional to velocities, with highest velocities toward the head being black and toward the feet, white. Note high velocities in opposing directions in the ascending aorta *(solid black arrow)* and descending aorta *(open black arrow)*. High velocities are also evident in the central pulmonary arteries *(white arrows)* in this systolic image.

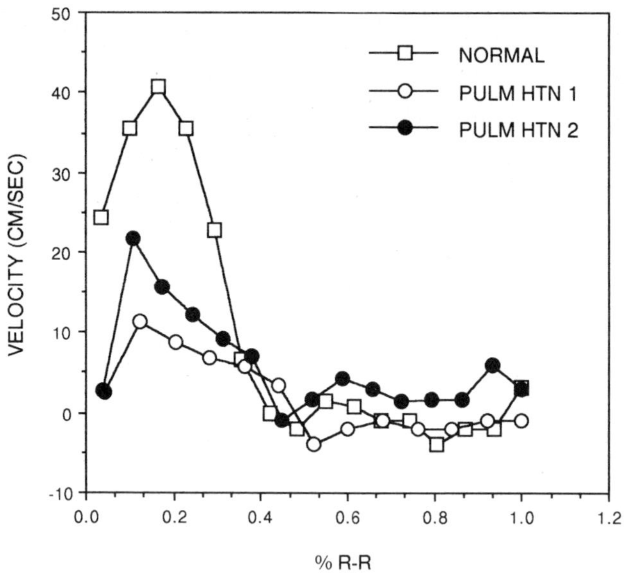


**FIGURE 9** Velocity-encoded cine MRI measurements obtained from the main pulmonary artery. Velocities in a normal subject are compared with those of two patients with pulmonary hypertension. Note the decreased systolic velocities and the earlier time to peak velocity characterizing the patients with pulmonary hypertension.

images through multiple phases of the cardiac cycle. Using this technique, abnormal flow patterns, including heterogeneous flow distributions and large components of retrograde flow, have been detected and correlated with varying degrees of pulmonary hypertension. In addition, a decreased peak velocity as well as an earlier time to peak velocity (faster pulmonary artery acceleration time) have been identified and correlated with pulmonary hypertension (Fig. 9). By integrating flow volumes in the main pulmonary artery throughout the cardiac cycle, right ventricular stroke volume can be derived; likewise left ventricular stroke volume is derived from velocity sampling in the ascending aorta. Such measurements have been validated and have been used to accurately evaluate pulmonary/systemic blood flow ratios in cases of intracardiac shunts.

MRI flow measurements by velocity mapping have also been obtained and validated in the proximal right and left pulmonary arteries. In this way total blood flow to each lung through the cardiac cycle can be derived. The technique can be used to quantitate flow to each lung in cases in which there is abnormal distribution of flow including lung transplantation, congenital or acquired pulmonary artery stenosis, and so on. It is hoped that with the coupling of such flow encoding with ultrafast techniques, such as echo-planar imaging, together with high-resolution methods as described for pulmonary MRA, it might be possible to accurately measure regional pulmonary artery flow even at the level of individual pulmonary lobes and segments.

## Suggested Reading

Berthezene Y, Vexler V, Clement O, et al. Contrast-enhanced MR imaging of the lung: Assessments of ventilation and perfusion. Radiology 1992; 183:667–672.

Berthezene Y, Vexler V, Kuwatsuru R, et al. Differentiation of alveolitis and pulmonary fibrosis with a macromolecular MR imaging contrast agent. Radiology 1992; 185:97–103.

Brasch RC. New directions in the development of MR imaging contrast media. Radiology 1992; 183:1–11.

Foo TKF, MacFall JR, Hayes CE, Sostman HD. Pulmonary vasculature: Single breath-hold MR imaging with phased-array coils. Radiology 1992; 183:473–477.

Gefter WB, Hatabu H. Pulmonary vascular applications of magnetic resonance. J Thorac Imaging (in press).

Gefter WB, Kundel H, Hatabu H. Magnetic resonance imaging in chest medicine. In Fishman AP, ed. Update: Pulmonary Diseases and Disorders. New York: McGraw-Hill, 1992:299.

Hatabu H, Gefter WB, Konishi J, Kressel HY. Magnetic resonance approaches to the evaluation of pulmonary vascular anatomy and physiology. Magn Reson Q 1991; 7:208–225.

Mostbeck GH, Caputo GR, Higgins CB. MR measurement of blood flow in the cardiovascular system. AJR 1992; 159:453–461.

Webb WR, Sostman HD. MR imaging of thoracic disease: Clinical uses. Radiology 1992; 182:621–630.

Wielopolski PA, Haacke EM, Adler LP. Three-dimensional MR imaging of the pulmonary vasculature: Preliminary experience. Radiology 1992; 183:465–472.

# Radiology of Thoracic Trauma

*PAUL STARK, M.D.*

Trauma is the leading cause of death in people under the age of 40 and accounted for 147,912 deaths in 1986 in the United States alone. The cost of trauma in this country amounts to $84 billion per year. Close to 45,000 fatalities per year are a result of traffic accidents. Thoracic injuries play a major role in 50 percent of deaths. Potential life years lost exceed those caused by heart disease and cancer.

Blunt trauma, also called wide impact trauma, is a result of motor vehicle, home, and industrial accidents. Blunt trauma results from transfer of kinetic energy to the human body. Three mechanisms are responsible for this conversion. Inertial deceleration occurs because of the inherent difference in momentums of organs and tissues. It results in shearing forces. Spalling phenomena occur when a broad kinetic shock wave is partially reflected by gas-fluid interfaces. It leads to disruption of tissue. Implosion means rapid compression with rebound overexpansion of gas bubbles and subsequent rupture of organs. Penetrating trauma results primarily from missile and stab wounds.

Multisystem trauma is a characteristic of motor vehicle accidents. The extremities are involved most frequently (90 percent), followed by head trauma (70 percent), chest trauma (50 percent), abdominal (30 percent), and pelvic injuries (25 percent).

Modified from Stark P. Radiology of thoracic trauma. Invest Radiol 1990; 25:1265–1275; with permission.

## Rib Fractures

Rib fractures occur in over 50 percent of patients with significant chest trauma. They are frequently missed on the initial chest radiograph because of superimposition of structures or because the fracture line is not tangential to the central x-ray beam; nondisplaced fracture fragments and an intact periosteum can also prevent or complicate their detection. The fourth through the ninth ribs are most commonly fractured. Injuries to the first three ribs indicate major blunt trauma, yet their association with rupture of the aorta or the tracheobronchial tree is not as constant as previously believed. Fractures of the 10th through 12th ribs are frequently associated with liver, spleen, or kidney trauma.

## Flail Chest

Flail chest is a most severe form of chest trauma, resulting in a freely moving, unstable segment of rib cage (Fig. 1). Flail chest is a clinical diagnosis characterized by paradoxic respiratory motion and pendelluft. Together with associated lung contusions, it can have a grave prognosis, with a mortality of close to 30 percent. The radiologist can suspect a flail chest when more than five adjacent ribs are fractured or more than three segmental rib fractures are present. Bilateral rib fractures and accompanying sternal fractures increase the likelihood of a flail chest.

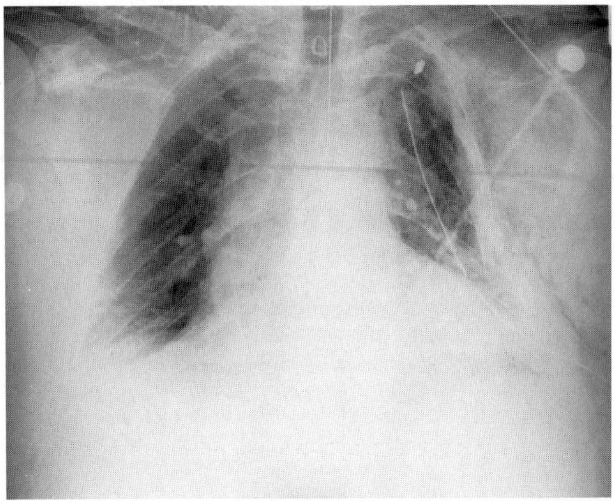

**FIGURE 1** Flail chest after car accident. Frontal view of the chest shows multiple displaced left-sided rib fractures producing significant deformity of the rib cage.

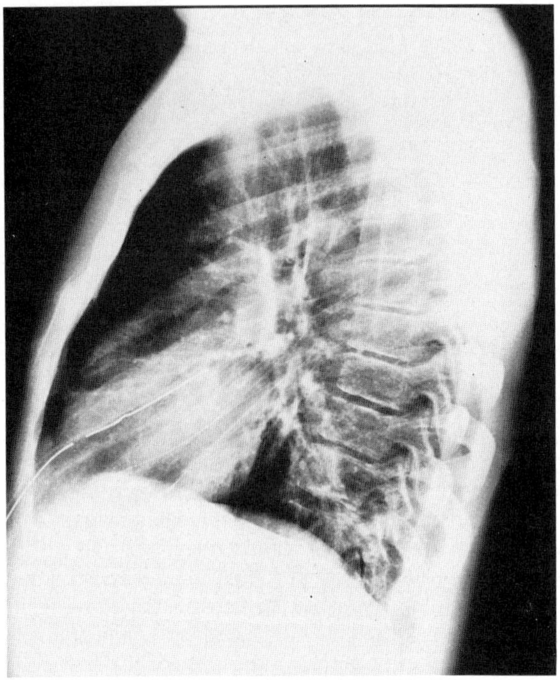

**FIGURE 2** Fracture of sternum after steering wheel injury. Lateral view of the chest shows a near horizontal, partially displaced fracture of the sternal body. Note the positive epicardial fat pad sign indicative of a pericardial effusion.

## Sternal Fractures

Sternal fractures occur in 8 to 10 percent of patients after violent blunt trauma (Fig. 2). They are more likely to occur in seat belt users and are usually located within 2 cm of the angle of Louis. Frequently, fractures of the anterior ribs, costal cartilages, retrosternal hematoma, and pericardial and cardiac injuries are associated. If the fracture fragments buckle posteriorly, they can avulse the innominate artery. A mortality of close to 25 percent has been reported in complicated sternal fractures. An initial diagnosis can be obtained with a lateral view of the anterior chest wall, but computed tomography (CT) is the imaging method of choice, particularly to assess the retrosternal soft tissues and the integrity of the rib cartilages.

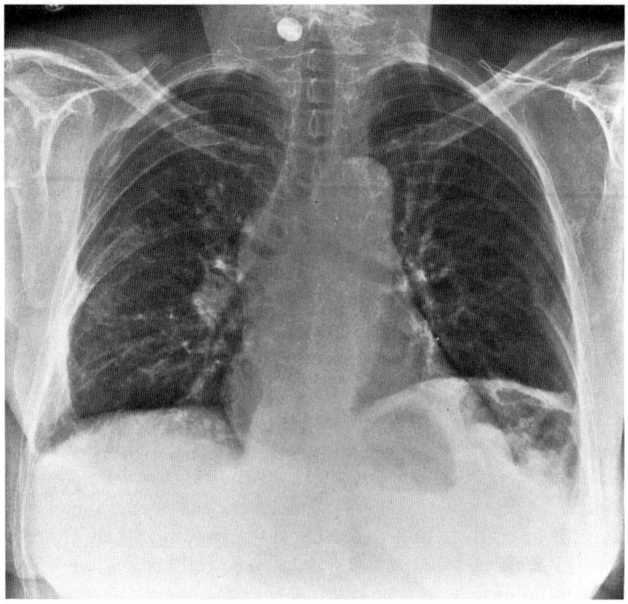

**FIGURE 3** Lung hernia after remote chest wall trauma. Chest radiograph shows lung protruding into the right axillary region through a deformed right rib cage.

## Post-traumatic Lung Hernias

Post-traumatic lung hernias (Fig. 3) can occur in the acute phase, but are more commonly found as a late sequela of rib fractures, tube thoracostomy, or thoracotomy. They protrude into the subcutaneous tissues during inspiration and can simulate a solid mass. Accidental puncture or even strangulation can occur.

## Sternoclavicular Joint Dislocation

Sternoclavicular joint dislocation accounts for 3 percent of all dislocations. Anterior dislocations are more common; posterior dislocations are more dangerous because they are easily missed and can compress the trachea and the brachiocephalic vessels.

## Lung Contusion

Lung contusion represents a bruise of the lung parenchyma. Extravasation of blood and edema fluid follows the traumatic event. It is the most common radiographic finding after blunt injury and is seen in 75 percent of such patients. Radiographically it presents as a nonsegmental consolidation adjacent to ribs, spine, heart, or liver. The time course is characteristic. The opacities appear within 6 hours of impact and clear within 3 to 10 days (Fig. 4). Contused lung is prone to pulmonary edema or superimposed pneumonia. Massive contusion can lead to the development of adult respiratory distress syndrome (ARDS). Massive contusions can have a mortality of up to 40 percent.

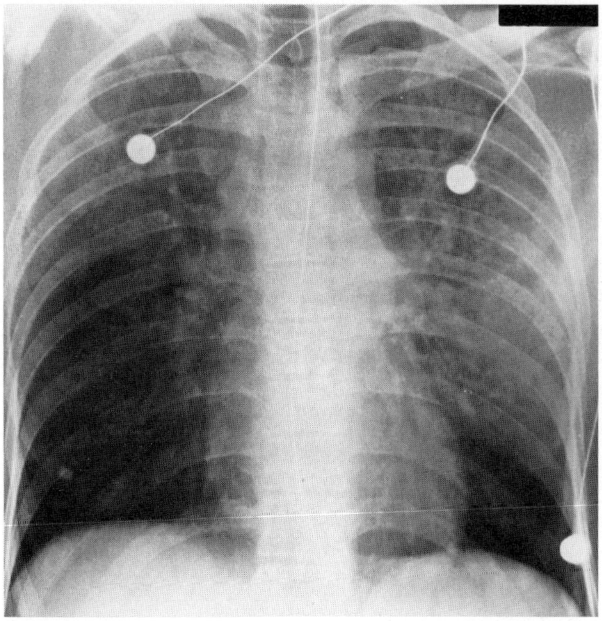

**FIGURE 4** Lung contusion after motor vehicle accident. Frontal chest film shows ill-defined consolidation of the entire left upper lobe.

## Blast Injury

Blast injury is a variant of contusion. It is a result of abrupt pressure changes after an explosion. The lungs are affected at pressures over 2 atm. Damage occurs at the gas-fluid interfaces, with resulting parenchymal hemorrhage, edema, and even laceration. The changes can be bilateral. Blast injury is reported to be a cause of death in 45 percent of explosion fatalities.

## Lung Laceration

Lung laceration leads to the formation of traumatic pneumatoceles. It results from a tear in the lung parenchyma. Because of the elastic recoil of the underlying lung, the linear laceration forms a spherical cavity. Its wall is composed of compressed alveoli. The cavity is initially filled with blood, which is usually expectorated. On early post-traumatic radiographs, the laceration can be masked by surrounding pulmonary contusion (Figs. 5, 6). Such cavities can persist for 3 to 7 weeks or even longer. Traumatic pneumatoceles have been described in the pulmonary ligament, but most of these probably are loculated medial pneumothoraces.

## Lung Hematomas

Lung hematomas (Figs. 7, 8) form in pre-existing cavities like lacerations or bullae. They appear as nodular opacities on the chest radiograph. If expectorated, they leave behind a cyst that corresponds to the previously described laceration. Otherwise, these nodules can persist for several months. Residual nodules or scars can mimic a bronchogenic carcinoma.

## Atelectasis

Atelectasis (Fig. 9) can be a result of obstruction by mucous plugs, foreign bodies, endobronchial thrombi, bronchial compression, or bronchial rupture. Relaxation or compression of lung leads to atelectasis in patients with pleural effusions or pneumothorax. Temporary lack of surfactant after pulmonary contusion leads to so-called "adhesive atelectasis."

## Fat Embolism Syndrome

Fat embolism syndrome (Fig. 10) occurs after major bone fractures combined with hypovolemic shock. Ninety percent of

A

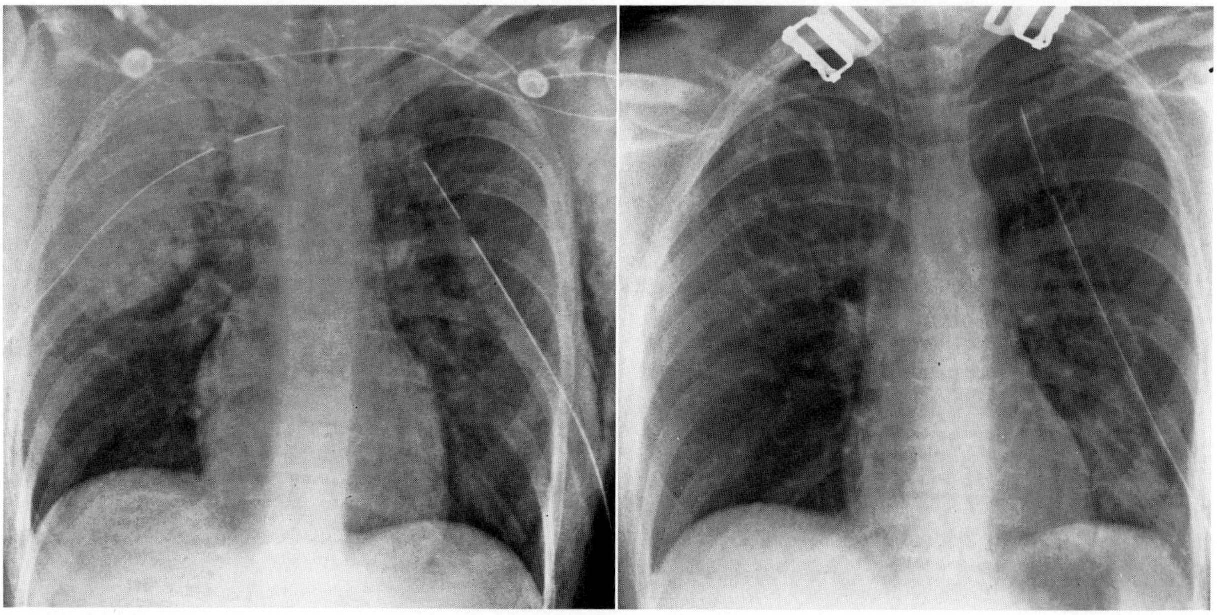

B

**FIGURE 5** *A,* Lung contusion and laceration after motor vehicle accident. Frontal chest film shows massive consolidation of the right upper lobe as well as a fractured right clavicle. *B,* One week later the contusion has cleared unmasking several thin-walled cavities in the right upper lobe, likely representing pulmonary lacerations.

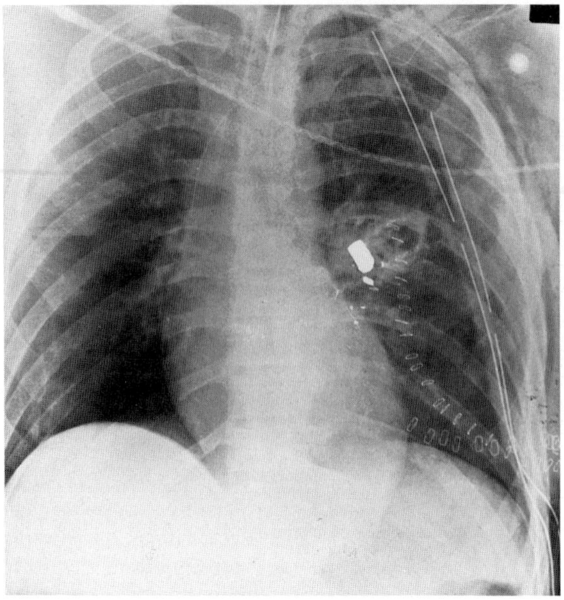

**FIGURE 6** Pulmonary laceration caused by bullet injury. Chest radiograph shows the missile over the left lung, adjacent to a round lucency that represents a tubular laceration. Note extensive subcutaneous emphysema.

A

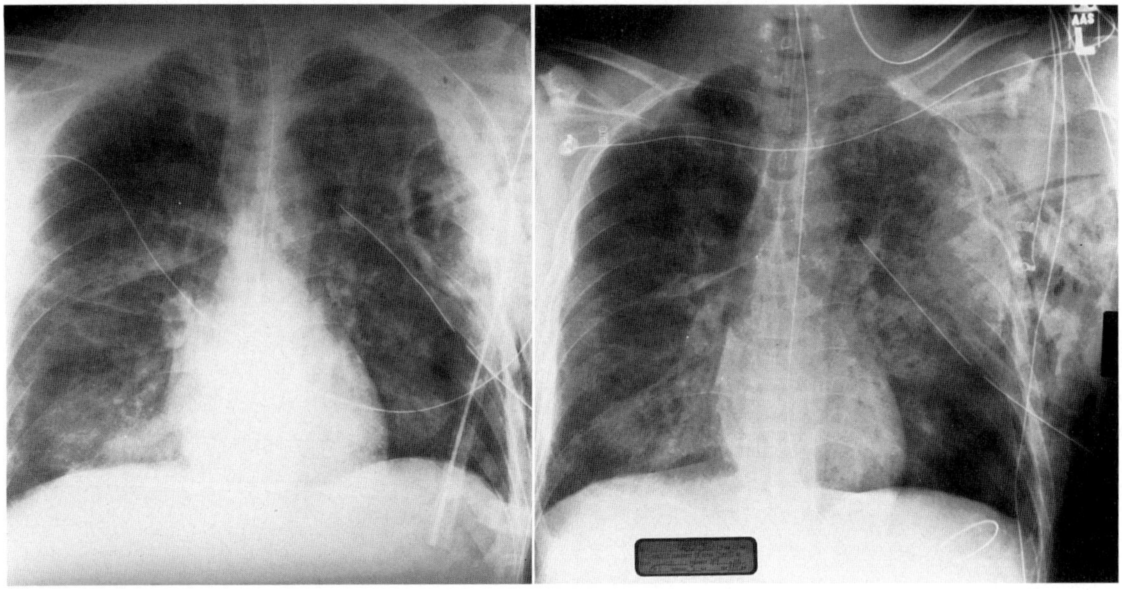

B

**FIGURE 7** *A,* Post-traumatic laceration of left lung. Chest radiograph shows subpleural ellipsoid cystic lucency in left lung laterally. *B,* Several days later, the previously described cavity has filled with blood, forming an intrapulmonary hematoma.

patients with bone trauma have fat emboli, yet only 10 percent develop the full-blown syndrome. The mortality of fat embolism syndrome has fallen to about 5 percent. The clinical picture consists of cerebral symptoms (headache, confusion, seizures), cutaneous signs (cyanosis, petechiae in 50 percent), and pulmonary symptoms (dyspnea, tachypnea). Fever, retinal hemorrhage, and fat in urine also are frequently found. The origin of fat emboli is disputed. The bone marrow is a likely source, although the chemical composition of emboli resembles chylomicrons rather than the bone marrow fat composition. Pulmonary dysfunction results from mechanical occlusion of arterioles by fat or platelets. Endothelial injury with subsequent capillary leak and pulmonary edema occurs by released fatty acids after saponification of embolized triglycerides in the pulmonary arterioles. In addition, vasospasm as a result of serotonin released from decaying platelets complicates the picture. Radiographically, a delay of 12 to 48 hours is typical. Patchy opacities that progress to increased permeability pulmonary edema are characteristic. Clearing takes 2 days to 2 weeks. Full-blown ARDS is rare.

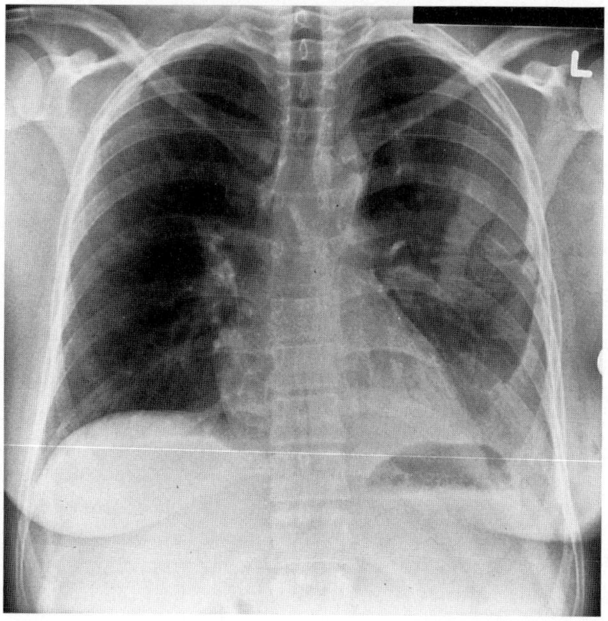

**FIGURE 8** Tubular pulmonary hematoma due to gunshot wound. Chest radiograph shows a broad band of opacity in the left mid lung and a left pleural effusion.

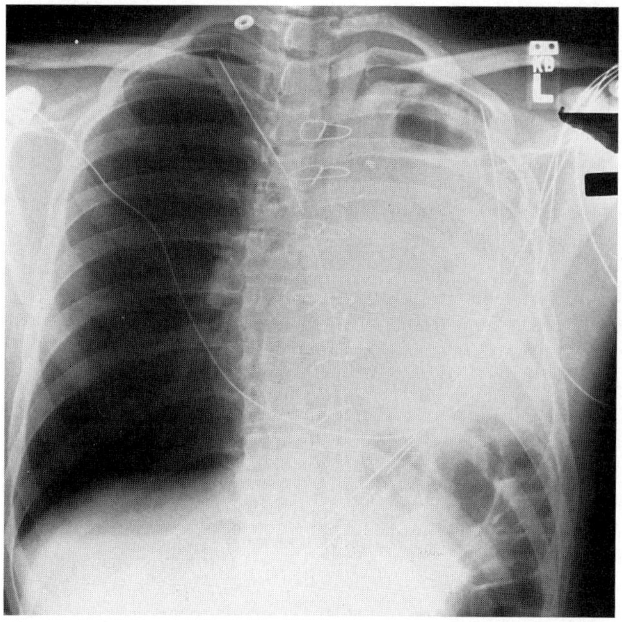

**FIGURE 9** Complete atelectasis of the left lung after trauma, from a clot in the left main bronchus. The chest radiograph shows complete opacification of left hemithorax with ipsilateral cardiomediastinal shift and a small left apical hydropneumothorax.

## ARDS

ARDS (Figs. 11, 12) is a syndrome characterized by clinical respiratory failure, severe hypoxemia, lung consolidation, and low compliance. At least 150,000 cases per year occur in the United States alone. The mortality of the full-blown syndrome is between 50 and 75 percent. Only 16 percent of these patients succumb to respiratory failure. The majority die of multiple organ failure. The pathogenesis of the syndrome is explained by sequestration and agglutination of neutrophils in the lung capillaries. Release of oxygen radicals, proteolytic enzymes, and activation of complement follow. These factors combine to damage the capillary endothelium and the type 1 pneumocytes. Pathologically, ARDS begins with an exudative phase that lasts 1 to 7 days. Vascular congestion, endothelial swelling, high protein content, hemorrhagic pulmonary edema, platelet aggregation with vascular obstruction, and hyaline membrane formation are found. In the subsequent 7 to 14 days, the proliferative phase ensues in an attempt to repair the damage. Proliferation of type 2 pneumocytes, collagen deposition in the alveolar and interstitial space with resulting fibrosis, microvas-

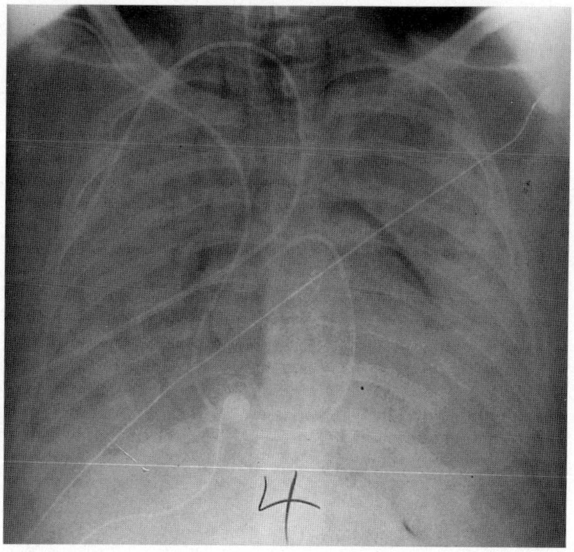

**FIGURE 10** Fat embolism. The chest radiograph shows diffuse pulmonary consolidation as well as pneumomediastinum.

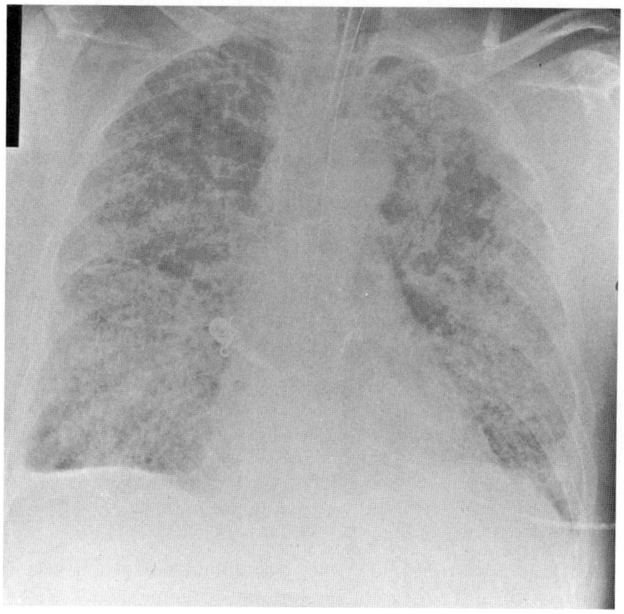

**FIGURE 11** ARDS after trauma. The chest radiograph shows diffuse consolidation of both lungs.

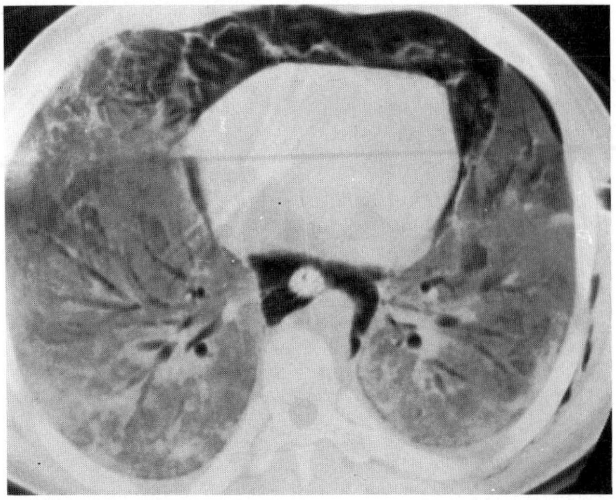

**FIGURE 12** ARDS after trauma. A CT scan shows homogenous opacification of both lungs, clearly visible air-bronchograms, extensive pneumomediastinum, and a small left pneumothorax.

cular destruction, and necrosis characterize this phase.

ARDS is most likely to develop after sepsis (38 percent), aspiration of gastric content (30 percent), multiple emergency transfusions (24 percent), pulmonary contusion (17 percent), and multiple major fractures (12 percent). Most cases of ARDS declare themselves within 72 hours of the traumatic or inciting event. Clinically the patients develop dyspnea or severe hypoxemia, with oxygen tension in the arterial blood measuring only one-third of the alveolar oxygen pressure. Patients have to be mechanically ventilated, with peak inspiratory pressures frequently exceeding 35 mm Hg.

Several phases are evident radiologically: in the first 12 to 24 hours the latent phase predominates. The lungs are still clear, although poorly expanded. Lung consolidation follows either with confluent homogeneous opacities (70 percent) or with patchy peripheral opacification (30 percent). Air bronchograms are frequently present and, particularly on CT, cysts are found in 50 percent of affected patients. Peribronchial cuffing and Kerley's lines are uncommon. Accompanying pleural effusions can be seen in up to 30 percent of cases. After 7 days ground glass opacification can supervene. Lung consolidation shows no tendency to resolve for several weeks.

The differential diagnosis of early ARDS includes hypoventilation, pulmonary embolism, and airway obstruction. In the later stages, cardiogenic edema, aspiration pneumonia, or pulmonary hemorrhage have to be considered.

## Post-traumatic Pulmonary Edema

Post-traumatic pulmonary edema can be categorized according to the time of appearance. Early pulmonary edema at presentation is usually a result of neurogenic factors, massive lung contusion, aspiration or inhalation of toxic gases. Edema in the first 24 hours can result from overhydration, transfusion reaction, or progressive chemical pneumonitis from aspiration or inhalation of noxious substances. Beyond 24 hours pulmonary edema is usually the result of ARDS, fat embolism, or overhydration.

## Pleural Effusions After Trauma

Pleural effusions after trauma are usually a result of blood in the pleural space. Hemothorax is found in 50 percent of trauma victims. They are small if the blood originates from the low-pressure pulmonary circulation subsequent to lung contusion or laceration. Large effusions originate from lacerated systemic vessels like intercostal or mediastinal vascular structures. Blood loss, not respiratory compromise, is the most common cause of death after chest trauma. Drainage is important to avoid lung compression, empyema, or delayed fibrothorax. Chylothorax is a rare cause of post-traumatic pleural effusion. It can result from crushing injury, penetrating trauma, or surgery. A delay of 2 to 10 days between the traumatic event and the appearance of the effusion is typical, likely because of gradual formation and perforation of a chylous duct cyst. On radiographs a large effusion is visible. The pleural fluid accumulates in the right hemithorax with low thoracic injuries and in the left hemithorax with high chest injuries. This is explained by the sinuous course of the thoracic duct, which swings from the lower right into the upper left hemithorax. The clinical course of a chylothorax can be life-threatening because of malnutrition, fluid depletion, and compromise of the immune system, as up to 2,000 ml of chyle can be lost per day.

The differential diagnosis of early post-traumatic pleural effusion includes a pre-existing pleural process, infusion of fluid into the pleural space through a central line, diaphragmatic rupture, or total atelectasis of one lung. Delayed manifestations can be caused by chylothorax, empyema, biliary pleural or subarachnoid pleural fistula.

## Pneumothorax

Pneumothorax can result from closed chest trauma. In 70 percent of such cases rib fractures are also present, but 30 percent of pneumothoraces occur without rib fractures. Penetrating injuries can also lead to a pulmonary air leak. Contrecoup injuries elicit a pneumothorax on the side opposite the impact. Stab wounds are more likely to produce a pneumothorax than missiles, because the latter can coagulate the visceral pleura because of their intense heat. A pneumothorax can be closed or open. A closed pneumothorax can be either simple or under expiratory tension. The visceral and parietal pleura are uncoupled. If the expiratory intrapleural pressure exceeds the atmospheric pressure, the contralateral lung is compressed. Yet, contrary to popular belief, the venous return to the heart is not impeded, because of the tremendous, negative, inspiratory intrapleural pressure generated by the dyspneic patient.

Open pneumothorax occurs once a large defect in the chest wall is present. In inspiration, outside air is rushing into the pleural space and competes with the inspired intratracheal air. The mediastinum is displaced toward the normal side. In expiration, the pneumothorax air exits through the chest wall defect, the mediastinum swings back, the end-expiratory air from the normal lung enters the collapsed lung. This so-called pendelluft, or pendulum air, combined with the mediastinal flutter, leads to rapid respiratory failure. It is imperative to close the chest wall defect and convert the open pneumothorax into a closed one.

The radiologic findings of a pneumothorax in an upright

A B C

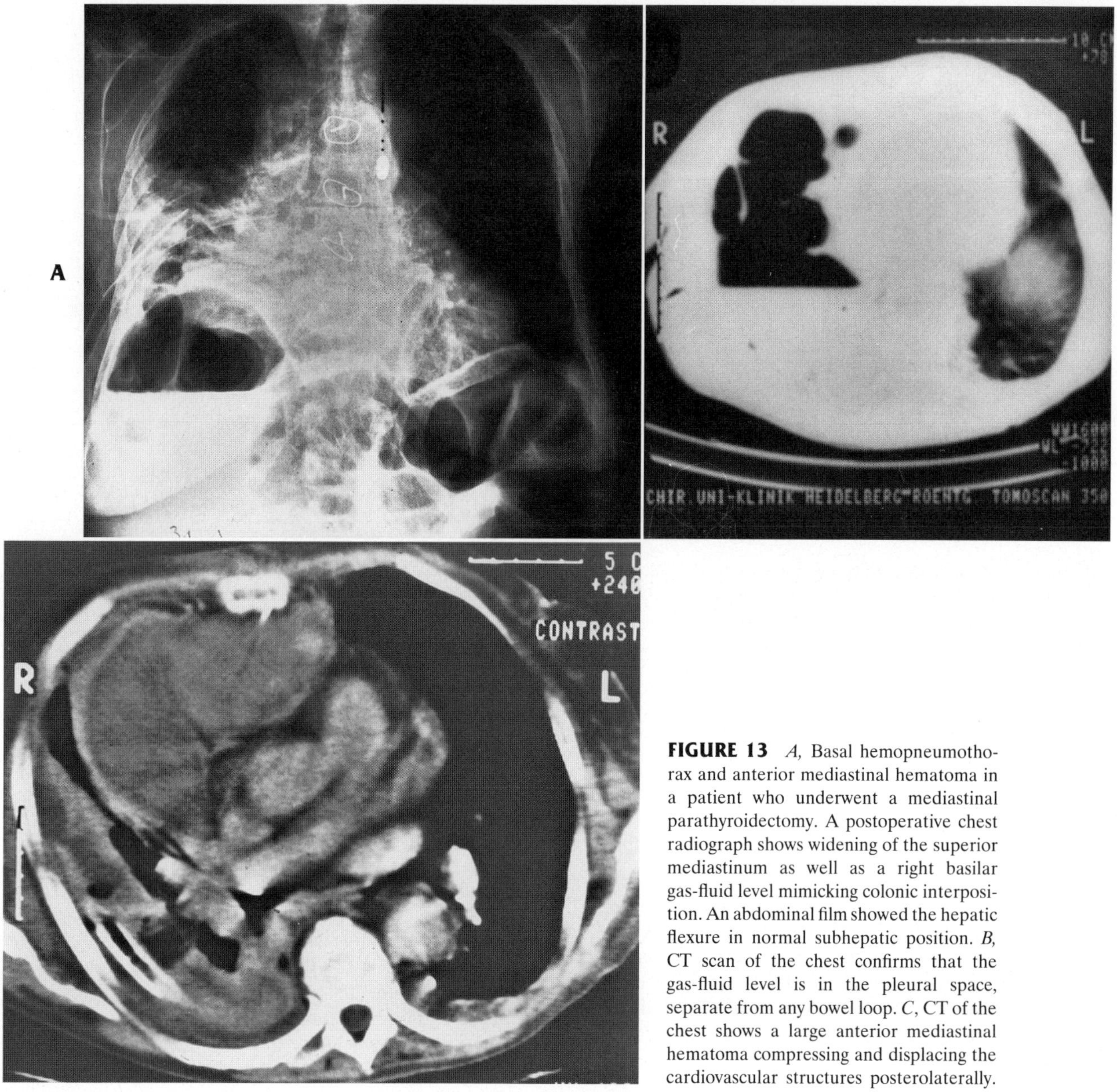


**FIGURE 13** *A,* Basal hemopneumothorax and anterior mediastinal hematoma in a patient who underwent a mediastinal parathyroidectomy. A postoperative chest radiograph shows widening of the superior mediastinum as well as a right basilar gas-fluid level mimicking colonic interposition. An abdominal film showed the hepatic flexure in normal subhepatic position. *B,* CT scan of the chest confirms that the gas-fluid level is in the pleural space, separate from any bowel loop. *C,* CT of the chest shows a large anterior mediastinal hematoma compressing and displacing the cardiovascular structures posterolaterally.

person include apicolateral accumulation of pleural air and a visible visceral pleural line. A lateral width of 1 cm for the air collection corresponds to approximately a 10 percent pneumothorax. On supine films, the pneumothorax collects in anteromedial, subpulmonic, or costophrenic locations. Skin folds should be differentiated from pneumothorax by their different density profile, with a black Mach band instead of the white visceral pleural line; the skin fold frequently extends beyond the rib cage or stops short of the ribs and vessels extend beyond it. Bullae can mimic a pneumothorax, yet their inner wall is convex toward the hilus, whereas a visceral pleural contour is either straight or convex laterally. Problems can arise with subpulmonic collections (Fig. 13) of air, because the lung base is convex upward and can behave like a bulla. Upright or decubitus films clarify the issue.

## Tracheobronchial Fractures

Tracheobronchial fractures occur in 3 percent of patients with chest trauma. At least 30 percent are missed initially, and these result in a 30 percent mortality. The mechanism is a sudden chest compression, as in crush or steering wheel injuries. In 90 percent the tear is in a mainstem bronchus, and in 10 percent in the trachea within 2 cm of the carina.

The radiographic findings are (1) those of an air leak with pneumomediastinum, deep cervical emphysema, subcutaneous emphysema, retropneumoperitoneum, or tension pneumothorax uncontrolled by chest tubes; (2) findings pertinent to the bronchial tree such as obstruction, disruption, and deformity of the involved bronchus; and (3) findings in the subtended lung, including atelectasis or the so-called falling lung sign. Associated fractures of the first three ribs are seen in 40 to 90 percent

A 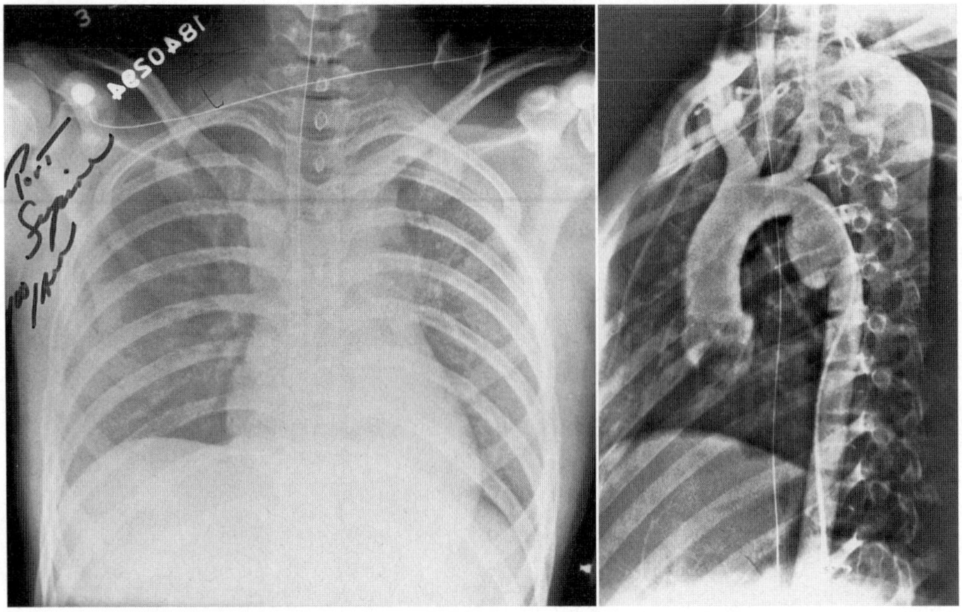 B

**FIGURE 14** *A,* Ruptured aorta from a motor vehicle accident. The chest film shows several features of mediastinal hematoma; widening of the superior mediastinum, left apical pleural cap, widening of right paratracheal and left paraspinal stripe, deviation of the nasogastric tube to the right and downward displacement of left mainstem bronchus. *B,* Aortogram shows a pseudoaneurysm distal to the origin of the left subclavian artery.

of patients over 30 years of age. If the diagnosis is initially missed, bronchial stenosis with atelectasis, pneumonia, and bronchiectasis results.

## Traumatic Rupture of the Thoracic Aorta

In 90 percent of cases traumatic rupture of the thoracic aorta occurs at the aortic isthmus, distal to the take-off of the left subclavian artery. In 10 percent the ascending aorta or descending aorta are involved. In 4 to 10 percent of cases, the aortic arch branches are also involved, either alone or in combination with a ruptured aorta. The mechanism involved is horizontal or vertical deceleration with injury of the relatively fixed segments of the aorta, or osseous pinch by the clavicles, ribs, and spine.

Rupture of the aorta is a common cause of death in the coroner's office: 16 percent of motor vehicle accident fatalities have succumbed to such an injury. Eighty-five percent of aortic rupture victims die at the scene of the accident. Fifteen percent reach the hospital, and of these, 30 percent die in 6 hours, 50 percent by 24 hours, and 90 percent are dead by 4 months if not discovered and treated. Eighty percent survive with prompt surgical repair.

The radiologist relies on the presence of a mediastinal hematoma on plain chest radiographs to suspect the diagnosis of aortic rupture. In survivors the adventitia holds the aortic tear together, even though the ends of the intima and media might be distracted several centimeters. The blood in the mediastinum originates from smaller injured vessels, not from the aorta. Only 12 to 20 percent of aortograms performed for clearly visible mediastinal hematomas indicate a ruptured aorta. This relatively high number of negative aortograms is warranted to detect the few patients with an aortic tear. A normal chest radiograph in a patient with an acute aortic rupture is extremely unusual. A normal CT scan of the mediastinum excludes a ruptured aorta, even if a mediastinal hematoma is suggested on the initial chest radiograph.

Multiple chest radiographic signs of mediastinal hematoma have been described, and include (Fig. 14):

1. Featureless, wide superior mediastinum measuring more than 8 cm at the level of the aortic arch
2. Partial obliteration of the aortic-pulmonic (AP) window and the descending aorta
3. Left apical cap
4. Downward displacement of the left bronchus
5. Tracheal deviation to the right
6. Nasogastric tube deviation to the right
7. Obscuration of the aortic arch
8. Right paratracheal stripe thickening
9. Enlarged or abnormal aortic contour
10. Left hemothorax
11. Wide left paraspinal stripe
12. Wide right paraspinal stripe
13. First rib fracture (as an isolated finding, no indication for aortography)

## Diaphragmatic Injuries

About 3 percent of patients with chest trauma develop a ruptured diaphragm (Fig. 15). Traumatic rupture accounts for 5 percent of all diaphragmatic hernias but for 90 percent of all strangulated diaphragmatic hernias. With blunt trauma, the left hemidiaphragm is affected 10 times more often than the right, accounting for 90 percent of ruptures. This is explained by the cushioning of the right hemidiaphragm by the liver. With penetrating injuries the situation is different: gunshot wound injuries do not have any preference for either side, but stab wounds preferentially involve the left hemidiaphragm, as 95 percent of the population is right-handed. The tears can be surprisingly large and have an average length of 10 cm. The

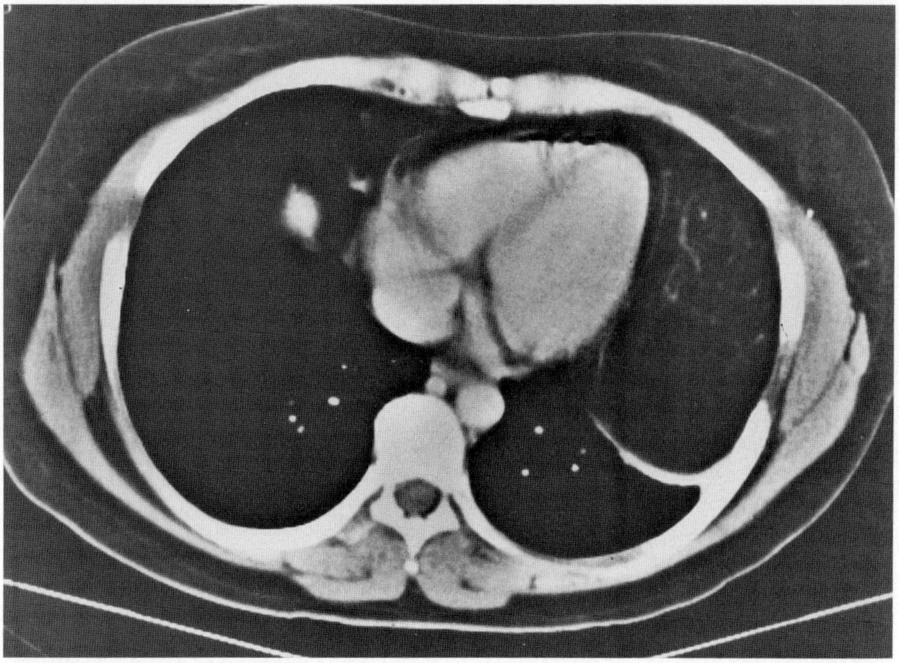

**FIGURE 15** Ruptured left hemidiaphragm after a gunshot wound. The CT scan through the lower chest shows herniated omentum in the left hemithorax. A small anterior pneumomediastinum is also present.

defect is located in the centrum tendineum or at its transition to the muscular portion of the diaphragm.

Seventy percent of diaphragmatic tears are initially missed because of the lack of early herniation of organs into the chest, and because of associated injuries that divert the physician's attention. Bergquist described a triad of rib fractures, pelvic fractures, and diaphragmatic rupture. Aortic tears and abdominal visceral injuries are also frequently present. Complications of a delayed diagnosis include strangulation, intestinal obstruction, and respiratory impairment. Radiographic findings include an irregular diaphragmatic contour and a markedly elevated lung base, which can mimic an elevated diaphragmatic leaflet (pseudodiaphragm effect). Gas-filled structures like the stomach, small bowel, or colon frequently occupy large portions of the thoracic cavity. If a nasogastric tube is inserted, it descends into the abdomen and then coils in the chest. A markedly distended stomach can be mistaken for a pneumothorax and chest tube insertion can have disastrous consequences. Fluid levels can mimic hydropneumothorax; herniated liver or spleen can mimic loculated pleural effusions or solid pleural and lung masses. Pleural effusions can be the first indication of strangulated bowel. Strangulated colon can have a characteristic bird-beak shape on barium enema.

With CT the interrupted diaphragmatic contour can be detected, the nature of the herniated viscera can be easily determined, and small amounts of pleural fluid can be identified. Abdominal viscera are normally located centrally on cross-sectional images of the thoracoabdominal junction. With rupture of the diaphragm, the abdominal viscera occupy the outer margin formed by the thoracic cavity.

## Esophageal Trauma

Injuries to the esophagus can be caused by intraluminal or extraluminal events. Intraluminal injuries are most common and are usually due to iatrogenic interventions, which account for 75 percent of esophageal ruptures: 0.1 percent of all endoscopies, 5 percent of esophageal dilatations, and 10 to 35 percent of Sengstaken-Blakemore tube placements result in perforation. The sites of predilection for perforations are below the cricopharyngeus muscle, at the level of the left mainstem bronchus and just above the gastroesophageal junction.

Ingestion of foreign bodies and chemical burns, particularly lye ingestion, can cause esophageal trauma. Vomiting injuries, which result from a rapid increase in intraluminal pressure, may produce a Mallory-Weiss mucosal tear with massive hematemesis, or the Boerhaave's syndrome with a complete tear of the esophageal wall. In 90 percent of Boerhaave cases, the linear vertical tear, about 4 cm in length, occurs first in the outer longitudinal muscle layer of the left posterolateral aspect of the distal esophagus, 2 to 3 cm proximal to the gastroesophageal junction. The most frequent radiographic findings include a left-sided pleural effusion (91 percent) and left pneumothorax or hydropneumothorax. Pneumomediastinum and deep cervical emphysema are visible in 66 percent of cases. Mediastinal widening and gas-fluid levels also can be present. A crescentic collection of gas separating the diaphragmatic pleura from the actual diaphragm, and connected with gas along mediastinal fascial planes, has been described as Naclerios' V-sign. With high esophageal rupture, the pleural abnormalities are more likely to occur on the right side. The prognosis of Boerhaave's syndrome is guarded. Without treatment the mortality is virtually 100 percent. With prompt diagnosis and surgical intervention, the mortality is still 30 to 50 percent.

Extraluminal esophageal injuries are infrequent. Gunshot wounds, stab injuries, or surgery, particularly during a pneumonectomy, can involve the esophagus. Blunt trauma can lead to compressive tracheoesophageal fistulas, particularly in patients with a tracheostomy balloon cuff and a nasogastric tube in place.

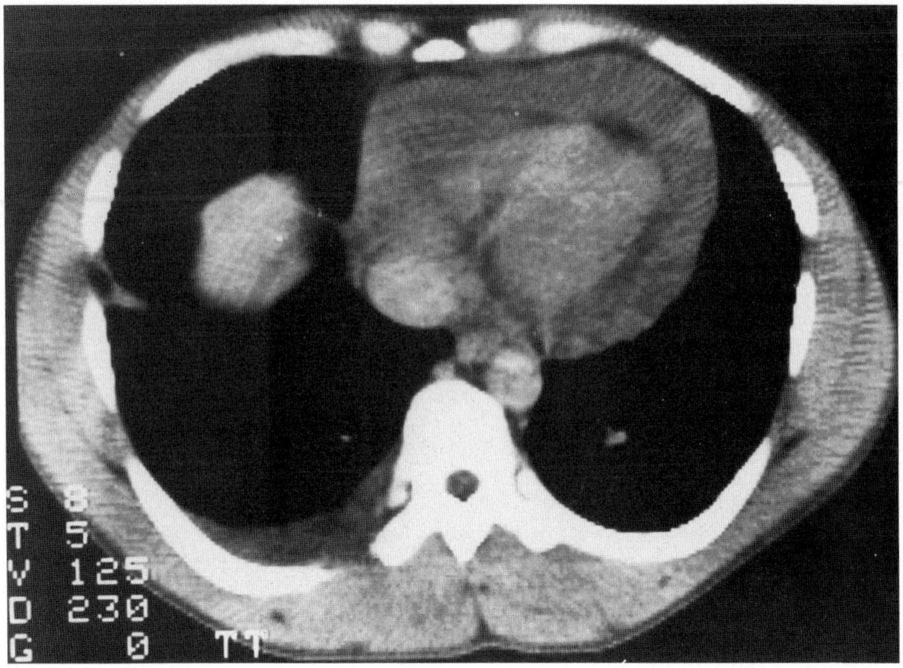


**FIGURE 16** Hemopericardium after sternal fracture due to a steering wheel injury. The CT scan shows a large pericardial effusion.

## Trauma to Cardiac Structures

### *Pericardial Injuries*

Pericardial injuries can produce hemopericardium (Fig. 16) and cardiac tamponade. Rupture of the pericardium can lead to herniation of atrial appendages or, particularly after a right pneumonectomy, to cardiac torsion. Tension pneumopericardium has been described after blunt or penetrating trauma.

### *Myocardial Contusion*

Myocardial contusion can be present in up to 20 percent of severe chest injuries and represents the most common manifestation of cardiac trauma. It results in myocardial edema, hemorrhage, and necrosis, and an increase in the MB fraction of the enzyme creatine phosphokinase. Electrocardiographic changes are similar to those of myocardial infarction. Right ventricular tardokinesis on gated blood pool scans has also been observed.

Myocardial lacerations can result from penetrating or blunt injuries. Late sequelae of penetrating trauma are myocardial pseudoaneurysms, which represent contained perforations. Blunt trauma can lead to the formation of true myocardial aneurysms.

The coronary arteries can be injured in 4 percent of penetrating thoracic injuries. Injury is manifested as thrombosis and myocardial infarction or laceration and hemopericardium.

### *Endocardial Injuries*

Endocardial injuries result in atrial or ventricular septal defects and in valve injuries. The right-sided valves are more likely to be affected because of their proximity to the anterior chest wall. Rupture of chordae tendineae, papillary muscles, valve cusps, or leaflets, as well as a cracked valve annulus, can result in tricuspid, pulmonic, mitral, or aortic regurgitation.

Foreign bodies like bullets, knives, or nails can be lodged in the heart without lethal outcome.

## Radiologic Triage in Thoracic Trauma

Phase I is the critical emergent evaluation: life-threatening injuries have to be excluded and little time is available for imaging procedures.

Phase II, the stabilization-emergent evaluation, concerns itself with the evaluation and exclusion of aortic, airways, lung, rib cage, diaphragmatic and cardiac trauma, plus the monitoring of therapeutic procedures.

During phase III, the stabilization-recovery period, injury resolution is evaluated and fluid balance, therapeutic interventions, the declaration of ARDS, and cardiac and diaphragmatic injuries are monitored.

In phase IV, the delayed-urgent period, recognition of sequelae of trauma, such as aortic pseudoaneurysms, lung herniations, pneumatoceles, delayed diaphragmatic herniation, and bronchial stenosis is imperative.

## Suggested Reading

Aronchick JM, Epstein DM, Gefter WB, Miller WT. Chronic traumatic diaphragmatic hernia: The significance of pleural effusion. Radiology 1988; 168:675–678.

Batra P. The fat embolism syndrome. J Thorac Imaging 1987; 2:12–17.

Bergquist D, Dahlgran S, Hedelin H. Rupture of the diaphragm in patients wearing seatbelts. J Trauma 1978; 18:781–783.

Bhalla M, Leitman BS, Forcade C, Stern E, et al. Lung hernia: Radiographic features. AJR 1990; 154:51–53.

Curci JJ, Horman MJ. Boerhaave's syndrome: The importance of early diagnosis and treatment. Ann Surg 1976; 183:401–408.

Dennis LN, Rogers LF. Superior mediastinal widening from spine fractures mimicking aortic rupture on chest radiographs. AJR 1989; 152:27–30.

Godwin JD, Merten DF, Baker ME. Paramediastinal pneumatocele: Alternative explanations to gas in the pulmonary ligament. AJR 1985; 145:525–530.

Godwin DJ, Tolentino CS. Thoracic cardiovascular trauma. J Thorac Imaging 1987; 2:32–44.

Greene R. Adult respiratory distress syndrome: Acute alveolar damage. Radiology 1987; 163:57–66.

Greene R. Lung alterations in thoracic trauma. J Thorac Imaging 1987; 2:1–11.

Greene R, McLoud TC, Stark P. Pneumothorax. Semin Roentgenol 1977; 12:313–325.

Greene R, Stark P. Trauma of the larynx and trachea. Radiol Clin North Am 1977; 16:309–320.

Henry DA. Thoracic trauma: Radiologic triage of the chest radiograph. ARRS Categorical Course on Chest Radiology Syllabus 1986; 13–22.

Kerns SR, Gay SB. CT of blunt chest trauma. AJR 1990; 154:55–60.

Kleinman PK, Marks SC, Adams VG, Blackbourne BD. Factors affecting visualization of posterior rib fractures in abused infants. AJR 1988; 150:635–638.

Mirvis SE, Indeck M, Schorr RM, Diaconis JN. Posttraumatic tension pneumopericardium: the "Small Heart" sign. Radiology 1986; 158:663–669.

Mirvis SE, Kostrubiak J, Whitley WO, et al. Role of CT in excluding major arterial injury after blunt thoracic trauma. AJR 1987; 149:601–605.

Perlman SJ, Rogers LF, Mintzer RA, Mueller CF. Abnormal course of nasogastric tube in traumatic rupture of left hemidiaphragm. AJR 1984; 142:85–88.

Rogers LF, Ruiz AW, Dooley BN, Cuello L. Diagnostic considerations in mediastinal emphysema: A pathophysiologic roentgenologic approach to Boerhaave's syndrome and spontaneous pneumomediastinum. AJR 1972; 115:495–511.

Silverberg E, Boring CC, Squires TS. Cancer statistics 1990. Ca – A Cancer Journal for Clinicians 1990; 40:9–26.

Stark P. Traumatic rupture of the diaphragm – A problem in radiological diagnosis. Radiologe 1982; 22:22–25.

Stark P. Traumatic rupture of the thoracic aorta – A review. Crit Rev Radiol 1984; 2:229–255.

Stark P. Right subclavian artery aneurysms – role of CT. Comp Radiol 1986; 10:253–258.

Stark P. CT of the sternum. CRC Press 1987; 27:321–350.

Stark P. Traumatic rupture of the diaphragm. ACR Chest Disease IV Syllabus 1989; 526–524.

Stark P. The pleura. In: Taveras JM, Ferrucci JT, eds. Radiology: Diagnosis, Imaging, Intervention, vol. 1, chapter 80. Philadelphia: JB Lippincott, 1990:1.

Stark P, Ben-Menachem Y. Traumatic occlusion of the left common carotid artery. ROFO 1983; 138:752–753.

Stark P, Cook M, Vincent A, Smith D. Traumatic rupture of the thoracic aorta: A review of 49 cases. Radiologe 1987; 27:402–406.

Stark P, Greene R, Kott MM, et al. CT-findings in ARDS. Radiologe 1987; 27:367–369.

Stark P, Jaramillo D. CT of the sternum. AJR 1986; 147:72–77.

Stark P, Jasmine J. CT of pulmonary edema. Crit Rev Diagn Imaging 1989; 29:245–255.

Stark P, Oglevie S. Roentgenographic findings of bronchial trauma. Radiologe 1989; 29:224–227.

Stark P, Phillips JM. Rupture of the esophagus as a complication of Sengstaken-Blakemore tube. Radiologe 1985; 25:76–77.

Tocino J. Pneumothorax in the supine patient. Radiographic anatomy. Radiographics 1985; 5:557–586.

Tocino J, Miller MH. Computed tomography in blunt chest trauma. J Thorac Imaging 1987; 2:45–59.

Tocino J, Miller MH, Fairfax WR. Distribution of pneumothorax in the supine and semirecumbent critically ill adult. AJR 1985; 144:901–905.

Wagner RB, Crawford WO, Schimpf PP. Classification of parenchymal injuries of the lung. Radiology 1988; 167:77–82.

# Imaging of the Pleura: Ultrasonography, CT, and MRI

*JAMES C. REED, M.D.*

The plain chest radiograph is the starting point for evaluation of most chest diseases and is often the first indicator of a wide variety of pleural diseases. Analysis of the plain film on occasion permits the radiologist to make a confident diagnosis, but evaluation of pleural diseases often presents serious diagnostic challenges for the radiologist. Difficulty in detection and precise localization are two frequently encountered limitations of the plain film, and distinguishing between peripheral lung abnormalities and pleural or even-chest wall lesions can be troublesome. In fact, Fleischner's original description of the air bronchogram emphasized the importance of the sign for differentiating parenchymal lung disease from pleural effusion. Chest-wall lesions may be diagnosed easily when there is obvious bone destruction, but they are difficult to distinguish from pleural lesions by plain film in the absence of bone abnormality. This chapter concentrates on the choice of ultrasonography, computed tomography (CT), and magnetic resonance imaging (MRI) for confirmation, precise localization, and diagnosis of diseases of the pleura. It also emphasizes the utility of the techniques for biopsy and therapeutic interventions.

The most common indication for pleural ultrasonography, CT, or MRI is confirmation of the presence of an abnormality suggested by the plain film. These procedures are rarely indicated in patients whose plain films are normal unless there is a high index of clinical suspicion, as, for example, in patients with occupational exposure to asbestos or patients with primary neoplasms that have a high rate of thoracic metastases.

Pleural abnormalities that may require these advanced imaging procedures include the general categories of pleural effusions, scarring either from infections, trauma, or occupational diseases, and neoplasms. Metastases are clearly the most common cause of pleural neoplasm, but malignant mesothelioma and even benign tumors of the pleura, such as benign fibrous tumors, are not rare.

## Ultrasonography

The chest radiologist tends to overlook ultrasonography as a useful procedure in the evaluation of chest disease. Ultrasonography is limited by the fact that the sound signal is

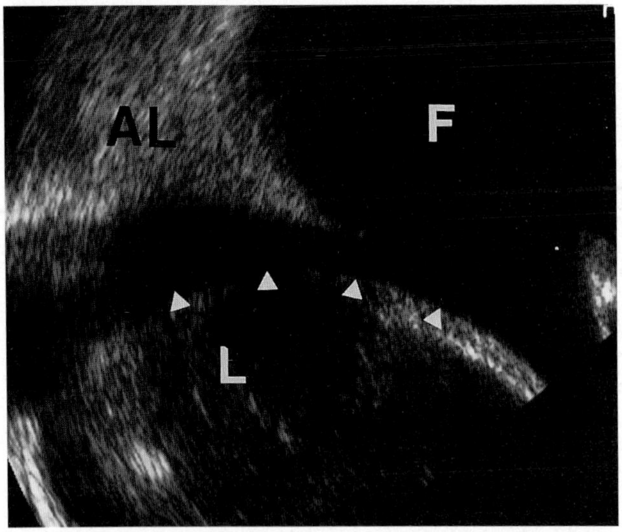


**FIGURE 1** Ultrasonography performed by an experienced technician paying careful attention to orientation is a reliable method for localizing peripheral pleural fluid collections. In this study the sonolucency of the pleural fluid contrasts with the echogenic atelectatic lower lobe (AL = atelectatic lung, L = liver, F = fluid, *arrowheads mark diaphragm*).

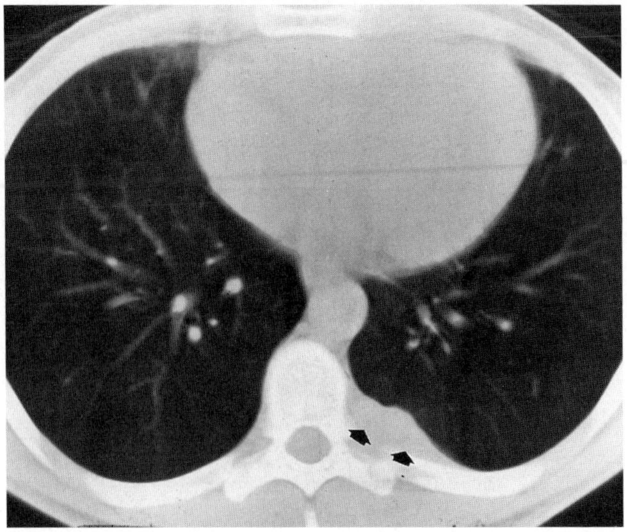

**FIGURE 2** Chest CT scan was performed for staging of primary testicular seminoma in a young man with an apparently normal plain film. The left posterior soft-tissue opacity *(arrows)* has smooth, tapered borders that appear to extend from the paraspinous area around the posterior pleura. CT guidance was used for fine-needle aspiration of the pleural mass, which confirmed the diagnosis of metastatic seminoma.

blocked by bones and is not transmitted through air-containing lung. Since pleural lesions are usually contiguous with the chest wall, the transducer can be placed between the ribs to image the pleural space without interference from intervening lung. This imaging procedure is highly effective for confirmation and localization of pleural effusions and masses. Pleural effusions suggested on plain films may easily be located and marked for thoracentesis (Fig. 1). Thoracentesis with ultrasonography guidance is far superior to thoracentesis performed without imaging guidance, especially if the effusions are small or loculated. This technique also may be used for placement of pleural catheters. It has the advantage of being portable and less expensive than either CT or MRI. One disadvantage of using ultrasonography to diagnose loculated effusions is that the absence of transmission through aerated lung may limit detection of fluid collections within the fissures. The success of ultrasonography is also highly dependent on the experience of the ultrasonographer. Further, for most chest radiologists, orientation requires careful attention to identify normal structures, especially the diaphragm, a fact that probably explains why ultrasound evaluation of pleural effusions is an underused procedure.

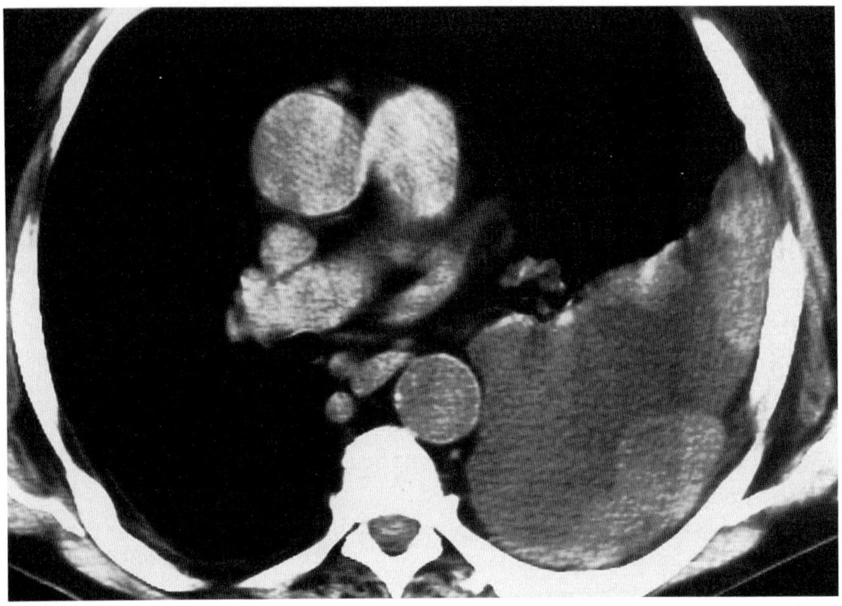

**FIGURE 3** A patient with malignant fibrous histiocytoma of the femur presented with a left-sided pleural effusion and a lateral smooth, tapered, soft-tissue opacity that suggested either loculated malignant effusion or pleural mass. CT scan shows a large low-density effusion with multiple higher-density pleural masses. CT-guided biopsy confirmed pleural metastases.

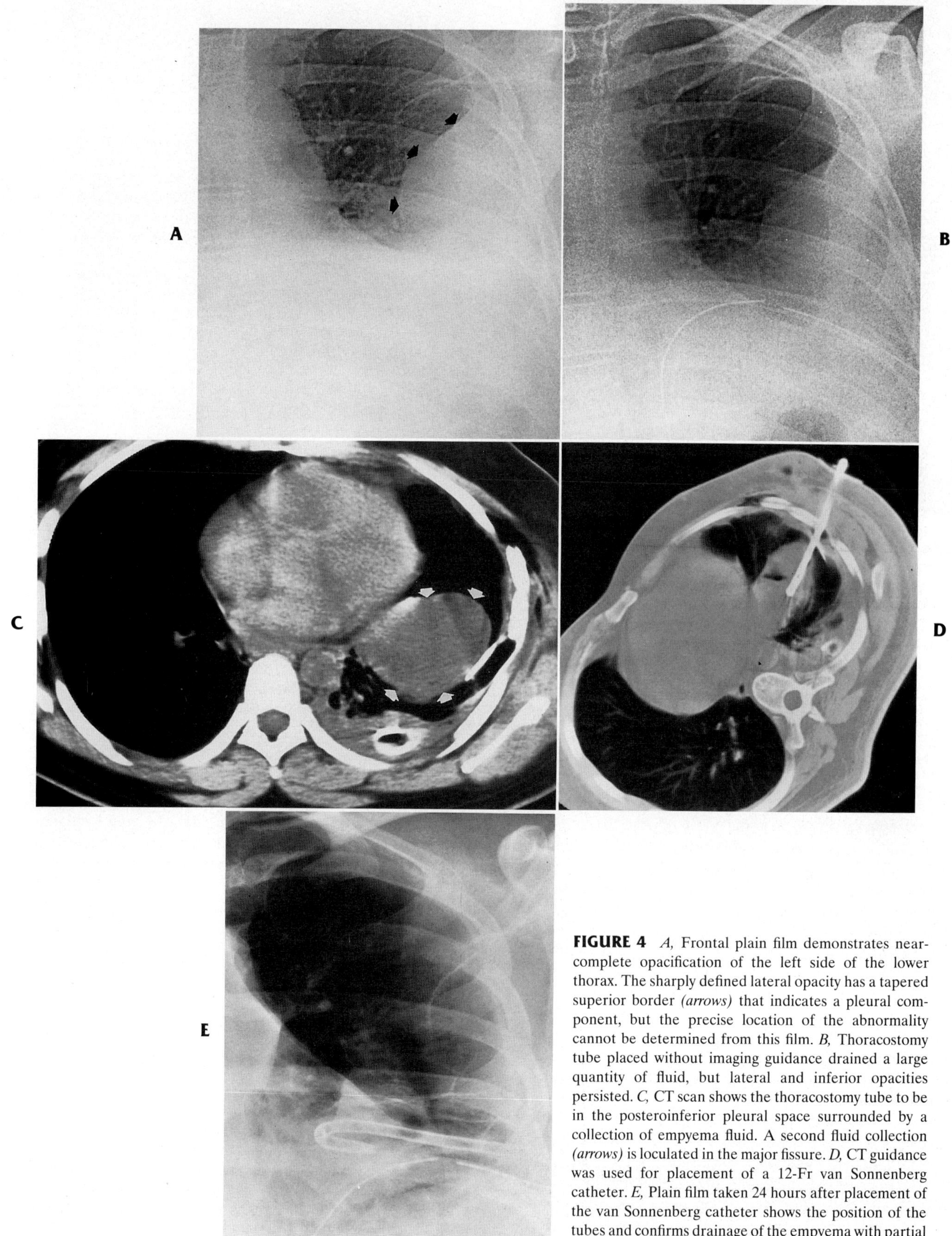


**FIGURE 4** *A,* Frontal plain film demonstrates near-complete opacification of the left side of the lower thorax. The sharply defined lateral opacity has a tapered superior border *(arrows)* that indicates a pleural component, but the precise location of the abnormality cannot be determined from this film. *B,* Thoracostomy tube placed without imaging guidance drained a large quantity of fluid, but lateral and inferior opacities persisted. *C,* CT scan shows the thoracostomy tube to be in the posteroinferior pleural space surrounded by a collection of empyema fluid. A second fluid collection *(arrows)* is loculated in the major fissure. *D,* CT guidance was used for placement of a 12-Fr van Sonnenberg catheter. *E,* Plain film taken 24 hours after placement of the van Sonnenberg catheter shows the position of the tubes and confirms drainage of the empyema with partial reexpansion of the left lower lobe.

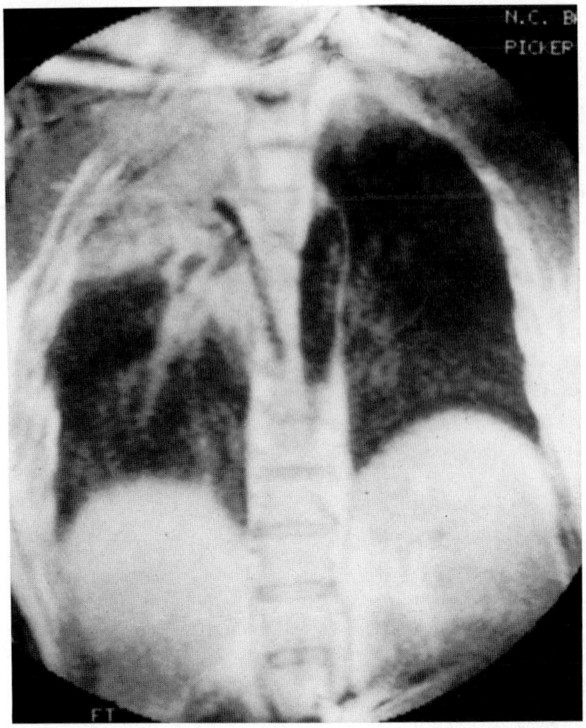

**FIGURE 5** T1-weighted coronal image of a large right-sided apical mass shows extension through the pleura and chest wall. Optimal imaging of the brachial plexus should also be done with a small field of view for more detail of the vessels and the brachial plexus.

## CT of the Pleura

CT is the primary imaging modality for evaluation of complicated abnormalities of the pleural space. It provides excellent resolution without motion artifact and permits detection of abnormalities not suspected on the basis of plain films. CT is also reliable for differentiating among pulmonary, pleural, and chest wall abnormalities. It is the most reliable method for distinguishing lung abscesses from empyemas with bronchopleural fistulas. The efficacy of CT for detection of peripheral pulmonary and pleural metastases that are not suggested by plain films is well established. Initial staging and follow-up of tumors with a high frequency of thoracic metastases should include chest CT scan, even if the plain film appears normal. CT-guided fine-needle aspiration biopsy is a highly accurate technique for histologic confirmation of metastasis and should be considered when the CT appearance is not characteristic for an unequivocal diagnosis of metastasis (Fig. 2). CT also provides detailed anatomic information in the axial plane about the relation of fluid collections to the fissures, lung, and chest wall. It can reliably discriminate between soft-tissue and pleural fluid collections (Fig. 3) and is extremely useful for guiding needles into pleural masses that are surrounded by fluid. Additionally CT guidance permits precise localization of fluid collections for percutaneous drainage of empyemas and metastatic effusions (Fig. 4). CT is more expensive than ultrasonography but has the advantage of better delineating the relationship of fluid collections to the fissures and identifying loculated collections that may be partially surrounded by air and therefore in difficult locations for ultrasonographic guidance. The advantages of CT over MRI are its excellent spatial resolution, good cross-sectional anatomic detail, absence of motion artifacts, and lower cost. CT also is better suited for percutaneous needle biopsy and pleural drainage.

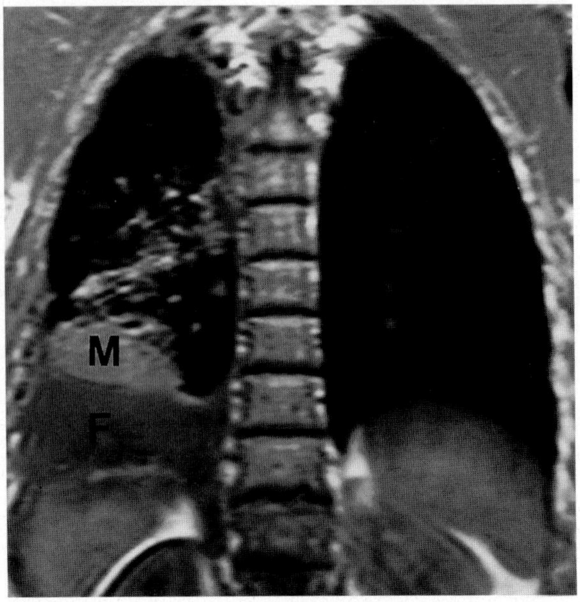


**FIGURE 6** T1-weighted coronal image of a patient with a large area of opacification in the lower right hemithorax clearly distinguishes homogeneous soft-tissue mass (M) from the heterogeneous signal pattern of atelectatic lung and the lower signal intensity of the pleural fluid (F).

## MRI of the Pleura

MRI is an exciting new technology that yields precise anatomic information. The images provide high soft-tissue contrast and may be obtained in multiple planes. Because of its cost, MRI is not usually the technique of choice for studying loculated pleural effusion. However, it appears to be the most sensitive and precise method for detection of abnormalities that involve both pleura and chest wall. One of the best-documented effective uses of this technology is in the evaluation of peripheral lung cancers that extend through the pleura and into the chest wall (Fig. 5). MRI is now an established technique for staging apical tumors that extend into the soft tissues of the chest wall and involve the brachial plexus. It is also effective for isolating components of complex abnormalities such as atelectasis, pleural effusion, and mass lesions (Fig. 6).

## Suggested Reading

Fleischner FG. The visible bronchial tree: A roentgen sign in pneumonic and other pulmonary consolidations. Radiology 1948; 50:184–189.

McLoud TC, Flower CDR. Imaging the pleura: Sonography, CT, and MR imaging. AJR 1991; 156:1145–1153.

Pugatch RD, Faling LJ, Robbins AH, et al. Differentiation of pleural and pulmonary lesions using computed tomography. J Comput Assist Tomogr 1978; 2:601–606.

Stark DD, Federle MP, Goodman PC. CT and radiographic assessment of tube thoracostomy. AJR 1983; 141:253–258.

Ulmer JL, Choplin RH, Reed JC. Image-guided catheter drainage of the infected pleural space. J Thorac Imaging 1991; 6:65–73.

van Sonnenberg E, Nakamoto SK, Mueller PR, et al. CT- and ultrasound-guided catheter drainage of empyemas after chest-tube failure. Radiology 1984; 151:349–353.

# Digital Radiography of the Chest

*HEBER MACMAHON, M.D. · MARYELLEN L. GIGER, Ph.D.*

Although digital radiography may be viewed as just one of several new diagnostic modalities, it has uniquely important implications for the future practice of radiology. For instance, digital archives will eventually replace film libraries, enabling clinicians to access and review radiographs of their patients on remote video displays throughout the hospital and beyond. Comparison with previous studies will be expedited, and computer-aided diagnosis will become feasible. But for now, many radiologists and hospital administrators face an urgent practical problem: how to take full advantage of the existing technology during its present developmental phase, and how to use commercially available digital radiography systems to solve specific problems within the radiology department. In this brief overview, we attempt to throw some light on these issues.

When digital chest radiography was introduced more than 10 years ago, many believed that it would offer immediate diagnostic advantages compared with conventional film-screen systems. This impression was based on various novel aspects of the technology, such as increased latitude of the digital receptors and the ability to enhance digital images by windowing and processing. The possible operational advantages of digital imaging received less attention. Now, after many years of rigorous observer tests and clinical experience, digital chest radiographs from existing commercial systems are generally regarded as only diagnostically adequate and even marginally inferior to a high-quality conventional radiograph in certain applications. The spatial resolution and contrast of film-screen radiographs have proven to be surprisingly difficult to match. At the same time, the speed of computers and the capacity of digital archival media have vastly increased while the cost of these components has continued to fall. Consequently the arguments in favor of introducing digital radiography at present tend to be based more on practical operational issues of service and economy than on assumptions of improved diagnostic accuracy.

## Digital Radiography Systems

Although many different techniques for digital chest radiography have been described, only two are in routine clinical use. The more established of the two is storage phosphor computed radiography (SPCR). SPCR systems employ a reusable flexible plastic plate, instead of film, coated with a stimulable phosphor to record the image. The plates are loaded into special cassettes and are exposed to x-rays with conventional equipment. However, unlike film, which must be developed in chemical solutions to bring out the latent image, a phosphor plate is unloaded into a special digital processing device. The plate is scanned by a fine laser beam that causes it to release energy, in the form of light, in proportion to the amount of x-ray energy absorbed. The emitted light is measured, the signal is digitized, and the image data are recorded permanently on an optical disc. These systems are configured to produce a final image on film using a laser printer, though video displays are also available. Most commercially available SPCR systems print two reduced-size images side-by-side on a single sheet of film, with differing degrees of image processing. The image matrix is approximately 2,000 × 2,000 with at least 1,024 shades of gray. When combined with edge enhancement, this results in an image quality that is adequate for most clinical applications. One of the attractive features of these systems is the large range of x-ray exposures that can be accommodated.

The second approach to digital chest radiography, which is enjoying a new wave of popularity, is film digitization. As the name implies, this method uses the conventional x-ray film as the image receptor. Although special wide-latitude films have been developed specifically for this purpose, conventional moderately wide-latitude film can produce excellent results. After exposure and chemical processing in the usual way, the film is transferred to a digitizer device. The least expensive systems for film digitization use a television (TV) camera to record the image, the video signal being subsequently digitized. This is adequate for some teleradiology and teaching applications, although the image quality is limited by the characteristics of the TV system. For most clinical applications, laser-scanning digitization is the preferred method, because it provides superior spatial and contrast resolution. As in the case of SPCR, the digital data can be stored, processed, and transmitted to a display device such as a laser printer. A typical laser-scanning digitizer provides a pixel size and number of shades of gray comparable to SPCR. The original radiograph is scanned in 30 seconds or less and immediately returned to the operator. Production of a final digital image may take several minutes, depending on the speed of the computer and whether image processing is performed. Very-high-resolution laser digitizers are now available, providing a matrix of approximately 4,000 × 5,000, corresponding to a pixel size of 0.1 mm on a 14 × 17 inch image, with up to 4,096 shades of gray. This level of image quality can be virtually indistinguishable from the original radiograph. Thus the image quality characteristics of these film digitizers exceed those of current SPCR devices. At the University of Chicago, we have developed software that automatically analyzes the original radiograph to determine whether the x-ray exposure is correct. If under- or over-exposure is detected, the system alters the optical density of the recorded image accordingly. Depending on the characteristics of the original radiograph, considerable amounts of under- or over-exposure can be accommodated. Undoubtedly such automated exposure correction software will become available commercially for film digitizers in the near future.

Generally speaking, both of these digital radiography systems can provide the following immediate benefits: (1) relatively consistent image quality compared with conventional film radiographs; (2) reduced retakes as a result of automatic correction for exposure errors; (3) inexpensive duplicates, each of which is completely identical to the initial digital image; and (4) the ability to reprint lost radiographs by retrieving digital data from a disc, months or even years after the examination has been performed.

Therefore most institutions that use digital radiography have applied it in clinical situations such as portable examinations, where these features are most useful. At the University of Chicago Hospitals, we use both SPCR and film digitization in our routine clinical work. In common with other institutions, we have used these systems predominantly for portables in order to take full advantage of their wide exposure latitude. We have also found it useful to provide inexpensive digital duplicates to intensive care unit and emergency room physicians. In situations where the need for duplicate images can be anticipated, digital radiography certainly provides a distinct advantage. Not only is the quality of the duplicate consistently high, but it can be less expensive than a conventional duplicate (depending on the film format used) and more convenient to produce.

## Display Options

Once a radiograph has been converted to a digital format it can be displayed in various ways. One option is to print the image on film, using a laser printer. Presently clinical digital chest radiography systems are used almost exclusively with hard copy for primary diagnosis. Depending on the printer used, the image may be altered in size (usually reduced 50 percent) and processed to enhance diagnostic information.

Another option is to view the image on a video monitor. Use of a video ("soft") display has advantages and disadvantages. The ability to manipulate the image during viewing is a possible diagnostic advantage. For instance, a chest radiograph can be displayed at different window levels to optimize lung or mediastinal detail, and different types of digital processing can be selected depending on the subject matter. In practice, however, windowing of radiographs on a video display is time-consuming and of limited diagnostic value, especially when the image has been reasonably optimized at a standard "default" setting. On the other hand, there are significant operational advantages in using video displays, such as allowing radiologists and clinicians in different parts of a hospital or even in distant locations to review a patient's images. The familiar frustrations associated with lost films, and the logistics of storing and signing out film radiographs, can be reduced in the short term and potentially eliminated in the long term. However, video displays presently have some practical limitations. For instance, reliable detection of subtle detail, such as pneumothorax, requires a high-resolution display, in the range of a 2,000 × 2,000 matrix. Therefore a conventional 512 line video monitor is not adequate for primary diagnosis in the chest. High-resolution video displays with 1,000 or 2,000 lines of resolution are available, though their adequacy for primary diagnosis remains to be proved. In addition, the cost of 2000 line monitors is prohibitively high. In clinical practice video displays are generally used by clinicians in locations remote from the radiology department, such as the intensive care unit, where rapid access to the images is of greater importance than the highest possible image quality. However, it is likely that the technology will improve to the point where digital workstations are accepted for primary diagnosis of chest radiographs. At the University of Chicago we have used only hard copy display for our digital radiography systems, though we have started to experiment with a high-speed workstation for possible use in primary diagnosis.

## Image Processing

The most popular type of image processing in chest radiography is digital unsharp mask filtering, which produces an edge enhancement effect. Based on observer tests and clinical experience, it is apparent that this type of processing can improve detectability of certain abnormalities such as pneumothorax and increase the conspicuity of catheters and other internal devices. However, excessive unsharp mask processing in the lungs can interfere with the detection of various types of infiltrates. Also, the effect of digital unsharp masking can vary from case to case, depending on the inherent image contrast and the presence or absence of certain types of pathology. A practical consideration is the need to compare processed digital images with conventional chest radiographs that may have been performed on the same patient. Clearly use of a heavily processed image as the only basis for interpretation would be undesirable. On the other hand, deletion of all processing from a digital image results in a subjective lack of sharp definition, which is less pleasing and probably less diagnostic than an image with a mild degree of unsharp mask processing. The standard display format for SPCR systems employs dual images on a single sheet of film. One image is mildly processed to appear similar to a conventional radiograph, and the second is more heavily processed. Although use of two complementary images in this way seems logical, it has not yet been convincingly demonstrated that this dual-image format is optimal from either a diagnostic or operational point of view. We have chosen to implement a new single-image format for both SPCR and film digitization. This incorporates a form of nonlinear image processing such that the lungs are relatively mildly processed, while low-density areas such as the mediastinum receive more aggressive enhancement. Before implementing this single-image format on a routine basis, we performed an observer test which confirmed our impression that it was diagnostically equivalent, for practical purposes, to the standard dual-image format.

One advantage of using this single-image format is that two identical images can be printed side-by-side on the standard film, which is then divided with a film cutter. We have used this strategy to provide diagnostic-quality films to the clinicians in the intensive care unit or emergency room at no additional cost. An alternative approach is to print a single image of considerably larger size than the standard digital hard copy radiograph. The necessary software to achieve this is now available from commercial SPCR vendors. At least one of the newer SPCR systems is configured to produce full-size 14 × 17 inch digital hard copy. This may be more readily accepted by radiologists and clinicians, because the size is similar to a conventional radiograph. However, this format is considerably more expensive than using reduced-size hard copy.

## Portable Radiography

Many radiologists have become frustrated with the poor quality of portable radiographs, and digital radiography is sometimes viewed as a possible solution. Digital radiography does provide more consistent quality, in that under- or over-exposure can be corrected, and consequently repeat examinations can be reduced. The principal cause of poor image quality in portable radiography, however, is scattered radiation, and use of a digital system does not address this problem. In fact, back-scatter can be somewhat increased in the case of storage phosphor radiography due to the absence of lead backing in SPCR cassettes. The only reliable way to achieve consistently high quality in portable radiography is by using a grid, and this remains equally important with digital systems. Although we have developed experimental grid alignment devices, virtually all of our portable work is still performed using 6:1 ratio grids without any special alignment aids. As a result of training and practice by the technologists, results are generally good. The average image quality is far superior to nongrid radiographs, regardless of whether a conventional or a digital system is employed. We have found that interference patterns, which might be a concern because of possible coincidence of the grid line spacing with digital sampling distances, have not occurred when the grid lines are oriented perpendicular to the direction of digital scanning. If unusual grids are used, such that grid lines are oriented across the short axis of the film or plate, or if a cross-hatched or other nonlinear grid is employed, interference patterns are a possibility, depending on the individual grid and digital device.

Although a theoretical argument can be made for using a lower kilovoltage for storage phosphor plates, we have achieved good results using the same exposure factors as for our film-screen radiographs. Our portable chest examinations are performed at 90 kV using a 6:1 grid with a 48 inch distance. For standard upright chest evaluations we use 125 kV with a 12:1 grid at a 72 inch distance.

## Interpreting Digital Radiographs

Interpreting digital radiographs is not fundamentally different from interpreting conventional films, but two aspects of digital images can cause problems for the inexperienced reader. First, the size is usually reduced. This requires using a closer viewing distance. Glare from the uncovered portion of the view box is annoying and can impair the viewer's ability to detect subtle findings. We have addressed this by placing a packet of precut squares of discarded overexposed film at each viewing station. When digital radiographs are mounted on the alternator by a clerk, a section of the masking material is placed above each digital film to block the excess light.

The small size of digital images can also cause confusion when comparing them with conventional full-size radiographs. This need not be a problem, because the standard format produces a 50 percent reduction, and a correspondingly reduced centimeter scale is printed on the margin of the film. Intermediate degrees of reduction are also possible with some digital systems but, provided the image size is standardized and that the amount of reduction is known, this issue is easily solved.

The second common source of error in interpreting digital radiographs relates to image processing. As explained, the intensity, or weighting factor, for digital unsharp mask processing can be varied throughout the image. When this type of processing is applied in the lung areas, it can accentuate normal bronchovascular markings to the point where an interstitial abnormality may be diagnosed erroneously. In other instances, actual interstitial disease may be accentuated. For this reason, we have chosen to employ an algorithm that applies only mild processing in the lungs, with greater processing in the mediastinal and upper abdominal areas. Pronounced processing can also produce an excessive edge enhancement effect, such that a dark line can appear alongside dense structures such as the heart or hemidiaphragm. This can simulate the appearance of pathology such as a subpulmonic pneumothorax. However, these processing artifacts are readily recognized with experience and do not negate the advantages of moderate degrees of image enhancement by this technique.

Finally, storage phosphor digital radiographs are more noisy (i.e., grainy) for a given dose than conventional film images. When an SPCR plate is badly underexposed, the image can become extremely noisy to the point where it is uninterpretable, although the density is within the acceptable range. Again, with experience this problem can be readily identified. Technologists must be educated to recognize this phenomenon, so that the examination can be repeated if necessary. In practice, because image quality is not adversely affected by overexposure up to extremely high levels, technologists have a tendency to err on the side of overexposure when using SPCR systems.

## Reliability

Although SPCR has been in clinical use for many years, reliability is still a significant issue. We have found that most downtime occurs from relatively trivial causes, which can be corrected quickly by an experienced technologist. More serious mechanical problems can also occur in the system, and these may take more time to correct. The reported downtime for SPCR systems is in the range of 5 to 15 percent, and most users consider this to be a substantial limitation. This is particularly the case when only one processing system is available. We have found reliability to be less of an issue with film digitization in the sense that, although minor computer malfunctions may occur frequently, the original radiograph is still available for interpretation, and therefore clinical service is not seriously disrupted.

## Discussion

In summary, digital chest radiography has both short-term and long-term advantages. In the immediate short term, digital systems can reduce retake rates by correcting for exposure errors and provide more consistent image quality than conventional film-screen systems. For most clinical purposes, the diagnostic content is comparable to conventional radiographs. In a few demanding applications, such as evaluation of diffuse interstitial disease, a high-quality conventional radiograph is slightly superior to a standard 2,000 × 2,000 matrix digital radiograph. In situations where conventional radiography is not always optimally performed, such as at the bedside, the more consistent quality of digital images may provide a diagnostic advantage.

In radiology departments where the quality of portable

radiographs is the primary concern, the existing film-screen system should be reviewed to determine that it has been reasonably optimized. This should include use of a low-ratio grid with moderately wide-latitude film for all adult chest radiography, as well as standardized kilovoltage and distance for each type of examination. Routine quality assurance procedures should be implemented also to reduce variations in chemical film processing. These measures can markedly improve image quality while reducing variations in film density from one day to the next. Digital radiography systems can also eliminate these density variations, but optical density is only one aspect of image quality. Digital systems should not be used solely to compensate for careless technique; an SPCR unit is an expensive exposure control device. However, if practical needs exist, such as a requirement to issue high-quality duplicates, to transmit images to a remote location, or to implement digital archiving, purchase of a storage phosphor system is a possible solution. A reasonable alternative is to adopt a wait-and-see attitude with the expectation that increasingly sophisticated and reasonably priced systems for film digitization will become available commercially within the next few years.

## Suggested Reading

Aberle DR, Hansell D, Huang HK. Current status of digital projectional radiography of the chest. J Thorac Imaging 1990; 5:10–20.

Fraser RG, Sanders C, Barnes GT, et al. Digital imaging of the chest. Radiology 1989; 171:297–307.

Huang HK. Three methods of implementing a picture archiving and communication system. Radiographics 1992; 12:131–139.

MacMahon H, Doi K, Chan H, et al. Computer-aided diagnosis in chest radiology. J Thorac Imaging 1990; 5:67–76.

Sagel SS, Jost RG, Glazer HS, et al. Digital mobile radiography. J Thorac Imaging 1990; 5:36–48.

# GASTROINTESTINAL RADIOLOGY

## Abdominal Imaging in AIDS

*MICHAEL P. FEDERLE, M.D.*

The gastrointestinal (GI) and genitourinary tracts are commonly affected by opportunistic infections and neoplasms as manifestations of acquired immunodeficiency syndrome (AIDS) and are major sources of morbidity and mortality. Imaging plays an important role in evaluation, though sensitivity and specificity of findings rarely are optimal.

### Indications

Generalized symptoms such as abdominal pain, weight loss, fever, and night sweats are nonspecific but suggest disseminated disease such as lymphoma or mycobacterial disease. If tests such as blood and bone marrow analysis are nondiagnostic, or if an objective marker of abdominal disease is desired, I have found computed tomography (CT) to be most valuable. Dysphagia or odynophagia are best evaluated by barium esophagography, while barium studies are also useful to diagnose causes of intermittent bowel obstruction or GI bleeding. Clinical signs and symptoms of hepatobiliary dysfunction are best addressed first with sonography or CT, with cholangiography (endoscopic or transhepatic) reserved for those needing more detailed analysis of biliary pathology. I believe that barium studies are of little value when the principal complaint is diarrhea or hemotochezia. These symptoms are extremely common, affecting at least 80 percent of AIDS patients at some point, and are usually a result of bowel infection or infestation. Radiographic findings are rarely definitive, and proper therapy requires isolation of the offending organism by endoscopic biopsy or laboratory analysis of bowel contents.

Complaints of dysuria, flank pain, and fever, often with accompanying pyuria and elevated levels of urea and creatinine, suggest renal infection or obstruction. Renal ultrasonography or CT can provide valuable information affecting patient management. Excretory urography is insufficiently sensitive or specific in most cases.

No special equipment or techniques are necessary for imaging evaluation of the abdomen in AIDS patients. Double-contrast barium studies are essential for detection of early mucosal and submucosal processes. Optimal CT technique includes complete bowel opacification and scanning during a bolus administration of intravenous contrast medium.

Mention should be made, however, of the necessity to use precautions to protect patients and health-care personnel from infection and contamination. Universal precautions, as advised by the Centers for Disease Control, mandate barriers to prevent contamination of the skin or mucous membranes by the secretions or body fluids of all patients, not just those suspected of being human immunodeficiency virus (HIV) positive.

### Diagnostic Approach

My approach is to discuss the most common abdominal symptom complexes and the radiographic differential diagnosis of potential causes.

#### *Dysphagia and Odynophagia*

Odynophagia (pain on swallowing) usually is indicative of mucosal ulceration. Dysphagia is a less specific complaint potentially caused by inflammatory or neoplastic processes in the pharynx, mediastinum, or stomach. A barium swallow, or esophagram, reliably displays esophagitis, helps distinguish *Candida* esophagitis from other less common causes, obviates endoscopy in many cases, and allows a noninvasive means of monitoring therapy.

*Candida* infection is the most common cause of esophagitis in AIDS patients and frequently the first manifestation of immunosuppression. Radiographic findings vary but almost always include clusters of mucosal plaques over a considerable length of the esophagus. In more advanced cases, the esophagus appears diffusely shaggy with a "tree bark" appearance caused by innumerable ulcers, plaques, and thickened mucosal folds. Such findings are characteristic enough to initiate antifungal medication. Only if the patient fails to respond are esophagoscopy and biopsy generally indicated.

Viral esophagitis has been diagnosed with increasing frequency. Cytomegalovirus (CMV) is the most common pathogenic organism and typically causes large shallow ulcers with normal intervening esophageal mucosa (unlike the more diffuse plaques and ulcers of *Candida* esophagitis). The ulcers tend to be circular or diamond-shaped, discrete, surrounded by an edematous submucosal halo, and may extend into the gastroesophageal junction (Fig. 1).

Herpes simplex esophagitis may be indistinguishable from CMV esophagitis but tends to produce more numerous ulcerations. Recently the HIV organism itself has been reported to cause esophagitis. Scattered reports of mycobacteria, pyogenic bacteria, actinomycosis, and other causes of esophagitis underscore the necessity to obtain microbiological documentation in atypical or unresponsive cases.

Neoplasm may cause dysphagia by encasement or submucosal infiltration of the proximal GI tract. Assessment of the pharynx by double-contrast barium studies and maneuvers such as the modified Valsalva is essential along with similar views of the stomach. Kaposi's sarcoma (KS) commonly affects the hypopharynx, appearing as scattered submucosal nodules or infiltrating masses. Similar submucosal masses, sometimes with mucosal ulceration causing a "target" or "bull's-eye" appearance, are virtually diagnostic of KS in the esophagus or stomach. Lymphoma tends to be more diffuse but is indistinguishable from advanced cases of KS with marked encasement or infiltration.

## Obstruction and Bleeding

Bowel obstruction and GI bleeding require radiographic assessment, because these symptoms may have various causes, and surgeons are reluctant to intervene unnecessarily. Bleeding may result from infectious or neoplastic breakdown of mucosa at any point in the GI tract. Obstruction occurs most commonly in the small bowel, and I have found both CT and barium studies useful in diagnosis. KS is the most likely diagnosis, particularly in homosexual AIDS patients with submucosal nodules evident. Either KS or lymphoma may encase the bowel or may cause obstruction by intussusception, the characteristic findings of which are recognized easily by CT or barium studies. Both CT and barium studies accurately depict symptomatic bowel neoplasms, and the homogeneous soft-tissue density masses should not be confused with the generally widespread bowel wall thickening typical of infectious enteritis or colitis.

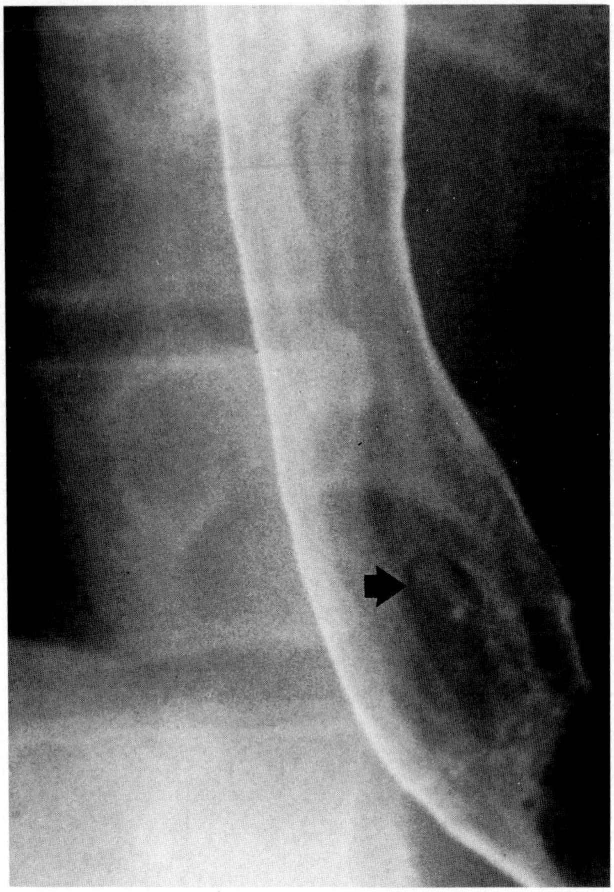

**FIGURE 1** CMV esophagitis. Discrete large ulcer *(arrow)* with surrounding edema near the gastroesophageal junction. Remaining esophageal mucosa is normal.

## Abnormal Liver Function

Hepatomegaly and abnormal liver function tests are found in most AIDS patients at some point in their disease. Extensive radiographic evaluation, however, is usually not necessary, particularly in the terminal phases of the disease or when disseminated opportunistic infection and/or neoplasm has been documented. Nevertheless, I must stress the importance of prompt and complete evaluation of rapidly deteriorating liver function, particularly if this is the initial or primary clinical sign. Ultrasonography or CT accurately detects most infiltrative and focal hepatic masses and biliary pathology. Although sonographic or CT findings are often nonspecific, guided biopsies have proven accurate.

AIDS-related lymphoma is a common cause of hepatomegaly, vague upper quadrant pain, and altered liver function. Typical findings include hypodense or sonolucent masses that may simulate abscesses or metastases (Fig. 2). Diffuse involvement is also encountered through subtle focal lesions and can usually be detected in such cases. Hepatic lymphoma is much more common in AIDS than in the general population with lymphoma.

KS can be detected in the liver in about one-third of patients with KS who come to autopsy. However, KS rarely causes hepatomegaly or significant alteration of function, and most

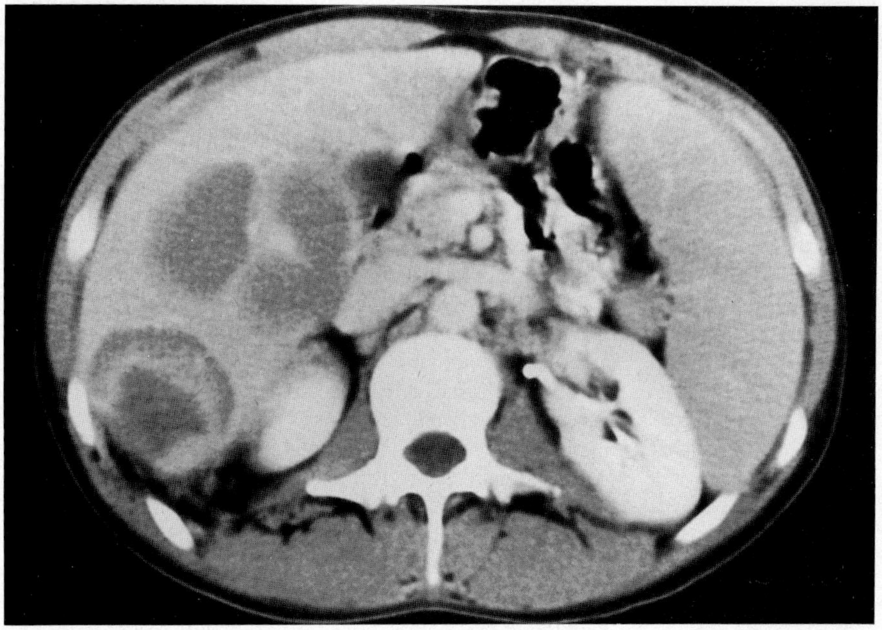

**FIGURE 2** AIDS-related hepatic lymphoma. Large discrete hepatic masses may simulate abscesses or metastases.

hepatic lesions are small foci along the portal tracts that usually are not detected by CT or sonography. Microscopic foci of hepatic KS are indistinguishable from lymphoma, metastases, or certain infections.

Almost every opportunistic organism has been recognized as a cause of acute hepatic pathology. CMV and mycobacterial infections are commonly diffuse and may simulate fatty liver (steatosis). Pyogenic bacteria tend to cause clustered or coalescent abscesses, while *Candida* typically produces innumerable microabscesses as reported in other patient populations. Many viral, fungal, mycobacterial, and bacterial organisms can produce multiple small focal abscesses. The main value of CT and sonography is to identify the lesions and to guide diagnostic needle aspiration.

A nihilistic attitude about detecting hepatic disease is not warranted unless the patient is near terminal. Hepatic lymphoma and many infections respond to therapy, and many months or even years of relatively symptom-free life are possible.

The bile ducts and gallbladder may be obstructed by neoplasm, usually lymphoma, or infection. AIDS-related cholangitis is characterized by right upper quadrant pain, fever, and laboratory evidence of biliary obstruction. CT and sonography demonstrate thickened biliary mucosa with submucosal edema and segmental strictures and dilatations of ducts. Involvement of the proximal ducts may closely simulate features of sclerosing cholangitis, while predominant involvement of the distal common bile duct resembles papillary stenosis or even neoplasm radiographically. Endoscopy, with cholangiography and biopsy, is definitive; infestation of the biliary mucosa by *Cryptosporidium* and/or CMV is almost always found (Fig. 3). Acalculous cholecystitis may accompany cholangitis or occur separately, but is likely due to the same infectious agent. Wall thickening and pericholecystic fluid are the imaging hallmarks, along with focal tenderness on palpation.

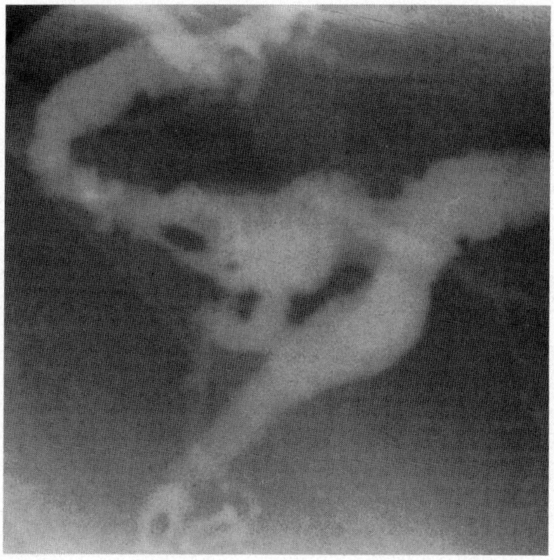

**FIGURE 3** AIDS-related cholangitis. Cholangiogram shows severe biliary mucosal ulceration with intermittent strictures and areas of dilatation.

### *Generalized Constitutional Symptoms*

Fever, night sweats, malaise, and weight loss are extremely common, but nonspecific, symptoms in HIV-infected patients. When generalized infection or tumor is known, additional radiographic evaluation may not be warranted. I must stress, however, that opportunistic infections may coexist with neoplasms, and KS and lymphoma also may affect the same patient.

AIDS-related lymphomas (ARLs) differ in several important respects from lymphoma in the general population, including a strikingly increased incidence (up to 100 times).

ARLs are highly aggressive B-cell lymphomas presenting in advanced clinical stage with a poor clinical prognosis. There is a clear predilection for extranodal sites, and abdominal visceral involvement is extremely common. While one-third of patients have adenopathy, typically retroperitoneal and mesenteric, up to half may demonstrate focal or diffuse hepatic involvement. Renal, bowel, and even omental masses of lymphoma are encountered regularly. In an HIV patient with an abdominal soft-tissue mass (nodal or visceral), lymphoma is the presumptive diagnosis and can be confirmed with needle biopsy. Experienced pathologists can even classify lymphomas for treatment based on percutaneous aspiration or core biopsy in over 80 percent of cases.

Splenomegaly is detected in the great majority of HIV patients and even in those patients with risk factors who are HIV negative. As an isolated finding, therefore, it is of no value. Focal splenic lesions may reflect infarcts, spontaneous lacerations and/or hematomas, neoplasm, or infection. Infarction and laceration can usually be confidently diagnosed, while neoplasm and infection have features in common. Infarcts usually appear as wedge-shaped peripheral defects with volume loss (chronic) and capsular enhancement. Lacerations are generally linear or rounded and are associated with perisplenic hemorrhage. A pattern of massive splenomegaly with diffuse low density has been reported recently as characteristic of disseminated histoplasmosis. As with renal infection, described later, disseminated *Pneumocystis carinii* may cause focal lucent abscesses in the spleen, later replaced by focal or diffuse calcification.

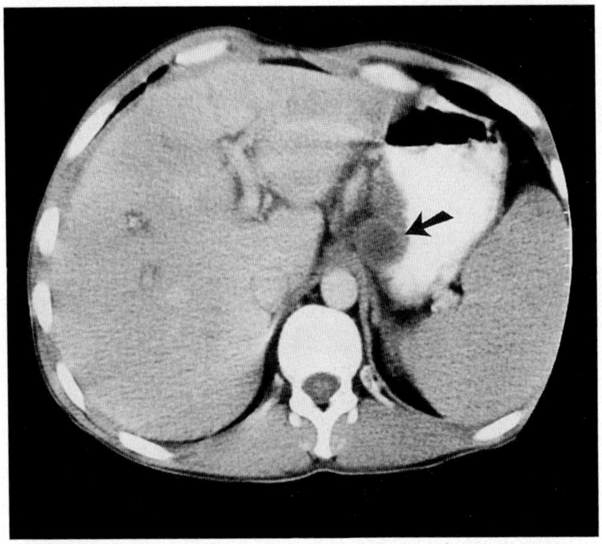

**FIGURE 4** *Mycobacterium avium-intracellulare* infection. Enlarged gastrohepatic node *(arrow)* has low density centrally, characteristic of mycobacterial infection.

Abdominal lymphadenopathy is an important and common finding on CT scans. Many homosexual male patients have persistent generalized lymphadenopathy with enlarged palpable nodes present in many sites. Similar clusters of normal-size to slightly enlarged nodes are seen in the retroperitoneum and mesentery. Biopsy of such nodes is not warranted in my experience, showing only reactive hyperplasia. Matted nodes or nodes greater than 1.5 cm in diameter command greater scrutiny. Soft-tissue density nodes are nonspecific; we usually biopsy such nodes and can easily distinguish between lymphoma, KS, and mycobacterial disease, the most common causes. Enlarged nodes with central or diffuse low density are highly suggestive of mycobacterial infection (Fig. 4) (*Mycobacterium tuberculosis* or *M. avium-intracellulare* [MAI]) or disseminated histoplasmosis. Most of these patients have systemic disease confirmed by blood, bone marrow, or peripheral node biopsy, obviating retroperitoneal node biopsy.

## Acute Abdominal Pain

The HIV patient with acute abdominal pain is a diagnostic and therapeutic challenge. Diagnostic evaluation must be quick, preferably noninvasive, and must identify those patients requiring urgent surgical or medical therapy. Symptoms are usually nonspecific and multiple processes may coexist. CT has

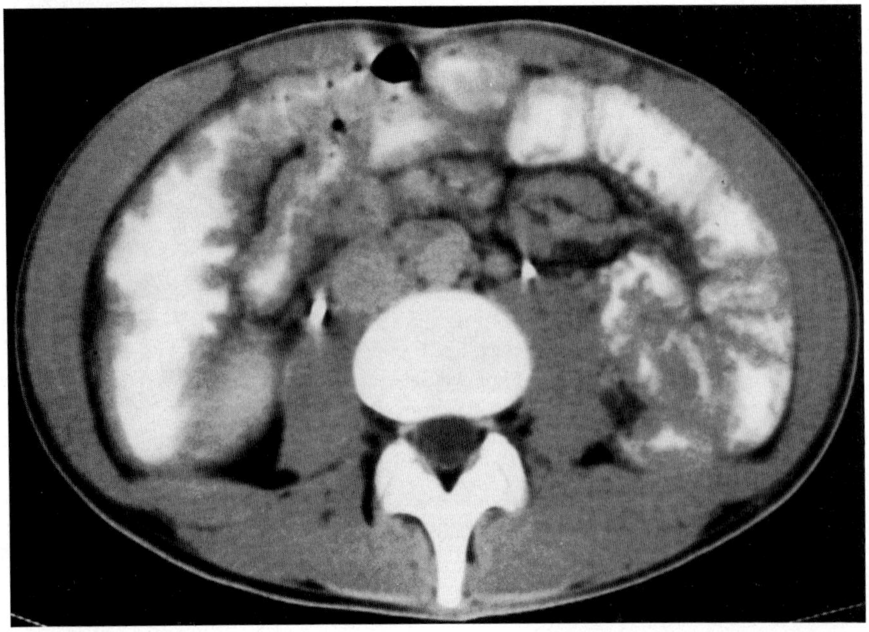

**FIGURE 5** CMV colitis. In a patient presenting with nonspecific acute abdominal pain, CT scan demonstrates diffuse moderate thickening of the colonic wall.

proven most useful as the initial imaging tool. Bowel perforation, obstruction, or infection can be diagnosed or suggested by CT evaluation with appropriate confirmatory studies as necessary (Fig. 5). Infections, infarctions, and acute neoplastic involvement of liver, kidney, spleen, or biliary tract have all been reliably diagnosed using CT as the primary triage tool.

### *Renal Disease*

Renal insufficiency and proteinuria are present in up to 40 percent of hospitalized AIDS patients and may be multifactorial (e.g., dehydration, drugs). Focal segmental glomerulosclerosis is a common renal manifestation of AIDS and leads to death within months. Characteristic sonographic findings are diffusely increased cortical echogenicity with preservation of corticomedullary differentiation. Renal cortical and medullary calcifications have been reported to result from opportunistic infections, including *Pneumocystis carinii* and MAI. MAI has also been reported to cause nephrocalcinosis. *Pneumocystis carinii* may cause focal hypodense lesions of all solid abdominal viscera, later giving way to punctate, rimlike, or linear calcifications within the viscera or along peritoneal surfaces.

Pyelonephritis from common bacterial pathogens is also more common in AIDS, having familiar and characteristic features best depicted by CT as striated or multiple wedge-shaped renal defects on enhanced scans.

The incidence of renal lymphoma is increased markedly over the general population. Multifocal or infiltrative masses are identified, often bilateral, and obstruction of the collecting system may occur. Absence of retroperitoneal adenopathy cannot be considered evidence against renal lymphoma.

As in other presentations, the main value of imaging patients with renal disease is to identify treatable pathology (e.g., pyelonephritis or an obstructing renal lymphoma) or to identify lesions that may first suggest the underlying diagnosis of HIV disease.

## Suggested Reading

Federle MP. A radiologist looks at AIDS: Imaging evaluation based on symptom complexes. Radiology 1988; 166:553–562.

Federle MP, ed. Radiology of the immunocompromised patient. Radiol Clin North Am, May 1992.

Federle MP, Megibow AJ, Naidich DP, eds. Radiology of AIDS. New York: Raven Press, 1988.

Jeffrey RB Jr. Abdominal imaging in AIDS. Curr Probl Diag Radiol 1988; 17:109–117.

Kuhlman JE, Fishman EK. Acute abdomen in AIDS: CT diagnosis and triage. Radiographics 1990; 10:621–634.

Wall SD, Olcott EW, Gerberding JL. AIDS risk and risk reduction in the radiology department. AJR 1991; 157:911–918.

# Radiologic Evaluation of Esophageal Dysphagia

*DAVID W. GELFAND, M.D.*

Because of the wide spectrum of disorders capable of causing esophageal dysphagia, the examination of the esophagus in these patients must be somewhat elaborate. However, if the examination is pursued with thoroughness, the cause can be demonstrated in the great majority of cases.

The following description of my method of examining patients with dysphagia includes contrast media, equipment, motion-recording techniques, single-contrast techniques, and double-contrast technique. I believe that a complete, accurate examination of the esophagus cannot be achieved by a single-technique, simplistic approach.

## Contrast Media

A high-density, 250 percent weight per volume barium sulfate suspension (HD, E-Z-EM, Inc., Westbury, N.Y.) is used throughout the esophageal examination and is employed for the barium-filled, mucosal relief, and double-contrast views. In addition to liquid barium suspension, half of a standard marshmallow may be employed as a semisolid bolus for evaluation of subtle constricting lesions or motility disorders. In conjunction with the marshmallow, a dilute 30 to 40 percent weight per volume barium suspension is used to wash down the semisolid bolus and to outline it during its passage through the esophagus.

## Equipment

All fluoroscopic examinations are performed on remote-control equipment (Siregraph D1, Siemens Medical Systems, Iselin, N.J.). The equipment provides complete radiation protection for our personnel and allows full-length spot films of the esophagus to be obtained under direct fluoroscopic control. The machine incorporates a 1,023 line high-resolution television chain for accurate fluoroscopic viewing.

A wide band pass video recorder is employed for motion recording (Sony WBS-700 H videocorder). The video recorder is compatible with the 1,023 line television system and incorporates a digital freeze-frame device. The recorder is capable of forward, reverse, slow motion, and frame-by-frame playback. Individual video frames can be sent from the freeze-frame device to a hard-copy camera for a permanent film record.

## Motion Recording

The procedure begins with an examination of the pharynx and cervical esophagus using motion recording via the videotape recorder. Because a swallowed bolus traverses the pharynx and cervical esophagus rapidly, it is difficult to obtain barium-filled views of these regions by synchronizing swallowing and conventional spot filming. Video recording of the swallow, with subsequent generation of hard copy from the videotape, circumvents this difficulty and uniformly provides satisfactory images of the barium-distended oropharynx and cervical esophagus.

The examination begins with the patient upright and with his or her back to the table. The image intensifier is first centered on the patient's cervical region. The patient is then asked to take a mouthful of high-density barium suspension and to elevate the chin to prevent superimposition of the mandible on the cervical structures. The tape recorder is started, and the patient is instructed to swallow (Fig. 1). After recording the swallow on videotape, a conventional spot film of the cervical region is obtained that shows the pharynx in double contrast (Fig. 2). The patient is then turned to the lateral position and the swallow, with tape recording and a subsequent spot-film, is repeated.

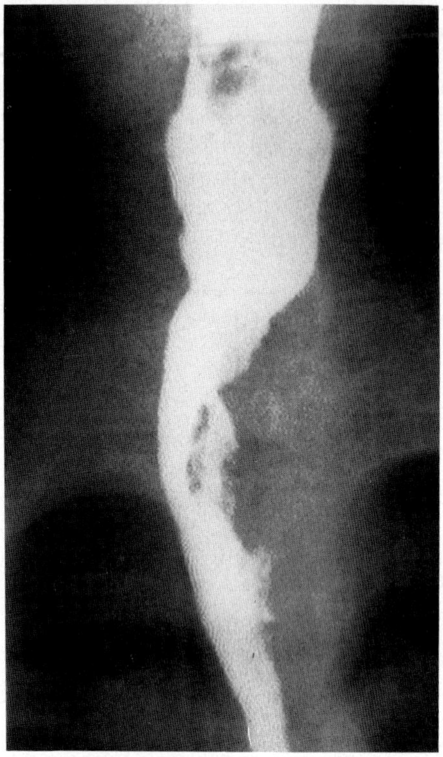

**FIGURE 1** Hard copy of videotaped swallow showing carcinoma of the cervical esophagus.

The foregoing procedure is designed to show a variety of abnormalities. Distention of the cervical esophagus during swallowing shows any web, stricture, carcinoma, or other constricting lesion (see Fig. 1). Pharyngeal diverticula, either lateral diverticula or Zenker's type, also are demonstrated. Muscular abnormalities, such as cricopharyngeus achalasia, are recorded during the passage of the bolus. The subsequent spot-films of the pharynx are used primarily to show pharyngeal neoplasms (see Fig. 2). The lateral spot-film also documents large cervical spine osteophytes that may be a source of dysphagia. After the examination, a hard copy is generated of any abnormality recorded on videotape.

## Double-Contrast Examination

The double-contrast examination of the thoracic esophagus is the next phase of the examination. The patient is examined in the upright position with his or her back to the table and turned 30° to his or her left. The image intensifier and spot-film device are centered on the region of the thoracic esophagus before any contrast material is given to the patient. The patient ingests the carbon dioxide–producing granules with a small amount of water (15 ml). The gas generated by the carbon dioxide–producing granules distends the esophageal lumen for a short period. The patient then drinks the high-density barium suspension as quickly as possible, so that the esophageal mucosa is thoroughly coated while the lumen remains distended by gas (Fig. 3). Filming must be rapid and properly timed if the esophagus is to be filmed in double contrast and fully distended.

Several limitations of the double-contrast technique should

A

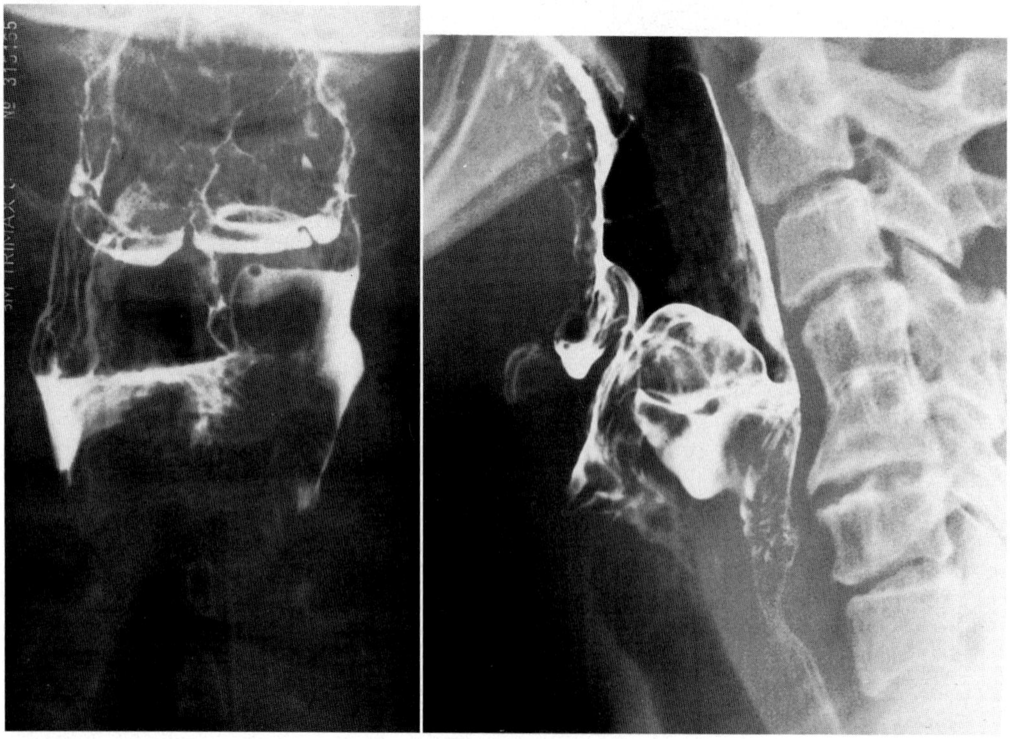

B

**FIGURE 2** *A* and *B*, Spot-films of the pharynx taken after swallowing high-density barium suspension showing pharyngeal carcinomas.

be mentioned. First, double-contrast films of the esophagus are often obtained without achieving full distention of the esophageal lumen by gas. Second, a barium pool may fill the distal esophagus, obscuring its mucosa. Finally, some patients with dysphagia have sufficient swallowing difficulties that the cooperation needed for double-contrast filming cannot be achieved. As a result, only about 75 percent of attempts at double-contrast filming are completely successful. Also, 15 to 20 percent of lower esophageal rings and strictures are not seen on double-contrast films, mainly because of failure to achieve adequate distention of the esophagogastric region.

The unique strength of double-contrast filming in patients with dysphagia is its ability to show the subtle mucosal irregularities associated with infectious esophagitis (Fig. 4). In this era of acquired immunodeficiency syndrome (AIDS), increasing numbers of patients with possible infectious esophagitis must be examined, often presenting with symptoms of dysphagia and odynophagia. Moniliasis is demonstrated radiologically as plaques and ulcers lining the esophagus (Fig. 3, *A*). Herpetic esophagitis is seen as small punctate ulcers separated by normal intervening mucosa (Fig. 3, *B*). The lesions found in association with cytomegalic inclusion virus and with the AIDS virus itself usually present as broad, shallow ulcerations.

## Single-Contrast Examination

The single-contrast examination is performed next; it remains a basic method of examining the esophagus in patients with dysphagia. Since the examination requires minimal cooperation and is performed with the patient in the recumbent position, it can be performed on any patient able to drink the barium suspension. The single-contrast method shows most causes of dysphagia including carcinomas, strictures, lower esophageal rings, and esophageal dysmotility (Fig. 4).

### *Full-Column Technique*

This phase of the examination is conducted with the patient in the right prone oblique position drinking through a straw. My technique is to ask the patient to drink six large swallows as rapidly as possible. The repeated swallows inhibit esophageal peristalsis and provide the volume of barium suspension necessary to achieve distention of the entire thoracic esophagus. When the esophagus is maximally distended, a full-length spot-film of the esophagus is obtained. For maximum distention of the esophagogastric junction region, the patient can be asked to perform a Valsalva maneuver after the esophagus is filled with barium suspension. The downward motion of the diaphragm also helps reveal lower esophageal rings and small hiatal hernias.

### *Mucosal Relief Technique*

The mucosal relief technique provides a view of the collapsed esophageal folds coated with barium. Normal esophageal folds are smooth and in the completely collapsed esophagus

A 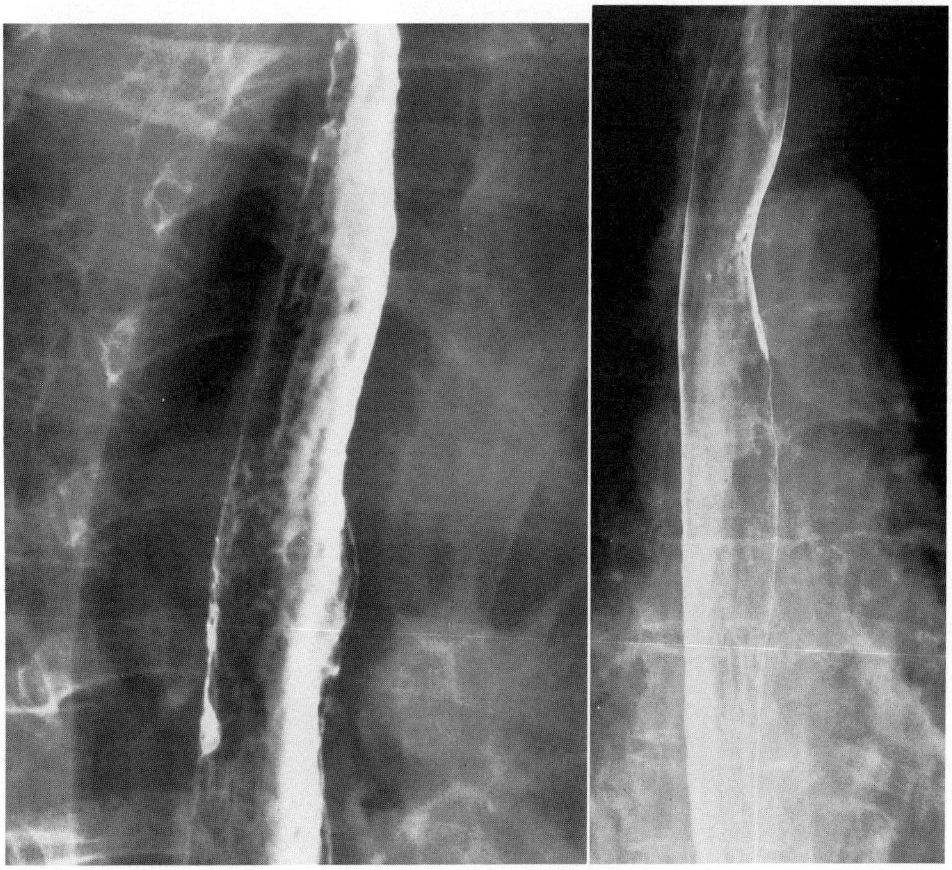 B

**FIGURE 3** Double-contrast films of the thoracic esophagus demonstrating moniliasis *(A)* and herpetic esophagitis *(B)* in patients with dysphagia.

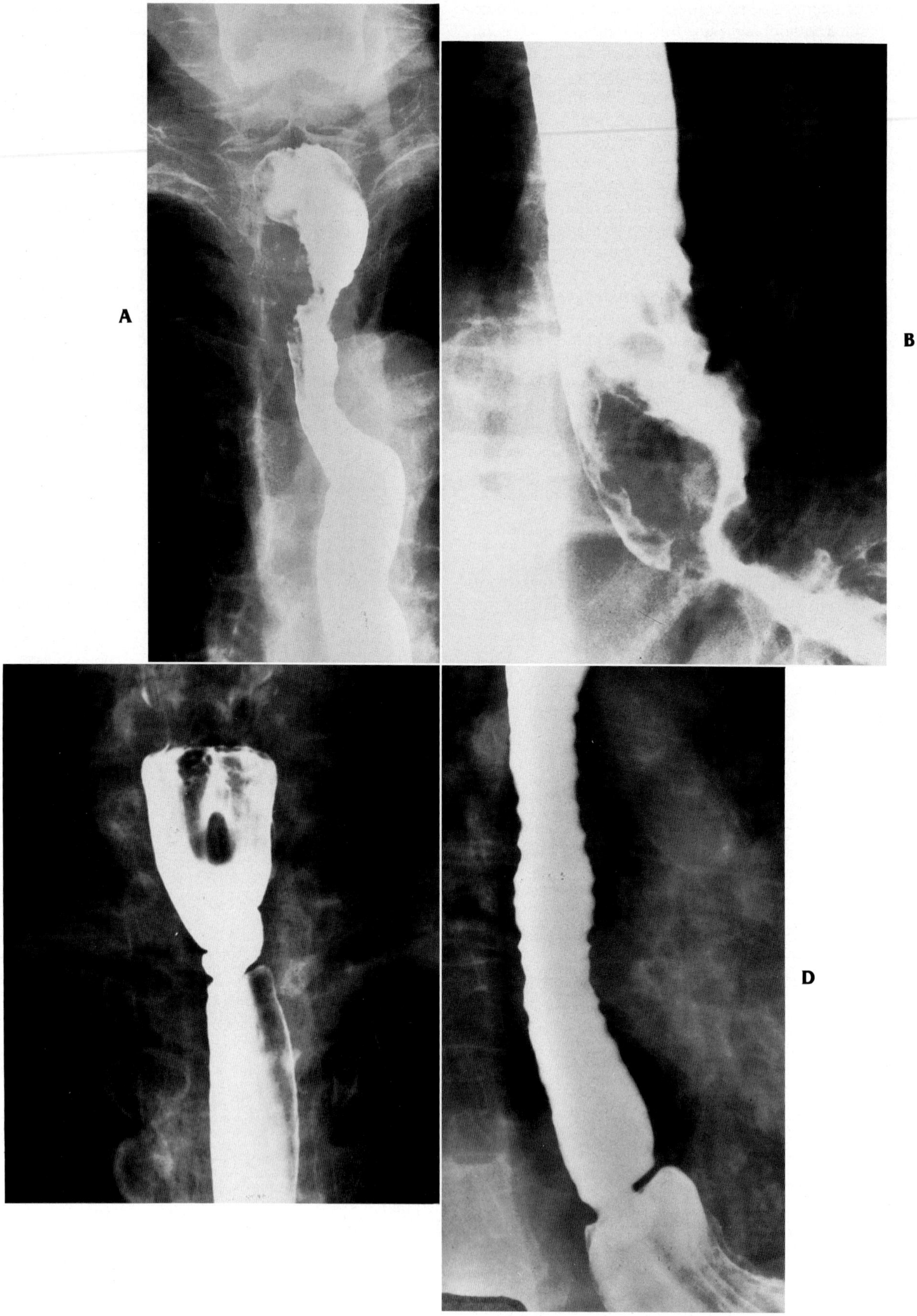


**FIGURE 4** Full-column examinations revealing carcinomas of the cervical esophagus and esophagogastric junction (*A* and *B*) and webs and rings of the cervical and distal esophagus (*C* and *D*).

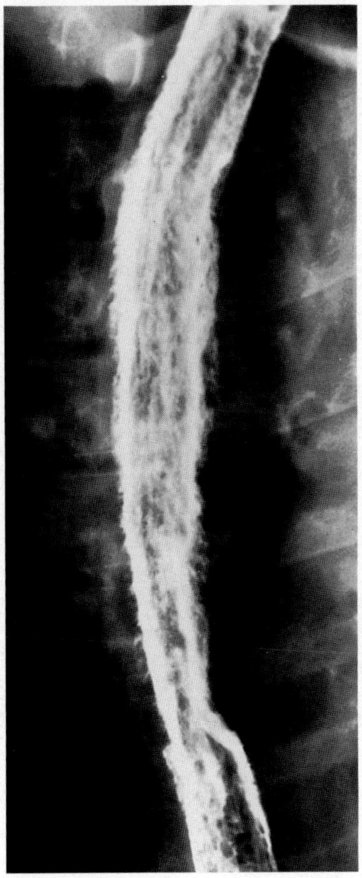

**FIGURE 5** Granular, ulcerated appearance of esophageal moniliasis as shown by the mucosal relief technique.

measure approximately 2 mm in maximum thickness.

Mucosal relief films are obtained by having the patient ingest high-density barium suspension and waiting until peristalsis strips most of the barium into the stomach. The barium suspension left behind coats the collapsed folds of the esophagus. As with the full-column views, an advantage of the mucosal relief technique is that it can be obtained in virtually any patient who can swallow.

Mucosal relief films are a sensitive indicator of esophagitis. Because esophagitis causes inflammation of mucosal and submucosal tissues, there almost always is an accompanying thickening and/or irregularity of the esophageal folds. These findings are very common in reflux esophagitis and are also seen in infectious esophagitis. Mucosal relief films present a typical granular, ulcerated picture in patients with esophageal moniliasis (Fig. 5). However, mucosal relief films do not reliably demonstrate the punctate ulcers of herpetic esophagitis nor clearly delineate the large shallow ulcerations associated with cytomegalic inclusion virus or the AIDS virus. For best demonstration of these entities, double-contrast filming is required.

### *Motion Recording in the Thoracic Esophagus*

Esophageal dysmotility is a significant cause of dysphagia in elderly patients. For its documentation, the radiologic examination should be performed in a manner similar to esophageal manometry. Radiologic demonstration of esophageal dysmotility on videotape is more easily understood by referring physicians than the abstract graphs produced by manometry.

The examination is conducted in the right prone oblique position with the patient taking single swallows of barium at intervals of 10 to 15 seconds. Sufficient time is allowed for the primary wave of each swallow to progress from the pharynx to the stomach. Double swallows or quickly repeated swallows should be avoided, since they cause reflex inhibition of primary peristalsis and thus give an inaccurate assessment of motility. Five individual swallows are recorded on videotape. The recordings are retained for several days for review by the referring physician.

Several esophageal motility disorders may produce symptoms of dysphagia. These disorders can be accurately detected and identified if a systematic functional examination is performed as previously described (Fig. 6). Achalasia presents as an absence of normal peristalsis, failure of the distal esophageal sphincter to relax, dilatation of the thoracic esophagus, and a "rat tail" appearance at the esophagogastric junction (Fig. 6, *A*). Diffuse esophageal spasm is seen as an intense spasm of the distal esophagus that does not allow the passage of a liquid or solid bolus (Fig. 6, *B*). The esophageal spasm may or may not be accompanied by chest pain. Elderly patients often develop a nonspecific esophageal dysmotility that entails failure of primary peristalsis accompanied by tertiary contractions (Fig. 6, *C*). This may be severe enough to cause difficulty in transporting food from the pharynx to the stomach.

## The Marshmallow Swallow

When the examination using liquid barium suspension does not clearly reveal the cause of dysphagia, it is useful to employ a marshmallow swallow to evaluate the response of the esophagus to a semisolid bolus. The marshmallow swallow is performed using half of a standard marshmallow and a dilute barium suspension of 30 to 40 percent weight per volume density. The patient is asked to swallow the marshmallow unchewed, using the dilute barium suspension to wash it down intact. Passage of the marshmallow through the thoracic esophagus and esophagogastric junction is monitored fluoroscopically and recorded on videotape or spot-films. Although hesitation at the esophagogastric junction for a few seconds is normal, obstruction of the bolus or its retention in the esophagus for a prolonged period is abnormal.

The marshmallow swallow is helpful in demonstrating two types of abnormalities. First, subtle strictures or rings may be shown by wedging of the semisolid bolus into the constricted area. Second, failure of transport of the semisolid bolus through the thoracic esophagus may be seen in patients in whom liquid barium suspension is easily transported. In these patients the semisolid bolus may elicit strong tertiary contractions or diffuse esophageal spasm not observed in response to liquid barium suspension.

## Discussion

Many techniques are available for the radiologic examination of the esophagus in patients with dysphagia. I employ all of these techniques as necessary. With this approach, the cause of the patient's dysphagia can be identified in the great majority

A B C

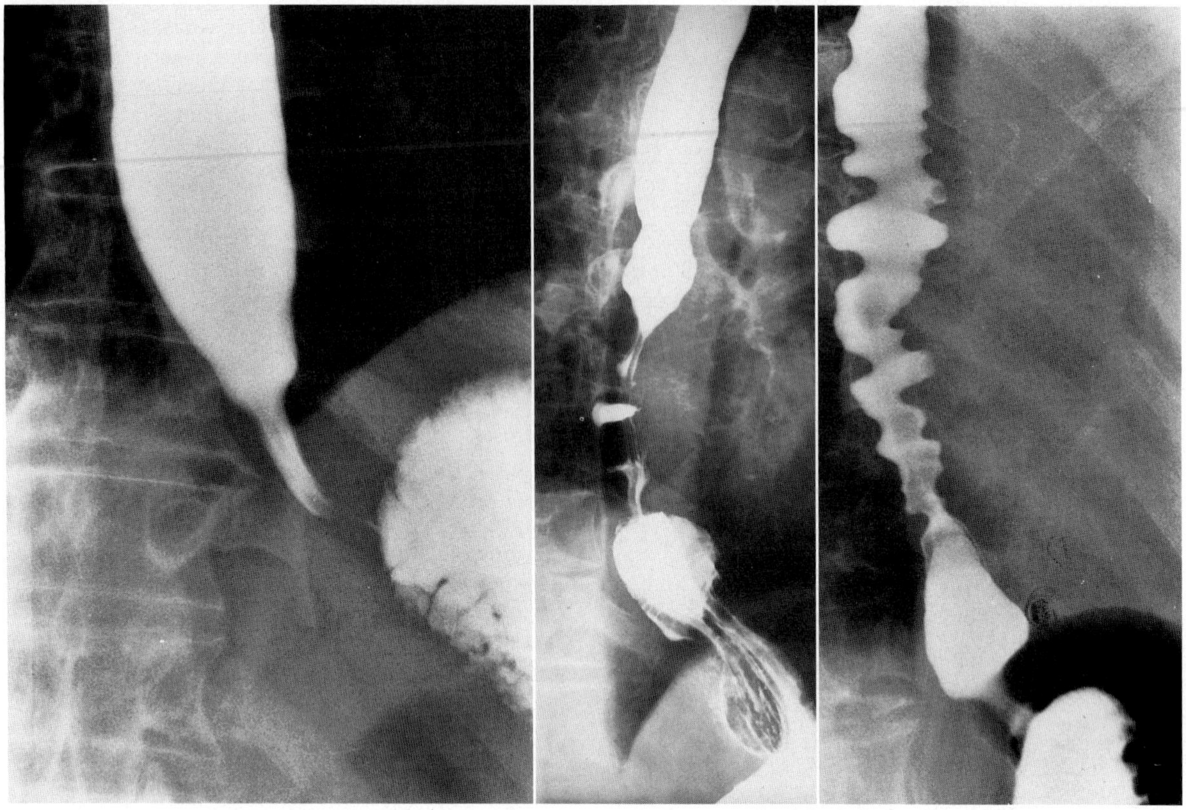

**FIGURE 6** Motility disorders diagnosed radiologically include achalasia *(A)*, diffuse esophageal spasm *(B)*, and marked tertiary contractions *(C)*.

of cases. Because patients with dysphagia have such a high yield of positive examinations, the examining radiologist should not stop the examination until the cause of the patient's symptoms has been demonstrated or every available technique has been exhausted.

## Suggested Reading

Chen YM, Ott DJ, Gelfand DW, Munitz HA. The multiphasic examination of the esophagogastric region for strictures, rings and hiatal hernia: Evaluation of individual techniques. Gastrointest Radiol 1985; 10:311–316.

Gelfand DW, Ott DJ. Anatomy and technique in evaluating the esophagus. Semin Roentgenol 1981; 16:168–182.

Laufer I. Double contrast gastrointestinal radiology. Philadelphia: WB Saunders, 1979:79.

Levin MS, Woldenberg R, Herlinger H, Laufer I. Opportunistic esophagitis in AIDS: Radiographic diagnosis. Radiology 1987; 165:815–825.

Ott DJ, Chen YM, Hewson EG, et al. Esophageal motility: Assessment with synchronous videotape fluoroscopy and manometry. Radiology 1989; 172:419–422.

Somers S, Stevenson GW, Thompson G. Comparison of endoscopy and barium swallow with marshmallow in dysphagia. J Can Assoc Radiol 1986; 37:73–75.

# Double-Contrast Upper Gastrointestinal Evaluation

*VINCENT H. S. LOW, M.B.B.S. · IGOR LAUFER, M.D.*

Our radiologic evaluation of the upper gastrointestinal (GI) tract remains a mainstay of radiologic practice. In general terms the upper GI tract can be examined by single- or by double-contrast techniques. In our view the improved mucosal detail visible by double contrast makes it the radiologic evaluation of choice for patients with symptoms referable to the upper GI tract. In modern medical practice, with upper GI endoscopy widely available and practiced, only those radiologic techniques capable of accuracy approaching that of endoscopy remain viable. Although modern cross-sectional imaging techniques such as ultrasonography, computed tomography (CT), and magnetic resonance imaging (MRI) have a limited role in the evaluation of the upper GI tract, the major methods of evaluation of the hollow viscera remain radiology and endoscopy.

## Indications and Clinical Utility

There are many indications for double-contrast upper GI radiology. The largest group consists of patients presenting with nonspecific epigastric distress or "dyspepsia." A variety of disorders affecting the upper GI tract including gastroesophageal reflux, gastritis, and peptic ulcer disease can usually not be differentiated by symptoms alone. The upper GI is also useful for various other indications including dysphagia, upper GI bleeding, nausea, vomiting, or weight loss.

## Technical Approach

The routine double-contrast upper GI should be performed as a biphasic study with single- and double-contrast views of the esophagus, stomach, and duodenum. In the double-contrast phase, we try to coat the mucosal surface with a thin layer of high-density barium while the lumen is distended with gas. We use fluoroscopy to achieve optimal coating, distention, and projection. Pharmacologically induced hypotonia with glucagon, 0.1 mg IV, improves the examination and can be used routinely or selectively.

Mucosal coating is achieved by washing the mucosal surface with high-density barium. This can be recognized at fluoroscopy when the mucosal surface is outlined by a thin uniform line of barium. The patient should be required to fast overnight before the examination and should also be discouraged from smoking.

The optimal degree of distention should just efface the normal mucosal folds. In the esophagus adequate distention can be achieved with rapid gulping of barium. For the stomach and duodenum, gas is introduced by the ingestion of granules, liquid, or tablets that release carbon dioxide on contact with the fluid in the stomach.

An adequate number of projections should be obtained to show each area free of overlap. This is of particular importance for the evaluation of the gastric antrum and pylorus to ascertain that they are free of overlapping duodenum.

## Normal Appearances

### *Esophagus*

When observed in double contrast, the normal mucosal surface of the esophagus is smooth and featureless. As it collapses, the normal longitudinal folds are observed. Occasionally, fine transverse folds may also be observed (Fig. 1, *A*). These folds are a transient phenomenon caused by contraction of the longitudinal muscularis mucosae. They may be observed with increased frequency in patients with gastroesophageal reflux, but they may also occur in the absence of any esophageal abnormality.

In older patients small nodules may be observed on the esophageal mucosa. These are a result of glycogenic acanthosis (Fig. 1, *B*) and should be considered a degenerative phenomenon with no pathologic significance.

A

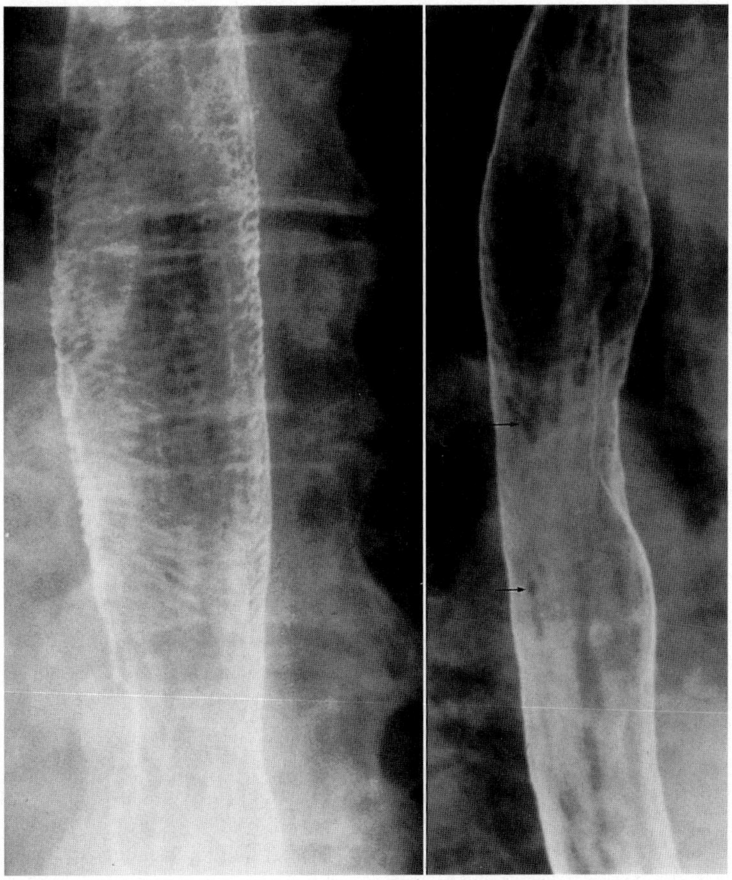

B

**FIGURE 1** Normal appearances in the esophagus. *A,* Transverse folds are seen in the midesophagus. These fine folds are a transient phenomenon, no longer present a few seconds later. *B,* Glycogenic acanthosis manifested as mucosal nodularity (*arrows*) in the midesophagus in this asymptomatic patient. Candidiasis may appear similar, but the patient would be symptomatic with dysphagia or odynophagia.

**FIGURE 2** Normal appearances in the stomach. *A,* Areae gastricae in the gastric antrum are seen as a mucosal pattern of 2–4 mm polygonal structures. Their visualization indicates adequate mucosal coating. *B,* Normal cardia appearing as centrally radiating folds (the cardiac "rosette").

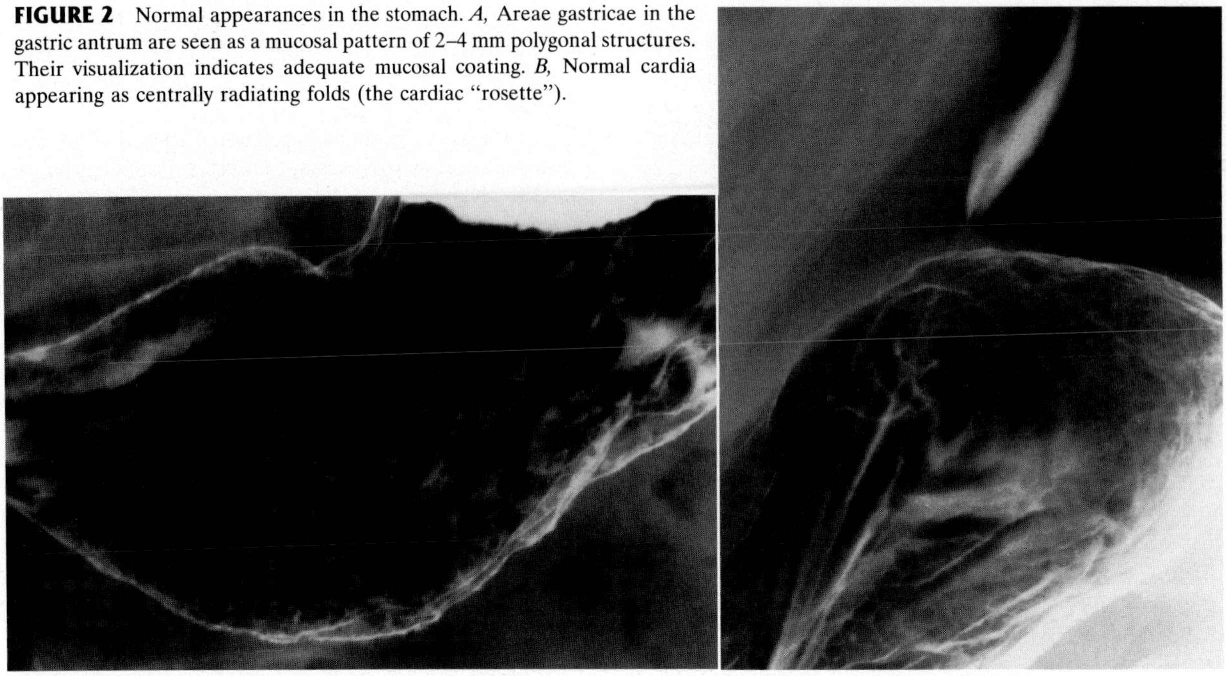

## Stomach

The double-contrast examination is particularly valuable for the demonstration of minute detail in the surface of the stomach. In addition to the rugal pattern, the areae gastricae pattern is routinely observed and serves as a barometer of good mucosal coating (Fig. 2, *A*).

The gastric cardia has a distinctive appearance on double-contrast evaluation. The constellation of findings includes a filling defect and radiating folds (cardiac rosette) (Fig. 2, *B*). This distinctive appearance should not be mistaken for an ulcer or mass.

## Duodenum

The distended, coated duodenal bulb has a smooth, featureless surface. In some patients a fine reticular pattern representing the villi can be observed (Fig. 3, *A*). In other patients a stippled mucosal surface is seen as a normal variant. This appears to represent trapping of barium in normal mucosal pits and should not be mistaken for erosive duodenitis (Fig. 3, *B*).

In the descending duodenum, the complex anatomy of the major and minor papillae and their associated folds can often be demonstrated (Fig. 3, *C*).

# Key Diagnostic Features

## Esophagus

### Esophageal Ulcers

The double-contrast technique is well suited to the detection of esophageal ulcers. The ulcers of gastroesophageal reflux disease may be punctate, linear, or irregular. Regardless of the mucosal changes, reflux may be implicated as the cause of the ulcer by the distal location of the lesion, the presence of gastroesophageal reflux, and the presence of a hiatus hernia (Fig. 4, *A*).

Viral esophagitis has become a major cause of esophageal ulceration. This is particularly common in patients with acquired immunodeficiency syndrome (AIDS), where multiple small ulcers are characteristic of herpes esophagitis. Giant esophageal ulcers may also be observed as a result of infection with either cytomegalovirus (CMV) or human immunodeficiency virus (HIV) (Fig. 4, *B*). A cluster of small ulcers in the midesophagus is also characteristic of drug-induced esophagitis usually due to tetracycline or doxycycline (Fig. 4, *C*).

### Esophageal Plaques

Candidal esophagitis should be diagnosable by double-contrast examination in at least 90 percent of cases. The classic picture is that of irregular linear longitudinally oriented plaquelike filling defects with intervening normal mucosa (Fig. 5, *A*). In AIDS patients the disease is usually advanced, resulting in a "shaggy" contour caused by coalescent plaque formation (Fig. 5, *B*).

Early esophageal carcinoma may appear as a plaquelike lesion. These often have central ulceration and irregular ill-defined surface and margins. The superficial spreading type of esophageal cancer, a potentially curable form, is manifested by tiny coalescent nodules or plaques that may be associated with shallow areas of ulceration. These lesions may simulate candidal esophagitis, but may be differentiated because the carcinoma occurs as a continuous area of disease without intervening normal mucosa.

## Stomach

### Gastric Ulcers

Radiological diagnosis of a gastric ulcer requires demonstration of an ulcer crater, preferably both in profile and en face. The profile appearance is similar to that seen in conventional single-contrast technique. However, ulcers have a variable en face appearance, ranging from a barium-filled pocket to a ring shadow to a partial crescent. Ulcers are not always round, but may be linear or have unusual shapes. Occasionally the

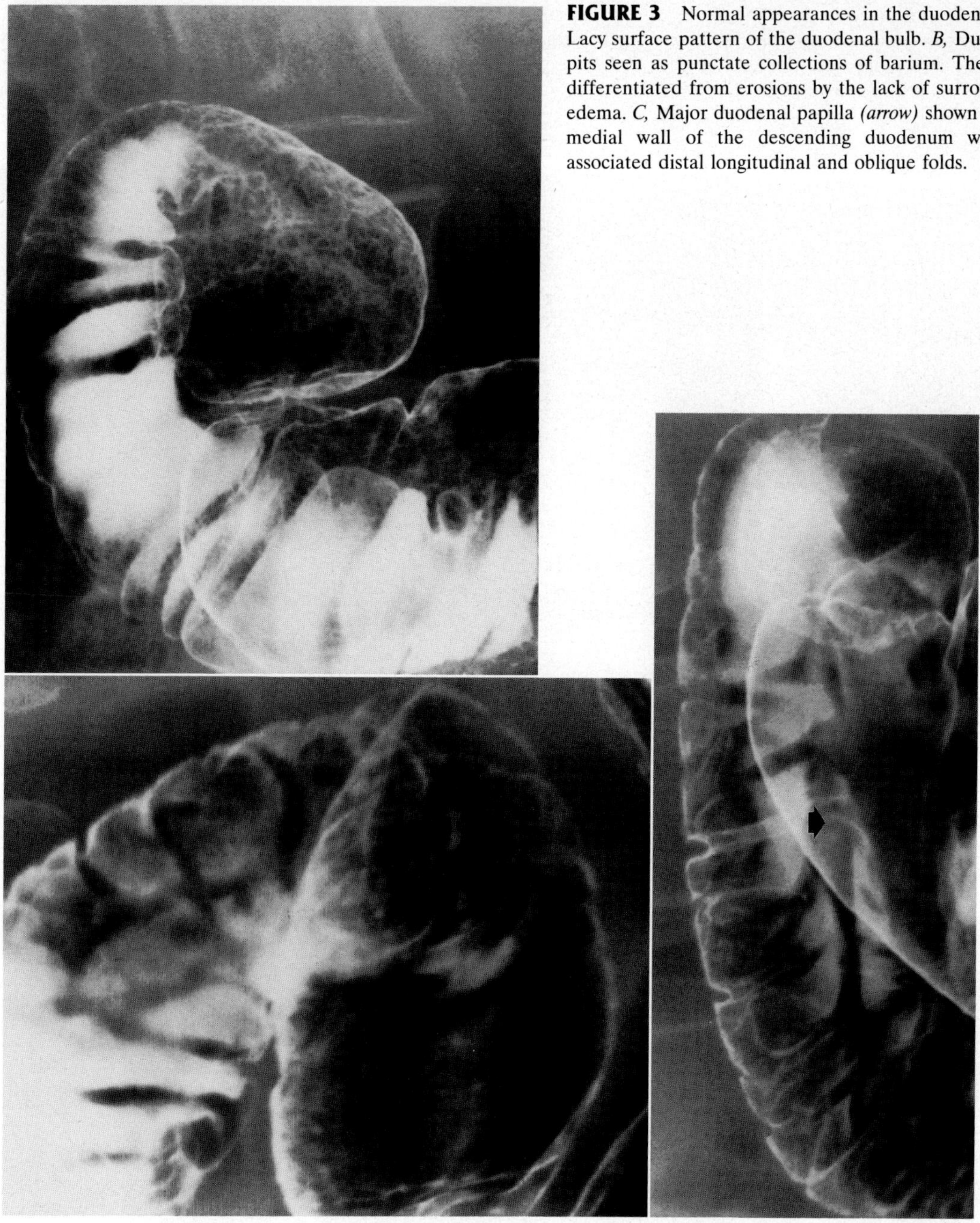


**FIGURE 3** Normal appearances in the duodenum. *A,* Lacy surface pattern of the duodenal bulb. *B,* Duodenal pits seen as punctate collections of barium. These are differentiated from erosions by the lack of surrounding edema. *C,* Major duodenal papilla *(arrow)* shown on the medial wall of the descending duodenum with its associated distal longitudinal and oblique folds.

radiating folds and edema may be more prominent than the ulcer itself.

The radiologically benign ulcer crater can be described as a hole punched out of normal mucosa. The surrounding mound of edema should be smooth. The radiating folds should be regular, symmetric, smooth, and extend to the edge of the crater (Fig. 6, *A*). Malignancy should be suspected if the ulcer shows nodularity; if there is a surrounding mass effect or rigidity; if there is destruction of the surrounding mucosa or distortion of the areae gastricae; or if the surrounding radiating folds show clubbing, amputation, or nodularity (Fig. 6, *B*). Therefore the mucosa surrounding the ulcer requires careful scrutiny.

Most benign gastric ulcers are located on the lesser curve or posterior wall of the gastric antrum or body. The occasional benign ulcer on the greater curvature of the distal stomach is almost always due to ingestion of aspirin or nonsteroidal anti-inflammatory drugs. Ulcers on the proximal greater curvature are rarely benign and should be evaluated endoscopically.

## Infiltration

The distention provided by the double-contrast technique is valuable in the detection of infiltrating tumors, since distention accentuates localized areas of rigidity or decreased distensibility.

Infiltrating lesions of the stomach may be due to primary carcinoma of the scirrhous type (Fig. 7), metastatic cancer (particularly primary breast cancer), or lymphoma. Endoscopic biopsy occasionally fails to diagnose the lesion, because the tumor cells are located in the submucosa, requiring a deep biopsy.

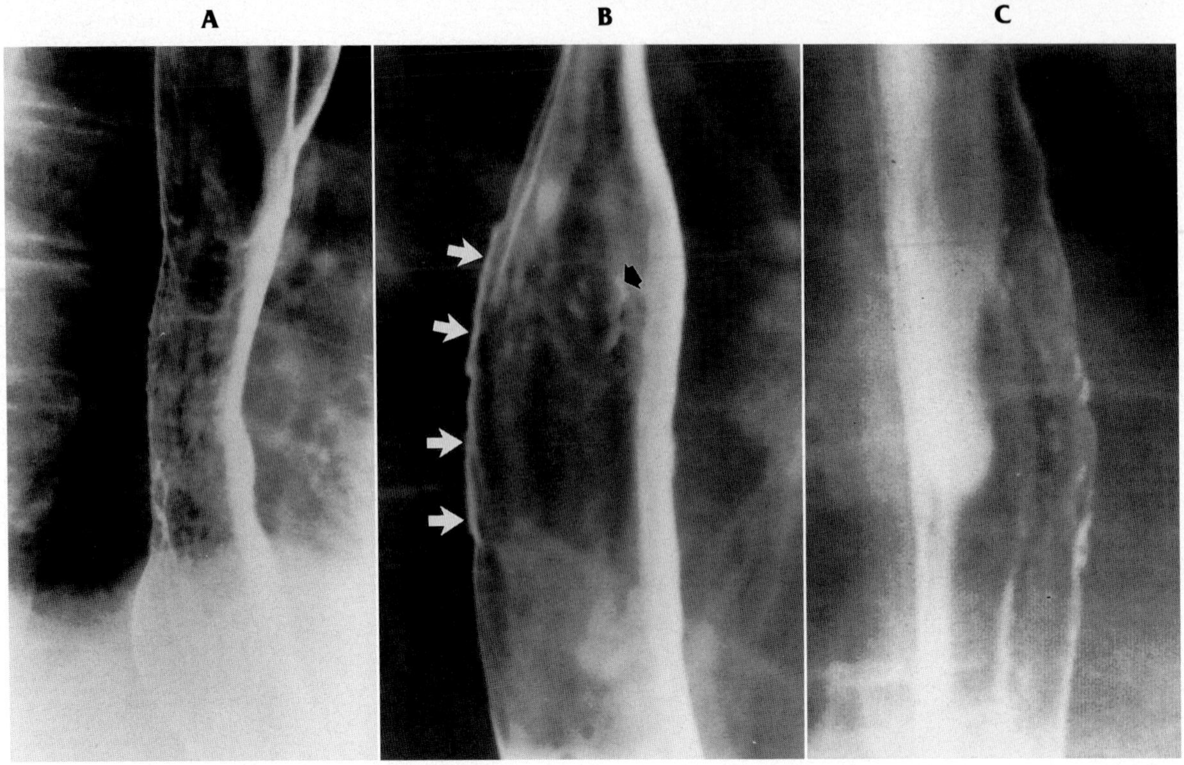


**FIGURE 4** Esophageal ulcers. *A,* Gastroesophageal reflux disease. There are superficial ulcers, asymmetric retraction, and narrowing (scarring) in the distal esophagus, extending up from the gastroesophageal junction. Note the hiatus hernia. *B,* CMV esophagitis shown as extensive midesophageal shallow ulceration. An ulcer is seen in profile as a depression in the mucosal line of the esophageal wall *(white arrows).* Another is seen en face as barium outlines the irregular edge of the ulcer *(black arrow). C,* Tetracycline ulcerative esophagitis with a cluster of tiny, superficial ulcers at the level of the aortic arch impression.

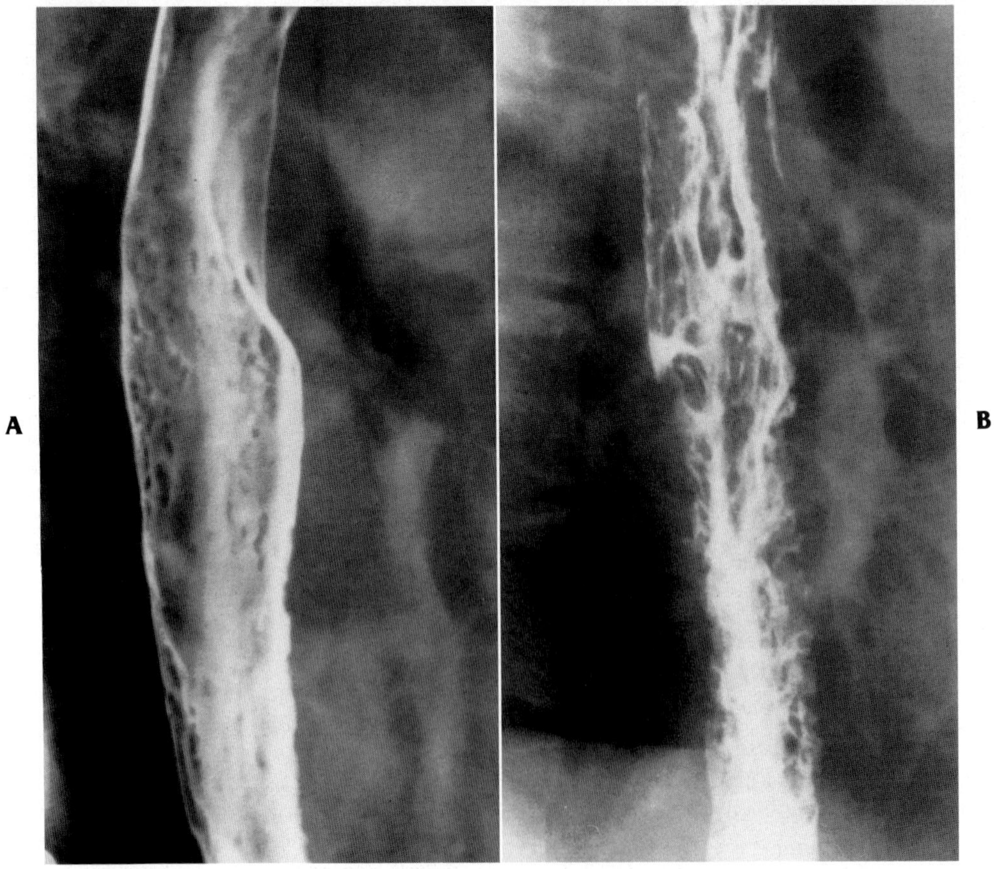


**FIGURE 5** Monilial esophagitis. *A,* Plaques are the usual manifestation of *Candida* esophagitis. They appear as well-defined, irregular-contoured, filling defects, longitudinally oriented with intervening normal mucosa. *B,* Shaggy esophagus is used to describe advanced *Candida* esophagitis, usually seen in patients with AIDS. Numerous coalescent plaques and pseudomembranes result in this grossly irregular esophageal contour.

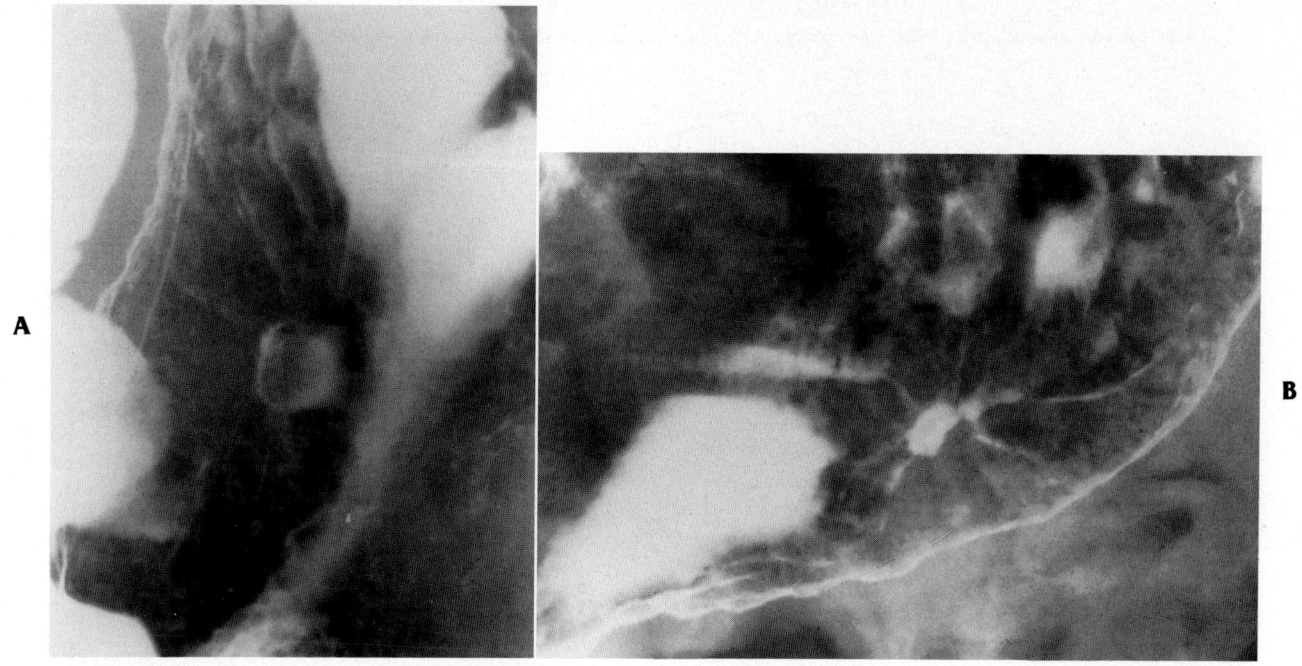

**FIGURE 6** Gastric ulcers. *A,* Typical benign gastric ulcer with a well-defined ulcer niche *(arrow)* and smooth surrounding radiating folds. *B,* Malignant gastric ulcer. The ulcer has an irregular shape, and the radiating folds are clubbed.

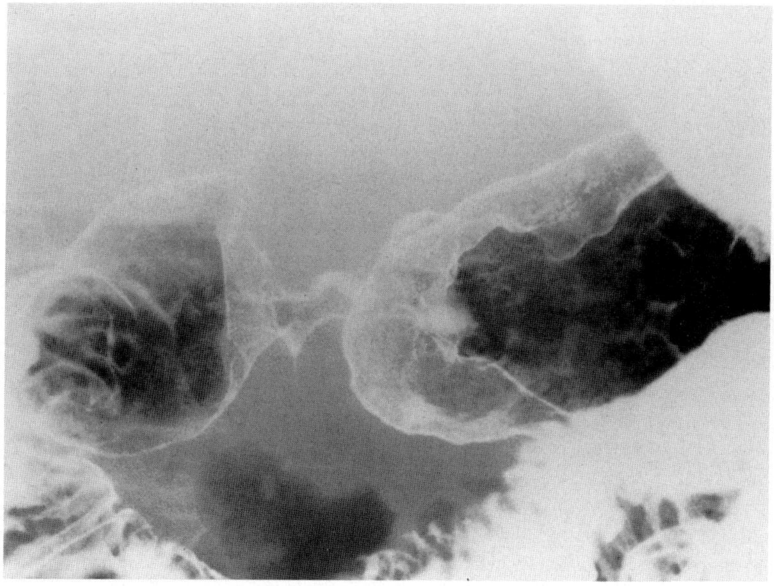

**FIGURE 7** Infiltration of the stomach in scirrhous cancer. There is marked nondistensibility of the gastric antrum with irregular narrowing and distortion of the surface pattern.

## Gastric Polyps

The double-contrast technique has increased the detection of polyps to 1 to 2 percent of examinations. A polyp is recognized en face on the dependent wall as a round filling defect in the barium pool and on the nondependent wall as a ring shadow as the barium etches the edge of the polyp in white (Fig. 8).

The vast majority of gastric polyps are hyperplastic polyps and appear as smooth, small ($\leq 1$ cm diameter), and often multiple lesions, most frequently in the body and fundus. These lesions are not premalignant and do not need endoscopic biopsy or removal.

Ten percent of gastric polyps are adenomas. These may progress to carcinoma with the risk reaching significance when they are 2 cm in diameter or greater. Adenomatous polyps are usually solitary, antral, lobulated, and occasionally pedunculated.

A submucosal polyp in the stomach is most commonly a leiomyoma or lipoma. These lesions are characterized by the intact overlying mucosa and right angles or obtuse angles created by the borders of the polyp when viewed in profile. Although these lesions are usually discovered incidentally, they occasionally ulcerate and cause hemorrhage (Fig. 9, *A*). Leiomyomas may undergo sarcomatous degeneration when they enlarge (Fig. 9, *B*).

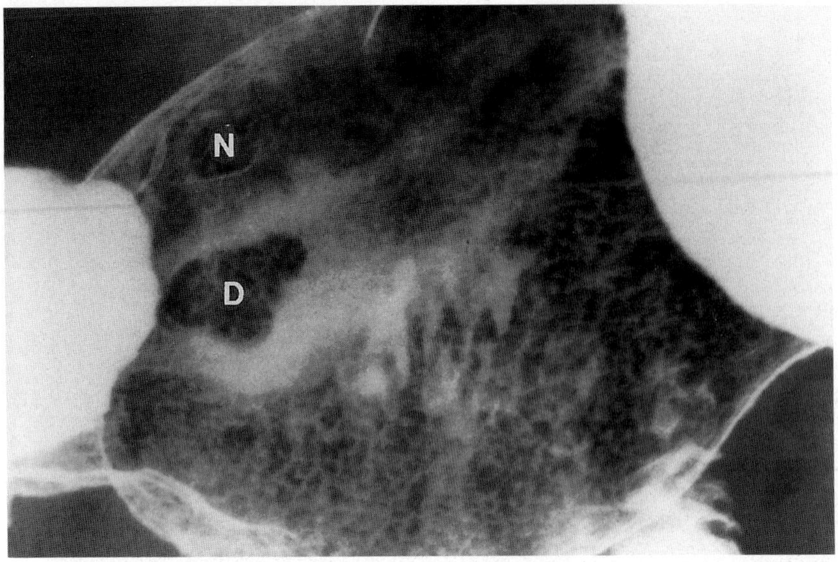


**FIGURE 8** Gastric polyps. Gastric polyps are seen on the dependent surface as a filling defect (D) in the shallow barium pool and on the nondependent surface as a ring shadow (N). These were submucosal polyps due to Kaposi's sarcoma.

A

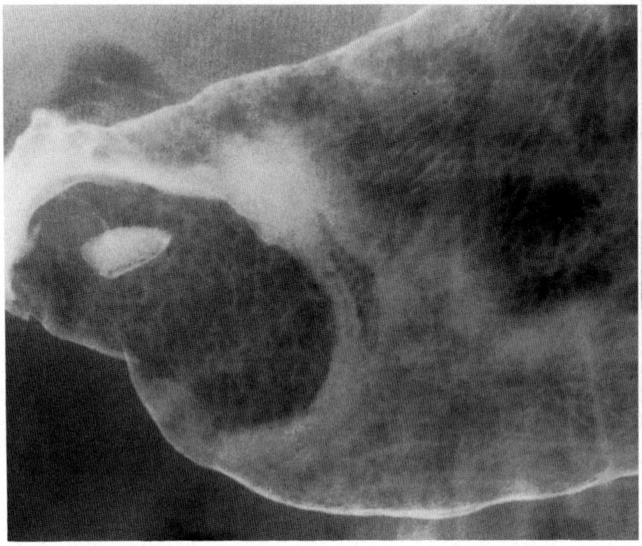

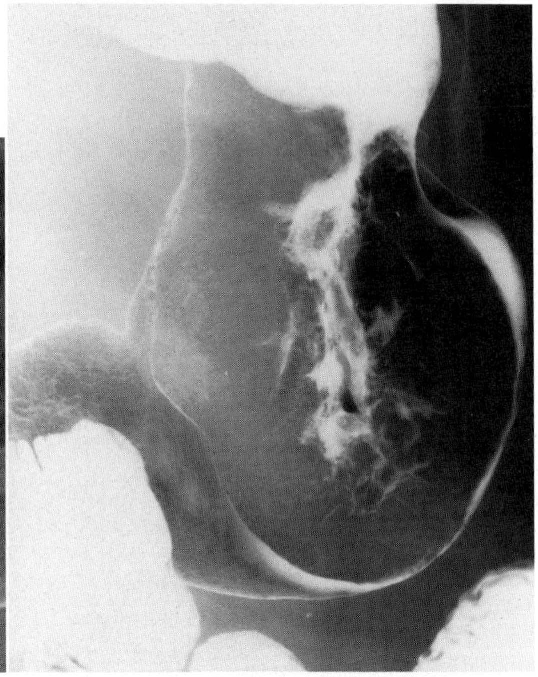

B

**FIGURE 9** Submucosal tumors of the stomach. *A,* Ulcerated leiomyoma. The tumor has a smooth surface with intact areae gastricae, indicating its submucosal location. The central collection of barium indicates ulceration. *B,* Leiomyosarcoma seen as a huge submucosal mass with a large cavitation. (*B* from Laufer I, Levine MS. Double Contrast Gastrointestinal Radiology. 2nd ed. Philadelphia: WB Saunders, 1992; with permission.)

## *Duodenum*

### Duodenal Ulcer

Duodenal ulcers are essentially always benign. Diagnosis of a duodenal ulcer is made by demonstration of an ulcer niche. This crater is usually surrounded by a smooth radiolucent mound of edematous mucosa and radiating folds. Ninety-five percent occurs in the duodenal bulb. These ulcers are best shown by double-contrast studies in the supine position (Fig. 10, *A*). Prone compression study is most useful to demonstrate ulcers on the anterior wall of the duodenal bulb, whereas the prone or upright position is needed to demonstrate ulcers on the medial wall of the descending duodenum above the papilla of Vater, with its associated radiating folds and indentation of the opposite wall of the duodenum (Fig. 10, *B*). Ulcers distal to the papilla of Vater should raise the possibility of Zollinger-Ellison syndrome.

## Pitfalls and Artifacts

The double-contrast technique makes it easier to distinguish true pathology from artifacts. This is done by the use of gravity and horizontal-beam films, which allow artifacts to be observed to flow away. However, the radiologist should be aware of some artifacts peculiar to this technique. Precipitation and floccu-

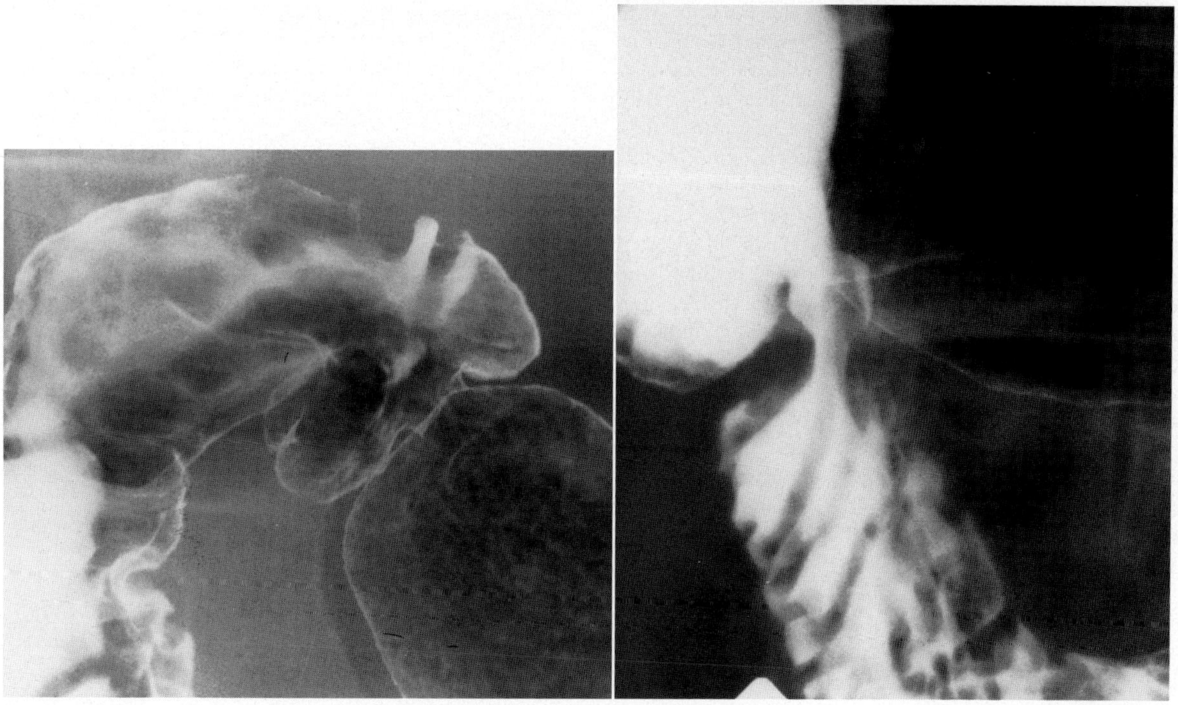


**FIGURE 10** Duodenal ulcer. *A,* Posterior wall ulcer of the duodenal bulb by double contrast is seen as an ovoid crater with radiating folds. *B,* Typical postbulbar ulcer *(arrow)* on the medial wall of the proximal descending duodenum. Note the indentation of the opposite wall.

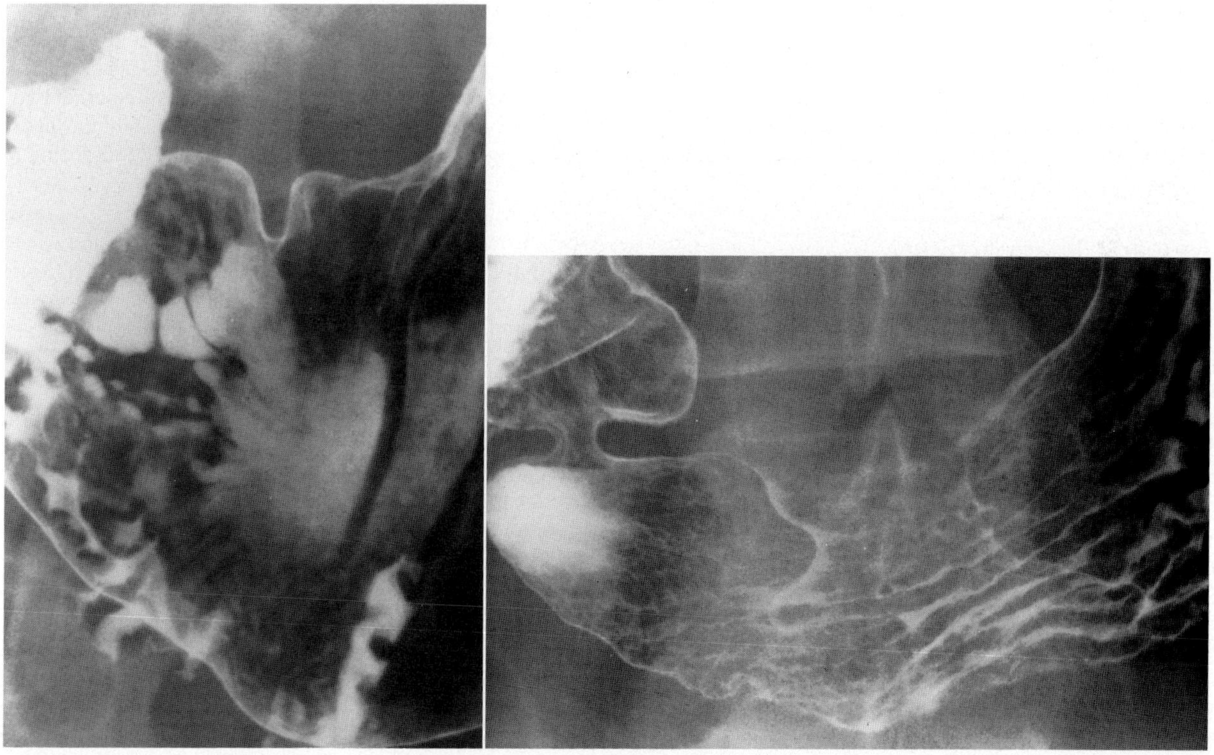


**FIGURE 11** Artifacts. *A,* Barium flocculation due to mucus within the stomach. *B,* Kissing artifact as a result of apposition of anterior and posterior walls in a slim patient.

lation of the barium suspension occurs in patients with excessive fluid and/or debris or in prolonged examinations (Fig. 11, *A*). The result simulates diffuse shallow ulceration but can be differentiated by the lack of edema or marginal irregularity, and barium is seen to lie on the mucosal surface rather than projecting beyond the luminal contour when viewed in profile.

Where there is insufficient gaseous distention to separate the anterior from the posterior walls, the region of contact is outlined by barium, producing an impression of an ulcer or polypoid lesion (Fig. 11, *B*). This is the "kissing artifact" and is readily recognized, because it disappears when the region is adequately distended. This artifact is particularly likely in examinations of slim patients.

The ability of the double-contrast technique to render the GI tract transparent produces a further problem. Any opacity (skeletal or other calcified structures and contrast-filled structures) may be projected within the GI tract and so simulate a lesion. Such artifacts are diagnosed by other projections showing the "lesion" in question to be projected outside the GI tract.

## Suggested Reading

Bova JG, Kamath V, Tio FO, et al. The normal mucosal surface pattern of the duodenal bulb: Radiologic-histologic correlation. AJR 1985; 145:735–738.

Glick SN, Teplick SK, Goldstein J, et al. Glycogenic acanthosis of the esophagus. AJR 1982; 139:683–688.

Gohel VK, Edell SL, Laufer I, et al. Transverse folds in the human esophagus. Radiology 1978; 128:303–308.

Gohel VK, Kressel HY, Laufer I. Double contrast artifacts. Gastrointest Radiol 1978; 3:139–146.

Herlinger H, Grossman R, Laufer I, et al. The gastric cardia in double-contrast study: Its dynamic image. AJR 1980; 135:21–29.

Laufer I, Levine MS. Double Contrast Gastrointestinal Radiology. 2nd ed. Philadelphia: WB Saunders, 1992.

Levine MS. Evaluation of dyspepsia or epigastric pain. Radiol Rep 1990; 2:347–352.

Levine MS, Kong V, Rubesin SE, et al. Scirrhous carcinoma of the stomach: Radiologic and endoscopic diagnosis. Radiology 1990; 175:151–154.

MacKintosh CE, Kreel L. Anatomy and radiology of the areae gastricae. Gut 1977; 18:855–864.

# Glucagon: Principles of Use and Adverse Reactions

*DEAN D. T. MAGLINTE, M.D. · STANLEY M. CHERNISH, M.D.*

The need to show greater detail in abdominal and gastrointestinal (GI) imaging procedures has required a pharmacological agent that abolishes peristalsis and relaxes the smooth muscle of the GI tract. Because of its predictable onset and duration of action, as well as its minimal side effects, glucagon has replaced anticholinergic agents as the drug of choice for this purpose in the United States. Its ability to decrease resistance in certain sphincters has extended its use to some therapeutic applications.

## History and Pharmacology

In early studies of insulin in humans, scientists noted that there was a short temporary rise in the blood sugar before insulin took effect. More than 30 years later (1953), research scientists isolated and then crystalized glucagon. Glucagon was determined to be another hormone, which, in conjunction with insulin, served to maintain the blood sugar within a normal range. About 1960 glucagon was marketed for the treatment of hypoglycemia in diabetic patients.

In 1972, while investigating the effects of glucagon on the human gallbladder, Chernish and Miller noted a hypotonic effect on the duodenum. Randomized, double-blinded, crossover studies on volunteers were then done, evaluating the effect of glucagon on the duodenum, stomach, small bowel, and colon. From that point on, the use of glucagon to relax the GI tract during radiologic procedures is history. In the initial studies of glucagon, the large doses used were known to be safe, because these doses were safe and effective when given to diabetics for the treatment of hypoglycemia. Clinical studies have since shown that smaller doses of glucagon are effective in producing hypotonia or atonia with few adverse effects.

Physically glucagon is a white powder; chemically it is a single-chain polypeptide secreted by the alpha cells of the islets of Langerhans and contains 29 amino acid residues with a molecular weight of 3,484. It is relatively insoluble in water but soluble at a pH of less than 3 or more than 9.5. It is stable in lyophilized form at room temperatures. Glucagon for injection, USP, contains 1 mg (1 U) of glucagon and 49 mg of lactose. The diluent that comes with glucagon contains 1.6 percent glycerin with 0.2 percent phenol as a preservative. Sodium hydroxide and/or hydrochloric acid may have been added during manufacture to adjust the pH.

When glucagon is given parenterally, there is increased blood sugar concentration in both the diabetic patient and in normal people. Glucagon acts on liver glycogen, converting it to glucose. The half-life of glucagon in plasma is approximately 3 to 6 minutes, which is similar to that of insulin. Late effects occur because of stimulation of insulin production.

Glucagon relaxes the duodenal sweep, duodenal bulb, small bowel, stomach, and the large bowel, in that order of effectiveness. It appears to act directly on smooth muscle by enhancing adenyl cyclase activity, rather than by neuromuscular transmission.

## Applications

### *Studies of the Esophagus*

In studies of the esophagus in patients with esophageal varices, glucagon did not relax the esophagus but has been reported to relax the gastroesophageal junction. An anticholinergic agent is therefore needed if relaxation of the esophageal body is desired to demonstrate esophageal varices.

In radiologic practice the effect of glucagon on the lower esophageal sphincter is used in the treatment of acute esophageal food impaction. Following identification of the impacted foreign body by single-contrast esophagography, we

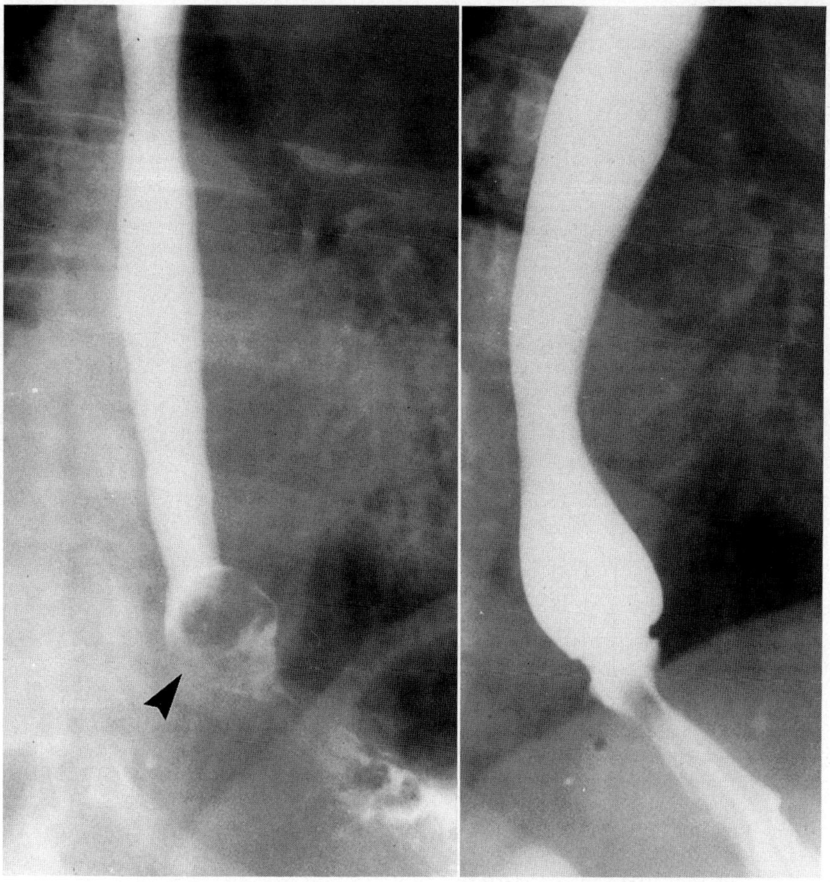


**FIGURE 1** Glucagon to relieve food impaction in distal esophagus. *A*, Esophagogram showing foreign body (meat) impacted in distal esophagus *(arrow)*. Nonpropulsive contractions were seen in lower esophagus fluoroscopically. *B*, Repeat esophagogram following administration of 1 mg glucagon IV. A packet of effervescent agent and a half glass of water were given by mouth 5 minutes after glucagon infusion. The gastroesophageal junction is relaxed. The impacted foreign body has passed. A small axial hiatus hernia and a nonstenotic ring are noted. A 13 mm barium tablet passed unimpeded.

inject 1 mg of glucagon IV with the patient supine. A packet of effervescent agent and water is then given with the patient in the upright position. If the patient feels that the impacted food has passed, a multiphasic esophageal study is performed to determine the etiology of the impaction (Fig. 1). If the first administration of effervescent agent and water is unsuccessful, we allow the patient to rest for 20 to 30 minutes and then repeat the administration of gas and water. Although not uniformly successful, this approach is efficient, safe, and cost-effective, but it should be avoided if the impacted foreign body is sharp (bone fragments suspected) or if pneumomediastinum is observed. Glucagon is ineffective if the foreign body is impacted in other segments of the esophagus.

## *Studies of the Stomach and Duodenum*

Abolishment of gastric peristalsis is an essential part of the modern biphasic upper GI evaluation (Fig. 2). In our practice we use a small dose of intravenous glucagon routinely. For upper GI studies, 0.25 mg IV allows us about 5 to 8.5 minutes to study the stomach and 7.5 to 12.5 minutes to study the duodenal bulb and the sweep (Fig. 3). The glucagon is injected slowly before ingestion of the effervescent granules. The lag time of intravenously administered glucagon (45 seconds) allows us to perform the esophageal survey while waiting for its effect on the stomach and duodenum. The use of remote-control fluoroscopic units has allowed us to examine simultaneously the stomach and duodenum. The overlap of the duodenum on segments of the stomach is erased by angled radiography and by positioning. This has decreased our total procedure time. If the patient moves slowly, a larger dose of glucagon is administered to allow more time for the procedure. When a known or suspected lesion requires further evaluation, the patient can be given a second dose of glucagon. Postgastrectomy patients require a larger dose to distend and coat the gastric remnant and to fill the afferent loop.

A similar dose of glucagon is given for tubeless hypotonic duodenography (see Fig. 3). Radiographs of the esophagus and stomach are not done if these areas have already been examined.

Because glucagon is not inexpensive and can occasionally prolong examination time of the upper GI tract, the minimum effective dose should be used.[1] Table 1 gives the average

[1] Glucagon is marketed in 1 mg ampules, which can hold only 3 ml of solution. After mixing the glucagon with 1 ml diluent, this is brought to 3 ml by removing 2 ml of air and adding 2 ml of 0.9 percent sodium chloride or 5 percent dextrose in water. At this dilution 0.3 ml is equivalent to 0.1 mg. This ampule should be discarded when the GI studies are completed that day.

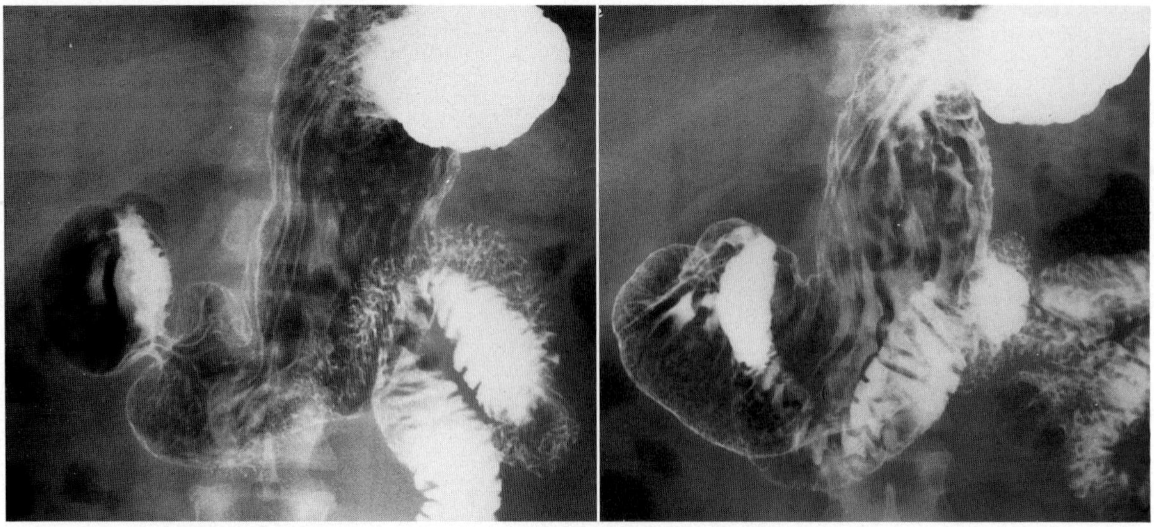


**FIGURE 2** Effect of minidose glucagon on the stomach and duodenum. *A,* Before glucagon administration. *B,* Same patient 1 minute following IV injection of 0.1 mg glucagon. Note improved visualization of area gastricae. The added effect of glucagon in diminishing hydrochloric acid and peptic gastric secretions allow better visualization of small surface lesions as erosions, polyps, ulcers, and early gastric cancer. The myorelaxant effect allows the high-density low-viscosity barium mixture longer contact with the sulci gastricae and gastric pits, thus improving surface coating. Note improved filling of duodenal sweep and better fold depiction compared with *(A).*

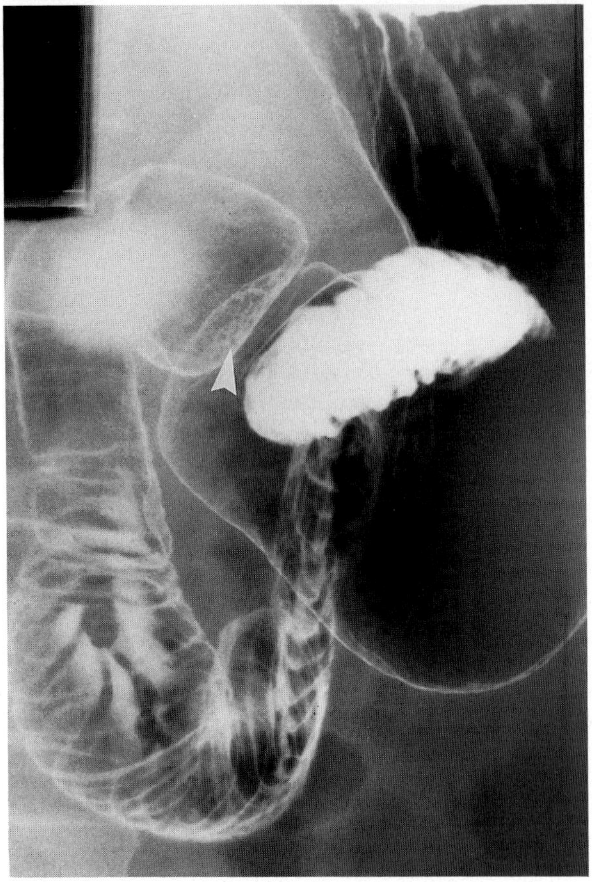

**FIGURE 3** "Tubeless" hypotonic duodenography with glucagon. The entire duodenum can be examined in detail without intubation as part of a hypotonic biphasic upper GI examination using 0.2 mg glucagon IV. Normal anatomical structures at level of ampulla should be discernible with proper technique. Note details of small amount of heterotopic gastric mucosa at the base of the duodenal bulb *(arrow).*

duration of action of glucagon on the upper GI tract and small bowel. The speed of the examiner and the ability of the patient to move determine the optimal dose.

### Small Bowel Studies

Since our adoption of enteroclysis as the primary method of examining the small bowel, we have not found glucagon to be necessary. Adjustment of the rate of infusion of contrast renders the small bowel hypotonic during the methylcellulose double-contrast phase of a biphasic enteroclysis. However, if enteroclysis is performed per ileostomy, we administer 0.5 mg glucagon IV before intubation. This abolishes peristalsis and diminishes discomfort during the retrograde examination (Fig. 4). We have also used glucagon as advocated by Dr. R. E. Miller when performing the occasional retrograde small bowel enema. It relaxes the bowel and ileocecal valve, thus making the examination more acceptable to the patient. The use of enteroclysis has markedly decreased the use of the retrograde small bowel enema in our practice.

### Studies of the Colon

The lowest effective dose of glucagon on the colon is 0.75 mg IV. For ease of preparation, we use 1 mg.

In studies of the colon, hypotonic agents have been recommended for patients with (1) lesions with diffuse painful spasm, ulcerative or granulomatous colitis, or functional disorders; (2) areas of localized narrowing—spasms versus constricting lesion, colonic valves or sphincters, or evaluation of strictures in colitis; (3) diverticular disease with sigmoid spasm; (4) decrease in smooth muscle tone for adequate distention during air-contrast study; and (5) functional inability to retain the enema, observed especially in aged patients. In these cases 1 mg IV of glucagon is usually given slowly, just before the barium is given or at the time of the spasm (Fig. 5).

**TABLE 1** Average Duration in Minutes of Atonicity and Moderate Hypotonicity of the Stomach, Duodenal Bulb, Duodenum, and Proximal and Distal Small Bowel in 15 Subjects Given Placebo and Glucagon

| Gastrointestinal Tract | | Placebo | Glucagon Dose 0.25 mg | 0.5 mg | 1 mg | 2 mg |
|---|---|---|---|---|---|---|
| Stomach | Atonic | 0.0 (2)* | 4.9 (11) | 8.7 (14) | 10.1 | 15.1 |
| | Moderately hypotonic | 0.6 (2) | 8.5 | 13.1 | 14.7 | 21.7 |
| Duodenal bulb | Atonic | 0.0 (0) | 7.5 | 10.1 | 12.5 | 16.7 |
| | Moderately hypotonic | 1.3 (3) | 12.5 | 16.2 | 18.3 | 24.0 |
| Duodenum | Atonic | 0.0 (0) | 7.8 | 10.1 | 12.5 | 16.1 |
| | Moderately hypotonic | 1.4 (3) | 12.2 | 16.5 | 18.7 | 23.7 |
| Proximal small bowel | Atonic | 0.0 (0) | 8.3 | 9.4 | 13.7 | 19.7 |
| | Moderately hypotonic | 0.1 (1) | 11.5 | 14.9 | 19.7 | 25.0 |
| Distal small bowel | Atonic | 0.0 (0) | 8.6 | 9.4 | 14.0 | 19.7 |
| | Moderately hypotonic | 0.1 (1) | 11.9 | 14.7 | 20.3 | 24.3 |

*( )Number of subjects who achieved response. All are 15 unless otherwise noted.
From Miller RE, Chernish SM, et al. Double-blind radiographic study of dose response to intravenous glucagon for hypotonic radiography. Radiology 1978; 127:555–559; with permission.

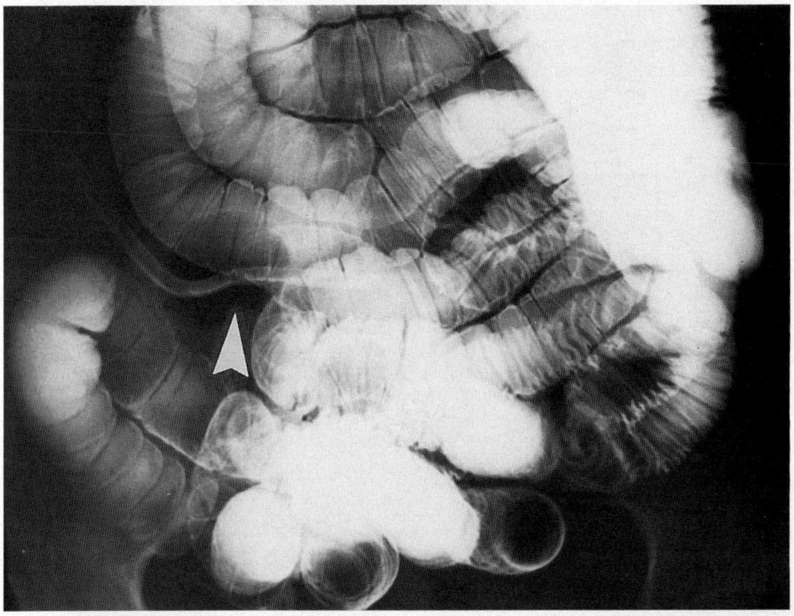

**FIGURE 4** Per ileostomy enteroclysis. The use of 0.5 mg glucagon IV results in diminished discomfort to patient and uniform distention of the small bowel from prestomal ileum to proximal jejunum. Note the balloon of the enteroclysis catheter *(arrow)* occluding stoma from within, below the level of peritoneal lining.

A 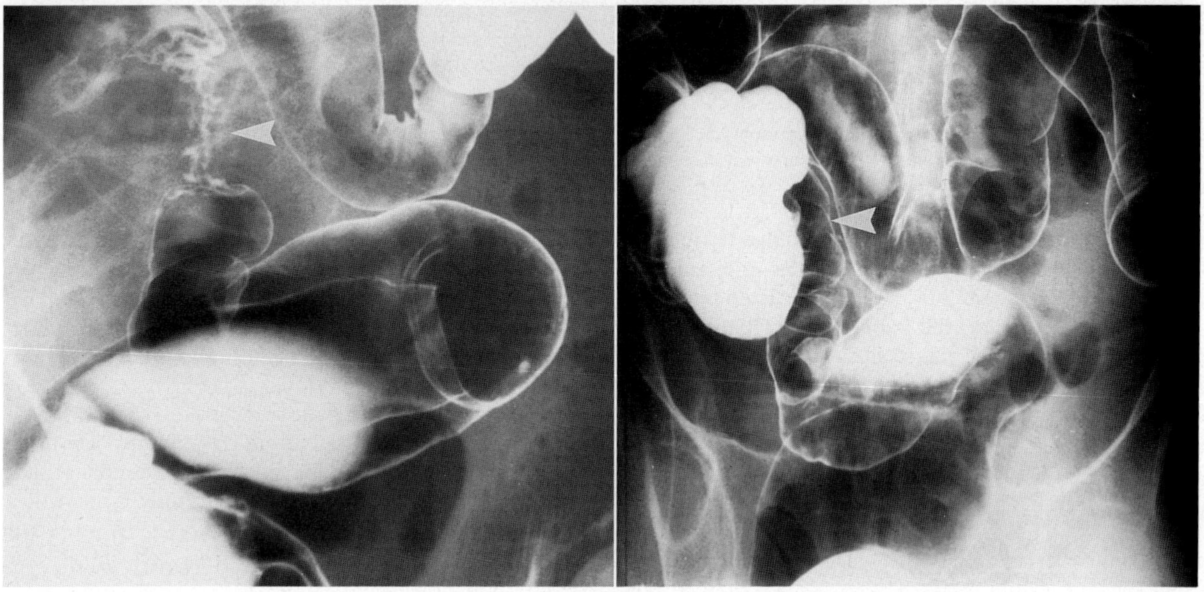 B

**FIGURE 5** Use of glucagon to relieve colonic spasm. *A,* Spot radiograph of a double-contrast examination showing an area of narrowing in sigmoid *(arrow),* simulating an infiltrating lesion. *B,* Area of narrowing disappeared *(arrow)* following IV administration of 1 mg glucagon, indicating spasm as the cause of the pseudolesion.

A

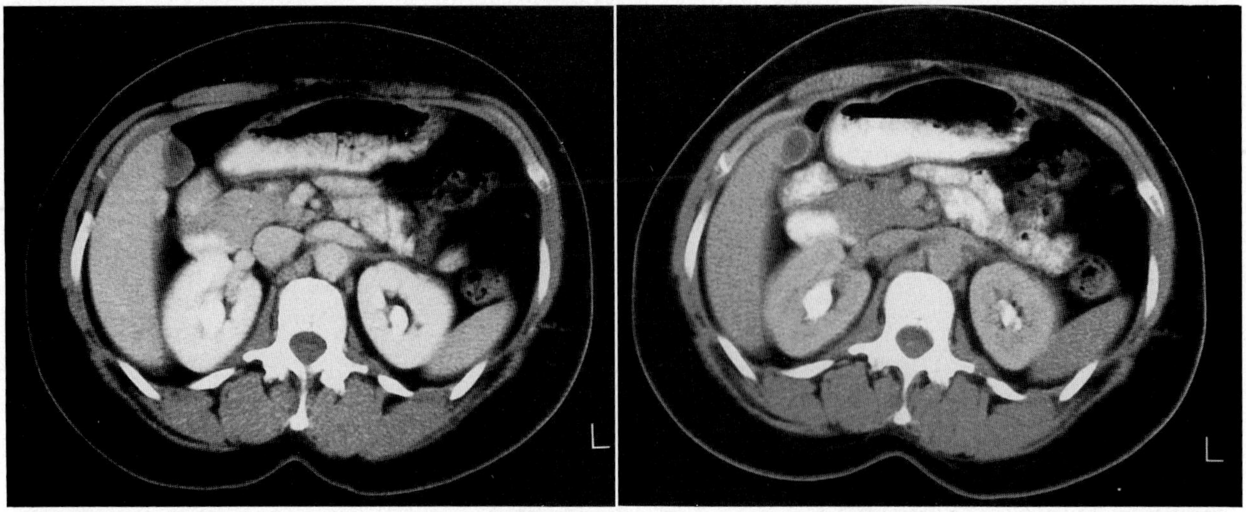

B

**FIGURE 6** Glucagon in abdominal CT. *A,* Section through upper abdomen, 2 second scanning time, before glucagon administration. *B,* Repeat scan through the same level following 1 mg of glucagon IV. Abolition of peristalsis and the resulting hypotonicity have improved delineation of the gastric walls, providing a better filling of the descending duodenum including segments of the small bowel. Also note the effect of glucagon on the gallbladder. (Courtesy of Thomas N. Vahey, M.D., Methodist Hospital of Indiana, Indianapolis, IN.)

A

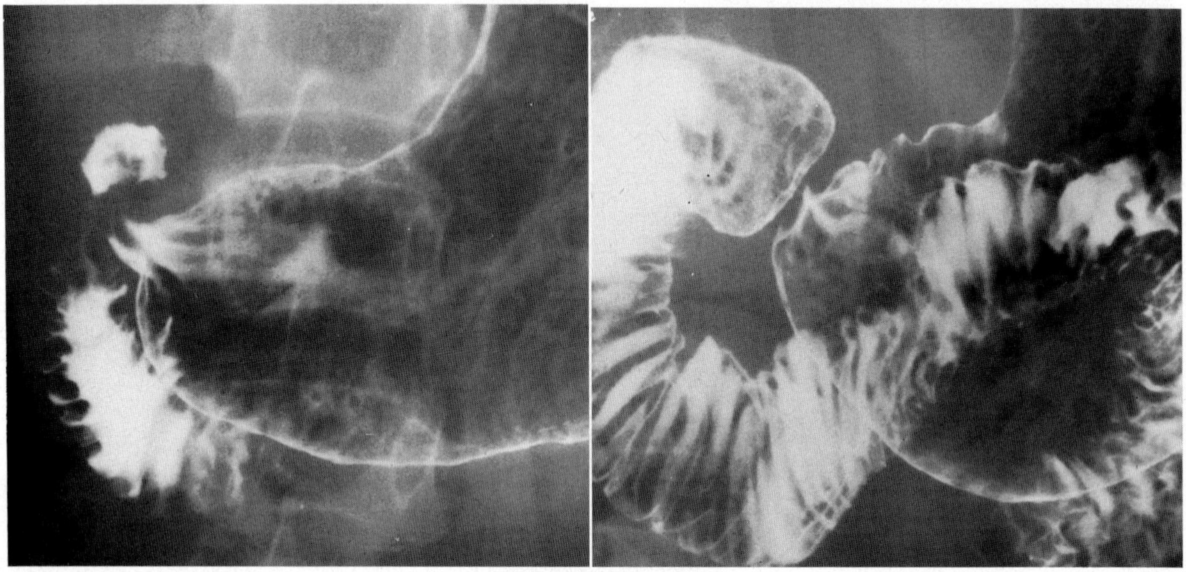

B

**FIGURE 7** Glucagon in pediatric hypotonic radiography. *A,* Spot radiograph (before glucagon administration) of distal stomach and duodenum during a double-contrast examination of 7-year-old patient. *B,* Spot radiograph of same area following 0.05 mg glucagon IV. Surface details of the stomach and duodenum are shown better after glucagon administration. The duodenal bulb and sweep are better filled.

Because most of our patients fit the above categories and, in our experience, the onset of action of glucagon appears unpredictable when spasm has already occurred and the patient appears to tolerate the barium enema better when glucagon is given, we give 1 mg of glucagon IV before rectal intubation for both single- and double-contrast barium enema studies.

## *Abdominal Computed Tomography or Magnetic Resonance Imaging*

When abdominal imaging is to be performed, the dose of glucagon selected should relax all areas of the GI tract. For abdominal computed tomography (CT), even with current 2 second scanning times, the diagnostic value of glucagon is apparent (Fig. 6). For ease of preparation and to allow for rescans, 1 mg is optimal for abdominal CT. This is not necessary with barium studies or endoscopy where the dose to be used can be tailored to the segment of the GI tract to be examined. One must remember, when tailoring the dose how much is minimally effective.

For abdominal magnetic resonance imaging (MRI), 1 mg of glucagon is needed with current pulse sequences. When more is given, the effect is prolonged. With doses greater than 1 mg, the side effects are increased significantly.

## *Glucagon in Infants and Children*

Glucagon has been used in infants and children during GI radiologic examinations. A dose of 0.5 to 1.0 μg/kg body weight

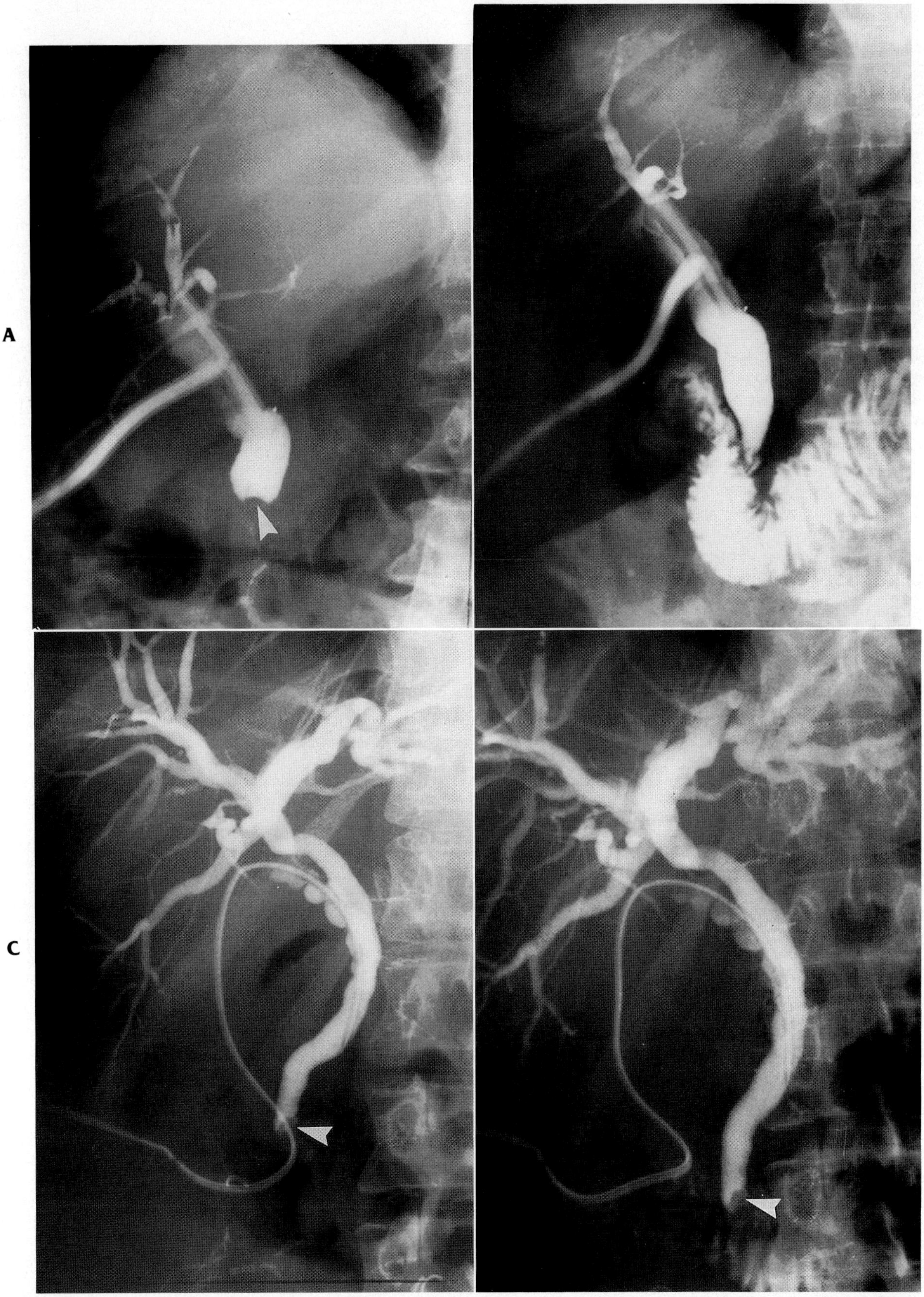

**FIGURE 8** Value of glucagon in differentiating pseudocalculus defect from retained distal common duct calculus. *A,* Initial radiograph of a T-tube cholangiogram showing a defect *(arrow),* simulating a distal common duct calculus. *B,* Following IV administration of 1 mg glucagon, the defect has disappeared, indicating a pseudocalculus defect. Unobstructed egress of contrast into the descending duodenum is now seen. This is caused by the decreased resistance at the sphincter of Oddi and the increased bile flow induced by glucagon. *C,* Initial radiograph of a postoperative cholangiogram, showing a defect in the distal common duct *(arrow)* suggestive of a retained stone. Note the lack of contrast drainage into duodenum. *D,* Defect persists *(arrow)* after IV administration of 1 mg glucagon, indicating retained calculus. Drainage into the duodenum is now seen.

given intravenously produces satisfactory atonicity for 3 to 5 minutes using double-contrast meals. For barium enema studies, doses of 0.8 to 1.25 μg/kg IV to produce atonicity for 5 to 10 minutes have been recommended. The benefits of these small doses of intravenous glucagon are as follows: (1) atony of stomach and duodenum, permitting a good double contrast examination (Fig. 7); (2) rapid return to normal, permitting motility to be examined; (3) relief of painful and obstructive spasm in barium enemas; (4) quieting of angry, hungry infants; and (5) probable shortening of the total examination time. No undesirable side effects have been observed.

### *Cholangiography*

Because of its effect on the sphincter of Oddi, glucagon is of value in cholangiography in the differentiation of a pseudocalculus defect from retained distal common duct calculus (Fig. 8).

The distal common bile duct can be difficult to visualize, especially if it is not dilated, despite the increase in resolution of modern gray-scale ultrasonography equipment. The use of water in the duodenum and glucagon given intravenously, to stop duodenal motion, has improved the ability to demonstrate the distal common bile duct during ultrasonography. This may have current relevance in the screening for common bile duct stones before laparoscopic cholecystectomy.

### *Expulsion of Biliary Calculi*

Impacted calculi in the distal common bile duct are difficult to engage with a basket and can be responsible for the failure of the steerable catheter technique. When ampullary spasm is relieved with 1 mg of glucagon given IV, small and even large (6 mm) stones can be pushed through the ampulla of Vater into the duodenum. This method has proved successful when percutaneous stone removal has failed.

### *Hysterosalpingography*

The myorelaxant effect of glucagon has been used to differentiate between tubal spasm and occlusion from organic strictures. Tubal patency is more obvious when there is more visible free peritoneal spill, which may be facilitated by glucagon given intravenously.

## Adverse Effects

The most common complaint, from all doses of glucagon given intravenously to volunteers and all symptoms reported for 4 hours after drug was given, was nausea and/or vomiting. In practice, nausea is not uncommon when 0.5 to 1 mg of glucagon is injected (IV) quickly. This dose should be injected slowly (over a period of 1 minute) to prevent or decrease this complication. When one gives 2 mg, one gains about 3 to 5 minutes of hypotonicity at the expense of almost twice the number of adverse effects. During double-blind studies in volunteers, there were no changes in the respirations, pulse, systolic or diastolic blood pressure as compared with placebo.

Glucagon should be administered cautiously to patients with a history suggestive of insulinoma and/or pheochromocytoma. In patients with insulinoma, intravenous glucagon produces an initial increase in blood glucose; however, because of the insulin-releasing effect of glucagon, it may cause the insulinoma to release its insulin and subsequently cause hypoglycemia. A patient developing hypoglycemia after a dose of glucagon should be given glucose orally, intravenously, or through a nasogastric tube. Exogenous glucagon can stimulate the release of catecholamines. In the presence of pheochromocytoma, glucagon can cause the tumor to release catecholamines, resulting in a sudden and marked increase in blood pressure. If a patient suddenly develops hypertension, 5 to 10 mg of phentolamine mesylate may be administered IV in an attempt to control the blood pressure.

There are virtually no contraindications to glucagon in small doses of 0.1 to 0.2 mg given IV. It is contraindicated in patients with a known hypersensitivity or in patients with pheochromocytoma. Generalized allergic reactions, including urticaria, respiratory distress, and hypotension, have been reported in patients who have received glucagon by injection but are rare.

## Discussion

The ability of glucagon to abolish peristalsis and allow full distention of the stomach, duodenum, small bowel, and colon, combined with its ability to decrease resistance or tone of certain sphincters, have made it the main pharmacologic agent in abdominal and GI radiology. Radiologists are currently among the major users of glucagon in the United States.

## **Suggested Reading**

Chernish SM, Miller RE, Rosenak BD, Scholz NE. Hypotonic duodenography with the use of glucagon. Gastroenterology 1972; 63:392–398.

Chernish SM, Miller RE, Rosenak BD, Scholz NE. Effect of glucagon on size of visualized human gallbladder before and after a fat meal. Gastroenterology 1972; 62:1218–1226.

Ferrucci JT Jr, Benedict KT Jr. Anticholinergic-aided study of the gastrointestinal tract. Radiol Clin North Am 1971; 9:23–39.

Kreel L. Glucagon in radiology. In Picazo J, ed. Glucagon in Gastroenterology. Baltimore: University Park Press, 1979:61.

Latshaw RF, Kadir S, Watt WS, et al. Glucagon-induced choledochal sphincter relaxation: Aid for expulsion of impacted calculi into the duodenum. AJR 1981; 137:614–616.

Maglinte DDT, Caudill LD, Krol KL, et al. The minimum effective dose of glucagon in upper gastrointestinal radiography. Gastrointest Radiol 1982; 7:119–122.

Maglinte DDT, Chernish SM. The optimal dose of glucagon: What is enough? Radiology 1992; 183:326–327.

Pons MS, Cooperberg PG. Technical note: Oral water and intravenous glucagon – to aid ultrasonic visualization of the common bile duct. J Can Assoc Radiol 1979; 30:173–174.

Ratcliffe JF. Glucagon in barium enema examination in infants and children: Special reference to dosage. Br J Radiol 1980; 53:860–862.

Taylor I, Duthie HL, Cumberland DC, Smallwood R. Glucagon and the colon. Gut 1975; 16:973–978.

# Double-Contrast Barium Enema

*PETER J. FECZKO, M.D.*

The last two decades have seen a revolutionary change in the diagnosis of colorectal disease. The impetus for this has been the development of the fiber-optic endoscope. With the detail and flexibility allowed by these instruments, the threshold of pathology now detected is measured in millimeters and not centimeters. Unfortunately the radiologic community has been slower to adapt, and it is only in the last decade that studies have shown a shift from the older single-contrast colon evaluation (single-contrast barium enema [SCBE]), with limited detection of luminal and mucosal abnormalities, to the more sensitive double-contrast colon examination (double-contrast barium enema [DCBE]), with its inherent ability to detect more subtle pathologic changes in the colon (Fig. 1). Despite this, it is well documented that there has been a rather sharp decrease in radiologic studies of the colon during this same period.

Certainly the shift in examination methodology reflects a need for a highly detailed evaluation of the colon. The DCBE is designed to assess two of the three major pathologic entities in the colon: neoplasia and inflammation. Colorectal carcinoma is now one of the most common malignancies in industrialized nations, representing the third leading cause of cancer deaths in the United States in both men and women. It is also recognized that carcinoma arises from a precursor lesion, the adenomatous polyp. Thus the thrust of colon evaluation in all its forms involves not only carcinoma detection, but polyp detection and removal as well. Another diagnostic category well suited for the DCBE is inflammatory bowel disease (IBD). IBD is now detected in all age and ethnic groups. With the increasing prevalence of human immunodeficiency virus, the incidence of infectious colitides is increasing.

Although this is beyond the scope of this chapter, endoscopy and DCBE are complementary in their diagnostic ability, with some areas of weakness apparent in both methods. Controversy surrounds the issue of which method is most desirable, and this may never be resolved. From the radiologist's point of view, however, it is apparent that the DCBE is currently the only radiologic imaging modality that can hope to remain competitive with endoscopy.

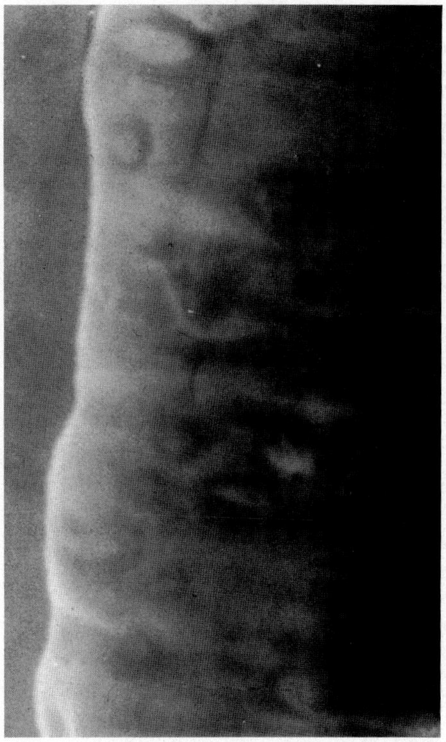

**FIGURE 1** The DCBE has the ability to show fine mucosal detail. Close-up view of colonic mucosa shows tiny aphthous ulcers measuring only a few millimeters in diameter.

## Indications for DCBE

Perhaps this can best be answered by indicating which patients should not have a DCBE. Most outpatient colon evaluations are performed for reasons (i.e., anemia, bleeding, diarrhea, occult blood) that warrant a DCBE. It is my policy that the standard outpatient radiographic evaluation of the colon is the DCBE.

Patients who do not receive a DCBE are usually those with suspected bowel obstruction of any type, ischemic bowel, and acute diverticulitis. Patients with an acute toxic colitis or suspected bowel perforation should not have a barium enema study performed. Although it has been shown that the DCBE can be consistently performed on the elderly, I admit that age and physical considerations are factors in the selection of the type of examination. Because of the slow growth of neoplastic polyps, high prevalence of diverticular disease, and frequent physical disability, patients over the age of 80 usually receive a SCBE. Of course, each patient should be evaluated individually, and clinical information is still the most important guide in selecting the type of examination.

One difficult area concerns patients with abdominal pain. If the patient has vague symptoms and no fever or elevated white blood cell (WBC) count, I still perform a DCBE. However, if the pain is highly specific, or if the patient has a fever or elevated WBC count, computed tomography should probably be performed, and then possibly a SCBE. Another problematic area concerns patients who have had recent biopsy. If a large tumor or mass has been biopsied, I usually proceed with the study even if the patient is sent to us directly from endoscopy. If the patients have a superficial mucosal biopsy through a fiber-optic endoscope, it is permissible to proceed with a DCBE, but I prefer to wait 48 hours. Biopsies through the rigid proctoscope are usually much deeper and it is wise to wait 5 to 7 days before proceeding with a DCBE.

## Bowel Preparation

Since the time of the first barium enemas, radiologists have appreciated the importance of thorough bowel cleansing. Even in the presence of some fecal contamination, the DCBE is still preferable over a SCBE because the positional views (decubitus, upright) demonstrate movement of the fecal material and make it easier to differentiate polyps from feces.

There are numerous methods for bowel cleansing, and several commercial packages are available, usually at a reasonable cost. Regardless of which method is chosen, two fundamental procedures should be applied: (1) low-residue (liquid) diet for 24 hours preceding the examination, and (2) high oral fluid intake during bowel preparation.

Cleansing enemas are acceptable as part of the bowel preparation, but it is wise to wait at least 1 hour after an enema so that excess fluid is resorbed by the colon and does not diminish mucosal coating by the barium.

## Technical Aspects of Examination

After many years of performing the DCBE, I still have great satisfaction in personally doing the examination. No matter what method of DCBE you employ, your goal should be to consistently produce a good diagnostic study with as little patient discomfort as possible. Attention to the "atmosphere" of the fluoroscopy section can be more important than bowel preparation or what barium is used. For that reason, I would like to address some issues that are never discussed by the "experts."

### *Technical Support*

The importance of having your technologists dedicated to producing high-quality DCBEs cannot be overemphasized. Not only does the quality of the study improve, the work is more enjoyable, and patient satisfaction is higher. If possible, you should have a core of full-time gastrointestinal (GI) technologists who spend the majority of their time in fluoroscopy. Admittedly this is not always feasible, and a substitute for this is to have the general technicians rotate on a weekly (not daily) basis. You will be surprised at how the work improves during the week. I have used GI technologists to perform DCBEs, and they consistently outperform residents and non-GI radiologists.

### *Positive Mental Attitude*

All personnel in the department should be instructed to be as positive and "upbeat" as possible. From the patient viewpoint, this is one of the most distasteful examinations to undergo, and the patient has already gone through the rigors of the bowel preparation. Any negative comments or experiences will further complicate the examination. Receptionists, technologists, and other personnel should maintain a cheerful, reassuring attitude with the patient.

### *Communication*

The importance of good communication must be emphasized. Throughout the examination either I or the technician will ask the patient how he or she is feeling. This not only reassures patients, but distracts them from what is occurring. It is helpful to take their mind off the examination, particularly when you are placing liters of air and fluid into their bowel. Many technicians emphasize slow, deep breathing as a form of relaxation for the patient, and I have found this to be successful.

### *Fluoroscopy Room*

The type of equipment is dependent on many factors, but given a choice, I prefer remote-controlled fluoroscopy. Its advantages include the ability for tube angulation, larger selection of cassette sizes, and ability to obtain "overhead" films rapidly. Equipment is readily available to control the enema remotely, and for the DCBE, compression is not critical. In a busy outpatient setting, other studies are easily performed with remote-controlled fluoroscopy when the GI schedule is done. Another detail is to keep the fluoroscopy room clean and orderly, and if possible there should be wallpaper and pictures.

### *Enema Equipment*

A variety of commercially available equipment exists for the DCBE. I always use an enema tip with an inflatable retention cuff in case it is necessary, but I do not inflate it routinely, and only inflate under fluoroscopy.

## Method of Examination

A variety of methods have been described for the DCBE and no particular method is ideal for all circumstances. I am a strong advocate of a "tailored" DCBE. That is, a few basic principles should be followed, and then other aspects of filling, filming, and so on should depend on the clinical situation and pathologic/anatomic considerations. The importance of fluoroscopic observation cannot be overemphasized, since one must be ready to adjust the examination to what is encountered. What follows is my preferred technique in performing the DCBE.

### *Enema Tip Insertion*

The enema tip should be inserted with the patient in the left lateral position. The use of a retention cuff is recommended even if it is not inflated. The cheeks of the buttock should be taped together so that the tip does not slip out. Simply taping the enema tip to the buttock does not seem to help. A female should insert the tip into a female patient, and all patients should be properly covered to put them at ease.

### *Barium Instillation*

I start the patient in the left lateral position and introduce the barium until it reaches the splenic flexure. I then turn the patient prone, and barium usually passes readily into the transverse colon. At that point I drain the barium from the rectum by putting the bag down and tilting the table upward. I try to put barium across the midline before draining if I observe that the transverse colon is particularly redundant. One thing to note is that I do not start the patient in a prone position, which increases abdominal pressure and is very difficult on elderly patients. Also, gravity is the only force I use to instill the barium. *Never* compress the bag to increase the pressure of the barium column.

### Air Insufflation

After draining the barium slightly, air is then insufflated while the patient is slightly RAO or prone. Air should be instilled slowly, with interruptions when the patient feels uncomfortable. The colon must adapt to the increased distention, and patients will evacuate if air is insufflated too rapidly. Fluoroscopy should be concentrated on the transverse colon to make sure that the barium is traversing across to the ascending colon. The patient is always then turned on the right side so that barium continues to the right colon. Once sufficient barium has reached the right side, the patient may then be turned supine. A major mistake I often see is that the fluoroscopist becomes mesmerized with the rectosigmoid and fails to observe the advancement of the barium column.

### Spot Filming

A sufficient number of spot films should be obtained to adequately demonstrate key areas, particularly the rectosigmoid, flexures, and cecum. The number should vary on the redundancy of the bowel, presence of diverticula, patient age, and pathology (Table 1). There is no magic to the number or sequence of spot filming. Both prone and supine filming is recommended (sigmoid and cecum) to ensure movement of the barium pool (Fig. 2). *Never* use camera spots: they minify subtle pathology so that it is barely perceptible.

**TABLE 1** Recommended Views for a Routine DCBE

| Overhead Films | Spot Films |
|---|---|
| Supine* | Rectosigmoid |
| Left lateral decubitus* | (2–5 views) |
| Right lateral decubitus* | Cecum |
| Cross-table prone rectum* | (1–3 views) |
| Left posterior oblique | Splenic flexure |
| Right posterior oblique | Hepatic flexure |
| Upright | |

*These limited number of views are recommended for patients under 35 years of age.

### Overhead Films

The list of overhead films is given in Table 1. The main views are the decubitus and cross-table rectum views. I believe this is all that is necessary in a younger patient, whereas I prefer several more views in older patients.

### Views to Delete

Several studies have indicated the lack of value of scout films in detecting either adequacy of bowel preparation or significant pathology. Also, postevacuation films are unnecessary unless there is an area of concern needing further evaluation. For routine studies, scout and postevacuation films should not be obtained unless you have time and money to waste.

### Hypotonic Agents

Glucagon is the main agent of choice to induce colonic hypotonia. One milligram must be given for adequate effect on

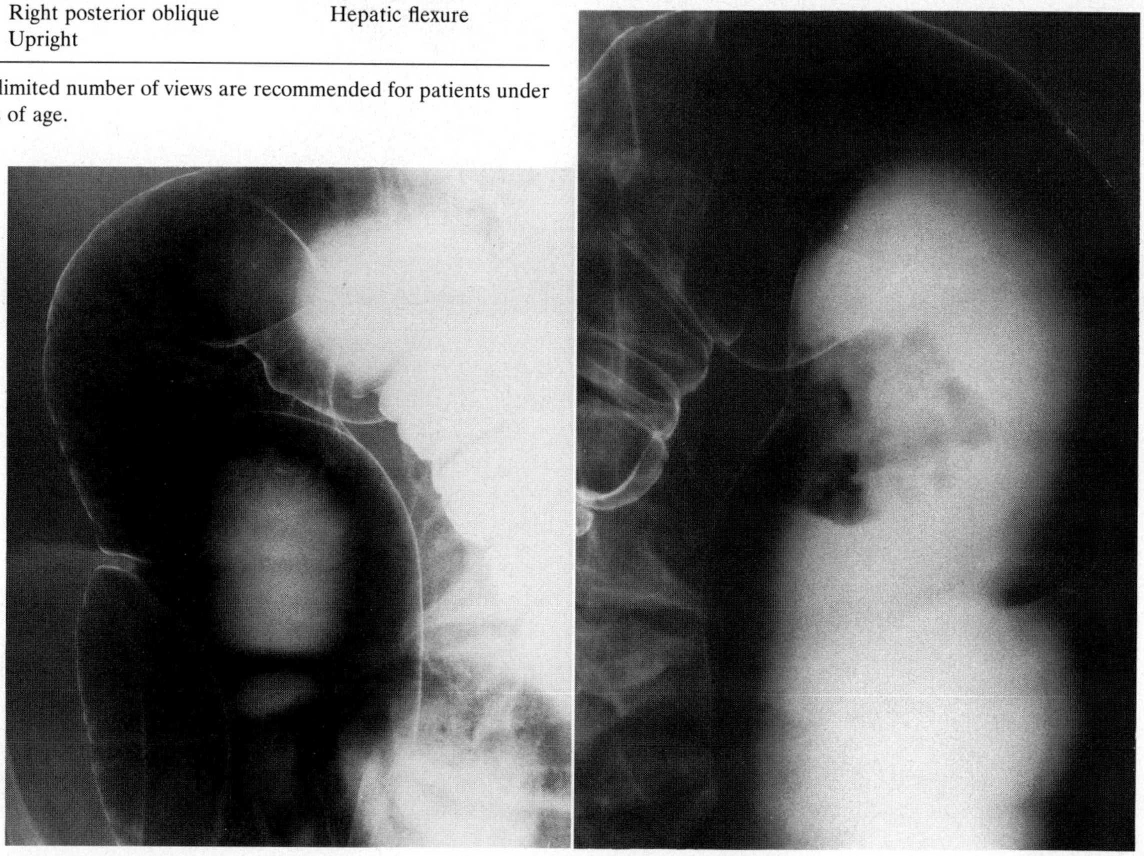

A

B

**FIGURE 2** Varying position and movement are important in obtaining maximum diagnostic yield. *A,* An adequate view of the ascending colon shows only a faint suggestion of pathology. *B,* Prone view of same portion of bowel, with shift of barium pool, demonstrates a large villous adenoma.

A

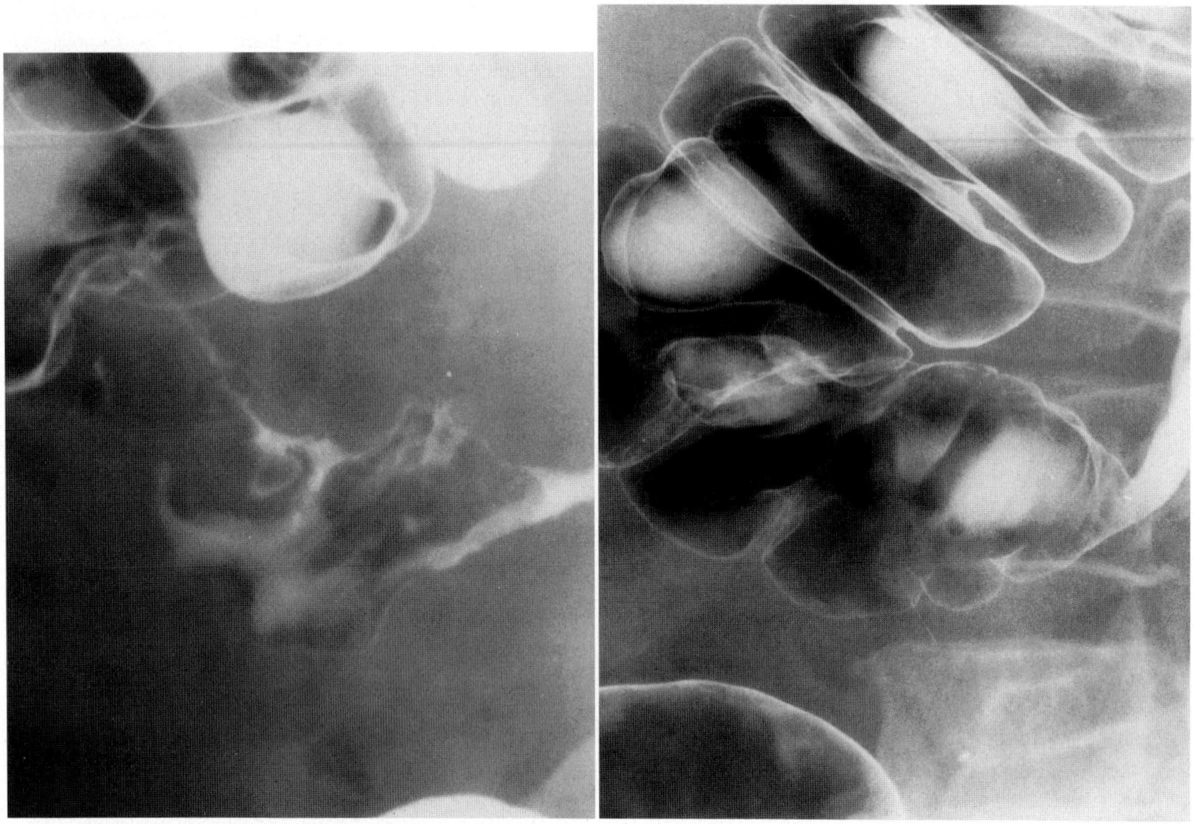

B

**FIGURE 3** Hypotonic agents can be useful in selected circumstances. *A,* View of the cecum shows an apparent constriction lesion. *B,* After injection of 1 mg of glucagon, the area dilates, indicating that this narrowing was just due to spasm.

A

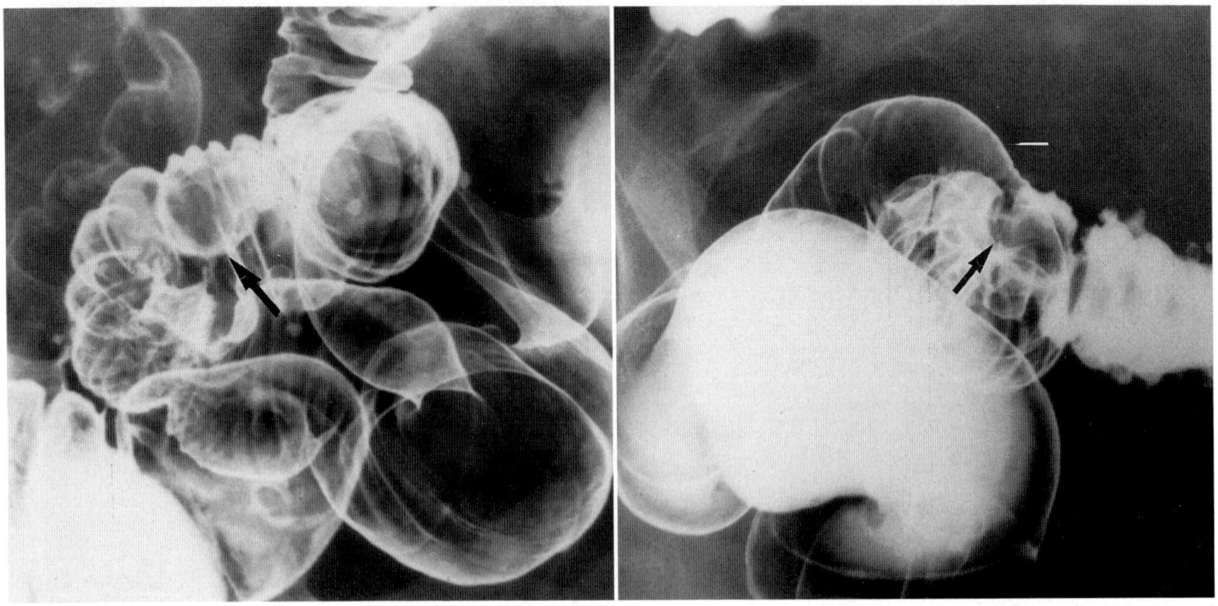

B

**FIGURE 4** The differentiation between polyps and diverticula can be extremely difficult. *A,* View of the sigmoid colon shows a circular lesion amongst diverticula *(arrow)*. *B,* Another view shows a large filling defect in the barium pool, indicating it is a polyp *(arrow)*.

the colon, and one should expect it to last only 5 to 10 minutes. I see no reason to use it on a routine basis, but it is helpful in circumstances of severe spasm or to evaluate strictures of the colon (Fig. 3).

#### *Failed Examinations*

When properly performed, a DCBE should fail only rarely. On those occasions, it is certainly proper to refill the colon as in a SCBE. The patient should be allowed to go to the bathroom to evacuate as much air and high-density barium as possible before the SCBE.

### Interpretation

Pathology of the large bowel is limited in its appearance, usually consisting of diverticula, strictures, polyps, or ulceration. The major difficulties associated with interpretation are perceptive errors or confusion with diverticula/feces. Although the DCBE has inherently greater sensitivity, even with an adequate examination significant pathology may not be detected by the radiologist. There is no definitive method to improve accuracy, but some general concepts may reduce missed lesions.

#### *Review All Films*

Admittedly the fluoroscopist is often quite busy performing examinations. It is important to design a system where all radiographs are reviewed before the patient leaves the department. In that way suspicious areas may be rechecked. The best way to accomplish this is to have every film developed as soon as possible after it is exposed. In an ideal system, the radiologist is able to review the spot films right after leaving the fluoroscopy suite to ensure adequate distention and coating as well as assess for troublesome areas.

#### *Double Reading*

Few departments can afford to have studies evaluated by two different radiologists. An easier substitution for this is self double-reading. As the study is being developed, I make an attempt to review every film and inspect for pathology. I highlight any suspicious areas with a removable marker. Later, I review all the studies and make a final interpretation. *Do not* attempt to dictate studies between fluoroscopic examinations, since this will certainly increase your "miss" rate.

#### *Rely on Endoscopy*

Frequently, pathology can be seen on only a few films. It is important to realize that significant pathology may be demonstrated on just a single view. If any doubt exists, I recommend an endoscopic procedure to further evaluate a suspicious area.

Certainly the most difficult portion of DCBE interpretation lies in distinguishing polyps from feces/diverticula (Fig. 4). My suggestion is to obtain a sufficient number of views, particularly upright and decubitus, to determine if a lesion persists.

## Suggested Reading


de Roos A, et al. Colon polyps and carcinoma: Prospective comparison of the single- and double-contrast examination in the same patient. Radiology 1985; 154:11–13.

Feczko PJ, Halpert RD. Reassessing the role of radiology in hemoccult screening. AJR 1986; 146:697–701.

Gelfand DW, Laufer I, directors. Colon cancer: Diagnosis in an era of cost containment. Proceedings of a professional conference. American College of Radiology, 1990.

Harned RK, et al. Clinical application of in vitro studies for barium-enema examination following colorectal biopsy. Radiology 1985; 154:319–321.

Kelvin FM, et al. Colorectal carcinoma missed on double contrast barium enema study: A problem in perception. AJR 1981; 137:307–313.

Laufer I. Double contrast enema: Technical aspects. In Laufer I, Levine MS. Double Contrast Gastrointestinal Radiology. 2nd ed. Philadelphia: WB Saunders, 1992:423.

Schwab FJ, et al. The barium enema scout film: Cost effectiveness and clinical efficacy. Radiology 1986; 160:615–622.

Thoeni RF, et al. Effect of glucagon on the diagnostic accuracy of double-contrast barium enema examinations. AJR 1984; 142:111–114.

Wolf EL, et al. Feasibility of double-contrast barium enema in the elderly. AJR 1985; 145:47–48.


# Colorectal Carcinoma: Diagnosis and Staging

*FRANK P. McGRATH, M.B., M.Sc. · GILES W. STEVENSON, B.M.*

Colorectal cancer is now the most common noncutaneous malignancy and has a mortality close to 50 percent. The lifetime risk for an individual to develop this cancer in industrialized countries is between 2.5 and 6 percent and increases with age. Fortunately almost all colon cancers arise from adenomas that have grown to 1 cm or more in size, raising the hope that prevention of colon cancer could be achieved by detection and removal of these lesions. However, around 35 percent of the elderly have adenomas, although only 6 percent have adenomas over 1 cm in diameter.

## Diagnosis of Colon Cancer

### *Symptomatic Patients*

#### Nonimaging Methods

*Digital rectal evaluation* detects most rectal cancers and should be part of the routine physical examination of patients over age 40, but it has no value in excluding colonic or even rectal cancer. *Evaluation of the stool for occult blood* with Hemoccult, on a modified diet, fails to detect 75 percent of adenomas and approximately 30 to 50 percent of colorectal cancers, and has a high number of false positives. As a screening tool, it does identify an increased proportion of early cancers. It may thus be a useful test for case detection, but is unsuitable for ruling out the disease. Newer immunochemical tests of higher sensitivity and specificity may change this. *Carcinoembryonic antigen* (CEA) in the blood is a marker for colon cancer, but is more useful for detection of recurrence, especially hepatic, than for primary diagnosis. Evaluation of colonic effluent by cytological methods, genetic markers in blood, flow cytometry on rectal and colon biopsies, and examination of the retina for hypertrophy of pigment epithelium are in research development for identification of subsets of patients at risk, but none are ready for routine clinical use.

## Imaging Methods

*Bowel Preparation.* A clean colon is essential for endoscopy or barium enema study. Unfortunately the amount of stool present in the North American adult human colon varies from a 12 hour food supply to 2 weeks' ingestion, because of the variation in colonic transit time. Therefore a bowel preparation should be selected that succeeds in 95 percent of patients, without excessive discomfort, and fails in 5 percent. Patients in this 5 percent should be re-examined after further preparation if the examination does not rule out cancer and if this diagnosis would affect their management. Appropriate regimens have been well described. We use Dulcolax and a 4 L polyethylene glycol (PEG) preparation for both colonoscopy and barium enema study, with the PEG given the morning of the study for colonoscopy patients but on the evening before for barium enema study patients.

*Barium Radiology.* Both single- and double-contrast methods exist. The *single-contrast method* readily misses lesions in the cecum and rectum. It has only three indications: (1) for examination of the unprepared colon mainly in suspected obstruction, (2) for examination of debilitated patients (e.g., those unable to climb on the table and lie prone unaided and in whom overlooking a small neoplasm might not be relevant), and (3) in those few centers, such as the Mayo Clinic, in which a high volume and dedicated gastrointestinal (GI) radiologists have elevated the technique to an art form. Non-GI radiologists, outside such a center, should not use single-contrast examinations in mobile patients to detect colon neoplasms. Overdistention of the bowel should be avoided in the early stages, and the flow of barium has to be carefully observed. Subsequently the colon is drained of as much barium as possible, and the patient goes to the washroom. A post-evacuation radiograph should always be performed, because this may on occasion be the only radiograph to demonstrate an abnormality.

*Double-contrast barium enema* (DCBE) is the radiological method of choice to detect colon tumors and is capable of detecting 97 percent of colon cancers.

*Sigmoid colon.* A digital rectal examination is performed first to assess anal sphincter tone because this is important in deciding whether an inflatable cuff is required. Barium is run into the colon, with the patient in the prone position, until the splenic flexure is reached, which usually requires between 400 and 700 ml. Carbon dioxide is then insufflated, pushing the barium column forward as long as the $CO_2$/barium interface is maintained in a vertical segment of bowel. Making full use of $CO_2$ insufflation, gravity, and patient movements it should be possible to obtain views of the sigmoid loop devoid of barium puddles.[1] An average of four spot views is sufficient for the sigmoid colon; for these the patient is rotated into the supine oblique right-side-up, left lateral, prone, and prone left-side-up positions, with occasionally a supine left-side-up position being helpful for long or complex sigmoid loops. We have shown that the use of $CO_2$, rather than air, significantly reduces the amount of discomfort experienced by patients.

*Examination of the remainder of the colon.* Once an adequate examination of the rectosigmoid colon has been achieved, the patient is turned from supine, slightly head down to a right-side-down position, while additional puffs of $CO_2$ are given to push the barium column across the transverse colon and into the ascending colon. The patient is then moved to a supine, table, semierect position so that the barium will flow into the cecum. To allow the cecum to fill completely, the patient is then placed in the left-side-down position and then turned prone. The table position is moved to the horizontal and the patient is asked to roll completely around to achieve optimal coating of the hepatic flexure. The patient is brought erect and radiographs of both flexures are obtained in the left-side-forward (splenic) and right-side-forward (hepatic) positions. Standard spot radiographs of the cecum are taken, first with the right side down and the table head lowered to 10° to 15°, and then gradually moving supine, left side down and then prone, the next spot radiograph is taken (a compression paddle may be of benefit in this position). Six overhead radiographs are then performed in the following positions: supine; prone; prone angled view of the sigmoid; right and left lateral decubiti; and also, especially if an inflated rectal cuff has been used, a lateral view of the rectum with the enema tip removed. If coating of the right colon is poor initially after barium has been maneuvered into the cecum, the spots of the flexures and cecum may be deferred until after the overhead films have been taken.

At McMaster we perform flexible sigmoidoscopy before the barium enema study in patients between 40 and 80 years old. Since the sigmoid has been well seen, we then use a larger volume of barium to optimize right-sided colon coating, accepting a small chance of early ileal filling, which might compromise the sigmoid films.

Irritable bowel, diverticular disease, and inflammatory bowel disease may all cause visible spasm, and IV glucagon 0.5 mg, or Buscopan 20 mg, will ease patient discomfort, allow the contrast to run more freely, and improve the films.

*Errors in Recognition of Colon Cancer.* The radiographic appearances of colon cancer are well described, but errors continue. Neoplasms are rarely flat, and detection relies on perception of the edge of a raised lesion that may be straight (Fig. 1) or more often curved (Figs. 2, 3). If the edge involves a barium puddle, it produces a concave margin to the puddle; if there is no puddle, the edge produces a curvilinear line as a result of the meniscus effect (Fig. 4). A central ulcer may show as a ring or puddle of barium. If the lesion is over about 12 mm in diameter, it produces an indentation of the margin of the bowel when seen tangentially, whether benign or malignant (Figs. 2, 5). Diluted barium coats poorly and fails to demon-

[1] The interested reader is referred to the work by Dobranowski and co-workers for a more comprehensive review of our method of sigmoid clearance.

A

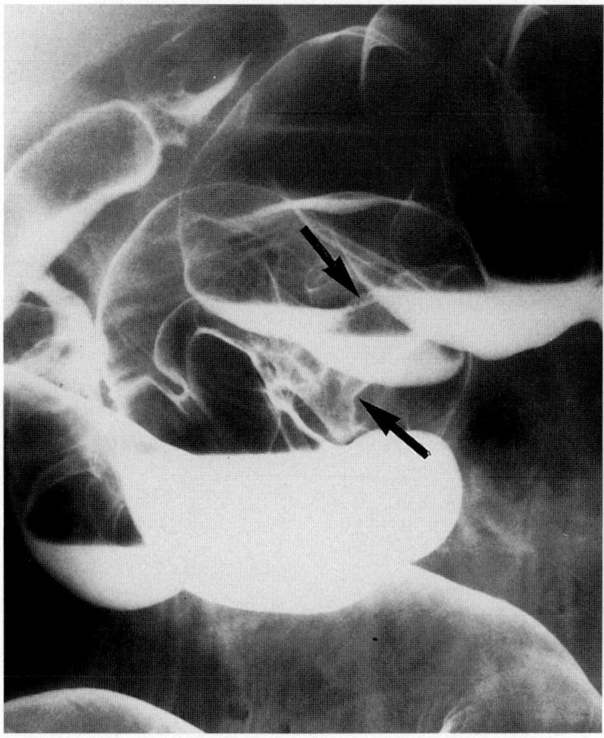

B

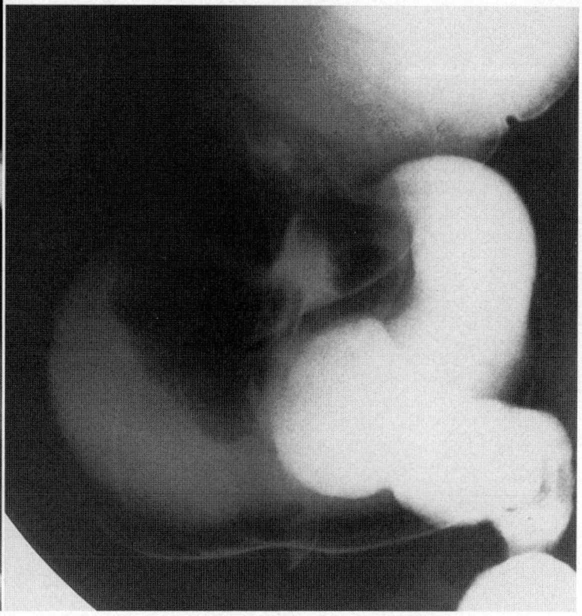

**FIGURE 1** *A,* A coned view of the cecal pole from a double-contrast examination of this patient with an annular carcinoma shows too many parallel lines *(arrows)*, which may be easily overlooked and attributed to overlying small bowel loops. *B,* A single-contrast view of the cecum in the same patient improves the perceptibility of the large polypoid cancer.

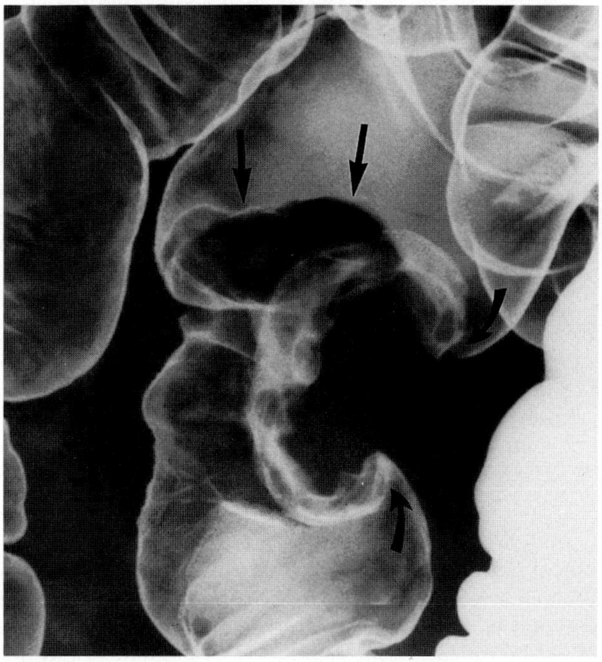

**FIGURE 2** Sigmoid carcinoma in a 40 year old female. The curved edge of the tumor *(arrows)* is well outlined by the adjacent barium puddle. The mass is approximately 5 cm in diameter and is indenting the margin of the bowel wall *(curved arrows)*.

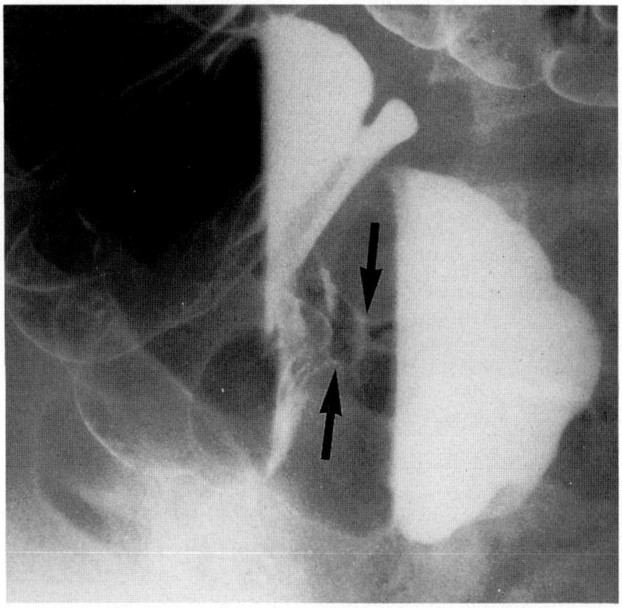

**FIGURE 3** Cecal pole cancer. The well-distended lower pole of cecum is superimposed on the tight annular stricture, which was not perceived at the time of initial reporting. Note again the importance of perceiving the additional linear edges *(arrows)* as a clue to the presence of an underlying neoplasm.

A

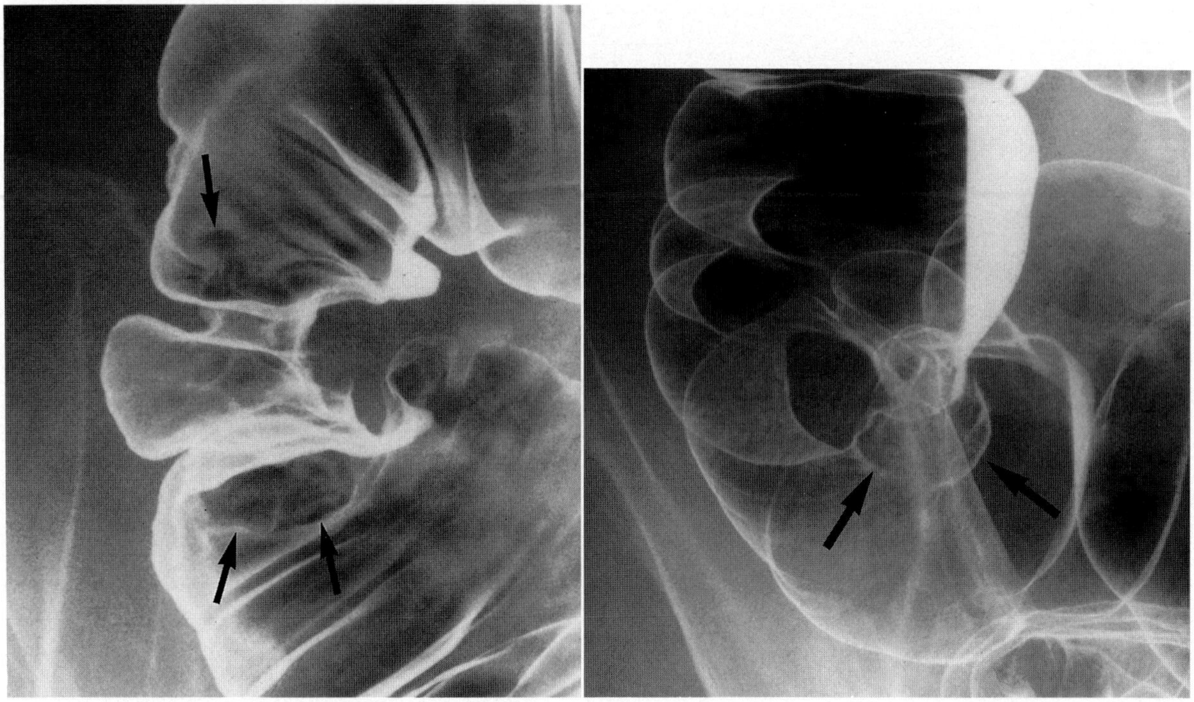

B

**FIGURE 4** *A,* Ascending colon cancer. *B,* Cecal pole carcinoma. When there are no adjacent barium puddles present, the edges of a tumor are shown as a curved line *(arrows)* because of the meniscus effect.

A

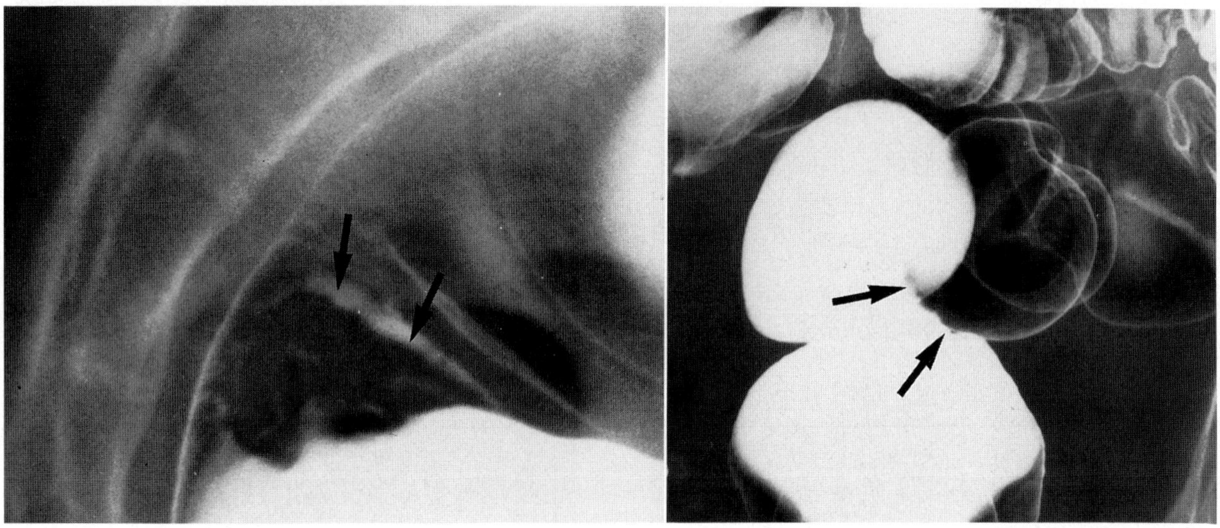

B

**FIGURE 5** Rectal cancer. *A,* An overexposed coned lateral double-contrast view of the rectum shows a subtle poorly defined convex tumor margin *(arrows). B,* The single-contrast view shows some puckering and indentation of the rectal wall *(arrows).*

strate edges (Fig. 6), whereas stool, diverticular disease (Fig. 7), or other tumors act as distractors to perception. Particular attention to the lower rectum at the site of tube insertion is also necessary to see a small tumor that may have avoided detection by the digital examination (Fig. 8). Large puddles of barium may cause overexposure, and carcinomas may escape detection in the darker areas of these radiographs (Fig. 5).

Flat villous adenomas are a particular problem, because their meniscal edge is subtle, and detection of their villous surface pattern requires particularly good coating (Fig. 9). There is a suggestion that they are more common in the right colon of cancer family syndrome patients, including those who have had a relative with colon cancer before the age of 55. Extra efforts should be made to ensure optimal coating in the right colon for such individuals.

Quality control of barium enemas should ideally be monitored regularly. In adult patients polyps should be detected on over 10 percent of barium enema studies. There is evidence that double reporting can optimize detection. Simpkins has suggested that we indicate which segments of the colon have been optimally demonstrated and in which segments a neoplasm might have been overlooked in order to facilitate

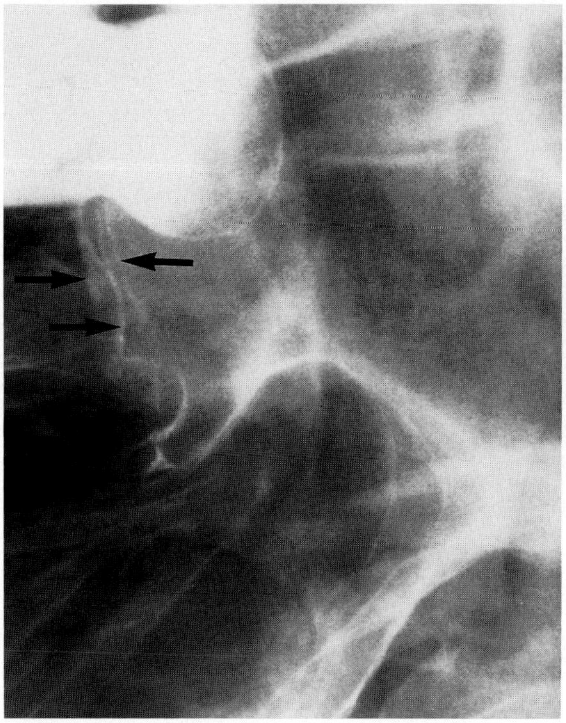

**FIGURE 6** Cecal carcinoma. Poor coating of the right part of the colon in this 41 year old male was thought to be a significant contributing factor in the lack of perception of this cancer, although three subtle linear edges can be seen *(arrows)*.

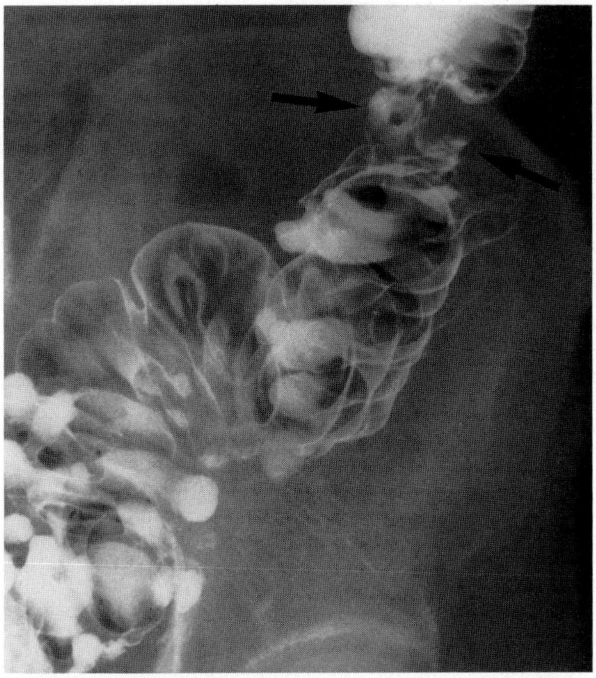

**FIGURE 7** Diverticulosis, which is most common in the sigmoid colon, may act as a distractor to the perception of additional lesions. A double-contrast barium enema from a 73 year old male shows extensive diverticular changes in the sigmoid colon. The short concentric asymmetrical narrowing representing a cancer more proximally was overlooked *(arrows)*.

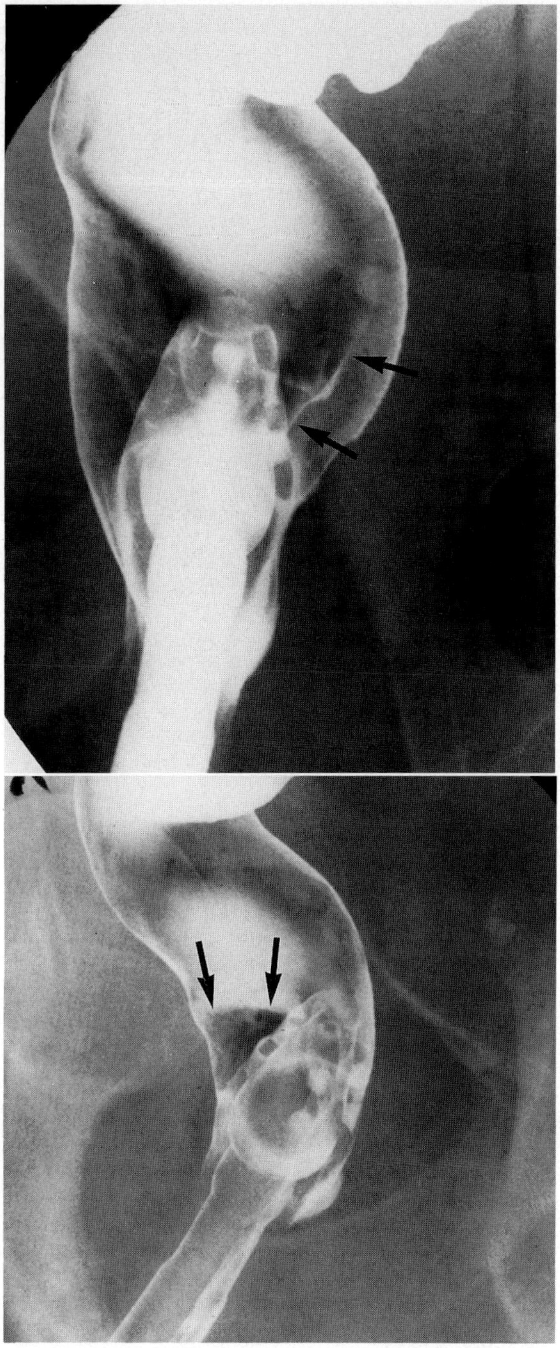

A

B

**FIGURE 8** Low rectal carcinoma. *A,* The tip of the enema tube obscures most of the cancer, with only a subtle line providing a clue as to its presence *(arrows)*. *B,* A further view taken at a slightly different degree of obliquity shows the lesion outlined by a concave margin on a small pool of barium *(arrows)*.

decisions by our clinical colleagues on when to proceed to endoscopy.

*Endoscopy. Flexible sigmoidoscopy* is most often an office procedure following a Fleet enema. It has no place as the only diagnostic imaging test for patients with large bowel symptoms. We perform small biopsies (2.8 mm channel forceps) of small polypoid lesions immediately before a barium enema study.

*Colonoscopy*—The bowel preparation is similar to that for

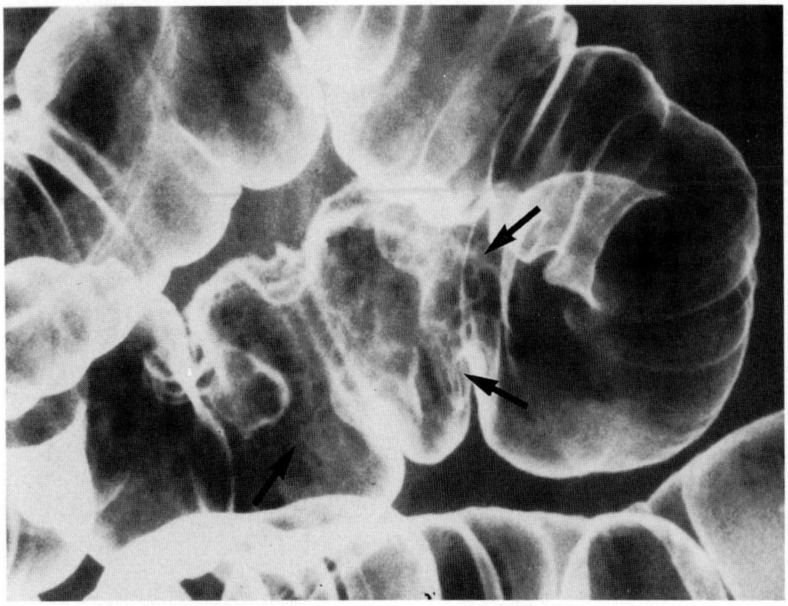

**FIGURE 9** Villous adenoma of the sigmoid colon in an 80-year-old male. Note the poorly defined area of abnormal mucosal coating in the sigmoid loop *(arrows)*. The smoother coating of the normal adjacent bowel segments facilitated the detection of this subtle villous adenoma.

A

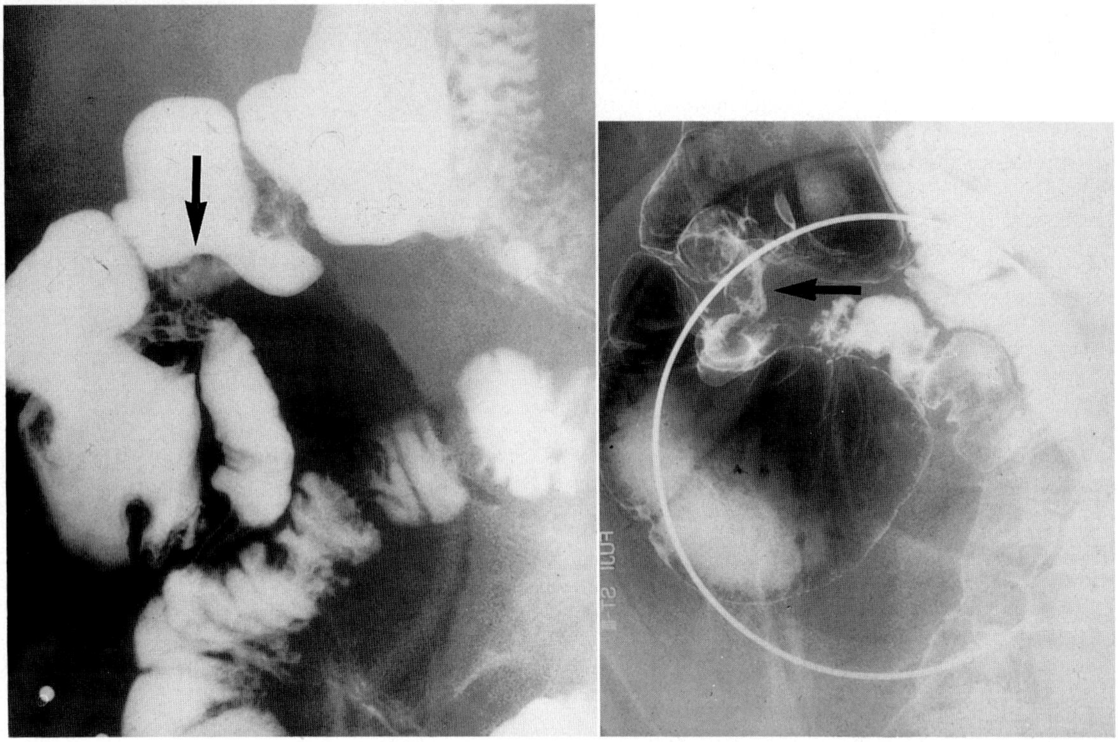

B

**FIGURE 10** Carcinoma of the ascending colon that was overlooked on colonoscopy. The upper end of the annular carcinoma *(arrow)* was thought at colonoscopy to represent the ileocecal valve. A small bowel meal was next performed. *A,* The single-contrast view is hard to interpret, but rectal insufflation of gas (*B*) demonstrated the annular carcinoma just above the ileocecal valve *(arrow)*.

DCBE. With 5 to 40 percent of colonoscopies incomplete, there should be large numbers of patients having a barium enema study immediately after failed colonoscopy, yet these numbers are small. We are now beginning to see numbers of patients with colon cancer who have had a negative colonoscopy within the past 3 years. The absence of hard copy makes quality control of colonoscopy difficult, and review of videotape is more suitable for occasional peer review rather than routine quality control. Radiologists should encourage and facilitate arrangements for barium enema studies immediately after failed or incomplete colonoscopy.

*Endoscopic findings of colon cancer and reasons for error*—An annular tumor may mimic the ileocecal valve (Fig. 10), as may an area of spasm that leads to false confidence that the cecum has been reached. Diverticular disease, poor preparation, and previous pelvic surgery make the examination technically more difficult.

*Ultrasonography.* Early reports of abdominal ultrasonography after filling the colon with fluid suggest that it might have great sensitivity for detection of both colon cancer and polyps, with no radiation and no morbidity. Further experience with this exciting development is urgently required.

*Colonoscopy versus DCBE.* Ideally patients with polyps require colonoscopy, and flexible sigmoidoscopy is one way to select such patients. Otherwise, a barium enema study is a cheaper and safer way to begin colonic evaluation. Patients who should be selected for colonoscopy probably include those at high risk for adenomas, those elderly patients with persistent iron deficiency anemia (to look for angiodysplasia), and those with major acute rectal bleeding.

### *Screening*

The rationale for screening is that benign adenomas grow in the colon for 5 to 20 years before some of them develop invasive characteristics and that removal of the larger adenomas would prevent the development of colorectal cancer. Since 35 percent of elderly adults harbor adenomas, strategies need either to offer everyone a reliable inexpensive test that excludes bowel cancer (such a test does not yet exist) or to identify those at highest risk who can be offered the existing more expensive and dangerous screening tests of barium enema study and colonoscopy with polypectomy. Such individuals include those with polyposis coli (risk 100 percent), those in Lynch I or Lynch II families (risk approaching 30 percent), those with a first-degree relative who developed colon cancer under the age of 55 (risk 15 to 20 percent), and those with one first-degree relative with colon cancer (risk around 10 percent), as well as those surviving a previous colon cancer and those with previous large adenomas. Colonoscopy is inappropriate as a screening test, because of its morbidity and mortality, as well as its cost, but is required for those with polyps. For high-risk patients, flexible sigmoidoscopy is an excellent way to identify those who should go straight on to colonoscopy; patients with negative flexible sigmoidoscopy findings should have a DCBE. In patients with long-standing ulcerative colitis, however, colonoscopy is the screening method of choice (Fig. 11). Screening of the whole adult population should not be advocated as a public health measure until we have effective programs screening those at highest risk, and have more evidence to show benefit.

## Staging of Colon Cancer

### *Preoperative Staging*

#### Computed Tomography

Computed tomography (CT) may depict tumor extension into the perirectal fat, adjacent organs or lymph nodes, and liver. Recent reports of preoperative staging with CT have been disappointing, revealing much lower accuracy rates (41 to 64 percent) than earlier studies. This is chiefly because of poor identification of lymph node metastases and inability to determine the extent of local tumor spread. Lymph nodes over 1 cm are often malignant, but biopsy or lymphangiography provides greater certainty than CT.

The imaging plane should extend from the dome of the liver to the anal verge, because a significant portion of patients (25 percent) have extracolonic disease. Patients drink 500 ml of dilute Gastrografin 1.5 to 2 hours before the examination. Oral metoclopramide 20 mg is given to hasten the passage of contrast to the right colon. An additional 500 ml of Gastrografin is given 30 minutes before the CT scan. In addition, a rectal contrast agent (either dilute Gastrografin or rectal air) is also administered. Preliminary bowel preparation and a vaginal tampon may both be useful. Intravenous contrast medium (70 ml of iohexol 350 administered at 1 ml per second) is also given.

Caution must be used when assessing for local invasion in thin or cachectic patients and should only be diagnosed when the tumor almost surrounds or clearly invades the organ (i.e., prostate, ovaries, uterus, bladder, ureters, or sciatic nerves). Invasion of bone structures (e.g., the sacrum) is easily appreciated on the bone window settings. The presence of scarring, inflammation, or congestion can mimic the streaking of the pericolonic fat that may be found in early extracolonic tumor spread, and conversely, apparently localized lesions may have spread into adjacent lymph nodes without alteration of size or appearance on CT scanning.

#### Magnetic Resonance Imaging

Despite early optimism, magnetic resonance imaging (MRI) does not presently seem to offer accurate determination of extent of tumor infiltration and lymph node involvement.

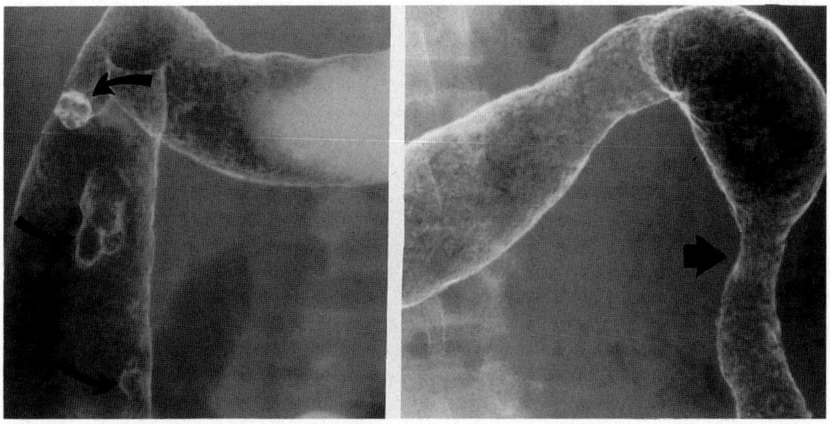

**FIGURE 11** Long-standing ulcerative colitis in an 18-year-old female. The stricture in the proximal descending colon *(arrow)* prevented passage of the colonoscope. A double-contrast barium enema was subsequently performed and demonstrated one large and two smaller polypoid lesions in the ascending colon *(curved arrows)* that required biopsy to exclude malignant change.

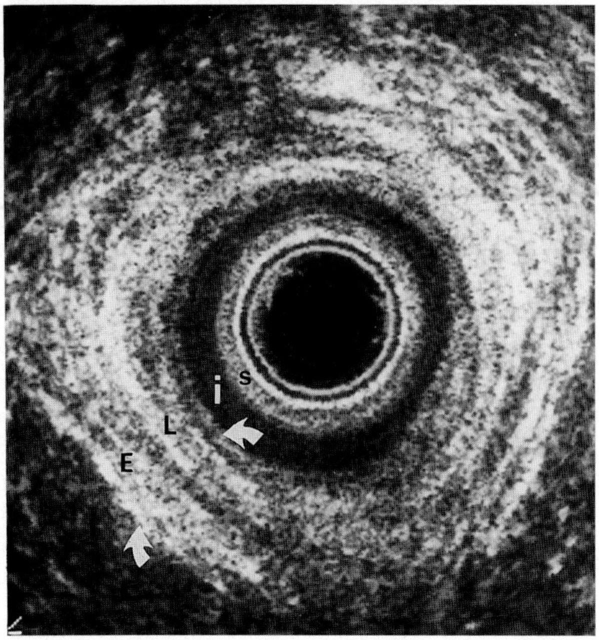


**FIGURE 12** Normal endosonographic anatomy of the anal canal. The cone creates two bright inner concentric echoes. The subepithelial tissues (s) are relatively hyperechoic, the internal sphincter (i) a clearly defined hypoechoic ring, and the longitudinal muscle (L) combined with the external sphincter (E) forms an outer hyperechoic ring (*arrows*). There is often some variation in the echogenicity of the external sphincter. In males it is commonly hypoechoic, whereas in females the echogenicity of the two layers is similar and indistinguishable sonographically, as illustrated. (Courtesy C. Bartram, M.D.)

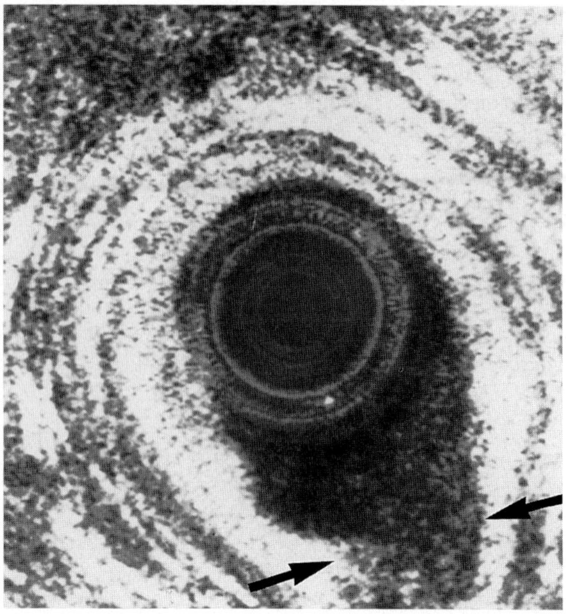

**FIGURE 13** Anal cancer. Endorectal ultrasonography shows an irregular hypoechoic mass invading the posterior aspect of the internal anal sphincter into the intersphincteric space *(arrows)*. The external sphincter is spared. (Courtesy of C. Bartram, M.D.)

### Endorectal Sonography

Transrectal ultrasonography (TRUS) shows excellent delineation of the layers of the gut wall (Fig. 12). Rigid intrarectal transducers with rotating crystals that allow a full 360° plane are optimal for tumor identification.

Rectal cancers appear as regions of decreased echogenicity that disrupt the alternating hypo- and hyperechoic layers making up the normal bowel wall (Fig. 13). Unfortunately features of malignancy in lymph nodes are not easily or reliably depicted with TRUS. Nevertheless, it is the best method currently available for assessment of transmural spread of tumors within 15 cm of the anal margin, and for confirmation of the suitability of low early rectal cancers for local radiotherapy as definitive treatment.

## *Postoperative Tumor Recurrence*

### Follow-up for Colonic Recurrence or New Tumors

Follow-up for detection of anastomotic recurrence is not useful for cure, since such recurrence is caused by reinvasion from adjacent local disease. However, there should be follow-up for the bowel to detect and remove synchronous tumors, since 3 percent develop a second carcinoma. Further, the likelihood of developing further colon cancers is 20 percent over 25 years.

### Detection and Assessment of Noncolonic Metastases

*CT.* Radiologic authors recommend a baseline CT scan at 2 to 3 months to establish the normal postsurgical appearances to facilitate differentiation of tumor recurrence from scar formation. More recent accuracy rates quoted for staging with CT range from 69 to 88 percent. A postoperative mass suggests tumor recurrence, but this appearance can also be found with postsurgical granulation tissue. In general, however, a postoperative mass decreases in size between the 2 to 3 month baseline CT scan and a follow-up study performed at 4 to 9 months. It is not known whether the baseline study is cost-effective, or whether it is simpler to carry out routine serum CEA levels, and only do CT, with biopsy if necessary, in patients with rising CEA levels.

*MRI.* As with preoperative evaluation, initial enthusiasm has been replaced by the recognition that the allegedly specific high signal intensity on T2-weighted sequences may be found with scar, inflammation, and tumor.

*TRUS.* TRUS may be used when sphincter-saving surgery has been performed. Because rectal tumor recurrence is normally extraluminal, a pericolic hypoechoic mass or focal wall thickening may be found. A baseline study is helpful in the interpretation of later images.

*Positron Emission Tomography.* Positron emission tomography combined with monoclonal antibodies against CEA is undergoing intensive research. The early results are encouraging for both preoperative colon cancer staging and postoperative tumor recurrence.

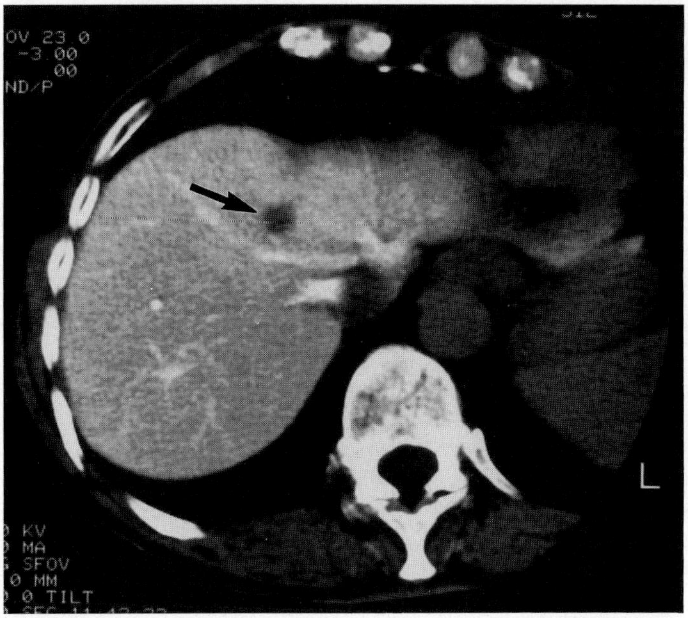


**FIGURE 14** CT portography in a 64-year-old female with a history of bowel resection for colon cancer. The patient had a known large metastatic deposit in the right lobe of the liver (not shown). The CT portogram demonstrated a second smaller deposit in the left lobe *(arrow)*, thereby excluding the patient from hepatic resectional surgery. The left lobe lesion was not identified on previous ultrasonography or standard CT evaluations.

*Resectable liver metastases* – Distant metastases (Duke's D) commonly involve the liver. At McMaster, patients considered for potentially curable hepatic resections have both ultrasonography and bolus dynamic-contrast CT (140 ml iohexol 350 administered at 2 ml per second). If the disease still appears resectable after these tests, an MRI and subsequently a CT portogram (Fig. 14) are obtained to exclude disease in the liver segments to be left behind. Research on destruction of small liver metastases by ultrasonography-guided laser may, if successful, greatly expand the relevance of such detailed hepatic imaging.

### Overview of Staging for Colorectal Cancer

For preoperative staging CT should not be used as a primary imaging method. Rather it should be reserved for those patients in whom locally extensive or widespread disease is suspected, so that if the tumor is too extensive, alternative treatment can be instituted. Because CT has poor sensitivity for local tumor extent, TRUS should be used to evaluate focal bowel wall involvement in the rectum and to detect adjacent lymph nodes, but is not specific for malignancy in the latter, and biopsy may be required. MRI may be used to determine involvement of the pelvic floor musculature. A case can be made for no preoperative staging by imaging if the patient is clearly fit for surgery.

For colon cancer recurrence, if an abdominoperineal resection and colostomy have been performed, a choice may be made between following with CEA levels or following with CT or MRI as baseline studies at 2 to 3 months. If a primary rectal resection and reanastomosis have been performed, then TRUS, if available, should be used for the perianastomotic area, with CT or MRI with percutaneous biopsy reserved for those with rising CEA levels. In patients who do not clearly have secondary disease, a follow-up program for synchronous and metachronous bowel tumors should be instituted.

## Suggested Reading


Coblentz CL, Frost RA, Molinaro V, Stevenson GW. Pain after barium enema: Effect of $CO_2$ and air on double-contrast study. Radiology 1985; 157:35–36.

Darmon E, Tobi M, Rozen P. Newer tests, on colonic effluent, for identifying persons with colorectal neoplasia. In: Rozen P, Reich CB, Wianawer SJ, eds. Large Bowel Cancer: Policy, Prevention, Research and Treatment. Vol. 18. Front Gastrointest Res. Basel: Karger, 1991:236.

Dobranowski J, Stringer DA, Somers S, Stevenson GW. Procedures in Gastrointestinal Radiology. New York: Springer-Verlag, 1990:61.

Dunlop MG. Screening for large bowel neoplasms in individuals with a history of colorectal cancer. Br J Surg 1992; 79:488–494.

Fitzsimons P, Shorvon P, Frost RA, et al. A comparison of Golytely and standard preparation for barium enema. J Can Assoc Radiol 1987; 38:109–112.

Fork FT, Lindstrom C, Ekelund GR. Reliability of routine double contrast examination (DCE) of the large bowel in polyp detection: A prospective clinical study. Gastrointest Radiol 1983; 8:163–172.

Limberg B. Diagnosis of large bowel tumours by colonic sonography. Lancet 1990; 335:144–146.

Lynch HT, Kimberling WJ, Albano W, et al. Hereditary nonpolyposis colorectal cancer; parts I, II. Cancer 1985; 56:934–951.

McGrath FP, Malone DE, Dobranowski J, Stevenson GW. CT portography and delayed high dose iodine CT. Clin Radiol (article in press).

Seidman H, Mushinski MH, Gelb SK, Silverberg E. Probabilities of eventually developing or dying of cancer – United States: 1985. Ca-A Cancer J Clin 1985; 35:36–56.

Thoeni RF. Colorectal cancer: Cross-sectional imaging for staging of primary tumor and detection of local recurrence. AJR 1991; 156:909–915.

Tio TL, Coene PP, van Delden OM, Tytgat GNJ. Colorectal carcinoma: Preoperative TNM classification with endosonography. Radiology 1991; 179:165–170.

Wargovich MJ, Lynch PM, Roubein LD, Levin B. Biomarkers of increased risk for large bowel neoplasia. In: Rozen P, Reich CB, Winawer SJ, eds. Large Bowel Cancer: Policy, Prevention, Research and Treatment. Vol. 18. Front Gastrointest Res. Basel: Karger, 1991:225.

# Plain Film Radiography of the Acute Abdomen

*STEPHEN R. BAKER, M.D.*

In recent years the plain film of the abdomen has received little attention in imaging journals, radiology textbooks, and the teaching curricula of many residency programs. The insights provided by computed tomography (CT), ultrasonography, and magnetic resonance imaging have deflected attention from the plain film in circumstances in which it still has enduring merit. There is a danger that this time-honored examination will become neglected and our interpretation skills will wither as we become accustomed to selecting cross-sectional studies for every clinical situation.

It is my contention that the plain film still occupies a vital place in our imaging armamentarium, but its territory should become restricted to only a few abnormal conditions for which it can play a crucial role. There is no need to obtain a survey radiograph of the abdomen if the presenting symptom is mild-to-moderate pain because, almost always, the plain film is nondiagnostic. Diarrhea or vomiting alone should not stimulate a request for an abdominal film unless it is part of a clinical context suggestive of obstruction. The presence and site of bleeding anywhere in the gastrointestinal tract rarely is elucidated by noncontrast abdominal radiographs. Further, in blunt or abdominal trauma, the plain film has little to offer and is therefore wasteful of precious time before more definitive procedures can be performed.

On the other hand, a scout film is helpful before a barium enema study. Although it does not determine that a colon is feces-free, it can alert the radiologist when a patient is poorly prepared, which may be obscured on subsequent images with contrast in the bowel. The preliminary plain film is an essential part of an intravenous urography examination, because it helps identify calculi and other densities in the genitourinary tract before they become hidden by excreted contrast material. In selected cases, when history and physical findings are equivocal, plain film recognition of a stone in the appendix can substantiate the diagnosis of acute inflammation of that hollow viscus.

## Indications

The two urgent abnormal conditions for which the plain film should always be the first imaging study are intestinal obstruction and perforated viscus. A feature of both is acute abdominal distress accompanied by the abnormal accumulation of air or gas. In perforated viscus even small amounts of free air can be observed on plain films. Similarly, in bowel obstruction, it is the distention of intestinal air in segments proximal to an occlusion that provides the clue to the diagnosis. Both conditions can be assessed with exquisite sensitivity by CT and, in skilled hands, by ultrasonography. Yet compared with these cross-sectional techniques, the plain film is nearly as sensitive as well as less expensive, universally available, and always readily repeatable. Moreover, it is not invasive or operator independent. Its efficacy and accessibility at all hours mandate that radiologists become knowledgeable about its subtleties.

## Technical Approach

An appreciation of the capabilities and complexities of abdominal plain films is hampered not only by a lack of interest in interpretation, but also by diffidence about technique. The same meticulousness that one routinely brings to the assessment of chest films should be applied to radiographs centered below the diaphragm. A chest examination that excludes the lung apex or costophrenic angles is considered inadequate, but a supine abdominal film that cuts off the lower half of the pelvis or fails to reveal a margin of lung at its superior border is often accepted without criticism. The span of the abdomen extends from the obturator foramina below to the apex of the higher diaphragm above. A truncated view that does not include the uppermost edge of the liver shadow can fail to demonstrate a small lucency that might be the only sign of free intraperitoneal air. By the same token, gas in bowel trapped in an inguinal hernia, a telling finding in obstruction, is seen only if the entire pelvis is visualized. If necessary, two overlapping supine views should be done to encompass a long abdomen, even if it entails extra time and diligence.

An undue reliance is placed on erect abdominal views. The assumption is that the upright projection can disclose abnormalities unseen on recumbent films. In fact, the upright abdomen view has little value in the detection of perforation. Erect and decubitus views use a horizontal beam that can depict fluid levels both within and outside the bowel lumen. It is true that horizontal-beam films are more sensitive for the evaluation of air-liquid interfaces than standard supine and prone films, which are obtained with a vertically oriented beam. Yet for the recognition of free air, an erect abdomen film is not as sensitive as an erect chest film. To discern small aggregations of free air, the central ray should be directed just above the diaphragm. In a properly positioned upright abdominal view, the central beam passes through the umbilicus. Therefore only oblique rays intersect the subdiaphragmatic fluid levels characteristic of pneumoperitoneum. In contrast, an erect chest view has its central beam directed just above the diaphragm, almost parallel to the gas-liquid interface of free air and intraperitoneal fluid.

An appropriate series of films for the detection of free air is a supine abdominal film and an upright chest film. When the patient cannot assume a sitting or standing position, a left lateral decubitus view is valuable. It is probably just as sensitive as the erect chest view in patients who have had no previous surgery. In fact, it may be the best view when postoperative adhesions restrict the upward migration of free air. A limitation of the left lateral decubitus view is the time it takes for small volumes of free air to migrate laterally; an adequate study requires placing the patient with the left side down for 15 or 20 minutes before an exposure is made. Many individuals cannot tolerate such prolonged immobility on a hard tabletop. Moreover, preparation for a lateral decubitus view must take place in the radiography suite. Routine use of this view lengthens examination time and, in a busy department, may cause unacceptable delays in throughput.

## Diagnostic Approach

Often the diagnosis of free air depends exclusively on the interpretation of the plain supine radiograph. It may be the only film obtained in patients too sick to stand or lie on one side. Moreover, if pneumoperitoneum is unsuspected there may be no upright or decubitus film to help secure the diagnosis. Therefore a careful assessment of the supine film is imperative in these patients. Unfortunately the best-known indicators of free air are unreliable because they are insensitive, often nonspecific, and infrequent. For example, the bas-relief sign (so-called because it depends on visualization of both sides of the gut wall, intraluminal air within and intraperitoneal gas outside) is rarely positive unless there is a liter or more of free air. Thus it usually just confirms what is obvious clinically.

To appreciate the less obvious radiographic manifestations of pneumoperitoneum, we must look at the right upper quadrant. The liver occupies this space and imparts a homogeneous gray shadow. Any lucency superimposed on it that cannot be identified as stomach, small bowel, or colon must be viewed with suspicion if the diagnosis of spontaneous pneumoperitoneum or pneumoretroperitoneum is under consideration. We have identified four patterns of minimal free air accumulation in the right upper quadrant that stand out against the hepatic background. The largest is an anterior bubble of lucency that usually resides just beneath the apex of the diaphragm. Another configuration is an obliquely oriented slit several centimeters in length located outside bowel. A third finding is a vertically directed thin band of gas positioned to the right of the midline, which represents free air in the fissure for the ligamentum teres. The fourth pattern is ill-defined periduodenal lucencies , either solitary or multiple, which are seen just lateral to the descending duodenum. Such an intraperitoneal conglomeration is identical in appearance to the bubbles of retroperitoneal gas often present after acute duodenal rupture. All these subtle signs of free air can be overlooked if the liver shadow is evaluated casually. Thus, to detect pneumoperitoneum, the right upper quadrant must be scrutinized carefully and any lucency, no matter how seemingly inconsequential, must be explained.

The plain film diagnosis of intestinal obstruction does not suffer from a paucity of signs. Rather, the limitations of this technique relate to a lack of rigor with respect to the significance of distributional differences in the intraluminal accumulation of intestinal gas. Probably no other area of radiologic interpretation is so haunted by traditional misconceptions and unjustifiable assumptions. Moreover, close coordination is necessary between the referring physician and the radiologist, because intestinal obstruction cannot be ascertained definitively on plain film without corroborating clinical information. Because many nonocclusive conditions also cause dilatation of sections of the gut resembling obstruction, the history and physical examination provide essential information that must be available before a diagnosis can be suggested.

Often dependence is placed on the presence and configuration of fluid levels demonstrated on erect or decubitus projections. Several recent studies have questioned the usefulness of the upright abdomen view in the assessment of obstruction. Each has shown that supine views need not be routinely supplemented by horizontal-beam views. Except for the unusual circumstance of a nearly gasless abdomen, for which upright and decubitus films are valuable, adequate information about bowel pattern is usually available on supine and prone projections.

The diagnosis of small and large bowel obstruction relies on the demonstration of dilated intestine proximal to the site of blockage. There is often a temptation to assign an actual point of obstruction on the basis of plain film findings alone. Because the length of liquid-filled bowel loops interposed between the most distal gas-filled loop and the actual site of obstruction is variable and can range from a few inches to many feet, an estimate of the exact location of an obstruction is usually incorrect, and most often the putative site is placed too proximal in the intestinal tract. Mechanical obstruction close to the ligament of Treitz may be missed, because only a few centimeters of bowel are available for dilatation in response to nearby blockage. A jejunal obstruction can often be mistaken for a localized ileus induced by adjacent inflammation from nearby organs such as the pancreas and kidney. On occasion, massive air swallowing may appear transiently with dilated proximal loops, a configuration reminiscent of obstruction. Large bowel occlusions may sometimes present with small bowel dilatation alone, because an incompetent ileocecal valve permits colonic decompression by the reflux of flatus from cecum to ileum.

Another cause of imprecision in the plain film analysis of obstruction is an impetus to read too much into the film beyond the finding of obstruction itself. Terms such as early, incomplete, or partial obstruction are frequently used in radiologic reports, but by and large are not justifiable from evidence supplied by conventional radiography. The temporal course of obstruction requires a series of studies; thus the notion of recent onset or protracted course cannot be construed from one film alone. Colonic gas in nondilated loops distal to an intestinal obstruction is often present initially and persistently, even with total, uninterrupted bowel blockage. Consequently there are no plain film criteria allowing one to say that the lumen is only partially or intermittently occluded. It is best to report only that an obstruction exists, which is, of course, the essential clinical question the plain film is called on to answer. If more information about site, severity, and constancy of luminal blockage is needed, then additional studies such as CT, enteroclysis, or surgery should be performed.

The plain film diagnosis of bowel obstruction depends on the accumulation of bowel gas or swallowed air proximal to the obstruction. Removal of intestinal contents may remove the lucent markers of obstruction, but need not open the lumen. Hence the gas pattern may improve after vomiting or following the placement of a nasogastric or long tube. Is the obstruction relieved? Certainly the patient can feel better and the film may appear improved, but it is only the antegrade passage of feces and flatus that signals relief of obstruction, not the retrograde departure of intestinal gas by tube suction or vomiting.

Two nonobstructing conditions that engender small bowel gas accumulation are urinary retention and mesenteric ischemia. A dilated bladder should be looked for whenever numerous air-filled fluid loops with prominent valvulae conniventes dominate plain film findings. It is amazing how quickly a nonobstructed air-filled bowel returns to normal once the bladder is evacuated. The most common appearance of the abdomen in small bowel ischemia is a nonspecific arrangement of bowel gas. The second most frequent appearance is dilated jejunal and ileal loops, a configuration easily mistaken for distal obstruction. In elderly patients and in those with heart and vascular disease, mesenteric ischemia must be ruled out clinically before obstruction can be diagnosed with reasonable assurance on plain films.

If the limitations and pitfalls of plain film interpretation are recognized, and close interaction between referring physicians and clinical radiologists is achieved, the noncontrast supine view of the abdomen can be a powerful tool for the recognition of bowel obstruction. In most cases no other imaging studies aside from follow-up supine views need to be done.

## Suggested Reading

deLacey BO, Wignall BK, Bradbrooke S, et al. Rationalizing abdominal radiography in the accident and emergency department. Clin Radiol 1980; 31:453–455.

deLacey B, Wilkins R, Cramer B, et al. The accuracy of plain film radiography in assessing colonic faecal contamination. Clin Radiol 1983; 34:73–74.

Eisenberg RL, Heincken P, Hedgcock MV, et al. Evaluation of plain radiographs in the diagnosis of abdominal pain. Ann Surg 1983; 197:464–469.

Gammill SL, Nice CM Jr. Air fluid levels: Their occurrence in normal patients and their role in the analysis of ileus. Surgery 1972; 71:771–780.

Han SY, Witten DM, Prim HS. Plain film findings in massive gastrointestinal bleeding. Am J Roentgenol 1977; 129:437–439.

Mievis SE, Young JWR, Keramati B, et al. Plain film evaluations of patients with abdominal pain: Are three radiographs necessary? Am J Roentgenol 1986; 147:501–503.

Miller RE, Nelson SW. The roentgenographic demonstration of tine amounts of free intraperitoneal gas: Experimental and clinical studies. Am J Roentgenol 1971; 112:574–585.

Simeone JF, Novelline RA, Ferrucci JT Jr. Comparison of sonography and plain films in evaluations of acute abdomen. Am J Roentgenol 1985; 144:49–52.

# Radiology of the Diaphragm and Lesser Sac

*ROBERT E. MINDELZUN, M.D. · JAMES J. McCORT, M.D.*

## The Diaphragm

The diaphragm is composed of three primary muscle groups (sternal, costal, lumbar) that converge centrally into a strong aponeurosis of interwoven and decussating fibers called the central tendon of the diaphragm. It is pierced by three major apertures: the aortic, vena caval, and esophageal hiatuses. Additional potential regions of thoracoabdominal communication exist at sites of diaphragmatic weakness anteriorly (foramina of Morgagni) and posteriorly (foramina of Bochdalek) (Fig. 1). The diaphragm is the primary barrier between the abdominal and thoracic cavities and is the major muscle of inspiration. It is innervated by the phrenic nerve, which arises from C4 nerve roots with variable contributions for C3 and C5. Contraction of the diaphragm increases the intrathoracic volume by downward movement of the diaphragm and by elevation of the rib cage.

### *Intrinsic Abnormalities of Position and Function*

On the erect posteroanterior (PA) chest radiograph, the right hemidiaphragm lies at the level of the posterior ninth to tenth

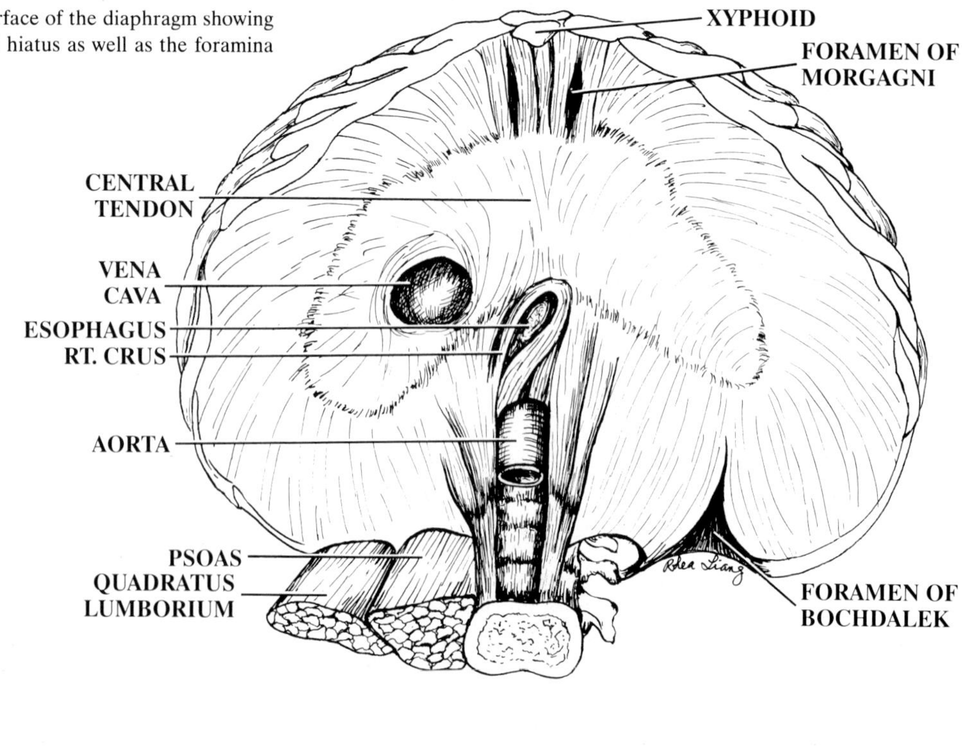


**FIGURE 1** Anatomy of the undersurface of the diaphragm showing the aortic, vena caval, and esophageal hiatus as well as the foramina of Morgagni and Bochdalek.

rib. The left hemidiaphragm is usually one-half to one interspace lower. In up to 9 percent of normal individuals, the left hemidiaphragm is at the same level as the right hemidiaphragm, or it may actually be higher. The average diaphragmatic excursion is 3 to 4 cm. Radiographic evaluation of the diaphragm begins with a PA and a lateral chest film. Potential abnormalities are best evaluated by comparison with prior examinations. Fluoroscopy remains an important tool in the evaluation of the diaphragm, providing both anatomic and functional information. The central portion of the diaphragm and the peripheral zone should be evaluated separately for symmetrical motion. Minimal dyssynchrony is commonly observed and is of little clinical significance. Fluoroscopy should be first performed during quiet respiration, in the upright position if possible, with progressively increasing respiratory effort to accentuate abnormalities. Paradoxical hemidiaphragmatic motion is best seen during a "sniff test," which is performed by forceful rapid inspiration through the nose. In the decubitus position, the dependent diaphragm shows the greatest excursion, which thus accentuates any abnormality. A useful supplement to the foregoing is a "double-exposed" chest radiograph, taken alternately in full inspiration and full expiration, which provides a permanent record of diaphragmatic motion.

Intrinsic abnormalities of diaphragmatic position and function have two major causes: (1) congenital or acquired loss of muscle tissue and (2) defective innervation.

### Eventration

Loss of muscle substance followed by fibrous tissue replacement is commonly called *eventration.* Congenital eventration, which is believed to be a result of defective myoblast migration, can involve all or any portion of the diaphragm. It is most commonly right sided, partial, and located anteromedially. Acquired eventration usually follows trauma or may develop secondary to diaphragmatic paralysis with progressive loss of tone, muscle atrophy, and fibrosis. The process is usually unilateral. Radiographic differentiation of eventration from paralysis is often impossible.

### Defective Innervation

Neuronal control of diaphragmatic contraction extends from the respiratory center through the spinal cord to the phrenic nerve. Direct phrenic nerve invasion by tumor, especially bronchogenic carcinoma, represents a common cause of phrenic paralysis. Idiopathic paralysis may be caused by viral- or bacterial-induced toxic neuritis and involves both leaves with equal frequency. A third cause is actual neural trauma, which includes direct nerve injury and C3 to C5 cervical cord injury. Birth injuries as well as chest, mediastinal, and neck surgery occasionally result in phrenic paralysis. More unusual causes are brain stem lesions, Guillain-Barré syndrome, multiple sclerosis, diabetes, aortic aneurysm, goiter, and mediastinal lymph node enlargement. In the absence of a specific history that would explain the phrenic injury, it is most important to exclude the presence of a malignant tumor in the chest, mediastinum, or neck. This is best done with chest radiographs, computed tomography (CT), magnetic resonance imaging (MRI), and occasionally angiography.

## *Diaphragmatic Hernias*

Exclusive of the post-traumatic type, there are three primary types of hernias that affect the diaphragm: (1) esophageal or paraesophageal hernias, (2) Bochdalek's hernias, and (3) Morgagni's hernias. The first is rarely congenital, whereas Bochdalek and Morgagni hernias are most often congenital.

### Esophageal and Paraesophageal Hernias

These hernias, which are usually seen in adults, especially the elderly, result from an acquired widening of the esophageal hiatus with stretching of the phrenicoesophageal membrane. They are commonly seen on chest radiographs as round or oblong masses that usually demonstrate a prominent air-fluid level located immediately behind the heart.

Sliding hernias are characterized by a gastric fundus that protrudes through the esophageal orifice. They are most commonly seen in elderly or obese patients and may be associated with esophageal dysmotility. Chronic reflux esophagitis may lead to esophageal scarring and retraction, resulting in a hiatus hernia.

Paraesophageal hernias are much less common than sliding hernias and are characterized by an esophagogastric junction that lies at or below the esophageal orifice. When an esophageal hiatus is especially capacious, it may allow protrusion of a segment of transverse colon or omentum into the chest, resulting in a combined hernia.

### Bochdalek's Hernia

The diaphragm is normally formed during the sixth to tenth fetal weeks. Development begins in the septum transversus, which incompletely separates the thoracic and abdominal cavities. Posteromedially the last areas to close are the pleuroperitoneal canals, also known as the foramina of Bochdalek. When there is defective or delayed closure of these canals, abdominal organs may enter the thorax. Bochdalek's hernias have an incidence of 4.8 cases per 10,000 live births. Ninety percent are left sided. Small hernias cause few or no symptoms and are often discovered incidentally on chest radiographs. During routine CT scanning, minimal protrusion through the foramen of Bochdalek has been reported in 6 percent of patients. In these situations subdiaphragmatic fat or occasionally kidney or other organ may herniate through the opening. Only 10 to 20 percent of hernias possess a pleural peritoneal sac.

The neonate with a Bochdalek's hernia presents with progressive respiratory distress, unilateral absent breath sounds, shift of cardiac dullness, and a scaphoid abdomen. Twenty-five percent of these patients have other congenital anomalies, especially intestinal malrotations and central nervous system (CNS) and cardiac anomalies. The chest radiograph reveals stomach and bowel loops that extend into the thorax, compressing the ipsilateral lung, resulting in contralateral mediastinal shift (Fig. 2). When these characteristic findings are present, the infant requires no further investigation before surgery. Staphylococcal pneumonia or adenomatoid malformation of the neonatal lung can mimic a Bochdalek's hernia. When direct extension of bowel loops is not seen, the diagnosis can be elucidated by introducing a nasogastric tube and injecting air or barium.

### Morgagni's Hernia

At the anterior muscle insertion into the xiphoid, two slitlike openings (foramina of Morgagni) transmit the continuations of the internal mammary arteries. Herniations are usually seen in adults, often as a result of increased intra-abdominal pressure associated with obesity or trauma. Rarely defective develop-

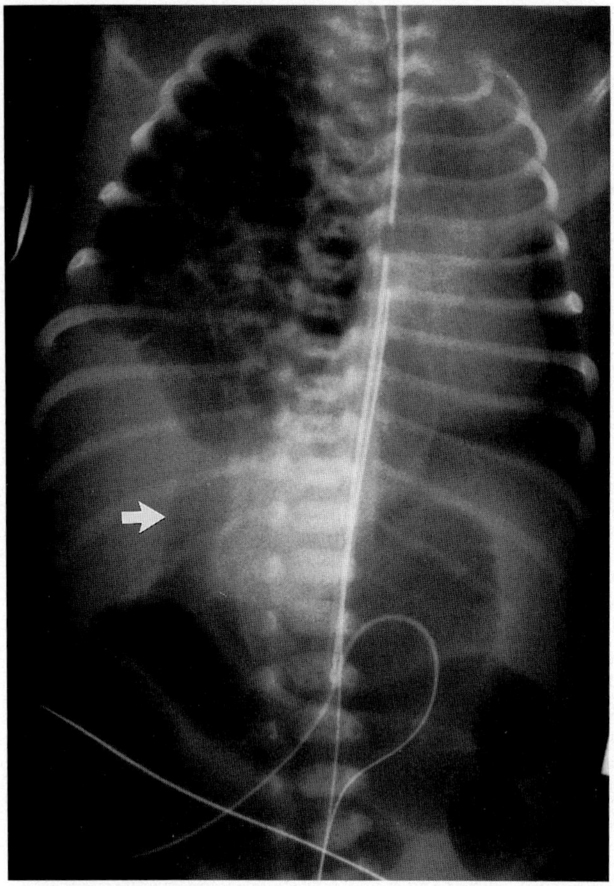

**FIGURE 2** Bochdalek's hernia. Newborn with difficulty breathing. Herniation of multiple loops of small and large bowel into the right hemithorax with displacement of the mediastinum to the contralateral side. Continuity of bowel loops *(arrow)* readily establishes the correct diagnosis. This Bochdalek's hernia is unusual in that it involves the right hemidiaphragm.

ment of the anterior muscle allows intrathoracic herniation of the omentum and/or transverse colon. The hernia, most often right sided, is identified as a solid mass behind the xyphoid and may contain gas if the colon is contained within the sac (Fig. 3). A barium enema study demonstrates a herniated transverse colon, which appears constricted as it extends through the diaphragmatic orifice (Fig. 4). Differential diagnosis possibilities include pericardial cyst, bronchogenic cyst, esophageal duplication, or solid tumor and are best evaluated with CT.

### Peritoneopericardial Hernia

These rare hernias are congenital or occasionally post-traumatic. Bowel or omentum most commonly herniates into the pericardial cavity.

## *Diaphragmatic Tumors*

Primary tumors are equally divided between benign and malignant. The most common malignant tumor is the fibrosarcoma, followed in frequency by fibrous histiocytoma, hemangiopericytoma, and leiomyosarcoma. Lipomas are the most common benign tumors, with other reported tumors representing angiofibroma, neurofibroma, neurilemoma, leiomyoma, ectopic hepatic tissue, congenital or acquired cyst, endometrioma, and teratoma. Direct extension of abdominal or thoracic malignancy accounts for most secondary lesions. The early detection and evaluation of the rare diaphragmatic tumor presents considerable difficulty. The chest radiograph depicts only the pleural surfaces of the diaphragm, hence the initial finding may be just an abnormal diaphragmatic bulge (Fig. 5). Differentiation of a tumor from a focal eventration, fat herniation, or an ectopic kidney may be difficult. Ultrasonography represents the least invasive and least expensive imaging modality and can often evaluate the full thickness and continuity of the diaphragms. In addition, most of the time it is sufficiently diagnostic to suggest fat interposition and renal ectopia. Thin-section CT scans or sagittal MRI provide excellent anatomic detail, although the exact nature of the

A

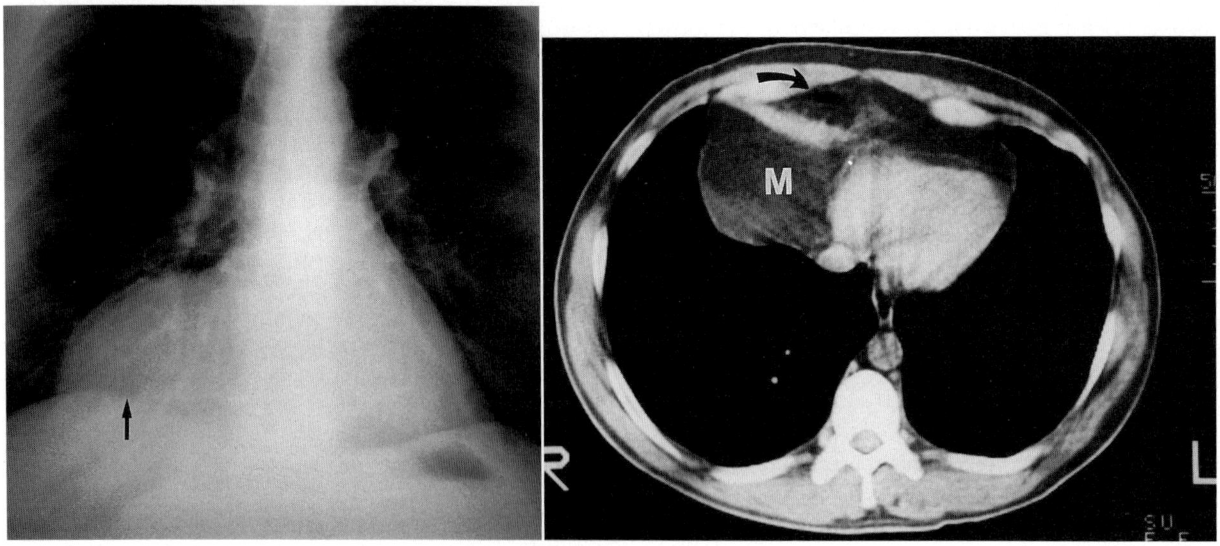


B

**FIGURE 3** *A,* Post-traumatic Morgagni's hernia. Competitive weight lifter who suddenly felt retrosternal pain after strenuous exercise. Prior chest films were normal. Large right-sided cardiophrenic mass *(arrow)*. *B,* The mass (M) is primarily composed of omental fat. Small collection of gas *(arrow)* noted anteriorly representing the transverse colon.

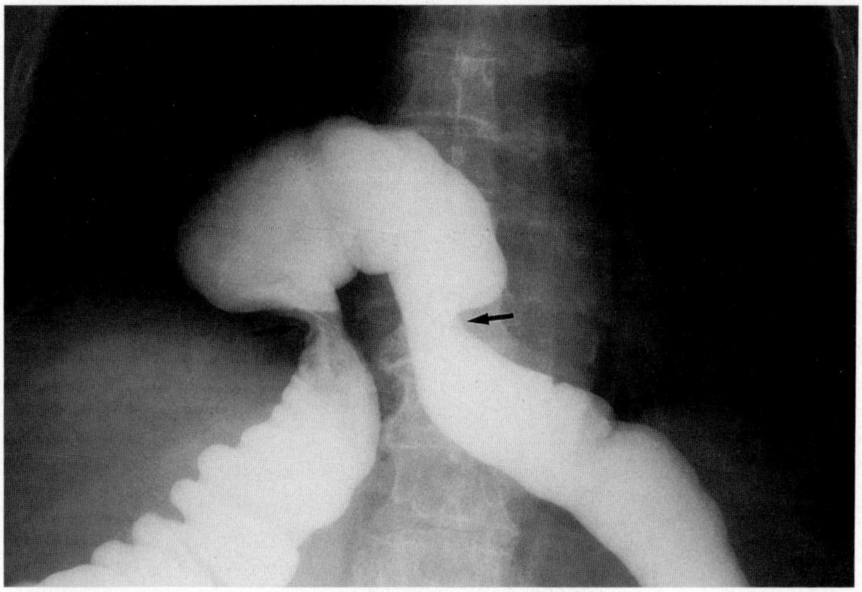

**FIGURE 4** Morgagni's hernia. Barium enema study demonstrated herniation of the transverse colon, with constriction of the colonic contour *(arrows)*.

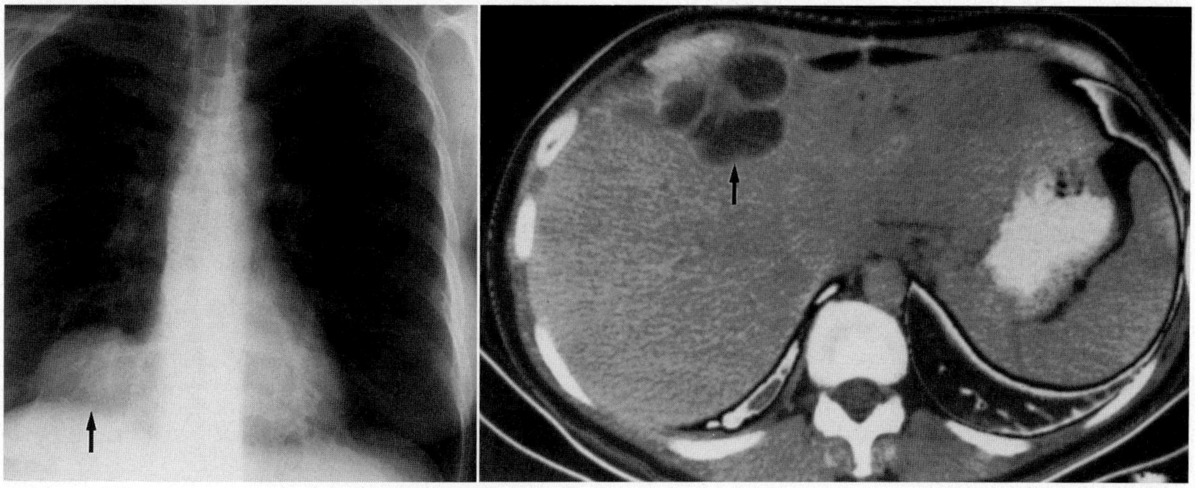


**FIGURE 5** *A,* Anaplastic primary tumor of the diaphragm. Middle-aged woman noted to have an incidental mass on a routine chest film. Large right-sided cardiophrenic mass *(arrow)* without specific diagnostic characteristics. *B,* Multiloculated mass *(arrow)* with enhancing periphery. At surgery the mass was extrahepatic and arising from the diaphragm.

mass often requires tissue analysis. Although not commonly employed, a diagnostic pneumoperitoneum with either $CO_2$ or air is excellent for visualization of the peritoneal surface of the diaphragm and can help the surgeon plan a thoracic or abdominal approach to the lesion.

## *Juxtadiaphragmatic Fluid Collections*

### Supradiaphragmatic Fluid

Fluid above the diaphragm may be pulmonary or pleural and is readily identified on an erect chest radiograph. Most pleural fluid collections are easily characterized on decubitus views with CT and ultrasonography reserved for the cryptic fluid collection. Increasing accumulation of fluid within the pleural cavity, especially on the left side, may cause inversion of the hemidiaphragm. This is recognized on chest radiography by caudal displacement of the gastric air bubble and can be confirmed by ultrasonography.

### Infradiaphragmatic Fluid

Most loculated subdiaphragmatic fluid collections are inflammatory and intraperitoneal. Retroperitoneal fluid collections rarely extend to the diaphragm, and lesser sac fluid collections are kept from extending to the diaphragm by the inferior coronary ligament on the right side and the gastrophrenic ligament on the left side. In the usual circumstance, infected intraperitoneal fluid extends from the pelvis along the lateral peritoneal gutters to the subdiaphragmatic spaces. This occurs more readily on the right side, because the left subphrenic space is somewhat protected by the phrenicocolic ligament. Subphrenic abscesses are common complications of prior surgery, gastroduodenal or colonic perforations, intraperitoneal or visceral abscesses, and peritoneal carcinomatosis. Any of the foregoing conditions associated with a fixed or elevated diaphragm should suggest a subphrenic abscess, which usually necessitates ultrasonography or CT for diagnosis.

The differentiation of pleural from peritoneal fluid on CT scans can be difficult. Most signs described have a relative accuracy of 60 to 70 percent, but a combination of signs should result in a correct diagnosis in most cases. The most helpful signs are as follows:

1. *Displaced crus sign*—Pleural fluid in the posterior sulcus displaces the ipsilateral crus anteriorly and laterally.
2. *Interface sign*—Peritoneal fluid produces a sharp interface with the liver and spleen, whereas pleural fluid results in a hazy interface.
3. *Diaphragm sign*—Pleural fluid lies outside the contour of the diaphragm, whereas ascites lie within the diaphragmatic contour.
4. *Bare area sign*—Pleural fluid can extend posterior to the bare area, whereas peritoneal fluid cannot.
5. *Inferior pulmonary ligament sign*—Identification of the inferior pulmonary ligament indicates that the fluid is pleural and usually associated with pulmonary atelectasis.
6. *Split pleura sign*—Fluid separates the two adjacent pleural surfaces.
7. *Subdiaphragmatic structure sign*—Identification of an intra-abdominal structure, such as the spleen or falciform ligament, surrounded by fluid indicates that the fluid is subdiaphragmatic. In the presence of an inverted diaphragm fluid centrally lies within the thorax, whereas fluid peripherally is peritoneal. This can be recognized by noting that the central fluid collections represent rings of progressively decreasing diameter as the images extend rostrally.

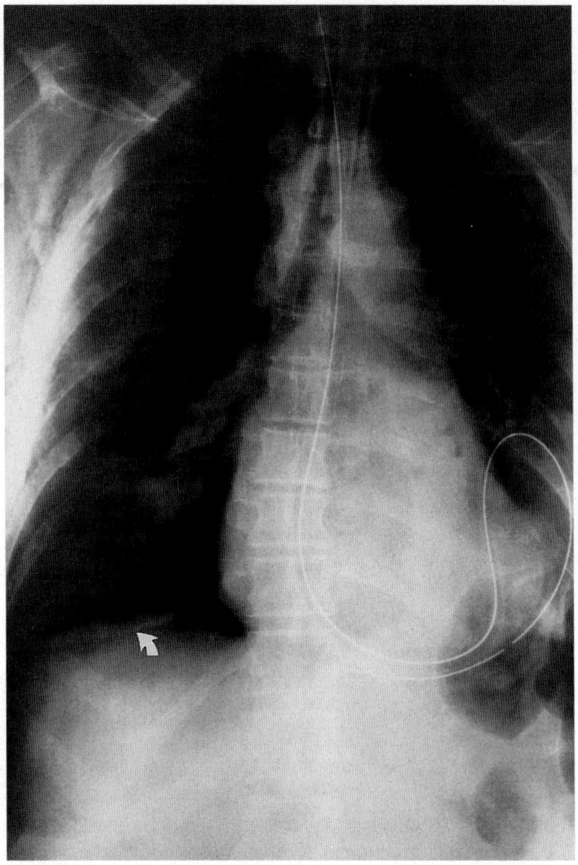

**FIGURE 6** Rupture of the left hemidiaphragm. Diagnosis is readily established by the ectopic cephalically placed nasogastric tube, which conforms to the position of the stomach. Note the associated right-sided subcutaneous emphysema and right-sided pneumothorax *(arrow)*.

## *Trauma to the Diaphragm*

Injuries of the diaphragm may be caused by penetrating injury, blunt abdominal or thoracic trauma, surgery, and forceful vomiting. In blunt trauma a general "rule of 90 percent" helps to highlight the cogent features. Thus 90 percent of reported injuries involve the left hemidiaphragm, 90 percent of injuries are overlooked initially, and 90 percent of strangulated diaphragmatic hernias are of traumatic origin. Supposedly the liver lessens the likelihood of a right hemidiaphragmatic injury.

The diagnosis of diaphragmatic rupture requires a high index of suspicion and attention to even the most minor of diaphragmatic abnormalities. The following findings have been noted on chest radiographs in diaphragmatic injuries:

1. Irregularity and/or elevation of the diaphragm.
2. A masslike density above the diaphragm caused by either fluid-filled bowel, omentum, liver, kidney, spleen, or pancreas.
3. Gas or contrast-containing stomach or bowel above the diaphragm.
4. An ectopic cephalic course of the nasogastric tube into the left side of the hemithorax (Fig. 6).
5. Contralateral mediastinal shift.
6. Widening of the cardiac silhouette with identification of peritoneal contents.
7. Pleural effusion. Large pleural effusions are uncommon with diaphragmatic rupture, because fluid is likely to drain through the laceration.
8. When the right side of the diaphragm is lacerated, a portion of the liver may result in a mushroom-shaped right-sided supradiaphragmatic density.
9. Fractures of the lower ribs, pulmonary contusions, splenic, pancreatic, renal, and liver injuries as well as foreign bodies are occasionally noted in association with diaphragmatic injuries.

In most patients with diaphragmatic injuries, the chest film shows progressive loss of the diaphragmatic outline, with protrusion of either solid or gas-containing viscera into the thorax. A normal diaphragm on the initial examinations does not eliminate the possibility of diaphragmatic injury.

In addition to the chest films, the diaphragm can be studied by several other imaging modalities. Barium can be introduced either with a nasogastric tube or by drinking and may demonstrate a gastric or a small bowel herniation. On barium enema study, the afferent and efferent colonic loops undergo focal tapered narrowing as they pass through the laceration (the double-beak sign). This constriction will be absent in colonic interposition due to diaphragmatic eventration or paralysis. CT can be helpful in evaluating discontinuity of the diaphragm, especially on the left side where the diaphragm interfaces with intra- or extra-peritoneal fat. On the right side, contact of the diaphragm with the liver usually precludes the diagnosis of diaphragmatic tear. Occasionally sagittal or

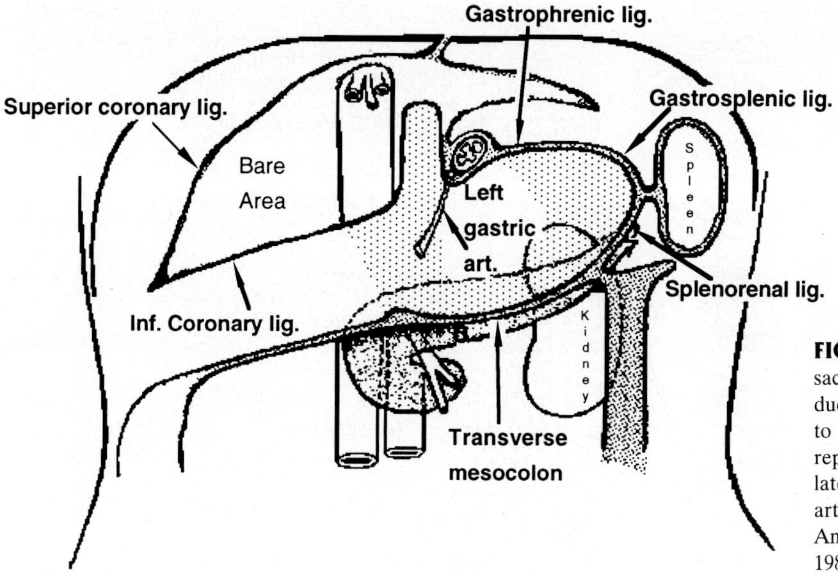


**FIGURE 7** Coronal depiction of the lesser peritoneal sac showing the "right-hand projection method" introduced by Dodds and co-workers. The right hand is noted to be lying within the lesser sac. The extended thumb represents the superior recess. The medial and the lateral compartments are divided by the left gastric artery. (Modified from Dodds WJ, Foley WD, et al. Anatomy and imaging of the lesser peritoneal sac. AJR 1985; 144:567–575.)

coronal reformatted images can clarify the diagnosis. Ultrasonography can readily identify the diaphragm because of its strongly echogenic character and movement and is most helpful in the evaluation of right-sided diaphragmatic injury. Injection of 20 to 50 ml of $CO_2$ intraperitoneally can confirm a diaphragmatic injury by demonstrating a small pneumothorax on the side in question after the patient has been brought into an upright position. Nuclear liver imaging has occasionally been used to demonstrate liver herniation through a diaphragmatic rent.

Most diaphragmatic injuries are overlooked at the time of the original evaluation. With time, lacerations of the diaphragm enlarge because of the pressure gradient between the abdominal and thoracic cavities. The stomach, small bowel, transverse colon, omentum, spleen, kidney, liver, and tail of pancreas may herniate through the opening. With an increase in the size of the diaphragmatic rent, the herniated structure may undergo strangulation, obstruction, or volvulus. Clinical manifestations may not occur for years after the original injury, which may have been forgotten by the patient. Herniation of viscera into the chest may lead to pulmonary compression (tension enterothorax), resulting in life-threatening respiratory distress.

## The Lesser Peritoneal Sac

The anatomy of the lesser peritoneal sac can be best understood by using the "right-hand projection method" introduced by Dodds et al (Fig. 7). The right hand is visualized as lying within the lesser peritoneal sac, with the fifth finger paralleling the pancreas. A wrist bracelet approximates the position of the free margin of the hepatoduodenal ligament. The extended thumb indicates the position of the superior recess. The course of the left gastric artery parallels the thenar crease and divides the lesser peritoneal sac into a medial and a lateral compartment. The medial compartment is further divided into a superior recess and an inferior space. The lateral compartment consists of a suprapancreatic, prepancreatic, and occasionally an infrapancreatic space.

The superior border of the lesser sac on the right side is the inferior reflection of the right coronary ligament (Fig. 8) and on the left side the gastrophrenic ligament, which extends from the stomach to the postero-inferior surface of the diaphragm. Because of these barriers, gas within the lesser sac always projects inferior to the apex of the diaphragm, an important differential consideration when evaluating plain films. The left border of the lesser sac is found at the hilus of the spleen at the junction of the splenorenal and the gastrosplenic ligaments. The right border of the lesser sac is located at the portocaval junction, which lies just to the right of the thoracolumbar spine. The lesser sac is open to the peritoneal cavity at the foramen of Winslow (see Fig. 12). This opening, which averages 2 to 5 cm in size is located posterior to the free margin of the lesser omentum. The posterior boundary of the lesser sac is the peritoneal reflection over the anterior pararenal space. The anterior border is comprised of the posterior surface of the liver, the gastrohepatic ligament, the stomach, and the gastrocolic ligament. The inferior border is the most variable, because of differential fusion of the anterior and posterior leaves of the greater omentum (see Fig. 8, *A*). This may result in a short gastrocolic ligament or in unfused anterior and posterior leaves of the greater omentum, which extend to the pelvis. Posteriorly the inferior border is delineated by the transverse colon and mesocolon. After surgical resection of the stomach, duodenum, transverse colon or spleen, the normally confined recesses of the lesser sac will be open to the greater peritoneal cavity.

Abnormalities of the lesser peritoneal sac can be divided into four categories: internal herniations, abnormal gas accumulations, fluid collections and masses.

### *Internal Herniations*

The most common structure to herniate into the lesser sac is the gallbladder, which usually represents an incidental finding without clinical significance. The small bowel and the large bowel can also herniate into the lesser sac. Herniation of the cecum into the lesser sac necessitates an elongated mesentery and a capacious foramen of Winslow. Herniation of the cecum into the lesser sac usually results in an obstruction that can involve either the right colon or the small bowel. Diagnosis is established by identification of a cephalically placed, dilated

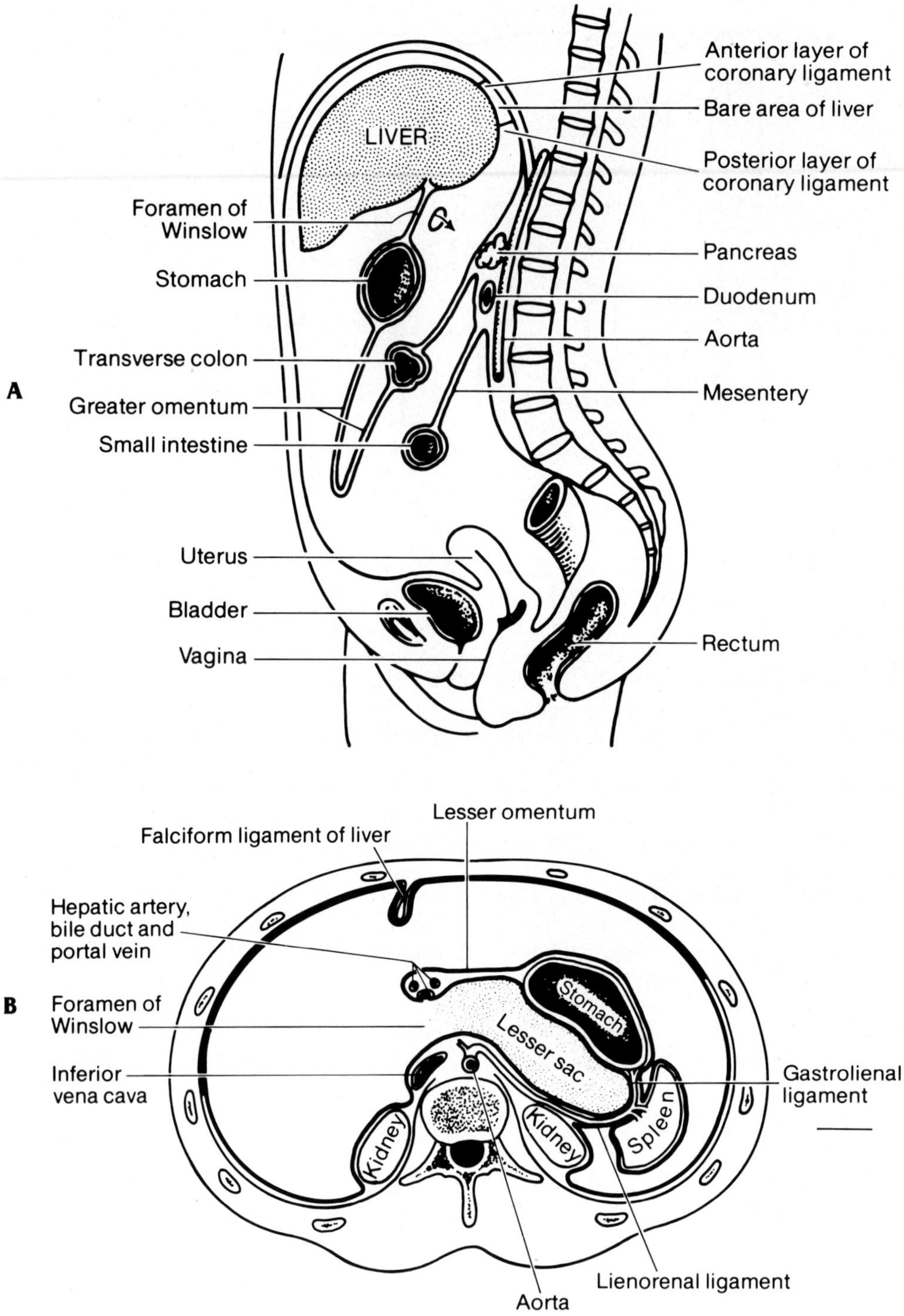


**FIGURE 8** *A,* Sagittal diagram through the lesser sac showing the foramen of Winslow and the unfused leaves of the greater omentum. *B,* Transverse diagram through the lesser sac and the foramen of Winslow. (From Mindelzun RE. Abnormal gas collections. In: McCort JJ, et al., eds. Abdominal Radiology. Baltimore: Williams & Wilkins, 1981:181–249; with permission.)

cecum posterior to the stomach. The stomach is displaced anteriorly and to the left. The diagnosis is confirmed on barium enema study by identification of a cecal obstruction characterized by an inferior "hook," resulting from entrapment of the cecum at the inferior margin of the foramen of Winslow (Fig. 9).

### Abnormal Gas Accumulations

Gas may collect in the lesser sac in the presence of a pneumoperitoneum, but usually the collection in the greater peritoneal cavity is greater in volume and dominates the radiographic findings. Collections of gas that are limited to the lesser sac are usually a result of perforations of the posterior

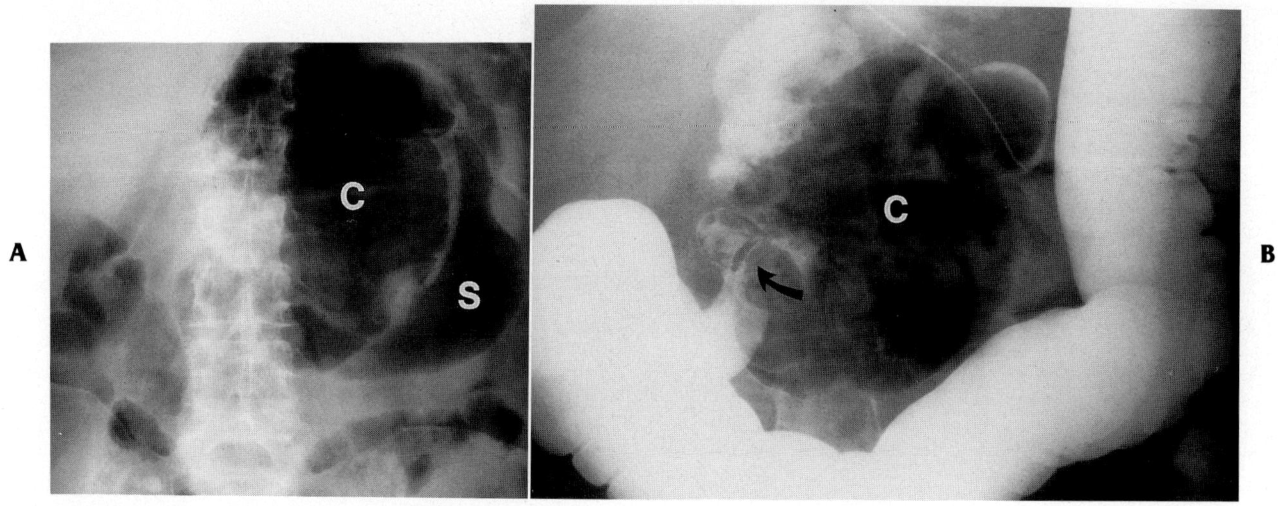


**FIGURE 9** *A,* Herniation of the cecum into the lesser peritoneal sac. Note the displacement of the stomach (S) inferiorly and to the left by the dilated cecum (C). *B,* Barium enema study demonstrating the herniated cecum within the lesser peritoneal sac with a prominent "hook sign" *(arrow).* C= cecum.

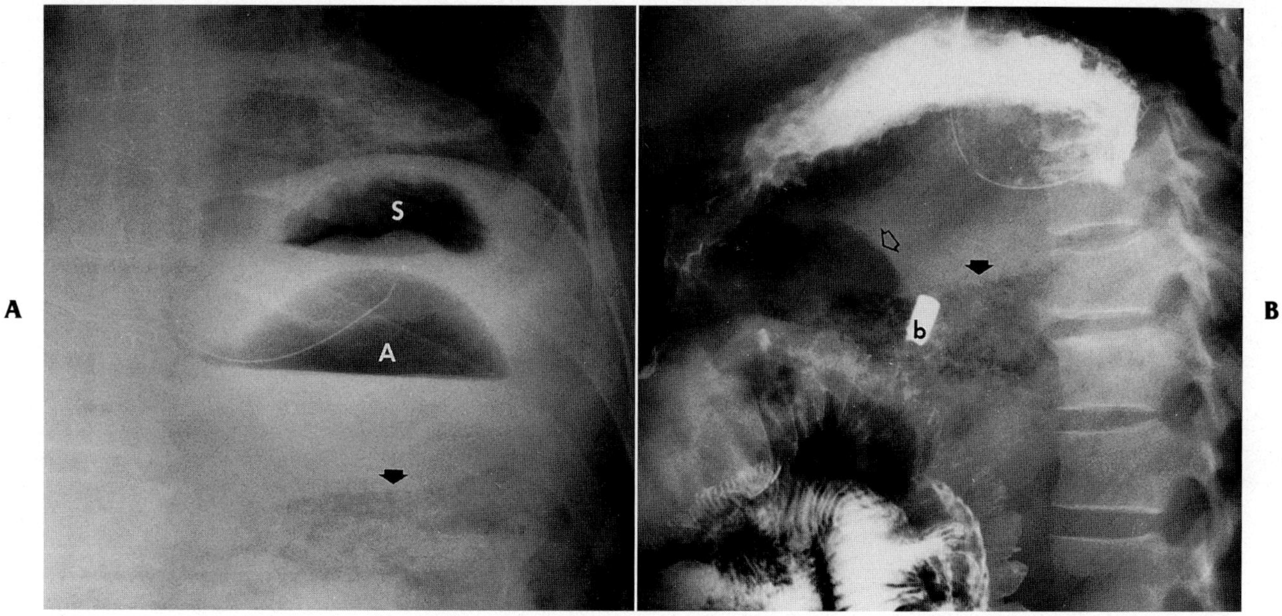


**FIGURE 10** *A,* Large lesser sac abscess (A) demonstrating a prominent air-fluid level on this upright abdominal film. Multiple small gas bubbles *(arrow)* are shown in the pancreatic bed secondary to emphysematous pancreatitis. S= stomach. *B,* Post-traumatic emphysematous pancreatitis *(black arrow)* with a large gas collection in the lesser peritoneal sac *(open arrow).* A bullet (b) is lying in the pancreas. The stomach is draped over the lesser sac mass. (From Mindelzun RE. Abnormal gas collections. In: McCort JJ, et al., eds. Abdominal Radiology. Baltimore: Williams & Wilkins, 1981:181–249; with permission.)

wall of the stomach, duodenum, or colon. With perforations the foramen of Winslow often closes, and gas is absent from the greater peritoneal cavity. Collections caused by perforation usually consist of a single collection of gas, often with an air-fluid level. When multiple small collections of gas are present within the lesser sac, the etiology is more likely to be due to an infection that has extended from adjoining processes such as emphysematous pancreatitis (Fig. 10).

### Fluid Collections

Fluid collections in the lesser sac include ascites (benign or malignant), inflammatory exudates, bile, blood, and rarely lymph. In the presence of ascites, there is often a small amount of fluid noted within the lesser sac. This is also true in the setting of a large hemoperitoneum. With these large fluid collections, it is important to remember that fluid posterior to the gastrohepatic ligament is in the lesser sac and fluid anterior to the ligament is in the peritoneal cavity. The distribution of fluid collections within the lesser sac, especially inflammatory exudates, largely depends on a fold of peritoneum raised by the left gastric artery. This natural barrier divides the lesser sac into a lateral compartment that is primarily retrogastric and a medial compartment that extends cephalad to surround the caudate lobe of the liver. Fluid collections within the lateral compartment separate the stomach from the pancreas and

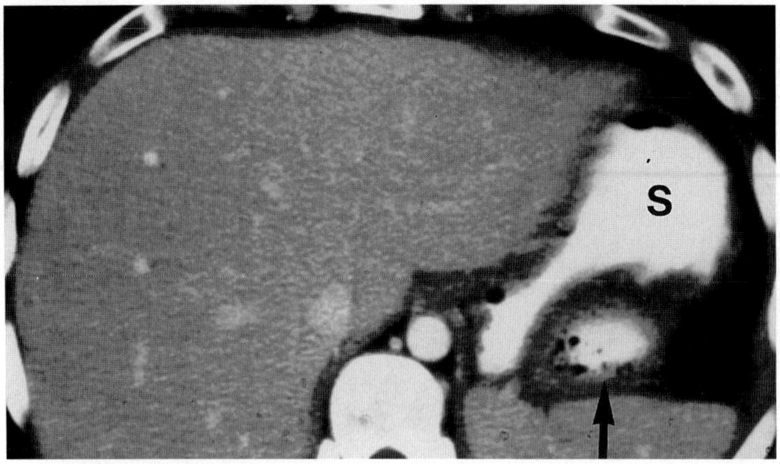


**FIGURE 11** Postgunshot gastric perforation into the lesser peritoneal sac. Contrast material has leaked into the lesser sac *(arrow),* indenting the posterior wall of the stomach (S).

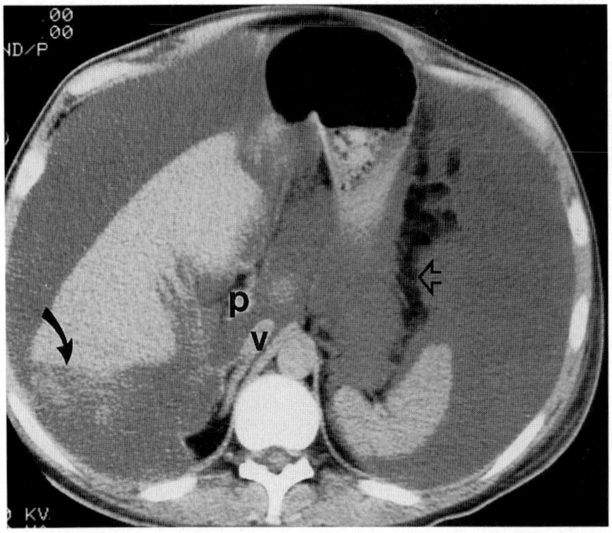


**FIGURE 12** Post-traumatic laceration of the right lobe of the liver *(black arrow).* Massive hemoperitoneum with blood present within the peritoneal cavity as well as in the lesser sac. The gastrosplenic ligament *(open arrow)* marks the left border of the lesser sac. Blood is noted to be entering the lesser sac at the foramen of Winslow between the portal vein (p) and vena cava (v).

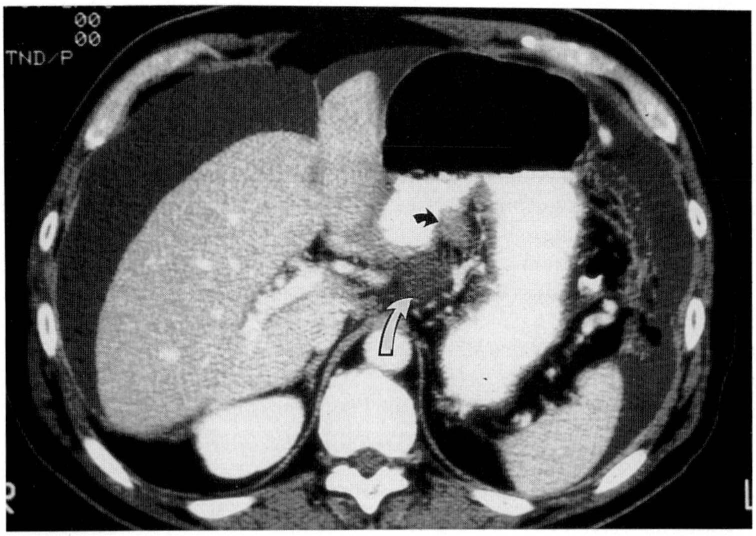

**FIGURE 13** Diffuse intraperitoneal ovarian carcinomatosis with involvement of the lesser peritoneal sac. A surgically proven tumor nodule is noted within the lesser sac *(black arrow)* adjoining the left gastric artery. In addition, there is a small amount of fluid in the medial compartment of the lesser sac *(white arrow).* Ascites and diffuse enhancement of the peritoneum are also present.

displace the stomach anteriorly and to the right (Fig. 11). Occasionally, when the gastrosplenic ligament is redundant, a fluid collection may insinuate itself anterior to the stomach and then displace the stomach posteriorly and to the right. The spleen is most often displaced to the left and posteriorly. Fluid collections within the lesser sac should not be found lateral to the spleen. Most fluid collections within the lesser sac are a result of inflammatory exudates, which are usually secondary to pancreatitis, perforated duodenal and gastric ulcers, left perinephric inflammation, and inflammation of the transverse colon. On occasion appendicitis or sigmoid diverticulitis reaches the lesser sac via the unfused omental leaves. Most inflammatory processes within the lesser sac do not secondarily involve the greater peritoneal cavity, because the foramen of Winslow is readily closed by adhesions. Bile commonly collects in the lesser sac after gallbladder surgery, with formation of localized bilomas most often in the medial recess. Blood is recognized in the lesser sac by its increased density with CT numbers of 50 to 60 (Fig. 12). The most common causes of blood in the lesser sac are hepatic lacerations, splenic lacerations, splenic artery aneurysm rupture, hemorrhagic pancreatitis, hemoperitoneum, and hemorrhage from an adjacent neoplasm.

### *Masses*

The most common masses found in the lesser peritoneal sac are fat, pseudocyst, abscess, and primary or secondary neoplasms. Accumulation of fat is recognized readily by its low CT numbers. A fluid collection within the lesser sac with a well-defined wall is most commonly a pseudocyst, but may also represent a biloma or an abscess. Aspiration is necessary for proper characterization. When gas is seen within a fluid collection, it is usually secondary to an abscess or to an enteric communication. Primary neoplasms involving the lesser sac are rare and consist primarily of mesotheliomas, liposarcomas, and other mesenchymal tumors. Secondary tumors that affect the lesser sac usually extend from adjacent organs such as the pancreas, stomach, duodenum, jejunum, left kidney, or left adrenal. Tumors that spread primarily via ascitic fluid, such as ovarian neoplasms, will on occasion involve the lesser peritoneal sac, especially the medial compartment (Fig. 13).

## Suggested Reading


Cullen ML, Klein MD, Philippart AI. Congenital diaphragmatic hernia. Surg Clin North Am 1985; 65:1115–1134.

Dodds WJ, Foley WD, Lawson TL, et al. Anatomy and imaging of the lesser peritoneal sac. AJR 1985; 144:567–575.

Gale MN. Bochdalek hernia: Prevalence and CT characteristics. Radiology 1985; 156:449–452.

Halversen RA, Fedyshin PJ, Korobkin M, et al. CT differentiation of pleural effusion from ascites: An evaluation of four signs using blinded analysis of 52 cases. Invest Radiol 1986; 21:391–395.

Jeffrey RB, Federle MB, Goodman TC. Computed tomography of the lesser peritoneal sac. Radiology 1981; 141:117–122.

Mindelzun RE. Abnormal gas collections. In: Abdominal Radiology. McCort JJ, Mindelzun RE, Filpi, Rennell, eds. Baltimore: Williams & Wilkins, 1981.

Mindelzun RE. Diaphragmatic trauma. In: McCort JJ, ed. Trauma Radiology. New York: Churchill-Livingstone, 1990.

Panicek DM, Benson CB, Gottlieb RH, et al. The diaphragm: Anatomic, pathologic, and radiologic considerations. Radiographics 1988; 8:385–425.

Tarver RD, Conces EJ, Cory DA, Vix VA. Imaging the diaphragm and its disorders. J Thorac Imaging 1989; 1:1–18.

Walker LA, Weens HS. Radiologic observations on the lesser peritoneal sac. Radiology 1963; 80:727–737.

Wienchek RG, Wilson RF, Steiger Z. Acute injuries of the diaphragm: An analysis of 165 cases. J Thorac Cardiovasc Surg 1986; 92:989.

Zirinsky K, et al. Portacaval space: CT with MR correlation. Radiology 1985; 156:453.


# CT in Abdominal Trauma

*RICHARD SACKNOFF, M.D.*

Trauma is the leading cause of death in America in persons under 38. The trauma patient often has combined injuries to the head, spine, abdomen, chest, pelvis, and extremities that all require prompt treatment. With the availability and increased sophistication of computed tomography (CT), imaging has assumed a major role in the initial diagnosis and management of these patients. With a single test, CT imaging of the abdomen can provide information as to the nature and severity of abdominal, retroperitoneal, pelvic, and skeletal injury, which together with head CT and pertinent plain films assist in immediate triage of the patient to the most appropriate treatment modality. For trauma patients we equip our CT scanners with an accessible crash cart, remote blood pressure cuff, and pulse oximeter to monitor blood oxygen saturation during the procedure. A clinician or nurse is present for patients potentially unstable or who are monitored or sedated.

## Indications and Alternative Technologies

As CT has become readily available to trauma patients, the radiologist has assumed a role in triage of these patients. CT is recommended for hemodynamically stable patients with evidence of significant blunt trauma to the abdomen alone or in combination with other injury. In addition, trauma patients with neurological impairment as a result of head or spine injury, alcohol, or drug ingestion are candidates for CT, because the abdominal physical examination may be unreliable. CT is helpful in screening the abdomen and pelvis in patients with skeletal injury requiring prompt or extensive surgery. Also, hemophiliacs or patients receiving anticoagulants who are at risk of retroperitoneal hemorrhage from even trivial trauma are candidates for CT evaluation.

More and more, CT has become the evaluation of choice

instead of diagnostic peritoneal lavage. The advantages of CT include better localization of injury, as well as evaluation of renal and retroperitoneal injuries that are not well evaluated by lavage. CT is better able to evaluate the abdomen in patients with pelvic fractures that can bleed into the abdomen and result in a false-positive lavage. In fact, at many hospitals CT may be less expensive than diagnostic peritoneal lavage. Because CT provides better analysis of the location and extent of injury, fewer exploratory laparotomies are required.

As a practical matter, CT has become generally preferred to lavage if performed expeditiously with 24 hour availability. Many trauma patients require CT scanning for head injury. It takes only a few minutes more to perform an abdominal CT evaluation. CT is not recommended in hemodynamically unstable patients. Also patients who require immediate treatment or surgery are not CT candidates. Children with severe trauma who are hemodynamically stable are CT candidates.

Ultrasonography is not routinely performed as the initial evaluation for the trauma patient. However, some hospitals are using ultrasonography as an alternative to diagnostic peritoneal lavage in unstable patients. Ultrasonography is limited in its ability to visualize the entire abdomen and retroperitoneum. Also it is operator dependent and more time consuming and less accurate than CT. For similar reasons intravenous urography is not usually performed for evaluation of trauma. CT provides superior demonstration of the extent of renal injury. Equally important is the ability of CT to evaluate these patients for extrarenal injury.

## Technical Approach

Before CT evaluation the radiologist is consulted and helps to coordinate the imaging evaluations. A portable lateral view of the cervical spine in cervical collar and a portable chest radiograph are initially obtained and reviewed. Relevant plain films may be obtained before or after CT, depending on clinical condition. Until the patient's cervical spine has been cleared with a complete cervical spinal series, the cervical collar remains on the patient. If injury to the spine is suspected, the patient is left on the trauma board during transport to the CT suite. When indicated, the head CT is performed before the abdominal CT evaluation to maximize the detection of intracranial hemorrhage because intravenous contrast material, which is required for abdominal CT for trauma, may obscure intracranial hemorrhage.

Attention to CT technique is critical to realizing the high overall accuracy of CT for trauma (Table 1). A contemporary CT scanner gives better overall results and is more forgiving of patient motion. Our protocol calls for obtaining a digital scout view and scanning using 10 mm contiguous slices from above the top of the hemidiaphragms to the pubic symphysis. The lung bases should be included to evaluate for pneumothorax and lung contusion that may not be evident on the supine chest radiograph. Scanning the pelvis is routinely performed to demonstrate the often large intra-abdominal hemorrhage that may collect in the dependent lower abdomen and pelvis in a supine patient. Related fractures and pelvic injuries are often demonstrated. If a pelvic injury is evident or suspected, thinner sections through the pelvis are obtained.

Before scanning the digital scout image is obtained and evaluated for metallic leads and buckles that may cause artifact. On current scanners it is usually not necessary to partially withdraw the nasogastric tube. The Foley catheter if present should be clamped before scanning to allow the bladder to fill with contrast material, optimizing detection of bladder injury. If the bladder is sufficiently distended, a cystogram may be unnecessary to exclude bladder injury. The patient's arms should be placed outside the gantry whenever possible.

**TABLE 1** CT Technique for Abdominal Trauma

Preparation
- Clamp Foley catheter to maximize bladder distention.
- Position patient's arms above head; if not possible position arms on lower chest.
- Obtain digital scout view; inspect for and remove potential artifacts (metallic buckles, e.g., pads) from area to be scanned.

Contrast
- Oral contrast agent optional: give 10–20 oz of Gastrografin solution (¼ oz of Gastrografin in 10 oz of water).
- IV contrast agent: inject 120–140 ml of 60% iodinated IV contrast solution with power injector at 1–1.5 ml/second. After 45 second delay, begin dynamic scanning. Monitor IV site for possible extravasation during first few seconds of infusion.

Mechanics:
- Obtain 10 mm thick contiguous slices from above hemidiaphragms to pubic symphysis. Minimal exposure time (half scanning) recommended for patients on ventilator or nonsedated children. Thinner sections used through pelvis if pelvic fractures suspected.
- Photograph entire abdomen and pelvis with soft-tissue and bone windows. Photograph liver and spleen with liver windows. Photograph lung bases with lung windows.

In adults an oral contrast agent is optional, but may facilitate diagnosis of bowel or pancreatic injury. In a seriously injured patient, CT of the abdomen should not be delayed to administer oral contrast material. However, if time permits, a patient is given one or two 10 oz cups of Gastrografin solution 20 minutes before the scan and an additional cup when positioned on the scanner. The Gastrografin solution consists of ¼ oz of Gastrografin in 10 oz of water. In children oral contrast material is strongly recommended, because the paucity of intraperitoneal and retroperitoneal fat makes detection of bowel and retroperitoneal injury more difficult. If patients with penetrating injuries are evaluated with CT, oral and rectal contrast agents with dilute Gastrografin solution are recommended to supplement the intravenous contrast agent.

Intravenous contrast material and dynamic scanning are required to maximize the detection of liver and spleen injury. For adults 100 to 150 ml of iodinated contrast solution is administered via a low-pressure mechanical injector at the rate of 1 to 1.5 ml/sec. To minimize extravasation of the contrast agent, a 20 gauge or larger soft intravenous catheter is used and the injection site monitored during the first few seconds of injection. For children, we use a hand injection of nonionic contrast material, using 2 to 3 mg per kilogram of weight followed by dynamic scanning.

After a 40 second delay following initiation of intravenous contrast infusion, dynamic scanning is performed through the abdomen to the bottom of liver and spleen, using short interscan delays (i.e., 4 to 7 seconds). Then the remainder of the lower abdomen and pelvis is scanned. Scanning the lower abdomen and pelvis nondynamically allows the bladder to fill and may increase detection of bladder injury. Two second scan times are used on most patients. Patients on respirators and patients unable to hold still are scanned with 1.3 second half scans to minimize motion. Scans with obvious motion artifact are repeated or electronically postprocessed (segmented) at the end of the evaluation. The evaluation is monitored on the console and additional thin sections are obtained if needed.

The entire evaluation is photographed using soft-tissue windows (level 10, window 300) and bone windows (level 500, window 2,000). Liver windows (level 55, window 250) photographed through the liver, spleen, and kidneys may reveal subtle contusions. Lung windows (level −500, window 500) photographed through the lung bases are required to evaluate for contusion or pneumothorax (Fig. 1). In addition to detecting skeletal fractures, the bone windows are helpful in the evaluation of free intraperitoneal air. The CT evaluation is reviewed with the clinician on completion.

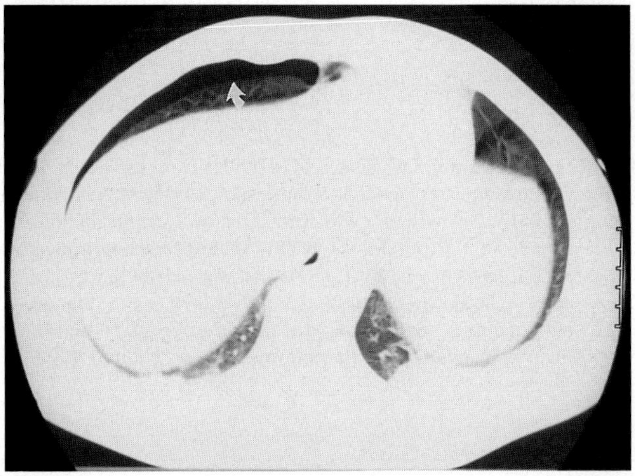

**FIGURE 1** CT image of the upper abdomen viewed on lung window settings reveals a right-sided pneumothorax (*arrow*) This pneumothorax was not visible on the supine chest radiograph.

## Diagnostic Approach

### *Hemoperitoneum*

The key image sign of abdominal injury is the presence of free blood or hemoperitoneum. Blood under 48 hours old has a CT density of greater than 30 HU. It can readily be separated from simple ascites by measuring its CT density. On a contrast-enhanced CT scan, the blood appears less dense than adjacent liver or spleen. Intra-abdominal blood usually collects in the dependent portions of the abdomen, such as in Morrison's pouch between the lower margin of the liver and right kidney. Blood may also be observed in the pericolic gutters (Fig. 2, *B*) and pelvis. It is particularly important to survey the pelvis, because large amounts of hemorrhage may collect there with little hemorrhage in the upper abdomen. Blood often is of higher CT density closer to the site of injury than on the contralateral side. If substantial intraperitoneal blood is present, it is useful to evaluate for contraction of the inferior vena cava and aorta. In young children severe volume loss may be associated with abnormal enhancement of the bowel wall, kidneys, gallbladder, and great vessels with dilated fluid-filled bowel termed the *hypovolemic complex*. This is often associated with liver or spleen injury and carries a poor prognosis.

Because free intraperitoneal hemorrhage may be the only sign of abdominal injury, I prefer not to perform diagnostic peritoneal lavage before CT. Residual lavage fluid may obscure blood from a bowel or mesenteric injury. However, scanning the abdomen may be helpful in patients who have had prior lavage that is borderline positive or for further characterization of injury of patients with positive lavage who have stabilized sufficiently with conservative management to not require immediate surgery. It is rare to find a major organ injury without a component of intraperitoneal or retroperitoneal hemorrhage.

A

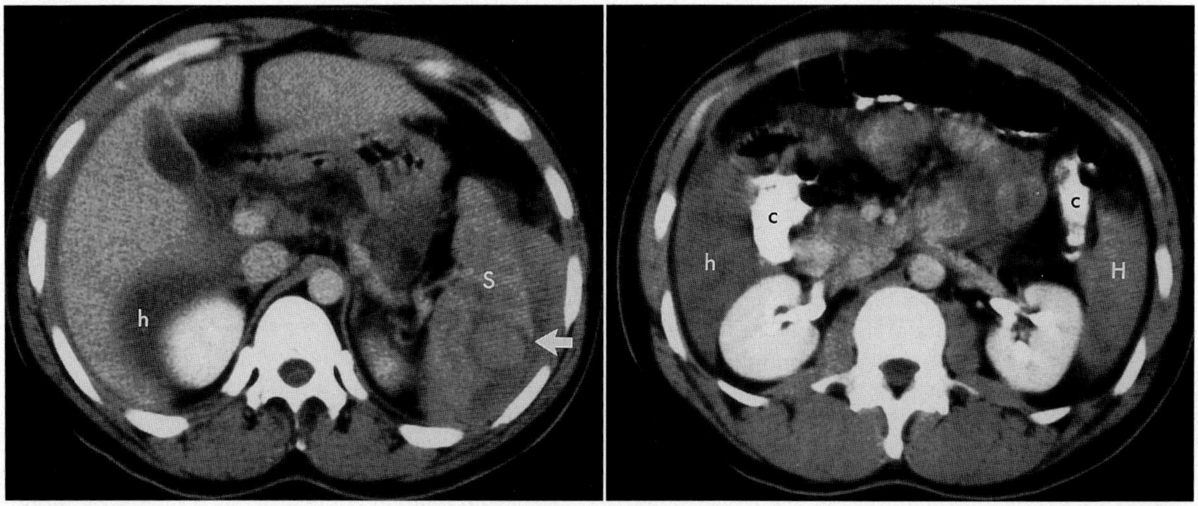


B

**FIGURE 2** *A,* CT image of splenic rupture. After intravenous bolus, the complex splenic laceration (*arrow*) appears lower in density than the intact portion of the spleen (S). Hemoperitoneum (h) is present in Morrison's pouch, as well as around the liver and spleen. *B,* In the lower abdomen of the same patient, hemorrhage from the ruptured spleen is present adjacent to the colon (c) in the right and left pericolic gutters. Hemorrhage (h) adjacent to the injured spleen has higher CT density than hemorrhage (H) on the contralateral side.

A B

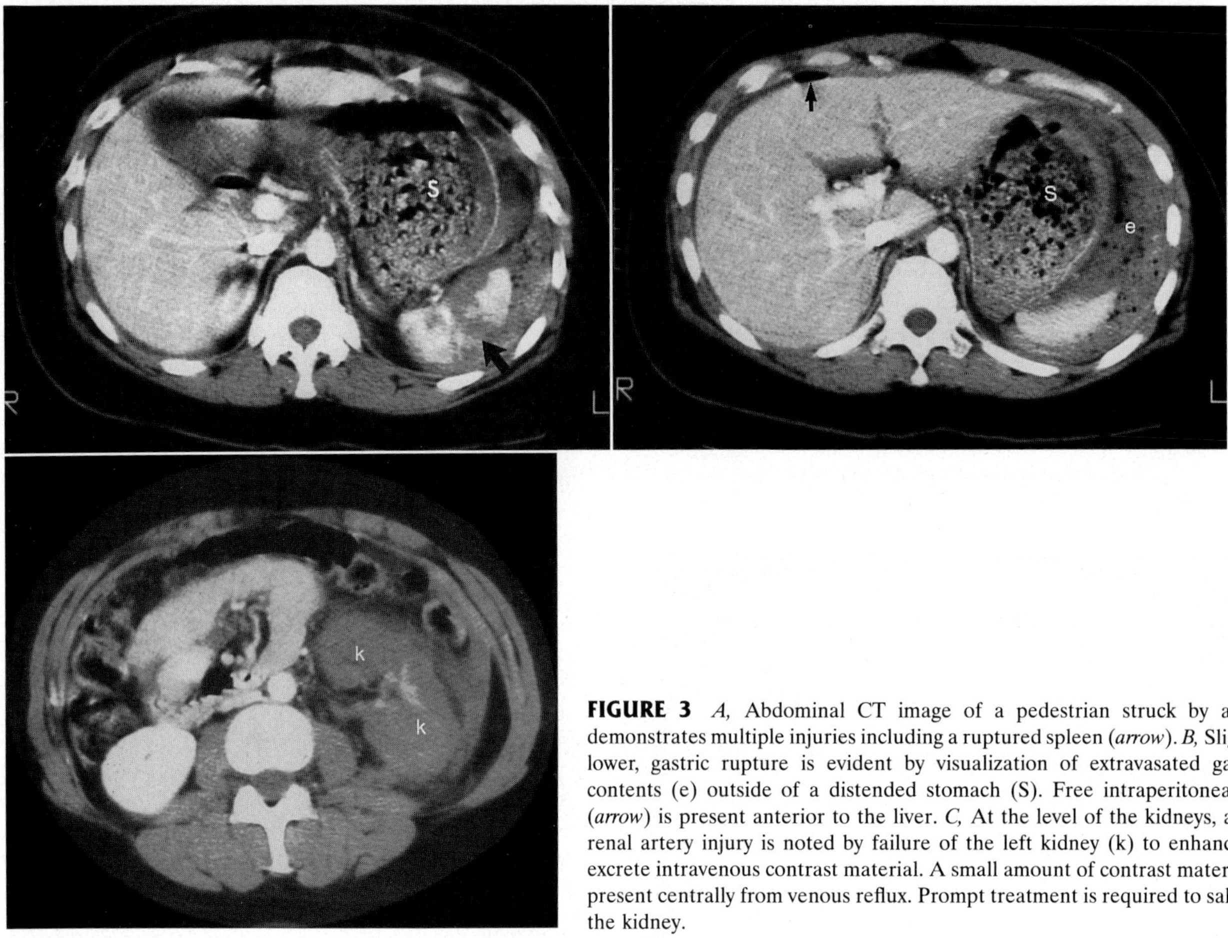


C

**FIGURE 3** *A,* Abdominal CT image of a pedestrian struck by a car demonstrates multiple injuries including a ruptured spleen (*arrow*). *B,* Slightly lower, gastric rupture is evident by visualization of extravasated gastric contents (e) outside of a distended stomach (S). Free intraperitoneal air (*arrow*) is present anterior to the liver. *C,* At the level of the kidneys, a left renal artery injury is noted by failure of the left kidney (k) to enhance or excrete intravenous contrast material. A small amount of contrast material is present centrally from venous reflux. Prompt treatment is required to salvage the kidney.

## *Spleen*

The spleen is the most commonly injured abdominal organ. Because the spleen is prone to severe hemorrhage from injury, attention to the spleen is important. Quantitative classification of splenic injury is not widely accepted or used at our hospital because it has not been a reliable predictor as to which patients require surgery. However, a general classification based on description together with an estimation of the amount of intraperitoneal blood is useful. Injury to the spleen (Fig. 2) may consist of laceration, a linear lower density within the spleen. Mottled low-density regions are characterized as contusion or hematoma. Splenic fractures, a shattered spleen, pedicle injury, or extensive vascular injury to the spleen more often requires surgery. CT provides an accuracy of approximately 95 percent for evaluation of splenic injury.

Because of the protective nature of intact spleen from rapid overwhelming sepsis from bacterial infection, every effort is now made to preserve the spleen whenever possible. This is particularly true in the pediatric population. CT is helpful together with clinical signs in the initial decision process and in subsequent management of patients treated conservatively.

Pitfalls are present in the performance and interpretation of CT scans. Artifacts from adjacent ribs and motion are often present and often require repeat thin sections to clarify. Some newer scanners have electronic segmentation that may be performed as a postprocessing technique to reduce artifact from motion. If intravenous contrast material is not administered or not given in combination with rapid dynamic scanning, lacerations, contusions, and subcapsular hematomas may appear isodense with the spleen and not be detected. Bolus contrast administration and review of the scan on a monitor with optimal window settings minimizes this. On many CT scanners, artifact is present from the nasogastric tube. If this is the case, the nasogastric tube should be withdrawn to the distal esophagus before scanning. An important pitfall of interpretation is overlooking associated injuries (Fig. 3). A substantial number of patients have multiple injuries. Care must be taken to search for associated abdominal and bony injuries once one injury is found. Similarly abnormalities not related to trauma are often present on CT scans, and scrutiny of the scan for incidental findings is helpful.

## *Liver*

With blunt abdominal trauma, the liver is second only to the spleen in frequency of injury. The types of injury to the liver are contusions, fractures, and lacerations—which may be stellate, subcapsular, or intrahepatic hematomas. Most often liver injury is associated with hemoperitoneum. The right lobe is most often injured and may be associated with injury to the right kidney (Fig. 4) or right adrenal gland. Low-density areas of hemorrhage may track along perivascular regions. Careful scrutiny on bone windows is helpful to distinguish periportal hemorrhage from periportal fat. In general most liver injuries

A

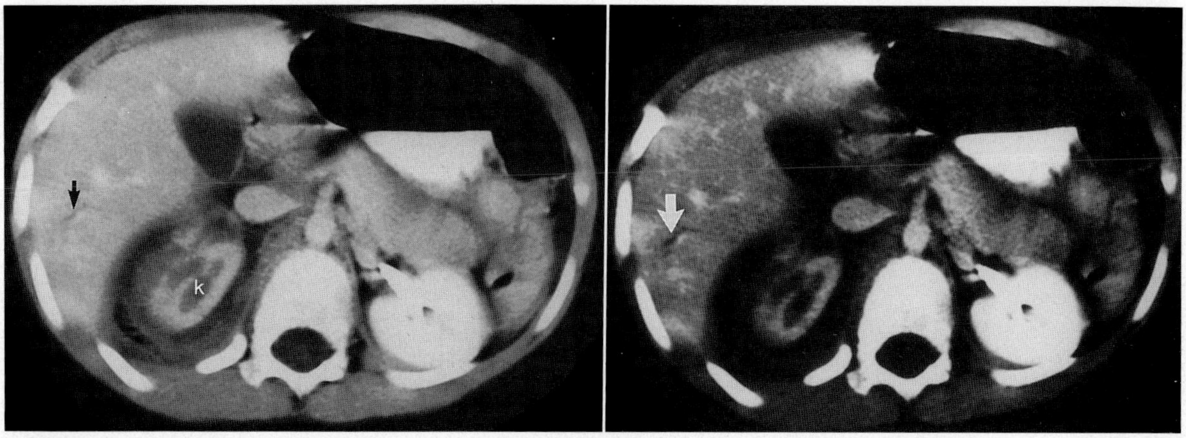


B

**FIGURE 4** *A,* CT image of the midabdomen demonstrates contusion of the right kidney (k) in association with a right lobe liver laceration (*arrow*). *B,* The liver laceration (*arrow*) is more apparent on liver window settings.

A

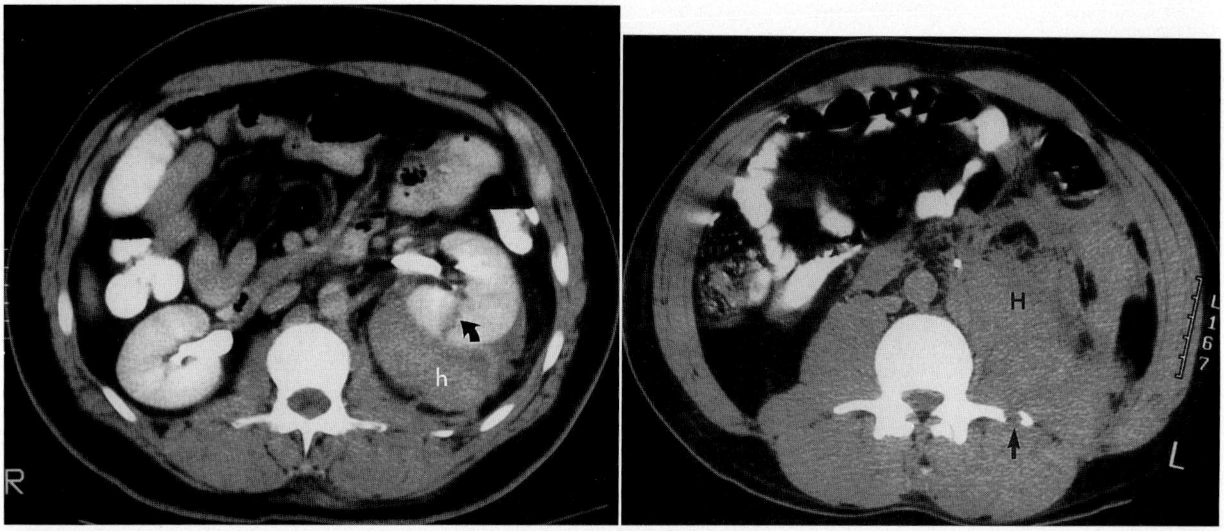


B

**FIGURE 5** *A,* CT image of the left kidney demonstrates a fracture (*arrow*) and adjacent perinephric hemorrhage (h). *B,* Extensive hemorrhage (H) extends down the retroperitoneum adjacent to the left psoas muscle. Even extensive retroperitoneal hemorrhage may not be detected by a diagnostic peritoneal lavage. A left transverse process fracture (*arrow*) is present.

may be managed conservatively. The grading of liver injury includes the extent of injury, evaluation for perihepatic blood or bile, and estimate of amount of hemoperitoneum. The CT accuracy for liver injury is about 90 percent.

## *Kidneys*

CT is the imaging modality of choice for renal trauma. Renal trauma is reported as mild, moderate, or severe. Mild injury consists of contusion and small laceration not extending into the collecting system. Subcapsular hematomas are included in this class. Moderate injuries include larger lacerations (Fig. 5) and those injuries extending into the collecting system with extravasation of urine. Severe injuries include shattered or fractured kidney or renal pedicle injury characterized by partial or complete absence of contrast excretion on the side of injury. Delayed images are helpful to distinguish blood from urine. Extravasated urine is initially low in CT density but becomes high in CT density on delayed images as intravenous contrast material is excreted into the urine (Fig. 6). Follow-up

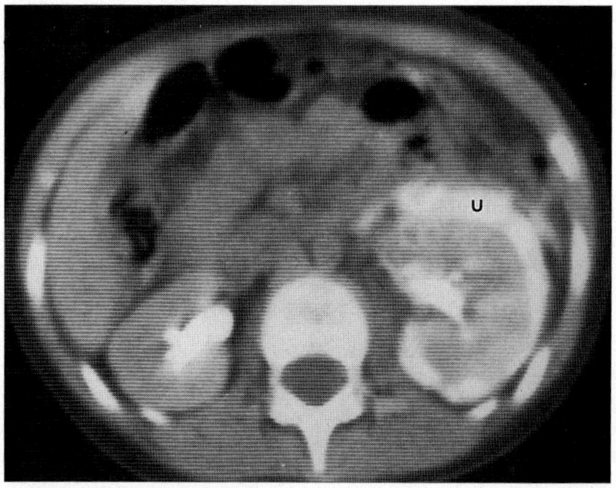


**FIGURE 6** Delayed CT image of kidneys in a patient with bladder perforation demonstrates high-density urine (u) tracking up and surrounding the left kidney. Initially the extravasated urine may be low density because contrast material has not reached the bladder.

A 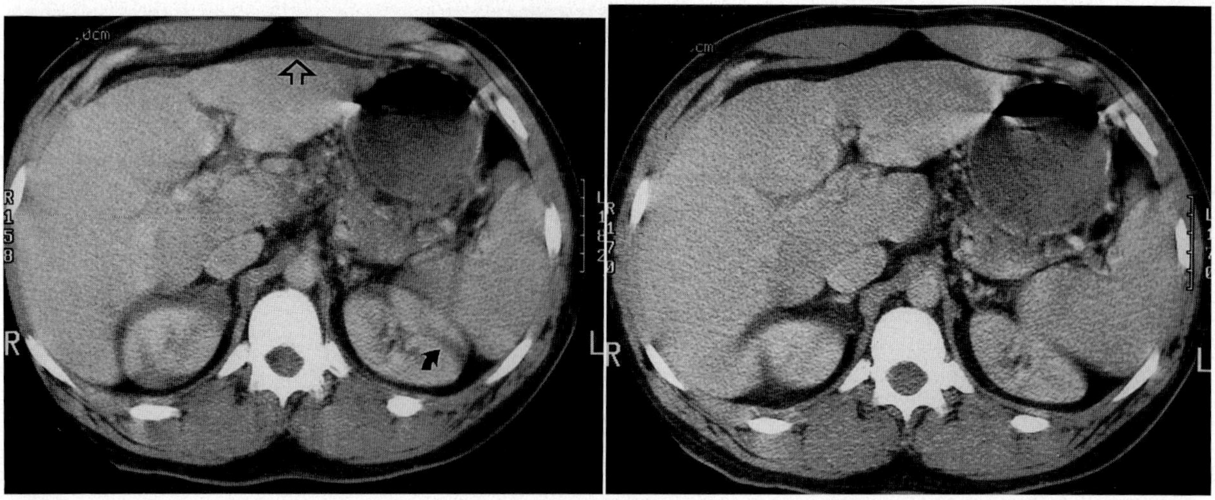 B

**FIGURE 7** *A,* Artifact from respiratory motion may simulate injury to the kidney (*arrow*), as well as perihepatic fluid (*open arrow*). *B,* Most of this artifact is eliminated by segmenting the image.

A 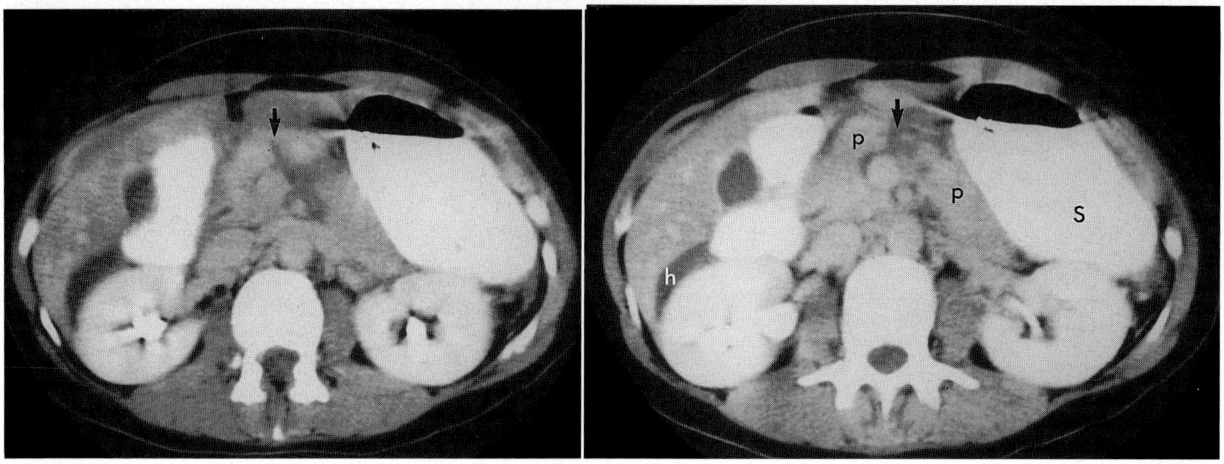 B

**FIGURE 8** *A and B,* CT demonstration of a fracture (*arrow*) of the pancreas (p). Intraperitoneal hemorrhage (h) is present in Morrison's pouch. The stomach (s) is filled with oral contrast material. Thin sections after administration of oral contrast material may aid in visualization of pancreatic injury.

CT or ultrasonography is often used for mild and moderate renal injuries, which most often are treated without surgery. Prompt treatment is required to salvage kidneys with absence of perfusion from renal vascular injury. The kidney is prone to artifacts from motion that may simulate subcapsular hematoma. Usually the artifact can be distinguished from real injury by the same artifact on the anterior abdominal wall and by a normal appearance on slices just above and below the slice in question (Fig. 7).

### *Pancreas*

Pancreatic injury carries a high mortality if not promptly treated. The morbidity is high, because complications such as pancreatitis and pseudocyst often develop. CT is less accurate for detection of pancreatic injury than for the liver, spleen, and kidneys. Identification of fracture (Fig. 8), contusion, or signs of pancreatitis provide CT diagnosis. If pancreatic injury is suspected on the initial CT scan, delayed 5 mm contiguous slices after administration of oral contrast material often help demonstrate the abnormality. Pancreatic fractures are often associated with injury to the left lobe of the liver. Because CT is less sensitive in the evaluation of pancreatic injury, a follow-up scan in 24 hours as well as endoscopic retrograde cholangiopancreatography (ERCP) may also be performed to aid in the diagnosis and management of patients with suspected pancreatic injury.

### *Bowel and Mesentery*

Bowel injury may be difficult to diagnose, because many of the key imaging signs are nonspecific. The most common finding with bowel injury is intraperitoneal blood or fluid. Free intraperitoneal air is more specific, but present less than half of the time. The free air may be subtle and often collects anterior to the liver and posterior to the adjacent abdominal

A

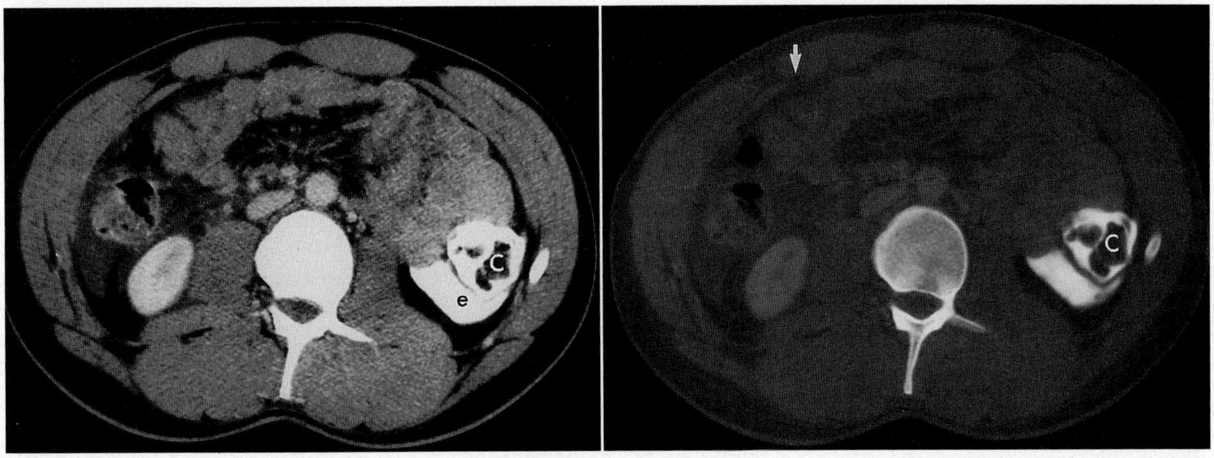


B

**FIGURE 9** *A,* CT image of the lower abdomen in a patient with penetrating injury following administration of triple (oral, intravenous, and rectal) contrast material reveals left-sided colon perforation with extravasation (e) of colonic contrast material adjacent to the perforated descending colon (c). Hemorrhage is present in the right pericolic gutter. *B,* A tiny amount of free intraperitoneal air (*arrow*) at this level of the abdomen can be distinguished from fat on bone window settings.

wall. Specific signs include extraluminal retroperitoneal air, extraluminal bowel contents, and extravasated oral contrast material. Small amounts of air are best detected on bone or lung windows. Free intraperitoneal air can also be due to bladder rupture, prior lavage, or occasionally abdominal extension of pneumomediastinum. Other CT findings in bowel injury are hemoperitoneum, mesenteric hemorrhage, and higher-density clot or stranding immediately adjacent to the bowel injury (Fig. 9). Focal bowel thickening is often present. Mesenteric injury is characterized by focal mesenteric hemorrhage and infiltration of blood and fluid. Nearly all CT evaluations of patients with bowel injury are abnormal.

## Suggested Reading

Dodds WJ, Taylor AJ, Erickson SJ, Lawson TL. Traumatic fracture of the pancreas: CT characteristics. J Comput Assist Tomogr 1990; 14:375–378.

Federle MP. CT of abdominal trauma. In Federle MP, Brant-Zawadzki M, eds. Computed Tomography in the Evaluation of Trauma. 2nd ed. Baltimore: Williams & Wilkins, 1986:191.

Gay SB, Sistrom CL. Computed tomographic evaluation of blunt abdominal trauma. Radiol Clin North Am 1992; 30:367–388.

Himmelman RG, Martin M, Gilkey S, Barrett JA. Triple-contrast CT scans in penetrating back and flank trauma. J Trauma 1991; 31:852–901.

Pollack HM, Wein AJ. Imaging of renal trauma. Radiology 1989; 172:297–308.

Rizzo MJ, Federle MP, Griffiths BG. Bowel and mesenteric injury following blunt abdominal trauma: Evaluation with CT. Radiology 1989; 173:143–148.

Wolfman NT, Bechtold RE, Scharling ES, Meredith JW. Blunt upper abdominal trauma: Evaluation by CT. AJR 1992; 158:493–501.

# CT in Acute Small Bowel Obstruction

*JACK WITTENBERG, M.D. · G. SCOTT GAZELLE, M.D.*

The identification, confirmation, and/or anatomic definition of intestinal obstruction in the acutely ill patient are everyday problems in a busy radiologic practice. The multitude of pathophysiologic problems associated with nausea and vomiting challenges even the most veteran surgeon's confidence in the definitive diagnosis of mechanical intestinal obstruction. This is particularly highlighted in the recent postoperative patient in whom paralytic ileus and mechanical obstruction are likely contenders, since vomiting can be caused by obstruction or distention of a hollow viscus and auscultation of bowel sounds is notoriously unreliable. Radiology has traditionally played an important analytic role for this condition, and recent experience indicates computed tomography (CT) increases the accuracy with which this problem can be solved.

## Indications

The key screening radiographic evaluation remains the plain film evaluation of the abdomen (PFA), which should always include an upright projection. The latter permits a search for both pneumoperitoneum and the presence of fluid in bowel loops. The diagnostic usefulness of the latter finding is often overlooked in assessing obstruction, but may be as valuable as the analysis of the degree of intestinal distention by gas. Distention with both gas and fluid is much more commonly a sign of mechanical obstruction than is distention by gas alone. Analytically it is convenient to assign patterns of obstruction (intestinal distention with both air and fluid) into the following four categories:

1. Colonic distention without small bowel dilation and the

cecum more dilated than the dilated transverse colon.
2. Small bowel and colonic distention with the cecum more dilated than the dilated transverse colon.
3. Small bowel and colonic distention with the cecum less dilated than the dilated transverse colon.
4. Distended small bowel without distention of the colon.

The first two patterns are consistent with the colon as the source of obstruction, although a nonobstructive ileus (paralytic ileus) may alternatively produce these appearances. Under the appropriate clinical circumstance, a barium enema study should be performed. LaPlace's law argues that pattern 3 is unlikely to be colonic obstruction, unless some congenital, pathologic, or surgical procedure has caused the cecum to be intrinsically smaller in diameter than the rest of the colon. This appearance may be observed in small bowel obstruction, although is it more common with paralytic ileus. Pattern 4 is most consistent with small bowel obstruction. It is the radiologic algorithm of the latter two potentially obstructive small bowel patterns with which we deal in the remainder of this chapter.

As with all radiologic decisions to proceed to more complex imaging, the clinical context is critical. Mechanical obstructive patterns so commonly overlap with the radiographic appearance of paralytic ileus (and its close cousin, hyperaerophagia) that clinical correlation is critical. The radiologist's responsibility can terminate at the point at which an interpretation of small bowel obstruction is made, since this may be sufficient confirmation of the clinician's opinion to precipitate surgical intervention. Alternatively a number of indications may precipitate further radiographic evaluation as follows:

1. Clinician's unwillingness to accept the radiographic diagnosis.
2. Clinician's desire to have 100 percent confirmation, definition of site, and/or etiology.
3. Clinician's desire to have clear-cut anatomic information in a complex patient with previous surgery and/or inflammatory bowel disease.
4. Radiologist's inability to offer an unequivocal diagnosis.

The traditional approach to a PFA suggesting distal small bowel obstruction is the barium enema study with attempted reflex into the terminal ileum, or beyond if possible. The colonic evaluation permits exclusion of unsuspected diseases that may coexist with small bowel obstruction (diverticulitis predominantly) or discovery of the proximal right-sided colonic obstructing tumor masquerading as small bowel obstruction. However, rarely in our experience is there sufficient small bowel reflex (before the patient involuntarily evacuates) to permit an unequivocal assessment of small bowel obstruction. A small bowel follow-through study with barium is certainly the next consideration, the success of this being inversely related to the degree of obstruction. In patients whose PFA evidence is that of lower-grade obstruction (diameter of small bowel loops less than 4 cm and moderate fluid retention and the presence of bowel sounds) progress of the barium and maintenance of its continuity may be sufficient to define the problem. In more severe degrees of small bowel obstruction, slowness of barium transit, dilution of barium, and time requirements all make small bowel follow-through studies less desirable. It is certainly in the latter, more common, group of patients (and possibly also eventually in the former) that CT scans for suspected small bowel obstruction has become useful.

The superior density discrimination of CT allows the considerable intraluminal fluid characteristic of high-grade obstruction to act as an intrinsic small bowel contrast agent (Fig. 1), circumventing the previously noted problems related to barium follow-through studies. The examination can be done immediately, without the need for ingestion of an intestinal opacifying agent. In less profound obstructions, the advantages of CT are not as clear-cut, although arguable. A conventional antegrade barium study is superior for defining mucosal-based abnormalities, whereas the advantage of CT lies in defining intramural or mesenteric processes (Fig. 2). Since most acute small bowel obstructions are not mucosal based, a theoretical argument exists for preferring CT in all suspected small bowel obstruction. If the CT is nonrevealing or

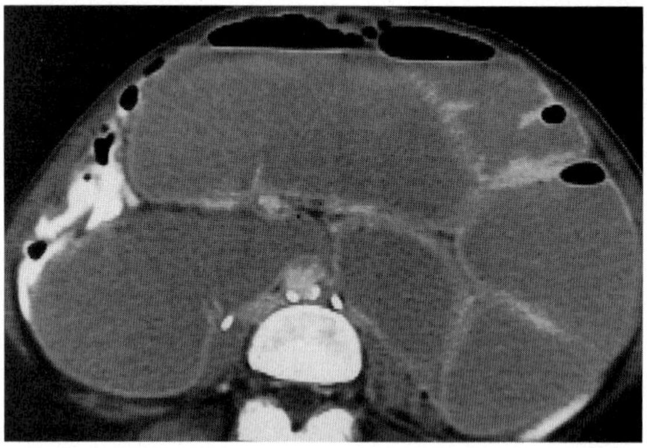

**FIGURE 1** High-grade obstruction. The small intestine is very dilated with unopacified, retained small bowel secretions. There is a small amount of opaque fluid remaining in the colon from a previous enema that failed to define the cause of the small bowel obstruction. Both "contrast agents" provide sufficient information of intestinal diameter to classify this pattern as suspicious for small bowel obstruction (category 4). The width of normal small intestinal wall is evident, in part because of its highlighting through the use of intravenous contrast material.

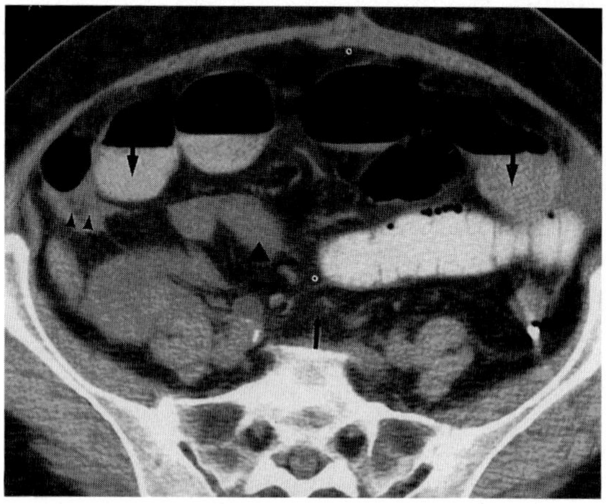

**FIGURE 2** Low-grade obstruction. Iodinated contrast material has progressed to an abrupt cutoff in the midileum in a patient who 7 days previously had undergone a laparotomy. More dilute contrast is present in proximal dilated loops of small intestine (*large arrows*). More distal ileum is less dilated and contains no contrast material (*arrowhead*) and the nondilated colon (*double arrowheads*) is relatively fluid-free. Linear densities (*small arrows*) at point of obstruction may represent the adhesions found at surgery.

**TABLE 1** Approach to Acute Intestinal Obstruction

| Plain Film Finding | Subsequent Study |
|---|---|
| Colonic obstruction | Barium enema |
| Severe small bowel obstruction | CT |
| Mild small bowel obstruction | (?) CT or small bowel follow-through |

alternatively suspicious for a colon abnormality in patients whose PFA suggested small bowel obstruction, one can immediately perform a barium enema study. If one begins with a barium enema study, the density of retained barium in the colon precludes doing a satisfactory, immediate CT evaluation.

Table 1 is a summation of our current approach to the PFA that suggests intestinal obstruction.

## Technique

The critical decision of whether to give oral contrast material (OCM) prior to initiating a CT scan is keyed to the PFA and clinical signs. Fluid-filled, dilated (>4.0 cm diameter) small bowel loops and poor or absent bowel sounds are strong indicators that OCM will not be effective. Less severe dilation, particularly with only partial fluid-filled loops and/or active bowel sounds, argue for a trial of OCM. If there is any question, one should try to give 15 to 25 ounces of OCM over a period of 60 to 90 minutes or as much as the patient can tolerate. Since iodinated contrast material is considered to have a faster intestinal transit time than barium, we routinely use it as a 10 percent solution. Duration to actual scanning is similarly tied to previous observations. The patients with severely dilated, fluid-filled intestinal loops (see Fig. 1) can be scanned immediately; patients receiving OCM should, and more likely clinically can, tolerate several hours to scanning, thereby allowing the OCM to maximally progress (see Fig. 2). Intravenous contrast material is preferable since mucosal highlighting (see Fig. 1) improves density discrimination of native fluid-filled loops of bowel and may make unexpected pathology more apparent. The radiologist must review the scan before terminating the examination. Equivocal findings, such as a questionable area of obstruction or an unclear etiologic process, can be studied with additional sections, perhaps more closely spaced. Manipulation of window settings at the console may allow one to appreciate subtle mesenteric changes not readily apparent on routinely windowed hard copy. Finally, if OCM has not progressed sufficiently through the small bowel and if an obstructive diagnosis is suggested, but not yet unequivocal, follow-up scanning several hours later should be arranged (Fig. 3). In the interim, treatment of the patient with nasogastric tube suction should not interfere with the diagnostic process.

## Interpretive Analysis

Fortunately the rules for CT diagnosis of small bowel obstruction are simply a reinvention of the "wheels" we have always used with the PFA or a small bowel follow-through study for analysis of obstruction. The CT analysis may be more demanding than these since it requires a mental "coronal three-dimension (3D) reconstruction" of all the transverse sections to have the best perspective of the entire course of

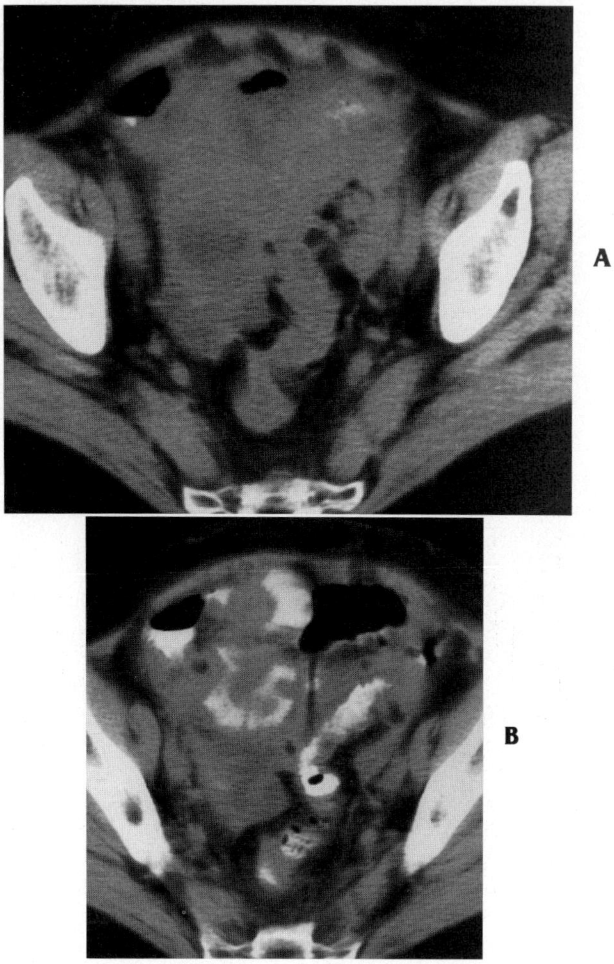


**FIGURE 3** Utility of follow-up scanning. *A,* Initial scanning of this patient 4 hours after receiving oral contrast material demonstrates little opacification of any ileal loops. More proximal findings suggested small intestinal obstruction. *B,* Repeat scanning 4 hours later demonstrates opacification of narrowed terminal ileum, cecum, and sigmoid colon. The ileum is surrounded by masslike tissue consistent with the patient's known ovarian carcinoma. The demonstrated bulk of the tumor influenced the surgical decision to perform an ileocolostomy.

both small bowel and colon. There should be a disproportion of diameters of large and small bowel loops, as well as the amount of fluid they contain. That is, small bowel obstruction, particularly if severe, should be accompanied by a relative lack of colonic distention with gas and fluid. Depending on the severity of the small bowel obstruction, the small bowel is variably dilated, more likely containing a proportionately small-to-moderate amount of fluid. It is important to keep in mind that almost all "radiographic" obstructions are incomplete, so that some gas and fluid distal to an obstruction are expected (see Fig. 3). Intestinal loops in paralytic ileus tend to have intervening non-dilated or less dilated segments (a "linked-sausage" appearance) (Fig. 4, *A*) as opposed to mechanically dilated small bowel loops, which tend to be continuously dilated (Fig. 4, *B*). In mechanical obstruction, fluid retention parallels the severity of gaseous dilation, whereas in ileus the amount of dilation may be out of proportion to the amount of fluid. However, severe paralytic ileus may simulate

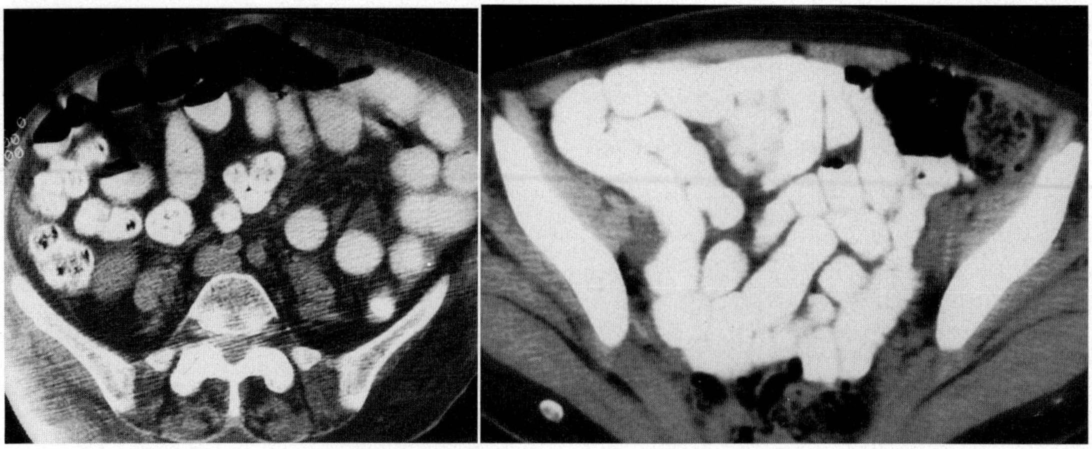


**FIGURE 4** Paralytic ileus versus mechanical obstruction. *A,* The small intestine is mildly dilated in a noncontinuous fashion ("linked-sausage appearance"). *B,* Mildly dilated loops of distal ileum demonstrate none of the segmentation seen in *A*. Rather they have a continuous tubular appearance.

all the foregoing characteristics of mechanical obstruction. The key to their differentiation is, as with a small bowel barium follow-through study, demonstration of a persistent transition zone, i.e., the point at which the bowel goes from dilated (often the most dilated point of the entire dilated small bowel) to a narrower segment, with the loops beyond this point appearing less dilated and less fluid filled than the more proximally dilated small bowel segments (see Fig. 2). This dynamic should be apparent whether or not the bowel has been opacified with intraluminal contrast material. In more severe obstructions, much of the OCM may still be proximal to this transition point (see Fig. 3, *A*); in the less severe, depending on the duration from ingestion to scanning, there may be considerable contrast material distal to the obstruction, but the distal loops should remain nondilated. All the foregoing findings may be mimicked by paralytic ileus (presumably a nondistended segment simulating a transition point), but occur in fewer than 5 percent of patients that we have examined. If the signs are equivocal, repeat scanning over the area of interest, sometimes within 15 to 20 minutes, demonstrates persistence of the findings in mechanical obstruction, or alternatively, in ileus, less narrowing at the suspected transition zone and/or considerable passage of OCM beyond that point.

The sine qua non of obstruction is the demonstration of an etiologic factor. Intraluminal (Fig. 5), intramural (Fig. 6), and mesenteric processes (see Fig. 3, *B*) are readily demonstrated. Primary tumors originating in the wall of the bowel or metastatic implants in the mesentery, extrinsically invading the bowel, are usually the bulkiest pathology and therefore the easiest to distinguish. Inflammatory processes thickening the intestinal wall as a consequence of such conditions as Crohn's disease or radiation enteritis (see Fig. 6) are readily identified. Not only can one identify the presence of internal and superficial hernias, but also assess the presence and degree of potential obstruction by monitoring the progress of contrast material. The definitive identification of an adhesion may be more challenging. Although occasionally one can identify a linear band crossing the bowel at a transition zone, more often the appearance is simply tiny wisps of irregular linear densities (see Fig. 2), giving the accompanying mesentery a heterogeneous appearance. On occasion there may be no discernible abnormality caused by adhesions, and the radiographic diagnosis needs to be made as one of exclusion in a patient who has previously undergone a laparotomy.

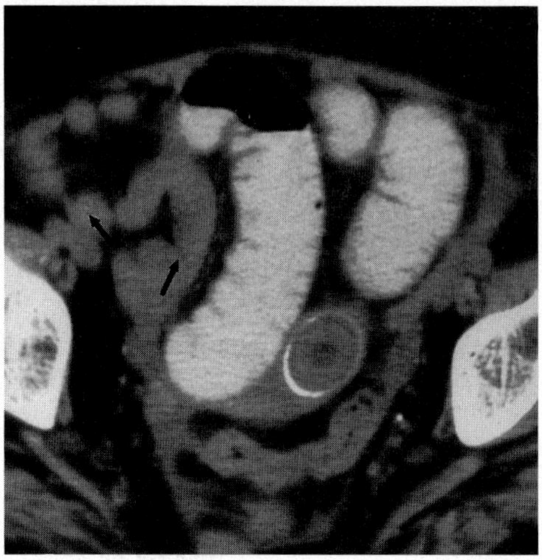

**FIGURE 5** Gallstone ileus. Dilated opacified ileal loops are identified proximal to an obstructing gallstone. Note nondilated nonopacified loops (*arrows*) of more distal ileum beyond the stone. Images of the liver demonstrated gas in intrahepatic bile ducts and contrast material to have entered the gallbladder by way of the duodeno-cholecystic fistula.

## Pitfalls

As previously indicated, the local signs of small bowel obstruction may be mimicked by paralytic ileus, but it is uncommon. Since these equivocal findings often occur in patients without evidence of high-grade obstruction and therefore under less urgent clinical circumstances, the patient with an uncertain transitional point can have progressive scanning. Our routine is to ask the patient to drink more OCM while waiting in a radiology holding area and then to repeat the examination within an hour, focused only in the area of interest.

The decision to use OCM is subjective. Patients with high-grade obstruction often sort themselves out by being unable to drink and retain the material. Fortunately it is the

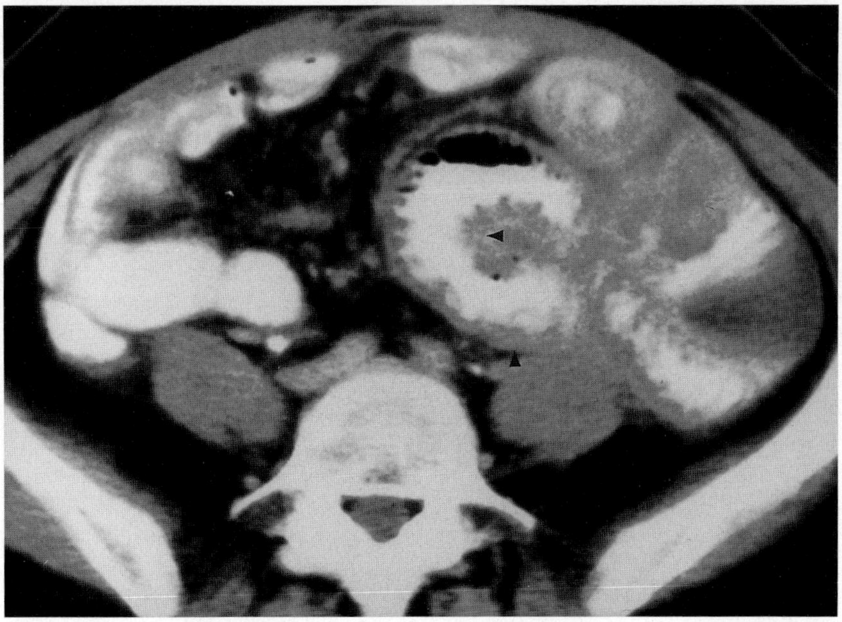

**FIGURE 6** Radiation enteritis. Oral contrast material demonstrates angulated narrowed loops of jejunum with mural thickening (*arrowhead*). At surgery both radiation enteritis and adhesions were present.

more challenging patients with lesser grades of obstruction who are able to tolerate ingestion of OCM, and one should err on the side of giving too much rather than too little OCM (see Fig. 3). Subtle transition points may only be detected by maximally challenging the obstructing area, which does not necessarily occur without OCM.

The diagnosis of the presence of more than one obstructed point is challenging, more so since it often occurs with adhesive etiologies whose specific identification is difficult. If one is to recognize this event, it will occur in the setting of a definitive high-grade, more proximal obstruction with the paradox of fluid and dilation being additionally present more distally. Again progressive scanning can be confirmatory, and/or the observation of an etiologic factor responsible for the downstream second obstruction may be apparent (see Fig. 3).

The inability to consistently and specifically identify the offending structure with adhesive obstruction can be disturbing. This lack of a convincing etiologic agent at a presumed transition point always raises the issue of the presence of one of the uncommon false positives occurring in a setting of paralytic ileus. In the immediate postoperative state, the presence of paralytic ileus is so common as to be a less useful clinical clue in differential diagnosis as it would be in the patient remotely operated. Careful inspection of the adjacent mesentery may provide a clue to diagnosis (see Fig. 2), and this analysis can be enhanced by obtaining additional thinner slices at the site of question during progressive scanning.

Finally, the well-known entity of right-sided colonic obstruction presenting clinically or radiographically as distal small bowel obstruction may potentially be overlooked. This can occur either because the examination is prematurely terminated when the OCM has reached the ileocecal area or because the colon etiology is less evident or mistaken, in the case of tumor, for feces. Although we have identified right-sided colonic obstructing cancers, the sensitivity of CT for so doing is completely unknown. If the clinical conviction persists that mechanical obstruction is present and the focus now becomes the colon, an immediate barium enema can be performed. However, keep in mind that if the traditional approach of performing a barium enema in the setting of a PFA suggesting a distal small bowel fails in diagnosis it is likely that retained colonic barium will delay the performance of a CT for many hours if not days.

## Suggested Reading


Balthazar EJ. CT of the gastrointestinal tract: Principles and interpretation. AJR 1991; 156:23–32.

Megibow AJ, Balthazar EJ, Kyunghu CC, et al. Bowel obstruction: Evaluation with CT. Radiology 1991; 180:313–318.

Nemak AA Jr. CT of acute gastrointestinal disorders. Radiol Clin North Am 1989; 27:773–786.

Rattner DW. Case records of the Massachusetts General Hospital (Case 28-1991). N Engl J Med 1991; 325:118–122.

Rubesin SE, Herlinger H. CT evaluation of bowel obstruction: A landmark article–implications for the future. Radiology 1991; 180:307–308.

# Scintigraphic Diagnosis of Focal Inflammatory Disease in the Abdomen

*I. ROSS McDOUGALL, M.D., Ph.D.* · *LEE R. LISKEY, M.D.*

The diagnosis of certain abdominal infections or inflammatory diseases may be obvious in some patients by the history and physical examination. However, in some patients, focal signs and symptoms are less obvious and imaging tests are necessary to localize the site of infection. Computed tomography (CT), magnetic resonance imaging (MRI), and ultrasonography provide noninvasive high-resolution images that can help in the diagnosis of intra-abdominal infection or occult abscess. Nuclear medicine scintigraphy has the advantage over other noninvasive tests in that it is not necessary a priori to know specifically the area of interest, since whole-body scanning is obtained routinely. The two standard nuclear medicine approaches are gallium and indium white blood cell scintigraphy.

Gallium, like iron, binds to plasma transferrin. It concentrates in normal tissues that have a high content of lactoferrin (i.e., salivary and lacrimal glands) and the nasopharnyx. It also concentrates in the liver, because both transferrin and lactoferrin are found there. Renal activity is observed within the first 24 hours, since this is the early route of excretion. Gut activity is observed after 24 hours, as approximately 10 to 20 percent of gallium is excreted by the colon.

Indium is similar to gallium, because it also binds to transferrin. When labeled to white blood cells, the distribution is that of the cells. Normal activity is observed mostly in the spleen, liver, and bone marrow. Renal and gut activity are not observed in normals, because white blood cells are not normally excreted through the kidneys or into the gastrointestinal tract.

An advantage of gallium is that no preparation is required. The patient is simply injected with the dose, usually in the range of 3 to 6 mCi, and the scan is performed 24 or 48 hours later. It usually shows uptake in infections or inflammatory conditions; however, intense uptake is observed in wounds healing normally and in several cancers, especially Hodgkin's and non–Hodgkin's lymphomas. Another disadvantage of gallium is that the uptake in diseased tissue is nonspecific. Also, some abdominal infections may be missed because of normal kidney and gut activity.

Indium white blood cell scanning requires preparation, which is described in the following section, but in general it provides both high sensitivity and specificity. This chapter reviews the methods, normal and abnormal findings, pitfalls including false-positive and false-negative scans, and overall conclusions for the role of this test in practice.

## Methods

It is generally accepted that indium in the form of indium oxine provides the most reliable method of labeling white blood cells. Although indium tropolone and technetium labeling using technetium HMPAO have been described in the literature, these approaches are not fully approved for routine clinical use.

Our method is based on the approach by Thakur. We use 40 ml of the patient's blood. This is heparinized and 3 ml of hydroxyethyl starch and 3 ml of saline are added under sterile conditions. The blood is allowed to sit for 1 hour, which allows gravity centrifugation to bring down the red blood cells, leaving white blood cells and platelets in the supernatant. The supernatant is gently centrifuged to produce a pellet of white blood cells. The platelet-rich plasma is removed and spun at a sufficiently high rate to bring down the platelets, leaving cell-free plasma that is used to resuspend the labeled cells. The button of white blood cells obtained at an earlier stage is resuspended in 5 ml of saline, and approximately 700 to 1,000 μCi of indium oxine is added. The cells are incubated for 30 minutes, spun down, and resuspended in 5 ml of platelet-free plasma. In general, we try to inject 500 μCi of labeled cells. Studies have shown that the majority of labeled cells are polymorphonuclear leukocytes (PMLs), and in general the labeling technique does not damage their function.

It is critical that the patient receives his or her own labeled cells. There are reports of patients being injected with the wrong blood, and transmission of the human immunodeficiency virus has been documented. We take extreme precautions, identical to those that would be used for a blood transfusion, to ensure that this could not happen unless our protocol is breached.

For this labeling method, it is necessary that the patient have adequate circulating PMLs. When they have less than $1{,}500/mm^3$, we use donor blood. This requires coordination with the blood bank to obtain an appropriate ABO donor whose blood meets all the requirements for a regular blood transfusion. The blood bank provides us with a buffy coat, and we then subject it to the same steps previously described.

The patients are generally imaged 18 to 24 hours after injection of labeled cells, although earlier imaging can be done, a point that is described later. We prefer to use a dual-headed whole-body camera that obtains simultaneous anterior and posterior images. Spot views can be made of areas that are equivocal.

## Results

At approximately 20 hours after injection of labeled white blood cells, the distribution shows that the spleen is the most intense organ on scintiscan, followed by liver, and then bone marrow. The half-life of the labeled cells in the circulation is usually about 5 to 7 hours; therefore background activity is low and blood pool is not observed at the time of imaging. This makes most abnormalities in the abdomen or chest easily interpretable. Figure 1, *A* and *B*, shows normal anterior and posterior whole-body scintiscans. However, if the suspected lesion is in or adjacent to the liver or spleen, a technetium-99m sulfur colloid subtraction scan may be required for a more accurate diagnosis. This technique is described later.

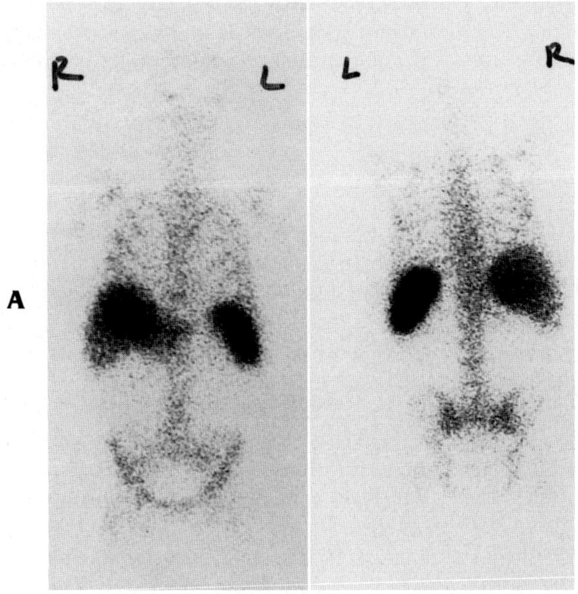


**FIGURE 1** *A,* Anterior and *(B)* posterior scans. Normal whole-body indium-111–labeled white blood cell scan. The spleen shows the highest concentration of radioactivity, followed by the liver and bone marrow. There is virtually no background activity, and the renal tract and gut are not visualized. (NOTE – All images in this chapter were made 18 to 24 hours after the injection of 400 to 500 μCi of $^{111}$In–labeled white blood cells.)

Most of the published series do not address the question of focal uptake in the abdomen as an isolated finding, but consider the diagnosis of abscess and occult infection anywhere in the body. Several series demonstrate a sensitivity and a specificity of approximately 90 percent. Figure 2 shows a right-sided diverticular abscess. One large study that we conducted comparing the white blood cell scan with the clinical findings and with ultrasonography demonstrated a higher sensitivity for the white blood cell scan, and the benefit of evaluating the whole body, since many patients were at risk for infection in multiple sites. Surprisingly, the key unsuspected area of abnormality was often the lung, even when the clinician suspected the problem to be in the abdomen.

One of the most important uses of indium-labeled white blood cells is for the diagnosis of suspected infection of vascular grafts. In our hands, the sensitivity has been perfect, but the specificity is approximately 85 percent, with false positives being found in grafts that had been placed within 4 weeks before the scan was done. Some of the false-positive scans were in areas such as infected wounds, but since the lesion was not truly an infected graft per se we did not designate them as true positives.

White blood cell scanning has been useful in the evaluation of inflammatory bowel disease, pseudomembranous colitis, necrotic bowel, and appendicitis. The pathology of inflammatory bowel disease, such as ulcerative colitis, is the crypt abscess. As expected, in these disorders the bowel lights up intensely on the white blood cell scan. The scan can be used as an index of extent and severity of disease. This is one of the few situations in which an early scan at 2 to 4 hours is recommended, since the white blood cells are excreted into the lumen of the colon and are lost from the body. In almost every other situation, as previously described, the cells remain at the abnormal site and are not excreted. In a double-blind study comparing the accuracy of labeled cells with conventional tests like barium enema studies and colonoscopy, we were surprised to learn that we could not differentiate ulcerative colitis from Crohn's colitis; however, the test was extremely sensitive and predictive of severity and extent of inflammatory bowel disease. These findings have been confirmed by others. Figure 3 shows a scan with inflammatory bowel disease.

In the evaluation of suspected appendicitis, indium-labeled white blood cells may provide a prompt and accurate diagnosis. In most cases, history and physical examination, laboratory results, abdominal plain films, and ultrasonography establish a diagnosis. When ultrasonography demonstrates an appendix with an enlarged thickened wall, the diagnosis can be made. However, if the appendix is not visualized, the diagnosis should not be excluded. In the past surgical false-positive rates have been reported to be around 25 percent. White blood cell scans provide sensitivity and specificity of approximately 90 percent and can aid the clinician in a more accurate diagnosis. The initial imaging can be performed at approximately 3 hours after the injection of the labeled cells.

Infections of the urinary tract such as acute pyelonephritis, perinephric abscess, or infected cyst in a polycystic kidney can

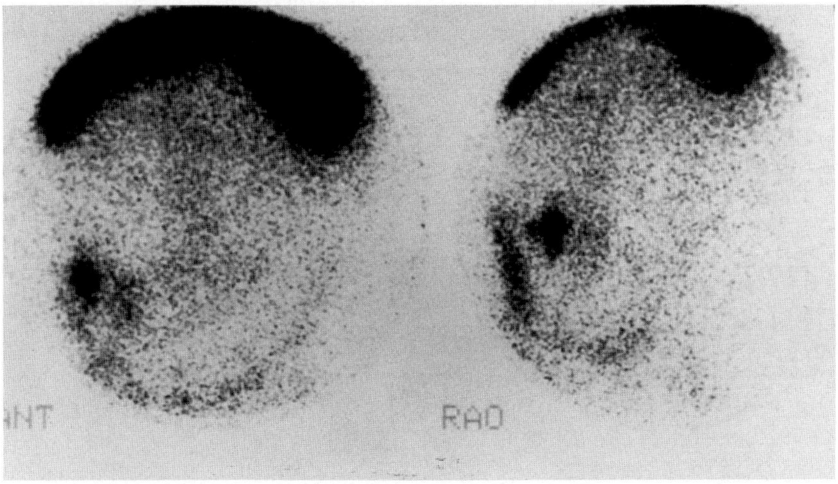


**FIGURE 2** Anterior and right anterior oblique spot views of the abdomen in a patient with a diverticular abscess.

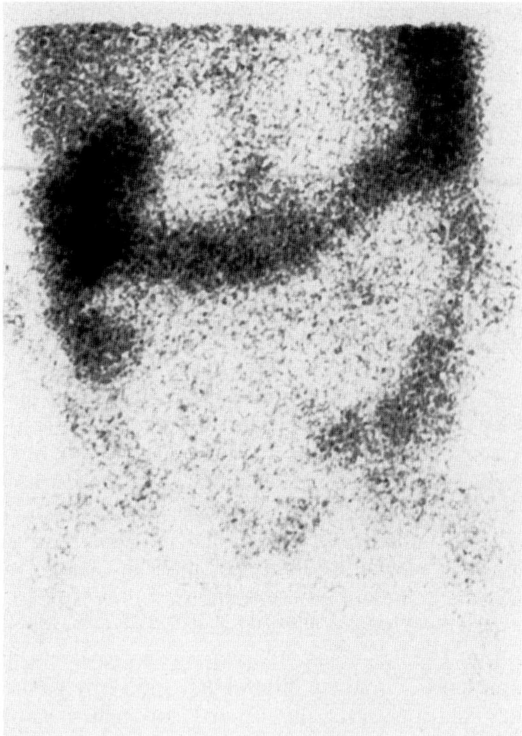

**FIGURE 3** Spot views of the abdomen in acute inflammatory colitis.

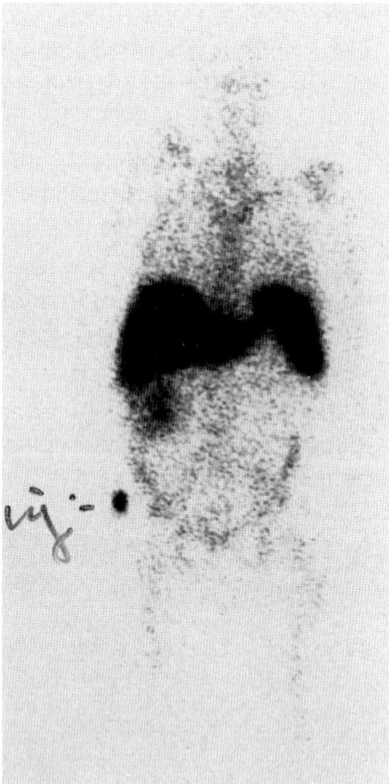

**FIGURE 4** Anterior scan in a patient with a right-sided perinephric abscess.

be diagnosed (Fig. 4). The fact that labeled white blood cells are not normally excreted in the kidney is stressed. A white blood cell scan does not have the high resolution of CT or ultrasonography, and an abnormality that appears in the abdomen may actually be in soft tissue, and the precise anatomic localization may be difficult to define. A good example of this would be a psoas abscess. However, by obtaining anteroposterior spot views, lateral views, or oblique views, it is usually possible to make an appropriate diagnosis.

## Problems

### *Technical*

Occasionally the percentage of radioactivity attaching to the white blood cells is low. In general, we like to achieve more than 80 percent of added indium labeling to the cells, and usually we achieve more than 90 percent. When the percentage is less than this, we review whether the patient had sufficient circulating white blood cells and determine if the protocol was done correctly. If so, it is worth obtaining an additional 40 ml of blood and relabeling. It is important to ensure that the camera is set appropriately for the two gamma peaks of indium (179 and 249 keV), which are of higher energy than technetium (140 keV). A medium-energy collimator is necessary. Although it is difficult to damage PMLs by the labeling technique previously described, if the cells are damaged, there is preferential uptake in the liver with much less uptake in spleen and marrow. This should be a clue to that problem.

### *False-Positive Scans*

Any disease in which there is intense collection of inflammatory cells gives a positive result on the white blood cell scan. Examples include gouty arthritis and acute rheumatoid arthritis, where joints "light up" on the scan, but are not necessarily infected. Fortunately these conditions tend to be uncommon in the abdomen. If a hematoma forms when labeled white blood cells are in the circulation, that hematoma appears "hot" on scan and can be interpreted as an abscess. Therefore, if arteries are punctured for test purposes during the 24 hours between injection of white blood cells and imaging, that area can appear as a hot focus. Sometimes the abnormal cells accumulate in one area, which is the diseased organ, but then migrate to a normal site that is imaged and interpreted as abnormal. A good example of this is the patient with pneumonia who coughs up radioactive sputum and swallows it, and that sputum is observed as an abnormal focus in the abdomen (Fig. 5). When we observe a combination of uptake above the diaphragm, and a focus of uptake below the diaphragm, we generally repeat the scan after a further 12 to 24 hours to ascertain that the focus below the diaphragm is interpreted correctly. If it moves, it is in the gut. If it remains in the same spot, it is likely to be an abscess.

Since many large solid tumors become necrotic in the center, it has been hypothesized that such a lesion would appear hot on the scan. The number of reports of this finding are extremely limited; we have imaged hundreds of patients with solid cancers and encountered this in only one case.

False-positive scans also may be observed in patients with bleeding ulcers, diverticula, or an accessory spleen.

### *False-Negative Scans*

If the scanning is done early, for example, 2 to 4 hours after injection of labeled cells, the sensitivity of the procedure is dramatically reduced. There are false negatives that turn to true positives on imaging at the standard time at approximately

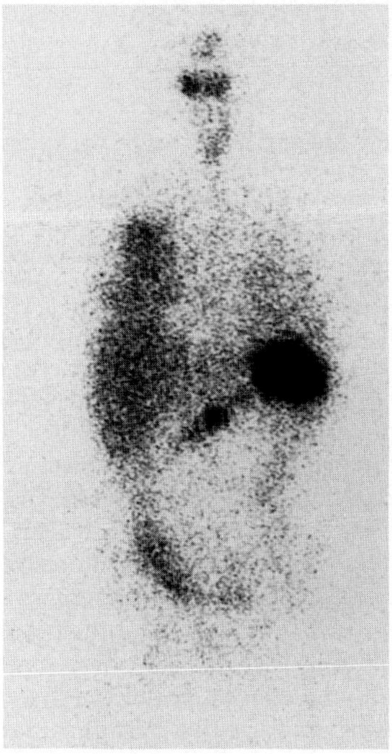

**FIGURE 5** Anterior whole-body scan shows abnormal uptake in both lungs (more on right), oropharynx, and colon. The labeled cells in the colon are likely to be due to swallowed radioactive white blood cells; this can be confirmed by repeating the scan at 48 hours.

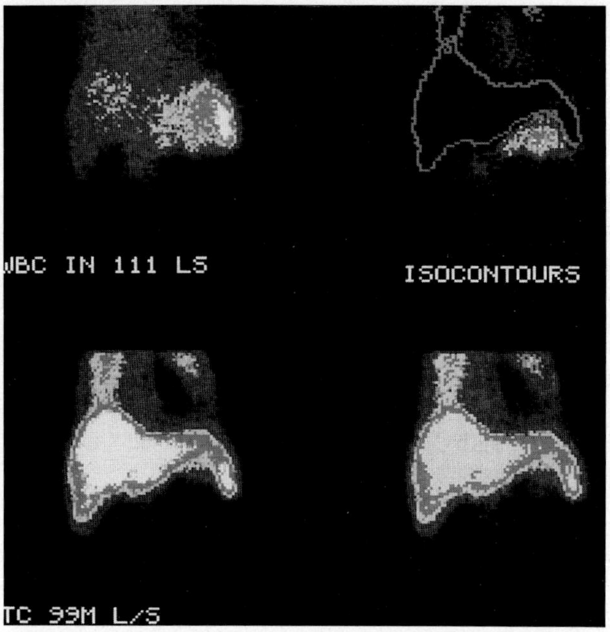


**FIGURE 6** White blood cell scan *(upper left)* and $^{99m}$Tc liver/spleen scan *(bottom)*. The subtraction scan *(upper right)* shows the focal abscess.

24 hours. This has been well documented by Datz and colleagues. Therefore if an early study is requested, and is positive, a diagnosis can be made. However, if that scan is negative, it is imperative that the delayed scan be conducted. A scan may also be negative in the case of hepatic or splenic abscess, because the lesion is masked by activity in normal liver. If suspected, 2 to 5 mCi of Tc-99m sulfur colloid should be given and a liver/spleen subtraction scan performed (Fig. 6). Therefore an abscess in or adjacent to liver and/or spleen can be easily identified.

A second area of concern relates to chronic abscesses. The pathology of a chronic abscess is different. There are fewer PMLs, and the predominant cells are leukocytes, plasma cells, and giant cells. Often chronic abscesses have fibrous capsules that are impervious to labeled cells. The sensitivity of the procedure for diagnosing chronic abscess is low. In general, if the lesion is of 6 weeks' duration or less, we recommend a white blood cell scan. If it is more than 6 weeks' duration, consideration should be given to a gallium scan.

Osteomyelitis in the spine has been an area reported to give false negatives, but on review of the reports, they are often chronic lesions. In general, most investigators have not found that antibiotics, steroids, or underlying hepatic and renal disease affect the sensitivity of the procedure.

## Discussion

The indium-111 white blood cell scan is a robust test with high sensitivity and specificity for diagnosing intra-abdominal infections or inflammatory diseases. It can be done in patients with illnesses of all degree of severity. We have imaged patients postoperatively, on ventilators, and patients with bandages and tubes who might not be imaged easily by other techniques. It is extremely important that the labeled cells injected into the patient are the correct ones, whether these are autologous labeled cells or appropriately chosen donor cells. The scan is excellent where multiple areas could be at risk.

## Suggested Reading

Biello DR, Levitt RG, Melson GL. The roles of gallium-67 scintigraphy, ultrasonography and computed tomography in the detection of abdominal abscesses. Semin Nucl Med 1979; 9:58–65.

Datz FL, Morton KA. Radionuclide detection of occult infection: Current strategies. Cancer Invest 1991; 9:691–698.

Lannto EH, Lantto TJ, Vorne M. Fast diagnosis of abdominal infections and inflammations with technetium-99m-HMPAO labeled leukocytes. J Nucl Med 1991; 32:2029–2034.

McDougall IR: The use of white blood cell scanning techniques in infectious disease. In: Remington JS, Schwartz MN, eds. Current Clinical Topics in Infectious Diseases. Vol 4. New York: McGraw-Hill, 1983:130.

Mountford PJ, Kettle AG, O'Doherty MJ, Coakley AJ. Comparison of technetium-99m-HM-PAO leukocytes with indium-111-oxine leukocytes for localizing intraabdominal sepsis. J Nucl Med 1990; 31:311–315.

Navarro DA, Weber PM. Indium 111 imaging in appendicitis. Semin Ultrasound CT MR 1989; 10:321–325.

Palestro CJ, Kim CK, Swyer AJ, et al. Radionuclide diagnosis of vertebral osteomyelitis: Indium-111-leukocyte and technetium-99m-methylene diphosphonate bone scintigraphy. J Nucl Med 1991; 32:1861–1865.

Peters AM. Imaging inflammation: Current role of labeled autologous leukocytes. J Nucl Med 1992; 33:65–67.

Pike MC. Imaging of inflammatory sites in 1990's: New horizons. J Nucl Med 1991; 32:2034–2036.

Segal AW, Thakur ML, Arnot RN, Lavender JP. Indium-111 labeled leukocytes for localization of abscesses. Lancet 1976; 2:1056–1058.

# Scintigraphic Diagnosis of Acute Cholecystitis

*WILLIAM C. KLINGENSMITH III, M.D.*

In the last few years, I have changed my approach to the role of cholescintigraphy in the diagnosis of acute cholecystitis. Previously I took the approach, prevalent in the literature, of focusing on the sensitivity and specificity of cholescintigraphy and its chief competitor, ultrasonography, in the diagnosis of acute cholecystitis. Thus it was primarily a question of which modality had a higher accuracy (sensitivity and specificity combined) for diagnosing acute cholecystitis.

However, I noticed whenever I recited the published sensitivities and specificities of cholescintigraphy and ultrasonography to my surgical colleagues that there was a certain lack of resonance in their response. After a while I began to realize that the question they were asking was different from the one I was answering, even though the question was never explicitly stated. The clinically relevant question was not simply "Does the patient have acute cholecystitis?" but rather "Does the patient have acute gallbladder disease that will benefit from a cholecystectomy?"

Notice that the clinically relevant question refers to "acute gallbladder disease" and not to "acute cholecystitis." Acute gallbladder disease is used to refer to both acute cholecystitis and acute biliary colic secondary to chronic cholecystitis. Cholecystectomy is the generally accepted treatment for acute biliary colic secondary to chronic cholecystitis, just as it is for acute cholecystitis.

## Indications, Clinical Utility, and Alternative Technologies

It is generally recognized that ultrasonography is highly accurate in the diagnosis of gallstones and thus for chronic cholecystitis, and that it is also moderately accurate in the diagnosis of acute cholecystitis. On the other hand, although cholescintigraphy is generally considered more accurate than ultrasonography for the diagnosis of acute cholecystitis, it is not capable of detecting gallstones and, therefore, is of little use in the diagnosis of chronic cholecystitis.

Although performing both cholescintigraphy and ultrasonography in every patient might give the best diagnostic results, economic constraints dictate that we follow a more cost-effective algorithm. The algorithm that I currently use requires the clinician to first decide whether he has a low or high threshold for performing a cholecystectomy (Fig. 1). A low threshold implies that a cholecystectomy would be performed if the patient has just gallstones, even if he does not have acute cholecystitis. On the other hand, a high threshold implies that a cholecystectomy would be performed only if the patient has acute cholecystitis. In general, the former patient is a good surgical risk and the latter one is a poor surgical risk.

If the imaging study that is performed first is inconclusive, the other imaging study can be performed secondarily. For example, if ultrasonography is performed first and no gallstones are seen, cholescintigraphy can be performed to better evaluate the possibility of acalculous acute cholecystitis. And if cholescintigraphy is performed first and no tracer is excreted, ultrasonography can be performed to evaluate both the gallbladder and the extrahepatic biliary tract.

Because most patients are good surgical candidates, the approach described here means that most patients with acute gallbladder disease are studied first with ultrasonography, and if gallstones are identified, proceed to cholecystectomy without undergoing additional imaging studies of the gallbladder. Clinicians tend to use ultrasonography primarily for other reasons as well. It allows evaluation of other structures such as the extrahepatic bile ducts and pancreas, and it can be performed in a shorter period. The somewhat lower cost of ultrasonography and its lack of ionizing radiation are of lesser importance.

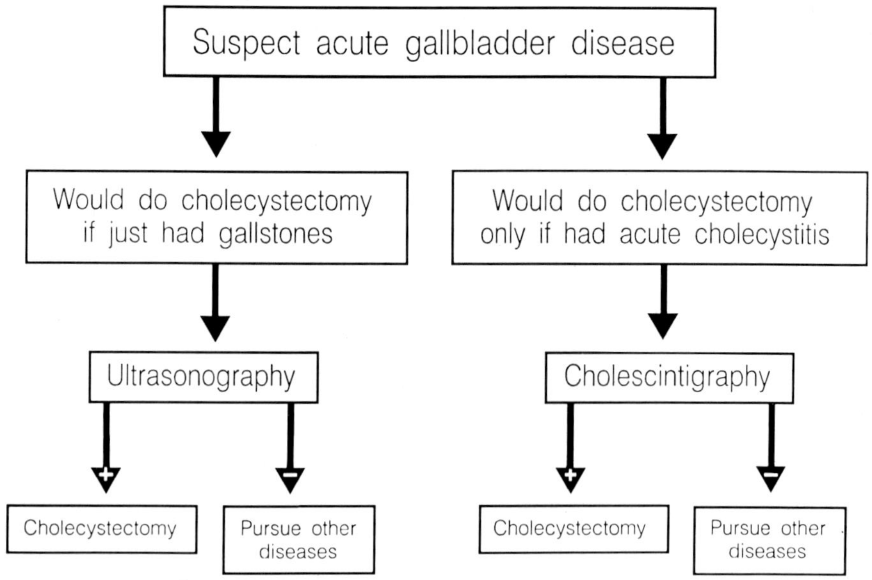


**FIGURE 1** An algorithm for imaging patients suspected of acute gallbladder disease. The clinician must first decide whether he has a low or high threshold for performing a cholecystectomy. In other words, whether he would operate if just gallstones were found or whether he would operate only if acute cholecystitis were present. With a low threshold for operating, ultrasonography is performed first. If gallstones are present, a cholecystectomy is done; if gallstones are not present, other disease possibilities are pursued. With a high threshold for operating, cholescintigraphy is performed first. If the gallbladder does not visualize, cholecystectomy is done; if the gallbladder visualizes, other disease possibilities are pursued.

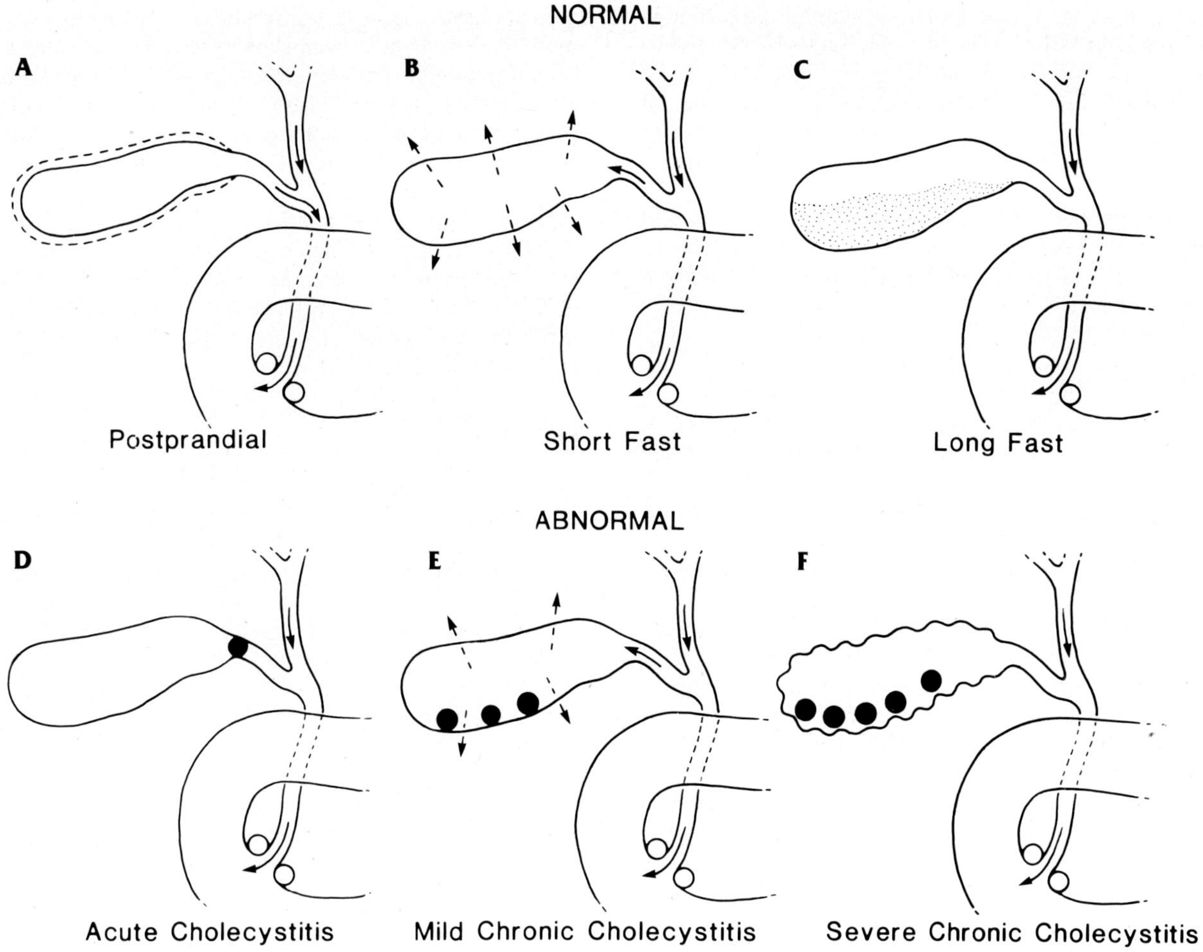


**FIGURE 2** Diagrams of several normal and abnormal gallbladder states. The top row depicts the flow of bile in normal subjects who *(A)* have recently eaten, *(B)* have fasted for a short period, e.g., 2-14 hours, or *(C)* have fasted for a prolonged period. Patients studied in the first and last of these normal states may give false-positive results, because of a contracting gallbladder wall and hyperconcentrated gallbladder contents with sludge, respectively. The second row depicts the flow of bile in patients with *(D)* acute cholecystitis, *(E)* mild chronic cholecystitis, and *(F)* severe chronic cholecystitis. The gallbladder usually visualizes by 1 hour in mild chronic cholecystitis because the gallbladder wall still functions, but often fails to visualize in severe chronic cholecystitis because the gallbladder wall is unable to reabsorb water.

## Technical Approach

In performing cholescintigraphy, it must first be determined whether evaluation of the gallbladder is of interest. If not, no special patient preparation is necessary. Usually, however, evaluation of the gallbladder is desired and one must ensure that the gallbladder is in a state conducive to visualization. This means that the gallbladder must not be contracting during the study, and it must not have already concentrated its contents to the point where the gallbladder wall can no longer transport ions against the osmotic gradient (Fig. 2).

If the gallbladder is contracting during the study, the bulk flow of bile is out of the gallbladder and the radiopharmaceutical does not enter the gallbladder, even if the gallbladder is perfectly normal. If the patient has recently eaten, cholescintigraphy should be delayed until 2 hours following the meal. In most cases, however, the patient is sufficiently ill that he or she has not eaten for at least 2 hours before reaching the nuclear medicine department.

The more common problem is the patient who has been fasting for so long that nonvisualization of the gallbladder secondary to overly concentrated gallbladder contents is a possibility. In this situation I give kinevac, an analog of cholecystokinin, by intravenous injection 20 minutes before injecting the radiopharmaceutical. I currently inject the kinevac over 3 minutes, but there is evidence that a more consistent and complete contraction of the gallbladder could be obtained if the kinevac were infused over 45 minutes. Because of the inconvenience of the longer injection time, I have not yet changed my protocol. All patients who have been fasting for more than 14 hours are pretreated with kinevac.

In general, the best radiopharmaceutical for studying a particular pathway or function is one that exhibits the highest extraction efficiency for that pathway and has the lowest extraction efficiency for all other pathways—radiopharmaceutical sensitivity and specificity. In addition, for pathways that involve multiple steps, such as the hepatobiliary pathway, it is desirable for the radiopharmaceutical to pass through the steps quickly and in a bolus fashion. Radiopharmaceuticals that meet these criteria give the greatest number of useful photons per radiation dose to the patient. In the case of cholescintigraphy, technetium-99m trimethylbromo-IDA best meets these criteria and is the current radiopharmaceutical of choice.

Images routinely are acquired in the anterior projection at 5 and 10 minutes after injection of the radiopharmaceutical and in the anterior and right lateral projections at 15, 30, 45, and 60 minutes. The initial anterior image is acquired for counts, e.g., 500 to 750 thousand counts, and all subsequent images are obtained for the same time as the initial image. Acquiring most images as anterior and right lateral image pairs allows the interpreter to localize activity by triangulation, and acquiring all images for equal time allows the interpreter to evaluate change in activity within the visualized structures from change in film density.

## Diagnostic Approach

The hallmark of acute cholecystitis by cholescintigraphy is nonvisualization of the gallbladder in the face of relatively normal excretion of the tracer. The normal gallbladder in the properly prepared patient will visualize by 1 hour. If the gallbladder does not visualize, and the radiopharmaceutical is not excreted in significant quantities, the study is indeterminate for acute cholecystitis.

Nonvisualization of the gallbladder by 1 hour is not totally specific for acute cholecystitis. The most common cause of nonvisualization of the gallbladder at 1 hour, other than acute cholecystitis, is chronic cholecystitis. Some patients with chronic cholecystitis, whose gallbladders do not visualize by 1 hour, will demonstrate visualization of the gallbladder in delayed images. Delayed visualization allows differentiation of chronic cholecystitis from acute cholecystitis. Delayed imaging is usually continued until the gallbladder visualizes or until 4 hours.

In my experience relatively few patients with chronic cholecystitis, whose gallbladders do not visualize by 1 hour, show visualization between 1 and 4 hours. In addition, it has been shown that whether or not a gallbladder with chronic cholecystitis visualizes at 1 hour correlates strongly with the severity of chronic cholecystitis at histologic evaluation. Gallbladders with mild chronic cholecystitis are likely to visualize by 1 hour and be indistinguishable from normal gallbladders. Conversely, gallbladders with severe chronic cholecystitis are unlikely to visualize even with delayed imaging through 4 hours.

One of my colleagues has found some evidence (unpublished) that patients with relatively severe chronic cholecystitis and nonvisualization of the gallbladder at 1 hour are more likely to benefit from cholecystectomy than those with relatively mild chronic cholecystitis and visualization of the gallbladder by 1 hour. One of my colleagues conducted a phone survey of patients who had undergone cholecystectomy and who had only chronic cholecystitis at histologic evaluation. The patients' statement as to whether they had benefited from surgery tended to correlate with the severity of the chronic cholecystitis.

Because relatively few patients with chronic cholecystitis, whose gallbladders do not visualize at 1 hour, show visualization in delayed images, and because there is evidence that these patients have relatively severe chronic cholecystitis and are more likely to benefit from cholecystectomy, I usually do not prolong my cholescintigraphic studies beyond 2 hours. For the same reasons, I have not instituted the practice of injecting the patient with morphine at 45 to 60 minutes with an additional 1 hour of imaging. The reduction in false-positive studies for acute cholecystitis attributed to morphine injection may represent patients with relatively severe chronic cholecystitis.

The foregoing findings raise the possibility that many cholescintigraphic studies that are false positive for acute cholecystitis are not false positive for acute gallbladder disease that will benefit from cholecystectomy. This hypothesis requires additional evaluation.

## Discussion

In the patient suspected of acute gallbladder disease, and in whom there is no contraindication to surgery, ultrasonography is probably the primary imaging test because of its ability to evaluate a variety of diseases of the gallbladder and biliary tract. However, in the patient who is not a good surgical candidate, cholescintigraphy is a highly sensitive test for acute cholecystitis and represents the imaging study of choice. Not infrequently both tests are needed to completely elucidate the patient's condition.

## Suggested Reading


Fig LM, Wahl RL, Stewart RE, et al. Morphine-augmented hepatobiliary scintigraphy in the severely ill: Caution is in order. Radiology 1990; 175:467–473.

Fink-Bennett D, Balon H, Robbins T, et al. Morphine-augmented cholescintigraphy: Its efficacy in detecting acute cholecystitis. J Nucl Med 1991; 32:1231–1233.

Hermann RE. Surgery for acute and chronic cholecystitis. Surg Clin North Am 1990; 70:1263–1275.

Klingensmith WC, Fritzberg AR, Spitzer VM, et al. Clinical evaluation of Tc-99m-trimethylbromo-IDA and Tc-99m-diisopropyl-IDA for hepatobiliary imaging. Radiology 1983; 146:181–184.

Klingensmith WC, Spitzer VM, Fritzberg AR. The normal fasting and postprandial Tc-99m-diisopropyl-IDA hepatobiliary study. Radiology 1981; 141:771–776.

Klingensmith WC, Turner WM. Cholescintigraphy for acute cholecystitis: False positive results caused by chronic cholecystitis. Gastrointest Radiol 1990; 15:129–132.

Larsen MJ, Klingensmith WC, Kuni CC. Radionuclide hepatobiliary imaging: Nonvisualization of the gallbladder secondary to prolonged fasting. J Nucl Med 1982; 23:1003–1005.

Marton KI, Doubilet P. How to image the gallbladder in suspected cholecystitis. Ann Intern Med 1988; 109:722–729.

Sarva RP, Schreiner DP, Van Thiel D, et al. Gallbladder function: Methods for measuring filling and emptying. J Nucl Med 1985; 26:140–144.

Weissmann HS, Badia J, Sugarman LA, et al. Spectrum of Tc-99m-IDA cholescintigraphic patterns in acute cholecystitis. Radiology 1981; 138:167–175.

Weissmann HS, Berdowitz D, Fox MS, et al. The role of technetium-99m iminodiacetic acid (IDA) cholescintigraphy in acute acalculous cholecystitis. Radiology 1983; 146:177–180.

# Scintigraphic Detection of Acute Gastrointestinal Bleeding

*MICHAEL F. HARTSHORNE, M.D. · NANCY WOLF, M.S., R.Ph.*

Gastrointestinal (GI) hemorrhage is a common medical problem with mortality rates of 10 to 20 percent. Many different sources of hemorrhage are possible as are various etiologies. The proximal bleeds are more frequently massive and life-threatening. Lower GI bleeds tend to be more intermittent and less often pose an immediate threat to life. However, upper GI bleeding from peptic ulcer disease, gastritis from any cause, esophageal varices, Mallory-Weiss syndrome, and occasional tumors may be initially confused with lower sources such as diverticula, angiodysplasia, inflammatory bowel diseases, and tumors. This chapter details the role of scintigraphy in detection of GI hemorrhage.

## Indications, Clinical Utility, Alternative Technologies

Concurrent with initial stabilization of a patient with GI bleeding, a rapid evaluation of the bleeding site requires separation of those occurring above and below the ligament of Treitz. Hematemesis usually means a site above that location, and this can be confirmed by gastric aspiration followed by upper endoscopy. If the immediate evaluation proves a proximal source, it usually also dictates therapy. In the majority of patients, upper GI hemorrhage ceases irrespective of an early diagnosis and choice of therapy.

When a proximal site of bleeding is excluded we prefer immediate radionuclide evaluation of the patient. Emergent lower endoscopy in an inadequately prepared colon is unlikely to be successful in detecting the site of bleeding. Contrast radiographic examinations of the upper and lower GI system have no place in the acutely bleeding patient and should be reserved for the investigation of a patient who has stopped bleeding. Neoplastic and inflammatory lesions in the small bowel may be detected with enteroclysis techniques. Barium enema studies may find incidental lesions, such as diverticula, that may or may not be the cause of hemorrhage. Arteriography and exploratory surgery are not particularly successful in the detection of bleeding sites. Both are reserved for last-ditch efforts to localize hemorrhage. The window of opportunity for detection of a bleeding site with angiography is extremely limited, since the bolus of contrast lasts only seconds. The correct vessel must be injected and filmed at the same time that bleeding occurs. Both angiography and surgery have a better role as therapies once another technique has found the source.

## Technical Approach

The scintigraphic evaluation of the gastrointestinal bleeder is the product of experimental work with dogs, in which bleeding was detected as the extravasation of technetium-99m sulfur colloid (TcSC) into the lumen of the bowel at a surgically created arterial hemorrhage. The window of opportunity for this technique is rather brief, since the intravenously injected TcSC is cleared from the blood with a half-life of 2 to 3 minutes by the normal reticuloendothelial system. The theoretical advantage of this technique is that complete removal of the background activity allows even small target hemorrhages (0.05 to 0.1 ml/min) to be detected in animal experiments. However, given the intermittent nature of most lower GI bleeding, the TcSC study requires serendipitous timing or a rapid continuous hemorrhage to be routinely successful.

A definite improvement in the scintigraphic GI bleeding study required the perfection of Tc-99m red blood cell ($^{99m}$TcRBC) labeling techniques. Heat-damaged TcRBC preparations last longer in circulation than TcSC before the spleen removes the background activity. The window of opportunity is extended, but the study requires additional time and technical expertise to prepare the heat-damaged TcRBCs.

Schemes to label TcRBCs have evolved to limit the physiologic stomach excretion of free $^{99m}$Tc pertechnetate (TcO4). If a simple in vivo labeling of the RBCs is done with sequential intravenous injections of stannous pyrophosphate and TcO4, there is a high percentage of stomach excretion of TcO4. This activity peristalses through the gut and becomes indistinguishable from hemorrhage. Pure in vitro methods of labeling can achieve almost pure TcRBC labels, but may require the use of investigational new drugs or in-house compounding by a radiopharmacist.

A modification of the pure in vivo and in vitro techniques was in vogue for a few years and has been called the "in vivtro" technique. This strategy for high-efficiency labeling calls for injecting the patient with intravenous stannous pyrophosphate and then withdrawing blood from the patient into a heparinized syringe loaded with TcO4 and taped to the patient's arm. After 10 minutes the contents of the syringe are injected. Initial reports of experiments with microcurie amounts indicated that in vivtro labeling produced little free TcO4, but there is reasonable doubt that clinically used millicurie amounts label RBCs as completely as advertised. Difficulties with shielded TcO4 syringes and temporary intravenous lines attached to the patient's arm require extra attention with this technique.

A technique elegant for its simplicity and effectiveness was first published by Benedetto and Nusynowitz. We routinely use a minor modification of this technique (Table 1). The patient is injected with stannous pyrophosphate as soon as the imaging service is alerted to the need for a GI bleeding study. After about 15 minutes, blood is withdrawn into a heparinized tube. Both of these steps can be conducted at a site remote from the nuclear medicine laboratory. The contents of the tube are labeled with an excess of TcO4, and after simple centrifugation the plasma layer (which contains any unwanted free TcO4) is discarded. The remaining TcRBCs suspended in saline are then used for the GI bleeding study.

A new alternative for high-efficiency TcRBC labeling is now available as the ULTRATAG RBC kit from Mallinckrodt Medical, Inc. Labeling efficiency greater than 95 percent is accomplished by mixing 1 to 3 ml of anticoagulated whole blood with stannous ion. The stannous ion is allowed to

**TABLE 1** RBC Labeling

1. Prepare a stannous pyrophosphate solution by reconstituting a kit with 2 ml of sterile saline. Draw up the entire 2 ml (approximately 1.8 mg of stannous chloride) and inject into a peripheral vein.
2. After 15 minutes, collect 6 ml of blood into an evacuated, sterile, heparinized collection tube. Use no smaller than a 22 gauge needle to withdraw the blood.

**Perform the remaining steps behind lead shielding**

3. Inject 35–40 mCi of $^{99m}$Tc sodium pertechnetate into the collection tube containing the blood.
4. Mix gently by inverting the collection tube several times and incubate at room temperature for 5 minutes.
5. After allowing the blood to incubate, centrifuge the collection tube stopper down for 5 minutes to separate the RBCs from the plasma.
6. Gently remove the collection tube from the centrifuge, keeping the stopper end down. The RBC layer should be packed against the stopper.
7. Using a 10 ml syringe with a 20 gauge 1.5 inch needle, gently insert the needle into the collection tube to the needle hub. While inserting the needle, exert a slight pulling pressure on the syringe plunger until the needle tip is above the RBC layer. This helps avoid disturbing the RBC layer with an air jet.
8. Slowly aspirate the entire plasma layer, withdrawing the needle slightly if needed. Approximately 2 ml of RBCs will remain in the tube.
9. Withdraw the needle from the collection tube while maintaining a firm grip on the plunger to prevent the syringe contents from being inadvertently sucked back into the tube.
10. Add 2–4 ml of sterile saline to the remaining RBCs in the collection tube and gently invert several times to resuspend the cells.
11. Place the collection tube carefully in the dose calibrator to measure the amount of activity in the cells.
12. Withdraw 30 mCi of TcRBCs and reinject this amount into the patient.

*Note:* We have found that approximately 70% of the initial activity will remain in the RBC fraction. Therefore if a 20 mCi dose of TcRBC is desired, approximately 25–30 mCi of TcO4 should be added to the blood initially.
Modified from Benedetto AR, Nusynowitz ML. A technique for the preparation of TC-99m red blood cells for the evaluation of gastrointestinal hemorrhage. Clin Nucl Med 1983; 8:160–162.

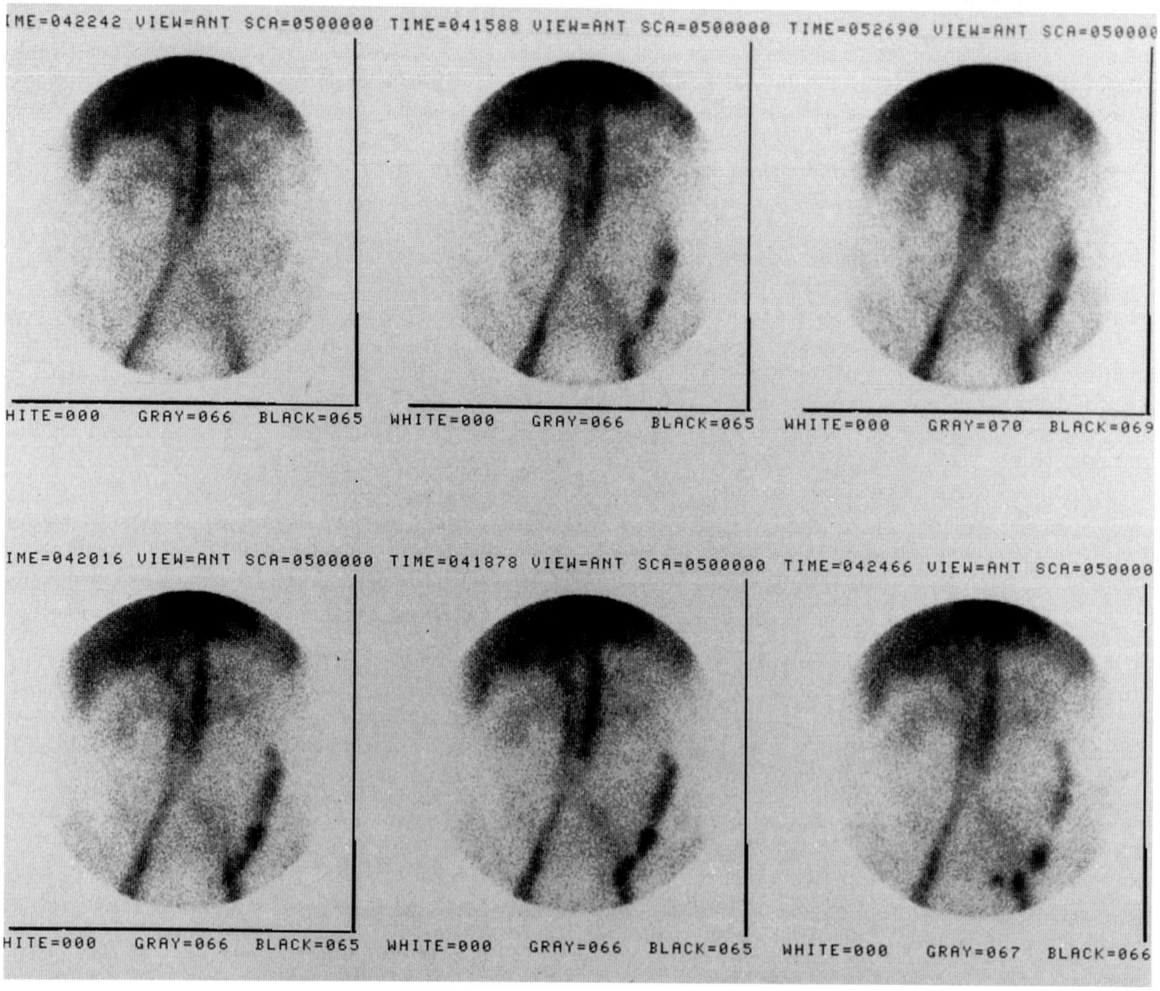


**FIGURE 1** Images taken immediately and every 5 minutes after the injection of 30 mCi of TcRBCs show the early appearance of a GI bleeding study in the descending colon. A bleeding diverticulum briefly pumped blood into the lumen of the bowel that peristalsed proximally as well as distally away from the bleeding site. Computer cine replay of these studies is persuasive in discussions with referring clinical physicians.

passively diffuse across the RBC cell membrane. Sodium hypochlorite is then added to oxidize any extracellular stannous ion. Thus only the intracellular stannous ions are able to reduce the subsequently added TcO4. The total time for this labeling procedure is 25 to 30 minutes.

We prefer to start the scintigraphic evaluation with the TcSC technique only when TcSC is already prepared for routine daily use and the patient appears to have an emergent, massive, and possibly continuous bleed. In that situation it may be possible to quickly obtain a diagnosis ($<15$ minutes) without delaying the steps in Table 1 for the more sensitive TcRBC study. The studies can be done one after the other if the TcSC technique is negative after 15 minutes.

The camera-computer acquisition of the GI bleeding study depends on dynamic imaging. The patient's abdomen and pelvis should be positioned under a large-field-of-view camera with a low-energy collimator before injection with either TcSC (10 mCi) or TcRBC (20 to 30 mCi) techniques. In mobile situations with the smaller standard-field-of-view camera, a diverging collimator is used to image the whole abdomen and pelvis simultaneously. With the high photon flux available, we prefer high-resolution collimation. Film acquisition should be backed up by a dynamic computer acquisition. A $128 \times 128$ matrix is optimal, but a $64 \times 64$ will serve if the computer has a limited memory capacity. Computer images at 1 minute intervals allow a study to be performed for a minimum of 90 minutes. The acquisition can be terminated early if a bleeding site is detected. Lower GI bleeding rates of about 0.1 ml/min with total hemorrhaged volumes of 2 to 3 ml of blood are routinely localized with this technique. Optimal interpretation of this study is provided by fast cine replay of the computer acquisition. Small intermittent hemorrhages will appear to flash into existence and then wiggle away and perhaps disperse as they dilute into nonlabeled gut fluids. These may not be confidently seen on film acquisitions (Fig. 1).

## Diagnostic Approach

"When GI bleeding is the game, you get no points for a nuclear guaiac test." Localization of the bleeding site is the purpose of the scintigraphic study. To qualify as a bleeding site, the extravasation into bowel must superimpose itself on the blood pool background activity, become more intense with time, and flow away from its origin in either direction (Table 2). If a suspected lesion is observed on the first and the last image of a study unchanged, it is undoubtedly a concentration of TcRBCs in a vascular structure such as an aneurysm, arteriovenous malformation, uterus, dilated vein, or abscess. Care must be taken not to mistake excretion into the genitourinary system of TcRBC fragments. Voiding the urinary bladder during or after the study may be helpful if the patient does not have the bladder catheterized.

If GI bleeding is not detected after 90 minutes, we stop the study. The patient is returned to the clinical service with a request that in the next 24 hours (while TcRBCs continue to circulate) he return to the imaging service immediately if there is clinical suspicion that he is bleeding again. Sometimes this strategy works and the rules in Table 2 allow a diagnosis. Sometimes the patient has bled into the bowel and peristalsed activity to and fro in a manner that makes it impossible to detect the site of bleeding. If the patient is not suspected of rebleeding in 24 hours, a repeat acquisition consisting of one static image is requested for quality assurance purposes. Localized hemorrhages detected are expressed as a percentage of the localized hemorrhages plus the hemorrhages found but not localized. About 85 percent of those who bleed in this 24 hour period will be localized within the first 90 minutes, making possible a quantitative evaluation of the imaging service's performance.

**TABLE 2** Rules for GI Bleed Interpretation*

| Bleeders must: |
|---|
| 1. Come out of nowhere. |
| 2. Get more intense. |
| 3. Move away through gut. |

*No points for nuclear guaiacs.

## Suggested Reading

Alavi A, Dann RW, Baum S, et al. Scintigraphic detection of acute gastrointestinal bleeding. Radiology 1977; 124:753–756.

Benedetto AR, Nusynowitz ML. A technique for the preparation of Tc-99m red blood cells for the evaluation of gastrointestinal hemorrhage. Clin Nucl Med 1983; 8:160–162.

Bunker SR, Brown JM, McAuley RJ, et al. Detection of gastrointestinal bleeding sites: Use of in vitro technetium Tc 99m-labeled RBCs. JAMA 1982; 247:789–792.

Bunker SR, Lull RJ, Tanascu DE, et al. The superiority of 99mTc RBC over 99mTc sulfur colloid in the detection and localization of gastrointestinal hemorrhage. AJR 1984; 143:543–548.

Landry A, Hartshorne MF, Bunker SR, et al. Optimal technetium-99m RBC labeling for gastrointestinal hemorrhage study. Clin Nucl Med 1985; 10:491–493.

Smith R, Copley DJ, Bolen FH. 99mTc RBC scintigraphy: Correlation of bleeding rates with scintigraphic findings. AJR 1987; 148: 869–874.

Som P, Oster ZH, Atkins HL, et al. Detection of gastrointestinal blood loss with 99mTc-labeled heat-treated red blood cells. Radiology 1981; 138:207–209.

Steer ML, Silen W. Diagnostic procedures in gastrointestinal hemorrhage. N Engl J Med 1983; 309:646–650.

Thorn DA, Datz FL, Remley K, Christian PE. Bleeding rates necessary for detection of acute gastrointestinal bleeding with technetium 99m-labeled red blood cells in an experimental model. J Nucl Med 1987; 28:514–520.

Winzelberg GG, McKusick KA, Froelich JW, et al. Detection of gastrointestinal bleeding with 99mTc-labeled red blood cells. Semin Nucl Med 1982; 12:139–146.

# CT in Acute Pancreatitis: Diagnosis, Staging, and Prognosis

*EMIL J. BALTHAZAR, M.D.*

Acute pancreatitis is a relatively common illness characterized by nonspecific pancreatic inflammation triggered by a variety of etiologic factors. The most common etiologies found in over 80 percent of patients are repeated bouts of heavy alcohol intake and cholelithiasis.

The ability to diagnose and evaluate patients with acute pancreatitis has improved dramatically with the recent development of fast, high-resolution computed tomography (CT) scanners. The need for a reliable imaging modality in this group of patients becomes evident when the limitations of the clinical examination and laboratory evaluation are known. Based only on the clinical examination, before the introduction of CT, the diagnosis of hemorrhagic pancreatitis was missed in up to 30 to 40 percent of patients. This was occurring because hyperamylasemia associated with acute abdominal symptoms is suggestive but not pathognomonic of pancreatitis. In fact hyperamylasemia can be triggered by other acute abdominal conditions such as bowel infarction, small bowel obstruction, acute cholecystitis, and peptic ulcers. Conversely the serum amylase level can be normal in patients with acute pancreatitis, especially a few days following the initial attack. Further, there is no correlation established between the degree of elevated serum amylase and severity of pancreatitis. For this reason, exploratory laparotomy was performed often in the attempt to properly diagnose patients presenting with acute abdominal symptoms and hyperamylasemia.

To circumvent these shortcomings, conventional imaging modalities (plain abdominal films, barium enema studies, ERCP) have been used for many years with relatively limited success. They have a low sensitivity and specificity and today should be considered complementary modalities used mainly in special circumstances. Sonography is more commonly used because it can visualize an enlarged and abnormal gland and mainly because it can detect gallstones, which are a common cause of acute pancreatitis. Compared with CT however, sonography has a lower sensitivity in visualizing the entire pancreatic gland and is inferior in detecting the full range of peripancreatic inflammatory changes (the hallmark of pancreatitis). CT must be considered the primary and most reliable imaging modality for evaluating patients clinically suspected of acute pancreatitis.

## Indications

The role of CT in the evaluation of patients suspected of having acute pancreatitis is threefold:

1. CT plays a significant role in the early diagnosis, having a reported sensitivity of 77 to 92 percent and a specificity of over 95 percent. Further, by evaluating the entire abdomen, CT is able to detect a variety of other acute abdominal conditions, elucidating the clinical presentation and the possible need for emergency surgical interventions.
2. Together with the multiple objective laboratory risk factors developed by Ranson (Table 1), CT plays a dominant role as a prognostic indicator of the severity of the acute inflammatory disease.
3. Finally, CT plays a crucial role in the detection of local complications such as abscesses, retroperitoneal bleeding, and pseudocyst formation, and should be used in the follow-up evaluation of patients with severe forms of necrotizing pancreatitis.

**TABLE 1** Early Objective Prognostic Signs Used to Estimate the Risk of Death or Major Complications from Acute Pancreatitis

| At Admission or Diagnosis | During Initial 48 Hours |
|---|---|
| Age >55 years | Hematocrit fall >10 percentage points |
| White blood cell count >16,000/mm³ | Blood urea nitrogen rise >5 mg/dl |
| Blood glucose >200 mg/dl | Serum calcium level <8 mg/dl |
| Serum lactic dehydrogenase >350 IU/L | Arterial $Po_2$ <60 mm Hg |
| Serum glutamic oxaloacetic transaminase >250 sigma Frankel units (%) | Base deficit >4 mEq/L |
| | Estimated fluid sequestration >6,000 ml |

Mild clinical forms of edematous acute pancreatitis that spontaneously resolve in 24 to 48 hours do not require routine CT evaluations. In our institution, however, CT evaluation is performed early in almost all patients suspected of having acute pancreatitis. I believe that except for medical contraindications and emergency time requirements, CT evaluation should be performed as early as possible when (1) the clinical diagnosis is in doubt; (2) there is no response to medical treatment within 48 to 72 hours; (3) there are acute abdominal symptoms (severe distention, tenderness), leukocytosis, or fever; or (4) patients present with or develop more than two of Ranson's grave signs (see Table 1).

## Technical Considerations

The use of high-resolution CT technique is crucial in the early diagnosis and evaluation of patients with acute pancreatitis. Unless contraindicated (allergy, renal failure, congestive heart failure), intravenous contrast material should be administered in all patients, and the pancreatic gland should be imaged rapidly during its arterial phase of parenchymal enhancement. To achieve this objective, a rapid bolus intravenous injection of 50 ml of 60 percent iodinated contrast material is given at a rate of 3 ml per second using a 20 gauge Angiocath, followed by 100 ml at 1 ml/sec. Rapid scan time (1 to 2 seconds) and incremental dynamic sequential scanning technique are essential. Scanning starts at the end of the bolus phase of injection at the level of the L2 to L3 intervertebral space and proceeds cephalad to the level of the vertebral body T11. Dynamic sequential 5 x 5 mm or 5 x 8 mm transaxial images over the pancreas are initially obtained, and the rest of the abdomen is scanned subsequently with 10 mm collimation. Diluted 2

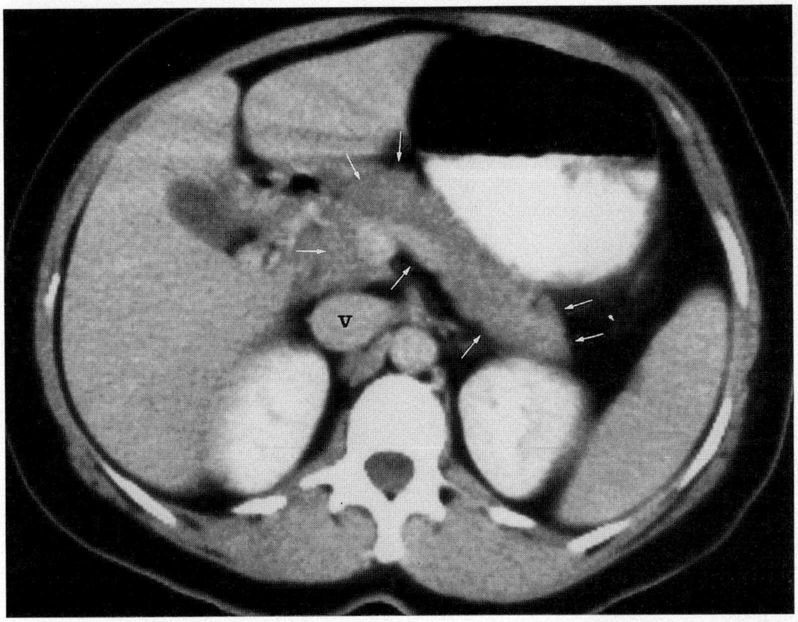


**FIGURE 1** Normal pancreas. Pancreas is sharply defined, homogeneous in density, and normal sized (*arrows*). Uncinate process is triangular and it is located anterior to the inferior vena cava (v) at the confluence with the left renal vein. CT scan was performed because of abdominal pain and hyperamylasemia. Grade A staging, normal enhancing gland, severity index 0.

percent barium sulfate solution (800 ml) is given orally in small increments starting 30 to 60 minutes before the evaluation to promote adequate visualization of the gastronintestinal tract.

## Normal Pancreas and Terminology

On CT scans, the pancreas enhances homogeneously and appears as a sharply defined structure with a smooth outer contour or an undulating acinar configuration (Fig. 1). The gland is visualized in the upper abdomen, and in most individuals it is obliquely located with the tail cranial in the hilum of the spleen and the head caudal and to the right of the spine, within the duodenal sweep. The most caudal segment of the gland is the uncinate process. It is located at the level of the confluence of the left renal vein with the inferior vena cava and has a triangular configuration. The gland varies slightly in size in normal individuals and often atrophies to a variable extent in the aging population. The head of the pancreas is the largest segment, measuring about 3 cm in the anteroposterior diameter. The body measures about 2 cm and the tail 1 cm, with a gradual transition between segments. On a high-resolution examination, segments of the pancreatic duct measuring 1 mm wide can be detected in up to 50 percent of patients. The surrounding peripancreatic fatty tissue that envelops the gland has a homogeneous low-attenuation value, and the peripancreatic vascular channels are distinctly observed.

CT terminology is important for the goal of employing a common language that can properly define the wide spectrum of abnormalities present in patients with acute pancreatitis. The pathologic changes include mild interstitial edema, extravasation of pancreatic secretion, secondary inflammatory reaction, hemorrhage, and necrotic tissue. In the initial stages of the disease, there is an ill-defined, indurated, spongy, inflamed and necrotic retroperitoneum, but usually there is no drainable free fluid. Different amounts of free fluid, originally poorly defined and later partially encapsulated, develop later. The retroperitoneal fluid can spontaneously resolve; it can persist and encapsulate, forming a pseudocyst; or it can become infected, producing an abscess. To portray these pathologic changes, the following terminology should be used:

1. *Peripancreatic inflammation*—slight increase in the density of fatty tissue with a dirty, hazy, or lacelike appearance
2. *Phlegmon*—ill-defined area of heterogeneous soft-tissue densities intermixed with lower-attenuation values (20 to 40 HU) in or around the pancreatic gland
3. *Fluid collections*—nonencapsulated or partially and poorly encapsulated homogeneous collections of water density (10 to 20 HU) in the retroperitoneum
4. *Pseudocyst*—sharply defined round or oval fluid collection with a clearly identifiable circumferential capsule
5. *Abscess*—retroperitoneal extraluminal air collection associated with phlegmon or fluid collection
6. *Pancreatic necrosis*—absence of contrast enhancement with liquefaction and loss of normal glandular texture of a portion of, or the entire, pancreas

## CT Diagnosis

The CT findings in acute pancreatitis are similar, irrespective of etiology, with the exception of traumatic pancreatitis in which fresh hematomas and lacerations can be detected. In milder forms of interstitial pancreatitis, the CT scan may show a normal gland or a slight-to-moderate increase in the size of the gland associated with a shaggy contour and hazy and dirty peripancreatic fat (Fig. 2). The inflammatory process is usually diffuse, involving similarly the entire gland. Segmental forms of acute pancreatitis occur in as many as 18 percent of patients, and the segment most often involved is the head of the pancreas. In these cases CT detects an asymmetric pattern, with involvement of only a part of the gland either exclusively or predominantly. A morphologically normal pancreas is seen in about 20 percent of patients clinically diagnosed as having pancreatitis. This presentation is always associated with a mild and self-limiting clinical course, and its frequency varies in different series depending on the severity of disease in the population examined. Its exact prevalence is not known, and I

A

B

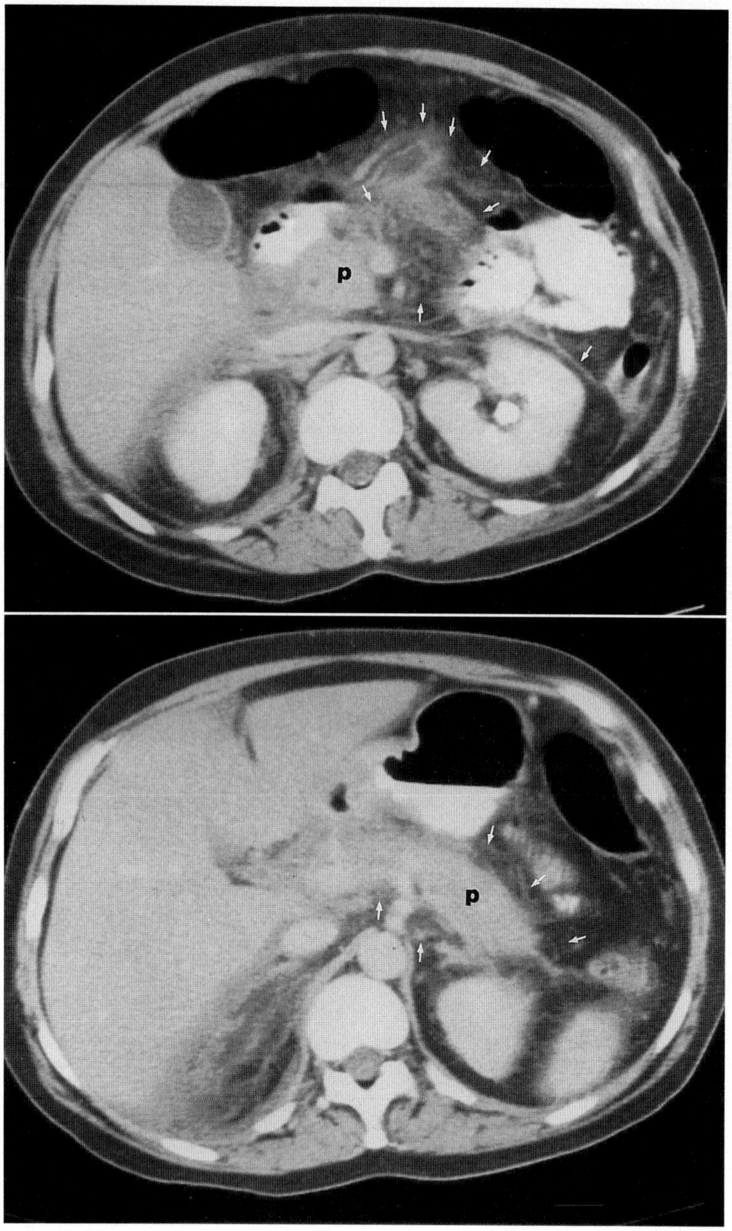


**FIGURE 2** *A* and *B,* Pancreas is enlarged (p) and there are extensive peripancreatic inflammatory changes (*arrow*). There is normal enhancement of the entire gland without necrosis. Grade C staging, severity index 2.

suspect it to be significantly lower if one defines pancreatitis as a gross morphologic and/or histologic alteration of the pancreas, rather than a temporary functional abnormality.

In the more severe forms of pancreatitis, the gland may be enlarged, irregular in contour, and heterogeneous in density; peripancreatic phlegmons and fluid collections rapidly develop (Fig. 3). The inflammatory exudates obliterate the peripancreatic fat and dissect into peripancreatic fascial planes, violating peritoneal surfaces and compartments. The most common locations of the fluid collections are left anterior pararenal space and the lesser peritoneal sac. Within a few days after the initial attack, these collections decrease in density, become poorly encapsulated, and begin to resolve (see Fig. 3). When massive, phlegmons can extend inferiorly into the pelvis, may involve the small bowel mesentery, transverse mesocolon, posterior pararenal spaces, perirenal space, and even the greater peritoneal cavity, producing pancreatic ascites.

## *Local Complications*

The most common and clinically significant local complications of acute pancreatitis are pancreatic abscess, pancreatic pseudocyst, and retroperitoneal hemorrhage.

Pancreatic abscess can be defined as an infected phlegmonous or fluid collection in or around the pancreatic gland (Fig. 4). Abscesses occur usually within 2 to 3 weeks after an episode of acute pancreatitis in anywhere from 3 to 21 percent of patients. They are considered the major cause of death in acute pancreatitis. CT has a high sensitivity to detect a pancreatic abscess, but it has a limited specificity since it cannot differentiate infected from noninfected fluid collections unless they contain air bubbles. Poorly defined or partially encapsulated fluid collections (10 to 40 HU) that persist for more than 2 or 3 weeks in a septic patient should be considered infected, unless proven otherwise. In our institution, if there is no adequate alternative explanation for the sepsis, these patients undergo extensive retroperitoneal debridement and drainage.

C

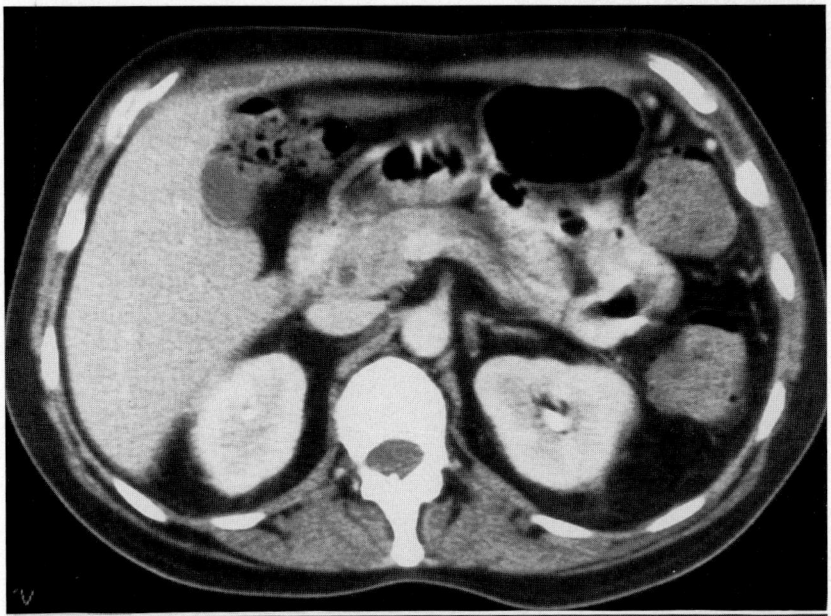

D

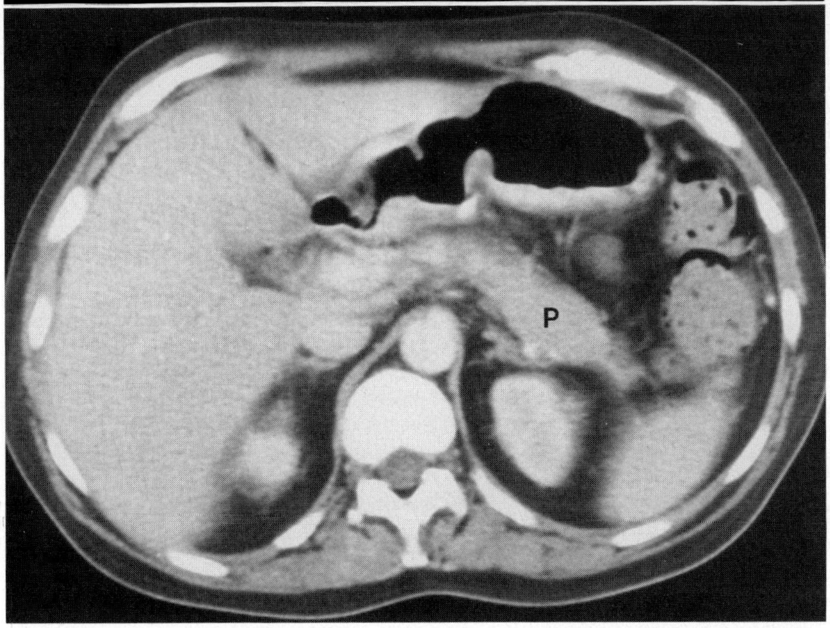


**FIGURE 2, cont'd** *C* and *D,* Follow-up evaluation 3 weeks later. Tail of the pancreas (p) remains enlarged, but all the peripancreatic inflammatory changes have resolved. Patient had an uneventful clinical course without complications.

In equivocal clinical cases, CT-guided aspiration of fluid can reliably distinguish infected from noninfected fluid collections. After an attack of acute pancreatitis, the great majority of developing fluid collections resolve spontaneously or become infected and form abscesses. In about 1 to 3 percent of patients, however, encapsulated fluid collections persist for more than 6 to 7 weeks, whereas the remaining acute inflammatory pancreatic and peripancreatic reaction resolves (Fig. 5).

Pseudocysts tend to be more stable, although spontaneous resolution can still occur. They have a sharp contour, are oval or round, and can vary greatly in size (Fig. 6). They are located usually within the pancreas or peripancreatic retroperitoneum, but can dissect fascial planes and erode into adjacent organs. It is not unusual to detect pseudocysts in the lower mediastinum, lower abdomen and pelvis, and within the spleen and liver. Many pseudocysts are detected in relatively asymptomatic individuals with evidence of chronic pancreatitis or history of heavy alcohol abuse. Their clinical significance appears to correlate with their size. Dangerous complications such as rupture with peritonitis, abscess formation, and bleeding occur more often in pseudocysts larger than 3 to 4 cm in diameter. For this reason, in asymptomatic individuals I recommend internal drainage for large pseudocysts and clinical and radiographic follow-up for patients with pseudocysts smaller than 3 cm.

Retroperitoneal hemorrhage can occur as a complication of pseudocyst formation or as a consequence of the extravasated proteolytic enzymes eroding the peripancreatic vessels. Bleeding can occur in the acute phase of pancreatitis or later, with the spontaneous rupture of a developing pseudoaneurysm. CT demonstrates the high-attenuation fluid, representing fresh blood (40 to 60 HU) in the retroperitoneum, as well as extravasated intravascular contrast material in patients actively bleeding (see Fig. 6). When the exact site of bleeding is not

A

B

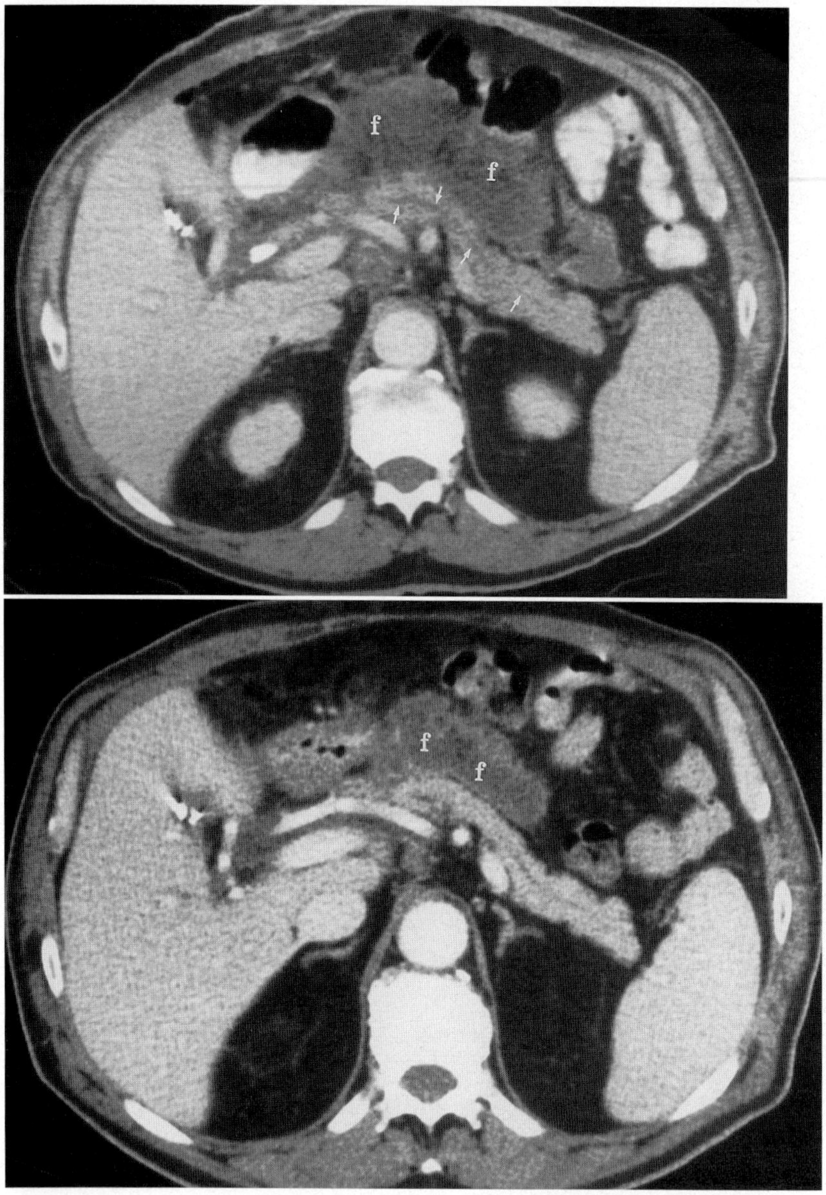


**FIGURE 3** *A,* Normal-sized pancreas shows a slightly distended pancreatic duct (*arrows*). A large ill-defined fluid collection is present anterior to the body and tail of the pancreas (f). The gland is enhancing normally without evidence of necrosis. Grade D pancreatitis, severity index 3. *B,* Follow-up evaluation 4 weeks later shows significant resolution of the fluid collection, with a residual smaller collection (f) still present. Patient did not develop complications.

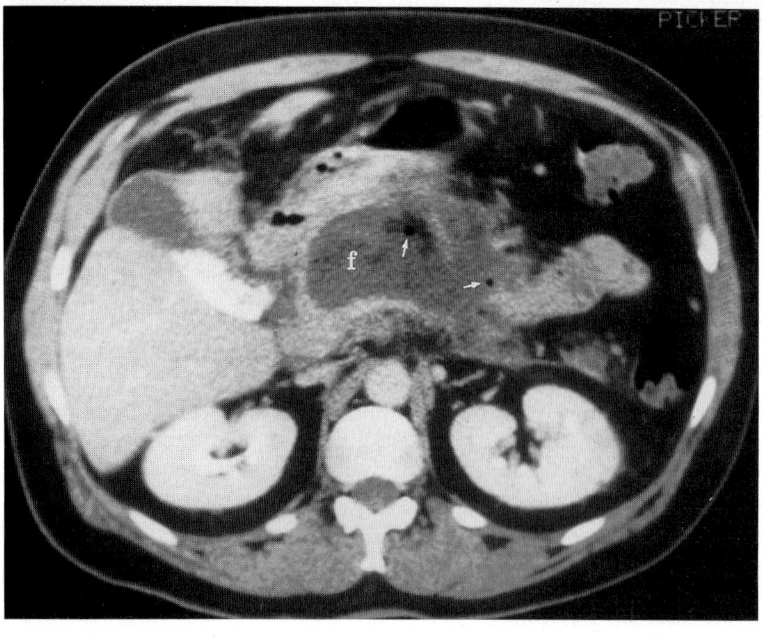


**FIGURE 4** Abscess in the lesser sac associated with previous grade E pancreatitis and pancreatic necrosis. Partially encapsulated fluid collection (f) containing a few bubbles of air (*arrows*) is present. Abscess was proven at surgery.

A

B

C

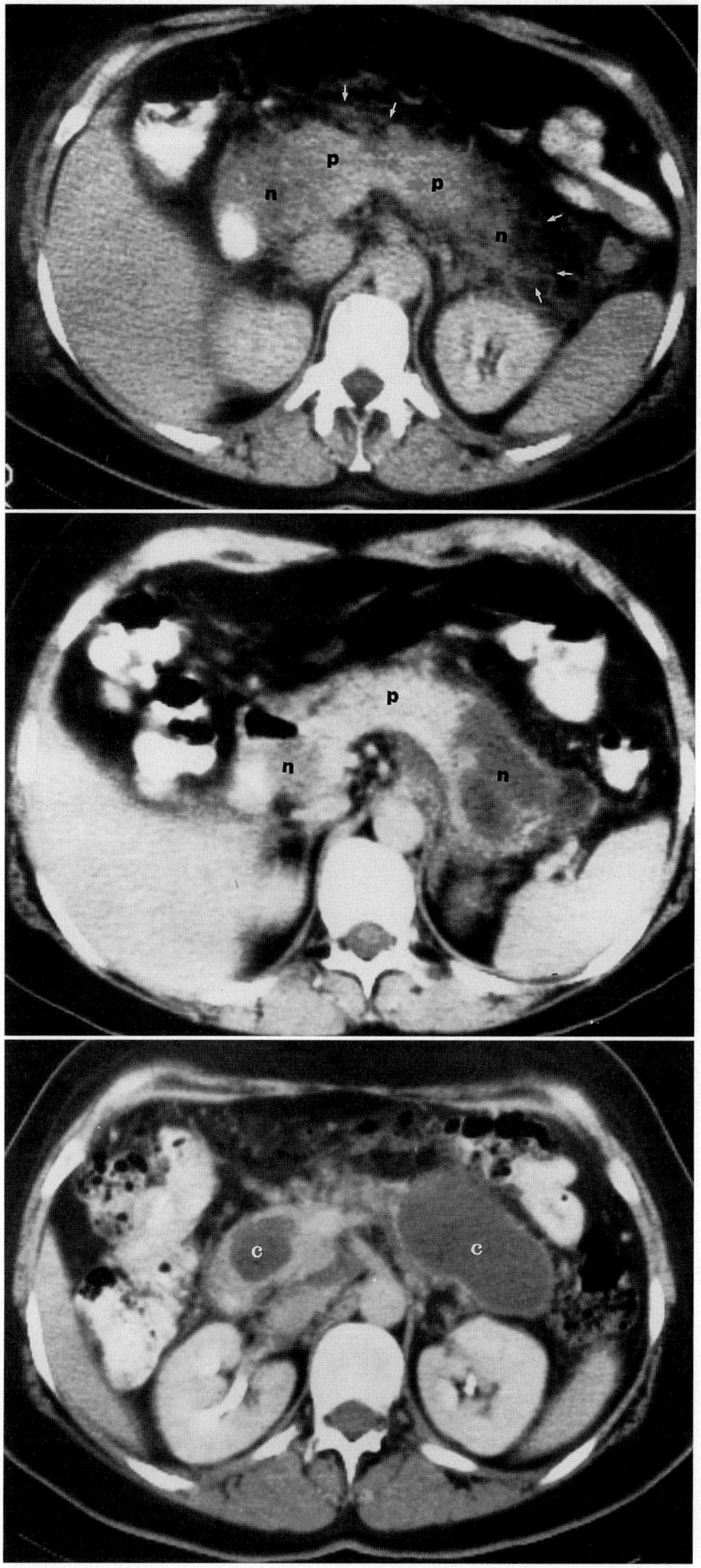


**FIGURE 5** *A,* Pancreas is enlarged, heterogeneous (p), and is enveloped by peripancreatic inflammation and fluid collections (not seen at this level). Grade D pancreatitis. There is lack of enhancement of the tail and head of pancreas (n) consistent with about 50 percent necrosis. Grade D pancreatitis with necrosis, severity index 7. *B,* Ten days later the liquefied necrotic areas in the tail and the head of the pancreas are better delineated (n). Patient underwent surgical drainage of necrotic infected fluid collections with clinical improvement. *C,* One month after surgery, CT reveals large, well-defined, encapsulated fluid collections in the tail and head of the pancreas (c) consistent with pseudocysts.

A

B

C

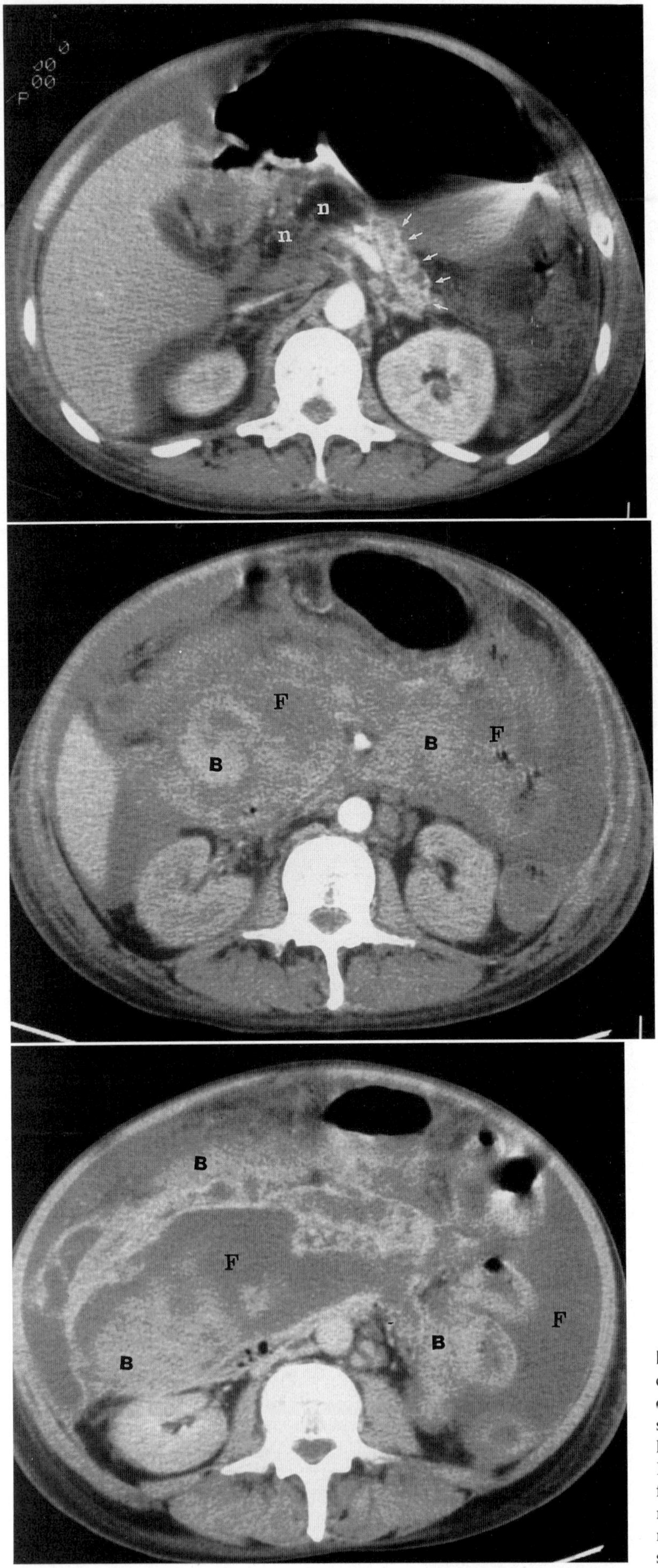


**FIGURE 6** *A*, Pancreatitis with peripancreatic fluid collections and necrosis of the head and part of the body of pancreas (n). Stage E with over 50 percent necrosis, severity index 10. *B* and *C*, Sudden drop in hematocrit level led to emergency follow-up CT 8 days later. Retroperitoneum and peritoneal cavity are filled with fluid (F) containing large areas of high attenuation (B), representing fresh hemorrhage and blood clots. Surgery revealed extensive retroperitoneal bleeding that subsided to surgical packing.

seen on CT scans, emergency angiography is recommended. Angiography may be a life-saving procedure, because therapeutic arterial embolization of the bleeding artery may be performed at the same time.

## CT Staging

Staging of acute pancreatitis was initially performed based on a variety of clinical and laboratory parameters. Among them, the statistical analysis of multiple risk factors (see Table 1) has been more commonly used in the last decade. The reported mortality associated with 0 to 2 prognostic signs is less than 1 percent, 3 to 4 signs is 16 percent, 5 to 6 signs is 40 percent, and 7 signs or over is approaching 100 percent. It should be emphasized, however, that these prognostic indicators have no diagnostic value and should be applied only in patients with proven acute pancreatitis. Further, the risk factors (see Table 1) adequately reflect systemic abnormalities related to cardiovascular, renal, pulmonary, and liver failure. The correlation with the extent and degree of local retroperitoneal involvement is more limited. I have observed patients with extensive pancreatic disease, including pancreatic abscesses, with only 1 to 3 grave signs. For these reasons, CT evaluation must be performed early (within the first 48 hours) to confirm the suspected clinical diagnosis and to assess the degree and severity of local disease.

The CT staging is accomplished by (1) estimating the presence and degree of pancreatic and peripancreatic inflammation, phlegmon, and fluid accumulation and (2) evaluating for the presence and extent of pancreatic necrosis via bolus contrast CT.

Our original grading system, which can be performed without a rapid bolus injection, divides patients with pancreatitis into five distinct groups: grade A, normal (see Fig. 1); grade B, focal or diffuse enlargement of the gland; grade C, pancreatic abnormalities associated with haziness and streaky densities in the peripancreatic fat (see Fig. 2); grade D, single phlegmonous collection (see Fig. 3); and grade E, two or more phlegmonous collections and/or the presence of gas in or adjacent to the pancreas.

Pancreatic necrosis, detected by the appearance of the gland during a contrast-enhanced bolus injection, is used to categorize patients into four groups: normal parenchymal gland enhancement (see Figs. 1, 2, 3), and lack of enhancement of about one-third, one-half (see Fig. 5), or greater than one-half of the gland (see Fig. 6).

In our experience, all deaths and most complications occur in patients with peripancreatic phlegmons and fluid collections (grades D and E) and in patients with pancreatic necrosis. The correlation between CT grading, mortality, and local morbidity (abscess and pseudocyst formation) is presented in Figure 7. In half of the patients initially diagnosed of having phlegmons (grades D and E), the collections resolve spontaneously. In the other half they persist, liquefy, partially encapsulate and eventually develop into abscesses or pseudocysts. Which half resolves spontaneously and which half develops complications cannot be predicted. This limitation has initiated clinical investigations focusing on the potential prognostic contribution of pancreatic necrosis to the original grading system.

A good correlation between lack of pancreatic enhancement (bolus CT) and the presence and degree of pancreatic necrosis has been documented at surgery and experimentally. CT has shown an overall sensitivity of 77 to 85 percent in detecting pancreatic necrosis, with 100 percent sensitivity for detecting extended areas of necrosis (see Figs. 5, 6), and 50 percent sensitivity if only minor necrotic areas are developing. An excellent correlation between pancreatic necrosis (lack of enhancement on CT), length of hospitalization, development of complications, and death has been documented (Fig. 8). Although patients without necrosis had no mortality and only a 6 percent complication rate, patients with CT evidence of necrosis exhibited a 23 percent mortality and 82 percent morbidity (see Fig. 8). Further, the degree of necrosis has a major prognostic significance. Patients with mild necrosis exhibit no mortality and 40 percent morbidity, whereas large areas of necrosis are associated with 75 to 100 percent morbidity and 11 to 25 percent mortality. There is no significant statistical difference in prognostic value among patients with 50 percent and those with more than 50 percent necrosis. The combined morbidity in patients with more than 30 percent necrosis is 94 percent, and the mortality is 29 percent.

Although most patients with pancreatic necrosis exhibit CT signs of necrosis at the initial CT evaluation (24 to 48 hours),

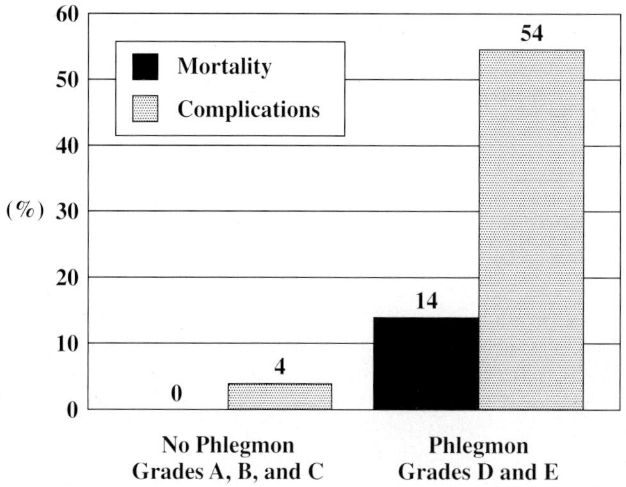


**FIGURE 7** CT grading versus morbidity and mortality in 88 patients with acute pancreatitis.

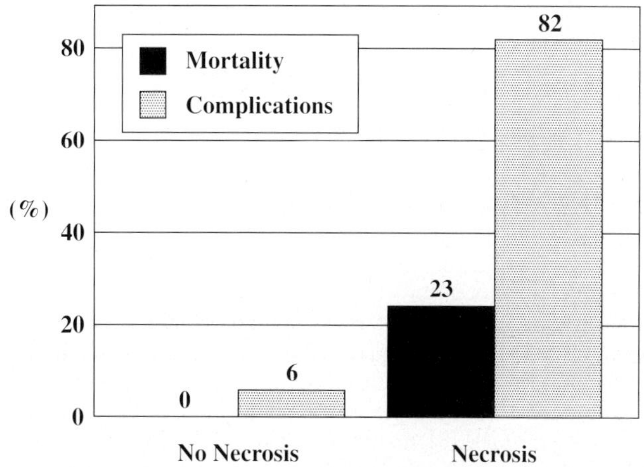


**FIGURE 8** Early- and late-onset necrosis versus morbidity and mortality in 88 patients with acute pancreatitis.

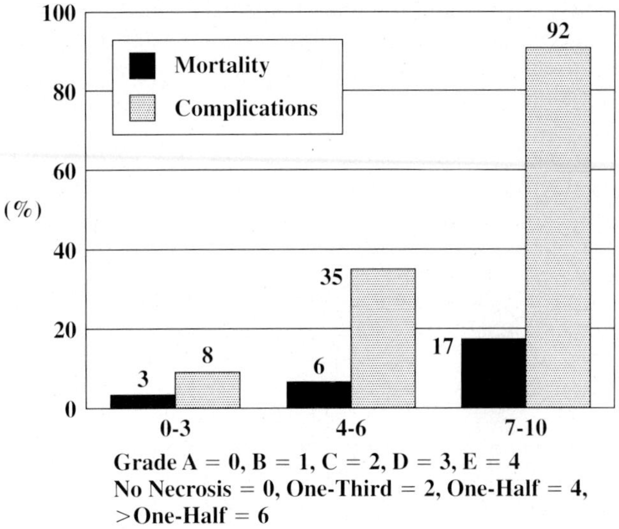


**FIGURE 9** CT severity index versus morbidity and mortality in 88 patients with acute pancreatitis: grade A = 0 points, grade B = 1 point, grade C = 2 points, grade D = 3 points, and grade E = 4 points. No necrosis = 0 points, one-third necrosis = 2 points, 50 percent necrosis = 4 points, and over 50 percent necrosis = 6 points.

a few patients develop necrosis later, during the first 2 weeks of hospitalization. This curious phenomenon represents a minor but definite limiting factor for using necrosis alone as a prognostic indicator at the initial CT evaluation. I have seen this phenomenon occurring in only four patients and only in individuals in whom the initial CT evaluation detected peripancreatic inflammation, phlegmons, and/or fluid collections. For this reason, follow-up CT evaluations should be performed in patients with grades D or E pancreatitis at about 2 weeks or earlier if the clinical presentation deteriorates.

CT severity index is an attempt to improve the early prognostic value of CT in acute pancreatitis by combining in a single grading system the two previously mentioned prognostic indicators (Fig. 9). Grade A to E patients have been assigned 0 to 4 points plus 2 points for 30 percent, 4 points for 50 percent, and 6 points for more than 50 percent necrosis. A severity index grading into three categories, 0 to 3, 4 to 6, and 7 to 10 points, more accurately reflects the prognostic value of CT as judged by the initial CT evaluation (see Fig. 9). Patients with a severity index of 0 or 1 exhibit 0 percent mortality and 0 percent morbidity, whereas patients with a severity index of 2 had no mortality and only 4 percent morbidity. In contrast, a severity index of 7 to 10 yielded 17 percent mortality and 92 percent morbidity.

## Discussion

Over the past decade, CT has become the primary and most important imaging modality in evaluating patients with acute pancreatitis. CT has a high sensitivity and specificity in diagnosing forms of moderate and severe pancreatitis, as well as in detecting serious complications often clinically unsuspected. In addition, CT plays a prominent role as an early predictive indicator of disease severity. Patients with pancreatic phlegmonous collections, and particularly those with pancreatic necrosis, are at high risk for developing local complications. CT evaluation should be performed early, and barring medical contraindications, it should be done by employing the high-resolution technique.

## Suggested Reading

Balthazar EJ, Ranson JHC, Naidich DP, et al. Acute pancreatitis: Prognostic value of CT. Radiology 1985; 156:767–772.

Balthazar EJ, Robinson DL, Megibow AJ, et al. Acute pancreatitis: Value of CT in establishing prognosis. Radiology 1990; 174:331–336.

Beger HG, Maier W, Block S, et al. How do imaging methods influence the surgical strategy in acute pancreatitis? In: Malfertheiner P, Ditschuneit H, eds. Diagnostic procedures in pancreatic disease. Berlin: Springer-Verlag, 1986:54.

Clavien PA, Hauser H, Meyer P, et al. Value of contrast-enhanced computerized tomography in the early diagnosis and prognosis of acute pancreatitis: A prospective study of 202 patients. Am J Surg 1988; 155:457–466.

Kivisaari L, Kalevi S, Standertskjold-Nordenstam CG, et al. A new method for the diagnosis of acute hemorrhagic-necrotizing pancreatitis using contrast-enhanced CT. Gastrointest Radiol 1984; 9:27–30.

Ranson JHC. Etiological and prognostic factors in human acute pancreatitis: A review. Am J Gastroenterol 1982; 77:633–638.

Ranson JHC, Pasternak BS. Statistical methods for qualifying the severity of clinical acute pancreatitis. J Surg Res 1977; 22:79–91.

# Ultrasound Imaging of Rectal and Perirectal Abnormalities

*ROBERT L. BREE, M.D.*

Endorectal sonography of the rectum and perirectal space is emerging as an important diagnostic and staging modality in the evaluation of rectal neoplasms and rectal and perirectal inflammatory processes. In addition, a transrectal approach can be used to evaluate extrarectal masses that may be palpated through the rectum or documented adjacent to the rectum by other imaging modalities such as computed tomography (CT). With the considerable experience obtained from transrectal evaluation of the prostate and its accompanying biopsy techniques, transrectal interventional procedures outside of the prostate gland are also included in this discussion.

The bulk of literature on endorectal sonography centers on rectal cancer and the ability of sonography to accurately stage this disease. Most of the literature is confined to the gastroenterology and surgical journals, but a few articles have appeared in the radiology literature. Acceptance of the validity of the technique depends on the significance of the findings and the confidence that the results can be used to alter therapeutic protocols. Alternative methods to evaluate the rectum and perirectal regions include barium enema studies, CT, magnetic resonance imaging (MRI) using surface coils and MRI using endorectal coils. The availability of the endorectal coil challenges the accuracy of sonography, but the differential diagnostic criteria may be similar, particularly when attempting to separate neoplasm from inflammation in invasive carcinoma. This subject is discussed in depth in a later section.

## Techniques of Endorectal Sonography

Generally patients who are candidates for this evaluation need no preparation other than a single disposable enema. This can be self-administered before or after arrival in the department. The level of discomfort is minimal, and the procedure usually takes less than 30 minutes. Occasionally patients with large carcinomas may experience significant pain and may need mild sedation.

Equipment most commonly used for endorectal sonography are probes that can also perform evaluations of the prostate. These include mechanical sector scanners, which rotate 360° in a straight axial plane, mechanical sector scanners, which rotate from an end-fire position 90° to 120° for sagittal or coronal imaging, and phased array probes, which may have the sound beam emanating from the end or side of the probe for both coronal or sagittal imaging. Additionally, a system is available that is coupled with an endoscope such that the lesion can be visualized endoscopically along with the sonography evaluation. This is most useful in high rectal lesions or in performing colonoscopic evaluations accompanied with sonography. This system uses a 360° radial scanner. Minimum frequencies of 5 MHz are necessary to adequately examine the detailed anatomy of the rectum.

The patient is usually examined in a left decubitus position, and the probe is placed into the rectum after adequate lubrication. The probe is always covered with a condom and often requires placement of a water path between the probe and the sheath. This can be accomplished using the hardware that is available with the probe. The sheath should be discarded between uses and the probe carefully sterilized with an antimicrobial agent, typically glutaraldehyde, for at least 10 to 15 minutes between patients. Additionally, the tubing used to place the water in the water path should be discarded between patients, since there is potential for contamination of this fluid if the sheath does not remain intact. Alternatively, water may be instilled into the rectum and the probe placed into the water-filled rectum such that a water path is not necessary. This has been advocated by some as a more natural way to visualize the anatomy, since the pressure of the water-filled sheath on the lesion can cause distortion. In my experience this has not been a problem in diagnosis. Attention should be paid to the potential for latex allergy and, if possible, condoms made out of another material should be preferentially used.

The evaluation should be accompanied by a digital examination of the rectum. Endorectal sonography is not useful as a screening technique, but is most used to evaluate a known abnormality. Following identification of a lesion, images can be obtained in axial, coronal, or sagittal planes. This imaging can be recorded on videotape as well as hard copy using a multiimage camera. It is usually wise to magnify the image such that fine detail can be observed.

## Normal Anatomy

The gastrointestinal tract has a fairly uniform anatomic appearance from the esophagus through the rectum. There are typically five layers that can be seen with standard ultrasound probes. With very high frequency, seven to eight layers can be seen. These five layers are as follows, beginning at the rectal surface:

1. *Inner echogenic layer*—interface between probe cover and mucosa
2. *Inner echolucent layer*—mucosa and muscularis mucosae
3. *Echogenic*—submucosa
4. *Outer echolucent*—muscularis propria
5. *Outer echogenic*—perirectal fat

A transverse 360° radial image of this normal anatomy is illustrated in Figure 1. Note that with the water balloon, one can define the anatomic layers, despite the degree of distention. Unfortunately, except for using the prostate and seminal

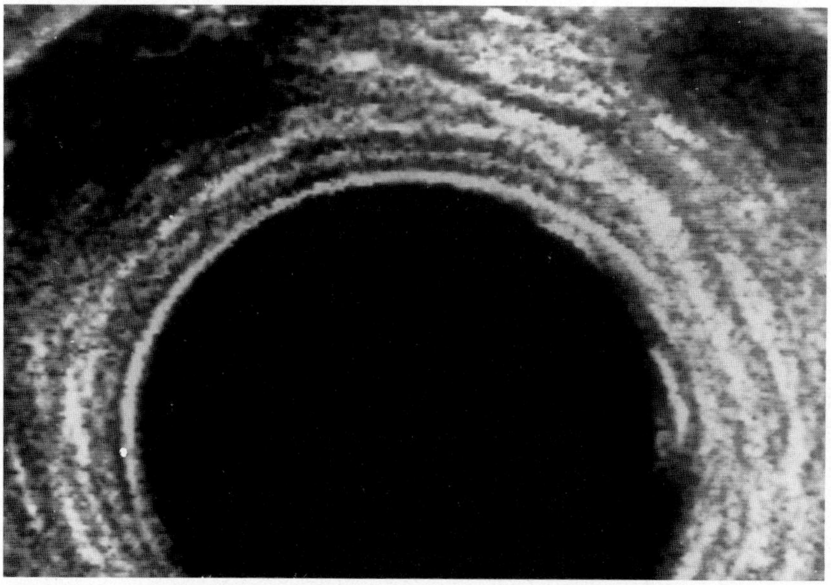

**FIGURE 1** Normal rectal sonography. Three hundred sixty degree radial scan of the rectal wall. The anechoic center is the water-filled balloon. The five layers are well demarcated as outlined in the text.

vesicles or the uterus and ovaries as landmarks, exact location of the anatomic structures is difficult to define with this imaging technique. It is useful to label the images relative to each other to better define the location within the rectum.

## Sonography in the Evaluation and Staging of Rectal Neoplasms

Colorectal carcinoma represents a significant health problem in the United States and around the world. Typically these cancers are found incidentally and late in their course, and only a small percentage are found by various screening techniques, the most popular being detection of occult fecal blood. It has been common practice that preoperative staging of colorectal carcinoma be limited to cursory evaluation of liver function studies and general health status, without significant preoperative staging procedures. More recently, CT has been used for local staging and detection of metastases; however, local staging is not highly successful with CT. Recently MRI has also been used, but this is expensive, time-consuming, and may not be cost-effective on a widespread basis. In the rectum, sonography has gained favor as a staging technique. The general indications for staging rectal carcinoma with sonography are (1) to help assess the depth of local invasion in sphincter-preserving local excision, (2) to evaluate the extent of tumor for low rectal anastomosis, and (3) to evaluate for the necessity of preoperative radiation.

There are two major staging systems for colorectal cancer. Dukes' classification listed in Table 1 evaluates local extension as well as lymph nodes. The International Union Against Cancer TNM classification may be a more appropriate technique to correlate with endorectal sonography, since it relates more to the features identifiable on the sonography evaluation and separately assess lymph nodes. This classification is listed in Table 2.

Based on the TNM classification, management of rectal carcinoma using sonography criteria can be altered using local excision surgical techniques, sonography, and preoperative radiation as outlined in Table 3.

**TABLE 1** Dukes' Staging of Colorectal Cancer

| Stage | Penetration | Lymph Nodes |
|---|---|---|
| A0 | Mucosa only | − |
| A1 | Submucosa | − |
| B1 | Into muscularis propria | − |
| B2 | Through muscularis propria into fat | − |
| B3 | Involves adjacent structure | − |
| C1 | Into muscularis propria | + |
| C2 | Through muscularis propria into fat | + |
| C3 | Involves adjacent structure | + |
| D | Distant metastasis | +/− |

**TABLE 2** TNM Staging of Colorectal Cancer

| | |
|---|---|
| T1 | Tumor in mucosa or submucosa |
| T2 | Tumor confined to rectal wall |
| T3 | Tumor penetrating perirectal fat |
| T4 | Tumor involving surrounding organs |
| N0 | No tumor in lymph nodes |
| N1 | Metastatic carcinoma in 1–3 perirectal lymph nodes |
| N2 | Metastatic carcinoma in more than 3 perirectal lymph nodes |

**TABLE 3** Sonography Criteria for Management of Rectal Carcinoma

| Stage | Treatment |
|---|---|
| T1 N0 | Local excision |
| T2 N0 | Abdominoperineal resection (APR) |
| T2 N1 or T3 N0 | APR<br>Preoperative radiation sometimes used |
| T3 N1 | Preoperative radiation often followed by APR |
| T4 N0 or T4 N1 | Preoperative radiation sometimes followed by APR |

### *Sonography Criteria for Staging Rectal Cancer*

The depth of invasion of rectal cancer can be accurately assessed with transrectal sonography. A tumor that is located in the mucosa or submucosa is classified as T1 (Fig. 2). In this

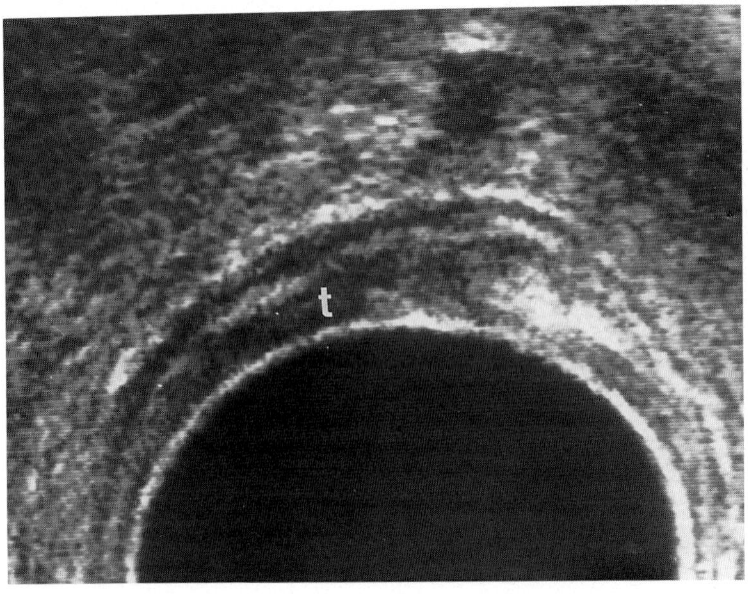


**FIGURE 2** T1 (mucosal) carcinoma. A superficial carcinoma was palpated. Scan demonstrates thickening of the mucosa, which is replaced by neoplasm (t). The echogenic line representing the submucosa is intact.

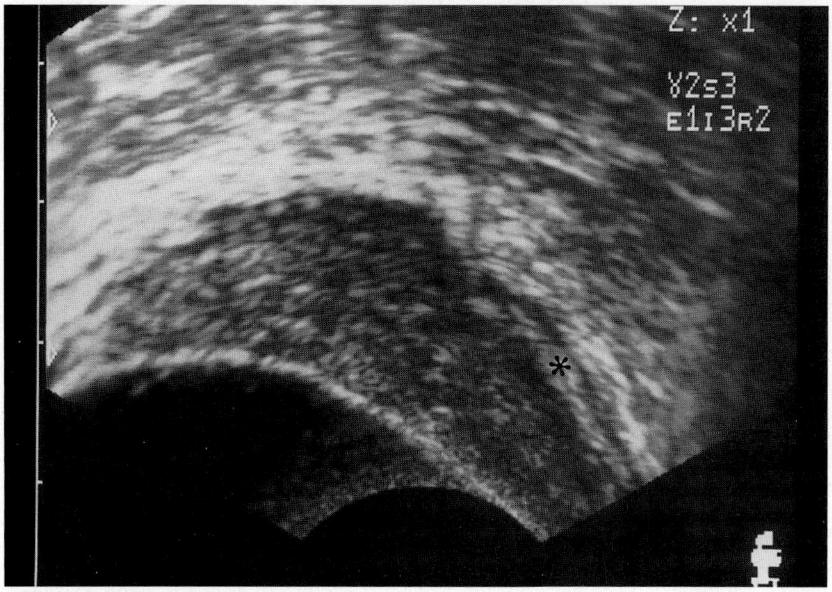


**FIGURE 3** T2 cancer. A neoplasm is identified and is evaluated with an end-fire probe in the sagittal plane. The neoplasm extends through the submucosal layer (*). The muscularis propria layer is involved, but the border between the neoplasm and the perirectal fat is smooth, indicating that the tumor is confined to the muscularis propria.

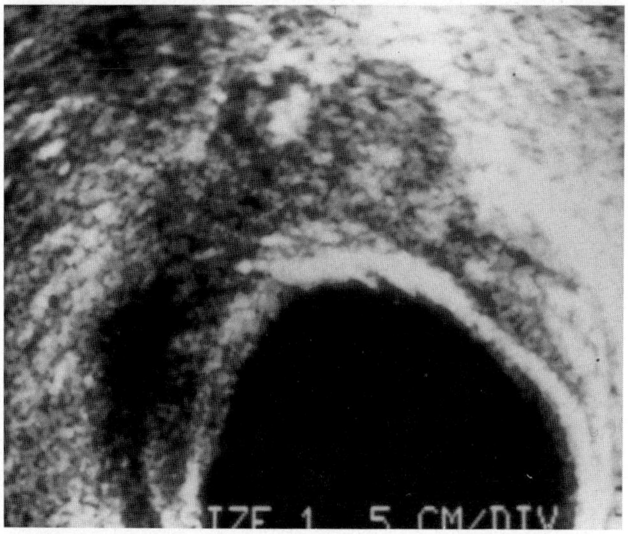

**FIGURE 4** T3 carcinoma. A large tumor encompasses much of the anterolateral aspect of the rectum. There is lobulation and irregular margin between the inner extent of the tumor and the perirectal fat. This tumor invaded extensively into perirectal fat. The normal layers are not identified.

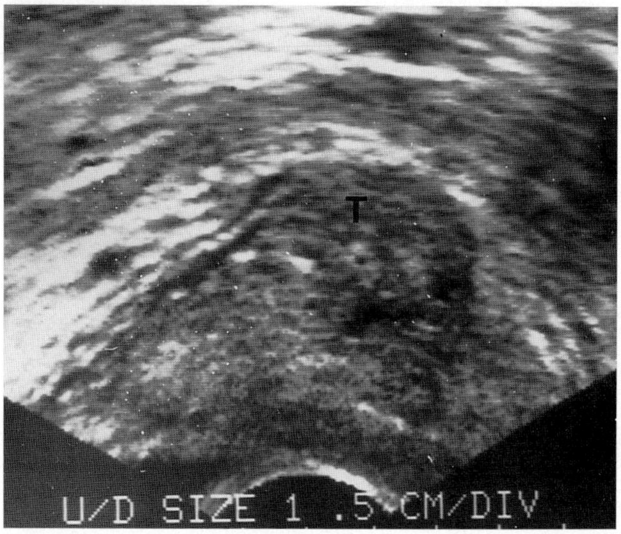


**FIGURE 5** T3 carcinoma with fixation on sagittal image. The sagittal scan performed for tumor evaluation and identification of fixation demonstrates obliteration of the submucosal line and extension of the tumor (T) through the muscularis propria layer. The exact depth of invasion was difficult to assess with standard imaging, but with pressure techniques, the mass was fixed, indicating invasion through the muscularis propria. This was confirmed at surgery.

case the muscularis propria layer is intact. The submucosal hyperechoic layer should also be present, although it could be thin if tumor is within this histologic layer. If the discrete echogenic line of the submucosal layer is interrupted, a T2 lesion is likely (Fig. 3). Irregular borders suggest invasion into the perirectal fat and a T3 carcinoma (Fig. 4).

When assessing tumor invasion, imaging in the parasagittal plane allows evaluation of movement of the layers of the rectum and the degree of fixation of the tumor into the perirectal fat. This can be elicited by a gentle pressure on the mass and evaluating the ability of the layers to move relative to one another. The T3 lesion illustrated in Figure 5 demonstrates invasion through the muscularis propria, and during real-time scanning, this relationship was fixed.

The accuracy of staging of rectal carcinoma has been evaluated in several series in the literature. In general, the ability to identify a T1 lesion has been excellent, with accuracy of 80 to 90 percent. This has been our experience as well, and local excision techniques typically are performed on these patients. Since the rectum is not removed, absolute histologic proof of deeper invasion cannot always be obtained, and it is only if the tumor recurs that inaccuracy can be proven. The ability to separate T2 lesions from T3 lesions is less important for surgical planning, since both of these levels of invasion require rectal excision, typically with abdominoperineal resection (APR). The information, however, could be used to separate patients into those with high versus low probability of cure such that a surgeon could perform a palliative sphincter-

A 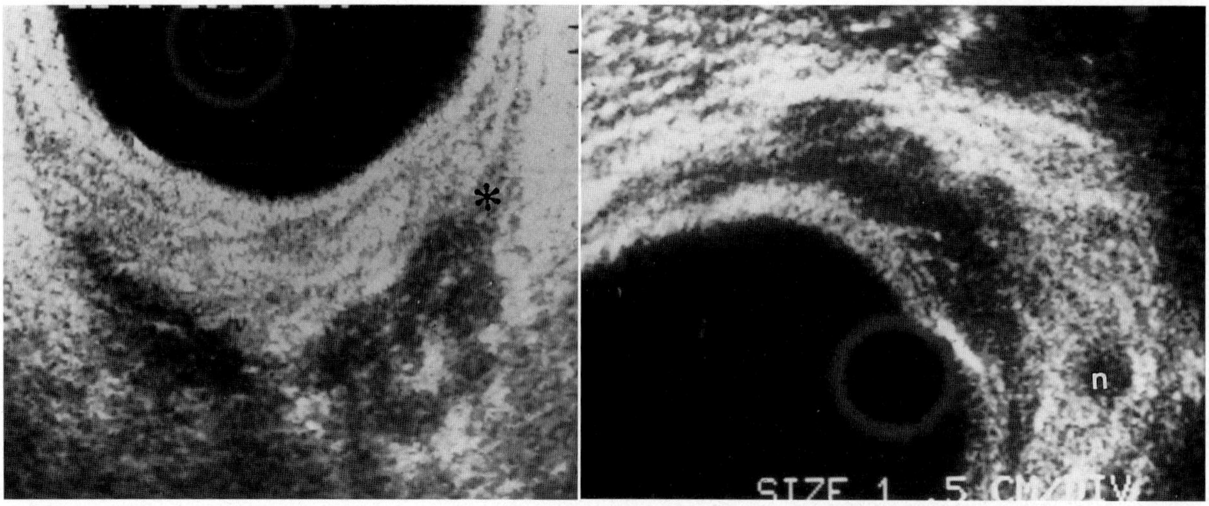 B


**FIGURE 6** False-positive sonography evaluations. *A,* Perirectal inflammation. A large neoplasm was palpated and the examination demonstrated hypoechoic mass effect extending beyond the muscularis propria layer (*). At surgery, this tumor did not invade through the muscularis propria but there was extensive perirectal inflammation causing the ultrasonographic abnormality. *B,* Thick muscle and false-positive lymph node. This neoplasm appears to extend beyond the muscularis propria with irregular nodular invasion into the perirectal fat. At surgery, the muscularis propria was markedly thickened and nodular but the tumor did not extend into the perirectal fat. A 7 mm lymph node (n) was rounded and hypoechoic suggesting metastatic disease. At surgery no abnormal lymph nodes were identified.

sparing procedure on a patient with a T3 lesion, whereas it would be more appropriate to perform a radical curative procedure on a patient with a T2 lesion. The accuracy for determining invasion into the perirectal fat suffers from the inability of sonography to separate invasion into fat from perirectal inflammation, a common phenomenon accompanying rectal cancer. The generally accepted sensitivity for sonography in evaluating fat invasion is over 90 percent, but the specificity may be as low as 50 percent. Some series have higher percentages of T3 lesions, leading to higher specificity as a result of the decreased number of false-positive evaluations.

## False-Positive Invasive Tumors

In our experience, as well as in the literature, a number of false-positive invasive cancers have been recognized. Generally these have been thought to be secondary to perirectal inflammation. We have also seen marked thickening of the muscularis propria layer, without significant inflammation, which has also been sonographically suggestive of perirectal neoplasm (Fig. 6).

## Lymph Node Assessment

Criteria that have been used to evaluate lymph nodes include size, shape, and echogenicity. High-resolution transrectal sonography is able to identify small lymph nodes in a large number of patients. Sonography is not able to identify all of the possible lymph nodes that can be seen by the pathologist. Lymph nodes smaller than 4 mm have a low probability of containing metastatic carcinoma. Lymph nodes that are hyperechoic are more typically inflammatory, and hypoechoic nodes suggest carcinoma. Lymph nodes that maintain their oval shape are more likely to be benign. Those that are rounded strongly suggest neoplasm. If a thorough evaluation of the entire rectum fails to reveal an enlarged lymph node in a patient with known rectal cancer, the incidence of lymph node involvement is extremely small. When nodes are identified, there can be overlap between inflammatory and neoplastic nodes (Fig. 6*B,* 7).

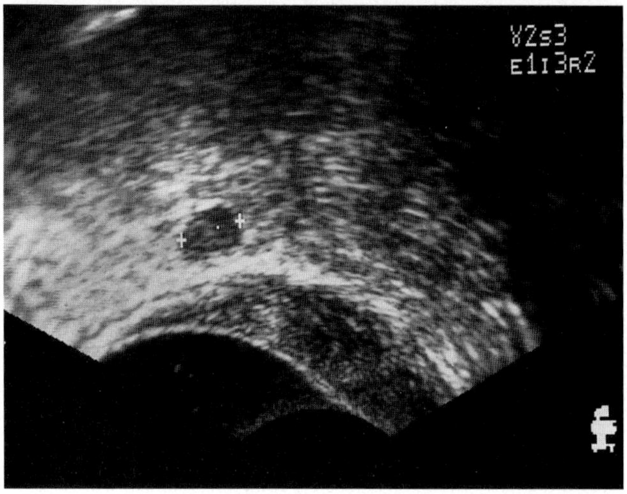

**FIGURE 7** T3 carcinoma with positive lymph node. A rectal carcinoma extends through the muscularis propria layer. A large lymph node (between cursor marks) has lost its oval shape and is hypoechoic. At surgery, metastatic lymphadenopathy was present.

## Evaluation with Other Imaging Modalities

CT and MRI have been used for evaluation of local spread of rectal cancer as well as metastatic disease. Accuracy for local invasion with CT is less than that with sonography because of the lower resolution of CT. Evaluation of the rectal wall with endorectal MRI shows some promise in separating perirectal inflammation from neoplasm, but this conclusion is based on preliminary results. General availability, as well as the expense, may not prove to be cost-effective in the evaluation of rectal

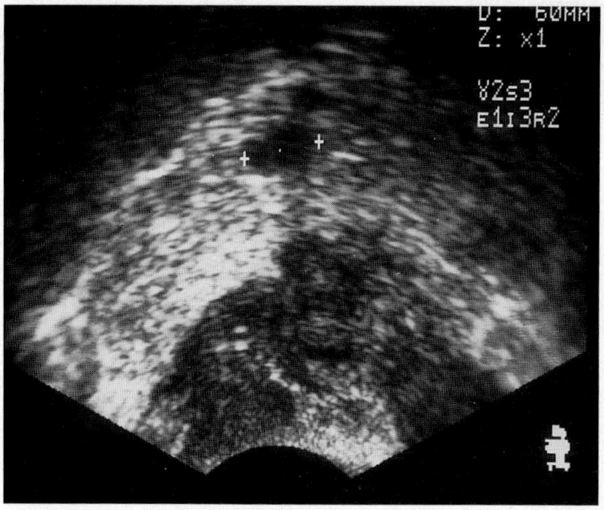


**FIGURE 8** Large deeply invasive T3 cancer with positive lymph node. This patient underwent radiation therapy before definitive surgery. The tumor did not respond significantly to radiation. Lymph node measuring 1 cm (between cursor marks) is hypoechoic but oval. Positive nodes were present at surgery.

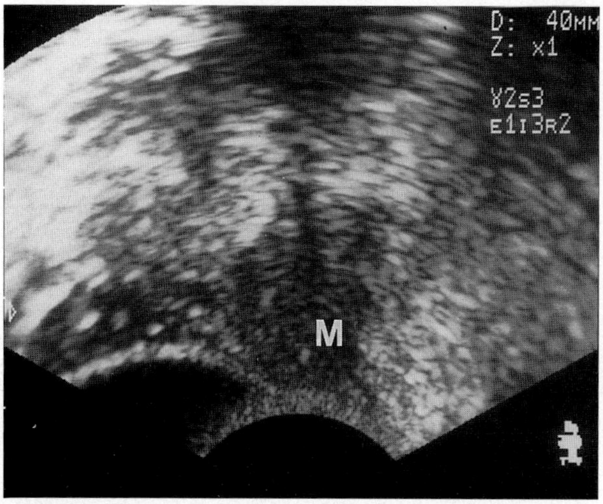


**FIGURE 9** Recurrent rectal cancer. A mass (M) is identified in a submucosal location near the anastomosis following resection of rectal carcinoma. Tumor recurrence was suggested and biopsy proven. Radiation therapy to this area was successful in significant reduction in tumor bulk. Subsequently, a radical resection was performed.

cancer. Competitive imaging techniques to evaluate the remainder of the abdomen for metastases include abdominal sonography, CT, and MRI. These three imaging modalities all suffer from lower sensitivity because of the inability to resolve small superficial liver lesions. More sophisticated techniques, including CT arterial portography and intraoperative sonography, have a high sensitivity for detecting metastatic lesions to the liver.

### *Evaluation of Success of Radiation Therapy and Detection of Local Recurrence*

Some high-risk patients, because of the size of the tumor or risk of surgery, undergo radiation therapy before or instead of surgery. A useful objective way to follow the success of this

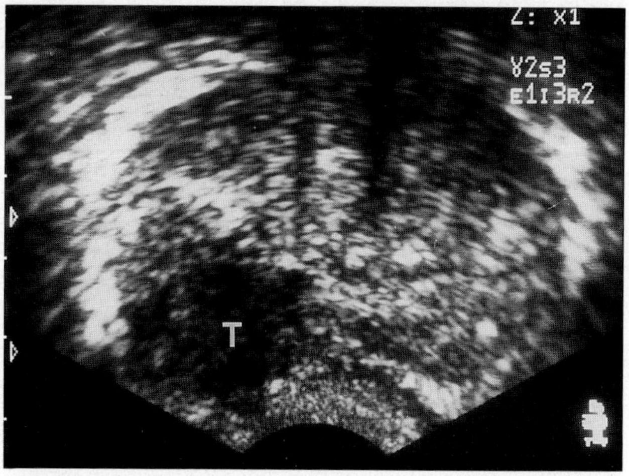


**FIGURE 10** Incidentally discovered prostate cancer in patient with T1 rectal carcinoma. The rectal mass was correctly staged as T1 with sonography. Evaluation of the prostate performed at the time of the endorectal sonography demonstrated a large, otherwise unsuspected, hypoechoic tumor (T) in the right peripheral zone, appearing to penetrate the capsule. This was a clinical stage C prostate cancer and was treated with radiation therapy.

procedure is with endorectal sonography. The patients benefit from palliation to control bleeding and relieve obstruction. Tumor growth or involution is easily assessed (Fig. 8).

Patients who have had sphincter-sparing resections for rectal carcinoma can be assessed with endorectal sonography to search for recurrence. When the recurrence is in the mucosa, identification can be established endoscopically. Occasionally, however, the recurrence is in the wall of the rectum or in an extrarectal site. In this situation sonography can define a mass, although it is unable to differentiate postoperative fibrosis from neoplasm. Follow-up evaluation or biopsy using sonographic guidance can be helpful in this differentiation (Fig. 9).

### *Evaluation of the Prostate in Patients with Rectal Cancer*

In men who have rectal cancer and are candidates for APR, endorectal sonography gives an opportunity to evaluate the prostate. Although prostate sonography is not typically considered a screening procedure, the prostate should not be ignored in these patients. Figure 10 illustrates a patient with a rectal mass and a large prostate lesion that was discovered incidentally during the evaluation of the rectum. The rectal lesion was a T1 villous adenocarcinoma. The prostate cancer was clinically and sonographically stage C and was treated with radiation therapy.

## Rectal and Perirectal Inflammatory Conditions

Infections and abscesses confined to the rectal wall are sometimes difficult to assess by physical examination. Sonography can guide needle aspiration to determine the offending organism. Usually an abscess in the rectal wall does not require drainage, and aspiration followed by appropriate antibiotic coverage is adequate treatment (Fig. 11).

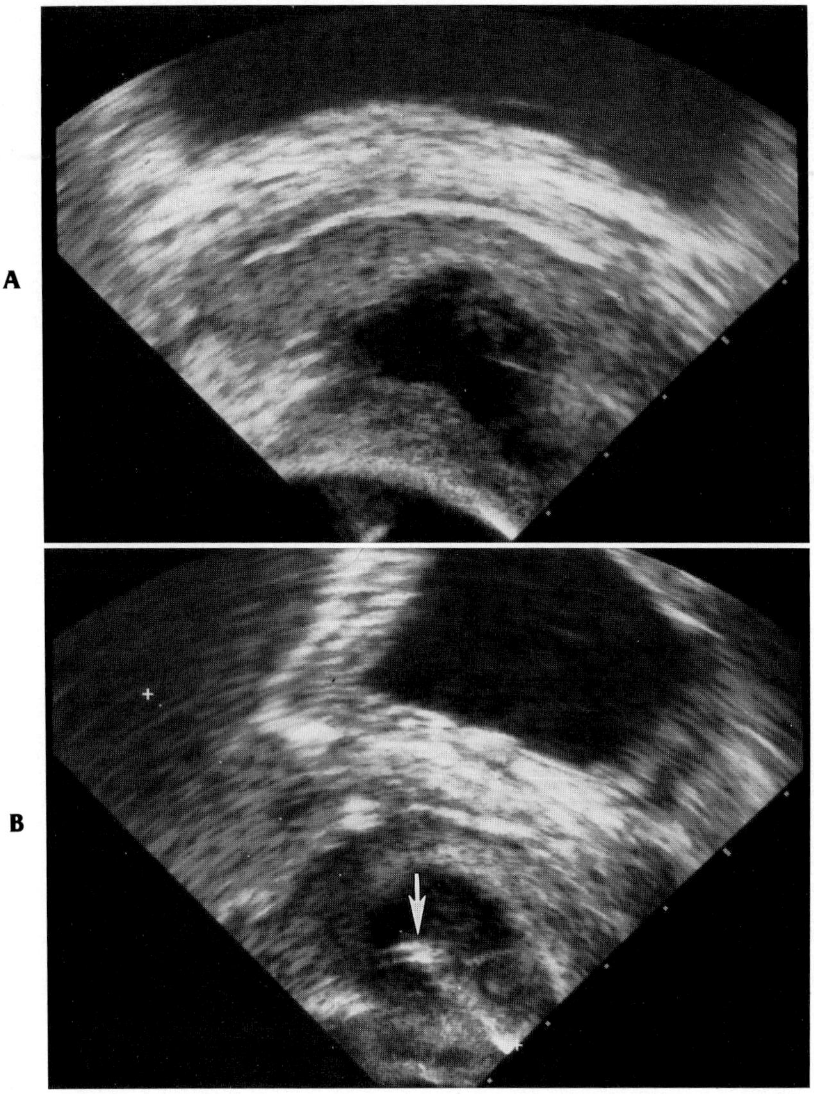


**FIGURE 11** Perirectal abscess. *A,* A thick-walled anechoic mass is located in the rectal wall in a patient with inflammatory bowel disease suspected of having a perirectal abscess. *B,* Image obtained during needle aspiration identifies the needle tip (*arrow*) in the abscess. Purulent material was removed and the abscess completely drained. Appropriate antibiotic coverage was begun.

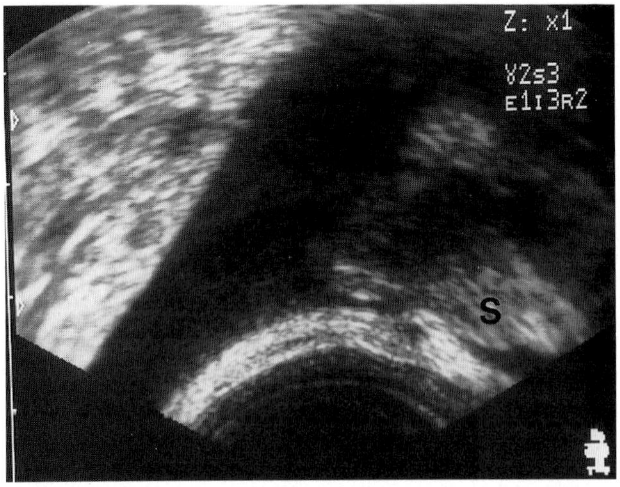


**FIGURE 12** Perirectal free fluid. Endorectal evaluation demonstrates moderate amount of echogenic fluid in the sacral cul-de-sac surrounding the rectum. Small intestinal loops (S) are noted within the fluid. Transrectal needle aspiration yielded purulent material.

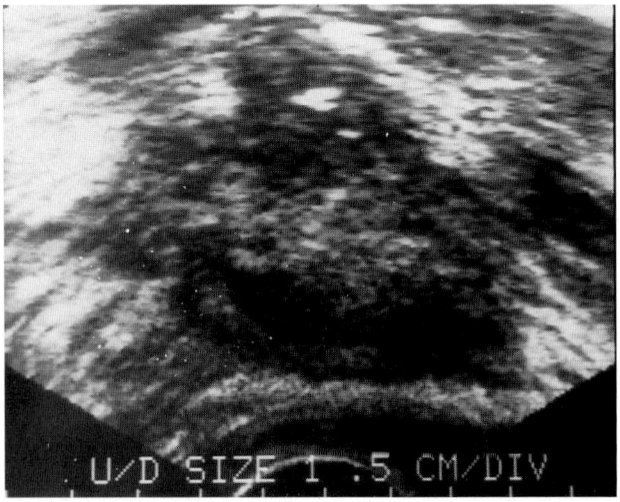


**FIGURE 13** Diverticular abscess. A mixed echogenic, primarily hyperechoic irregular mass is seen in the proximal rectal wall. Needle aspiration yielded inflammatory tissue. A chronic diverticular abscess was removed surgically.

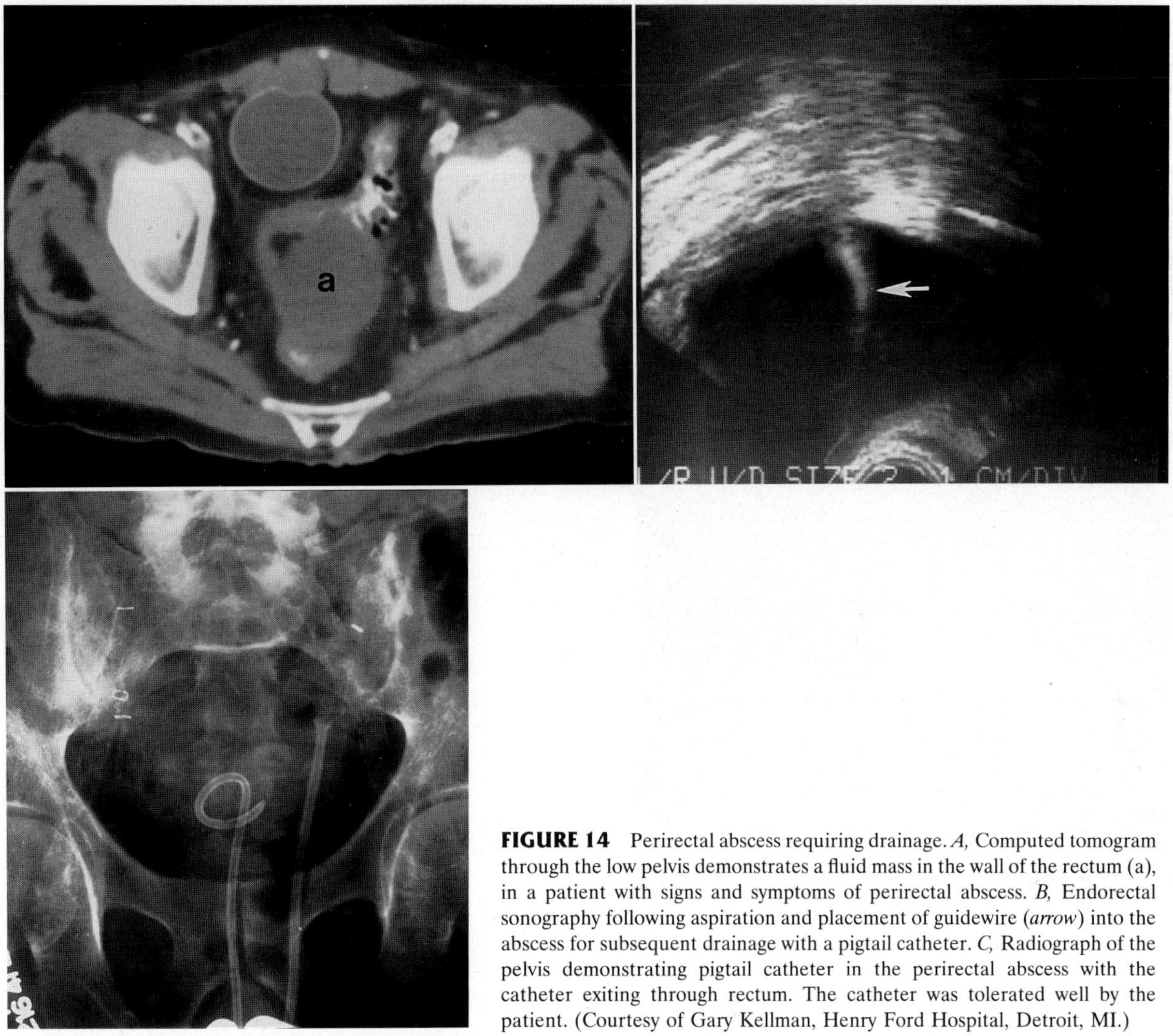


**FIGURE 14** Perirectal abscess requiring drainage. *A,* Computed tomogram through the low pelvis demonstrates a fluid mass in the wall of the rectum (a), in a patient with signs and symptoms of perirectal abscess. *B,* Endorectal sonography following aspiration and placement of guidewire (*arrow*) into the abscess for subsequent drainage with a pigtail catheter. *C,* Radiograph of the pelvis demonstrating pigtail catheter in the perirectal abscess with the catheter exiting through rectum. The catheter was tolerated well by the patient. (Courtesy of Gary Kellman, Henry Ford Hospital, Detroit, MI.)

Perirectal inflammation can consist of phlegmon or abscess in addition to free pus in the peritoneal cavity near the rectum. A transrectal approach to diagnosis and needle aspiration is useful in many of these patients. Etiologies may include diverticulitis, Crohn's disease, peritonitis, or opportunistic organisms in patients with acquired immunodeficiency syndrome (AIDS). The sonographic appearance of inflammation varies with the consistency and location. Free fluid is typically hypoechoic with internal echoes (Fig. 12), but chronic abscesses such as might be observed with diverticulitis can be echogenic and mimic a solid mass. Needle aspiration may be necessary for differentiation (Fig. 13).

Occasionally a perirectal abscess may need to be drained because of its size and location. Using a combination of transrectal sonography and fluoroscopy, a catheter may be inserted through the rectum into the abscess. This technique is preferable over transcutaneous procedures, which require CT guidance and have associated problems with patient acceptance and necessity to traverse the area of the sciatic nerve (Fig. 14).

## Miscellaneous Rectal and Perirectal Masses and Interventions

### *Rectal Adenomas*

Adenomas are typically benign; however, villous adenomas may have severe dysplasia or malignant degeneration. Sonography can help in the assessment of these lesions by evaluating the size, since villous adenomas larger than 2 cm have a 50 percent malignant potential. Using the echo pattern alone, the histologic differentiation can not be made sonographically. Sonography can clearly be used to assess depth of invasion, as well as involvement of lymph nodes as with frankly malignant tumors.

### *Rectal Wall Masses*

The most common rectal wall masses include endometriosis and smooth muscle neoplasms, primarily leiomyoma or leiomyosarcoma. These lesions can be small and difficult to differentiate from one another.

## *Perirectal Masses*

A commonly identified perirectal mass is a teratoma or dermoid cyst, which can be found anywhere in the perirectal soft tissues, particularly posteriorly. These can be palpated clinically and transrectal sonography with subsequent needle aspiration can be used to confirm the diagnosis (Fig. 15). A sacrococcygeal teratoma is a more extensive variant of the perirectal dermoid. Other perirectal masses that have been evaluated with sonography include extensive prostate or seminal vesicle carcinoma, melanoma, pelvic lipomatosis, and chordoma. I have also evaluated a retroperitoneal cystic hamartoma (tail gut cyst) that was found in a perirectal location.

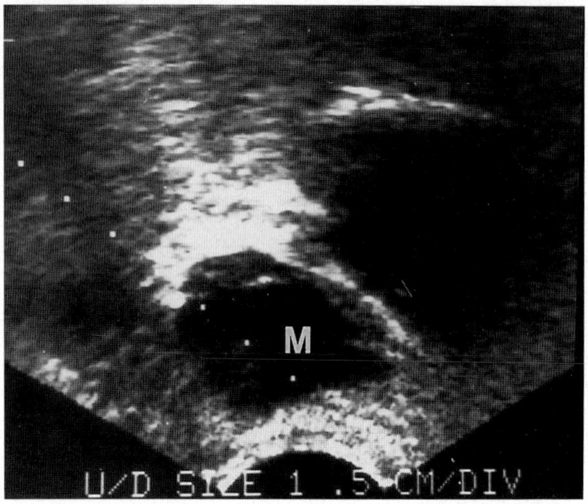


**FIGURE 15** Perirectal dermoid. A mass was palpable through the rectum in the posterior perirectal space. Endorectal sonography demonstrated a hypoechoic mass (M). This was subsequently aspirated with sonographic guidance, and thick sebaceous material was removed consistent with a dermoid.

Occasionally masses that are found on other imaging modalities such as CT or MRI may be situated near the rectum. If a biopsy is deemed necessary, a transrectal approach is safe and effective and typically less painful than a transcutaneous approach. An example of the use of this technique is illustrated in Figure 16.

## Discussion

Endorectal sonography is a new and exciting emerging technique used primarily for the evaluation of rectal cancer. Indications and limitations have been discussed. Overall, the accuracy of the procedure is high when one understands the difficulty in separating invasive carcinoma from inflammation. The use of endorectal sonography to evaluate rectal wall masses and perirectal inflammation and masses continues to grow in popularity. An internal approach to interventions in this area is safer and more comfortable for the patient. With the increasing use of endoluminal probes for endovaginal and prostate procedures, this facet of rectal evaluation should become more popular among radiologists. Additionally, newer equipment is rapidly becoming available to perform endoscopic sonography that can be extended into the colon and rectum for more extensive evaluation of colorectal cancer.

## Suggested Reading

Beynon J, Mortensen NJ McC, Foy DMA, et al. The detection and evaluation of locally recurrent rectal cancer with rectal endosonography. Dis Colon Rectum 1989; 32:509–517.

Hildebrandt U, Feifel G. Endorectal sonography. Surg Annu 1990; 22:169–183.

Holdsworth PJ, Johnston D, Chalmers AG, et al. Endoluminal ultrasound and computed tomography in the staging of rectal cancer. Br J Surg 1988; 75:1019–1022.

Rifkin MD, Ehrlich SM, Marks G. Staging of rectal carcinoma: Prospective comparison of endorectal US and CT. Radiology 1989; 170:319 322.

A

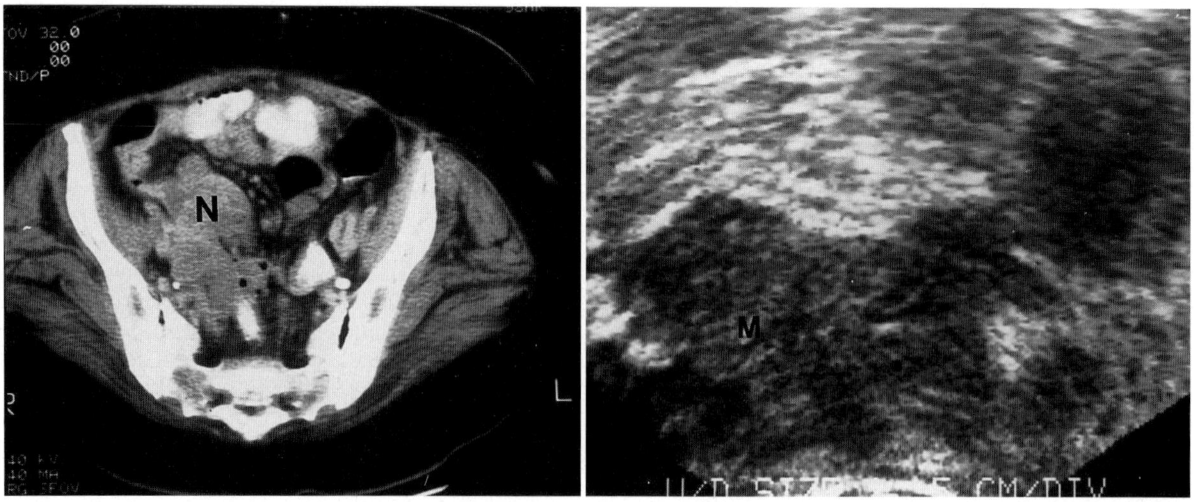


B

**FIGURE 16** Metastatic carcinoma to pelvic lymph nodes with transrectal biopsy. *A*, Transverse computed tomogram in the midpelvis demonstrates extensive adenopathy in the right internal iliac nodal chain (N). Transcutaneous access would require traversing bowel. *B*, Transrectal evaluation demonstrates a lobulated mass (M) corresponding to the mass seen on the CT. Transrectal biopsy with histologic technique yielded metastatic adenocarcinoma.

Rösch T, Lorenz R, Classen M. Endoscopic ultrasonography in the evaluation of colon and rectal disease. Gastrointest Endosc 1990; 36:33–39.

St. Ville EW, Jafri ZH, Madrazo BL, et al. Endorectal sonography in the evaluation of rectal and perirectal disease. AJR 1991; 157:503–508.

Tio TL, Coene PPLO, van Delden OM, Tytgat GNJ. Colorectal carcinoma: Preoperative TNM classification with endosonography. Radiology 1991; 179:165–170.

Wang KY, Kimmey MB, Nyberg DA, et al. Colorectal neoplasms: Accuracy of US in demonstrating the depth of invasion. Radiology 1987; 165:827–829.

Zainea GG, Lee F, McLeary RD, et al. Transrectal ultrasonography in the evaluation of rectal and extrarectal disease. Surg Gynecol Obstet 1989; 169:1553–1556.

# Doppler Sonography in Liver Transplantation: Pre- and Post-transplant Evaluation

*M. LEON SKOLNICK, M.D. · GERALD D. DODD III, M.D.*

Doppler ultrasonography plays a significant role in the management of patients before and after transplant surgery through the assessment of blood flow in the hepatic artery (HA), portal vein (PV), hepatic veins (HVs) and retrohepatic vena cava (VC).

Among the pretransplant group, vessel patency is the key concern. Postoperatively detecting a hemodynamically significant stenosis is as important as detecting a thrombosed vessel.

## Normal Hepatic Vascular Anatomy and Doppler Imaging Techniques

We routinely examine the three HVs (right, middle, left), the retrohepatic VC, the HA, and PV in the portahepatis, first with gray-scale real-time imaging, then with spectral Doppler to record blood velocity profiles. Color Doppler helps us to rapidly locate these vessels for spectral Doppler study, especially when they are of small caliber or have slow flow. Color Doppler is also invaluable to locate focal stenosis (a major concern in the transplant recipient) before more quantitative study with spectral Doppler.

The patient is initially studied in the supine position. However, rotating the patient to the left lateral decubitus position may be helpful. The liver moves below the costal margin and away from the VC, exerting less pressure on it, which is helpful when a large liver compresses the VC in the supine position and makes it difficult to detect VC flow. The portahepatis may also become easier to image as the liver projects further below the rib cage.

### *Hepatic Veins*

All three veins may be imaged in the transverse plane as they drain into the VC. The probe is oriented transversely and placed either subcostal on the anterior abdominal wall or intercostally in the flank and angled cephalad toward the diaphragm. Individual HVs may also be observed in the sagittal or coronal plane as the VC is imaged. Blood normally flows toward the heart and exhibits a triphasic waveform indicative of cyclic variations of intracardiac pressures (Fig. 1).

### *Inferior Vena Cava*

This vessel is best delineated in its long axis, either in the sagittal plane approached with the probe subcostally or in the coronal plane with the probe intercostally along the axillary line. In the proximal VC, close to the right atrium, one normally observes a fluctuating waveform similar to that observed in the hepatic veins (Fig. 2). However, more caudally, the caval waveform is less affected by the heart and has more continuous cephalad flow.

### *Portal Vein and Hepatic Artery*

These vessels lie adjacent to each other in the portahepatis as they enter the liver. The portahepatis is most readily examined in the long axis, either in the coronal plane through intercostal spaces or sagittally via a subcostal approach, the former being favored in small livers. In both, blood flow is toward the liver (hepatopedal) (Figs. 3, 5, 6, *A*, and Color Plate 1). The normal PV Doppler waveform is usually of constant velocity, though it may show mild velocity variations either from respiratory or cardiac cycle variations (Fig. 4). Preliminary imaging with color Doppler provides overall assessment of flow direction and helps the examiner choose optimal locations for spectral Doppler interrogation.

Since the HA may be spiraled around or cross back and forth over the PV, one may observe apparent hepatopedal or hepatofugal flow (flow away from the liver) depending on the orientation of the Doppler beam to the artery (see Fig. 5). However, hepatic arterial flow is always hepatopedal.

If no HA flow is detected in the portahepatis, the presence of flow is sought in the branch vessels. Occasionally flow is present in branch arteries but not in the main HA in the portahepatis because of an anomalous entry of the HA into the liver.

## General Pitfalls of the Doppler Examination

When no Doppler signal is detected in a vessel, even though the vessel is well visualized and echo-free on the real-time

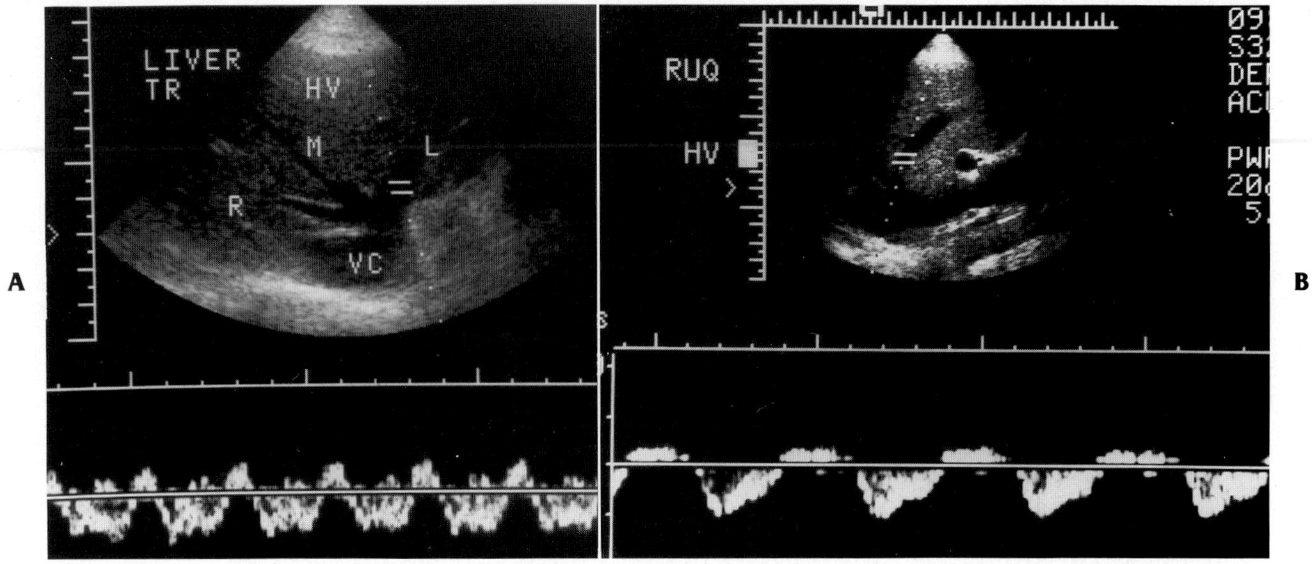


**FIGURE 1** Hepatic veins (normal imaging and spectral Doppler). *A,* Transverse plane. Right (R), middle (M), left (L) veins enter vena cava. Spectral Doppler tracing from left hepatic vein. *B,* Sagittal plane. Single hepatic vein enters vena cava. Doppler velocity profile shows normal variations in direction and velocity of flow reflecting physiologic changes in blood flow during the cardiac cycle.

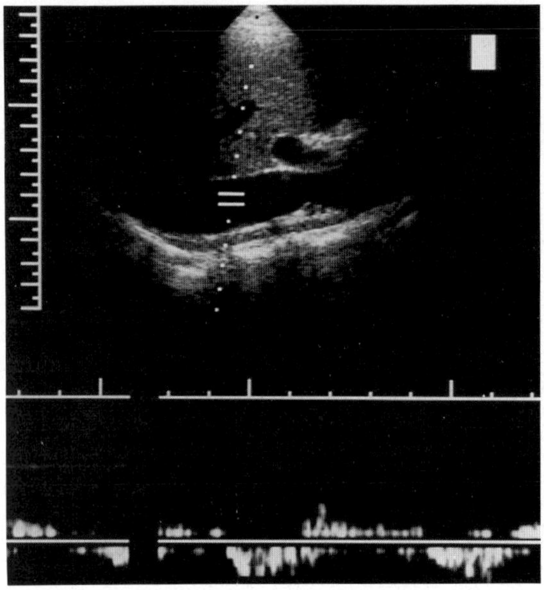

**FIGURE 2** Vena cava. Normal imaging and spectral Doppler. Sagittal view. Intracaval Doppler velocity measurements close to the right atrium show velocity variations similar to those observed in hepatic veins.

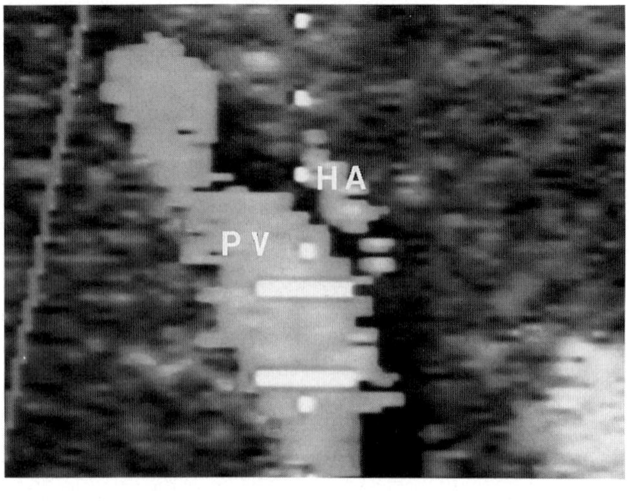


**FIGURE 3** Normal hepatic artery (HA) and portal vein (PV), long-axis view. Flow in both vessels is hepatopedal. See also Color Plate 1.

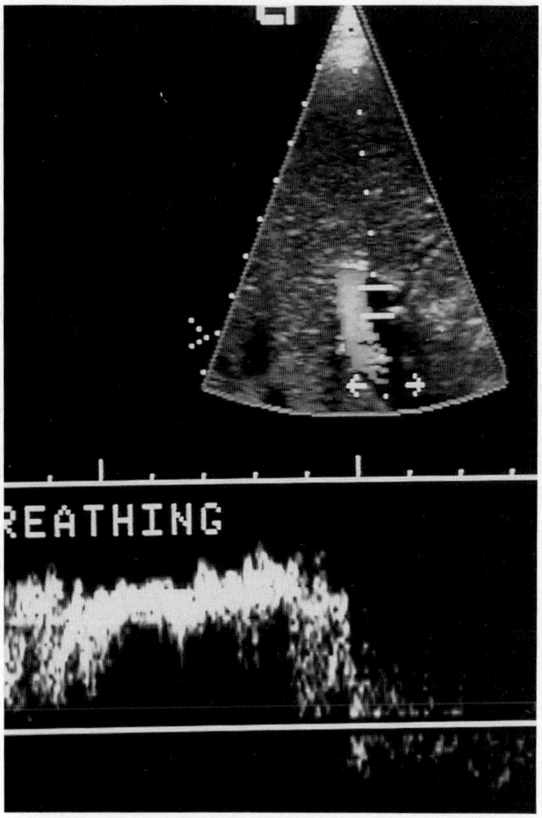


**FIGURE 4** Normal portal vein. Variations in velocity occur secondary to respiratory movements of the liver. Flow velocity is greater in the center than at the margins of a vein. As the portal vein moves across the Doppler gate during breathing, regions of different flow velocity are detected. Increasing the width of the Doppler gate and having the patient suspend respiration minimize such effects.

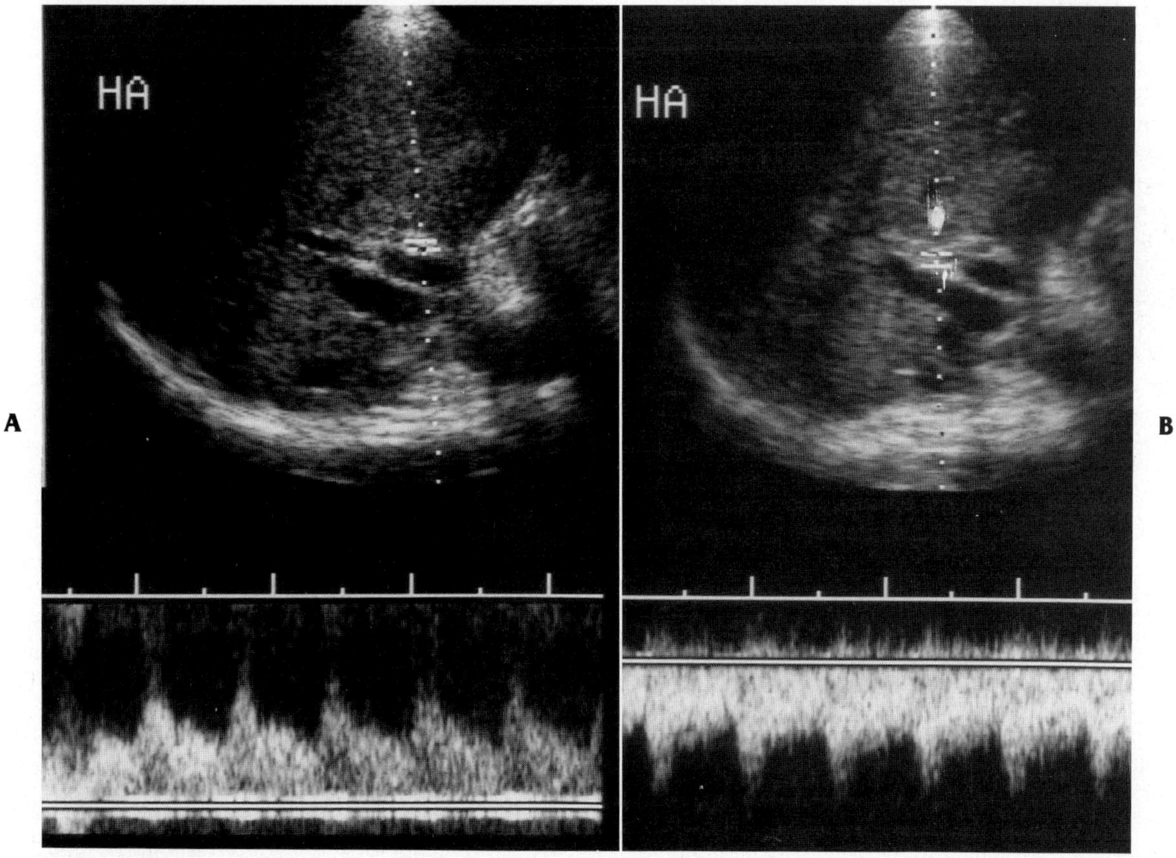


**FIGURE 5** Normal hepatic artery. Although blood flow is always hepatopedal, the hepatic artery may zig-zag around the portal vein. Depending on the orientation of a particular region of the artery to the Doppler beam, direction of flow may be recorded as *(A)* hepatopedal (above the baseline) or *(B)* hepatofugal (below the baseline).

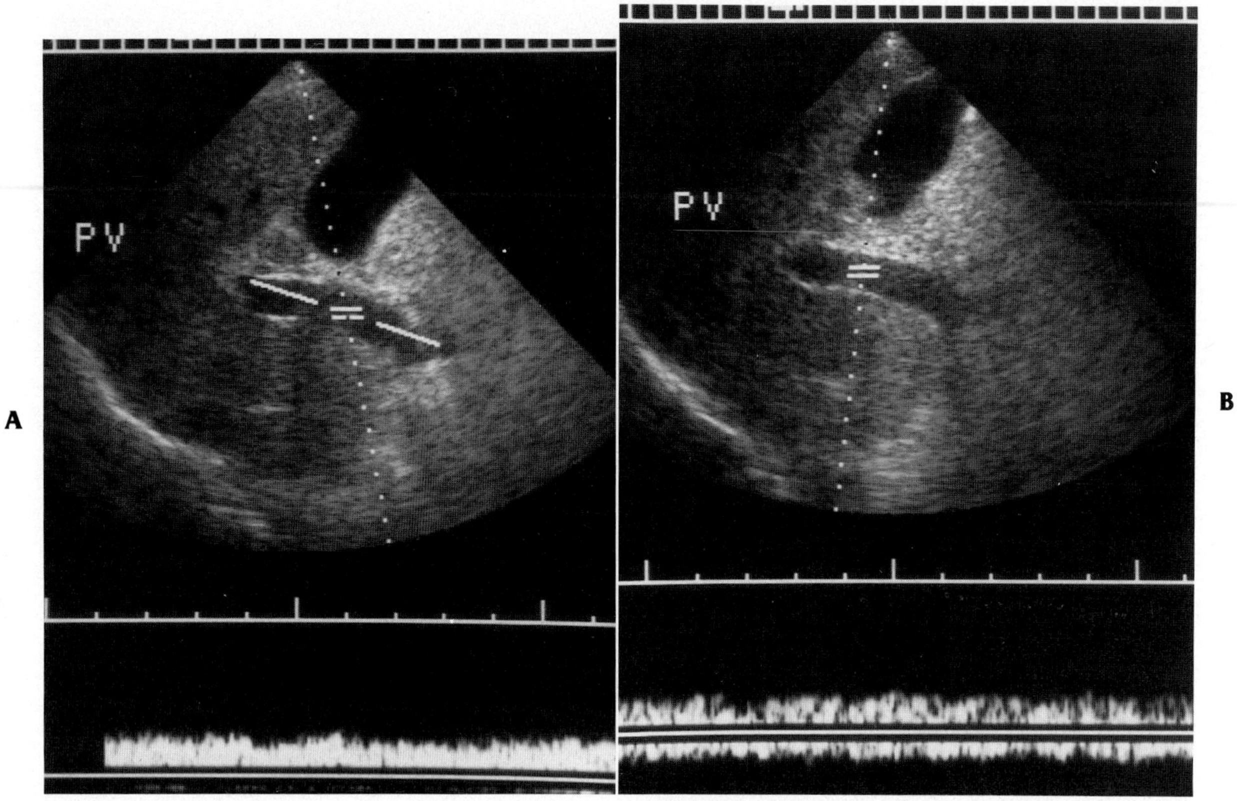


**FIGURE 6** Normal portal vein (sagittal view). *A,* Blood flow is displayed as hepatopedal when the Doppler beam intersects the vein at an angle between 30 and 60°. *B,* Blood flow appears artifactually bidirectional when the Doppler beam is perpendicular to the vein.

imaging study, one must determine if the absence of a Doppler signal is indicative of absence of blood flow or from technical causes.

For a given depth in tissue, gray-scale imaging may be more sensitive than Doppler, and spectral Doppler may be more sensitive than color Doppler. If two similar vessels (vein vs. vein or artery vs. artery) are at the same depth and same orientation as the Doppler beam and blood flow can be detected in one, then the absence of the other Doppler signal in a vessel presumes the absence of flow.

If flow is present in an artery but not in an adjacent vein, then the Doppler sensitivity setting may not be low enough to detect venous flow, the wall filter may be too high (rejecting low-flow Doppler signals), or the angle at which the Doppler beam intersects the vessel may be such that Doppler sensitivity is reduced. Doppler sensitivity and determination of direction of flow is best between 30 and 60°. Sensitivity significantly decreases as 90° is approached. When the Doppler beam is perpendicular to a vessel, no flow or a bidirectional flow pattern may be displayed (see Fig. 6). If the vessel is deep, a lower Doppler frequency may produce greater penetration and thus record flow not detected with a higher-frequency beam.

The Valsalva maneuver, which may occur when a patient is asked to stop breathing, can produce a brief cessation of blood flow in the PV. This effect is more common in patients with severe liver disease in whom hepatopedal portal vein flow is already reduced. Occasionally in the same patient group, the Valsalva maneuver may produce a transitory reversal in PV flow. Re-examining the patient during quiet respiration may more accurately demonstrate the direction of blood flow.

## Vascular Complications of the Native Liver

### *Hepatic Veins*

#### Unidirectional Nonvarying Flow Toward the Heart

As the liver becomes increasingly rigid in cirrhosis, the multiphasic flow pattern observed in normal HVs in compliant liver tissue is damped and becomes unidirectional (Fig. 7).

#### No Flow

Absence of flow indicates HV thrombosis, a part of the Budd-Chiari syndrome (Fig. 8). All three HVs should be examined because occasionally the absence of flow may be limited to one or two veins. Other findings may be caval thrombosis, especially the region adjacent to the entrance of the HVs, and PV thrombosis (no flow), or reversed PV flow. Alternate paths develop for the splanchnic venous flow that can no longer enter the liver via the PV. Thus there is usually reversed flow in the retropancreatic splenic vein connecting with gastric esophageal or splenic varices.

### *Portal Vein*

#### No Flow

Visible thrombus may be observed within the lumen and the vessel may be dilated. In the presence of thrombus one should consider hepatocellular carcinoma invading the PV and look for masses within the liver parenchyma (Fig. 9). Occasionally,

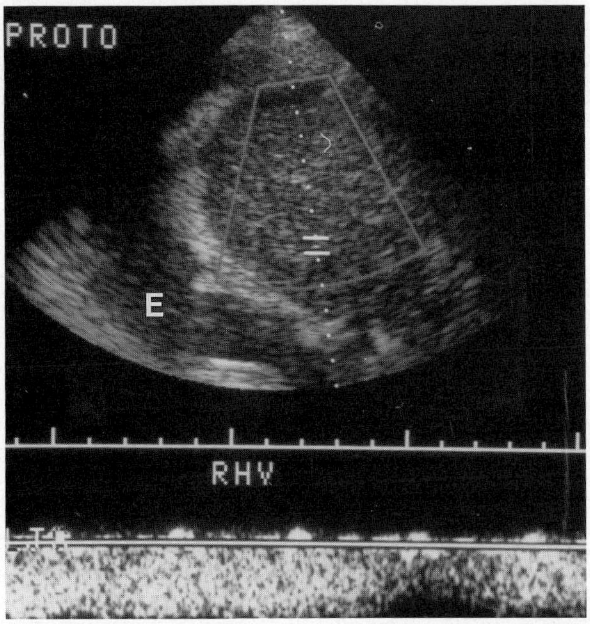


**FIGURE 7** Hepatic vein (sagittal view). Loss of normal cardiac cyclic variation in blood flow. Flow is nonvarying and unidirectional because increased rigidity of the diseased liver dampens cyclic changes. Incidental right-sided pleural effusion (E).

A

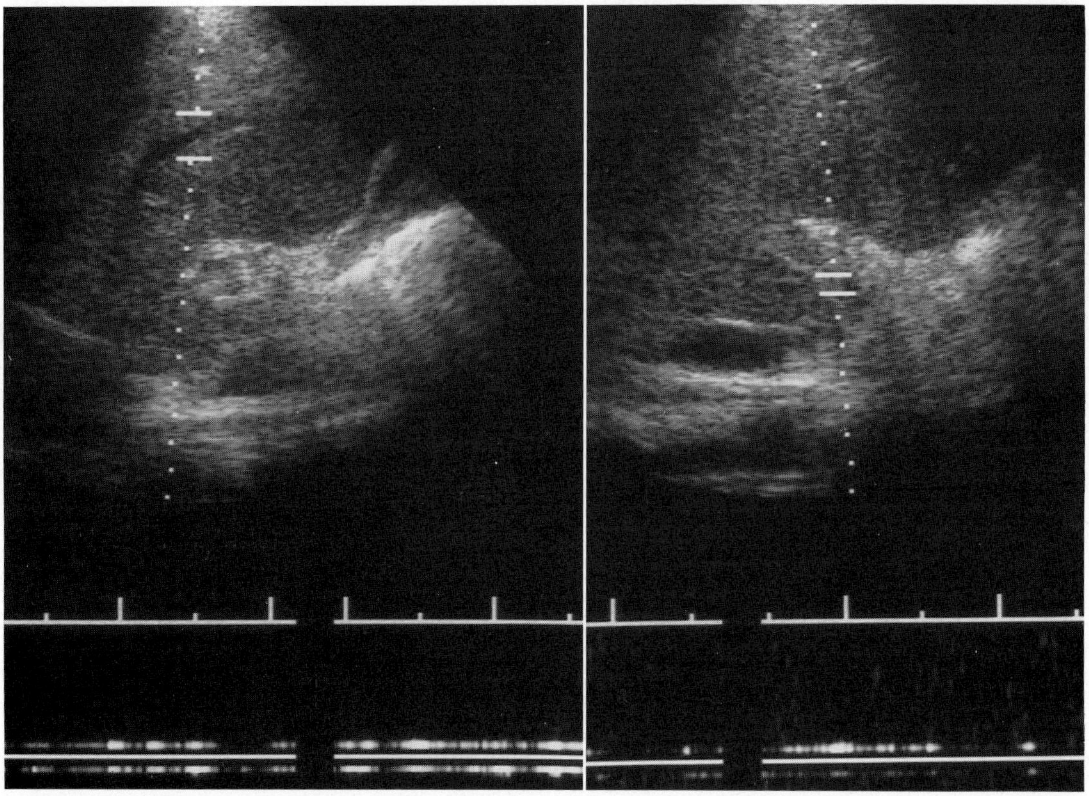

B

**FIGURE 8** Budd-Chiari syndrome (sagittal view). No flow in *(A)* hepatic veins or *(B)* portal vein. Vena cava remains patent.

A

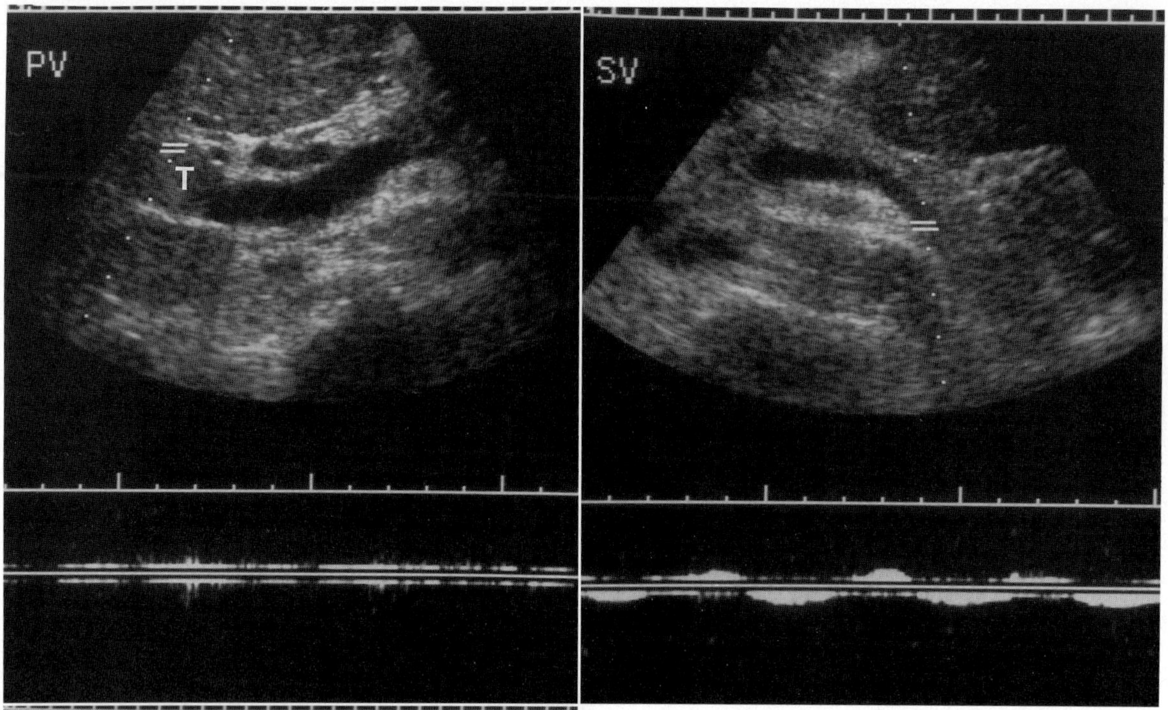


B

C

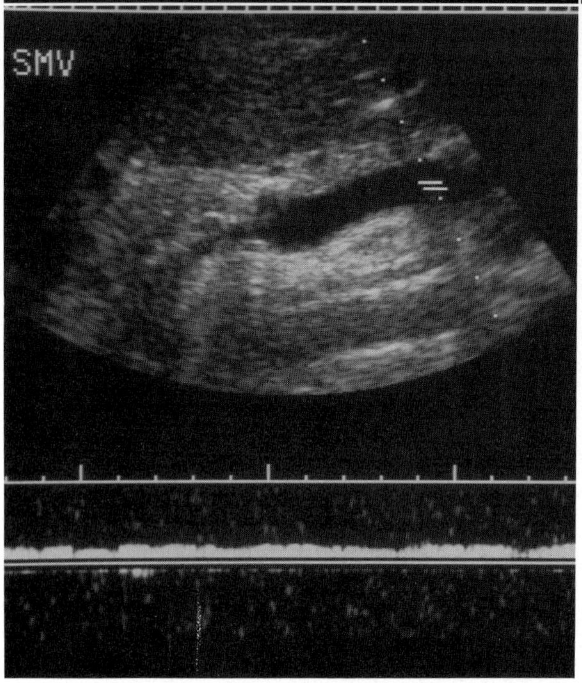


**FIGURE 9** Portal vein (occluding thrombus secondary to hepatocellular carcinoma). *A,* Thrombus (T) in the portal vein with no flow (sagittal view). *B,* Associated findings; reversed flow in splenic vein (transverse view) (waveform below baseline). *C,* Normal hepatopedal flow in superior mesenteric vein (sagittal view), which then reverses direction when it drains into the splenic vein.

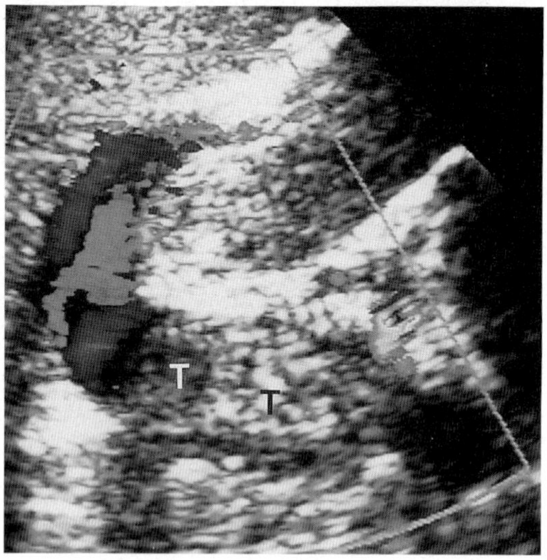


**FIGURE 10** Portal vein (sagittal view). Nonoccluding thrombus (T) in patient with hepatocellular carcinoma. Color Doppler sonogram (*reproduced here in black and white*) shows flow distal to thrombus. Localized regions of reversed flow are present, although overall flow direction is hepatopedal. When reversed flow is detected by spectral Doppler in the portal vein, multiple regions of the vein should be evaluated to prevent misinterpreting a localized region of reversed flow as representative of the overall flow direction in the vein. See also Color Plate 2.

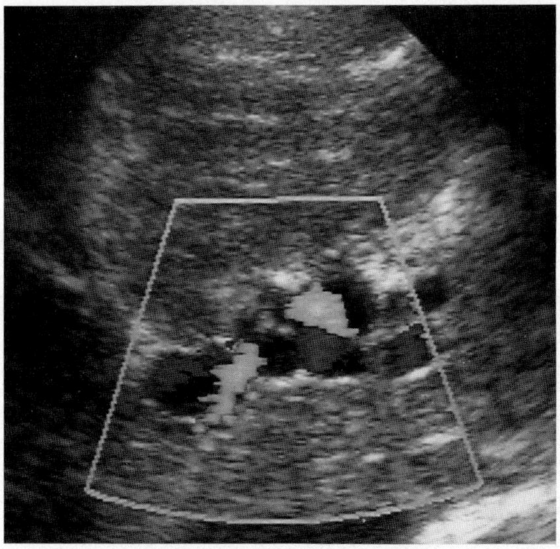

**FIGURE 11** Portal vein (transverse view). Cavernous transformation. Multiple tortuous collateral venous channels adjacent to thrombosed portal vein. See also Color Plate 3.

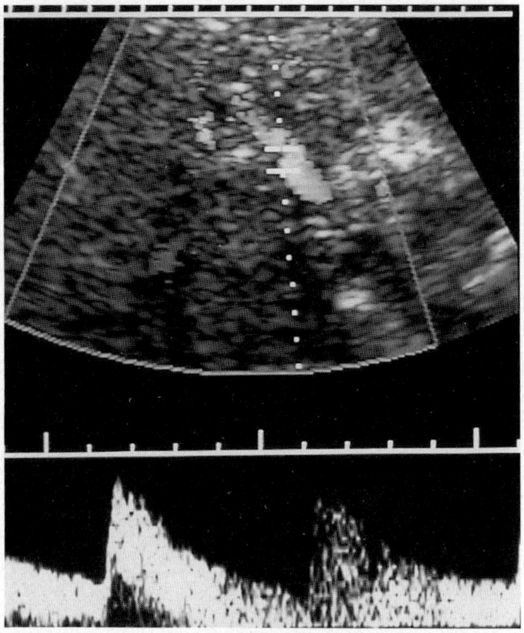

**FIGURE 12** Portal vein occlusion (sagittal view). No portal vein is observed. Single vessel in portahepatis is a prominent HA.

hepatocellular carcinoma may diffusely involve the liver and PV thrombosis may be its only sign. Fresh thrombus may show no intravascular echoes; however, no flow is demonstrated by Doppler. PV thrombosis may also occur in end-stage liver disease. Even when thrombus appears to fill the lumen of the vein, it may not actually completely obstruct the vein since Doppler may show blood flowing distal to the thrombus (Fig. 10 and Color Plate 2).

When there is no flow in the PV, it is important to determine what major mesenteric veins are patent to assist the surgeon in planning the anastomosis to the donor liver PV. Therefore one examines the retropancreatic splenic and superior mesenteric veins. The former is best visualized in transverse plane behind the pancreas and the latter in sagittal plane.

Usually in PV thrombosis, there is reversed flow in the splenic vein while the normal cephalad flow is maintained in the superior mesenteric vein (see Fig. 9). In the splenic hilum, splenic vein flow is in its normal splenofugal direction. To account for reversed splenic vein flow in the retropancreatic segment of the PV, and normal direction of flow in the splenic hilum, there must be collateral channels from the splenic vein to systemic circulation (i.e., gastroesophageal or perisplenic varices). Those around the spleen may be appreciated by Doppler as dilated venous channels. Rarely, a spontaneous splenorenal shunt may be present and detected with color Doppler.

Occasionally multiple small collateral venous channels may develop adjacent to the thrombosed PV to carry portal blood to the liver (cavernous transformation of the PV) (Fig. 11 and Color Plate 3). If one of these channels becomes prominent, one should be careful not to mistake it for a normal main PV.

When the PV is thrombosed, all blood entering the liver is supplied by the HA. The HA may be larger than usual in the portahepatis and HA velocity of flow is greater, making it easy to detect both the main HA and its branches. Rarely a single vessel may be observed in the porta that resembles the PV by real-time imaging, but is characterized by Doppler as a large HA (Fig. 12). The PV may be reduced to an echogenic cord. PV thrombosis may be an isolated finding or associated with HV and vena caval thrombosis.

#### Reversed Flow

Blood flows in a hepatofugal instead of hepatopedal manner (Fig. 13 and Color Plate 4). It may be observed in end-stage liver disease or in a patient with Budd-Chiari syndrome. As in PV thrombosis, there is reversed flow in the splenic vein and splenic systemic varices. Normal direction of flow is usually present in the superior mesenteric vein.

### *HA*

Preoperatively we have not observed HA thrombosis. However, occasionally, the position of the HA may be anomalous so that it is not adjacent to the PV in the portahepatis. Color Doppler may help locate the main artery, and detecting flow in peripheral branch arteries confirms the presence of arterial flow into the liver.

## Vascular Complications of the Liver Transplant

The hepatic transplant is susceptible to pseudoaneurysms of the HA and thromboses and stenoses of the HA, PV, HVs, and inferior vena cava (IVC). All of these vascular complications can lead to graft failure. However, if detected early, some can be repaired by radiologic or surgical intervention. Although angiography is the definitive imaging method for the diagnosis of these abnormalities, most can be detected by sonography. At our institution sonography is used as the primary screening technique, with angiography performed to confirm sonographically detected abnormalities and evaluate patients in whom the sonographic study was suboptimal.

Sonographic screening for vascular complications includes

A

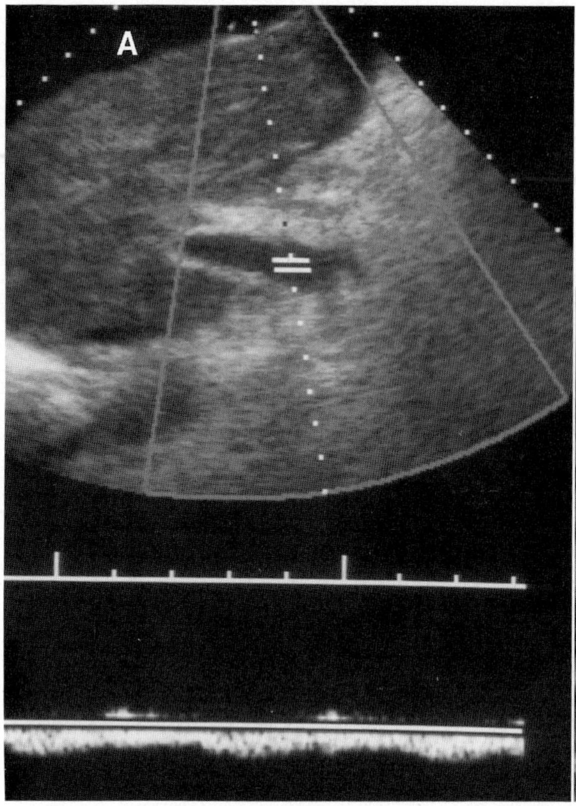


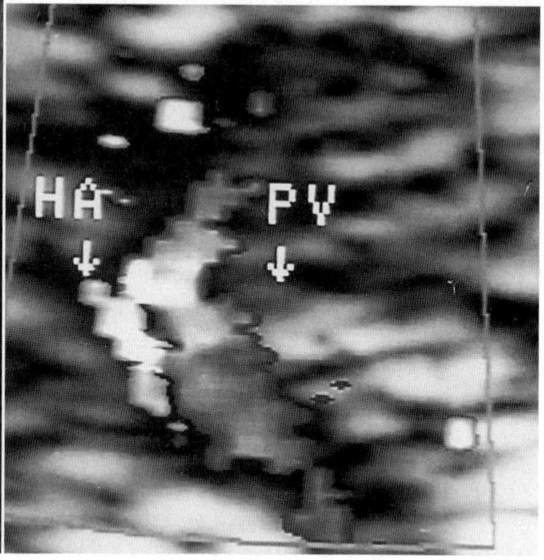


B

**FIGURE 13** Portal vein (sagittal view). Reversed flow. Small cirrhotic end-stage liver. *A,* Spectral Doppler shows portal vein flow is hepatofugal (below baseline). Note ascites (A) above the liver. *B,* Color Doppler sonogram (*reproduced here in black and white*). HA is hepatopedal and PV is hepatofugal. See also Color Plate 4. Compare with Figure 3 (Color Plate 1).

gray-scale, duplex Doppler and color Doppler imaging. Gray-scale sonography is used to identify the major hepatic vessels and detect obvious stenoses and echogenic thromboses of the larger vessels. Color Doppler is used to screen all of the hepatic vessels and IVC for patency, direction of flow, and focal alterations in velocity. It is also used to evaluate fluid collections suspicious for pseudoaneurysms. Duplex Doppler is used to confirm, decipher, and quantitate the abnormalities identified by gray-scale and color Doppler.

## Hepatic Artery Stenosis and Thrombosis

Hepatic artery stenoses most commonly occur at the anastomosis of donor and recipient artery. Therefore effective screening for arterial stenoses must be centered on the site of anastomosis, most commonly the portahepatis. Because of its small size, the HA is commonly invisible to gray-scale sonography and thus difficult to evaluate by duplex Doppler. Color Doppler, however, can usually depict the full extent of the portal segment of the HA. With the pulse repetition frequency appropriately set, stenoses are detected by color Doppler as focal regions of aliasing (representing areas of increased velocity) (Fig. 14, *A,* and Color Plate 5). Once found, aliasing must be evaluated with duplex Doppler to quantitate the severity of stenosis (Fig. 14, *B*). Duplex Doppler evaluation of a stenosis includes insonation above, at, and below the stenosis. A significant arterial stenosis has a peak velocity in excess of 2 m/s or a greater than threefold increase in velocity at the stenosis relative to the prestenotic vessel. Significant stenoses may also be suspected by alterations of the intrahepatic arterial flow consisting of peak velocities less than 0.4 m/s, a slow rise to peak systole, and a decrease in the pulsatility of the waveform (Fig. 14, *C*). If this type of waveform is identified in the intrahepatic arterial vessels, the main HA must be extensively evaluated for possible stenosis.

HA thromboses, like HA stenoses, most commonly occur at the level of the vascular anastomosis. Therefore HA thrombosis is usually detected as absence of arterial flow in the region of the portahepatis. In rare instances intrahepatic flow can be detected in the presence of complete HA thrombosis (Fig. 15). The intrahepatic arterial flow exists by virtue of arterial collaterals that form about the portahepatis. The intrahepatic arterial flow has a characteristic waveform of low velocity and low resistance, similar to that observed with significant HA stenoses.

## Hepatic Artery Pseudoaneurysms

HA pseudoaneurysms are uncommon. They can occur either intrahepatically or extrahepatically. Intrahepatic pseudoaneurysms are almost exclusively caused by trauma from percutaneous liver biopsy. Extrahepatic pseudoaneurysms almost always occur at the anastomosis of the donor and recipient arteries and are the result of a failed suture. Both intra- and extrahepatic pseudoaneurysms appear as spherical fluid collections that exhibit internal pulsatile flow on Doppler evaluation (Fig. 16 and Color Plate 6). Direct insonation of the neck of a simple arterial pseudoaneurysm reveals a classic to-and-fro flow. To prevent catastrophic hemorrhage, all small periportal and intrahepatic fluid collections should be evaluated by Doppler to exclude the possibility of a pseudoaneurysm before percutaneous aspiration.

## Portal Vein Stenosis and Thrombosis

Stenosis of the PV is most commonly located in the portahepatis at the anastomosis of the donor and recipient vessels. Most stenoses are visible by gray-scale sonography as a focal

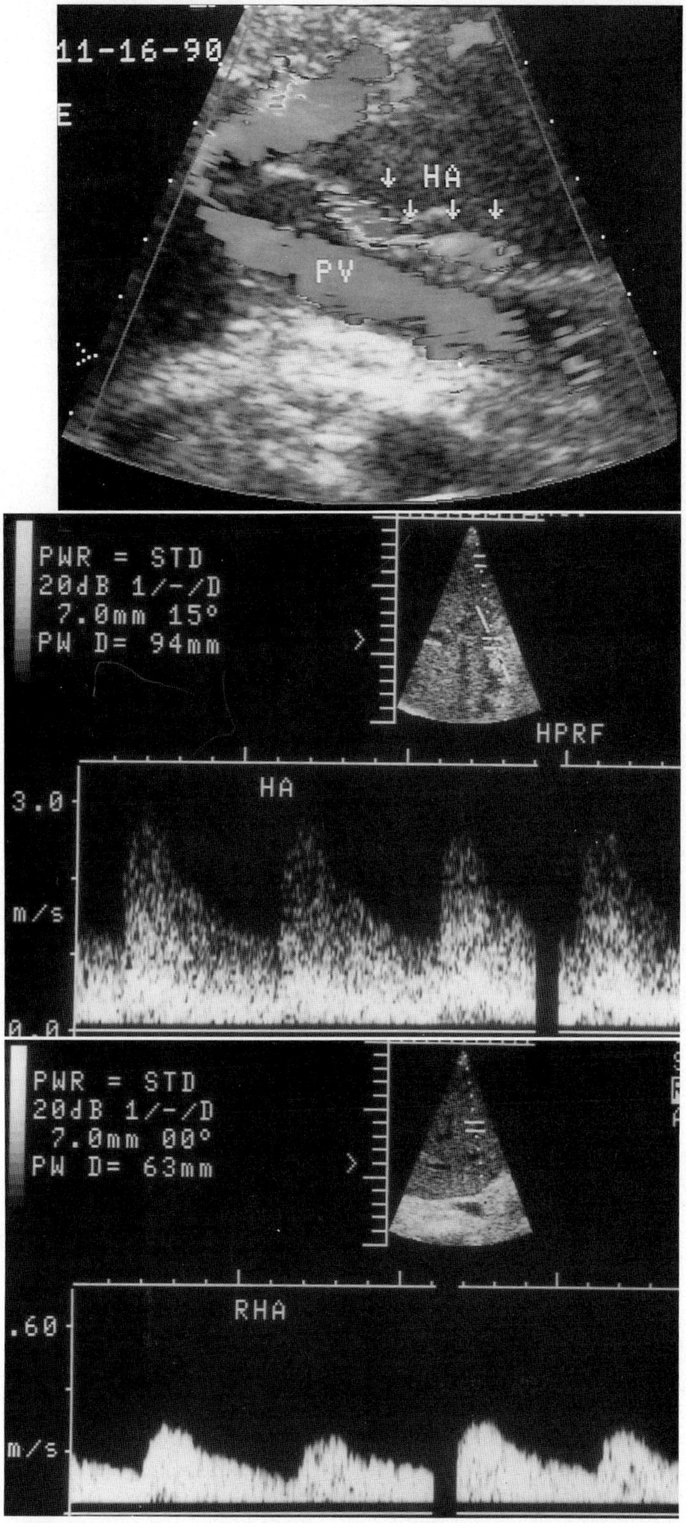


A

B

C

**FIGURE 14** Hepatic artery stenosis. *A,* Color Doppler sonogram of the proper hepatic artery in portahepatis shows abrupt alteration in arterial flow depicted as color aliasing (*reproduced here in black and white*). See also Color Plate 5. *B,* Duplex Doppler evaluation of the region of color aliasing shows a marked increase in velocity up to 3 m/s, which is highly suggestive of a significant arterial stenosis. *C,* Duplex Doppler evaluation of the left hepatic artery in the same patient shows a low-velocity, low-resistance waveform with a slow rise to peak systole. This type of waveform is highly suggestive of a significant proximal arterial stenosis.

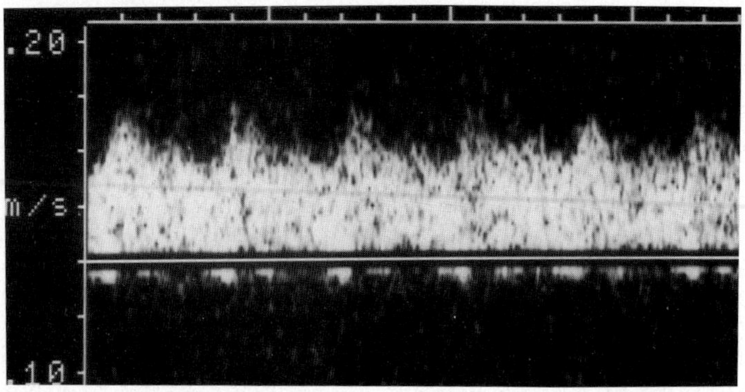


**FIGURE 15** Hepatic artery thrombosis. Duplex Doppler spectral waveform of the left hepatic artery shows a low-velocity, low-resistance configuration similar to that observed with hepatic artery stenosis. The two can only be differentiated by identification of flow in the proper hepatic artery.

A

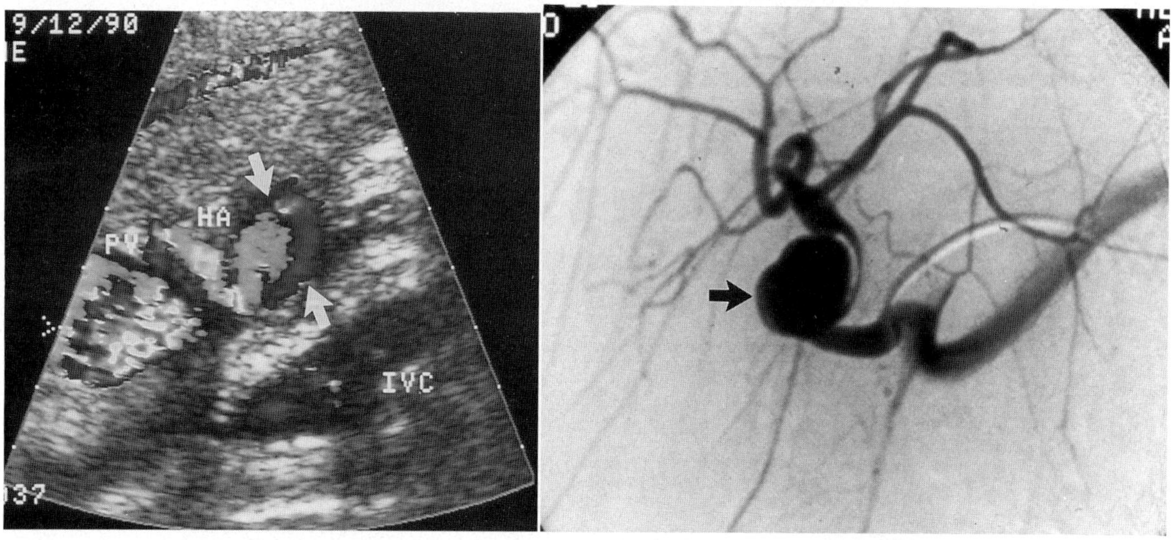


B

**FIGURE 16** Hepatic artery pseudoaneurysm. *A,* Color Doppler sonogram (*reproduced here in black and white*) shows a periportal spherical region of flow *(arrows)* adjacent to the proper hepatic artery (HA). Duplex Doppler evaluation of the spherical region demonstrated pulsatile arterial flow highly suggestive of a pseudoaneurysm. See also Color Plate 6. *B,* Celiac artery arteriogram shows a spherical extravascular mass *(arrow)* that fills with contrast material during the arterial injection phase. The mass is located at the hepatic artery anastomosis and exerts mass effect on the proper hepatic artery. The appearance of this mass is diagnostic of a pseudoaneurysm.

narrowing (Fig. 17). Color Doppler identifies significant stenoses as regions of aliasing. Duplex Doppler at, above, and below a significant stenosis reveals a three- to fourfold increase in velocity at the stenosis relative to the prestenotic vessel. To prevent false-negative evaluations, it is imperative that angle-corrected velocities be obtained about the region of a stenosis.

PV thrombosis can be complete or incomplete. Most PV thromboses are visible by gray-scale sonography as echogenic material within the vessel lumen. Hypoechoic PV thrombi are difficult to detect by gray-scale sonography. With acute complete thromboses, no flow is detected by color or duplex Doppler. Chronic complete thromboses may have flow in or around them as a result of recanalization of the thrombus.

## Hepatic Vein Stenosis and Thrombosis

Stenosis of the HVs is uncommon, because they are usually undisturbed in the transplantation technique. However, stenoses of the HVs may occur in patients in whom it was necessary to anastomose the donor HVs to the recipient's IVC or right atrium. High-grade stenosis of the HVs causes a decrease in hepatic venous flow, with associated loss of the normal hepatic venous periodicity (cardiac pulsations).

Hepatic venous thrombosis produces loss of all Doppler detectable flow in the HVs.

## Inferior Vena Cava Stenosis and Thrombosis

Stenoses of the IVC almost always occur at the cephalad (superior) or caudal (inferior) anastomosis of the donor and recipient IVC (Fig. 18, *A*). Superior caval stenoses produce Budd-Chiari–type symptoms, whereas inferior caval stenoses cause edema of the lower extremities. Irrespective of site, a significant caval stenosis produces at least a threefold to fourfold increase in velocity at the stenosis relative to the prestenotic cava and loss of the normal caval periodicity proximal to the stenosis (Fig. 18, *B* and *C*). Significant stenoses of the upper caval anastomosis can produce changes in the

A B

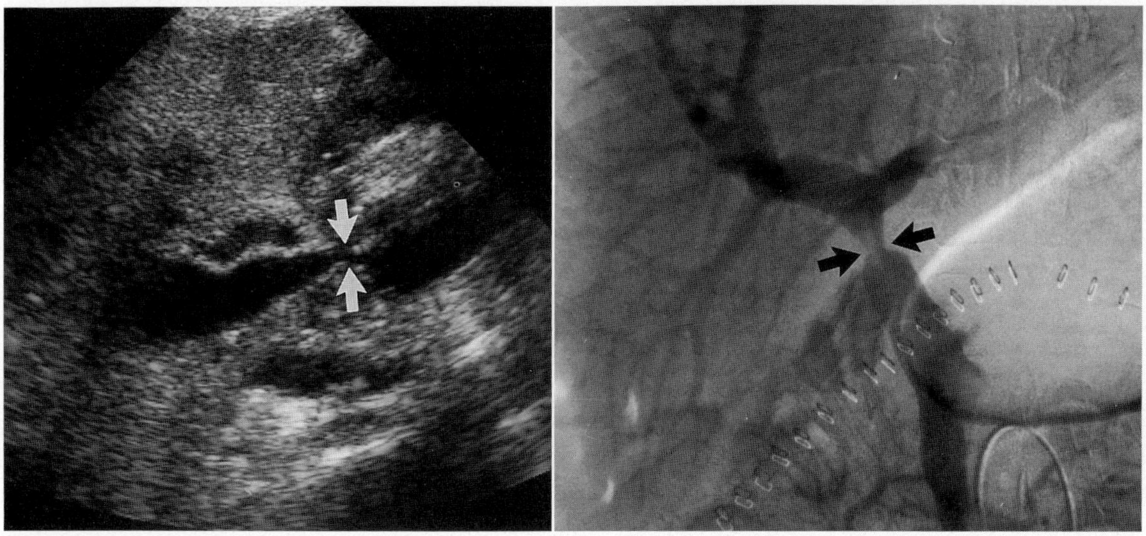

**FIGURE 17** Portal vein stenosis. *A,* Gray-scale sonogram of the portal vein shows a marked narrowing *(arrows)* in the region of the surgical anastomosis. Duplex Doppler evaluation of the portal vein revealed a fivefold increase in velocity through the stenosis relative to the velocity in the prestenotic portal vein. These findings are highly suggestive of a significant portal vein stenosis. *B,* Angiogram of the portal vein in the same patient confirms the presence of a high-grade stenosis *(arrows).*

A B C

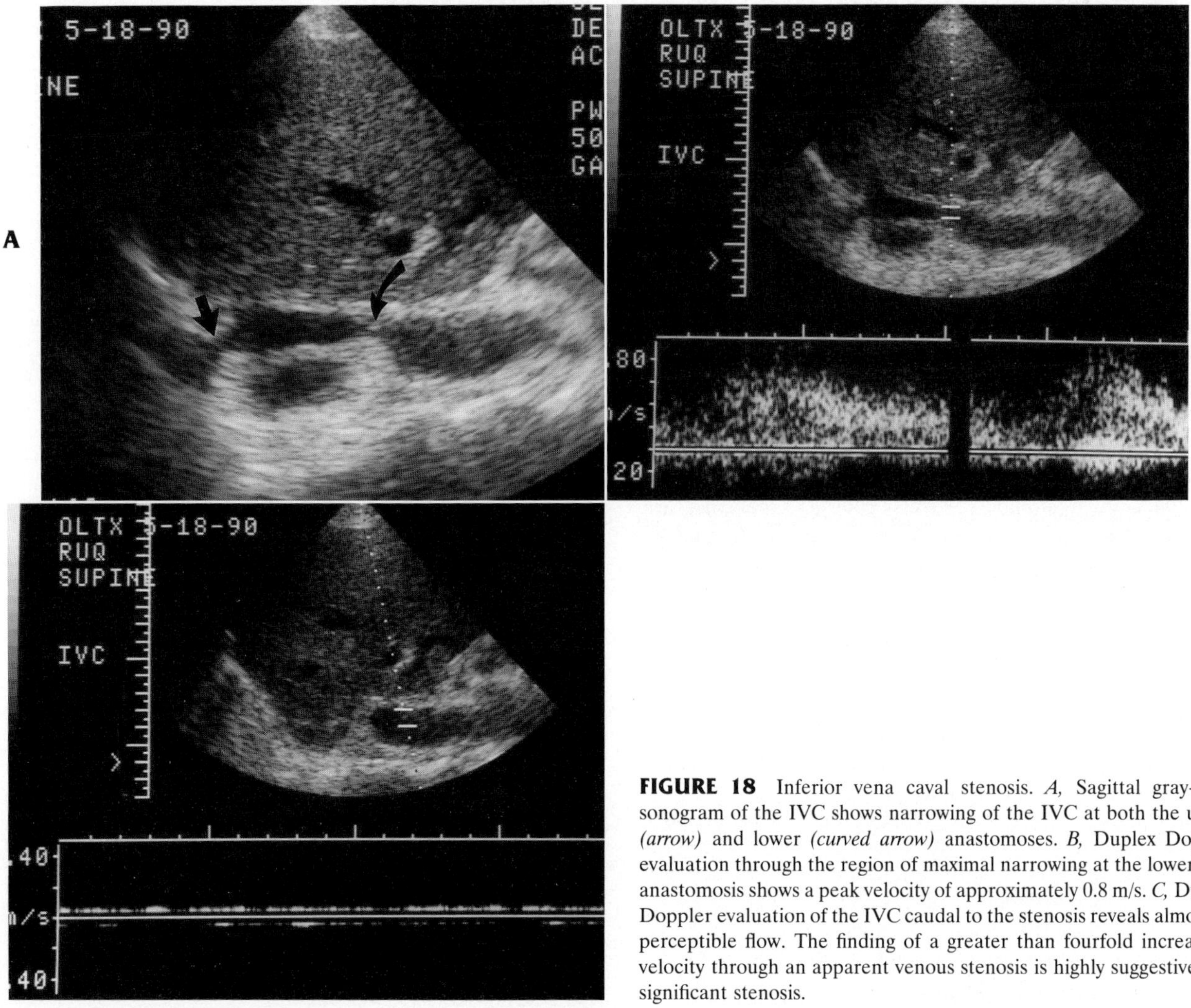


**FIGURE 18** Inferior vena caval stenosis. *A,* Sagittal gray-scale sonogram of the IVC shows narrowing of the IVC at both the upper *(arrow)* and lower *(curved arrow)* anastomoses. *B,* Duplex Doppler evaluation through the region of maximal narrowing at the lower IVC anastomosis shows a peak velocity of approximately 0.8 m/s. *C,* Duplex Doppler evaluation of the IVC caudal to the stenosis reveals almost no perceptible flow. The finding of a greater than fourfold increase in velocity through an apparent venous stenosis is highly suggestive of a significant stenosis.

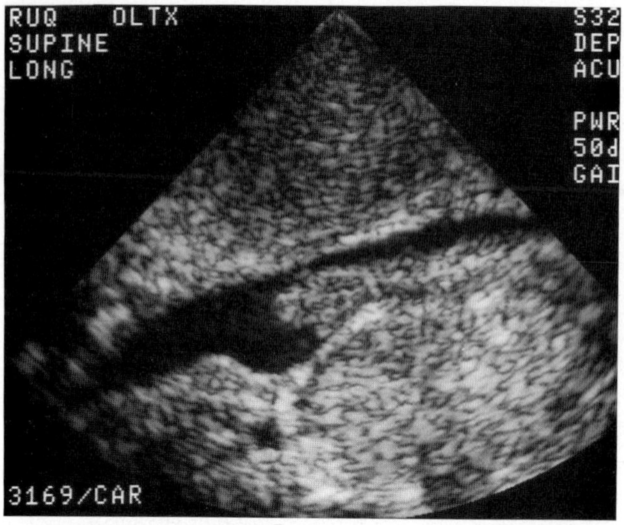


**FIGURE 19** Inferior vena caval thrombosis. Sagittal sonogram of the IVC shows an echogenic nonocclusive thrombus in the region of the lower anastomosis.

hepatic venous flow, consisting of loss of the normal hepatic venous periodicity and reversal of flow in some of the HVs.

IVC thromboses are usually visible by gray-scale sonography as internal echogenic debris (Fig. 19). The thromboses may be complete or partial. If complete, they cause Doppler findings similar to those observed with significant caval stenoses.

## Suggested Reading

Bolondi L, Li Bassi S, Gaiani S, et al. Liver cirrhosis: Changes of Doppler waveform of hepatic veins. Radiology 1991; 178:513–516.

Hall TR, Diarmid SV, Grant EG, et al. False-negative duplex Doppler studies in children with hepatic artery thrombosis after liver transplantation. AJR 1990; 154:573–575.

Longley DG, Skolnick ML, Zajko AB, Bron KM. Duplex Doppler sonography in the evaluation of adult patients before and after liver transplantation. AJR 1988; 151:687–696.

Taylor KJW, Morse SS, Weltin GG, et al. Liver transplant recipients: Portable duplex US with correlative angiography. Radiology 1986; 159:357–363.

Wozney P, Zajko AB, Bron KM, et al. Vascular complications after liver transplantation: A 5-year experience. AJR 1986; 147:657–663.

# Oral Contrast Agents for Abdominal MRI

*PETER F. HAHN, M.D., Ph.D.*

Many substances have been proposed and investigated as gastrointestinal (GI) contrast agents for abdominal magnetic resonance imaging (MRI). In fact, the first exogenous contrast agent applied to human MRI was introduced into the GI tract. Nevertheless, after nearly 10 years of clinical experience with MRI, no GI contrast agent is approved for marketing by the United States Food and Drug Administration, and there is no agreement among practitioners or investigators as to what an ideal GI contrast agent should be.

For abdominal computed tomography (CT) scans, exogenous contrast agents are routinely given to mark and distend the bowel. The principal goal for a CT contrast agent is to differentiate bowel from nonbowel structures such as pancreatic masses or lymph nodes. Most GI contrast agents increase x-ray absorption from the intestinal lumen; these include dilute barium and iodinated derivatives of benzoic acid. Low-density materials, including fatty material and water, have also been used.

For MRI a similar dichotomy exists between bright-bowel (positive) contrast agents and dark-bowel (negative) ones. This classification is complicated by the diversity of imaging techniques employed in MRI. Water provides a simple example—bright on T2-weighted images and dark on T1-weighted images.

A second classification of GI MRI contrast agents asks whether the agent is intended to mix with or to replace natural GI contents. The first type, sometimes called "dispersed" or "miscible" contrast agents, changes the signal intensity of succus entericus so that it can be recognized as intraluminal. Nondispersed contrast agents do not mix with bowel contents. Air introduced by rectal tube is a simple example of this type.

**TABLE 1** Classification of GI Contrast Agents for MRI

| | Positive | Negative |
|---|---|---|
| Dispersed | Paramagnetic ions (gadolinium, iron)<br>Readicat 2 (aqueous carrier) | Superparamagnetic iron oxide<br>Clay minerals (Kaopectate)<br>Concentrated barium sulfate |
| Nondispersed | Fats and oils | Perfluorochemicals<br>Gas and gas granules |

Examples of dispersed and nondispersed, positive and negative, GI contrast agents are categorized in Table 1.

The optimal imaging parameters for their intended use constitute a third division among GI MRI contrast agents. T1 contrast agents, such as those producing paramagnetic T1 shortening, work best on T1-weighted images. T2 agents, such as superparamagnetic iron oxides that act by local distortion of the imaging magnetic field, are effective at lower concentrations on T2-weighted images than T1-weighted images. Perfluoro-octyl bromide (PFOB), which has no hydrogen protons, appears dark on both T1- and T2-weighted images. Extremely short transit time, together with the feeling of distention that it induces, may limit PFOB to rapid-scan techniques.

GI contrast agents can introduce noise into MRI. Moving structures with high signal intensity, including bowel, tend to produce phase artifacts. Positive contrast agents can contribute noise by this mechanism. A distended patient breathes deeply and irregularly, a source of noise whatever contrast agent produces the distention. Magnetic susceptibility artifacts, such

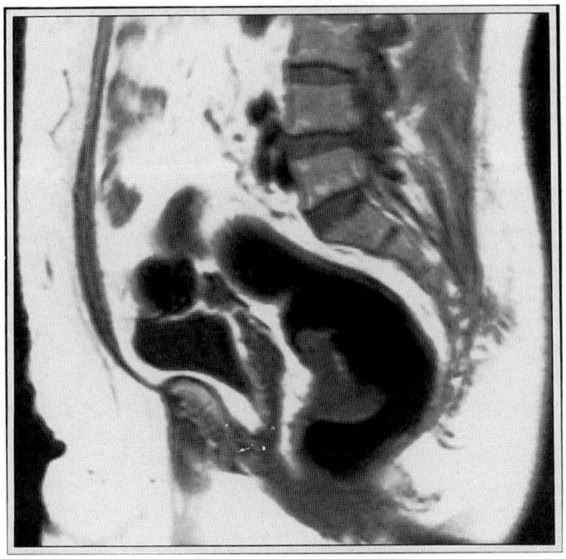

**FIGURE 1** Rectal air insufflation to evaluate rectal carcinoma. Mildly T1-weighted sagittal image (SE500/30; 1.5 T Signa) shows a large, polypoid tumor arising from the anterior rectal wall. Linear strands extending into perirectal fat from the base of the tumor indicate transmural invasion. After bowel preparation, air is instilled through a rectal catheter until the patient feels full. Between pulse sequences the patient is encouraged to squeeze the air bulb insufflator (E-Z-Em) on the end of the tube to maintain distention.

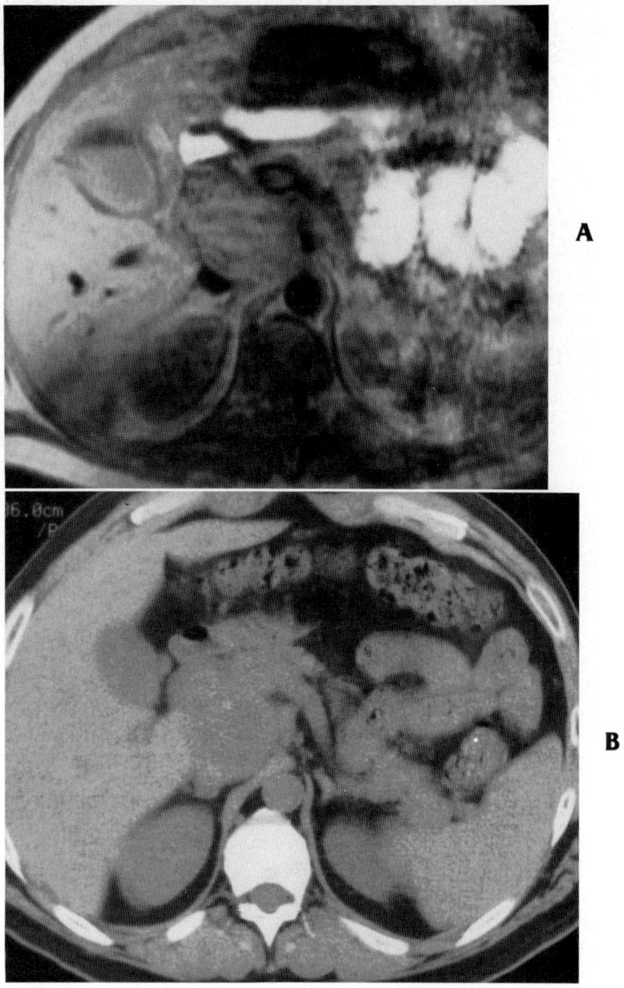

**FIGURE 2** Ferric ammonium citrate to evaluate a peripancreatic lymph node metastasis. *A,* Fat-saturated T1-weighted spin-echo image after ingestion of 12 oz of a 1:10 aqueous dilution of Geritol. High signal intensity contrast material is present in the stomach, proximal jejunum, and duodenal bulb, which is displaced anteriorly by the mass. Note phase artifacts arising from jejunal loops moving during the 3.5 minute acquisition. *B,* Corresponding radiographic CT image, without oral contrast material.

as at air-fluid interfaces or from overconcentration of magnetic particles, also can result in image degradation. Inhibition of peristalsis by injection of glucagon or scopolamine has been recommended; but passive motion of the bowel from respiration or transmitted vascular pulsations also contributes noise.

Status of GI contrast agents is linked to development of new imaging technologies. For example, rectal air insufflation is a convenient method for distending the rectum in local staging of rectal carcinomas (Fig. 1). Dissemination of purpose-built endorectal coils diminishes the importance of this technique.

Oral administration of contrast agents is limited in the United States to protocol agents and materials already available for other purposes. Among the latter, four agents are discussed: Geritol, Kaopectate, infant-feeding formula, and Readicat 2. No agent is perfect. In most cases I use no contrast agent at all, relying on CT for its anatomic resolution.

The hematemic and magnetically active ingredient in Geritol (Beecham; Bristol, TN) is ferric ammonium citrate (FAC). FAC is paramagnetic; potency of T1 shortening is about one-fifth that of gadolinium chelates. An aqueous 1:10 dilution of Geritol ingested immediately before positioning in the magnet marks the stomach and duodenum on T1-weighted images (Fig. 2). Distention of the duodenum is improved by imaging in the right decubitus position. Geritol contains ethanol and should not be used in patients receiving the antibiotic metronidazole. FAC has been reformulated as a protocol drug in an effort to get better marking of the small bowel. This is analogous to the use of the nonabsorbable sugar mannitol with gadolinium-DTPA to promote better distribution in the small bowel, a result demonstrated in European trials.

The nonprescription antidiarrhea agent Kaopectate (Upjohn; Kalamazoo, MI) contains the clay attapulgite. An earlier formulation uses kaolin. Both minerals produce diamagnetic enhancement of relaxation (T1 and T2 shortening). Except on extremely T1-weighted pulse sequences, Kaopectate acts as a negative bowel contrast agent. In motivated patients willing to ingest 8 oz (one bottle) or more of this unappetizing material, good bowel marking can be achieved.

Infant-feeding formulas increase the signal intensity of gut lumen. Iron-supplemented formulas are particularly effective on T1-weighted images. These materials distribute well throughout the small bowel of very young children and have the additional advantage of quieting the subject during imaging.

Readicat 2 (E-Z-Em; Westbury, NY) is an oral contrast agent intended for CT use. Although concentrated barium has been investigated as a negative MRI contrast agent, the 2 percent barium sulfate in Readicat 2 has negligible effect on signal intensity. One bottle of Readicat 2 (450 ml) produces uniform mild distention of the upper GI tract and appears bright on T2-weighted images. Because of artifacts induced by

A

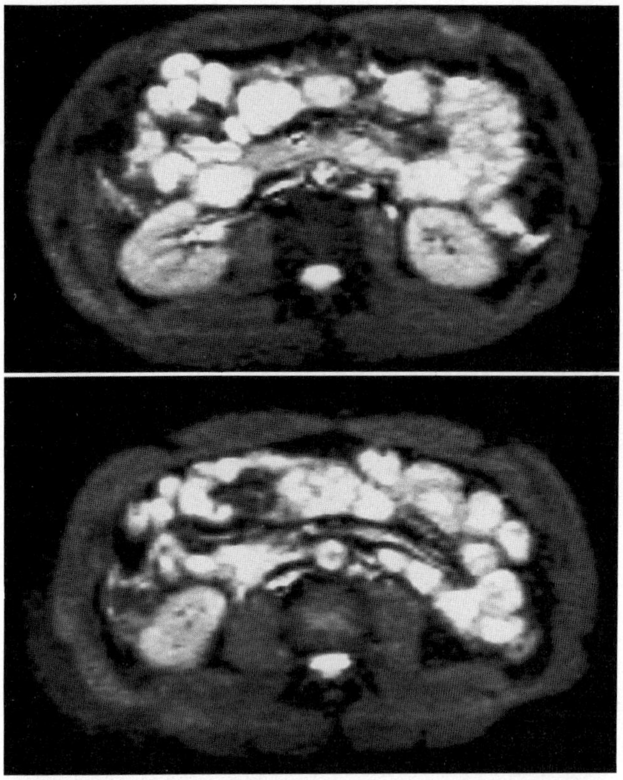

B

**FIGURE 3** Ultrafast echo-planar images, showing bowel marking in a normal volunteer. Single excitation spin-echo image with TE at 26 milliseconds, acquired on the Instascan (Advanced NMR Systems; Wilmington, MA) modification of a Signa imager. Orally ingested long T2 fluid (Readicat 2) appears as high signal. Sixty millisecond image acquisition freezes motion, so no increase in noise is associated with increased signal in the gut lumen.

high signal, Readicat 2 is not recommended for conventional imaging. Ultrafast echo-planar imaging is an ideal setting for an aqueous, long T2 contrast agent. Image acquisitions in under 100 msec freeze biological motion, providing clear and reliable bowel marking without phase artifacts (Fig. 3).

## Suggested Reading

Gerscovich EO, McGahan JP, Buonocore MH, et al. The rediscovery of infant feeding formula with magnetic resonance imaging. Pediatr Radiol 1990; 20:147–151.

Hahn PF, Saini S, Cohen MS, et al. An aqueous gastrointestinal contrast agent for use in echo–planar MR imaging. Magn Reson Med 1992; 25:380–383.

Mitchell DG, Vinitski S, Mohamed FB, et al. Comparison of Kaopectate with barium for negative and positive enteric contrast at MR imaging. Radiology 1991; 181:475–480.

Patten RM, Moss AA, Fenton TA, Elliot S. OMR, a positive bowel contrast agent for abdominal and pelvic MR imaging: Safety and imaging characteristics. J Magn Reson Imaging 1992; 2:25–34.

Ros PR, Steinman RM, Torres GM, et al. The value of barium as a gastrointestinal contrast agent in MR imaging: A comparison study in normal volunteers. AJR 1991; 157:761–767.

Saini S, Modic MT, Hamm B, Hahn PF. Advances in contrast-enhanced MR imaging. AJR 1991; 156:235–254.

# Targeted Contrast Agents for Abdominal MRI

*RALPH WEISSLEDER, M.D., Ph.D.*

Gadolinium (Gd) chelate contrast agents (such as Gd-DTPA) currently in clinical practice have only limited use for abdominal imaging, because of their broad distribution and the need to perform sequential dynamic imaging for the majority of imaging tasks. Two classes of contrast agents currently in clinical trials have a more restricted distribution volume: hepatobiliary agents (e.g., Mn-DPDP, Gd-EOB-DTPA, Gd-BOPTA) and iron oxides. After an initial vascular phase, both types of agents accumulate to some degree in liver (within hepatocytes or phagocytic cells, respectively), thus improving liver lesion detectability. Although these agents hold promise for liver imaging, the wish list of magnetic resonance imaging (MRI) contrast agents for abdominal imaging is more extensive (Table 1).

Target-specific MRI contrast agents optimally accumulate in either normal or abnormal tissue, but not both. The more specific the accumulation of a contrast agent within the target tissue, without distribution to surrounding tissue, the better the resulting lesion-tissue contrast. Specific contrast agents commonly are complex macromolecules consisting of a carrier molecule with target specificity and a magnetic label detectable by MRI. Magnetic labels may be either T1-type agents (i.e., polylanthanide chelates, other paramagnetic compounds) or T2-type agents (i.e., iron oxides).

The focus of this chapter is to summarize the attempts of drug targeting in abdominal MRI. It will become obvious that target selectivity and receptor and/or antigen specificity are important if the diagnostic accuracy of abdominal MRI is to be improved.

## Lymph Nodes

Evaluation of regional and distant lymph nodes provides critical information for treatment planning for cancer patients. Currently used size criteria for computed tomography (CT) and MRI are insensitive indicators for the presence of metastases within lymph nodes. Although it was initially hoped that MRI signal intensities of normal, metastatic, and hyperplastic lymph nodes would be different, considerable overlap has been well documented. Because of this overlap, lympho-

**TABLE 1** Contrast Agents for Abdominal MRI

| Problem Area | Comments |
|---|---|
| Abdominal lymph nodes: | |
| Cancer staging<br>Residual vs. active disease | Lymphotropic T2 agents (MION) and T1 agents have been developed. Agents accumulate in macrophages of normal nodes. |
| Liver: | |
| Detection of tumors<br>Differentiation of tumors<br>Primary tumors in cirrhotic liver | Hepatobiliary agents are in clinical trials. Efficacy of hepatocyte receptor–directed agents has been proven for tumor detection and differential diagnosis. |
| Adrenal glands: | |
| Differential diagnosis of tumors<br>Evaluation of pheochromocytoma | Only one class of aminated polymeric agents has been described. Further studies are required. |
| Pancreas: | |
| Detection of small tumors | A T2 label has been used as an experimental MRI probe. Mn-DPDP is in clinical trials. |
| Abdominal vasculature: | |
| Preoperative mapping of tumor vascularity<br>Abdominal aortic aneurysm, renal artery stenosis<br>Detection of bleeding sites<br>Intestinal ischemia | Several agents are in preclinical evaluation. Agents with long blood half-life (MPEG polymers) have been developed. |
| Tumor imaging: | |
| Improved detection of ovarian, prostate, and colorectal cancer | No specific agents have been developed or systematically evaluated. Some MRI contrast agents have nonspecific tumor accumulation. |

tropic contrast agents are necessary if MRI is to improve detection of lymph node metastases in cancer patients. Preferably such agents should be administrable intravenously.

We have recently synthesized prototypic T1- and T2-type MRI contrast agents that accumulate in lymph nodes to a high degree after intravenous use. The mechanism by which these agents accumulate in lymph nodes is currently under investigation. It has been shown that these compounds leave the vascular compartment, and that they escape rapid removal by macrophages of the liver and the spleen. Once in the interstitium, re-entry into the vascular system appears to be limited, so that agents are primarily cleared via the lymphatic route and are subsequently taken up by lymph node macrophages.

The T1-type agent consists of a poly-L-Lysine Gd-DTPA core to which are grafted polysaccharides. These T1 compounds show a remarkable accumulation in retroperitoneal lymph nodes of up to 140% dose/g tissue after IV injection. The T2-labeled lymphotropic compound consists of a unique monocrystalline iron oxide (MION). Up to 44%/g tissue of the IV injected dose of this agent accumulates in lymph nodes. IV administrations of doses of as low as 20 μmol Fe/kg are thus expected to change nodal MRI signal intensity. The blood half-life of both agents is approximately 2 to 3 hours, and maximum nodal concentration occurs within 12 to 24 hours after injection, the optimal time for imaging.

Successful early feasibility studies have prompted the need for clinical trials to demonstrate the ultimate use of these agents. Along with the development of magnetopharmaceuticals, MRI techniques must be perfected to facilitate high-resolution imaging of small lymph nodes. This appears feasible with surface coils, high-resolution 512 × 512 matrices, and thinner slice thickness.

## Liver

The most commonly encountered problems in liver imaging (ultrasonography, CT, and MRI) are the inability to detect early metastases and difficulties in differentiating between benign and malignant hepatic neoplasms. These problems are aggravated in livers with underlying medical disease such as cirrhosis. Animal experiments and clinical trials of hepatobiliary and reticuloendothelial contrast agents have shown that detection of hepatic mass lesions can be significantly improved after administration of liver-specific contrast agents. The more specific the agent is for normal liver tissue and the less accumulation in tumors, the more efficient is the compound. Specificity can be achieved, for example, by directing the magnetic label to a variety of normal hepatocyte receptors.

One of the useful hepatocyte receptors for drug targeting is the asialoglycoprotein (ASG) receptor, because of the large number of sites per cell and rapid cell internalization of the receptor. Hepatocyte-directed magnetopharmaceuticals have three potential advantages over Kupffer cell–directed iron oxides: (1) improved tumor-liver contrast-to-noise ratios at equimolar doses (i.e., lower dose requirements), (2) ability to assess organ function, and (3) the potential for tumor differential diagnosis. For example, asialofetuin (ASF) bound to MION has been shown to increase hepatic uptake 1.8-fold when compared with the parent compound MION. In addition to the increased hepatic accumulation, the different spatial distribution of MION-ASF to hepatocytes, rather than MION to Kupffer cells, increases liver relaxivity, thereby decreasing the amount of contrast agent needed.

Although clinical trials have not yet been conducted, the utility of some ASG targeted agents for the differentiation of liver tumors has been demonstrated in human specimens. These specimens demonstrated high ASG activity and binding of receptor agents to normal liver tissue, focal nodular hyperplasia, adenoma, hepatitis liver, and cirrhotic liver tissue (Fig. 1). Neither primary hepatic tumors (hepatocellular carcinoma, hemangioma) nor metastatic tumors to the liver (colon, renal cell carcinoma) showed significant accumulation of receptor agents. Similar results have been obtained in animal models of liver metastases and primary hepatocellular carcinoma.

Further refinements of new hepatocyte-specific agents are expected to continue over the next few years. The development of a T1 hepatocyte-specific agent seems intuitively preferable with current imaging technology, because T1-weighted imaging of the liver results in higher signal-to-noise ratios and improved anatomic resolution compared with T2-weighted imaging. There are two approaches to improving hepatocyte delivery: (1) develop agents that undergo high hepatobiliary excretion (the excretion rate should also be sufficiently slow to allow imaging of the liver with as little blood pool or tumor activity

A B

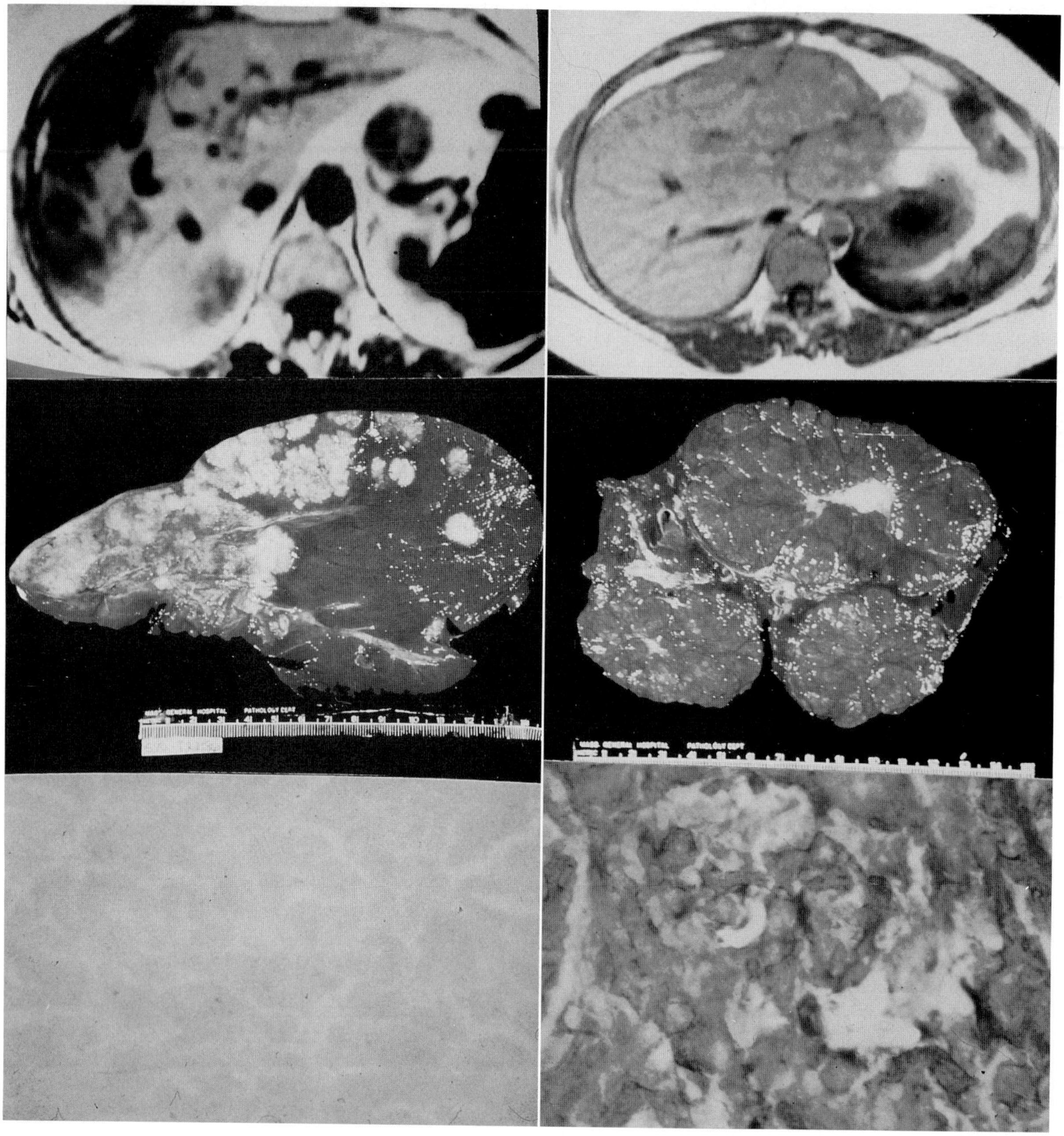

**FIGURE 1** Receptor assays in human liver tumors. *A,* Hepatocellular carcinoma. SE 275/14/4 (*top*) demonstrates a hepatocellular carcinoma in the right lobe of the liver. The surgical specimen (*middle*) demonstrates additional multiple lesions in the left liver lobe invisible on the MR image. Histologic receptor labeling was performed by incubating the human specimen with the iron-containing receptor agent and counterstaining for iron. There is no attachment of the receptor agent to HCC tissue. *B,* Focal nodular hyperplasia. The T1-weighted images demonstrate an isointense focal nodular hyperplasia in the left liver lobe (*top*). Surgical specimen (*middle row*). The histologic receptor labeling demonstrates specific attachment of the receptor agent (*dark areas, bottom*). (From Reimer P, Weissleder R, et al. Receptor-directed contrast agents for MR imaging: Preclinical evaluation with affinity assays. Radiology 1992; 182:565–569; with permission.)

as possible) or (2) design T1 agents that recognize hepatocyte surface receptors and are internalized into the lysosomal compartments where they would undergo degradation. For the second class of agents, the intracellular pathway of the T1 labels will have to be studied in detail and labels other than Gd or Mn may have to be used because of potential de-chelation, re-chelation, and cellular toxicity. Iron seems a logical choice as a biocompatible paramagnetic T1 label; however, only preliminary feasibility studies have been conducted.

## Adrenal Glands

Common indications for adrenal imaging include (1) workup of metastatic disease to the adrenal glands, (2) workup of incidental adrenal mass lesions detected during routine ultrasonography or CT imaging of the abdomen, and (3) pheochromocytoma evaluation. Previous clinical studies have evaluated the use of perfusion markers (Gd-DTPA) for the differentiation of benign and malignant adrenal mass lesions. Because of the overlap of perfusion patterns, quantitative studies are not performed routinely in a clinical setting. An adrenospecific MRI agent that would accumulate in normal adrenal glands, but not malignant tissue, would therefore be extremely useful. Various adrenal imaging agents have been used in nuclear medicine, including pharmaceuticals for adrenocortical imaging (iodocholesterols) or adrenomedullary imaging (metiodobenzylguanidine).

We have previously observed accumulation of certain macromolecules in the adrenal glands. One of the agents consists of a poly-L-lysine conjugate, which had 70 percent free epsilon amino groups and 30 percent diethylene-triamine-pentaacetic acid (DTPA)-derivatized amino groups for Gd binding. One hour after IV administration of this compound, adrenal uptake was as high as $10.1 \pm 0.7$ percent of the injected dose per gram of tissue. When all free epsilon amino groups of the poly-L-lysine were completely substituted with DTPA, adrenal uptake was 3.4 times lower, indicating the importance of free amino groups. MRI showed that a dose of 0.08 mmol Gd/kg was sufficient to enhance signal intensity of rodent adrenal glands 186 percent 3 hours after injection. Fluorescence microscopy and autoradiography demonstrated that the agent accumulated primarily in the adrenal cortex. The cellular uptake mechanism of this compound has not yet been fully determined.

Conceivable disadvantages of modified poly-L-lysine drug carriers are their relatively high cost and the uncertainty of the intracellular fate of the macromolecule. Although poly-L-lysine is thought to be degradable into lysine monomers, the in vivo function of the intact polymer is largely unexplored. Further studies are therefore required to investigate molecular pathways, intracellular degradation, excretion, and cellular toxicity. In parallel to the evaluation of poly-L-lysine derivatives, alternative agents targeted to the adrenal glands are being studied (e.g., carboxylic acid derivatives of polyethyleneimine).

## Pancreas

One of the most common problems encountered in pancreatic imaging is the inability to consistently detect small tumors in symptomatic patients. Therefore a MRI contrast agent is needed to improve tumor detection. Accumulation of MRI contrast agents in pancreatic tissue has been reported for two compounds: MION-CCK and Mn-DPDP.

Cholecystokinin (CCK) binds to pancreatic acinar cells and is subsequently internalized and transported to the endoplasmatic reticulum. MION-CCK hypothetically undergoes a similar uptake mechanism and thus accumulates in the pancreas. Preclinical studies have shown that pancreatic uptake of MION-CCK can be competitively blocked with proglumide, a CCK receptor antagonist. After IV administration of MION-CCK to rats, signal intensity of pancreas decreases in a dose-dependent fashion. MION-CCK is likely to remain an experimental MRI probe, because of its relatively low accumulation in pancreatic tissue.

Mn-DPDP, a label originally developed for hepatobiliary imaging, has been shown to increase signal intensity of the pancreas for a prolonged period (>6 hours after injection). The mechanism by which this enhancement occurs is largely unknown. Further clinical studies are required to determine the diagnostic value of Mn-DPDP for pancreatic imaging.

## Abdominal Vasculature

The most common indications for abdominal angiography are (1) preoperative evaluation of tumor neovascularity, (2) evaluation of abdominal aneurysms and atherosclerotic disease including renal artery stenosis, (3) detection of bleeding sites, and (4) workup of intestinal ischemia. Although MR angiography (MRA) without the use of contrast agents has made vast progress in the last years, the quality of evaluations has to improve considerably to be comparable to conventional angiography. One dramatic improvement can be achieved by decreasing blood T1 relaxation times through contrast agents whose distribution volume is limited to the vascular space. Various contrast agents have been tested: Gd-DTPA poly-L-lysine, Gd-DTPA dextran, or Gd-DTPA albumin. Unfortunately none of these agents seems perfect for angiographic purposes, either because of short blood half-life, high background activity (i.e., interstitial leakage), or because of tissue accumulation (liver, spleen).

An optimal intravascular MRI contrast agent should have (1) exclusive intravascular distribution volume with slow blood clearance, (2) high molecular relaxivity, and (3) low toxicity with no potential for immunogenicity. We have recently synthesized such macromolecular polymeric agents by shielding surface Gd-DTPA groups from opsonization and accumulation in the reticuloendothelial system (RES). This shielding was achieved by grafting methoxypolyethyleneglycol succinate (MPEG) onto poly-L-lysine Gd-DTPA. MPEG-derivatized conjugates were shown to retain high molecular relaxivities and have an extended blood half-life of 6 to 24 hours. Because these agents do not significantly accumulate in the interstitial space or the RES as unconjugated polylysine, dextran, or albumin, a significant difference in T1 between vessels and surrounding tissues can be achieved.

MRI feasibility studies have shown excellent retention of MPEG conjugates in the vascular space in rats and rabbits, and as a result small vessels could be consistently visualized by MRI. Compared with established MRA sequences, this class of contrast agent also consistently allowed visualization of renal arteries in rabbits, improved visualization of stenotic vessels in a model of femoral artery stenosis, and demonstration of tumor neovascularity and tumor supply. These results indicate that MRA with an optimal intravascular contrast agent greatly improves vessel delineation.

## Tumor-Specific Imaging

Imaging of pelvic and abdominal malignancies is of considerable clinical importance. MRI particularly lacks sensitivity for the detection of pelvic and colorectal tumors. Only initial feasibility studies have evaluated the use of tumor-specific contrast agents. Several studies have evaluated the use of porphyrins to improve tumor detection. Achievable tumor-to-surrounding-tissue ratios with these compounds are often low, and tumors do not seem to enhance uniformly. Similarly, accumulation of poly-L-lysine Gd-DTPA has been observed in some tumors.

Development of pharmaceuticals that would accumulate in tumor via binding to tumor-associated antigens has been pursued in nuclear medicine with mixed results. Development of similar labels for MRI of tumors is considerably more difficult. Although antibody MRI of tumors has been shown to be possible under ideal circumstances, considerable difficulties are expected in a clinical setting. First, the threshold of detectability of radionuclides is several orders of magnitude lower than that of magnetic labels, requiring large doses of antibodies. Second, expression of tumor-associated antigens is variable and may be absent in some malignancies. Third, motion artifacts often degrade the image quality of MR images; this is a particular concern for colorectal malignancies. Finally, concomitant nonspecific uptake of antibody compounds by the RES of liver, spleen, and lymph nodes would limit the use of these agents in the RES organs.

Despite the problems associated with tumor antibody imaging, MRI contrast agents labeled with antibodies for nontumor applications have been successfully used. Targeting of antibodies to normal tissues rather than to malignant tissues has the advantage of a more uniform antigen expression. For example, antimyosin antibodies attached to MION or T1 labels have been used for MRI of myocardial infarction.

## Suggested Reading

Brasch R. New directions in the development of MR contrast media. Radiology 1992; 183:1–11.

Weissleder R, Bogdanov A, Papisov M. Drug targeting in magnetic resonance imaging. Magn Reson Q 1992; 8:55–63.

Weissleder R, Lee AS, Fischman AJ, et al. MR antibody imaging: Polyclonal human IgG labelled with polymeric iron oxide. Radiology 1991; 181:245–249.

Weissleder R, Reimer P, Lee AS, et al. MR receptor imaging: Ultrasmall iron oxide particles targeted to asialoglycoprotein receptors. AJR 1990; 155:1161–1167.

# Imaging of Liver Cancer: CT, MRI, and Ultrasonography

*SANJAY SAINI, M.D.*

## Clinical Problem

Two major objectives of diagnostic imaging of the liver in the oncologic patient population are (1) detection of hepatic tumors (primary or metastatic) and (2) their tissue characterization. For example, detection of liver metastases from colon carcinoma is of critical importance in patient management, because surgical resection is considered if four or fewer metastases are present and are limited to one lobe of the liver. However, because of the high prevalence of benign liver tumors (estimated to be in excess of 20 percent in adults), the goal of diagnostic radiology cannot be limited to the detection of focal liver lesions. Therefore tissue characterization of liver tumors for differentiation of benign masses from malignant tumors is an equally important concurrent goal for diagnostic radiology.

This chapter provides an algorithm for the diagnostic workup of patients with known or suspected liver tumors.

## Survey Evaluation

Survey of the liver for metastases is commonly performed in patients with known malignancy (most commonly colon, breast, lung, and pancreas). However, in these patients detection of liver tumors and extrahepatic metastases is equally important. Therefore the goal of diagnostic imaging in this setting is to perform a global evaluation of the abdomen-pelvis, which includes the liver but is not limited to it. This evaluation should be undertaken with a contrast-enhanced computed tomographic (CT) scan. Although the sensitivity of CT, magnetic resonance imaging (MRI), and ultrasonography for the identification of patients with liver metastases is highly similar (~85 percent), CT is preferred because it is superior to both MRI and ultrasonography in evaluation of the extrahepatic peritoneal cavity (bowel, mesentery, retroperitoneum). Comparatively lower cost and wider availability are additional advantages of CT over MRI as a test for screening the abdomen-pelvis (including liver) in patients with cancer.

Adherence to proper CT technique is critical and requires incremental dynamic scanning so that the entire liver is imaged within 3 minutes of the initiation of contrast infusion (>150 ml of 60 percent contrast material given at 2 ml/sec with a 30 to 45 second delay). In patients with so-called hypervascular malignancies (carcinoid, melanoma, islet cell, breast, pheochromocytoma, and hepatocellular carcinoma), a noncontrast liver CT scan should precede the contrast-enhanced evaluation. For patients unable to undergo an incremental dynamic-contrast enhanced CT scan as a result of, for example, iodine allergy or renal insufficiency, an MRI should supplement the noncontrast CT study for evaluation of the liver. In addition, when fatty infiltration of the liver is observed with a CT scan, an MRI study is helpful for evaluation of the liver.

The liver MRI study is performed with both T1- and T2-weighted imaging techniques. The T1-weighted images are excellent for display of normal anatomy and lesion detection. These images are usually obtained with a spin-echo pulse sequence. The critical parameter that influences image quality and lesion detection is TE which must be kept as short as possible. If the $TE_{min}$ is longer than 15 msec, lesion-liver contrast will be limited and the ability to detect focal liver lesions will be lowered. Signal intensity difference between spleen and liver should be used to predict lesion-liver contrast. Increasingly the spin-echo T1-weighted images are being replaced with breath-hold gradient-echo (GE) images. GE pulse sequences provide equivalent if not superior lesion-liver contrast, much shorter scan time, and images that are nearly free of artifacts from gross physiologic motion (e.g., breathing). On GE pulse sequences, $TE_{min}$ and flip-angle are the important imaging parameters. TE must be kept under 5 msec and flip-angles of 60° to 90° can be used. T2-weighted images are useful for confirming lesions observed or suspected on T1-weighted images and, more importantly, for tissue characterization (discussed later).

## Staging Evaluation

The staging evaluation is different from the screening evaluation because the staging study is limited to the liver and is performed for a more accurate assessment of focal liver lesions (number and location). Invariably this evaluation is performed when surgical resection of extrahepatic (e.g., pancreatic cancer) or hepatic (e.g., metastases) malignancy is being contemplated. CT with arterial portography (CT-AP) is recognized to be the most sensitive test for detecting individual liver lesions. This imaging technique is based on the fact that liver neoplasms are perfused by neovascularity that arises from the hepatic artery. Therefore liver enhancement with contrast delivered to it via the portal vein (superior mesenteric artery injection of 75 to 120 ml of 60 percent contrast material given at 0.5 ml/sec with a 20 second delay) allows selective enhancement of normal liver, which increases tumor-liver density difference. The sensitivity for detection of liver metastases with CT-AP is approximately 85 percent. In comparison, noncontrast MRI detects about 67 percent of liver lesions and contrast-enhanced CT detects only 50 percent. When perfusion defects are suspected on the CT-AP evaluation, a 4 to 6 hour delayed CT study is required to clarify the CT-AP images to distinguish them from metastases. All these imaging techniques are particularly limited in detecting small surface and central hepatic metastases ($<0.5$ cm) for which surgical inspection and intraoperative ultrasonography are recommended.

## Liver Cancer Characterization

Metastases, hepatocellular carcinoma (HCC), hemangiomas, and cysts constitute the majority of liver tumors that need to be differentiated. Tissue characterization is most commonly required when evaluating incidental liver masses. However, this is an especially important function in patients with cancer in whom screening or staging evaluations show liver lesions. If patient management will change depending on the etiology of some or all liver lesions (i.e., cancer vs. incidental coexisting benign liver tumors), tissue characterization of focal liver masses is mandatory. For the characterization of liver lesions that are suspected of being simple liver cysts, liver ultrasonography should supplement the survey evaluation. For characterization of hemangiomas and solid primary liver tumors, MRI has emerged as the diagnostic modality of choice. However, if imaging characteristics are atypical, percutaneous biopsy (for suspected malignant lesions) or follow-up imaging (for suspected benign lesions) should be considered.

At MRI T2-weighted images are primarily used for tissue characterization of liver tumors. On heavily T2-weighted images (TR $>3{,}000$ msec; TE $>150$ msec) the signal intensity of hemangiomas (and cysts) is similar to that of the cerebrospinal fluid, whereas the signal intensity of solid liver tumors mimics splenic signal intensity. This differentiation is not possible on T1-weighted images (noncontrast), where hemangiomas and metastases appear similar, both being hypointense to normal liver. Administration of gadolinium chelates may also aid in differentiation of liver masses. On postgadolinium T1-weighted images, hemangiomas demonstrate nodular peripheral enhancement in the early post-bolus infusion period and complete enhancement in the delayed equilibrium phase (slow wash-in and slow wash-out). MRI can also aid in the diagnosis of focal nodular hyperplasia (FNH). Approximately 10 percent of these benign liver tumors appear isointense to normal liver on T1- and T2-weighted images and in addition have a central scar that is hypointense on T1-weighted images and hyperintense on T2-weighted images. Often these tumors are suspected when a central scar is noted, but nonisointensity on either or both T1- and T2-weighted images hinders a definitive diagnosis. In this situation dynamic imaging after gadolinium chelate injection is most useful, because these tumors show intense enhancement in the first 60 seconds, which disappears just as rapidly (fast wash-in and fast wash-out). The central scar enhances on equilibrium phase images.

Like FNH, malignant liver tumors, including hypervascular liver metastases and hepatocellular carcinoma, also show similar intense enhancement early after gadolinium chelate injection. However, their appearance on noncontrast images is different from that of FNH. The signal intensity of metastases mimics that of the spleen. Hepatocellular carcinomas generally arise in patients with cirrhosis and can appear isointense to liver or hyperintense to liver on T1-weighted images (from steatosis and/or copper deposition). Slow-growing hepatocellular carcinomas possess a peripheral scar that is hypointense on T1- and T2-weighted images, but does enhance on delayed post–gadolinium chelate–enhanced images.

## Future Directions

Contrast-enhanced MRI with tissue-specific contrast agents is likely to emerge as the preferred modality for the detection and characterization of focal liver tumors. For example, liver imaging with reticuloendothelial and hepatobiliary contrast agents has yielded diagnostic sensitivity (lesion detection rate) similar to CT-AP evaluations. In addition, these contrast agents can produce alteration in signal intensity of focal liver lesions when tumors possess reticuloendothelial (FNH) or hepatobiliary (FNH, HCC, liver cell adenoma) cellular function. Hence MRI contrast agents may add further diagnostic specificity to the diagnostic evaluation.

## Historical Perspective

During the last 10 to 15 years, ultrasonography has experienced a diminishing role for the evaluation of liver cancer. Although ultrasonography is an effective survey evaluation, it suffers from a limited potential to evaluate the extrahepatic abdomen and the inability to characterize solid liver tumors (even with color-flow Doppler). However, an equally important reason accounting for decreased usefulness of ultrasonography is the much greater demand on physician time associated with a careful ultrasonography evaluation (e.g., from 15 to 30 min for ultrasonography vs 3 to 5 min for CT).

The declining role of nuclear scintigraphy is due to other reasons: a much lower image resolution, inability to evaluate the extrahepatic abdomen, and the need for multiple imaging tests for tissue characterization.

## Discussion

A survey evaluation of the liver (and extrahepatic and hepatic abdomen-pelvis) should be performed with contrast-enhanced CT (incremental bolus dynamic technique). A preoperative staging evaluation of the liver requires CT-AP. In specific cases this may be supplemented with a delayed CT scan to distinguish tumors from perfusion defects and MRI to characterize newly discovered liver lesions. Characterization of primary liver tumors should be performed with MRI, with which gadolinium chelates may allow a more tissue-specific diagnosis. In the near future, MRI with tissue-specific hepatobiliary or reticuloendothelial contrast agents may replace the traditional survey and tissue characterization evaluations. Percutaneous liver biopsy should be performed when results of noninvasive imaging tests are inconclusive.

## Suggested Reading


Ferrucci JT. Liver tumor imaging: Current concepts. AJR 1990; 155:473–484.

Foley WD. Dynamic hepatic CT. Radiology 1989; 170:617–622.

Heiken JP, Weyman PJ, Lee JKT, et al. Detection of focal hepatic masses: Prospective evaluation with CT, delayed CT, CT during arterial portography, and MR imaging. Radiology 1989; 171:47–51.

Karhunen PJ. Benign hepatic tumours and like conditions in men. J Clin Pathol 1986; 140:695–700.

Lee MJ, Saini S, Hamm B, et al. Focal nodular hyperplasia: MR findings in 35 proven cases. AJR 1991; 156:317–320.

Nelson RC, Chezmar JL. Diagnostic approach to hepatic hemangiomas. Radiology 1990; 176:11–12.

Rifkin MD, Rosato FE, Baruck M, et al. Intra-operative ultrasound of the liver: An important adjunctive tool for decision making in the operating room. Ann Surg 1987; 205:466–471.

Rummeny E, Saini S, Wittenberg J, et al. Pictorial essay: Magnetic resonance imaging of the liver. AJR 1989; 152:63–72.

Saini S. Contrast enhanced MR imaging of the liver. Radiology 1992; 182:12–14.

Saini S, Modic MT, Hamm B, Hahn PF. Advances in contrast enhanced MR imaging. AJR 1991; 156:235–254.

# GENITOURINARY RADIOLOGY

## Transvaginal Ultrasonography in Gynecologic Disorders

*ARTHUR C. FLEISCHER, M.D.*

Transvaginal ultrasonography (TVS) affords detailed depiction of the uterus and ovaries. The proximity of the probe to these organs is usually advantageous, but in some situations lesions can be missed if TVS is used alone. Thus this chapter emphasizes the selective use of TVS to enhance evaluation of uterine and adnexal disorders. Those sonographic features that can be used for enhancing diagnostic accuracy are emphasized.

### Scanning Technique and Instrumentation

The transducer probes used for TVS utilize relatively high frequencies (>5 MHz) that afford detailed delineation but for only limited (within 10 cm) fields of view. The technique with which these probes are used varies from the standard transabdominal approach, which is usually used with a distended urinary bladder, to the transvaginal study, which is organ-oriented or focused on a particular area of interest. Images are optimized by exerting pressure with the vaginally introduced probe and with an abdominal palpating hand and/or by asking the patient to press on her lower abdomen (Fig. 1). For this maneuver, the patient's bladder should be completely nondistended. During the procedure, one should observe for appropriate movement of the pelvic organs when moderate pressure is exerted with the probe and abdominal palpation.

There are a variety of transvaginal transducer/probe configurations. These include those using a single-element oscillating transducer, curved phase array, or linear phased array (Fig. 2). TV transducer/probes vary according to their footprint size and scanning head configuration. For most applications, curved phased arrays are preferred, since they afford excellent fields of view and lateral and axial resolution (Fig. 3).

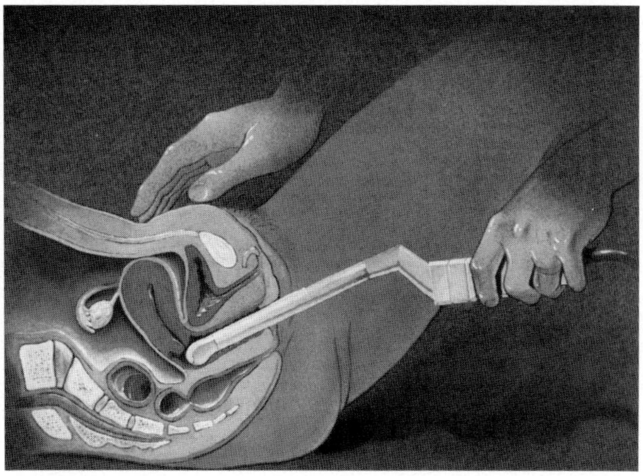

**FIGURE 1** Diagram shows use of TV probe with abdominal palpation (drawn by Paul Gross, M.S.).

TV transducer/probes capable of color Doppler sonography are also useful in several selected gynecologic evaluations. These probes afford delineation of vessels surrounding the uterus and ovaries as well as those within these organs. Color Doppler sonography allows identification of vessels for placement of the sample volume to obtain a Doppler frequency spectrum. The spectrum can be analyzed according to the relative resistance to forward flow by parameters such as the pulsatility index and resistance index. Improved waveform

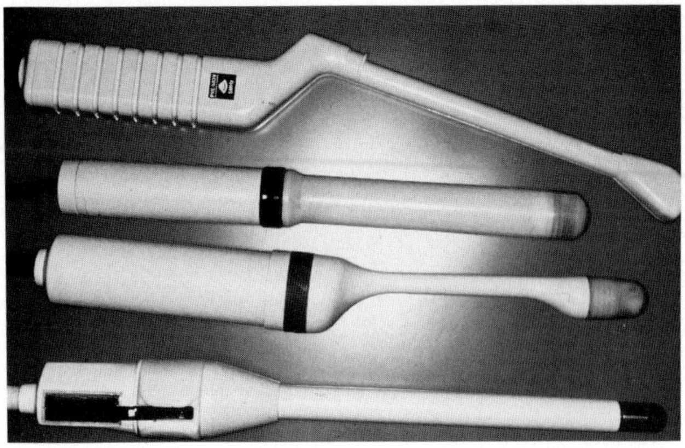

**FIGURE 2** Photograph of a variety of transvaginal transducer/probes; from top to bottom: Toshiba 5.0 MHz curvilinear probe; Siemens 5.0 and 6.5 MHz mechanical sector; Toshiba 7.5 MHz single-element oscillating probe; Diasonics 7.5 MHz single-element oscillating probe.

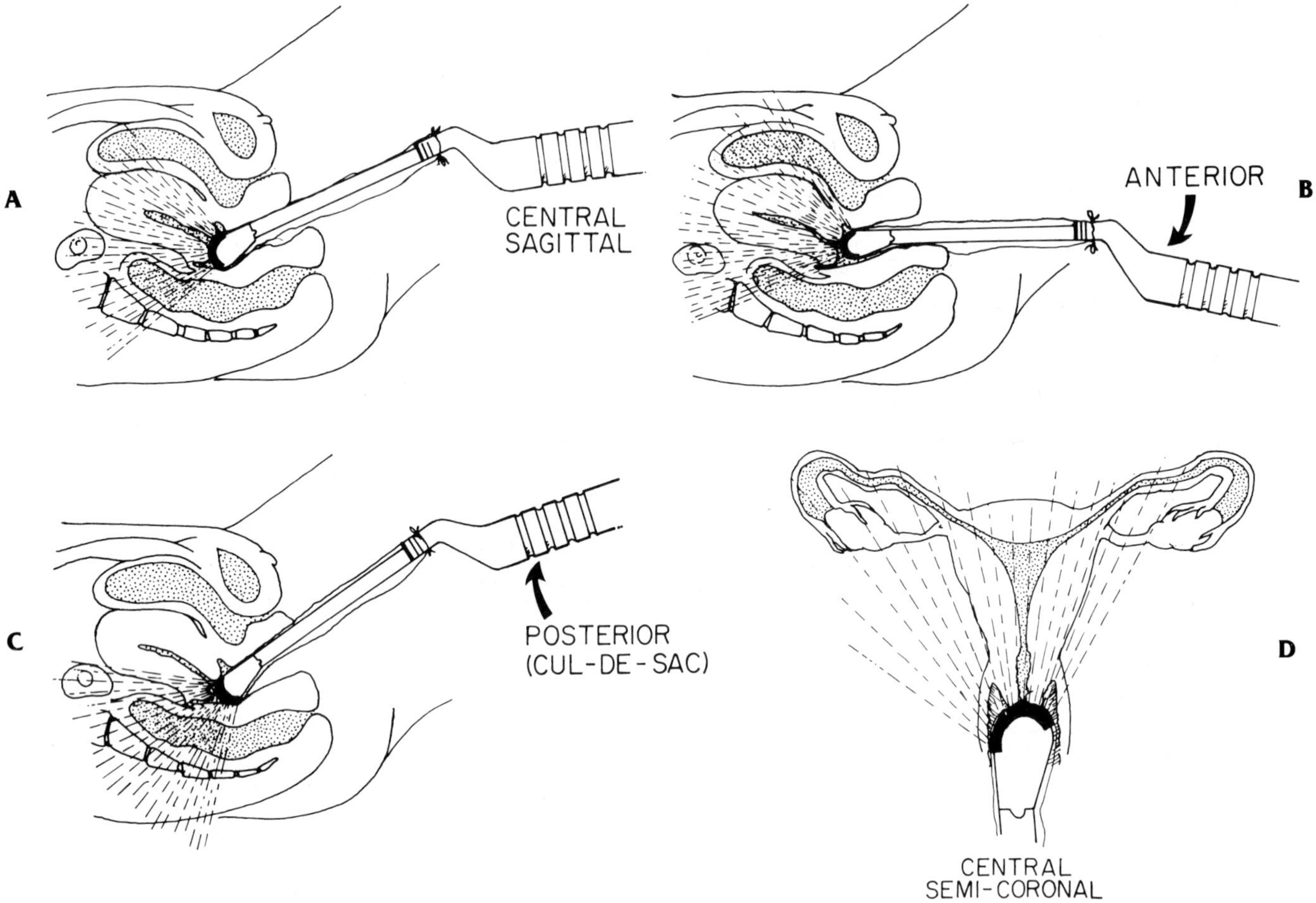


**FIGURE 3** Scan planes used in TVS. *A,* Sagittal midline. *B,* Anterior sagittal. *C,* Sagittal posterior (cul-de-sac). *D,* Coronal.

analysis may also yield better information about parenchymal flow.

## Differential Diagnosis of Pelvic Masses

TVS affords categorization of pelvic masses according to their

1. Location (uterine, ovarian, tubal, or other) and size (small [< 5 cm], medium [5 to 10 cm], and large [> 10 cm]).
2. Internal consistency (serous fluid, fluid with low-level echoes, smooth vs. nodular wall, complex, or solid).
3. Associated findings (such as intraperitoneal cul-de-sac fluid).

Utilizing these parameters and integrating clinical information can usually yield a sufficiently specific diagnosis.

I prefer using TVS as an adjunct to transabdominal scanning (TAS) (Fig. 4). TAS of the pelvis allows global depiction of the uterus and ovaries, whereas TVS is confined to the pelvis and may indeed miss lesions located superior to the urinary bladder (Fig. 5). Several studies have shown that use of TVS in this manner improves diagnostic accuracy in 60 to 70 percent of

E

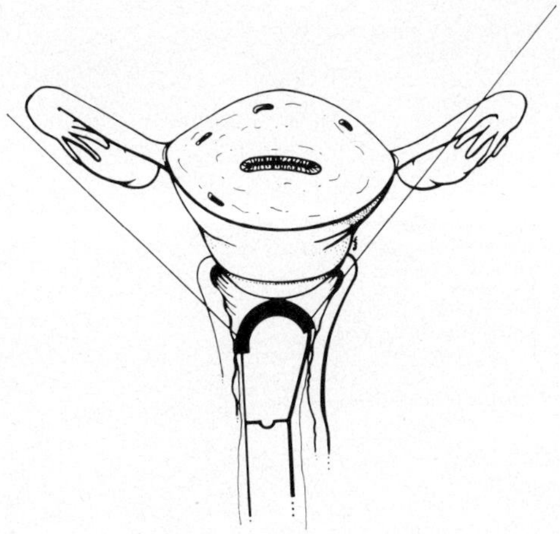

F

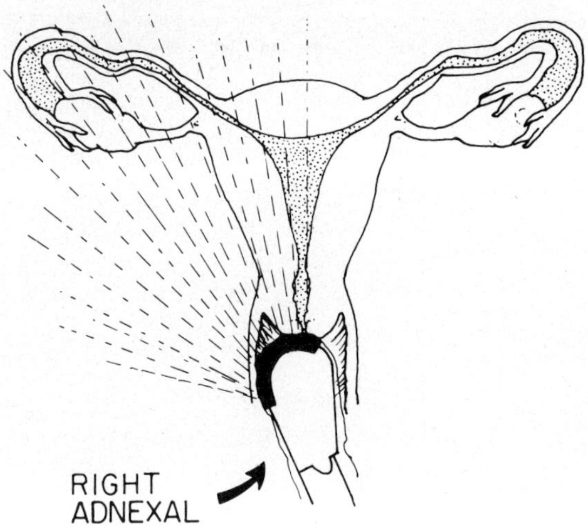


G

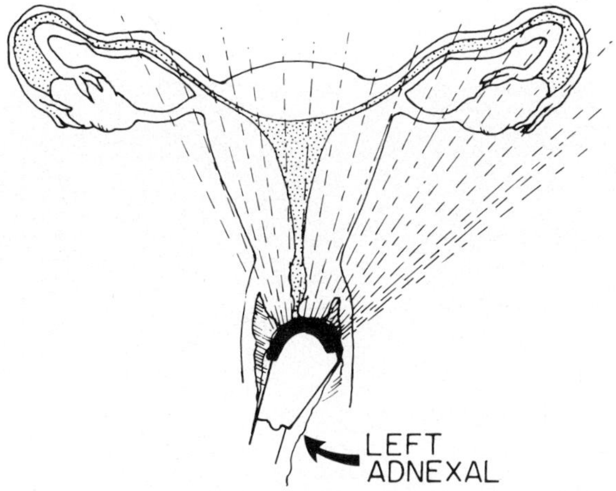


**FIGURE 3, cont'd** *E,* Short axis or semiaxial. *F,* Right adnexal. *G,* Left adnexal.

A

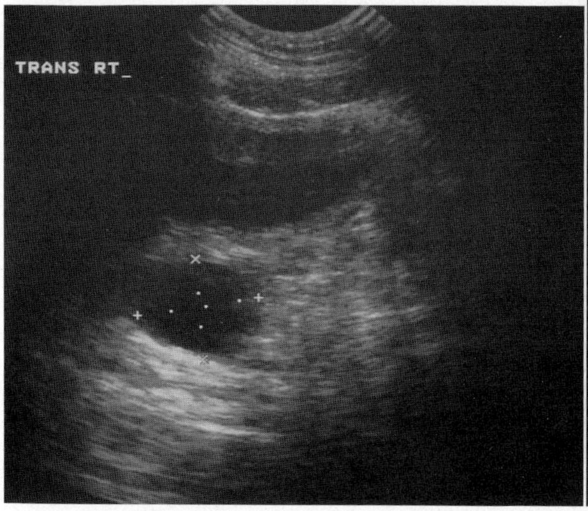


B

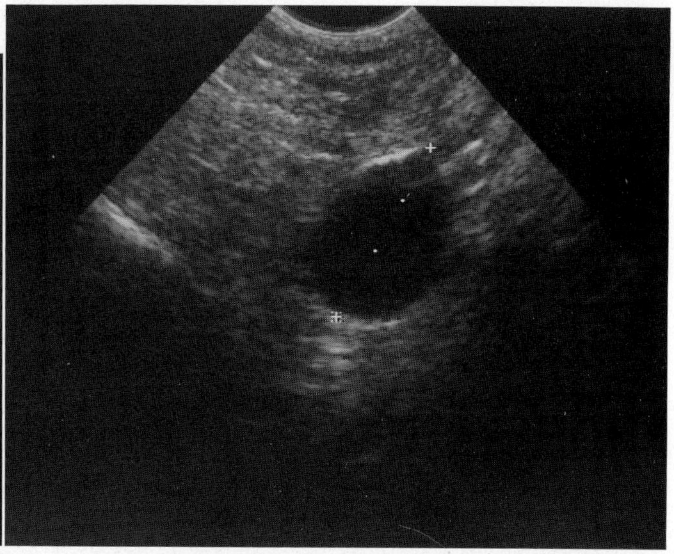

**FIGURE 4** TVS as adjunct to TAS. *A,* TAS shows a nonspecific 3 cm cystic right adnexal mass. *B,* TVS shows that the cyst (*between cursors*) is within the right ovary, thereby confirming the sonographic impression of a benign, simple ovarian cyst.

cases. TVS may not need to be used if the uterus and ovaries are adequately documented with TAS.

The specific areas where TVS is most helpful include evaluation of tubal disease, endometrial or myometrial disorders, and differentiation of bowel from adnexal pathology (Fig. 6).

Transvaginal color Doppler sonography (TV-CDS) has been shown to be accurate in distinguishing benign from malignant ovarian lesions and in the diagnosis of adnexal torsion (Figs. 7, 8). Thus it should be used in evaluating any adnexal mass thought to be ovarian or when adnexal torsion is

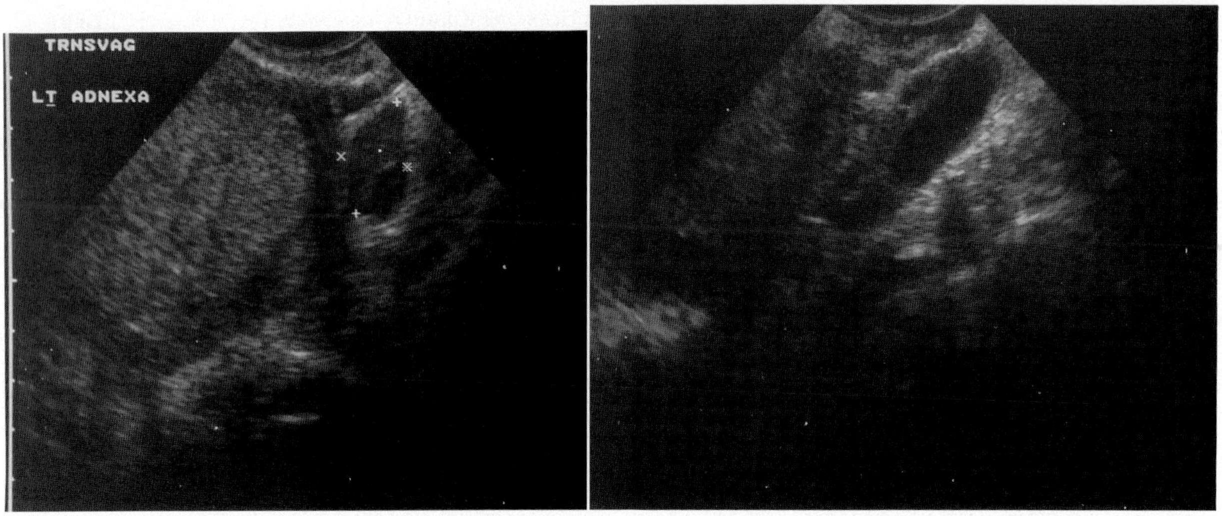


**FIGURE 5** TVS detection of lesion not observed on TAS. *A,* A 1 cm cystic area adjacent to the left ovary (*within cursor*). *B,* The same mass, imaged in long axis, shows the fusiform shape of this paratubal cyst.

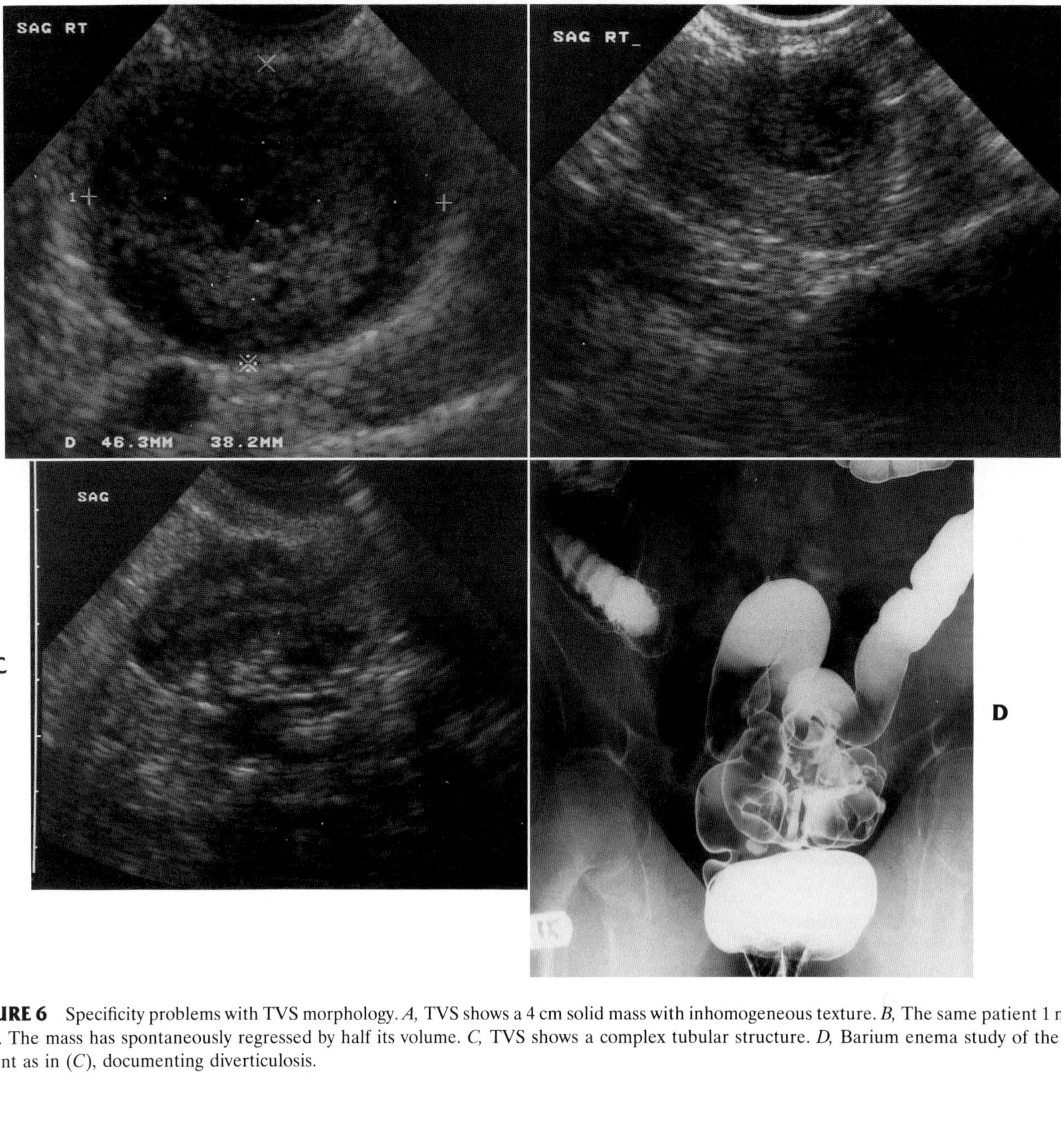


**FIGURE 6** Specificity problems with TVS morphology. *A,* TVS shows a 4 cm solid mass with inhomogeneous texture. *B,* The same patient 1 month later. The mass has spontaneously regressed by half its volume. *C,* TVS shows a complex tubular structure. *D,* Barium enema study of the same patient as in (*C*), documenting diverticulosis.

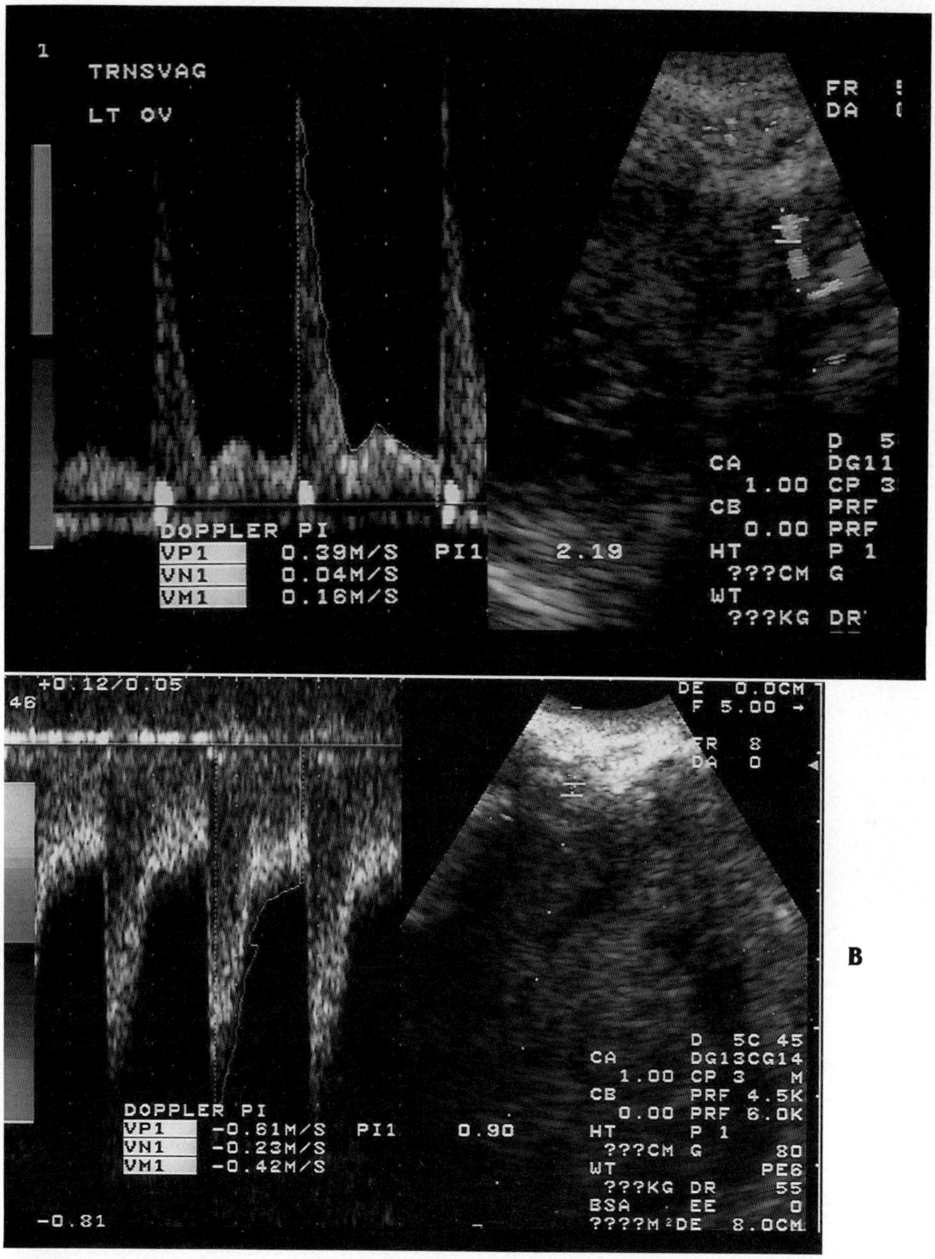


A

B

**FIGURE 7** Improved specificity with TV-CDS in morphologically similar masses (*reproduced in black and white*). *A,* Triplex TV-CDS shows high-impedance flow within a hemorrhagic endometrioma. *B,* A morphologically similar mass shows low-impedance high-velocity flow in a papillary serous cystadenocarcinoma.

A

B

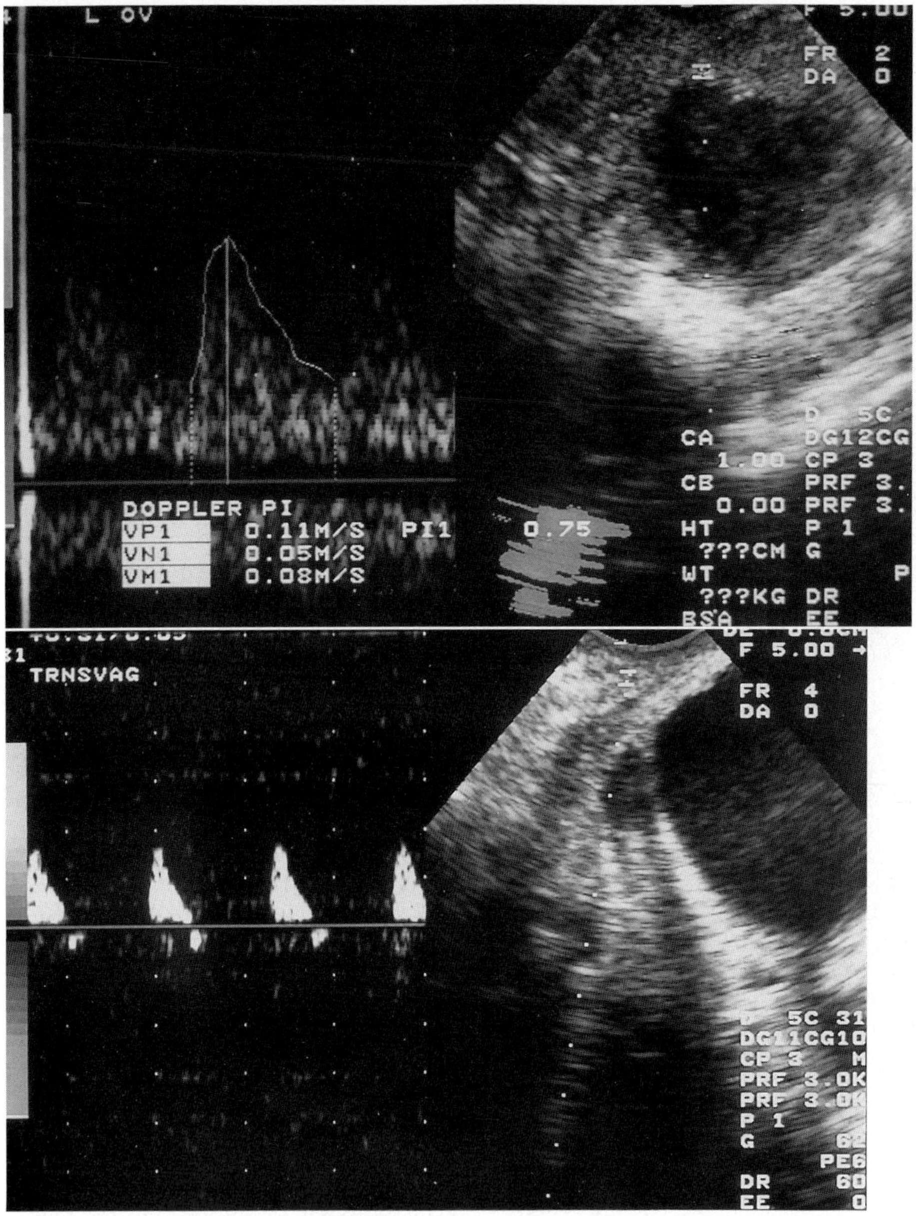


**FIGURE 8** Transvaginal color Doppler sonograms of small ovarian vessels (*reproduced in black and white*). *A,* A 3 cm papillary shows cystadenocarcinoma with low-impedance flow. *B,* This torsed hemorrhagic cyst shows a "spikey" systolic waveform and no diastolic flow.

suspected. Similarly, TV-CDS can be used to assess the vascularity of uterine fibroids and to evaluate patients with thickened endometrium.

## Endometrial and Myometrial Disorders

TVS affords detailed evaluation of the endometrium and myometrium. It is particularly helpful in evaluating the extent of tumor invasion in patients with known endometrial cancer or in evaluation of uterine fibroids before medical treatment (Fig. 9). It may be used to monitor women receiving hormone replacement therapy or tamoxifen. In general, an endometrial thickness (width) of over 6 mm should be considered abnormal, and endometrial biopsy should be performed to determine the histologic nature of the abnormality. If a patient with postmenopausal bleeding has an endometrium less than 5 mm, endometrial biopsy may be precluded, since these patients typically have an atrophic endometrium or senile endometritis.

Transvaginal CDS may be useful in evaluation of women with thickened endometria, since areas of increased vascularity typically indicate tumor. However, these patients should nevertheless undergo biopsy. As a generalization, the primary role of TVS of the endometrium is identification of women who may be spared endometrial biopsy. Thickened endometria detected by TVS usually require histologic confirmation.

## Early Detection of Ovarian Cancer

TVS has the potential for early detection of ovarian carcinoma. This can be accomplished by using either morphologic criteria or color Doppler detection of neovascularity. Up to 15 percent of postmenopausal women may have a cystic adnexal mass. The vast majority of these are benign and, in fact, may even regress. However, a significant percentage may also represent early-stage ovarian carcinoma, which, if detected, could be associated with an excellent prognosis.

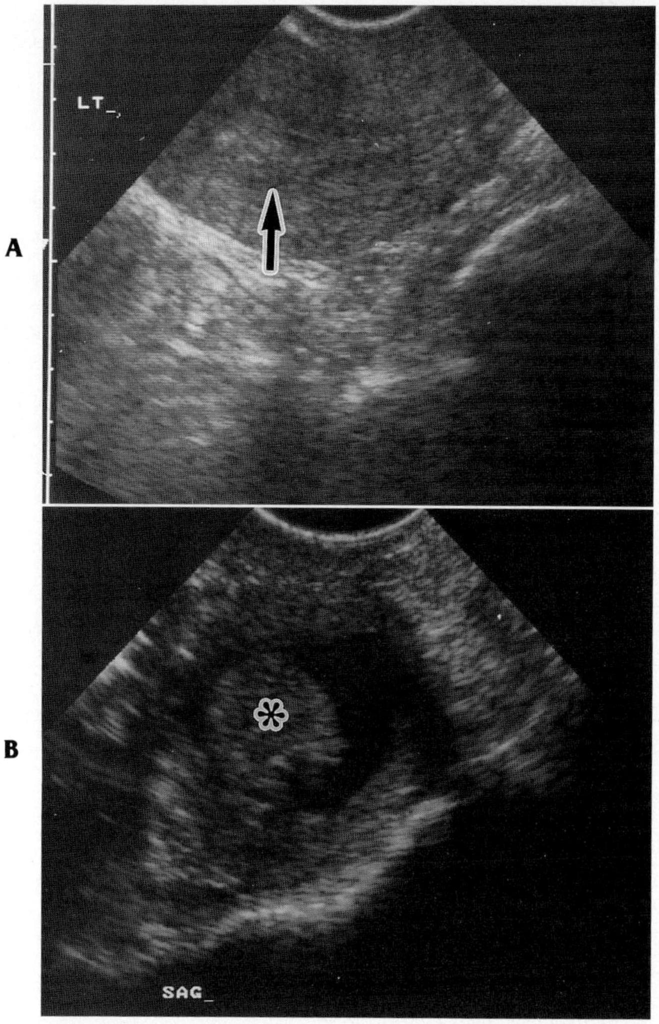


**FIGURE 9** TVS of endometrial disorders. *A,* Moderately invasive endometrial carcinoma shows disruption of the subendometrial halo (*arrow*). *B,* Polypoid tumor (∗) surrounded by fluid representing an exophytic endometrial cancer.

Screening with TVS of the general postmenopausal population, however, is impractical since the incidence of the disease is relatively low. However, evaluation of patients with risk factors with TVS as a primary test, followed by TV-CDS seems to be efficacious and practical. The detection of ovarian tumor by TV-CDS is based on the recognition of tumor neovascularity, which is characterized by relatively high diastolic flow (see Figs. 7, 8). This finding is thought to reflect the characteristics of tumor neovascularity, such as the lack of a muscular media and a sinusoid type of arrangement of vessels within tumors.

## Evaluation of Tubal Disease

Although the normal tube is only infrequently delineated with TVS, evaluation of certain tubal abnormalities is possible. Hydrosalpinges, which appear as fusiform cystic structures, can be differentiated from tubo-ovarian abscesses. With the injection of an albumin-like contrast agent into the tube, tubal patency can be assessed.

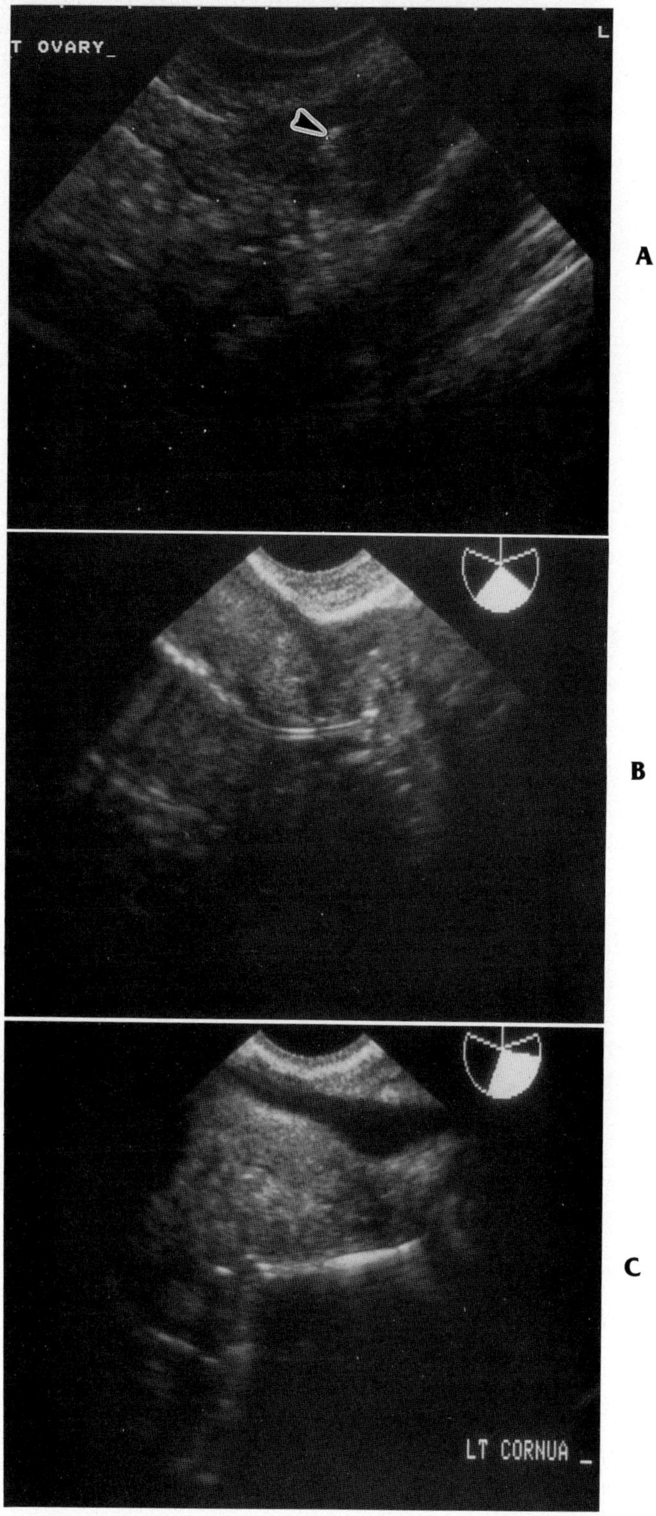


**FIGURE 10** TVS-guided procedures. *A,* Aspiration of a mature follicle. The needle tip (*arrowhead*) followed the projected needle path. *B,* Tubal cannulation for dilatation shows initial placement of the outer catheter within the cornual portion of the tube. *C,* Same as (*B*) after further introduction of the catheter into the proximal position of the left tube.

## TVS-Guided Procedures

TVS affords accurate guidance of ovarian follicle and cyst aspiration, abscess drainage, and other gynecologic procedures involving directed needle or catheter placement. This is accomplished using a needle guide placed over the shaft of a transvaginal transducer/probe (see Fig. 9). In some patients with medical problems who cannot undergo surgery, guided aspiration of the cystic mass is recommended (Fig. 10). Lesions that should not be aspirated include masses with internal septal or nodular walls, those containing echogenic material that may represent sebum, or mucinous material. A CA-125 serum test should also be drawn before the procedure to minimize the chance of inadvertent aspiration of an ovarian tumor.

Although there is *no* report of their spread after fine-needle aspiration of a malignant ovarian tumor, the possibility exists that fine-needle aspiration may precipitate eventual rupture. In addition, cytologic evaluation of the fluid may be misleading or inaccurate. Therefore one should carefully weigh the potential risks and benefits of such a procedure before deciding whether or not to aspirate under TVS.

## Suggested Reading


Andolf A, Jorgensen C. A prospective comparison of transabdominal and transvaginal ultrasound with surgical findings in gynecologic disease. J Ultrasound Med 1990; 9:71–75.

Bourne TH. Transvaginal color Doppler in gynecology. Ultrasound Obstet Gynecol 1991; 1:1–15.

Bourne TH, Campbell S, Steer CV, et al. Detection of endometrial cancer by transvaginal ultrasonography with color flow imaging and blood flow analysis: A preliminary report. Gynecol Oncol 1991; 40:253–259.

Bourne TH, Campbell S, Steer CV, et al. Transvaginal colour flow imaging: A possible new screening technique for ovarian cancer. Br Med J 1989; 299:1367–1370.

Bourne TH, Whitehead MI, Campbell S, et al. Ultrasound screening for familial ovarian cancer. Gynecol Oncol 1991; 43:92–97.

Coleman BG, Arger PH, Grumbach K, et al. Transvaginal and transabdominal sonography: Prospective comparison. Radiology 1988; 168:639–643.

Fleischer A, Gordon A, Entman S. Transabdominal and transvaginal sonography of pelvic masses. J Ultrasound Med Biol 1989; 15:529–533.

Fleischer AC, Rodgers WH, Rao BK, et al. Assessment of ovarian tumor vascularity with transvaginal color Doppler sonography. J Ultrasound Med 1991; 10:563–568.

Goldstein SR, Nachtigall M, Snyder JR, Nachtigall L. Endometrial assessment by vaginal ultrasonography before endometrial sampling in patients with postmenopausal bleeding. Am J Obstet Gynecol 1990; 163:119–123.

Gordon A, Fleischer A, Reed G. Depth of myometrial invasion in endometrial carcinoma: Pre-operative assessment by transvaginal sonography. Gynecol Oncol 1990; 34:321–327.

Granberg S, Norstrom A, Wikland M. Tumors in the lower pelvis as imaged by vaginal sonography. Gynecol Oncol 1990; 37:224–229.

Granberg S, Wikland M, Karlsson B, et al. Endometrial thickness as measured by endovaginal ultrasonography for identifying endometrial abnormality. Am J Obstet Gynecol 1991; 164:47–52.

Kurjak A, Zalud I, Alfirevic Z. Evaluation of adnexal masses with transvaginal color ultrasound. J Ultrasound Med 1991; 10:295–297.

Kurjak A, Zalud I, Jurkovic D, et al. Transvaginal color flow Doppler for the assessment of pelvic circulation. Acta Obstet Gynecol Scand 1989; 68:131–135.

Lande IM, Hill JC, Cosco FE, Kator NN. Adnexal and cul-de-sac abnormalities: Transvaginal sonography. Radiology 1988; 166:325–332.

Lin MC, Gosink BB, Wolf SI, et al. Endometrial thickness after menopause: Effect of hormone replacement. Radiology 1991; 180:427–432.

Matta WHM, Stabile I, Shaw RW, Campbell S. Doppler assessment of uterine blood flow changes in patients with fibroids receiving the gonadotropin releasing hormone agonist buserelin. Fertil Steril 1988; 49:1083.

Mendelson EB, Bohm-Velez M, Joseph N, Neiman HL. Gynecologic imaging: Comparison of transabdominal and transvaginal sonography. Radiology 1988; 66:321–324.

Sassone AM, Timor-Tritsch IE, Artner A, et al. Transvaginal sonographic characterization of ovarian disease: Evaluation of a new scoring system to predict ovarian malignancy. Obstet Gynecol 1991; 78:70–76.

Schlief R, Deichert U. Hysterosalpingo-contrast sonography of the uterus and fallopian tubes: Results of a clinical trial of a new contrast medium in 120 patients. Radiology 1990; 178:213–215.

Tessler F, Pervella R, Fleischer A, Grant E. Endovaginal sonography of dilated fallopian tubes. AJR 1989; 153:523–525.

Wolf SI, Gosink BB, Feldsman MR, et al. Prevalence of simple adnexal cysts in postmenopausal women. Radiology 1991; 180:65–71.


# MRI of the Female Pelvis

*HEDVIG HRICAK, M.D., Ph.D*

Magnetic resonance imaging (MRI) is gaining acceptance as an important problem-solving modality in the evaluation of the female pelvis. In the evaluation of congenital anomalies and benign pelvic disease, ultrasonography remains the most appropriate initial investigation, and MRI should be reserved for those patients in whom ultrasonography is technically suboptimal or results are equivocal. In the evaluation of malignant neoplasms—namely, endometrial, cervical, and vaginal carcinoma—MRI has become the primary imaging approach. Although computed tomography (CT) remains more widely used in the evaluation of ovarian carcinoma, the introduction of MRI contrast media has expanded the role of MRI in that disease as well.

## Indications, Clinical Utility, and Alternative Technologies

### *Congenital Anomalies*

Hysterosalpingography (HSG) and laparoscopy or surgery have, until now, been the mainstay for the diagnosis of müllerian duct anomalies (MDAs). Ultrasonography, particularly in the pregnant patient, has also been used. Both HSG and ultrasonography have limitations, particularly in the differentiation between septate and bicornuate uteri. MRI has been shown to be an accurate and noninvasive technique for the evaluation of MDAs. Because of its capability for tissue characterization, MRI is particularly useful for patients in whom surgical unification is anticipated. Bicornuate uterus (septum composed of myometrium) requires open-surgical repair, whereas uterus biseptus (septum composed of connective tissue) can be corrected hysteroscopically (hysteroscopic metroplasty). MRI is also helpful in elucidating the etiology of MDA complications (e.g., obstruction).

### *Leiomyomas*

Ultrasonography is the modality of choice in the evaluation of clinically suspected leiomyomas. However, sonography has been reported to result in false-negative results in 22 percent of cases. Ultrasonography is particularly limited when the tumor size is small ( < 2 cm in diameter) or very large, when the uterus is retroverted or duplicated, or when there is coexisting adnexal or pelvic pathology. MRI has been shown to be superior to ultrasonography in the evaluation of uterine leiomyomas, regardless of tumor location or size. The main indications for MRI include: limited or inconclusive ultrasonography evaluation (especially when the lesion origin, being either adnexal or uterine, needs to be clarified); infertile patient; before myomectomy (when the location and size of leiomyomas need to be known); and differentiation between leiomyomas and adenomyosis. Serial MRI can also facilitate assessment of response to hormone analog treatment.

### *Adenomyosis*

Before the advance of MRI, preoperative diagnosis of adenomyosis was not possible. In a patient with clinical suspicions for adenomyosis, MRI should be ordered (1) when the patient has dysfunctional bleeding and an enlarged but otherwise normal uterus on clinical examination and ultrasonography study or (2) when patient counseling concerning surgical treatment options (e.g., myomectomy vs. hysterectomy) is required. Although diffuse adenomyosis is accurately diagnosed with MRI studies, differentiation between adenomyoma (focal adenomyosis) and leiomyoma may be difficult.

### *Carcinoma of the Cervix*

The superiority of MRI over either the clinical examination or CT in the evaluation of cervical carcinoma has been documented. The main advantage of MRI is direct tumor visualization. This permits evaluation of important tumor prognostic factors such as tumor size, depth of stromal invasion, and stage of the disease. In the evaluation of lymph nodes, the accuracy of MRI is similar to that of CT; however, neither modality can differentiate hyperplastic from malignant nodes. The present indications for MRI are as follows: (1) on clinical examination, lesion size is greater than 3 cm in diameter; (2) lesions are located primarily within the endocervical canal, which is difficult to evaluate clinically; (3) possible parametrial extension, which influences the choice of therapy; (4) the patient is pregnant; and (5) before radiation therapy, when tumor volume assessment and locoregional extent are needed for radiation port planning.

### *Endometrial Carcinoma*

Routine surgical staging for patients with endometrial carcinoma is recommended. However, preoperative knowledge of the depth of myometrial invasion, advanced locoregional disease, or presence of lymph node metastasis may obviate surgical exploration, because in those patients primary radiation therapy is a better treatment option. Many studies document the inherent value of MRI in the evaluation of endometrial cancer, suggesting that MRI should be performed when (1) physical examination is limited (those patients are often obese and of short stature, making physical examination difficult); (2) there are concomitant uterine lesions (e.g., leiomyoma); (3) a histologic grade III lesion is diagnosed (with the increased likelihood of deep myometrial invasion), the histologic tumor type is papillary serous carcinoma; (4) advanced stage of the disease is suspected clinically, warranting initial treatment by radiation therapy rather than surgery; and (5) the patient is a poor medical risk for surgery.

### *Carcinoma of the Ovary*

Surgical staging is routinely performed for cancer of the ovary. The value of imaging is controversial, but many agree that preoperative assessment of tumor extent aids in the design of the surgical approach. CT is successfully used for preoperative evaluation. The value of MRI is emerging with the introduction of faster imaging and the use of contrast media. The current literature shows a similar accuracy for MRI and CT in lesion characterization and the evaluation of its extent. Because MRI is still a developing modality, its value in ovarian cancer needs further investigation.

## Techniques

For the evaluation of the uterus, both T1- and T2-weighted spin-echo images are routinely recommended. The exact TR and TE parameters for T1- and T2-weighted images are difficult to assign, because they vary between MRI devices. It is generally agreed that T1-weighted images should not have a TR greater than 500 msec nor a TE greater than 20 msec. T2-weighted images should have a minimum TR of 2,000 msec and a minimum TE of 60 msec. Longer TR and TE values are, however, often used. The change in the recommended TR and TE values is especially seen with the use of fast spin-echo techniques. Fast T2-weighted spin-echo images are gaining in popularity, and it has been suggested by many that they may replace conventional T2-weighted images. Although this may be true, it does need to be proven. T2-weighted spin-echo images are always needed for demonstration of the uterine zonal anatomy, and T1-weighted images are required for the detection of lymphadenopathy and tissue characterization. Contrast-enhanced images allow visualization of the uterine zonal anatomy on the T1-weighted image. The use of T1-weighted sequences results in shorter imaging time (thus less motion artifact); therefore contrast-enhanced images are currently used in patients who are seriously ill, uncooperative, claustrophobic, or who may not complete the long imaging time ( ~ 17 minutes) required for conventional T2-weighted images. Fast T2-weighted spin-echo images, however, in those patients may be an alternative. Although the use of contrast media is optional for the study of tumors of the cervix and myometrium, in the evaluation of endometrial abnormalities and ovarian tumors, the routine use of contrast media is recommended. The gradient recall echo technique is reserved for those patients in whom differentiation between blood vessels and lymph nodes is needed or when the patency of blood vessels needs to be determined. The other recommended imaging technique in the pelvis is fat-saturation imaging. Presently fat-saturation imaging is recommended routinely only for those patients in whom the characterization of ovarian lesions is required; namely, diagnosis of teratomas and differentiation between endometrioma and teratoma.

MRI offers three orthogonal planes of imaging, each of which has specific advantages in the assessment of the uterus. In the transverse plane, the uterus, cervix, and vagina are well demonstrated as is the region of the parametria, uterosacral ligaments, and presacral space. In the sagittal plane, the uterus is seen along its long axis. The uterovesical space is best visualized in this plane as is the relationship of the uterus and vagina to the bladder and rectum. The coronal plane is complementary in the evaluation of the uterus and vagina. It can be used as an adjunct in the assessment of uterine morphology, broad ligaments and parametria, cervix and vagina. It also offers the opportunity to identify lymphadenopathy.

Off-axis imaging may be of value in assessing the corpus uterus and cervix, where precise measurements are required or demonstration of contour abnormalities will aid in the diagnosis of suspected congenital anomalies.

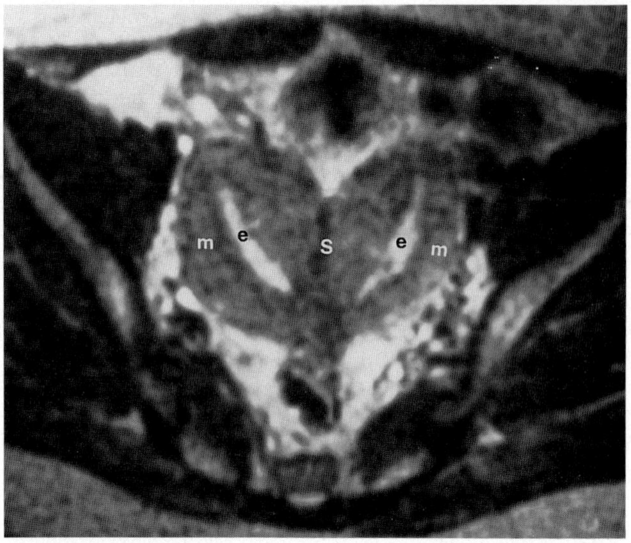


**FIGURE 1** Bicornuate uterus. Transaxial T2-weighted (2000/60) image. The septum (S) between the endometrium (e) of the right and left cornua is composed of myometrium. It demonstrates signal intensity similar to the myometrium (m) in the remaining corpus uteri.

## Diagnostic Approach

### *Uterine Anomalies*

#### Uterine Agenesis or Hypoplasia

In uterine agenesis there is no identifiable uterine tissue. Patients with uterine hypoplasia have a small endometrial cavity with a reduced intercornual diameter ($<2$ cm). In the hypoplastic uterus (uterus associated with hormonal dysfunction [infantile uterus]), not only is the uterus small, but it demonstrates abnormally low signal intensity with poorly differentiated zonal anatomy on T2-weighted images.

#### Unicornuate Uterus

The "banana"-shaped endometrial echo complex is a characteristic feature of the unicornuate uterus. Endometrial and myometrial width are normal. When there is incomplete development of the second müllerian duct, the unicornuate uterus has a rudimentary horn that either does or does not contain endometrium.

#### Didelphys Uterus

Two uteri, cervices, and a partially septate vagina are observed. The two uterine horns are widely separated. The endometrial and myometrial width are preserved.

#### Bicornuate Uterus

The main diagnostic feature is the presence of the myometrial septum between the two endometrial cavities (Fig. 1). Therefore, on T2-weighted images or unenhanced or contrast-enhanced T1-weighted images, the septal signal intensity is similar to the myometrium. The intercornual distance can be increased, and often there is an outward fundal concavity. The endometrial and myometrial widths and ratios are normal. In arcuate uteri, the mildest form of bicornuate uterus, the fundal surface is flattened or slightly concave.

#### Septate Uterus

The septum is composed of collagen tissue and demonstrates low signal intensity on both T1- and T2-weighted images (Fig. 2). If the septum reaches to the internal os, the result is uterus biseptus bicollis. If it terminates above the internal os, the anomaly is uterus biseptus unicollis. The fundal contour is normal, with an outward fundal convexity.

### *Benign Tumors of the Uterus*

#### Leiomyoma

Leiomyomas are divided into two categories based on their histologic characteristics: nondegenerative and degenerative. On T1-weighted images, nondegenerative leiomyomas demonstrate signal intensity similar to or slightly lower than the surrounding myometrium (Fig. 3, *A*). On T2-weighted images, nondegenerative leiomyomas demonstrate homogeneous low signal intensity with excellent contrast between the low signal intensity leiomyoma and the higher signal intensity myometrium or endometrium (Fig. 3, *B*). Degenerative leiomyomas demonstrate heterogeneous, often higher, signal intensity on T2-weighted scans (Fig. 3, *B*). The type of degeneration (hyaline, myxomatous, or fatty) cannot be differentiated with MRI. Benign degenerative leiomyoma and malignant leiomyosarcoma cannot be differentiated with MRI. The use of gadolinium-DTPA does not improve the characterization of uterine leiomyomas. Nondegenerative leiomyomas often do not enhance following Gd-DTPA injection, but enhancement of the tumors has been reported (Fig. 3, *C*). Degenerative leiomyomas demonstrate various degrees of enhancement (Fig. 3, *C*). The detection of tumor heterogeneity and the ability to differentiate viable tumor from necrosis or cystic degeneration are facilitated by the use of Gd-DTPA. Gd-DTPA is not helpful, however, in differentiating between benign leiomyoma and leiomyosarcoma.

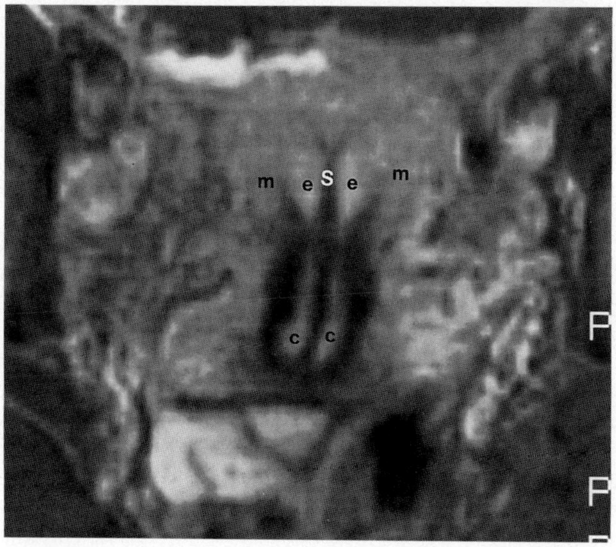


**FIGURE 2** Uterus biseptus bicollis. Transaxial T2-weighted (2000/60) image. The septum (S) between the endometrium (e) of the right and left cornua is of low signal intensity. The collagen septum extends to the external cervical os; therefore two endocervical canals (c) are seen. The myometrium (m) is of higher signal intensity than the collagen septum (S).

### Adenomyosis

There are two forms of adenomyosis: diffuse and focal. The MRI appearance of diffuse adenomyosis is characteristic. The uterine body and fundus are diffusely enlarged, and on T2-weighted images the low signal intensity junctional zone is increased in thickness and segmentally or diffusely extends through the myometrium (Fig. 4). In some patients high signal intensity foci can be detected within the adenomyosis. When these foci of high signal intensity are demonstrated on both T1- and T2-weighted images, they are thought to represent hemorrhage. When they are seen only on T2-weighted images, it is postulated that they represent endometrial nests.

MRI diagnosis of focal adenomyosis is more difficult. Focal adenomyosis is observed as a low signal intensity mass, which may appear similar to a leiomyoma. Differentiation between focal adenomyosis and leiomyoma depends on the configuration of the lesion (adenomyosis is often oval, whereas leiomyomas are usually round) and margin (adenomyosis has indistinct margins, whereas leiomyomas are sharply demarcated) (Fig. 5). Focal adenomyosis is more commonly present in the posterior part of the corpus uterus. The use of Gd-DTPA does not contribute to either detection or characterization of adenomyosis. Following Gd-DTPA injection, the area of adenomyosis may show homogeneous or heterogeneous enhancement with low signal intensity foci scattered throughout the lesion. The enhancement pattern of adenomyosis results in decreased lesion conspicuity as compared to T2-weighted images.

## *Carcinomas*

### Endometrial Carcinoma

With present MRI techniques, endometrial carcinoma cannot be consistently visualized or differentiated from blood clot, benign tumor (submucosal leiomyoma or endometrial polyp),

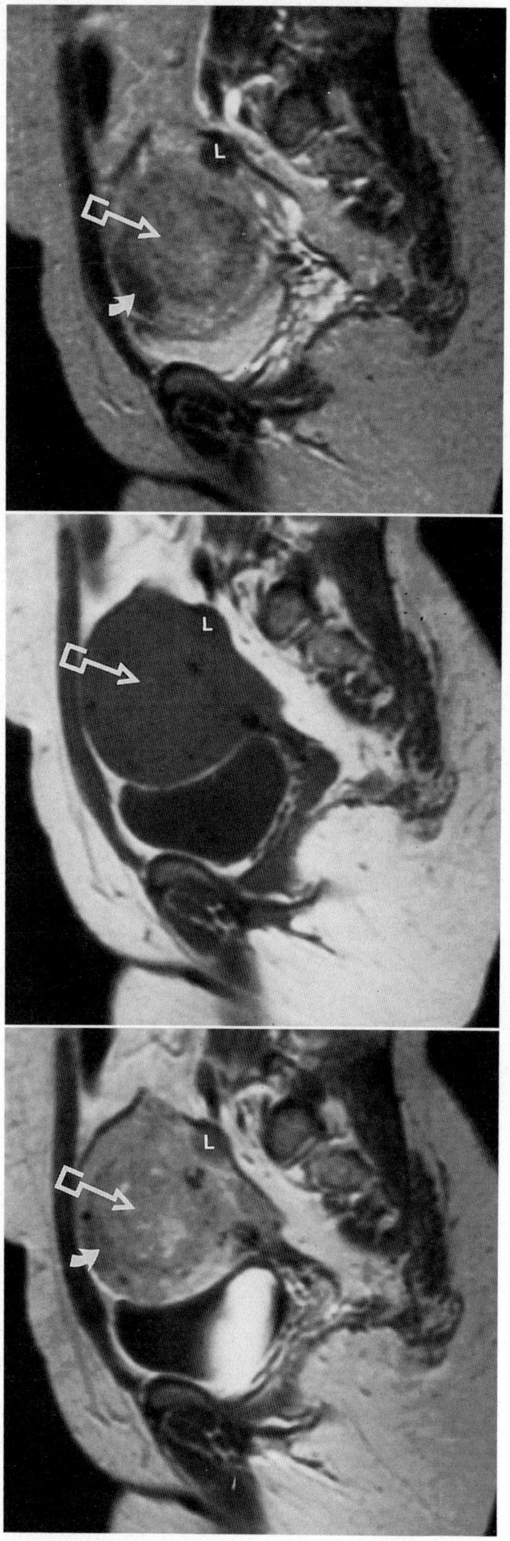


A

B

C

**FIGURE 3** Multiple uterine leiomyomas. *A,* Sagittal T2-weighted (2000/60) image; *B,* transverse T1-weighted (500/20) image; and *C,* contrast-enhanced T1-weighted (5000/20) image. The nondegenerative leiomyoma (L) demonstrates low signal intensity on unenhanced and contrast-enhanced images. The degenerative (hyaline degeneration) leiomyoma *(open arrowhead)* is of high signal intensity on T2-weighted image and shows enhancement on the contrast-enhanced study. A small smaller leiomyoma *(curved arrow)* anteriorly is well depicted on T2-weighted image, but the lesion conspicuity is diminished on contrast-enhanced studies.

or adenomatous hyperplasia. On unenhanced T2-weighted MRI, endometrial carcinoma and normal endometrium usually are of similarly high signal intensity; therefore lesions confined to the endometrium can be detected only by demonstration of an increased thickness or lobulation of the uterine cavity. In some cases, however, tumors are of a lower signal intensity than the remaining normal endometrium, facilitating their detection. This limitation of unenhanced T1- or T2-weighted spin-echo MRI can in part be overcome by the use of either increased resolution offered by high-resolution multicoils (multiphased array surface coils) or intravenous contrast application. On immediate postcontrast scans, the endometrial carcinoma demonstrates an enhancement similar to or lower than that of the myometrium and less than that of the endometrium. Further, although differentiation between retained debris (e.g., hematometra, pyometra) and tumor as a cause for the enlarged uterine cavity is often difficult on unenhanced scans, this distinction is possible on contrast-enhanced T1-weighted image. The use of contrast media thus leads to an overall improvement in tumor detection, staging, and assessment of the depth of myometrial invasion (Fig. 6).

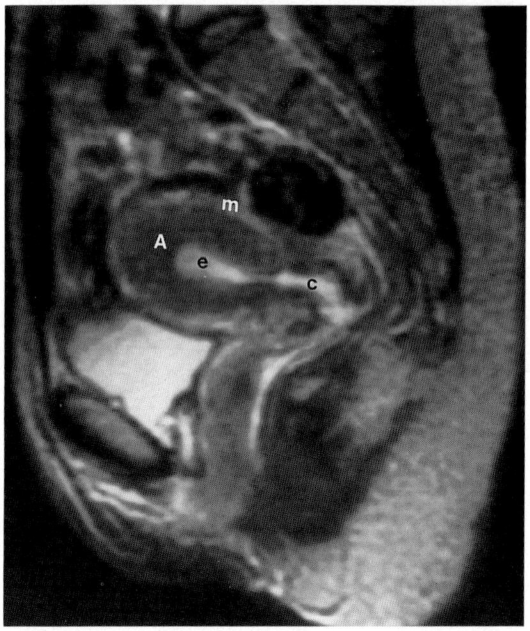


**FIGURE 4** Diffuse adenomyosis. Sagittal T2-weighted (2000/60) image. The junctional zone is widened and demonstrates low signal intensity, indicative of adenomyosis (A). The normal myometrium (m) is of higher signal intensity. Endometrium (e), cervix (c).

The MRI staging classification for endometrial carcinoma follows the guidelines of surgical staging. Imaging is not applicable to stage 0 (Tis) cancer. In stage I endometrial carcinoma, the tumor is confined to the uterine corpus. Stage I tumors are further divided into (1) stage Ia—tumor confined to the endometrium, (2) stage Ib—tumor invasion to the inner half of the myometrium, and (3) stage Ic—tumor invasion extending into the outer half of the myometrium. Tumors are considered to be confined to the endometrium when the junctional zone is preserved or there is sharp tumor-myometrium interface. Stage Ib disease is indicated by the disruption of the junctional zone, with an irregular myometrial-endometrial interface and/or by direct demonstration of tumor in the inner half of the myometrium. Deep myometrial invasion is suggested by the demonstration of the tumor extending into the outer half of the myometrium. An accuracy rate of 82 percent has been reported by the NCI multicenter study in the differentiation between superficial and deep myometrial invasion. The evaluation of myometrial tumor invasion is further improved when contrast-enhanced studies are analyzed (Fig. 7).

Stage II endometrial cancer is diagnosed when the tumor extends into the cervix. The differentiation between stage IIa disease (invasion of the glandular and epithelial surface only) and stage IIb disease (cervical stroma is invaded) is possible by MRI. The uninvolved cervical stroma in stage IIa disease remains of low signal intensity on T2-weighted images.

MRI can also be used in the evaluation of stage III and stage IV disease. The bladder or rectum is considered to be invaded when its wall demonstrates focal or diffuse loss of normal low

A

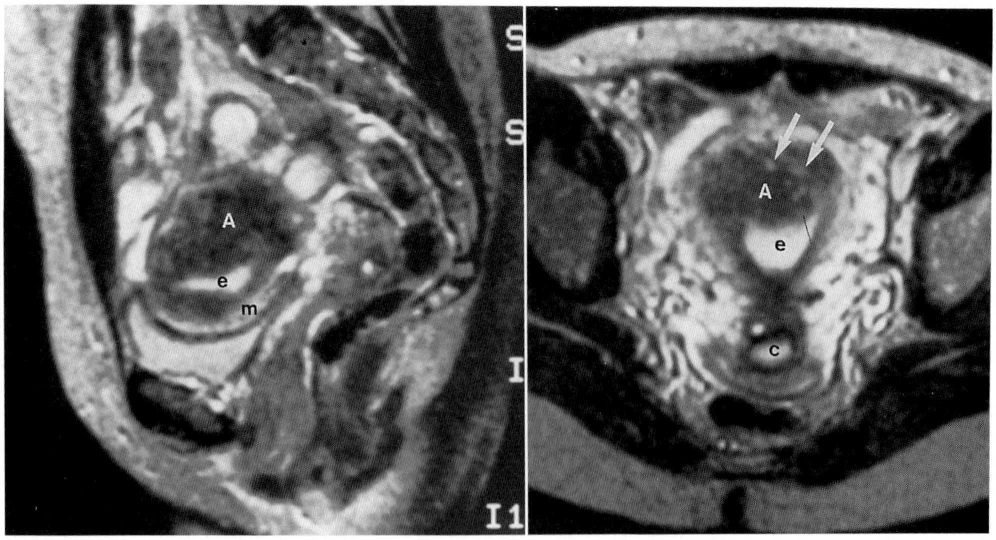


B

**FIGURE 5** Focal and diffuse adenomyosis. Sagittal *(A)* and transaxial *(B)* T2-weighted (2000/60) image. Focal adenomyoma (A) is oval. The margin towards the myometrium is indistinct and there are high signal intensity foci *(white arrows)*. Endometrium (e), myometrium (m), cervix (c).

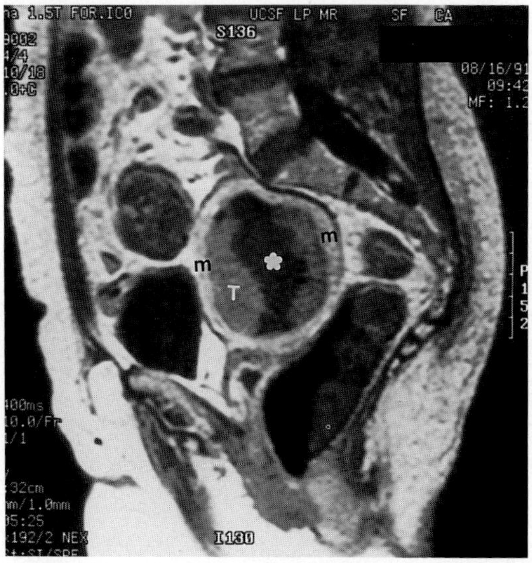


**FIGURE 6** Endometrial carcinoma, stage Ib. Sagittal plane contrast-enhanced T1-weighted (500/20) image. Myometrium (m) is of higher signal intensity than is the endometrial tumor (T). The irregular tumor-myometrial margin anteriorly indicates superficial myometrial invasion. Retained debris within the endocervical cavity *(asterisk)* shows no enhancement.

A

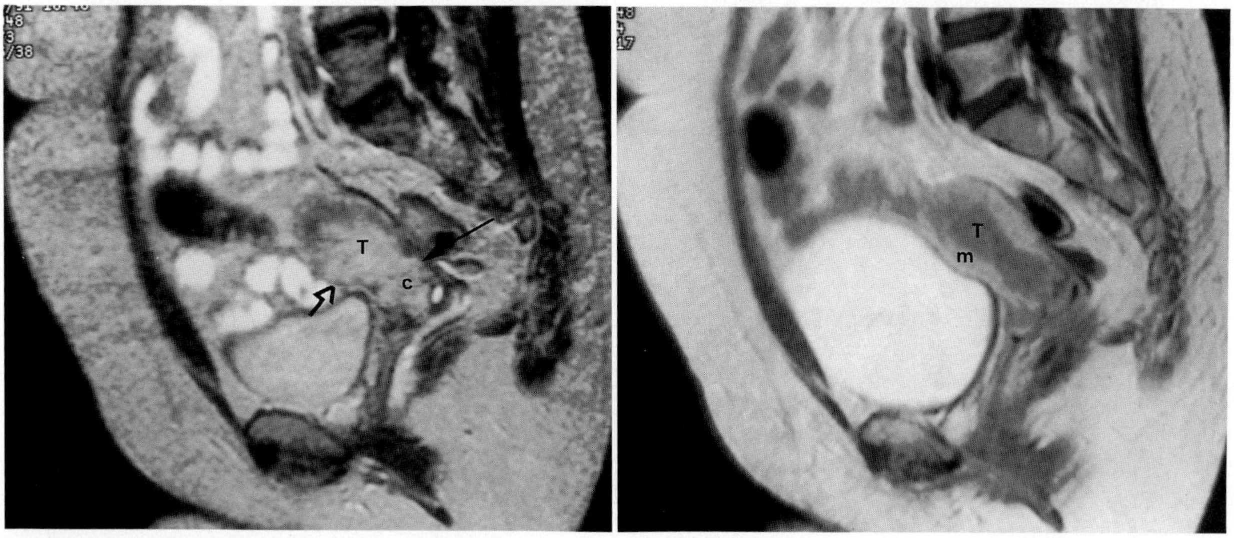


B

**FIGURE 7** Endometrial carcinoma, stage IIb. *A,* Sagittal T2-weighted (2000/60) image; *B,* contrast-enhanced T1-weighted (500/20) image. Large tumor (T) occupies the corpus uterus and extends into the endocervical canal (c). On noncontrast image, there appears to be deep myometrial invasion *(arrowhead)* as well as invasion of the cervical stroma *(solid arrow)*. On contrast-enhanced study, tumor (T) extends into the endocervical canal, and by its irregular tumor stromal margin indicates cervical stromal invasion. However, the normal thickness of the myometrium (m) is well observed, indicating that no deep invasion has occurred.

signal intensity on T2-weighted images. The accuracy of MRI in the detection of lymph nodes relies on assessment of nodal size; MRI cannot distinguish between malignant and hyperplastic nodes nor can it diagnose malignant disease within normal-size nodes (Fig. 8).

## Cervical Carcinoma

On T2-weighted images, cervical cancer appears as a high signal intensity mass that can be distinguished from the normal low signal intensity cervical stroma (Fig. 9). T1-weighted images provide contrast between cervical tumor and the surrounding pelvic fat. In combination, unenhanced T1- and T2-weighted images allow the precise delineation of tumor location, depth of cervical stromal invasion, and extension of tumor to the uterine corpus. The use of contrast media does not improve tumor depiction. Various degrees of tumor

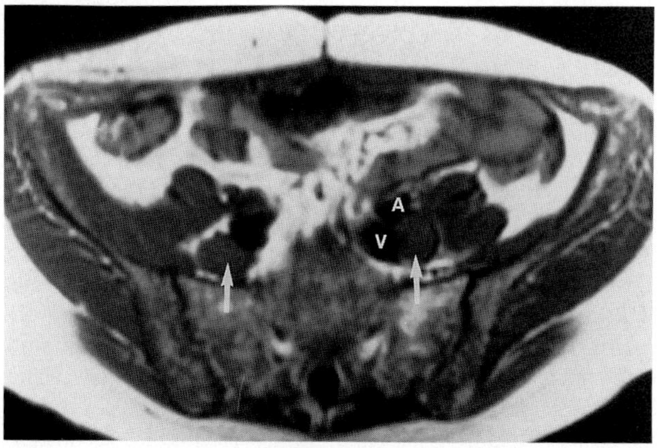


**FIGURE 8** Bilateral common iliac adenopathy. Transaxial T1-weighted (500/20) image shows enlarged lymph nodes *(arrows)* lateral to the common iliac artery (A) and vein (V).

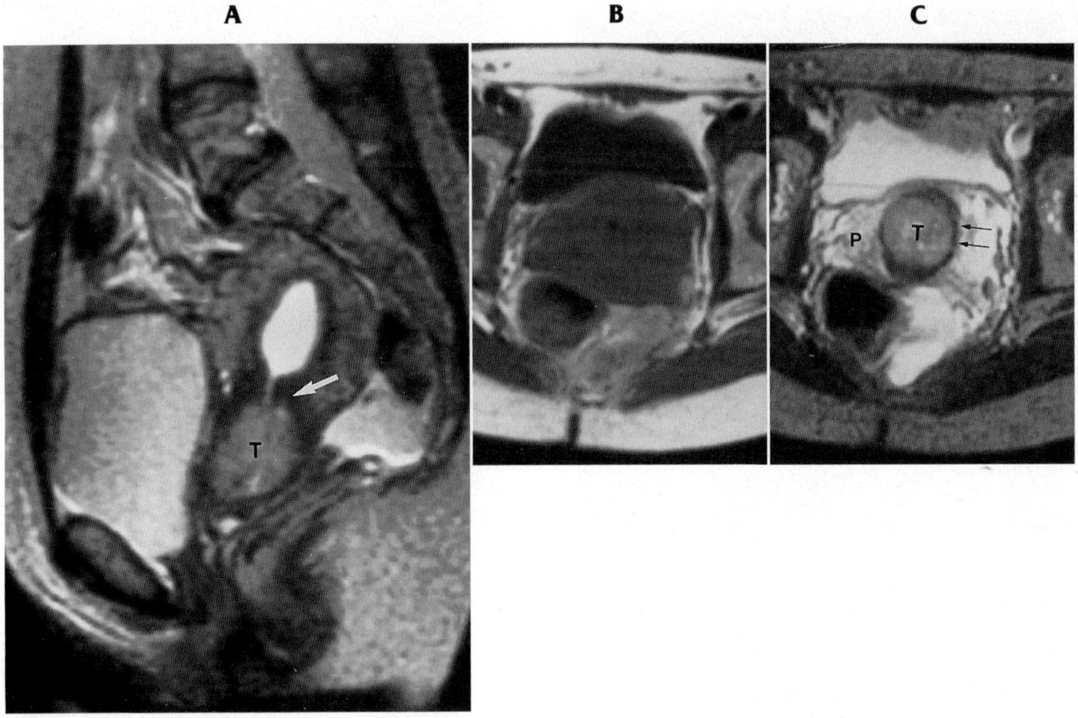


**FIGURE 9** Stage Ib carcinoma of the cervix. *A,* Sagittal T2-weighted (2000/60) image; *B,* transverse T1-weighted (500/20) image; and *C,* T2-weighted (2000/60) images. The carcinoma of the cervix (T) demonstrates higher signal intensity than the adjacent normal low signal intensity cervical stroma *(black arrows)* or the cervical stroma at the level of the internal os of the cervix *(white arrow).* The parametria (P) are not invaded. However, the evaluation of the parametrial extension can be performed only on the T2-weighted image (image B), because on the T1-weighted image the region of the cervix and parametria appears enlarged.

enhancement are observed, often making the tumor isointense with the surrounding cervical tissue. Further, the surrounding normal stroma often shows enhancement as well; therefore the use of contrast media may cause overestimation of tumor size. Tumor heterogeneity, however, is well demonstrated on contrast-enhanced scans, allowing the differentiation between viable tumor and necrosis. Tumor heterogeneity is better demonstrated on contrast-enhanced T1-weighted images than on either T1- or T2-weighted noncontrast-enhanced scans.

The MRI staging classification follows the guidelines of FIGO staging. Stage Ib disease are tumors confined to the cervix (see Fig. 9). Stage II disease—tumor extending outside the cervix—is divided into stage IIa tumor (a mass is seen extending into the upper two-thirds of the vagina) and stage IIb, where the tumor extends into the parametria. For detecting parametrial tumor spread, transverse or coronal plane sections are helpful. Both morphologic and signal alterations must be assessed. Criteria include an irregular lateral tumor margin, prominent parametrial strands, eccentric parametrial enlargement, and loss of periparametrial fat planes on T1-weighted images, or an abnormal high signal intensity tumor demonstrating direct extension into the parametria. Stage III lesions are usually bulky tumors. In stage IIIa disease, the tumor extends into the lower third of the vagina. In stage IIIb disease (extension to the pelvic side wall, with or without hydronephrosis), the normal low signal intensity of the pelvic wall muscles is disrupted on T2-weighted images. In stage IV disease, the tumor extends into the urinary bladder or rectum, and on T2-weighted images the normal low signal intensity wall of those organs is no longer intact (Fig. 10). The use of contrast-enhanced imaging is helpful in the evaluation of advanced disease, particularly when invasion of the bladder or rectum is suspected.

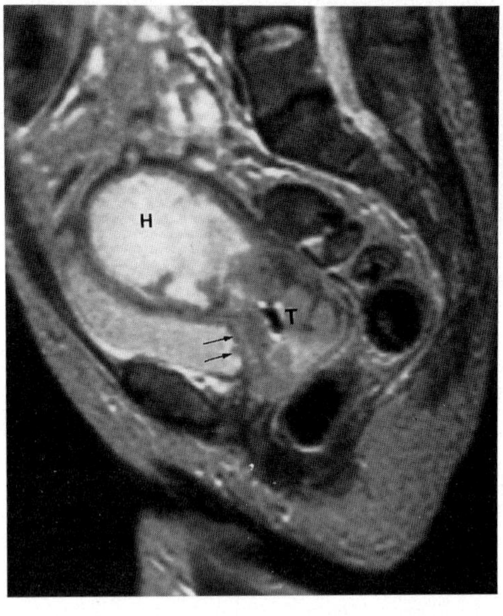


**FIGURE 10** Stage IVa carcinoma of the cervix. Sagittal T2-weighted (2000/60) image. The large cervical tumor (T) shows direct extension into the lower third of the vagina as well as extension into the urinary bladder *(arrows).* The tumor is obstructing the endocervical canal, and hematometra (H) is visualized.

MRI is considered an excellent modality in the evaluation of carcinoma of the cervix, with a reported accuracy in assessing tumor size of 70 to 100 percent, in determining

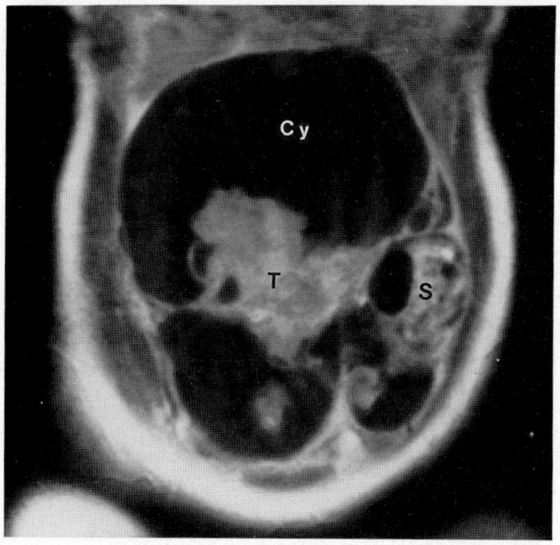


**FIGURE 11** Carcinoma of the ovary. Coronal plane contrast-enhanced T1-weighted (500/20) image. The large ovarian lesion is predominantly cystic (Cy), but also has a large, enhancing, solid component (T). The tumor is adherent to the sigmoid colon (S).

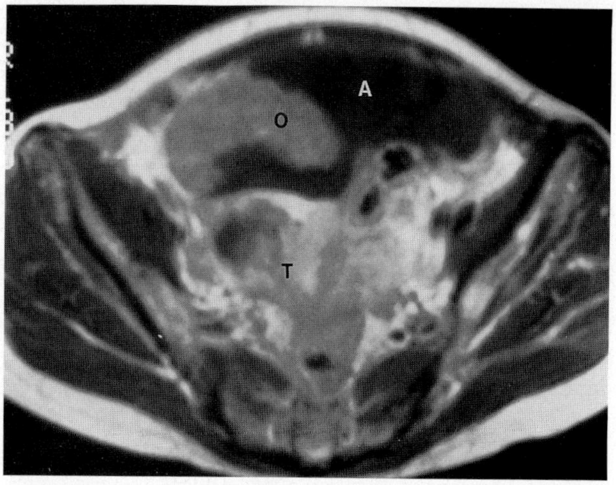


**FIGURE 12** Ovarian carcinoma, stage IIIc, with demonstration of omental cake. Transaxial contrast-enhanced T1-weighted (500/20) image. The enhancing omental cake (O) is seen in contrast to the low signal intensity ascites (A). Primary tumor (T).

parametrial and vaginal involvement of 85 to 100 percent; MRI excels also in detecting nodal disease.

### Ovarian Carcinoma

The role of MRI in the evaluation of ovarian cancer is still developing. Unenhanced MRI was felt, in the past, to be inferior to CT in detection, characterization, or staging of ovarian cancer. Technical advances and introduction of intravenous contrast media are redefining the value of MRI. With the use of contrast-enhanced T1-weighted image, lesion detection of 92 percent has been reported with superb ability to characterize the lesion as benign or malignant. The presence of nodularity or vegetations or presence of a solid mass are all features indicative of malignancy (Fig. 11). In addition, indirect signs such as ascites and peritoneal, mesenteric, or omental metastases further establish the nature of the disease (Fig. 12). Unlike CT, the detection of primary ovarian lesions on MRI is not hindered by the presence of ascites. The peritoneal metastases are diagnosed by the demonstration of thickening, irregularity, or nodularity of the peritoneal surface. Peritoneal metastases enhance following contrast injection. MRI is helpful in the demonstration of omental metastases. Omental metastases demonstrate medium signal intensity on T1-weighted images and usually decrease in signal intensity on T2-weighted images. On immediate postcontrast scans, the omental cake shows enhancement, further contributing to its detection (see Fig. 12). MRI is superior to CT in the evaluation of tumor extension into the uterus, bladder, or rectum and in all three, the diagnosis is facilitated by contrast-enhanced images and by the availability of multiplanar scanning.

## Suggested Reading

Carrington BM, Hricak H, Nuruddin R, et al. Müllerian duct anomalies: MR imaging evaluation. Radiology 1990; 176:715–720.

Dudiak CM, Turner DA, Patal SK, et al. Uterine leiomyomas in the infertile patient: Preoperative localization with MR imaging versus US and hysterosalpingography. Radiology 1988; 167:627–630.

Fedele L, Dorta M, Brioschi D, et al. Magnetic resonance imaging of unicornuate uterus. Acta Obstet Gynecol Scand 1990; 69: 511–513.

Hricak H, Finck S, Honda G, Göranson H. MR imaging in the evaluation of benign uterine masses: Value of gadopentetate dimeglumine-enhanced T1-weighted images. AJR 1992; 158:1043–1050.

Hricak H, Hamm B, Semelka RC, et al. Carcinoma of the uterus: Use of gadopentetate dimeglumine in the MR evaluation of carcinoma of the uterus. Radiology 1991; 181:95–106.

Hricak H, Rubinstein L, Gherman GM, Karstaedt N. MR imaging evaluation of endometrial carcinoma: Results of an NCI cooperative study. Radiology 1991; 179:829–832.

Kim SH, Choi BI, Lee HP, et al. Uterine cervical carcinoma: Comparison of CT and MR findings. Radiology 1990; 175:45–51.

Sironi S, Taccagni G, Garancini P, et al. Myometrial invasion by endometrial carcinoma: Assessment by MR imaging. AJR 1992; 158:565–569.

Stevens SK, Hricak H, Stern JL. Ovarian lesions: Detection and characterization with gadolinium-enhanced MR imaging at 1.5 T. Radiology 1991; 181:481–488.

Togashi K, Nishimura K, Sago T, et al. Carcinoma of the cervix: Staging with MR imaging. Radiology 1989; 171:245–251.

Togashi K, Ozasa H, Konishi I, et al. Enlarged uterus: Differentiation between adenomyosis and leiomyoma with MRI. Radiology 1989; 171:531–534.

Weinreb JC, Barkoff ND, Megibow A, et al. The value of MR imaging in distinguishing leiomyomas from other solid pelvic masses when sonography is indeterminate. AJR 1990; 154:295–299.

# Prenatal Diagnosis of Congenital Malformations with Obstetrical Ultrasonography

*LUÍS FLÁVIO GONÇALVES, M.D. · ROBERT L. LAPIDUS, M.D.*
*JOYCE KELLY, R.D.M.S. · PHILIPPE JEANTY, M.D., Ph.D.*

## Central Nervous System

Our approach to the prenatal diagnosis of central nervous system (CNS) malformations with ultrasonography consists of the following three steps:

1. Imaging of the brain:
   - Transventricular axial view, focusing on the atrium of the posterior horn
   - Transthalamic axial view—biparietal diameter
   - Transcerebellar view—posterior fossa
2. Imaging the face:
   - Sagittal view of the face (profile)
   - Coronal view through the mouth and nose
   - Axial view of the eyes
3. Careful scanning of other organs and systems, searching for associated malformations

Anomalies of the CNS can present in various forms. In this section we discuss the differential diagnosis for ventricular dilatation, intracranial cysts, intracranial neoplasms, and microcephaly.

### *Intracranial Cysts*

Intracranial cystic images may result from dilatation of normal intracranial structures or degeneration of cerebral tissue with replacement by fluid. They can be isolated or multiple, symmetrical or asymmetrical, and associated or not with CNS and extra-CNS anomalies.

### *Intracranial Masses*

Intracranial echogenic structures can represent a neoplasm, hemorrhage, infection, or ischemic brain necrosis. Neoplasms are generally large, heterogeneous, echogenic structures that grow remarkably fast in serial sonograms, with occasional calcifications, and are rarely cystic. They can deform the cranium and lead to hydrocephalus if they obstruct the cerebrospinal fluid (CSF) flow.

### *Microcephaly*

Microcephaly refers to a small head with concomitant reduction of brain mass and total cell number. It is defined by the majority of investigators as a decrease in the head circumference more than three standard deviations below the mean. It should always be suspected when the head circumference and biparietal diameter (BPD) are small for gestational age and when the head is smaller than expected for the size of the abdomen. Serial examinations demonstrate poor growth of the fetal head and confirm the diagnosis. Associated anomalies include: encephalocele, porencephaly, lissencephaly, holoprosencephaly, macrogyria, microgyria, agyria, Kellblattschadel, and intracranial calcifications.

### *Differential Diagnosis*

The following questions may help in orienting the differential diagnosis of a CNS anomaly:

#### 1. Is the Shape of the Head Normal?

A "lemon head" is characterized by flattening of the frontal bones, leading to a pointed appearance at the level of the metopic suture (Fig. 1). It is suggestive of an associated spinal defect (see Neural Tube Defects section).

#### 2. Are the Ventricles Dilated?

We recognize ventricular dilatation by the following signs (Fig. 2):

1. A transverse ventricular diameter at the level of the atrium greater than 10 mm between 15 and 35 weeks of gestation
2. Separation of the choroid plexus from the medial wall of the lateral ventricle
3. Sinking of the choroid plexus in the fluid-filled ventricle, also known as the "dangling choroid plexus sign"

Bear in mind that the head circumference and BPD are not necessarily increased and that many CNS malformations are associated with ventricular dilatation. For instance, 30 percent of fetuses with hydrocephalus have spina bifida as part of the Arnold-Chiari malformation (see the Neural Tube Defects

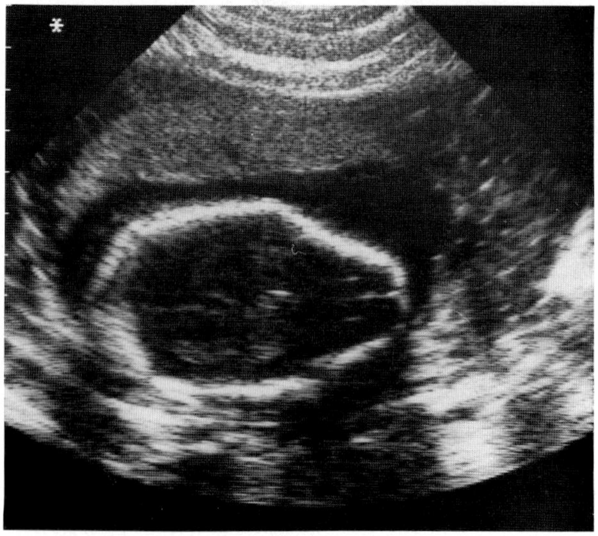

**FIGURE 1** Lemon head. Note the depression of the frontal bones. The depression can be flat or concave. When it is not bilateral, it is a result of an inappropriately oblique scan. This sign should prompt a thorough search for neural tube defects.

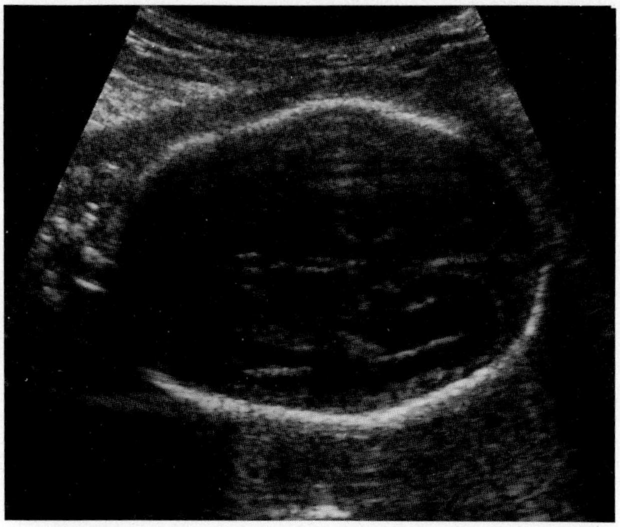

**FIGURE 2** Ventricular dilatation. The diagnosis is made by measuring the atrium (the junction of the occipital horns with the temporal and frontal horns). The measurement of the atrium should be less than 10 mm.

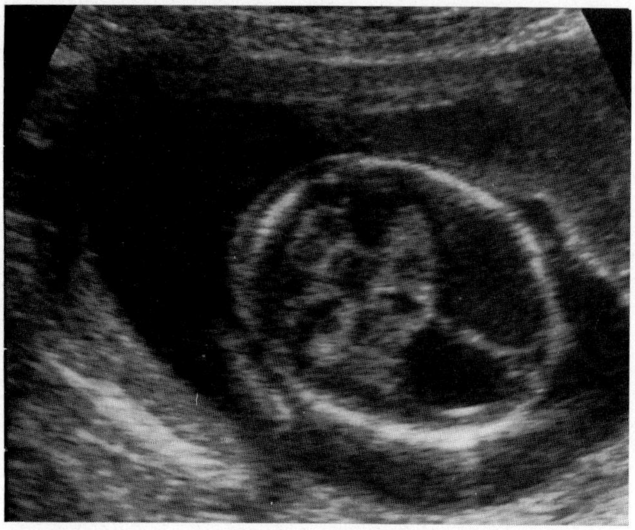

**FIGURE 3** Aqueductal stenosis. Distention of the lateral ventricles and third ventricle without enlargement of the fourth.

section). Hydrocephalus is associated not only with other CNS malformations but also with a number of multiple anomaly syndromes including, but not limited to, trisomy 13, trisomy 18, chromosomal deletions, translocations, and fragility.

### 3. Is the Ventricular Dilatation Asymmetrical?

Marked asymmetrical dilatation of the lateral ventricles is a common finding in porencephaly. This disorder results from vascular occlusion, inflammatory diseases, hemorrhage, or trauma leading to degeneration of the nervous system. Fluid-filled spaces replace the brain parenchyma. There are no associated anomalies.

### 4. Are There Abnormal Midline Structures?

The following structures are located in the midline: the falx cerebri, cavum septi pellucidi, third ventricle, cerebellar vermis, and posterior fossa.

*Aqueductal Stenosis.* The third ventricle is a small anechoic structure bordered by echogenic margins between the thalami. Aqueductal stenosis is an obstruction of the aqueduct of Sylvius, which is a narrow communication between the third and the fourth ventricles. Characteristic findings include marked and progressive enlargement of the lateral ventricles; dilatation of the third ventricle; cortical mantle present (Fig. 3). The male-female ratio is 1.8:1. The disease may result from intrauterine infection, intraventricular hemorrhage, extrinsic compression by adjacent masses, or as an X-linked trait in 25 percent of the affected males. Associated anomalies include a 30 percent association with spina bifida in Arnold-Chiari malformation and flexion abnormalities of the thumbs in male fetuses with X-linked inheritance.

*Communicating Hydrocephalus.* The characteristic findings in communicating hydrocephalus are dilatation of the lateral, third, and fourth ventricles. However, the dilatation of the fourth ventricle is often minimal; hence, the differential diagnosis with aqueductal stenosis may be impossible prenatally. The pathognomonic sign is the dilatation of the subarachnoid cistern, which is best imaged in the coronal view. The male-female ratio is 1:1. Communicating hydrocephalus was thought in the past to be a result of the obstruction of the foramina of Luschka and Magendie; a new theory proposes that it results from an overproduction of CSF by the fourth ventricle.

*Agenesis of the Corpus Callosum.* The corpus callosum is a bundle of white matter that decussates between the cerebral hemispheres. It forms the roof of the lateral ventricles. Agenesis of the corpus callosum can occur in two forms: with and without an interhemispheric cyst. This cyst represents a dilatation and superior displacement of the third ventricle. The characteristic findings are disproportional dilatation of the occipital horns and atrium of the lateral ventricles (colpocephaly) and increased separation of the lateral ventricles; an interhemispheric cyst is not always present. There is a 1:1 male-female ratio. The incidence is 68 per 100,000 in the Charlevoix–Saguenay–Lac St. Jean area of Quebec, Canada. Inheritance is autosomal recessive. Associated CNS anomalies include gyral anomalies, heterotopia, midline intracerebral lipomas, encephalocele, interhemispheric arachnoid cysts, Dandy-Walker malformation, Arnold-Chiari malformation, holoprosencephaly, hydrocephalus, and aqueductal stenosis. Extra-CNS anomalies include long, triangular, and asymmetric face with hypoplastic maxilla, low hairline, hypertelorism; and gastrointestinal, cardiovascular, genitourinary, respiratory, musculoskeletal, and chromosomal anomalies.

*Dandy-Walker Malformation.* A midline cyst in the posterior fossa is usually a sign of Dandy-Walker malformation. The disease is thought to result from cystic dilatation of the fourth ventricle, with compression and further aplasia of the cerebellar vermis. Characteristic of this disorder is the splaying of the cerebellar hemispheres and the communication between the

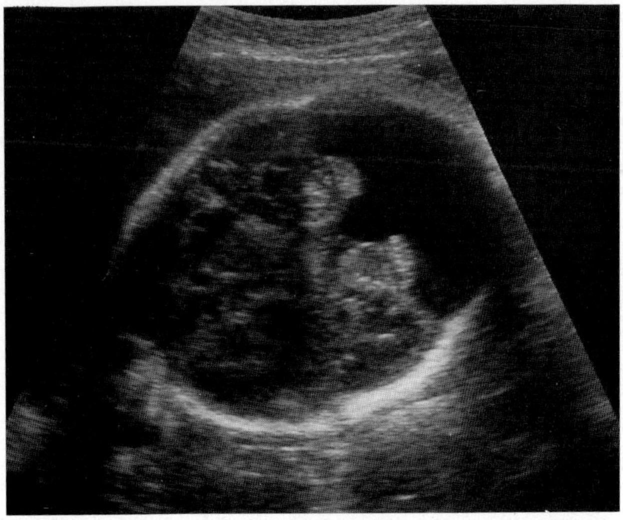

**FIGURE 4** Dandy-Walker malformation. A "cyst" between the lateral lobes of the cerebellum with hypoplasia of the vermis is typical of the disorder. This image is from a severe case with wide separation of the lateral lobes of the cerebellum.

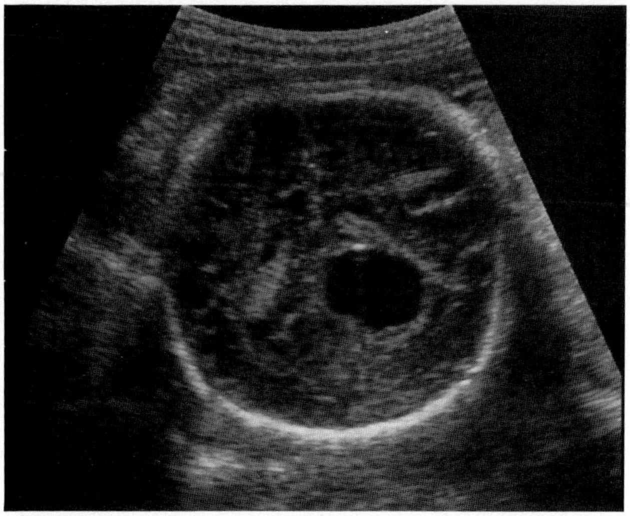

**FIGURE 5** A well-defined arachnoid cyst that displaces the lateral ventricle. It does not communicate with the lateral ventricles, since the choroid plexus is deflected. This differentiates the disorder from porencephalic cysts. (Reprinted with permission from The Fetus, p 7429-1.)

cyst and the fourth ventricle through the cerebellar vermis defect (Fig. 4). Hydrocephalus can be of any degree and is sometimes absent. Etiology includes autosomal recessive, autosomal dominant, X-linked dominant, single gene, chromosome, and multifactorial disorders. Dandy-Walker malformation is associated with CNS and extra-CNS anomalies, so a complete search is mandatory. CNS anomalies include microcephaly, encephalocele, aqueductal stenosis, lipomas, agenesis of the corpus callosum, and nonspecific gyral anomalies. Extra-CNS malformations include polydactyly and anomalies of the face, heart, and genitourinary system.

*Congenital Midline Porencephaly*. Congenital midline porencephaly is characterized by a midline intracranial cyst, midline scalp alopecia or encephalocele, and hydrocephalus. The disease is associated with polyhydramnios, macrocephaly, and absence of midline echo at the level of the cerebral hemispheres. There are no facial or other associated anomalies.

*Arachnoid Cyst.* Sometimes an arachnoid cyst may be identified in the midline. Arachnoid cysts are fluid-filled, thin-walled cystic masses derived from abnormal leptomeningeal formation or entrapment of CSF by arachnoid adhesions (trauma, infection, or hemorrhage). They usually displace adjacent brain structures and may be associated with hydrocephalus if it obstructs the CSF flow (Fig. 5).

*Aneurysm of the Vein of Galen.* An aneurysm of the vein of Galen is a tubular cystic structure located in the quadrigeminal plate cistern, superior and posterior to the thalami. Doppler studies demonstrate turbulent venous and/or arterial flow (Fig. 6). The carotid arteries and jugular veins as well as the right

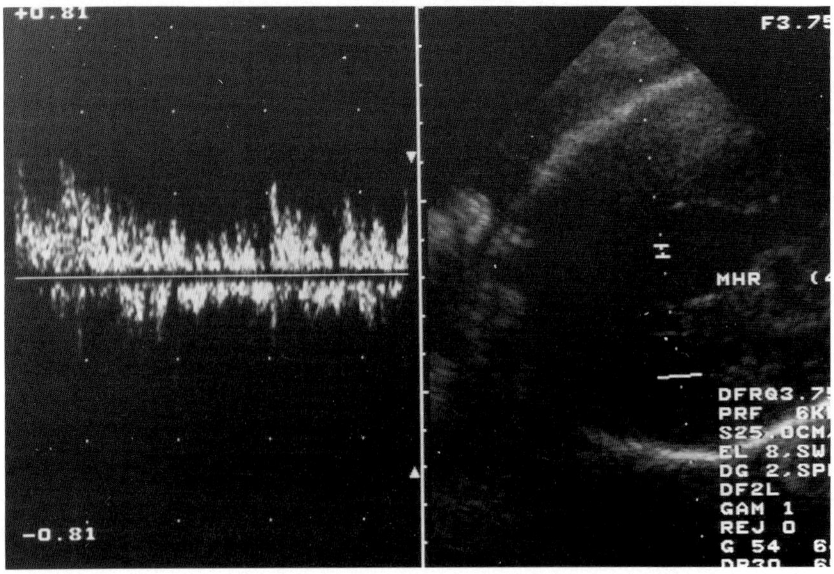


**FIGURE 6** A central fluid collection with high flow on pulsed-wave Doppler *(left side of the image)*. This is pathognomonic of aneurysm of the vein of Galen. (From Jeanty P, Kepple D, et al. In utero detection of cardiac failure from a vein of Galen aneurysm. Am J Obstet Gynecol 1990; 163:50–51; with permission.)

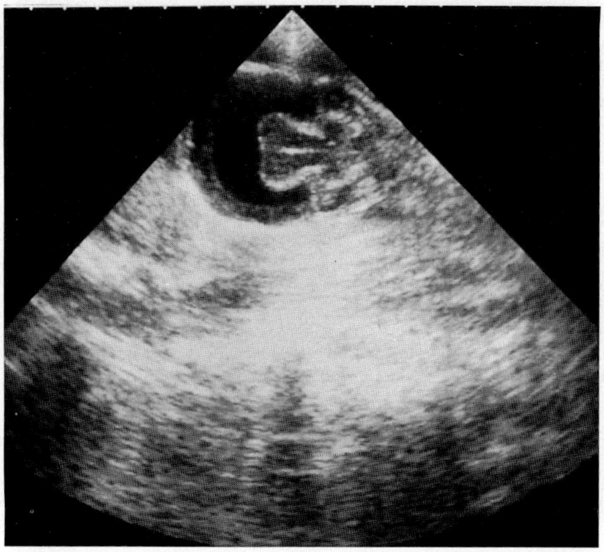

**FIGURE 7** Alobar holoprosencephaly. A large single ventricle occupies the head. The thalami are fused in the middle. Note the layer of cortex close to the skull that differentiates this disorder from hydranencephaly.

atrium are usually dilated. Areas of ischemia and infarction may be seen surrounding the aneurysm. Nonimmune hydrops may result from cardiac failure.

## 5. Are Normal Midline Structures Absent?

*Holoprosencephaly.* In alobar holoprosencephaly we usually see a large single collection of fluid denoting a single ventricle. The thalami are fused. The following structures are absent: third ventricle, neurohypophysis, corpus callosum, falx cerebri, optic tracts, and olfactory bulbs (Fig. 7). Anomalies of the face are frequently associated and include cyclopia, hypotelorism with high midline proboscis, hypotelorism with a single nostril in nose, median cleft, and bilateral facial cleft. When the diagnosis is made, one should also search for renal cysts and dysplasia, omphalocele, cardiovascular malformations, clubfoot, myelomeningocele, and intestinal anomalies.

In semilobar holoprosencephaly we have the same findings as above, except that there is partial segmentation of the ventricles and partial fusion of the thalami. Both forms of holoprosencephaly are strongly associated with chromosomal anomalies, mainly trisomy 13, 18, and triploidy, and multiple anomaly syndromes such as Meckel-Gruber, Kallmann's, camptomelic dysplasia, and Hall-Pallister and Vasadi syndromes.

*Hydranencephaly.* Hydranencephaly is thought to result from massive cerebral infarction following obstruction of the carotid arteries. Ultrasonography demonstrates a large anechoic area filling the cranium, no cerebral cortex, macrocephaly, and polyhydramnios. Preserved structures include the midbrain, thalami, cerebellum, basal ganglia, and choroid plexus. There are no associated anomalies.

## 6. Can You Identify the Cerebral Cortex?

Some disorders result in the degeneration of the cerebral cortex and replacement of the structures by fluid. Hydranencephaly and porencephaly have been previously discussed. In

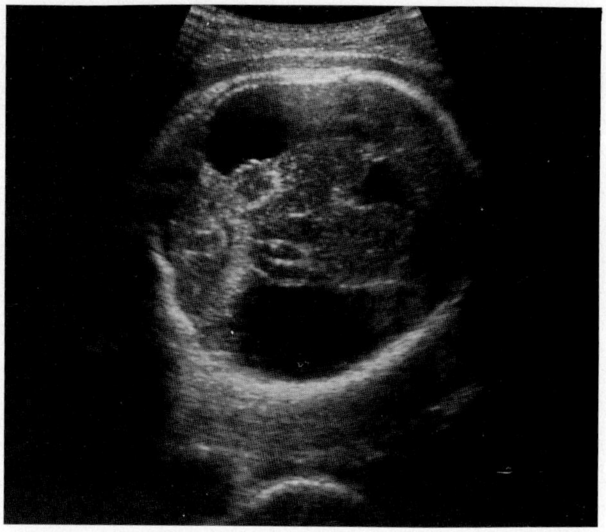

**FIGURE 8** Schizencephaly. A bilateral infarction of the middle cerebral arteries results in the loss of the cortex of the parietal region. The anterior, posterior, and superior aspects of the cortical mantle are preserved since they are perfused by the anterior cerebral arteries and the basilar system. The infarction leaves a line of cortex on the top of the head, which is given the nickname of "basket handle" configuration, because of its appearance similar to woven baskets. The lateral ventricles communicate with the subarachnoid space.

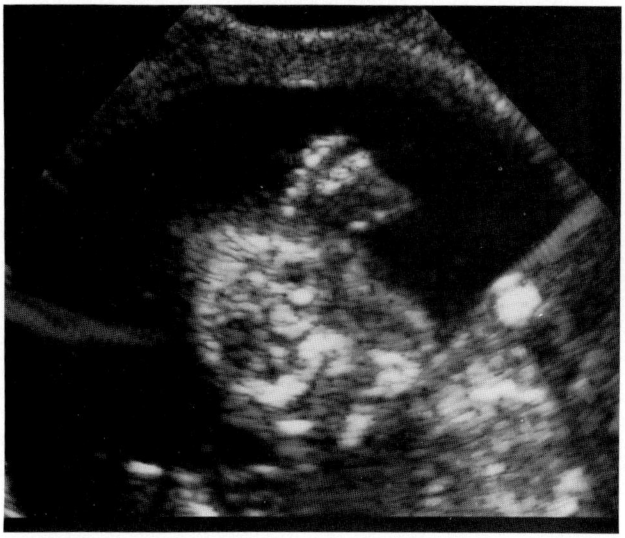

**FIGURE 9** Cebocephaly. The close proximity of the orbits is visible. The proboscis is more anterior and not demonstrated on this image.

schizencephaly there are full-thickness clefts in the cerebral hemispheres, usually bilateral and located in the expected distribution of the middle cerebral artery. There are no associated anomalies (Fig. 8).

## 7. Is the Face Abnormal?

Most of the CNS anomalies associated with an abnormal face have been previously discussed. Holoprosencephaly is the anomaly associated with the most bizarre anomalies: fused orbits with supraorbital proboscis (cyclopia), hypotelorism with high midline proboscis (ethmocephaly), hypotelorism with a single nostril in the nose (cebocephaly) (Fig. 9), premaxillary

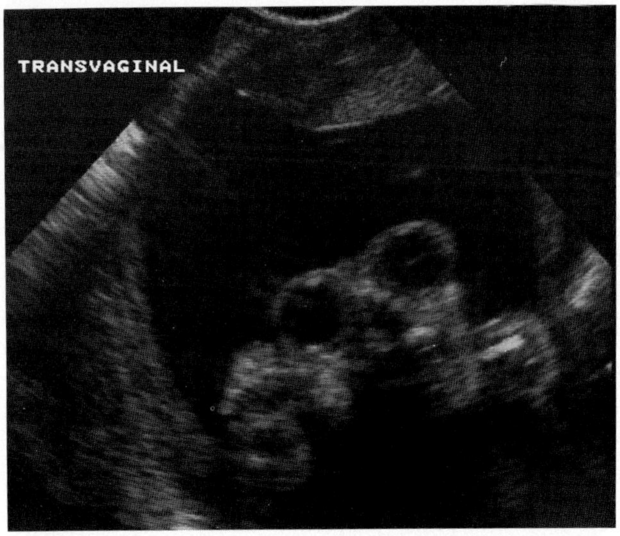


**FIGURE 10** Anencephaly. Anencephalic fetuses have a short neck, bulging eyes, and a large tongue, giving them the classic "froglike" appearance.

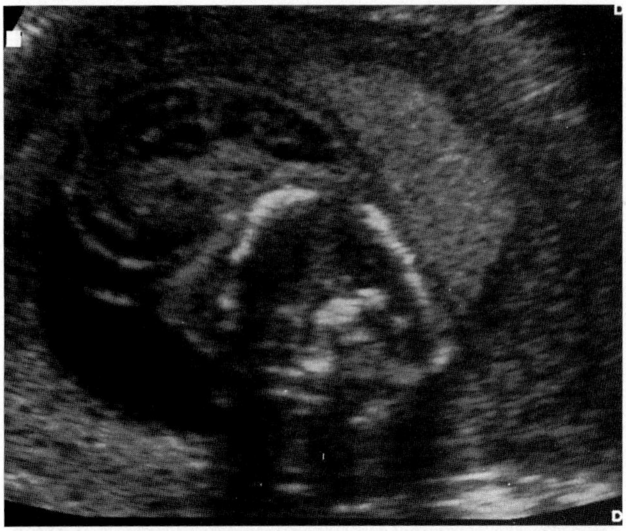

**FIGURE 11** Acrania. In acrania the neural tube has formed, but the calvarium has not formed, leaving the brain exposed. Further, because of the absence of induction, the brain does not develop properly. The brain floats in the amniotic fluid.

agenesis (median cleft), and bilateral face cleft. Other CNS anomalies associated with an abnormal face are Dandy-Walker malformation and agenesis of the corpus callosum.

## Neural Tube Defects

Neural tube defects (NTDs) are a group of disorders that have in common the failure of neural tube closure during embryogenesis. This group includes anencephaly, acrania, iniencephaly, encephalocele, and spina bifida. The incidence is higher in some parts of the United Kingdom such as Wales and Ireland. Risk factors include a family history, maternal diabetes, and teratogen exposure. The recurrence risk is around 4 percent.

Alpha-fetoprotein (AFP) is a glycoprotein produced by the fetal liver, kidneys, gastrointestinal tract, and the yolk sac. In open NTDs, AFP gains access to the amniotic fluid through exposed fetal capillaries. Maternal serum and amniotic fluid AFP are elevated in the presence of an NTD and have been successfully used as a screening tool for NTDs. Other conditions associated with elevated AFP are gastroschisis, omphalocele, amniotic band syndrome, pentalogy of Cantrell, body stalk anomaly, and esophageal defects.

### *Absence of the Cranial Vault*

The absence of the cranial vault occurs in two conditions: anencephaly and acrania. Anencephaly results from failure of fusion of the anterior neuropore around the twenty-fourth day of intrauterine life. The frontal and parietal bones are completely absent as well as the squamous part of the temporal and occipital bones. The diencephalic and mesencephalic structures are destroyed, but the hypophysis and rhombencephalic structures are preserved. Anencephalic fetuses have a short neck, bulging eyes, and a large tongue, giving them the classic "froglike" appearance with ultrasonography (Fig. 10). They are highly active, and their movements are sometimes described as painful by the patients. Polyhydramnios is a frequent finding. The association of anencephaly and spinal dysraphism is called craniorachischisis.

Acrania is not an NTD and is included in this section for differential diagnosis purposes only. It results from failure of mesenchymal migration after closure of the anterior neuropore. The cranial vault is completely or partially absent. The cerebral hemispheres are grossly abnormal and surrounded by a thin membrane (Fig. 11). Associated anomalies include cleft lip, cleft palate, and clubfoot.

### *Midline Paracranial Mass*

The identification of a paracranial mass is suspicious for a cephalocele (Fig. 12). A cephalocele is a combination of a midline mass associated with a skull defect. The term includes a spectrum of defects with a progressive degree of severity. Cranial meningocele is the herniation of the meninges alone; in cranial meningomyelocele there is associated neural tissue in the sac; encephalocele is used when there is herniated brain tissue; and encephalocystomeningocele denotes that the ventricles are partially included in the herniated sac. The presence of the skull defect is not always easily visualized with ultrasonography. The most common location is the occipital; other locations are the vertex and frontonasal positions. Associated anomalies include hydrocephalus, microcephaly, vertebral anomalies (craniorachischisis), microphthalmos, micrognathia, low-set ear, and lip and palate malformations. The main differential diagnosis is cystic hygroma of the neck. Cephaloceles are often associated with hydrocephaly and may contain identifiable brain tissue. Cystic hygromas are paracervical masses, usually with multiple septa, and have a paracervical origin.

### *Lemon Head*

The abnormal shape of the head characterized by a "concave or linear contour abnormality located at the expected position of the coronal sutures" is known as the lemon sign (see Fig. 1). The lemon sign constitutes indirect evidence of spina bifida. It

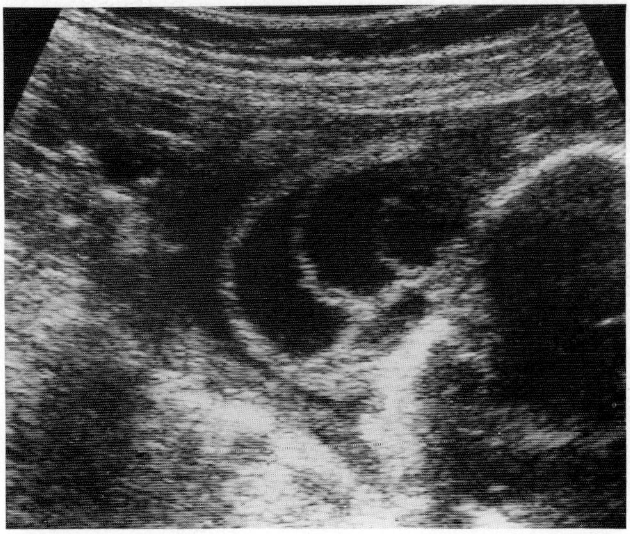

**FIGURE 12** Cephalocele. A herniated mass in the occiput, with acute angle of junction to the skin. This is typical of cephaloceles, and the acute angle of junction to the skin differentiates it from cystic hygroma (the same principle as that used to differentiate submucous leioma in the gastrointestinal tract). Search for associated hydrocephaly and microcephaly.

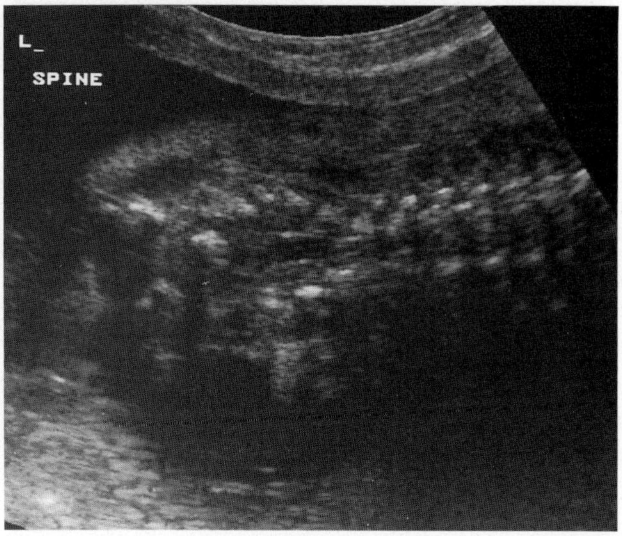


**FIGURE 13** Spina bifida. The separation of the lateral processes in spina bifida appears as a widening of the two external lines in the coronal plane.

is thought to result from decreased intraspinal pressure translated to the cranium and deforming the plastic fetal calvarium. It is highly predictive before 24 weeks, especially when associated with hydrocephalus (false-positive rate of 1 percent; positive predictive value of 81 to 84 percent).

### Abnormal Cerebellum ("Banana Sign")

The normal cerebellar hemispheres point posteriorly. The banana sign is the result of downward displacement of the cerebellum associated with spina bifida. In this instance, the cerebellar hemispheres point anteriorly and the cisterna magna is virtually obliterated. The reported sensitivity of the banana sign as an indirect marker of spina bifida is 96 percent and the negative predictive value is 100 percent.

### Abnormal Spine in Spinal Dysraphism

The fetal spine is evaluated in three basic scanning planes: sagittal, coronal, and transverse. We find the coronal and transverse sections the most useful for screening purposes.

An appropriate coronal scan of the spine demonstrates (1) two parallel lines corresponding to the lateral processes of the vertebrae, when the scanning plane is more posterior; (2) three lines, when the transducer is moved anteriorly and the vertebral bodies come into view; and (3) equal amounts of soft tissue on both sides of the vertebrae.

In transverse sections, the ossification centers of the posterior laminae and vertebral bodies encircle the neural canal. A variable amount of soft tissue and skin cover the posterior laminae.

In sagittal scans of the spine, two lines are observed. The posterior line corresponds to the laminae and the anterior line to the vertebral bodies.

### Spina Bifida

Spina bifida is a midline defect of the vertebra. In the majority of cases, the defect is posterior and is a result of the failure of fusion of the vertebral laminae. The herniation of meninges through the defect is called meningocele. The herniation of meninges and medulla is known as myelomeningocele. When skin covers the defect, the spinal dysraphism is known as spina bifida occulta. It happens in only 15 percent of cases, making the prenatal diagnosis extremely difficult. In rare instances the defect is anterior. The most common locations are the sacral and lumbar spine.

The association of spina bifida and herniation of the cerebellar vermis through the foramen magnum is known as Arnold-Chiari malformation type 2. This association is almost invariably present and results not only in the "lemon" and "banana" signs discussed above but also in some degree of obstructive hydrocephalus.

The separation of the lateral processes in spina bifida appears as a widening of the two external lines in the coronal plane (Fig. 13). In transverse sections the posterior laminae are absent and the lateral processes are set apart, giving the appearance of a V or U (Fig. 14). In open defects the skin and soft tissue are not identified. A cystic image covered by a membrane usually corresponds to a meningocele. The visualization of irregular echoes arising from the defect suggests the presence of a myelomeningocele. In longitudinal scans spina bifida is observed as an interruption of the posterior line, with absence of the overlying soft tissue and skin. A meningocele or a myelomeningocele can be identified by the same signs as previously described.

Loss of innervation leads to unopposed action of certain muscular groups of the legs. Associated anomalies include hip dislocation, clubfoot, and rocker-bottom foot.

### Spinal Lordosis

The association of short lordotic spine, imperfect formation of the base of the skull, and rachischisis is known as iniencephaly.

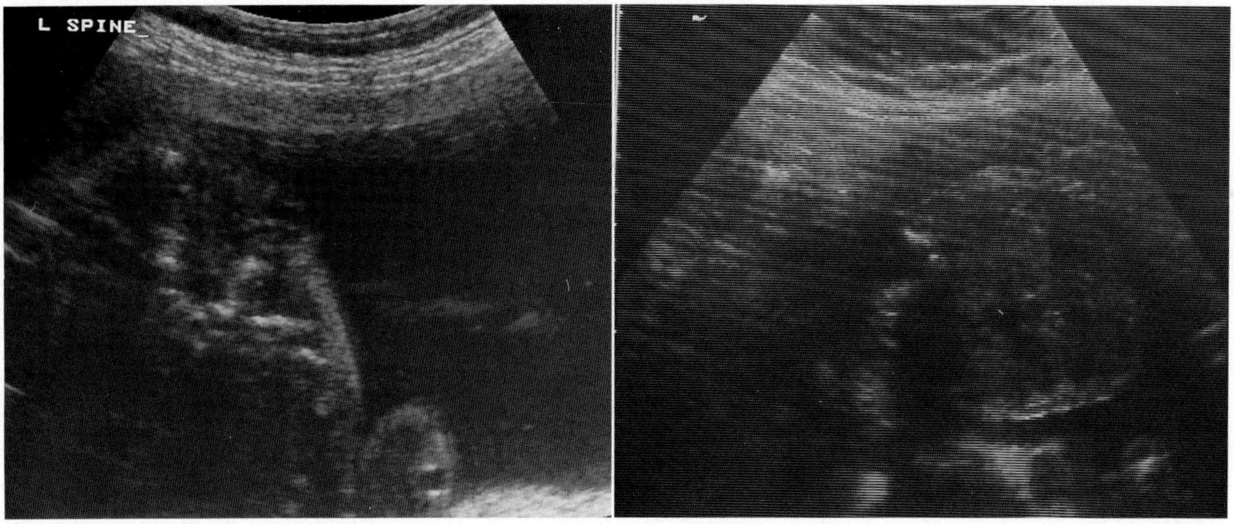


**FIGURE 14** *A* and *B*, Spina bifida. In transverse sections the posterior laminae are absent and the lateral processes are set apart, giving the appearance of a "V" or "U".

The head is extremely dorsoflexed. Associated anomalies include anencephaly, cephalocele, hydrocephaly, cyclopia, absence of mandible, cleft lip and palate, cardiovascular anomalies, diaphragmatic hernia, single umbilical artery, omphalocele, gastroschisis, situs inversus, polycystic kidneys, arthrogryposis, and clubfoot.

## The Heart

This section focuses on structural malformations of the heart. Cardiac arrhythmias are not covered, and the reader is referred to the Romero, Nyberg, and Rumack textbooks.

The incidence of congenital heart disease ranges from 2 to 6.5 percent. The five most common anomalies are ventricular septal defect (30.3 percent), patent ductus arteriosus (8.6 percent), pulmonary stenosis (7.4 percent), atrial septal defect (ASD) secundum type (6.7 percent), and coarctation of the aorta (5.7 percent).

### *Indications for Fetal Echocardiography*

Fetal echocardiography is indicated in the following circumstances:

1. Family history of congenital heart disease
2. Diabetes, lupus erythematosus, or phenylketonuria in the pregnant woman
3. Exposure to drugs, alcohol, or infections during pregnancy
4. Pregnancies complicated by polyhydramnios, nonimmune hydrops, dysrhythmias, extracardiac abnormalities, chromosomal abnormalities, and symmetrical intrauterine growth retardation (IUGR)

### *Examination Sequence*

#### 1. Determine Right and Left Sides of Fetus

By imaging the head and spine, one can establish the right and left sides of the fetus.

#### 2. Establish Heart Position Within Body

Observe the position of the heart with respect to the fetal head and spine. In levocardia (normal) the apex of the heart points to the left. The right ventricle is anterior and related to the sternum, whereas the left ventricle is posterior and close to the spine. In mesocardia the apex of the heart points anteriorly. In dextrocardia it points to the right. Dextroposition is the displacement of the heart to the right side by compressing structures such as abdominal organs in diaphragmatic hernia or lung tumors.

The evaluation of the visceral situs involves the comparison of the heart position within the thorax with the relative position of the abdominal structures. In transverse sections of the upper fetal abdomen, the stomach and spleen are normally located on the left side. The portal sinus is located to the right. The abdominal aorta in transverse sections is recognized as a pulsing round structure anterior and to the left of the spine. The inferior vena cava is found to the right of the spine, and it is more anterior than the aorta. Situs solitus is the normal situation, with the apex of the heart and stomach on the left side.

*Abnormal Situs.* Situs inversus is the mirror image of situs solitus. In isomeric situs (situs ambiguous), there is an abnormal arrangement of the thoracic and abdominal organs. Situs ambiguous can be divided in asplenic and polysplenic syndromes, and these are associated with a wide range of cardiac malformations (Fig. 15).

In asplenia syndrome or bilateral right-sidedness, left-sided organs are mirror images of the right-sided ones. As the name implies, the spleen is usually absent; the left lung is trilobed and has three main bronchi; the stomach is located either to the left, central, or to the right; the liver is central and symmetrical; and malrotation of the gut is frequent. The left atrium resembles the morphologic right, leading to bilateral superior vena cava. The hallmark of asplenia syndrome is the relationship between the aorta and inferior vena cava: they always run on the same side of the spine, either to the left or to the right. This can be easily identified in transverse sections of the fetal

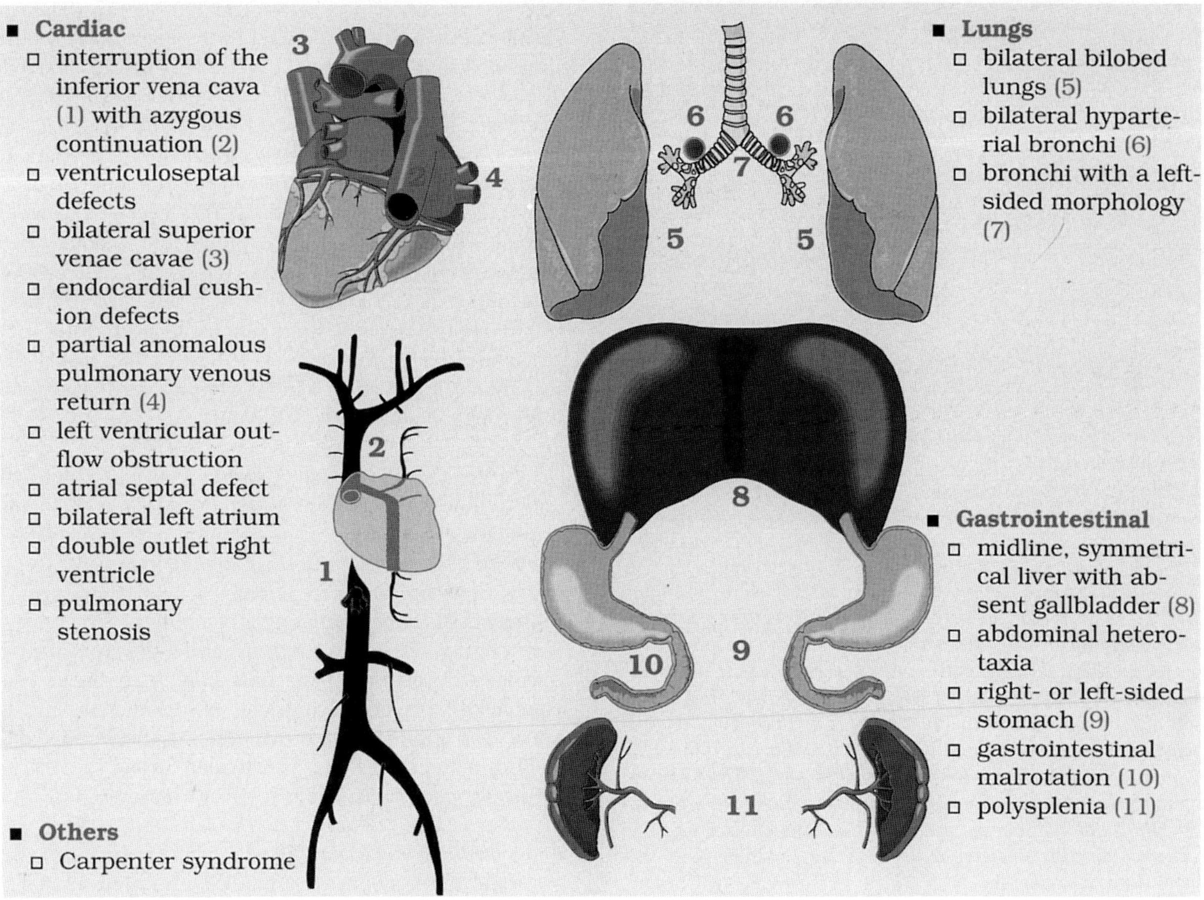


**FIGURE 15** Findings in situs ambiguous and cardiosplenic syndromes. (From Fedrizzi RP, Bruner JP, Jeanty P. Polysplenia syndrome. The Fetus 1992; 2(3):7590–7593; with permission.)

abdomen below the diaphragm. Associated cardiac malformations are total anomalous pulmonary venous return (almost 100 percent); endocardial cushion defects (85 percent); pulmonary stenosis or atresia (70 percent); transposition of the great arteries (58 percent); single ventricle (51 percent); and dextrocardia (42 percent).

Polysplenia syndrome or bilateral left-sidedness, on the other hand, is associated with two or more spleens on both sides of the mesogastrium. Both lungs are bilobed and have two stem bronchi in two-thirds of the affected individuals; the liver and stomach may be either on the right or on the left; malrotation of the gut is also frequent. The useful diagnostic hint is the frequent absence of the inferior vena cava. In this case the aorta is found anterior to the spine on the midline, and blood from the lower extremities drains through an azygous vein either on the right or the left side. The finding of an aorta and vena cava running on the same side of the spine has been reported in some cases of polysplenia. Cardiac malformations are less frequent in polysplenia than in asplenia syndrome. The most frequent are anomalous pulmonary venous return (70 percent); endocardial cushion defects (43 percent); ASDs (37 percent); dextrocardia (37 percent); double-outlet right ventricle (20 percent); and transposition of the great arteries (17 percent). Polysplenia syndrome is frequently associated with complete heart block.

### 3. Image the Four Chambers

The fetal heart is almost horizontal; therefore a four-chamber view can be obtained by a transverse section of the thorax just above the fetal diaphragm. The heart is observed on the left side of the chest, and the cardiac apex is noted pointing toward the left. The right atrium and ventricle are anterior to the left atrium and ventricle. The trabecular pattern of the morphologic right ventricle is coarse, and this ventricle has a pyramidal shape. It is also characterized by the presence of the trabecula septomarginalis of the moderator band, which appears as a thickening of the interventricular septum near the cardiac apex. Also of note is the fact that the tricuspid valve inserts in a more apical position than the mitral valve. The foramen ovale communicates between the right and left atrium. It is guarded by a valve, the foramen ovale flap, that opens toward the left atrium (Fig. 16). Using the four-chamber view, the sonographer can evaluate the integrity of the atrial and ventricular septum. A potential pitfall when scanning the fetal heart with an apical four-chamber view is that the lack of lateral resolution may lead to an artifactual dropout of echoes at the level of the ventricular septum and atrial septum secundum. An approach perpendicular for the septum should be used instead.

*Dropout of Echoes at Level of Interatrial Septum.* A dropout of echoes at the level of the interatrial septum may represent an

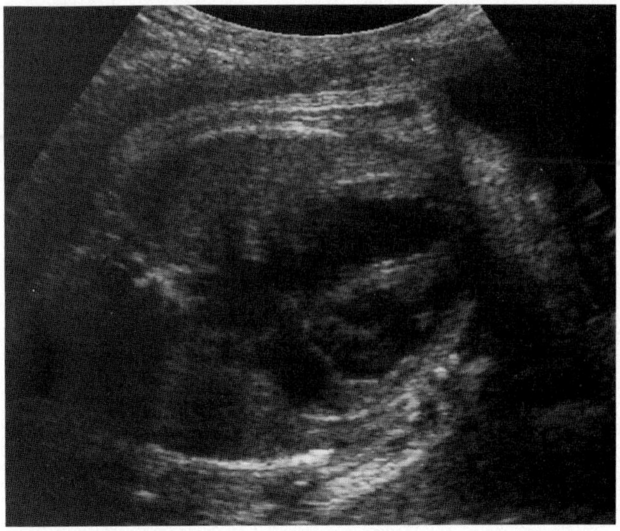

**FIGURE 16** Normal four-chamber view. A four-chamber view is obtained in a transverse section of the thorax, just above the fetal diaphragm. The heart is on the left side of the chest and the apex points to the left. The right atrium and ventricle are anterior to the left atrium and ventricle. The trabecular pattern of the right ventricle is coarse, and this ventricle has a pyramidal shape. It is also characterized by the presence of the moderator band, which is a thickening of the interventricular septum near the cardiac apex. The tricuspid valve inserts in a more apical position than the mitral valve. The foramen ovale communicates between the right and left atrium. It is guarded by the foramen ovale flap that opens toward the left atrium. Using the four-chamber view, the sonographer can evaluate the integrity of the atrial and ventricular septum.

ASD. According to the location, the defect is classified as follows:

- Sinus venosus ASD – high, close to the inlet of the superior vena cava and invariably associated with anomalous pulmonary return
- Ostium secundum ASD – central, characterized by a small or absent flap of the foramen ovale, and usually small and difficult to diagnose with prenatal ultrasonography
- Ostium primum ASD – posteroinferior, almost always associated with an abnormal left atrioventricular valve in the atrioventricular septal defect

An atrioventricular septal defect is visualized by ultrasonography as a combination of an ostium primum ASD, a single atrioventricular valve bridging both ventricles and a ventricular septal defect.

Associated cardiac malformations include asplenia and polysplenia syndromes, meso- and dextrocardia, coarctation of the aorta, tetralogy of Fallot, double-outlet right ventricle, transposition of the great arteries, pulmonary stenosis or atresia, and complete heart block. Endocardial cushion defects are frequently associated with Down's syndrome (see the Aneuploidy section).

*Dropout of Echoes at Level of Interventricular Septum.* The ventricular septum is divided into two parts: a membranous portion and a muscular portion. The muscular portion is further subdivided into inlet, trabecular, and outlet. The most common location for a ventricular septal defect is the membranous portion. A defect in the membranous portion of the ventricular septum can be missed in the four-chamber view. A complete search should include a long-axis view of the left ventricle, a long-axis view of the right ventricle, and an apex-to-base sweep across the short axis of the heart. Lack of lateral resolution of the ultrasound equipment may lead to an artifactual dropout of echoes at the level of the ventricular septum when scanning with an apical four-chamber view. The artifact is visualized as a fading out of the echo, whereas the true defect is recognized when the septum terminates as a bright spot. The best approach is to scan with the beam perpendicular to the septum. A ventricular septal defect is usually a component of a more complex cardiac anomaly, and a thorough evaluation is mandatory.

*Absence of Interventricular Septum.* Univentricular heart is a condition in which there is a single ventricle connected to two atrioventricular valves or a common atrioventricular valve. Absence of one atrioventricular connection results from mitral or tricuspid atresia. In 85 percent of cases, the ventricle has a left morphology. A rudimentary chamber may be present, and it may or may not have a connection with the great arteries. The diagnosis is made by demonstrating two atrial chambers connected to a single ventricle. Associated findings include aortic and pulmonic stenosis, and the differential diagnosis should include a large ventricular septal defect and an atrioventricular septal defect.

*Reduction in Size of Right Ventricle.* The normal ratio between the right and left ventricle should be no more than 1:3. The apex should be at the same level in the fetus. Nomograms can be used to assess normal dimensions, but the range of measurements is very wide and the anatomic landmarks may be altered in malformed hearts.

Pulmonary atresia with an intact ventricular septum and a competent tricuspid valve leads to obstruction of flow from the right ventricle to the pulmonary artery and ductus arteriosus. Because of the physiologic shunts during the fetal life, this obstruction leads to a hypoplastic right ventricle. A circular shunt is established between the dilated myocardial sinusoids and the coronary circulation, allowing blood to flow back from the right ventricle toward the right atrium and re-enter the blind ventricle through the tricuspid valve. This finding has been recently documented with color Doppler. Congestive heart failure can develop when the tricuspid valve is insufficient. In this case the right ventricle may be normal in size. A secundum-type ASD is a frequent associated anomaly.

Pulmonic stenosis results from fusion of the commissures of the pulmonary valve leaflets. Because of the distal obstruction, the right ventricle is frequently hypertrophic and reduced in size, whereas the pulmonary artery distal to the obstruction is enlarged. Associated anomalies include ASDs (common), total anomalous pulmonary venous return, and supravalvular aortic stenosis. Pulmonic stenosis is also associated with Noonan's syndrome and maternal rubella infection.

A reduction in the size of the right ventricle also occurs in Ebstein's anomaly (see opposite page).

*Reduction in Size of Left Ventricle.* Hypoplastic left ventricular syndrome results from aortic atresia and mitral hypoplasia or atresia. A large interatrial communication is present in the

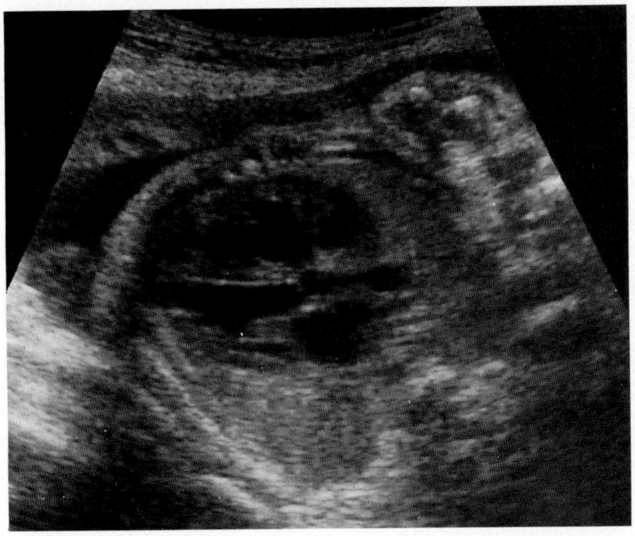

**FIGURE 17** The left ventricular outflow tract. The important landmarks to recognize are that the anterior wall of the aorta is in continuity with the interventricular septum and that the posterior wall is in continuity with the anterior leaflet of the mitral valve.

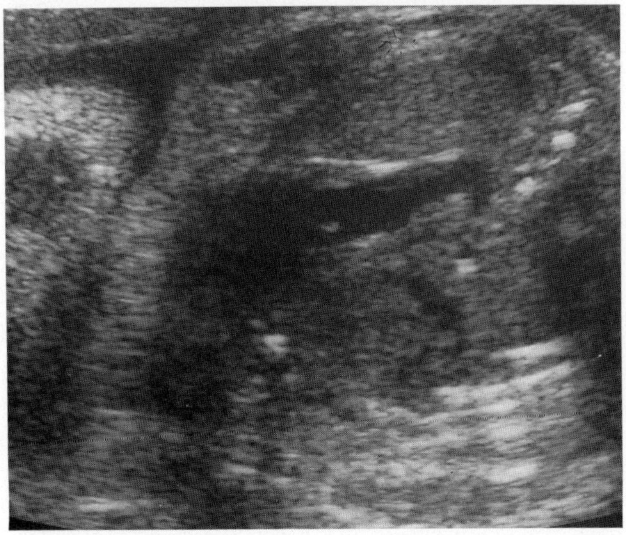

**FIGURE 18** The right ventricular outflow tract view continues in the main pulmonary artery, which divides in a large ductus and a small right pulmonary artery.

majority of cases. The decreased perfusion of the left ventricle and atrium leads to reduction in size of the left cardiac chambers. Herniation of the foramen ovale flap towards the right atrium allows for a left-to-right shunt. The right ventricle supplies the systemic circulation through the ductus arteriosus. Retrograde flow to the aortic arch and ascending aorta supplies the coronary circulation. The pulmonary venous return is diverted from the left to the right atrium through the shunt. In utero congestive heart failure can result from right ventricular work overload. (The evaluation of the size of the ventricular chambers was previously discussed.) Evaluation of the left outflow tract should demonstrate the hypoplastic ascending aorta. Coarctation of the aorta is associated in 80 percent of cases.

*Thickened Ventricular Walls.* Cardiomyopathies are caused by a variety of etiologic factors such as viruses, bacteria, glycogenosis, mucolipidosis, mucopolysaccharidosis, muscular dystrophies, endocardial fibroelastosis, maternal diabetes, and myocardial ischemia. A uniform finding is the hypertrophic myocardium leading to thickening of the ventricular walls, cardiomegaly, valvular insufficiency, poor contractility, and signs of congestive heart failure (hydrops).

*Apical Displacement of Tricuspid Valve.* Ebstein's anomaly is characterized by the apical displacement of the posterior and anterior leaflets and dysplasia of the tricuspid valve. The right ventricle is usually small as a result of "atrialization." Tricuspid insufficiency leads to blood regurgitation and enlargement of the right atrium. Regurgitation can be demonstrated with pulsed and color Doppler. Signs of in utero congestive heart failure are found in 50 percent of the cases and include cardiomegaly, hydrops, and arrhythmias. Associated anomalies include secundum-type ASDs, pulmonary atresia or stenosis, patent ductus arteriosus, tetralogy of Fallot, coarctation of the aorta, atrioventricular canal, and transposition of the great vessels.

*Enlargement of Right Atrium.* An enlarged right atrium can occur in Ebstein's anomaly (previously described) and also in vein of Galen aneurysm (see Central Nervous System section).

*Enlargement of Left Ventricle.* In aortic stenosis the left ventricle and aorta can be either hypoplastic or enlarged. The aortic valve may appear thickened. An hourglass deformity or membrane above the valve is difficult to visualize with fetal echocardiography. Asymmetric septal hypertrophy and cardiomyopathy can be demonstrated in the subvalvular types associated with maternal diabetes. Associated anomalies include the Williams syndrome in the supravalvular form. Turner's syndrome, Noonan's syndrome, and congenital rubella are associated with subaortic stenosis.

### 4. Image the Outflow Tracts

The outflow tracts are obtained by tilting the transducer in the direction of the outflow tracts of the ventricles.

The left ventricular outflow tract (Fig. 17) view demonstrates important landmarks: the mitral valve is observed between the left atrium and the left ventricle. Note that the posterior leaflet is shorter than the anterior leaflet. The anterior leaflet is in continuity with the posterior wall of the aorta. The anterior wall of the aorta is in continuity with the interventricular septum. The aortic valve can be observed at the base of the aorta.

The right ventricular outflow tract view (Fig. 18) demonstrates the main pulmonary artery originating from the right ventricle and trifurcating into a large vessel, the ductus going into the descending aorta, and two small vessels, the pulmonary arteries. The pulmonary valve is anterior and cranial to the aortic valve.

*Single Artery Over-riding the Ventricular Septum.* During the sixth and seventh weeks of embryonic development, the truncus conus segments, causing the separation of the aorta and pulmonary artery and formation of the ventricular outflow

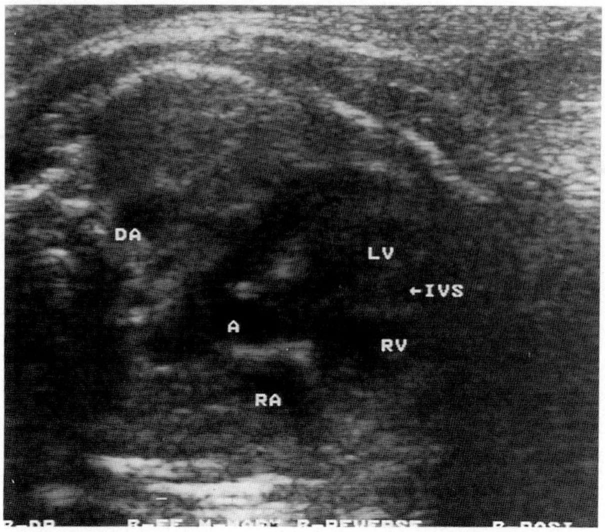


**FIGURE 19** Tetralogy of Fallot. The aorta (A) is over-riding the interventricular septum (IVS), and both ventricles feed the aorta.

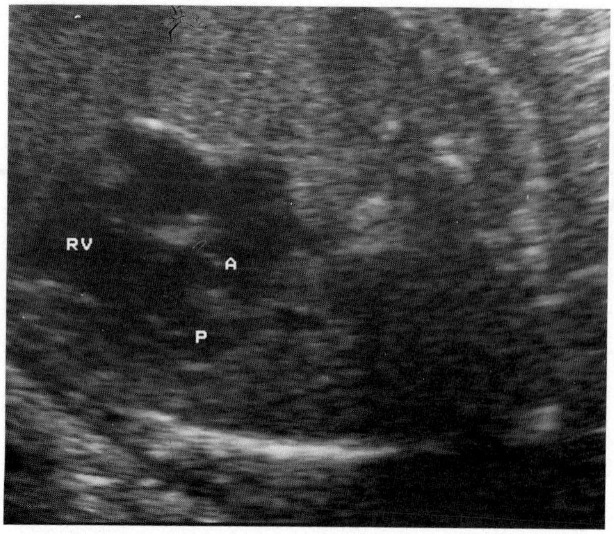


**FIGURE 20** Double-outlet right ventricle. The aorta (A) and pulmonary artery (P) arise from the right ventricle (RV).

tracts, as well as the muscular portion of the interventricular septum. Defective segmentation of the truncus conus may lead to several abnormalities including tetralogy of Fallot, truncus arteriosus, and double-outlet right ventricle.

Tetralogy of Fallot (Fig. 19) is characterized by an aorta over-riding the interventricular septum, a ventricular septal defect, and stenosis of the infundibulum of the pulmonary artery. Hypertrophy of the right ventricle usually occurs postnatally. Because of the unique shunts present during the intrauterine period, there should be no hemodynamic compromise of the fetus. Tetralogy of Fallot is usually diagnosed by imaging the left ventricular outflow tract and detecting a dilated aorta over-riding the interventricular septum. A potential artifact characterized by septo-aortic discontinuity in a normal fetus may happen with incorrect orientation of the transducer while imaging the left ventricular outflow tract. Differential diagnosis includes truncus arteriosus and double-outlet right ventricle.

In truncus arteriosus one great artery with one semilunar valve arises from both ventricles supplying the coronary, pulmonary, and systemic circulations. Depending on the presence or absence of a ventricular septal defect, the disorder is classified as A or B. According to Van Praagh, there are four possible combinations in type A as follows:

- A1 – a partially separated main pulmonary artery
- A2 – two pulmonary arteries arising from the truncus
- A3 – one pulmonary artery arising from the truncus supplying one lung and collateral arteries arising from the descending aorta supplying the other lung
- A4 – hypoplasia, coarctation, atresia, and interruption of the aortic arch

Truncus arteriosus is visualized as a single arterial vessel over-riding the ventricular septum, just as in tetralogy of Fallot. The differential diagnosis is possible only when the pulmonary arteries are observed arising from the truncus or by the identification of more than three leaflets in a truncal valve. Associated anomalies include mitral atresia, ASDs, univentricular heart, and aortic arch abnormalities.

In double-outlet right ventricle, both the pulmonary artery and most of the aorta (>50 percent) arise from the right ventricle (Fig. 20). It is usually associated with a ventricular septal defect. The diagnosis relies on the demonstration of the aorta over-riding the ventricular septum, with more than 50 percent on the right side. The disease may be easily confused with tetralogy of Fallot and corrected transposition of the great arteries. Associated defects include abnormal atrioventricular valves, anomalous venous return, coarctation of the aorta, and univentricular heart.

*Outflow Tracts Arising in Parallel from the Ventricles.* Complete transposition of the great arteries is another disorder resulting from abnormal development of the conus truncus. In this condition the atrioventricular connections are normal, the aorta arises from the right ventricle and supplies the systemic circulation, whereas the pulmonary artery arises from the left ventricle and supplies the pulmonary circulation. Three main types are distinguished, depending on the associated anomalies: (1) without a ventricular septal defect (it may or may not have an associated pulmonic stenosis), (2) with a ventricular septal defect, and (3) with a ventricular septal defect and pulmonic stenosis.

The defect can be demonstrated by imaging both ventricular outflow tracts in the long-axis view of the ventricles or short-axis views of the great vessels. Instead of the normal criss-crossing of the great vessels, they arise in parallel. Besides the aforementioned anomalies, atrioventricular septal defects, anomalies of the atrioventricular valves, and coarctation of the aorta can be associated with complete transposition of the great arteries.

The same diagnostic findings described for complete transposition apply for corrected transposition. The associated anomalies are responsible for the poor prognosis and include situs inversus, ventricular septal defect, pulmonic stenosis, and a pulmonary artery over-riding the ventricular septum. Ebstein-like malformations of the tricuspid valve and derangement of the conduction system lead to atrioventricular block.

*Narrowing of Aortic Arch.* Coarctation of the aorta is defined as a shelflike lesion present at any point along the aortic arch. The diagnosis is usually performed by demonstrating a narrowing on the isthmic region of the aortic arch. Coarctation of the aorta is associated with a wide range of intracardiac malformations including aortic stenosis, aortic insufficiency, ventricular septal defects, ASDs, transposition of the great arteries, atrioventricular canal, truncus arteriosus, and double-outlet right ventricle. Once the diagnosis is suspected, a careful search for signs of Turner's syndrome or chromosomal analysis is recommended.

### 5. Image the Inflow Tracts

The systemic venous return can be assessed easily by a right parasagittal scan, demonstrating the inferior and superior vena cava entering the right atrium.

*Failure to Demonstrate Pulmonary Veins Connecting to Left Atrium.* Total anomalous pulmonary return is a condition in which the pulmonary veins drain into the right atrium in one of the following ways:

- Draining into a right superior vena cava, azygous vein, and innominate vein and then to the right atrium
- Draining into a left superior vena cava and then to the coronary sinus
- Draining to a portal vein and then to the inferior vena cava and right atrium
- Draining directly into the inferior vena cava and right atrium

The diagnosis relies on the failure of visualizing the pulmonary veins entering a usually small left atrium. This anomaly is frequently associated with atrioventricular septal defects and cardiosplenic syndromes.

*Echogenic Masses Inside Heart.* The finding of an echogenic mass inside the cardiac cavities is highly suggestive of a cardiac tumor. The most frequent ones are rhabdomyomas, teratomas, and fibromas of the heart. Rhabdomyomas are singular or multiple and typically arise from the interventricular septum. They have a strong association with tuberous sclerosis. Another common tumor is fibroma.

## Skeletal Dysplasias

The fetal extremities are examined both for biometric purposes and to screen for anatomical abnormalities. The humerus and femur lengths are correlated with various tables to give more parameters in addition to the BPD to estimate gestational age. This is obtained by measuring the ossified diaphyses of these long bones. It is important to identify all segments of the fetal extremities, because limb reduction abnormalities are, for the most part, a nongenetic group of disorders. Of interest are three limb reduction abnormalities that are inherited on a genetic basis. These are Robert's syndrome, Holt-Oram syndrome, and thrombocytopenia with absent radius syndrome. Robert's syndrome is autosomal recessive and is characterized by tetraphocomelia with associated midfacial clefting or hypoplastic nasal alae. Holt-Oram syndrome is inherited as autosomal dominant, with variable penetrance, and is characterized by hypoplasia or aplasia of the radius with associated congenital heart disease, mainly secundum-type ASDs. Thrombocytopenia with absent radius syndrome is autosomal recessive and is characterized by thrombocytopenia and bilateral absence of the radii.

The differential diagnosis of skeletal dysplasias is complicated. The workup of a suspected fetus is time-consuming and involves a meticulous scanning of all organs and systems. The sonographer must know the normal skeletal anatomy and be able not only to obtain adequate measurements but also to identify deviations from normal in shape, integrity, and degree of mineralization of the bones. Once a skeletal anomaly is suspected, a thorough search for associated malformations should be performed.

Micromelia refers to shortening of the entire limb; rhizomelia is the shortening of the proximal segment; mesomelia refers to shortening of the intermediate segment; and acromelia is the shortening of the distal segment of the limb. The differential diagnosis of micromelic, rhizomelic, and mesomelic skeletal dysplasias involves the comparison of measurements of the bones of the thigh and leg as well as the arm and forearm.

Cloverleaf skull is a form of craniosynostosis resulting from premature closure of the coronal and lambdoid sutures. It is characterized by a prominent vertex of the calvarium in the middle and of the two temporal bones on the sides.

Platyspondyly is the flattening of the vertebral bodies with apparent widening of the intervertebral spaces.

Postaxial polydactyly refers to the presence of additional digits on the ulnar or fibular side of the limb. Preaxial polydactyly is the presence of additional digits on the radial or tibial side of the extremity. Syndactyly is the fusion of two or more digits. Clinodactyly is the deviation of one or more digits.

Clubfoot (Fig. 21) is characterized by medial deviation and inversion of the sole of the foot. It can be diagnosed by imaging both bones of the leg and the foot in the same plane at an angle to each other.

The following is a workup on the differential diagnosis of skeletal dysplasias. The process of learning skeletal dysplasias is lengthy and comes only with experience. We concentrate on features that lead to the suspicion of a skeletal anomaly, rather than the description of the diseases themselves. The tables provide a quick reference guide and diagnostic orientation. For a detailed discussion of specific anomalies, please refer to the textbooks by Romero, Nyberg, and Fleischer.

### *Biometry of the Long Bones*

Evaluation of fetal bone growth is one of the parameters used in the diagnosis of a skeletal dysplasia. We consider a measurement abnormal when it falls below the fifth percentile for gestational age. One must realize that 2.5 percent of the normal population falls below the fifth percentile for age, and that an abnormal measurement is not by itself diagnostic of a skeletal anomaly. Whenever there is a suspicion of a skeletal dysplasia, all bones in all extremities should be measured and examined to differentiate between micromelia, rhizomelia, and mesomelia and also to exclude the absence or hypoplasia of specific bones.

Preliminary results of a multicentric study in skeletal dysplasias indicate that some disorders affect growth more than others. For instance, fetuses with achondrogenesis are the most strikingly affected, with measurements always below one-half and sometimes below one-fourth of the mean for gestational age. Measurements for fetuses with thanatophoric

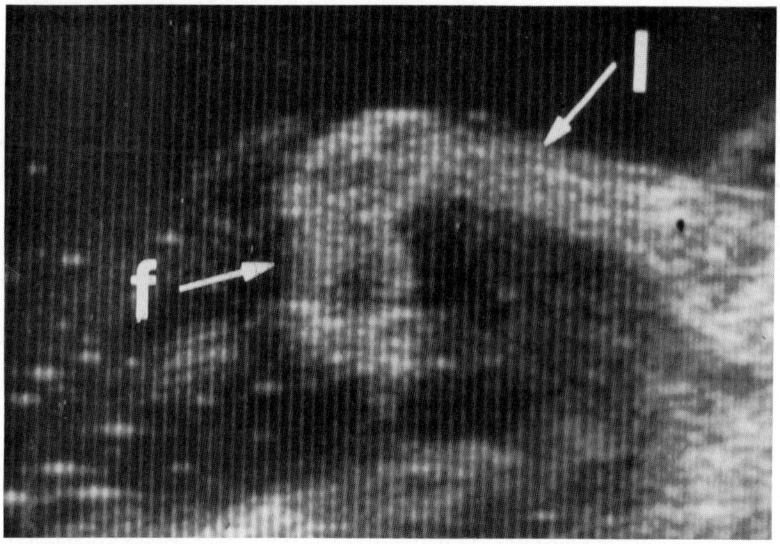


**FIGURE 21** Clubfoot. Observe both bones of the leg (l) and the foot (f) in the same plane at an angle to each other.

dysplasia tend to fall between one-quarter and three-fourths of the mean for gestational age. The measurements of the long bones in hypochondroplasia and achondroplasia usually fall between half of the mean and the fifth percentile for gestational age.

### *Chest Biometry*

Some disorders affect the growth of the ribs, leading to a narrow thorax. Chest dimensions are evaluated by the ratio between the chest circumference measured at the level of the four-chamber view of the heart and the abdominal circumference. It is useful to have both circumferences displayed on the same image to establish a visual comparison. The normal thoracic-to-abdominal circumference ratio ranges between 0.77 and 1.01.

Disorders associated with a narrow thorax are asphyxiating thoracic dysplasia, chondroectodermal dysplasia, metatropic dysplasia, fibrochondrogenesis, atelosteogenesis, camptomelic dysplasia, achondrogenesis, hypophosphatasia, short rib–polydactyly syndrome, thanatophoric dysplasia, and heterozygous achondroplasia. The differential diagnosis for these anomalies is presented in Tables 1 and 2.

### *Bowing of Bones*

There is no simple rule to establish the degree of curvature of the long bones. The difference between normal and abnormal comes only with experience.

The following skeletal dysplasias are characterized by bone bowing: camptomelic dysplasia (Fig. 22), osteogenesis imperfecta, dis-segmental dysplasia, otopalatodigital syndrome, thanatophoric dysplasia, Robert's syndrome, hypophosphatasia, and heterozygous achondroplasia. The differential diagnosis is presented in Tables 3 and 4.

### *Bone Fractures*

Bone fractures are found in osteogenesis imperfecta, hypophosphatasia, and achondrogenesis. The differential diagnosis for these conditions is listed in Table 5.

### *Absence or Hypoplasia of Bones*

The absence of a limb or limbs is known as amelia; hemimelia is the absence of a longitudinal segment of a limb; phocomelia refers to the hypoplasia of the limbs, with the hands and feet attached to the shoulder and hips; acheira is the absence of one or both hands, apodia is the absence of one or both feet, and acheiropodia is the absence of both hands and feet. The differential diagnosis of skeletal dysplasias associated with specific limb reduction anomalies is shown in Tables 6 and 7.

### *Other Skeletal Dysplasias*

The following diseases do not fit in the categories previously described: Larsen's syndrome, Kniest syndrome, spondyloepiphyseal dysplasia, diastrophic dysplasia, and chondrodysplasia puntacta. The differential diagnosis for these conditions is presented in Tables 8 and 9.

## Aneuploidy

Chromosomal abnormalities can be detected by different diagnostic modalities. Women at risk for a chromosome disorder are usually screened with a variety of tests including maternal serum α-fetoprotein, serum β-HCG, and fetal karyotype obtained at amniocentesis, chorionic villus sampling, or fetal blood sampling. However, screening all mothers at risk would probably identify only 20 percent of the fetuses currently born with trisomy 21, since 80 percent of affected newborns are the offspring of young mothers with no known risk factors.

Prenatal ultrasonography can aid in the diagnosis of a fetal aneuploidy in several ways. The first one is to establish a gestational age on which to rely while interpreting the results of the tests mentioned previously. The second one is to provide guidance for the invasive procedures necessary to obtain a fetal karyotype. The third one is to detect warning signs that may lead to a high degree of suspicion of a more complex syndrome in otherwise low-risk patients. The objective of this section is to review the findings suggestive of aneuploidy. Bear in mind that even though some anomalies are highly suggestive of a chromosome abnormality, no one is 100 percent specific.

*Text continued on p. 213.*

**TABLE 1** Differential Diagnosis of Skeletal Dysplasias Associated with a Narrow Thorax: Skeletal Findings

| | 1 | 2 | 3 | 4 | 5 | 6 | 7 | 8 | 9 | 10 | 11 |
|---|---|---|---|---|---|---|---|---|---|---|---|
| Acromesomelia | | | | | | + | | | | | |
| Bowed long bones | | + | + | + | | | | + | + | | |
| Cleft lip and palate | | + | | + | + | | | + | | | |
| Cleft of vertebral bodies | | + | | | | | | + | | | |
| Cloverleaf skull | | | + | | | | | | | | |
| Clubfoot | | | | + | | | | | | | + |
| Contractures | | | | | + | | | | | | |
| Demineralization of bones | | | | | | | | | + | | |
| Depressed nasal bridge | + | | + | + | | | + | + | | | |
| Disproportionally short fibula | | | | | + | | | | | | |
| Dumbbell-shaped metaphyses | | | | | + | | | | | | + |
| Frontal bossing | | | + | | + | | | | | | |
| Hypertelorism | | | + | | + | | | | | | |
| Hypoplastic scapulae | | | | | | | | + | | | |
| Hypoplastic vertebral bodies | | | | | | | | + | | | |
| Lack of vertebral ossification | + | | | | | | | | | | |
| Large head | | | + | | | | + | | | | |
| Long and thin clavicles | | | | | + | | | | | | |
| Low-set ears | | | | | + | | | | | | |
| Micrognathia | + | | | | | | | + | | | |
| Mildly shortened bones | | | | | | | | | | + | |
| Multiple fractures | + | | | | | | | | + | | |
| Platyspondyly | | | + | | | | | | | | |
| Polydactyly | | + | | | | + | | | | | |
| Radioulnar synostosis | | | + | | | | | | | | |
| Rhizomelia | | | + | + | + | | | | | | |
| Severe micromelia | + | + | + | + | + | | | | | | |
| Tail-like appendage at level of coccyx | | | | | | | | | | | + |
| Vertically narrowed iliac bones | | | | | | | | + | | | |

1. Achondrogenesis
2. Short rib–polydactyly syndrome
3. Thanatophoric dysplasia
4. Atelosteogenesis
5. Fibrochondrogenesis
6. Chondroectodermal dysplasia
7. Heterozygous achondroplasia
8. Camptomelic dysplasia
9. Hypophosphatasia
10. Asphyxiating thoracic dysplasia
11. Metatropic dysplasia

**TABLE 2** Differential Diagnosis of Skeletal Dysplasias Associated with a Narrow Thorax: Associated Anomalies

| | 1 | 2 | 3 | 4 | 5 | 6 | 7 | 8 | 9 | 10 | 11 |
|---|---|---|---|---|---|---|---|---|---|---|---|
| Agenesis of gallbladder | | + | | | | | | | | | |
| Aortic stenosis | | | | | | | | + | | | |
| Atrial septal defect | | | + | | | | | + | | | |
| Cryptorchidism | | | | | | + | | | | | |
| Cystic dilatation of collecting ducts | | | | | | | | | | + | |
| Defective tricuspid valve | | | + | | | | | | | | |
| Double-outlet right ventricle | | + | | | | | | | | | |
| Endocardial cushion defect | | + | | | | | | | | | |
| Horseshoe kidney | | | + | | | | | | | | |
| Hydrocephalus | | | + | | | | + | + | | | |
| Hydronephrosis | | | + | | | | | + | | | |
| Hyperplasia of bile ducts | | | | | | | | | | + | |
| Hypoplastic kidneys | | + | | | | | | | | | |
| Imperforate anus | | + | + | | | | | | | | |
| Interstitial fibrosis of pancreas | | | | | | | | | | + | |
| Intestinal atresia | | + | | | | | | | | | |
| Periglomerular fibrosis of kidneys | | | | | | | | | | + | |
| Periportal fibrosis | | | | | | | | | | + | |
| Polycystic kidneys | | + | | | | | | | | | |
| Polycystic liver disease | | | | | | | | | | + | |
| Polyhydramnios | + | | + | | | | | | + | | + |
| Tetralogy of Fallot | | | | | | | | + | | | |
| Transposition of great arteries | | + | | | | | | | | | |
| Tubular dysplasia of kidneys | | | | | | | | | | + | |
| Ventricular septal defect | | | | | | | | + | | | |

1. Achondrogenesis
2. Short rib–polydactyly syndrome
3. Thanatophoric dysplasia
4. Atelosteogenesis
5. Fibrochondrogenesis
6. Chondroectodermal dysplasia
7. Heterozygous achondroplasia
8. Camptomelic dysplasia
9. Hypophosphatasia
10. Asphyxiating thoracic dysplasia
11. Metatropic dysplasia

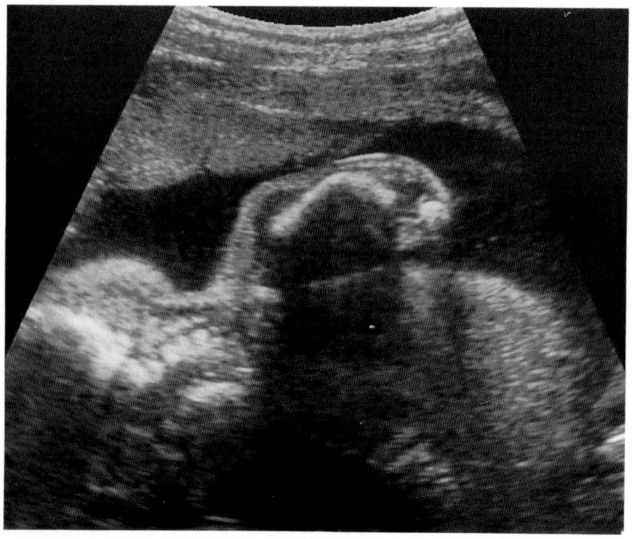

**FIGURE 22** Camptomelic dysplasia. Note the pronounced bowing of the humerus in this fetus.

**TABLE 3** Differential Diagnosis of Skeletal Dysplasias Associated with Bowing of the Long Bones: Skeletal Findings

| | 1 | 2 | 3 | 4 | 5 | 6 | 7 | 8 |
|---|---|---|---|---|---|---|---|---|
| Absent or hypoplastic fibula | | | | + | | | | |
| Cleft lip and palate | + | | + | + | | + | | |
| Cloverleaf skull | | | | | + | | | |
| Clubfoot | | | | | | + | | |
| Congenital hip dislocation | + | | | | | | | |
| Demineralization of bones | | + | | | | | + | |
| Depressed nasal bridge | | | | + | | | | + |
| Disorganization of vertebral bodies | | | + | | | | | |
| Fractures of long bones | | + | | | | | + | |
| Frontal bossing | | | | | + | | | + |
| Hypertelorism | | | | + | | + | | |
| Hypoplastic scapulae | + | | | | | | | |
| Hypoplastic vertebral bodies | + | | | | | | | |
| Macrocephaly | + | | | | + | | | |
| Metaphyseal flaring of long bones | | | + | | | | | |
| Microcephaly | | | | | | + | | |
| Micrognathia | + | | | + | | | | |
| Narrow intervertebral space | | | | | | | | + |
| Narrow thorax | + | | | | + | | | |
| Nonmineralized pedicles of spine | + | | | | | | | |
| Overlapping fingers | | | | + | | | | |
| Polydactyly | | | | + | | | | |
| Radioulnar synostosis | | | | | + | | | |
| Severe micromelia | | | + | | | | | |
| Short big toes | | | | + | | | | |
| Short bones of hands and feet | | | | | | | | + |
| Short thumbs | | | | + | | | | |
| Skull thinner than usual, compressible | | + | | | | | + | |
| Syndactyly | | | | + | | | | |
| Tetraphocomelia | | | | | | + | | |
| Trident hand | | | | | | | | + |
| Vertebral clefts | | | + | | | | | |
| Vertically narrow iliac wings | + | | | | | | | |

1. Camptomelic dysplasia
2. Osteogenesis imperfecta type 2
3. Dis-segmental dysplasia
4. Otopalatodigital syndrome
5. Thanatophoric dysplasia
6. Robert's syndrome
7. Hypophosphatasia
8. Heterozygous achondroplasia

**TABLE 4** Differential Diagnosis of Skeletal Dysplasias Associated with Bowing of the Long Bones: Associated Anomalies

| | 1 | 2 | 3 | 4 | 5 | 6 | 7 | 8 |
|---|---|---|---|---|---|---|---|---|
| Atrial septal defect | + | | | | + | | | |
| Cephalocele | | | + | | | + | + | |
| Defective tricuspid valve | | | | | + | + | | |
| Horseshoe kidney | | | | | + | + | + | |
| Hydrocephalus | + | | + | | + | | | + |
| Hydronephrosis | + | | + | | + | | | |
| Imperforate anus | | | | | + | | | |
| Inguinal hernia | | | + | | | | | |
| Ocular proptosis | | | | | | | + | |
| Patent ductus arteriosus | | | + | | | | | |
| Polycystic kidneys | | | | | | + | + | |
| Polyhydramnios | | | | | + | | + | |
| Spina bifida | | | | | | + | | |
| Tetralogy of Fallot | + | | | | | | | |
| Ventricular septal defect | + | | | | | | | |

1. Camptomelic dysplasia
2. Osteogenesis imperfecta type 2
3. Dis-segmental dysplasia
4. Otopalatodigital syndrome
5. Thanatophoric dysplasia
6. Robert's syndrome
7. Hypophosphatasia
8. Heterozygous achondroplasia

**TABLE 5** Differential Diagnosis of Skeletal Dysplasias Associated with Bone Fractures

| | 1 | 2 | 3 |
|---|---|---|---|
| Bowed bones | + | + | |
| Extreme micromelia | | | + |
| Lack of ossification of calvarium | + | + | + |
| Lack of ossification of spine | + | + | + |
| Large cranium | | | + |
| Narrow thorax | | | + |
| Polyhydramnios | | + | + |
| Skull thinner than usual, compressible | + | + | |

1. Osteogenesis imperfecta
2. Hypophosphatasia
3. Achondrogenesis

**TABLE 6** Differential Diagnosis of Skeletal Dysplasias Associated with Limb Reduction Abnormalities: Skeletal Findings

| | 1 | 2 | 3 | 4 | 5 | 6 | 7 | 8 | 9 |
|---|---|---|---|---|---|---|---|---|---|
| Absence of hypoplasia of the clavicle | | | + | + | + | + | | | |
| Absence or hypoplasia of radial structures (radius, thumb, first metacarpal and carpal bones) | | | | + | | | | | |
| Absent toes and fingers | | | + | | | | | | |
| Bilateral absence of radius | | | | | + | | | | |
| Bowed long bones | + | | + | | | | + | + | |
| Brachycephaly | | | | | + | | | | |
| Cleft lip and palate | + | + | + | | | | + | | + |
| Cleft of vertebral bodies | + | | | | | | | | |
| Clubfoot | | | + | | + | | + | + | |
| Depressed nasal bridge | + | | | | | | + | | + |
| Dumbbell-shaped metaphyses | | + | | | | | | | |
| Enlarged foramen magnum | | | | | | + | | | |
| Hemivertebra | | | | | | | | + | |
| Hypertelorism | | + | + | | | | | + | + |
| Hypoplastic nasal alae | | | + | | | | | | |
| Hypoplastic or absent fibula | | + | | | | | + | + | |
| Hypoplastic or absent humerus | | | | | + | | | | |
| Hypoplastic or absent ulna | | | | | + | | | + | |
| Hypoplastic scapulae | + | | | | | | | | |
| Hypoplastic vertebral bodies | + | | | | | | | | |
| Long and thin clavicles | | + | | | | | | | |
| Low-set ears | | + | | | | | | | |
| Mesomelia | | | | | | | | + | |
| Microcephaly | | | + | | | | | | |
| Micrognathia | + | | | | + | | | + | + |
| Narrow thorax | + | + | | | | + | + | | |
| Overlapping fingers | | | | | | | | | + |
| Polydactyly | | + | | | | | | + | + |
| Rhizomelia | | + | | | | | + | | |
| Severe micromelia | | + | + | | | | + | | |
| Short big toes and thumbs | | | | | | | | | + |
| Syndactyly | | | | | + | | | | + |
| Tetraphocomelia | | | + | | | | | | |
| Vertically narrowed iliac bones | + | | | | | | | | |
| Wide sutures and multiple wormian bones of skull | | | | | | + | | | |

1. Camptomelic dysplasia
2. Fibrochondrogenesis
3. Robert's syndrome
4. Holt-Oram syndrome
5. Thrombocytopenia with absent radius
6. Cleidocranial dysplasia
7. Atelosteogenesis
8. Mesomelic dysplasia
9. Otopalatodigital syndrome

**TABLE 7** Differential Diagnosis of Skeletal Dysplasias Associated with Limb Reduction Abnormalities: Associated Anomalies

| | 1 | 2 | 3 | 4 | 5 | 6 | 7 | 8 | 9 |
|---|---|---|---|---|---|---|---|---|---|
| Atrial septal defect | + | | | + | + | | | | |
| Cephalocele | | | + | | | | | | |
| Horseshoe kidneys | | | + | | | | | | |
| Hydrocephalus | + | | + | | | | | | |
| Hydronephrosis | + | | | | | | | | |
| Ocular proptosis | | | + | | | | | | |
| Polycystic kidneys | | | + | | | | | | |
| Polyhydramnios | | | + | | | | | | |
| Spina bifida | | | + | | + | | | | |
| Tetralogy of Fallot | + | | | + | + | | | | |
| Thrombocytopenia | | | | | + | | | | |
| Ventricular septal defect | + | | | + | | | | | |

1. Camptomelic dysplasia
2. Fibrochondrogenesis
3. Robert's syndrome
4. Holt-Oram syndrome
5. Thrombocytopenia with absent radius
6. Cleidocranial dysplasia
7. Atelosteogenesis
8. Mesomelic dysplasia
9. Otopalatodigital syndrome

## *Head*

Refer to the Central Nervous System section for the sonographic characteristics of the anomalies cited below. Signs of microcephaly, hydrocephalus, choroid plexus cysts, holoprosencephaly, agenesis of the corpus callosum, and the Dandy-Walker variant (a cyst in the posterior fossa and cerebellar hypoplasia without ventricular dilatation) are often associated with aneuploidy (Table 10).

1. Holoprosencephaly is suggestive of trisomy 13 (also trisomy 18, 5p+, 13q−, 18p−), especially when associated with facial anomalies, omphalocele, and renal cystic dysplasia.
2. The Dandy-Walker variant, with cerebellar hypoplasia and no ventricular dilatation, suggests trisomy 18 or 13.
3. Large, bilateral, choroid plexus cysts, especially if associated with other anomalies, suggest trisomy 18. The risk for small, isolated, choroid plexus cysts is around 1 percent.
4. Hydrocephalus and/or spina bifida: the risk of a chromosome anomaly associated with hydrocephalus alone is 3 percent; when hydrocephalus is associated with spina bifida it is 33 percent; for spina bifida alone the risk is estimated as 8 percent. The anomalies more commonly associated in decreasing order of frequency are trisomy 18, 13, and triploidy.
5. Agenesis of the corpus callosum is associated with trisomy 18, 13, and 8; triploidy; and translocations.
6. Changes of the shape of the head can be associated with aneuploidy. Dolichocephaly and brachycephaly can be recognized by the cephalic index (cephalic index = biparietal diameter/occipitofrontal diameter). The cephalic

**TABLE 8** Differential Diagnosis of Skeletal Dysplasias Not Associated with Either a Narrow Thorax, Bowing, Fractures, or Limb Reduction Abnormalities: Skeletal Findings

| | 1 | 2 | 3 | 4 | 5 |
|---|---|---|---|---|---|
| Abducted position of the thumbs (hitchhiker thumb) | | | | + | |
| Broad thorax | | + | + | | |
| Cleft of vertebral bodies | | + | | | + |
| Cleft palate | + | + | | | |
| Clubfoot | | | | + | |
| Depressed nasal bridge | + | + | | + | + |
| Dumbbell-shaped tubular bones | | + | | | |
| Flat face | + | + | | | + |
| Hypoplasia of odontoid process | | | + | | |
| Micrognathia | | | | + | |
| Micromelia (not necessarily severe) | | | | + | |
| Mild to no shortening of long bones | | | + | | |
| Multiple joint flexion contractures | | | | + | + |
| Multiple joint laxities, dislocations | + | | | | |
| Ovoid vertebral bodies | | | + | | |
| Platyspondyly | | + | + | | |
| Scoliosis | + | + | | + | |
| Supernumerary ossification center of calcaneus | + | | | | |
| Tubular bones not shortened | + | | | | |

1. Larsen's syndrome
2. Kniest syndrome
3. Spondyloepiphyseal dysplasia
4. Diastrophic dysplasia
5. Chondrodysplasia puntacta, rhizomelic type

**TABLE 9** Differential Diagnosis of Skeletal Dysplasias Not Associated with Either a Narrow Thorax, Bowing, Fractures, or Limb Reduction Abnormalities: Associated Anomalies

| | 1 | 2 | 3 | 4 | 5 |
|---|---|---|---|---|---|
| Cardiac defects | + | | | | |
| Cataract | | | | | + |
| Deafness | | + | | | |
| Ichthyosiform skin dysplasia | | | | | + |
| Inguinal hernia | | + | | | |
| Myopia | | + | | | |
| Retinal detachment | | + | | | |

1. Larsen's syndrome
2. Kniest syndrome
3. Spondyloepiphyseal dysplasia
4. Diastrophic dysplasia
5. Chondrodysplasia punctata, rhizomelic type

**TABLE 10** CNS Malformations Associated with Aneuploidy

| | Trisomy 13 | Trisomy 18 | Trisomy 21 | Triploidy | Monosomy 45,XO |
|---|---|---|---|---|---|
| Hydrocephalus | + | | * | + + | |
| Microcephaly | + + + | * | * | | |
| Holoprosencephaly | + + + + | * | | + + | |
| Cerebellar anomalies | + + | | | | |
| Agenesis of corpus callosum | + | * | | + | |
| Myelomeningocele | | + | | + | |
| Dolichocephaly | | * | | | |
| Brachycephaly | | | * | | |
| Choroid plexus cysts | | † | | | |

\+ Below 25%
\+ + Between 25 and 50%
\+ + + Between 50 and 75%
\+ + + + Above 75%
*The association is reported in the literature, but the incidence is unknown.
†Large and bilateral choroid plexus cysts have been reported in association with trisomy 18. The reported incidence of choroid plexus cysts in fetuses with trisomy 18 varies from 20 to 71%.

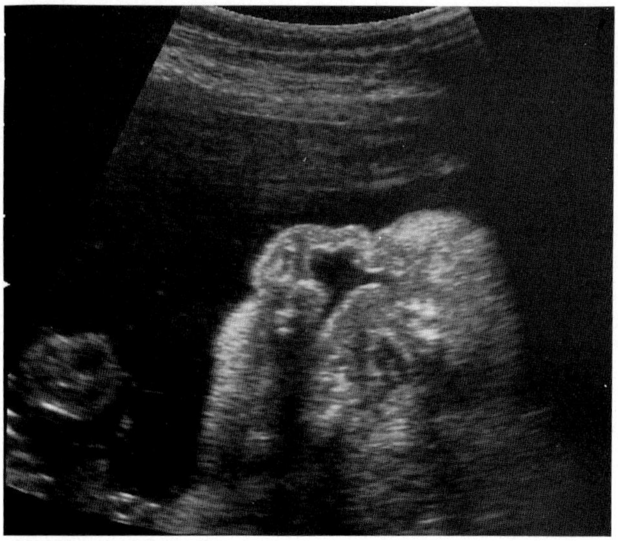

**FIGURE 23** Cleft lip. A defect extending from the mouth to the left nostril is visible.

index is below 75 percent in dolichocephaly, whereas in brachycephaly it is above 85 percent. Because of compression of the fetal head, dolichocephaly is usually a normal finding in breech presentation and oligohydramnios. However, it can be associated with trisomy 18. Brachycephaly is commonly associated with aneuploidy or craniosynostosis.

## *Face and Neck*

1. Facial clefts (Fig. 23) are identified using a coronal view through the lips and nose and axial scans of the palate. They can be unilateral, bilateral, or central. The association between median clefts and holoprosencephaly is known as the median cleft syndrome. The cleft involves the upper lip and the palate, and the tongue is usually higher than the normal position inside the oral cavity in axial scans. Facial clefts are associated with trisomy 13 and 18, particularly when CNS disorders or malformations are present (Table 11).
2. Ocular anomalies: hypertelorism, hypotelorism, cyclopia, and microphthalmia. Nomograms for the binocular distance, interorbital distance, and ocular diameter have been described in the literature. Hypertelorism (increased interocular distance) and hypotelorism (decreased interocular distance) can be identified using these nomograms. Cyclopia is a condition in which the two orbits merge to form a single cavity containing one eye; it is associated with a proboscis that projects from the lower forehead superior to the orbit; the nose is absent. Cyclopia and hypotelorism are associated with the holoprosencephaly sequence.
3. Proboscis is a trunklike structure, usually with a central

**TABLE 11** Facial Anomalies Associated with Aneuploidy

| | Trisomy 13 | Trisomy 18 | Trisomy 21 | Triploidy | Monosomy 45,XO |
|---|---|---|---|---|---|
| Facial clefts | + + + | + | | + | |
| Microphthalmia | * | | | | |
| Cyclopia | * | | | | |
| Hypotelorism | * | | | | |
| Hypertelorism | | | | * | |
| Micrognathia | | * | | + + | |
| Low nasal bridge | | | * | | |
| Macroglossia | | | * | | |
| Cystic hygroma of neck | | + | + | | + + + |
| Nuchal skin thickening | * | * | + + + | | * |

\+ Below 25%
\+ + Between 25 and 50%
\+ + + Between 50 and 75%
\+ + + + Above 75%
*The association is reported in the literature, but the incidence is unknown.

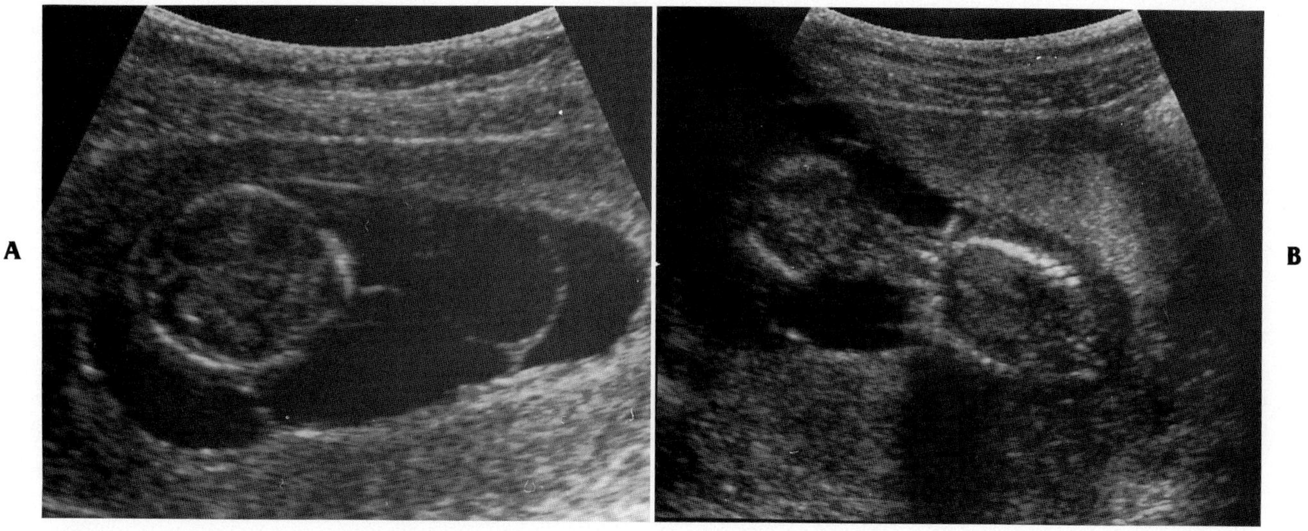

**FIGURE 24** Cystic hygroma. Large fluid-filled cyst around the neck, head, and back of the fetus: transverse *(A)* and longitudinal *(B)* views.

opening, either occupying the normal position of the nose or hanging above the orbits. It is usually associated with the absence of a nose. It is present in cyclopia, cebocephaly, and ethmocephaly and often is part of the holoprosencephaly sequence.

4. Micrognathia is diagnosed using a midsagittal scan of the face denoting hypoplastic mandible. It is associated with trisomy 18 and triploidy.
5. Macroglossia is defined as a resting tongue protruding beyond the teeth or alveolar ridge. Most prenatal case reports have depicted it in association with the Beckwith-Wiedemann syndrome. It may be found in association with trisomy 21.
6. Cystic hygroma of the neck (Fig. 24) suggests Turner's syndrome (45,XO). Other chromosome anomalies include trisomy 18 or 21.
7. A thick nuchal fold between 15 and 21 weeks of gestation is a warning sign for trisomy 21. It is measured in an axial view, passing through the thalamus and posterior fossa, from the outer edge of the occipital bone to the skin. Other anomalies have also been reported including trisomy 13, 18, and 45,XO.

## Heart

The presence of a cardiovascular anomaly increases the risk of an underlying chromosome anomaly. Over 90 percent of fetuses with trisomy 18 and 13, 40 to 50 percent of fetuses with trisomy 21, and 15 to 20 percent of fetuses with monosomy 45,XO have a cardiac anomaly (Table 12). The malformations most often associated with an aneuploidy are atrioventricular septal defects, double-outlet right ventricle, and hypoplastic left ventricular syndrome (see The Heart, earlier in this chapter).

**TABLE 12** Cardiac Anomalies Associated with Aneuploidy

| | Trisomy 13 (90%) | Trisomy 18 (99%) | Trisomy 21 (50%) | Triploidy (?) | Monosomy 45,XO (35%) |
|---|---|---|---|---|---|
| Ventricular septal defect | * | * | + + | * | * |
| Atrial septal defect | * | * | | | |
| Mitral or aortic stenosis | * | | | | * |
| Pulmonary stenosis | * | | | | |
| Anomalous pulmonary venous return | * | | | | |
| Double-outlet right ventricle | | * | | | |
| Bicuspid aortic valve | | * | | | |
| Bicuspid pulmonic valve | | * | | | |
| Atrioventricular septal defect | * | * | + + | | |
| Coarctation of aorta | | | | | * |
| Tetralogy of Fallot | | | * | | |

\+ Below 25%
\+ + Between 25 and 50%
\+ + + Between 50 and 75%
\+ + + + Above 75%
*The association is reported in the literature, but the incidence is unknown.

## *Thorax*

1. Hydrothorax is easily visualized as a fluid collection between the lungs and the chest wall in axial, coronal, and sagittal sections. It can be unilateral or bilateral and among the etiologies are chylothorax, hydrops fetalis, pulmonary lymphangiectasia, cystic adenomatoid malformation of the lungs, bronchopulmonary sequestration, diaphragmatic hernia, chest wall hamartoma, and pulmonary vein atresia. It has been occasionally associated with chromosome anomalies, particularly trisomy 21 and 45,XO.
2. Diaphragmatic hernia is usually recognized because of the mediastinal shift produced by herniated bowel or liver, more commonly on the left side. Intestinal peristalsis confirms the diagnosis. Associated anomalies include trisomy 18, 13, and 21 in 21 to 25 percent of cases diagnosed prenatally (Table 13).

## *Gastrointestinal Tract*

1. Duodenal atresia is characterized sonographically by the classic "double-bubble sign" (Fig. 25) and polyhydramnios. It is associated with trisomy 21 in 20 to 30 percent of cases (see Table 13).
2. Omphalocele (Fig. 26) is an abdominal wall defect characterized by herniation of the abdominal contents through the base of the umbilical cord. Loops of bowel, liver, and stomach are herniated most frequently. The defect is covered by an amnioperitoneal membrane. Unlike gastroschisis, omphalocele can be associated with aneuploidy, most often trisomy 13 and 18, followed by trisomy 21 and 45,XO. The risk is higher when only bowel is found in the omphalocele sac.

**TABLE 13** Thoracic, Gastrointestinal, and Genitourinary Anomalies Associated with Aneuploidy

| | Trisomy 13 | Trisomy 18 | Trisomy 21 | Triploidy | Monosomy 45,XO |
|---|---|---|---|---|---|
| Hydrothorax | | | * | | * |
| Diaphragmatic hernia | * | * | * | | |
| Duodenal atresia | | | + | | |
| Omphalocele | + + | * | * | + | |
| Bladder outlet obstruction | | + | | | |
| Renal cystic dysplasia | + + | * | | * | |
| Horseshoe kidney | | * | | | * |

\+ Below 25%
\+ + Between 25 and 50%
\+ + + Between 50 and 75%
\+ + + + Above 75%
*The association is reported in the literature, but the incidence is unknown.

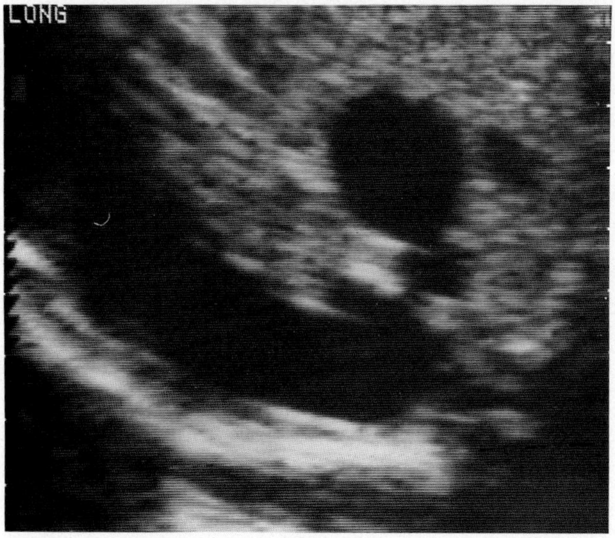

**FIGURE 25** Duodenal atresia. The typical double-bubble image with distention of the proximal portion of the second duodenum.

### Genitourinary Anomalies

1. The characteristic findings in urethrovesical obstruction are dilatation of the bladder with a thickened wall, dilatation of the posterior urethra (keyhole sign), dilatation of both ureters and kidneys with variable degrees of kidney dysplasia and oligohydramnios (Fig. 27). It can be associated with trisomy 18 in 23 percent of cases (see Table 13).
2. The sonographic criteria for the diagnosis of renal cystic dysplasia are hydronephrosis, renal cysts, and hyperechoic renal parenchyma. When other anomalies are present, the association of chromosome anomalies should be considered.
3. Mild hydronephrosis can be associated with trisomy 21.

### *Limb Anomalies* (Table 14)

Please refer to the section on the diagnosis of skeletal anomalies for the diagnostic criteria for the following disorders:

1. Clubfoot has been associated with multiple chromosome anomalies, including trisomy 18, 13, 4p−, and 18q−.
2. Limb reduction anomalies occur including micromelia, radial aplasia, and thumb aplasia.
3. Polydactyly is found in 80 percent of fetuses with trisomy 13.
4. Syndactyly of the third and fourth digits is a characteristic feature of triploidy.
5. Flexion deformities of the hands and overlapping fingers (more commonly the second overlapping the third and the fifth overlapping the fourth) are features of trisomy 18 (Fig. 28). The length of the middle phalanx of the fifth digit should be at least 70 percent of the length of the fourth. Hypoplasia of the middle phalanx of the fifth digit and clinodactyly are common in trisomy 21 (Fig. 29).
6. Widened space between the first and second toes and elevation of the first toe are also features of trisomy 21 (Fig. 30).
7. Shortened femurs and humeri as well as simian crease (Fig. 31) have been described in association with trisomy 21.

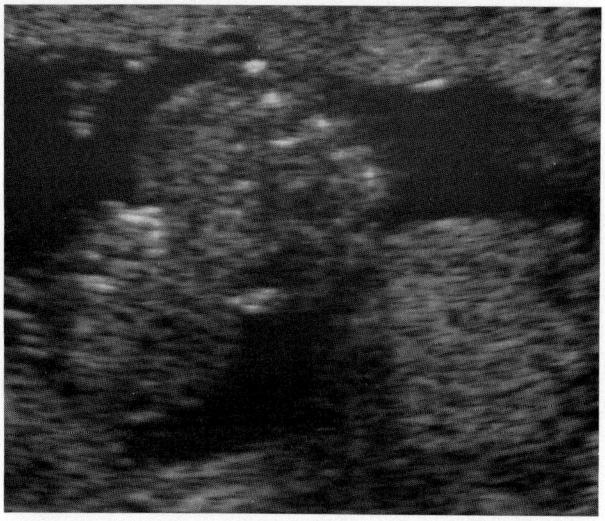

**FIGURE 26** Omphalocele. A smooth, liver-containing mass is in front of the abdomen.

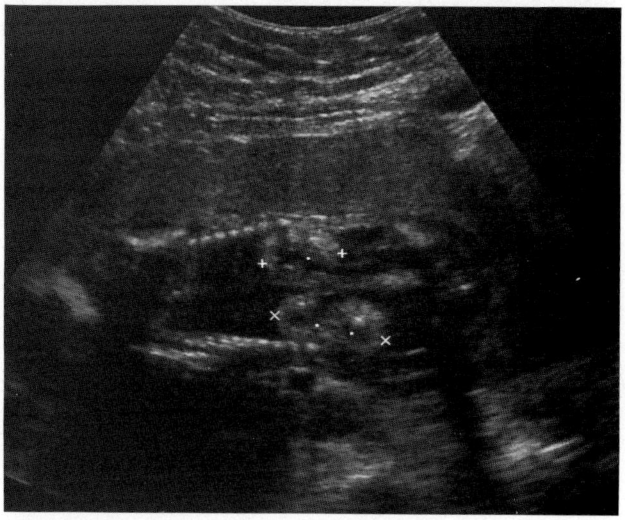

**FIGURE 27** Dysplastic kidneys. Kidneys that are submitted to increased pressure for long periods become echogenic.

### Single Umbilical Artery

1. A single umbilical artery is found in 50 percent of fetuses with trisomy 18 and 10 to 50 percent of fetuses with trisomy 13. Also associated are monosomy 45,XO, triploidy, and other chromosome anomalies (Table 15).
2. Cysts of the umbilical cord can be present in trisomy 13 and 18.

### Polyhydramnios

1. The association of polyhydramnios and IUGR suggests trisomy 18, 21, and triploidy.
2. The association of polyhydramnios and a fetal malformation should also raise the suspicion of a chromosome anomaly.

**TABLE 14** Limb Anomalies Associated with Aneuploidy

| | Trisomy 13 | Trisomy 18 | Trisomy 21 | Triploidy | Monosomy 45,XO |
|---|---|---|---|---|---|
| Polydactyly | +++ | | | | |
| Overlapping fingers | * | ++++ | | | |
| Rocker-bottom feet | * | * | | | |
| Clinodactyly | | | +++ | | |
| Hypoplasia of middle phalanx of fifth digit | | | ++++ | | |
| Simian crease | * | * | +++ | * | |
| Shortened femur | | | * | | |
| Separation between first and second toes | | | * | | |
| Syndactyly of third and fourth digits | | | | ++ | |

\+ Below 25%
\++ Between 25 and 50%
\+++ Between 50 and 75%
\++++ Above 75%
*The association is reported in the literature, but the incidence is unknown.

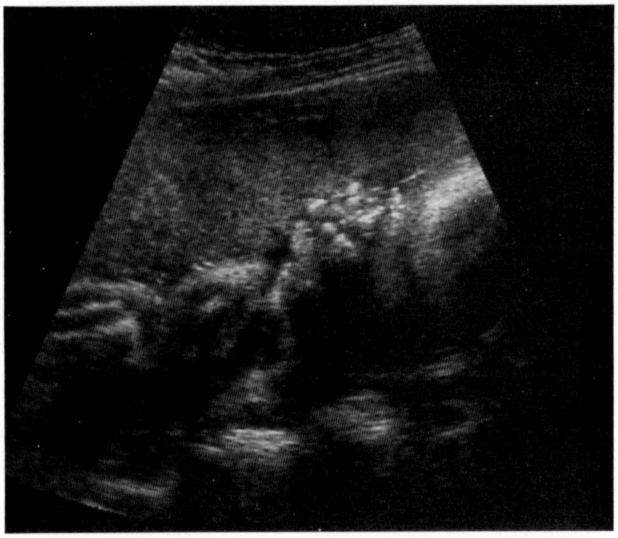

**FIGURE 28** Overlapping finger. The fingers are maintained in a permanently flexed position, with some of them overlapping others.

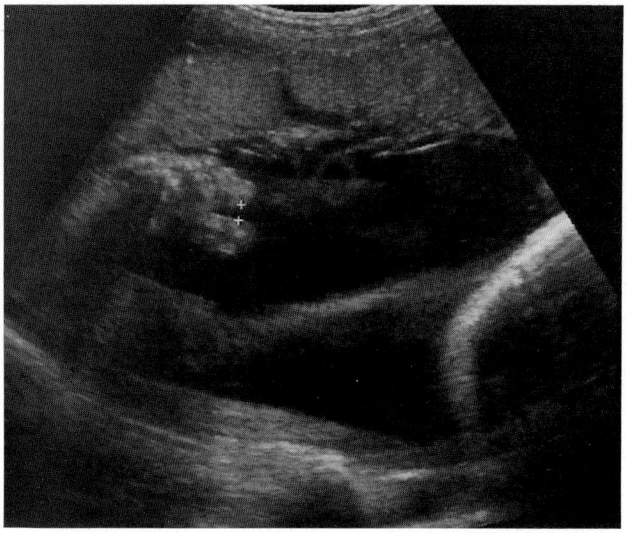

**FIGURE 30** Sandal gap. Widened space between the first and second toes and elevation of the first toe are also features of trisomy 21.

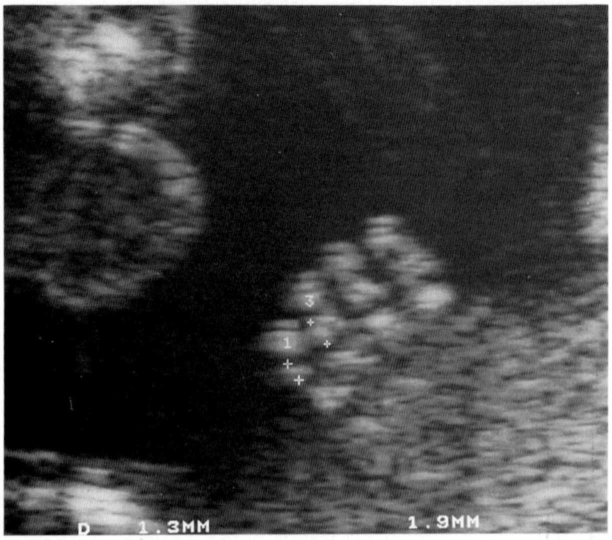


**FIGURE 29** Hypoplasia of the middle phalanx of the fifth digit.

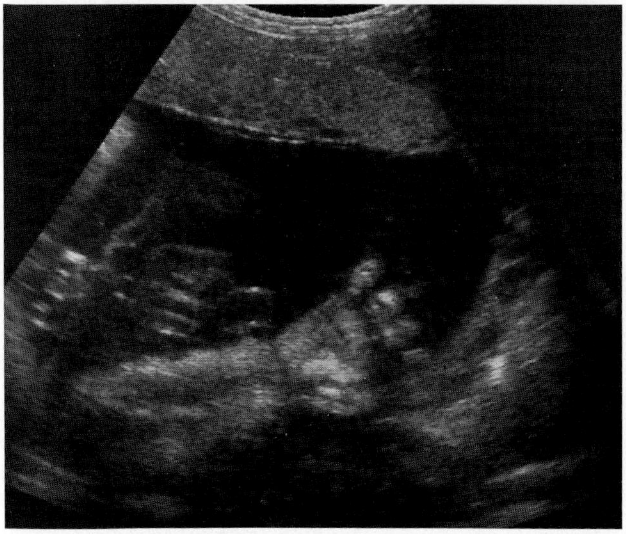

**FIGURE 31** Simian crease. A single palmar crease replaces the normal proximal and distal transverse crease. (From Jeanty P. Prenatal detection of simian crease. J Ultrasound Med 1990; 9:131–136; with permission.)

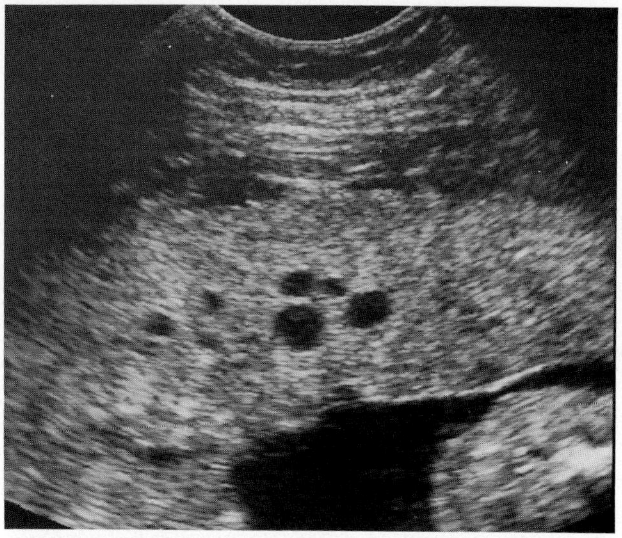

**FIGURE 32** Punched-out cysts out of the placenta are highly suggestive of triploidy.

**TABLE 15** Anomalies of Placenta, Cord, Amniotic Fluid, and Growth Associated with Aneuploidy

| | Trisomy 13 | Trisomy 18 | Trisomy 21 | Triploidy | Monosomy 45,XO |
|---|---|---|---|---|---|
| Single umbilical artery | + + | + + + | * | | * |
| Polyhydramnios | * | * | * | | |
| Symmetric IUGR | * | * | | * | |
| Small placenta | | + + + | | | |
| Single umbilical artery | | + + + + | | | |
| Hydatidiform degeneration of the placenta | | | | * | |

\+ Below 25%
\+ + Between 25 and 50%
\+ + + Between 50 and 75%
\+ + + + Above 75%
*The association is reported in the literature, but the incidence is unknown.

### *Symmetric IUGR*

Symmetric IUGR is associated with many anomalies including trisomy 18, 13, and triploidy.

### *Placental Anomalies*

Hydatidiform degeneration or hydropic changes suggest triploidy (Fig. 32).

## Suggested Reading


Benacerraf BR, Stryker J, Frigoletto FD Jr. Abnormal US appearance of the cerebellum (banana sign): Indirect sign of spina bifida. Radiology 1989; 171:151–153.

Campbell J, Gilbert WM, Nicolaides KH, et al. Ultrasound screening for spina bifida: Cranial and cerebellar signs in a high-risk population. Obstet Gynecol 1987; 70:247–250.

Cardoza JD, Goldstein RB, Filly RA. Exclusion of fetal ventriculomegaly with a single measurement: The width of the lateral ventricular atrium. Radiology 1988; 169:711–714.

Chitkara U, Cogswell C, Norton K, et al. Prenatal diagnosis of choroid plexus cysts: A benign anatomical variant or pathological entity? Report of 41 cases and review of the literature. Obstet Gynecol 1988; 72:185–189.

Fitzsimmons J, Wilson D, Pascoe-Mason J, et al. Choroid plexus cysts in fetuses with trisomy 18. Obstet Gynecol 1989; 73:257–260.

Fleischer AC, Romero R, Manning F, et al. The principles and practice of ultrasonography in obstetrics and gynecology. 4th ed. Norwalk, Conn: Appleton & Lange, 1991.

Hoffman JI, Christianson R. Congenital heart disease in a cohort of 19,502 births with long-term follow-up. Am J Cardiol 1978; 42:641.

Joffe G, Izquierdo LA, Del Valle GO, et al. Pulmonary valve atresia with intact ventricular septum, Type I. The Fetus 1992; 2: 7460.

Nyberg DA, Crane JP. Chromosome abnormalities. In: Nyberg DA, Mahony BA, Pretorius DH, eds. Diagnostic ultrasound of fetal anomalies. St. Louis: Mosby–Year Book, 1990:676.

Nyberg DA, Mack LA, Hirsch J, et al. Abnormalities of fetal contour in sonographic detection of spina bifida: Evaluation of the lemon sign. Radiology 1988; 167:387–392.

Nyberg DA, Mahony BS, Pretorius DA. Diagnostic ultrasound of fetal anomalies. St. Louis: Mosby–Year Book, 1990.

Penso C, Redline R, Benacerraf BR. A sonographic sign which predicts which fetuses with hydrocephalus have an associated neural tube defect. J Ultrasound Med 1987; 6:307–311.

Romero R, Pilu G, Jeanty P, et al. Prenatal diagnosis of congenital malformations. Norwalk, Conn: Appleton & Lange, 1988.

Stamm ER, Drose JA, Thickman D. The fetal heart. In: Rumack CM, Wilson SR, Charboneau JW, eds. Diagnostic ultrasound. St. Louis: Mosby–Year Book, 1991:800.

Van Praagh R, Ongley PA, Swan HJC. Anatomic types of single or common ventricle in man: Morphologic and geometric aspects of sixty necropsies cases. Am J Cardiol 1964; 13:367.

Van Praagh R, Van Praagh S. The anatomy of common aorticopulmonary trunk (truncus arteriosus communis) and its embryologic implications. A study of 57 necropsy cases. Am J Cardiol 1965; 16:406.

# Antenatal Detection of Fetal Abnormalities by MRI

*WILLIAM T.C. YUH, M.D., M.S.E.E. · E. TURGUT TALI, M.D.*

Ultrasonography remains the imaging modality of choice because of its low cost and easy accessibility. It is considered generally to be adequate for evaluation of fetal anomalies. Magnetic resonance imaging (MRI) is noninvasive, can provide multiplanar images, involves no ionizing radiation, and is considered safe for both the pregnant patient and the fetus. Because the potential adverse bioeffects have not been thoroughly evaluated, however, MRI is avoided during pregnancy, particularly in the first trimester. When the ultrasonographic diagnosis is unclear or antenatal intervention based on the knowledge of exact anatomic detail might be considered, the additional information provided by MRI in some cases may be helpful and outweigh the risk.

MRI examinations of the fetus can be challenging because of both maternal and fetal motion, which may be difficult to control. Fetal motion gradually increases and becomes more frequent and complex as the pregnancy progresses. In response to loud gradient coil, fetal motion increases during the data acquisition and degrades the images, obscuring the anatomic detail, particularly at long pulse sequences. The best approach to eliminate the degradation from motion is transient fetal paralysis, which may be achieved by injection of pancuronium bromide (0.3 mg/kg estimated fetal weight) into the umbilical vein during funipuncture for chordocentesis or directly into the fetal gluteal region. Pancuronium cannot cross the placenta and affect the mother. Complete transient fetal paralysis can be achieved for 30 to 60 minutes by adequate injection, while oxygenation of the fetus can still be maintained by the umbilical vessels. Placing the mother in the left lateral decubitus position also helps to minimize maternal aortic pulsation during the MRI. With adequate control of fetal motion, MRI appears to be a useful adjunct to ultrasonography in selected cases.

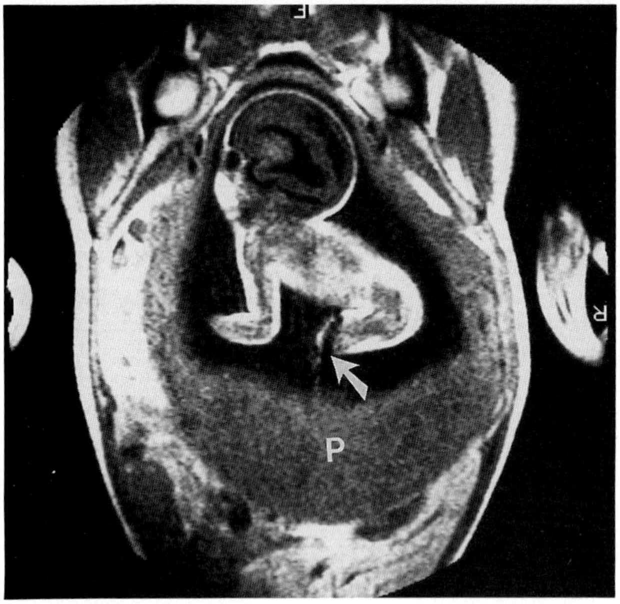


**FIGURE 1** Fetal sagittal T1-weighted image shows a fetus in a cephalic presentation with the head close to the maternal bladder. The dilated ventricle can be identified readily. Flow void phenomenon is also identified within the umbilical cord (*arrow*). The placenta (P) is shown as a crescent-shaped isointense structure. (From Weinreb JC, Yuh WTC. Obstetrics. In: Stark DD, Bradley WG Jr., eds. Magnetic Resonance Imaging. St. Louis: Mosby–Year Book, 1992:1987; with permission.)

The appropriate planes and pulse sequences for fetal imaging depend on the capabilities of the particular MRI unit used and the reason for the study. We prefer initially to obtain maternal axial T1-weighted images for determination of the fetal orientation and anatomy. Serial oblique images can be performed to obtain the approximate fetal coronal, sagittal (Fig. 1), or axial plane with respect to the area of interest (Fig. 2) after the initial scan. Section thickness can range from 3 to 5 mm, preferably without gaps. Fetal fast-scan imaging (GRASS) (Fig. 3) with breath-holding is generally not useful, because of the low signal-to-noise ratio, inferior anatomic detail, and poor tissue contrast.

## Intracranial Abnormalities

Hydrocephalus results from the excessive accumulation of cerebrospinal fluid (CSF) within the ventricles (Figs. 4, 5). Obstruction is most commonly seen in the aqueduct of Sylvius (43 percent). The prognosis of congenital hydrocephalus is frequently poor: fetal death occurs in 24 percent, and neonatal death occurs in 17 percent. The differentiation of hydrocephalus from holoprosencephaly can be difficult, and the useful findings of hydrocephalus include an identifiable cerebral mantle and midline structures such as the falx, as well as separation of the thalamus (see Fig. 5).

Alobar holoprosencephaly is an early, severe, developmental defect of the brain, in which there is failure of the prosencephalon to divide. The cerebrum is composed of a thin rim of brain tissue, the lateral ventricles are represented by a single midline cavity, and the thalamus may be fused (Fig. 6). Usually there is associated arhinencephaly (absence of olfactory bulbs and tracts, cleft lip, proboscis, and microphthalmia

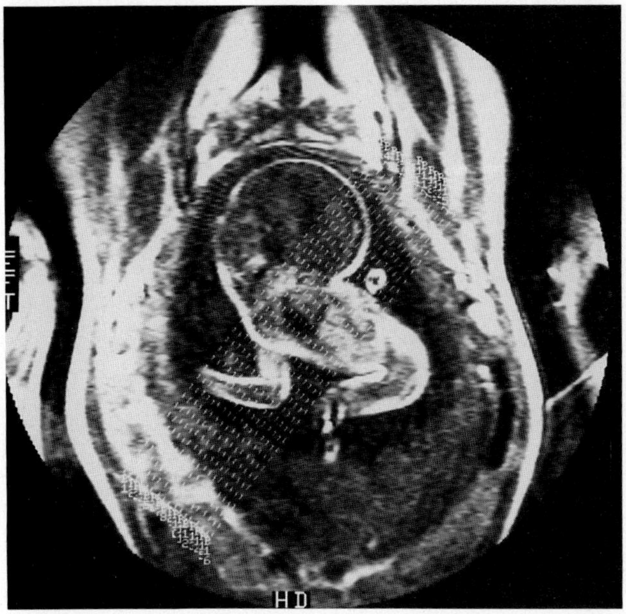

**FIGURE 2** Pilot scan with dotted parallel lines provides an example of how to obtain axial imaging through the fetal chest and abdomen. (From Weinreb JC, Yuh WTC. Obstetrics. In: Stark DD, Bradley WG Jr., eds. Magnetic Resonance Imaging. St. Louis: Mosby–Year Book, 1992:1987; with permission.)

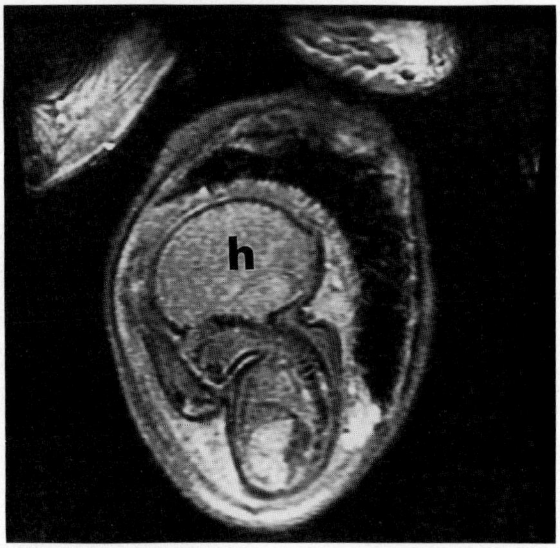


**FIGURE 3** Fetal parasagittal fast-scan image (GRASS) with breath-holding technique shows excellent fetal outline as a result of the susceptibility artifacts from the bony structures. However, in these particular pulse sequences, there is poor tissue contrast and anatomic detail, especially within the intracranial structures (h). (From Weinreb JC, Yuh WTC. Obstetrics. In: Stark DD, Bradley WG Jr., eds. Magnetic Resonance Imaging. St. Louis: Mosby–Year Book, 1992: 1987; with permission.)

A

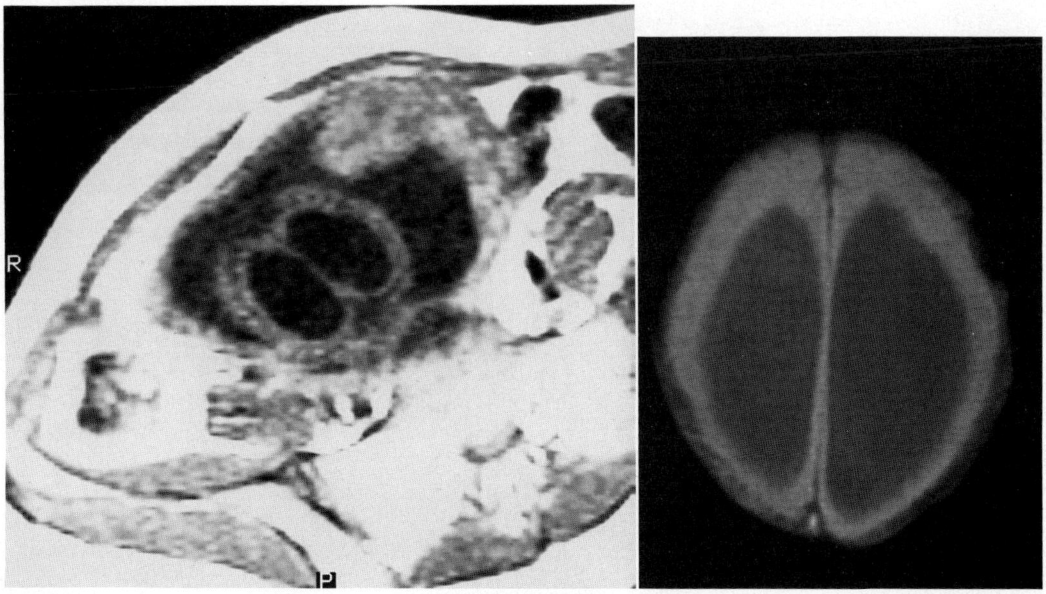


B

**FIGURE 4** Hydrocephalus. *A,* Fetal axial T1-weighted image shows dilated lateral ventricles. *B,* Neonatal proton density image corresponding to (*A*) demonstrates the dilated ventricular system. (From Weinreb JC, Yuh WTC. Obstetrics. In: Stark DD, Bradley WG Jr., eds. Magnetic Resonance Imaging. St. Louis: Mosby–Year Book, 1992:1987; with permission.)

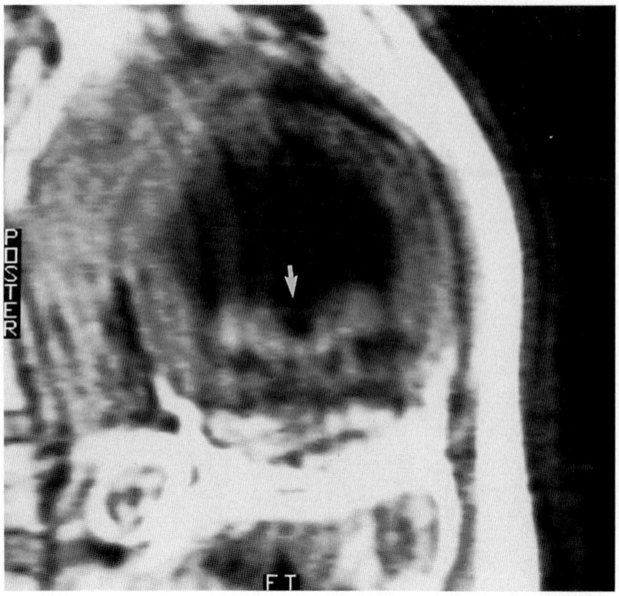


**FIGURE 5** Hydrocephalus. Coronal T1-weighted image clearly demonstrates the existence of a third ventricle (*arrow*) and a thick mantle, as well as a separate thalamus, suggesting the diagnosis of hydrocephalus rather than holoprosencephaly. This was confirmed postpartum. Pulsation artifact from the maternal aorta can be seen. Oligohydramnios is also present. (From Weinreb JC, Yuh WTC. Obstetrics. In: Stark DD, Bradley WG Jr., eds. Magnetic Resonance Imaging. St. Louis: Mosby–Year Book, 1992:1987; with permission.)

A

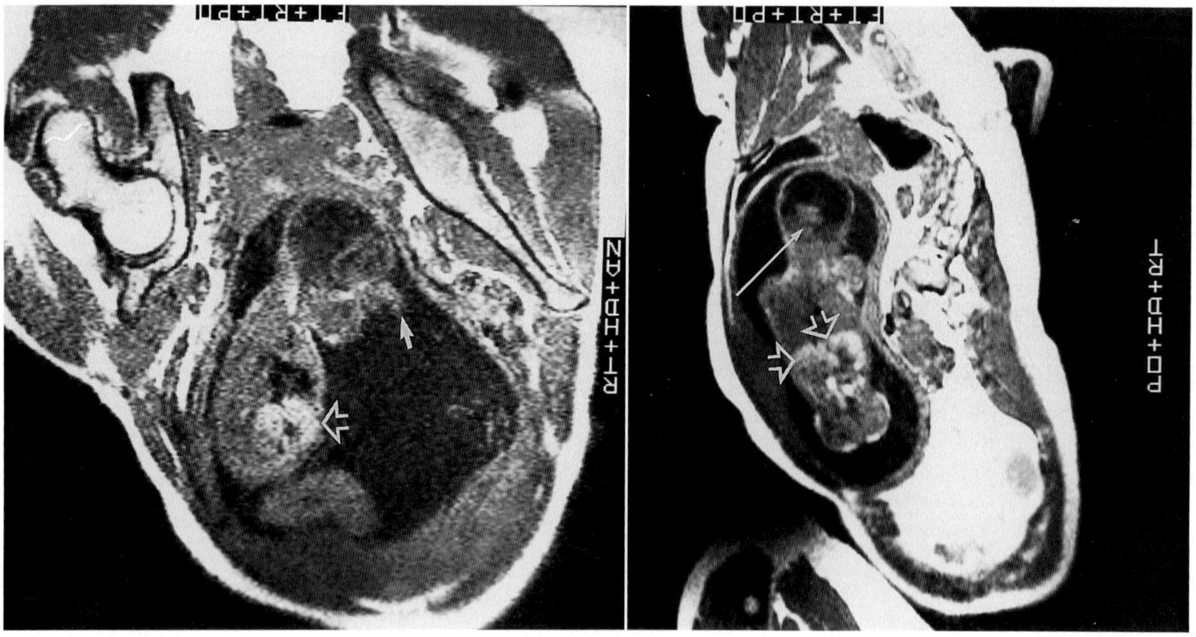

B

**FIGURE 6** Alobar holoprosencephaly. Fetal parasagittal (*A*) and coronal (*B*) T1-weighted images show normal fetal position. The fetus has a dilated single ventricle and proboscis (*A, small arrow*). A fused thalamus (*B, long arrow*) is also identified. High signal intensity (*A* and *B, open arrows*) in the intestines represents meconium. (From Wenstrom KD, Williamson RA, et al. Magnetic resonance imaging of fetuses with intracranial defects. Obstet Gynecol 1991; 77:529–532; with permission.)

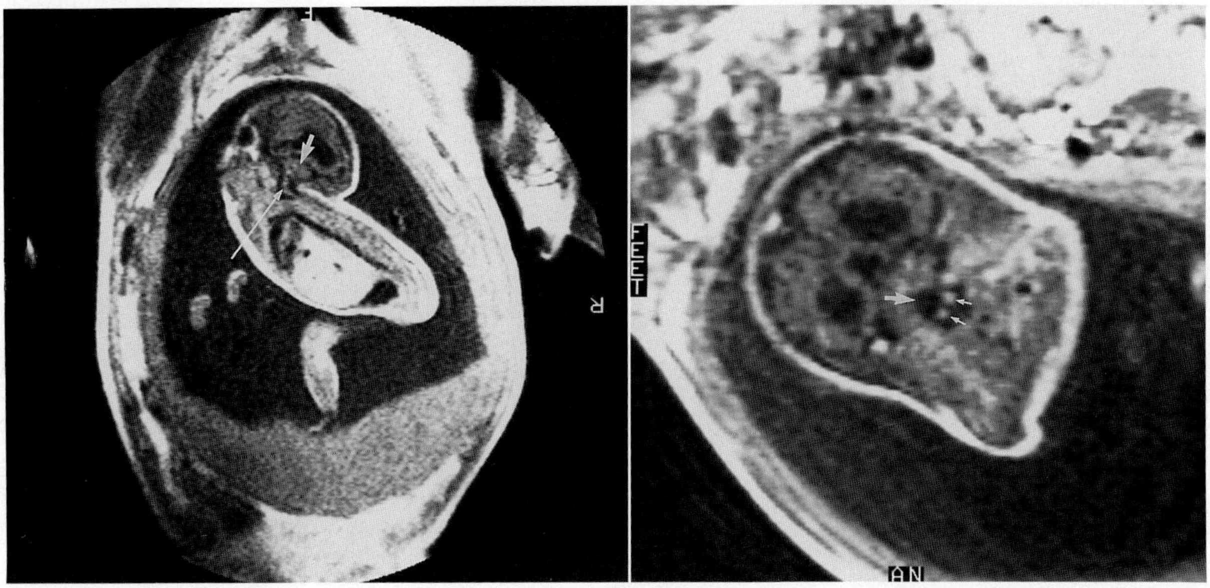


**FIGURE 7** Iniencephaly. *A,* Fetal parasagittal T1-weighted image shows normal fetal position, polyhydramnios, dilated ventricular system, and hyperextended neck (stargazer). The cerebellum (*short arrow*) and brain stem (*long arrow*) appear to be intact. *B,* Fetal axial T1-weighted image shows splitting of the cervical spinal cord. More cranially, a linear structure (*large white arrow*) between the two halves of the spinal cord (*small white arrows*) may represent a bony spicule or a fibrous band, supporting the diagnosis of diastematomyelia of the cervical cord. (From Williamson RA, Weiner CP, et al. Magnetic resonance imaging of anomalous fetuses. Obstet Gynecol 1989; 73:952–956; with permission.)

or cyclopia). Severe mental and motor deficits usually are present; affected children rarely survive past infancy.

Iniencephaly is a complex developmental anomaly that is characterized by the imperfect formation of the skull base at the foramen magnum, a rather wide cervical spina bifida, and marked backward flexion of the head and spine (Fig. 7, *A*). Diastematomyelia is a relatively uncommon condition in which there is splitting and transfixing of the spinal cord by an abnormal fibrocartilaginous or bony spicule extending from the dorsal aspect of a vertebral body to the corresponding neural arch (Fig. 7, *B*). The abnormality most frequently occurs in the lower thoracic and upper lumbar regions.

Megalencephaly is a rare developmental defect in which there is excessive, chaotic hyperplasia and hypertrophy of neuronal elements, resulting in an abundance of disorganized brain parenchyma and cerebral dysfunction (Fig. 8). It may be unilateral or bilateral in distribution. Affected newborns usually have considerable developmental delays and may present with early seizures or severe encephalopathy.

Agenesis of the corpus callosum results from a failure of formation of the corpus callosum, originating from the lamina terminalis at 7 to 13 weeks of gestation. Partial agenesis of the corpus callosum usually occurs at its posterior portion (Fig. 9).

Dandy-Walker syndrome results from congenital atresia of the foramina of Luschka and Magendie. The cerebellar hemispheres are separated by cystic dilation of the fourth ventricle, and the cerebellum is usually underdeveloped, dysplastic, and displaced anterosuperiorly by the enlarging fourth ventricle (Fig. 10).

Congenital arachnoid cysts are CSF-containing loculations in the arachnoid space without ventricular communication or brain maldevelopment (Fig. 11). They comprise 1 percent of all intracranial masses and arise from clefts or duplications of the arachnoid membrane. Arachnoid cysts are usually asymptomatic but may cause symptoms by compressing adjacent tissues.

Intracranial lipomas have the same signal characteristics as those of subcutaneous fat (Fig. 12) and represent less than 1 percent of all brain tumors. They are asymptomatic in 50 percent of cases and associated with agenesis of the corpus callosum in 50 percent. Usual locations include midline lesions at the genu of the corpus callosum (25 to 50 percent), tuber cinereum, quadrigeminal region, and cisterns.

Hydranencephaly is the congenital absence of the cerebral hemispheres, which are replaced by a thin membranous sac of leptomeninges and atrophic glial cells filled with CSF and necrotic debris (Fig. 13). The brain stem and basal ganglia are well formed, and rudiments of the frontal and occipital cortex may be present. The cause of this anomaly is unknown, but it may result from the failure of development of the cerebral arteries or severe intrauterine infections.

## Extracranial Abnormalities

Congenital diaphragmatic hernias result from an absence of closure of the pleuroperitoneal fold by the ninth week of gestation. They occur posterolaterally through the foramen of Bochdalek in 90 percent of cases and are found most commonly on the left side (80 percent) (Fig. 14, *A*). They may also occur through a congenitally absent hemidiaphragm, anteriorly through the foramen of Morgagni, or alongside the esophagus. These hernias vary in size, and large hernias may produce severe respiratory distress. If herniation occurs on the right, the intestine and liver or liver alone may fill the right-sided hemithorax (Fig. 14, *B* and *C*). Pulmonary hypoplasia results from long-standing intrauterine compression of the lungs by the hernia. Intrauterine surgical correction of this abnormality can be life-saving; however, if the herniation involves the liver, surgical correction is not indicated because of high mortality.

*Text continued on p. 228.*

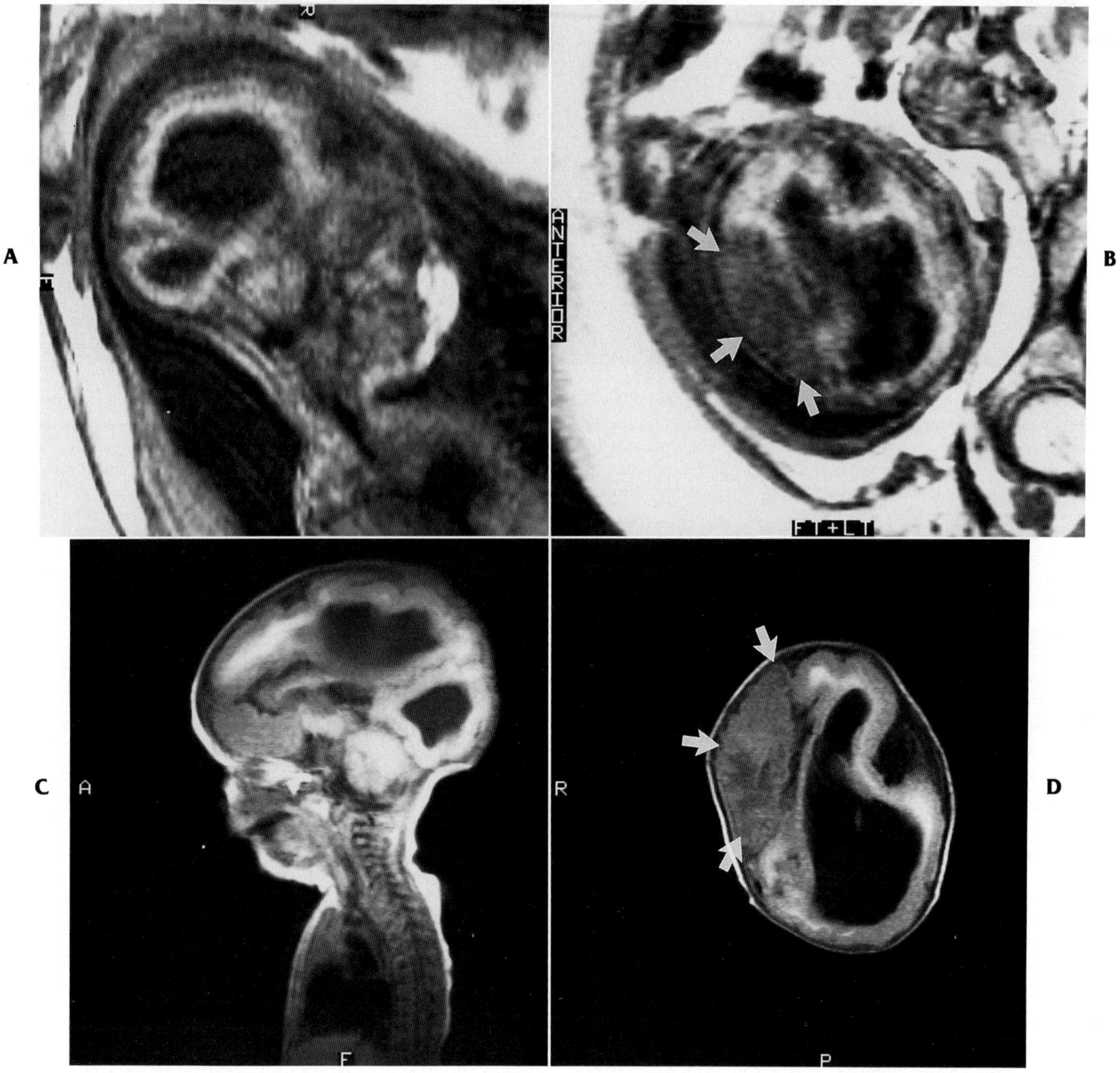


**FIGURE 8** Hemimegalencephaly. Fetal parasagittal (*A*) and axial (*B*) T1-weighted images show a dilated ventricular system of the left hemisphere. The white matter of the enlarged left hemisphere appears to have a much higher signal intensity than that of the normal parenchyma in the relatively normal-sized right cerebral hemisphere (*B, arrows*). This may represent hypermyelination or accelerated myelination of the white matter in the involved hemisphere. Pachygyria of the abnormal hemisphere is also noted. Neonatal parasagittal T1-weighted image (*C*) corresponding to (*A*) and axial T1-weighted image (*D*) corresponding to (*B*) show dilated ventricular system in the enlarged left cerebral hemisphere. Similar to the fetal brain (*B*), normal neonatal brain parenchyma (*D, arrows*) appears hypointense on the T1-weighted images, which is the typical finding during the first year of life because of excess water content. The parenchymal signal intensity of the abnormal left hemisphere (*C* and *D*) is similar to that of the typical adult brain on T1-weighted images. Again note the pachygyria of the left cerebral hemisphere. (From Weinreb JC, Yuh WTC. Obstetrics. In: Stark DD, Bradley WG Jr., eds. Magnetic Resonance Imaging. St. Louis: Mosby–Year Book, 1992:1987; with permission.)

A

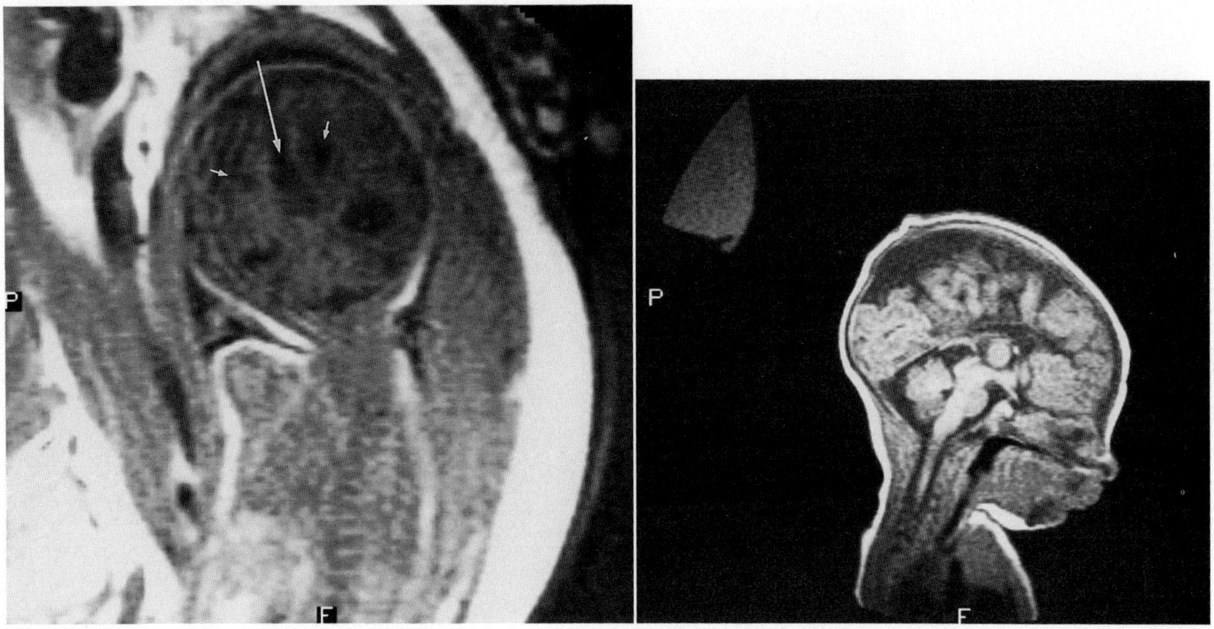

B

**FIGURE 9** Partial agenesis of the corpus callosum. *A,* Fetal coronal T1-weighted image shows the third ventricle (*long arrow*) interposed between the upward-tilted lateral ventricles (*short arrows*). This is consistent with partial or complete agenesis of the corpus callosum. *B,* Neonatal parasagittal T1-weighted image shows partial agenesis of the corpus callosum and enlarged massa intermedia. (From Weinreb JC, Yuh WTC. Obstetrics. In: Stark DD, Bradley WG Jr., eds. Magnetic Resonance Imaging. St. Louis: Mosby–Year Book, 1992:1987; with permission.)

A

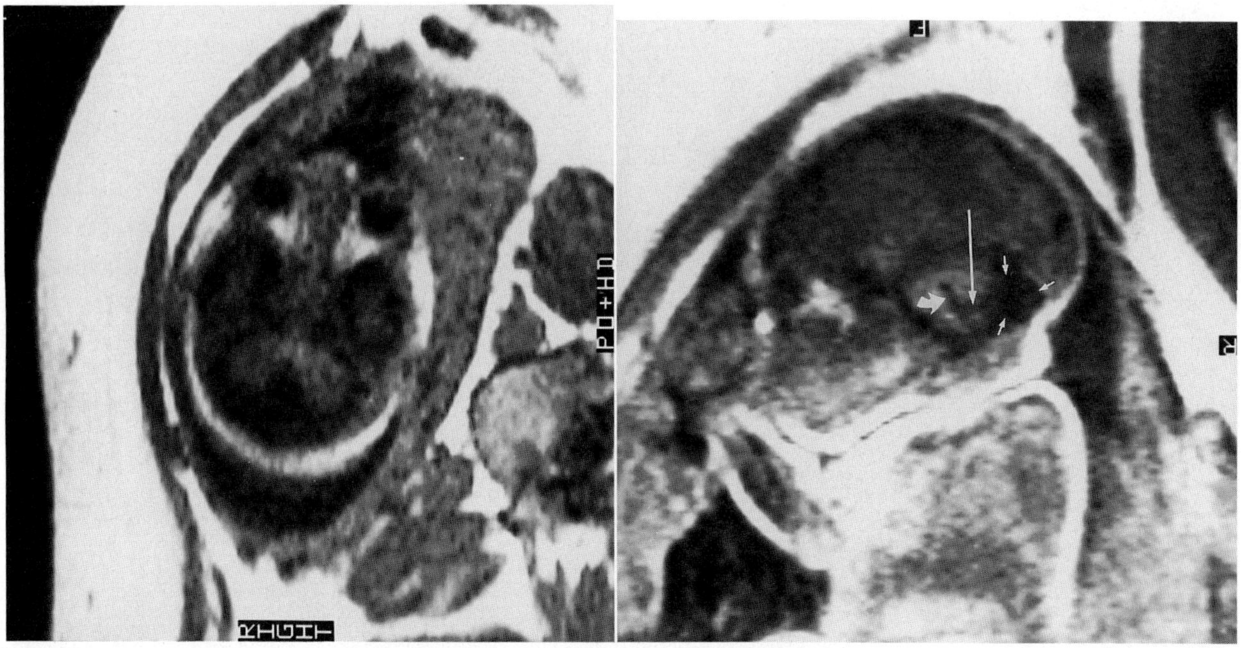

B

**FIGURE 10** Dandy-Walker syndrome. *A,* Fetal axial T1-weighted image demonstrates a hypoplastic inferior cerebellum and a connection between the fourth ventricle and the posterior fossa cyst. *B,* Fetal near-parasagittal T1-weighted image shows a posterior fossa cyst (*small arrows*) with a connection (*long arrow*) to the fourth ventricle (*curved arrow*). (From Weinreb JC, Yuh WTC. Obstetrics. In: Stark DD, Bradley WG Jr., eds. Magnetic Resonance Imaging. St. Louis: Mosby–Year Book, 1992:1987; with permission.)

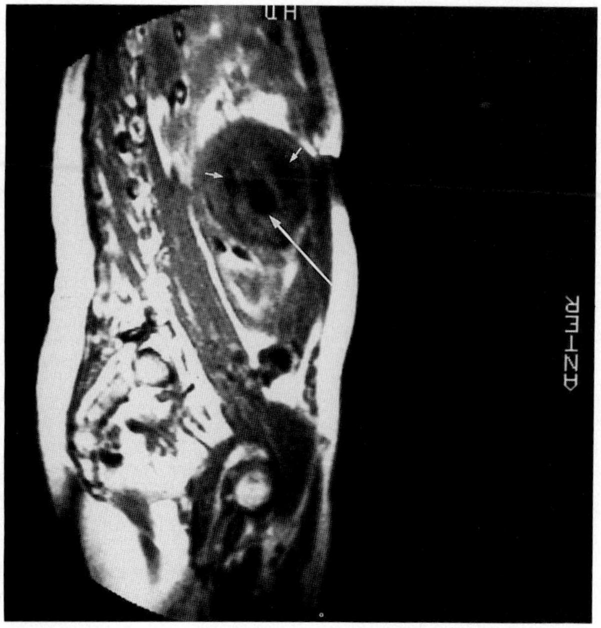

**FIGURE 11** Quadrigeminal plate cistern cyst. Fetal coronal T1-weighted image shows a quadrigeminal plate cistern cyst (*long arrow*) identified as a low signal intensity structure between the lateral ventricles (*small arrows*) and just above the cerebellum. (From Weinreb JC, Yuh WTC. Obstetrics. In: Stark DD, Bradley WG Jr., eds. Magnetic Resonance Imaging. St. Louis: Mosby–Year Book, 1992: 1987; with permission.)

A

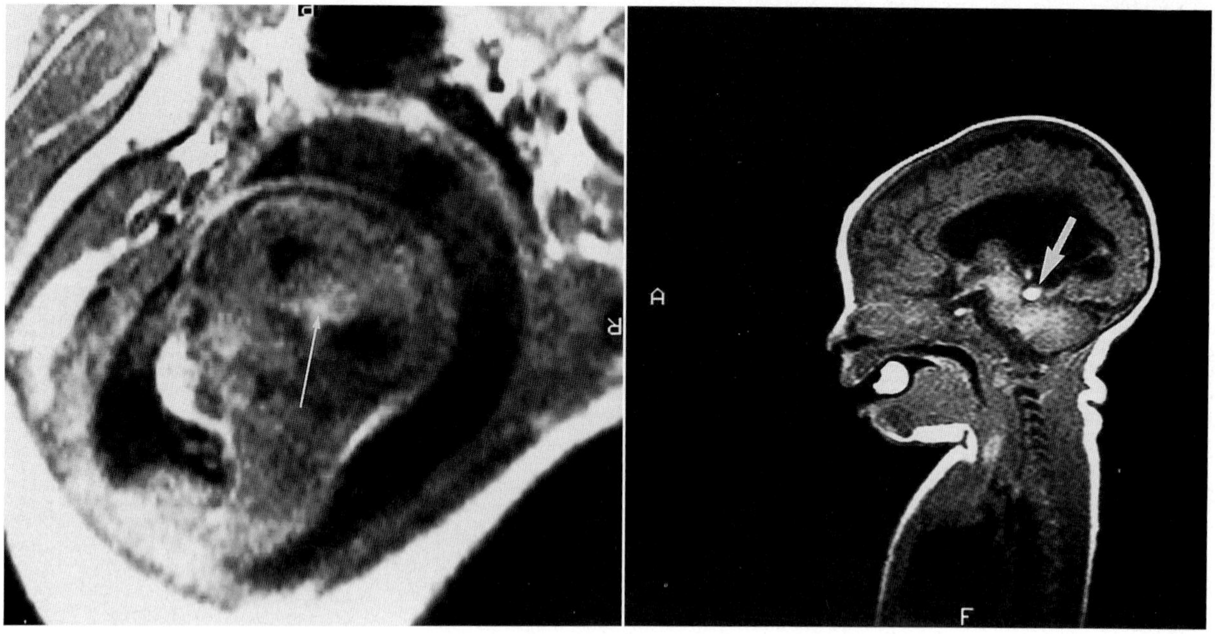

B

**FIGURE 12** Intracranial lipoma. *A,* Fetal near-parasagittal T1-weighted image with 1 cm slice thickness shows a dilated ventricular system and a small hyperintense lesion (*arrow*) just posteroinferior to the thalamus. This lesion has a signal intensity much brighter than that of normal fetal brain parenchyma and similar to that of fat, which is consistent with lipoma. *B,* Neonatal sagittal T1-weighted image confirms the diagnosis of intracranial lipoma (*arrow*). Note the worsening hydrocephalus. (From Weinreb JC, Yuh WTC. Obstetrics. In: Stark DD, Bradley WG Jr., eds. Magnetic Resonance Imaging. St. Louis: Mosby–Year Book, 1992:1987; with permission.)

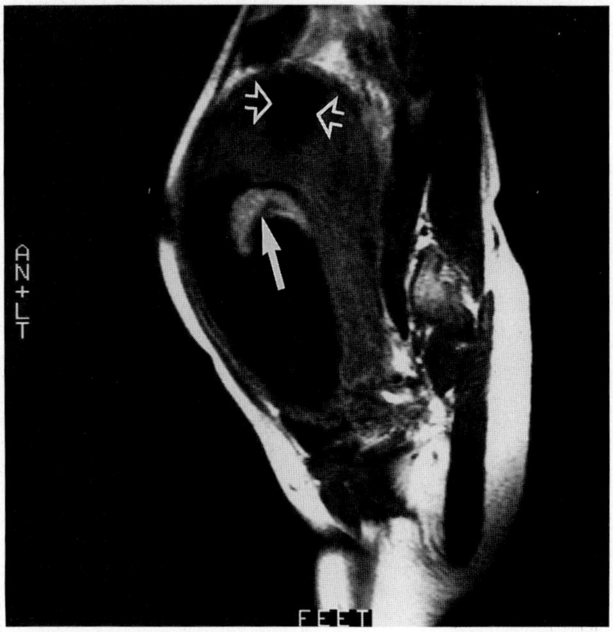


**FIGURE 13** Hydranencephaly. Fetal near-coronal T1-weighted image shows hydranencephaly as a low signal intensity region (*open arrows*) without identifiable intracranial structures. The fetal liver, shown as a high signal intensity structure (*large arrow*), is suspended in ascites. There is no identifiable amniotic fluid. The fetus is in a breech presentation. (From Weinreb JC, Yuh WTC. Obstetrics. In: Stark DD, Bradley WG Jr., eds. Magnetic Resonance Imaging. St. Louis: Mosby–Year Book, 1992:1987; with permission.)

A

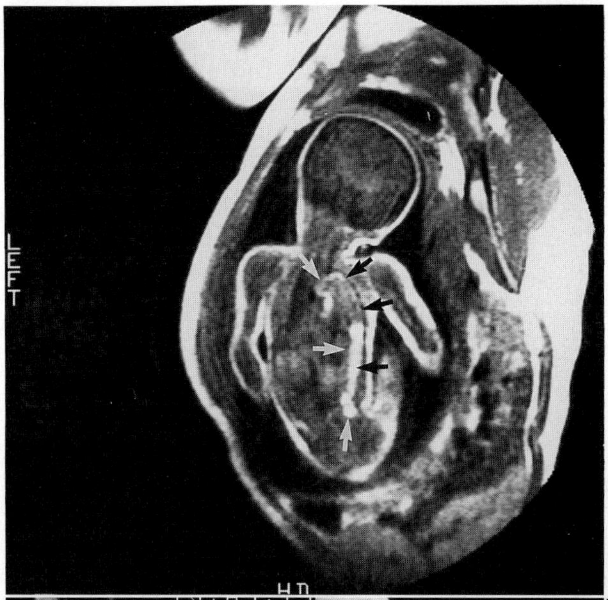


B

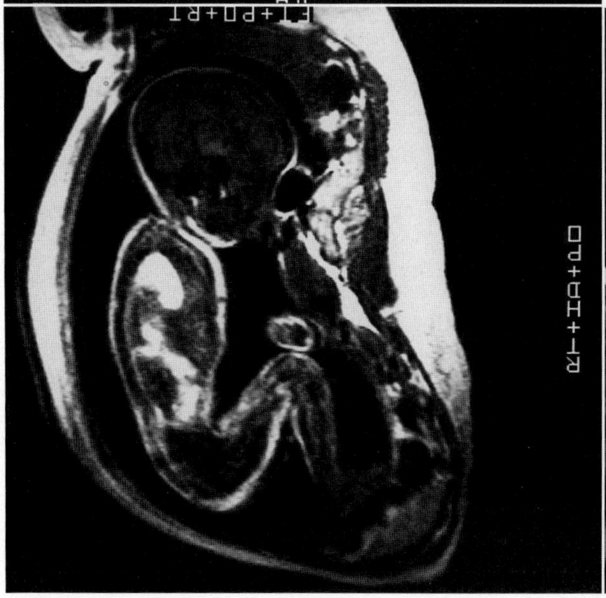

C

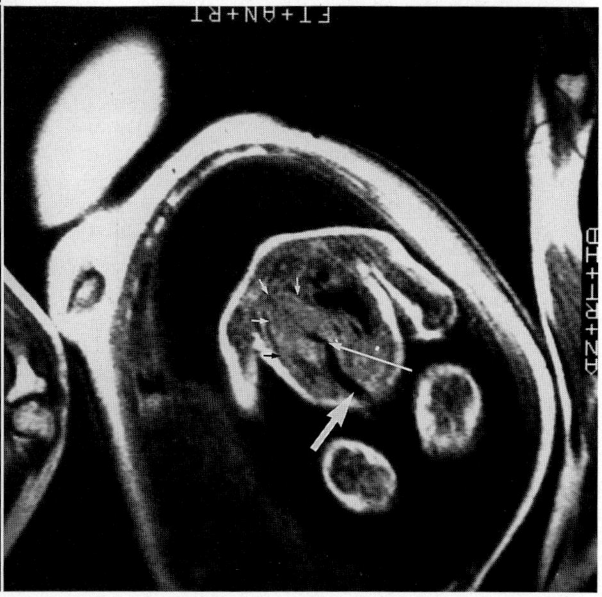

**FIGURE 14** Diaphragmatic hernia with and without liver involvement. *A,* Fetal near-coronal T1-weighted image shows bowel herniated into the chest cavity (*arrows*). The herniation is located posteriorly and toward the left side (Bochdalek). The meconium is shown as a high signal intensity area within the gastrointestinal tract. The liver is located anteriorly without evidence of herniation (not shown). *B,* Fetal parasagittal T1-weighted image shows another patient with high signal intensity intestine herniated into the chest. *C,* Fetal coronal T1-weighted image of the same patient in (*B*) shows the inverted liver (*small arrows*) herniated into the chest cavity. The flow void phenomenon is identified within the umbilical (*large arrow*) and portal (*long arrow*) veins. (From Weinreb JC, Yuh WTC. Obstetrics. In: Stark DD, Bradley WG Jr., eds. Magnetic Resonance Imaging. St. Louis: Mosby–Year Book, 1992:1987; with permission.)

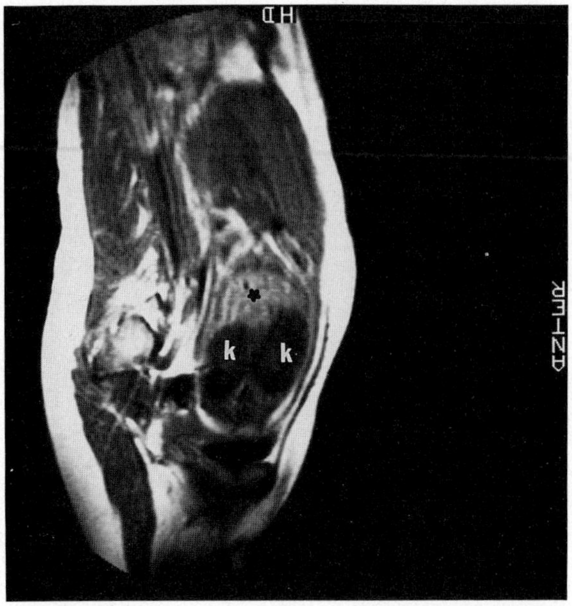


**FIGURE 15** Polycystic kidneys in a fetus with Meckel-Gruber syndrome. Fetal coronal T1-weighted image shows the enlarged bilateral polycystic kidneys as low signal intensity structures (k) just beneath the high signal intensity liver (*asterisk*). The fetus is in a breech presentation. Oligohydramnios is also present. (From Weinreb JC, Yuh WTC. Obstetrics. In: Stark DD, Bradley WG Jr., eds. Magnetic Resonance Imaging. St. Louis: Mosby–Year Book, 1992:1987; with permission.)

A

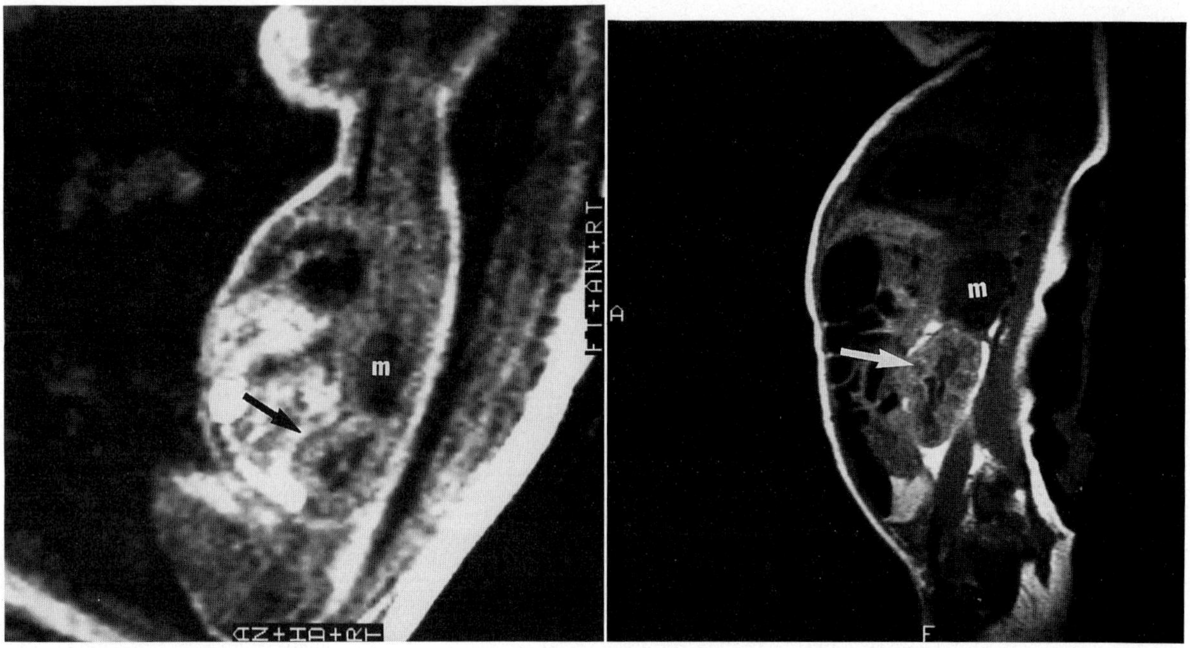


B

**FIGURE 16** Extrapulmonary sequestration (infradiaphragmatic). Fetal (*A*) and neonatal (*B*) parasagittal T1-weighted images show a low signal intensity suprarenal mass (m) with effacement of the kidney (*large arrow*). This mass was initially thought to be a neuroblastoma, but surgical excision showed an infradiaphragmatic extrapulmonary sequestration. (From Weinreb JC, Yuh WTC. Obstetrics. In: Stark DD, Bradley WG Jr., eds. Magnetic Resonance Imaging. St. Louis: Mosby–Year Book, 1992:1987; with permission.)

There are associated anomalies in 20 percent of liveborn and in 90 percent of stillborn fetuses. Morbidity and mortality are high, and 35 percent of cases may be stillborn and another 35 percent die in the neonatal period without intrauterine correction.

Multicystic kidneys represent about 20 percent of abdominal masses in neonates. In multicystic kidney disease, there is a lack of differentiation of both nephrotic and ductal elements and a replacement of collecting tubules by cystic dilation. Additionally, because there is no urine production, the fetal bladder is not visualized. Multicystic kidneys may be associated with Meckel-Gruber syndrome (multicystic kidneys, occipital encephalocele, eye abnormalities, cleft lip and palate, polydactyly, microcephalus, and congenital heart disease) (Fig. 15), which is invariably fatal at birth because of pulmonary hypoplasia and renal failure.

Fetal ascites is frequently secondary to urinary tract obstruction (usually from posterior urethral valves) (see Fig. 13). Other types include chylous ascites, probably resulting from congenital hypoplasia or obstruction of the lymphatic

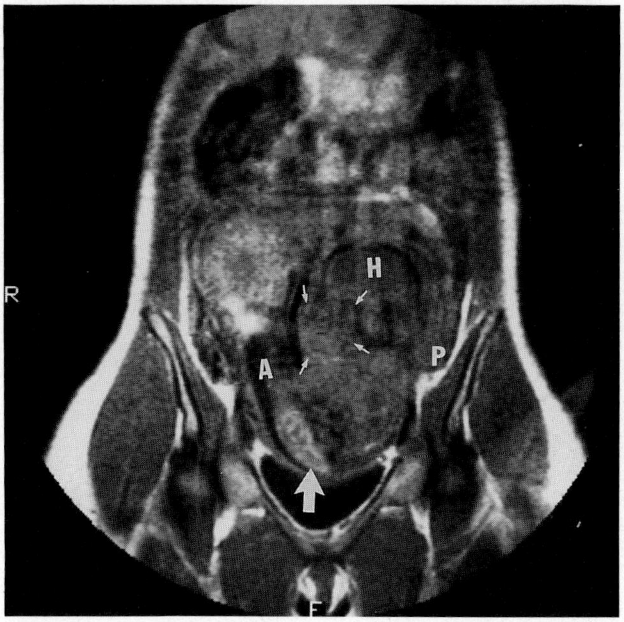


**FIGURE 17** Pentalogy of Cantrell. Fetal parasagittal T1-weighted image shows absence of amniotic fluid and breech presentation of the fetus. Anteriorly herniated fetal heart (*small arrows*) and liver (*large arrow*) are demonstrated. A = anterior aspect of the fetus; P = posterior aspect of the fetus; H = head. (From Weinreb JC, Yuh WTC. Obstetrics. In: Stark DD, Bradley WG Jr., eds. Magnetic Resonance Imaging. St. Louis: Mosby–Year Book, 1992:1987; with permission.)

system, and bile ascites, resulting from perforation of the common bile duct or cystic duct.

Pulmonary sequestration is a congenital bronchopulmonary foregut malformation consisting of a nonfunctioning lung segment with a systemic artery supply and no communication with the tracheobronchial tree. Intralobar pulmonary sequestrations classically are located in the lower lobes. Extralobar pulmonary sequestrations are located outside the pleura and are usually present in the left-sided hemithorax (80 percent). Rarely, they can occur below the diaphragm (Fig. 16).

Pentalogy of Cantrell is a rare abnormality in which there is a midline defect, including the supraumbilical abdomen and lower sternum, resulting in ectopia cardis (Fig. 17), deficiency of the diaphragm, and intracardiac abnormalities (atrial septal defect, 50 percent; ventricular septal defect, 18 percent; and tetralogy of Fallot, 11 percent).

## Suggested Reading

Hill MC, Lande IM, Larsen JW Jr. Prenatal diagnosis of fetal anomalies using ultrasound and MRI. Radiol Clin North Am 1988; 26:287–307.

Weinreb JC, Yuh WTC. Obstetrics. In: Stark DD, Bradley WG Jr, eds. Magnetic Resonance Imaging. St. Louis: Mosby-Year Book, 1992:1987.

Wenstrom KD, Williamson RA, Weiner CP, et al. Magnetic resonance imaging of fetuses with intracranial defects. Obstet Gynecol 1991; 77:529–532.

Williamson RA, Weiner CP, Yuh WTC, Abu-Yousef MM. Magnetic resonance imaging of anomalous fetuses. Obstet Gynecol 1989; 73:952–956.

# Diagnosis of Ectopic Pregnancy

*ROBERT S. PERRET, M.D. · M. KRISTIN THORSEN, M.D.*
*THOMAS L. LAWSON, M.D.*

Ectopic pregnancy continues to be the leading cause of first-trimester maternal mortality in the United States. It accounts for up to 25 percent of deaths associated with childbearing and affects young, otherwise disease-free women. The risk of death from an ectopic pregnancy is 10 times greater than for a vaginal delivery and 50 times greater than for a legal abortion. Besides mortality risks, women who have ectopic pregnancies have an increased incidence of infertility and 10 percent have a second ectopic pregnancy. The incidence of ectopic pregnancy is approximately 13 per 1000 live births. This reported incidence has quadrupled over the last 15 years; however, the death rate has fallen as a result of improved methods of diagnosis. Despite advances, the diagnosis of ectopic pregnancy remains difficult for the clinician as well as the ultrasonographer.

## Etiology

Ninety-five percent of ectopic pregnancies are tubal in origin, either in the ampulla or isthmus portion of the tube. Approximately 2 to 3 percent occur in the interstitial portion of the tube. The remaining 2 percent occur in the abdomen, ovary, and cervix (Fig. 1).

The etiology of ectopic pregnancy is secondary either to mechanical factors that prevent or retard the passage of the fertilized ovum into the uterus or to functional factors that lead to decreased transit of the ovum in the tube. Specific mechanical factors include: salpingitis, which leads to narrowing of the tube and/or reduced ciliary motion of the tubal mucosa; peritubal adhesions secondary to previous pelvic infections; previous tubal surgery; developmental anomalies of the tube; previous ectopic pregnancy; and tumors that distort the tube or the presence of an intrauterine device. Specific functional factors include altered tubal motility secondary to changes in estrogen and progesterone or secondary to diethylstilbestrol exposure in utero. Altered tube motility may also be encountered in women being treated for infertility.

## Clinical Presentation

The most frequent symptoms of ectopic pregnancy are pelvic and abdominal pain (100 percent) and abnormal vaginal bleeding (75 percent). Other symptoms and signs include amenorrhea, shoulder pain, gastrointestinal symptoms, vertigo, syncope, and shock. Commonly the patient has the signs and symptoms of early pregnancy. The uterus enlarges during the

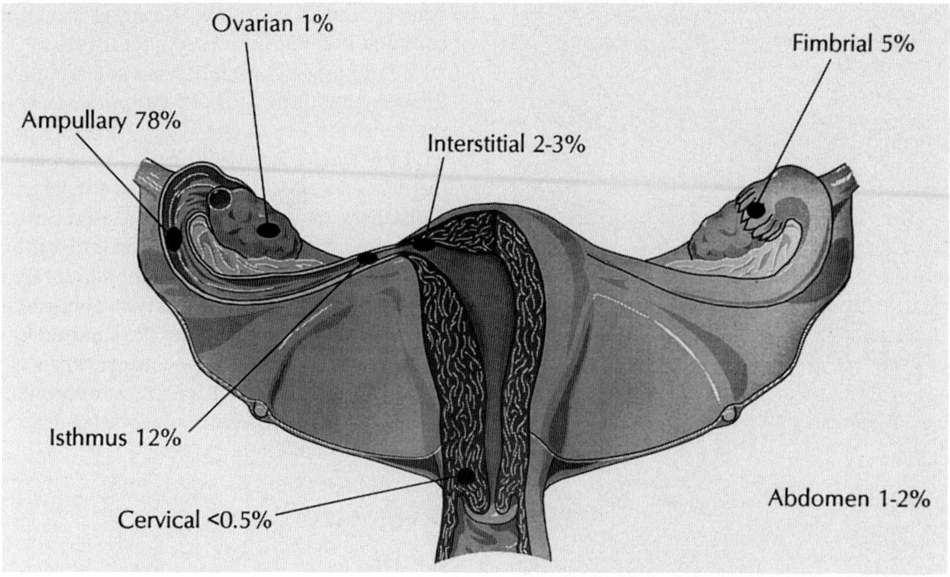


**FIGURE 1** Extrauterine sites of ectopic pregnancy.

first 3 months of gestation as for a normal pregnancy. On physical examination, the patient may have orthostatic hypotension due to tubal rupture and hemorrhage. Abdominal examination discloses tenderness on palpation. Motion of the cervix during the vaginal examination causes extreme pain. The posterior fornix of the vagina may be bulging secondary to blood (hemoperitoneum) in the vaginal fornix. Approximately 20 percent of patients may have a tender adnexal mass. The clinical question arising most frequently is whether the pain is due to an ectopic pregnancy or a leaking corpus luteal cyst encountered in a normal pregnancy. Other diagnoses that may be initially considered are missed or complete abortion, torsion of the fallopian tube, ruptured ovarian cysts, endometriosis, and pelvic inflammatory disease.

## Laboratory Tests

The serum radioimmunoassay for human chorionic gonadotropin (hCG) is the most sensitive method for detecting pregnancy. The antibodies in these tests are specific for the beta subunit of the hormone and can detect 1 to 2 mIU/ml of hCG. Currently two common assays are in use. The first was described in the 1960s and was defined as the Second International Standard (2nd IS). Later, a purer standard was developed that was termed the International Reference Preparation (IRP). Approximately 1.8 mIU/ml (IRP) is equal to 1.0 mIU/ml (2nd IS). These serum radioimmunoassay tests allow the diagnosis of pregnancy as early as 10 days after conception (3.5 postmenstrual weeks). Urine tests that assay for the whole hCG molecule are also extremely sensitive for detecting early pregnancy. These urine tests are sensitive to hCG levels of 30 mIU/ml (IRP). A negative serum or urine hCG determination essentially rules out an intrauterine or ectopic pregnancy.

The clinician and sonographer need to be familiar with the specific assays employed in their institution. Each assay has a particular "discriminatory" hCG zone that determines above which level a normal pregnancy should be visualized on transabdominal sonography (TAS) or transvaginal sonography (TVS). In virtually all cases, a viable intrauterine pregnancy should be detected above 3600 mIU/ml (2nd IS) or 6500 mIU/ml (IRP) using TAS. This corresponds to a 6.5 week gestation. TVS identifies a normal intrauterine pregnancy at approximately 5.5 postmenstrual weeks or above an 800 mIU/ml (2nd IS) or 1800 mIU/ml (IRP). These discriminatory zones may vary depending on the type and frequency of the equipment employed.

If no intrauterine pregnancy (IUP) is identified above these discriminatory hCG levels, the patient may have an ectopic pregnancy or an abnormal intrauterine pregnancy (missed, incomplete, or complete abortion). Below the discriminatory zone, patients with bleeding and pain may have a normal early intrauterine pregnancy, an ectopic pregnancy, or an abortion in progress. In these cases, a repeat serum hCG determination with sequential measurements 2 days apart and a follow-up ultrasonographic examination are suggested. Eighty-five percent of women with a normal IUP will have a 66 percent increase in the serum concentration of hCG between the first and second measurement. Serum concentrations in women with ectopic pregnancies will rise less than 66 percent in 2 days. A patient aborting will have decreasing serum hCG levels over time.

## Scanning Technique

When the patient with a suspected ectopic pregnancy presents to the Ultrasound Department, we assess bladder fullness using a transabdominal technique. If the bladder is full, a complete transabdominal pelvic sonogram is performed. If the bladder is not full, TVS is our initial study. If either study is diagnostic, the other study does not need to be performed. If either study is questionable or nondiagnostic, both studies should be done. The uterus, adnexal regions, both ovaries, and cul-de-sac must be carefully evaluated.

TVS can identify a normal intrauterine pregnancy approximately 1 week earlier than TAS and often provides better detail of the adnexal regions, providing a more confident diagnosis. However, TVS may miss an ectopic pregnancy if the ectopic gestation is located above the uterus beyond the transvaginal probe's field of view. We consider TVS and TAS complementary examinations.

## Sonographic Findings

### *Uterus*

For all practical purposes, the presence of an intrauterine pregnancy virtually excludes an ectopic pregnancy. The incidence of coexisting intra- and extrauterine pregnancy has been reported to be in the range of 1 in 30,000 pregnancies, although this ratio is lower in women receiving ovulation-inducing medication. All ectopic pregnancies have an "empty uterus" or no intrauterine gestation. The uterus may be enlarged. Most commonly the endometrium is thick and echogenic due to hypertrophy from increased hormone levels. A mixed echogenic picture of increased echoes peripherally with central low-level echoes can also be present. These two endometrial patterns usually have correspondingly higher hCG levels than in patients with the "pseudogestational sac" or an echogenic peripheral endometrium with a central fluid cavity. The pseudogestational sac, which is observed in approximately 20 percent of patients with ectopic pregnancy, represents decidual degeneration with bleeding (Fig. 2). These endometrial findings are nonspecific and can be seen in normal patients and in patients who have other causes of endometrial hypertrophy. The double decidual sign of a normal pregnancy is not seen in patients with an ectopic pregnancy.

Interstitial or cornual pregnancy is caused by implantation of the embryo in the intramural portion of the fallopian tube. These ectopic pregnancies rupture early and lead to acute life-threatening intraperitoneal hemorrhage. On sonography, these ectopic pregnancies are eccentrically located in the uterus, and there is splaying and thinning of the overlying myometrium. The endometrium should be identified as a separate structure from the ectopic gestation (Fig. 3).

### *Adnexa*

Sonographically the definitive diagnosis of an ectopic pregnancy can be made if an extrauterine gestation sac and fetal pole, with or without cardiac activity, are identified (Fig. 4). In our series of 60 surgically proven ectopic pregnancies, these findings were observed in 38 percent of patients with TVS. Another finding that can be observed on sonography is the presence of an adnexal ring or gestational sac without a yolk sac or fetal pole (Fig. 5).

A complex adnexal mass with an empty uterus in the presence of a serum hCG level above the discriminatory zone is also highly suggestive of an ectopic pregnancy (Fig. 6). Another nonspecific finding is the discrepancy in size of the adnexa, usually a difference greater than 2 cm.

### *Pelvic Fluid*

The absence of free pelvic fluid excludes active bleeding, but does not exclude an ectopic pregnancy. In our series 28 percent of proven ectopic pregnancies had no free fluid, whereas 47 percent had a small amount of fluid. Small amounts of pelvic fluid can be observed in normal patients. A large amount of pelvic fluid, with or without blood clots, in the presence of an empty uterus is suspicious for an ectopic pregnancy but is not specific. The presence of fluid with small echogenic particles should suggest hemoperitoneum and the possibility of an ectopic pregnancy in the appropriate clinical setting.

### *Color Doppler*

Duplex Doppler evaluation may increase the sensitivity of screening ultrasonography in patients with suspected ectopic pregnancies. With the increased use of TVS, adnexal masses are frequently seen in patients with positive serum hCG levels. These adnexal masses, often complex/cystic in appearance at sonography, most commonly represent a functioning corpus luteal cyst of a normal intrauterine pregnancy. If these women are examined early in their pregnancy, the absence of an intrauterine gestational sac immediately raises the possibility of an ectopic implantation. Duplex Doppler sonography may be able to define more clearly the etiology of these adnexal masses, reducing the need for laparoscopic or surgical intervention.

The functioning corpus luteum cyst is one of the most common cystic adnexal masses encountered in gynecologic sonography. Doppler evaluation of normal ovaries, with and without a functioning luteal cyst, shows a specific sonographic spectral pattern. The normal ovary has a low-amplitude, high-impedance spectral signal with minimal diastolic forward flow. Ovaries containing a functioning corpus luteum show a low-impedance waveform with continued forward flow in both systole and diastole.

Examination of placental blood flow in both normal intrauterine gestation and ectopic implantation shows a similar low-impedance spectral waveform but with significant high-velocity flow in both systole and diastole. Peak systolic frequencies are often greater than 2 kHz, with the average range between 2 and 4 kHz, and associated diastolic frequency greater than 1 to 2 kHz (Fig. 7 and Color Plate 7).

The high-velocity, low-impedance flow pattern seen at the site of placental development is thought to be secondary to the significant pressure gradient that exists between the maternal spiral arteries and the placental intervillous spaces. This pressure gradient, on the order of 60 mm Hg, generates a high-velocity spectral pattern similar to the abnormal signal seen in the neovascularity of ovarian tumors.

The detailed Doppler examination of the periphery of cystic adnexal masses is required for localization of a possible site of placentation. If the characteristic Doppler pattern is observed, the diagnosis of an ectopic pregnancy is further supported. Color duplex sonography significantly reduces the time necessary to acquire adequate spectral images. False-positive studies occur because of the overlap in Doppler shift patterns between luteal flow and ectopic placental flow. As a result of this overlap, the most significant sonographic finding in the evaluation of a possible ectopic pregnancy remains the presence of intrauterine gestation or sonographically visible adnexal ectopic implantation with fetal heartbeat (Fig. 8 and Color Plate 8).

## Suggested Reading

Cacciatore B, Stenman UH, Ylöstalo P. Comparison of abdominal and vaginal sonography in suspected ectopic pregnancy. Obstet Gynecol 1989; 73:770–774.

*Text continued on page 236.*

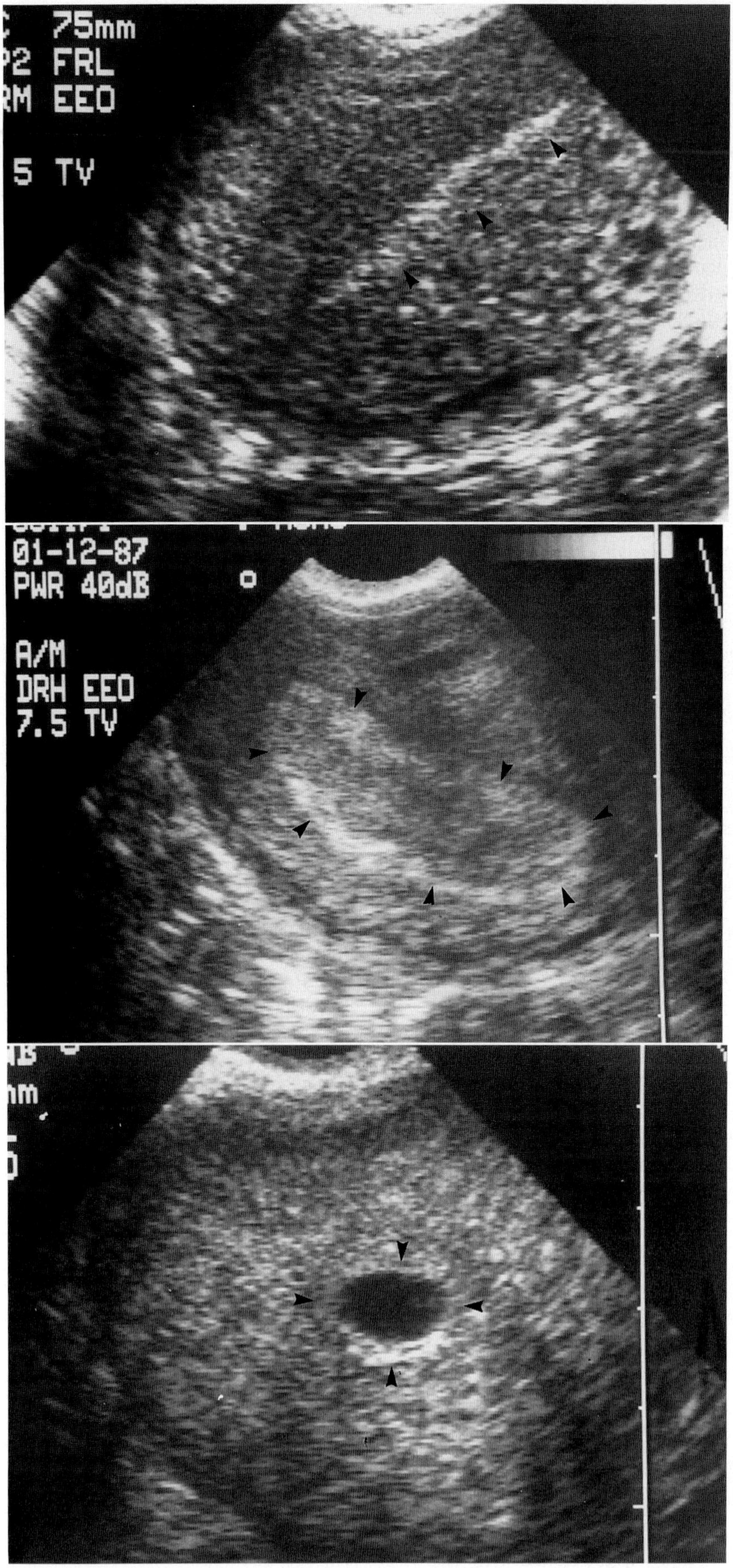


A

B

C

**FIGURE 2** Appearance of the endometrium in ectopic pregnancy. *A,* Echogenic endometrium *(arrowheads). B,* Mixed echogenic pattern *(arrowheads). C,* Pseudogestation sac *(arrowheads).* (From Thorsen MK, Lawson TL, Aiman EJ, et al. Diagnosis of ectopic pregnancy: Endovaginal vs. transabdominal sonography. AJR 1990; 155:307–316; with permission.)

A

B

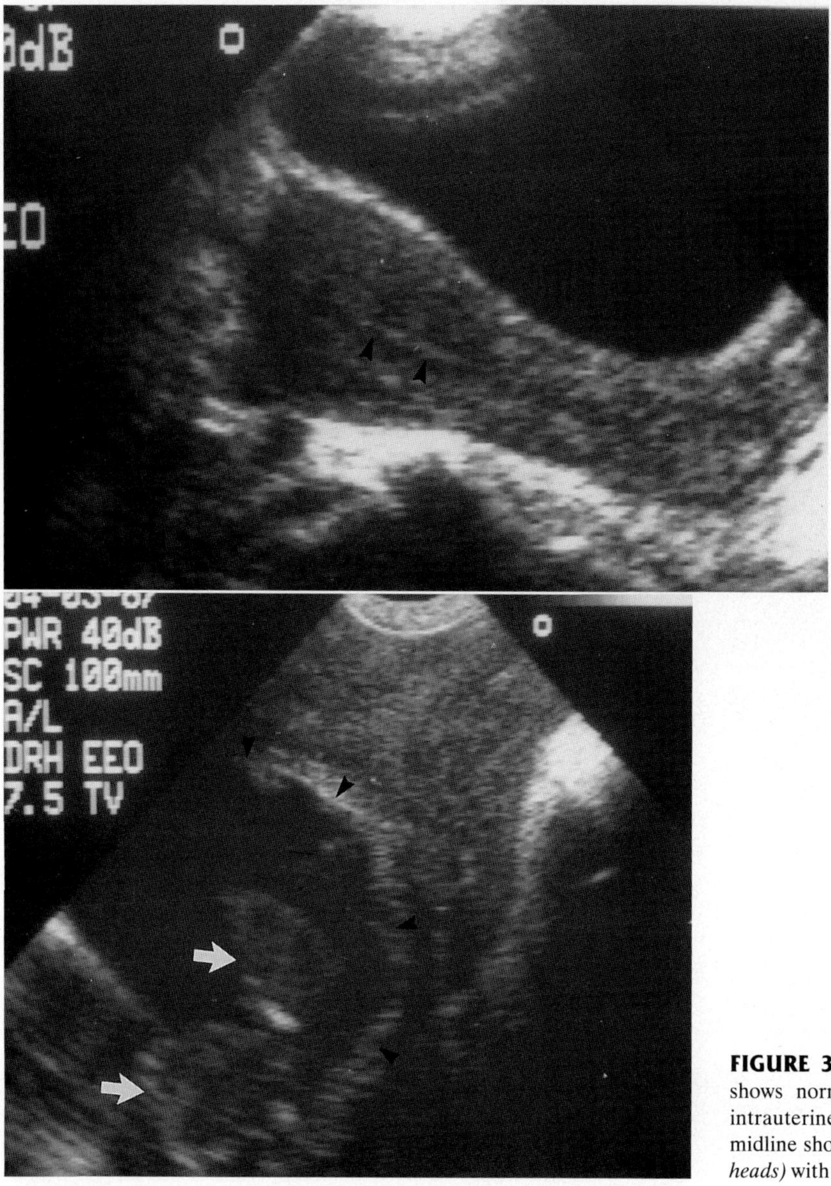


**FIGURE 3** Interstitial ectopic pregnancy. *A,* Sagittal scan shows normal endometrial stripe *(arrowheads)* without an intrauterine pregnancy. *B,* Sagittal scan slightly to the left of midline shows an 8 week interstitial ectopic pregnancy *(arrowheads)* with fetus *(arrows)*. There is splaying of the myometrium.

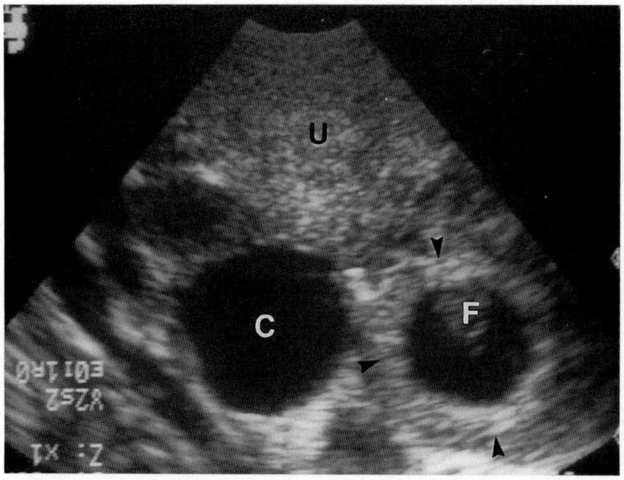


**FIGURE 4** Tubal ectopic pregnancy. An ectopic gestation sac *(arrowheads)* with viable fetus (F) is present. A corpus luteal cyst (C) is seen adjacent to the ectopic uterus (U).

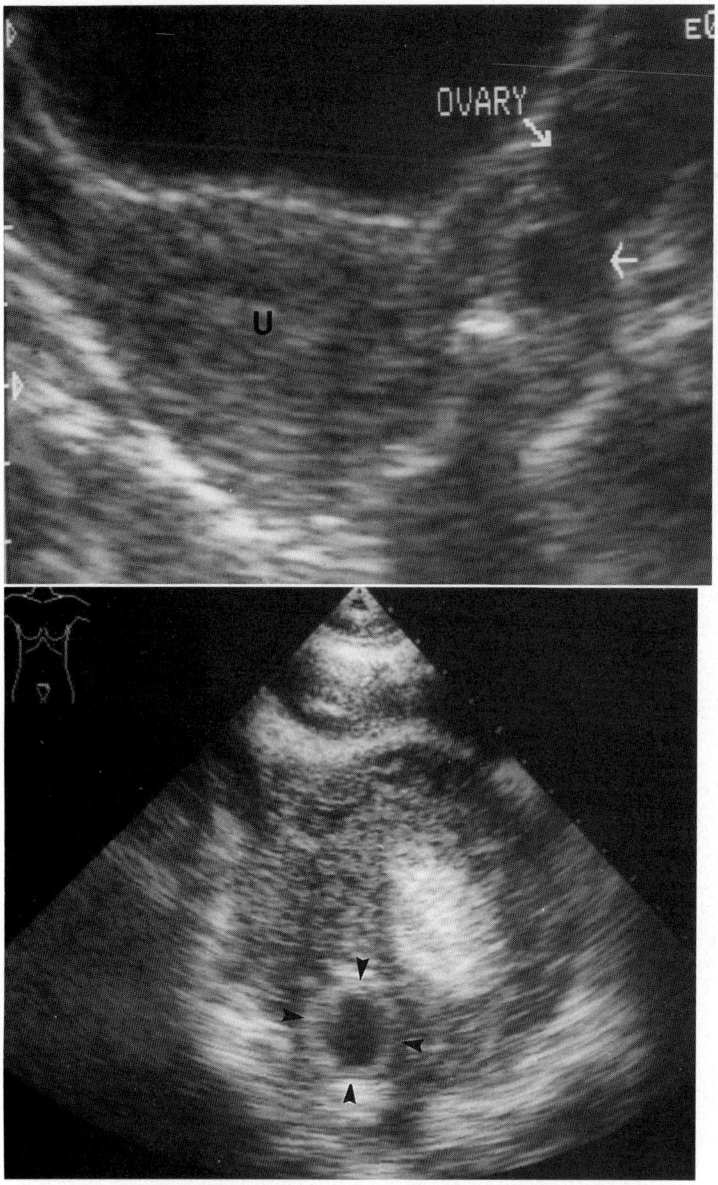


**FIGURE 5** Adnexal rings. *A,* Transverse scan using full bladder technique shows a gestational sac or adnexal ring *(arrow)* located in the ampullary region of the fallopian tube between the ovary and uterus (U). *B,* A transverse scan in another patient shows a gestational sac or adnexal ring *(arrowheads)* in the interstitial portion of the fallopian tube.

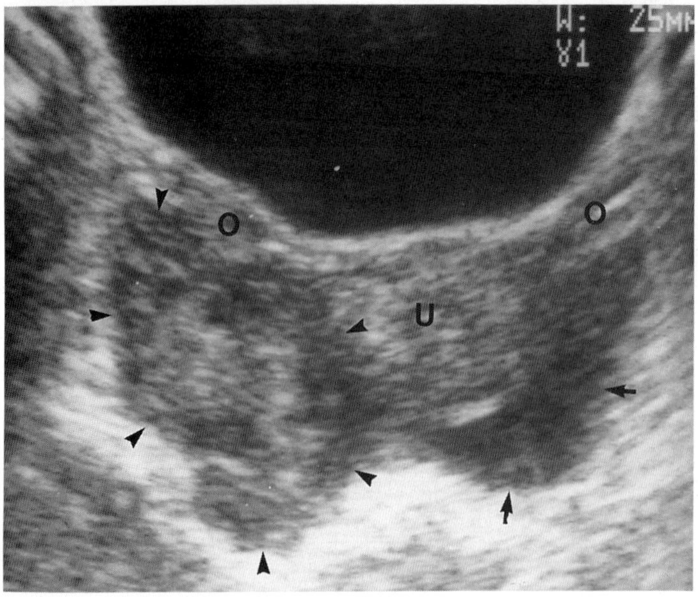


**FIGURE 6** Ruptured ectopic pregnancy. Transverse scan using TAS shows complex right-sided adnexal mass, which represents a ruptured ectopic pregnancy *(arrowheads).* There is also fluid in the cul-de-sac *(arrows).* Empty uterus (U), ovary (O).

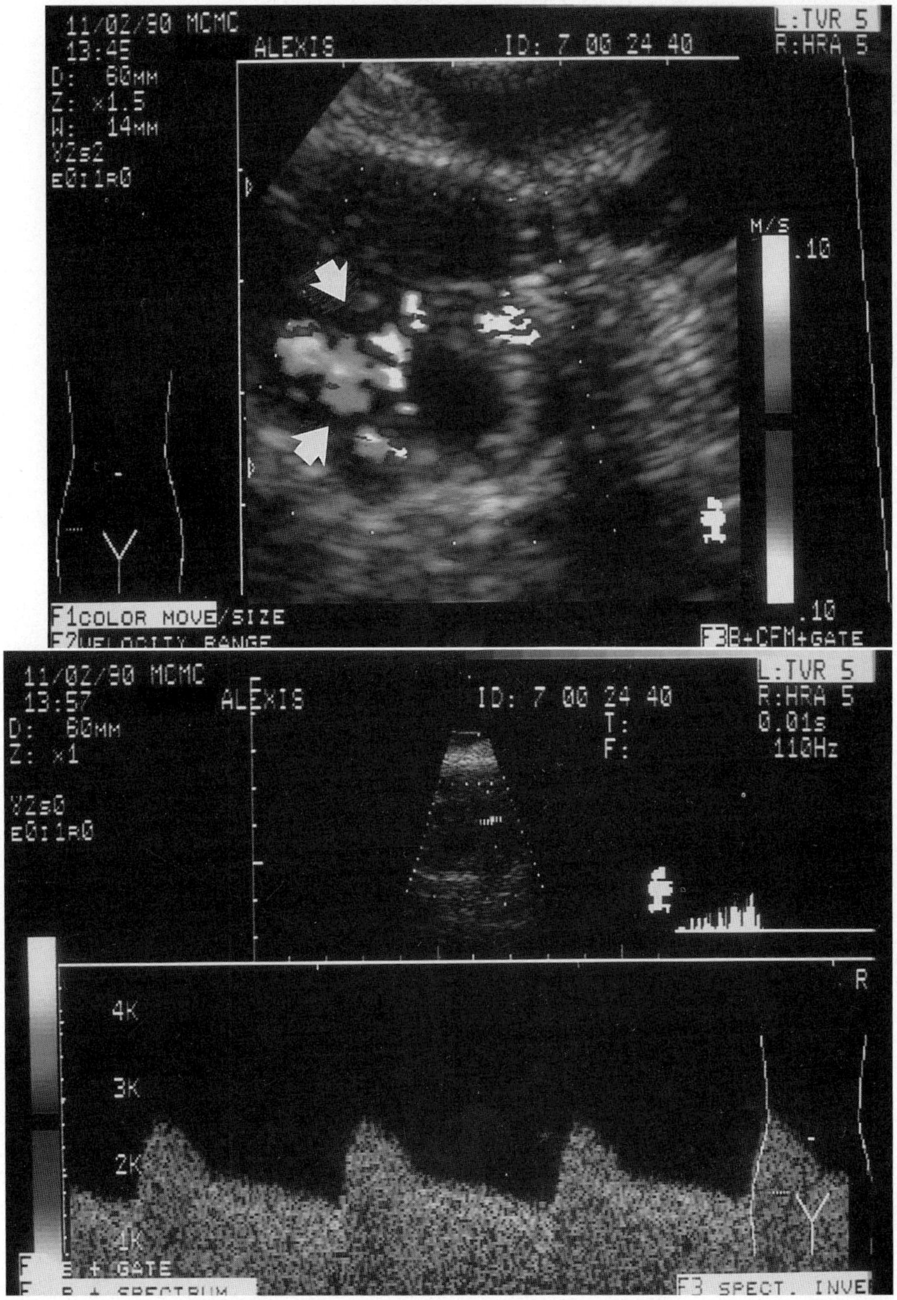


A

B

**FIGURE 7** Tubal ectopic pregnancy. Color Doppler sonograms *(reproduced here in black and white)* show *(A)* adnexal ring with increased blood flow at placentation site *(arrowhead)* and *(B)* low-impedance, high-velocity spectral pattern of placental blood flow. See also Color Plate 7.

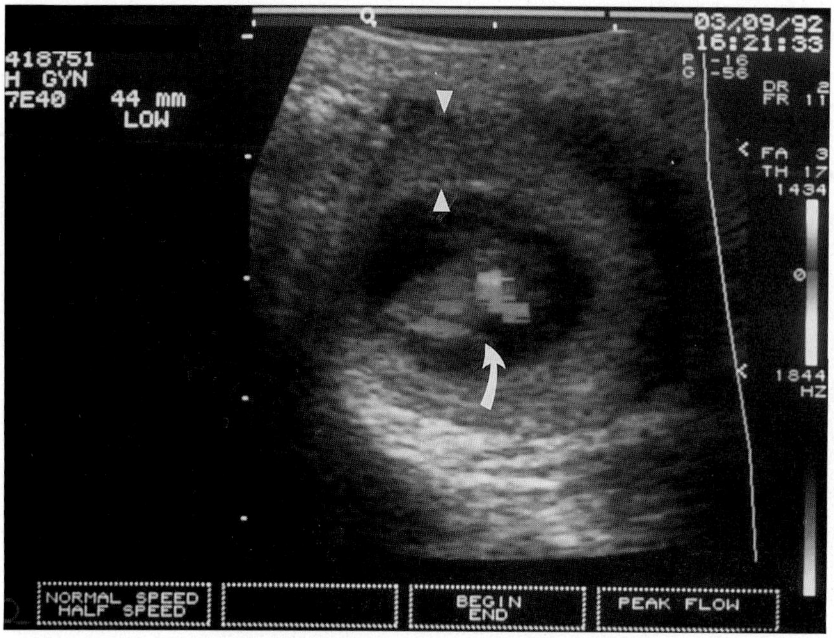


**FIGURE 8** Tubal ectopic pregnancy. Color Doppler sonogram *(reproduced here in black and white)* demonstrates dilated and thickened fallopian tube *(arrowheads)* and living ectopic fetus *(curved arrow)*. See also Color Plate 8.

Dillon EH, Feyock AL, Taylor KJW. Pseudogestational sacs: Doppler US differentiation from normal or abnormal intrauterine pregnancies. Radiology 1990; 176:359–364.

Dorfman SF. Deaths from ectopic pregnancy, United States, 1979 to 1980. Obstet Gynecol 1983; 62:334–338.

Filly RA. Ectopic pregnancy: The role of sonography. Radiology 1987; 162:661–668.

Jain KA, Hamper UM, Sanders RC. Comparison of transvaginal and transabdominal sonography in the detection of early pregnancy and its complications. AJR 1988; 151:1139–1143.

Kadar N, DeCherney AH, Romero R. Receiver operating characteristic curve analysis of the relative efficacy of single and serial chorionic gonadotropin determinations in the early diagnosis of ectopic pregnancy. Fertil Steril 1982; 37:542–547.

Lawson TL. Ectopic pregnancy: Criteria and accuracy of ultrasonic diagnosis. AJR 1978; 131:153–156.

Nyberg DA, Hughes MP, Mack LA, Wang KY. Extrauterine findings of ectopic pregnancy at transvaginal US: Importance of echogenic fluid. Radiology 1991; 178:823–826.

Nyberg DA, Mack LA, Jeffrey RB Jr, Laing FC. Endovaginal sonographic evaluation of ectopic pregnancy: A prospective study. AJR 1987; 149:1181–1186.

Nyberg DA, Mack LA, Laing FC, Jeffrey RB. Early pregnancy complications: Endovaginal sonographic findings correlated with human chorionic gonadotropin levels. Radiology 1988; 167:619–622.

Pellerito JS, Taylor KJW, Quedens-Case C, et al. Ectopic pregnancy: Evaluation with endovaginal color flow imaging. Radiology 1992; 183:407–411.

Schwartz RD, DiPietro DL. βhCG as a diagnostic aid for suspected ectopic pregnancy. Obstet Gynecol 1980; 56:197–201.

Taylor KJW, Ramos IM, Feyock AL, et al. Ectopic pregnancy: Duplex Doppler evaluation. Radiology 1989; 173:93–97.

Thorsen MK, Lawson TL, Aiman EJ, et al. Diagnosis of ectopic pregnancy: Endovaginal vs. transabdominal sonography. AJR 1990; 155:307–316.

Weckstein LN. Current perspective on ectopic pregnancy. Obstet Gynecol 1985; 40:259–272.

Weinstein L. Epidemiology of ectopic pregnancy. In: DeCherney AH, ed. Ectopic Pregnancy. Rockville, MD: Aspen, 1986:1–14.

# MRI Evaluation of Prostate Cancer

*LESLIE E. QUINT, M.D.*

Prostate cancer is the most commonly diagnosed malignancy and the second most common cause of cancer deaths in American men. Approximately 9 percent of men develop prostate cancer, and most of these are diagnosed after age 65. Treatment for tumors confined to the gland (primary tumor stages A and B) usually consists of radical prostatectomy, leading to potential cure. Tumors that have spread through the glandular capsule into adjacent tissues (primary tumor stage C) and those with distant metastatic spread are generally believed to be incurable via surgery, and patients with these tumors are usually treated with radiation and/or hormonal therapy.

Most prostate cancers are detected as an asymptomatic nodule found on routine digital rectal examination, although a patient may occasionally present because of symptoms of metastatic disease, especially bone pain. Some tumors are initially suspected as a result of abnormal screening serum assay levels, such as prostatic acid phosphatase (PAP) or prostatic-specific antigen (PSA). Screening endorectal ultrasonography (ERU) with random biopsy is also detecting an increasing number of clinically silent prostatic malignancies. However, these methods have many limitations for tumor detection and staging. Digital examination detects only those nodules in the posterior aspect of the gland, adjacent to the rectum, and cannot be considered a highly sensitive test for prostatic cancer detection. ERU demonstrates areas with different echogenicity as compared with the surrounding prostatic tissue. Unfortunately not all cancers show abnormal echogenicity and, conversely, other disease processes may simulate cancer, leading to limited sensitivity and specificity for tumor detection. Moreover, digital examination and ERU have both shown poor staging accuracy. Computed tomography (CT) has demonstrated extremely limited value in prostatic cancer detection and staging. None of these techniques is entirely reliable in distinguishing between cancer and benign prostatic hyperplasia (BPH). This is an important clinical consideration, since both diseases occur in the same patient population and in fact often coexist in the same patient.

When affected with cancer, the prostate is usually grossly enlarged, although it may be normal in size or even smaller than normal. Coexistent BPH, if present, often contributes to overall glandular enlargement. The majority of cancers (75 percent) are situated posteriorly and peripherally, in the so-called peripheral zone, and most of these are subcapsular in location, which predisposes to early capsular penetration and later spread to the urinary bladder and/or seminal vesicles. The tumors are often multifocal within the gland. Regional lymph node metastases occur in intrapelvic nodes, particularly in the periprostatic and obturator regions. Nodal disease can then spread to para-aortic, inguinal, and even mediastinal or supraclavicular regions. Prostate cancer also metastasizes hematogenously to bone, especially the pelvis and lumbar spine, and to lung.

## Clinical Utility of Prostate MRI

In patients with biopsy proven prostate cancer, magnetic resonance imaging (MRI) is sometimes used to stage the lesion and direct treatment planning. Published studies have shown that routine body coil MRI of the prostate is inaccurate in demonstrating and staging known prostate cancers. Most investigators are now performing MRI of the prostate using an endorectal, receive-only, surface coil. This affords a better signal-to-noise ratio and consequently better spatial resolution for evaluating the prostate, and preliminary results suggest that endorectal coil imaging may have higher accuracy for lesion detection and staging. A large clinical study is currently being conducted by the Radiology Diagnostic Oncology Group (RDOG 1), using endorectal probes, but the results are not yet known.

Occasionally MRI is indicated in patients with clinically suspected prostate cancer (e.g., as a result of elevated PSA) and negative prostatic biopsies. MRI may demonstrate an abnormal area that can be biopsied later with ultrasonographic guidance.

Features evaluated on MRI studies of the prostate include lesion detection, presence or absence of capsular penetration, invasion of the neurovascular bundles and seminal vesicles, pelvic lymphadenopathy, and skeletal metastases. If adenopathy is detected, it may be biopsied under CT guidance to prove involvement with neoplasm and resulting inoperability. If MRI findings suggest gross, direct tumor extension outside of the gland, surgery may be stayed. However, MRI findings are often nonspecific, and it is generally inadvisable to deny a patient a potentially curative surgical resection based on unproven imaging findings. Therefore biopsy proof of such findings should be obtained whenever possible.

## Technical Approach

Prostatic MRI is generally performed using a 1.5 T magnet. Techniques employed with the endorectal probe are as follows. After coil insertion, the balloon is inflated with 40 to 90 ml of air. Sagittal localizer images are obtained in the supine position to evaluate for coil position, and the patient is then given 1.0 mg glucagon IM or IV to reduce colonic peristalsis. Four mm thick, axial T2- and T1-weighted images are obtained through the prostate gland and seminal vesicles using an 8 to 14 cm field of view (FOV). The frequency-encoding direction must be anteroposterior to shift motion artifact from the colon away from the prostate gland. An image-processing filter is used to reduce the disparity in signal intensity between the near field and the far field. This facilitates visualization of structures throughout the prostate at one window setting. Prostatic MRI takes less than 25 minutes, and the procedure is usually well tolerated. The probe is then removed from the supine patient without significantly altering his position, and a T1-weighted axial body coil sequence is obtained through the entire pelvis to evaluate for pelvic lymphadenopathy.

It has been reported that fat-suppression pulse sequences are useful in eliminating the chemical shift artifact at the margins of the gland and in detecting extracapsular tumor spread. Some centers perform T2-weighted or other specialized types of fat-suppression techniques as part of their routine evaluation. In addition, some data suggest an advantage to the use of external phased array coils in conjunction with an endorectal coil. This combination avoids the problem of signal falloff in areas outside of the optimal sensitive range of the endorectal coil ($\sim$3 cm in depth), and is therefore useful in evaluating the anterior portions of the gland. This type of setup should be commercially available in the near future. For patients who refuse the endorectal probe, the external pelvic phased array coil used alone is a superior alternative to the body coil.

## Diagnostic Approach

### *Prostatic Anatomy*

The peripheral zone, the site of origin of most cancers, is located posterolaterally and predominantly at the apex (inferior aspect) of the gland. The central gland, including the central zone and the transitional zone, is located centrally and anteriorly, predominantly at the base (superior aspect) of the gland. This is where BPH is generally seen. The seminal vesicles are paired, symmetric, bow-tie–shaped structures posterior to the base of the gland.

### *Normal MRI Appearance*

The normal gland is fairly homogeneous and similar to muscle in intensity at T1 weighting. With T2 weighting, the peripheral zone is hyperintense and the central gland is mildly hyperintense compared with muscle (Fig. 1). The seminal vesicles are overall low in signal intensity, similar to muscle, at T1 weighting and high in intensity at T2 weighting because of their fluid content (Fig. 2). The convoluted nature of the tubules leads to a "bunch of grapes" appearance in cross section at T2 weighting. The neurovascular bundles are usually identified as small, low-intensity tubular structures in the periprostatic fat posterolateral to the gland at T1 weighting (see Fig. 1). The

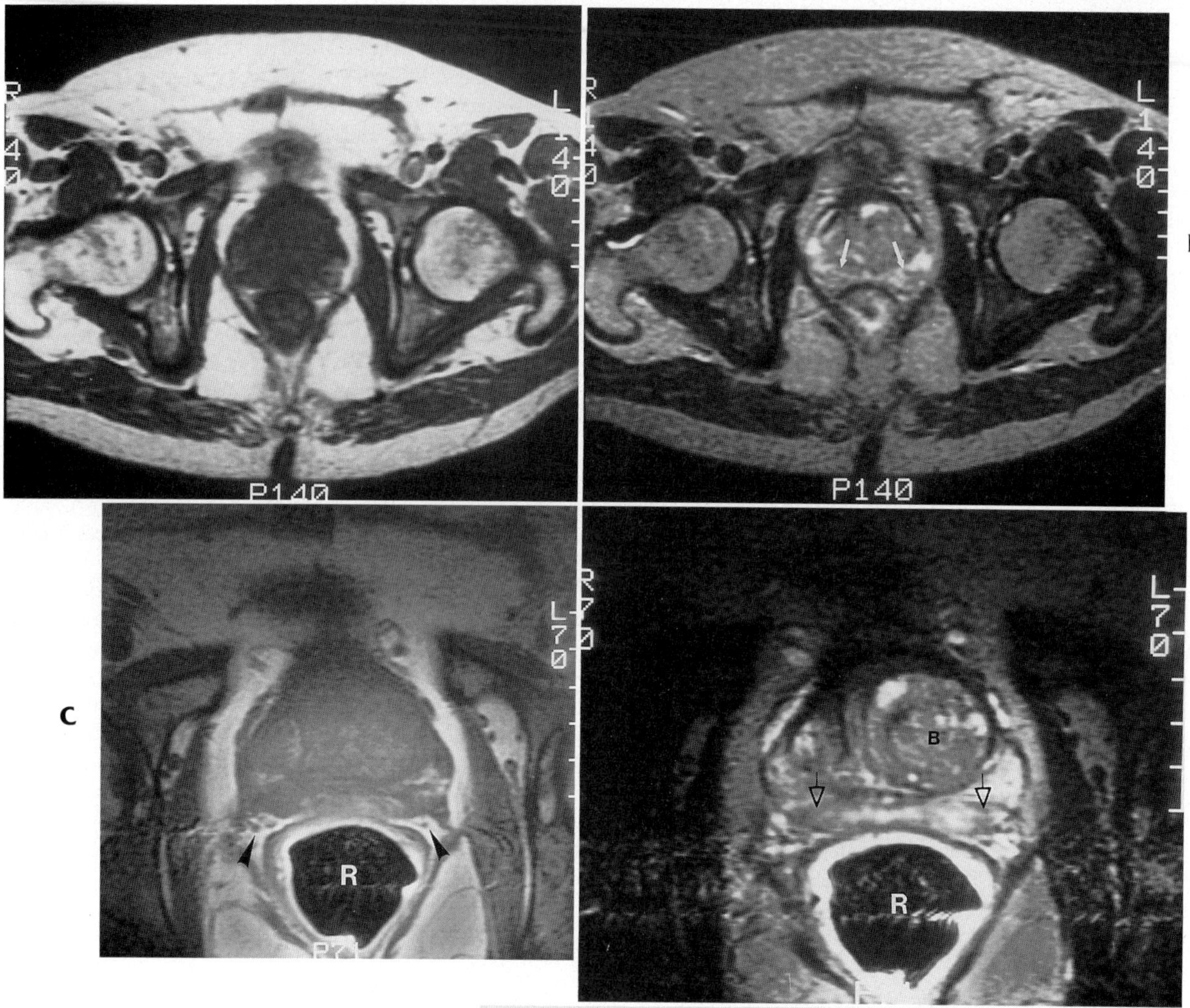


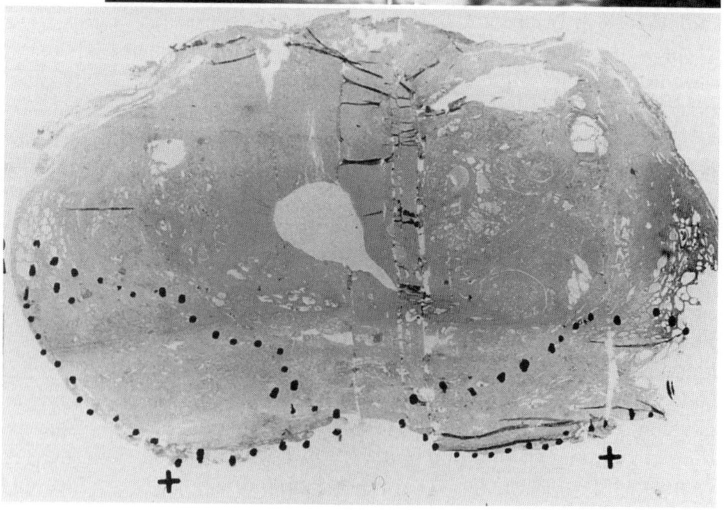


**FIGURE 1** Bilateral prostate cancers demonstrated on body coil (*A* and *B*) and endorectal coil (*C* and *D*) images. The cancers are isointense at T1 weighting (*A* and *C*) and hypointense at T2 weighting (*B* and *D*) (*arrows*). Extracapsular tumor spread is difficult to appreciate. Matching pathological whole mount section (*E*) shows cancers outlined by dots; "+" marks indicate bilateral, microscopic, extracapsular tumor spread. R = rectum; arrowheads = neurovascular bundles; B = BPH.

A

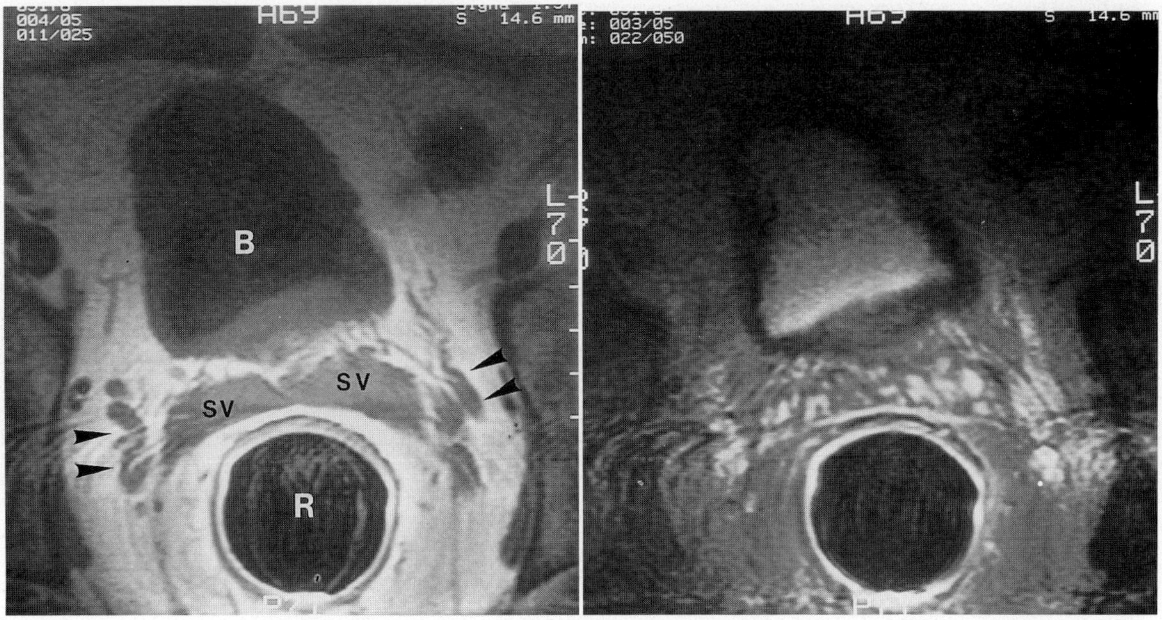


B

**FIGURE 2** Normal seminal vesicles (SV) on T1-weighted (*A*) and T2-weighted (*B*) endorectal coil images (same patient as in Fig. 1). B = thick-walled urinary bladder; R = rectum; arrowheads = periprostatic venous plexus.

periprostatic venous plexus is composed of slightly larger, tortuous, tubular structures at the lateral aspects of the gland and the seminal vesicles; these are hyperintense at T2 weighting (see Fig. 2).

## *MRI Appearance of Prostate Cancer and Benign Prostatic Hyperplasia*

The majority of prostate cancers appear as focal areas of decreased signal intensity within the normally high signal intensity peripheral zone at T2 weighting (Figs. 1 and 3). Extracapsular tumor spread may be demonstrated by abnormal soft tissue in the periprostatic fat with or without focal obliteration of the neurovascular bundle or of the periprostatic venous plexus. Seminal vesicle invasion may be suspected if there is abnormal soft tissue filling the normally fluid-containing spaces of the vesicles and/or if the tubules show thickened walls or are enlarged or abnormally lobulated.

Depending on the underlying histology, BPH may have a variety of appearances, ranging from low to high signal intensity at T2 weighting; it is usually isointense with the remainder of the gland at T1 weighting. BPH often results in enlargement of the central gland, sometimes showing a whorled or nodular appearance, occasionally with pseudocapsules (see Fig. 1). The hyperplastic central gland may severely distort, compress, and obscure the surrounding peripheral zone.

Signal intensity characteristics of lymph nodes are not helpful in distinguishing benignancy from malignancy; therefore nodal metastases can only be suggested if there is obvious lymph node enlargement. There are no established size criteria for lymphadenopathy in the setting of prostate cancer, although 10 to 15 mm is probably a reasonable threshold.

## Pitfalls

There are many pitfalls in the performance and interpretation of MRI scans of patients with prostate cancer. Images may be degraded because of motion artifact, particularly in a patient who is unable to cooperate fully. In addition, although artifact from bowel peristalsis is greatly reduced by administration of glucagon and by assigning the frequency-encoding direction to be anteroposterior, it is still sometimes problematic. Imperfect placement of the endorectal coil may lead to signal drop-off in areas of interest. I have found that inflation of the coil balloon with more than 50 ml of air often leads to superior coil migration, so that the apex (inferior aspect) of the gland lies outside the optimal sensitive range of the coil. This can be remedied by repositioning the coil after visualization of incorrect coil placement on the initial sagittal localizer images.

Although the classic prostate cancer is demonstrated as a low-intensity defect surrounded by normal high-intensity peripheral zone tissue, many cancers do not show this appearance, leading to false-negative studies. In addition, other prostatic processes, including BPH, may simulate cancers, leading to false-positive studies (see Fig. 3). Occasionally high signal intensity, postbiopsy hemorrhage within the prostate may obscure an underlying focus of cancer on T2-weighted images, although this is not a frequent problem (see Fig. 3). On the other hand, it is likely that the cancer is commonly obscured as a result of heterogeneity within the tumor, within the surrounding peripheral zone tissue, or both. Although BPH arises in the central portions of the gland, advanced hyperplastic changes may extend into or severely compress the peripheral zone. The signal intensity of such tissue depends on the exact tissue composition of the hyperplastic changes; low-intensity hyperplastic areas (generally sclerotic or fibromuscular hyperplasia) that appear to lie in the peripheral portion of the gland may simulate a cancer, or lead to overestimation in size of an adjacent cancer, or even obscure an adjacent malignant focus. Hyperplastic changes may also be intermingled with areas of malignancy, further hindering detection of the malignant focus. Prostate cancers tend to grow in irregular shapes rather than spherically, and the margins often infiltrate into surrounding tissue; this blurring of the tumor edges may lead to difficulty in visualization and volume

A

C

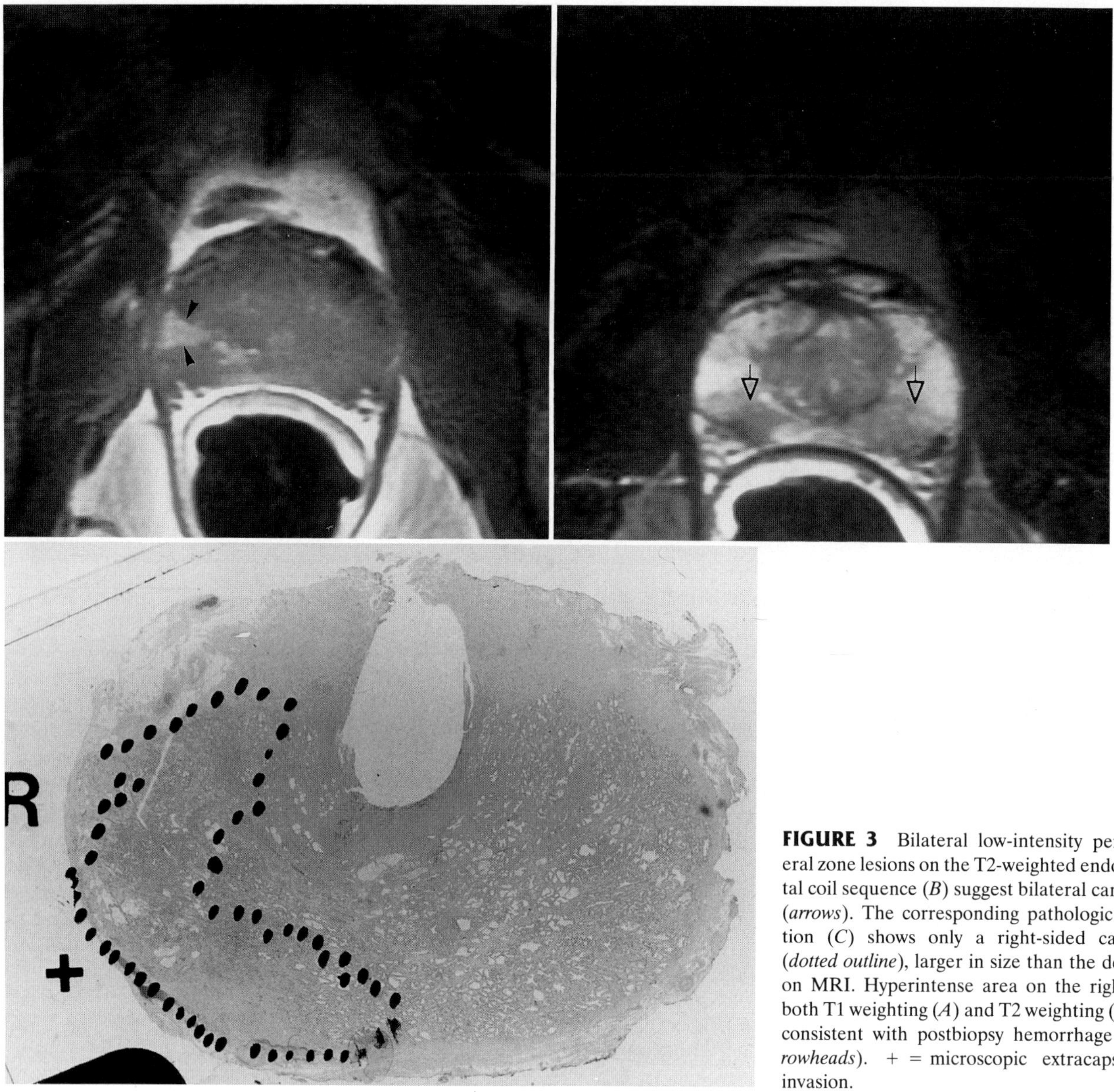


**FIGURE 3** Bilateral low-intensity peripheral zone lesions on the T2-weighted endorectal coil sequence (*B*) suggest bilateral cancers (*arrows*). The corresponding pathologic section (*C*) shows only a right-sided cancer (*dotted outline*), larger in size than the defect on MRI. Hyperintense area on the right at both T1 weighting (*A*) and T2 weighting (*B*) is consistent with postbiopsy hemorrhage (*arrowheads*). + = microscopic extracapsular invasion.

estimation on imaging studies. Cancers that arise in the anterior portions of the gland are particularly difficult to detect and are easily confused with central BPH.

Tumor detection is also difficult in large, bilateral cancers with no adjacent, normal peripheral zone tissue to frame the cancer and reveal its boundaries. Not surprisingly, previous body coil MRI studies have shown that the small cancers (<1 cm diameter) are especially hard to detect. Unfortunately it is these small tumors that need early detection, before the cancer has spread through the gland capsule and become unresectable.

Just as there are many pitfalls in MRI detection of prostate cancer, there are also difficulties in MRI tumor staging. Abnormal soft tissue extending through the capsule into the periprostatic fat adjacent to a tumor in the gland is the hallmark MRI finding of capsular penetration. Unfortunately this finding is often difficult to appreciate. First, the prostatic capsule is not a well-defined anatomic structure. Instead it consists of a zone of relatively hypocellular fibromuscular stroma of varying thickness, often less than 1 mm. At the prostatic apex, it blends with the skeletal muscle of the urogenital diaphragm, and it is particularly difficult to define in this region. The capsule is usually not directly visualized at MRI, and the location of the capsule in the region of a tumor must often be extrapolated from the contour of adjacent glandular tissue. In addition, at our institution, most radical prostatectomy specimens with extracapsular tumor spread show only microscopic invasion into the periprostatic fat; this invasion is not grossly evident, and one should not expect to see this at MRI using currently available techniques (see Figs. 1 and 3). Similarly, microscopic tumor invasion of the seminal vesicles is generally invisible at MRI. Conversely, the seminal vesicles can appear to contain low signal intensity areas on T2-weighted images that do not represent true tumor invasion.

Lymph nodes involved with metastatic disease in the pelvis do not appear to show any unique signal intensity characteristics, and therefore MRI evaluation of lymph nodes is performed using only a size threshold for diagnosing abnormality. Thus MRI will misdiagnose enlarged, benign nodes as well as microscopic tumor foci in normal-sized nodes. Therefore visualization of enlarged pelvic nodes at MRI should be considered suggestive of metastatic disease, and tissue biopsy proof should be obtained before using this information to alter treatment planning.

## Suggested Reading

Carrol CL, Sommer FG, McNeal JE, Stamey TA. The abnormal prostate: MR imaging at 1.5 T with histopathologic correlation. Radiology 1987; 163:521–525.

Quint LE, Van Erp JS, Bland PH, et al. Prostate cancer: Correlation of MR images with tissue optical density at pathologic examination. Radiology 1991; 179:837–842.

Quint LE, Van Erp JS, Bland PH, et al. Carcinoma of the prostate: MR images obtained with body coils do not accurately reflect tumor volume. AJR 1991; 156:511–516.

Rifkin MD, Zerhouni EA, Gatsonis CA, et al. Comparison of magnetic resonance imaging and ultrasonography in staging early prostate cancer: Results of a multi-institutional cooperative trial. N Engl J Med 1990; 323:621–626.

Schiebler ML, Tomaszewski JE, Bezzi M, et al. Prostatic carcinoma and benign prostatic hyperplasia: Correlation of high-resolution MR and histopathologic findings. Radiology 1989; 172:131–137.

Schnall MD, Imai Y, Tomaszewski J, et al. Prostate cancer: Local staging with endorectal surface coil MR imaging. Radiology 1991; 178:797–802.

# Radiographic Contrast Media–Induced Renal Dysfunction

*EVERETT MARC LAUTIN, M.D.* · *JEFFREY LEWIS LAUTIN, M.D.*

Radiographic contrast media (RCM) are a fundamental part of diagnostic radiology with an essential role in urography, angiography, computed tomography (CT), and myelography. Although considered relatively safe substances, RCM still must be viewed and dispensed with the same caution that one would afford any pharmaceutical. There are no absolute contraindications for the use of RCM; however, there exist certain patient profiles that confer on the patient an increased risk for complications, one of which is RCM-induced acute renal dysfunction. It has been estimated that 10 percent of cases of acute renal failure result from the administration of RCM and that these agents are more commonly the cause of hospital-acquired renal insufficiency than are the aminoglycoside antibiotics. Although the new lower-osmolar contrast agents offer increased safety for many higher-risk patients, the availability of other diagnostic tests that do not call for RCM should always be considered as alternatives in these patients. This chapter discusses contrast-induced nephropathy as it relates to higher-risk patients, presents an approach to avoiding RCM in these patients, and discusses diagnosing renal impairment when it does occur.

## Risk Factors and Pathophysiology

Many patients suffer some degree of renal impairment after administration of contrast material, although, for most, the effect is only mild and transient, and probably of no consequence. However, in a small minority of patients, especially those with certain underlying medical conditions, the consequent renal injury can be marked and sometimes irreversible. Patients at increased risk for contrast-induced nephropathy include diabetics and those with elevated precontrast serum creatinine levels, dehydration, and multiple myeloma; other risk factors may include age greater than 70 years, proteinuria, peripheral vascular disease, hyperuricemia, hypertension, and a prior episode of contrast-induced renal failure (Table 1).

Risk factors for contrast-induced nephropathy can be additive. Insulin-dependent diabetics have a greater chance of developing contrast-induced nephropathy than non–insulin-dependent diabetics. Therefore an elderly insulin-dependent diabetic who is dehydrated (with an elevated blood urea nitrogen to serum creatinine ratio greater than 20:1) and has an elevated creatinine level would be at significantly increased risk for contrast-induced nephropathy. Although somewhat controversial, the volume of RCM administered has also been correlated with an increased risk of contrast-induced nephropathy; therefore a smaller volume (e.g., a half-dose) can be administered to certain higher-risk patients, such as those with elevated serum creatinine levels. (Note that some studies show no increased risk of higher doses of contrast material and contrast-induced renal damage.) This must be weighed against the possible loss of diagnostic information that a smaller contrast dose provides. Multiple studies using RCM should be separated by as much time as is reasonably possible, because there is evidence that a short separation between studies using RCM places the patient at increased risk of contrast-induced nephrotoxicity (e.g., an excretory urogram followed a day later by an angiogram or contrast-enhanced CT).

When one is presented with a patient that falls within any of the foregoing categories, it is advisable to consider alternative tests that do not require RCM, such as nonenhanced CT, ultrasonography, magnetic resonance imaging (MRI), and nuclear medicine imaging. However, these evaluations may not be readily available or have the diagnostic value of a study using RCM. In such situations the diagnostic benefit of intravenous contrast material may outweigh the risk of renal damage, and in these circumstances the necessity of administering RCM and the risk of renal damage should be discussed with the patient.

The definition of and the pathophysiological mechanism of contrast-induced nephropathy are controversial. Changes in serum creatinine levels are a useful measure of changes in renal function. The definition of a significant rise in the serum creatinine level, as well as the definition of elevation of baseline creatinine level, have varied considerably in the literature. This probably accounts for the wide variation in the incidence of RCM-induced nephropathy as reported in the literature (Table 2). Multiple possible mechanisms of RCM-induced renal damage have been proposed. The marked hyperosmolarity of RCM is suggested as a cause of renal toxicity. Hemodynamic changes induced by RCM, character-

**TABLE 1** Risk Factors for Contrast-Induced Nephropathy

| Risk factor |
|---|
| Increased risk for contrast-induced nephropathy |
| Elevated baseline serum creatinine level |
| Insulin-dependent diabetes |
| Dehydration |
| Multiple myeloma |
| RCM study within the past few days |
| History of RCM–induced renal failure |
| Possible increased risk of contrast-induced nephropathy |
| Advanced age (>70 years) |
| Proteinuria |
| Peripheral vascular disease |
| Crystalluria (hyperuricemia) |
| Non–insulin-dependent diabetes |
| Cardiovascular disease |
| Diuretic use |
| Hypertension |

ized by an initial rise in renal perfusion, followed by a decline, with an eventual return to baseline, also may play a role. Another suspected mechanism is direct toxicity of the RCM on the renal tubules. RCM injection also results in a marked increase in blood viscosity secondary to mechanical red blood cell changes; these are probably caused by fluid outflow from the red blood cells secondary to the marked hyperosmolarity of RCM. It is also suspected that RCM causes precipitation of Tamm-Horsfall protein (the substance that makes up much of the hyaline casts seen during the diuretic phase of acute tubular necrosis), which could conceivably obstruct flow through the tubules.

## Guidelines for Administration of RCM

Whatever the specific pathophysiology of contrast-induced renal impairment, it is generally agreed that decreasing the transit time of the contrast material through the kidney is advantageous. This is most commonly achieved by adequate

**TABLE 2** Definitions of RCM-Associated Renal Dysfunction (Racard) and Pre-existing Creatinine Elevation Used in the Literature

| Reference | Definition of Pre-existing Renal Insufficiency (serum creatinine level) | Definition of a Significant Change in Serum Creatinine Level | Time for Increase (days) | Type of Contrast Study | Incidence of Racard |
|---|---|---|---|---|---|
| Shafi Arch Intern Med (1978) | Not given | Creatinine increase ≥25% | 5 | IVP (prospective) | Prior azotemic patients only<br>Nondiabetic 17/28 (61%)<br>Diabetic 11/12 (92%) |
| Cochran AJR (1983) | ≥1.5 mg/dl | Creatinine increase >0.3 mg/dl and >20% | 5 | Renal angiography (retrospective) | All patients 45/266 (16.9%)<br>Prior nonazotemic 2/54 (3.7%)<br>Prior azotemic 43/212 (20.3%) |
| Van Zee Annals of Int Med (1978) | >1.5 mg/dl | Creatinine increase ≥1.0 mg/dl | 7 | IVP (retrospective) | All patients 18/377 (4.8%)<br>Nonazotemic<br>Nondiabetic 1/169 (0.6%)<br>Diabetic 0/19 (0.0%) |
| Byrd Medicine (1979) | ≥1.6 mg/dl | Creatinine increase ≥2.0 mg/dl | 2 | All contrast studies (retrospective) | All nephrology consultations: 18/12,000 (0.15%) |
| Eisenberg AJR (1981) | ≥1.8 mg/dl or BUN ≥30 mg/dl | BUN increase of 50% or 20 mg/dl or creatinine increase of >1.0 mg/dl | 1 | All angiography (prospective) | All patients—500 ml NS/hour given as prophylaxis: 0/537 (0.0%) |
| Harkonen Am J Med (1977) | ≥2.0 mg/dl | Creatinine increase ≥1.0 mg/dl | 5 | IVP (retrospective) | Diabetics with elevated baseline creatinine: 22/29 (76%) |
| D'Elia Am J Med (1982) | ≥1.5 mg/dl and BUN ≥30 mg/dl | Creatinine increase ≥1.0 mg/dl | 3 | Nonrenal angiography (prospective) | Prior nonazotemic, nondiabetic 1/199 (0.5%)<br>Prior nonazotemic, diabetic 1/95 (1%)<br>Prior azotemic, nondiabetic 1/10 (10%)<br>Prior azotemic, diabetic 3/13 (23%) |
| Kumar Arch Intern Med (1981) | ≥1.5 mg/dl | Creatinine increase ≥0.5 mg/dl | 2 | All noncardiac angiography (prospective) | All patients 1/100 (1%) |
| Parfrey N Engl J Med (1989) | ≥1.7 mg/dl | Two criteria: creatinine increase >50% and >1.4 mg/dl [>25% and >1.4 mg/dl] | 2 | All intravascular contrast studies (prospective) | Diabetic, nonazotemic 0/85 (0%)—[2/85 (2.4%)]<br>Diabetic, azotemic 3/34 (8.8%)—[3/34 (8.8%)]<br>Nondiabetic, azotemic 4/101 (4.0%)—[6/94 (6.4%)] |

After Lautin EM, Freeman NJ, et al. Radiocontrast-associated renal dysfunction. AJR 1991; 157:49–65; with permission.

hydration of the patient both before and after the test. However, the amount of hydration must be tailored in patients with poor cardiac function, pre-existing renal impairment, and before excretory urography. Excretory urography, unlike other imaging studies using contrast media, has a trade-off: mild dehydration may improve renal opacification, while overhydration may result in a poor nephrogram. Therefore in this situation mild dehydration may be justified. In our opinion, except possibly before an excretory urogram, virtually all patients should be well hydrated before and/or after contrast material administration. Patients undergoing excretory urography should be in a homeostatic state of hydration or mildly dehydrated before the study (typically nothing by mouth after midnight for an early morning study); they then should receive fluids liberally immediately after the study.

The new lower-osmolar contrast agents (so called 3:1 agents) are gaining more of a role and are gradually replacing the standard high-osmolar contrast agents (3:2 agents). The term *low-osmolar,* however, is a misnomer. This new generation of contrast agents, which includes Omnipaque 300 (iohexol, 672 mOsm/kg $H_2O$), Optiray 320 (ioversol, 702 mOsm/kg), Isovue 300 (iopamidol, 616 mOsm/kg), and Hexabrix 320 (ioxaglate sodium/meglumine, 600 mOsm/kg), still has a higher osmolality than human serum (290 mOsm/kg). However, when compared to standard ionic compounds such as Hypaque 50% (sodium diatrizoate, 1515 mOsm/kg), the osmolality of this generation is significantly closer to that of serum. The non-ionic class has many other advantages aside from lower osmolality, including fewer somatic and allergic complications. Further, a significant decrease in the incidence of contrast-induced nephropathy has been shown with lower-osmolar compounds, notably in patients that are at increased risk for renal impairment. Unfortunately this margin of safety comes at a significant increase in cost. Lower-osmolar contrast material costs approximately one dollar per milliliter, compared with standard ionic contrast, which typically costs five cents per milliliter. Therefore at many institutions financial considerations commonly dictate that the use of nonionics must be rationed to high-risk patients. Currently available only on a research basis are the 6:1 agents, with approximate isoosmolarity to serum at typical concentration; the nephrotoxicity of these have yet to be evaluated (Iotrol 300, 360 mOsm/kg).

After RCM has been administered to a patient who is considered to be at increased risk of contrast-induced nephropathy, it is important to monitor the patient for signs of renal failure. A rise in the serum creatinine level of more than 0.3 mg/dl within 2 to 3 days after the study may indicate that some renal damage has occurred. Greater increases in serum creatinine level indicate more severe renal damage. Other signs include a decrease in the creatinine clearance and oliguria or anuria. Because the nephrogram normally peaks within a few minutes after the administration of RCM, a delayed or persistent bilateral nephrogram suggests possible renal damage. The nephrogram at 20 minutes should be of a density less than or equal to that at 5 or 10 minutes, and films at 1 hour should demonstrate a further decrease in the nephrogram. If the nephrogram is not decreasing bilaterally with time, the possibility of RCM-induced renal damage should be considered. To this end, an abdominal film obtained at approximately 24 hours may be particularly useful. If there is still contrast material in the renal parenchyma, then contrast-induced toxicity should be strongly suspected and serum creatinine levels obtained and compared with the serum creatinine level before the study, if available. In addition, one may observe so-called "vicarious excretion of contrast media" in the gallbladder or in the colon. These findings do not, however, indicate irreversible damage to the kidneys, and vicarious excretion of contrast material may occasionally be seen normally, especially after the administration of a large volume of contrast material. Vicarious excretion of RCM results when there is a prolonged circulation of RCM, with resultant excretion by the secondary and tertiary pathways (the liver via the bile with concentration in the gallbladder; the small bowel mucosa with concentration in the colon). Because CT is much more sensitive to small changes in radiographic contrast, the finding of vicarious excretion of RCM on CT is less suggestive of renal damage than the same finding on plain film.

## Management of RCM-Induced Nephropathy

The management of a patient with contrast-induced renal failure centers on careful fluid management. It is important to prevent dehydration, but in the face of renal dysfunction, overhydration can easily occur. Therefore the patient's fluid status must be monitored including urine output, weight, blood pressure, and physical signs of cardiac decompensation (e.g., presence of jugular venous distention or extremity edema).

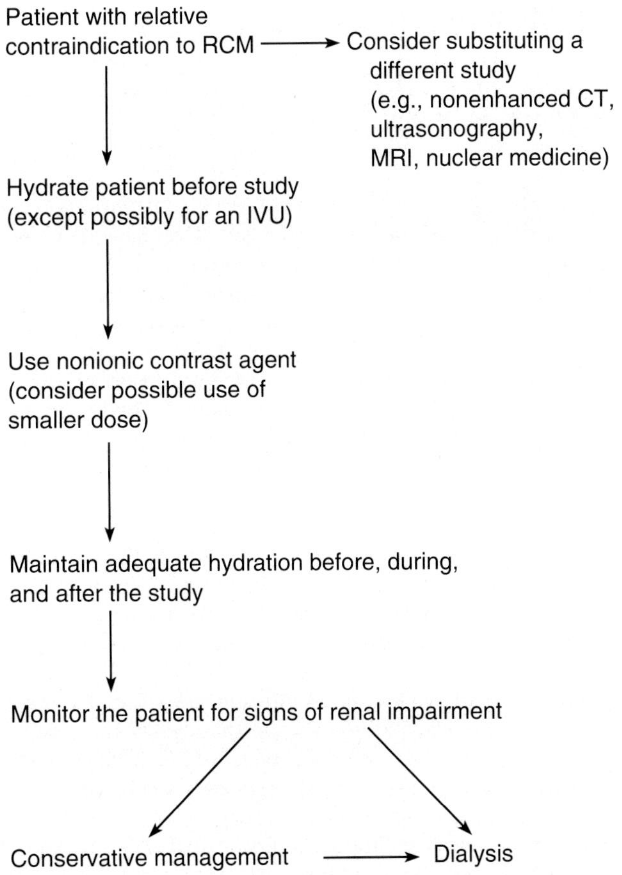


**FIGURE 1** Guidelines for administration of RCM.

Electrolyte abnormalities frequently complicate renal dysfunction, especially hyperkalemia, acidosis, and uremia. Hyperkalemia can be treated by limiting the intake of potassium and administering potassium-binding resins. Acidosis can be treated with the addition of sodium bicarbonate. However, with severe renal impairment dialysis can address both volume and electrolyte problems. If the kidneys regain some or all of their function, these measures can be stopped.

In most cases RCM-induced renal toxicity appears to be entirely, or at least partially, reversible. However, it should be noted that if RCM must be given to a patient with multiple myeloma and renal failure ensues, it has a significant likelihood of being irreversible.

## Discussion

The most important rule to remember is that if there is a question about the safety of injecting RCM in a patient who is at increased risk for contrast-induced nephropathy—do not. The benefit of the contrast study may easily be overshadowed by kidney damage. Alternative tests must first be considered; however, if the decision is made that the administration of RCM is justified, certain guidelines should be observed. The patient must be well hydrated; a nonionic agent should be considered, keeping the dose as low as possible (commensurate with an adequate study); and the kidney function should be monitored for three days or more after the test. This scheme selects patients at increased risk for renal failure and attempts to minimize the possibility that they will suffer renal complications (Fig. 1).

## Suggested Reading

Dawson P. Contrast agent nephrotoxicity—an appraisal. Br J Radiol 1985; 58:121–124.

Katzberg RW. New and old contrast agents: Physiology and nephrotoxicity. Urol Radiol 1988; 10:6–11.

King BF, Hartman GW, Williamson B, et al. Low-osmolality contrast media: A current perspective. Mayo Clin Proc 1989; 64:976–985.

Lautin EM, Freeman NJ, Schoenfeld AH, et al. Radiocontrast-associated renal dysfunction: Incidence and risk factors. AJR 1991; 157:49–58.

Lautin EM, Freeman NJ, Schoenfeld AH, et al. Radiocontrast-associated renal dysfunction: A comparison of lower-osmolality and conventional high-osmolality contrast media. AJR 1991; 157:59–65.

Miller DL, Chang R, Wells WT, et al. Intravascular contrast media: Effect of dose on renal function. Radiology 1988; 167:607–611.

Older RA, Miller JP, Jackson DC, et al. Angiographically-induced renal failure and its radiographic detection. AJR 1976; 126:1039–1045.

Schwab SJ, Hlatky MA, Pieper KS, et al. Contrast nephrotoxicity: A randomized trial of a nonionic and an ionic radiographic contrast agent. N Engl J Med 1988; 320:149–153.

# Endoluminal Sonography of the Urinary Tract

*JI-BIN LIU, M.D. · DEMETRIUS H. BAGLEY, M.D.*
*BARRY B. GOLDBERG, M.D.*

Ultrasonography has been used almost since its inception for the evaluation of the urinary tract. The most common approach is to apply the transducer on the flanks to visualize the kidneys and suprapubically to visualize the urine-filled bladder. With this technique, it has been possible to demonstrate such abnormalities as masses (differentiating tumors from cysts), hydronephrosis, and filling defects, especially stones within the kidneys and urinary bladder. The ureters are not routinely visualized unless they are dilated and, even then, only the most proximal or distal portions. Rigid ultrasound probes have been inserted through the urethra into the urinary bladder to detect tumors and evaluate their degree of invasion. Endorectal sonography has been used to image the prostate, seminal vesicles, and urethra. An endovaginal approach has also been used to evaluate the lower urinary tract. Beyond this, there has not been an attempt to use endoluminal sonography to evaluate the urologic system.

At present, the following nonultrasonographic endoluminal techniques are available to evaluate the urinary tract: retrograde or antegrade catheterization with injection of an iodinated contrast agent, rigid or flexible cystoscopes, and ureteroscopes. The ureteroscope is particularly important in mucosal evaluation and the identification of stones and tumors projecting into the lumen of the ureter. However, the extent of tumor beyond the surface and stones embedded within the mucosa cannot be evaluated. In addition, the cause of an area of narrowing or dilatation may not be clearly demonstrated.

Endoluminal sonography is ideally suited to supply this type of important additional information. The concept of endoluminal sonography was first successfully used in specially designed ultrasound transducer-containing gastroscopes for the upper gastrointestinal tract. Advanced through the esophagus into the stomach, the ultrasound transducer-containing endoscopes have proven effective in producing either cross-sectional or linear images to visualize the structures within the walls and beyond. Submucosal masses, tumor invasion, and enlarged adjacent lymph nodes have been clearly demonstrated.

With technical developments, specially designed high-frequency miniature ultrasound transducers housed in flexible catheters have been inserted into arteries to analyze atherosclerotic plaque. Initial investigations have been carried out in the peripheral vessels to monitor the effectiveness of angioplasty and atherectomy. During the past three years, we have used these catheter-based ultrasound transducers in nonvascular lumina including the urethra, urinary bladder, ureters, renal pelvis, endometrial canal, fallopian tubes, esophagus, bowel, bile, and pancreatic ducts. Initial work in animal models showed the feasibility of imaging these structures and in detecting a variety of abnormalities. There has been close correlation between the cross-sectional ultrasound measurements of the thickness of the mucosa and mural structures and actual anatomical specimens. Adjacent structures have also been accurately identified. Because of this initial success, these specially designed catheter-based ultrasound transducers were used in human subjects for a variety of urologic abnormalities.

Several manufacturers make endoluminal ultrasound equipment, and a variety of catheter-based ultrasound transducers are available. In our investigations we used the Diasonics IVUS unit (Milpitas, CA). This equipment uses a single-element transducer that revolves at more than 30 frames per second, producing a real-time cross-sectional image. The 20 MHz ultrasound transducer provides axial resolution of 0.1 mm and a maximum penetration of approximately 2 cm. The 6 Fr (2 mm diameter), 95 cm long catheters (Medi-Tech/Boston Scientific, Watertown, MA) are either blunt-tipped or worked over a guidewire that facilitates the advancement of the catheter into smaller lumina (Fig. 1). For procedures in humans, the catheter is used only once and then disposed. The catheters and inner core transducers are sterilized using standard gas sterilization techniques. The inner core transducer can be resterilized. The catheter is made so that a 27 gauge needle can be inserted through the tip and sterile water injected to displace any trapped air near the transducer that might interfere with the propagation of the ultrasound beam. In most cases the ultrasound equipment is taken into the operating room, where the urologist proceeds with the indicated urologic endoscopy.

## Indications and Clinical Utility

Many features of endoluminal sonography make it attractive to the urologist. Since the ultrasound transducer-containing catheters are no more than 2 to 3 mm in diameter, they can be easily passed into the urethra without the need for dilatation. When positioned within the urethra, it is possible to visualize various anatomical structures and to demonstrate areas of abnormality such as plaque or fibrosis. Endoluminal urethral sonography in conjunction with transrectal sonography has been used to guide Teflon injection into the external urinary sphincter in men with urinary incontinence after radical prostatectomy. This technique allows the urologist to inject Teflon precisely at the region of the sphincter and to measure the exact depth and volume of the injected material. Transurethral sonography has also been used to assess the deployment of the intraprostatic and intrasphincter urethral stent placement. It can precisely identify the proximal and distal margins of the stent deployment and measure the stent diameter (Fig. 2). Follow-up endoluminal sonography can be used to determine if there is any breakage in the stent wires, alteration in the stent diameter, abscess or calculi formation, and/or neoepithelium growth along with the stent. Thus these miniature catheter-based transducers have been able to provide important information to the urologist for the long-term follow-up of intraurethral stents. In addition, transure-

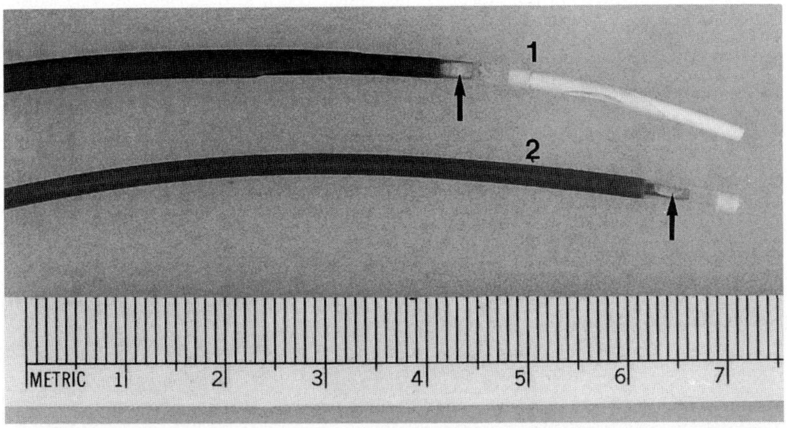


**FIGURE 1** Twenty MHz ultrasound transducers (*arrows*) housed in 6 Fr flexible catheters (1: over a guidewire, 2: blunt-tipped).

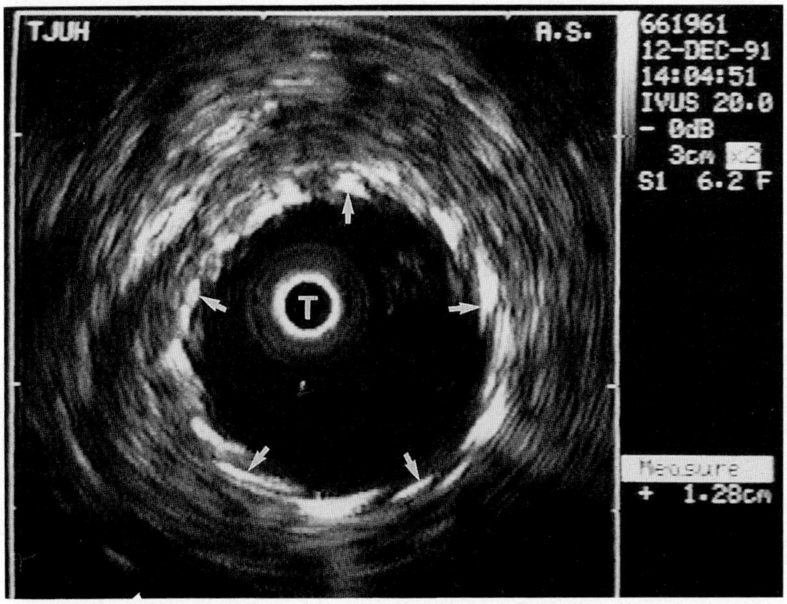


**FIGURE 2** Cross-sectional ultrasound image demonstrates the urethral stent in a patient with neurogenic bladder. The diameter of the stent (*arrows*) can be precisely measured. T = ultrasound transducer.

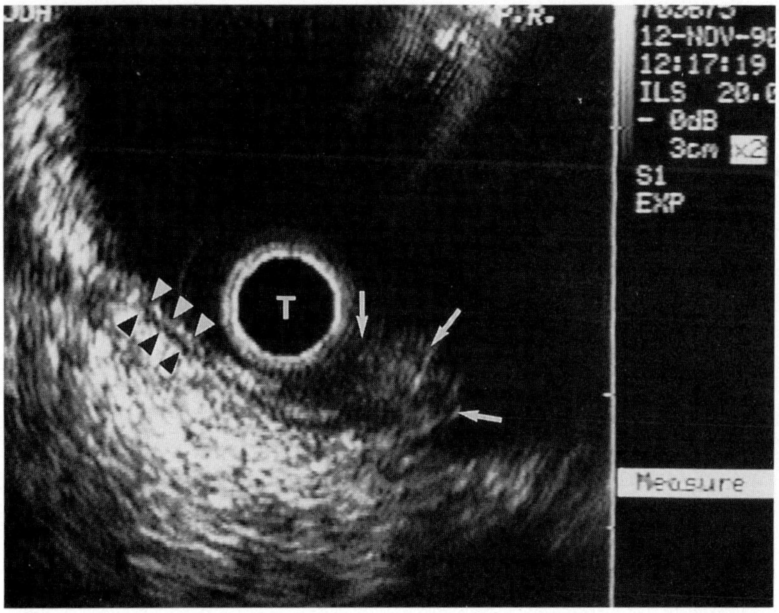


**FIGURE 3** Cross-sectional ultrasound image of the saline-filled bladder demonstrating a mass (*arrows*) arising from the posterior wall. Cystoscopic biopsy confirmed the presence of transitional cell carcinoma. The normal three layers of the bladder wall representing the mucosa (hyperechoic), media (hypoechoic), and adventitia (hyperechoic) can be seen in noninvolvement region (*arrowheads*). T = ultrasound transducer.

thral sonography should be ideal for the delineation of urethra diverticulum, which can be difficult to visualize using either cystoscopy or urethrography.

Although rigid transurethral ultrasound transducers have been used to assess the urinary bladder, these small, flexible, transducer-containing catheters can also be used to evaluate the urinary bladder. It is possible to visualize all the layers of the bladder wall including the hyperechoic mucosa, hypoechoic muscular media, and hyperechoic adventitia. Small tumors are clearly identified and their degree of invasion evaluated (Fig. 3). It is therefore helpful in urinary bladder tumor staging, aiding the urologist in clinical management decisions.

Endoluminal sonographic evaluation of the ureter is easily performed during endoscopic procedures. The flexible 6 Fr catheter is stabilized by its passage through the channel of an endoscope, and a guidewire is used to stabilize the probe as it is directed into the ureter, thus minimizing the risk of perforation. However, the catheter-based transducer can also be passed with the aid of fluoroscopic monitoring without the necessity for simultaneous cystoscopy. It can also be placed through a nephrostomy into the renal pelvis and ureter and positioned under direct nephroscopic observation. A smaller 4.8 Fr ultrasound catheter-based probe can be passed through the lumen of some rigid ureteroscopes.

These ultrasound catheters have been used to evaluate the ureters in 80 patients undergoing endoscopic procedures with no complications. Using high-frequency catheter-based sonography, the ureteral wall was imaged (Fig. 4). Extramural structures adjacent to the ureter, such as blood vessels, lymph nodes, and muscles, also were delineated (Figs. 5, 6). These transducer-containing catheters have proven useful for detecting stones located beneath the surface of the mucosa in both the ureter and renal pelvis (Figs. 7, 8). Stones that can be seen radiographically but not detected endoscopically can be

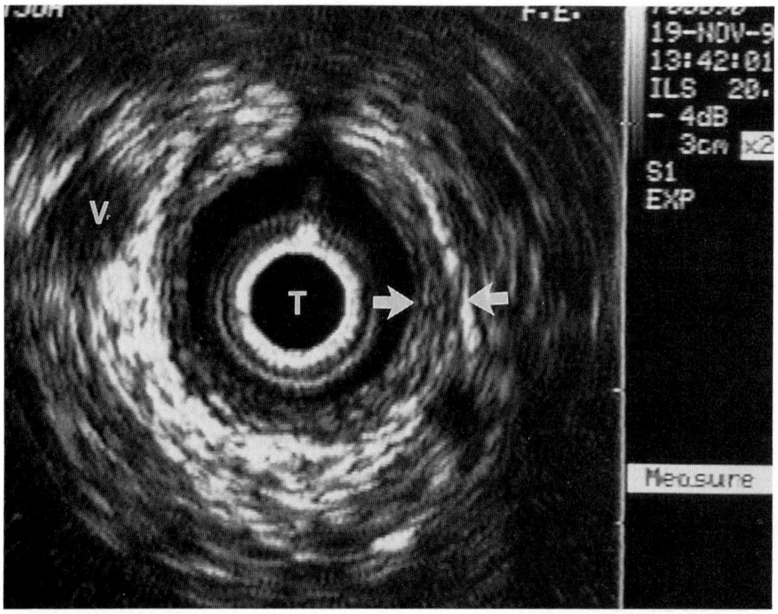


**FIGURE 4** Cross-sectional ultrasound image of the distal left ureter showing normal ureteral wall thickness (*arrows*). Note the guidewire as a bright reflector at 12 o'clock associated with distal acoustic shadowing. T = ultrasound transducer; V = vessel.

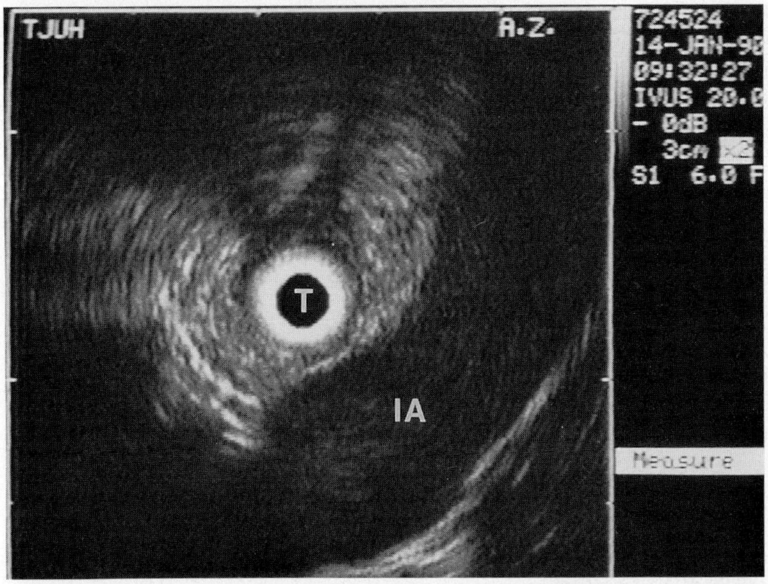


**FIGURE 5** Cross-sectional ultrasound image obtained from region of the distal ureter demonstrates the iliac artery (IA) crossing behind the ureter. T = ultrasound transducer.

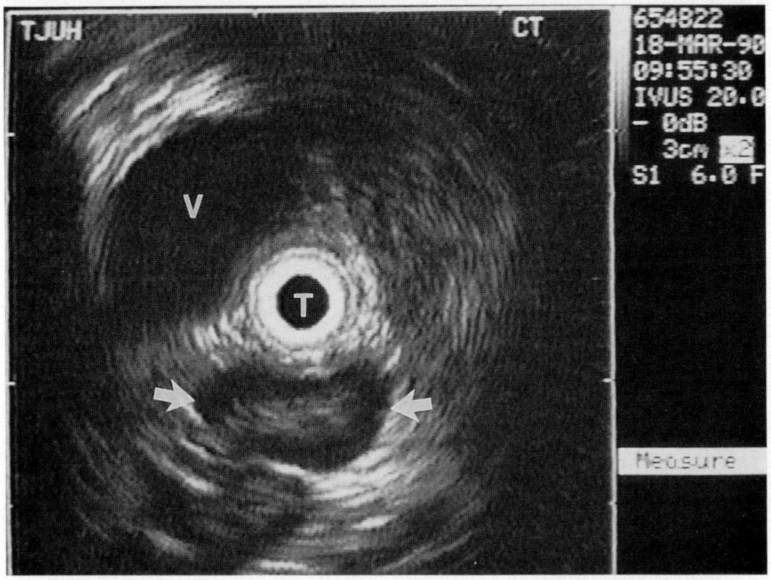


**FIGURE 6** Cross-sectional ultrasound image obtained from within the ureter demonstrates the presence of a normal-sized lymph node (*arrows*). T = ultrasound transducer; V = blood vessel.

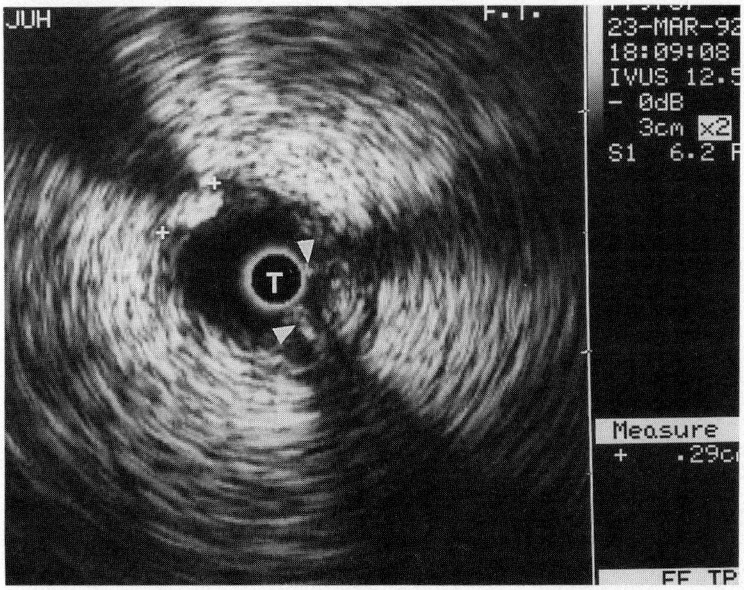


**FIGURE 7** Cross-sectional ultrasound image of the distal right ureter in a patient with hydronephrosis demonstrated a hyperechoic area (+'s) with distal acoustic shadowing located within the thickened mucosa corresponding to embedded submucosal stone. Note two bright reflectors from the guidewires (*arrowheads*). T = ultrasound transducer.

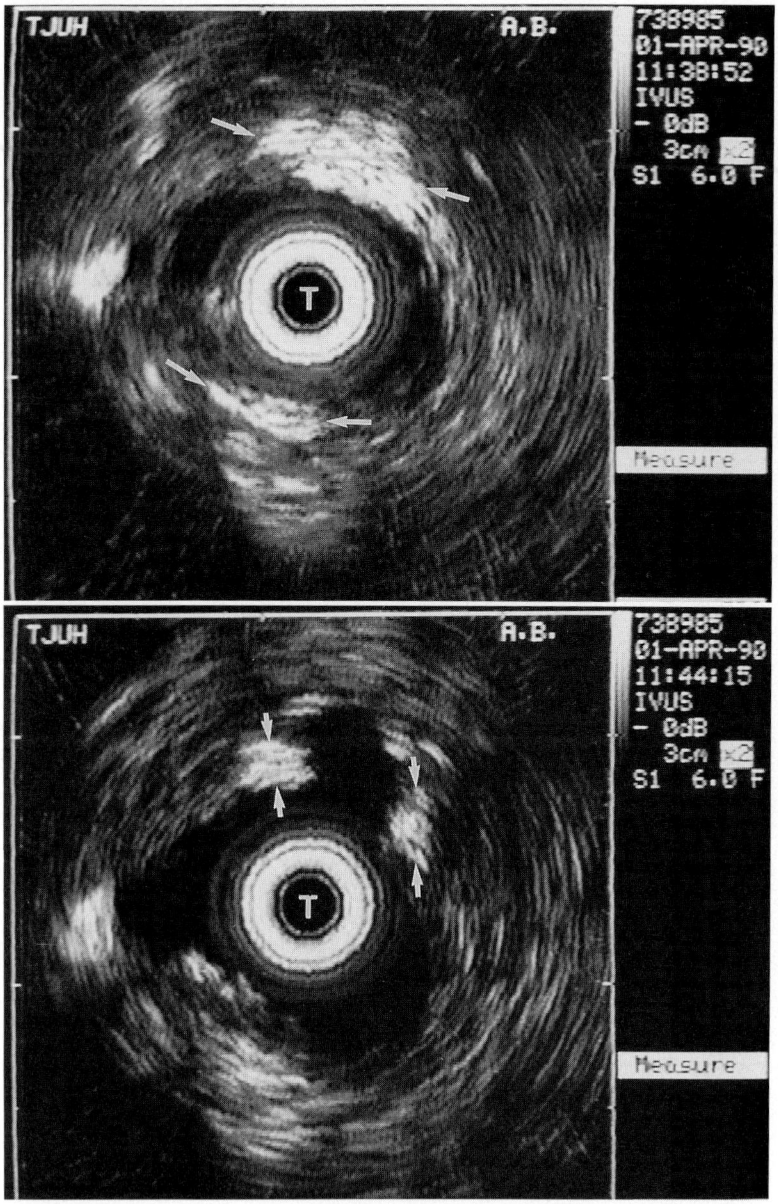


**FIGURE 8** *A,* Cross-sectional ultrasound image obtained from the renal pelvis in a patient with hydronephrosis evaluated via nephroscopy. Multiple stones embedded within the renal parenchyma were demonstrated (*arrows*). T = ultrasound transducer. *B,* A defect can be seen after partial removal of the embedded stones. Note residue stones (*arrows*). T = ultrasound transducer.

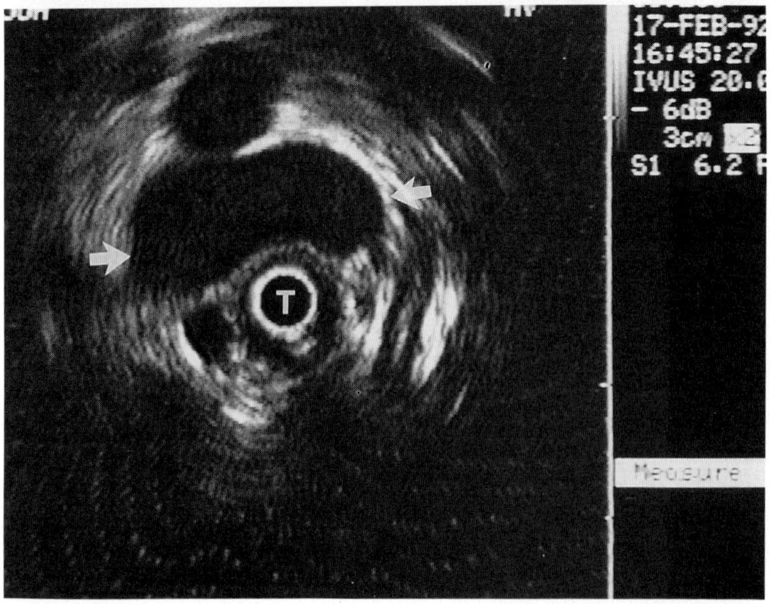


**FIGURE 9** A crossing vessel (*arrows*) is seen just adjacent to the course of the proximal ureter. T = ultrasound transducer.

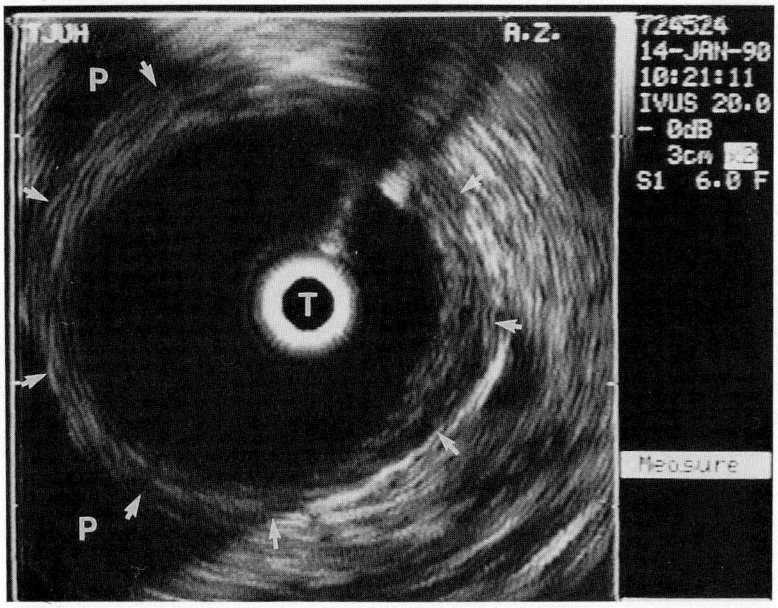


**FIGURE 10** Cross-sectional ultrasound image demonstrates a dilated ureter (*arrows*) inserting into the dilated renal pelvis (P). T = ultrasound transducer.

located and their exact size and depth beneath the surfacc clearly documented and measured. The information provided by this sonographic approach has proven of value in assisting the urologist in making surgical decisions concerning stone removal. One of the drawbacks with the present technique is that the site of the lumen being scanned cannot be simultaneously visualized endoscopically because of the size of the instruments. However, catheter modification is under development.

Localization of blood vessels outside the ureter by endoluminal sonography has also proven to be clinically useful. The size of the vessel and its exact location can be accurately delineated (Fig. 9). This information has proven helpful before endopyelotomy to define the location and size of the crossing vessel. Pulsatile arteries and nonpulsatile veins can be easily differentiated. Endoluminal sonography has also been successful in demonstrating ureters invaginating into the renal pelvis (Fig. 10). Thus this technique has proven to be of considerable value in determining the cause of ureteropelvic junction obstruction, particularly when treatment by endopyelotomy is contemplated.

## Technical Approach

Orientation during endoluminal sonography may be difficult. However, some landmarks can be identified, such as the level of the urinary bladder, the iliac vessels, the psoas muscle, and the renal pelvis. In order to know the exact anteroposterior and lateral position of these transducer-containing catheters within the urinary tract, it has been necessary to use several different techniques. With the ultrasound catheter in the urine-filled bladder, pressure on the anterior abdominal wall will cause distortion of the anterior wall of the bladder, helping to determine the position of the ultrasound image relative to its true anatomical placement. Within the ureter and renal pelvis, the reflection from the adjacent guidewire visualized as a bright reflector with a distal acoustic shadowing is used to determine the orientation. The guidewire is then imaged fluoroscopically and localized to the medial or lateral aspect of the ultrasound probe. With this information the relationship of the bright reflection (guidewire) on the ultrasound image relative to its true anatomical location can then be determined and the ultrasound image appropriately oriented. This is important when documenting the exact location of stones embedded within the mucosa of the ureter or renal parenchyma, as well as the orientation of crossing vessels relative to the ureter or renal pelvis before any intraluminal surgical procedures.

## Diagnostic Approach

High-resolution endoluminal sonography has been able to detect the presence and extent of ureteral and renal pelvis neoplasms, providing information not available with such other imaging techniques as conventional ultrasonography, computed tomography (CT), magnetic resonance imaging (MRI) and intravenous urography (Fig. 11). Even ureteroscopy

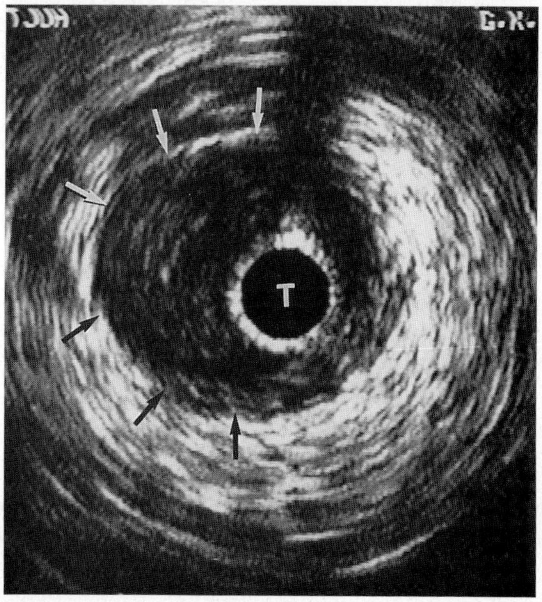


**FIGURE 11** The endoluminal ultrasound transducer (T) located within the midportion of the ureter demonstrates a hypoechoic solid mass (*arrows*) arising from a portion of the ureteral wall. This was proven to be a transitional cell carcinoma.

cannot provide this information, since it can only visualize lesions that involve the luminal surface and cannot image beyond the surface. This technique has also been able to differentiate between areas of focal thickening or extrinsic mass. However, complete staging of ureteral and renal pelvic malignancies has been limited by the lack of significant penetration from the high-frequency transducer.

In other urological clinical situations, the value of endoluminal sonography remains unexplored. Although ureteral strictures have demonstrated differences in echogenicity along the ureteral wall and in the adventitia, it has been difficult to maintain distention of the ureter above and below the narrowing, preventing adequate evaluation of the extent of the abnormality. Theoretically this difficulty can be overcome by irrigating with a catheter adjacent to the ultrasound probe while simultaneously obstructing the distal ureter. Alternatively it could be achieved by placing a small ultrasound transducer-containing catheter through an endoscope with irrigation through the normal channel. With this approach there would be the potential for differentiating intrinsic versus extrinsic fibrosis as the cause of the stricture.

## Discussion

High-resolution endoluminal sonography has proven useful in the evaluation of the urinary tract. In most cases significant additional information was provided to the urologist, aiding in appropriate treatment decisions. Although there are other methods to image the kidneys, ureters, urinary bladder, and urethra, including standard ultrasonography, intravenous urography, CT, and MRI, as well as approaches for direct visualization through endoscopy, these flexible catheter-based miniature ultrasound probes permit evaluation, not only of the mucosal surface, but also of the walls and adjacent structures. Overall, the application of endoluminal sonography for ureteral lesions has proven to be the most beneficial. When used as an adjunct to endoscopy, this approach has provided more information than other conventional external imaging modalities.

## Suggested Reading

Dake MD. Intravascular ultrasound. Curr Opin Radiol 1991; 3:181–187.

Devonec M, Chapelon JY, Codas, et al. Evaluation of bladder cancer with a miniature high frequency transurethral ultrasonography probe. Br J Urol 1987; 59:550–553.

Goldberg BB, Bagley D, Liu JB, et al. Endoluminal sonography of the urinary tract: Preliminary observations. AJR 1991; 156:99–103.

Goldberg BB, Liu JB, Kuhlman K, et al. Endoluminal gynecologic ultrasound: Preliminary results. J Ultrasound Med 1991; 10:583–590.

Goldberg BB, Liu JB, Merton DA, Kurtz AB. Endoluminal US: Experiments with nonvascular uses in animals. Radiology 1990; 175:39–43.

Holm HH, Northeved AA. A transurethral ultrasonic scanner. J Urol 1974; 111:238–241.

Huffman JL, Bagley DH, Lyon ES. Extending cystoscopic techniques into the ureter and renal pelvis: Experience with ureteroscopy and pyeloscopy. JAMA 1983; 250:2002–2005.

Murata Y, Suzuki S, Hashimoto H. Endoscopic ultrasonography of the upper gastrointestinal tract. Surg Endosc 1988; 2:180–183.

Quinn MJ, Beynon J, Mortensen NJM, Smith PJB. Transvaginal endo-sonography: A new method to study the anatomy of the lower urinary tract in urinary stress incontinence. Br J Urol 1988; 62:414–418.

Tio TL, Coene PPLO, Schouwink MH, Tytgat GNJ. Esophagogastric carcinoma: Preoperative TNM classification with endosonography. Radiology 1989; 173:411–417.

# Ultrasound Imaging of Renal Disease

*MICHAEL J. LEE, M.D. · NICHOLAS PAPANICOLAOU, M.D.*

Improvements in design of ultrasound transducers and equipment have facilitated the widespread use of this modality for imaging patients with renal abnormalities. New electronically focused transducers permit increased morphologic detail to be visualized within the normal and abnormal kidney. In addition, the recent development of duplex and color Doppler ultrasound technologies has improved the capability of ultrasonography to display the vascular anatomy and perfusion of both the native and transplant kidney.

## Normal Anatomy

The normal kidney consists of the central renal sinus and the peripheral renal pyramids and cortex. The renal sinus appears as a central zone of increased echogenicity due to varying amounts of fat and fibrous tissue within the central renal sinus complex. The peripheral renal cortex was originally described as having an echogenicity less than that of liver or spleen. However, with the improved image quality generated by the more modern electronically focused transducers, this relationship has been re-evaluated, and it is now apparent that renal cortical echogenicity may be similar to that of liver, but should not exceed it. The medullary pyramids are defined by the junction of the renal cortex and renal sinus and are echo-poor structures.

Normal variants, such as junctional parenchymal defects and duplicated collecting systems, are important to recognize in order to differentiate them from other echogenic masses such as angiomyolipomas (Fig. 1). The scanning technique should be optimized so that the kidneys are evaluated in true sagittal and transverse planes. Scanning in oblique planes may produce pseudomasses, particularly where there is associated fetal lobulation or indentation of the renal cortex (Fig. 2).

## Indications

Renal sonography is indicated for evaluation of patients with acute renal failure, obstructive uropathy, chronic renal disease, transplant kidney abnormalities, and renal mass identification and characterization.

A B

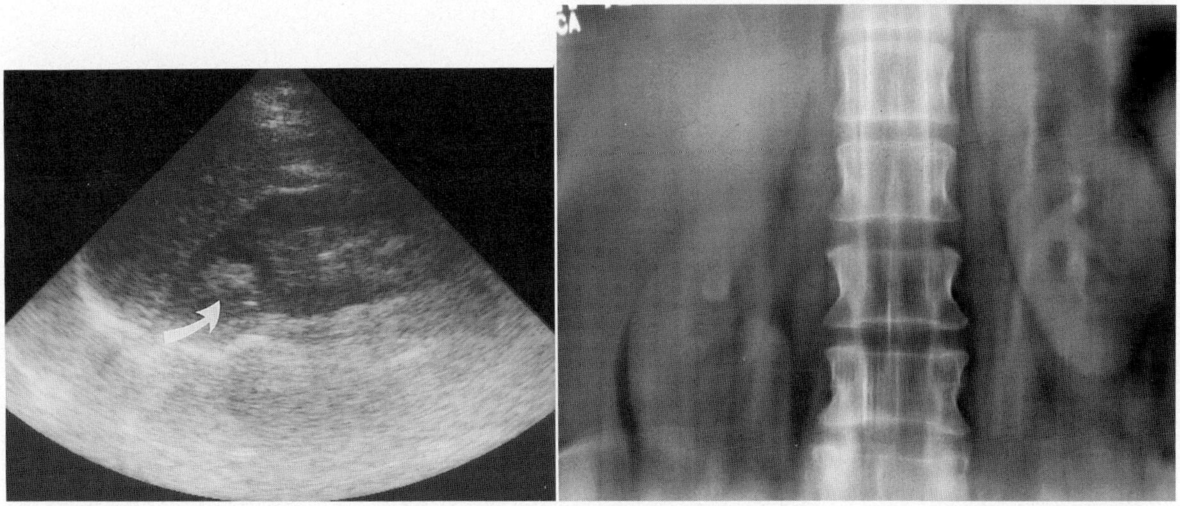

**FIGURE 1** Duplex collecting system gives the appearance of a renal pseudomass. *A,* Sagittal sonogram of left kidney with duplicated collecting system shows echogenic pseudomass *(arrow)* in upper pole, representing renal sinus of upper pole moiety cortex. This could be mistaken for an angiomyolipoma. *B,* Nephrotomogram confirms the presence of a duplex collecting system.

A B

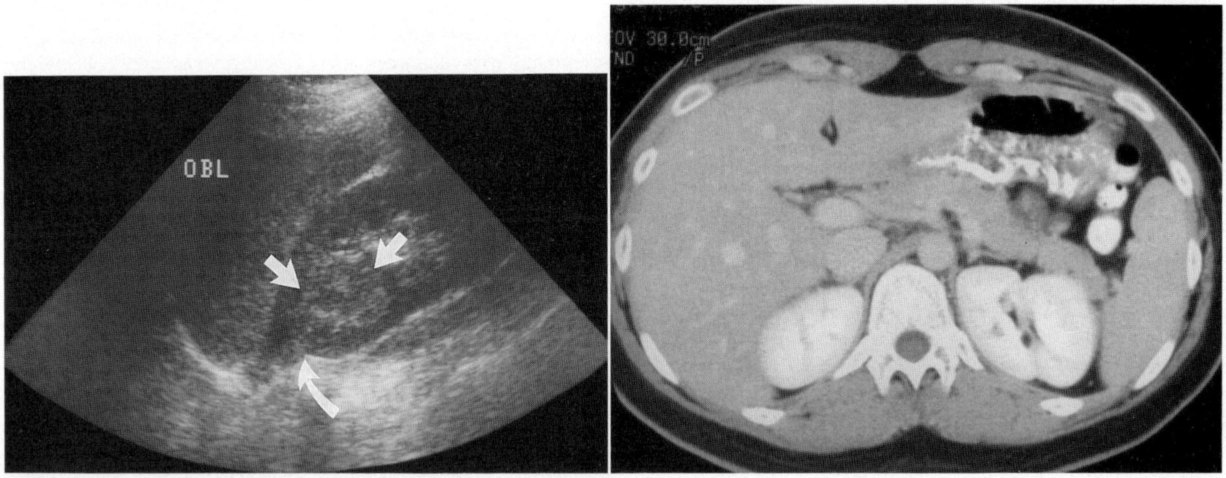


**FIGURE 2** Pseudomass caused by scanning in oblique planes. *A,* Sonogram of left kidney shows pseudomass *(straight arrows)* in upper pole observed only on oblique sonograms. This is caused by scanning obliquely through the renal sinus and cortex, with concurrent fetal lobulation *(curved arrow)* giving the appearance of margins to the pseudomass. *B,* Renal CT scan with intravenous contrast material in the same patient shows no evidence of a mass. Fetal lobulation is evident in the upper pole.

## *Obstructive Uropathy*

Exclusion of hydronephrosis is one of the most common indications for renal sonography. Hydronephrosis is identified as an anechoic zone within the bright echoes of the central renal sinus complex. Although the accuracy of ultrasonography in detecting hydronephrosis approaches 100 percent, some pitfalls exist. The false-negative rate is approximately 1 percent, the most common causes including misinterpretation of hydronephrosis as peripelvic cystic disease (Fig. 3) and the presence of nondilated collecting systems early on in acute renal obstruction and chronically in retroperitoneal fibrosis.

At the other end of the spectrum, a false-positive diagnosis of hydronephrosis occurs in approximately 7 percent of examinations. Causes of false-positive diagnoses are listed in Table 1. Some correctable pitfalls that may lead to a false-positive diagnosis of hydronephrosis include the presence of a full bladder and renal vessels simulating mild caliectasis. The former can be excluded by rescanning the patient after the bladder has been emptied. In the case of mild caliectasis, color Doppler imaging of the kidneys should be performed to exclude the possibility of renal vessels simulating caliectasis (Fig. 4 and Color Plate 9).

A number of methods can be used to increase the specificity of ultrasonography in diagnosing obstructive uropathy. Scanning the urinary bladder and paying close attention to the ureterovesical junction occasionally reveals an obstructing stone or tumor (Fig. 5). Identification of a stone in this region obviates the need for future urography. Recently Doppler ultrasonography has been proposed as an aid to differentiate between obstructive and nonobstructive uropathy. Clinical studies have shown that a renal resistive index (RI) greater than 0.7 is suggestive of obstructive uropathy. However, we

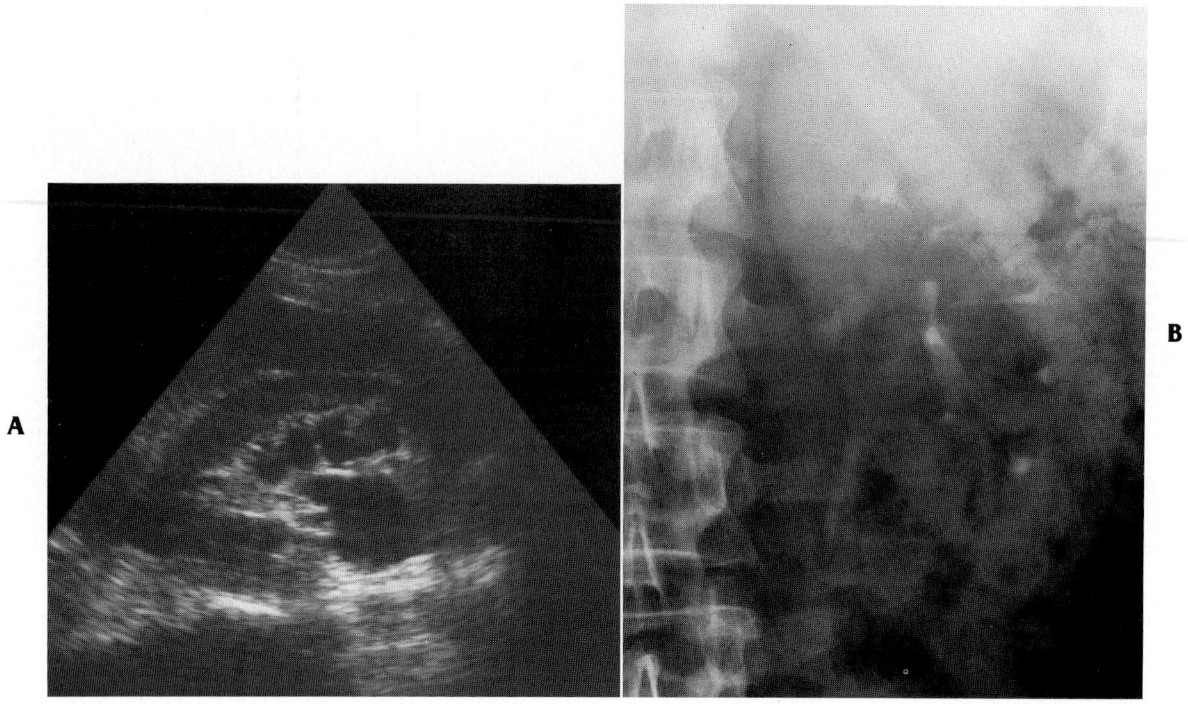

**FIGURE 3** Peripelvic cystic disease mistaken for hydronephrosis. *A,* Ultrasonographic examination of the left kidney shows multiple anechoic areas within the renal sinus, simulating a dilated collecting system. *B,* Intravenous urography in the same patient reveals a nondilated collecting system, which, however, was attenuated because of compression from adjacent peripelvic cystic disease.

**TABLE 1** Pitfalls in the Sonographic Diagnosis of Obstructive Hydronephrosis

| | |
|---|---|
| Normal Variants | Inflammatory Disease |
| Full bladder | Acute or chronic pyelonephritis |
| Prominent renal vessels | Tuberculosis |
| Extrarenal pelvis | Other Causes |
| Congenital megacalyces | Peripelvic cysts |
| Increased Urine Flow | Adult polycystic disease |
| Overhydration | Vesicoureteric reflux |
| Diuretic medication | Postobstructive dilatation |
| Diabetes insipidus | |

Data from Amis ES, Cronan JJ, et al. Ultrasonic inaccuracies in diagnosing renal obstruction. Urology 1982; 19:101–105.

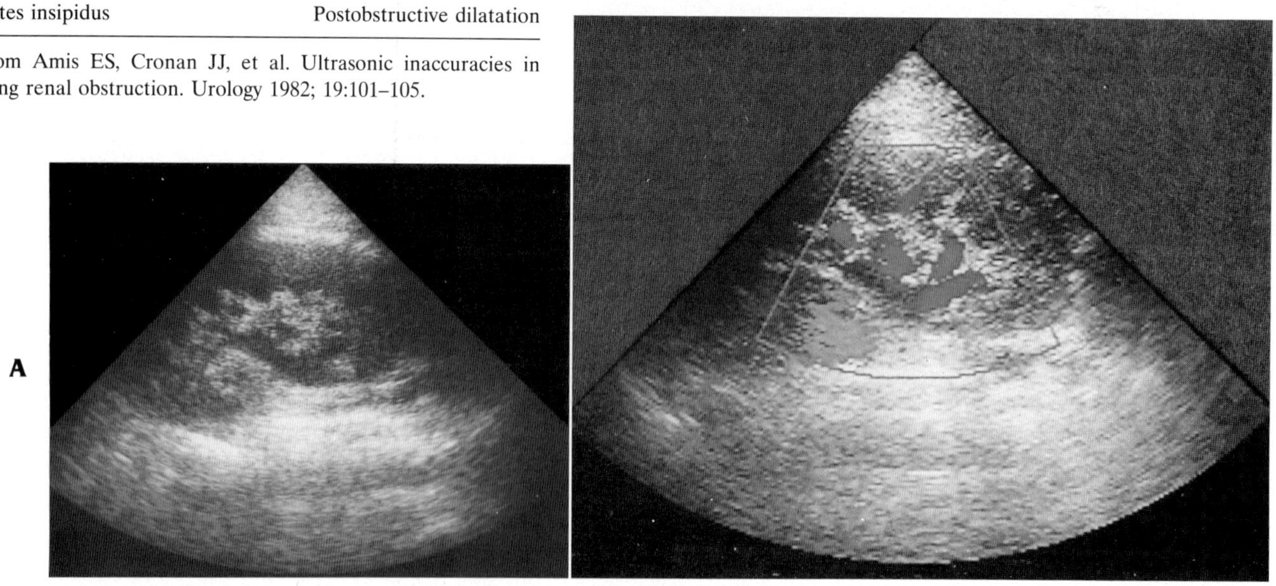

**FIGURE 4** False-positive hydronephrosis due to large renal sinus blood vessels. *A,* Branching hypoechoic structures in hilum of left kidney, giving the appearance of hydronephrosis. A dilated upper ureter could not be visualized. *B,* Color-flow Doppler sonogram (*reproduced here in black and white*) of the same kidney confirms the appearance of large, branching renal sinus vessels, giving the appearance of hydronephrosis. See also Color Plate 9.

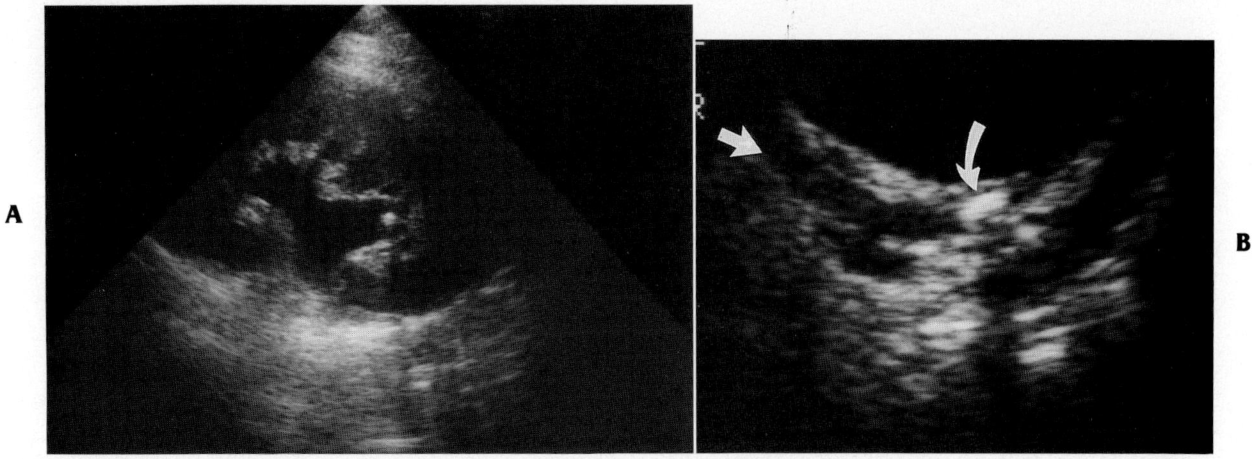

**FIGURE 5** A 24-year-old pregnant woman with left flank pain. *A,* Sagittal sonogram of left kidney shows hydronephrosis and hydroureter and a small stone with posterior acoustic shadowing in the lower pole. *B,* Sagittal sonogram through the left ureterovesical (UV) junction shows a dilated lower left ureter *(straight arrow)* and an obstructing stone *(curved arrow)* at the UV junction.

have not found this technique completely reliable. False-negative and positive results can be explained by the fact that the RI may be normal in partial or mild obstructive uropathy, and it may be raised in a wide range of medical renal diseases as well as some other extrarenal disease states. Color Doppler ultrasonography, used to evaluate the presence or absence of ureteric jets in the bladder, has also been proposed as a method of confirming or excluding the presence of obstruction. The theory is that in patients with urinary obstruction the ureteric jet on the affected side is absent or reduced in frequency. In practice it is recommended that continuous evaluation for up to 30 minutes is necessary to assess jet frequency and symmetry.

Currently we do not recommend replacing intravenous urography with sonography. However, in patients who are not candidates for urography, such as pregnant patients, those with renal failure, and those who are allergic to contrast media, particular attention should be paid to the RI, ureteric jet phenomenon, and the search for a stone at the ureterovesical junction, during renal sonography. The extra time involved in performing the sonographic examination is probably worthwhile in these patient groups.

## *Renal Masses*

Sonography is the technique of choice to determine whether indeterminate mass lesions observed on urography represent solid or cystic masses. The typical cyst demonstrates enhanced through transmission, is anechoic, and has a barely discernible wall or no wall. Evidence of internal echoes, thick wall, mural nodules, calcification or septations indicates a complex cyst (Fig. 6). Evidence of one or any of the previous criteria implies that the patient should have computerized tomographic (CT) scanning of the kidneys with and without intravenous contrast material for further characterization. Occasionally reverberation echoes can be observed in the anterior third of simple cysts, which should be recognized as an artifact. In general, cysts that are minimally complicated, such as lesions with thin septations (< 1 mm) without mural nodules, minimally calcified cysts, and high-density cysts observed on CT scans may be followed-up with serial ultrasonography or CT to document stability in appearance. On the other hand, cysts that have thickened septations, mural nodules, heavy or irregular calcification, or solid elements require needle aspiration, biopsy, and/or surgical exploration.

Tumors of the kidneys, such as angiomyolipomas, are recognized by their fat content on CT scans; a clue to their diagnosis is given by their high echogenicity on ultrasonographic examination (Fig. 7). Increased echogenicity, however, is not sufficient to make the diagnosis on sonographic examination. An artifact called the *speed propagation artifact* can be used to make a more specific diagnosis of an angiomyolipoma. Because the speed of sound in fat is slower than in soft tissue, structures behind a fat-containing lesion, such as an angiomyolipoma, appear artifactually distal to their actual position. If the lesion is large enough, structures behind the renal mass, such as the diaphragm, are displaced distally due to this artifact. If any doubt exists, CT or magnetic resonance imaging (MRI) is recommended for specific diagnosis.

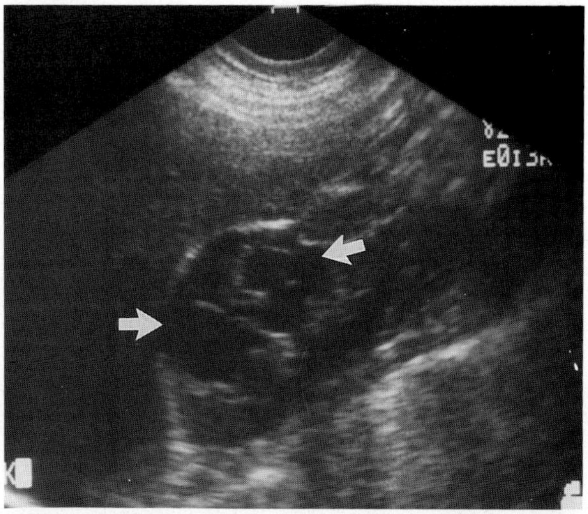

**FIGURE 6** A 39-year-old woman with an incidentally discovered complex cystic mass on upper pole of right kidney *(arrows)*. A multilocular cystic mass is observed with internal thick septations. This mass was surgically removed and proved to be benign.

A

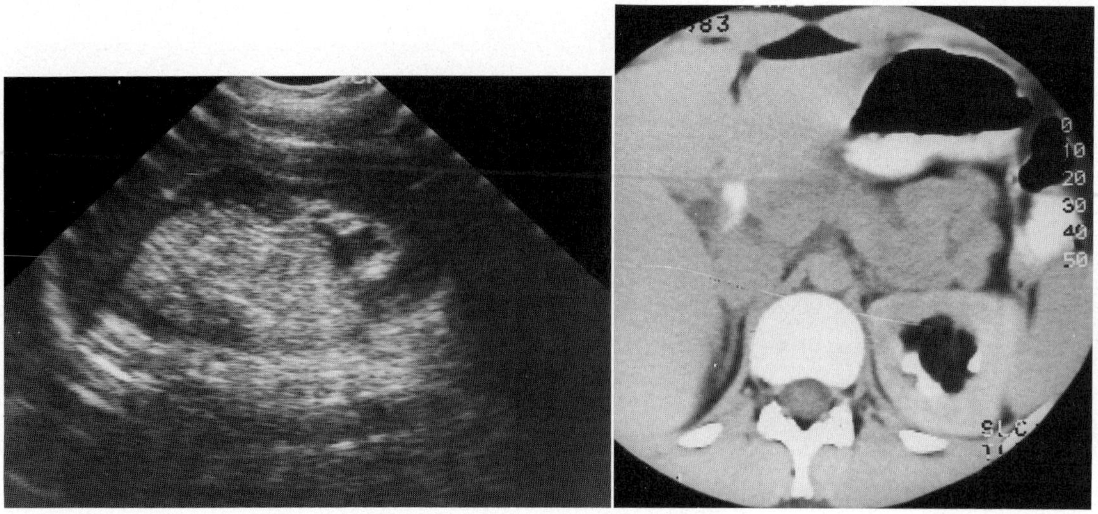


B

**FIGURE 7** Angiomyolipoma of the kidney. *A,* Large echogenic mass in upper pole of left kidney involving the renal sinus and cortex suggests an angiomyolipoma. *B,* A specific diagnosis of angiomyolipoma was made by CT scanning, where the attenuation of the mass is consistent with fat.

While CT and MRI are the preferred modalities for staging of renal cell carcinoma, much information can be gained by a thorough sonographic examination. Most hypernephromas tend to be hypervascular on angiographic examination with extensive neovascularity, arteriovenous anastomoses, and low-impedance flow. These features can be recognized on color Doppler and pulsed Doppler sonograms. Tumor vessels have relatively thin walls with a deficiency of vessel musculature, giving rise to low-impedance flow shown as a high diastolic component on pulsed Doppler sonograms. Frequent arteriovenous anastomoses are also present, producing high peak velocities that are often well over 100 cm per second (Fig. 8 and Color Plate 10). Doppler shifts in the range of 2.5 to 10 kHz have been documented in renal cell carcinomas. Color Doppler ultrasonographic examination of renal masses may therefore aid in characterization of benign versus malignant masses.

Hypernephromas also tend to invade the renal vein and vena cava, and color Doppler imaging can be helpful in identifying tumor thrombus in both these structures (Fig. 9 and Color Plate 11). However, the renal vein may not always be visualized, depending on the amount of overlying bowel gas and the patient's body habitus.

## *Diffuse Renal Disease*

Using current state-of-the-art equipment, the echogenicity of the normal renal parenchyma tends to be equal to that of the liver in healthy patients. Renal failure due to medical renal

A

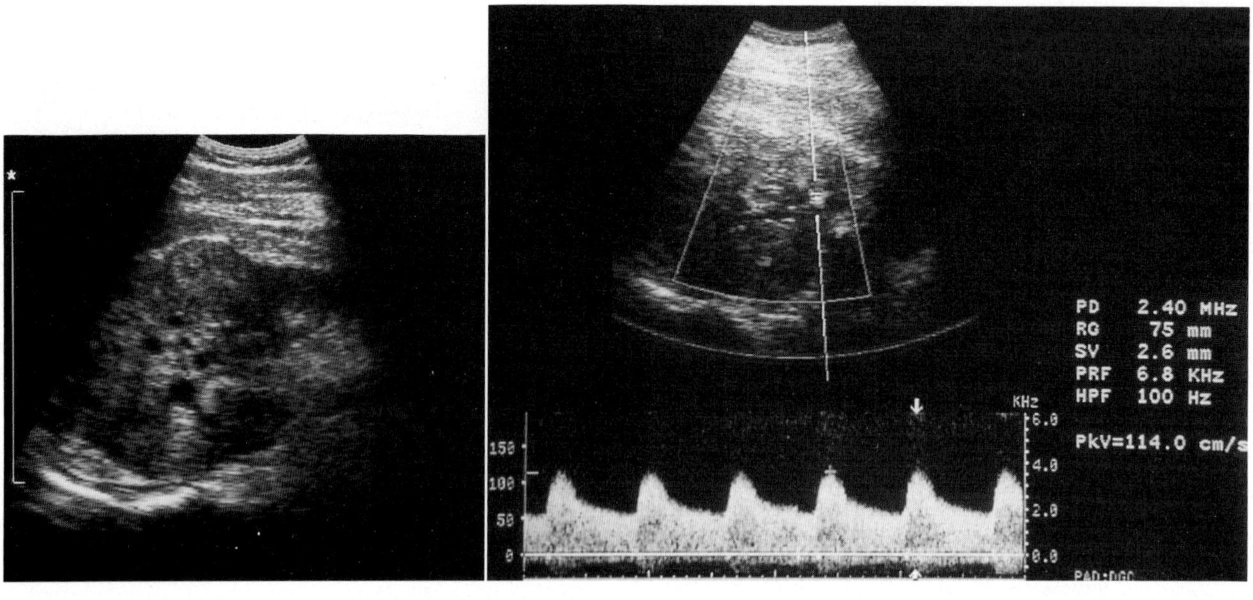


B

**FIGURE 8** Incidentally discovered renal cell carcinoma in 41-year-old male. *A,* Sagittal image of the right kidney reveals a large right upper pole mass. *B,* Transverse view of mass on color Doppler sonogram (*reproduced here in black and white*) shows chaotic neovascularity. Pulsed Doppler sonogram confirms the low-impedance flow of tumor neovascularity with a Doppler shift of 4 kHz. See also Color Plate 10.

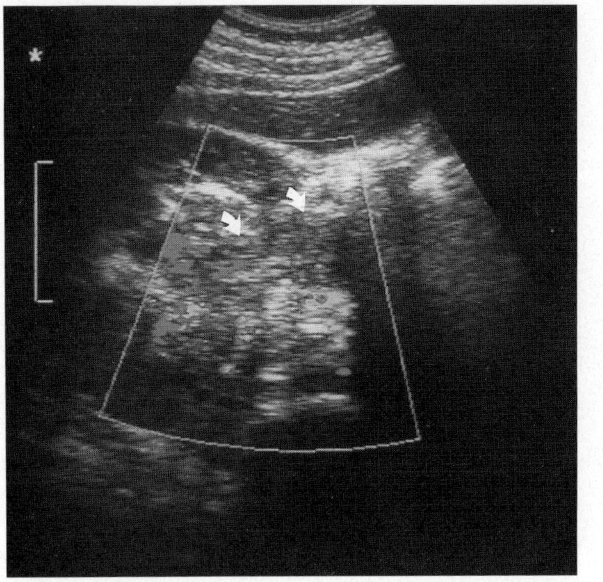

**FIGURE 9** Color Doppler sonogram (*reproduced here in black and white*) reveals no flow in the renal vein of this patient with a hypernephroma. Tumor thrombus can be observed within the renal vein *(arrows)*. See also Color Plate 11.

diseases and infiltrative diseases leads to an increase in cortical echogenicity relative to adjacent organs with preservation of the cortico-medullary definition (Fig. 10). Categories of diseases that cause this bilateral diffuse increase in echogenicity are listed in Table 2. Diffuse medical renal diseases such as acute glomerulonephritis, chronic glomerulonephritis, lupus nephritis, and acquired immunodeficiency syndrome (AIDS) nephropathy may cause this pattern. Renal manifestations of AIDS are becoming increasingly common. It has been estimated that a renal abnormality is present in more than one-third of patients with AIDS. Renal involvement indicates a poor prognosis, with reported mortality of 100 percent within 6 months in patients with persistent uremia despite dialysis.

Bilateral cortical nephrocalcinosis in early stages may show increased cortical echoes before dense calcification has laid down in sufficient amounts to cause acoustic shadowing. This appearance may be identified before visualization of calcification of the cortex on plain radiographs. Infiltrative diseases

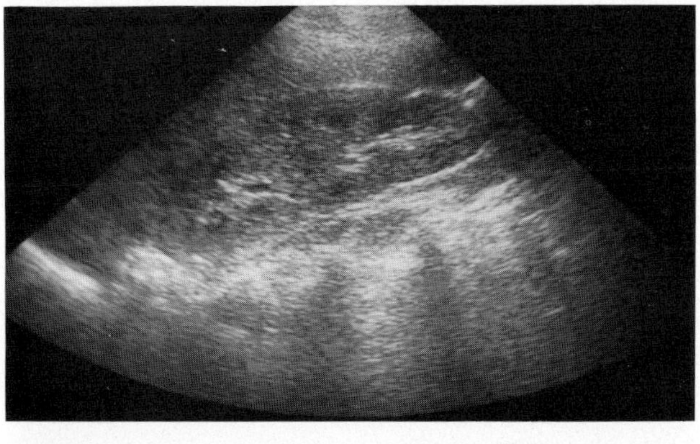

**FIGURE 10** Sagittal image of the right kidney in a patient with AIDS nephropathy. Diffusely increased cortical echoes with preservation of the corticomedullary junction is evident when compared with the adjacent liver.

**TABLE 2** Causes of Bilateral Increased Cortical Echogenicity

| | |
|---|---|
| Diffuse Medical Renal Diseases | Cortical Nephrocalcinosis |
| Acute glomerulonephritis | Chronic glomerulonephritis |
| Chronic glomerulonephritis | Renal cortical necrosis |
| Lupus nephritis | Alport's syndrome |
| AIDS | Oxalosis |
| Infiltrative Diseases | Unilateral Diseases |
| Leukemic infiltration | Subacute renal vein thrombosis |
| Amyloid | Suppurative pyelonephritis |

causing this appearance include leukemic and amyloid infiltrations. Acutely, renal vein thrombosis produces a global decrease in cortical echogenicity. However, in the subacute stage, an increase in cortical echogenicity is observed (1 week to 10 days after the acute situation).

## *Renal Transplant Sonography*

Because of the proximity of the renal transplant to the anterior abdominal wall, the transplant kidney is ideally suited to sonographic evaluation. Ultrasonography has long been used to diagnose perirenal collections and to provide guidance when drainage is indicated. Pulsed and color Doppler sonograms can be used to document perfusion of the transplanted kidney, to ensure arterial and venous patency, to diagnose vascular abnormalities such as pseudoaneurysms and arteriovenous fistulas resulting from biopsy, to recognize abnormal renovascular impedance, and to document transplant arterial stenoses.

The gray-scale appearances of acute transplant rejection include an enlarged kidney with increased cortical echogenicity, prominent pyramids, mild hydronephrosis, and thickening of the uroepithelium due to edema (Fig. 11). These gray-scale changes, however, are nonspecific and in an effort to increase the specificity of ultrasonography in diagnosing rejection, measurement of the renovascular impedance (resistive index [RI]) has been proposed. Early studies revealed markedly increased renovascular impedance in patients with acute vascular rejection in the early postoperative period; however, subsequent studies of patients at various intervals after transplantations have shown poor sensitivity and specificity of this technique for acute rejection. Currently this technique of measuring the RI is useful only when there is loss or reversal of diastolic flow in the transplanted kidney (RI $> 0.9$) (Fig. 12).

Pulsed or color Doppler imaging can be used to demonstrate arterial and venous flow to all segments of the kidney. Occlusion of either renal artery or vein can occur in the early postoperative period due to technical problems with vascular anastomosis at surgery. Prompt recognition of this may enable graft-sparing surgery to be performed. Early in the postoperative period, if the artery is patent but the vein is obstructed a very high RI may be observed ($>0.9$). When this pattern is observed early in the postoperative period, the venous drainage of the transplanted kidney should be evaluated with color Doppler or pulsed Doppler sonograms.

Renal artery stenosis occurs in approximately 12 percent of renal transplant recipients. Significant stenoses of the transplanted renal artery include a focal high-velocity jet through the area of stenosis followed by poststenotic turbulence. This can be identified with color Doppler sonograms and confirmed by using pulsed Doppler sonograms. Peak systolic velocities

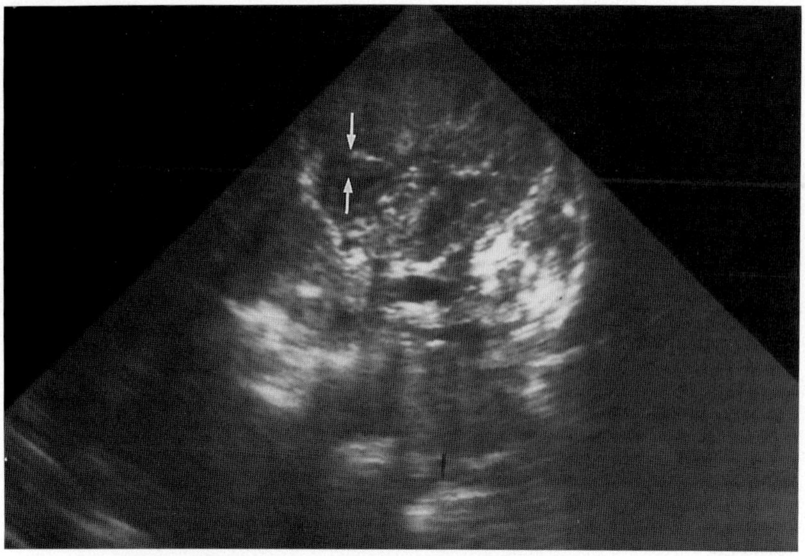

**FIGURE 11** Transverse sonogram of a transplanted kidney with biopsy-proven rejection. Mild hydronephrosis is evident with thickening of the uroepithelium *(arrows)*.

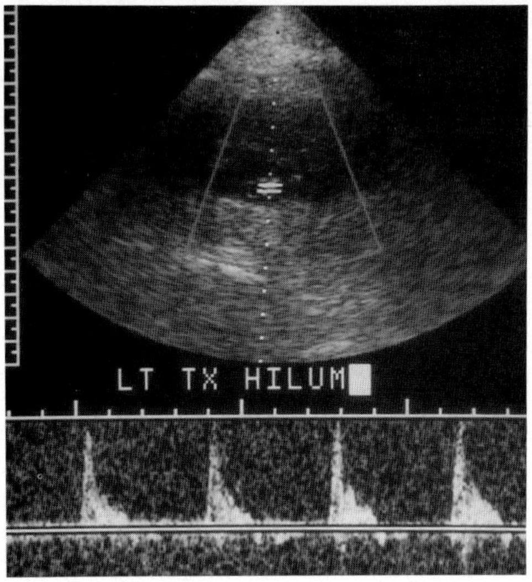


**FIGURE 12** Pulsed Doppler sonogram confirms the clinical diagnosis of rejection in this patient with a renal allograft. There is no diastolic flow and a high RI of 0.98.

greater than 250 cm/s are usually indicative of a significant stenosis. However, high velocities may be observed in the early postoperative period, possibly related to edema at the anastomotic site. Therefore, if turbulent flow is noted in the early postoperative period, the examination should be repeated at a later date.

Arteriovenous shunts and/or pseudoaneurysm may occur in renal allografts after renal biopsy. Both of these entities are easily diagnosed on color Doppler sonograms and can be differentiated using pulsed Doppler. In pseudoaneurysms examined by pulsed Doppler, a characteristic to-and-fro motion is observed across the neck of the pseudoaneurysm, whereas continuous forward flow from the artery to the vein is observed with arteriovenous fistulas.

## Suggested Reading

Amis ES, Cronan JJ, Pfister R, et al. Ultrasonic inaccuracies in diagnosing renal obstruction. Urology 1982; 19:101–105.

Bosniak MA. The current radiological approach to renal cysts. Radiology 1986; 158:1–10.

Cox IH, Erickson SJ, Foley WD, Dewire DM. Ureteric jets: Evaluation of normal flow dynamics with color Doppler sonography. AJR 1992; 158:1051–1055.

Desberg AL, Paushter DM, Lammert GK, et al. Renal artery stenosis: Evaluation with color Doppler flow imaging. Radiology 1990; 177:749–753.

Genkins SM, San Filippo FP, Carroll BA. Duplex Doppler sonography of renal transplants: Lack of sensitivity and specificity in establishing pathologic diagnosis. AJR 1989; 152:535–539.

Haddad MC, Sharif HS, Abomelha MS, et al. Management of renal colic: Redefining the role of the urogram. Radiology 1992; 184:35–36.

Haddad MC, Sharif HS, Shahed MS, et al. Renal colic: Diagnosis and outcome. Radiology 1992; 184:83–88.

Kier R, Taylor KJW, Feyock AL, Ramos IM. Renal masses: Characterization with Doppler US. Radiology 1990; 176:703–707.

Platt JF, Rubin JM, Ellis JH, DiPietro MA. Duplex Doppler US of the kidney: Differentiation of obstructive from nonobstructive dilatation. Radiology 1989; 171:515–517.

Schaffer RM, Schwartz GE, Becker JA, et al. Renal ultrasound in acquired immune deficiency syndrome. Radiology 1984; 153:511–513.

Taylor KJW, Marks WH. Use of Doppler imaging for evaluation of dysfunction in renal allografts. AJR 1990; 155:536–539.

# Contrast-Enhanced MRI Evaluation of Renal Masses

*PHILIP J. KENNEY, M.D.*

Radiologic evaluation of renal masses requires that three tasks be accomplished: (1) detection – determining if a pathologic mass is present (true tumors must be distinguished from pseudotumors); (2) diagnosis – determining the nature of a pathologic mass, specifically deciding whether a mass is malignant or benign; and (3) staging – determining if a mass is resectable, since renal carcinoma at present is curable only if it can be resected.

Unenhanced magnetic resonance imaging (MRI) has been shown to have fair ability to depict large renal masses, and the staging accuracy of MRI is at least as good as, if not better than, that of computed tomography (CT) with iodine-contrast enhancement. This advantage of MRI is largely because of its better ability to detect and distinguish nodal disease and venous invasion, and to a lesser degree, because of its multiplanar imaging capability. Without contrast enhancement, however, the usefulness of MRI for detection and diagnosis of small renal masses is limited.

## MRI Indications and Alternatives

The role of MRI of renal masses can only be defined in the context of other available diagnostic methods. Because of its cost and limited availability, MRI is not, and may never be, the initial study for detection of a renal mass. That role is best served by intravenous urography and increasingly by sonography. Both of these procedures, however, have limited sensitivity and specificity in that small masses are often missed, and benign masses often cannot be distinguished from malignant ones (e.g., on sonography a hemorrhagic cyst commonly has an appearance similar to a renal carcinoma). The most accurate method at present for detection and diagnosis of renal masses is CT done before and after injection of an iodinated contrast agent. This is the procedure of choice for further evaluation of a mass detected by intravenous urography or sonography, or for evaluation of a patient with signs strongly suggestive of a renal tumor (such as hematuria) even if prior studies have been negative. Arteriography and needle biopsy are rarely needed, since diagnosis and staging can nearly always be done noninvasively.

Although CT is the mainstay of evaluation of renal masses at present, its high accuracy requires use of an iodinated contrast agent. In some patients this may be problematic because of either a history of contrast reaction or renal insufficiency. Although a patient may be given premedication and/or a low-osmolality contrast agent, risk cannot be completely eliminated, and the patient may refuse. Pre-existing renal insufficiency is one of the strongest risk factors for contrast-associated nephrotoxicity, and low-osmolality contrast agents have not been proven to be safer in this regard. Although a patient who is receiving dialysis may have a contrast study coordinated with a dialysis treatment, patients who are not yet receiving dialysis could be significantly harmed by contrast. However, preservation of renal tissue is imperative in such patients, and removal of a kidney because of a lesion that proves benign must be avoided at all costs. In my experience, both patients and clinicians, especially nephrologists, are happy to have a safe and effective alternative to contrast-enhanced CT when a patient with renal failure or contrast reactivity is discovered to have a suspicious mass. This is currently the most valuable role for contrast-enhanced MRI. CT also requires rapid scanning in a brief time window after contrast injection to get good vascular enhancement; if this is not accomplished, diagnostic and staging accuracy may be diminished. MRI may be useful in cases in which CT is indeterminate for diagnosis or staging. I believe contrast-enhanced MRI is useful as a second-echelon test to further evaluate a mass, usually detected by sonography, in lieu of contrast-enhanced CT in high-risk patients, or a third-echelon test for further evaluation of a patient in whom CT is not adequate.

Gadolinium DTPA (Gd-DTPA) is a paramagnetic agent that rapidly equilibrates in the extracellular fluid space. It speeds T1 relaxation, resulting in increased signal intensity on T1-weighted images. Outside the brain, any perfused organ or tissue will enhance after Gd-DTPA. This agent, although developed primarily for neurologic uses, has peculiar advantages for evaluating renal masses. Gd-DTPA equilibrates in the extracellular fluid space so that any vascularized organ or mass will enhance. Conveniently, the commonest benign masses in the kidney are cysts, which are avascular and do not enhance. Because it is eliminated purely by glomerular filtration, the renal parenchyma becomes enhanced for several minutes after injection of Gd-DTPA. While renal tumors also enhance, they do so less brightly than the normal parenchyma in which the contrast agent is more concentrated because of tubular resorption of water. If one performs rapid sequential scans after injection of Gd-DTPA (e.g., with the TurboFLASH method), an early cortical phase can be seen, followed by a tubular phase, and there may be a seemingly paradoxical decrease in signal intensity, because of the nonlinear relationship of signal intensity to Gd-DTPA at high concentrations. Because of these factors, it is easier to evaluate renal masses by beginning scanning 2 to 3 minutes after injection and acquiring imaging data during the plateau period of renal parenchymal enhancement. The standard dose of Gd-DTPA (0.1 ml/lb) is effective. Other paramagnetic agents, such as Gd-BOPTA, may be useful, but only Gd-DTPA is currently FDA approved and widely marketed. Although Gd-DTPA has not been approved for renal diagnosis, it may be used at the discretion of the physician.

Enhancement after Gd-DTPA can be effectively shown by both spin-echo and gradient recalled echo (GRE) methods with T1 weighting. Respiratory artifact must be controlled, and respiratory-ordered phase encoding is usually effective on spin-echo scans. GRE methods have the advantage of "bright blood" vessels. GRE scans can be done during suspended respiration, eliminating motion artifact, but thin slices may

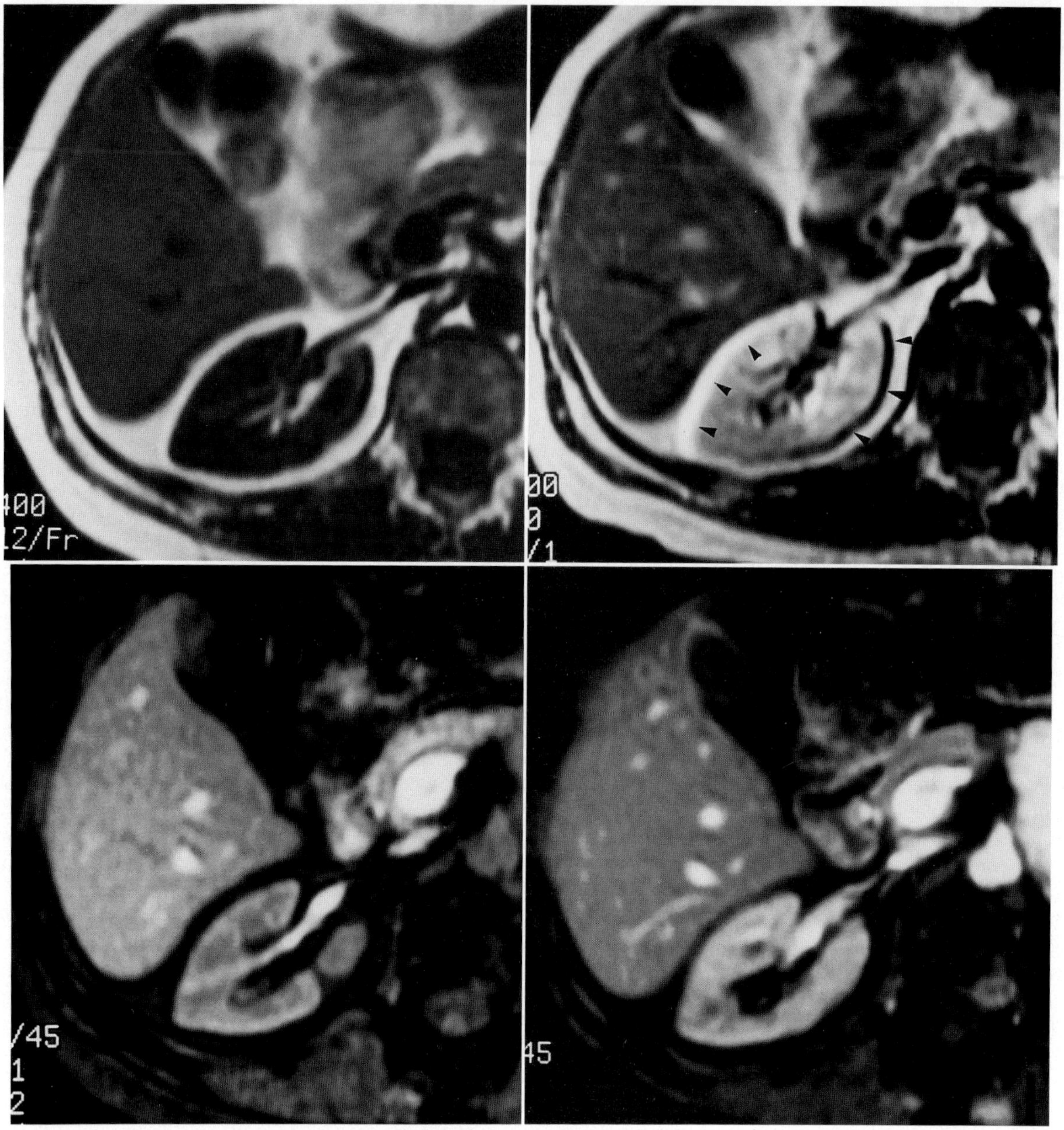


**FIGURE 1** Normal kidney. *A,* On T1-weighted spin-echo image (TR400, TE12), the relatively dark kidney is surrounded by very bright fat. The pyramids are slightly darker than the cortex. *B,* After Gd-DTPA, the kidney is bright, similar to the fat. Note the chemical shift artifact *(arrowheads)*. *C,* A T1-weighted GRE image (SPGR, flip 45, TR51, TE12) with fat suppression done during a 10 second breath-hold shows the kidney brighter than the retroperitoneal fat. Corticomedullary junction is visible. Note the bright appearance of the normal vessels. *D,* After Gd-DTPA, the same sequence shows the kidney is bright, with no corticomedullary differentiation. Note the high contrast between the enhanced kidney and suppressed fat and lack of chemical shift artifact.

have limited signal-to-noise ratio (SNR) compared with spin echo. Section thickness must be appropriate to the size of the mass, especially if measurement of signal intensities is to be done to determine enhancement and avoid volume averaging. If a mass is 2 cm or less, 5 mm slices should be done; if the mass is over 5 cm, 10 mm slices may be sufficient. If thin sections are used, more signal averages may be needed to provide acceptable SNR.

Whether spin-echo or GRE methods are used, fat suppression is useful. On unenhanced T1-weighted images, the low signal kidney is surrounded by bright fat, but after Gd-DTPA, both kidney parenchyma and fat are bright (Fig. 1). Suppressing fat increases contrast-to-noise ratio (CNR) between enhanced kidney tissue and the retroperitoneum. This can be accomplished by selective radiofrequency suppression of the fat resonance at only a small time penalty. Because of the floating point scale system used on most MRI scanners, if fat (usually the brightest substance on T1 scans) is suppressed, the scanner presents other tissues as relatively brighter, making enhancement clearer. However, use of fat suppression carries some penalties. If the wrong peak is selected for suppression, scan quality is degraded; if the field is heterogeneous, fat suppression will be heterogeneous; if a fat-suppressed scan is done after Gd-DTPA, there should be a precontrast scan of the same type to compare with for certain determination of increase in signal intensity after contrast. A fat-suppressed T1-weighted scan without Gd-DTPA, however, is useless except as a baseline for enhancement evaluation. Therefore, if contrast is given, two additional sequences are required in addition to the usual T1 and multiecho scans. Fat suppression is also useful to improve T2-weighted spin-echo scans. This also improves the CNR between the bright tumor and surrounding retroperitoneal fat and allows use of variable bandwidth to increase SNR on the second echo.

## Diagnostic Approach

### *Imaging Protocol*

In general, renal mass evaluation can be well done using a T1 coronal sequence as a localizer, followed by axial unenhanced T1 and then fat-suppressed multiecho (proton density and T2-weighted) spin-echo scans done with coverage from the diaphragm to the lower poles of the kidneys. Either a fat-suppressed T1-weighted spin-echo or GRE (e.g., spoiled GRASS, SPGR, FLASH) sequence should be done before and then after Gd-DTPA injection. These sequences need only cover the kidneys themselves. At least one GRE sequence should be done for vascular evaluation, with coverage from the renal vein to the right atrium. Coronal or sagittal sequences may be added as needed; these are most useful for evaluation of possible superior extension of upper pole masses or for definition of the extent of caval tumor thrombus.

### *Simple Cyst*

MRI is not indicated for evaluation of a mass that is shown to be a simple cyst by sonography or CT. If scanned, however, the cyst will be homogeneous with very low signal on T1-weighted images and homogeneously bright on T2-weighted scans. There is no enhancement after Gd-DTPA. The wall is very thin; assessment of wall thickness is aided by fat suppression, which reduces the chemical shift artifact that otherwise can impede this assessment.

### *Complicated Cyst*

Cysts that contain protein or hemorrhage can have variable appearance, depending on the exact contents and the age of the hemorrhage. On T1-weighted images, the cyst may have signal similar to or greater than renal parenchyma and may be very bright (Figs. 2, 3). Typically the lesion is hyperintense on T2-weighted images, brighter than either simple cyst or tumor. The cyst may be homogeneous or heterogeneous, and the wall may be thick with septations possible (although perhaps difficult to resolve on MRI). The key to diagnosis is documentation of the lack of any enhancing components. The usual diagnostic pattern is a mass isointense or hyperintense to renal parenchyma on T1- and hyperintense on T2-weighted images with no enhancement. Of 26 masses evaluated at my institution, 9 had these findings on enhanced MRI, and all have been proven to be cysts.

A mass that is hyperintense on both T1- and T2-weighted images presents special problems. A fat-containing lesion must be excluded. Fat or water suppression is useful for this: if the signal drops after fat suppression, or conversely remains after water suppression, fat must be present and the lesion is presumably an angiomyolipoma. To document or exclude enhancement, pre– and post–Gd-DTPA scans of the same type (preferably fat-suppressed T1 spin echo) must be carefully compared (see Fig. 3). Without a baseline, the brightness of the lesion on the post–Gd-DTPA T1 image may be misconstrued as enhancement.

### *Renal Carcinoma*

The MRI appearance of renal carcinoma varies with the degree of differentiation, presence of cystic or necrotic areas or hemorrhage, and with size since larger tumors are more often heterogeneous, with central necrotic areas. The neoplastic tissue itself usually is nearly isointense with renal cortex on both T1- and T2-weighted images. Cystic or necrotic areas are variably hyperintense. The neoplastic tissues enhance, although somewhat less brightly than renal parenchyma when imaged 2 to 5 minutes after injection (Fig. 4). The tumor may show homogeneous enhancement if small and well differentiated or heterogeneous enhancement if there is central necrosis. Any enhancing component within a renal mass indicates it is a vascularized lesion, not a cyst, and most often a renal carcinoma. Fat suppression not only aids detection of enhancement, but also helps define extent of the tumor if it extends beyond the renal outline; since the enhanced tumor is bright, if fat is bright as on standard T1 scans, there is little contrast between tumor and surrounding tissue. This is also true on unenhanced T2-weighted scans.

Since large, necrotic masses do not present a diagnostic challenge (they clearly are malignancies, not cysts), enhanced MRI is most useful for evaluating small renal masses, especially in patients who cannot tolerate iodinated contrast material. When MRI is done to evaluate a large, clearly malignant mass, Gd-DTPA enhancement is probably not necessary, because it does not aid in staging. Staging criteria include local extension of the tumor, adenopathy, venous invasion, and bone or liver metastases. These can be accurately evaluated by unenhanced MRI. Instead of taking the time to do two or more sequences (including pre– and post–Gd-DTPA) to determine enhancement, additional unenhanced sequences, perhaps in coronal or sagittal planes, would be more efficacious for staging.

The greatest use of Gd-DTPA enhancement is to decide whether a suspicious small renal mass is tumor or complicated cyst. In my experience with 26 such cases, 16 showed definite enhancement. Eleven were proven to be renal carcinoma; two patients with presumed carcinomas refused surgery or biopsy. One oncocytoma, one angiomyolipoma, and one myofibroma also showed enhancement. No mass showing apparent enhancement has been found to be a cyst; none of the nine with characteristics of a cyst has been found to be a neoplasm (in one case of spontaneous renal hemorrhage, no mass was found on MRI). None of the 26 patients had any adverse effect, including the 10 with chronic renal failure or the 2 with previous reactions to iodinated contrast material. No change in renal function occurred after Gd-DTPA in any of the patients.

### *Other Tumors*

Angiomyolipoma is a benign renal mass containing variable amounts of fat, smooth muscle, and vessels. Because of the

A

B

C

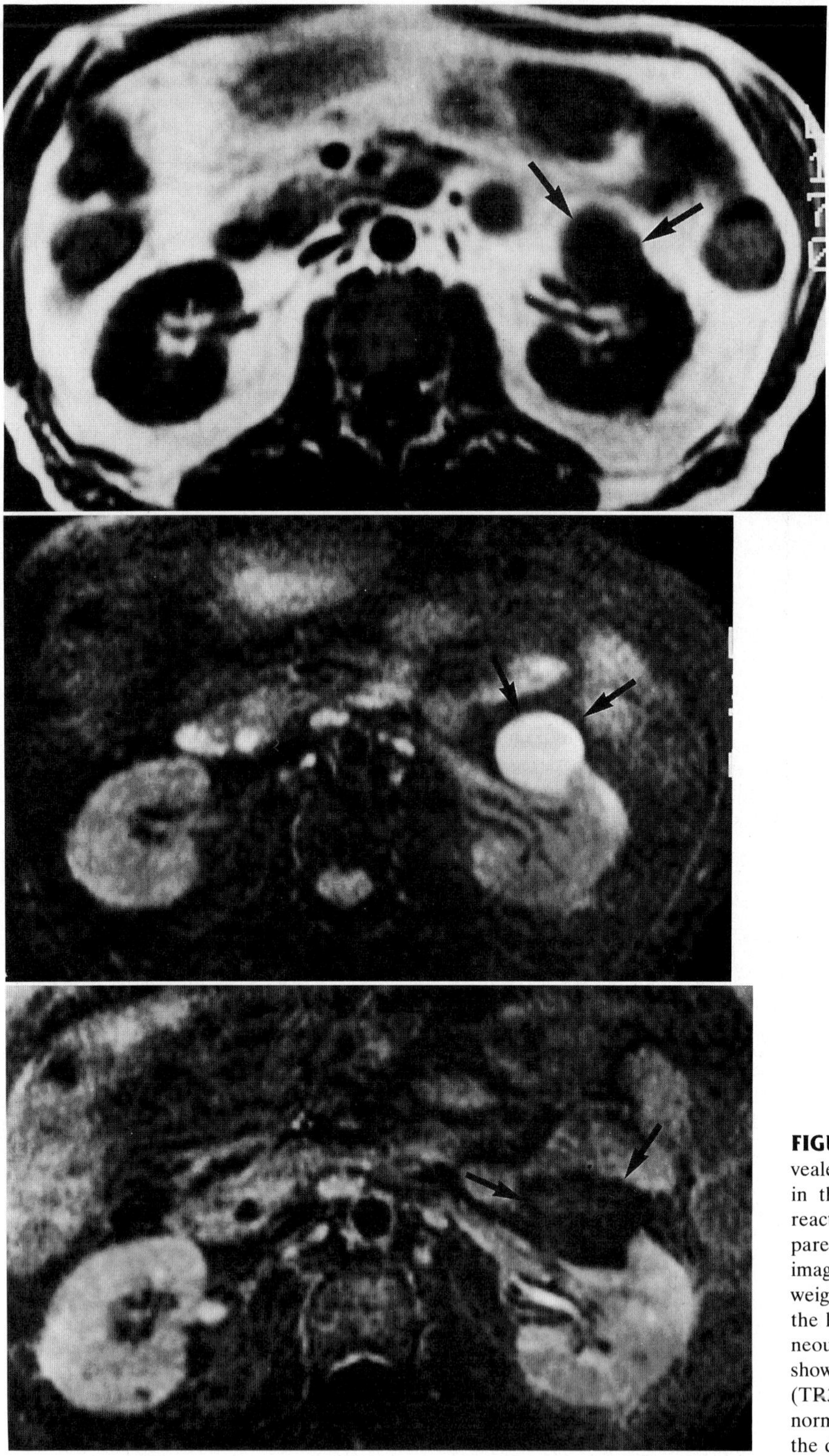

**FIGURE 2** Complicated cyst. Sonogram revealed a left-sided renal mass containing echoes in this 64-year-old man with a prior contrast reaction. *A,* A mass *(arrows)* isodense with renal parenchyma is seen on the T1-weighted spin-echo image (TR300, TE12). *B,* Fat-suppressed T2-weighted spin-echo scan (TR2500, TE60) shows the lesion *(arrows)* is hyperintense but homogeneous. *C,* The mass *(arrows)* did not enhance as shown by the fat-suppressed T1 spin-echo scan (TR300, TE15). Note the enhancement of the normal renal parenchyma is well shown against the dark perirenal fat.

A

B

C

D

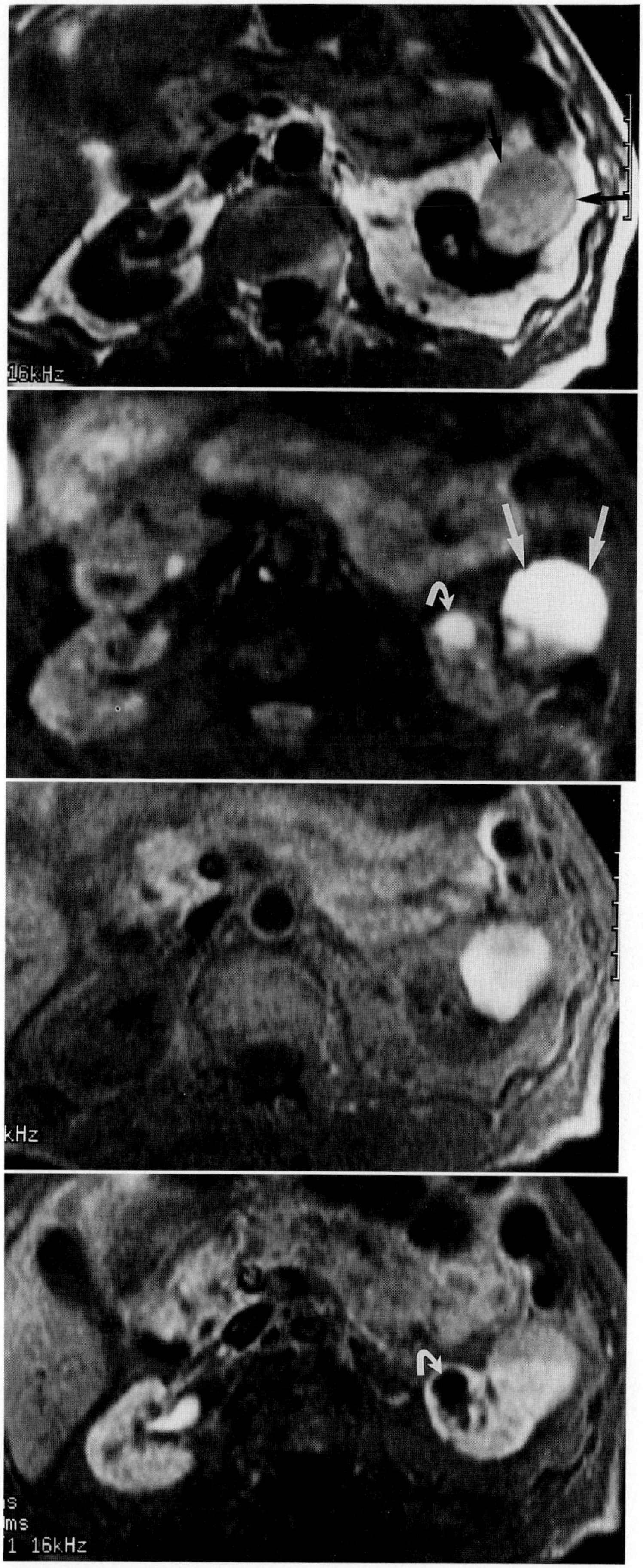


**FIGURE 3** Hemorrhagic cyst. Sonogram revealed a complex mass in this 68-year-old man with renal insufficiency not yet requiring dialysis. Unenhanced CT showed the mass had density of 23 Hounsfield units. *A,* T1-weighted spin-echo scan (TR500, TE11) shows the mass *(arrows)* is hyperintense. *B,* The mass *(arrows)* is very hyperintense and heterogeneous on fat-suppressed T2-weighted sequence (TR2200, TE80). Note another less intense lesion *(curved arrow)* difficult to identify on T1. *C,* On fat-suppressed T1-weighted spin-echo scan (TR550, TE11), the signal intensity of the hyperintense mass was 291. *D,* After Gd-DTPA, the signal intensity of the mass was 290. It now has similar brightness as the renal cortex due to enhancement of the cortex. Note the other lesion *(curved arrow)* is also nonenhancing: this is a typical simple cyst (proven by sonography).

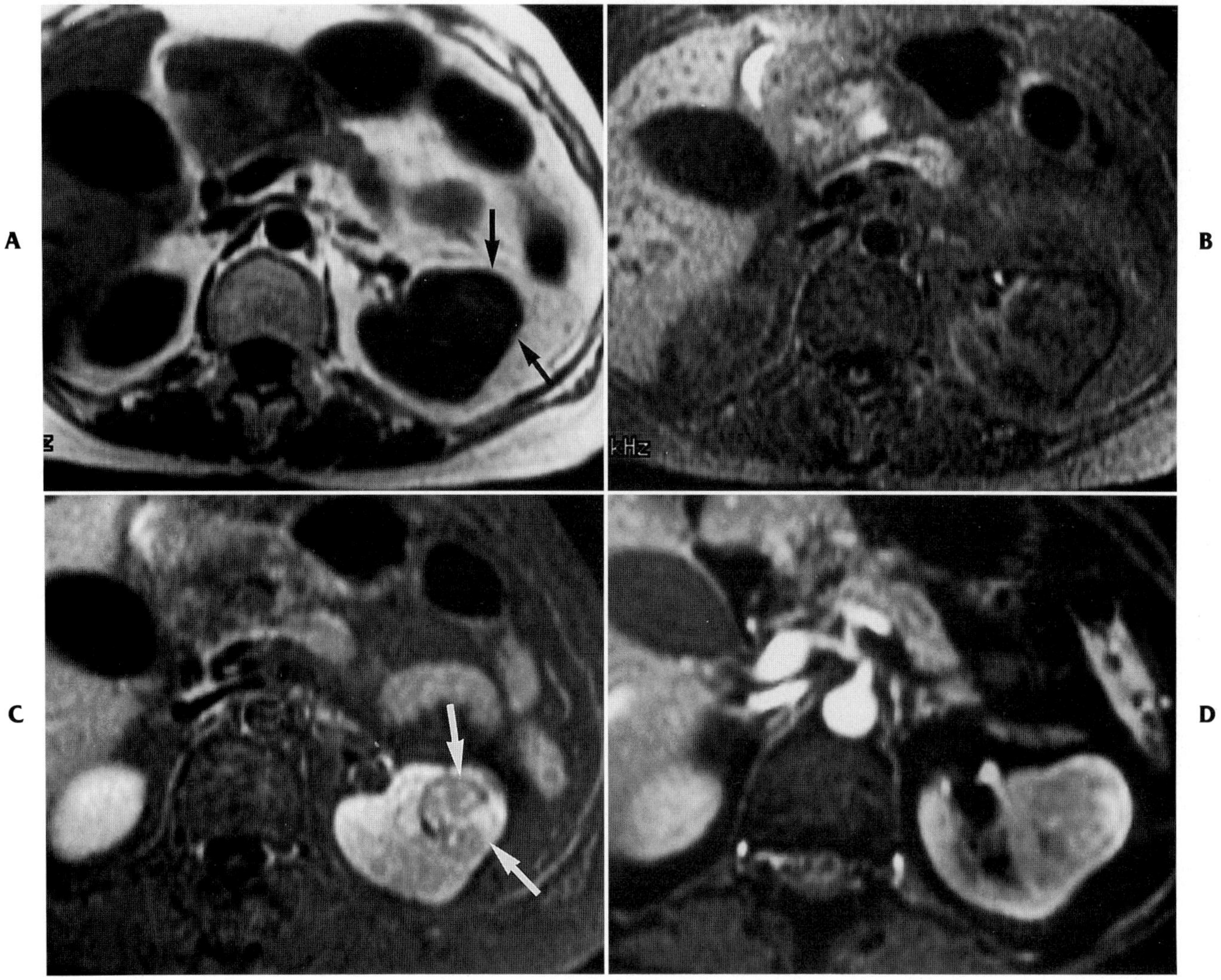

**FIGURE 4** Renal carcinoma. A 62-year-old female presented with hematuria; stage I renal carcinoma proven by nephrectomy. *A,* T1-weighted spin-echo image (TR300, TE11) shows a bulge in the left kidney *(arrows)* of similar signal to renal tissue. *B,* Fat-suppressed T1-weighted spin-echo scan (TR500, TE10) is useful only as a baseline, since there is very poor contrast-to-noise ratio between various tissues. *C,* The mass *(arrows)* shows heterogeneous enhancement after Gd-DTPA, yet is distinguishable from renal parenchyma. *D,* Fat-suppressed SPGR (TR50, TE12, flip 35) also shows lesion enhancement. Note the normal blood vessels are well shown.

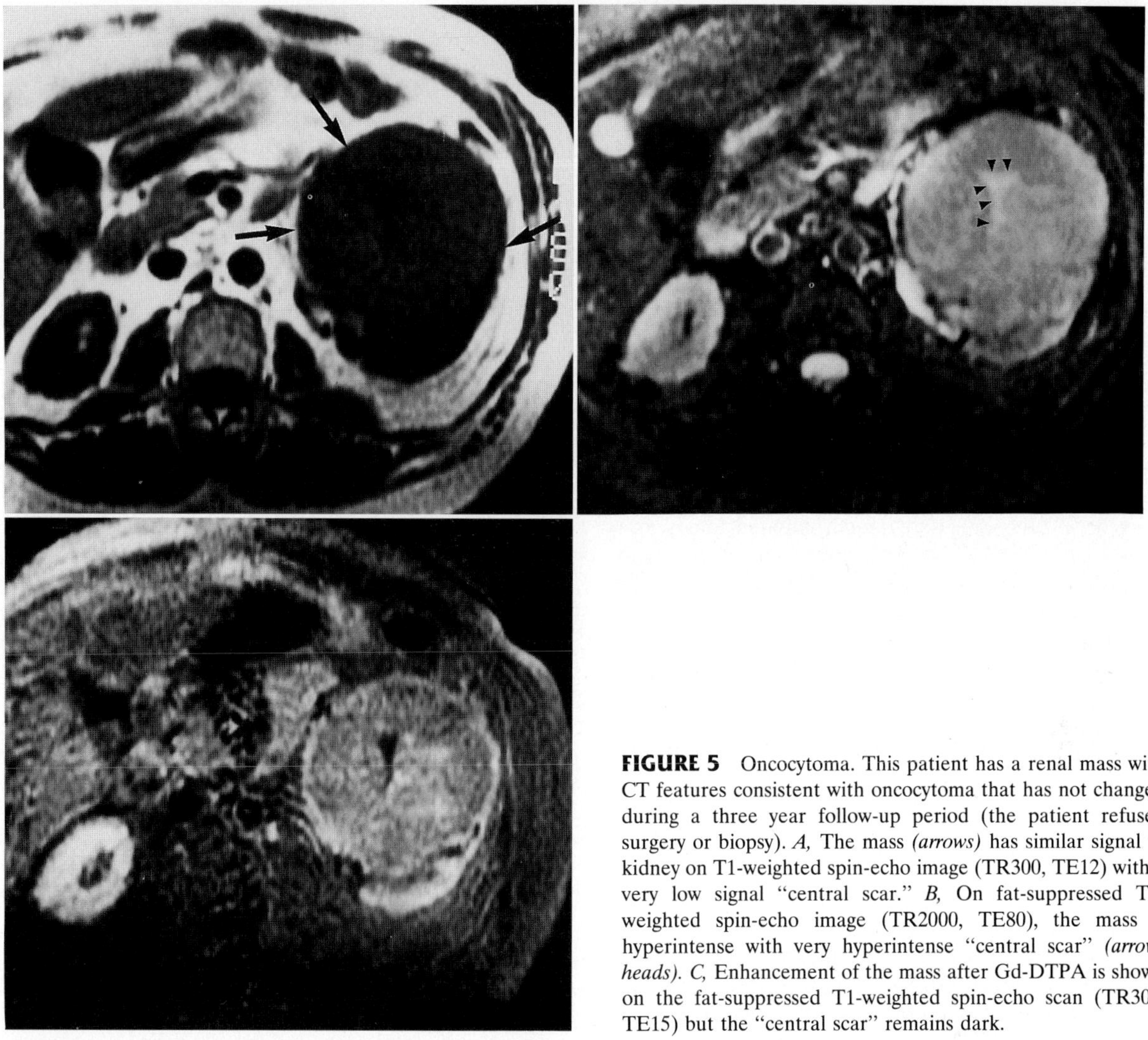


**FIGURE 5** Oncocytoma. This patient has a renal mass with CT features consistent with oncocytoma that has not changed during a three year follow-up period (the patient refused surgery or biopsy). *A,* The mass *(arrows)* has similar signal to kidney on T1-weighted spin-echo image (TR300, TE12) with a very low signal "central scar." *B,* On fat-suppressed T2-weighted spin-echo image (TR2000, TE80), the mass is hyperintense with very hyperintense "central scar" *(arrowheads). C,* Enhancement of the mass after Gd-DTPA is shown on the fat-suppressed T1-weighted spin-echo scan (TR300, TE15) but the "central scar" remains dark.

vascularity, this lesion can show enhancement after Gd-DTPA. The key to diagnosis is documentation of fat with the lesion, as discussed previously. In fact, while although MRI can accurately diagnose this lesion, CT is the preferred method since even unenhanced CT can detect fat.

Oncocytoma is a type of renal adenoma, believed by most experts to be a benign lesion with no malignant potential. When large, there may be features suggestive of the diagnosis, particularly the central scar that can be seen on CT scans and MRI (Fig. 5). Because these are vascularized lesions, they enhance after Gd-DTPA, as would be expected since they do so on CT scans after injection of iodinated contrast material. It may not be possible to distinguish oncocytoma from renal carcinoma in many cases.

A variety of other benign and malignant renal tumors occur including leiomyoma, leiomyosarcoma, transitional carcinoma, adenoma, and metastases. At present, experience with these is so limited it is not known if there are criteria that differentiate these from renal carcinoma on enhanced MRI. It is doubtful that this is the case, since it can be expected that most will enhance. Thus caution must be exercised when faced with a clearly enhancing renal mass—cyst is excluded and renal carcinoma is most likely (partly because renal carcinoma is statistically the commonest renal tumor by far), but other tumors, including benign ones, may be present. Nevertheless, this is no different than the situation with CT.

## Suggested Reading

Carvlin MJ, Arger PH, Kundes HL, et al. Use of Gd-DTPA and fast gradient-echo and spin-echo MR imaging to demonstrate renal function in the rabbit. Radiology 1989; 170:705–711.

Choyke PL, Frank JA, Girton ME, et al. Dynamic Gd-DTPA–enhanced MR imaging of the kidney: Experimental results. Radiology 1989; 170:713–720.

Eilenberg SS, Lee JKT, Brown JJ, et al. Renal masses: Evaluation with gradient-echo Gd-DTPA–enhanced dynamic MR imaging. Radiology 1990; 176:333–338.

Haustein J, Niendorf HP, Krestin G, et al. Renal tolerance of gadolinium-DTPA/dimeglumine in patients with chronic renal failure. Invest Radiol 1992; 27:153–156.

Hricak H, Thoeni RF, Carroll PR, et al. Detection and staging of renal neoplasms: A reassessment of MR imaging. Radiology 1988; 166:643–649.

Mirowitz SA, Gutierrez E, Lee JKT, et al. Normal abdominal enhancement patterns with dynamic gadolinium-enhanced MR imaging. Radiology 1991; 180:637–640.

Quint LE, Glazer GM, Chenevert TL, et al. In vivo and in vitro imaging of renal tumors: Histopathologic correlation and pulse sequence optimization. Radiology 1988; 169:359–362.

Rofsky NM, Weinreb JC, Bosniak MA, et al. Renal lesion characterization with gadolinium-enhanced MR imaging: Efficacy and safety in patients with renal insufficiency. Radiology 1991; 180:85–89.

Roubidoux MA, Dunnick NR, Sostman HD, et al. Renal carcinoma: Detection of venous extension with gradient-echo MR imaging. Radiology 1992; 182:269–751.

Semelka RC, Hricak H, Stevens SK, et al. Combined gadolinium–enhanced and fat-saturation MR imaging of renal masses. Radiology 1991; 178:803–809.

Vogl TJ, Pegios W, McMahon C, et al. Gadobenate dimeglumine – a new contrast agent for MR imaging: Preliminary evaluation in healthy volunteers. AJR 1992; 158:887–890.

# CT and MRI of the Adult Adrenal Gland

*JEFFREY H. NEWHOUSE, M.D.*

Two decades ago, imaging diagnosis of adrenal diseases was difficult. Noninvasive detection was possible only for large or calcified masses visible on radiographs. Smaller masses could be demonstrated only by the uncomfortable and risky angiography or retroperitoneal pneumography. But the simultaneous development of ultrasonography and computed tomography (CT), and the subsequent emergence of magnetic resonance imaging (MRI), permitted the detection of smaller lesions and allowed differential diagnosis to a degree previously impossible. The ability of CT to detect smaller masses more reliably than ultrasonography has led to the acceptance of the former as the primary imaging tool for depicting and characterizing adrenal abnormalities. More recently MRI has become capable of demonstrating most adrenal masses and performing differential diagnosis among certain masses hitherto not possible by imaging alone. MRI is beginning to rival CT as the primary way to search for adrenal disease.

## Indications and Technique

The indications for adrenal CT are numerous. Patients with clinical or biochemical evidence of Cushing's syndrome, hyperaldosteronism, or inappropriate virilization should have adrenal hyperplasia, adenoma, or carcinoma sought by CT. Those with clinical or biochemical evidence of medullary hyperfunction should be subjected to CT to search for pheochromocytoma. Patients with hypoadrenocorticism who are not known to have abnormalities of the pituitary-adrenal axis should have adrenal CT to exclude neoplastic, hemorrhagic, or inflammatory processes that might destroy the glands. Patients with a malignancy that might metastasize to the adrenals certainly require adrenal CT. Adrenal CT is frequently used in follow-up for patients who have a mass discovered at urography, ultrasonography, or abdominal scintigraphy which may have arisen from the adrenal. Finally, patients who are known to have MEN II (multiple endocrine neoplasia) syndrome, neurofibromatosis, or von Hippel-Lindau syndrome, and who may therefore have adrenal masses, require adrenal CT.

Most adrenal screening by CT can be done with 8 or 10 mm contiguous slices, but since some adrenal masses may be less than 1 cm in diameter, thinner contiguous slices (~5 mm) may also be used. More small adrenal masses are probably missed because of respiratory misregistration, however, than because of partial volume averaging. This problem can be overcome by using a rapid dynamic scanning technique and a single breathhold, by using overlapping slices, or by careful analysis of serial images to ascertain that the level of the diaphragm does not change between slices.

Sometimes intravenous contrast material is necessary. Contrast enhancement may be useful in distinguishing adrenal cysts from hypodense adrenal adenomas. In patients at risk for metastases to the adrenal, a contrast agent should certainly be added for simultaneous CT evaluation of the liver. The rare large adrenal malignancy that may be associated with venous thrombosis may require a contrast agent to demonstrate the thrombus. But much adrenal CT screening can probably be done without intravenous contrast material. Certainly, when normal adrenals are visualized, the addition of a contrast-enhanced evaluation has little to offer. Although many solid adrenal masses may enhance with varying degrees of homogeneity or heterogeneity, and the enhancement patterns may be visually striking, the differential diagnosis of the mass is critically affected by the enhancement pattern only rarely.

The indications for employing MRI in the investigation of adrenal diseases are several. MRI is useful to characterize masses detected by radiography, ultrasonography, and CT, and in the differential diagnosis of adrenal masses from each other and from masses in adjacent organs. MRI is useful in screening the trunk and neck for pheochromocytomas in patients who may have multiple tumors or metastases. It is valuable in screening patients with Cushing's or Conn's syndromes who may have adrenal adenomas. Finally, it is of use in searching for metastases to the adrenal gland, especially when the upper abdomen is being investigated for hepatic metastases. Although most of the available literature suggests that CT should precede MRI in the search for adrenal pathology since the spatial resolution of CT is high, current MRI devices have good spatial resolution and have the advantage of permitting multislice imaging, which makes failure to detect an adrenal mass as a result of respiratory misregistration unlikely.

The technique for investigating the adrenals with MRI is straightforward. Transverse T1-weighted spin-echo images through the region of the adrenals should be used first. The TR is not critical; the TE should be as short as possible. Slices should be contiguous or nearly so. If the sought-for adrenal mass might be small, slices 5 or 6 mm thick should be used; otherwise 1 cm slices suffice.

If normal adrenal morphology is observed on T1-weighted images, the evaluation may be terminated. Otherwise, T2-weighted images should be obtained. For these, the TR should be relatively long (1,800 to 2,500 msec) and a long (70 to 120 msec) TE should be used. Since tissue characterization, rather than anatomy, is the important information on T2-weighted images, the orientation of the slices is usually not critical. However, if the borders of the investigated mass with adjacent organs or tissues are important, coronal or sagittal views may be required instead. Of course, whatever tissue is intended to be used to compare intensities with the adrenal lesion should be included in the image.

## Pheochromocytoma

Pheochromocytomas are infrequently found tumors of the adrenal medulla, which appear most frequently in the fourth or fifth decade of life. They are often associated with hypertension, but are responsible for much less than 1 percent of all cases of hypertension, so that CT or MRI screening of all hypertensive patients is much too expensive to be practical. Although autopsy studies suggest that a significant number of small adrenal pheochromocytomas may be present throughout life and never come to clinical attention, a pheochromocytoma is only rarely the diagnosis when an adrenal mass is discovered incidentally by imaging techniques.

The possible locations of these tumors determine imaging strategy. About 10 percent of these tumors are found in extra-adrenal sites. They usually appear in the sympathetic ganglia of the abdomen and pelvis, but have been encountered as far cephalad as the base of the skull and as far caudad as the epididymis. The organ of Zuckerkandl is an occasional site for an extra-adrenal pheochromocytoma. About 10 percent of all pheochromocytomas are multiple, and the pattern of multiplicity is important. In the MEN syndromes, the tumors are multiple, frequently bilateral, and almost always confined to the adrenal gland. About 10 percent of all pheochromocytomas are malignant. Extra-adrenal pheochromocytomas are more likely to display malignant behavior than are intra-adrenal tumors. If multiple tumors are found, but all exist in sites of known sympathetic ganglia, the tumors are likely to be multiple but benign. Malignant pheochromocytomas tend to metastasize to bone, lung, liver, and local nodes.

The association of these tumors with other conditions also determines imaging decisions. Although most adrenal pheochromocytomas are encountered as isolated lesions, they appear with markedly increased prevalence in patients who have von Hippel-Lindau disease, neurofibromatosis, or renal artery stenosis. Pheochromocytomas are also part of some of the MEN syndromes. MEN IIA (Sipple's syndrome) consists of medullary thyroid carcinoma and parathyroid hyperplasia or adenomas, as well as pheochromocytomas. MEN IIB (which is sometimes called MEN III) consists of marfanoid facies and mucosal neuromas of the mouth in addition to adrenal pheochromocytomas.

In the past few years, CT has been the primary imaging method for detecting pheochromocytomas. It is capable of finding most, if not all, intra-adrenal pheochromocytomas, although careful scanning with thin contiguous slices may be necessary to demonstrate the small tumors seen in the MEN syndromes. In patients who have biochemical evidence of a pheochromocytoma but normal-appearing adrenals, CT can also be used to image the other potential sites. The abdominal and pelvic retroperitoneal areas should be scanned first. If these regions fail to reveal a mass, the mediastinum and neck should be scanned subsequently. Radioisotope scanning using iodine-131 metaiodobenzylguanidine (MIBG) is a reasonably sensitive and efficient way of scanning the entire body for pheochromocytomas, but this is not a technique that enjoys widespread availability.

When visualized at CT, pheochromocytomas most frequently appear as soft-tissue–density masses (Fig. 1). They may be relatively homogeneous or, if necrotic, appear with irregular low-density central regions. When most of the tumor is necrotic, the lesion may appear as a primarily cystic abnormality with a relatively discrete wall. The soft-tissue portions of the lesion enhance with intravenous contrast material; enhancement may therefore be homogeneous, heterogeneous or, in the case of cystic lesions, confined to the wall. In the absence of clinical information, the CT appearance of the lesions may not permit a histologic diagnosis. The CT characteristics may overlap to a certain degree with those of primary adrenocortical carcinomas, metastases to the adrenal, and even adrenal hematomas at certain stages in their evolution.

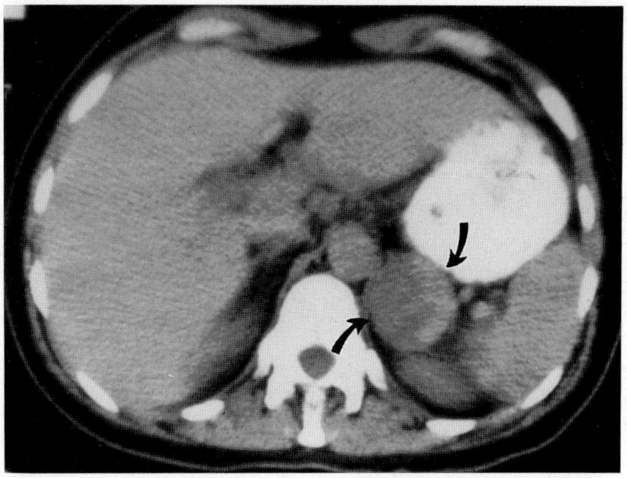

**FIGURE 1** Left adrenal pheochromocytoma. CT reveals a round, slightly heterogeneous left adrenal mass (*arrows*); intravenous contrast material has not been used.

At MRI the appearance of the lesion depends on the pulse sequence used. On T1-weighted spin-echo images (Fig. 2, *A*), the lesions may appear similar in intensity to some of the lower-intensity soft tissues such as spleen or renal medulla. If the lesion is solid throughout, it may appear relatively homogeneous, but lesions with necrotic portions may have focal regions of even lower intensity. On T2-weighted images (Fig. 2, *B*), the lesions are, as a group, the brightest of solid-tissue adrenal masses. They may also appear homogeneous or heterogeneous. Lesions that are heterogeneous in composition may tend to appear homogeneous, however, because they are so bright that they occupy an extreme end of the contrast scale of the image. The degree of brightness on T2-weighted images may give strong indication that a particular adrenal lesion is a pheochromocytoma. Unfortunately absolute accuracy and histologic prediction are usually not possible, both because the lesions may be heterogeneous and because other lesions, including metastases and primary adrenal carcinomas, may be sufficiently bright to overlap the brightness range of pheochromocytomas.

MRI may be used to search for pheochromocytomas in patients who have biochemical evidence of the tumor and whose adrenals appear normal. However, despite the fact that the strong contrast provided by T2-weighted images is an advantage, searching the entire region of sympathetic chains is time-consuming. When the search is limited to the adrenal, MRI may be competitive with CT.

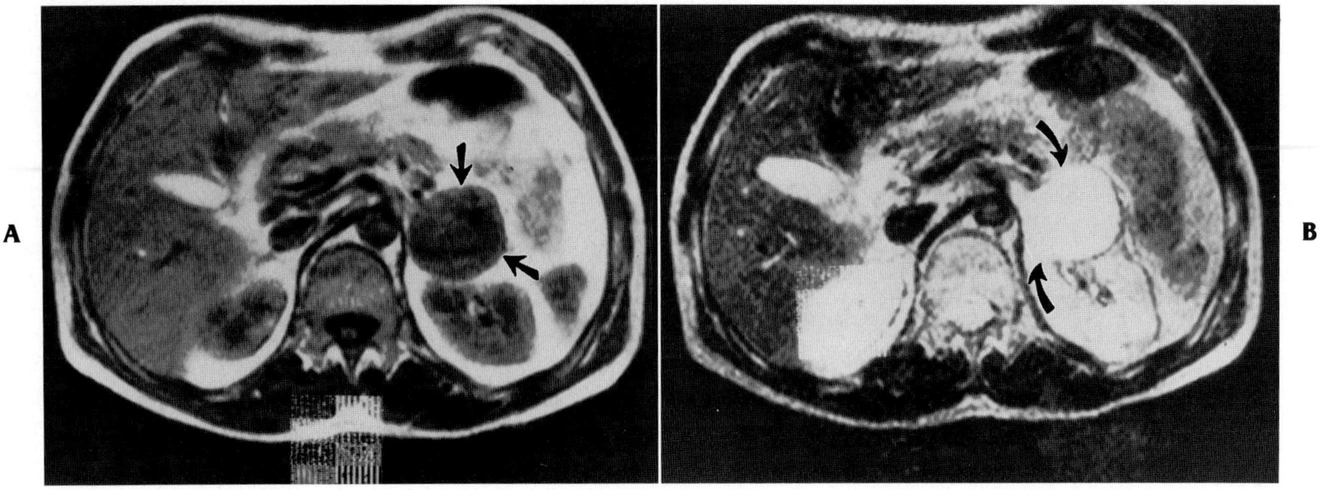


**FIGURE 2** MRI of left adrenal pheochromocytoma. *A,* T1-weighted image. The left adrenal mass (*arrows*) is slightly heterogeneous and approximately the intensity of renal medulla. *B,* T2-weighted image. The lesion (*arrows*) is bright. (From Newhouse JH. MRI of the adrenal gland. Urol Radiol 1990, 12:1–6; with permission.)

## Adrenocortical Carcinoma

Adrenocortical carcinoma is relatively rare. It may appear at any age, but is most frequently encountered in the fourth to sixth decade. It may be diagnosed serendipitously by imaging or may produce symptoms, which may either be reflections of excess production of hormones (Cushing's syndrome, virilization or feminization, Conn's syndrome) or because of pain or other symptoms produced by metastases. These tumors, especially the nonfunctional ones, are often large when diagnosed and may reach 25 cm or more in diameter. Their size and aggressiveness may be the clue to their malignancy. Although histologic criteria exist to distinguish carcinomas from adrenal adenomas, the distinction may be difficult if the tumor is small and relatively well differentiated. Surgical resection offers the only hope for cure; radiotherapy and chemotherapy are relatively ineffective.

The tumors are often heterogeneous, because of internal necrosis and/or hemorrhage, and frequently display gross calcification. They may invade or displace any adjacent organ or tissue that they encounter. When they metastasize, they may spread to local nodes or to the liver, lungs, brain, or peritoneal cavity. They may generate malignant thrombi in the adrenal vein, left renal vein, or inferior vena cava; occasionally venous compression by the tumor may produce bland venous thrombosis.

CT images reflect the gross pathology of the tumor. They may be of any size, but are frequently large. When small, they may look similar to adrenocortical adenomas. Larger masses may displace the ipsilateral kidney inferiorly; masses on the right may displace the liver superiorly, whereas those on the left may displace the splenic vessels and pancreas anteriorly, the stomach anterolaterally, and the spleen in a similar direction. Larger masses often display irregular calcification. The larger the mass, the more likely it is to be relatively heterogeneous, and the more likely it is to enhance heterogeneously with intravenous contrast material. Masses encountered at CT that may be adrenocortical carcinomas should prompt a CT search to reveal local extent and metastases. Dynamic scanning should be performed as needed to demonstrate any venous thrombi. The scan should be inspected for local nodal invasion, and, at the very least, the liver should be evaluated with contrast-enhanced images to reveal any metastatic lesions. Although common practice often consists of evaluating only the abdomen with CT, leaving the search for thoracic metastases to chest radiography, an argument can be made for extending CT to the chest.

T1-weighted MR images (Fig. 3) reveal the typical adrenocortical carcinoma to be heterogeneous, with the necrotic regions of relatively low intensity. Small homogeneous tumors probably have tissue intensities approximating that of other solid viscera in the upper abdomen. On T2-weighted images, the tumors tend to be bright (their intensity is similar to that observed with metastases) and somewhat heterogeneous, although, as with other highly intense tissues, the heterogeneity may be masked if the image of the lesion appears so bright as to be at the upper end of the contrast scale. Differentiation

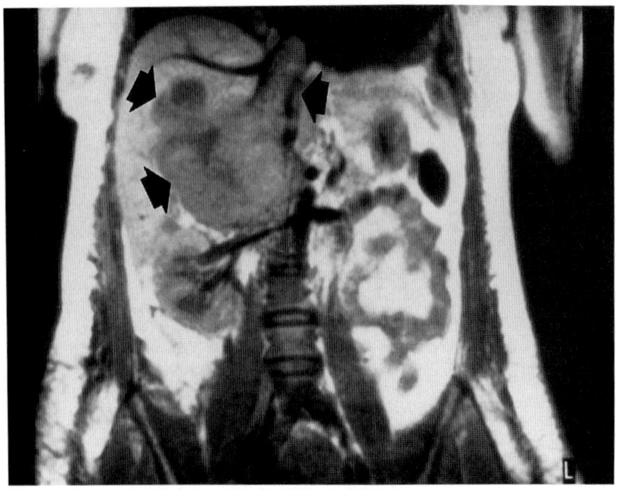


**FIGURE 3** MRI of right adrenal carcinoma; T1-weighted coronal image. The tumor (*arrows*) has extended into the inferior cava and invaded the inferior surface of the right hepatic lobe.

from pheochromocytomas may be difficult using imaging information alone. Small tumors may have an appearance that approximates that of adenomas. Calcified regions, if large enough to be observed, appear of extremely low intensity on all images. Sagittal and coronal images, when added to the standard transverse images, may aid in establishing whether the lesion has invaded adjacent organs or tissues, and may more dramatically demonstrate the extent of any venous involvement.

## Adrenal Adenoma

Although clinical syndromes produced by adrenal adenomas are uncommon, adenomas themselves are encountered with surprising frequency, as attested both by autopsy studies and the development of modern CT. The prevalence in autopsy studies has ranged up to 8 percent, although this figure is clearly higher than that revealed by CT evaluations, and is achieved only if extremely small adenomas are included. Most adenomas do not produce syndromes of inappropriate secretion of hormones during life, and are primarily discovered serendipitously during CT evaluations of the abdomen. These are whimsically entitled "incidentalomas" by some practitioners, and their major clinical importance stems from the procedures required for their differential diagnosis from more serious adrenal tumors. Adenomas may cause Conn's syndrome; these adenomas are often quite small. They may also cause about 20 percent of all cases of Cushing's syndrome. If biochemical tests suggest these syndromes, and CT or MRI evaluations are equivocal with regard to whether a focal mass is present, venous sampling may be of great help in diagnosis and for planning possible surgery.

The most frequently described adrenal adenomas encountered during imaging procedures are solitary, but adenomas may be multiple. Indeed, they may be so small and numerous that a continuum can be constructed that ranges from single adenomas to multiple adenomas to nodular hyperplasia to hyperplasia without macroscopically visible nodularity. At any point along this spectrum, the lesions may or may not produce syndromes of adrenocortical hyperfunction.

The most common appearance of these tumors on CT scans (Fig. 4) is that of small, solid, relatively homogeneous, and well-marginated masses that are circular or ovoid in cross section and that measure 1 to 5 cm in diameter. They may occasionally be larger and heterogeneous and rarely may display calcification. Frequently they have CT attenuation values considerably less than other soft tissues, with densities measuring from 0 to 30 Hounsfield units. When intravenous contrast material is used, these tumors usually enhance slightly and homogeneously; occasionally a fine punctate pattern of enhancement may be visualized. If a lesion does not enhance, or if intravenous contrast material is not used and the lesion is of relatively low density, there may be difficulty in differential diagnosis between adenomas and small cysts; ultrasonography may be used to resolve the issue. Adenomas may have their diagnosis confirmed by radionuclide scintigraphy, using NP-59 as an agent.

MRI detects most of these lesions. On T1-weighted spin-echo images (Fig. 5, *A*), the lesions are usually homogeneous and of an intensity approximately equal to that of liver. On T2-weighted spin-echo images (Fig. 5, *B*), the lesions do not appear particularly bright. Their intensity has been compared with a number of solid tissues in the upper abdomen. They are often approximately isointense to liver and considerably less intense than spleen or fat. Small lesions tend to be relatively homogeneous; heterogeneity is more frequently encountered in larger lesions.

## Adrenal Metastases

Malignant disease frequently metastasizes to the adrenal gland. One study has found that 27 percent of all patients dying with malignancies had adrenal metastases, and a similar figure has been quoted for patients dying of lymphomas. Carcinomas of the breast, lung, kidney, gut, and ovary metastasize to the adrenal, as do melanomas and carcinomas of other primary sites. The adrenals may be the first detectable site of metastasis. The metastases to the adrenal may be unilateral or bilateral. They may be sufficiently small that no gross morphologic abnormality is produced in the gland at all. At the other extreme, the metastases may produce masses many centimeters in diameter. Bilateral involvement of the adrenals with metastatic disease may, in unusual cases, destroy sufficient adrenal tissue to produce Addison's syndrome.

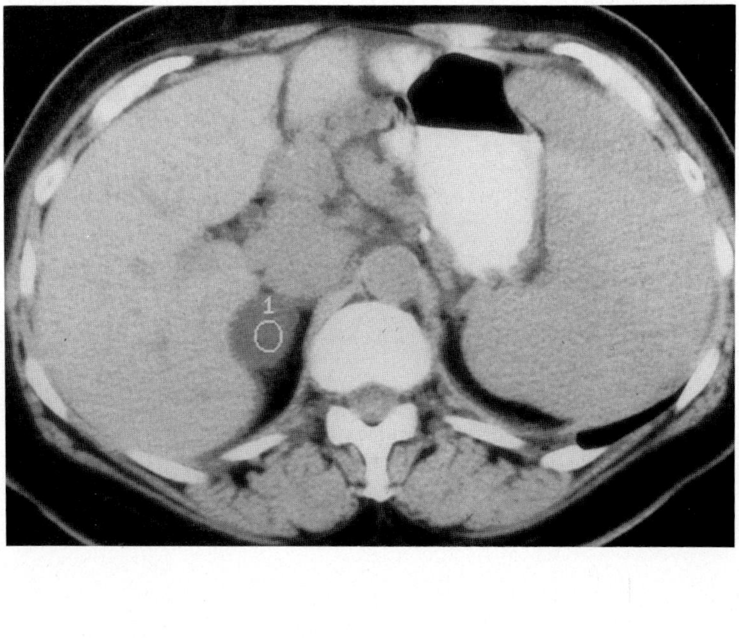


**FIGURE 4** Right adrenal adenoma. CT reveals the lesion to be nearly spherical and homogeneous. The region of interest within it revealed its density to be minimally greater than water.

A

B

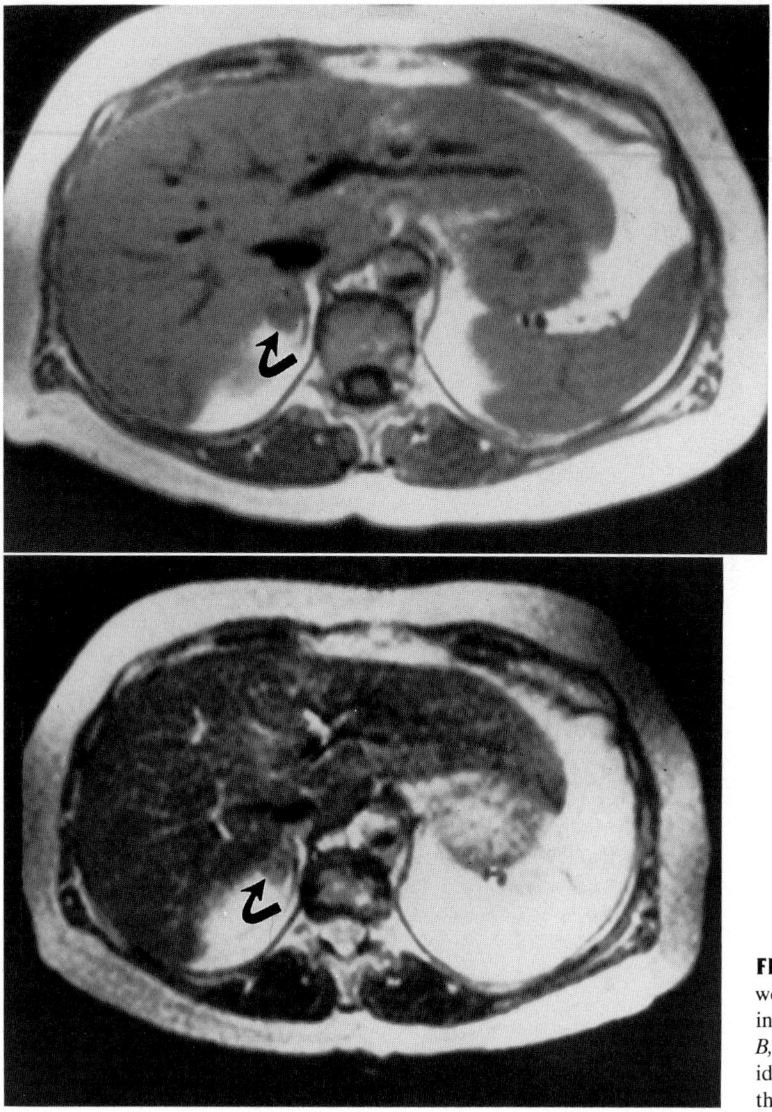

**FIGURE 5** MRI of right adrenal adenoma. *A,* T1-weighted image. The lesion (*arrow*) is of intermediate intensity, similar to other nonfatty tissues in the image. *B,* T2-weighted image. The lesion (*arrow*) is almost identical in intensity to the liver; it is considerably darker than the spleen.

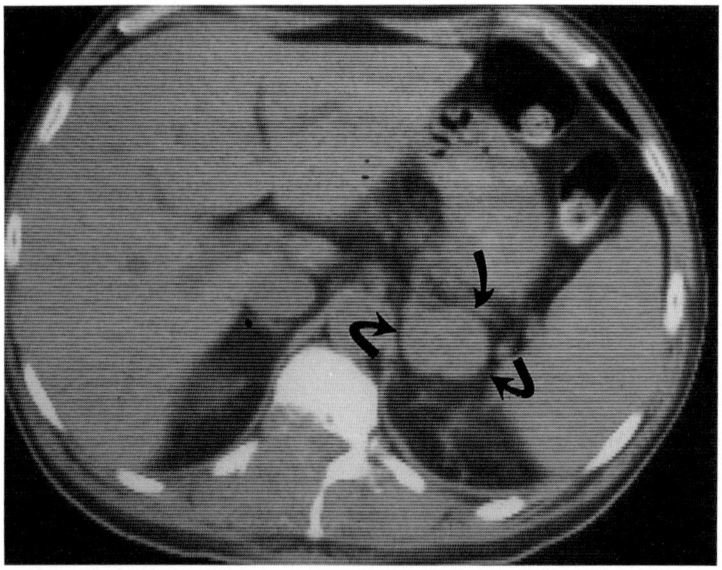

**FIGURE 6** CT of left adrenal metastasis. The lesion (*arrows*) is lobular and minimally heterogeneous (another metastasis has destroyed part of the vertebra). (From Amis ES, Newhouse JH. Essentials of Uroradiology. Boston: Little, Brown, 1991; with permission.)

A

B

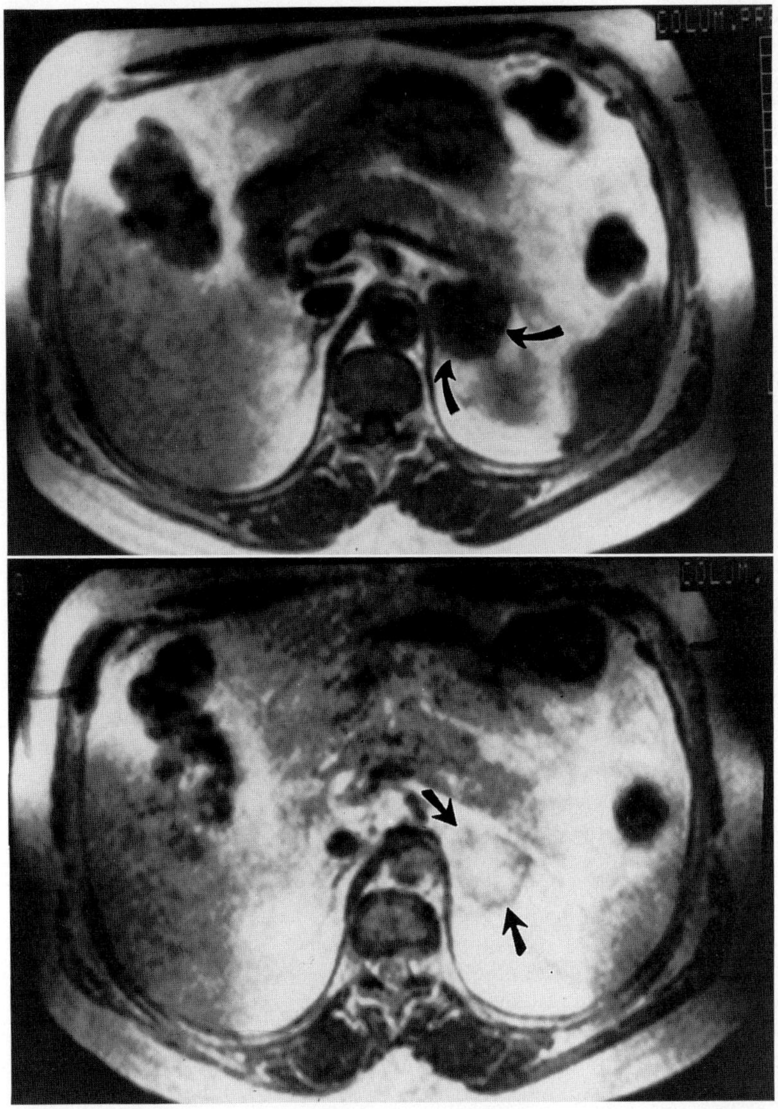

**FIGURE 7** MRI of left adrenal metastases. *A,* T1-weighted image. The lesion (*arrows*) is slightly less intense than liver and approximately the same intensity as spleen. *B,* T2-weighted image. The lesion (*arrows*) is heterogeneous and considerably brighter than liver. (From Newhouse JH. MRI of the adrenal gland. Urol Radiol 1990; 12:1–6; with permission.)

At CT, the appearance of adrenal metastatic disease is variable (Fig. 6). Microscopic metastases may be present in adrenal glands that appear normal. Masses of almost any size may be observed that tend to appear homogeneous when they are small (and to enhance relatively homogeneously) and tend to become more heterogeneous when they are larger (and enhance more heterogeneously). They often have irregular infiltrating margins. Infrequently they may undergo internal hemorrhage and present with high-density regions consistent with blood; they calcify only rarely.

At MRI, spin-echo T1-weighted sequences usually reveal the masses to be of similar intensity to liver and spleen; with strong T1-weighting, the spleen and adrenal metastases may appear slightly less intense than liver (Fig. 7, *A*). With T2-weighted spin-echo imaging, metastases are usually considerably brighter than liver (Fig. 7, *B*) and again approximate the intensity of spleen.

The specific issue of the differential diagnosis of nonfunctioning adrenal adenomas and metastases to the adrenal is difficult. The adrenal glands are a relatively frequent site of metastasis from a number of primary sources, so that an incidentally discovered adrenal mass in a patient not known to have a primary carcinoma raises the possibility that the adrenal mass may be the first indication of malignant disease. Conversely, nonfunctioning adenomas are also sufficiently common so that even in the patient group with malignancies that can metastasize to the adrenal, an adrenal mass may represent an adenoma rather than a metastasis. Since the decision to attempt curative therapy often rests on whether or not an adrenal metastasis is present, differential diagnosis is important.

The relative frequency of the two kinds of masses is of considerable assistance in the differential diagnosis. In patients not known to have a primary malignancy, an incidentally discovered adrenal mass is many times more likely to be an adenoma than a metastasis from an occult malignancy. In patients with cancers known to metastasize to the adrenal, however, there is not an overwhelming preponderance of one cause of adrenal mass. From a statistical point of view, an adrenal mass in such patients could be of either etiology.

Certain morphologic characteristics help the differential diagnosis on any imaging evaluation. Large adrenal masses, especially if bilateral, are more likely to be metastases, as are masses with heterogeneous enhancement and indistinct or irregular margins. Small masses with crisp margins are more likely to be adenomas. Specific CT criteria favoring adenoma are precontrast density of 0 to 30 Hounsfield units, without heterogeneity or evidence of liquefaction, and faint homogeneous or punctate enhancement with contrast.

At MRI, the appearance of the mass on a T2-weighted image is helpful: as a general rule, adenomas are approximately the intensity of liver, whereas metastatic lesions are more often approximately the intensity of spleen.

Differential diagnosis therefore can be made reasonably accurate by considering the likelihood of the two lesions, given the patient's clinical history. Combining these likelihoods with those acquired from CT and/or MRI characteristics may yield likelihoods so strong as to be sufficient. However, if the clinical situation is such that an absolute diagnosis must be approached as closely as possible, CT-guided percutaneous biopsy may be required.

## Myelolipoma

These rare adrenal tumors are benign nonfunctioning neoplasms composed of mixtures of fat and myeloid tissue. They are usually asymptomatic, are most frequently diagnosed in the fourth to sixth decades of life, show no sex or lateralizing predilection, and do not metastasize. They may range from 2 to 3 cm in size to 12 cm or more. The proportion of fatty and myeloid tissues varies from tumor to tumor; rarely they may undergo internal hemorrhage or produce calcified regions.

CT reveals these masses to be well circumscribed. A proportion of the lesion may have attenuation values consistent with fat (−20 Hounsfield units or less). When fat is unequivocally identified within a lesion that clearly arises in the adrenal, the diagnosis of a myelolipoma can be made with certainty. Confusion may arise if the fatty regions are so small that they cannot be detected by CT. In this case the soft-tissue density of a myeloid tissue lesion does not permit specific diagnosis, and resection or histologic evaluation of a biopsy is necessary for a specific diagnosis. When fat is observed, it is usually possible to distinguish it from the low-attenuation tissue of an adenoma, since the latter virtually never is as lucent as −20 Hounsfield units. Difficulties may also arise in cases of infiltrating or hemorrhagic adrenal tumors of any type. These occasionally entrap small regions of retroperitoneal fat that may masquerade as fatty tumor tissue. Large myelolipomas may be difficult to distinguish from upper pole renal angiomyolipomas. Sagittal or coronal images obtained by MRI or ultrasonography may be necessary to make the distinction. Finally, differential diagnosis from retroperitoneal fatty tumors, such as liposarcomas arising near the adrenal, may be difficult.

Few of these lesions have been subjected to MRI evaluation. When the fatty regions of the tumor are sufficiently large to be visualized, MRI reveals the fat to be relatively bright on T1- (Fig. 8) as well as T2-weighted images. Care must be taken, however, not to mistake a region of hemorrhage, which may also appear relatively bright on T1-weighted and T2-weighted sequences, for fat. This distinction can be made because regions of hemorrhage are often brighter than fat on T2-weighted images, or by using fat-suppression sequences.

There are other highly unusual benign tumors of the adrenal. These consist of hemangiomas, which may demonstrate phleboliths when evaluated by CT, and fibromas, leiomyomas, and lipomas.

## Adrenal Cysts

Adrenal cysts are relatively rare lesions. They may appear at any age, and there seems to be a female predominance. They are often asymptomatic, but occasionally may be palpable or produce pain if they become large. They have been classified as endothelial (angiomatous or lymphangiomatous), epithelial, parasitic (primarily echinococcal) cysts and pseudocysts (which may represent old hematomas).

CT evaluations reveal adrenal cysts as looking like cysts encountered elsewhere in the body. They are usually thin walled; the wall occasionally calcifies, especially if the cysts are echinoccal in origin, and may enhance. The fluid within them is usually not greatly different in attenuation from water, but occasionally hemorrhage or proteinaceous debris may cause the fluid to be denser.

No large series of cysts evaluated by MRI has been reported. As with cysts elsewhere in the body, the fluid is usually low intensity on T1-weighted images and relatively bright on T2-weighted images.

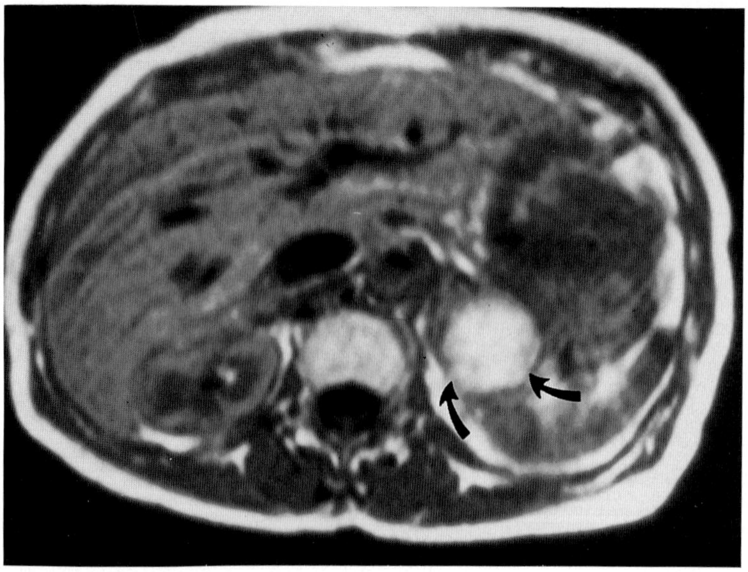

**FIGURE 8** T1-weighted MRI of left adrenal myelolipoma. The lesion (*arrows*) is slightly heterogeneous and is bright, approximating the intensity of normal fat.

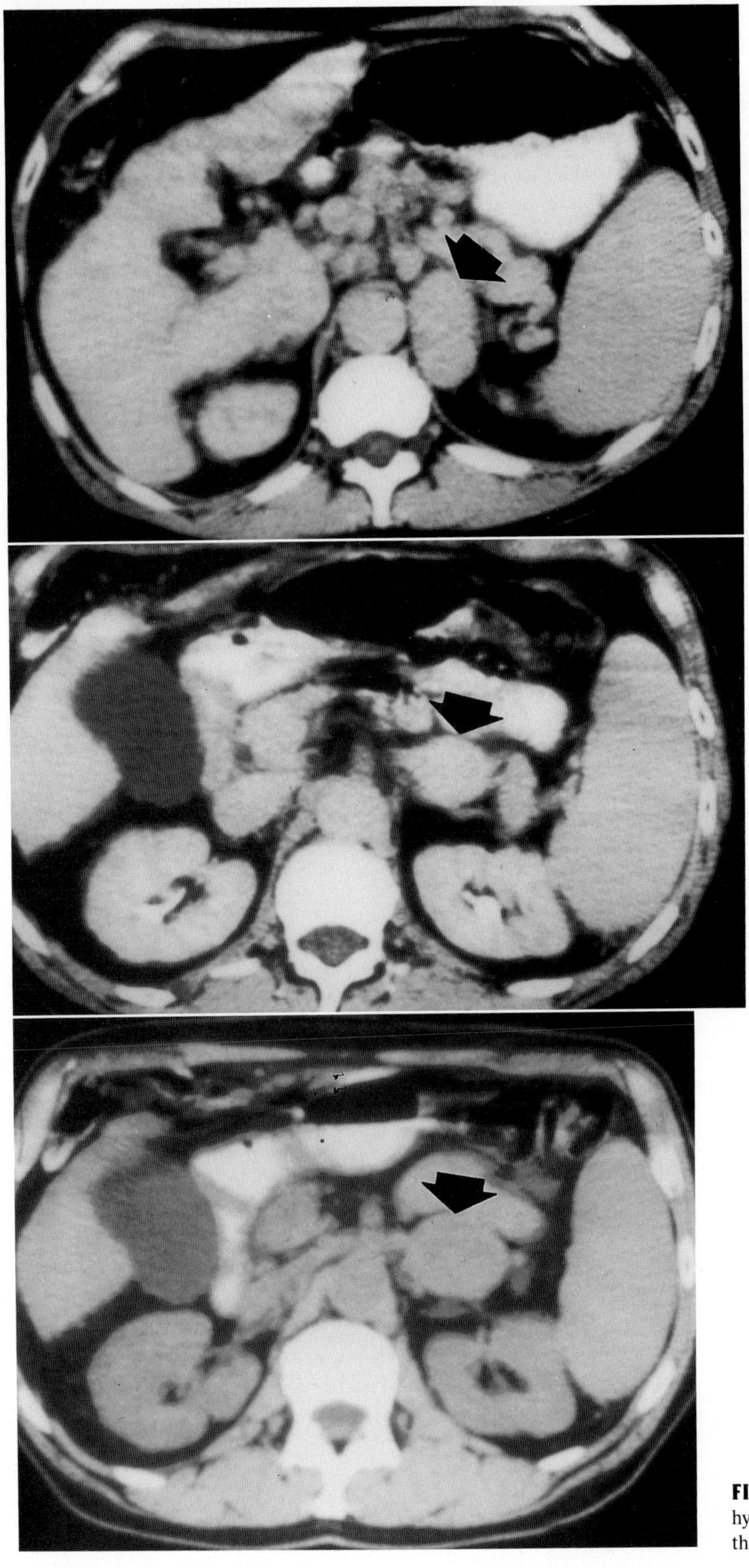

**FIGURE 9** CT of left adrenal varix in a patient with portal hypertension. The enlarged vein (*arrows*) extends inferiorly to the left renal vein.

## Adrenal Hemorrhage

Adrenal hemorrhage is more commonly encountered in neonates than in adults, but adult adrenal hemorrhage may occur under certain circumstances including major surgery, sepsis, widespread burns, hypotension, coagulopathies, or trauma. In the last case, there is a predilection for the right adrenal to be affected. Adrenal hemorrhage with adrenal insufficiency from meningococcemia occasionally occurs; this is called the Waterhouse-Friderichsen syndrome.

CT scans of adrenal hemorrhage reveal the adrenal to be enlarged; margins of the involved gland may be relatively crisp or, if the hematoma invades adjacent fat, irregular. Relatively early in the evolution of the hematoma, the blood may be of soft-tissue density or somewhat denser. Resolution of the hematoma may involve return of the adrenal gland to normal morphology, or the formation of a persistent pseudocyst with relatively low-density fluid in the center. MRI evaluation reveals the evolution of an adrenal hematoma to produce similar appearances to hematomas elsewhere in the body. Relatively early after the hemorrhage, the bloody fluid may appear bright on both T1- and T2-weighted images. Later, a bright ring with a darker center may appear, sometimes surrounded by a thin black line caused by hemosiderin at the margins of the lesions.

## Adrenal Vein Varices

An enlarged or vericeal adrenal vein may, when first encountered on an imaging evaluation, masquerade as an adrenal mass. Adrenal vein varices may be idiopathic or form as portosystemic shunts in patients with portal hypertension. In the latter case, the inferior phrenic and adrenal veins may be continuous with the splenic vein.

Distinction of varices from adrenal masses may be made by either MRI or CT (Fig. 9). MRI may reveal a flow void or other flow phenomenon within the structure, and CT may demonstrate the abnormality to be a vein if a rapid contrast bolus and dynamic scanning are performed.

## Suggested Reading

Amis ES Jr, Newhouse JH. The adrenal. In: Essentials of Uroradiology. Boston: Little, Brown, 1991:85.

Bosniak MA. Neoplasms of the adrenal medulla. In: Pollack HM, ed. Clinical Urography. Vol 3. Philadelphia: WB Saunders, 1990:2344.

Bosniak MA, Rumancik WM. Metastatic neoplasms to the adrenal glands and adrenal lymphoma. In: Pollack HM, ed. Clinical Urography. Vol 3. Philadelphia: WB Saunders, 1990:2388.

Doppman JL. Diseases of the adrenal cortex (causing hypofunction). In: Pollack HM, ed. Clinical Urography. Vol 3. Philadelphia: WB Saunders, 1990:2313.

Dunnick NR. Diseases of the adrenal cortex; hyperfunctioning and nonfunctioning neoplasms. In: Pollack HM, ed. Clinical Urography. Vol 3. Philadelphia: WB Saunders, 1990:2313.

Dunnick NR, McCallum RW, Sandler CM. The adrenal gland. In: Textbook of Uroradiology. Baltimore: Williams & Wilkins, 1991:254.

Korobkin M. Pheochromocytoma. In: Pollack HM, ed. Clinical Urography. Vol 3. Philadelphia: WB Saunders, 1990:2347.

Mitty HA. Adrenal embryology, anatomy and imaging techniques. In: Pollack HM, ed. Clinical Urography. Vol 3. Philadelphia: WB Saunders, 1990:2291.

Rumancik WM, Bosniak MA. Miscellaneous conditions of the adrenals and adrenal pseudotumors. In: Pollack HM, ed. Clinical Urography. Vol 3. Philadelphia: WB Saunders, 1990:2399.

# MUSCULOSKELETAL RADIOLOGY

## Musculoskeletal Ultrasonography

*JOHN F. MATHEWS, M.B., Ch.B.* · *RONALD S. ADLER, Ph.D., M.D.*

The development and dissemination of quality ultrasound equipment, with the capacity to achieve high-resolution images, has broadly paralleled the growth in interest in sports medicine. It is not surprising therefore that increased attention is being paid to imaging muscles, tendons, and other soft-tissue structures using this increased capability.

This chapter is intended as a general guide to principles employed in sonographic evaluation of the musculoskeletal system in adults, with emphasis placed on traumatic and inflammatory lesions. Special attention is paid to imaging of the adult shoulder, because this is a commonly requested evaluation requiring detailed knowledge of the relevant anatomy and potential pitfalls.

### Tendons

Our understanding of tendon pathology and nomenclature is still largely based on its historical development in which assessment is largely by clinical means. A tendon that develops focal tenderness on use, possibly clinically detectable swelling and pain on resisted active movement of the relevant muscle, has been traditionally called a tendonitis. We now know a variety of lesions can produce this picture, including tendonitis, tenosynovitis, bursitis, tears of the tendon or musculotendinous junction, and intramuscular hematoma. For the purposes of this chapter, terms are defined as follows. *Tendonitis* refers to focal or diffuse thickening of the tendon that may be associated with changes in internal organization. Although this terminology implies an active inflammatory component, histologic evaluation may reveal only mucoid degeneration, hyalinization, foci of necrosis, and microtrauma. Tendonitis can be associated with bursitis, and both may resolve with steroid injection of the involved bursa, suggesting that the tendon has been involved with secondary inflammatory changes. The term *tenosynovitis* is used to describe the condition of increased fluid within the synovial sheath of a tendon. This may be inflammatory, traumatic, or even infective. *Bursitis* refers to an abnormal quantity of fluid within the bursa, which unless hemorrhagic in origin is presumably associated with inflammation.

#### *Normal Appearances*

Tendons may be surrounded by a synovial sheath. This may not be apparent as a separate structure sonographically or appear as a thin hypoechoic region paralleling the tendon, presumably the small amount of synovial fluid normally present. This is typically 1 mm or less, although several authors accept up to a couple of millimeters. Tendons without a synovial sheath have a relatively dense connective tissue layer adherent to them, the epitendineum. This is brightly echogenic and sharply demarcates the tendon. The tendon itself consists of dense connective tissue in which collagen fibrils are arranged in bundles surrounded by loose connective tissue. These bundles are further arranged in a parallel linear fashion (Fig. 1). The resultant gray-scale ultrasound image reflects this anatomic configuration by displaying marked anisotropy; the tendon is remarkably echogenic when scanned perpendicular to its long axis with a linear array transducer. Reduction of the angle by as little as 2° to 7° produces isoechogenicity relative to muscle, and further reduction produces hypoechogenicity (Fig. 2). It is this fact that makes a linear array transducer so useful for imaging tendons and makes assessment of echogenicity in a curving tendon (e.g., the shoulder) so difficult. Alternatively use of a sector scanner, in which only a small portion of the central beam falls within this angular range, results in a hypoechoic appearance in the more peripheral parts of the tendon. Because of its fibrillar nature, the tendon is not

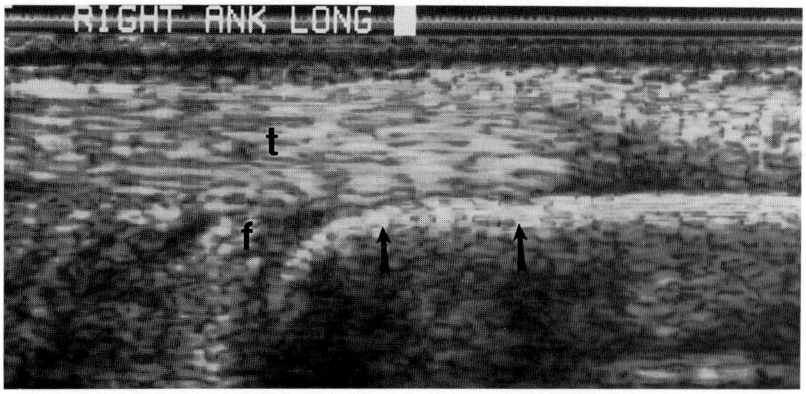


**FIGURE 1** Normal Achilles tendon. Sagittal sonogram obtained over the distal right Achilles tendon. The echogenic fibrillar nature of the tendon (t) is evident. The adjacent retrocalcaneal fat (f) has a more speckled appearance. The posterior calcaneal surface forms a strong specular reflector (*arrows*).

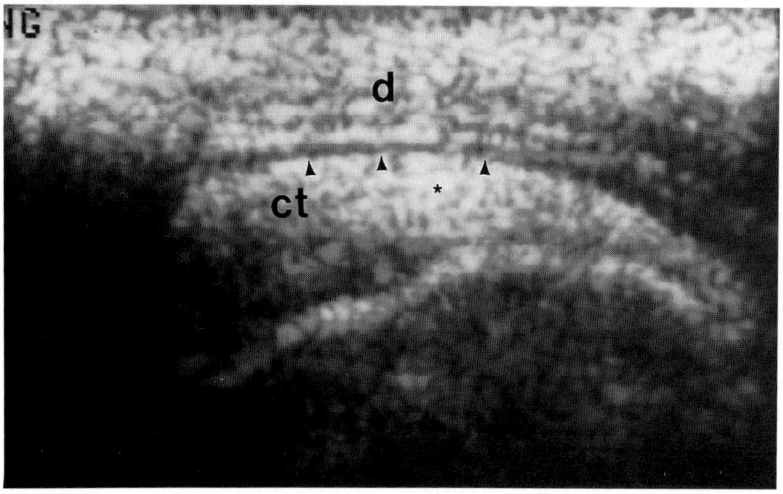


**FIGURE 2** Normal supraspinatus tendon. Oblique coronal scan over the shoulder. The subdeltoid bursa appears as a thin hypoechoic band (*arrowheads*) situated between the normal convex tendon (ct) and the overlying deltoid muscle (d). The tendon appears more echogenic centrally (*) as a result of the inherent tendon curvature relative to the transducer.

diffusely echogenic but appears as a series of echogenic parallel linear bands. These features make tendons easy to recognize ultrasonographically. Nerves can display a similar appearance but are easily differentiated on real-time evaluation while the appropriate muscle is exercised. The movement of the tendon is usually obvious.

At the insertion of a tendon, the parallel bundles of collagen give way to fibrocartilage. This usually images as a hypoechoic structure (e.g., the insertion of the Achilles tendon). However, such attachments are not always hypoechoic. The origin of the extensor tendons of the elbow appears hyperechoic.

Because of their close relation anatomically and functionally, bursae are discussed here. A bursa refers to a synovial lined structure that normally contains a small amount of fluid. Some bursae appear as saclike extensions of the joint on arthrography (e.g., the subscapular bursa). Others are present in areas of potential friction between a tendon and adjacent structures, and they can develop adventitiously at pressure points, apparently in response to the development of friction or pressure. When evident, their normal ultrasonographic appearance is a linear or crescentic hypoechoic band, usually 1 mm or less. They may display a hyperechoic boundary.

## *Pathological Findings*

### Tendonitis

Tendonitis can be diffuse or nodular. A diffuse tendonitis is visualized sonographically as diffuse thickening and hypoechogenicity of the tendon. Measurements of various tendons have been suggested, but it must be remembered that gender, size, and training contribute to tendon thickness and the final arbiter often relies on comparison with the opposite side. Edema and possibly increased ground substance within the tendon may increase the distance between the fascicles, and the echogenicity may be decreased on this basis. The tendon may lose its normal sharp outline, displaying indistinct margins (Fig. 3).

Focal tendonitis displays localized areas of thickening and hypoechogenicity (Fig. 4). Sometimes discrete hypoechoic clefts are present across which the linear echogenic bands cannot be traced. It seems a moot point whether these constitute tiny intratendinous tears or degenerative changes with focal necrosis; either condition would be expected to be associated with increased risk of rupture. We are not aware, however, of any data quantitating rupture risk in such patients with respect to the size of the apparent discontinuity.

A chronic tendonitis may slowly calcify. Alternatively patients can present with acute pain and focal tenderness in a previously asymptomatic lesion, and have a focal deposit of calcium at the site of tenderness. Calcium can be present in asymptomatic tendons. Calcification is easily recognized sonographically when it appears as a discrete echogenic area with posterior acoustic shadowing; an apparent discontinuity in the underlying cortex can be helpful (Fig. 5). Alternatively posterior shadowing is not always present, and the calcification may appear as an amorphous echogenic mass.

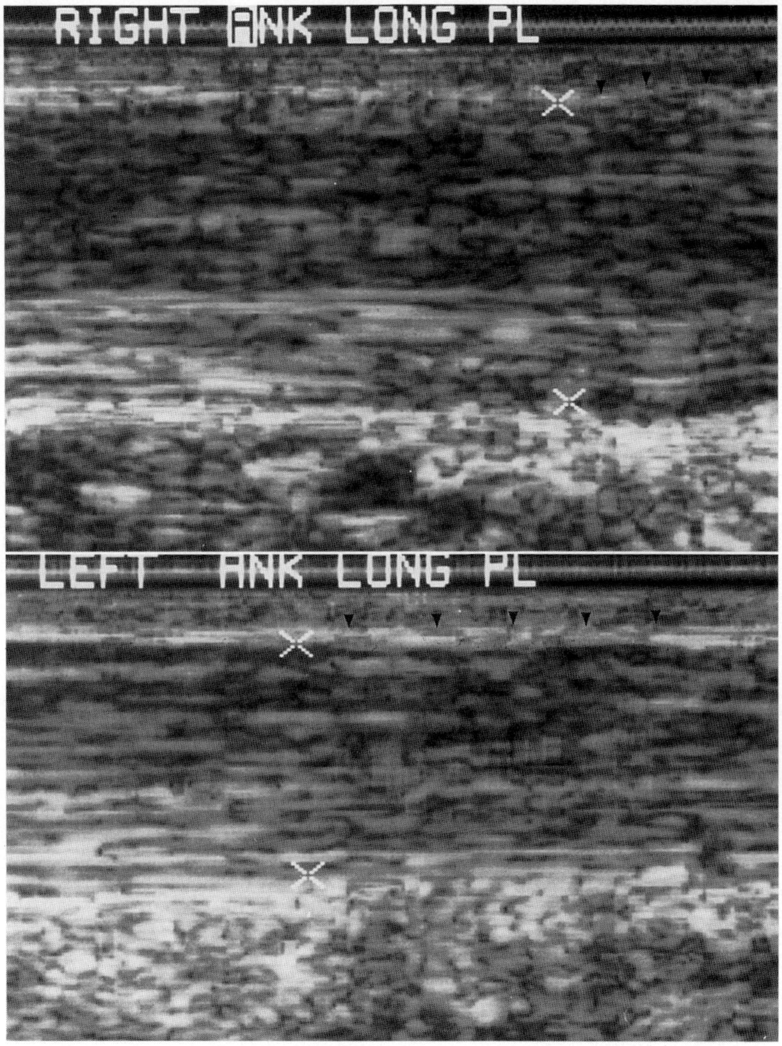


A

B

**FIGURE 3** Peroneus longus tendonitis. Coronal scans over the lateral aspect of each ankle. *A,* The peroneus longus tendon on the symptomatic right side is enlarged, measuring 8.5 mm in diameter, and is mildly heterogeneous with slightly indistinct margins (*arrowheads*). *B,* The asymptomatic left peroneus longus tendon measures 6 mm in diameter with greater uniformity in its fibrillar appearance. Compare the distinct margins (*arrowheads*) with (*A*).

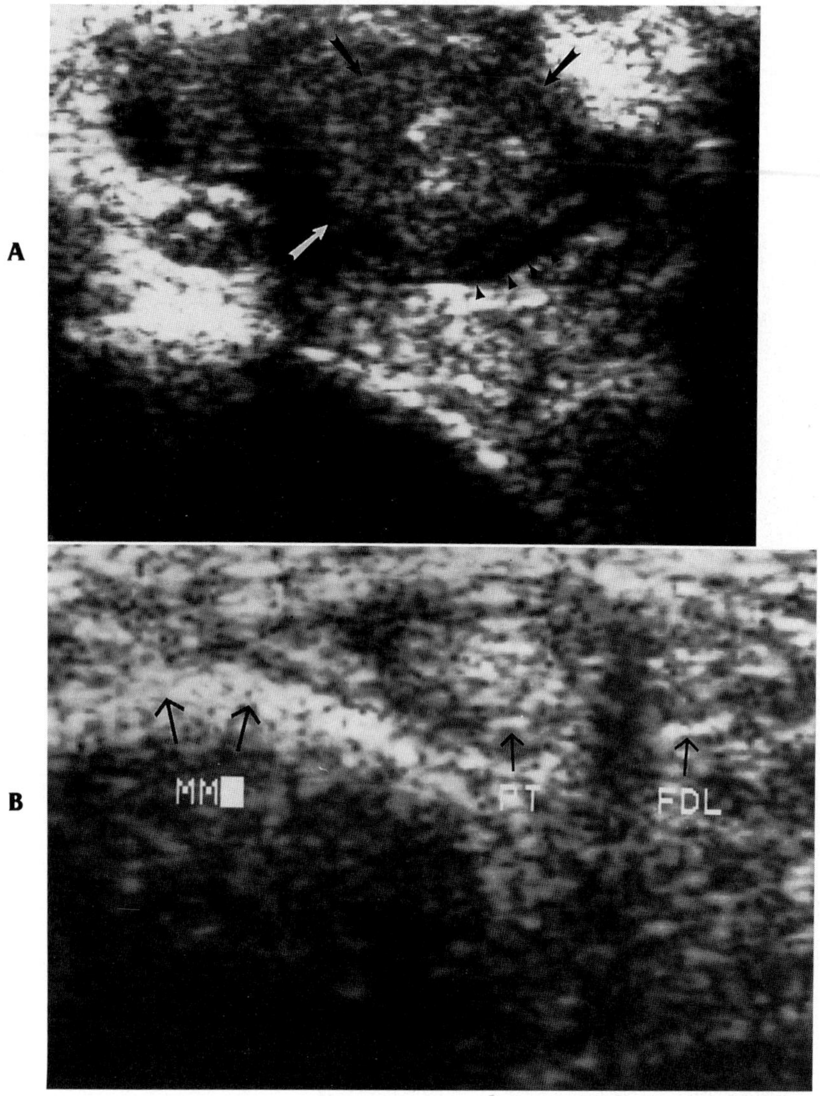


**FIGURE 4** Chronic tibialis posterior tendonitis. *A,* Transverse section at the level of the medial malleolus. The tibialis posterior tendon is markedly enlarged and hypoechoic (*arrows*). There is adjacent fluid (*arrowheads*) within the distended tendon sheath. *B,* Comparison section of the unaffected side shows the normal size and echogenicity of the tendon. MM = medial malleolus; PT = tibialis posterior tendon; FDL = flexor digitorum longus tendon.

### Tenosynovitis

An acute tenosynovitis is observed as a pathological quantity of fluid within the sheath of an otherwise sonographically normal tendon. This may be secondary to inflammation, infection, acute trauma, or in the case of the biceps tendon, caused by an effusion within the joint. A chronic tenosynovitis may be associated with diffuse synovial thickening and secondary inflammation of the tendon, which appears thickened and hypoechoic.

### Tendon Rupture

Complete rupture is easily recognized in the acute phase both clinically and sonographically. The tendon retracts, and the gap between the retracted ends is filled with hematoma, producing complex echoes. The relevant muscle may contract to produce a masslike lesion. The tendon itself may appear diffusely thickened, heterogeneous, and nodular in contour (Fig. 6).

Partial rupture is similar in that there is a discontinuity in the parallel linear echoes of the tendon, with the gap filled by material of variable, but usually decreased, echogenicity. This is generally easier to detect in tendons that have a course perpendicular to the beam over long intervals, thus explaining one of the difficulties in imaging tears in the shoulder. Because of the number of intact fibrils, there can be only minimal retraction in a partial tear. This is manifested as a contour deformity or focal thinning (Fig. 7), a particularly helpful sign in the shoulder.

### Bursitis

Distention of a bursa with fluid is described as bursitis, unless the bursa communicates with the joint and the fluid is secondary to an effusion. In this way the distended gastrocnemius/semimembranosus bursa is not thought of as bursitis but is given the title of Baker's cyst. Such distended bursae are perhaps best thought of as synovial cysts. In acute bursitis the fluid is anechoic. With chronicity, infection, hemorrhage or if due to rheumatoid disease, low-level echoes, septations, and nodular masses may be identified (Fig. 8). Chronic bursitis may contain calcification, producing hyperechoic foci with shadowing.

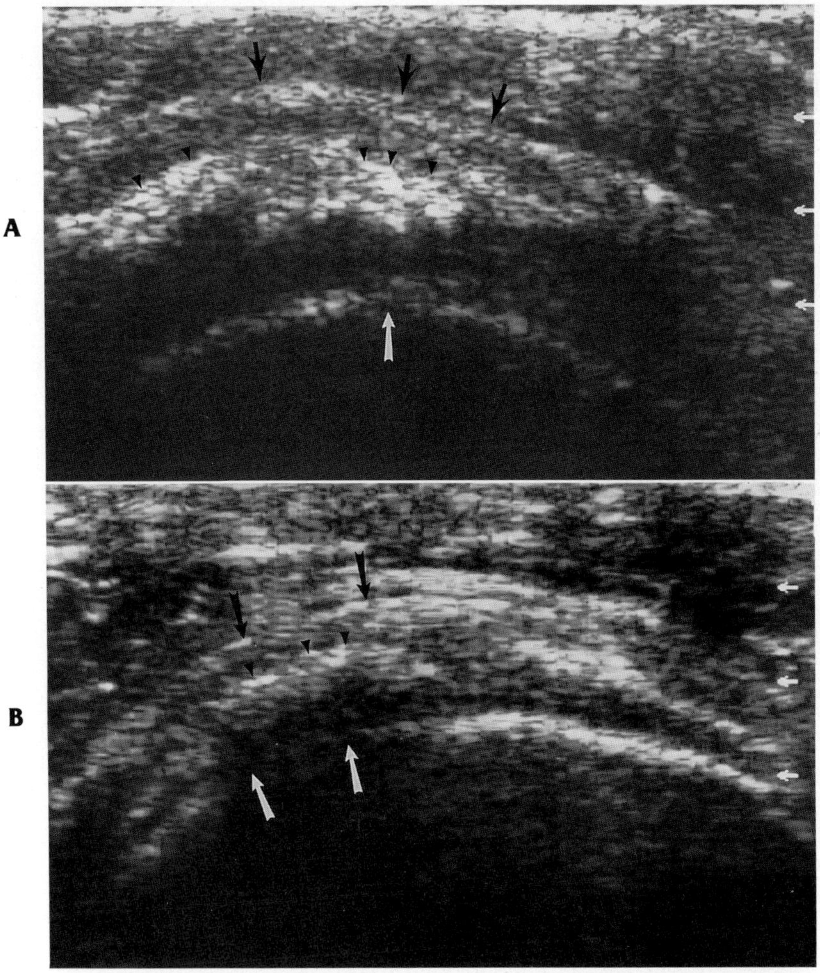


**FIGURE 5** Calcific tendonitis in supraspinatus. *A,* Sagittal section of the left supraspinatus tendon depicts it as enlarged, hypoechoic, and containing centrally amorphous nodular calcification. Arrows = thickened tendon; arrowheads = foci of calcification; white arrows = partial shadowing of cortical margin of humerus. *B,* Sagittal section of the right supraspinatus tendon. This side was asymptomatic. Arrows = supraspinatus tendon; arrowheads = heavy deposit of calcium. Note the complete obliteration of the cortical margin of the humerus by posterior shadowing (*white arrows*).

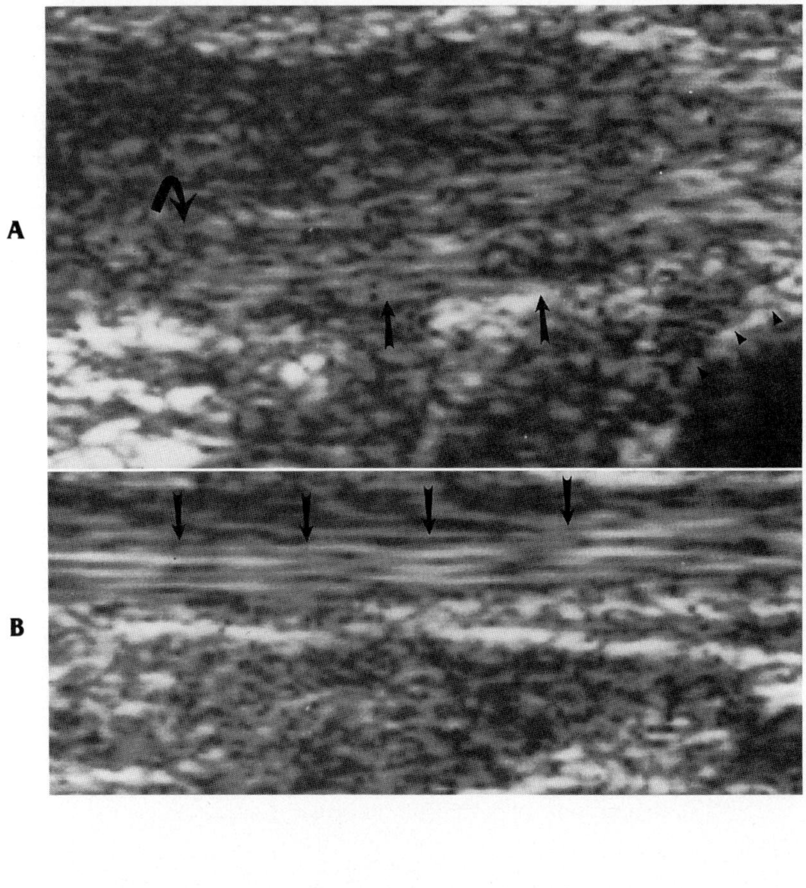


**FIGURE 6** Tendon rupture. *A,* Longitudinal section of the Achilles tendon (*arrows*). Note the separation of fibrils when compared with normal (*B*) and complete discontinuity of fibrils (*curved arrow*). The tendon is thickened, buckled, and displays indistinct margins. Arrowheads = calcaneal cortex. *B,* Note the fibrillar structure of the normal tendon for comparison (*arrows*).

A

B

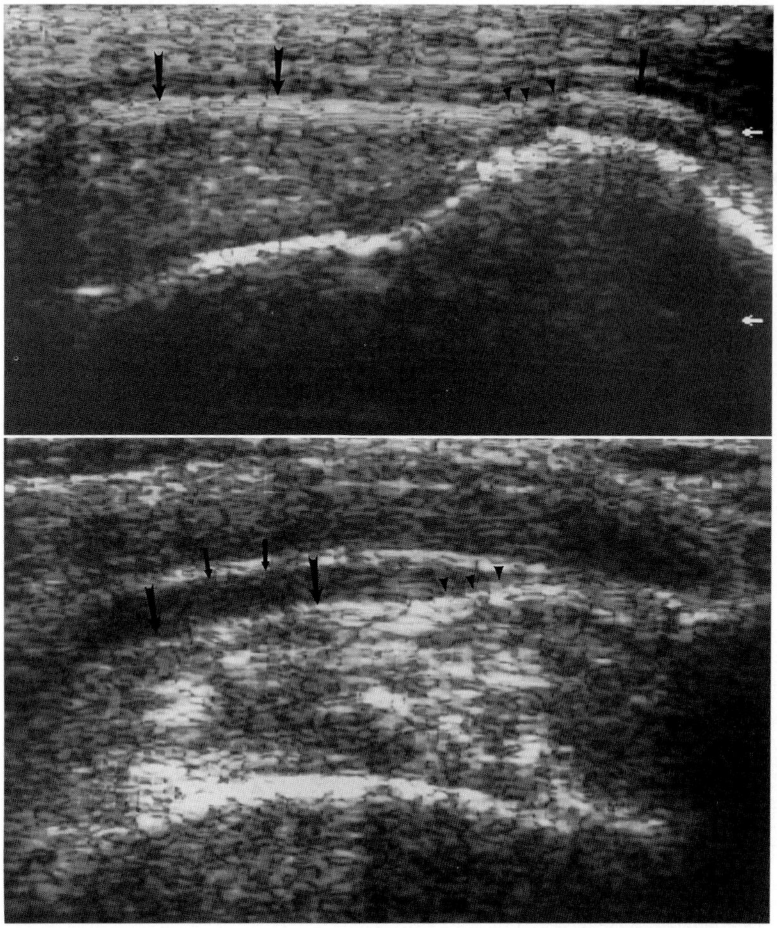

**FIGURE 7** Tendon tears without retraction (partial tears). *A,* Coronal section of the right supraspinatus tendon (*arrows*). Note the focal contour deformity *(arrowheads)* along the outer margin of the tendon, near its insertion. The tendon should be smoothly convex. *B,* Transverse image of the supraspinatus tendon (*arrows*) in a different patient. Note the contour deformity (*arrowheads*), fluid in the subacromial/subdeltoid bursa (*small arrows*), and the heterogeneous tendon echogenicity and thickening. The tear was confirmed at arthrography.

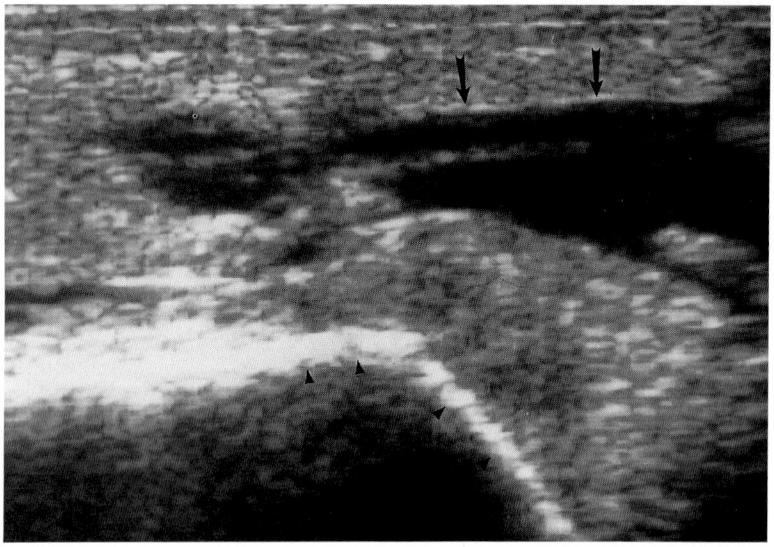

**FIGURE 8** Bursitis. Longitudinal image of the elbow. A fluid collection (*arrows*) is demonstrated in the expected position of the olecranon bursa, superficial to the triceps insertion. Arrowheads = cortex of ulna (olecranon).

## Muscles

Normal muscle is hypoechoic on gray-scale ultrasound imaging. The fibroadipose septa are identified as relatively bright dots if imaged in cross section and as echogenic lines if imaged longitudinally.

### *Pathological Findings*

#### Trauma

This is by far the most common pathology of muscle imaged by ultrasonography. The two basic mechanisms of injury are compression and forceful muscular contraction across an

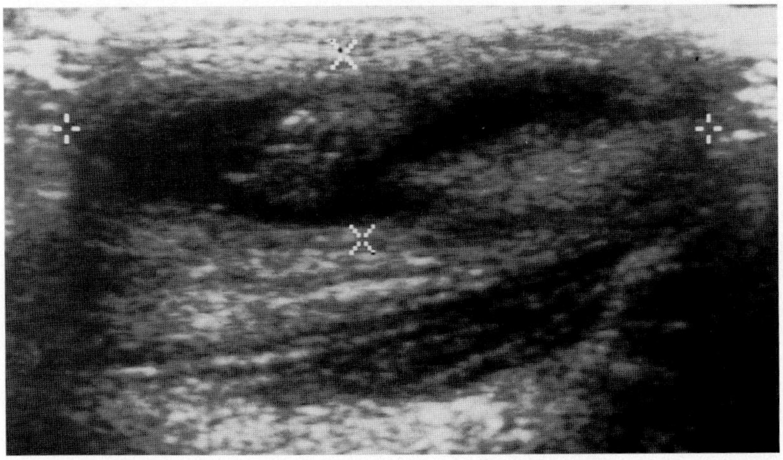

**FIGURE 9** Intramuscular hematoma. Longitudinal scan of the right deltoid. A complex fluid collection (within cursors) is observed within the deltoid muscle. This hematoma followed a direct blow.

immobilized joint. Compression forces can produce diffuse infiltrative hematoma, resulting in diffuse enlargement without a focal collection of blood. Blood can also dissect between muscles, producing a fusiform hematoma (Fig. 9). Further force produces blood-filled cavities within the muscle, secondary to bleeding, direct rupture, and necrosis. Similar changes may be observed in adjacent muscles that may or may not have the same action. When large, these lesions display an irregular cavity with shaggy borders. The sonographic appearance is dominated by the hematoma and follows typical evolutionary changes with time. Initially the blood is hypoechoic but clots within several hours producing internal echogenicity and possibly fluid levels. By 48 to 72 hours the hematoma is anechoic.

Distraction injuries differ in that the hematoma is confined usually to a single muscle and torn fragments of muscle are more likely to be identified within the cavity, producing the "bell-clapper" sign.

Ultrasonography can be useful to assess healing of these lesions. The cavity gradually decreases in size, and hypoechoic granulation tissue in the margins of the cavity advances to fill in the defect. Eventually organization can be demonstrated with the reappearance of fibroadipose septa. It has been stated that recommencement of activity before organization is associated with a worse functional outcome and reinjury.

#### Chronic Injuries

A scar within muscle is brightly echogenic. Myositis ossificans can be diagnosed on ultrasonography before the characteristic appearances are visible radiographically. A "triple zone" phenomenon is said to be diagnostic and consists of a thin echo-poor zone surrounding a broader, more reflective zone with an amorphous echo-poor zone centrally. With progressive mineralization, acoustic shadowing develops. A persistent cyst is a rare complication of muscle hemorrhage.

#### Miscellaneous

Other muscle disorders are less commonly imaged. Pyomyositis appears as a complex collection within the muscle. The presence of punctate echogenic foci, with associated "dirty" shadowing in the nondependent portions of the collection, may indicate a gas-forming organism. Although malignant fasciculations may be evident on real-time evaluation, ultrasonography has generally been disappointing when applied to neuromuscular disease. Grossly abnormal areas are evident, so that ultrasonography may be helpful in localizing areas for biopsy.

## Joints

### *Normal Appearances*

Collateral ligaments are hyperechoic and relatively homogeneous; these lack the fibrillar appearance typical of tendons. The subchondral bone is a strong specular reflector, with the overlying articular cartilage presenting as a thin hypoechoic band, typically 2 to 3 mm thick. The ability to which the latter may be visualized depends largely on acoustic access, as well as other overlying structures (e.g., subcutaneous fat) that may distort the beam. Synovial fluid may measure at maximum 2 to 3 mm in a dependent recess.

### *Pathological Findings*

#### Joint Effusions

Perhaps the most widely used application of ultrasonography in evaluation of joint disease is that of the infant hip. This is discussed elsewhere and will not be reviewed here. Effusions are easily detected sonographically (Figs. 10 and 11). This reflects both the exquisite sensitivity of ultrasonography in detection of fluid collections and the tendency for effusions to be many times the volume of fluid normally found within the joint. The presence of low-level echoes, septations, or solid material within the joint fluid may suggest infection, hemarthrosis, or other noninfective inflammatory debris such as fibrin. Fine echoes within the fluid can be observed following intra-articular corticosteroid administration. An anechoic effusion does not necessarily imply a simple synovial collection, and although its exact incidence is not well documented, infection can not be excluded in such a case. Similarly, differentiating the various causes of a complex effusion is not usually possible based on sonographic appearances alone. The major usefulness of ultrasonography in these circumstances is the demonstration of an effusion and to provide localization for aspiration. If a prosthesis is in place, ultrasonography may be the only modality to demonstrate the nature and extent of fluid, because both computed tomography (CT) and magnetic resonance imaging (MRI) are limited by artifact (see Fig. 11). Osteochondral bodies are usually suggested by their sharp definition and shape. If ossified, there is posterior shadowing.

Proliferation and edema of the synovium are most prominent in the pannus of rheumatoid arthritis, but a similar appearance can be observed in other inflammatory arthritides (Fig. 12), chronic infections, pigmented villonodular synovitis,

A

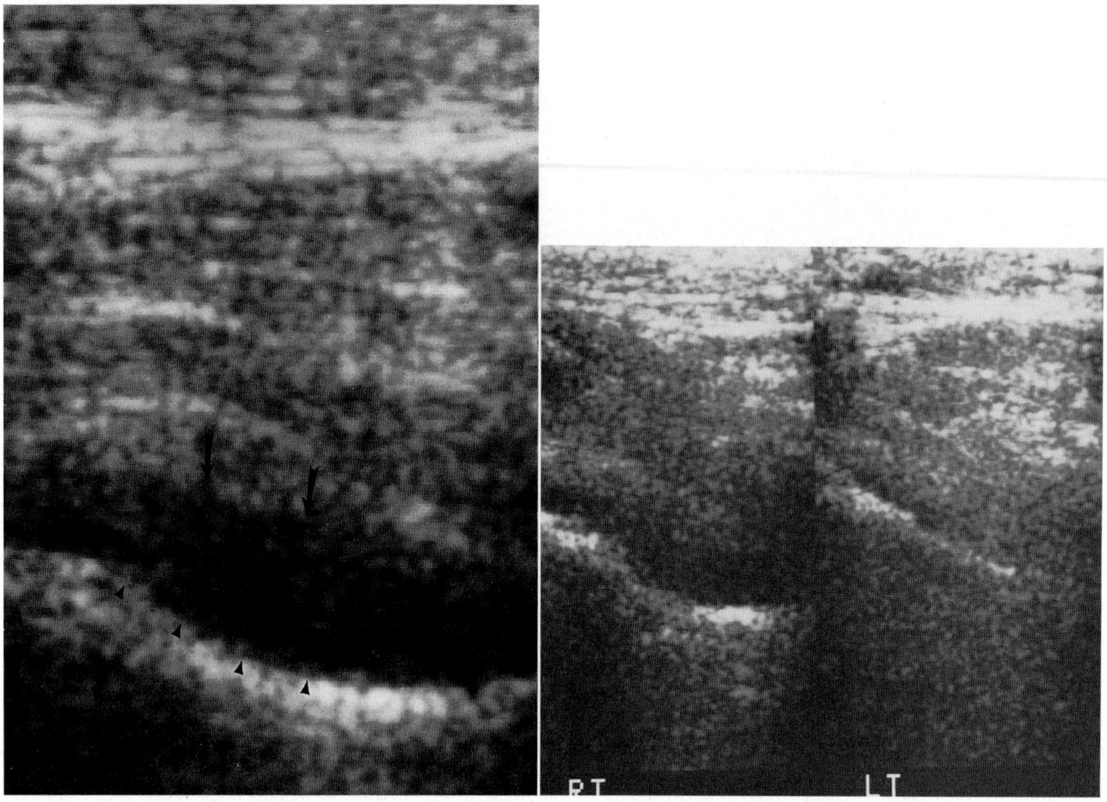


B

**FIGURE 10** Joint effusion. *A,* Longitudinal scan of the right hip. A complex fluid collection (*arrows*) distends the joint capsule. Arrowheads = femoral cortex. Ultrasound-guided aspiration made the diagnosis of septic arthritis. *B,* Same patient as in (*A*). Similar views of the right and left hips have been juxtaposed for comparison.

A

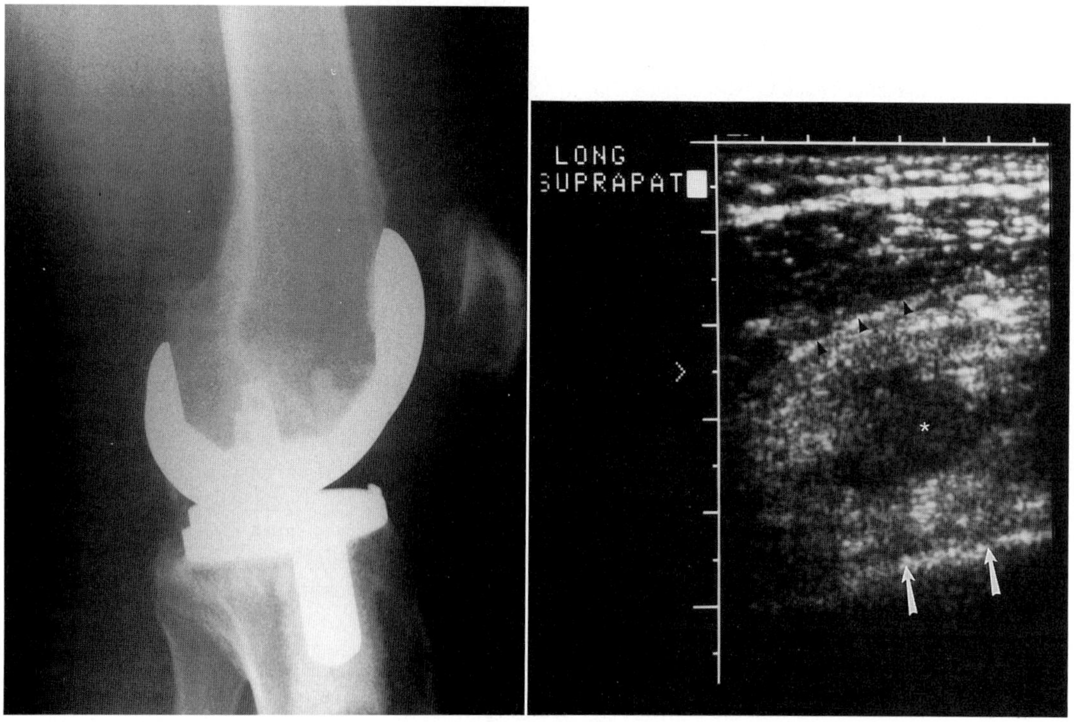


B

**FIGURE 11** Septic joint, postarthroplasty. *A,* Radiograph following right knee replacement. *B,* Same patient, longitudinal scan of the suprapatella region. The quadriceps muscle (*arrowheads*) is bowed by a complex purulent collection (*). Arrows = femoral cortex.

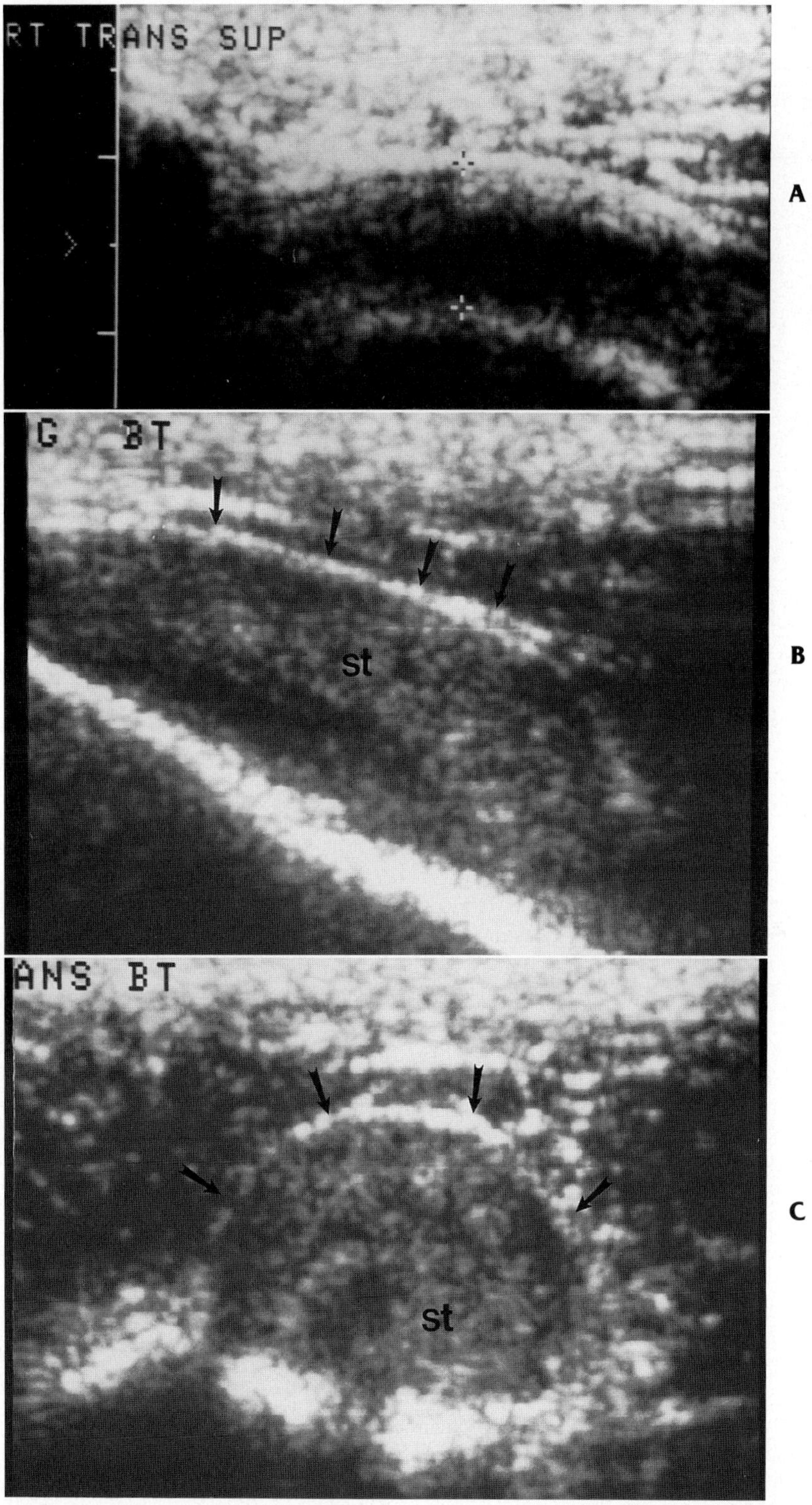


**FIGURE 12** Follow-up in proliferative tenosynovitis. *A,* Sagittal image through an enlarged hypoechoic supraspinatus tendon. Longitudinal *(B)* and transverse (*C*) scans through the biceps tendon sheath showing grossly proliferative synovium (st) distending the sheath (*arrows*). The tendon appears ill-defined and hypoechoic. The patient was a young man with a seronegative arthropathy.

*Continued.*

D

E

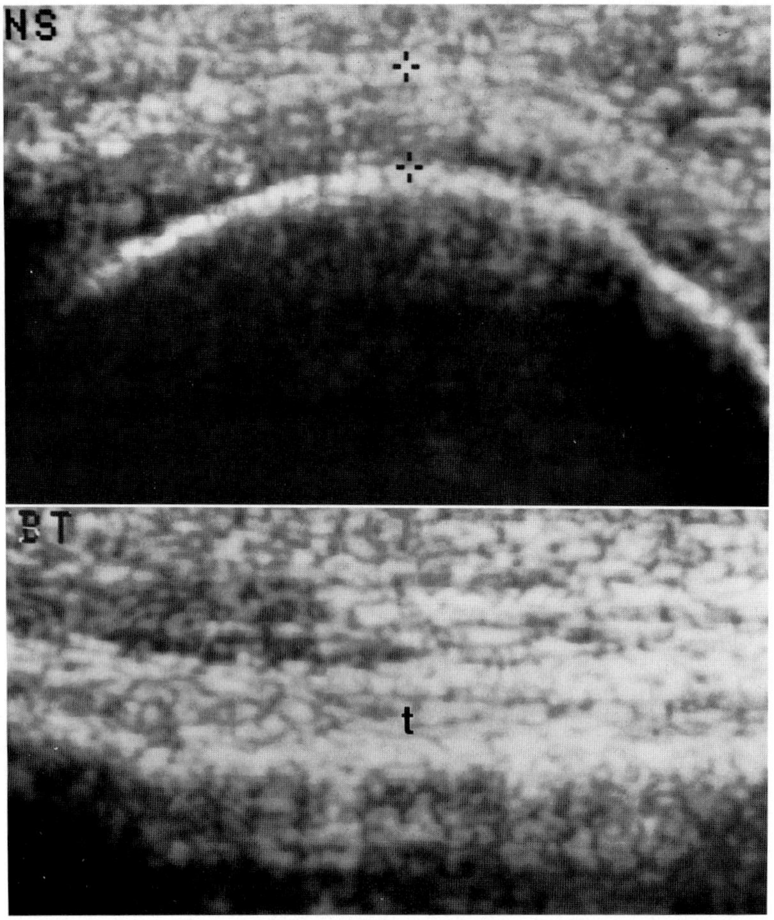


**FIGURE 12, cont'd** *D,* Sagittal image through the supraspinatus following treatment (compare with *[A]*). *E,* Longitudinal image through biceps tendon (t) following treatment (compare with *[B]*). The tendons have resumed a normal size and echotexture.

synovial osteochondromatosis, and amyloid. Hemophilia might also be expected to produce a similar picture. The synovium in these cases is markedly hypoechoic.

## Synovial Cysts

Special mention is made here of the fluid-filled gastrocnemius-semimembranosus bursa, referred to as a Baker's cyst, because this is the most frequently studied synovial cyst. The clinical presentation is usually that of a mass behind the knee in a child (Fig. 13) or adult with degenerative disease or rheumatoid arthritis. The key to diagnosis is the demonstration of communication with the joint. The cystic mass usually extends superficial to gastrocnemius, but especially in rheumatoid disease, may extend in a deep plane between gastrocnemius and soleus. The neck of the bursa should be identifiable between the gastrocnemius and semimembranosus tendons. With rupture of the cyst, fluid may be identified extending along the fascial planes. Cyst contents are highly variable, depending on etiologic factors and superimposed complications (e.g., infection, hemorrhage).

Synovial cysts can be observed in many other locations and in association with other arthropathies. The palpable mass can be so hard that clinically it may be confused with bone. Ultrasonography is ideal for evaluation of such a mass, demonstrating its cystic nature and enabling a firm diagnosis by demonstrating communication with the joint. Differentiation of these from other cystic masses (e.g., meniscal or ganglion cysts) may sometimes be difficult. The availability of duplex and color-flow Doppler in many real-time units allows one to distinguish between transmitted and arterial pulsations in the case of a pseudoaneurysm.

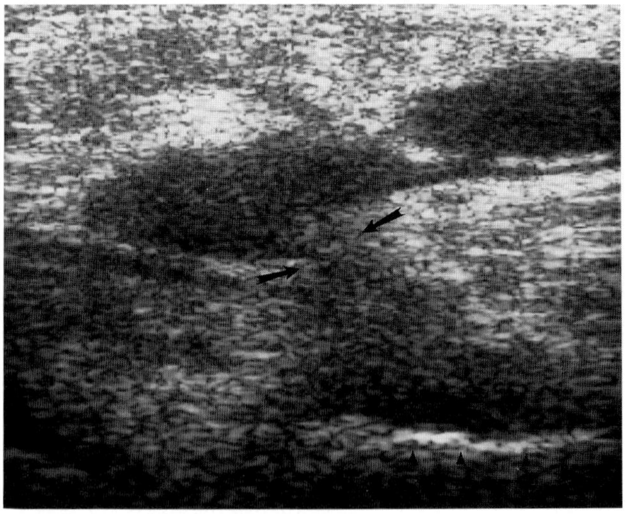

**FIGURE 13** Baker's cyst in a child. Longitudinal image of the posterior knee joint. Note the communication of the fluid collection via a narrow neck (*arrows*) with the knee joint. Arrowheads = tibial cortex.

## Intra-articular Structures

As the range of motion of a joint increases, the amount of cartilage that can be evaluated increases. The potential use of

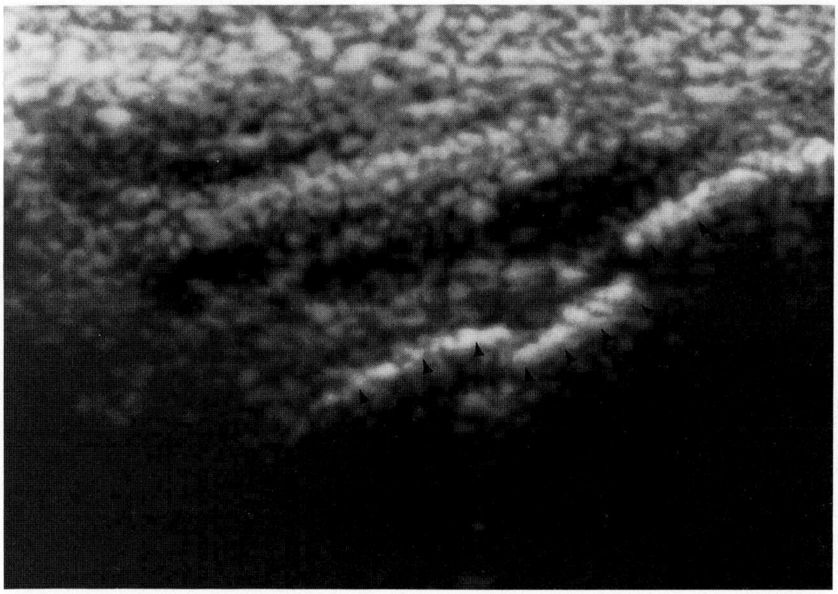

**FIGURE 14** Shoulder trauma. Coronal scan of the shoulder demonstrates cortical discontinuity, with slight depression of a central fragment in the humeral head. Arrowheads = humeral cortex.

ultrasonography in the evaluation of early degenerative change, osteochondral fractures, and osteochondritis dissecans has been described. Such indications have not found widespread clinical acceptance and have not formed an established part of our practice of musculoskeletal ultrasonography. Similar comments apply to the assessment of menisci and the cruciate ligaments in the knee and the triangular fibrocartilage in the wrist.

#### Extra-articular Structures

The assessment of collateral ligaments with ultrasonography is well described, particularly the collateral ligaments of the knee and ankle. Similar criteria for tears pertain here as are applied to tendons, although the ligaments are not as easily identifiable as tendons, and a thorough knowledge of the expected anatomy is required. A complete rupture is demonstrated as ligamentous discontinuity with hematoma between the torn ends and in the surrounding tissue. A partial tear may only show focal thickening as will a chronic tear with granulation tissue at the site of discontinuity.

## Bones

### *Normal Appearances*

The cortical margin of bone is essentially a total specular reflector with acoustic shadowing posteriorly, preventing imaging of the underlying medullary bone. The normal periosteum is closely adherent to bone and is not normally visible as a separate structure.

### *Pathological Findings*

#### Infection

Ultrasonography has been shown to be a sensitive modality in the detection of osteomyelitis. Inflammatory exudate elevating the periosteum, periosteal edema, and/or inflammation of the adjacent soft tissue may be detected well before there are plain film changes. The periosteum becomes visible as a brightly echogenic line separated from the bone by the hypoechoic fluid. Direct contiguity of the bone and fluid is an important differentiating point from other soft-tissue collections, where soft tissue separates the fluid and the bone. Hematoma, joint effusion, and rarely tumor can produce a similar appearance. Again the ability of ultrasonography to guide aspiration is invaluable.

#### Trauma

Because of its tomographic nature and ability to image in any plane, cortical discontinuity in a subtle or previously unrecognized fracture may occasionally be well observed on ultrasonograms. It is unlikely that ultrasonography is more sensitive than radiography in detection of acute fractures. However, if imaged incidentally, a fracture should be recognized (Fig. 14).

#### Tumor

The characteristic appearances of an aneurysmal bone cyst on cross-sectional imaging have been described on ultrasonograms when the cortex is sufficiently thinned to allow beam penetration. However, the specificity of fluid-fluid levels has been questioned recently, and ultrasonography finds little use in the assessment of tumors. One possible exception is the assessment of cartilage thickness on an osteochondroma, since increasing thickness correlates with malignancy. The soft-tissue extension of tumor at sites of cortical disruption may be evaluated, but as with other modalities, separation of tumor from the secondary inflammation that it may elicit may be difficult.

#### Inflammatory Disease

Erosions are well demonstrated as areas of cortical discontinuity on ultrasonograms (Fig. 15), and in a bone with a complex surface such as the shoulder, ultrasonography can show erosions with greater sensitivity than radiography. The clinical utility of this is unclear, but again, if imaged incidentally, erosions should be recorded.

### *Soft-Tissue Masses*

The major role of sonography in evaluating soft-tissue masses remains that of differentiating cystic versus solid lesions. Although some soft-tissue masses have a characteristic appear-

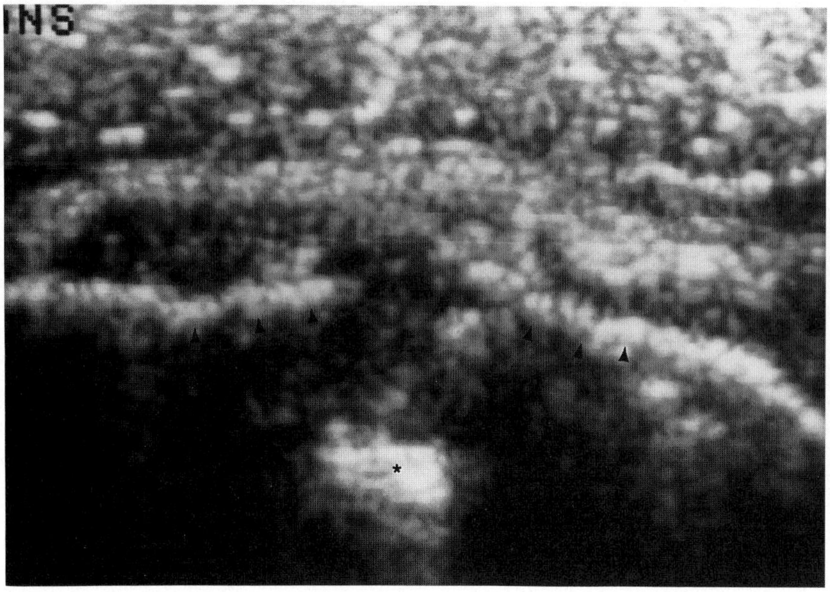


**FIGURE 15** Erosions. Sagittal scans of the shoulder demonstrate an erosion in an acute exacerbation of a seronegative arthropathy. This is manifested as discontinuity of the cortex with enhancement in the marrow space (✻). Arrowheads = humeral cortex.

A

B

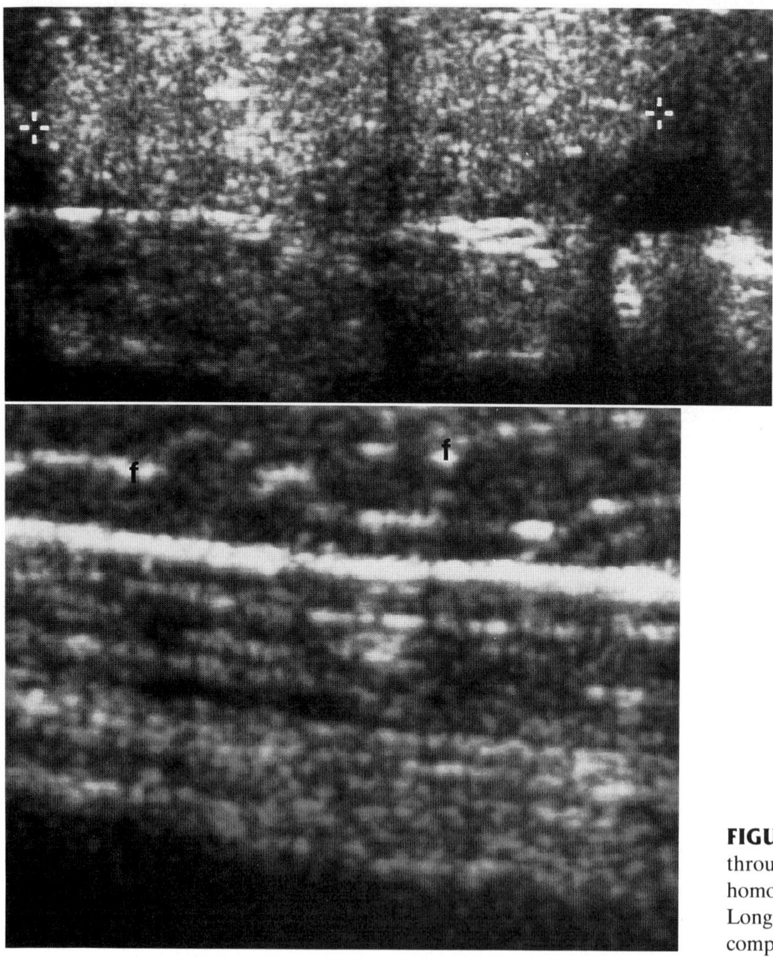


**FIGURE 16** Lipoma. *A,* Longitudinal scan through a lipoma (between cursors). Note the homogeneous diffusely increased echo texture. *B,* Longitudinal scan over the contralateral arm for comparison shows the normal subcutaneous fat (f).

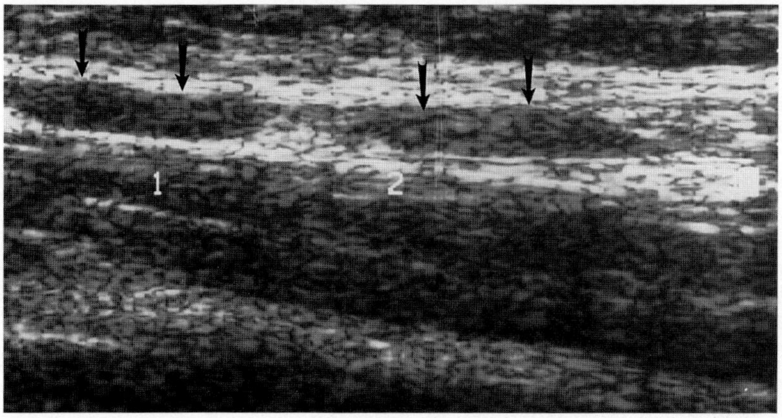

**FIGURE 17** Multiple neurofibromata in a patient with neurofibromatosis. Longitudinal scan along the length of the ulna nerve displays fusiform expansion of the nerve by hypoechoic masses (*arrows*).

ance, in general a tissue diagnosis is not possible. Lipomas (Fig. 16), for example, are circumscribed, diffusely echogenic, and easily deformable. Occasionally the direct contiguity of a mass with a nerve sheath can be demonstrated and be a pointer toward neurofibroma or schwannoma (Fig. 17). As is true with fluid collections, ultrasonography provides a simple and direct means of guidance for aspiration of these lesions.

### *Foreign Bodies*

Foreign bodies are echogenic, usually linear structures that may show a comet-tail artifact. This application is especially useful if the foreign body is radiolucent.

## General Principles of Technique

Many of the principles basic to ultrasound imaging elsewhere are of even more importance in musculoskeletal ultrasonography. The highest-frequency probe available that provides adequate penetration to image the area of interest should be employed. A 7.5 MHz probe is adequate for most purposes. For imaging of deep structures, or in obese patients, a 5 MHz or even a 3.5 MHz probe may be appropriate. It is important that the object of interest lies within the focal zone of the chosen transducer. Gain settings should provide an adequate level of echoes without excessive noise and be approximately even in imaged echo intensity over the field. When imaging an extremely superficial structure, the use of an acoustic standoff is helpful. The 10 MHz probe can be useful for superficial structures, but in practice adds little to musculoskeletal sonography and the small field of view is somewhat limiting. Muscle and tendons are best imaged with a linear array transducer, in part because of the anisotropy of tendons discussed earlier, and in part because of the greater field of view in the superficial region.

When performing the evaluation, remember the following principles:

1. The markedly anisotropic nature of tendons. This has already been discussed, but cannot be emphasized too strongly. Loss of anisotropy in an appropriately scanned tendon is an indicator of pathology.
2. Musculoskeletal ultrasonography is a dynamic evaluation. If in doubt about an abnormality, and even if not, view it in multiple planes, from different positions, and in different extremes of motion.
3. Know the normal anatomy. Even what seems to be a reasonable knowledge of anatomy can prove inadequate when confronted by the unfamiliar planes of a dynamic evaluation. Comparison with the asymptomatic side can be invaluable.
4. Analyze appropriate radiographs before beginning the ultrasonographic study. Plain films often provide useful correlation with the ultrasonographic appearances.

## The Shoulder

Specific mention is made of the shoulder, because it is among the most difficult joints to image well using ultrasonography, and this may contribute to the wide range of reported success of ultrasonography in comparison with other modalities. The following is a synopsis of our technique.

The patient is imaged seated in a rotating chair, allowing easy repositioning of the patient to evaluate the anterior and posterior shoulder. We start by evaluating the anterior structures. Slight external rotation puts the subscapularis under a little tension and makes it easier to image. If the probe is held horizontally, an axial section is obtained and the bicipital groove is easily identified. Slight movement of the probe medially brings the coracoid into view with its strong posterior shadowing. Having identified these two landmarks, the tendon of the subscapularis can be traced throughout its length from muscle belly to insertion. Rotation of the probe through 90° permits parasagittal evaluation of the subscapularis. We then return to the bicipital groove to obtain transverse and longitudinal images of the biceps tendon and sheath. The arm is then internally rotated, so that the forearm crosses the lower thorax with the arm remaining vertical. Axial and sagittal scans are then obtained of the infraspinatus (superiorly) and teres minor (inferiorly). The rotator cuff is normally thinner posteriorly, and no significance should be ascribed to this. For the evaluation of the supraspinatus (see Fig. 2), we have the patient internally rotate as far as is comfortable to bring the supraspinatus out from beneath the acromion. If possible, the arm is placed behind the back. It may be helpful to have the patient lean forward a little. The bony margin of the acromion is identified and the tendon traced from this point to its insertion on the humerus. Sagittal and coronal images are obtained.

The indicators of rotator cuff pathology are similar to signs used elsewhere in the musculoskeletal system. Special attention must be given to the potential pitfalls (see below) due to tendon curvature and the somewhat complex anatomy. The most reliable diagnostic feature of tears relates to complete absence, focal discontinuity, or contour deformity (see Fig. 7) within the tendon substance. Echogenic areas that may relate to tears may also indicate focal calcification, scar, normal anatomy, or be artifactual.

One particular pitfall of note is the intra-articular biceps tendon. When evaluating in this region, carefully trace the tendon from the bicipital groove to evaluate a possible area of altered echogenicity in the superior rotator cuff to ensure that this is not related to the tendon. Similarly, intertendinous junctions should not be confused with tears. Occasionally in elderly patients the supraspinatus tendon is relatively hypoechoic and can be difficult to differentiate from diffuse tendonitis, and comparison with the other side can be helpful. Tendinous calcification can be misinterpreted, and inferior subluxation of the humeral head can produce apparent thickening of the rotator cuff. These two features should be recognized by prior scrutiny of the radiographs, which is strongly recommended. Another possible pitfall is the postoperative rotator cuff. This may maintain abnormal echogenicity, documented as long as six years after repair, and in such cases discontinuity or complete absence is the only reliable sign of tear.

Although sonography can be highly useful in evaluation of the shoulder, its limitations must be recalled. Close communication with the referring physician is appropriate. The sensitivity of detection of a tear has been highly variable in the reported series, and the most experienced can miss small tears. Consequently, if the ultrasonographic study is negative in the face of strong clinical evidence for a tear, it may be appropriate in some instances to move to an alternative modality. In most cases, however, a normal sonogram indicates a trial of conservative therapy. It must also be remembered that the sonogram does not exclude an instability syndrome.

## Discussion

Because of its noninvasive nature, availability, cost-effectiveness, and exquisite ability to image the soft tissues, ultrasonography has much to offer in imaging of the musculoskeletal system. Its full potential is only just being appreciated by clinicians, and the time spent by a radiologist in becoming familiar with the technique is well spent.

## Suggested Reading


Abiri M, Kirpekar M, Ablow R. Osteomyelitis: Detection with US. Radiology 1989; 172:509–511.

Crass J, Craig E, Feinberg S. Sonography of the post-operative rotator cuff. AJR 1986; 146:561–564.

Crass J, Van deVegte G, Harkavy L. Tendon echogenicity: Ex vivo study. Radiology 1988; 167:499–501.

Fornage B. Current status of musculoskeletal sonography. Appl Radiol 1991; 29–42.

Kaplan P, Matamoros A, Anderson J. Sonography of the musculoskeletal system. AJR 1990; 155:237–245.

Lischi D. L'ecografia nella diagnosi di cisti ossea aneurismatica. Radiol Med (Torino) 1991; 81:249–252.

Maffulli N, Regine R, Carrillo F, et al. Tennis elbow: An ultrasonographic study in tennis players. Br J Sports Med 1990; 24:151–155.

Middleton W. Status of rotator cuff sonography. Radiology 1989; 173:307–309.

Middleton W, Reinus W, Melson G, et al. Pitfalls of rotator cuff sonography. AJR 1986; 146:555–560.

Van Holsbeeck M, Introcaso J. Musculoskeletal Ultrasound. St. Louis: Mosby–Year Book, 1991.


# MRI of Bone Marrow

*SHEILA G. MOORE, M.D.*

Radiologists have attempted to evaluate bone marrow using radiographic and scintigraphic techniques. All of these imaging modalities, however, have had significant limitations. Plain film radiography is of limited usefulness in the evaluation of bone marrow, since significant amounts of trabecular bone and/or cortical bone must be destroyed before there is plain film evidence of bone marrow abnormality. Computed tomography (CT) represented a significant advancement in the interpretation of bone abnormalities over plain film radiography, since attenuation differences of 0.5 percent for cortical bone could be resolved. For marrow analysis, however, comparison with contralateral "normal" marrow is needed to recognize focal marrow abnormalities, a technique that is less useful when diffuse processes involve all or most of the marrow. In addition, beam-hardening artifacts from cortical bone can obscure marrow detail and limit CT in interpretation of marrow abnormalities. Osseous blood flow and metabolic activity can be assessed using technetium-99m ($^{99m}$Tc)-labeled diphosphonate; however, this method of imaging is often insensitive to aggressive or diffuse marrow processes. Technetium-labeled sulphur colloid more directly evaluates bone marrow but is nonspecific and shows neither the distribution of fatty marrow nor marrow anatomic detail.

Magnetic resonance imaging (MRI) has evolved as the noninvasive modality of choice for the investigation of bone marrow disorders. This is primarily because of differences in proton density, T1, and T2 relaxation times of hematopoietic and fatty marrow on spin-echo MR images. Chemical shift and gradient recalled echo (GRE) images exploit proton resonant frequency and magnetic susceptibility as additional parameters of MR image contrast. T2-weighted spin-echo, fast spin-echo (FSE), fat-suppressed images, and short tau inversion recovery (STIR) images provide increased lesion conspicuity. Diagnosis of focal and diffuse marrow disorders, determination of disease stage in hematopoietic malignancies, assessment of treatment efficacy, and quantitation of marrow reconversion phenomena are all potential roles for MRI in the evaluation of marrow.

Marrow is composed of stromal cells, fat cells, hematopoietic stem cells, and a cancellous bony matrix of primary and secondary bridging trabeculae. The trabecular matrix provides architectural support for the cellular marrow elements, and influences marrow appearance on GRE images. Triacylglycerol contains two distinct fatty components that can be spectroscopically separated and is the primary lipid found in marrow fat cells. This characteristic of marrow fat cells may influence marrow signal intensity on chemical shift and GRE images. Additionally, these distinct fatty compounds may be apparent on proton spectroscopy of the marrow.

## Marrow-Imaging Techniques

T1-weighted and T2-weighted spin-echo images are the most frequently used images in the MRI evaluation of marrow. Most of the fat protons in fatty marrow are in the form of hydrophobic $CH_2$ groups, and spin-lattice relaxation is therefore efficient. Fatty marrow therefore has a relatively short T1 relaxation time (approximate range 350 to 550 msec). Spin-spin relaxation of fat is less efficient; therefore the T2 relaxation time of fat is somewhat longer than the T2 relaxation time of water. Fatty marrow appears as increased signal intensity on T1-weighted images, similar to the signal intensity of subcutaneous fat, and decreases slightly on T2-weighted images.

In contrast to fatty marrow, hematopoietic marrow contains relatively large amounts of cells, protein, and water. The interaction of these marrow components is complex and incompletely understood at this time. The relatively long T1 and T2 relaxation times of the protein and water in hematopoietic marrow will be averaged with the short T1 and long T2 relaxation times of fat, since some component of hematopoietic marrow signal will usually be derived from fat. To differentiate hematopoietic and fatty marrow on spin-echo MR images, marrow signal intensity is compared with that of surrounding muscle. Marrow signal intensity, which is less than that of adjacent muscle, is referred to as "low" signal intensity. In general, the lower the marrow signal intensity when compared with muscle, the greater the percentage of hematopoietic marrow. Marrow that has been infiltrated by abnormal cells can also be observed as "low" signal intensity. Hematopoietic marrow, which is "intermediate" signal intensity (equal to muscle) or "increased" signal intensity (between that of muscle and subcutaneous fat), contains varying percentages of microscopic fatty marrow. The greater the percentage of fatty marrow, the closer the marrow signal intensity appears to that of subcutaneous fat. Therefore marrow signal intensity similar to that of subcutaneous fat reflects primarily fatty marrow, although microscopic hematopoietic marrow may still be present. When compared with the gross anatomic (hematopoietic or fatty) appearance of marrow, marrow signal intensity on spin-echo MR images appears more "fatty" than might be expected for the percentage of macroscopic red marrow actually present. Spin-echo MR images therefore appear to more accurately reflect the percentage of microscopic yellow marrow than the percentage of macroscopic red marrow.

In the newborn, hematopoietic marrow signal intensity on T1-weighted images usually appears as low signal intensity, reflecting the large percentage (in many cases close to 100 percent) of hematopoietic cells in newborn marrow. Hematopoietic marrow in children, adolescents, and adults has a range of signal intensity depending on the relative percentages of red and yellow marrow. The greater the percentage of red marrow, the more intermediate the signal intensity of marrow will appear on T1-weighted spin-echo images. As a patient ages, and the red marrow is converted to yellow marrow, the appearance of the hematopoietic marrow will change and the marrow signal intensity will increase and ultimately approach that of subcutaneous fat. The signal intensity of hematopoietic marrow remains unchanged or increases slightly on T2-weighted images. Infiltration of marrow by abnormal or neoplastic cells will, in general, be seen as decreased signal intensity on T1-weighted images and increased signal intensity on T2-weighted images. Depletion of marrow cellular elements with a proliferation of fat cells can result in an overall increased (fatty) marrow signal intensity on both T1- and T2-weighted images. On the other hand, replacement of depleted cellular elements by fibrosis results in an overall decreased marrow signal intensity on both T1- and T2-weighted images.

Unlike spin-echo sequences, marrow signal intensity on GRE images is dependent on the effective transverse relaxation time (T2*). This technique is sensitive to field inhomogeneities arising either intrinsically (tissue differences in chemical shift frequency or magnetic susceptibility) or extrinsically. Marrow in contact with trabecular bone produces local field gradients, resulting in inhomogeneous susceptibility and T2* dephasing where mineralized trabecular matrix interfaces with marrow. This T2* dephasing and shortening results in the loss of marrow signal intensity on GRE images and is greatest in regions of marrow with the highest content of trabecular bone (epiphyses, epiphysoid bones, vertebral bodies, metaphyses). Dephasing does not occur in the diaphysis, where there is little or no trabecular bone (Fig. 1). This loss of marrow signal will be even more pronounced in hematopoietic marrow, where the presence of iron results in further T2* dephasing and magnetic susceptibility effect. Therefore GRE images of the marrow are most sensitive to trabecular bone content and the presence of iron, reflecting the underlying cellular composition of marrow (whether fatty or hematopoietic) primarily in regions of marrow without trabecular bone or iron.

These magnetic susceptibility effects can influence the appearance of marrow lesions on GRE images. Blastic lesions in heavily trabeculated bone may not be readily apparent, while lytic lesions cause loss of trabecular bone and increased lesion conspicuity. In the diaphysis lesions may or may not be appreciated, depending on the technique used to obtain the GRE image. Magnetic susceptibility effect, image resolution, and detection of marrow lesions may be improved by decreasing TE and pixel size for a given GRE sequence.

By exploiting the distinct resonant frequencies of aliphatic protons and water protons in the marrow, marrow signal can be separated into a fat component (fatty marrow) and a water component (hematopoietic marrow). Chemical shift imaging has been used in both the qualitative and quantitative assessment of patients with leukemia and aplastic anemia. Water fraction marrow signal intensity increases and the fat fraction marrow signal intensity decreases in patients with leukemia when compared with patients with no marrow disease. These changes are most obvious in adults, where the predominance of fatty marrow facilitates recognition of hypercellular marrow. In children signal intensity changes may not be qualitatively obvious, given the higher percentage of red marrow. Linear suppression of lipid signal independent of the relative abundance of water or lipid contribution results in fat-saturation images. This suppression of fat signal, including fatty marrow signal, results in increased conspicuity of bright signal intensity hematopoietic marrow and marrow lesions.

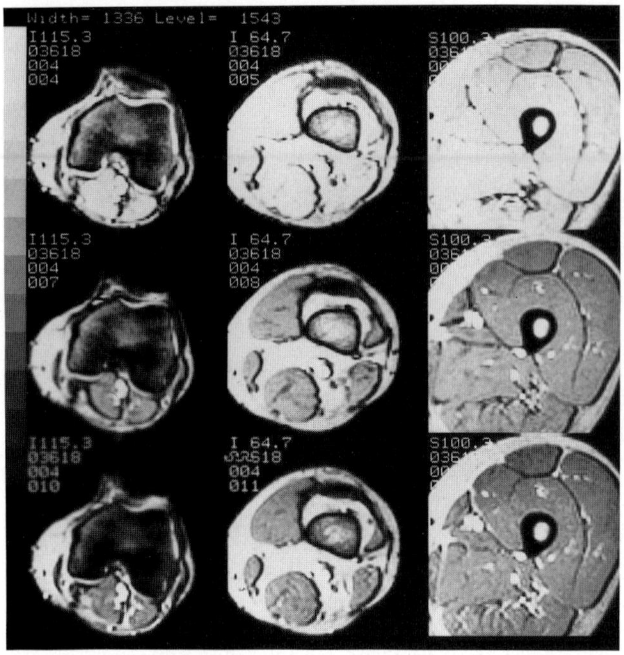


**FIGURE 1** Effect of trabecular bone on marrow signal intensity. GRE (TR60/30°) images through the femoral epiphyses (first column), femoral metaphyses (second column), and femoral diaphyses (third column) in a normal 28-year-old male. In the first transverse row, images are acquired at a TE of 12 msec; TE of 16 and 20 msec were used for the second and third rows, respectively. Note the increasing marrow magnetic susceptibility effect with increasing TE in the trabecular-rich epiphyses, whereas no marrow magnetic susceptibility effect is seen in the trabecular-poor diaphyses. An intermediate susceptibility effect is seen in the femoral metaphyses, which contains mild-to-moderate amounts of trabecular bone. (From Sebag G, Moore SG. Effect of trabecular bone on the appearance of gradient-echo imaging of the appendicular skeleton. Radiology 1990; 174:855; with permission.)

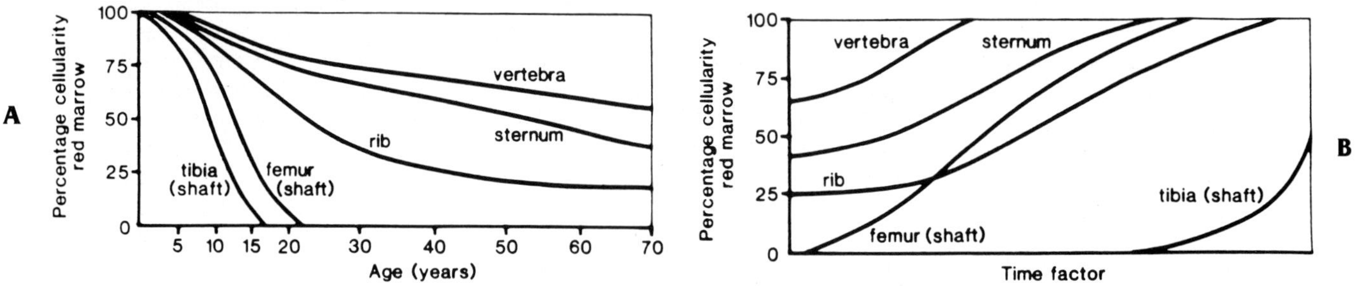


**FIGURE 2** Conversion and reconversion of marrow. *A,* Normal conversion of hematopoietic to fatty marrow. The relative amounts of macroscopic hematopoietic and fatty marrow in different anatomic sites are plotted against age. The percentage of hematopoietic marrow decreases with age but remains the greatest in the vertebral bodies and flat bones. *B,* Reconversion of fatty to hematopoietic marrow generally occurs in a pattern converse to that of hematopoietic to fatty marrow conversion. (Adapted from Kricun ME. Red-yellow marrow conversion: Its effects on the location of some solitary bone lesions. Skeletal Radiol 1985; 14:10; with permission.)

STIR imaging of the marrow results in increased lesion conspicuity. Fat, fatty marrow, air, fibrosis, calcification, and paramagnetic substances (Gd-DTPA and hemorrhage) are all suppressed and observed as low signal intensity on STIR images. Muscle, hematopoietic marrow, and mild marrow infiltration by abnormal cells are observed as intermediate signal intensity, while most musculoskeletal lesions, moderate-to-marked marrow infiltration by abnormal cells, fluid, edema, and nodes are observed as bright signal intensity. When evaluating STIR images for marrow abnormality, the signal intensity of muscle adjacent to marrow can be used as a control. In general, normal hematopoietic marrow is observed as isointense to surrounding muscle, while marrow with a signal intensity that is brighter than that of adjacent muscle is more likely abnormal.

## Normal Marrow Conversion

Progressive conversion of hematopoietic (red) to fatty (yellow) marrow is a normal part of the aging process. Marrow conversion occurs first in the distal long bones, then the proximal long bones, and finally in the flat bones and spine. In the long bones, the conversion process begins in the diaphyses, followed by the distal metaphyses, and finally the proximal metaphyses (Fig. 2). Fatty marrow forms a large reserve, potentially available for the formation of blood cells, which is not used in normal conditions. However, stress, anemia, or infiltration of red marrow by abnormal cells will initiate the "reconversion" of yellow marrow to red marrow, resulting in repopulation of fatty marrow by active hematopoietic cells. Marrow reconversion generally occurs in a pattern converse to that of red to yellow marrow conversion (see Fig. 2).

Four MRI patterns of bone marrow signal intensity and homogeneity on T1-weighted images in the femur have been described. These four recognizable conversion patterns are (1) the infant, (2) the child, (3) the adolescent, and (4) the adult. Homogeneous low-to-intermediate femoral marrow signal intensity during the first year of life constitutes the MRI infant pattern. Between the ages of 1 and 5, there is apparent initiation of the conversion process in the femoral diaphysis.

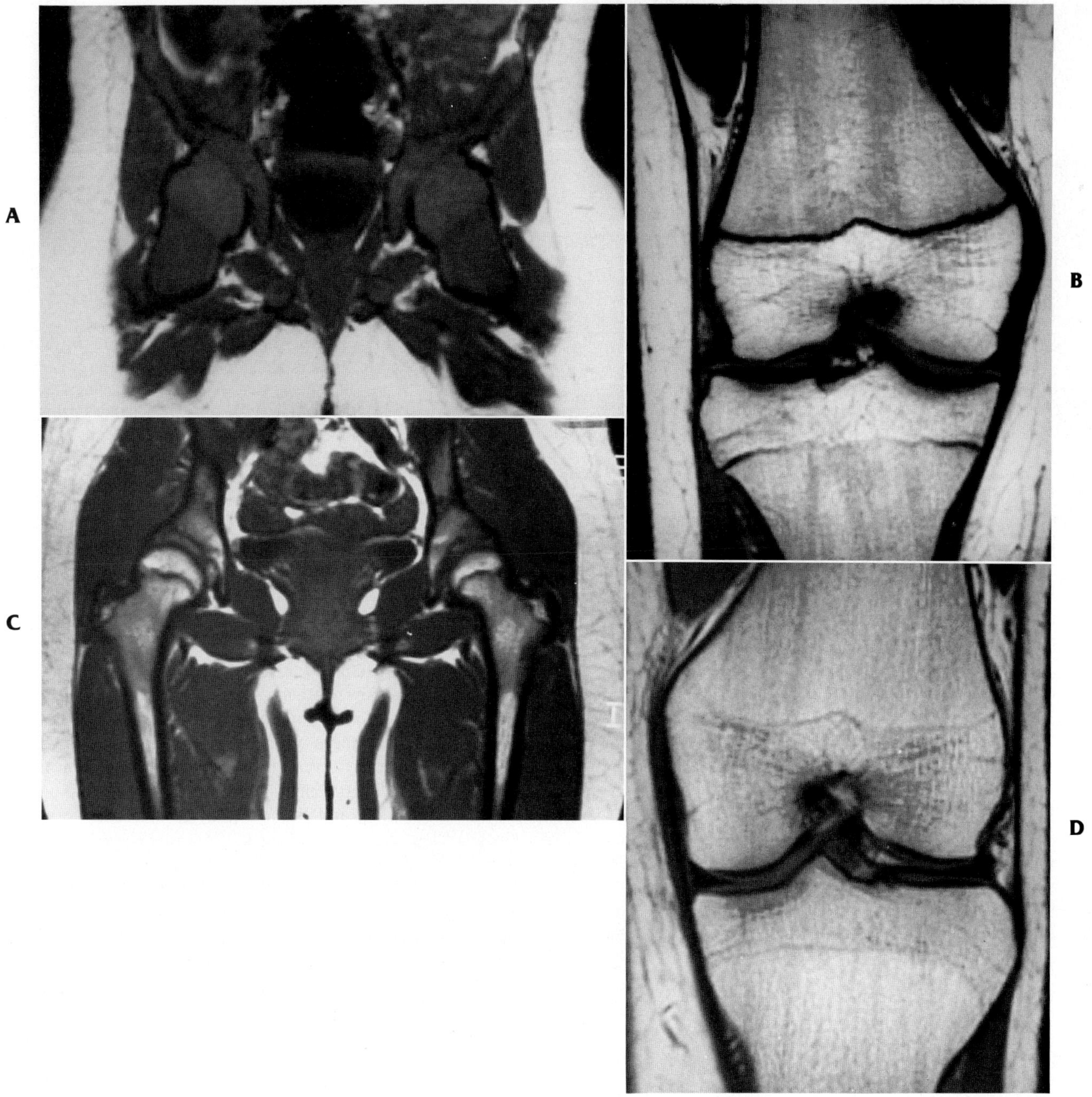


**FIGURE 3** Conversion of marrow in the pelvis and femur. *A,* Coronal T1-weighted (TR300/15) image through the pelvis and proximal femora in a newborn. Note the intermediate signal intensity (equal to muscle) red marrow in the iliac crest and proximal femoral metaphyses. The cartilaginous femoral epiphyses have a signal intensity slightly greater than that of the proximal femoral metaphyses. *B,* Coronal T1-weighted (TR300/15) image in a normal 14-year-old girl. Note the increased signal intensity fatty marrow in the anterior acetabulum, as well as the intermediate signal intensity red marrow in the proximal femoral metaphyses. Increased signal intensity yellow marrow is seen in the femoral epiphyses, greater trochanters, and diaphyses. *C,* Coronal T1-weighted (TR800/20) image through the knee in a normal adolescent. Patchy distal femoral and proximal tibial metaphyseal marrow is shown. *D,* Coronal T1-weighted (TR800/20) image through the knee in an adult, showing yellow marrow in both the metaphyses and epiphyses.

Between the ages of 6 and 10, this conversion process appears "complete" on MR images, and the diaphysis usually appears as increased signal intensity yellow marrow. Between the ages of 10 and 20, the distal femoral metaphysis becomes heterogeneous, with patchy regions of red and yellow marrow. The conversion of this adolescent pattern to the adult pattern occurs when the distal metaphyseal marrow has a primarily fatty appearance (Fig. 3).

Conversion of red to yellow marrow in the pelvis occurs first in the anterior iliac crest and acetabulum (Fig. 3, *B*). The pubic symphysis, posterior iliac crest, and sacral alae maintain varying percentages of hematopoietic marrow with increasing patient age. Marked pelvic heterogeneity most likely represents focal islands of cellular marrow within fatty marrow (particularly in the anterior pelvis), or foci of fatty marrow within regions of predominantly cellular marrow (particularly

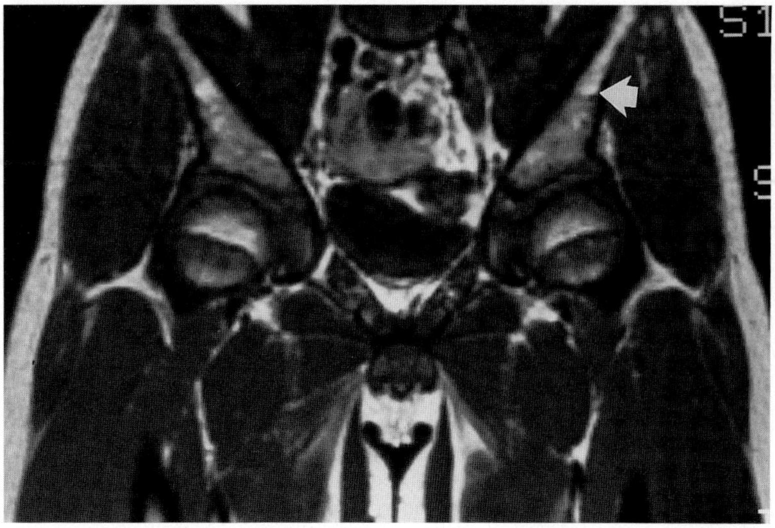

**FIGURE 4** Normal pelvic marrow. Coronal T1-weighted (TR800/30) image through the pelvis in a 13-year-old girl. Note the marked heterogeneity of the pelvic marrow. Increased signal intensity yellow marrow is seen in the anterior and superior iliac crest. There is a sharp demarcation between the anterior fatty marrow and the mottled hematopoietic marrow *(arrow)*. (From Moore SG. Pediatric musculoskeletal imaging. In: Stark DD, Bradley WG, eds. Magnetic Resonance Imaging. St. Louis: Mosby–Year Book, 1992:22–40; with permission.)

in the posterior pelvis). This heterogeneity is especially prominent in adolescents and young adults (Fig. 4). Occasionally this normal marrow heterogeneity can be problematic in evaluating MR images of the pelvis, where it can be confused for diffuse metastatic disease or marrow fibrosis. Because the signal intensity of fatty marrow tends to decrease on T2-weighted images and the signal intensity of hematopoietic marrow tends to increase slightly on T2-weighted images, normal bone marrow signal intensity often looks more homogeneous on T2-weighted images than on T1-weighted images. The T2-weighted image can therefore be used to screen the marrow in cases of marked marrow heterogeneity noted on the T1-weighted image. If the marrow looks more homogeneous on the T2-weighted image, one is likely looking at normal marrow heterogeneity. On the other hand, if the marrow continues to look fairly heterogeneous on the T2-weighted images, specific areas of low signal intensity on the T1-weighted image must be compared with these same regions on the T2-weighted image. Increase in signal intensity on a T2-weighted or STIR image suggests metastatic disease. If these areas remain low signal, this may represent diffuse marrow fibrosis. STIR imaging has an added advantage over spin-echo images in this determination, since hematopoietic marrow is isointense in signal intensity to muscle on STIR images and metastatic disease is bright.

Another normal marrow pattern in the pelvis is that of posterior intermediate signal intensity red marrow with anterior increased signal intensity yellow marrow. This pattern often first appears in adolescence and can persist in adults. It reflects the normal predominance of hematopoietic marrow in the posterior aspect of the pelvis and should not be mistaken for abnormal cells in the posterior iliac crest. The demarcation between these two regions of marrow can often be distinct and therefore alarming if one does not recognize this as a normal finding (see Fig. 4).

MRI patterns of marrow conversion with age in the spine have not been established, although recent studies have shown age-related trends of marrow signal intensity and examples of normal vertebral marrow variants on spin-echo MR images. The lack of specific age-related progression of vertebral marrow signal intensity is likely due to the fact that the spine is the primary hematopoietic reservoir in the skeletal system, and therefore amounts of hematopoietic and fatty vertebral marrow may vary greatly for each individual. Marked marrow heterogeneity, focal fibrosis, and vertebral sclerosis can be observed in children, is common in adults, and is of no known clinical significance. At birth, hematopoietic vertebral marrow appears as low signal intensity (less than that of muscle). The cartilaginous unossified portions of the vertebral body form an intermediate signal intensity border surrounding this low signal intensity red marrow. With age, there is progressive increase in marrow signal intensity, so that marrow signal intensity on T1-weighted MR images begins to approximate that of muscle in early childhood. Recent studies have shown that at 0.5 T, vertebral marrow signal intensity is similar to or lower than that of adjacent cartilage and disk in 87 percent of children less than 1 year of age. Between the ages of 5 and 15 years, vertebral marrow signal intensity is greater than that of adjacent disks in 90 percent of cases. As an overall trend, there is a tendency toward higher signal intensity with age, although at any age the signal intensity of vertebral marrow is variable and can be similar to that of surrounding muscle or more closely approximate that of fat. Since adult vertebral marrow signal intensity should be brighter than that of the adjacent disk on T1-weighted images, vertebral marrow signal intensity that is less than that of the adjacent disk on T1-weighted images is likely abnormal. Other criteria, such as abnormal low signal intensity marrow in the long bones or markedly increased signal intensity marrow on T2-weighted or STIR images, are useful adjunctive findings when the diagnosis of vertebral marrow abnormality is suspected.

There can be one of several patterns of fatty marrow deposition along vertebral end-plates, which may be a result of normal aging or the effect of local ischemia in marrow adjacent to degenerative lumbar disks. The "polka dot" spine, focal regions of fat surrounding the basivertebral vein observed on sagittal or coronal T1-weighted MR images, is another normal finding. This can be observed in both children and adults and is the consequence of the unique blood supply of the vertebral body. In the vertebral body, blood supply is via a nutrient artery that enters the posterior aspect of the vertebral body and parallels the course of the basivertebral vein. Branches of the nutrient artery decussate at the vertebral end-plates, forming endosteal sinusoids (Fig. 5). These sinusoids provide an

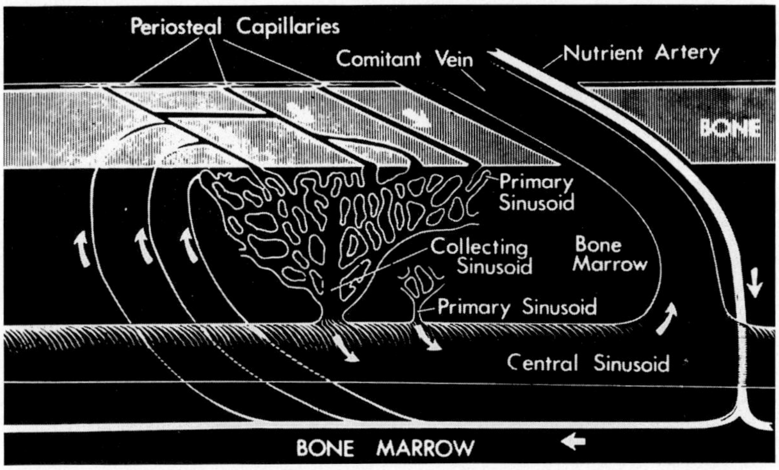


**FIGURE 5** Vertebral circulation. Schematic drawing of the vertebral circulation illustrates the peripheral sinusoids, the primary site of vertebral hematopoiesis within vertebral bodies. (From Trubowitz S, Davis S. In: Trubowitz S, Davis S, eds. The Human Bone Marrow. Boca Raton: CRC Press, 1982: 53; with permission.)

environment conducive to the presence and activity of hematopoietic cells, and the majority of hematopoietic cells are found in these endosteal sinusoids. The central region of the vertebral body is normally populated with fatty marrow, which surrounds the basivertebral vein, and is observed as bright signal intensity on T1-weighted images. Hematopoietic marrow may be observed as intermediate signal intensity in the periphery (endosteal) regions of the vertebral body. Malignant cells do not respect these normal cellular locations, and therefore malignant infiltration of vertebral marrow often results in obliteration of fatty marrow surrounding the basivertebral vein. If the signal intensity of vertebral marrow is lower than that of the adjacent disk, and the fatty marrow surrounding the basivertebral vein is preserved, infiltration of a vertebral body by malignant cells is less likely and proliferation of hematopoietic cells more likely. On the other hand, abnormally low vertebral marrow signal intensity, coupled with obliteration of the peribasivertebral fat, is suggestive of malignant marrow infiltration.

The largely hematopoietic marrow present in the vertebral bodies during the first year of life may enhance markedly with gadolinium. This enhancement of normal hematopoietic marrow should not be confused for abnormal marrow processes, such as infiltration by malignant cells, during the first year of life. Enhancement of vertebral marrow in adults and older children should, however, be considered abnormal.

Throughout life the calvarium is a site of active hematopoiesis. Therefore hematopoietic disorders may affect the marrow of the calvarium, clivus, and face, and these regions of marrow must be evaluated whenever MR images of the head and neck are obtained. The clivus and calvarium have uniformly low-to-intermediate signal intensity marrow on T1-weighted images in most infants less than 1 year of age. The marrow signal intensity increases with age, so that by the age of 7 clival marrow is seen as patchy low and high signal intensity. Less than 10 percent of children between the ages of 3 and 7 years have the homogeneous low signal intensity marrow seen during the first year of life, so that homogeneous low signal intensity clival marrow is likely abnormal in children over the age of 3, and definitely abnormal in children over the age of 7. High signal intensity homogeneous fatty marrow is present in both the clivus and calvarium by the age of 15, although intermediate signal intensity marrow can occasionally persist in the calvarium. Marrow signal intensity in the sphenoid sinus is uniformly low in children less than 6 months of age, since this marrow is predominantly hematopoietic. This hematopoietic marrow may enhance with gadolinium, particularly in newborns, and should not be misinterpreted as an enhancing lesion. Between 7 months and 2 years, apparent fatty conversion of this marrow is observed on spin-echo images. Between the ages of 3 and 6 years, pneumatization of the sphenoid sinus occurs.

The process of marrow conversion continues until the adult marrow pattern is reached. This pattern consists of intermediate signal intensity hematopoietic marrow in the spine, flat bones, proximal humeral and femoral metaphyses, and calvarium (Fig. 6). Although prospective studies to refine patterns of normal and abnormal marrow are currently in progress, the following guidelines can be useful in the interpretation of spin-echo MR images of marrow. First, marrow signal intensity that is decreased in regions of expected increased signal intensity fatty marrow for age is likely abnormal. The lower the marrow signal intensity when compared with that of muscle, the more likely a marrow abnormality exists. This is especially true in the distal long bones and diaphyseal regions in an adult, where intermediate signal intensity hematopoietic marrow is definitely abnormal. Further evidence that decreased signal intensity marrow on T1-weighted images is abnormal includes increasing marrow signal intensity on T2-weighted spin-echo, STIR, and fat-saturation images. Intermediate signal intensity marrow in the ossified epiphyses, which should contain only increased signal intensity fatty marrow, should be considered abnormal. The only exception to this would be in a newborn, where hematopoietic marrow can occasionally be observed in ossifying epiphyses. Symmetric, intermediate signal intensity marrow in regions of expected hematopoiesis (e.g., proximal femoral and humeral metaphyses, flat bones, and vertebral bodies) likely represents normal hematopoietic marrow or physiologic conversion of marrow, and significant detectable underlying hematopoietic disorder will likely be absent.

Finally, it is not unusual to see intermediate signal intensity foci in the distal femoral metaphyses on MR images of adult knees. Several studies have been designed to determine the relationship of this finding and the presence of hematopoietic abnormality. These studies have shown that although some adults with foci of distal femoral hematopoietic marrow may be anemic, there is no statistically significant correlation between the presence or extent of patchy distal femoral hematopoietic marrow and anemia. Although these studies analyze periph-

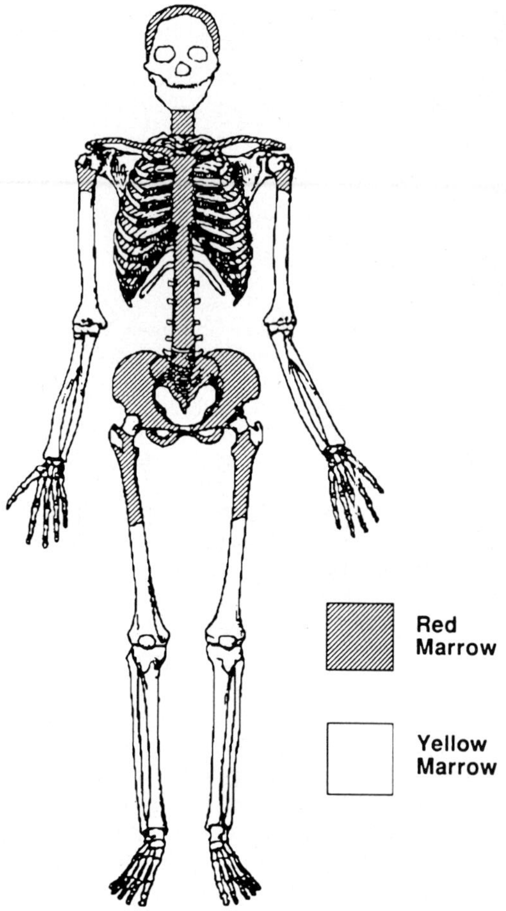


**FIGURE 6** Distribution of red and yellow marrow in an adult. Schematic drawing of the distribution of normal adult hematopoietic and fatty marrow. Macroscopic red marrow is observed in the vertebral bodies, flat bones, skull, and proximal femoral and humeral metaphyses in adults.

eral blood count, and not bone marrow aspirate or biopsy data, it seems likely that this finding should be considered a normal variant that is more prevalent in young adults. Conversion of distal femoral epiphyseal marrow, however, should be considered abnormal and should be reported to the ordering physician.

## Marrow Edema

Marrow edema is observed on spin-echo MR images as decreased signal intensity on T1-weighted images and increased signal intensity on T2-weighted images. Edema can appear either as well defined and geographic or less well defined and feathery (Fig. 7). It is a nonspecific generalized marrow response to stress or injury and is therefore observed in a variety of musculoskeletal disorders. The stimulus and controlling factors for the initiation of edema are uncertain; however, it is known that extracellular water increases as a result of hypervascularity and hyperperfusion. When marrow edema is identified on MR images, the differential diagnosis includes "transient" edema as a result of stress or osteoporosis, trauma, acute and chronic infection, ischemia, infarction, tumor, osteoid osteoma, and reflex sympathetic dystrophy. Although there have been no prospective studies to establish criteria for distinguishing these entities, the following guidelines can be useful.

The clinical history, physical examination, and radiograph aid in the interpretation of marrow edema observed on MRI evaluation. Diffuse, well-defined edema can be observed with infection and osteoid osteoma, and must be distinguished from medullary tumor. Evaluation of the cortex is essential. If the cortical bone is normal, marrow edema confined to medullary bone marrow most likely represents transient edema (i.e., aggressive osteoporosis), infarction, trabecular microfracture, or reflex sympathetic dystrophy. Surrounding soft-tissue edema may or may not be present. Transient marrow edema, such as that observed in young children with hip pain or in patients with aggressive osteoporosis, will likely not be accompanied by soft-tissue edema. Trabecular microfracture and reflex sympathetic dystrophy, on the other hand, may often be associated with surrounding soft-tissue edema. Low signal intensity, thickened cortical bone is observed with osteoid osteoma, stress fracture, and chronic infection, whereas intermediate signal intensity suggesting cortical edema or infiltration is observed with tumor, infection, osteoid osteoma, and aggressive osteoporosis. The presence or absence of soft-tissue edema and/or mass can also aid in the differential diagnosis of marrow edema. Soft-tissue edema has been reported in inflammatory and acute processes, while tumors and less aggressive processes are reportedly accompanied by less soft-tissue edema. Marrow edema in the presence of extensive soft-tissue edema suggests acute trauma and acute inflammation including infection. A small-to-moderate amount of edema surrounding the marrow abnormality is more

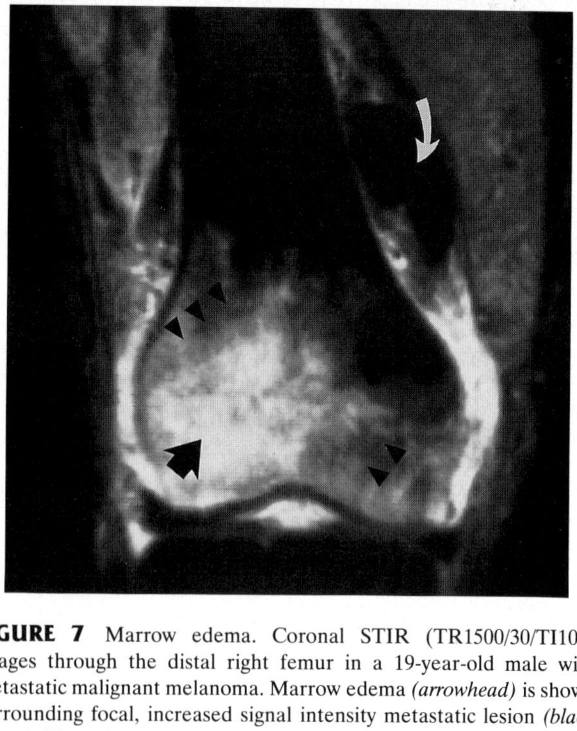

**FIGURE 7** Marrow edema. Coronal STIR (TR1500/30/TI100) images through the distal right femur in a 19-year-old male with metastatic malignant melanoma. Marrow edema *(arrowhead)* is shown surrounding focal, increased signal intensity metastatic lesion *(black arrow)*. Note the suppression of the fatty marrow in the unaffected femur and proximal tibia in this STIR image. A low signal intensity mass is shown adjacent to the medial distal femur, and represents a benign lipoma *(white arrow)*. (From Moore SG, Sebag GH. Primary disorders of bone marrow. In: Cohen MD, Edwards MK, eds. Magnetic Resonance Imaging of Children. Philadelphia: BC Decker, 1990:765; with permission.)

likely observed with slow-growing tumor, chronic infection, or subacute trauma. A soft-tissue mass associated with marrow abnormality makes tumor and infection more likely. Hemorrhage from acute trauma can also result in a soft-tissue mass.

## Marrow Disorders

Marrow infiltration by malignant cells usually is observed as decreased signal intensity on T1-weighted images and increased signal intensity on T2-weighted images. These changes can be diffuse or focal, depending on the underlying disorder. Indications for the use of MRI in the evaluation of marrow disease include identification of marrow abnormality, characterization and assessment of disease extent, evaluation of focal bone pain, assessment of marrow response to treatment, and localization of biopsy site.

Acute leukemia is observed in both pediatric and adult populations. Acute lymphocytic leukemia (ALL) is observed primarily in children; it is most frequently appreciated on MR images as diffuse decreased signal intensity on T1-weighted images and increased signal intensity on T2-weighted images. Vertebral marrow is most frequently affected, followed by marrow in the flat bones, and less frequently, the long bones. Although marrow findings in acute myelogenous leukemia (AML) can be similar, AML frequently is observed as a focal rather than a diffuse process; signal intensity is decreased on T1-weighted images and is isointense to slightly increased on T2-weighted images. Chronic myelogenous leukemia (CML) is more frequently observed in adults. It is characterized by a chronic phase lasting up to 10 years or more. This chronic phase invariably is followed by an acute phase of the disease, usually referred to as a "blast crisis." MRI marrow signal intensity in patients with CML is remarkable; there is diffuse replacement of all marrow spaces by decreased signal intensity malignant cells. Marrow may be either isointense or increased in signal intensity on T2-weighted images. Acute and chronic infarct in the medullary and periarticular spaces is common (Fig. 8).

Bone marrow involvement in lymphoma is not uncommon; 25 to 40 percent of patients with non-Hodgkin's lymphoma and up to 15 percent of patients with Hodgkin's lymphoma have involvement of the bone marrow. This is often observed on MRI evaluation as either focal or regional abnormalities of marrow occurring primarily in vertebral bodies, flat bones, and proximal humeri and femora. Marrow involvement by lymphoma is typically observed as intermediate-to-low signal intensity on T1-weighted images, and isointense-to-increased signal intensity on T2-weighted images. Focal lymphoma in the periarticular regions has been reported.

Quantitative MRI measurements of marrow relaxation time in leukemia and lymphoma have been successful in determining disease stage. Marrow T1 relaxation times have been calculated from both spin-echo and chemical shift images. Spin-echo studies show a significant prolongation of vertebral marrow T1 relaxation time in children with active disease (newly diagnosed and relapse leukemia) compared with children without active disease (remission and age-matched normal controls) (Fig. 9). T2 relaxation times are not significantly different. Calculation of marrow fat fraction using vertebral chemical shift imaging in adults also appears to correlate with disease stage.

Multiple myeloma is a plasma cell malignancy that has a variable clinical presentation. Clinical symptoms include bone pain, weakness, fatigue, and normocytic anemia. Serum or urine immunoelectrophoresis is abnormal. Multiple myeloma does not cause an osteoblastic bone response; therefore there is a high false-negative rate in bone scintigraphy. Marrow abnormalities can be either diffuse or focal and are most frequently observed in the lower thoracic and lumbar spine, flat bones, and skull. Untreated myeloma is intermediate signal intensity on T1-weighted images and tends to be intermediate signal intensity on T2-weighted images. In those patients treated with radiation therapy, marrow signal intensity may be decreased on both T1- and T2-weighted sequences secondary to post-therapeutic osteosclerosis and myelofibrosis. The

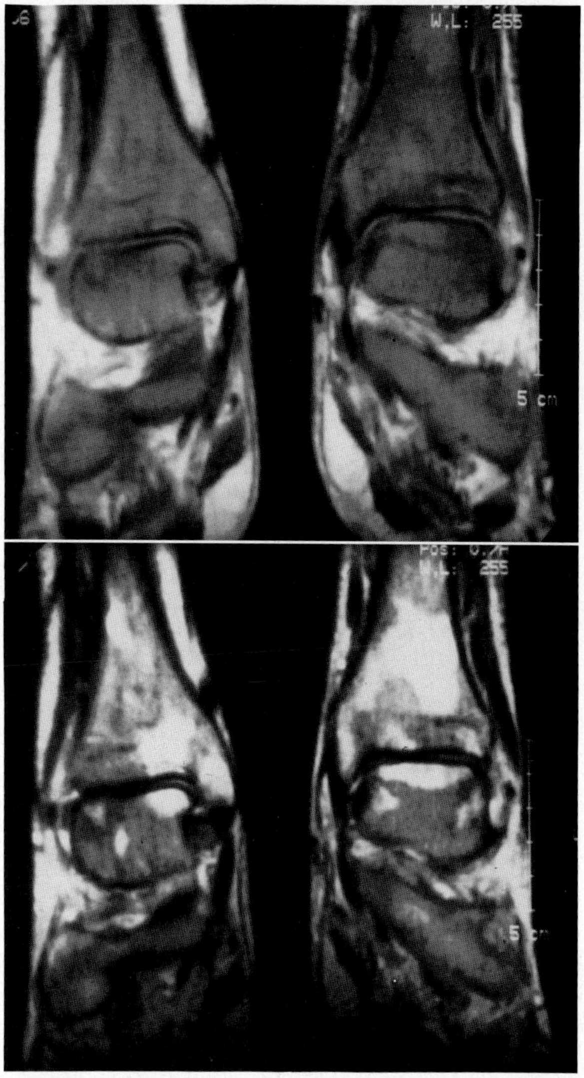


A

B

**FIGURE 8** CML with acute bone infarct. *A,* Coronal T1-weighted (TR600/20) and *B,* T2-weighted (TR2000/80) images through the ankle in a 19-year-old female with CML. Note the diffuse intermediate signal intensity marrow in the ankles. This is distinctly abnormal for the patient's age, when fatty marrow should be observed only in the distal long bones. *B,* Well-defined, focal areas of increased signal intensity are shown in the periarticular regions. This represents subacute medullary infarct as a sequela of the patient's disease and treatment. (From Moore SG, Sebag GH. Primary disorders of bone marrow. In: Cohen MD, Edwards MK, eds. Magnetic Resonance Imaging of Children. Philadelphia: BC Decker, 1990:765; with permission.)

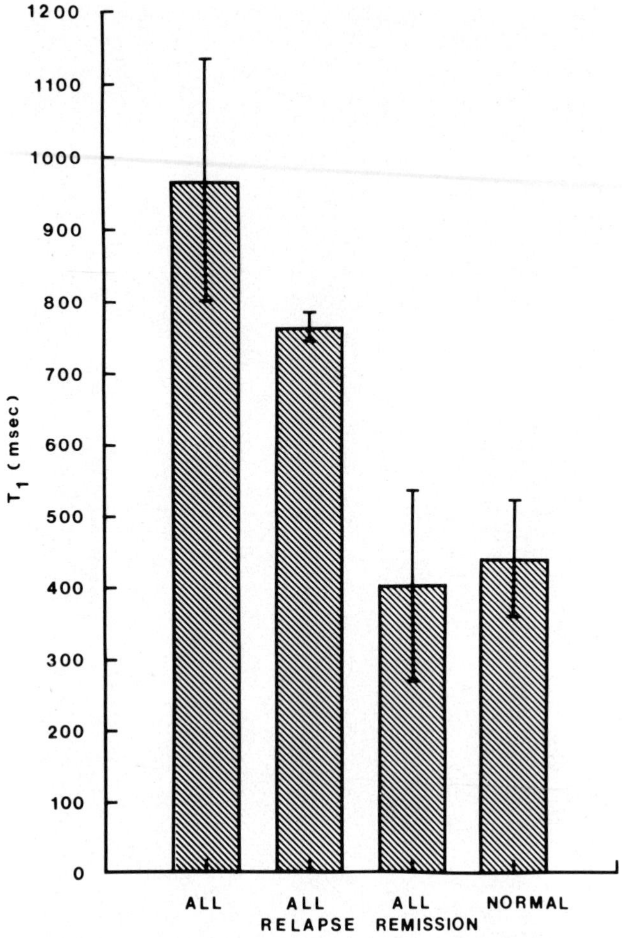


**FIGURE 9** T1 relaxation times in leukemia. Histogram of mean vertebral T1 relaxation times in each of four groups: (1) newly diagnosed ALL, (2) leukemia in relapse, (3) leukemia in remission, and (4) normal age-matched controls. T1 relaxation time is significantly prolonged in children with disease compared with children in remission and age-matched normal controls. (From Moore SG, Gooding CA, et al. Bone marrow in children with acute lymphocytic leukemia: MR relaxation times. Radiology 1986; 160:237; with permission.)

development of diffuse low signal intensity marrow in patients treated for multiple myeloma may herald the onset of CML as a sequela of myeloma therapy.

The differentiation of malignant and benign vertebral collapse can be problematic. Preservation of fatty marrow in the posterior aspect of a collapsed vertebral body generally favors the diagnosis of nonmalignant collapse. Malignant cells, such as the plasma cells in multiple myeloma, tend to involve the entire vertebral body and may or may not involve the pedicle. Of importance is the presence or absence of marrow fat surrounding the basivertebral vein. If this is preserved, the vertebral collapse is more likely secondary to benign disease than if this marrow fat is not preserved, since malignant cells may not respect normal anatomic barriers within the vertebral body. As a result, malignant cells may infiltrate and replace the fatty marrow normally surrounding the basivertebral vein. Vertebral compression accompanied by homogeneous low marrow signal intensity changes, a convex anterior and posterior vertebral contour, destruction of the cortex, multiple levels of abnormal marrow signal intensity without fracture, and paraspinal masses are additional findings that favor the diagnosis of malignant infiltration.

Caution must be used in the interpretation of marrow signal intensity in the presence of degenerative disk disease. Vertebral marrow edema observed as decreased signal intensity on T1-weighted images and increased signal intensity on T2-weighted images has been described in patients with severe degenerative disease. The edema usually does not extend beyond the adjacent vertebral bodies. However, in instances of multiple levels of degenerative disk disease, it is possible to see marrow edema at multiple levels.

Vertebral fractures at multiple levels with preservation of normal (usually fatty) bone marrow signal intensity are the hallmark of chronic, nonmalignant, vertebral collapse. Vertebral body fragmentation and disk rupture are more indicative of traumatic than malignant disease. Recently collapsed vertebral bodies from benign disease, however, can show signal intensity that is indistinguishable from that of metastatic disease. Although paraspinal masses are more conspicuous in malignant than benign disease, they can be observed in acute collapse secondary to trauma or osteoporosis.

Gd-DTPA may increase the specificity of MRI in distinguishing benign from malignant vertebral collapse. Metastatic deposits of vertebral bodies generally exhibit diffuse enhancement on T1-weighted images, whereas bandlike enhancement may be observed in osteoporotic collapse. It should be noted, however, that gadolinium may actually decrease the sensitivity of MRI to the detection of abnormal marrow, since low signal intensity marrow is not appreciated on T1-weighted images, and abnormal marrow can be isointense with surrounding marrow on T2-weighted images. It is therefore important to use fat-saturation techniques when using Gd-DTPA to evaluate for vertebral marrow disease. Leptomeningeal spread of tumor is more conspicuous on Gd-DTPA enhanced MR images; therefore Gd-DTPA is recommended in any patient in whom malignant disease is suspected.

Disorders of hematopoiesis (sickle cell anemia, thalassemia) eventually result in the "reconversion" of yellow marrow to red marrow. This reconversion is observed on T1-weighted images as diffuse intermediate signal intensity red marrow. Those regions of marrow that comprise the "reservoir" of hematopoietic marrow (spine, flat bones, proximal metaphyses), are affected first; the long bones and epiphyses are affected only when there is severe disease (Fig. 10). This hyperplastic cellular marrow is observed on T1-weighted images as patchy, segmental, or diffuse intermediate signal intensity. Typically the hyperplastic marrow does not get particularly bright on T2-weighted images. In addition to the MRI finding of hyperplastic marrow, metadiaphyseal infarction and avascular necrosis of the femoral and humeral heads also are observed. Low signal marrow intensity may be observed in severe cases of sickle cell anemia, reflecting the hemosiderosis observed in patients with repeated blood transfusions. The findings seen in thalassemia and other disorders of hematopoiesis are similar. The marrow of patients with thalassemia is routinely observed as low signal intensity, since hemosiderosis is a common complication as a result of the repeated transfusions required for treatment. In addition to hemosiderosis of the marrow, hemosiderosis of the liver and spleen is expected. Intermediate signal intensity posterior mediastinal masses with a fatty rim are observed in those patients with extramedullary hematopoiesis.

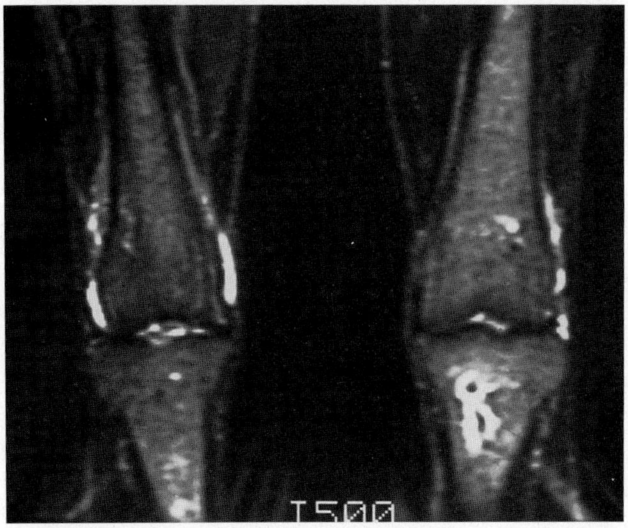

**FIGURE 10** Sickle cell anemia. Coronal T2-weighted (TR2500/120) image through the knees of a woman with sickle cell anemia. Diffuse intermediate signal intensity hyperplastic marrow is observed throughout the medullary space including the epiphyses. Foci of medullary increased signal intensity, observed especially in the proximal left tibia, represent acute bony infarcts. (Courtesy V Rao and R Steiner. From Moore SG. In: Stark DD, Bradley WG, eds. Magnetic Resonance Imaging. St. Louis: Mosby–Year Book, 1992; with permission.)

The MRI findings in aplastic anemia are variable. In some cases increased signal intensity marrow on both T1- and T2-weighted images reflect the diffuse replacement of hematopoietic marrow by fatty marrow. In others aplastic anemia is accompanied by regions of marrow fibrosis. This results in patchy intermediate or low signal intensity on both T1- and T2-weighted images.

## Response of the Marrow to Therapy

Post-therapeutic MRI evaluation of patients with a variety of malignancies is becoming increasingly common. Current therapies for patients with tumors include radiation therapy, chemotherapy, and bone marrow transplantation. Knowledge of the expected appearance of marrow as a result of these therapies is important when evaluating for residual or recurrent disease. For each mode of therapy, there may be changes in signal intensity in both abnormal and normal bone marrow as a result of therapeutic intervention.

Knowledge of the signal intensity changes in both the marrow and soft tissues during and following radiation therapy aids in the interpretation of postradiation therapy MR images. Pathologic changes in the spine in the first 2 weeks following fractionated radiation therapy include acute edema and cell death. Decreased cellularity and the migration of fat are seen at 1 month, whereas replacement of the marrow by fat and fibrosis characterize the marrow response at 3 months. In the first 2 weeks following radiation therapy, there are no appreciable vertebral marrow MRI signal changes on spin-echo images. However, increased signal intensity is observed on STIR images, reflecting the acute marrow edema known to occur at this time. Changes in vertebral marrow on spin-echo images are observed by 3 weeks after radiation therapy, when the vertebral marrow becomes increasingly mottled and heterogeneous, and central migration of increased signal intensity fatty marrow is noted. "Late" marrow patterns following radiation therapy include the "band" pattern (peripheral intermediate marrow signal intensity surrounding central fatty marrow signal intensity) (see Fig. 12) and homogeneous fatty replacement of vertebral marrow. Soft-tissue edema can still be observed 18 months following radiation therapy in children, and in both children and adults the development of soft-tissue edema in a pattern that reflects the radiation port can develop 6 to 9 months after completion of radiation therapy and does not necessarily reflect recurrent disease (Fig. 11). Reports describing the response of abnormal marrow and marrow lesions to radiation therapy are anecdotal, but resolution of the marrow abnormality, formation and

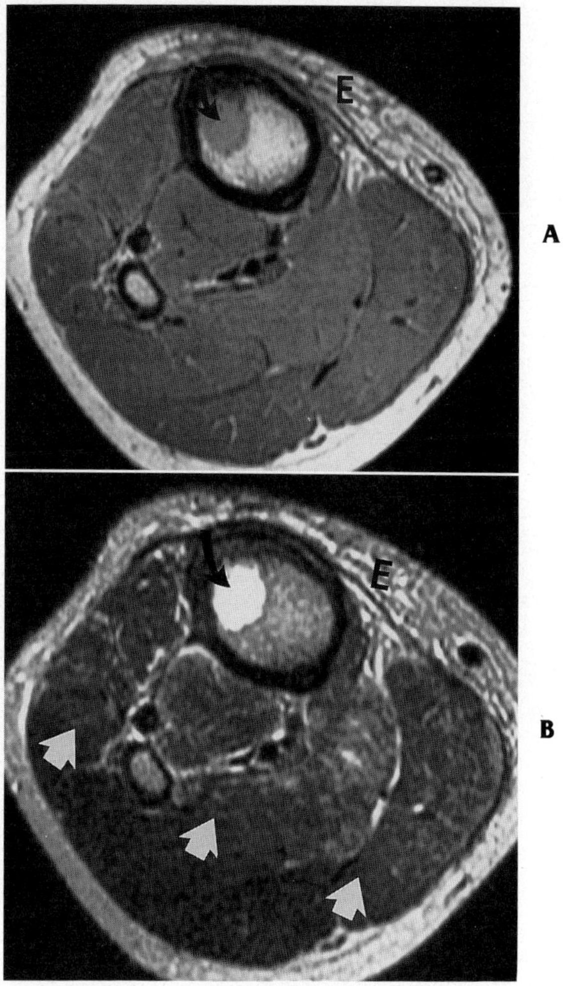


**FIGURE 11** Radiation therapy. Transverse images through the midcalf in a patient 16 months after radiation therapy for soft-tissue and intraosseous hemangiopericytoma. *A,* T1-weighted (TR600/20) and *B,* T2-weighted (TR2500/80) images show a bone cyst, the residua of the treated intraosseous tumor *(curved arrow).* This cyst is the same size as the original tumor and is observed as intermediate signal intensity on T1-weighted images and increased signal intensity on T2-weighted images. Note the increased signal intensity edema, corresponding to the radiation port, on the T2-weighted image *(white arrows).* The edema is not readily discernible on the T1-weighted image, although there is a subtle difference in muscle signal intensity. (From Moore SG. In: Stark DD, Bradley WG, eds. Magnetic Resonance Imaging. St Louis: Mosby–Year Book, 1992; with permission.)

A

B

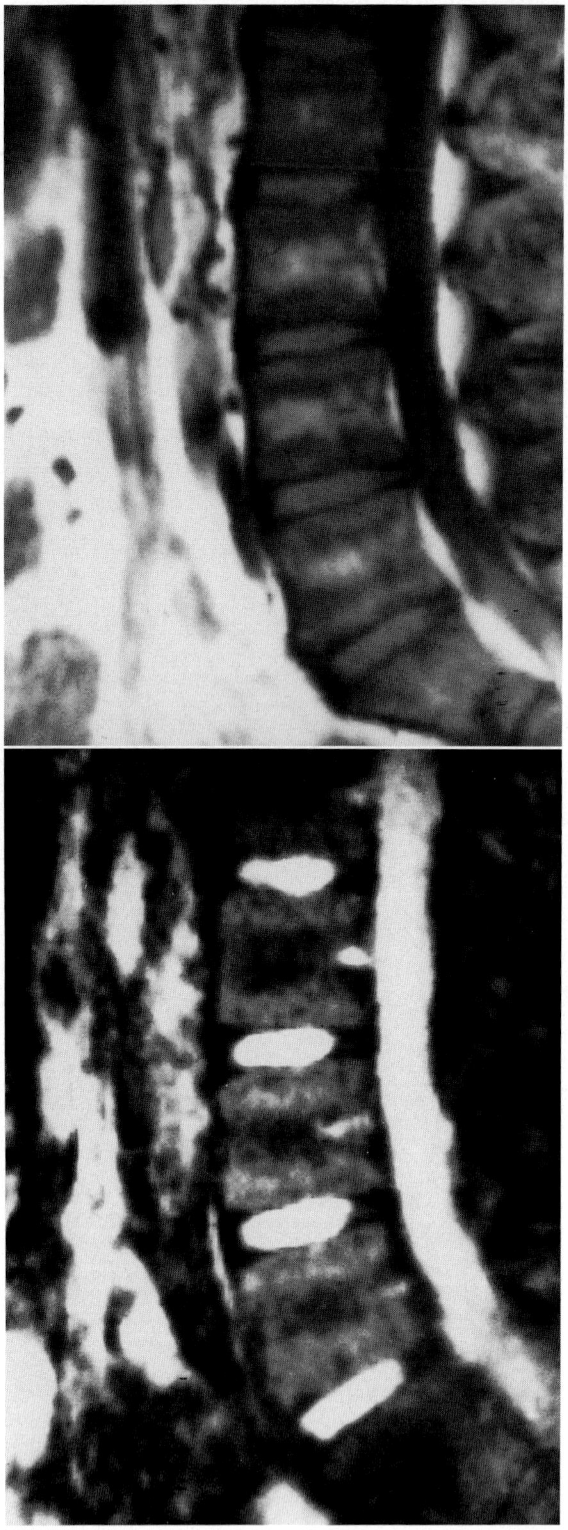

**FIGURE 12** Band pattern following marrow transplantation. Sagittal *(A)* T1-weighted (TR300/30) and *(B)* STIR (TR1500/30/TI100) images of the lumbar spine obtained on day 156 after transplantation. On spin-echo image, note the central band of increased signal intensity (fatty marrow surrounding the basivertebral vein) and the endosteal intermediate signal intensity hematopoietic marrow. On STIR image reciprocal marrow changes reflect the suppressed central fatty marrow and the increased signal intensity endosteal hematopoietic marrow. (From Stevens SK, Moore SG, Amylon MD. Repopulation of marrow after transplantation: MR imaging with pathologic correlation. Radiology 1990; 175:213–218; with permission.)

persistence of sterile cystic lesions, and low signal intensity "sclerosis" have all been described.

Anecdotally, marrow signal intensity following chemotherapy can be normal, decreased, or increased when compared with pretreatment scans. Decreased signal intensity on T1-weighted images can represent either marrow fibrosis or reconversion of yellow to red marrow as a response to the chemotherapeutic assault on marrow. Fatty replacement (aplastic anemia) as a result of chemotherapy is observed either as increased (fatty) marrow signal intensity or as patchy low and high signal intensity (fat and fibrosis). Bony lesions may either resolve or become cystic following treatment.

The response of vertebral marrow to marrow transplantation has been described. The typical pattern observed in vertebral bodies following marrow transplantation includes intermediate signal intensity in the endosteal region of vertebral body that surrounds a central zone of bright signal intensity on T1-weighted images. This marrow pattern is referred to as the band pattern and is usually observed within 3 months of autologous marrow transplantation (Fig. 12). Pathologic correlation of this pattern with excised vertebral bodies shows that the endosteal zone of intermediate signal intensity corresponds to a zone of repopulating hematopoietic cells, while the central zone of bright signal intensity corresponds pathologically to a central zone of fatty marrow. This pattern of repopulation reflects the unique blood supply of the vertebral body. The vascular sinusoids, the site of marrow hematopoiesis, are found along the endosteal surface of the vertebral body and infused hematopoietic cells "home" to this region of the vertebral body. Therefore it is not surprising that after both radiation therapy and marrow transplantation, hematopoietic cells repopulate the periphery of the vertebral body to give the band appearance.

In conclusion, MRI evaluation of the bone marrow is becoming increasingly useful in the identification, staging, and follow-up of marrow disorders. As the first imaging modality that accurately reflects cellular composition and infrastructure of bone marrow, MRI promises to play an increasingly important role in marrow evaluation over the next decade.

## Suggested Reading


Algra PR, Bloem JL. Magnetic resonance imaging of metastatic disease and multiple myeloma. In: Bloem H and Sartoris D, eds. MRI and CT of the Musculoskeletal System: A Text-Atlas. Baltimore: Williams & Wilkins, 1992:218.

Aoki S, Dillon WP, Barkovich AJ, et al. Marrow conversion before pneumatization of the sphenoid sinus: Assessment with MR imaging. Radiology 1989; 172:373–375.

Dawson KL, Moore SG, Rowland J. Age-related marrow changes in the pelvis: MR and anatomic findings. Radiology 1992; 183:47–51.

Fletcher BD, Hanna SL, Kun LE. Changes in MR signal intensity and contrast enhancement of therapeutically irradiated soft tissue. Magn Reson Imaging 1990; 8:771–777.

Jaramillo D, Laor T, Hoffer FA, et al. Epiphyseal marrow in infancy: MR imaging. Radiology 1991; 180:809–812.

Jensen KE, Thomsen C, Henriksen O, et al. Changes in T1 relaxation processes in the bone marrow following treatment in children with acute lymphoblastic leukemia. Pediatr Radiol 1990; 20:464–468.

Kaplan PA, Asleson RJ, Klassen LW, et al. Bone marrow patterns in aplastic anemia: Observations with 1.5T MR imaging. Radiology 1987; 164:441–444.

Kricun ME. Red-yellow marrow conversion: Its effect on the location of some solitary bone lesions. Skeletal Radiol 1985; 14:10–19.

Moore SG. Pediatric marrow and musculoskeletal MRI. Syllabus for 1991 categorical course: Magnetic resonance imaging. AJR 1991; 145–157.

Moore SG. Pediatric musculoskeletal imaging. In: Stark DD, Bradley WG, eds. Magnetic Resonance Imaging. St. Louis: Mosby–Year Book, 1992:2223.

Moore SG, Bisset GS, Siegel MJ, Donaldson JS. Pediatric musculoskeletal MR imaging. Radiology 1991; 179:345–360.

Moore SG, Dawson KL. Red and yellow marrow in the femur: Age related changes in appearance at MR imaging. Radiology 1990; 175:219–223.

Moore SG, Gooding CA, Brasch RC, et al. Bone marrow in children with acute lymphocytic leukemia: MR relaxation times. Radiology 1986; 160:237–240.

Moore SG, Sebag GH. Primary disorders of bone marrow. In: Cohen MD, Edwards MK, eds. Magnetic Resonance Imaging of Children. Philadelphia: BC Decker, 1990:765.

Okada Y, Aoki S, Barkovich AJ, et al. Cranial bone marrow in children: Assessment of normal development with MR imaging. Radiology 1989; 171:161–164.

Ramsey RG, Zacharias CE. MR imaging of the spine after radiation therapy: Easily recognizable effects. AJR 1985; 144:1131–1135.

Rao VM, Fishman M, Mitchell DG, et al. Marrow infarction in sickle cell anemia: Correlation with marrow type and distribution by MRI. Magn Reson Imaging 1989; 7:39–44.

Ricci C, Cora M, Kang YS, et al. Normal age-related patterns of cellular and fatty bone marrow distribution in the axial skeleton: Magnetic resonance imaging study. Radiology 1990; 177:83–88.

Rosen BR, Fleming DM, Kushner DC, et al. Hematologic bone marrow disorders: Quantitative chemical shift MR imaging. Radiology 1988; 169:799–804.

Sebag GH, Moore SG. Effect of trabecular bone on the appearance of marrow in gradient-echo imaging of the appendicular skeleton. Radiology 1990; 174:855–859.

Steiner RM, Mitchell DG, Rao VM, et al. Magnetic resonance imaging of bone marrow: Diagnostic value in diffuse hematologic disorders. Magn Reson Q 1990; 6:17–34.

Steiner RM, Mitchell DG, Rao VM, Rifkin MD. Magnetic resonance imaging of bone marrow disorders. In: Bloem H, Sartorius D, eds. MRI and CT of the Musculoskeletal System: A Text-Atlas. Baltimore: Williams & Wilkins, 1992:108.

Stevens SK, Moore SG, Amylon MD. Repopulation of marrow after transplantation: MR imaging with pathologic correlation. Radiology 1990; 175:213–218.

Stevens SK, Moore SG, Kaplan I. Early and late bone marrow changes following radiation: Magnetic resonance evaluation. AJR 1990; 154:745–750.

Sze G, Bravo S, Baierl P, et al. Developing spinal column: Gadolinium enhanced MR imaging. Radiology 1991; 180: 497–502.

Thomsen C, Sorensen PG, Karle H, et al. Prolonged bone marrow T1-relaxation in acute leukemia: *In vivo* tissue characterization by magnetic resonance imaging. Magn Reson Imaging 1987; 5:251–257.

Vogler JB, Murphy WA. Bone marrow imaging. Radiology 1988; 168:679–693.

# Trauma to the Cervical Spine

*JOHN H. HARRIS, Jr., M.D., D.Sc.*

The radiographic evaluation of a patient suspected of acute injury to the cervical spine is determined by the patient's condition, which not only determines the imaging modality(s) to be used but also the site within the hospital where the examination is optimally performed.

Patients suspected of having acute cervical spine injuries may fall into one of four groups depending on their clinical findings: group I—clinically stable and neurologically stable; group II—clinically stable and neurologically unstable; group III—clinically unstable and neurologically stable; and group IV—clinically unstable and neurologically unstable. Clinical instability usually refers to hemodynamic lability, but may also include a potentially life-threatening injury such as suspected acute traumatic aortic injury, grossly positive peritoneal lavage, or multiple long-bone fractures. Neurologic instability means any patient with a GCS of 1 to 4 or signs of acute post-traumatic myelopathy or radiculopathy.

The radiologic evaluation of all patients suspected of acute traumatic cervical spine injury begins with the plain-film evaluation.

## Group I: Clinically Stable, Neurologically Stable

This group constitutes the largest number of patients requiring radiologic evaluation of the cervical spine. Because they are clinically and neurologically stable, the radiographic examination of the cervical spine is optimally performed outside the Emergency Center using fixed radiographic equipment. These patients are usually in a rigid cervical collar or some other type of cervical spine immobilization, which should not be removed. The initial radiologic examination should include horizontal-beam lateral, anteroposterior (AP), and if possible, open-mouth radiographs. If this evaluation reveals all seven cervical segments to be normally aligned and intact with normal prevertebral soft-tissue shadows, the examination may be concluded and the spine declared radiographically normal.

Usually the density of the shoulders obscures the cervicothoracic junction. In this circumstance, and assuming the AP examination to be normal, the cervical immobilization may be carefully removed and attempts to visualize the lower cervical segments in lateral projection obtained by applying traction to the upper extremities only. Simultaneous countertraction through the head must be avoided so that an unsuspected injury is not distracted. If all seven segments are visualized by this maneuver and are normally aligned and intact, the cervical spine may be declared radiographically normal.

In the event that upper-extremity traction does not result in visualization of the lower cervical segments in lateral projection, "trauma" oblique views should be obtained. These views are made with the patient recumbent and the x-ray tube off-centered approximately 45° in each direction, with the central beam centered at the level of the thyroid cartilage and approximately 2.0 cm lateral to the midline. The trauma oblique projections demonstrate the posterolateral aspect of the cervical vertebrae, the pedicles, intervertebral foramina,

A

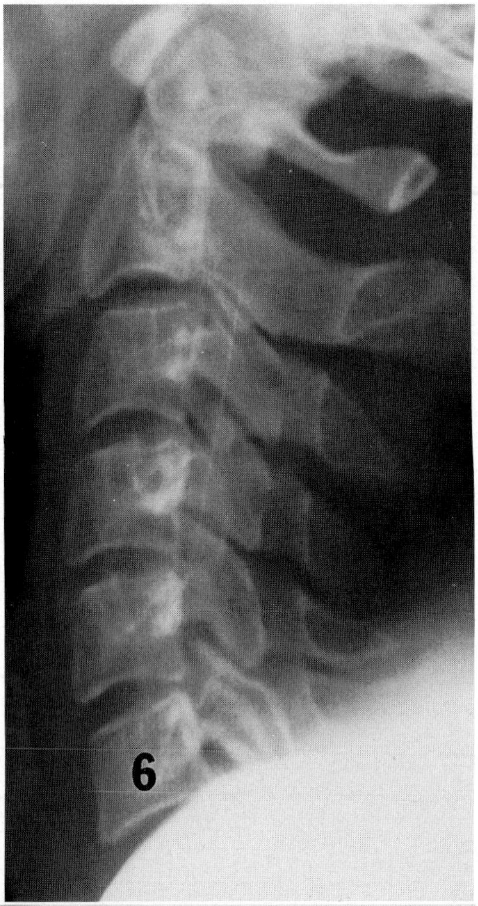


**FIGURE 1** Left C6 unilateral interfacetal dislocation (*curved arrow*) demonstrated on the left "trauma" oblique radiograph (*C*).

B

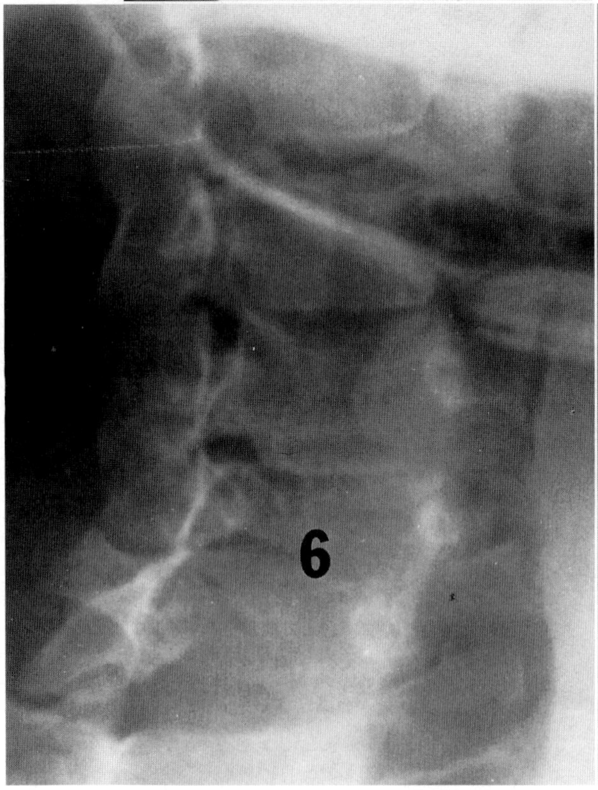


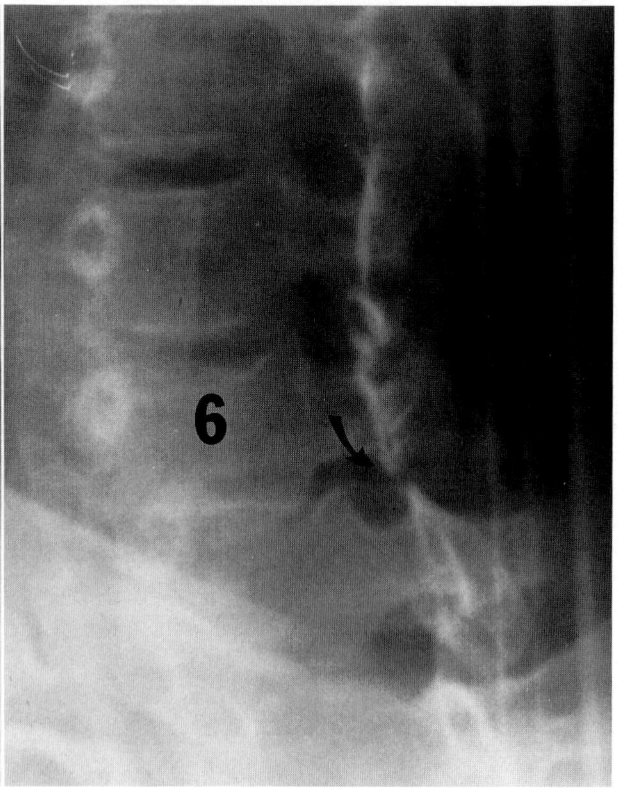


C

and the alignment of the laminae which reflect the position of the articular masses. Mental integration of the data from the AP and each oblique projection is usually sufficient to "clear" the lower cervical segments or identify major injury (Fig. 1).

The "swimmer's" view is sometimes advocated to demonstrate the lower cervical and upper thoracic vertebrae. I have found the swimmer's view to be of little practical value in the patient suspected of having an acute lower cervical or upper thoracic injury. The positioning required to obtain a swimmer's view is obviously contraindicated in an unconscious patient, a patient with a neurologic deficit or upper-extremity fractures or dislocations. Even in more optimal clinical circumstances, the swimmer's view is difficult, if not impossible, to obtain with cervical spine immobilization, including just a hard collar, in place. Under the best of circumstances, the lower cervical and upper thoracic segments are obscured by the superimposed density of the extended arm, the clavicles, and upper ribs (Fig. 2). For these reasons, I prefer the AP and the trauma oblique projections as the plain-film studies to clear the cervicothoracic junction.

Obviously the cervicothoracic junction can be cleared by computed tomography (CT), if the patient's condition permits and if CT is readily available. CT is not indicated to evaluate the cervicothoracic junction in a patient who is alert, cooperative, communicative, and has no symptoms referable to that area.

The only indication for lateral flexion and extension views of the cervical spine is inconclusive evidence of anterior subluxation on the neutral lateral radiograph. The signs of anterior subluxation are accentuated in hyperflexion and reduced in hyperextension. Lateral flexion and extension radiographs are not warranted as a test for mechanical stability of a known cervical spine injury.

The pillar view is indicated when the frontal and lateral radiographs suggest a fracture of the articular mass.

If the initial study demonstrates either a fracture or fracture-dislocation, CT with three-dimensional (3D) reformation is indicated to determine the position and alignment of fracture fragments and their possible relationship to the spinal canal.

Magnetic resonance imaging (MRI) is not indicated in this group of patients who have no neurologic deficit, with the single exception of providing the definitive imaging evaluation for anterior subluxation. Sagittal T2-weighted images demonstrate a high intensity signal of edema and hemorrhage in the presence of an acutely disrupted posterior ligament complex.

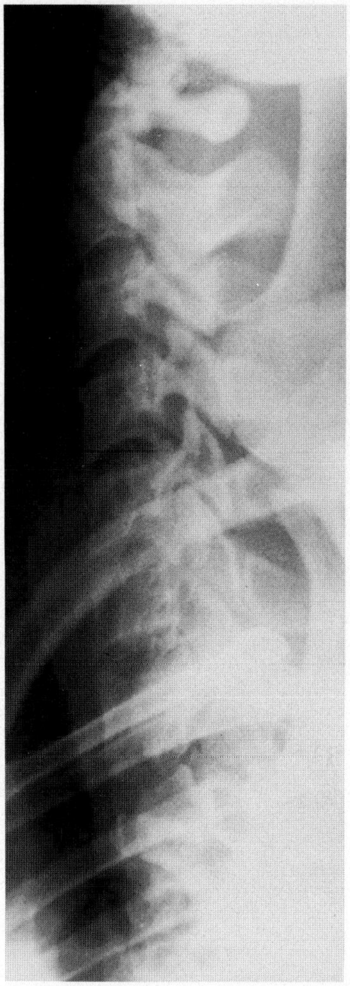

**FIGURE 2** The lower cervical and upper thoracic vertebrae are partially obscured by superimposed skeletal parts in this nearly perfect "swimmer's" projection.

## Group II: Clinically Stable, Neurologically Unstable

In this group of patients in whom the cervical spine injury is characterized by either a myelopathy or radiculopathy, the radiographic examination should be performed in the Emergency Center with portable or fixed equipment, whichever is available. The examination should be performed with whatever type of cervical immobilization device is in place and should consist of horizontal-beam lateral and AP projections. If possible, open-mouth projection of the atlantoaxial articulation is desirable. If not possible, the cervicocranium must be evaluated, initially at least, by the lateral projection only.

If the limited examination just described demonstrates a fracture or fracture dislocation, CT is indicated for the purposes previously stated, and MRI is indicated to evaluate the soft tissues of the cervical spine, particularly the disk, and the spinal cord itself.

If the horizontal-beam lateral radiograph reveals normally aligned and intact cervical vertebrae with diffuse prevertebral soft-tissue swelling (Fig. 3) in the presence of clinical signs of the acute central cervical cord syndrome, the diagnosis of hyperextension dislocation of the cervical spine is established. CT is not indicated in this injury, because hyperextension dislocation of the cervical spine is a predominantly soft-tissue injury and a CT scan does not provide any more information than is already available from the plain radiographs.

MRI is the essential subsequent imaging examination to demonstrate the location and extent of the soft-tissue injuries at the level of the hyperextension dislocation as well as the level, extent, and the MR characteristics of the cord injury, which are reflective of its histopathology.

## Group III: Clinically Unstable, Neurologically Stable

Patients who are clinically unstable but neurologically intact should have only a horizontal-beam lateral and AP radiograph of the cervical spine obtained in the Emergency Center, using

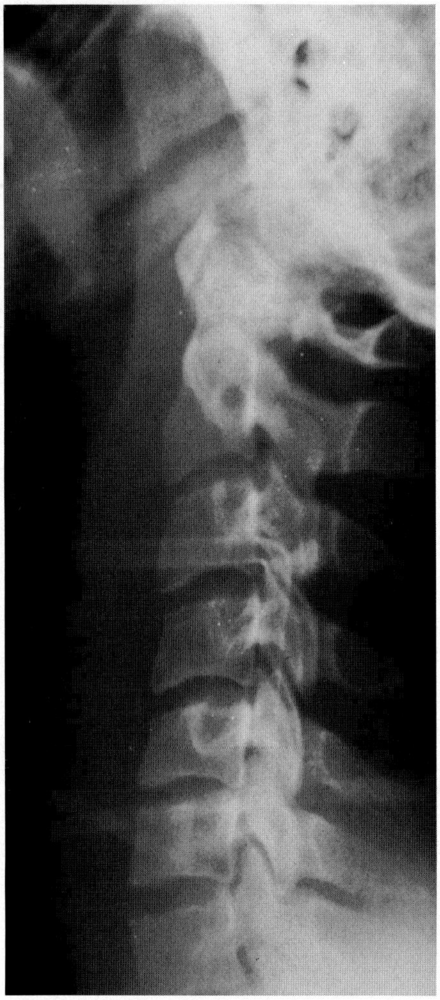

**FIGURE 3** Hyperextension dislocation of the cervical spine characterized by diffuse prevertebral soft-tissue swelling and normally aligned, intact cervical vertebrae.

whatever type of equipment is available, with the cervical restraint in place. The radiographic examination of the cervical spine is an integral part of the initial evaluation of this group of patients, and the necessary views may be obtained during the clinical evaluation. The purpose of the radiographic examination is to either "clear" the cervical spine or to identify a cervical spine injury that has not caused a neurologic deficit. Demonstration of an acute cervical injury concludes the radiographic evaluation of these patients. The cervical spine should remain immobilized until the patient is stabilized, at which time the radiographic evaluation of the cervical spine injury should be definitively concluded by the appropriate imaging modality. If the cervical spine cannot be cleared and a specific diagnosis cannot be established by this limited radiographic evaluation, the cervical spine must be considered potentially unstable and remain immobilized until the patient's condition has been stabilized and a definitive radiographic examination completed.

## Group IV: Clinically Unstable, Neurologically Unstable

In this most critical group of patients with cervical spine injury, the radiographic examination must be performed in the Emergency Center with whatever type of equipment is available. The evaluation should consist only of a horizontal-beam lateral and AP view, which should be obtained during the initial clinical evaluation of the patient. The sole purpose of the radiographic evaluation is to identify the level and type of cervical spine injury. If this purpose cannot be achieved with this limited study, the cervical spine must remain immobilized until the patient's condition has been stabilized sufficiently that the imaging evaluation may proceed to a definitive conclusion.

An algorithmic approach to the radiographic evaluation of patients with acute cervical spine trauma based on findings on the initial cervical spine examination is presented in Figure 4.

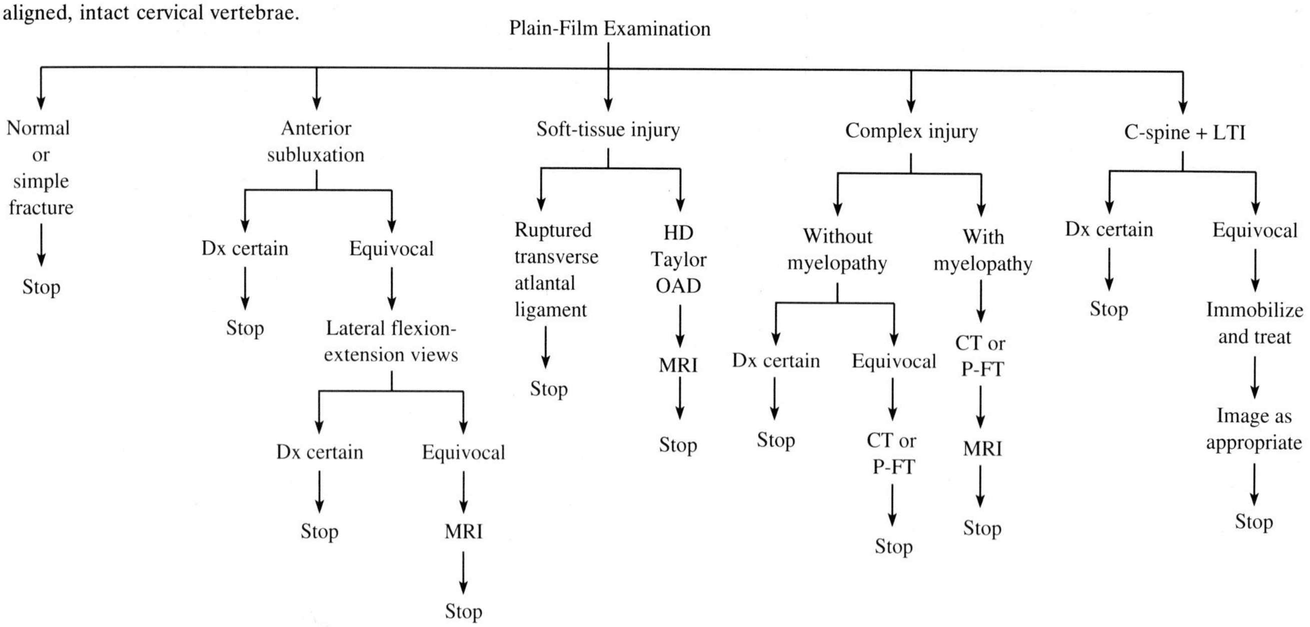


**FIGURE 4** Imaging acute cervical spine injury. Simple fractures include the following: *flexion* – simple wedge, clay shoveler's; *extension* – anterior arch of C1, posterior arch of C1, extension tear drop. Complex injuries include fracture of the neural arch, dislocations, and fracture-dislocations. Dx = diagnosis, HD = hyperextension dislocation, OAD = occipito-atlantal dislocation, P-FT = plain-film tomography, LTI = life-threatening injury.

**Suggested Reading**

Harris JH Jr. Radiographic evaluation of spine trauma. Orthop Clin North Am 1986; 17:75–86.

Harris JH Jr. Imaging the acutely injured spine. ACR Radiology Syllabus 1990; 95–104.

Harris JH Jr. Spinal imaging. In: Browner BD, Jupiter JB, Levine AM, Trafton PG, eds. Skeletal Trauma. Philadelphia: WB Saunders, 1992:605.

Harris JH Jr, Edeiken-Monroe B. The Radiology of Acute Cervical Spine Trauma. 2nd ed. Baltimore: Williams & Wilkins, 1987.

Mirvis SE, Young JWR. Imaging in Trauma and Critical Care. Baltimore: Williams & Wilkins, 1991.

# Soft-Tissue Evaluation in Trauma to the Hand and Wrist

*DAVID J. CURTIS, M.D.*

## Technique of Filming

Soft-tissue cassettes tend to provide adequate imaging of both bone and soft tissue. Two views are required to obtain 360° information. I use the posteroanterior (PA) and lateral (LAT) views, because they are easiest to interpret. Other views mainly enhance bone detail.

There are nine separate areas on the PA and LAT views to evaluate. The LAT has the pronator (P) and dorsal wrist (DW) as well as the dorsal hand (DH) and dorsal forearm (DF). Each of the last three is superficial and demonstrates superficial swelling, because of skin and subcutaneous fat, and they are separated from each other by perpendicular fascial sheets (Fig. 1).

The PA view shows five areas with only one deep: the navicular or scaphoid (S). The other four areas are the hypothenar (HT) adjacent to the base of the fifth metacarpal; the thenar (T) lateral to the base of the first metacarpal at the insertion of the abductor pollicis longus (APL); the pararadial (PR), lateral to the radial styloid and APL; and the paraulnar (PU), medial to the ulnar styloid.

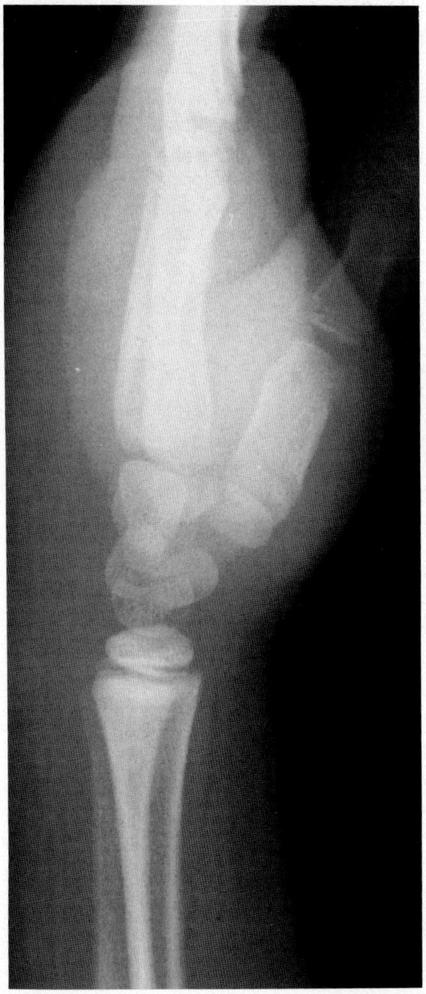

**FIGURE 1** Lateral view (LAT) of the hand and wrist demonstrates a normal pronator fat plane (P) in spite of massive swelling of the dorsal forearm. The subcutaneous fat is edematous, not fluid filled, in this hemophiliac. Note normal alignment of the radius and ulna, lunate, capitate, and metacarpals. This excludes most dislocations that should be considered because of the number of abnormal fat planes.

## Interpretation

A fat pad or skin region is considered positive if it cannot be demonstrated or it is pushed away from adjacent structures. The most commonly positive fat pad is the pronator fat pad, because radius fractures are the most common wrist fractures. The most subtle fractures are those of the scaphoid, because its fat pad is complex and only about 3 cm long (Fig. 2). It contains the wrist fat, the wrist capsule, the lateral collateral ligament, the APL, subcutaneous fat, and skin. Fat separates the capsule and lateral collateral ligament as well as the ligament and the APL. Each or all of these fat soft-tissue planes may disappear as the fat contrasts with the soft tissue only as long as it is not filled with fluid and "soft tissue" as well. Realize that only a part of the fat plane may disappear and still be positive. If the DW fat plane demonstrates a uniform whitening (fluid in the wrist capsule) and dorsal bowing with no problem in the S fat plane, I look even more carefully at the scaphoid, with my finger obscuring parts of the scaphoid, and finally consider a stress view if the ulnar side of the wrist also shows no problem.

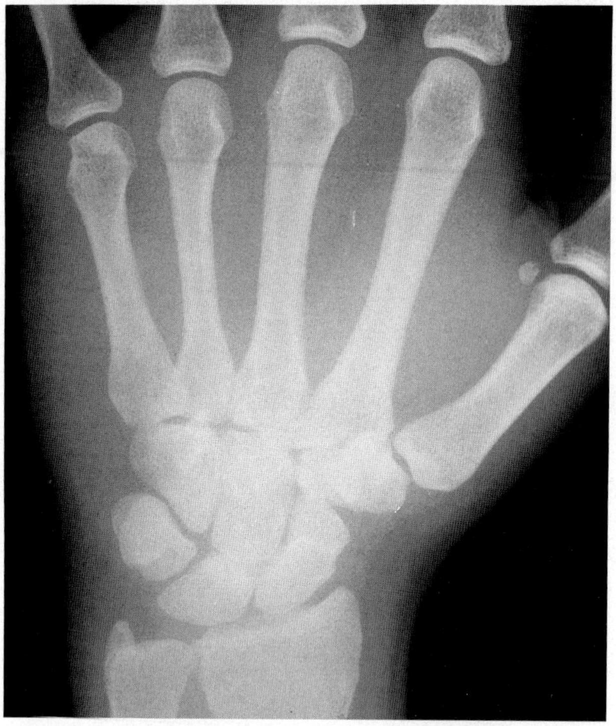

**FIGURE 2** Posteroanterior view of the hand and wrist demonstrates an abnormal scaphoid fat plane (S). The abductor pollicis longus (APL) is poorly outlined by fat between the base of the first metacarpal and obscured at the styloid before normal subcutaneous fat is observed more proximally. There is a torus cortical buckle just proximal to the normal subcutaneous fat. A punch fracture fragment appears to be present in the medial radius. Multiple joints in the wrist are not parallel, suggesting an acute, severe sprain centering on the scaphoid bone. In the S itself, hints are made to other parts of it being abnormal. We should see the lateral collateral ligament outlined by fat as it runs from the radial styloid to the greater tuberosity of the trapezium. Its density should be close to that of the subcutaneous fat observed more proximally.

## Mechanism of Injury

Many injuries are associated with each other in the hand and wrist, probably because dorsiflexion of the wrist is the most common type of injury, violently placing the weight of the whole body on the wrist and forearm. Hence one can suspect that radius and carpus injuries may occur simultaneously. Finger and metacarpal injuries are more frequently jamming forces along the axis of the individual bones. Hence there is low association between hand and wrist and forearm injuries, and if they are present, multiple injuries may have occurred in a short time, as in a motorcycle accident. The thumb is not protected like the other metacarpals and is abducted violently or fractured more easily with a jamming injury, because it creates an associated abduction. All metacarpals are subject to direct blow fractures.

## Sprains

Sprains of the wrist are common because of the orientation of the capitate as a wedge pointed at the scapholunate joint; there are few data concerning actual frequency. Sprains may be more significant than a fracture and require more healing time. A sprain is identified as an absence of a parallel joint, with a wider or narrower joint than its neighbors (see Fig. 2). The soft tissue of a joint is the cartilage. If swelling occurs adjacent to the joint space which is not parallel to itself, there is probably a sprain, and a stress view is indicated if there is any clinical question. Pain without any demonstrable fracture is another indication for a stress view. Any loss of parallel is abnormal. "Is it new or old?" is the only question, and it is answered with stress views.

### *Stress Views*

Stress views are easy to perform and are relatively painless for the patient. The easiest to perform is a clenched fist PA view. Clenching the fist exerts simultaneous contractions of all flexors and extensors, creating intrajoint pressure that in turn creates a driving apart of the intercalating segment joints. The other commonly considered stress view is a hanging PA, which pulls the wrist apart from the joint rather than pushing apart. Finally, a delayed view is performed in 10 days to 2 weeks to allow healing osteoporosis to demonstrate fracture lines. This last helps less with sprains.

## Fractures

Fractures are like pseudojoints and show themselves as lucencies through the bony cortex, the lamina dura of the bones (Figs. 3, 4). The most subtle include fractures of the scaphoid bone and punch fractures of the medial radius. These latter fractures are incomplete in the AP dimension, making them difficult to observe.

When the bony cortex is incomplete around a chip of bone, it confirms the avulsion nature of the bone. The triquetrum provides most of these avulsions. Occasionally when fractures are present, stress views or other views are required to demonstrate the existing fracture with its soft-tissue–filled interspace.

Beside the fracture line itself being visible, encroachment on the 11° palmar angle of the distal radius is an excellent indicator of a radius fracture. If there is no soft-tissue abnormality in the pronator, or pain, the injury is probably old.

## Dislocations

The last feature of my approach to trauma is to evaluate for dislocations. A dislocation is a completed sprain. The malalignment requires immediate reduction or aseptic necrosis may occur. The necrosis may occur anyway, but the fault will be considered ours if we do not describe and transmit the information to our colleagues. This is true of S fractures and is the reason this soft-tissue means of evaluation was undertaken initially. Approximately 95 percent of dislocations center around the lunate; these are the perilunate and lunate dislocations. The former is frequently associated with fractures, while the latter is less complicated. Both dislocations are caused by severe dorsiflexion of the wrist. The lunate dislocation completes the reflex toward the palm. The perilunate dislocation is impeded in some way in its reflex.

Alignment in the lateral view requires the radius to align with the lunate and capitate. In the foregoing dislocations discussed, the joint that is always widened and not parallel is the capitolunate. The perilunate dislocation maintains some association, whereas it is lost in lunate dislocations. The radius-lunate association is also abnormal in the palmar aspect.

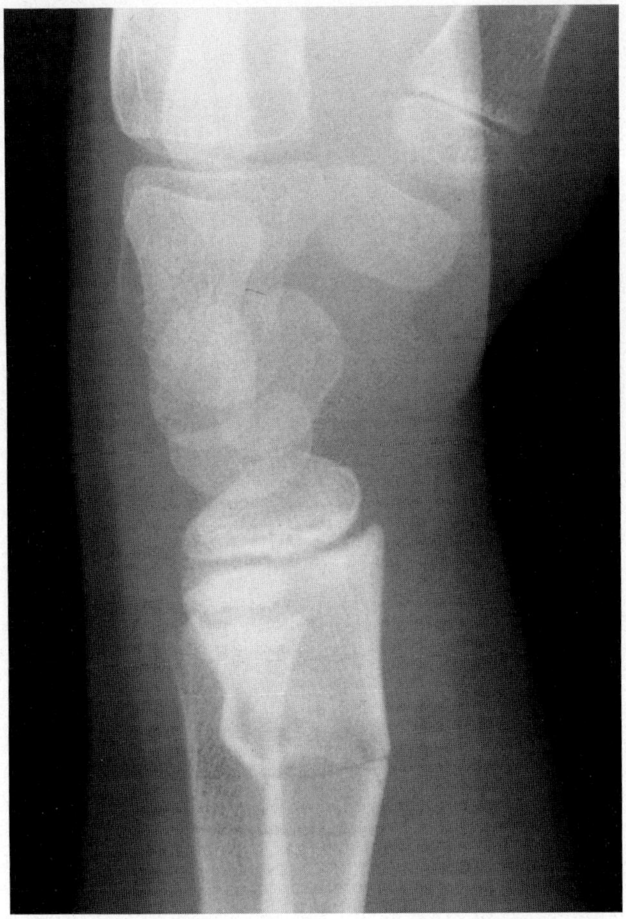

**FIGURE 3** LAT view of the radius shows an obvious distal diaphyseal fracture of the radius. The P is bowed and indistinct at the level of the fracture. It is thickened as well, suggesting fluid within the muscle. The lunatocapitate joint is widened dorsally, suggesting an acute sprain as the reason for the swelling in the DW. DF swelling is visible distal to the radius fracture.

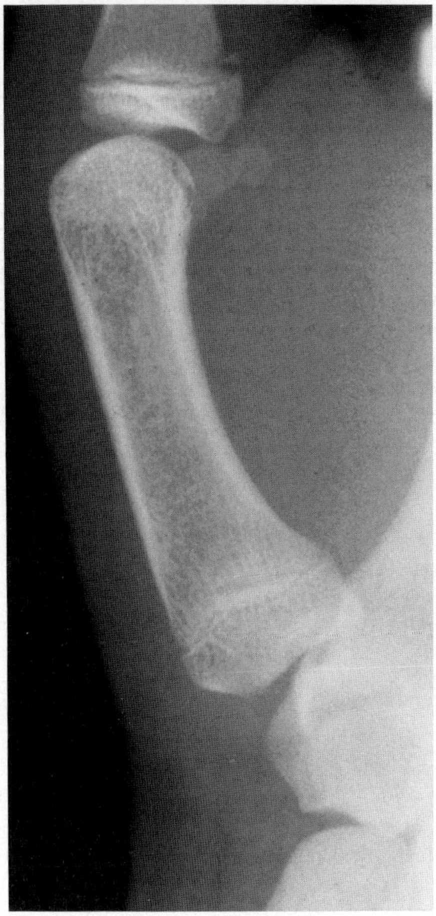

**FIGURE 4** LAT view of the thumb. Swelling makes the T interface between APL and subcutaneous fat indistinct for about 1 cm. Comparison with other subcutaneous fat proximal and distal makes this difference more apparent. Cause of this swelling is the Salter-Harris 2 fracture of the palmar aspect of the first proximal phalanx.

## Evaluation Summary

1. Check the P, DR, and APL portion of the DR to exclude radius fractures. Check PU to exclude ulna fractures (< 1 percent of solo injuries).
2. Check DW and S to exclude scaphoid fracture. If S is normal but DW positive, evaluate the rest of the wrist carefully.
3. Check APL of T to exclude metacarpal and proximal first phalangeal injuries.
4. Check DH and HT to exclude second through fifth metacarpal injuries.
5. Use a delayed view (7 to 10 days) to exclude a suspected fracture when the search for injury has been unsuccessful.
6. Exclude sprains by applying the principle of joints parallel and equal in width. Use compression and distraction views as necessary.
7. If five or more fat planes are distorted, check the alignment of the radius, lunate, capitate, and metacarpal bases to exclude dislocations.

## Suggested Reading

Carver RA, Barrington NA. Soft-tissue changes accompanying recent scaphoid injuries. Clin Radiol 1985; 36:423–425.

Curtis DJ. Injuries of the wrist: An approach to diagnosis. Radiol Clin North Am 1981; 19:625–644.

Curtis DJ, Downey EF Jr, and Brahman SL. Letter to the editor. Compartmentalized swelling in hand and wrist trauma. AJR 1985; 145:195.

Curtis DJ, Downey EF Jr, Brower AC, et al. Importance of soft-tissue evaluation in hand and wrist trauma: Statistical evaluation. AJR 1984; 142:781–788.

Downey EF Jr, Curtis DJ. Soft tissue radiography of the wrist. In: Lichtman DM, ed. The Wrist and Its Disorders. Philadelphia: WB Saunders, 1988:96.

MacEwan DW. Changes due to trauma in the fat plane overlying the quadratus muscle: A radiologic sign. Radiology 1964; 82:879–886.

Melon GL, Staple TW, Evans RG. Soft tissue radiographic technique. Semin Roentgenol 1973; 8:19–24.

Terry DW Jr, Ramish JE. The navicular fat stripe: A useful roentgen for evaluating wrist trauma. AJR 1975; 124:25–28.

# MRI of Rotator Cuff Tears

BARBARA N. WEISSMAN, M.D. · PIRAN ALIABADI, M.D.

Clinical assessment of patients with shoulder pain may leave doubt as to the cause of the pain and the appropriate clinical course. Differential considerations often include complete or partial rotator cuff tears, tendinitis, impingement, and instability or a combination of these disorders. Imaging procedures should allow differentiation among these possibilities. In addition to confirmation of the presence of a rotator cuff tear, the method optimally should allow assessment of the location and extent of the tear, the status of the torn edges of the cuff, the presence or absence of muscular atrophy, and the presence of arthritic changes of the glenohumeral joint.

## Indications, Clinical Utility, and Alternative Technologies

Standard radiographs are mandatory before other imaging modalities are used. Radiographs allow immediate exclusion or inclusion of some diagnoses (e.g., fracture, bone destruction from tumor, posterior dislocation). In addition, radiographs are important adjuncts to magnetic resonance imaging (MRI), particularly since calcification may be overlooked or misinterpreted on MRI, but is easily seen on standard radiographs. When radiographs show severe upward subluxation of the humeral head, a thinned or massively torn rotator cuff is likely, and additional studies may be unnecessary. Impingement of the rotator cuff is suggested by the presence of osteophytes from the inferior margin of the acromion process or from the acromioclavicular (AC) joint.

Three techniques are currently available for evaluation of the rotator cuff: MRI, ultrasonography, and arthrography. At the Brigham and Women's Hospital, ultrasonography has largely been abandoned in favor of MRI and arthrography.

### *Magnetic Resonance Imaging*

MRI is the preferred method of most physicians at the Brigham and Women's Hospital for studying the rotator cuff. Aside from the usual advantages of MRI anywhere in the body (the lack of ionizing radiation, the ability to image in any plane, high spatial resolution), MRI offers particular advantages in the assessment of the rotator cuff. For example, the location, size of the tear, and the quality of the tendon edges can be demonstrated with this noninvasive examination. Impingement can be documented, the status of involved muscles can be assessed, and abnormalities related to instability and arthritic changes of the glenohumeral joint can be studied.

In addition to the usual contraindications to MRI, patient size and claustrophobia are prominent problems when studying the shoulder. In comparison to arthrography, interpretation of MR images is more complex and evaluation more costly.

### *Arthrography*

Double-contrast arthrography remains the method of choice for some referring orthopedists. Although the double-contrast arthrographic method allows rotator cuff tears to be demonstrated, the presence of muscle atrophy and impingement of the cuff by soft tissue cannot be evaluated. Partial tears involving the superior surface of the cuff or intrasubstance tears also are not detected with this method.

At the Brigham and Women's Hospital, double-contrast arthrography is employed as the primary procedure when preference of the referring physician so indicates, when the least expensive examination is desired, when the results of MRI evaluation are equivocal, or when MRI is contraindicated.

Contraindications to arthrography include allergy to contrast material and skin infections overlying the shoulder. In comparison to the relatively noninvasive studies of ultrasonography or MRI, the shoulder arthrogram carries the potential risks (although uncommon) of contrast reaction or infection and the more common sequela of postprocedural pain.

### *Ultrasonography*

Initial enthusiasm for ultrasonography of the rotator cuff has waned as recent studies have not confirmed the high sensitivities and specificities at first reported. Despite the noninvasive nature of the procedure, and its low cost, the test has several drawbacks: (1) it is highly operator dependent, (2) only portions of the rotator cuff can be evaluated, and (3) it is unable to assess the glenoid labrum or impingement.

## Technical Approach for MRI of Rotator Cuff

Standard radiographs are reviewed whenever possible when MR images are interpreted. Thus, if radiographs have not been taken previously, they are obtained at the time of the MRI evaluation. Imaging is postponed for at least 2 weeks after corticosteroid injection or arthrography to avoid artifacts that may be produced by these procedures.

Imaging is performed on a 1.5 T Signa scanner (General Electric) or on a 0.5 T MAX scanner (General Electric) with the parameters listed in Tables 1 and 2. With the patient lying supine or slightly oblique toward the affected side, a 5 inch general-purpose coil or the 7 inch heart-shaped coil is positioned over the shoulder. The arm is at the side and in neutral rotation, since internal rotation has been found to produce overlap of tendons and potentially interfere with interpretation.

Images are routinely obtained in three planes, the coronal oblique (parallel to the supraspinatus tendon), the sagittal oblique (perpendicular to the supraspinatus tendon), and the axial (perpendicular to anterior and posterior labra). The coronal oblique is the most important plane for evaluating the rotator cuff and is obtained by choosing a plane along the axis of the supraspinatus muscle from a high scout axial image (Fig. 1). The sagittal oblique images are also chosen from the axial scout to be perpendicular to the supraspinatus muscle.

**TABLE 1** Imaging Protocol on 0.5 T Magnet

| Plane | TR | TE1/TE2 | Flip Angle | FOV | Slice Thickness/Skip | Matrix | NEX | Acquisition Time |
|---|---|---|---|---|---|---|---|---|
| Coronal oblique | 200 | 20 | | 42 | 15/10 | 128 | 1 | :20 |
| Axial | 500 | 25 | | 20 | 4/1 | 192 | 2 | 6:32 |
| Coronal oblique | 2,000 | 25/80 | | 16 | 5/0 | 192 | 2 | 13:12 |
| Axial | 600 | 28 | 30 | 16 | 5/0 | 192 | 2 | 4:33 |
| Sagittal oblique | 550 | 25 | | 16 | 5/0 | 192 | 2 | 5:50 |

FOV = field of view; NEX = number of excitations.

**TABLE 2** Imaging Protocol on 1.5 T Magnet

| Plane | TR | TE1/TE2 | Flip Angle | FOV | Slice Thickness/Skip | Matrix | NEX | Acquisition Time |
|---|---|---|---|---|---|---|---|---|
| Axial | 600 | Minimum | | 20 | 5/1 | 192 | 2 | 3:58 |
| Coronal oblique | 2,000 | Minimum | | 16 (20) | 5/0 | 192 | 1 | 7:08 |
| Sagittal oblique | 600 | Minimum | | 16 (20) | 5/0 | 192 | 2 | 3:58 |
| Axial | 300 | 13 | 30 | 16 | 5/0 | 192 | 4 | 3:54 |

A B C

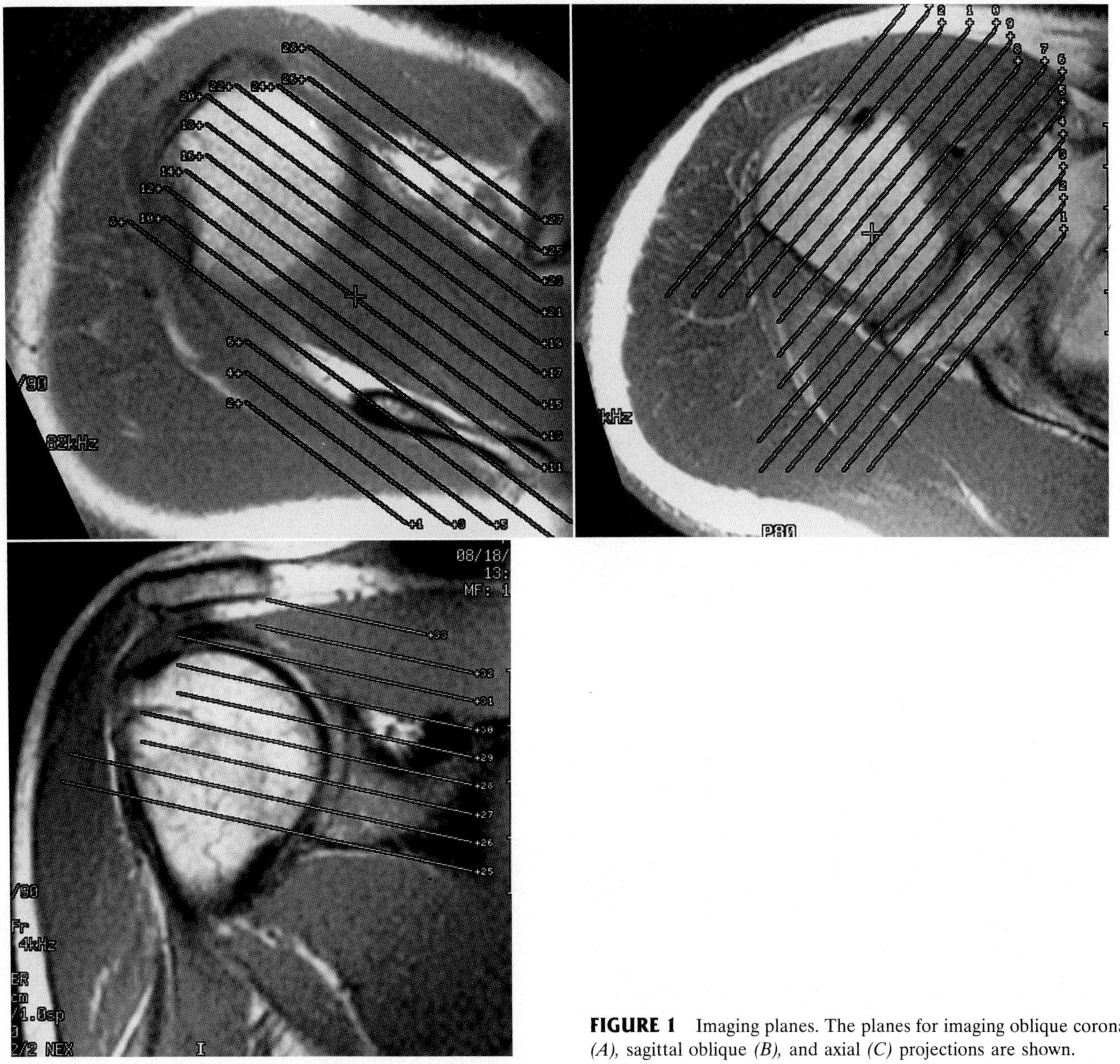

**FIGURE 1** Imaging planes. The planes for imaging oblique coronal *(A)*, sagittal oblique *(B)*, and axial *(C)* projections are shown.

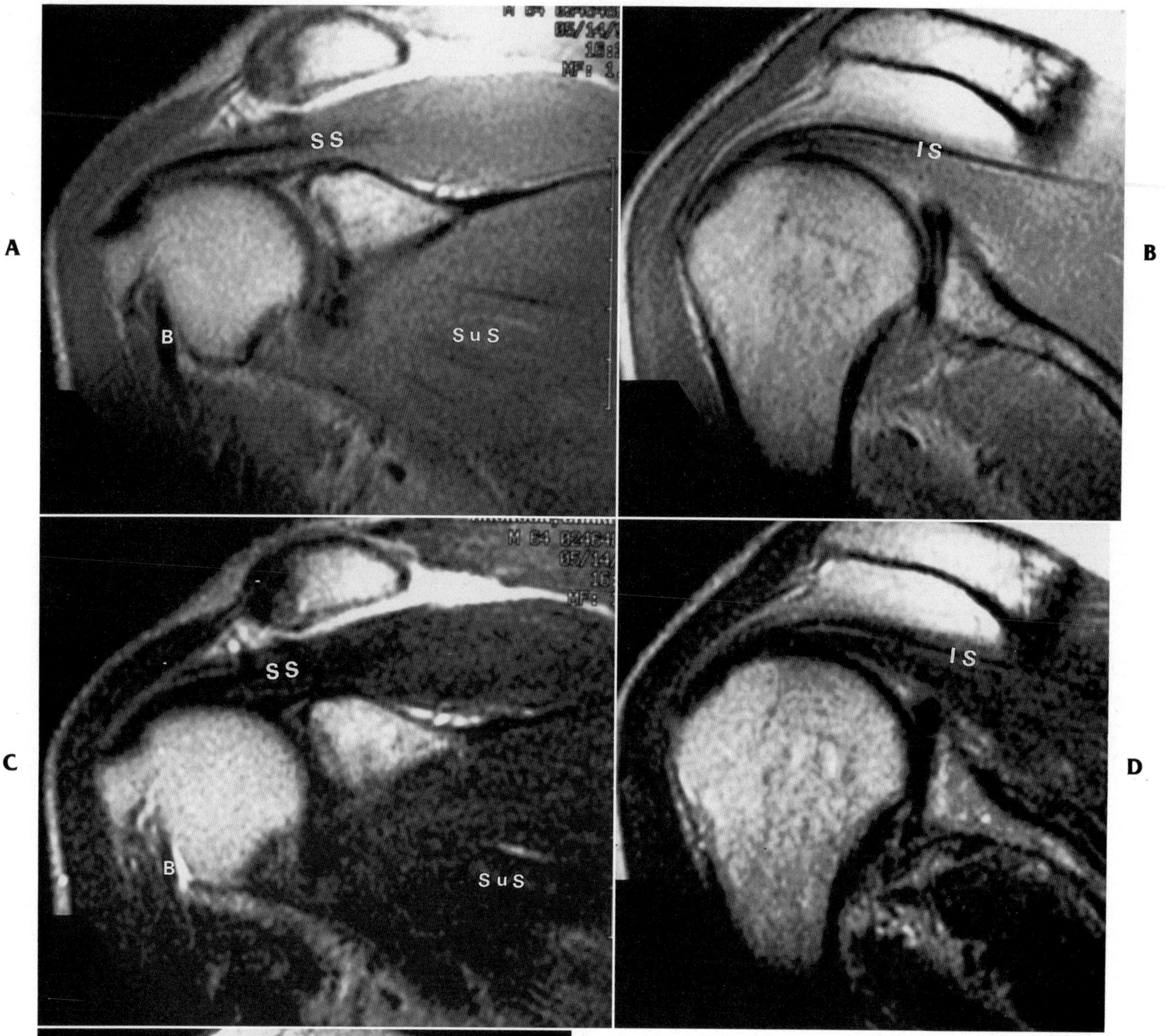


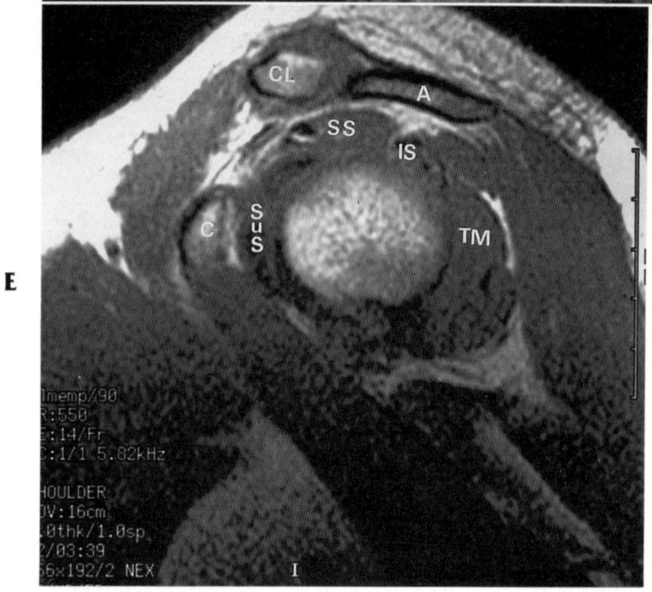


**FIGURE 2** Normal shoulder MRI. *A,* The normal supraspinatus muscle and tendon are shown in the coronal oblique projection. Proton density *(A)* and T2-weighted *(B)* images. Proton density *(C)* and T2-weighted *(D)* images show the intact infraspinatus muscle and tendon. *E,* The sagittal oblique view shows the rotator cuff in cross section. SS = supraspinatus muscle and tendon, IS = infraspinatus muscle and tendon. SuS = subscapularis. B = biceps tendon, CL = clavicle, C = coracoid, A = acromion.

## Diagnostic Approach

### *Normal Anatomy*

The rotator cuff consists of the supraspinatus, infraspinatus, and teres minor muscles and tendons that insert on the greater tuberosity, and the subscapularis that inserts on the lesser tuberosity. The supraspinatus tendon, particularly the "critical area" (the region from 0.5 cm proximal to the greater tuberosity to the musculotendinous junction over the long head of the biceps) is the most common region to be torn. The coronal oblique projection allows excellent visualization of the course of the supraspinatus tendon, the AC joint, and acromion (Fig. 2). The tendon appears uniformly low in signal (dark) and continuous with the muscle at about the 12 o'clock position. A thin crescent of bright signal on T1- and T2-weighted images represents fat associated with the subacromial subdeltoid bursa and is often observed in normal shoulders. The anterior (subscapularis) and posterior (infraspinatus and teres minor) portions of the rotator cuff may be observed on axial or sagittal images. The sagittal plane also allows assessment of the shape of the acromion, the coracoacromial ligament, the humeral head, and the rotator cuff tendons.

### *Impingement Syndrome*

Two major theories have been postulated to explain the cause of rotator cuff tears: primary degenerative disease of the cuff and secondary degeneration due to impingement. Neer supports the latter view and feels that 95 percent of cases of chronic rotator cuff tear are due to impingement of the supraspinatus tendon by the coracoacromial arch. In this condition impingement occurs in forward elevation of the arm; the supraspinatus tendon and often the biceps tendon are compressed against the anterior edge and undersurface of the anterior third of the acromion, the coracoacromial ligament, and sometimes the AC joint. Osteophyte formation from the undersurface of the acromion or the AC joint or a hooked anterior acromion process have been associated with impingement syndrome. Neer described a sequence of injury from reversible edema and hemorrhage to fibrosis and tendinitis to rotator cuff and/or biceps tears and bone spurs, and remodeling and narrowing of the acromiohumeral interval.

### *Criteria for Diagnosis of Rotator Cuff Tear (Table 3)*

#### Abnormal Tendon Signal

Full-thickness tears typically display abnormal signal involving the entire thickness of the tendon, with marked brightening of the abnormal area on T2-weighted images (Fig. 3). Fluid is present within the joint, and the subdeltoid bursa and joint effusion communicate through the tear.

In some cases the brightening on T2 images is not apparent and only moderate increase in signal is observed on T2-weighted images or there is low signal (scar) present. In these cases the diagnosis may be suggested by the attenuated irregular appearance of the tendon. In practice, however, we have found the diagnosis of complete tear difficult when high signal is not present in the tendon on the T2-weighted images.

#### Displacement of Musculotendinous Junction

Normally the musculotendinous junction of the supraspinatus tendon lies beneath the AC joint or the acromion. In moderate or large tears, retraction may produce media displacement of this zone.

#### Abnormal Fat Planes and Bursae

Zlatkin and co-workers pointed out the importance of studying the periarticular structures, the subacromial-subdeltoid fat plane and bursa as well as the tendon itself, when deciding whether or not a rotator cuff tear was present. Thus the proposed diagnostic criteria for rotator cuff tear included loss of the normally bright signal of the subacromial subdeltoid fat plane on T1- or proton density–weighted images, with or without fluid in the bursa on the T2-weighted images. An abnormal tendon (abnormal signal and thinning or irregularity) with intact periarticular tissues was thought to represent tendinitis. In practice the evaluation of the fat planes is more difficult than the easily identified fluid in the bursa. The presence of fluid in the bursa, although not normal, may be observed without a rotator cuff tear and is nonspecific. This finding should therefore be correlated with other signs of rotator cuff tear.

### *Criteria for Diagnosis of Partial Tears*

Partial rotator cuff tears theoretically display focal areas of increased signal on T1-weighted images that do not involve the entire thickness of the tendon. An increase in signal intensity is observed in these regions on T2-weighted images. In our experience the differentiation of partial tears from tendinitis is difficult.

Recently we have employed the method of Farley and co-workers for describing the rotator cuff (Table 4). Most cases can be categorized using this system, and correlation of findings with the probability of full- or partial-thickness tears has been made.

**TABLE 3** Typical Features of Rotator Cuff Abnormalities

| Status | T1 Signal of Cuff | T2 Signal of Cuff | Fat Along SDB | Fluid in SDB | Position of Musculotendinous Junction |
|---|---|---|---|---|---|
| Normal | Low | Low | Normal | Absent | Normal |
| Tendinitis | Increased | No brightening | Normal | Present | Normal |
| Partial tear | Focal increase | Moderate or marked increase | | Present in superior surface tear | Normal |
| Full-thickness tear | Increased, involves entire width | Marked increase | Absent | Present | May be displaced |

SDB = subdeltoid bursa.

A B C

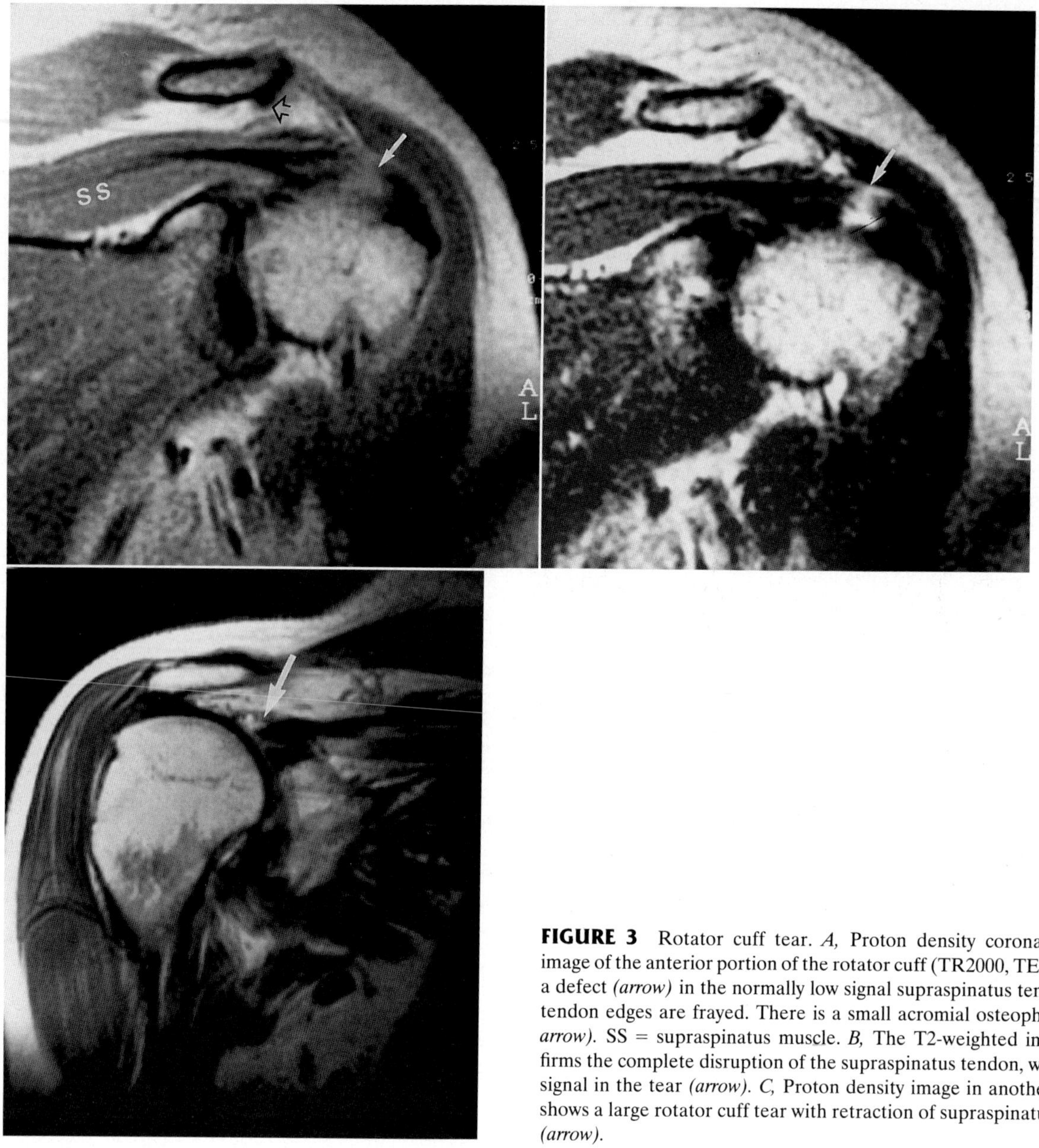


**FIGURE 3** Rotator cuff tear. *A,* Proton density coronal oblique image of the anterior portion of the rotator cuff (TR2000, TE80) shows a defect *(arrow)* in the normally low signal supraspinatus tendon. The tendon edges are frayed. There is a small acromial osteophyte *(open arrow).* SS = supraspinatus muscle. *B,* The T2-weighted image confirms the complete disruption of the supraspinatus tendon, with bright signal in the tear *(arrow). C,* Proton density image in another patient shows a large rotator cuff tear with retraction of supraspinatus tendon *(arrow).*

**TABLE 4** MRI Grading of Rotator Cuff Signal

| Grade | Characteristics | Meaning |
|---|---|---|
| Grade 0 | Normal, no increased signal | Normal |
| Grade 1 | Increased signal < water or fat on T2WI | Tendinitis |
| Grade 2 | Focal or partial-thickness increased signal of water intensity on T2WI | Grade 2 and 3, 89% sensitive and 77% specific for full-thickness SS tears |
| Grade 3 | Full-thickness, 1 cm long defect of water intensity on T2WI | 70% sensitive and 96% specific for full-thickness SS tears |

SS = supraspinatus; T2WI = T2-weighted images.
Modified from Farley TE, Neumann CH, et al. Full-thickness tears of the rotator cuff of the shoulder: Diagnosis with MR imaging. AJR 1992; 158:347–351; with permission.

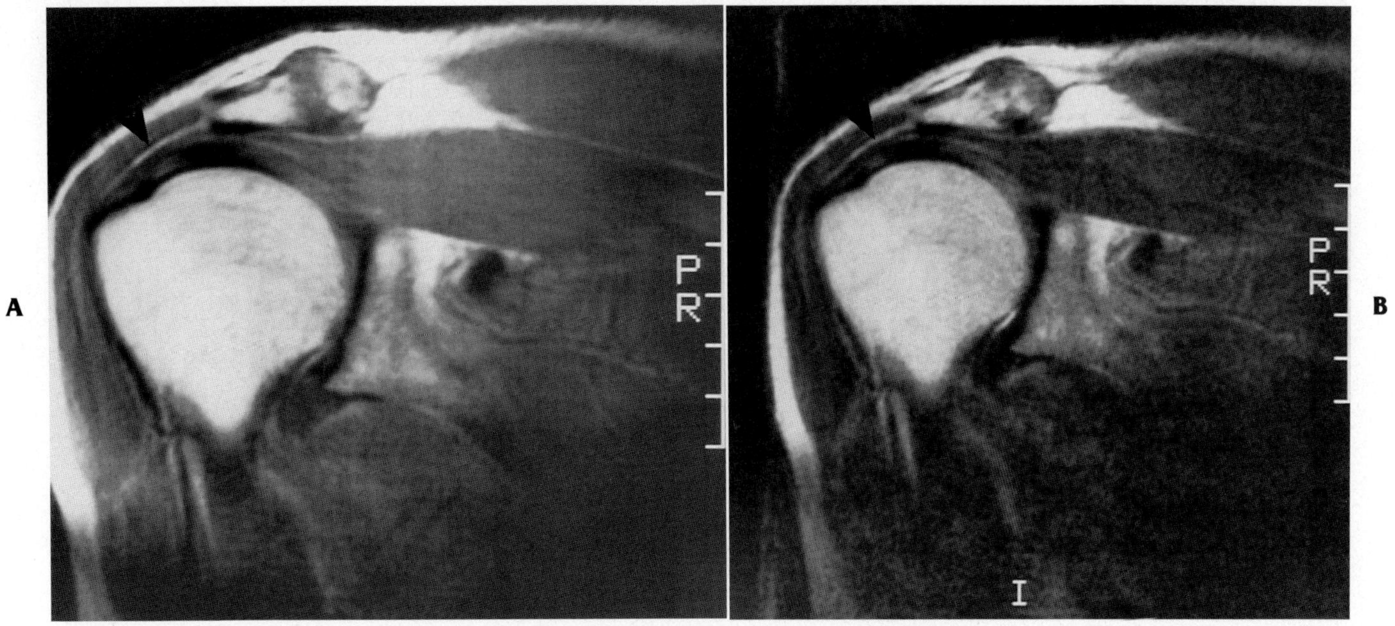


**FIGURE 4** Tendinitis/partial tear. *A,* Proton density image. There is abnormal signal within the supraspinatus tendon without brightening on the T2-weighted *(B)* sequence (grade 2). The deltoid fat plane *(arrow)* is intact.

**TABLE 5** MRI Evaluation of Rotator Cuff Tears: Sensitivity and Specificity

| | Full-thickness Tears | | All Tears | |
|---|---|---|---|---|
| Study | Sensitivity | Specificity | Sensitivity | Specificity |
| Burk et al. | | | 0.92 | 1.00 |
| Iannotti et al. | 1.00 | 0.95 | | |
| Raffii et al. | 0.97 | 0.94 | | |
| Traughber and Goodwin | 1.00 | 1.00 | | |
| Zlatkin et al. | | | 0.91 | 0.88 |

### *Criteria for Diagnosis of Tendinitis*

Patients with tendinitis demonstrate abnormally high signal within the tendon, but this area does not become highly bright on T2-weighted images (Fig. 4). Enlargement of the tendon may be present.

### *Criteria for Diagnosis of Impingement*

Impingement may be caused by bony or soft-tissue structures. Osteophytes from the inferior acromion process or the AC joint are well demonstrated on MR images as low signal projections or, if large and containing marrow, as high signal projections from the adjacent bone, with a low signal cortical margin. Deformity of the underlying muscle and absence of interposed fat between the osteophyte and the muscle or tendon suggest that impingement is present. Developmental variations in the acromion may also be responsible for impingement and are identifiable on MR images.

Soft-tissue hypertrophy causing impingement also may be demonstrated on MRI. Hypertrophy of the AC joint capsule producing impingement may be well observed on either the oblique sagittal or oblique coronal images. The description by Seeger and colleagues of increased bright signal material on T1-weighted images in the region of the subacromial, subdeltoid bursa has been attributed to an increase in fibrofatty tissue observed in patients with impingement and presumably reflects bursitis. Until further study is done, we have not used this finding as indicative of impingement.

## Accuracy of MRI for Diagnosis of Rotator Cuff Tears

Zlatkin and co-workers found MRI to offer greater sensitivity and specificity than arthrography for the diagnosis of rotator cuff tear. The size of the cuff tear demonstrated on the MR image correlated well with the size of tears demonstrated at surgery. The sensitivities and specificities of several series for the diagnosis of rotator cuff tears are shown in Table 5. Assessment of individual signs of rotator cuff tear have shown that discontinuity of the tendon with a 1 cm gap that becomes bright on T2-weighted images and atrophy of the supraspinatus muscle are highly specific indicators of a full-thickness tear. The presence of fluid in the subacromial bursa is a highly sensitive but rather nonspecific sign of a rotator cuff tear, whereas absence of fluid within the bursa appears to be an excellent sign that no full-thickness tear is present.

## Suggested Reading

Boorstein JM, Kneeland JB, Dalinka MK, et al. Magnetic resonance imaging of the shoulder. Curr Probl Diagn Radiol 1992; 1:3–27.

Brandt TD, Cardone BW, Grant TH, et al. Rotator cuff sonography: A reassessment. Radiology 1989; 172:323–327.

Burk DL, Karasick D, Kurtz AB, et al. Rotator cuff tears: Prospective comparison of MR imaging with arthrography, sonography and surgery. AJR 1989; 153:87–92.

Davis SJ, Teresi LM, Bradley WG, et al. Effect of arm rotation on MR imaging of the rotator cuff. Radiology 1991; 181:265–268.

Farley TE, Neumann CH, Steinbach LS, et al. Full-thickness tears of the rotator cuff of the shoulder: Diagnosis with MR imaging. AJR 1992; 158:347–351.

Hall FM, Rosenthal DI, Goldberg RP, Wyshak G. Morbidity from shoulder arthrography: Etiology, incidence and prevention. AJR 1981; 136:59–62.

Iannotti JP, Zlatkin MB, Esterhai JL, et al. Magnetic resonance imaging of the shoulder. Sensitivity, specificity and predictive value. J Bone Joint Surg 1991; 73A:17–29.

Neer CS: Impingement lesions. Clin Orthop 1983; 173:70–77.

Nelson MC, Leather GP, Nirschl RP, et al. Evaluation of the painful shoulder. A prospective comparison of magnetic resonance imaging, computerized tomography, arthrography, ultrasonography and operative findings. J Bone Joint Surg 1991; 73A:707–715.

Rafii M, Firooznia H, Sherman O, et al. Rotator cuff lesions: Signal patterns at MR imaging. Radiology 1990; 177:817–823.

Seeger LL, Gold RH, Bassett LW, Ellman H. Shoulder impingement syndrome: MR findings in 53 shoulders. AJR 1988; 150:343–347.

Traughber PD, Goodwin TE. Shoulder MRI: Arthroscopic correlation with emphasis on partial tears. J Comput Assist Tomogr 1992; 16:129–133.

Zlatkin MB, Iannotti JP, Roberts MC, et al. Rotator cuff tears: Diagnostic performance of MR imaging. Radiology 1989; 172:223–229.

# CT in Pelvic Trauma

*J. NASH LAWRASON, M.D.*

Motor vehicle accidents and falls are the major causes of fractures and dislocations of the pelvic ring and acetabula. Associated injury to the abdominal and pelvic viscera, including the bladder, are common. Pelvic fractures are the second leading cause of death associated with trauma (head injuries are the most common cause). Hemorrhage is one of the most life-threatening complications of pelvic fractures and may have a fatality rate as high as 30 percent. If an open pelvic fracture is present (i.e., bone fragments protrude through lacerated skin or into vagina or rectum), the mortality rate approaches 50 percent. Plain radiographs and computed tomography (CT) of the pelvis are important tools for the radiologist and trauma surgeon in establishing a rapid and accurate diagnosis of pelvic fracture and associated soft-tissue injury. They are also highly useful in determining the stability of pelvic fractures. Stability depends on the integrity of the posterior bony arch and tension band of posterior pelvic ligaments (Fig. 1).

There are many classification schemes of pelvic fractures, and most of them fall into one of two major categories: (1) classification as to "stable" and "unstable" injuries, depending on the number and position of fractures within the pelvic ring; and (2) classification based on the "mechanism of injury" into anteroposterior (AP) compression, lateral compression, and vertical shear fractures.

Regardless of which classification system is used, CT permits classification of pelvic and acetabular injuries based on true pathologic anatomy.

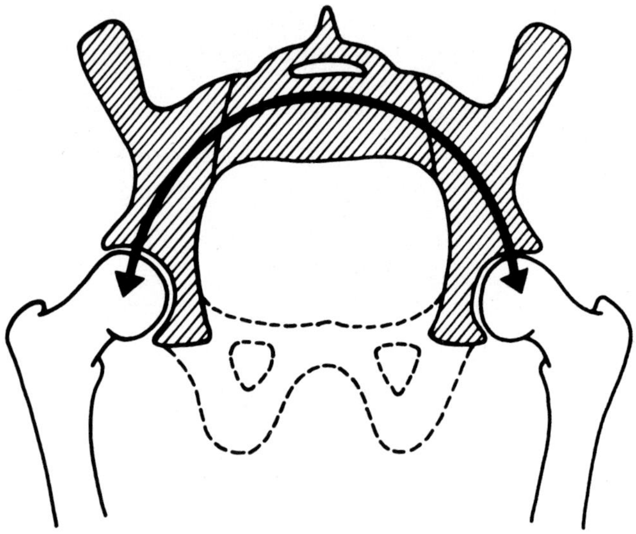

**FIGURE 1** Shaded area demonstrates the posterior bony arch of the pelvis, which along with the major pelvic ligaments, makes up the major weight-bearing pathway responsible for stability. Dotted lines represent the weaker anterior arch. It is more frequently fractured, but less important in pelvic stability. (From Rockwood CA, Green DP. Fractures in Adults, 3rd ed. Philadelphia: JB Lippincott, 1991:1401; with permission.)

## Indications and Clinical Utility

At my institution, patients with pelvic trauma are initially assessed with AP and angled (i.e., outlet view: 45° cephalic angulation of x-ray tube) plain film views. Judet views (bilateral 45° oblique views with the x-ray tube angled 15° cephalad) are occasionally obtained for more acetabular detail. When used in conjunction with these standard trauma radiographs, CT is superior to the sole use of plain films in detection of pelvic and acetabular injuries.

The following are indications for obtaining CT scans of pelvic trauma:

1. For more complete evaluation of virtually all complex pelvic and acetabular fractures.
2. If there is a question of pelvic fracture(s) that cannot be answered by plain films alone.
3. Simple or isolated pelvic fractures of the pubic or iliac bones or distal sacrum may be excluded unless there is concern of underlying hematoma or soft-tissue injury.

4. All patients receiving abdominal CT for blunt trauma will have CT images of the pelvis to search for free blood and occult pelvic fractures.

The basic components of most pelvic fractures will be detected by plain films. CT should not be used as a replacement for careful, correct analysis of plain films. Depending on the clinical situation and condition of the patient, however, CT will often demonstrate fractures that are undetectable or equivocal on plain films. I have often found CT helpful in detection of subtle sacral fractures and diastasis of the sacroiliac (SI) joints. In retrospect, these abnormalities were not observed on the plain films because of overlying bowel contents, osteopenia, underlying trauma board artifacts, or because the abnormality was simply too small or too subtle to be detected. CT is more sensitive in detection and orientation of fractures in the acetabular roof, acetabular columns, and quadrilateral plate. It is also useful in hip joint trauma, especially for detection and orientation of fracture fragments in and about the joint space.

Aside from bony trauma, pelvic CT is helpful in evaluating a pelvic hematoma, the presence of gas within the soft tissues, and the extent of intra- and retroperitoneal visceral injury. CT also shows free blood from abdominal injuries tracking into dependent portions of the pelvis. In patients with severe, complex pelvic fractures and extensive pelvic hemorrhage, imaging with CT may actually be safer than additional oblique radiographs. Rolling a patient for these additional plain films risks disruption of a pelvic tamponade and exsanguination.

Once the axial CT scan has been completed, most modern-generation scanners have computer programs that allow two-dimensional (2D) (i.e., sagittal or coronal) and three-dimensional (3D) reformatted images. These 2D and 3D reformations are not meant to be "high-tech" diagnostic replacements for conventional axial scans. However, they complement the axial images in demonstration of location, size, and displacement of fracture fragments. Radiologists and orthopedic surgeons are finding 3D CT to be an especially useful display of spatial orientation if the pelvic fractures are displaced. In many cases of pelvic and acetabular fracture, treatment is modified on the basis of information provided by CT.

## Technical Approach

Most patients scanned for pelvic trauma in our Emergency Ward are studied within minutes to a few hours of arrival. Those patients that are too hemodynamically unstable to spend 10 to 20 minutes in the CT scanner are surgically or medically stabilized and scanned at a later time. Most of the pelvic CT scans are performed as continuations of abdominal scans on multiple trauma patients. If there is no obvious clinical or plain radiographic evidence of pelvic fracture, 10 mm contiguous axial images from the iliac crest to just below the ischial tuberosities will suffice as a good screening study. These abdomen-pelvis studies are performed with intravenous contrast material and, if a bladder catheter is present, it should be clamped for optimal bladder evaluation. Before proceeding with any pelvic CT scan, it is best to remove as many potential causes of artifact as possible (i.e., place patient's arms above head, remove metal buckles, move monitoring hardware out of scan range, and, if possible, substitute plastic backboard for one that contains metal). Occasionally, artifact from traction splints, surgical hardware, or MAST trousers cannot be avoided. Once the scan is completed, all axial images of the pelvis should be photographed on soft-tissue and bone window settings. Maximum bone detail is offered by some of the latest modern-generation scanners equipped with special software to redisplay the scan data using bone or edge enhancement algorithms.

When evaluating a specific pelvic or acetabular fracture, or an equivocal area on the plain film, I usually obtain 3.0 mm contiguous axial sections through the area in question. If the area is small or fine detail is needed, 1.5 mm contiguous axial sections are obtained; 1.5 and 3.0 mm sections yield optimal 2D and 3D reformatted images.

## Diagnostic Approach

A thorough understanding of pelvic CT anatomy is key to accurate diagnosis of pelvic and acetabular trauma (Fig. 2).

### *Pelvic Fractures*

As briefly mentioned at the beginning of this chapter, there are two major classification schemes for pelvic fractures:

1. *Stable and Unstable*—This scheme is based on the number and position of fractures in the pelvic ring. Stable fractures consist of single breaks in the pelvic ring or fractures of the peripheral margins that do not disrupt the pelvic ring. Unstable fractures are those that disrupt the pelvic ring in two or more places and usually consist of fracture and/or diastasis in both the posterior and anterior arch (Fig. 3).
2. *Mechanism of Injury*—This scheme takes into account the disruptive forces of injury and how they relate to corrective management. It classifies pelvic fractures into AP compression, lateral compression, and vertical shear injuries (Figs. 4, 5, and 6). Pelvic fractures often result from a combination of these force vectors, but one should look for a predominant pattern of injury.

The majority of pelvic fractures (about two-thirds) are stable and result from moderate trauma such as falls. The patient shown in Figure 7 has a fracture that involves only the periphery of the pelvic ring. There is no disruption of the major weight-bearing pathway; therefore this is a stable injury. Both stable and unstable fractures can be the result of any of the aforementioned mechanism of injury forces. However, these disruptive forces are more commonly applied to the unstable injuries, because they provide information about what corrective forces should be used and whether external fixation is required.

The majority of pelvic fractures are caused by lateral compressive forces. Many different stable and unstable patterns can occur. When applied to one side of the pelvis, lateral compressive forces rotate that side inward. If severe enough, the superior and inferior pubic rami are fractured (most often horizontally), and in the posterior pelvis, the ipsilateral sacrum, SI joint, or ilium is involved. After being hit by a car, the patient shown in Figure 8 shows signs of lateral compression injury including inward, medial rotation of the left innominate bone, horizontal fracture of left superior pubic ramus, and fracture of the posterior pelvic arch near the left SI joint. These findings indicate that the proper therapy should include some form of lateral distraction of the innominate bone.

*Text continued on p. 316.*

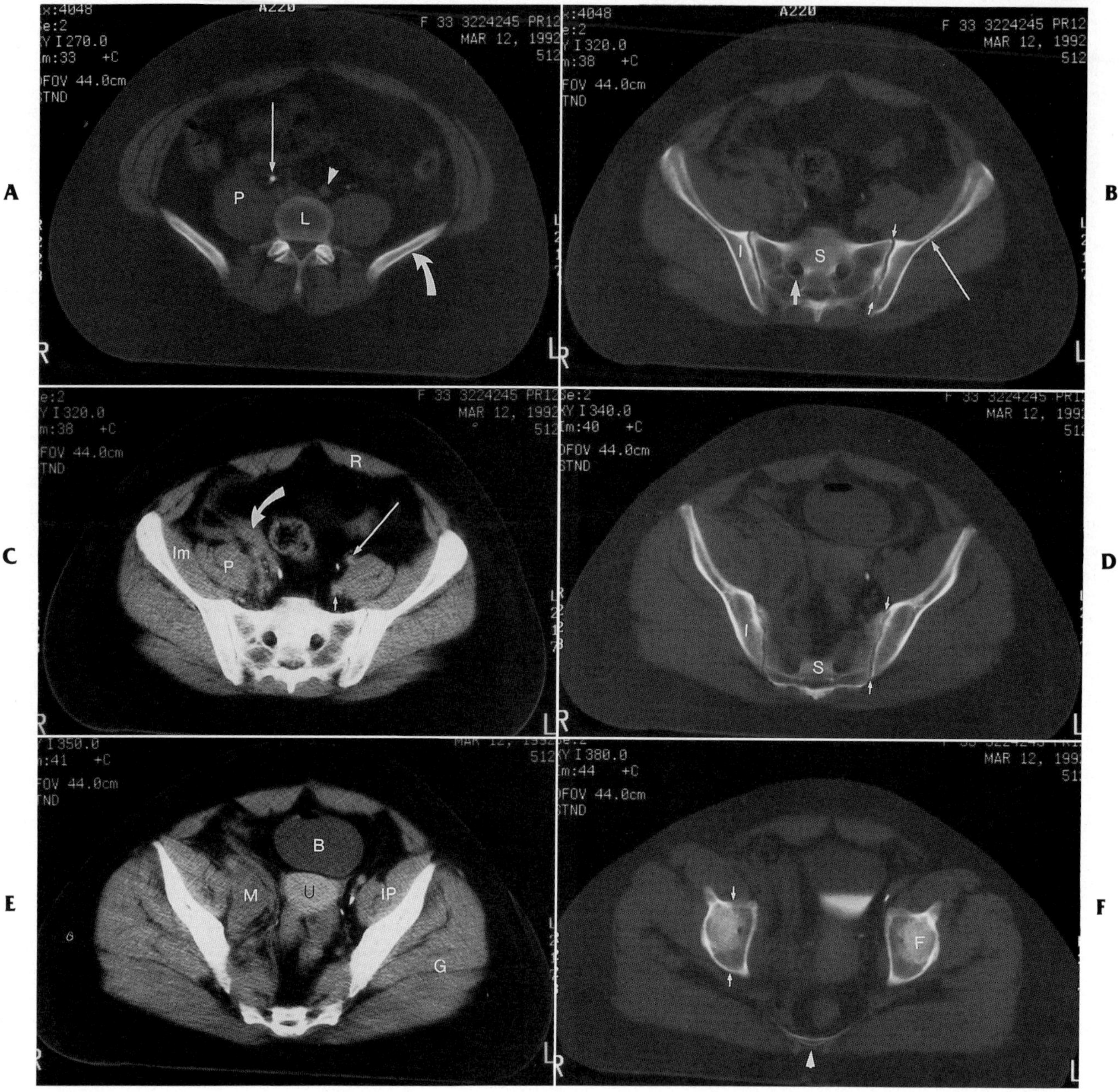


**FIGURE 2** Axial CT scan from superior to inferior of female pelvis showing normal bony anatomy. Soft-tissue injury is present at some levels on the right, secondary to a motor vehicle accident. *A,* Axial CT of iliac crest (*curved arrow*), psoas muscle (P), lumbar vertebra (L), left common iliac artery (*arrowhead*), ureter (*straight arrow*). *B,* Axial CT of superior SI joint (*short arrows*), iliac bone (I), upper horizontal portion of sacrum (S), sacral neural foramen (*large arrow*), groove for nutrient artery (*long arrow*). *C,* Soft-tissue window of (*B*). Rectus muscle (R), psoas muscle (P), iliacus muscle (Im). Left common iliac artery has divided into external (*long arrow*) and internal (*short arrow*) iliac arteries. Note the right-sided mesenteric hematoma (*curved arrow*). *D,* Axial CT of lower SI joints (*arrows*) and more vertical portion of lower sacrum (S). Iliac bone (I). *E,* Soft-tissue window 1 cm below (*D*). Bladder (B), uterine fundus (U). Psoas and iliacus muscles are fusing to form the iliopsoas muscle (IP). Gluteal muscles (G). Note the mesenteric hematoma (M) extending into the pelvis on the right. Compare with the normal left side. *F,* Axial CT of acetabular roof (*arrows*), top of femoral head (F), inferior tip of sacrum (*arrowhead*).

*Continued.*

G H I

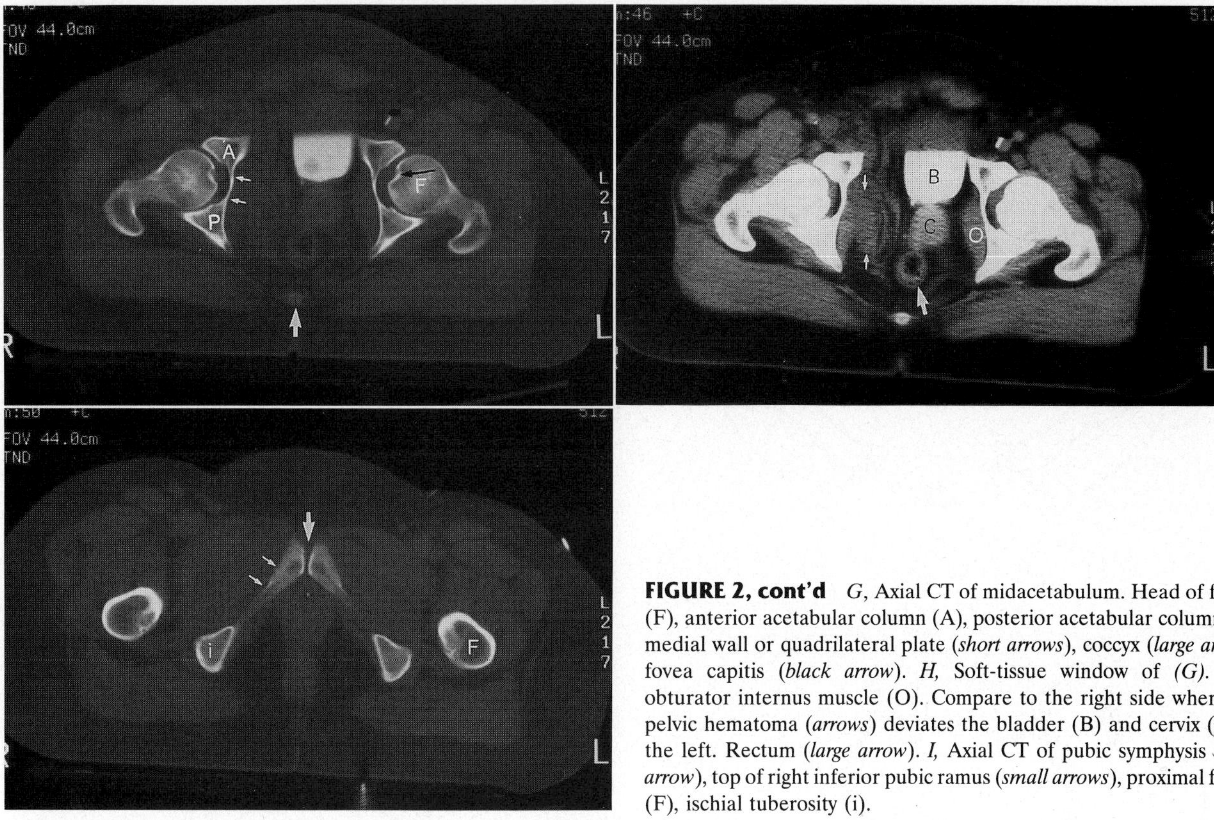


**FIGURE 2, cont'd** *G*, Axial CT of midacetabulum. Head of femur (F), anterior acetabular column (A), posterior acetabular column (P), medial wall or quadrilateral plate (*short arrows*), coccyx (*large arrow*), fovea capitis (*black arrow*). *H,* Soft-tissue window of *(G)*. Left obturator internus muscle (O). Compare to the right side where the pelvic hematoma (*arrows*) deviates the bladder (B) and cervix (C) to the left. Rectum (*large arrow*). *I,* Axial CT of pubic symphysis (*large arrow*), top of right inferior pubic ramus (*small arrows*), proximal femur (F), ischial tuberosity (i).

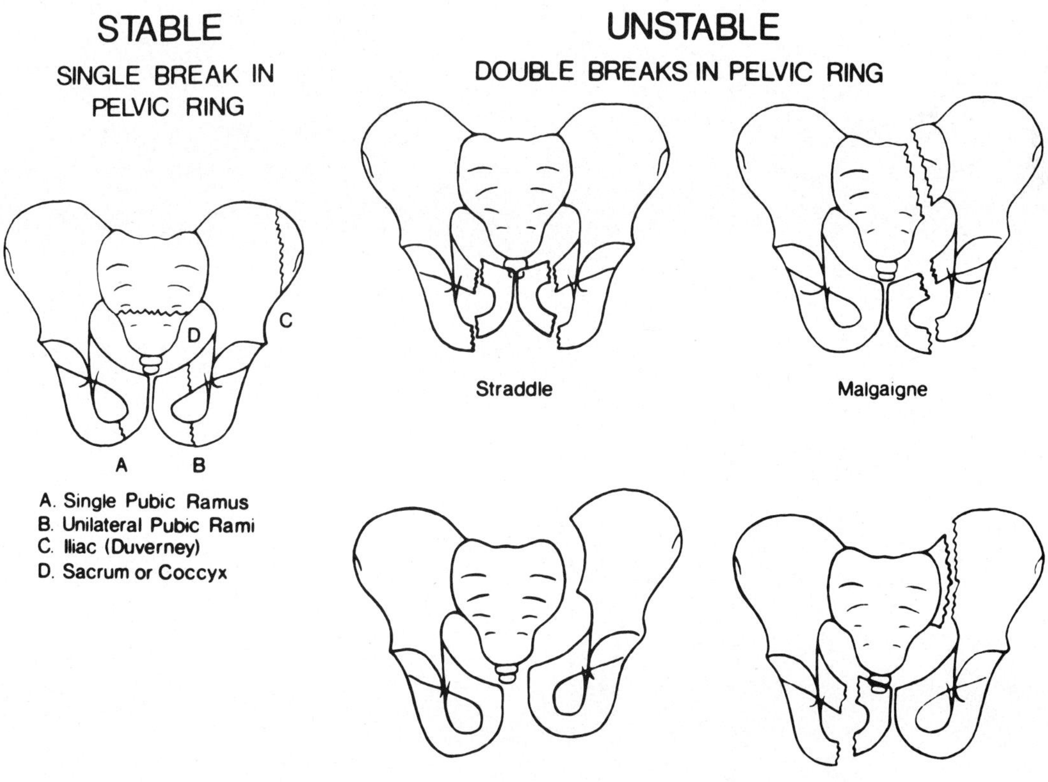


**FIGURE 3** Stable and unstable fractures of pelvis. (From Rogers LF. Radiology of skeletal trauma. New York: Churchill Livingstone, 1982; with permission.)

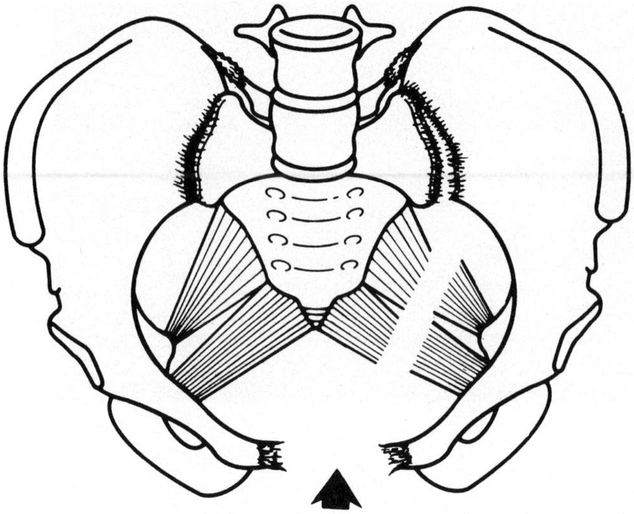

**FIGURE 4** AP compression injury. (From McCort JJ. Trauma Radiology. New York: Churchill Livingstone, 1990:362; with permission.)

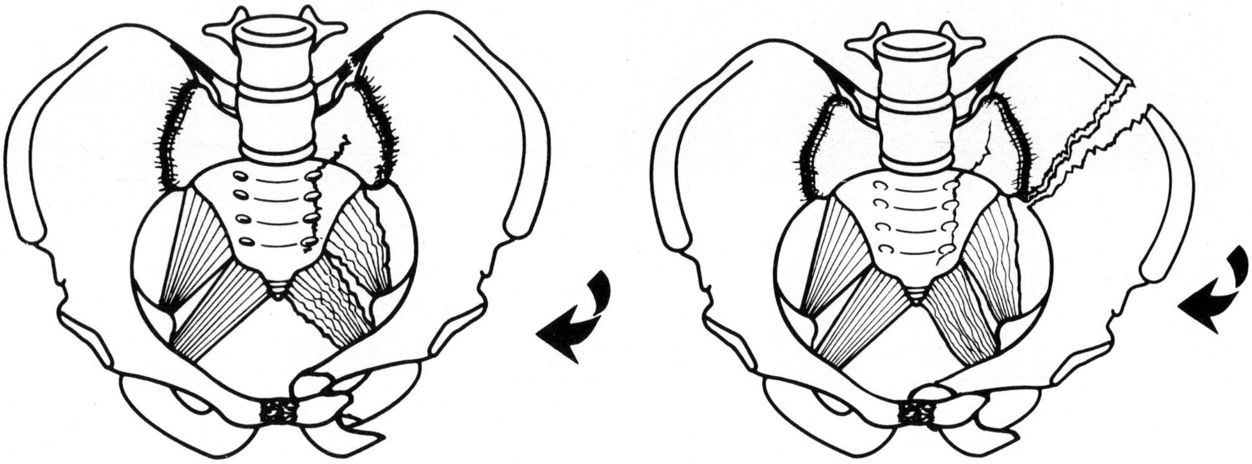

**FIGURE 5** Lateral compression injuries. (From McCort JJ. Trauma Radiology. New York: Churchill Livingstone, 1990; with permission.)

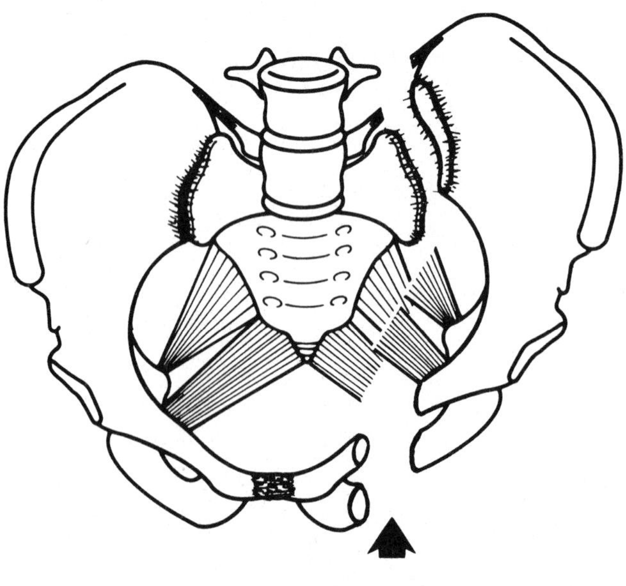

**FIGURE 6** Vertical shear injury. (From McCort JJ. Trauma Radiology. New York: Churchill Livingstone, 1990:364; with permission.)

A

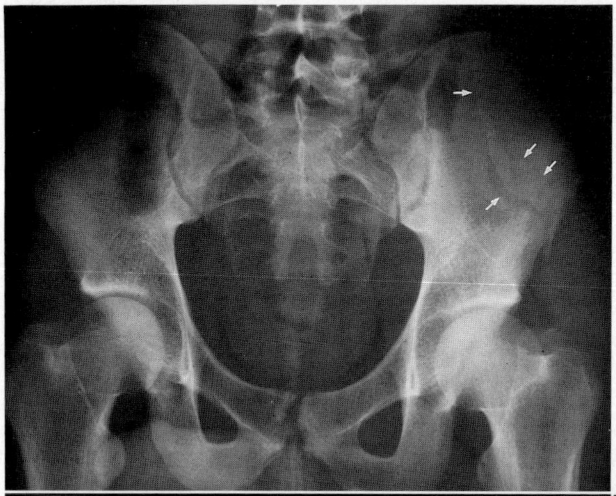

**FIGURE 7** Stable fracture of pelvis. A young intoxicated male fell from a balcony landing on his left side. *A,* AP view of pelvis demonstrates isolated fracture of left iliac crest *(arrows).* SI joints appear intact. This fracture is peripheral to the pelvic ring and does not disrupt the major weight-bearing pathways in the posterior pelvic arch. Thus it is a stable injury. *B,* Axial CT scan at level of upper sacrum confirms isolated fracture of left iliac crest (*short arrow*). Do not mistake groove for nutrient artery (*long arrow*) for a fracture. *C,* Axial CT scan at level of lower sacrum demonstrates intact SI joints (*black arrows*) with no diastasis. Note large pelvic hematoma (H).

B

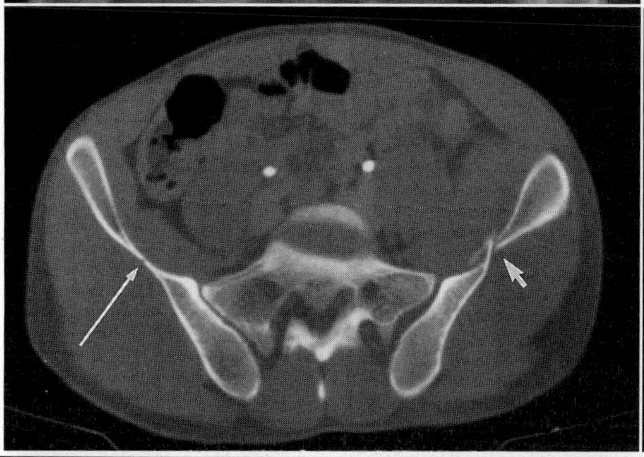

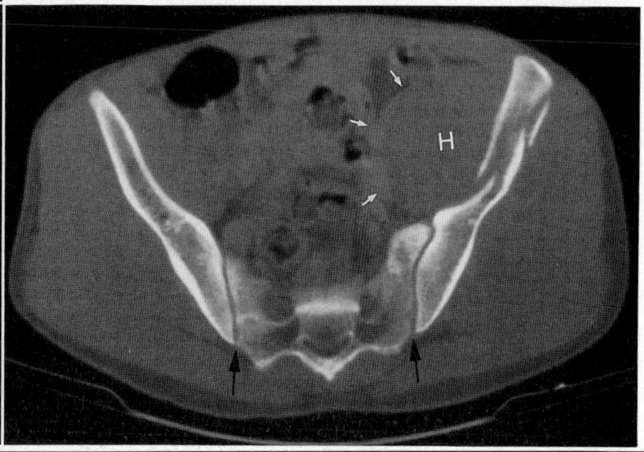


C

A

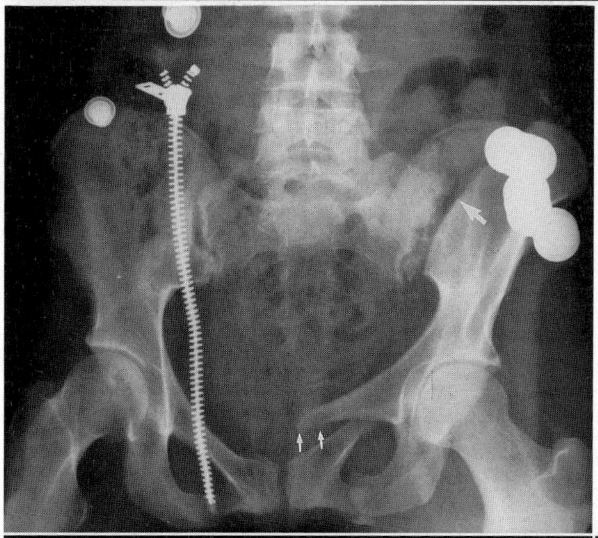

**FIGURE 8** Lateral compression injury. This pedestrian was hit on the left side by a car. *A,* AP view of the pelvis shows a fracture of the left iliac crest that appears to involve the left SI joint (*large arrow*). Note fractures of the left superior and inferior pubic rami, with medial rotation of the entire left innominate bone. The left superior pubic ramus fracture is horizontally oriented (*small arrows*), typical of lateral compressive injuries. *B,* Axial CT at the level of the midsacrum confirms fracture of the left iliac bone (*small arrow*) extending into left SI joint, which is diastatic (*long arrow*). *C,* Soft-tissue window of axial CT scan of the lower pelvis demonstrates a right-sided collection of intraperitoneal hemorrhage (H) from a splenic rupture.

B

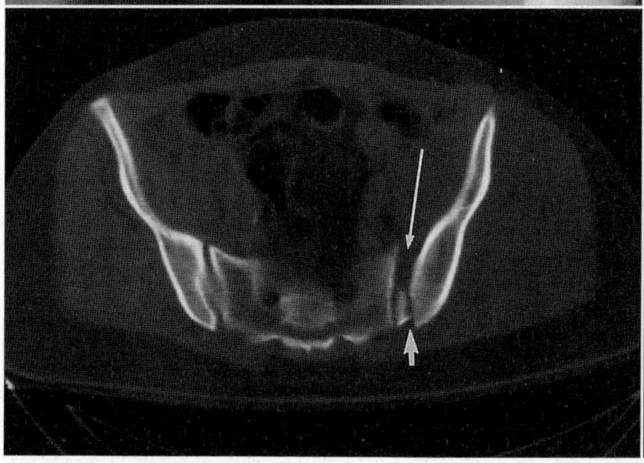

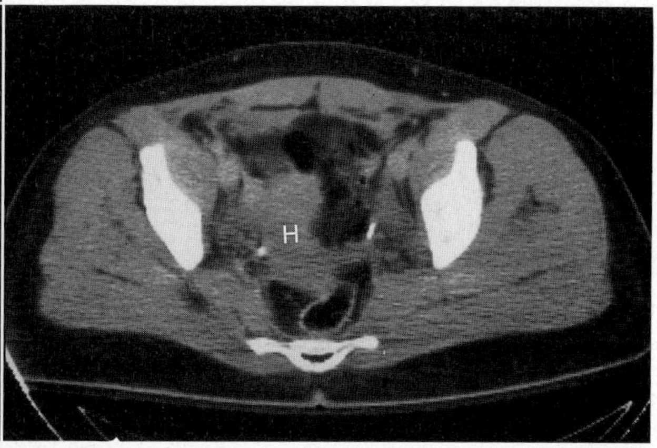


C

A

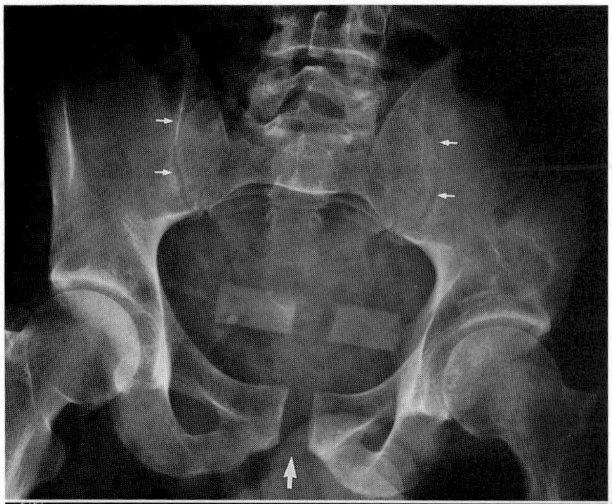

B C

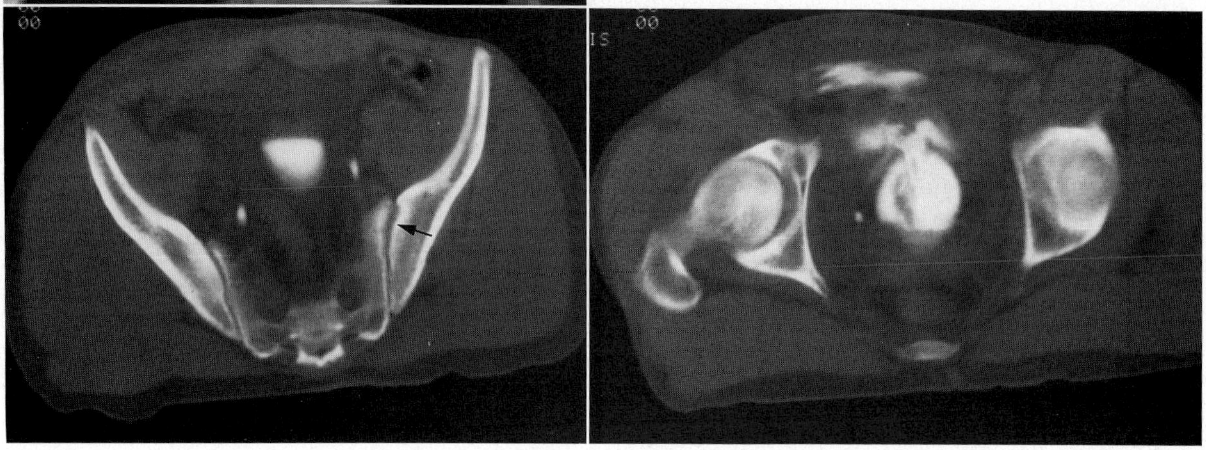

**FIGURE 9** AP compression injury. Patient was hit in front of pelvis by a car. *A,* AP plain film of pelvis shows minimal widening of the pubic symphysis *(large arrow)* and normal-appearing SI joints (*small arrows*). *B,* Axial CT scan shows minimal diastasis of the left SI joint (*arrow*). *C,* Note intrapelvic extravasation of contrast material from bladder rupture. Given the minor amount of bony disruption, a significant amount of pelvic stability is maintained. Conservative closed treatment may suffice.

AP compression fractures occur from disruptive forces in the sagittal plane. This is usually a blow to the front of the pelvis during a motor vehicle accident (Fig. 9). This force injures the anterior pelvis by separating the pubic symphysis, which is normally no more than 5 mm in width, or fracturing the pubic rami. In AP compression and vertical shear injuries, the pubic rami fracture lines are usually vertical. In lateral compression injuries, the pubic rami fracture lines are almost always horizontal – an important differentiating point. If the pubic symphysis is separated by more than 2.5 cm (Fig. 10), there is almost always damage to the posterior pelvic ligaments and SI diastasis. Since one or both sides of the pelvis are rotated externally, treatment is inward rotation of the affected parts or "closing the book."

Vertical shear fractures are usually all unstable and result from a major displacement of bony structures in the vertical plane. These injuries result from falls from heights, motor vehicle accidents, or crushing trauma. Radiographically the fracture lines are vertical and involve the sacrum, SI joint, or medial iliac bone. These are accompanied anteriorly by vertical fractures of the pubic rami or disruption of the pubic symphysis (Fig. 11).

## *Acetabular Fractures*

Acetabular fractures most commonly result from forces driving the femoral head into the pelvis. They are often described in the literature as a separate entity from pelvic fractures. However, they are found in as many as 20 percent of pelvic fractures. Once an acetabular fracture has been detected, one should carefully search the pelvis for additional injuries.

A thorough understanding of acetabular anatomy (Figs. 12, 13) is necessary for adequate description and classification of these fractures. The most commonly used classification system of acetabular fractures is that of Letournel and Judet (Fig. 14), which is based on the anterior and posterior acetabular columns supporting the acetabular dome. This system divides the acetabular fractures into a variety of groups including posterior wall fractures (24 percent), posterior column fractures (4 percent), anterior wall fractures (2 percent), anterior column fractures (4 percent), transverse fractures (9 percent), and T-shaped fractures (7 percent). There is also a variety of mixed patterns that involve two or more of the above. One frequent mixed pattern is the combination of transverse and posterior wall fracture (21 percent). Why so many groups in this system? There are several different surgical approaches used for treatment. The one chosen depends on the type of fracture. Therefore it is important that the radiologist and orthopedic surgeon be familiar with this classification of acetabular fractures.

One of the most common acetabular injuries is the posterior wall fracture during a motor vehicle accident. Typically an unrestrained passenger's knee hits the dashboard, posteriorly dislocates the femoral head, and fractures the posterior acetabular wall (Fig. 15). In fracture dislocations of the hip and acetabulum, CT is highly useful in determining the presence and donor site of fracture fragments in the joint space (Fig. 16). With fractures involving the quadrilateral plate, such as

*Text continued on p. 323.*

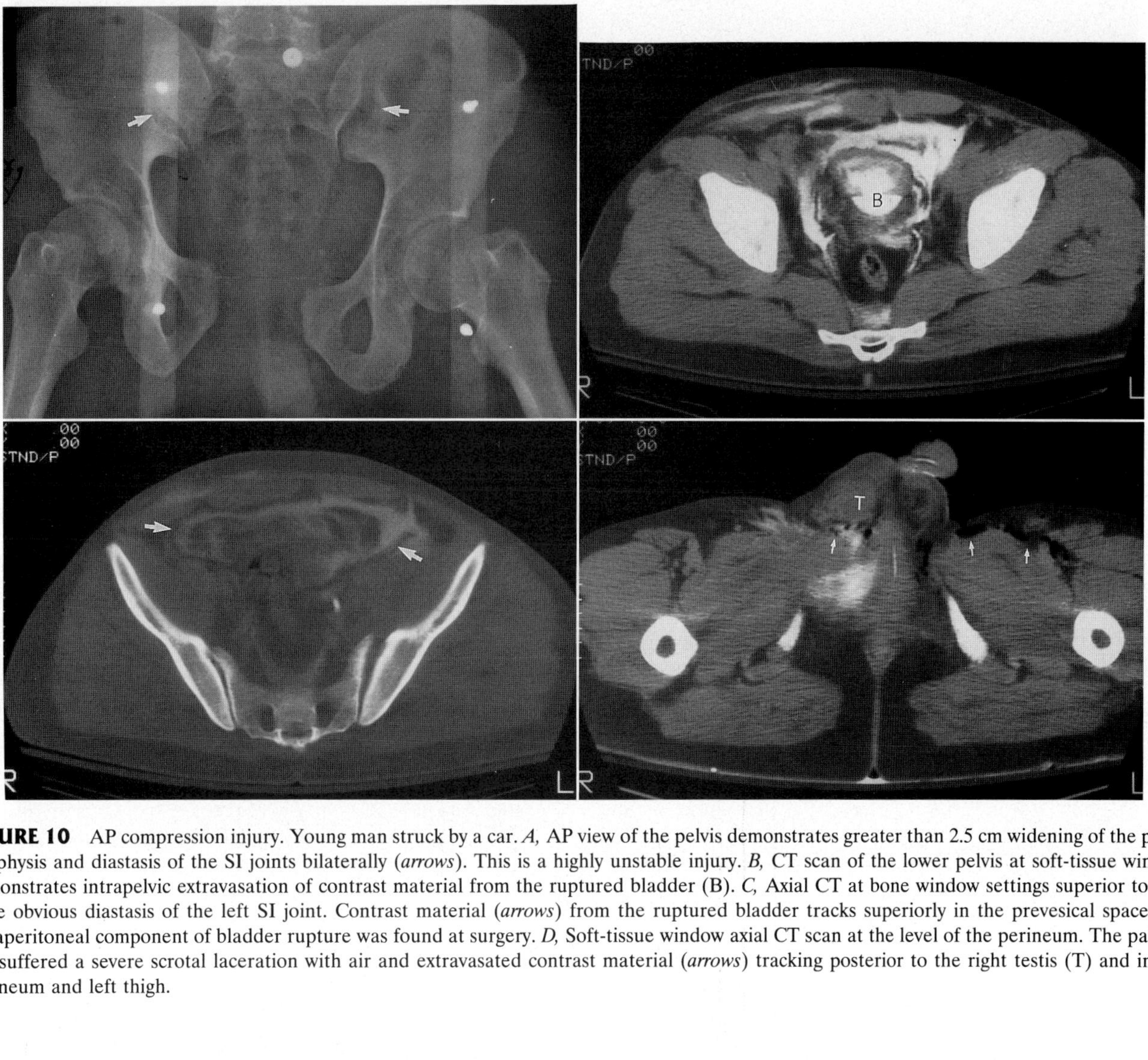


**FIGURE 10** AP compression injury. Young man struck by a car. *A,* AP view of the pelvis demonstrates greater than 2.5 cm widening of the pubic symphysis and diastasis of the SI joints bilaterally (*arrows*). This is a highly unstable injury. *B,* CT scan of the lower pelvis at soft-tissue window demonstrates intrapelvic extravasation of contrast material from the ruptured bladder (B). *C,* Axial CT at bone window settings superior to *(B).* Note obvious diastasis of the left SI joint. Contrast material (*arrows*) from the ruptured bladder tracks superiorly in the prevesical space. No intraperitoneal component of bladder rupture was found at surgery. *D,* Soft-tissue window axial CT scan at the level of the perineum. The patient has suffered a severe scrotal laceration with air and extravasated contrast material (*arrows*) tracking posterior to the right testis (T) and in the perineum and left thigh.

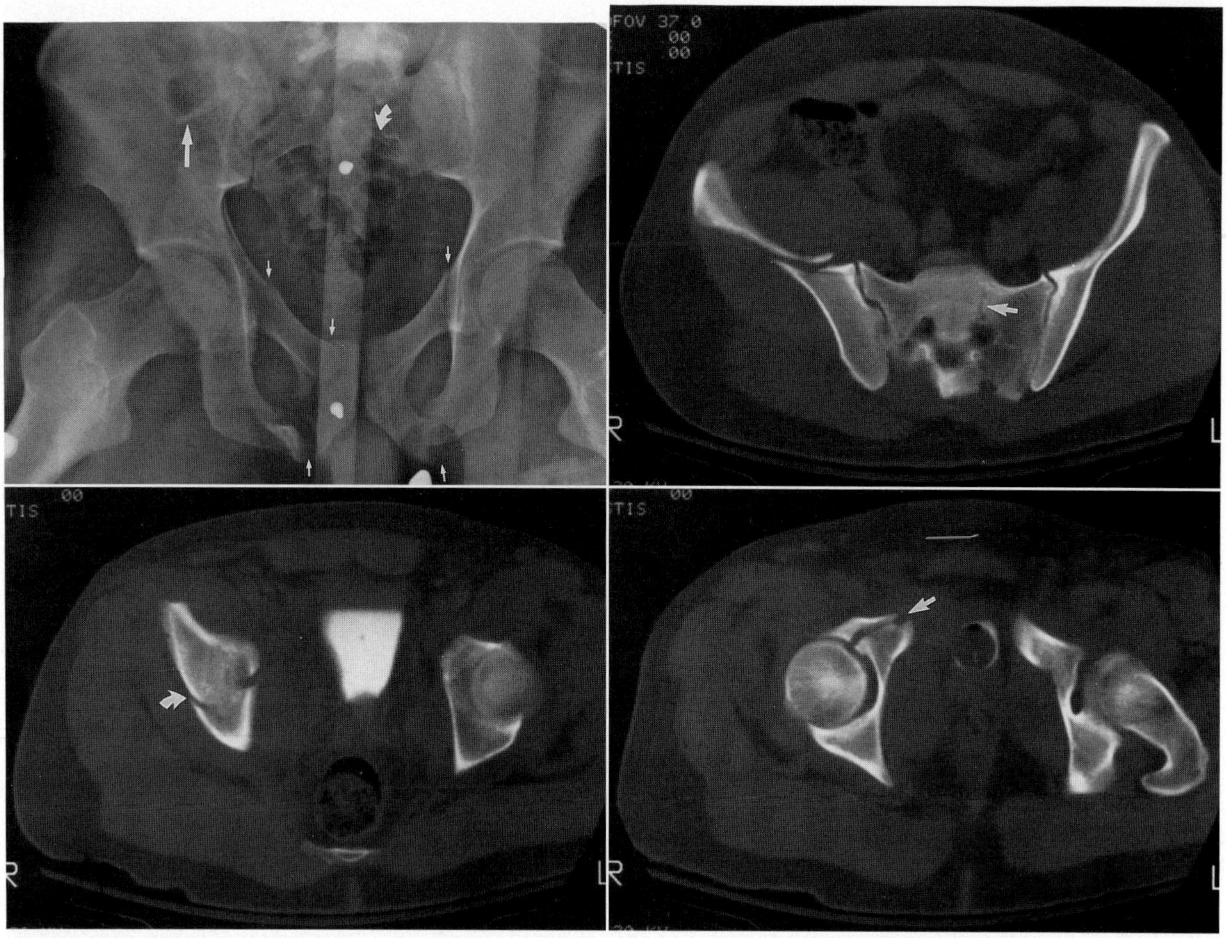


**FIGURE 11** Vertical shear injury. Patient jumped six stories out of a building. *A,* AP view of the pelvis demonstrates multiple vertically oriented fractures involving the superior and inferior pubic rami (*small arrows*). Wedge-shaped opacity (*large arrow*) is suspicious for overlapping fracture fragments in the right iliac bone vs. haustral shadow in the bowel. Left sacral fracture is indicated by subtle disruption of a left sacral neural arch *(curved arrow)*. Compare with the opposite normal side. *B,* Axial CT scan at the level of the SI joints confirms fracture of the right iliac bone. Fracture of the left sacrum (*arrow*) is more clearly visualized than on plain film. *C* and *D,* Fracture of the right iliac bone extends inferiorly to involve the right acetabular roof *(curved arrow)* and right anterior column (*straight arrow*). Note teardrop configuration of the bladder in (*C*), indicating pelvic hematoma.

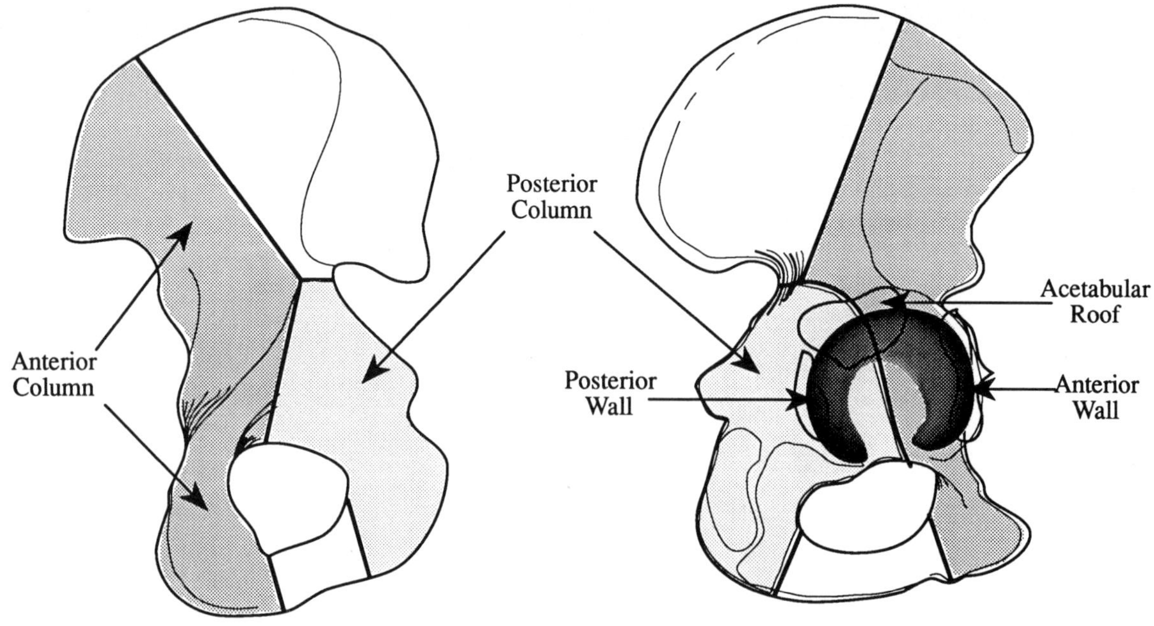


**FIGURE 12** Medial (*A*) and lateral (*B*) view of hemipelvis demonstrating extent of anterior and posterior acetabular columns.

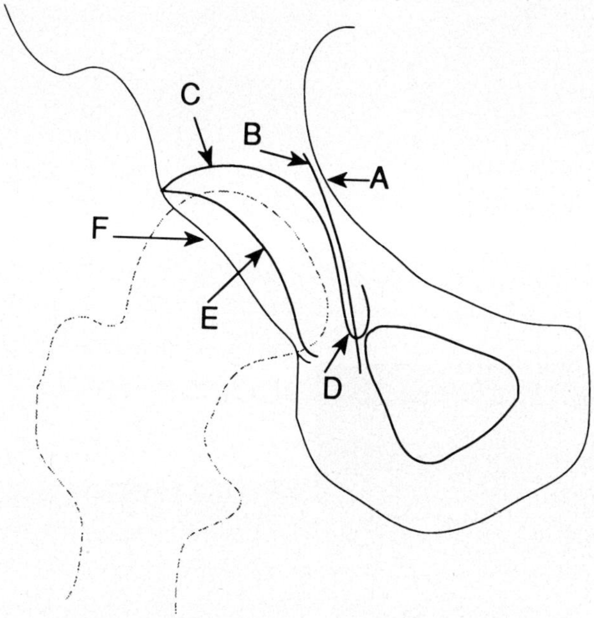


**FIGURE 13** Plain film anatomy of acetabulum. Iliopubic line (A) extends from the sciatic notch downward to the pubic tubercle. A break in this line suggests fracture of the anterior column. Ilioischial line (B) is formed by the posterior quadrilateral surface of the iliac bone. A break in this line suggests a fracture of the posterior column. Acetabular roof (C). Roentgenographic "U" (D) represents anterior-inferior portions of the acetabular fossa and quadrilateral surface of the iliac bone. Anterior lip or wall (E) of the acetabulum. Posterior lip or wall (F) of the acetabulum.

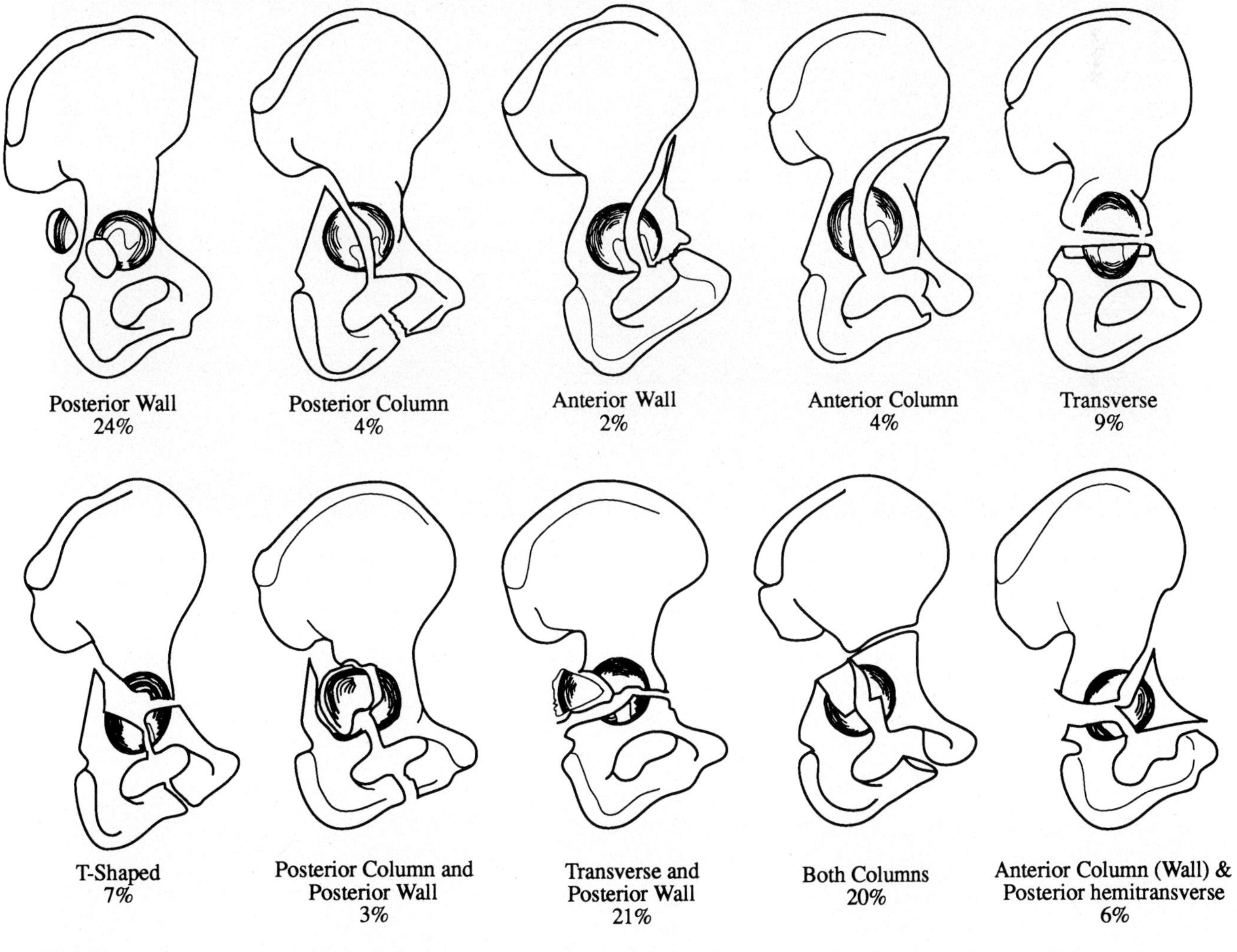


**FIGURE 14** Classification system of acetabular fractures of Letournel and Judet. (Modified from Martinez CR, DiPasquale TG, et al. Evaluation of acetabular fractures with two- and three-dimensional CT. Radiographics 1992; 12:227–242; with permission.)

A B C D

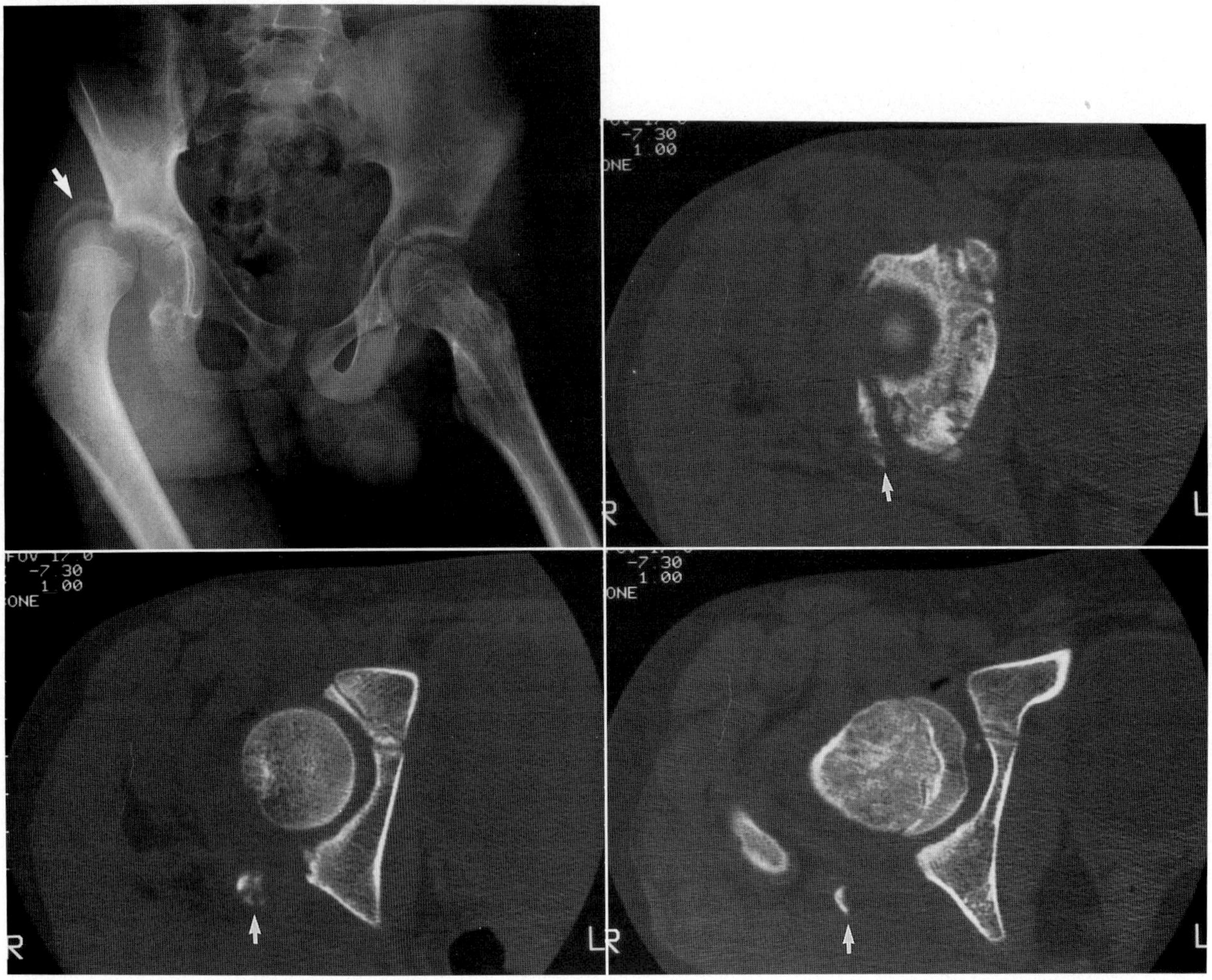

**FIGURE 15** Fracture of posterior wall of acetabulum. A 15-year-old male involved in motor vehicle accident. *A,* AP view of the pelvis demonstrates obvious right posterior hip dislocation. Caplike piece of bone (*arrow*) projected above the femoral head is the posterior wall fracture fragment. This is a typical appearance of a posterior wall fracture with posterior hip dislocation. *B, C,* and *D,* Axial CT images of the right hip from the acetabular roof to the midacetabulum. The hip has been reduced and the extent of the posterior wall fracture fragment (*arrow*) is observed from superior to inferior. After hip reduction, the fracture fragment has moved into a more anatomic position. In (*B*) note the usual mottled appearance of an ununited ossification center in this 15-year-old.

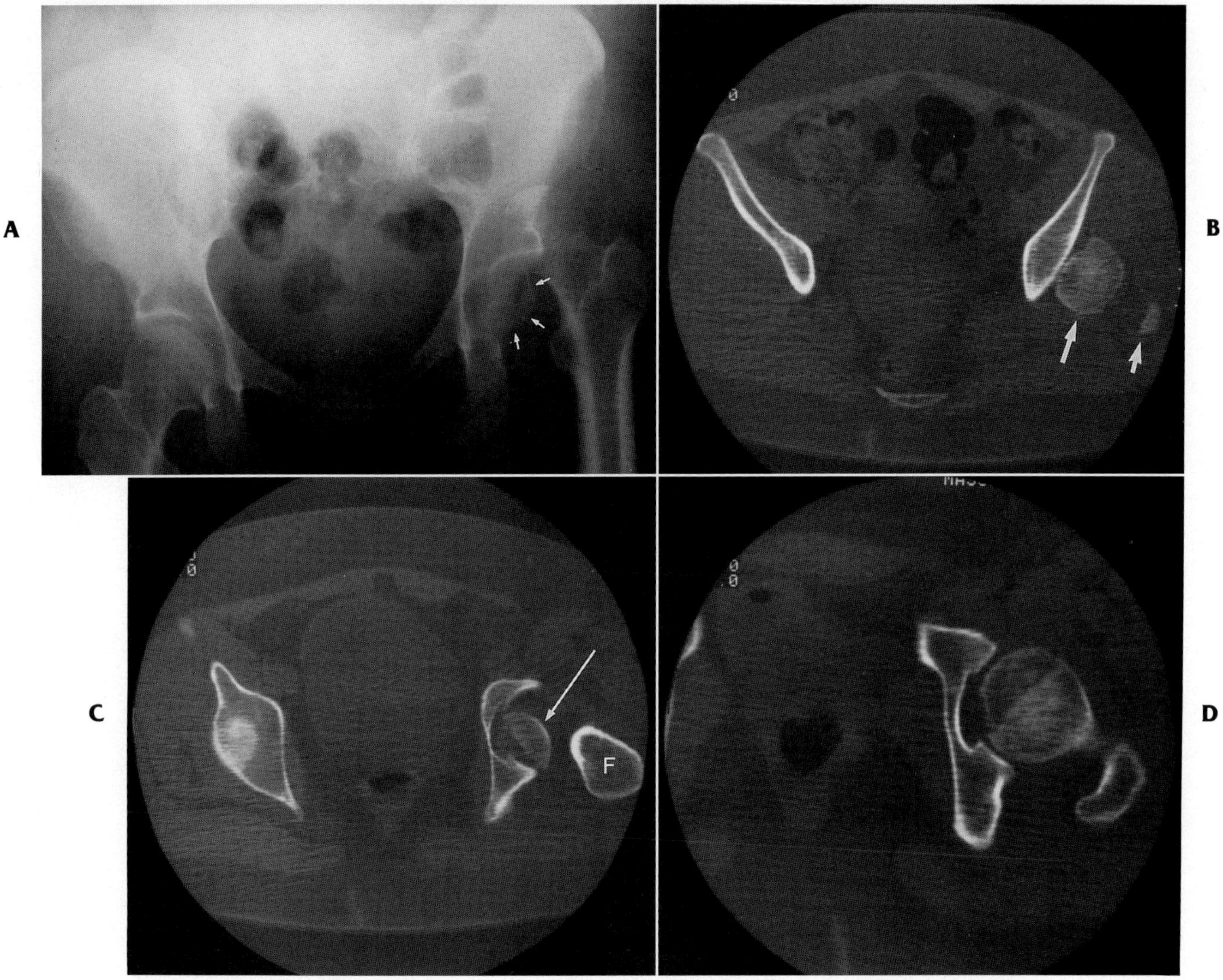


**FIGURE 16** Posterior fracture dislocation of left hip. A 38-year-old woman injured her left hip in a motor vehicle accident. CT was performed because of the unusual-appearing left acetabulum and inability to reduce the left hip. *A,* AP view of the pelvis demonstrates obvious posterior dislocation of the left hip and unusual convex appearance of the left acetabulum (*arrows*). The acetabulum should normally have a concave appearance. *B,* Axial CT scan superior to acetabulae demonstrates posteriorly, superiorly dislocated left femoral head (*large arrow*). Superior tip of the greater trochanter (*small arrow*). *C,* Axial CT scan at the level of the midacetabulum demonstrates sheared-off femoral head fragment (*arrow*) in the acetabular fossa. Intertrochanteric region of the femur (F). *D,* Repeat axial CT scan after a second attempt at closed reduction demonstrates alignment of fracture fragment with native femoral head.

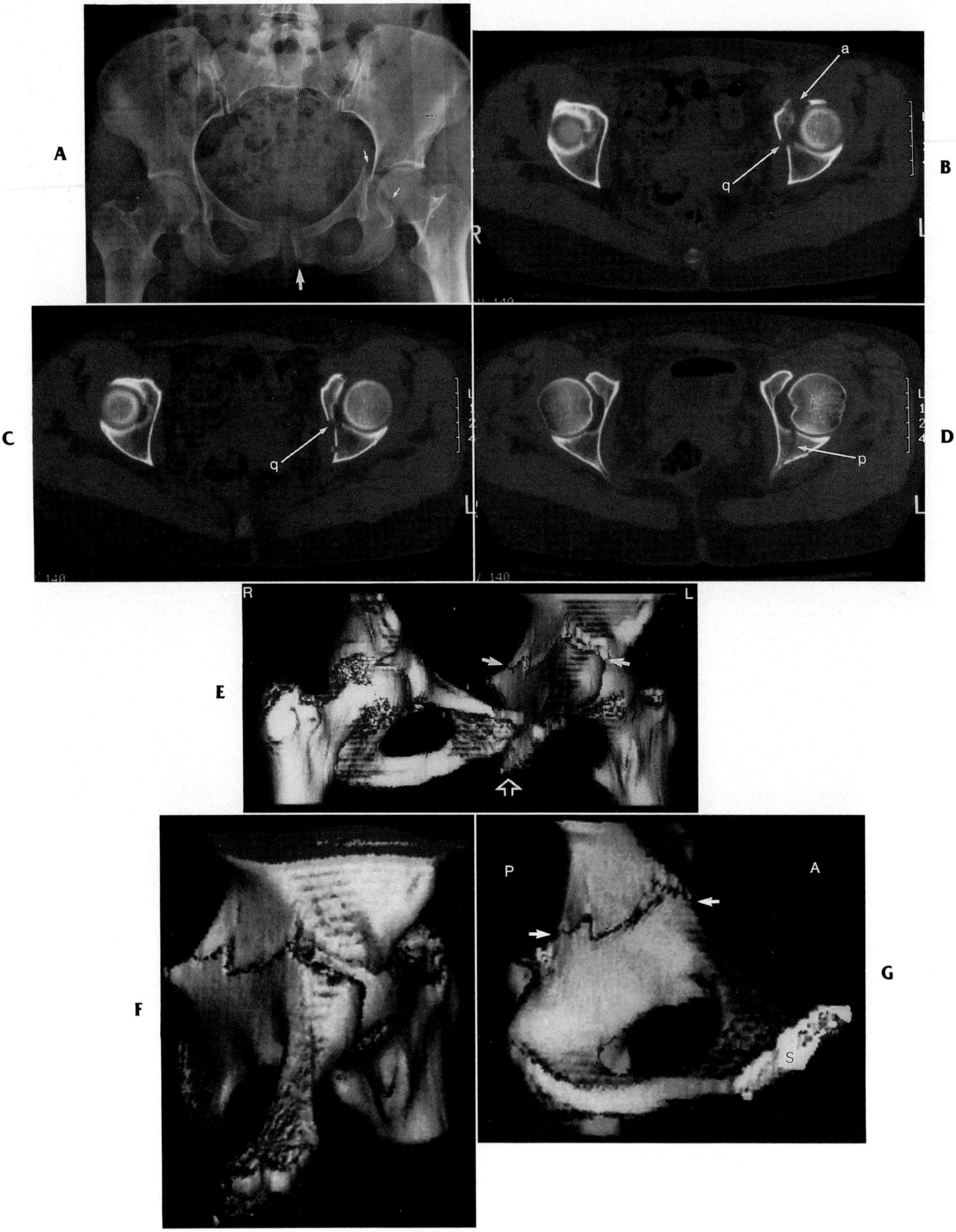


**FIGURE 17** Transverse fracture of left acetabulum. A 43-year-old female involved in a motor vehicle accident. *A,* AP view of the pelvis demonstrates extensive fracture of the left acetabulum (*small arrows*). There is disruption of the iliopubic and ilioischial lines. Note some widening of the pubic symphysis and downward displacement of the left pubic bone (*large arrow*). *B, C,* and *D,* Axial CT scan from superior to midacetabulum demonstrates transverse fracture extending from the anterior column (a) through the quadrilateral plate (q) and through the posterior column (p). *E,* 3D CT of the pelvis rotated into LPO position more clearly shows extent of the left transverse acetabular fracture (*arrows*) and spatial orientation of the inferiorly displaced left pubic bone (*open arrow*). *F,* 3D CT of the left hemipelvis in shallow LPO position and mild inferior tilt. The computer has removed the right hemipelvis. *G,* 3D CT of the left hemipelvis viewed as if the observer is standing in the midline of the pelvis and looking laterally at the medial wall of the left acetabulum. Transverse acetabular fracture (*arrows*), anterior (A), posterior (P), pubic symphysis (S).

transverse or T-shaped fractures, the fracture lines invariably extend into the anterior and posterior columns. Good-quality 3D CT (Fig. 17) is useful in demonstrating the full extent of the fracture and may alter the surgical approach if repair of both columns is needed.

## Suggested Reading

Daffner RH. Pelvic trauma. In: McCort JJ, ed. Trauma Radiology. New York: Churchill Livingstone, 1990.

Dalinka MK, Arger P, Coleman B. CT in pelvic trauma. Orthop Clin North Am 1985; 16.3:471–480.

Federle MP, Brant-Zawadszki M. Computed Tomography in the Evaluation of Trauma. Baltimore: Williams & Wilkins, 1986.

Iverson LD, Clawson DK. Manual of Acute Orthopedic Therapeutics. Boston: Little, Brown, 1987.

Letournel E. Acetabulum fractures: Classification and management. Clin Orthop 1980; 151:81–93.

Martinez CR, DiPasquale TG, Helfet DL, et al. Evaluation of acetabular fractures with two- and three-dimensional CT. Radiographics 1992; 12:227–242.

Tile M. Fractures of the Pelvis and Acetabulum. Baltimore: Williams & Wilkins, 1984.

Young JW, Burgess AR. Fractures of the pelvis. In: Mirvis SE, Young WR, eds. Imaging in Trauma and Critical Care. Baltimore: Williams & Wilkins, 1992.

Young JW, Resnik CS. Fractures of the pelvis: Current concepts of classification. AJR 1990; 155:1169–1175.

# Three-Dimensional CT of Facial Trauma

*ROBERT A. NOVELLINE, M.D.*

The facial skeleton comprises one of the most complex arrangements of curving bony surfaces in the body. Accordingly the diagnosis of facial fractures has proven to be a challenge for plain film radiography, on which these curving surfaces are compressed into two-dimensional images of many superimposed bony and soft-tissue structures. For each plain film, the viewer must mentally sort out the complex of overlapping structures to identify normal bony anatomy and diagnose fractures when present. In the trauma patient this task is further complicated by overlying soft-tissue edema and hemorrhage, which degrade the fine detail of the facial bones.

Facial imaging has been significantly advanced by the advent of computed tomography (CT), which can display curving bony contours with exquisite detail on cross-sectional images. CT has revolutionized the imaging workup of the facial trauma patient. More fracture lines and fragments can be shown by CT than plain films or by the combination of plain films and conventional tomography. CT can better display the position and orientation of fracture fragments and array of fracture lines for most accurate fracture classification and optimal treatment planning. CT can also delineate soft-tissue facial injuries. Consequently it has become routine to perform CT at our hospital on nearly all patients with clinically detected or plain film–demonstrated facial fractures.

The most recent advance in facial trauma imaging is three-dimensional computed tomography (3DCT). As CT acquires anatomic data as a volume of contiguous axial slices, it is possible to create a simulated 3D image of the face by computer stacking of adjacent axial slices (Fig. 1). Commercially available computer technology now permits the 3D reformation of axial CT scans into 3D images in routine clinical practice. This capability may be installed on the CT scanner computer itself, or 3D images may be generated on a free-standing workstation. With current technology, 3D reformations may be generated in minutes; software features allow rotation of images, shading alterations, and slicing mechanism for optimal viewing of interior facial structures (Fig. 2).

As with other types of reformations (e.g., coronal and sagittal), the resolution of 3DCT is inferior to the resolution of the original axial reconstructions (2DCT). In fact, nondisplaced fractures may be overlooked by 3DCT. Therefore the exact number of fracture lines and fracture fragments is best determined on the primary reconstructions (original axial and coronal slices). However, the ability of 3DCT to depict the position and orientation of displaced fractures is so exceptional that surgeons planning treatment enthusiastically request 3D reformations when displaced fractures are present. Their preferred sequence for viewing is to review the 3D images first to get the "big picture" (position and alignment of major fracture fragments), after which they review the individual primary axial and coronal slices to identify each of the individual fracture lines and fragments. Thus 3DCT has become recognized as an excellent display tool for communicating CT data of displaced fractures to referring physicians.

## Indications for Facial CT

At our hospital the initial imaging examination for facial trauma patients is a plain film facial series, consisting of Water's, Caldwell, lateral, and base views. All are taken upright, if possible, to demonstrate any air-fluid levels in the paranasal sinuses, which may serve as important indirect signs of facial fracture. If a polytrauma or other patient cannot be examined upright, the lateral film is taken with cross-table lateral technique. The base view may not be possible in all trauma patients, including those with a definite or suspected cervical spine fracture.

A routine facial series is generally inadequate for the detection of nasal fractures, because a correctly exposed lateral facial film overexposes the nasal bones. Our routine nasal series consists of coned, bilateral views of the nose, a Water's view of the face, and an occlusal view of the nose. Similarly evaluation of suspected mandible trauma generally requires a separate mandible series, consisting of a lateral, Towne's, posteroanterior, and bilateral oblique mandibular views.

After review of the plain films patients are referred for facial CT if (1) the plain films show one or more definite facial fractures; (2) the plain films show a secondary or indirect sign of a facial fracture, such as a paranasal sinus fluid level or orbital emphysema; (3) the plain films show a suspicious sign of a facial fracture such as an unexplained lucency, density, or variation in bony contour; (4) a soft tissue injury of the face is

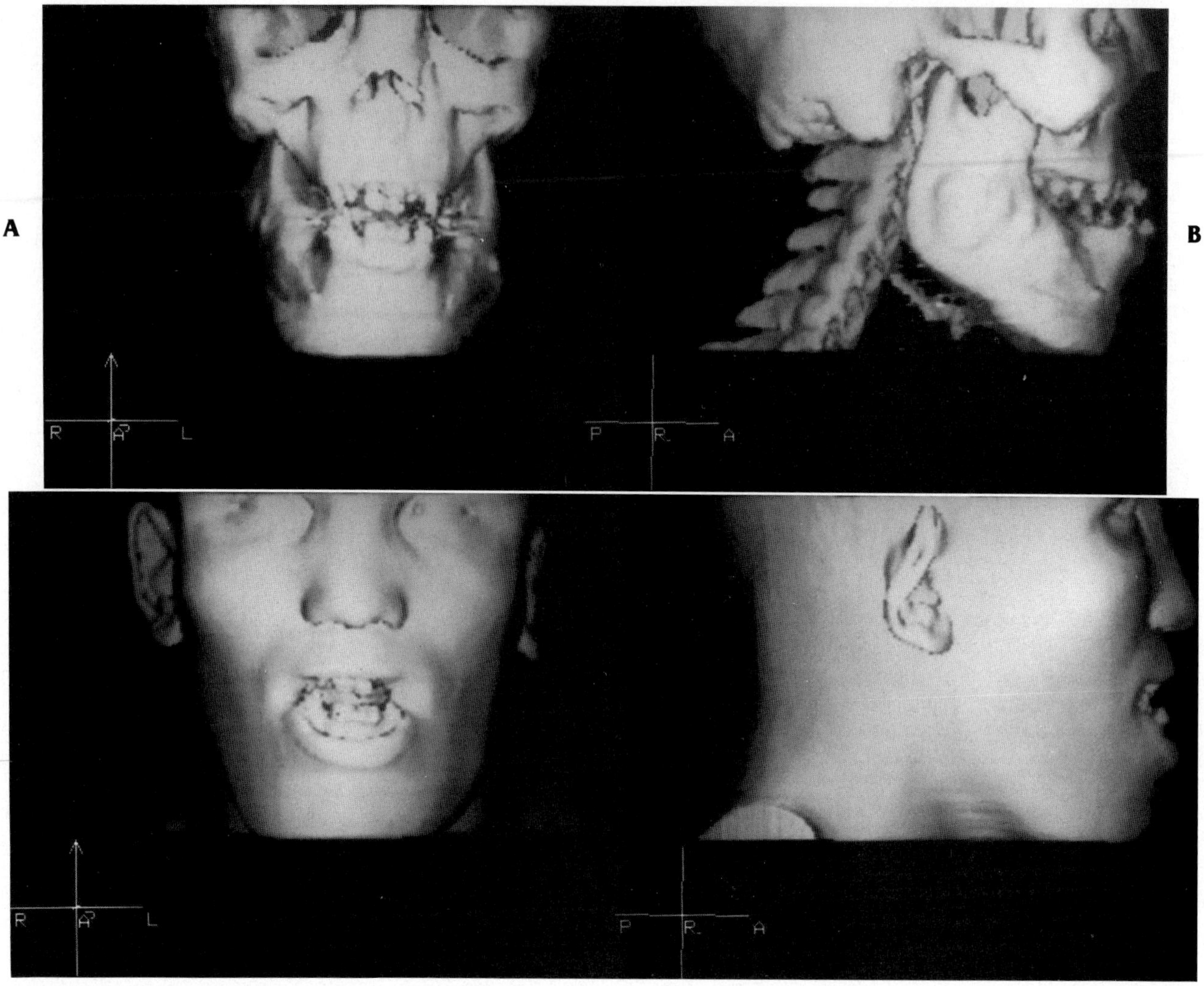

**FIGURE 1** 3DCT of a young man with fibrous dysplasia of the mandible. *A,* Frontal view, bone rendered image. *B,* Side view, bone rendered image. *C,* Frontal view, soft-tissue rendered image. *D,* Side view, soft-tissue rendered image. Note the enlargement of the mandible (bone images), which produces elongation of the face and prognathism (soft-tissue images). The 3D appearance is easier to comprehend with a computer 3D simulation than by mental stacking of a series of axial CT scans.

suspected; or (5) an orbital foreign body is clinically suspected. A multiple trauma patient with clinically obvious facial fractures who is taken directly to CT for an emergency examination of the head or abdomen may undergo an initial facial CT while already on the CT scanner table. A future direction might be the elimination of plain films of the face altogether in patients with obvious fractures who are evaluated by CT.

Three-dimensional reformations (3DCT) are performed when displaced fractures are depicted on the plain films or primary axial or coronal CT slices. After computer generation they are displayed and filmed in positions corresponding to a conventional plain film facial series (e.g., lateral, Water's, Caldwell, Towne's views). Special oblique or other views may be photographed that better display the anatomy of a particular fracture. Based on the clinical and CT findings, the 3D complex may then be sliced to show interior anatomic structures, such as within the orbits, paranasal sinuses, or other facial cavities.

## Technique for Facial CT

I routinely perform facial CT with 3.0 mm thick contiguous direct axial and coronal scans of the face, beginning above the frontal sinuses and extending inferiorly to the bottom of the mandible in the axial plane, and beginning just anterior to the nasal bones and extending posteriorly to the sphenoid sinuses in the coronal plane. Direct coronal imaging requires hyperextension of the neck, which may not be possible in certain trauma patients. If a patient cannot be positioned for direct coronal imaging, 1.5 mm contiguous axial scans are performed over the same portion of the face and coronal reformatted images are computer generated. Filming is obtained of all slices with bone and soft-tissue windows. Other planes of reformation (e.g., sagittal, oblique) may be performed as indicated clinically.

The rendering technique is the computer algorithm for converting axial CT imaging data into 3D images. It is, perhaps, the most important determinant of the quality of the 3D image. The most common involves a thresholding or surface-based

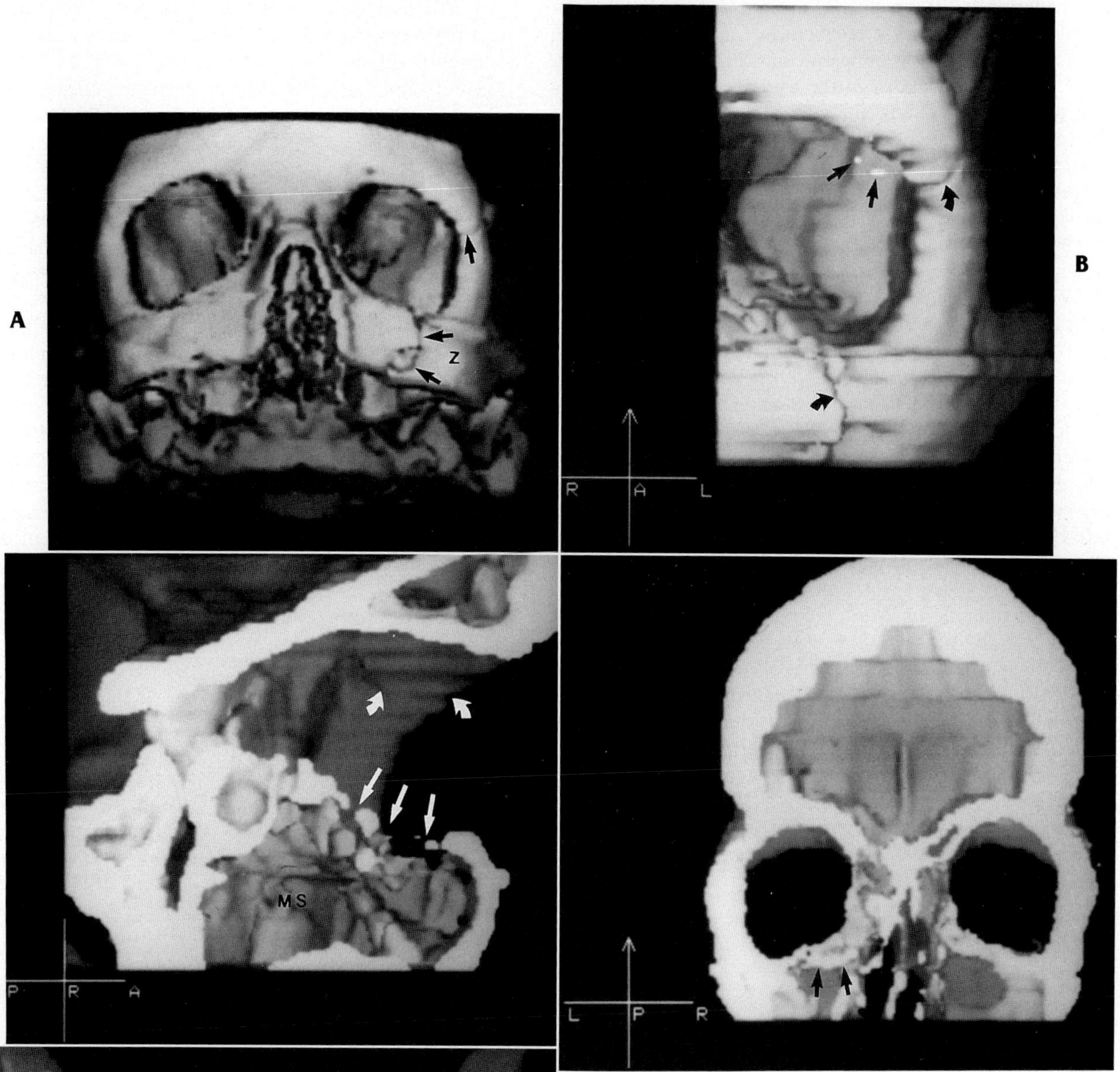


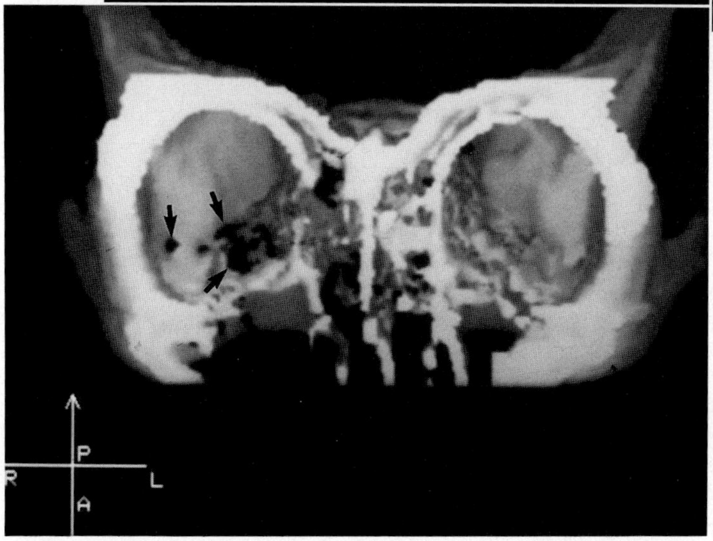


**FIGURE 2** 3DCT of zygoma fracture showing slicing possibilities and artifacts. *A,* Frontal view of face with image tilted upward to simulate a Water's view. Black arrows indicate zygoma (Z) fracture lines. *B,* Slicing through left orbit in sagittal plane to study lateral orbital segment. Curved arrows indicate fracture lines. Straight arrows indicate artifacts simulating bone fragments ("floaters"). *C,* Lateral orbital segment rotated to show interior of lateral orbital wall and fragmented left orbital floor *(straight white arrows).* Curved white arrows indicate fracture of the zygomaticofrontal suture. *D,* Coronal slicing with anterior portion of face removed and rotated so viewer is looking out through patient's orbits. Arrows indicate depressed segment of left orbital floor. *E,* Coronal slicing with anterior portion of face removed. Viewer is looking at posterior orbits. Arrows indicate pseudoforamina in right orbit, where the bony floor is particularly thin. Pseudoforamina can be observed elsewhere, in both orbits and in the walls of the maxillary and ethmoid sinuses.

rendering technique; the alternative is a semitransparent volume-based technique. Either technique requires three steps for rendering the 3D image: (1) volume formation, (2) classification, and (3) image projection. In the volume formation step, the computer is given instructions regarding the specific axial slices to be included in the final 3D image; the area of interest to be coned; and any resizing, image smoothing, and data editing (e.g., removing the CT cradle from the final image) to be performed. The classification step determines the type of tissue to be visualized on the final 3D image, whether fat, soft tissue, or bone (see Fig. 1). The projection step involves the display of volume data such that a 2D representation of the 3D volume is formed and allowed to rotate for hard copy filming.

For a good-quality 3D reformation, several requirements must be followed. The slice thickness of the original 2D scans must be appropriate for the specific anatomic part. For the face 1.5 to 3.0 mm thick slices are required. Thicker 5 mm or 10 mm slices would result in 3D images with steplike artifacts and poor detail. In addition, the slices should be contiguous, without any gaps. Patient motion should be eliminated or minimized, and any overlying radiopaque extraneous objects should be removed if possible. The radiologist must know what the referring physician needs to see and make certain that the 3D images will optimally display the particular injury.

There are a variety of artifacts associated with 3DCT. Pseudoforamina occur where bone is very thin and produce images of holes or absent bone (see Figs. 2 and 6). Incorrect thresholding when producing the 3D image may produce artifacts in the soft tissues that resemble bony fragments (see Fig. 2); these have been referred to as "floaters." Radiopaque nasogastric and endotracheal tubes and dental fillings may also be a cause of major artifact involving the lower half of the face (see Figs. 6 and 8). Artifacts generated by 3D reformation programs may even mimic signs of trauma. Consequently injuries suggested by 3D images should be confirmed on the original 2D axial scans.

## Facial Fractures by Classification

### *Orbital Fractures*

Orbital fractures are common among facial injuries and are often associated with other facial fractures. Orbital wall blow-out fractures may occur as an isolated (pure blow-out) fracture, or they may be associated with a break in the orbital rim (impure blow-out fracture). The latter are more often associated with other facial fractures such as a zygoma (see Fig. 2) or Le Fort II or III fractures. Pure blow-out fractures most frequently involve the orbital floor and less commonly the medial wall. The cause of a pure blow-out fracture is generally a blow to the orbit by an object that does not fit within the orbital rim. The blow suddenly increases intraorbital pressure and fractures a portion of the bony orbital lining. Three-dimensional CT may be helpful in displaying the increase in orbital volume associated with these fractures.

Orbital floor fractures occur with zygoma fractures (see Fig. 2) and Le Fort II fractures (see Fig. 9). Medial wall fractures may occur with nasal-orbital-ethmoid (NOE) fractures (see Fig. 7), which involve the nasal, lacrimal, and ethmoid bones. Lateral orbital wall fractures are usually associated with zygoma (see Fig. 4) or Le Fort III fractures (see Fig. 10). Orbital roof fractures (see Figs. 3, 8, and 11) are most often associated with a severe facial injury, such as a Le Fort III fracture or frontal fracture.

With orbital blow-in fractures, a fragment of bone lining the orbit is displaced within the orbital space itself. Most commonly they involve the orbital roof and occur with blows to the superior orbital rim or frontal bone. 3DCT is particularly useful showing orbital blow-in fragments (Figure 3). Orbital roof fractures are often associated with intracranial injury.

### *Zygoma Fractures*

The zygoma occupies a prominent and vulnerable position in the facial skeleton and is frequently fractured in motor vehicle accidents, assaults, sporting injuries, and falls. Zygoma fractures are present in nearly two-thirds of all facial fractures. The body of the zygoma is rarely fractured; rather, the zygoma disarticulates from its neighbors with fracture and/or dislocation at its suture lines with the maxillary, sphenoid, frontal, and temporal bones.

Zygoma fractures may be displaced and/or rotated. Displacement frequently occurs inferiorly and posteriorly, but may occur medially and laterally. Rotation may occur on either an anteroposterior, transverse, or craniocaudad axis. 3DCT is particularly helpful in depicting both displacement and rotation of zygoma fracture fragments (Fig. 4). Medially displaced zygoma fractures decrease orbital space volume and are often associated with injuries to orbital contents (Fig. 5).

### *Nasal Fractures*

The nose is the most frequently fractured facial structure. In adults the majority of nasal fractures (Figs. 4, 6, and 7) result from lateral blows. A mild-to-moderate lateral force may fracture only one nasal bone and frequently, also, the ipsilateral frontal process of the maxilla. More severe lateral forces may fracture both nasal bones and both frontal processes of maxillae. With lateral blows the septal cartilage is frequently dislocated and displaced laterally. We may see this dislocation with occlusal view plain films or CT. The nose is more resistant to trauma with direct anterior blows, which cause inferiorly displaced fractures of the distal portions of both nasal bones (see Fig. 9).

3DCT is helpful in showing the degree of bony displacement and alterations in nasal contour. Soft-tissue images may provide good correlation between the bony fracture and the cosmetic appearance of the patient (see Fig. 6).

### *NOE Fractures*

NOE fractures result from severe blows to the upper nose. They often involve multiple fractures of the maxillary, nasal, ethmoid, and lacrimal bones. There are two types: (1) a telescoped version, in which the nasal bones and central portion of the frontal processes of the maxillae are displaced posteriorly as a unit; and (2) the more common laterally spread type of NOE fracture, with severe comminution of the nasal, lacrimal, and ethmoid bones. NOE fractures may be unilateral; when they are, they may be associated with ipsilateral orbital blow-out and zygoma fractures (see Figs. 4 and 7).

### *Frontal Sinus Fractures*

Frontal sinus fractures are among the least common facial injury. They result from direct blows associated with assaults

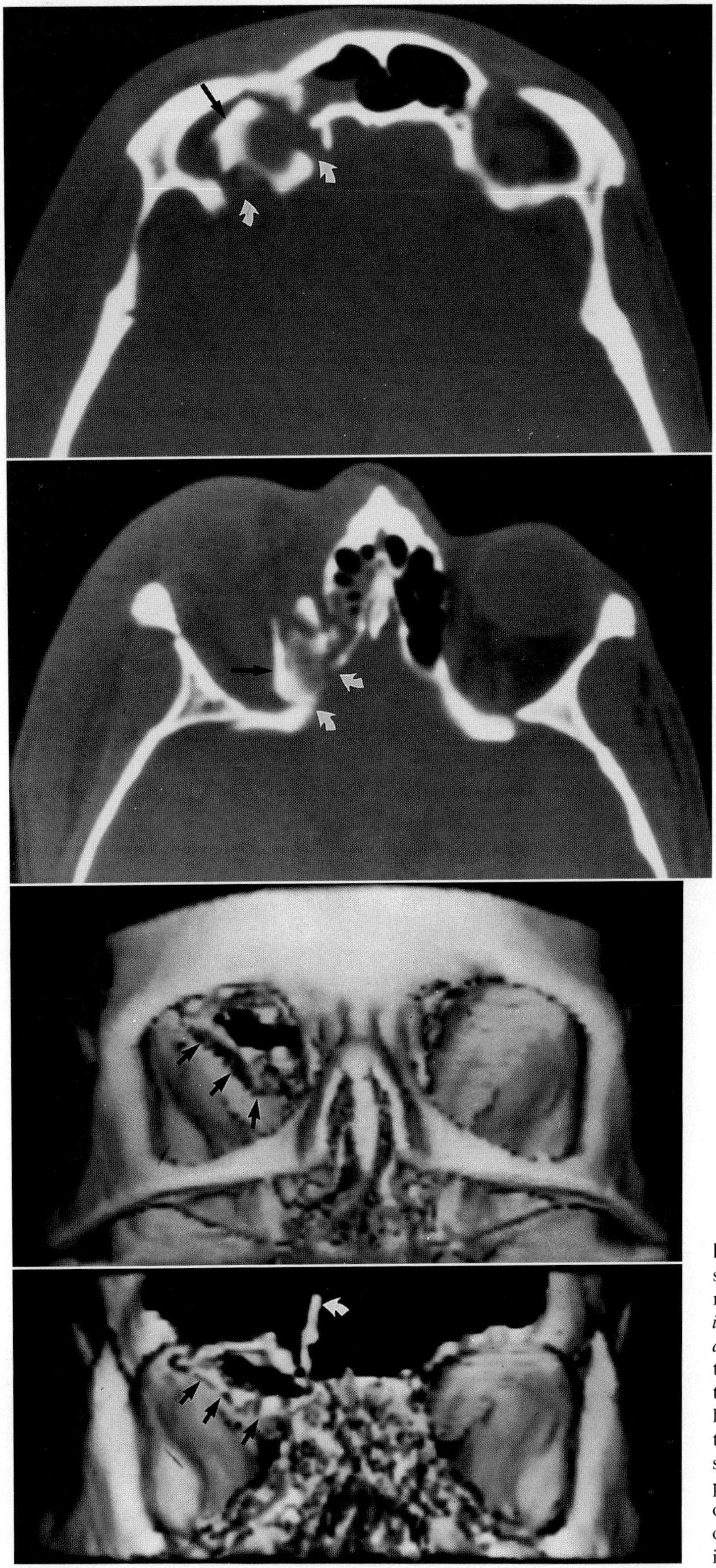


**FIGURE 3** Right orbital blow-in fracture. *A,* Axial slice through the extreme upper orbits and orbital roofs reveals a fracture of the right orbital roof *(curved arrows indicate fracture lines),* with bone fragment *(straight arrow)* within the superior orbital space. *B,* Axial slice through upper midorbit shows that the fracture involves the upper aspect of the medial orbit *(curved arrows).* A large bony fragment *(straight arrow)* is observed within the orbit itself. *C,* 3DCT in simulated Water's projection shows orbital blow-in fragment *(arrows). D,* View of posterior orbits after slicing off anterior face. Note the orbital blow-in fragment *(straight arrows)* and vertically oriented fragment *(curved arrow)* extending superiorly into the frontal lobe of brain.

A

B

C

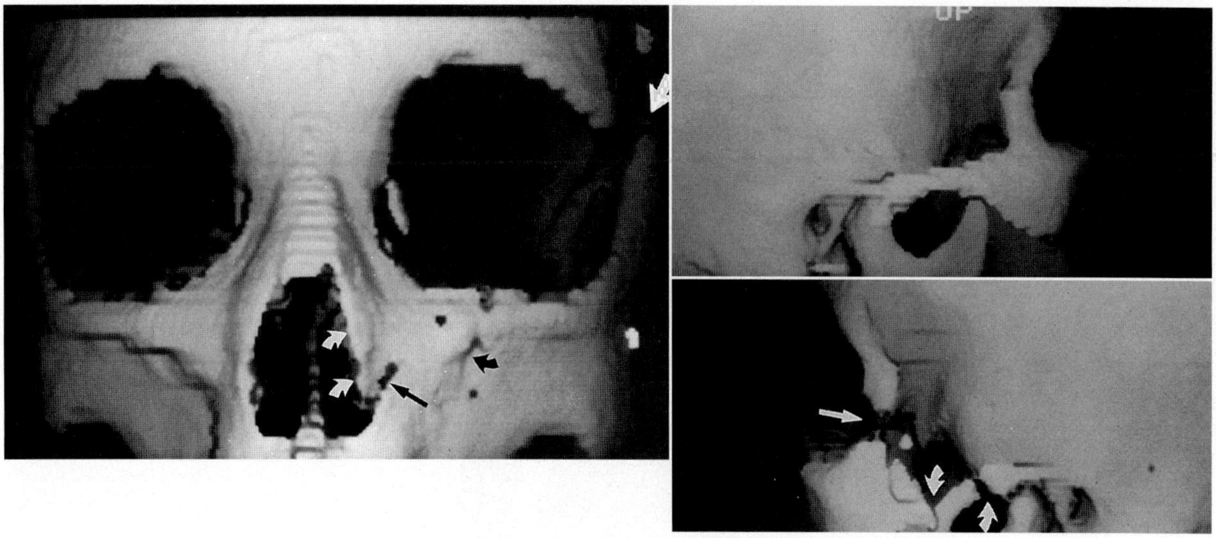

**FIGURE 4** Left zygoma fracture associated with unilateral left NOE fracture. *A,* Frontal view 3DCT shows lateral displacement of the left zygoma *(straight white arrow)* at the left zygomaticofrontal suture. Curved black arrow indicates a fracture line along the left maxillo-zygomatic suture. Straight black arrow indicates fracture of left frontal process of maxilla. Curved white arrows indicate flattening and slight medial displacement of left side of nose – all components of left unilateral NOE fracture. *B,* Right lateral 3DCT shows a normal right zygoma. *C,* Left lateral 3DCT shows a left zygoma fracture with inferior displacement of the main zygoma fragment. Comminution is observed at the zygomaticofrontal (*straight white arrow*) and zygomaticotemporal (*curved white arrows*) suture lines.

A

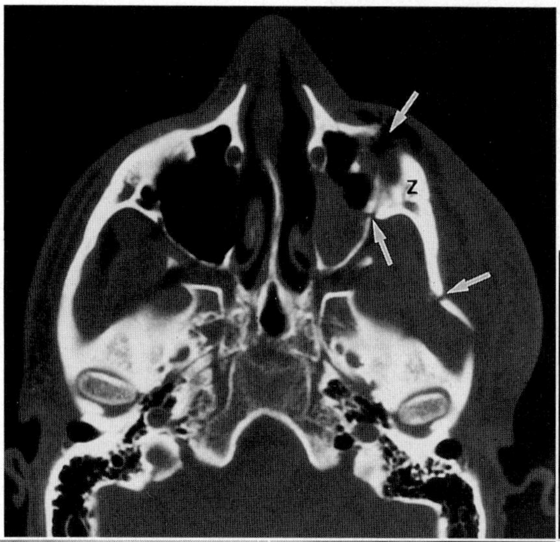


C

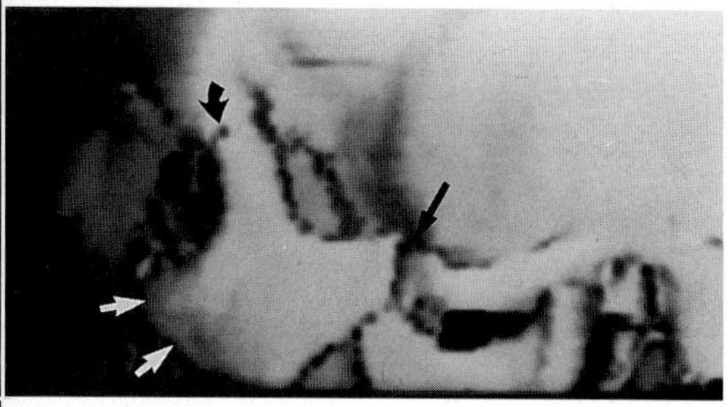

B

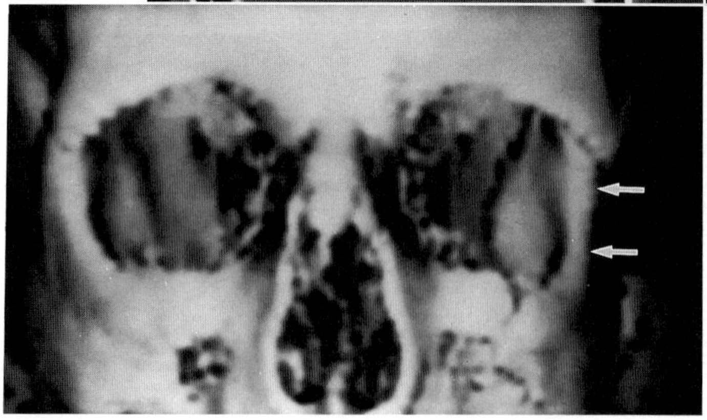

**FIGURE 5** Medially displaced left zygoma fracture. *A,* Axial CT scan through zygomatic arches shows a left zygoma fracture *(arrows),* with medial and posterior displacement of the major zygoma fragment (Z). *B,* Frontal view 3DCT shows medial displacement of the left zygoma *(arrows),* with decrease in size of the bony orbit. *C,* Lateral view 3DCT shows a fracture of the left zygomaticofrontal arch *(curved black arrow)* and zygomaticotemporal arch *(straight black arrow).* The left zygoma is posteriorly displaced and rotated *(white arrows).*

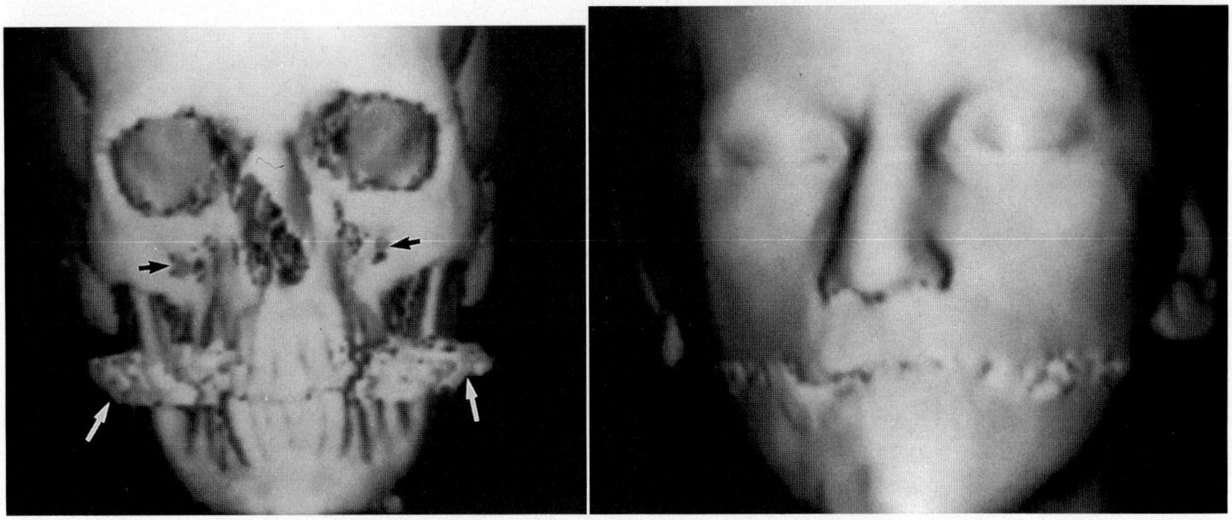


**FIGURE 6** Laterally displaced nasal fracture caused by a blow by a right-handed assailant. *A,* Frontal view 3DCT with bone rendering shows lateral displacement of both nasal bones and both frontal processes of maxillae (sides of nose). White arrows indicate artifacts from metallic dental fillings. Black arrows indicate pseudoforamina, where maxillary bone forming the anterior walls of the maxillary sinuses is particularly thin. *B,* Frontal view 3DCT with soft-tissue rendering shows displacement of the nose to the right. This rendering closely approximated the actual appearance of the patient. Metallic dental filling artifacts have produced skin irregularities at the level of the patient's mouth.

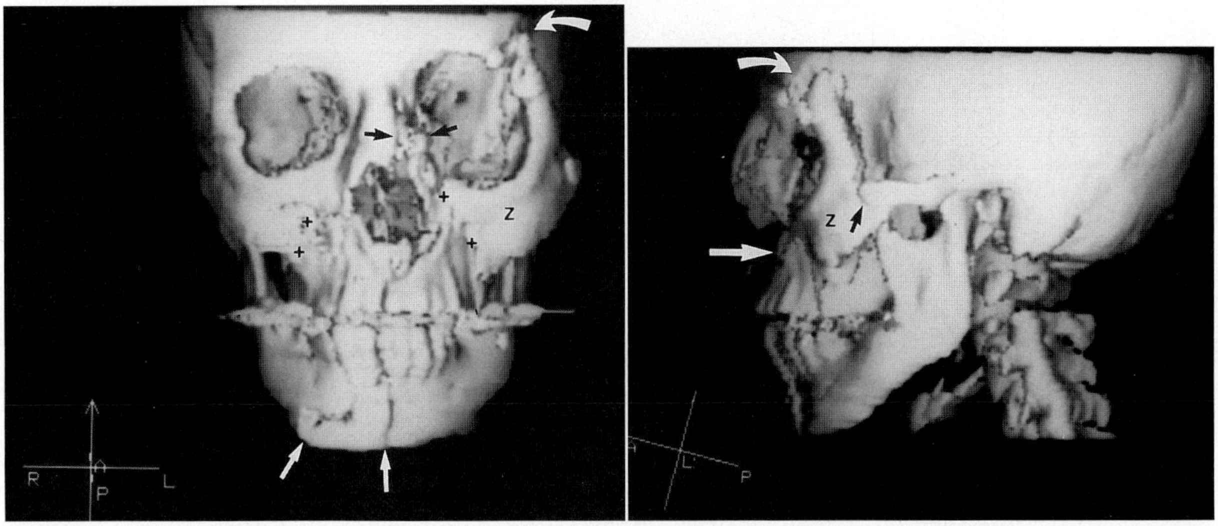


**FIGURE 7** Le Fort II fracture associated with a left zygoma fracture, left unilateral NOE fracture, and mandible fractures. *A,* Frontal view 3DCT. The left zygoma (Z) is displaced inferiorly and laterally. Note the increased size of the left orbit as compared with the right. Curved white arrow indicates site of zygomaticofrontal fracture. The Le Fort II fracture lines are delineated by +'s. Black arrows indicate a comminuted unilateral left NOE fracture. Straight white arrows indicate two mandibular fractures. *B,* Lateral view 3DCT. The left zygoma (Z) is displaced posteriorly and inferiorly. Curved white arrow indicates diastasis of left zygomaticofrontal junction. Short black arrow indicates fracture of zygomaticotemporal arch. Straight white arrow indicates posterior displacement of the maxilla associated with the Le Fort II fracture. Note the comminuted nasal fracture involving both the left nasal bone and left frontal process of maxilla.

or motor vehicle accidents (Figs. 8 and 11). They are classified according to the sinus wall involved. Anterior wall fractures are the least severe. Those that involve the posterior wall usually require a neurosurgical exploration. Those that involve the sinus floor or roof of orbits may result in orbital injuries (Fig. 8). 3DCT may be helpful in demonstrating fragment displacement and alterations in contour of the bony orbit.

### *Maxillary Fractures*

Maxillary fractures are common and three types are recognized: (1) dentoalveolar fractures, (2) Le Fort fractures, and (3) maxillary sagittal fractures. Dentoalveolar fractures are caused by a blow to the alveolar portion of the maxilla. Clinically this may manifest to the examining physician as one or more adjacent loose teeth.

Anatomic details of Le Fort fractures were described in

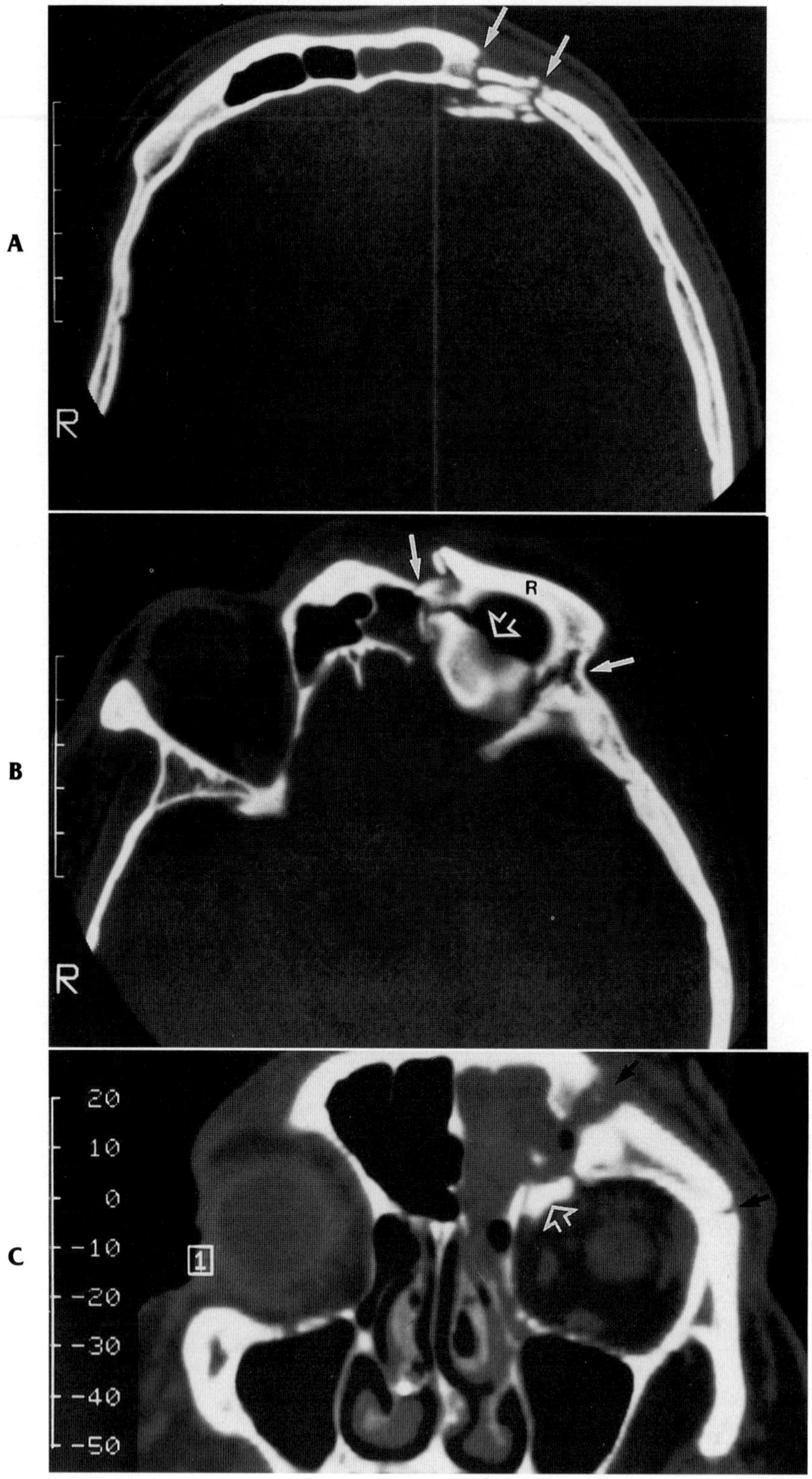


**FIGURE 8** Left depressed frontal fracture involving the left superior orbital rim and orbital roof with orbital blow-in fragments. The victim had been struck over the left eye with a tire iron. *A,* Axial CT scan through the frontal sinuses shows a depressed fracture of the left frontal bone *(white arrows).* The left frontal sinus is opacified with blood. *B,* Axial CT scan through upper orbits shows fractures of the left superior orbital rim *(white arrows),* with inferior and anterior displacement of the rim itself (R). The open arrow points to a blow-in fragment within the superior orbit. *C,* Coronal CT scan shows frontal fracture lines *(black arrows).* Open arrow indicates blow-in fragment. The orbital roof is slightly depressed and the volume of the left orbit is decreased.

D

E

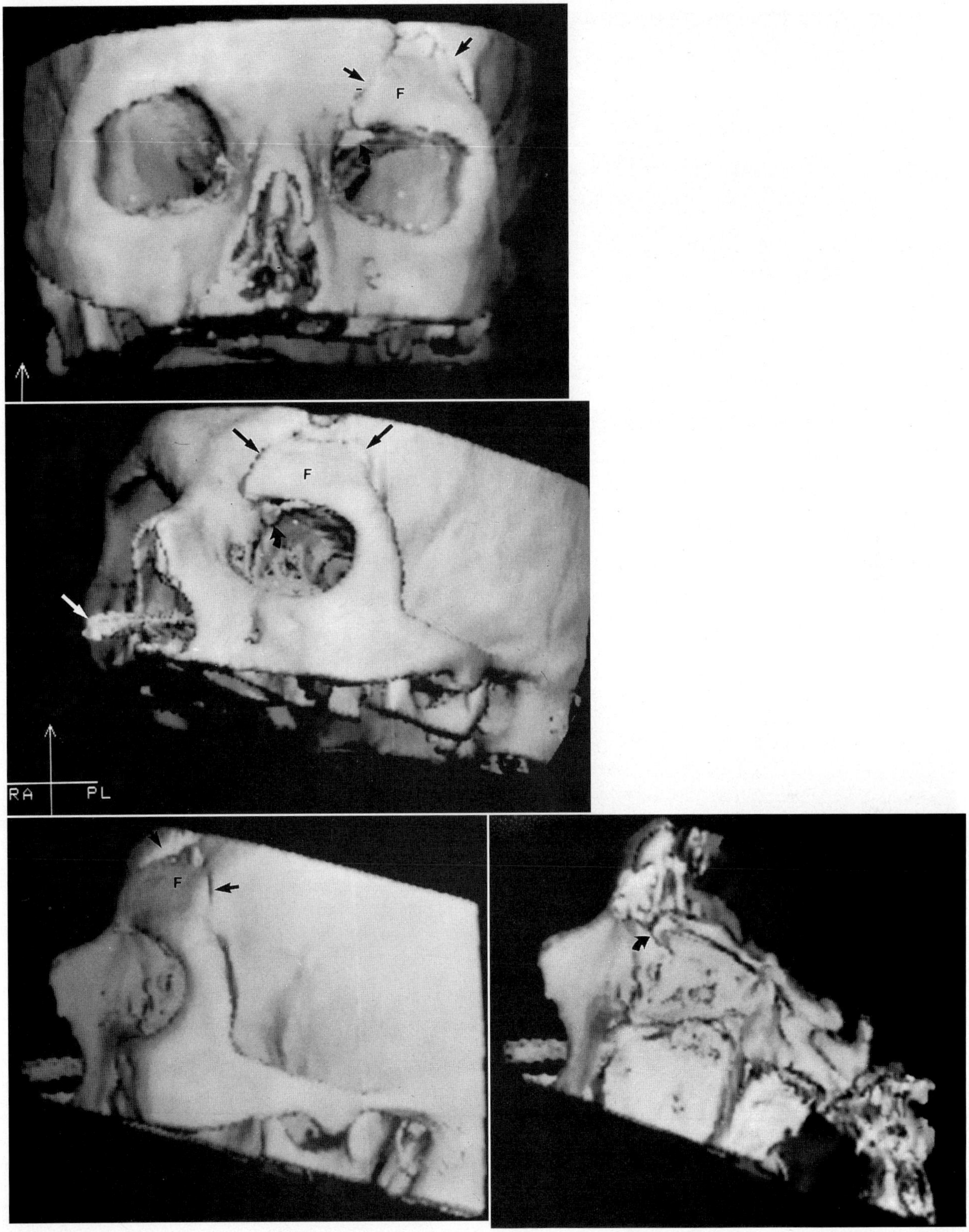


F

G

**FIGURE 8, cont'd** *D,* Frontal view 3DCT shows fracture line *(arrows)* around the depressed frontal fracture (F). Note the inferior displacement of the left orbital rim. Curved arrow indicates blow-in fragment. *E,* Oblique view 3DCT shows fracture line *(black arrows)* around depressed left frontal fracture (F). Again note the low position of superior orbital rim. Curved arrow indicates orbital blow-in fragment. White arrow indicates nasogastric tube. *F,* Lateral view 3DCT. Black arrows indicate fracture lines around depressed left frontal (F) fracture. *G,* 3DCT with lateral half of orbit removed. Curved arrow indicates orbital blow-in fragment.

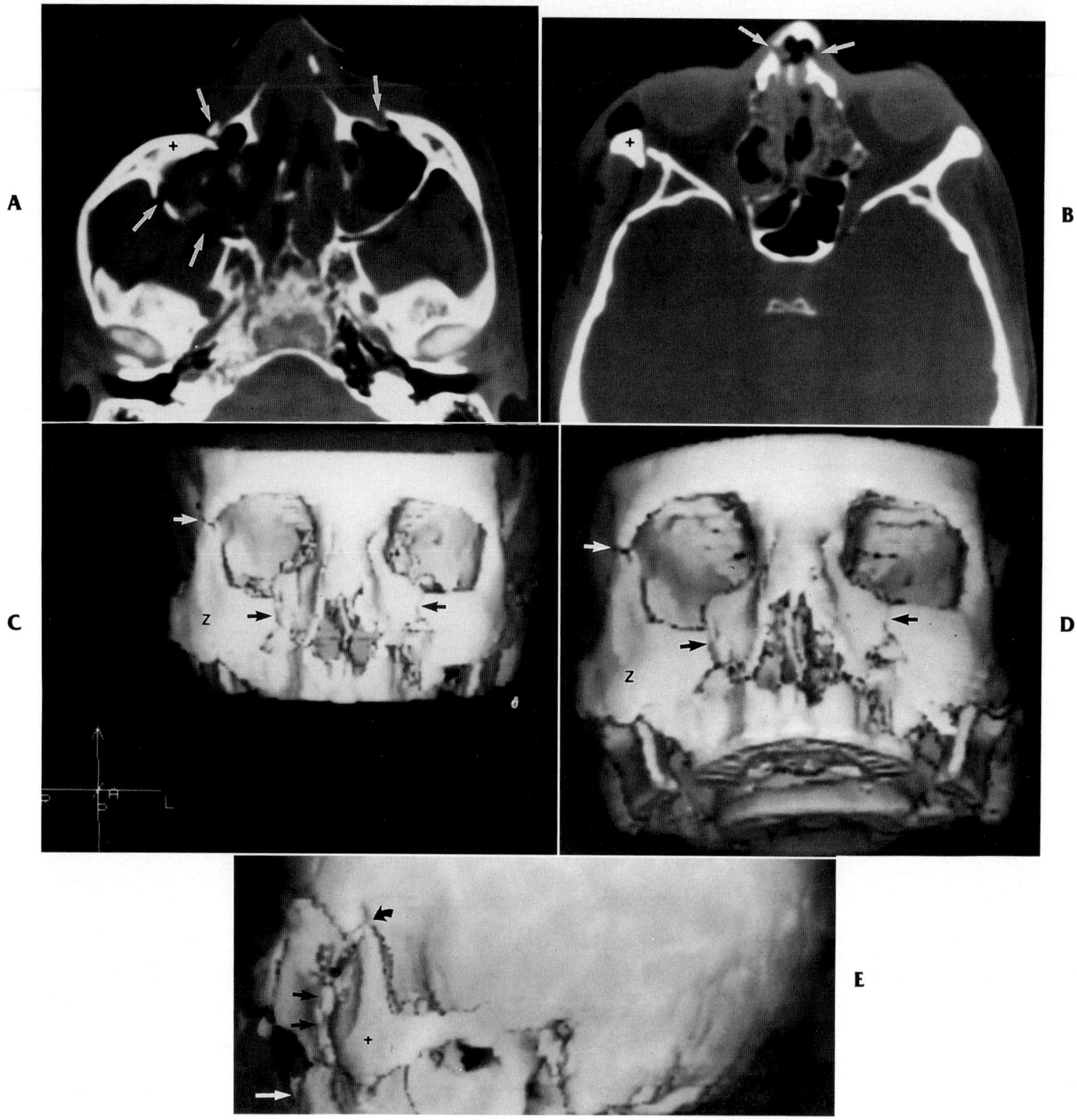


**FIGURE 9** Le Fort II fracture with right zygoma fracture. *A,* Axial CT scan through zygomatic arches and maxillary sinuses show Le Fort II fracture line *(arrows)* through the anterior walls of both maxillary sinuses and posterolateral wall of the right maxillary sinus. The right zygoma (+) is displaced posteriorly. Subcutaneous emphysema is present anterior to the zygoma. Nasal fractures are also present. *B,* Axial CT scan through orbits shows bilateral nasal fractures *(arrows)* and posterior displacement of the right zygoma (+) from its articulation with the greater wing of sphenoid bone, which forms the remainder of the posterior lateral wall of orbit. *C,* Frontal view 3DCT showing Le Fort II fracture lines *(black arrows).* The right zygoma (Z) is fractured and displaced inferiorly. Note the step in the contour of the right inferior orbital rim associated with inferior displacement of the zygoma. The white arrow points to the fracture at the right zygomaticofrontal suture. Multiple depressed nasal fractures can also be observed. *D,* Frontal view 3DCT tilted to simulate a Water's projection. Black arrows indicate Le Fort II fracture lines. White arrow indicates fracture at right zygomaticofrontal suture. The right zygoma (Z) is again noted to be depressed inferiorly. *E,* Lateral view 3DCT. The right zygoma (+) is noted to be displaced posteriorly from its normal level of articulation with the maxilla *(black arrows).* Curved arrow indicates the fractured right zygomaticofrontal suture. White arrow indicates posterior displacement of the maxilla associated with the Le Fort II fracture. Nasal fractures can also be observed.

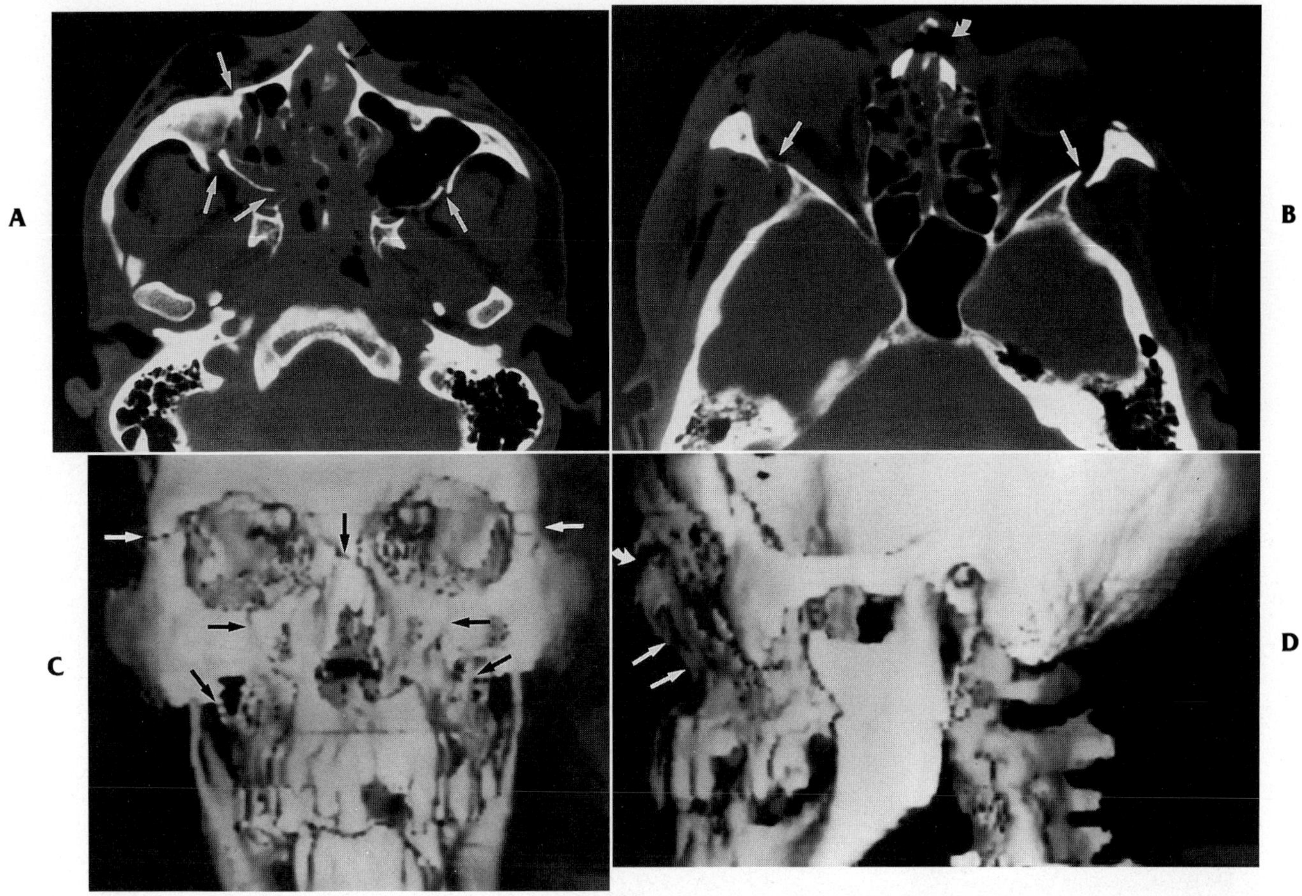


**FIGURE 10** Combined Le Fort II and III fracture. *A,* Axial CT scan through maxillary sinuses shows Le Fort II fracture lines in the anterior wall of the right maxillary sinus and the posterolateral wall of both maxillary sinuses *(white arrows).* Black arrow indicates a fracture of the left frontal process of maxilla. *B,* Axial CT scan through midorbits demonstrates fractures of both zygomaticosphenoid sutures *(straight white arrow)* along the Le Fort III fracture line. Curved white arrow indicates a fracture line at the upper portion of the nasal bones, where the nasal bones are separated from the frontal bone. *C,* Frontal view 3DCT shows fractures along the Le Fort III fracture line at both zygomaticofrontal sutures *(white arrows).* Black arrows indicate fractures along the Le Fort II fracture lines. Note also fractures of the mandible and nose. *D,* Lateral view 3DCT. Curved white arrow indicates fracture line at the top of the nose. Straight white arrows indicate posterior displacement of the maxillae. Note the overall flattening of the anterior face.

1901 by Rene Le Fort, a French surgeon who traumatized cadaver heads to identify lines of facial weakness. He described three lines of weakness along which Le Fort I, II, and III fractures occur. The Le Fort I fracture is a horizontal splitting of the maxillae just above the alveolar process, which extends posteriorly through the pterygoid plates. This injury may occur when an object with a small contact area, such as a tennis racquet or steering wheel, strikes the anterior face just below the nose. The plain film and CT findings are subtle, especially when the fracture is nondisplaced. Coronal CT is most helpful for diagnosed nondisplaced Le Fort I fractures.

A central blow may produce a Le Fort II fracture, resulting in a pyramid-shaped, fragment of midface. The nasal bones and frontal processes of maxillae are separated from the upper face, across the nasofrontal suture, with fracture lines extending down through the orbital rims, anterior and posterior walls of maxillary sinuses, and posteriorly through the pterygoid plates. This fragment, composed of upper teeth, maxillae, and nasal bones, is often displaced posteriorly and rotated upward (Figs. 7 and 9).

The Le Fort III fracture separates all the facial bones from the calvarial bones, resulting in craniofacial disarticulation. Beginning in the nasofrontal area, this fracture line extends through medial, lateral, and posterior walls of the orbits, the zygomaticofrontal sutures, zygomatic arches, and out posteriorly through the pterygoid plates. Le Fort II and Le Fort III fractures often occur together (Fig. 10).

The last category of maxilla fracture is the maxillary sagittal fracture. It usually results from a direct blow to the anterior surface of the maxilla (anterior wall of maxillary sinus) and runs in a sagittal plane through the maxilla.

## *Mandible Fractures*

Mandible fractures are most often caused by assaults and motor vehicle accidents. They are classified according to their location, and whether they are open or closed fractures. A mandible fracture may involve a condyle, subcondylar area or mandibular neck, coronoid process, ramus, angle, body, symphysis, or parasymphyseal area. Open mandibular fractures

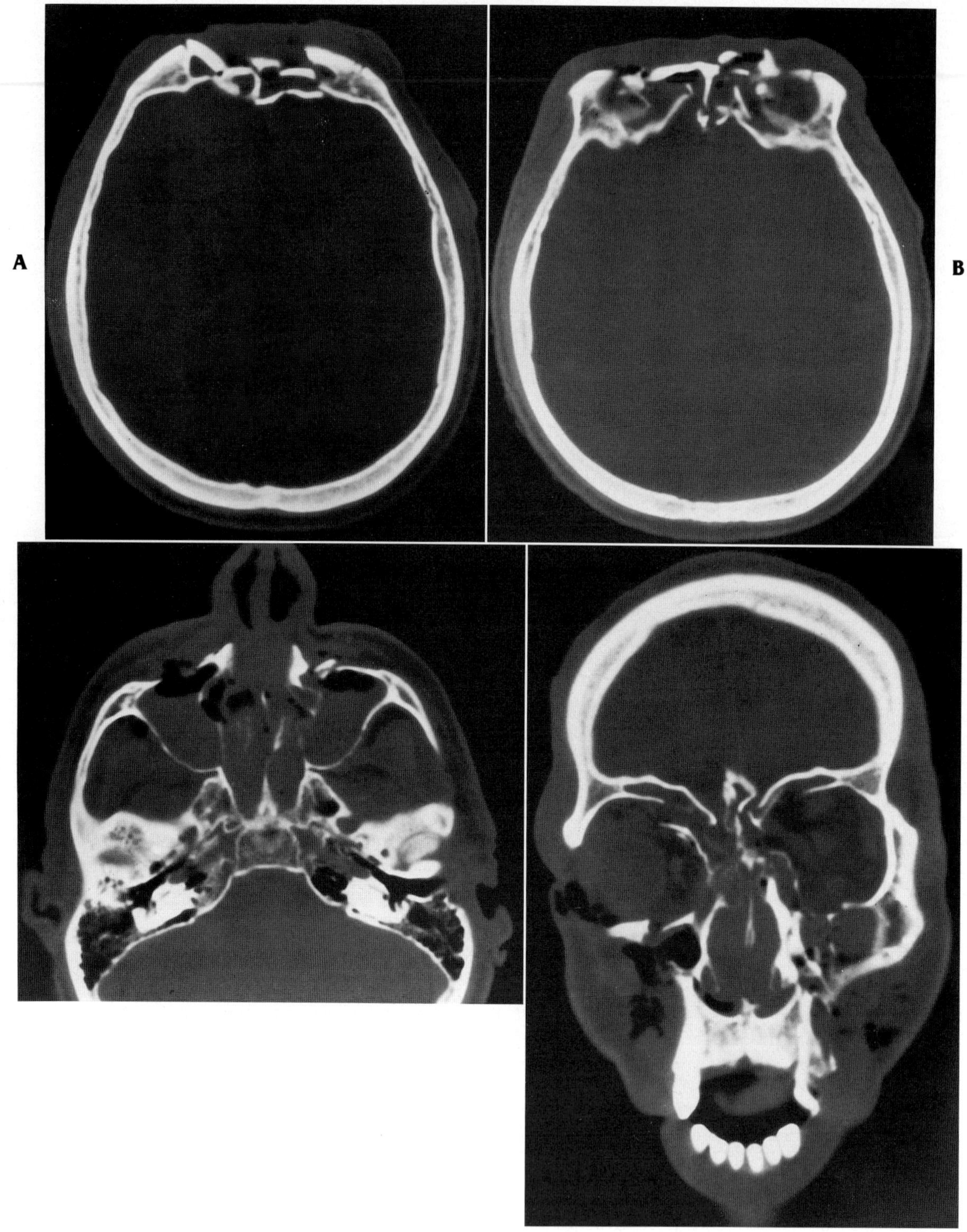


**FIGURE 11** Craniofacial fracture (smash fracture). *A,* Axial CT scan at level of frontal bone shows markedly comminuted and depressed fractures of the anterior frontal bone. *B,* Axial CT scan at level of orbital roofs shows comminuted fractures of the superior orbital rims, orbital roofs, and frontal sinuses. *C,* Axial CT scan at level of the maxillary sinuses shows fractures of the anterior walls of both maxillary sinuses. Note that the posterior lateral walls of the maxillary sinuses are intact, differentiating this anterior injury from a Le Fort fracture. *D,* Coronal CT scan through anterior orbits shows fractures of the roofs, medial walls, and floors of the anterior orbits.

E 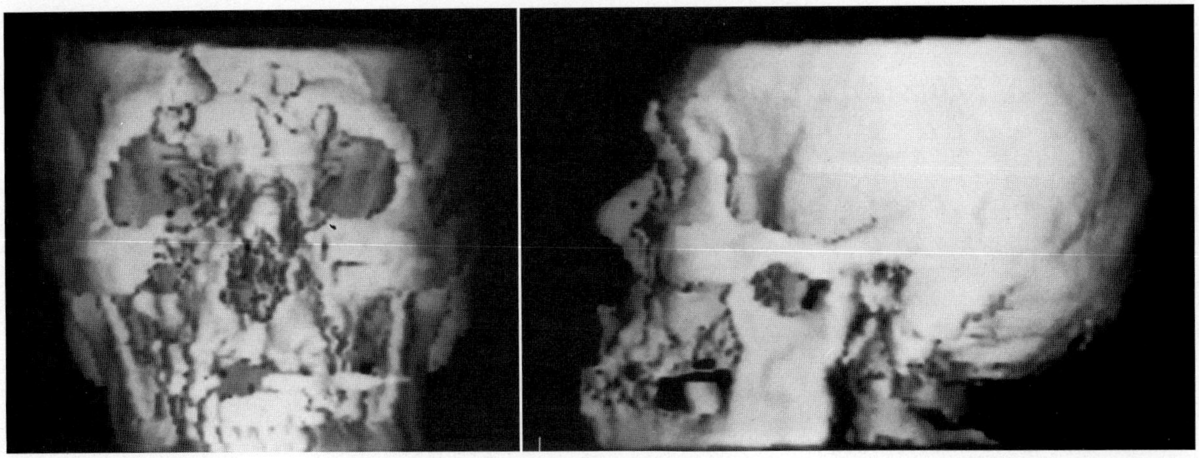 F

**FIGURE 11, cont'd** *E,* Frontal view 3DCT shows markedly comminuted fractures of the anterior portions of the forehead and face. *F,* Lateral view 3DCT shows comminuted fractures of the anterior face, with flattening of the face as well.

include any fracture exposed to the external environment by a tear in the skin or mucosa. Consequently any mandible fracture involving a segment that supports teeth is considered open because of exposure to the oral cavity.

A mandible series should include posteroanterior and lateral views, a Towne's view to show the condyles and infracondylar areas, and both oblique views. If a temporomandibular joint injury is suspected, then both closed- and open-mouth temporomandibular joint films may be useful. Because nondisplaced mandibular fractures are difficult to show on plain films, CT is indicated when a mandibular fracture is suspected clinically but not definitely observed on plain film or when the plain films are suspicious for fracture. 3DCT is particularly helpful in demonstrating the position and alignment of displaced mandibular fracture fragments (see Fig. 7).

### Craniofacial and Panfacial Fractures

Craniofacial and panfacial fractures are sometimes referred to as smash fractures. They often occur in patients who have suffered combined injuries of the cranium, face, and mandible. Central craniofacial fractures result from blows to the frontonasal region and involve nasal, vomer, maxillary, ethmoid, and frontal bones. The orbital rims and orbital walls, as well as the frontal sinuses, may also be involved. Lateral craniofacial fractures result from blows in the frontozygomatic region, leading to fractures in the lateral cranium and face. Frontal, sphenoid, zygomatic, and maxillary bones are often involved. With combined central and lateral fractures, there is severe instability and dislocation of multiple fracture fragments involving both the central and lateral face and skull. CT is essential in the workup of these patients, and 3DCT has proved highly useful in delineating the position and orientation of major fracture fragments associated with these injuries (Fig. 11).

## Discussion

Three-dimensional CT offers a simplified technique for viewing and interpreting facial CT data. It provides improved depth perception for viewers and shows continuity of structures and spatial relationships. The biggest advantage of 3D imaging is its ability to communicate with referring physicians. 3DCT is most helpful in displaying the position and alignment of the major fracture fragments of displaced fractures. However, its utility at diagnosis is limited. The resolution of 3D reformation is significantly inferior to the 2D axial and coronal CT slices, and 3D reformations are often degraded by artifacts. Most radiologists do not believe that 3D reformations improve the CT diagnoses of facial trauma. Nondisplaced fractures may be overlooked by 3DCT, and artifacts associated with current technology may even mimic facial injuries. Consequently 3DCT must also be reviewed in conjunction with the convential (2D) axial and coronal CT images. In only a limited number of cases has 3D been shown to alter the diagnosis made by plain films combined with conventional CT images. With future improvements in scanning equipment and software technology, the resolution of 3DCT should be improved, artifacts diminished, and diagnostic capability increased.

## Suggested Reading

Alling CC, Osbon DB. Maxillofacial Trauma. Philadelphia: Lea & Febiger, 1988.

Delbalso AM. Maxillofacial Imaging. Philadelphia: WB Saunders, 1990.

Dolan KD, Jacoby CG, Smoker WRK. Radiology of Facial Injury. 2nd ed. New York: Macmillan, 1988.

Foster CA, Sherman JE. Surgery of Facial Bone Fractures. New York: Churchill Livingstone, 1987.

Fishman EK, Magid D, Ney DR, et al. Three-dimensional imaging. Radiology 1991; 181:321–337.

Gerlock AJ, Sinn DP, McBride KL. Clinical and Radiographic Interpretation of Facial Fractures. Boston: Little, Brown, 1981.

Lawrason JN, Novelline RA. Diagnostic Imaging of Facial Trauma. In: Mirvis SE, Young JWR, eds. Imaging in Trauma and Critical Care. Baltimore: Williams & Wilkins, 1992.

# Quantitative CT in Osteoporosis

CORNELIS VAN KUIJK, M.D., Ph.D. · HARRY K. GENANT, M.D.

Computed tomography (CT) scanners are designed for imaging the human body. The images obtained show the anatomy in cross section and provide volumetric information to the radiologist. Although CT scanners are primarily dedicated to diagnostic imaging, they can be used to provide quantitative information on human body composition and physiology. This feature of CT scanning, called quantitative CT (QCT), has been used primarily for estimation of bone mineral density within the skeleton. The analysis of trabecular bone mineral density within the vertebral body of the lumbar spine with single-energy QCT (SEQCT) has become a well-established method for monitoring changes caused by aging, disease, and therapeutic interventions. The information obtained by CT can also be used to assess bone strength. Models used for strength estimation in engineering, such as finite element analysis, have been evaluated using CT data of the vertebral body and of the femur. Currently QCT is performed primarily at the lumbar spine. Some research centers have reported three-dimensional densitometric analysis of the proximal femur. Also special-purpose CT systems have been developed for bone mineral density measurements in the peripheral skeleton (radius, tibia). Until now, however, these systems were not widely used.

The main topic of interest within the field of noninvasive bone mineral assessment is osteoporosis. This syndrome of diminishing bone content and subsequent atraumatic fracturing of skeletal parts is a major health problem in Western society, with its increasingly aging population. Two categories of osteoporosis exist: primary and secondary. In secondary osteoporosis the reduced bone content is caused by conditions or diseases known to affect bone such as hypogonadism, Cushing's syndrome, malabsorption syndromes, drug-induced osteoporosis, and lack of exercise or immobilization. Primary osteoporosis is an aging phenomenon. It is categorized in two types: postmenopausal osteoporosis (type 1) and senile osteoporosis (type 2).

## Indications and Clinical Utility

We currently consider the following four clinical applications valid for use of bone densitometry in osteoporosis:

1. *Establishing a diagnosis of primary osteoporosis or assessing its severity.* Bone strength is correlated with bone density. Declining levels of bone density correspond to increasing fracture risk. Therefore the absolute level of bone density is predictive of future fracture risk. Other factors leading to fracture include damage to trabecular architecture and decreased postural stability caused by aging or disease. Conventional spine radiography is insufficient for establishing the diagnosis of diminished bone mineral content and thus the early stages of osteoporosis. Vertebral deformation like wedging, concavity of the end-plates, and eventually crush fracture, that can be seen on plain radiographs, are in fact the final outcome of osteoporosis. Therefore we recommend performance of quantitative evaluation of the skeleton in individuals in whom osteoporosis is suspected on clinical or historical grounds or in whom atraumatic fracture is suspected on plain radiography.
2. *Establishing a diagnosis of secondary osteoporosis or assessing its severity.* In the secondary forms of osteoporosis, bone density measurements can influence clinical decision making. The knowledge of the level of bone density in corticosteroid-induced osteoporosis can lead to the decision to reduce corticosteroid dosage. It also can prompt the decision to perform subtotal parathyroidectomy in the case of hyperparathyroid bone disease.
3. *Assessing perimenopausal women for initiation of estrogen therapy.* Estrogen therapy has been proven to decrease postmenopausal bone loss and to reduce the incidence of osteoporotic fractures. However, a major problem is the selection of women who need preventive medication. It could be claimed that medication should be restricted to women with an increased fracture risk to maximize cost-effective use and to enhance compliance with preventive therapy.

   The absolute level of bone density at menopause and the magnitude of subsequent bone loss are important considerations in assessing fracture risk. The decision to begin prophylaxis against osteoporosis, therefore, can be facilitated with knowledge of the woman's bone density.
4. *Monitoring efficacy of treatment or disease course.* If applied properly, QCT measurements have precision errors in vivo that approach 2 percent. This precision level permits use of this method for longitudinal follow-up. It can be used to establish the rate of bone loss in aging (primary osteoporosis) and disease (secondary osteoporosis) and to monitor efficacy of treatment given to increase bone mass or to prohibit further bone loss (treatment and prevention of osteoporosis).

## Alternative Technologies

QCT is only one of the techniques available for noninvasive bone mineral measurements. Many other techniques have been developed such as single- and dual-photon absorptiometry (SPA, DPA), dual x-ray absorptiometry (DXA), and ultrasonic attenuation and velocity. QCT, however, is the only method that gives a true volumetric density estimation. Other techniques like SPA and DXA give an estimation of projected linear or areal density. Further, QCT is the only technique measuring purely trabecular bone within the vertebral body. The other techniques give a bone mineral estimate of the integral bone, meaning that it is a measurement of the cortical and trabecular parts of the skeletal part under investigation. A comparison of the different techniques is given in Table 1. QCT has a higher radiation dose compared with SPA, DPA, or DXA. However, the tissue-equivalent dose for QCT is small compared with plain radiography for the spine or abdomen. Dependent on the technique used, the effective dose equivalent of a lateral lumbar spine radiograph varies between 700 and 2,700 μSv, which is 10 to 30 times the effective dose equivalent of a QCT evaluation.

**TABLE 1** Techniques for Bone Densitometry

| Technique | Site of Measurement | Type of Measurement | Precision in Vivo (%) | Evaluation Time (min) | Effective Dose Equivalent (μSv) |
|---|---|---|---|---|---|
| QCT | Spine, (hip) | Trabecular; volumetric density | 2–4 | 10–15 | 50–100 |
| DXA | Spine, hip, total body, (radius) | Integral; areal density | 1–3 | 5–20 | 1–3 |
| DPA | Spine, hip, total body | Integral; areal density | 2–5 | 20–40 | 3–5 |
| SPA | Radius, heel | Integral; linear or areal density | 1–2 | 10–15 | < 1 |
| US | Heel, patella | Integral; attenuation or velocity | 2–3 | 5 | – |

QCT = quantitative computed tomography; DXA = dual x-ray absorptiometry; DPA = dual-photon absorptiometry; SPA = single-photon absorptiometry; US = ultrasonography.

# Technique

## *Basic Principles*

The CT image is a two-dimensional display of a map of attenuation values. This map can be used to determine the average attenuation value (expressed in CT numbers) of an object of interest. The CT number is given in Hounsfield units according to the following equation:

$$CT\# = 1{,}000 * (\mu_o - \mu_w)/\mu_w$$

where CT# is the CT number in Hounsfield units, $\mu_o$ is the energy-dependent linear-attenuation coefficient of the object of interest, and $\mu_w$ is the linear-attenuation coefficient of water.

In SEQCT, a calibration standard with different solutions of a material that mimics bone ($K_2HPO_4$ in water, or calcium hydroxyapatite in a water-equivalent plastic) is scanned simultaneously with the patient. The mean CT numbers of the solutions are plotted against their concentrations using linear regression. The mean CT number of the object of interest is then converted to the bone mineral equivalent value.

## *Procedure*

The patient is scanned supine with a support cushion under the knees to reduce the degree of lumbar lordosis. A calibration standard is placed under the lumbar spine of the patient. On a lateral scout scan of the lower spine (T12 to L5), a slice selection is made at the midvertebral levels of three consecutive vertebral bodies, typically L1 to L3. Scans are made perpendicular to the axis of the vertebra at 80 kVp, 140 mA, and a slice thickness of 10 mm at a fixed table height. Image reconstruction is done using standard algorithms. The scanning protocol should not be changed over time.

The images are analyzed using an automated procedure as follows:

1. The mean CT numbers of the solutions in the reference device are determined and used for calculation of the calibration line.
2. The mean CT number of a specific region of interest (ROI) within the trabecular part of the vertebral body is determined and converted to the bone-equivalent value using the calibration equation.

The results are expressed in milligrams per milliliter. Usually the bone mineral estimate is given as the average bone-equivalent value for all the vertebral levels scanned.

A typical QCT evaluation is given in Figure 1. A QCT study takes 10 to 15 minutes including the bone mineral analysis.

# Diagnostic Approach and Pitfalls

## *Assessment of Bone Mineral Content*

In the third or fourth decade of life, a normal young adult achieves maximal bone mass, called peak bone mass. Men achieve a higher peak bone mass than women. Further, racial differences exist: black men and women achieve a higher peak bone mass than white men and women. In further aging the bone mineral content of the vertebral body diminishes at a relatively constant rate. Women experience an accelerated bone loss in the first years after menopause. QCT measurements should therefore be compared with those of age-, sex-, and race-matched controls. A normative data base is mandatory for interpreting the level of bone mineral content. Usually the average QCT estimation is given also as a Z-score. The Z-score gives the patient's results as the deviation from the mean of matched controls divided by the standard deviation of this mean, which is an indication of the biologic variability. In fact, QCT results can be interpreted in a manner analogous with the curves used in pediatrics to assess a child's progress in growth and maturation. In addition to the Z-score, the bone density of a patient is compared with the peak bone mass of young normal adults; the QCT estimation then is given as the T-score. The T-score, like the Z-score, gives the patient's results as a deviation from the mean of young normal adults divided by the standard deviation of the mean. As indicated, the level of bone density is predictive for future osteoporotic fractures and can be a guideline for initiation of preventive action.

## *Assessment of Bone Loss or Bone Gain*

With the precision level of 2 percent that can currently be achieved with QCT, changes in bone mineral density can be monitored in the individual patient. With this precision level, a bone density change in an individual patient must be 5.5 percent to be detected with a 95 percent two-tailed confidence limit or 3.6 percent with a 90 percent one-tailed confidence limit. Annual losses of bone density are 5 to 10 percent in women undergoing surgical or natural menopause in the first years after menopause as measured with QCT. Annual gains of bone mass are 5 to 15 percent in patients taking preventive or therapeutic medication for osteoporosis (e.g., calcitonin, sodium fluoride, or parathyroid hormones). Follow-up QCT bone mineral measurements can be used to monitor physiologic and pathologic bone loss (e.g., corticosteroid-induced osteoporosis or premature menopause as a result of surgery or hormonal disbalance from anorexia nervosa). Also, QCT can

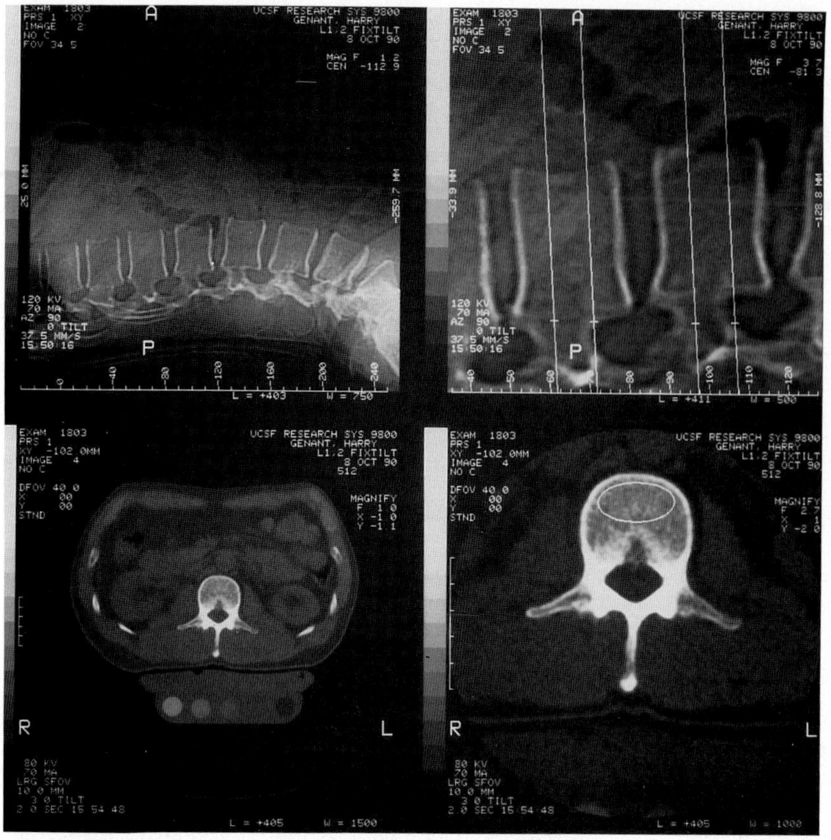

**FIGURE 1** Typical lateral scout view of lower spine *(upper left);* detail of volume scanned in vertebral body *(upper right);* typical QCT image: patient on top of calibration standard *(lower left);* QCT analysis: trabecular region of interest *(lower right).*

be used to monitor therapeutic intervention. Thus QCT can be used as a guideline in clinical decision making.

### *Pitfalls*

The accuracy, precision, and interpretation of bone mineral assessment with SEQCT are influenced by a number of factors as follows:

1. CT scanner variability (x-ray tube aging, detector stability, field nonuniformities)
2. Operator variability (midvertebral slice positioning, ROI positioning in analysis)
3. Patient variability (movement; changes in size and composition, especially marrow content changes as occur in myelofibrosis, hematopoietic disorders, and so forth)
4. Calibration variability (liquids in the reference device can cause problems because of air-bubble formation and change of concentrations)

CT scanner stability depends mainly on the scanner design. It must be monitored by quality assurance protocols. Usually a phantom is scanned on a regular basis. Newer CT systems claim a short-term stability within 1 Hounsfield unit. A fixed scanning protocol is mandatory.

Operator variability depends on the skill of the operator. It can be minimized by automation of as many steps in the QCT protocol as possible (midvertebral slice selection, automated ROI analysis).

Patient variability can hardly be controlled. Patient movement should be avoided by proper instructions. Pathologic changes in bone marrow composition can influence QCT measurements. One should be aware that a significant increase of fatty tissue within the marrow (like irradiation damage) could mimic a bone density decrease. On the other hand, myelofibrosis gives a high bone-equivalent value, suggesting a high bone density.

Calibration variability can be avoided by using solid-state phantoms instead of liquid solutions like $K_2HPO_4$ in water.

## Suggested Reading


Cann CE. Quantitative CT for determination of bone mineral density: A review. Radiology 1988; 166:509–522.

Faulkner KG, Glüer CC, Majumdar S, et al. Review. Noninvasive measurements of bone mass, structure and strength: Current methods and experimental techniques. AJR 1991; 157:1229–1237.

Genant HK, ed. Osteoporosis Update 1987. San Francisco: Radiology Research and Education Foundation, 1987.

Genant HK, Block JE, Steiger P, et al. Appropriate use of bone densitometry. Radiology 1989; 170:817–822.

Genant HK, Cann CE, Ettinger B, Gordan GS. Quantitative computed tomography of vertebral spongiosa: A sensitive method for detecting early bone loss after oophorectomy. Ann Intern Med 1982; 97:699–705.

Huddleston AL. Quantitative Methods in Bone Densitometry. Boston: Kluwer Academic, 1988.

Johnston CC Jr, Slemenda CW, Melton LJ III. Clinical use of bone densitometry. N Engl J Med 1991; 324:1105–1109.

Kalender WA, Klotz E, Suess C. Vertebral bone mineral analysis: An integrated approach with CT. Radiology 1987; 164:419–423.

Kanis JA, Geusens P, Christiansen C. Guidelines for clinical trials in osteoporosis. A position paper of the European Foundation for Osteoporosis and Bone Disease. Osteoporosis Int 1991; 1:182–188.

Tothill P. Methods of bone mineral measurement. Phys Med Biol 1989; 34:543–572.

# MRI Evaluation of Knee Trauma

*WILLIAM E. PALMER, M.D.*

Knee injury is the most frequent cause of sports-related disability. The role of magnetic resonance imaging (MRI) is to detect clinically occult soft-tissue and bony injuries that may be exacerbated by repeat trauma or lead to chronic instability and joint degeneration.

Structures of the knee are susceptible to injury because of their complex kinematic function and exposure to external forces. Although the knee moves primarily as a hinge joint in the sagittal plane, it is also designed for internal-external rotation and abduction-adduction. Multidirectional mobility is gained at the expense of stability.

Common mechanisms of trauma produce predictable patterns of knee injury. By using a pathophysiologic approach to knee trauma, identification of one injury may suggest the mechanism of trauma and lead to a directed search for associated injuries.

## Technical Considerations

A dedicated transmit-receive knee coil maximizes spatial and contrast resolutions and routinely shows all surgically important meniscal, ligamentous, tendinous, and osteocartilaginous elements of the knee joint. The entire anterior cruciate ligament (ACL) is often visible on a single sagittal image if the knee is externally rotated 15° to 20°. At Massachusetts General Hospital, the imaging protocol employs three sequences in orthogonal planes (Table 1).

The axial sequence is particularly valuable for diagnosing mild medial collateral ligament (MCL) and ACL sprains and for evaluating osteochondral fractures of the patella.

## Meniscal Injury

The menisci are precariously positioned between the femur and tibia. If the menisci fail to follow the excursion of the femoral condyles, they may be trapped, crushed, and torn. The lateral meniscus (LM) has fewer attachment sites than the medial meniscus (MM), moves more easily, and is injured less frequently.

The hallmark of a meniscal tear on MRI is focally increased signal intensity that extends through the articular surface. If extension through the articular surface is used as the only criterion for tear, MRI and surgical findings agree in over 90 percent of menisci. Homogeneously low meniscal signal virtually excludes the possibility of tear. Globular or linear intrameniscal signal is frequently observed on MR images, but at arthroscopy is rarely associated with tear.

Confidence in the MRI diagnosis of meniscal tear depends on differentiation between signal that approximates the articular surface and signal that passes through it. Although this differentiation is important in determining whether a meniscal abnormality can be located and treated at arthroscopy, MRI cannot always do it. The linear signal intensity of an equivocal tear is horizontally oriented and usually located in the posterior horn of the LM or MM.

Traumatic tears tend to be located in the posterior horn medial meniscus (PHMM). The cleavage plane courses vertically or obliquely toward the inferior articular surface and often extends anteriorly into the meniscal body and anterior horn. Longitudinal extension is important to detect, because the inner fragment can be repaired or resected before it becomes displaced and causes knee locking.

The bucket handle tear may be difficult to diagnose. On sagittal images, the stable peripheral meniscus is normal in appearance, diminished in height, or truncated centrally. If no cleavage plane is visible, the findings resemble degenerative or postmeniscectomy change. Coronal images suggest the diagnosis if a third focus of low signal is present in the intercondylar notch (Fig. 1). Only the horizontal portion of the posterior cruciate ligament (PCL) and more vertically oriented ACL should be present.

Locating the displaced meniscal fragment is important for the preoperative planning of arthroscopic surgery. The intercondylar segment should be followed to its attachment sites at the residual anterior and posterior meniscal horns. Posterior detachment is more common and permits anterior rotation of the free fragment. Sagittal images best demonstrate fragments that have rotated into the infrapatellar fat pad (Fig. 2).

## Ligamentous Injury

Normal collateral and cruciate ligaments are discrete, low signal intensity structures that should be continuous between their sites of origin and insertion.

**TABLE 1** MRI Protocol for the Knee

| | Localizer | Series 1 | Series 2 | Series 3 |
|---|---|---|---|---|
| Plane | SPGR Sagittal | MPGR Axial | T1 Coronal | T2 Sagittal |
| TR | 18 | 600 | 600–800 | 2,000–2,500 |
| TE | Minimum | 15 | Minimum | 15/80 |
| Flip-angle | 25° | 20° | 90° | 90° |
| Thickness | 10 mm | 3 mm | 4 mm | 3 mm |
| Spacing | 0 mm | 1 mm | 1 mm | 1 mm |
| Field of view | 20 cm | 16 cm | 16 cm | 16 cm |
| Matrix | 256 × 128 | 256 × 256 | 256 × 192 | 256 × 256 |
| NEX | 1 | 2 | 2 | 1 |
| Options | Freq S/I | Freq A/P | Freq S/I | NP, Freq A/P |

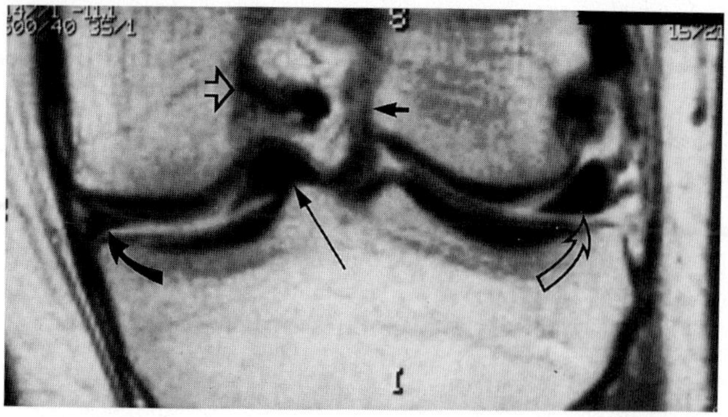

**FIGURE 1** Bucket handle tear. Coronal T1-weighted (TR700, TE20) MR image shows an abnormal low-signal focus (*long arrow*) in the intercondylar notch. The body of the MM (*curved black arrow*) is diminished in height and width. The LM (*curved open arrow*), PCL (*open arrow*), and ACL (*short arrow*) are normal.

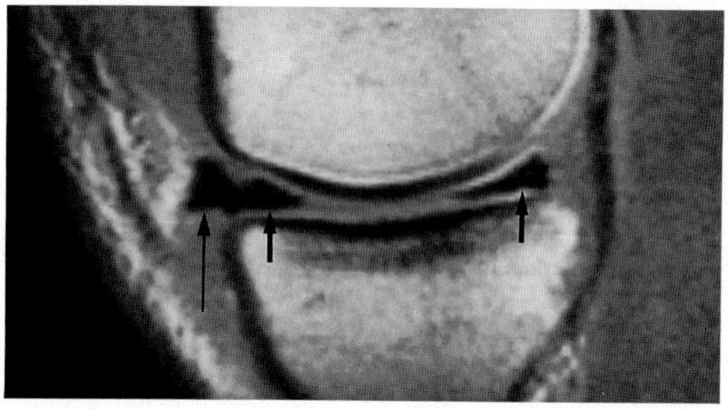

**FIGURE 2** Displaced meniscal segment. Sagittal balanced (TR2200, TE16) MR image shows a bucket handle fragment (*long arrow*) that has become detached from the PHMM and has rotated anteriorly. The residual anterior and posterior meniscal horns (*short arrows*) are diminished in height.

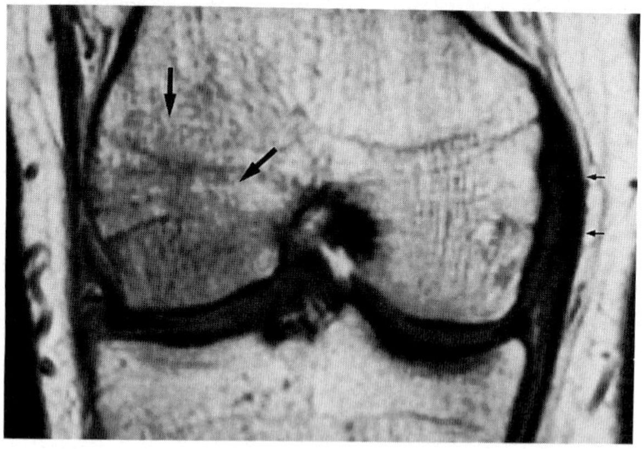

**FIGURE 3** MCL sprain. Coronal T1-weighted (TR800, TE20) MR image shows a lateral bone bruise (*large arrows*) resulting from valgus stress. The MCL is thickened and displaced from the femoral condyle (*small arrows*).

Acute ligamentous sprain is classified as mild, moderate, or severe. In mild sprain (stretching), MRI shows ligamentous thickening and edema in adjacent fat. In moderate sprain (partial tear), the ligament maintains gross continuity, but is increased in signal and surrounded by prominent hemorrhage

A

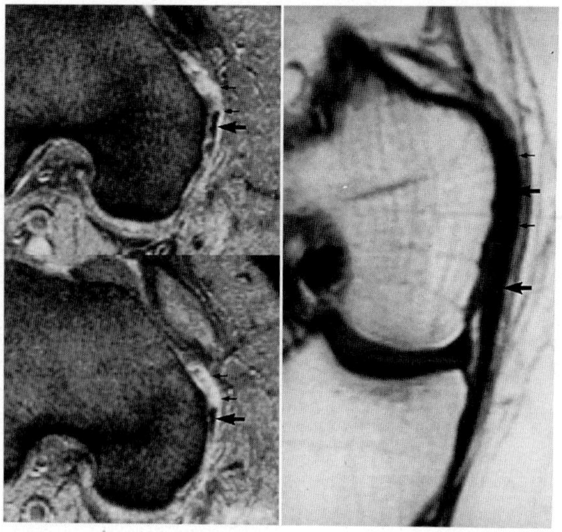

B

**FIGURE 4** Mild MCL sprain. Because of T2* contrast, surrounding edema (*small arrows*) is shown with greater conspicuity by axial MPGR (TR600, TE15, flip-angle 20°) MR images (*A*) than by a coronal T1-weighted (TR700, TE12) MR image (*B*). The MCL (*large arrows*) is otherwise intact.

and edema. Severe sprain (complete rupture) disrupts the continuity of the ligament. The torn end may be retracted and surrounded by fluid. The MRI appearance may simulate a soft-tissue mass.

## MCL Injury

The MCL stabilizes transverse alignment by reinforcing the joint capsule. Valgus force stresses the medial compartment and jeopardizes the MCL. A lateral bone bruise or fracture indicates valgus trauma and closely correlates with MCL sprain (Fig. 3). Because of T2* contrast, surrounding edema following mild MCL sprain is more conspicuous on gradient-echo axial than on T1-weighted coronal images (Fig. 4). As the degree of injury increases, the MCL is surrounded by greater edema and displaced further from the condyle (Fig. 5). In severe sprain the free ligamentous stump may become displaced into the joint.

## ACL Injury

ACL sprain is one of the most common knee injuries in sports. Hyperextension in internal rotation (IR) results from deceleration with quick pivoting and causes isolated sprain. Although both cruciates are wound up and stretched, the weaker ACL is at risk of injury.

The sagittal plane is best for evaluating ACL disruption and associated PCL buckling. However, when the sprain is mild and the fibers intact, volume averaging can obscure surrounding edema. The gradient-echo axial sequence shows this edema on multiple consecutive images. The axial plane is also valuable in identifying normal ACL fascicles when the ligament is oriented out of the sagittal plane as a result of improper positioning of the knee in the coil.

The ACL is torn in the majority of patients with acute hemarthrosis. Blood leaks into the joint after disruption of the thin layer of synovium lining the ACL. Because the hematocrit effect takes time to develop, no serum-cell level is visualized on the initial sequences of the study. On T1-weighted and

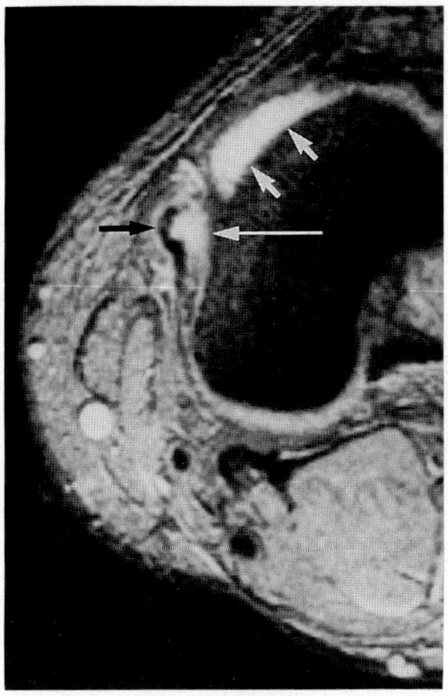

**FIGURE 5** Moderate MCL sprain. As the magnitude of stress increases, the axial MPGR (TR600, TE15, flip-angle 20°) image shows greater displacement of the MCL (*black arrow*) from the femoral condyle. Surrounding edema (*long white arrow*) is more prominent. Joint fluid (*short white arrows*) is separate from this edema.

balanced images, the dependent red blood cell (RBC) layer is increased in signal intensity compared with the serum layer as a result of T1 shortening caused by paramagnetic intracellular methemoglobin. These relative signal intensities become reversed on T2-weighted and gradient-echo images because of the susceptibility effect caused by the RBC layer (Fig. 6).

ACL atrophy and replacement by fat indicate an old injury that may predispose the knee to degenerative change. ACL deficiency causes anteroposterior instability. As the unrestrained femoral condyles skid posteriorly during flexion, repeated impact on the posterior meniscal horns causes tear and fragmentation. Loss of the meniscal cushion increases the load on a small area of articular cartilage. Cartilage thinning over the condyles is the earliest degenerative change and is best identified on T2-weighted sagittal images. High signal intensity fluid fills the space created by cartilage loss and contrasts sharply with intermediate and low signal intensity hyaline cartilage and subchondral bone.

### *PCL Injury*

PCL injury occurs less frequently than ACL injury and is more difficult to diagnose by physical examination. MRI often detects a PCL abnormality that otherwise remains clinically occult until the injury is exacerbated. Because of its strength, isolated injury of the PCL is rare but occurs when the tibia is subluxed posteriorly (dashboard injury or fall on a flexed knee). The medial and lateral ligaments are relatively lax in this position and have a large elastic reserve, whereas the PCL is taut and has exhausted its reserve.

### *LCL Injury*

The lateral collateral ligament (LCL) is protected by powerful musculotendinous synergists, explaining in part why lateral lesions account for only 5 to 10 percent of ligamentous injury. Varus stress usually fractures the medial tibial plateau before tearing the LCL. When LCL sprain occurs, associated injuries include cruciate sprain and bony avulsion of the tibial rim (Segond fracture) or fibular head.

## Combination Injury

Diagnosis of combination injury is important in determining prognosis and choosing treatment. Whereas bracing or rehabilitation is appropriate for most isolated ligamentous injuries, multiple sprains may require arthroscopic repair and reconstruction.

Knee trauma often produces predictable groupings of ligamentous and meniscal injuries. Structures that perform related kinematic functions are damaged by common traumatic mechanisms. When one supporting structure is disrupted, synergistic structures are jeopardized. For example, MCL or ACL sprain causes specific planar and rotational instabilities that permit tibial subluxation. The medial tibial plateau slides under the femoral condyle, which can trap, crush, and tear the PHMM.

Most combination injuries occur when stress limits are exceeded in one of two extreme positions. In flexion, full motion of the knee ranges from valgus–external rotation (ER) to varus-IR. Injury to the knee typically occurs when an additional valgus force acts on the knee that already is in extreme valgus-ER or when an additional varus force acts on the knee that is in extreme varus-IR. These injuries take the form of medial or lateral "unhappy triads." Excessive valgus

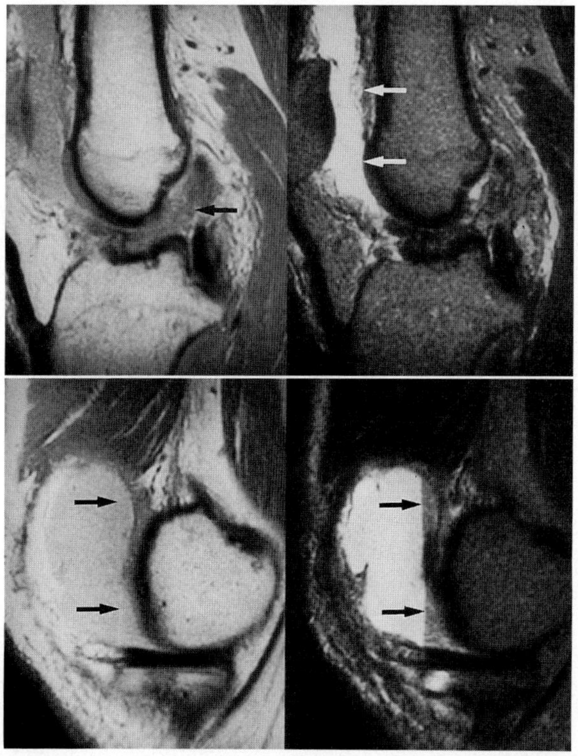

A

B

**FIGURE 6** ACL tear with hemarthrosis. *A,* Sagittal T2-weighted (TR2000, TE20(left) and 80(right)) MR images show an ACL tear (*black arrow*) and joint effusion (*white arrows*). *B,* The hemarthrosis and serum-cell layer (*arrows*) are more conspicuous on the second-echo (right) image.

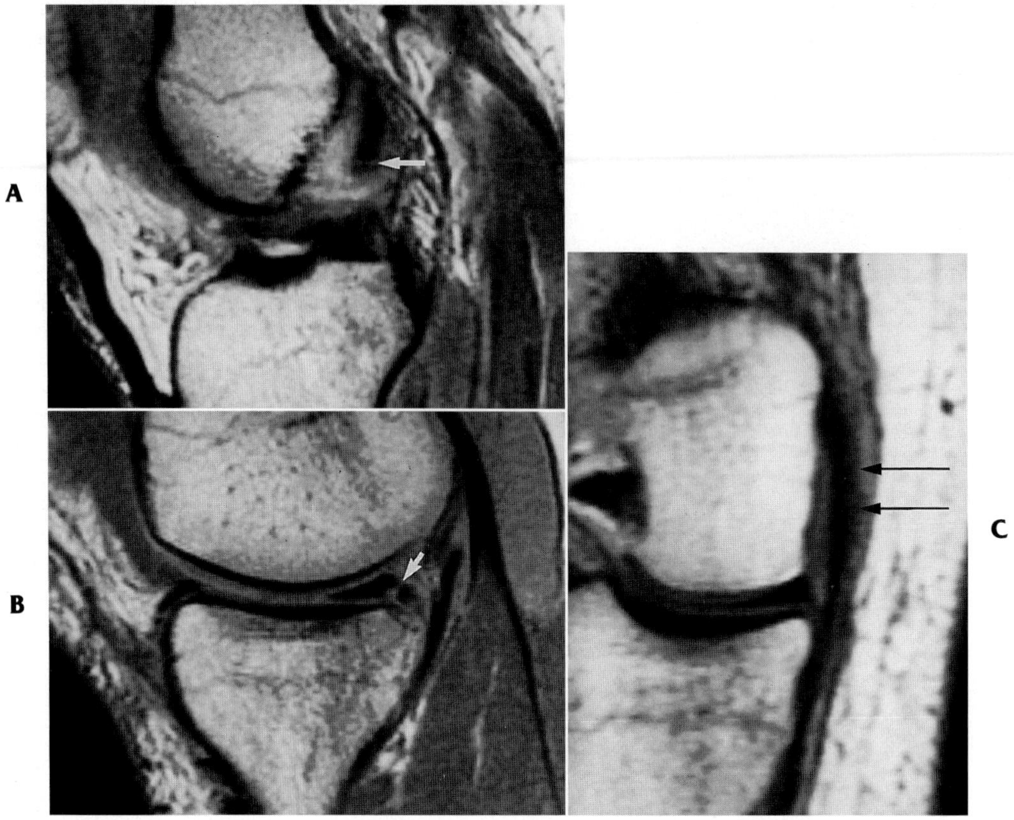


**FIGURE 7** Medial unhappy triad. Sagittal balanced (TR2200, TE16) MR images show (*A*) high signal intensity hemorrhage surrounding a torn ACL stump (*arrow*) and (*B*) a peripheral MM tear (*arrow*). *C,* On a coronal T1-weighted (TR700, TE12) image, the MCL (*arrows*) is thickened and surrounded by edema.

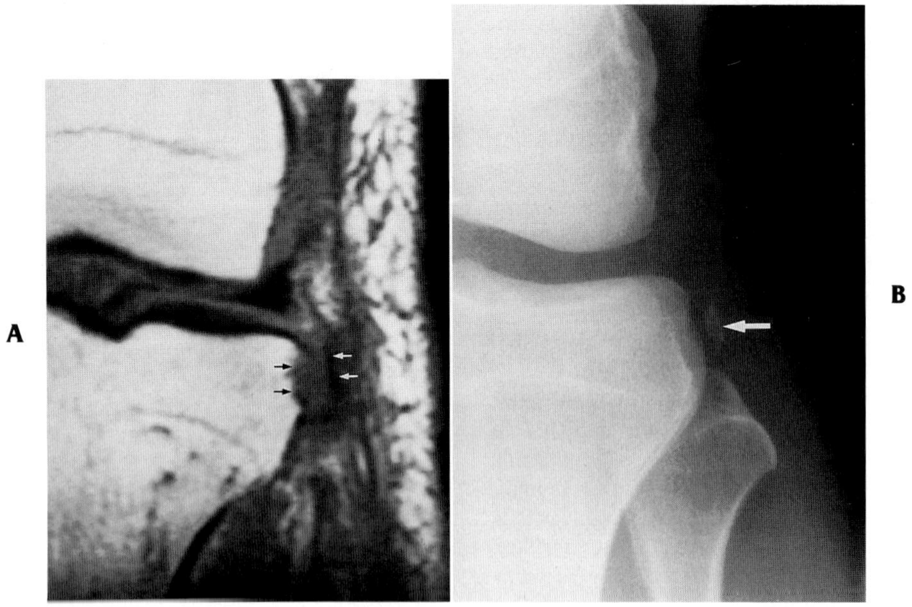


**FIGURE 8** Segond fracture. *A,* A coronal T1-weighted (TR800, TE12) MR image shows cortical discontinuity (*black arrows*) at the avulsion donor site without associated marrow edema. The linear fracture fragment (*white arrows*) is identified in retrospect. *B,* The avulsed cortical bone (*arrow*) is obvious on the plain radiograph.

stress in ER injures the MCL, ACL, and PHMM (Fig. 7), whereas varus stress in IR injures the LCL, PCL, and posterior horn lateral meniscus (PHLM).

Combined medial injuries are most common for two reasons. First, the lateral structures are relatively protected by powerful musculotendinous synergists. Second, the most common mechanisms of sports-related trauma involve valgus forces. For example, lateral stress results during the "clipping injury" when a football player is struck on the outside of a planted leg or during abduction when a skier catches the ski tip on ice.

Combined MCL, LCL, ACL, and PCL disruptions suggest previous knee dislocation that may have reduced spontaneously at the scene of the accident and remained unrecognized because of multiple trauma and life-threatening injuries. Dislocation results in planar and rotational instabilities that are extremely disabling and among the most serious of knee injuries. Evidence of knee dislocation alerts the referring clinician to the possibility of popliteal artery injury.

### Avulsion Injury

Sudden ligamentous tension tends to avulse bony attachment sites. In contrast to impaction forces, which cause a bone bruise or depressed fracture, distraction forces tend not to be associated with marrow edema (Fig. 8). As a result, avulsion fractures are difficult to identify by MRI unless the fracture fragment contains trabecular bone. In this case the high signal intensity of marrow fat is conspicuous against surrounding the lower signal intensity of edema and hemorrhage. If no marrow is avulsed, small bony fragments may not be detected even in retrospect. The only indication of fracture may be cortical discontinuity at the donor site. Lipohemarthrosis is a specific indicator of intra-articular fracture but is uncommon following avulsion injury.

The best way of identifying avulsion fractures is maintaining an index of suspicion and looking at the specific locations where they occur. Avulsions of the tibial eminence by the ACL or PCL are shown by coronal and sagittal images. Lateral avulsions are the most subtle and occur at the insertion site of the capsule on the lateral tibial rim (Segond fracture) and the conjoined LCL and biceps tendon on the fibula. Coronal and axial images show lateral fractures. Patients with injury to lateral structures should be studied by plain radiography to exclude cortical avulsions.

## Suggested Reading

Crues JV, Levy T, Laytysh M, Stoller DW. Meniscal tears of the knee: Accuracy of MR imaging. Radiology 1987; 164:445–448.

Herman LJ, Beltran J. Pitfalls in MR imaging of the knee. Radiology 1988; 167:775–781.

Kaplan PA, Nelson NL, Garvin KL, Brown DE. MR of the knee: The significance of high signal in the meniscus that does not clearly extend to the surface. AJR 1991; 156:333–336.

Kaplan PA, Walker CW, Kilcoyne RF, et al. Occult fracture patterns of the knee associated with anterior cruciate ligament tears: Assessment with MR imaging. Radiology 1992; 183:835–838.

Weber WN, Neumann CH, Barakos JA, et al. Lateral tibial rim (Segond) fractures: MR imaging characteristics. Radiology 1991; 180:731–734.

Zarins B, Adams M. Knee injuries in sports. N Engl J Med 1988; 318:950–961.

# Safety Considerations of MRI in Patients with Biomedical Implants and Devices

*FRANK G. SHELLOCK, Ph.D.*

Magnetic resonance imaging (MRI) may be contraindicated for a patient with a ferromagnetic metallic implant, material, or device primarily because of the risks associated with movement and/or dislodgement of the object as well as other possible hazards including the induction of electric current, excessive heating, and the misinterpretation of an artifact produced by the presence of the object as an abnormality. The potential for MRI to injure patients by inducing electric currents in conductive metallic materials or devices such as gating leads, unused surface coils, halo vests, or improperly used physiologic monitors has been discussed in other publications, and recommendations to protect the patient during MRI have been presented. Temperature elevations associated with MRI of implanted metallic implants, materials, and devices (with the exception of monitoring equipment, surface coils, or other externally applied equipment) have been studied, and there does not appear to be any significant hazard related to the minor temperature changes that have been measured. The type and extent of various artifacts caused by metallic implants, materials, and devices have also been described and are typically well recognized on MRI.

## Metallic Implants, Materials, and Devices

Numerous studies and investigations have assessed the ferromagnetic qualities of various metallic implants, materials, or devices by measuring deflection forces or movements associated with the static magnetic fields used for MRI. In general, these investigations have demonstrated that MRI may be performed safely in patients with metallic implants, materials, or devices if the object is nonferromagnetic or if it is only minimally attracted by the static magnetic field in relation to its in vivo application (i.e., the associated deflection force or attraction is insufficient to move or dislodge the implant or material in situ).

Since the prior knowledge of the relative degree of ferromagnetism that a specific type of metallic implant, material, or device possesses is essential for proper screening of patients before MRI, the articles pertaining to this topic have been reviewed and summarized. Table 1 lists data on over 260 different implants, materials, or devices that have been tested for ferromagnetism, whether or not the objects were deflected or attracted by static magnetic fields of the MRI

*Text continued on p. 356.*

**TABLE 1** Metallic Implants, Materials, and Devices Tested for Movement/Deflection Forces During Exposure to Static Magnetic Fields

| Metallic Implant, Material or Device | Movement/ Deflection | Highest Field Strength (T)* | Reference |
|---|---|---|---|
| *Aneurysm and Hemostatic Clips:* | | | |
| Drake (DR 14, DR 24)<br>Edward Weck, Triangle Park, NJ | Yes | 1.44 | New et al, 1983<br>Becker et al, 1988 |
| Drake (DR 16)<br>Edward Weck | Yes | 0.147 | New et al, 1983<br>Becker et al, 1988 |
| Drake (301 SS)<br>Edward Weck | Yes | 1.5 | Shellock and Crues, 1988A<br>Becker et al, 1988 |
| Downs multipositional (17-7PH) | Yes | 1.44 | New et al, 1983 |
| Gastrointestinal anastomosis clip, Auto Suture SGIA (SS)<br>United States Surgical Corp.<br>Norwalk, CT | No | 1.5 | Shellock and Crues, 1988A |
| Heifetz (17-7PH)<br>Edward Weck | Yes | 1.89 | Dujovny et al, 1985<br>Brown et al, 1987 |
| Heifetz (Elgiloy)<br>Edward Weck | No | 1.89 | Dujovny et al, 1985<br>Becker et al, 1988<br>Brown et al, 1987 |
| Hemoclip, #10 (316L SS)<br>Edward Weck | No | 1.5 | Shellock and Crues, 1988A |
| Hemoclip (tantalum)<br>Edward Weck | No | 1.5 | Shellock and Crues, 1988A |
| Housepian | Yes | 0.147 | New et al, 1983 |
| Kapp (405 SS)<br>V. Mueller | Yes | 1.89 | Dujovny et al, 1985<br>Becker et al, 1988 |
| Kapp curved (404 SS)<br>V. Mueller | Yes | 1.44 | New et al, 1983 |
| Ligaclip, #6 (316L SS)<br>Ethicon, Inc., Somerville, NJ | No | 1.5 | Shellock and Crues, 1988A |
| Ligaclip (tantalum)<br>Ethicon, Inc. | No | 1.5 | Shellock and Crues, 1988A |
| Mayfield (301 SS)<br>Codman, Randolph, MA | Yes | 1.5 | Shellock and Crues, 1988A |
| Mayfield (304 SS)<br>Codman | Yes | 1.89 | Dujovny et al, 1985 |
| McFadden (301 SS)<br>Codman | Yes | 1.5 | Shellock and Crues, 1988A<br>Becker et al, 1988 |
| Olivecrona | No | 1.44 | New et al, 1983 |
| Pivot (17-7PH) | Yes | 1.89 | Dujovny et al, 1985 |
| Scoville (EN58J)<br>Downs Surgical, Inc.<br>Decatur, GA | Yes | 1.89 | Dujovny et al, 1985<br>Becker et al, 1988 |
| Stevens (50-4190, silver alloy) | No | 0.15 | Barrafato and Henkelman, 1984 |
| Sugita (Elgiloy)<br>Downs Surgical | No | 1.89 | Dujovny et al, 1985<br>Becker et al, 1988 |
| Sundt-Kees (301 SS)<br>Downs Surgical | Yes | 1.5 | Shellock and Crues, 1988A<br>Becker et al, 1988 |

**TABLE 1** Metallic Implants, Materials, and Devices Tested for Movement/Deflection Forces During Exposure to Static Magnetic Fields—cont'd

| Metallic Implant, Material or Device | Movement/ Deflection | Highest Field Strength (T)* | Reference |
|---|---|---|---|
| Sundt-Kees Multi-Angle (17-7PH)<br>Downs Surgical | Yes | 1.89 | Dujovny et al, 1985<br>Becker et al, 1988 |
| Surgiclip, Auto Suture M-9.5 (SS)<br>United States Surgical Corp. | No | 1.5 | Shellock and Crues, 1988A |
| Vari-Angle (17-7PH)<br>Codman | Yes | 1.89 | Dujovny et al, 1985 |
| Vari-Angle McFadden (MP35N)<br>Codman | No | 1.89 | Dujovny et al, 1985<br>Becker et al, 1988 |
| Vari-Angle Micro (17-7PM SS)<br>Codman | Yes | 0.15 | Barrafato and Henkelman, 1984<br>Becker et al, 1988 |
| Vari-Angle Spring (17-7PM SS)<br>Codman | Yes | 0.15 | Barrafato and Henkelman, 1984<br>Becker et al, 1988 |
| Yasargil (316 SS)<br>Aesculap | No | 1.89 | Dujovny et al, 1985 |
| Yasargil (Phynox)<br>Aesculap | No | 1.89 | Dujovny et al, 1985<br>Becker et al, 1988 |
| *Carotid Artery Vascular Clamps:* | | | |
| Crutchfield (SS)<br>Codman | Yes† | 1.5 | Teitelbaum, Lin, et al, 1990 |
| Kindt (SS)<br>V. Mueller | Yes† | 1.5 | Teitelbaum, Lin, et al, 1990 |
| Poppen-Blaylock (SS)<br>Codman | Yes | 1.5 | Teitelbaum, Lin, et al, 1990 |
| Salibi (SS)<br>Codman | Yes† | 1.5 | Teitelbaum, Lin, et al, 1990 |
| Selverstone (SS)<br>Codman | Yes† | 1.5 | Teitelbaum, Lin, et al, 1990 |
| *Dental Devices and Materials:* | | | |
| Brace band (SS)<br>American Dental<br>Missoula, MT | Yes† | 1.5 | Shellock and Crues, 1988A |
| Brace wire (chrome alloy)<br>Ormco Corp<br>San Marcos, CA | Yes† | 1.5 | Shellock and Crues, 1988A |
| Castable alloy<br>Golden Dental Products, Inc.<br>Golden, CO | Yes† | 1.5 | Gegauff et al, 1990 |
| Cement-in keeper<br>Solid State Innovations, Inc.<br>Mt. Airy, NC | Yes† | 1.5 | Gegauff et al, 1990 |
| Dental amalgam | No | 1.44 | New et al, 1983 |
| Keeper, preformed post<br>Parkell Products, Inc.<br>Farmingdale, NY | Yes† | 1.5 | Gegauff et al, 1990 |
| GDP Direct Keeper, preformed post<br>Golden Dental Products, Inc. | Yes† | 1.5 | Gegauff et al, 1990 |
| Magna-Dent, large indirect keeper<br>Dental Ventures of America<br>Yorba Linda, CA | Yes† | 1.5 | Gegauff et al, 1990 |

(*Continued.*)

**TABLE 1** Metallic Implants, Materials, and Devices Tested for Movement/Deflection Forces During Exposure to Static Magnetic Fields—cont'd

| Metallic Implant, Material or Device | Movement/ Deflection | Highest Field Strength (T)* | Reference |
|---|---|---|---|
| Palladium clad magnet<br>Parkell Products, Inc. | Yes | 1.5 | Shellock, 1989A |
| Palladium/palladium keeper<br>Parkell Products, Inc. | Yes† | 1.5 | Shellock, 1989A |
| Palladium/platinum casting alloy<br>Parkell Products, Inc. | Yes† | 1.5 | Shellock, 1989A |
| Permanent crown (amalgam)<br>Ormco Corp. | No | 1.5 | Shellock and Crues, 1988 |
| Titanium-clad magnet<br>Parkell Products, Inc. | Yes | 1.5 | Shellock, 1989A |
| Stainless steel–clad magnet<br>Parkell Products, Inc. | Yes | 1.5 | Shellock, 1989A |
| Stainless steel keeper<br>Parkell Products, Inc. | Yes† | 1.5 | Shellock, 1989A |
| Silver point<br>Union Broach Co., Inc.<br>New York, NY | No | 1.5 | Shellock and Crues, 1988A |
| *Heart Valve Prostheses:* | | | |
| Beall<br>Coratomic Inc.<br>Indiana, PA | Yes† | 2.35 | Soulen et al, 1985 |
| Bjork-Shiley (convexo/concave)<br>Shiley Inc.<br>Irvine, CA | No | 1.5 | Shellock and Crues, 1988A |
| Bjork-Shiley (universal/spherical)<br>Shiley Inc. | Yes† | 1.5 | Shellock and Crues, 1988A |
| Bjork-Shiley, Model MBC<br>Shiley Inc. | Yes† | 2.35 | Hassler et al, 1987 |
| Bjork-Shiley, Model 25 MBRC 11030<br>Shiley Inc. | Yes† | 2.35 | Hassler et al, 1987 |
| Carpentier-Edwards Model 2650<br>American Edwards Laboratories<br>Santa Ana, CA | Yes† | 2.35 | Hassler et al, 1987 |
| Carpentier-Edwards (porcine)<br>American Edwards Laboratories | Yes† | 2.35 | Hassler et al, 1987 |
| Hall-Kaster,<br>Model A7700<br>Medtronic Inc.<br>Minneapolis, MN | Yes† | 1.5 | Shellock and Crues, 1988A |
| Hancock I (porcine)<br>Johnson & Johnson<br>Anaheim, CA | Yes† | 1.5 | Shellock and Crues, 1988A |
| Hancock II (porcine)<br>Johnson & Johnson | Yes† | 1.5 | Shellock and Crues, 1988A |
| Hancock extracorporeal, Model 242R<br>Johnson & Johnson | Yes† | 2.35 | Hassler et al, 1987 |
| Hancock extracorporeal, Model M 4365-33<br>Johnson & Johnson | Yes† | 2.35 | Hassler et al, 1987 |
| Hancock Vascor, Model 505<br>Johnson & Johnson | No | 2.35 | Hassler et al, 1987 |

**TABLE 1** Metallic Implants, Materials, and Devices Tested for Movement/Deflection Forces During Exposure to Static Magnetic Fields—cont'd

| Metallic Implant, Material or Device | Movement/ Deflection | Highest Field Strength (T)* | Reference |
|---|---|---|---|
| Inonescu-Shiley, Universal ISM | Yes† | 2.35 | Hassler et al, 1987 |
| Lillehi-Kaster, Model 300S<br>Medical Inc.<br>Inver Grove Heights, MN | Yes† | 2.35 | Soulen et al, 1985 |
| Lillehi-Kaster, Model 5009<br>Medical Inc. | Yes† | 2.35 | Hassler et al, 1987 |
| Medtronic Hall<br>Medtronic Inc. | Yes† | 2.35 | Hassler et al, 1987 |
| Medtronic Hall, Model A7700-D-16<br>Medtronic Inc. | Yes† | 2.35 | Hassler et al, 1987 |
| Omnicarbon, Model 3523T029<br>Medical Inc. | Yes† | 2.35 | Hassler et al, 1987 |
| Omniscience, Model 6522<br>Medical Inc. | Yes† | 2.35 | Hassler et al, 1987 |
| Smeloff-Cutter<br>Cutter Laboratories<br>Berkeley, CA | Yes† | 2.35 | Shellock and Crues, 1988 |
| Starr-Edwards, Model 1260<br>American Edwards Laboratories | Yes† | 2.35 | Soulen et al, 1985 |
| Starr-Edwards, Model 2320<br>American Edwards Laboratories | Yes† | 2.35 | Soulen et al, 1985 |
| Starr-Edwards, Model 2400<br>American Edwards Laboratories | No | 1.5 | Shellock and Crues, 1988A |
| Starr-Edwards, Model Pre 6000<br>American Edwards Laboratories | Yes | 2.35 | Soulen et al, 1985 |
| Starr-Edwards, Model 6520<br>American Edwards Laboratories | Yes† | 2.35 | Hassler et al, 1987 |
| St. Jude<br>St. Jude Medical Inc.<br>St. Paul, MN | No | 1.5 | Shellock and Crues, 1988A |
| St. Jude, Model A 101<br>St. Jude Medical Inc. | Yes† | 2.35 | Hassler et al, 1987 |
| St. Jude, Model M 101<br>St. Jude Medical Inc. | Yes† | 2.35 | Hassler et al, 1987 |
| *Intravascular Coils, Filters, and Stents:* | | | |
| Amplatz IVC filter<br>Cook<br>Bloomington, IN | No | 4.7 | Teitelbaum, Bradley et al, 1988 |
| Cragg nitinol spiral filter | No | 4.7 | Teitelbaum, Bradley et al, 1988 |
| Gianturco embolization coil<br>Cook | Yes | 1.5 | Teitelbaum, Bradley et al, 1988 |
| Gianturco bird nest IVC filter<br>Cook | Yes | 1.5 | Teitelbaum, Bradley et al, 1988<br>Watanabe et al, 1990 |
| Gianturco zig-zag stent<br>Cook | Yes | 1.5 | Teitelbaum, Bradley et al, 1988 |
| Greenfield vena cava filter, stainless steel<br>Meditech<br>Watertown, MA | Yes† | 1.5 | Teitelbaum, Bradley et al, 1988<br>Liebman et al, 1988 |

(*Continued.*)

**TABLE 1** Metallic Implants, Materials, and Devices Tested for Movement/Deflection Forces During Exposure to Static Magnetic Fields—cont'd

| Metallic Implant, Material or Device | Movement/ Deflection | Highest Field Strength (T)* | Reference |
|---|---|---|---|
| Greenfield vena cava filter, titanium alloy<br>Ormco<br>Glendora, CA | No | 1.5 | Teitelbaum, Bradley et al, 1988 |
| Gunther IVC filter<br>William Cook<br>Europe | Yes | 1.5 | Teitelbaum, Bradley et al, 1988 |
| Maas helical IVC filter<br>Medinvent<br>Lausanne, Switzerland | No | 4.7 | Teitelbaum, Bradley et al, 1988 |
| Maas helical endovascular stent<br>Medinvent | No | 4.7 | Teitelbaum, Bradley et al, 1988 |
| Mobin-Uddin IVC/umbrella filter<br>American Edwards Laboratories | No | 4.7 | Teitelbaum, Bradley et al, 1988 |
| New retrievable IVC filter<br>Thomas Jefferson University<br>Philadelphia, PA | Yes | 1.5 | Teitelbaum, Bradley et al, 1988 |
| Palmaz endovascular stent<br>Ethicon, Inc. | Yes | 1.5 | Teitelbaum, Bradley et al, 1988 |
| Strecker stent (tantalum)<br>Meditech | No | 1.5 | Teitelbaum, 1990<br>Teitelbaum et al, 1989 |
| *Ocular Implants:* | | | |
| Fatio eyelid spring/wire | Yes | 1.5 | Shellock et al, 1990 |
| Intraocular lens implant, Binkhorst, iridocapsular lens, platinium-iridium loop | No | 1.5 | DeKeizer and TeStrake, 1986 |
| Intraocular lens implant, Binkhorst, iridocapsular lens, platinum-iridium loop | No | 1.0 | DeKeizer and TeStrake, 1986 |
| Intraocular lens implant, Binkhorst, iridocapsular lens, titanium loop | No | 1.0 | DeKeizer and TeStrake, 1986 |
| Intraocular lens implant, Worst, platinum clip lense | No | 1.0 | DeKeizer and TeStrake, 1986 |
| Retinal tack (303 SS)<br>Bascom Palmer Eye Institute | No | 1.5 | Albert et al, 1990 |
| Retinal tack (titanium alloy)<br>Coopervision<br>Irvine, CA | No | 1.5 | Albert et al, 1990<br>Joondeph et al, 1987 |
| Retinal tack (303 SS)<br>Duke | No | 1.5 | Albert et al, 1990 |
| Retinal tack (cobalt/nickel)<br>Grieshaber<br>Fallsington, PA | No | 1.5 | Joondeph et al, 1987 |
| Retinal tack, Norton staple (platinum/rhodium)<br>Norton | No | 1.5 | Albert et al, 1990 |
| Retinal tack (aluminum tetraoxide)<br>Ruby | No | 1.5 | Albert et al, 1990 |
| Retinal tack (SS-martensitic)<br>Western European | Yes | 1.5 | Albert et al, 1990 |
| *Orthopedic Implants, Materials, and Devices:* | | | |
| AML femoral component bipolar hip prosthesis<br>Zimmer<br>Warsaw, IN | No | 1.5 | Shellock and Crues, 1988A |

**TABLE 1** Metallic Implants, Materials, and Devices Tested for Movement/Deflection Forces During Exposure to Static Magnetic Fields—cont'd

| Metallic Implant, Material or Device | Movement/ Deflection | Highest Field Strength (T)* | Reference |
|---|---|---|---|
| Cervical wire, 20 gauge (316L SS) | No | 0.3 | Lyons et al, 1989 |
| Cortical bone screw, large (titanium, Ti-6AL-4V alloy) Zimmer | No | 1.5 | Shellock, Mink et al, 1992 |
| Cortical bone screw, small (titanium, Ti6AL-4V alloy) Zimmer | No | 1.5 | Shellock, Mink et al, 1992 |
| Cotrel rods with hooks (316L SS) | No | 0.3 | Lyons et al, 1989 |
| DTT, device for transverse traction (316L SS) | No | 0.3 | Lyons et al, 1989 |
| Drummond wire (316L SS) | No | 0.3 | Lyons et al, 1989 |
| Endoscopic noncannulated interference screw (titanium) Acufex Microsurgical Norwood, MA | No | 1.5 | Shellock, Mink et al, 1992 |
| Fixation staple (Cobalt chromium alloy, ASTM F 75) Richards Medical Co. Memphis, TN | No | 1.5 | Shellock, Mink et al, 1992 |
| Harrington compression rod with hooks and nuts (316L SS) | No | 0.3 | Lyons et al, 1989 |
| Harris zip prosthesis Zimmer | No | 1.5 | Shellock and Crues, 1988A |
| Jewett nail Zimmer | No | 1.5 | Shellock and Crues, 1988A |
| Large staple plate Zimaloy (Zimmer) | No | 1.5 | Shellock, Mink et al, 1992 |
| Kirschner intermedullary rod Kirschner Medical Timonium, MD | No | 1.5 | Shellock and Crues, 1988A |
| Perfix interence screw (17-4 stainless steel, AL 630-17Cr) Instrument Makar Okemos, MI | Yes | 1.5 | Shellock, Mink et al, 1992 |
| Stainless steel plate Zimmer | No | 1.5 | Shellock and Crues, 1988A |
| Stainless steel screw Zimmer | No | 1.5 | Shellock and Crues, 1988A |
| Stainless steel mesh Zimmer | No | 1.5 | Shellock and Crues, 1988A |
| Stainless steel wire Zimmer | No | 1.5 | Shellock and Crues, 1988A |
| Zielke rod with screw, washer, and nut (316L SS) | No | 0.3 | Lyons et al, 1989 |
| *Otologic Implants:* | | | |
| Austin tytan piston (titanium) Treace Medical Nashville, TN | No | 1.5 | Shellock and Schatz, 1991 |
| Berger "V" bobbin ventilation tube (titanium) Richards Medical Co. | No | 1.5 | Shellock and Schatz, 1991 |
| Cochlear implant 3M/House | Yes | 0.6 | Mattucci et al, 1986 |

*(Continued.)*

**TABLE 1** Metallic Implants, Materials, and Devices Tested for Movement/Deflection Forces During Exposure to Static Magnetic Fields—cont'd

| Metallic Implant, Material or Device | Movement/ Deflection | Highest Field Strength (T)* | Reference |
|---|---|---|---|
| Cochlear implant<br>3M/Vienna | Yes | 0.6 | Mattucci et al, 1986 |
| Cochlear implant<br>Nucleus Mini 22-channel<br>Cochlear Corporation,<br>Engelwood, CO | Yes | 1.5 | Applebaum and Valvassori, 1990 |
| Cody tack | No | 0.6 | Mattucci et al, 1986 |
| Ehmke hook stapes prosthesis (platinum)<br>Richards Medical Co. | No | 1.5 | Shellock and Schatz, 1991 |
| Fisch piston (Teflon, SS)<br>Richards Medical Co. | No | 1.5 | Applebaum and Valvassori, 1990 |
| House single loop (ASTM A318-76 Grade 2 SS)<br>Storz<br>St. Louis, MO | No | 1.5 | Shellock and Schatz, 1991 |
| House single loop (tantalum)<br>Storz | No | 1.5 | Shellock and Schatz, 1991 |
| House double loop (tantalum)<br>Storz | No | 1.5 | Shellock and Schatz, 1991 |
| House double loop (ASTM A318-76 Grade 2 SS)<br>Storz | No | 1.5 | Shellock and Schatz, 1991 |
| House-type wire loop stapes prosthesis (316L SS)<br>Richards Medical Co. | No | 1.5 | Shellock and Schatz, 1991<br>Applebaum and Valvassori, 1990 |
| House-type stainless steel piston and wire (ASTM A318-76 Grade 2 SS)<br>Xomed-Treace Inc.<br>A Bristol-Myers Squibb Co. | No | 1.5 | Shellock and Schatz, 1991 |
| House wire (tantalum)<br>Otomed | No | 0.5 | White, 1987 |
| House wire (SS)<br>Otomed | No | 0.5 | White, 1987 |
| McGee piston stapes prosthesis (316L SS)<br>Richards Medical Co. | No | 1.5 | Shellock and Schatz, 1991<br>Applebaum and Valvassori, 1990 |
| McGee piston stapes prosthesis (platinum/316L SS)<br>Richards Medical Co. | No | 1.5 | Shellock and Schatz, 1991<br>Applebaum and Valvassori, 1990 |
| McGee piston stapes prosthesis (platinum/17Cr-4Ni SS)<br>Richards Medical Co.<br>(recalled by manufacturer) | Yes | 1.5 | Applebaum and Valvassori, 1990 |
| McGee shepherd's crook stapes prosthesis (316L SS)<br>Richards Medical Co. | No | 1.5 | Shellock and Schatz, 1991 |
| Plasti-pore piston (316L SS/plasti-pore material)<br>Richards Medical Co. | No | 1.5 | Shellock and Schatz, 1991<br>Applebaum and Valvassori, 1990 |
| Platinum ribbon loop stapes prosthesis (platinum)<br>Richards Medical Co. | No | 1.5 | Shellock and Schatz, 1991 |
| Reuter bobbin ventilation tube (316L SS)<br>Richards Medical Co. | No | 1.5 | Shellock and Schatz, 1991 |
| Richards bucket handle stapes prosthesis (316L SS)<br>Richards Medical Co. | No | 1.5 | Shellock and Schatz, 1991<br>Applebaum and Valvassori, 1990 |

**TABLE 1** Metallic Implants, Materials, and Devices Tested for Movement/Deflection Forces During Exposure to Static Magnetic Fields—cont'd

| Metallic Implant, Material or Device | Movement/ Deflection | Highest Field Strength (T)* | Reference |
|---|---|---|---|
| Richards platinum Teflon piston (0.6 mm) Richards Medical Co. | No | 1.5 | Applebaum and Valvassori, 1990 |
| Richards platinum Teflon piston (0.8 mm) Richards Medical Co. | No | 1.5 | Applebaum and Valvassori, 1990 |
| Richards piston stapes prosthesis (platinum/ fluoroplastic) Richards Medical Co. | No | 1.5 | Shellock and Schatz, 1991 |
| Richards shepherd's crook (platinum) Richards Medical Co. | No | 0.5 | White, 1987 |
| Richards Teflon piston Richards Medical Co. | No | 1.5 | Applebaum and Valvassori, 1990 |
| Robinson-Moon-Lippy offset stapes prosthesis (ASTM A318-76 Grade 2 SS) Storz | No | 1.5 | Shellock and Schatz, 1991 |
| Robinson-Moon offset stapes prosthesis (ASTM A318-76 Grade 2 SS) Storz | No | 1.5 | Shellock and Shatz, 1991 |
| Robinson incus replacement prosthesis (ASTM A318-76 Grade 2 SS) Storz | No | 1.5 | Shellock and Schatz, 1991 |
| Robinson stapes prosthesis (ASTM A318-76 Grade 2 SS) Storz | No | 1.5 | Shellock and Schatz, 1991 |
| Ronis piston stapes prosthesis (316L SS/ fluoroplastic) Richards Medical Co. | No | 1.5 | Shellock and Schatz, 1991 |
| Schea cup piston stapes prosthesis (platinum/ fluoroplastic) Richards Medical Co. | No | 1.5 | Shellock and Schatz, 1991<br>Applebaum and Valvassori, 1990 |
| Schea malleus attachment piston (Teflon) Richards Medical Co. | No | 1.5 | Applebaum and Valvassori, 1990 |
| Schea stainless steel and Teflon wire prosthesis (Teflon, 316 L SS) Richards Medical Co. | No | 1.5 | Applebaum and Valvassori, 1990 |
| Scheer piston stapes prosthesis (316L SS/ fluoroplastic) Richards Medical Co. | No | 1.5 | Shellock and Schatz, 1991 |
| Scheer piston (Teflon, 316L SS) Richards Medical Co. | No | 1.5 | Applebaum and Valvassori, 1990 |
| Schuknecht gelfoam and wire prosthesis, Armstrong style (316L SS) Richards Medical Co. | No | 1.5 | Leon and Gabriele, 1987 |
| Schuknecht piston stapes prosthesis (316L SS/ fluoroplastic) Richards Medical Co. | No | 1.5 | Shellock and Schatz, 1991 |
| Schuknecht Teflon wire incus attachment (ASTM A318-76 Grade 2 SS) Storz | No | 1.5 | Shellock and Schatz, 1991<br>Applebaum and Valvassori, 1990 |

(*Continued.*)

**TABLE 1** Metallic Implants, Materials, and Devices Tested for Movement/Deflection Forces During Exposure to Static Magnetic Fields—cont'd

| Metallic Implant, Material or Device | Movement/ Deflection | Highest Field Strength (T)* | Reference |
|---|---|---|---|
| Schuknecht Teflon wire malleus attachment (ASTM A318-76 Grade 2 SS)<br>Storz | No | 1.5 | Shellock and Schatz, 1991<br>Applebaum and Valvassori, 1990 |
| Schuknecht Teflon wire piston, 0.6 mm (Teflon, 316L SS)<br>Richards Medical Co. | No | 1.5 | Applebaum and Valvassori, 1990 |
| Schuknecht Teflon wire piston, 0.8 mm (Teflon, 316L SS)<br>Richards Medical Co. | No | 1.5 | Applebaum and Valvassori, 1990 |
| Sheehy incus replacement (ASTM A318-76 Grade 2 SS)<br>Storz | No | 1.5 | Shellock and Schatz, 1991 |
| Sheehy incus strut (316L SS)<br>Richards Medical Co. | No | 1.5 | Applebaum and Valvassori, 1990 |
| Sheehy-type incus replacement strut (Teflon, 316L SS)<br>Richards Medical Co. | No | 1.5 | Shellock and Schatz, 1991 |
| Silverstein malleus clip ventilation tube (Teflon, 316L SS)<br>Richards Medical Co. | No | 1.5 | Applebaum and Valvassori, 1990 |
| Spoon bobbin ventilation tube (316L SS)<br>Richards Medical Co. | No | 1.5 | Shellock and Schatz, 1991 |
| Tantalum wire loop stages prosthesis (tantalum)<br>Richards Medical Co. | No | 1.5 | Shellock and Schatz, 1991<br>Applebaum and Valvassori, 1990 |
| Tef-platinum piston (platinum)<br>Xomed-Treace Inc.<br>A Bristol-Myers Squibb Co. | No | 1.5 | Shellock and Schatz, 1991 |
| Total ossibular replacement prosthesis (TORP) (316L SS)<br>Richards Medical Co. | No | 1.5 | Applebaum and Valvassori, 1990 |
| Trapeze ribbon loop stapes prosthesis (platinum)<br>Richards Medical Co. | No | 1.5 | Shellock and Schatz, 1991 |
| Williams microclip (316L SS)<br>Richards Medical Co. | No | 1.5 | Shellock and Schutz, 1991 |
| Xomed stapes (ASTM A318-76 Grade 2 SS)<br>Xomed-Treace Inc.<br>A Bristol-Myers Squibb Co. | No | 1.5 | Shellock and Schatz, 1991 |
| *Pellets and Bullets:* | | | |
| BB's<br>(Daisy) | Yes | 1.5 | Shellock, 1989B |
| BB's<br>(Crosman) | Yes | 1.5 | Shellock, 1989B |
| Bullet 0.380 in. (copper, plastic, lead)<br>Glaser | No | 1.5 | Teitelbaum, Yee et al, 1990 |
| Bullet, 0.44 in. (Teflon, bronze)<br>North American Ordinance | No | 1.5 | Teitelbaum, Yee et al, 1990 |
| Bullet, 7.62 × 39 mm (copper, steel)<br>Norinco | Yes | 1.5 | Teitelbaum, Yee et al, 1990 |
| Bullet, 0.357 in. (copper, lead)<br>Cascade | No | 1.5 | Teitelbaum, Yee et al, 1990 |

**TABLE 1** Metallic Implants, Materials, and Devices Tested for Movement/Deflection Forces During Exposure to Static Magnetic Fields—cont'd

| Metallic Implant, Material or Device | Movement/ Deflection | Highest Field Strength (T)* | Reference |
|---|---|---|---|
| Bullet, 0.357 in. (lead)<br>Remington | No | 1.5 | Teitelbaum, Yee et al, 1990 |
| Bullet, 0.357 in. (aluminum, lead)<br>Winchester | No | 1.5 | Teitelbaum, Yee et al, 1990 |
| Bullet, 9 mm (copper, lead)<br>Remington | No | 1.5 | Teitelbaum, Yee et al, 1990 |
| Bullet, 0.380 in. (copper, nickel, lead)<br>Winchester | Yes | 1.5 | Teitelbaum, Yee et al, 1990 |
| Bullet, 0.357 in. (nylon, lead)<br>Smith & Wesson | No | 1.5 | Teitelbaum, Yee et al, 1990 |
| Bullet, 0.45 in. (steel, lead)<br>Evansville Ordinance | Yes | 1.5 | Teitelbaum, Yee et al, 1990 |
| Bullet, 0.357 in. (steel, lead)<br>Fiocchi | No | 1.5 | Teitelbaum, Yee et al, 1990 |
| Bullet, 0.357 in. (copper, lead)<br>Hornady | No | 1.5 | Teitelbaum, Yee et al, 1990 |
| Bullet, 9 mm (copper, lead)<br>Norma | Yes | 1.5 | Teitelbaum, Yee et al, 1990 |
| Bullet, 0.357 in. (bronze, plastic)<br>Patton-Morgan | No | 1.5 | Teitelbaum, Yee et al, 1990 |
| Bullet, 0.357 in. (copper, lead)<br>Patton-Morgan | No | 1.5 | Teitelbaum, Yee et al, 1990 |
| Bullet, 0.45 in. (copper, lead)<br>Samson | No | 1.5 | Teitelbaum, Yee et al, 1990 |
| Shot, 12 gauge, size 00 (copper, lead)<br>Federal | No | 1.5 | Teitelbaum, Yee et al, 1990 |
| Shot, 7½ (lead) | No | 1.5 | Teitelbaum, Yee et al, 1990 |
| Shot, 4 (lead) | No | 1.5 | Teitelbaum, Yee et al, 1990 |
| Shot, 00 buckshot (lead) | No | 1.5 | Teitelbaum, Yee et al, 1990 |
| *Penile Implants:* | | | |
| AMS Malleable 600<br>American Medical Systems<br>Minnetonka, MN | No | 1.5 | Teitelbaum, Yee et al, 1990 |
| AMS 700<br>CX Inflatable<br>American Medical Systems | No | 1.5 | Shellock et al, 1987 |
| Flexi-Flate<br>Surgitek, Medical Engineering Corp.<br>Racine, WI | No | 1.5 | Shellock et al, 1987 |
| Flexi-Rod (standard)<br>Surgitek, Medical Engineering Corp. | No | 1.5 | Shellock et al, 1987 |
| Flex-Rod II (firm)<br>Surgitek, Medical Engineering Corp. | No | 1.5 | Shellock et al, 1987 |
| Jonas<br>Dacomed Corp.<br>Minneapolis, MN | No | 1.5 | Shellock et al, 1987 |

(*Continued.*)

**TABLE 1** Metallic Implants, Materials, and Devices Tested for Movement/Deflection Forces During Exposure to Static Magnetic Fields—cont'd

| Metallic Implant, Material or Device | Movement/ Deflection | Highest Field Strength (T)* | Reference |
|---|---|---|---|
| Mentor Flexible<br>Mentor Corp.<br>Minneapolis, MN | No | 1.5 | Shellock et al, 1987 |
| Mentor Inflatable<br>Mentor Corp. | No | 1.5 | Shellock et al, 1987 |
| OmniPhase<br>Dacomed Corp. | Yes | 1.5 | Shellock et al, 1987 |
| *Vascular Access Ports:* | | | |
| Button (polysulfone polymer, silicone)<br>Infusaid Inc.<br>Norwood, MA | No | 1.5 | Shellock and Meeks, 1991 |
| Dome Port (titanium)<br>Davol Inc./Subsidiary of C.R. Bard, Inc.<br>Cranston, RI | No | 1.5 | Shellock and Meeks, 1991 |
| Dual MicroPort (polysulfone polymer, silicone)<br>Infusaid Inc. | No | 1.5 | Shellock and Meeks, 1991 |
| Dual MacroPort (polysulfone polymer, silicone)<br>Infusaid Inc. | No | 1.5 | Shellock and Meeks, 1991 |
| Hickman Port (316L SS)<br>Davol Inc./Subsidiary of C.R. Bard, Inc. | Yes† | 1.5 | Shellock and Meeks, 1991 |
| Hickman Port, Pediatric (titanium)<br>Davol Inc./Subsidiary of C.R. Bard, Inc. | No | 1.5 | Shellock and Meeks, 1991 |
| Implantofix II (polysulfone)<br>Burron Medical Inc.<br>Bethlehem, PA | No | 1.5 | Shellock and Meeks, 1991 |
| Infusaid, Model 400 (titanium)<br>Infusaid Inc. | No | 1.5 | Shellock and Meeks, 1991 |
| Infusaid, Model 600 (titanium)<br>Infusaid Inc. | No | 1.5 | Shellock and Meeks, 1991 |
| Lifeport, Model 6013 (Delrin)<br>Strato Medical Corporation<br>Beverly, MA | No | 1.5 | Shellock and Meeks, 1991 |
| Lifeport, Model 1013 (titanium)<br>Strato Medical Corp. | No | 1.5 | Shellock and Meeks, 1991 |
| MacroPort (polysulfone polymer, silicone)<br>Infusaid Inc. | No | 1.5 | Shellock and Meeks, 1991 |
| MicroPort (polysulfone polymer, silicone)<br>Infusaid Inc. | No | 1.5 | Shellock and Meeks, 1991 |
| MRI Port (Delrin plastic, silicone)<br>Davol Inc./Subsidiary of C.R. Bard, Inc. | No | 1.5 | Shellock and Meeks, 1991 |
| Norport-AC (titanium)<br>Norfolk Medical<br>Skokie, IL | No | 1.5 | Shellock and Meeks, 1991 |
| Norport-DL (316L SS)<br>Norfolk Medical | No | 1.5 | Shellock and Meeks, 1991 |
| Norport-LS (titanium)<br>Norfolk Medical | No | 1.5 | Shellock and Meeks, 1991 |
| Norport-LS (316L SS)<br>Norfolk Medical | No | 1.5 | Shellock and Meeks, 1991 |

**TABLE 1** Metallic Implants, Materials, and Devices Tested for Movement/Deflection Forces During Exposure to Static Magnetic Fields—cont'd

| Metallic Implant, Material or Device | Movement/ Deflection | Highest Field Strength (T)* | Reference |
|---|---|---|---|
| Norport-LS (polysulfone)<br>Norfolk Medical | No | 1.5 | Shellock and Meeks, 1991 |
| Norport-PT (titanium)<br>Norfolk Medical | No | 1.5 | Shellock and Meeks, 1991 |
| Norport-SP (polysulfone, silicione rubber, Dacron)<br>Norfolk Medical | No | 1.5 | Shellock and Meeks, 1991 |
| PeriPort (polysulfone, titanium)<br>Infusaid Inc. | No | 1.5 | Shellock and Meeks, 1991 |
| Port-A-Cath, P.A.S. Port Portal (titanium)<br>Pharmacia Deltec<br>St. Paul, MN | No | 1.5 | Shellock and Meeks, 1991 |
| Port-A-Cath, Titanium Dual Lumen Portal (titanium)<br>Pharmacia Deltec | No | 1.5 | Shellock and Meeks, 1991 |
| Port-A-Cath, Titanium Peritoneal Portal (titanium)<br>Pharmacia Deltec | No | 1.5 | Shellock and Meeks, 1991 |
| Port-A-Cath, Titanium Venous Low Profile Portal (titanium)<br>Pharmacia Deltec | No | 1.5 | Shellock and Meeks, 1991 |
| Port-A-Cath, Titanium Venous Portal (titanium)<br>Pharmacia Deltec | No | 1.5 | Shellock and Meeks, 1991 |
| Port-A-Cath, Venous Portal (316L SS)<br>Pharmacia Deltec | No | 1.5 | Shellock and Meeks, 1991 |
| Q-Port (316L SS)<br>Quinton Instrument Co.<br>Seattle, WA | Yes† | 1.5 | Shellock and Meeks, 1991 |
| S.E.A. (titanium)<br>Harbor Medical Devices, Inc.<br>Boston, MA | No | 1.5 | Shellock and Meeks, 1991 |
| Snap-Lock (titanium, polysulfone polymer, silicone)<br>Infusaid Inc. | No | 1.5 | Shellock and Meeks, 1991 |
| Synchromed, Model 8500-1 (titanium, thermoplastic, silicone)<br>Medtronic, Inc. | No | 1.5 | Shellock and Meeks, 1991 |
| Vasport (titanium/fluoropolymer)<br>Gish Biomedical, Inc.<br>Santa Ana, CA | No | 1.5 | Shellock and Meeks, 1991 |
| *Miscellaneous:* | | | |
| Artificial urinary sphincter, AMS 800<br>American Medical Systems | No | 1.5 | Shellock and Crues, 1988A |
| Cerebral ventricular shunt tube connector, Accu-Flow straight<br>Codman | No | 1.5 | Shellock and Crues, 1988A |
| Cerebral ventricular shunt tube connector, Accu-flow right angle<br>Codman | No | 1.5 | Shellock and Crues, 1988A |

*(Continued.)*

**TABLE 1** Metallic Implants, Materials, and Devices Tested for Movement/Deflection Forces During Exposure to Static Magnetic Fields—cont'd

| Metallic Implant, Material or Device | Movement/ Deflection | Highest Field Strength (T)* | Reference |
|---|---|---|---|
| Cerebral ventricular shunt tube connector, Accu-flow, T-connector<br>Codman | No | 1.5 | Shellock and Crues, 1988A |
| Cerebral ventricular shunt tube connector (type unknown) | Yes | 0.147 | Shellock et al, 1987 |
| Contraceptive diaphragm, All Flex<br>Ortho Pharmaceutical<br>Raritan, NJ | Yes† | 1.5 | Shellock and Crues, 1988A |
| Contraceptive diaphragm, Flat Spring<br>Ortho Pharmaceutical | Yes† | 1.5 | Shellock and Crues, 1988A |
| Contraceptive diaphragm, Koroflex<br>Young Drug Products<br>Piscataway, NJ | Yes† | 1.5 | Shellock and Crues, 1988A |
| Forceps (titanium) | No | 1.44 | Shellock et al, 1987 |
| Hakim valve and pump | No | 1.44 | Shellock et al, 1987 |
| Intrauterine contraceptive device (IUD), Copper T<br>Searle Pharmaceuticals<br>Chicago, IL | No | 1.5 | Mark and Hricak, 1987 |
| Shunt valve, Holtertype<br>The Holter Co.<br>Bridgeport, PA | Yes† | 1.5 | Go et al, 1989 |
| Shunt valve, Holter-Hausner type<br>Holter-Hausner, Inc.<br>Bridgeport, PA | No | 1.5 | Go et al, 1989 |
| Swan-Ganz thermodilution catheter‡<br>American Edwards Laboratories | No‡ | 1.5 | ECRI, 1988 |
| Tantalum powder | No | 1.44 | New et al, 1983 |
| Tissue expander with magnetic port<br>McGhan Medical Corp.<br>Santa Barbara, CA | Yes | 1.5 | Liang et al, 1989 |
| Vascular marker, O-ring washer (302 SS)<br>PIC Design<br>Middlebury, CT | Yes† | 1.5 | R.D. Becker, 1989, personal communication |

*Highest field strength refers to the highest intensity of the static magnetic field in Tesla (T) that was used for the evaluation of movement/deflection forces of the various implants, materials, and devices tested.

†Denotes that the metallic implants, materials, or devices were considered to be safe for MRI despite being moved/deflected by the static magnetic fields. For example, certain heart valve prostheses were moved/deflected by the static magnetic fields, but the forces were considered to be less than that exerted on the prosthetic valves by the beating heart.

‡Although there is no magnetic deflection associated with the triple-lumen thermodilution Swan-Ganz catheter, there has been a report of a catheter "melting" in a patient; therefore this would be considered a relative contraindication for MRI.

SS = stainless steel. Material(s) used to construct the object is indicated, if known. Manufacturer information is provided, if known.

scanners, and the highest static magnetic field strength (static magnetic field strengths ranged from 0.147 to 4.7 T) at which the objects were evaluated. It should be noted that, unless otherwise stated, this information specifically pertains to the safety aspects of imaging a patient with respect to the ferromagnetic qualities of a metallic implant, material, or device (i.e., its attraction to a static magnetic field). Other issues related to electrical conductivity, artifact production, and so forth are not discussed in this chapter.

Various factors influence the risk of performing MRI in a patient with a ferromagnetic implant, material, or device including the strength of the static and gradient magnetic fields, the relative degree of ferromagnetism of the object, the mass of the object, the geometry of the object, the location and orientation of the object in situ, and the length of time the object has been in place. These factors should be carefully considered before subjecting a patient with a ferromagnetic object to MRI, particularly if it is located in a potentially dangerous area of the body such as near a vital neural, vascular, or soft-tissue structure, in which movement or dislodgment could injure the patient.

All biomedical implants, materials, and devices, particularly those made from unknown materials should be evaluated using ex vivo techniques before performing MRI. By following this procedure, the presence and amount of ferromagnetism may be determined so that a competent decision can be made concerning the potential associated risks.

### Aneurysm and Hemostatic Clips

Nineteen of the twenty-six aneurysm clips previously tested displayed ferromagnetic qualities and therefore are considered a contraindication for patients undergoing MRI. Studies have demonstrated that there is a realistic hazard of subjecting ferromagnetic aneurysm clips to static magnetic fields insofar as these clips may be displaced and result in serious consequences to the patient. Therefore it is recommended that patients be evaluated by MRI only if the type of aneurysm clip is definitely known to be nonferromagnetic. Patients with nonferromagnetic or weakly ferromagnetic aneurysm clips have been scanned by MRI without incident.

None of the six hemostatic vascular clips evaluated were attracted by static magnetic fields used for MRI, up to field strengths of 1.5 T. These hemostatic clips are made from nonferromagnetic materials and therefore do not present a risk to patients during MRI.

### Carotid Artery Vascular Clamps

Each of the five carotid artery vascular clamps tested displayed magnetic deflection when in the presence of a 1.5 T static magnetic field. However, only the Poppen-Blaylock carotid artery vascular clamp was thought to be contraindicated for patients undergoing MRI, because of the tremendous ferromagnetism of this particular device. The others were believed to be safe due to the existence of only mild ferromagnetism. Patients with metallic carotid artery vascular clamps have been imaged by MRI systems with static magnetic fields ranging from 0.35 to 0.6 T without experiencing any discomfort or neurologic sequelae.

### Dental Devices and Materials

Of the 16 different dental devices and materials tested, 12 had measurable deflection forces but only 3 of these represent a potential problem for patients during MRI due to the fact that these are magnetically activated devices (also see the subsection Magnetically Activated Implants and Devices).

### Heart Valve Prostheses

Twenty-nine different heart valve prostheses have been evaluated for magnetic deflection related to exposure to a 1.5 or 2.35 T static magnetic field. Of these, 4 were nonferromagnetic and 25 had measurable deflection forces. Because the magnetic deflection of these heart valves is minimal compared with the force exerted by the beating heart, MRI is not considered to be hazardous for patients with these valvular prostheses (with the possible exception of performing MRI with a MRI system greater than 0.35 T on a patient that has a Starr-Edwards Pre 6000 valve when there is a concern regarding the integrity of the annulus or presence of valvular dehiscence).

### Intravascular Coils, Filters, and Stents

Fourteen different intravascular coils, filters, and stents have been assessed for ferromagnetic qualities. Five of these are ferromagnetic. However, these devices typically become firmly incorporated into the vessel wall after approximately 6 weeks; therefore it is unlikely that any of them would become dislodged by magnetic forces. In fact, patients with most of the intravascular coils, filters, and stents listed in Table 1 have been imaged with 1.5 T MRI scanners without incident. Therefore it is considered to be safe to image patients with any of the intravascular coils, filters, and stents listed after a suitable period has elapsed to ensure stable positioning and retention of the device. MRI should not be performed if there is any possibility that an intravascular coil, filter, or stent is not held firmly in place.

### Ocular Implants

Of the 12 ocular implants tested, the Fatio eyelid spring and the retinal tack made from martensitic stainless steel (Western European) were deflected by a 1.5 T static magnetic field. Both of these may be uncomfortable (i.e., the Fatio eyelid spring) or injure (i.e., the Western European retinal tack) the patient during MRI. The case of a ferromagnetic object damaging the eye of a patient undergoing MRI has been previously described, which underscores the need for special diligence when subjecting a patient with any type of ferromagnetic material located near the eye to this imaging procedure (also see the section Magnetically Activated Implants and Devices).

### Orthopedic Implants, Materials, and Devices

Most of the various orthopedic materials and devices tested are made from nonferromagnetic materials and are safe for MRI. Only the Perfix interference screw used for reconstruction of the anterior cruciate ligament (ACL) displayed a substantial deflection force and caused extensive signal loss. This screw was the only orthopedic implant tested to date that was substantially ferromagnetic and, more importantly, caused greater than the localized signal void typically observed with other metallic orthopedic implants. Images of the knee of one patient with two Perfix screws in place were not interpretable because of the image distortion caused by these implants. Therefore alternative nonferromagnetic implants should be considered for reconstruction of the ACL.

An additional concern of subjecting metallic orthopedic implants (which are typically large) to MRI is the potential heating that may develop as a result of exposure to the gradient and/or radiofrequency electromagnetic fields. However, studies have demonstrated that heating of these implants is relatively insignificant.

### Otologic Implants

The three cochlear implants tested are contraindicated for MRI because, in addition to being attracted by static magnetic fields, they are also activated by electronic or magnetic mechanisms. Of the remaining otologic implants, only one displayed magnetic deflection during testing with a 1.5 T static magnetic field. This implant, the McGee stapedectomy piston prosthesis, made from platinum and 17Cr-4Ni stainless steel (manufactured during mid-1987) has been recalled by the manufacturer. In addition, patients who received this implant have been identified and issued cards warning them not to undergo MRI.

### Pellets and Bullets

Most of the pellets and bullets tested are composed of nonferromagnetic materials. Ammunition that proved to be ferromagnetic tended to be manufactured in foreign countries and/or of military variety. Of note is that shrapnel typically contains steel and therefore presents a potential hazard for MRI. Because pellets, bullets, and shrapnel may be contaminated with ferromagnetic materials, the risk vs. benefits of performing MRI should be carefully considered, as well as whether the pellet, bullet, or shrapnel is located near a vital internal structure. Of further note is that, in an effort to reduce lead poisoning in "puddling"-type ducks, there is a requirement by the federal government in many of the eastern United States to use steel shotgun pellets instead of lead. This would present a potential hazard to patients undergoing MRI and cause severe artifacts.

### Penile Implants

Only one of the nine penile implants, the Dacomed Omniphase, had a significant deflection force measured when exposed to a 1.5 T static magnetic field. Although it is unlikely that this implant would severely injure a patient undergoing MRI because of the manner in which it is used, it would undoubtedly be uncomfortable for the patient; therefore scanning a patient with this implant is inadvisable.

### Vascular Access Ports

Two of the thirty-three implantable vascular access ports tested had measurable deflection forces, but the forces were thought to be insignificant relative to the in vivo application of these implants. Therefore it is safe to perform MRI in a patient that may have one of these implants. Future developments of this technology will include vascular access ports that are electronically activated and these, obviously, would be contraindicated for MRI.

### Miscellaneous

Of the miscellaneous metallic implants, materials, and devices tested, the cerebral ventricular shunt tube connector (type unknown) and tissue expander with magnetic port had significant deflection forces that may be hazardous to patients undergoing MRI. Another ferromagnetic implant, the O-ring washer vascular marker, displayed only slight ferromagnetic qualities and therefore does not represent a risk to patients undergoing MRI.

Contraceptive diaphragms were attracted strongly by the 1.5 T static magnetic field, but patients have been scanned with these devices who did not complain of any sensation related to movement of these objects. Accordingly the presence of a diaphragm is not believed to pose a hazard to a patient during MRI. There is, however, a remote possibility that the contraceptive properties of the diaphragm may be hindered if it is inadvertently moved during MRI.

Although the triple-lumen thermodilution Swan-Ganz catheter is constructed of nonferromagnetic materials, the presence of this device may be injurious to the patient during MRI. A report indicated that a portion of a thermodilution Swan-Ganz catheter that was outside the patient melted as a result of MRI. It was postulated that the high-frequency electromagnetic fields generated by the MRI system caused eddy current heating of either the wires within the thermodilution catheter or the radiopaque material inside the catheter. This incident suggests that patients with triple-lumen thermodilution Swan-Ganz catheters or other similar devices could be potentially injured during MRI.

### Magnetically Activated Implants and Devices

Certain ferromagnetic implants and devices such as cochlear implants, tissue expanders, ocular prostheses, and dental implants are activated by magnetic mechanisms. The majority of these are considered to be potentially hazardous to patients undergoing MRI. Besides dislodging these particular types of implants and devices, MRI may also alter or damage the operation of the magnetic component, possibly requiring surgery for replacement. Further, if the portion of the prosthesis that the magnet attracts is implanted in soft tissue (e.g., with certain ocular prostheses, the magnet is contained in the prosthesis and a ferromagnetic "keeper" is implanted in the subcutaneous tissue), it is inadvisable to perform MRI in a patient with this type of device, because of potential adverse effects associated with displacement of the "keeper." Magnetic resonance imaging may be performed safely in patients with dental magnet appliances that are properly attached to supporting structures after the magnet-containing portion of the device is removed.

## Electrically or Mechanically Activated or Electrically Conductive Devices

The United States Food and Drug Administration requires labeling of MRI systems to indicate that they are contraindicated for patients who have electrically, magnetically, or mechanically activated implants, because the magnetic and electromagnetic fields produced by MRI systems may interfere with the operation of these devices.

Patients with internal or external cardiac pacemakers, implantable cardiovascular defibrillators, cochlear implants, neurostimulators, bone-growth stimulators, implantable drug-infusion pumps, and similar devices that could be adversely affected by the electromagnetic fields used in MRI should not be examined with this modality.

The risks associated with MRI of patients with cardiac pacemakers are related to several factors. These include the possibility of movement of the devices, reed switch closure or damage, programming changes, inhibition or reversion to an asynchronous mode of operation, electromagnetic interference, and induced currents in lead wires or other conducting materials of the devices.

A "letter to the editor" recently indicated that a patient who was not dependent on a pacemaker had the device "disabled" during the MRI procedure. Although this patient experienced no apparent discomfort and the pacemaker was not damaged, it is inadvisable to perform this type of maneuver in patients with pacemakers, because of the potential to encounter any combination of the aforementioned hazards. Of particular concern is the possibility that the pacemaker lead wire(s) or other similar intracardiac wire configuration could act as an antenna in which the gradient and/or radiofrequency electromagnetic fields may induce sufficient current to cause cardiac fibrillation, thermal injury, or other potentially dangerous event. Because of this theoretically deleterious and unpredictable effect, potential risks are associated with MRI in patients with residual external pacing wires, temporary pacing wires, thermodilution Swan-Ganz catheters, and/or any other type of internally or externally positioned conductive wire or similar device.

All unnecessary and/or unused electrically conductive materials should be removed from the MRI scanner before the onset of imaging. For example, unused surface coils or gating leads should not be left within the MRI scanner even if disconnected from the system. Special care should be taken to ensure that no unnecessary loops are created in any electrically conductive materials within the MRI system. Further, surface coils, electrically activated gating equipment, monitoring devices, and other similar devices should be inspected and tested routinely to identify damaged or improperly operating equipment that could be hazardous to the patient undergoing MRI.

A patient with any other similar electrically, magnetically, or mechanically activated or electrically conductive devices should be excluded from MRI unless the particular device has been previously shown to be unaffected by the magnetic and electromagnetic fields used for clinical MRI, and there is no possibility of injuring the patient.

## Screening Patients with Metallic Foreign Bodies

Patients may present to MRI with a history of metallic foreign bodies such as bullets, shrapnel, or other types of metallic fragments. The relative risk of imaging these patients depends on multiple factors including the ferromagnetic properties of the object, the geometry and dimensions of the object, the strength with which the object is embedded in the tissue, the strength of the static and gradient magnetic fields of the MRI system, and whether the object is in or adjacent to a potentially hazardous site such as a vital neural, vascular, or soft-tissue structure.

Each imaging site should develop a standardized policy for screening patients with suspected metallic foreign bodies; the policy should include guidelines as to which patients require radiographic and/or CT examinations and the specific radiographic or CT techniques to be used (e.g., number of views, position of the anatomy to be examined). Each case should be considered individually on the basis of the relative risk of imaging this type of patient.

The foregoing precautions should be taken with regard to patients referred for MRI in any MRI system regardless of the field strength, magnetic type, and presence or absence of magnetic shielding.

## Patients with Halo Vests or Similar Externally Applied Devices

The use of MRI to assess cervical spine trauma in patients who require stabilization of the spine with a halo vest or similar device is usually not possible, because most of these devices are composed of metallic materials that may present risks and produce mild-to-severe artifacts. This is unfortunate because MRI frequently provides a useful evaluation of the spinal cord and associated soft-tissue structures that is not attainable with other diagnostic imaging techniques.

Investigators who evaluated the effect of various halo vests on image quality reported that these devices caused image distortion that depended on the type of material used to construct the halo rings and support uprights. Halo vests made from stainless steel resulted in the poorest image quality, followed by those made from aluminum, titanium, and graphite. This study did not directly assess deflection forces, heating, or induced currents, all of which potentially represent hazards to the patient if the halo vest is primarily composed of ferromagnetic and/or conductive materials.

Although some commercially available halo devices are composed of nonferromagnetic materials, there is still the theoretical hazard of inducing electric current in the ring portion of any halo device made from electrically conductive materials, according to Faraday's law of electromagnetic conduction, which states that a current can be induced in a closed-loop conductor as it moves through a magnetic field. The current within such a loop is of additional concern, because of eddy current induction and potential image degradation effects. Further, there is a potential for the patient to be involved in part of this current loop, so that there would be the concern of a possible burn or electrical injury to the patient.

Specially designed, commercially available halo vests have been developed recently that are made from nonferromagnetic and nonconductive materials that have little or no interaction with the electromagnetic fields used for MRI and therefore are not associated with safety-related problems or imaging artifacts. The advantages of using a nonferromagnetic, nonconductive halo device include (1) no associated deflection forces, (2) little or no heating, (3) no artifacts that distort the imaging area of interest, and (4) no likelihood of induction of electric current. To my knowledge, there have been no reports of injuries associated with MRI of patients with halo devices (although one incident of "electrical arcing" occurred with the use of a halo vest without injury to the patient was reported in the 1988 SMRI Safety Survey, Phase 1 Study).

Because of the known theoretical hazards associated with MRI in patients with halo vests or similar devices, it is prudent, from both safety and image artifact standpoints, to image only patients with halo vests and similar externally applied devices that are composed of materials that are both nonferromagnetic and nonconductive, especially since these devices are currently available from several commercial manufacturers.

## Discussion

According to the *Policies, Guidelines, and Recommendations for MR Imaging Safety and Patient Management* information issued by the Society for Magnetic Resonance Imaging Safety Committee, patients with electronically, magnetically, or mechanically activated devices or electrically conductive devices should be excluded from MRI unless the particular device has been previously shown (i.e., usually by ex vivo testing procedures) to be unaffected by the electromagnetic fields used for clinical MRI, and there is no possibility of injuring the patient. During the screening process for MRI, patients with these objects should be identified before examination by MRI or being exposed to the electromagnetic fields used for this imaging technique. In this chapter the numerous biomedical implants, devices, materials, and foreign bodies that are considered to be absolute contraindications, relative contraindications, or safe for MRI have been presented and discussed. It should be noted, however, that there are implants, materials, devices, or other foreign bodies that have yet to be evaluated for compatibility with MRI that may be encountered in the clinical setting. Patients that have untested objects should not be allowed to undergo MRI.

*Acknowledgments.* I wish to acknowledge the editorial contributions of Stacy M. Myers at the Department of Radiological Sciences, UCLA School of Medicine, Los Angeles, California.

## Suggested Reading

Alagona P Jr, Toole JC, Maniscalco BS, et al. Nuclear magnetic resonance imaging in a patient with a DDD pacemaker (letter). PACE 1989; 12:619.

Albert DW, Olson KR, Parel JM, et al. Magnetic resonance imaging and retinal tacks. Arch Ophthalmol 1990; 108:320–321.

Applebaum EL, Valvassori GE. Effects of magnetic resonance imaging fields on stapedectomy prostheses. Arch Otolaryngol 1985; 11:820–821.

Applebaum EL, Valvassori GE. Further studies on the effects of magnetic resonance fields on middle ear implants. Ann Otol Rhinol Laryngol 1990; 99:801–804.

Ballock RT, Hajek PC, Byrne TP, Garfin SR. The quality of magnetic resonance imaging, as affected by the composition of the halo orthosis. J Bone Joint Surg 1989; 71:431–434.

Barrafato D, Henkelman RM. Magnetic resonance imaging and surgical clips. Can J Surg 1984; 27:509–512.

Becker RL, Norfray JF, Teitelbaum GP, et al. MR imaging in patients with intracranial aneurysm clips. AJR 1988; 9:885–889.

Bellon EM, Haacke EM, Coleman PE, et al. MR artifacts: A review. Magn Reson Imaging 1984; 2:41–52.

Brown MA, Carden JA, Coleman RE, et al. Magnetic field effects on surgical ligation clips. Magn Reson Imaging 1987; 5:443–453.

Clayman DA, Murakami ME, Vines FS. Compatibility of cervical spine braces with MR imaging: A study of nine nonferrous devices. Am J Neuroradiol 1990; 11:385–390.

Davis PL, Crooks L, Arakawa M, et al. Potential hazards in NMR imaging: Heating effects of changing magnetic fields and RF fields on small metallic implants. AJR 1981; 137:857–860.

DeKeizer RJW, TeStrake L. Intraocular lens implants (pseudophakoi) and steelwire sutures: A contraindication for MRI? Doc Ophthalmol 1986; 61:281–284.

Dujovny M, Kossovsky N, Kossowsky R, et al. Aneurysm clip motion during magnetic resonance imaging: In vivo experimental study with metallurgical factor analysis. Neurosurgery 1985; 17:543–548.

ECRI, Health Devices Alert. A new MRI complication? 1988:1.

Erlebacher JA, Cahill PT, Pannizzo F, Knowles RJR. Effect of magnetic resonance imaging on DDD pacemakers. Am J Cardiol 1986; 57:437–440.

Fache JS, Price C, Hawbolt EB, Li DKB. MR imaging artifacts produced by dental materials. Am J Neuroradiol 1987; 8:837–840.

Fetter J, Abram G, Holmes D, et al. The effects of nuclear magnetic resonance imager on external and implanted pulse generators. PACE 1984; 7:720–727.

Gegauff, Laurell KA, Thavendrarajah A, Rosentiel SF. A potential MRI hazard: Forces on dental magnet keepers. J Oral Rehabil 1990; 17:403–410.

Go KG, Kamman RL, Mooyaart EL. Interaction of metallic neurosurgical implants with magnetic resonance imaging at 1.5 Tesla as a cause of image distortion and of hazardous movement of the implant. Clin Neurosurg 1989; 91:109–115.

Gold JP, Pulsinelli W, Winchester P, et al. Safety of metallic surgical clips in patients undergoing high-field-strength magnetic resonance imaging. Ann Thorac Surg 1989; 48:643–645.

Hassler M, Le Bas JF, Wolf JE, et al. Effects of magnetic fields used in MRI on 15 prosthetic heart valves. J Radiol 1986; 67:661–666.

Hayes DL, Holmes DR, Gray JE. Effect of 1.5 T nuclear magnetic resonance imaging on implanted permanent pacemakers. Am Coll Cardiol 1987; 10:782–786.

Holmes D, Hayes D, Gray J, Merideth J. The effects of magnetic resonance imaging on implantable pulse generators. PACE 1986; 9:360–370.

Joondeph BC, Peyman GA, Mafee MF, Joondeh HC. Magnetic resonance imaging and retinal tacks. Arch Ophthalmol 1987; 105:1479–1480.

Kanal E, Shellock FG, Sonnenblick D. MRI clinical site safety survey: Phase I results and preliminary data. Magn Reson Imaging 1988; 7(suppl 1):106.

Kanal E, Shellock FG, Talagala L. Safety considerations in MR imaging. Radiology 1990; 176:593–606.

Kelly WM, Paglan PG, Pearson JA, et al. Ferromagnetism of intraocular foreign body causes unilateral blindness after MR study. Am J Neuroradiol 1986; 7:243–245.

Kuethe DO, Small KW, Blinder RA. Non-ferromagnetic retinal tacks are a tolerable risk in magnetic resonance imaging. Invest Radiology 1991; 26:1–7.

Laakman RW, Kaufman B, Han JS, et al. MR imaging in patients with metallic implants. AJR 1985; 157:711–714.

Leon JA, Gabriele OF. Middle ear prosthesis: Significance in magnetic resonance imaging. Magn Reson Imaging 1987; 5:405–406.

Liang MD, Narayanan K, Kanal E. Magnetic ports in tissue expanders—A caution for MRI. Magn Reson Imaging 1989; 7:541–542.

Liebman CE, Messersmith RN, Levin DN, Lu CT. MR imaging of inferior vena caval filter: Safety and artifacts. AJR 1988; 150:1174–1176.

Lissac MI, Metrop D, Brugigrad J, et al. Dental materials and magnetic resonance imaging. Invest Radiol 1991; 26:40–45.

Lyons CJ, Betz RR, Mesgarzadeh M, et al. The effect of magnetic resonance imaging on metal spine implants. Spine 1989; 14:670–672.

Malko JA, Hoffman JC, Jarrett PJ. Eddy-current-induced artifacts caused by an "MR-compatible" halo device. Radiology 1989; 173:563–564.

Mark AS, Hricak H. Intrauterine contraceptive devices: MR imaging. Radiology 1987; 162:311–314.

Matsumoto AH, Teitelbaum GP, Barth KH, et al. Tantalum vascular stents: In vivo evaluation with MR imaging. Radiology 1989; 170:753–755.

Mattucci KF, Setzen M, Hyman R, Chaturvedi G. The effect of nuclear magnetic resonance imaging on metallic middle ear prostheses. Otolaryngol Head Neck Surg 1986; 94:441–443.

Mechlin M, Thickman D, Kressel HY, et al. Magnetic resonance imaging of postoperative patients with metallic implants. AJR 1984; 143:1281–1284.

New PFJ, Rosen BR, Brady TJ, et al. Potential hazards and artifacts of ferromagnetic and nonferromagnetic surgical and dental devices in nuclear magnetic resonance imaging. Radiology 1983; 147:139–148.

Pavlicek W, Geisinger M, Castle L, et al. The effects of magnetic resonance on patients with cardiac pacemakers. Radiology 1983; 147:149–153.

Persson BRR, Stahlberg F. Health and safety of clinical NMR examinations. Boca Raton, Fla: CRC, 1989.

Power W, Collum LMT. Magnetic resonance imaging and magnetic eye implants. Lancet 1988; 2:227.

Pusey E, Lufkin RB, Brown RKJ, et al. Magnetic resonance imaging artifacts: Mechanism and clinical significance. Radiographics 1986; 6:891–911.

Roberts CW, Haik BG, Cahill P. Magnetic resonance imaging of metal loop intraocular lenses. Arch Ophthalmol 1990; 108:320–321.

Shellock FG. MR imaging of metallic implants and materials: A compilation of the literature. AJR 1988; 151:811–814.

Shellock FG. Ex vivo assessment of deflection forces and artifacts associated with high-field strength of "mini-magnet" dental prostheses. Magn Reson Imaging 1989A; 7(suppl 1):38.

Shellock FG. Biological effects and safety aspects of magnetic resonance imaging. Magn Reson Q 1989B; 5:243–261.

Shellock FG. Biological effects and safety aspects of MRI. In: Stark DD, Bradley WG, eds. Magnetic Resonance Imaging. 2nd ed, St. Louis: Mosby, 1991.

Shellock FG, Crues JV. High field MR imaging of metallic biomedical implants: An in vitro evaluation of deflection forces and temperature changes induced in large prostheses. Radiology 1987; 165(abstr):150.

Shellock FG, Crues JV. High-field strength MR imaging and metallic biomedical implants: An ex vivo evaluation of deflection forces. AJR 1988A; 151:389–392.

Shellock FG, Crues JV. MRI: Safety considerations. Magn Reson Imaging Dec 1988B; 2:25–30.

Shellock FG, Crues JV. Safety aspects of MRI in patients with metallic implants or foreign bodies: Absolute and relative contraindications. Appl Radiol 1992;

Shellock FG, Crues JV, Sacks SA. High-field magnetic resonance imaging of penile prostheses: In vitro evaluation of deflection forces and imaging artifacts. (Abstract.) In: Book of Abstracts, Society of Magnetic Resonance in Medicine. Vol 2. Berkeley, Calif: Society of Magnetic Resonance in Medicine, 1987:915.

Shellock FG, Kanal E. SMRI Safety Committee. Policies, guidelines, and recommendations for MR imaging safety and patient management. J Magn Reson Imaging 1991; 1:97–101.

Shellock FG, Kanal E. Safety considerations of cardiovascular MR studies. In: Cardiovascular Applications of Magnetic Resonance Imaging and Spectroscopy. New York: Futura Publishing, 1992 (in press).

Shellock FG, Litwer C, Kanal E. MRI bioeffects, safety, and patient management: A review. Rev Magn Reson Imaging 1992; 4:21–63.

Shellock FG, Meeks T. Ex vivo evaluation of ferromagnetism and artifacts for implantable vascular access ports exposed to a 1.5 T MR scanner. J Magn Reson Imaging 1991; 1:243.

Shellock FG, Mink JH, Curtin S, Friedman MJ. MRI and orthopedic implants used for anterior cruciate ligament reconstruction: Assessment of ferromagnetism and artifacts. J Magn Reson Imaging 1992; 2:225–228.

Shellock FG, Schatz CJ. High-field strength MR imaging and metallic otologic implants. Am J Neuroradiol 1991; 12:279–281.

Shellock FG, Schatz C, Shelton C, Brown B. Ex vivo evaluation of ferromagnetism for metallic ocular and middle-ear prostheses exposed to a 1.5 T MR imager. Radiology 1990; 177(P):271.

Shellock FG, Slimp G. MRI-compatible halo vest for cervical spine fixation. AJR 1990; 154:631–632.

Soulen RL, Budinger TF, Higgins CB. Magnetic resonance imaging of prosthetic heart valves. Radiology 1985; 154:705–707.

Teitelbaum GP. Metallic ballistic fragments: MR imaging safety and artifacts. (Letter to the editor). Radiology 1990; 175:883.

Teitelbaum GP, Bradley WG, Klein BD. MR imaging artifacts, ferromagnetism, and magnetic torque on intravascular filters, stents, and coils. Radiology 1988; 166:657–664.

Teitelbaum GP, Lin MCW, Watanabe AT, et al. Ferromagnetism and MR imaging: Safety of carotid artery vascular clamps. Am J Neuroradiol 1990; 11:267–272.

Teitelbaum GP, Ortega HV, Vinitski S, et al. Low artifact intravascular devices: MR imaging evaluation. Radiology 1988; 168:713–719.

Teitelbaum GP, Raney M, Carvlin MJ, et al. Evaluation of ferromagnetism and magnetic resonance imaging artifacts of the Strecker tantalum vascular stent. Cardiovas Intervent Radiol 1989; 12:125–127.

Teitelbaum GP, Yee CA, Van-Horn DD, et al. Metallic ballistic fragments: MR imaging safety and artifacts. Radiology 1990; 175:855–859.

Watanabe AT, Teitelbaum GP, Gomes AS, Roehm JOF. MR imaging of the bird's nest filter. Radiology 1990; 177:578–579.

White DW. Interaction between magnetic fields and metallic ossicular prostheses. Am J Otol 1987; 8:290–292.

Williams S, Char DH, Dillon WP, et al. Ferrous intraocular foreign bodies and magnetic resonance imaging. Am J Ophthalmol 1988; 105:398–401.

Williamson MR, McCowan TC, Walker CW, Ferris EJ. Effect of a 1.5 Tesla magnetic field on Greenfield filters in vitro and in dogs. Angiology 1988; 12:1022–1024.

Yamanashi WS, Wheatley KK, Lester PD, Anderson DW. Technical artifacts in magnetic resonance imaging. Physiol Chem Phys Med NMR 1984; 16:237–250.

Yuh WTC, Hanigan MT, Nerad JA, et al. Extrusion of eye socket magnetic implant after MR imaging: Potential hazard to patient with eye prosthesis. J Magn Reson Imaging 1991; 1:711–713.

Zheutlin JD, Thompson JT, Shofner RS. The safety of magnetic resonance imaging with intraorbital metallic objects after retinal reattachment or trauma. (Letter.) Am J Ophthalmol 1987; 103:831.

Zimmerman BH, Faul DD. Artifacts and hazards in NMR imaging due to metal implants and cardiac pacemakers. Diagn Imaging Clin Med 1984; 53:53–56.

# Scintigraphic Detection of Osteomyelitis

*DONALD S. SCHAUWECKER, Ph.D., M.D.*

Multiple radiologic and scintigraphic procedures have been proposed to diagnose osteomyelitis. The fact that so many approaches are still advocated indicates that no single approach is optimal in all situations. The goal of this chapter is to describe the scintigraphic evaluation of osteomyelitis and show where it can be most useful.

## Indications and Utility of Alternative Technologies

Plain radiography should be the first study in every patient. If it is diagnostic, the workup is complete. However, most of the time it is not pathognomonic, since at least 10 to 14 days are required for the classic bone changes to develop. Even if the

A B C

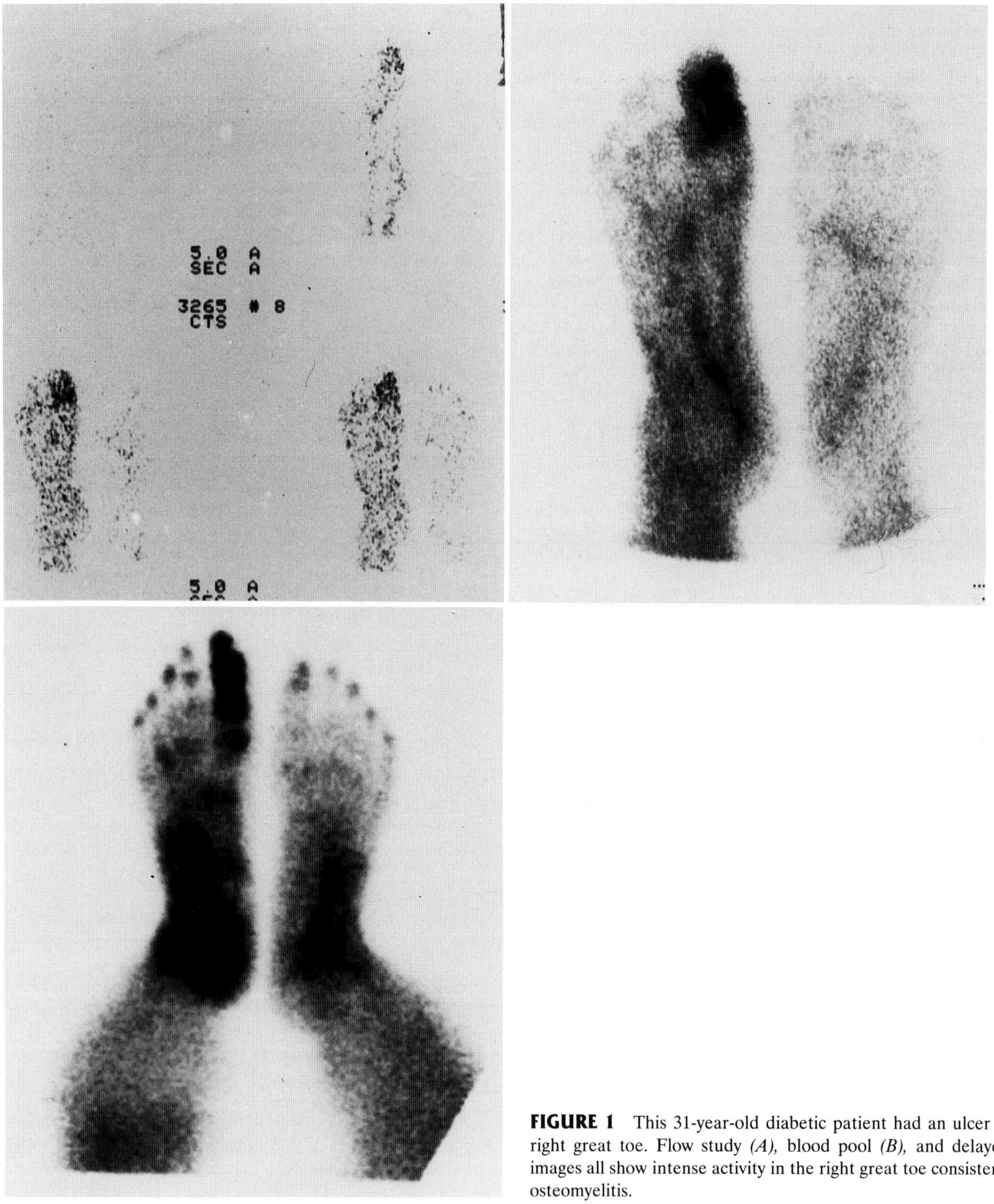


**FIGURE 1** This 31-year-old diabetic patient had an ulcer on his right great toe. Flow study *(A)*, blood pool *(B)*, and delayed *(C)* images all show intense activity in the right great toe consistent with osteomyelitis.

plain radiograph is not diagnostic, it is useful in directing further studies.

In adults with normal plain radiographs (i.e., no lesions present that cause increased bone remodeling), the three-phase bone scan has a sensitivity and specificity of about 95 percent. Usually osteomyelitis (Fig. 1) can be readily differentiated from cellulitis (Fig. 2). In routine clinical practice, most cases of osteomyelitis can be diagnosed using the three-phase bone scan.

In neonates imaged soon after the onset of osteomyelitis, the sensitivity of the three-phase bone scan is decreased. Falsely normal or "cold" defects occur as a result of subperiosteal abscess and/or disruption of the periosteal blood supply. In this situation gallium-67 citrate, indium-111 leukocytes, or a repeat three-phase bone scan have been recommended for the second study. Regardless of which scan is chosen, the time delay may make the second study more accurate. At our institution, most clinicians wish to avoid this delay and proceed immediately to bone biopsy based on high clinical suspicion.

If the plain radiograph reveals a fracture, prosthesis, neuropathic osteopathy, or other problem that causes increased bone remodeling, we perform an $^{111}$In leukocyte scan. If the suspected site of osteomyelitis is in the marrow-containing skeleton, we combine the $^{111}$In leukocyte scan with

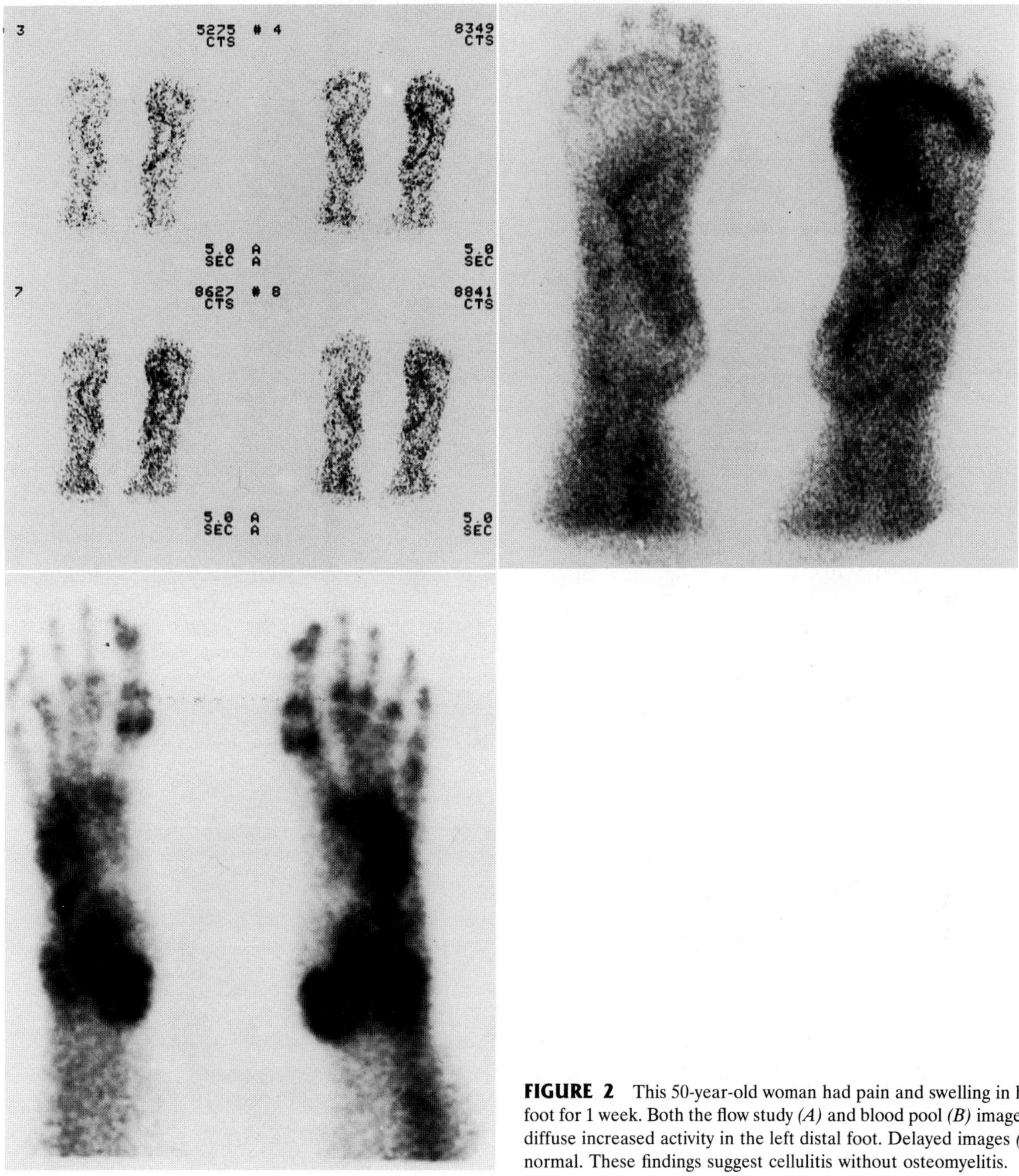


**FIGURE 2** This 50-year-old woman had pain and swelling in her left foot for 1 week. Both the flow study *(A)* and blood pool *(B)* images show diffuse increased activity in the left distal foot. Delayed images *(C)* are normal. These findings suggest cellulitis without osteomyelitis.

a bone marrow scan. This approach is discussed in the preceding chapter.

If the suspected osteomyelitis is not in the marrow-containing skeleton, and the plain radiograph reveals an abnormality that causes increased bone remodeling, we combine the $^{111}$In leukocyte scan with the three-phase bone scan. The sensitivity and specificity of the $^{111}$In leukocyte scan are both approximately 90 percent in the peripheral skeleton. Since there are no landmarks on the $^{111}$In leukocyte scan, the problem is to differentiate the soft-tissue infection from bone infection. By combining the three-phase bone scan with the $^{111}$In leukocyte scan, we are able to differentiate cellulitis (Fig. 3) from osteomyelitis (Fig. 4) in almost 90 percent of the cases.

Currently magnetic resonance imaging (MRI) has nearly supplanted computed tomography (CT) in the evaluation of osteomyelitis. At our institution, CT is used to detect foreign bodies, to determine the cortical extent of bone infection, and to guide biopsy in vertebral osteomyelitis and in other procedures when fluoroscopy is suboptimal.

For the diagnosis of osteomyelitis, MRI has a sensitivity and specificity of approximately 95 and 90 percent, respectively. However, any disease process that replaces bone marrow and causes increased tissue water (e.g., healing fracture or tumor) may resemble osteomyelitis. In addition, artifacts caused by a joint prosthesis may degrade the images sufficiently to make the diagnosis of infected joint arthroplasty impossible. For uncomplicated osteomyelitis, MRI gives results similar to the

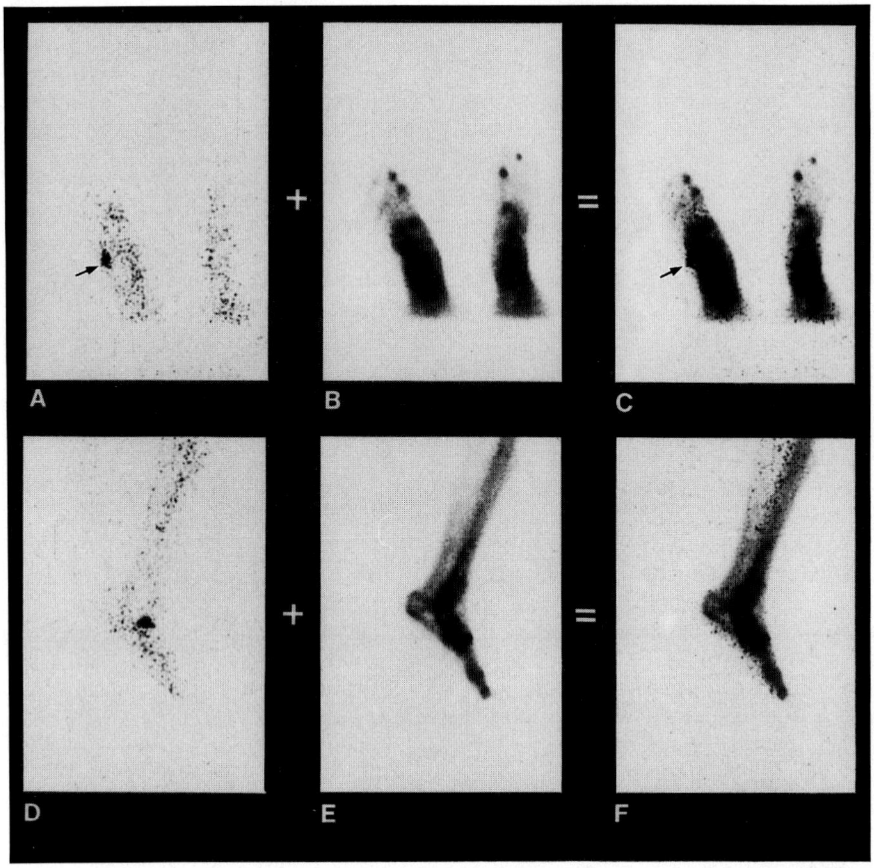


**FIGURE 3** This 74-year-old diabetic patient had pain, swelling, and redness of her right foot. *A* and *D* are the plantar and lateral $^{111}$In leukocyte images, respectively. *B* and *E* are the plantar and lateral 4 hour bone scan images, respectively. *C* is the superimposition of *A* on *B*, and *F* is the superimposition of *D* on *E*. The $^{111}$In activity *(arrow)* seems to be adjacent to, but not in, the bone on the plantar view *(C)*. (This was more apparent when the individual films were superimposed. Unfortunately this cannot be represented by a single print.) Thus this is cellulitis and not osteomyelitis. Notice in *B* and *E* that there is no focal uptake on the bone scan. Therefore osteomyelitis is ruled out. (If the bone scan results had been known ahead of time, the $^{111}$In leukocyte study was probably unnecessary.)

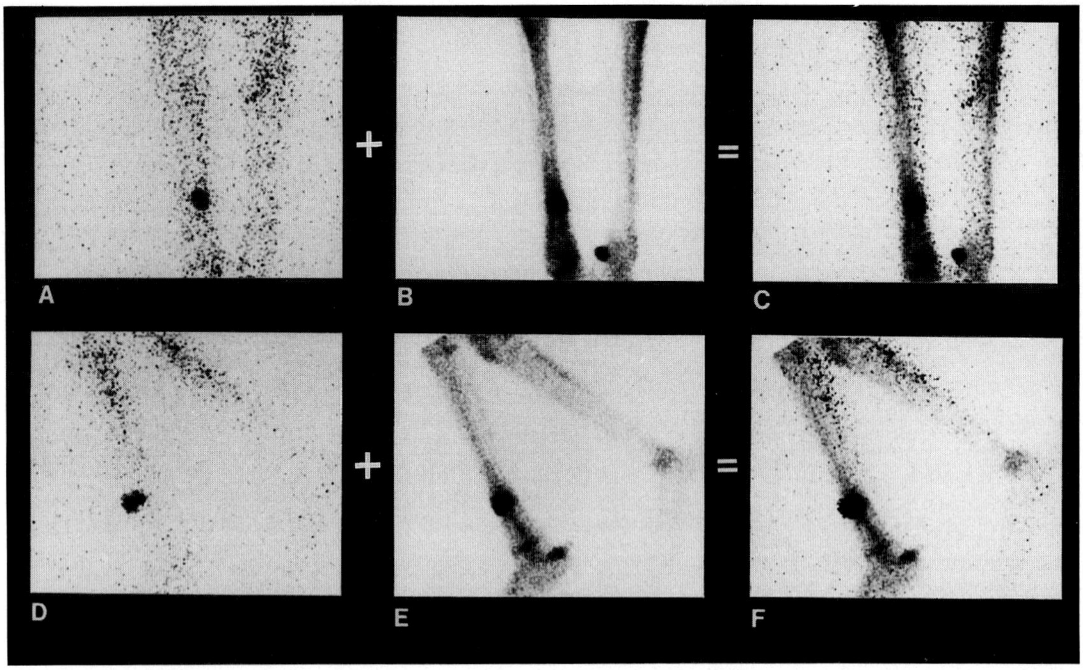


**FIGURE 4** This 65-year-old man had a traumatic injury to his right tibia. *A* and *D* are the anterior and lateral $^{111}$In leukocyte images, respectively. *B* and *E* are the anterior and lateral 4 hour bone scan images, respectively. *C* is the superimposition of *A* on *B*, and *F* is the superimposition of *D* on *E*. In both orthogonal views the $^{111}$In activity superimposes on the focal increased activity of the bone scan. Thus this represents osteomyelitis.

three-phase bone scan, but is considerably more expensive. At our institution, MRI is rarely used to diagnose osteomyelitis; however, its excellent resolution is often used to determine the extent of infection (e.g., possible soft-tissue abscess in a diabetic foot). Improved contrast agents or new pulse sequences may expand the future role of MRI in the evaluation of possible bone infection.

## Technical Approach

The three-phase bone scan is a well-established, routine study. Upon injection of 20 mCi (740 MBq) of technetium-99m MDP, serial 5 second images (flow or dynamic phase) are obtained in the projection chosen to best delineate the suspected site of osteomyelitis. The blood pool image is obtained in the same projection within 5 minutes of injection. We try to obtain the flow and blood pool images in a projection that includes the contralateral side for comparison. The blood pool image is obtained for a preset number of counts (500 K if both limbs, or 250 K if one limb is in the field of view, and 1,000 K when imaging the trunk). Approximately 3 hours later, the delayed bone image is obtained for the same number of counts as the blood pool image. Generally, orthogonal views of the affected area are obtained for both the blood pool and bone images.

For children the protocol of the three-phase bone scan is modified from the adult procedure. The Tc-99m MDP dose is reduced to the following scale: one-fourth of the adult dose for children under 5 years old, one-half of the adult dose for children 5 to 10 years old, and three-fourths of the adult dose for children 10 to 15 years old. Children over 15 should be given the adult dose. We deviate from this scale if the child is unusually large or small for his or her age. Total body images are obtained because hematogenous osteomyelitis may involve an unsuspected joint. Finally, images are obtained at two different intensities: one for a normal image and the other for a lighter image. The growth plate activity is often highly intense, and the lighter image allows one to see abnormalities in this region. Attention to detail is essential in children, because subtle changes may be the only findings.

There are multiple methods for separating and labeling leukocytes. We have used $^{111}$In tropolonate, because the separation and labeling are done in plasma and the cells are never exposed to saline. However, we have no data to show that our results are better than the more widely used $^{111}$In oxine approach. If I were starting today, I would probably use the $^{111}$In oxine approach, since it is commercially available and more widely accepted. In addition, labeled leukocytes are now available from commercial radiopharmacies. The Thakur approach for separation and labeling of the leukocytes is well discussed elsewhere. Care must be taken in the separation and labeling of the leukocytes: labeled viable leukocytes can produce excellent results; damaged leukocytes produce poor results.

We obtain our combined three-phase bone scan and $^{111}$In leukocyte scan on a camera that simultaneously captures and separates the 140 keV $^{99m}$Tc peak, and the 173 keV and 247 keV $^{111}$In peaks. We acquire an $^{111}$In leukocyte image for 50 K counts or 15 minutes, whichever comes first, at both 4 and 24 hours after injection of the $^{111}$In leukocytes. Care must be taken to prevent spectral overlap and possible misinterpretation. Using our equipment, a 10 percent window at the 140 keV $^{99m}$Tc peak and a 20 percent window at the 247 keV $^{111}$In peak are used for the 4 hour images. Intense $^{99m}$Tc localization often interferes with the 173 keV $^{111}$In peak at 4 hours. At 24 hours we use a 10 percent window at the 140 keV and 173 keV peaks and a 20 percent window at the 247 keV peak. By 24 hours the $^{99m}$Tc has mostly decayed, thus decreasing the interference, while the additional counts from the 173 keV $^{111}$In peak add significantly to the count-poor $^{111}$In leukocyte image. One needs to evaluate possible spectral overlap on each of the camera systems used for imaging, because there appears to be some variation among different types of equipment.

## Diagnostic Approaches

Classically the three-phase bone scan finding in osteomyelitis has intense focal accumulation of activity in the same location on the flow, blood pool, and bone phases (Fig. 1). Cellulitis has increased flow and diffuse blood pool activity that cannot be localized to a focal area of bone. The bone phase is either normal or has diffuse increased activity caused by increased blood flow, but no focal increased activity (Fig. 2).

Using the combined three-phase bone scan and $^{111}$In leukocyte scan, the $^{111}$In leukocytes produce the sensitivity and specificity, while the $^{99m}$Tc bone image provides the anatomic landmarks. We photograph the bone images and $^{111}$In leukocyte images on separate sheets of film. By carefully overlaying the films, we determine if the activity is within or outside of the bone. If the $^{111}$In leukocyte activity overlies the bone in both orthogonal projections, it is osteomyelitis (Fig. 4). If the $^{111}$In leukocyte activity is outside of the bone on either of the orthogonal projections, the diagnosis is cellulitis (see Fig. 3). Oblique views are obtained if the orthogonal views are not diagnostic.

Three minor points need to be considered when interpreting the combined three-phase bone scan and $^{111}$In leukocyte scan. First, if the $^{111}$In leukocyte activity is questionable, or minimal and diffuse, we call the study negative. I think this minimizes the false-positive results seen with fractures and the like. Generally osteomyelitis has definitely present, moderately intense, and focal $^{111}$In leukocyte activity. Second, the bone scan rarely is normal in the suspected area. If this occurs, it is unlikely to be osteomyelitis even if the $^{111}$In leukocyte activity is difficult to localize (see Fig. 3). Third, the more focal uptake observed at 4 hours is often better at localizing the infection to the bone or soft tissue than are the 24 hour images. However, slow migration of $^{111}$In leukocytes, usually in chronic infections, may result in $^{111}$In leukocyte activity that is clearly seen at 24 hours, but may be poorly seen or absent at 4 hours.

## Conclusion

Our diagnostic approach to osteomyelitis is summarized by the diagnostic decision tree (Fig. 5).

*Acknowledgment.* I wish to express my appreciation to Kathy Carlson for her help in the preparation of this manuscript. Her salary and the studies at Indiana University were supported in part by NIH 1R01 AR 36460.

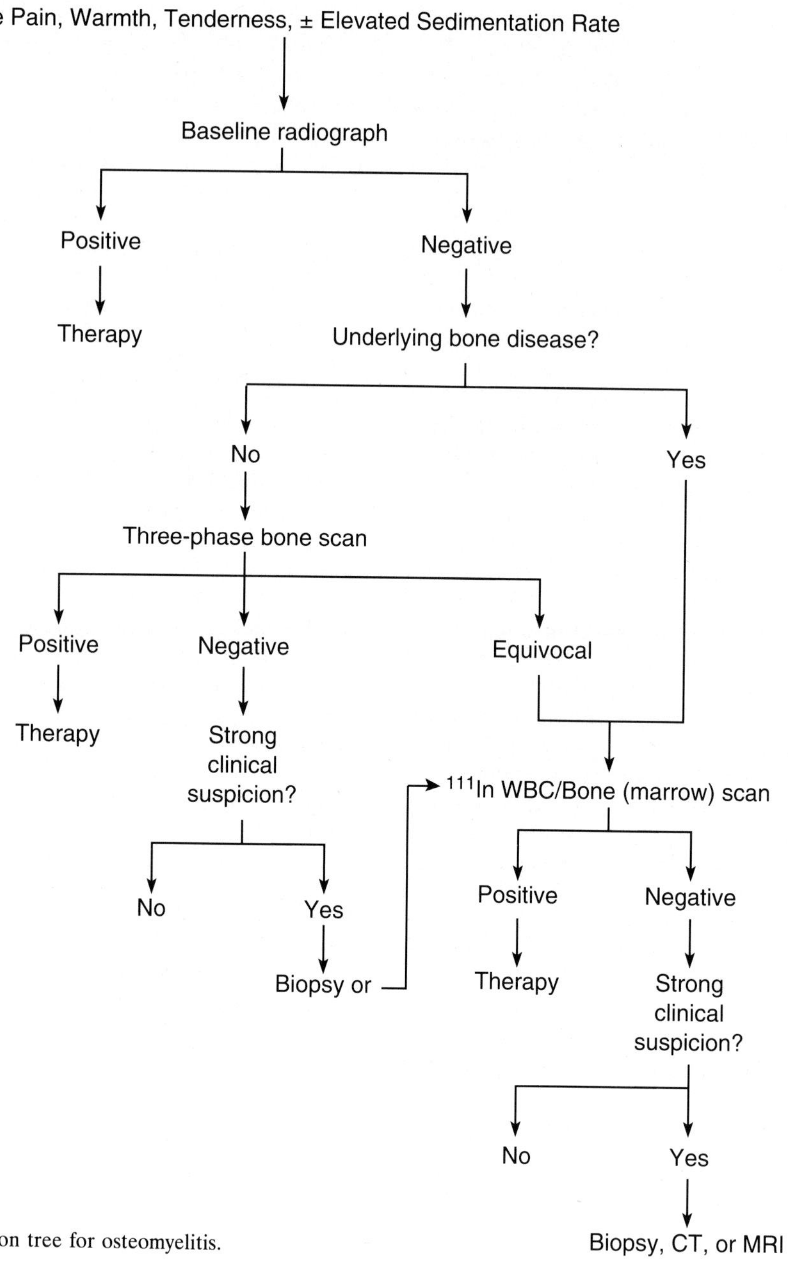


**FIGURE 5** Diagnostic decision tree for osteomyelitis.

## Suggested Reading


Esterhai JL, Goll SR, McCarthy KE, et al. Indium-111 leukocyte scintigraphic detection of subclinical osteomyelitis complicating delayed and nonunion long bone fractures: A prospective study. J Orthop Res 1987; 5:1–6.

Jacobson AF, Harley JD, Lipsky BA, Pecoraro RE. Diagnosis of osteomyelitis in the presence of soft tissue infection and radiologic evidence of osseous abnormalities: Value of leukocyte scintigraphy. Am J Roentgenol 1991; 157:807–812.

Kim EE, Haynie TP, Podoloff DA, et al. Radionuclide imaging in the evaluation of osteomyelitis and septic arthritis. Crit Rev Diagn Imaging 1989; 29:257–305.

McAfee JG, Thakur MC. Survey of radioactive agents for in vitro labeling of phagocytic leukocytes: I—Soluble agents. J Nucl Med 1976; 17:480–487.

Schauwecker DS. Osteomyelitis: Diagnosis with In-111 labeled leukocytes. Radiology 1989; 171:141–146.

Schauwecker DS. The scintigraphic diagnosis of osteomyelitis. Am J Roentgenol 1992; 158:9–18.

Schauwecker DS, Park HM, Burt RW, et al. Combined bone scintigraphy and indium-111 leukocyte scans in neuropathic foot disease. J Nucl Med 1988; 29:1651–1655.

Seabold JE, Nepola JV, Conrad GR, et al. Detection of osteomyelitis at fracture nonunion sites: Comparison of two scintigraphic methods. Am J Roentgenol 1989; 152:1021–1027.

# Scintigraphic Evaluation of Infected Hip and Knee Replacements

CHRISTOPHER J. PALESTRO, M.D.

Total hip replacement, which is performed approximately 120,000 times per year in this country, is the most successful surgery available for patients with advanced osteoarthritis and rheumatoid arthritis of the hip. The clinical results of total knee replacement, also performed about 120,000 times yearly, are similar to those achieved with hip replacements in terms of pain relief, function, and implant longevity. Despite the well-documented success of these procedures, however, complications including fracture, dislocation, loosening, and infection do occur. Although all of these complications are serious and may necessitate surgical intervention, none is more serious or more difficult to diagnose than prosthetic infection. To date no single diagnostic procedure has proven to be completely satisfactory for diagnosing the infected joint replacement. This is borne out by the fact that although the rate of infection following primary hip or knee arthroplasty is less than 5 percent, the rate of infection following revision arthroplasty has been reported to be as high as 38 percent. Therefore accurate preoperative diagnosis and treatment of the infected joint replacement is essential to the success of any contemplated revision.

Although overt sepsis may be diagnosed on clinical grounds, detection of occult sepsis remains a diagnostic challenge. The most common clinical presentation of a patient with an infected prosthesis is that of pain; however, this pain is indistinguishable from that caused by loosening or other postoperative complications of joint replacement and is of little value in the diagnosis of the patient's condition. Of the various modalities used to identify the infected joint replacement, most have met with mixed results. Laboratory tests such as the erythrocyte sedimentation rate, peripheral leukocyte count, and febrile response lack both sensitivity and specificity, as does plain radiography. Joint aspiration, although highly specific, is relatively insensitive.

## Alternative Technologies

Radionuclide studies that have been used to diagnose infected joint replacements include technetium-99m bone scintigraphy, gallium-67 citrate scintigraphy, and indium-111 leukocyte scintigraphy, performed alone and in various combinations. Bone scintigraphy, though exquisitely sensitive, suffers from a lack of specificity and cannot consistently differentiate infection from other causes of increased bone mineral turnover such as tumor, fracture, and arthritis. Moreover, in the case of hip arthroplasty, this study is particularly unreliable during the first 12 months following implantation; in the case of knee replacement, it may be necessary to perform serial studies over time if the results are to be meaningful. Sequential bone gallium imaging has been used in an effort to improve the accuracy of diagnosing joint replacement infection. Unfortunately gallium localizes in any region of increased osseous activity, and though better than bone imaging alone, the overall accuracy of this dual-tracer modality is only between 60 and 80 percent.

$^{111}$In-labeled leukocyte imaging would appear to be an ideal technique for identifying infected joint replacements, inasmuch as leukocytes do not generally accumulate at sites of increased bone mineral turnover in the absence of infection. However, the published results of labeled leukocyte imaging performed for joint replacement infection have varied greatly, with the reported sensitivity and specificity of the technique ranging from 50 to 100 percent and 23 to 100 percent, respectively. When leukocyte images are interpreted in isolation, they are typically classified as positive or negative for infection based on a comparison of uptake in the region of interest with uptake in some reference point; in the case of joint replacements, the reference point is typically an area of presumably normal bone marrow. The principal difficulty in using labeled leukocyte imaging alone is the inability of this procedure to differentiate labeled leukocyte activity in aberrant, but otherwise normal, marrow from activity caused by infection. Although the normal distribution of marrow in adults includes the axial skeleton, humeral and femoral heads, femoral trochanters, and proximal femoral shafts, there is considerable individual variation. Further, marrow distribution may be altered by underlying conditions such as tumor, previous radiation therapy, sickle cell disease, and Gaucher's disease, among others. Alterations in the normal distribution of marrow through surgical manipulation have been demonstrated in animals, and it is likely that the implantation of orthopedic hardware also produces alterations in the distribution of otherwise normal marrow. Consequently the selection of an appropriate reference point can be difficult, if not impossible. Therefore it is frequently not possible, on the basis of leukocyte imaging alone, to distinguish labeled leukocyte activity caused by marrow from labeled leukocyte activity caused by infection. This limitation to leukocyte imaging has been observed by several investigators, and two dual-tracer studies have been used in an effort to overcome this problem: combined leukocyte/bone and combined leukocyte/marrow imaging. I have had excellent results with the latter technique, and it is my opinion that among currently available procedures, leukocyte/marrow imaging should be the procedure of choice for diagnosing infected joint replacements.

The principle of leukocyte/marrow imaging is based on the fact that both labeled leukocyte and sulfur colloid images reflect radiotracer accumulation in the reticuloendothelial cells (fixed macrophages) of the bone marrow (Fig. 1). Alterations in the distribution of marrow that is otherwise normal produce similar, or congruent, images on both studies (Fig. 2). Infection, however, exerts opposite effects on leukocytes and sulfur colloid. While stimulating leukocyte accumulation, bony infection decreases sulfur colloid uptake. These inverse effects result in incongruent images and permit one to discriminate labeled leukocyte activity caused by infection from activity caused by aberrant, but not abnormal, marrow.

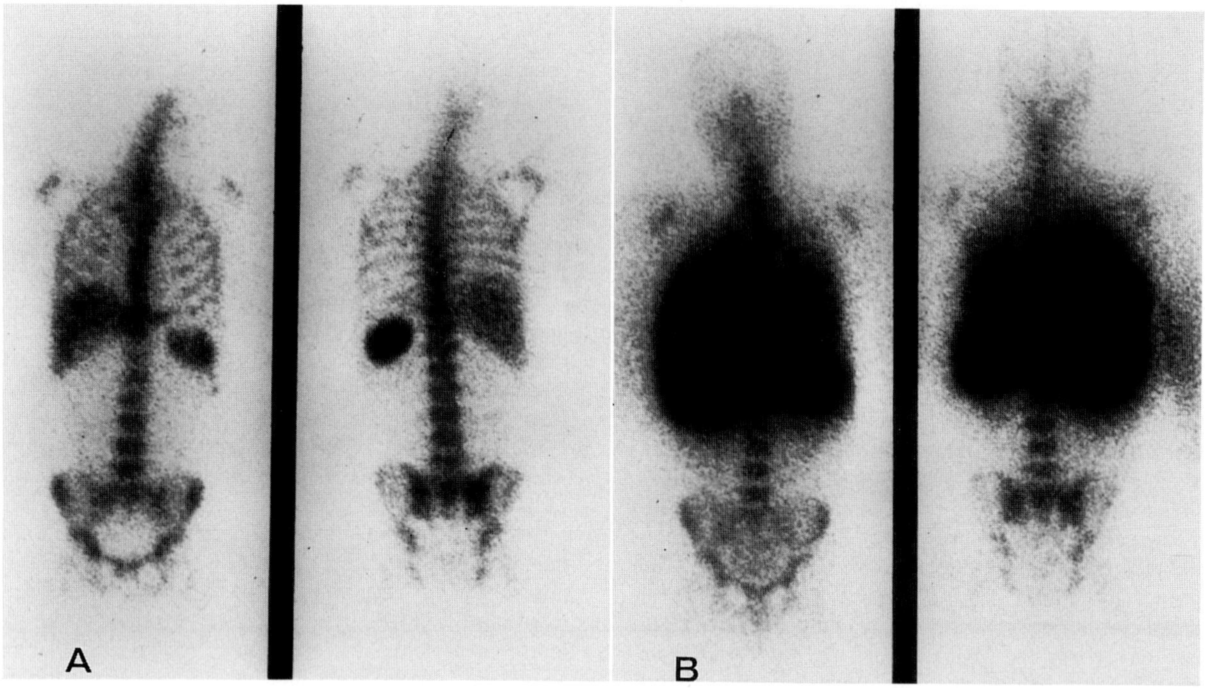


**FIGURE 1** *A,* Anterior and posterior whole-body images of a 38-year-old man performed 24 hours after injection of ~18.5 MBq of mixed autologous leukocytes labeled with $^{111}$In oxine. The distribution of marrow activity is normal. *B,* Anterior and posterior whole-body images performed on the same individual as in *(A),* 1 hour after injection of approximately 370 MBq of $^{99m}$Tc sulfur colloid. The spatial distribution of marrow activity in this study is similar or congruent with that in *(A)* (less liver-spleen activity actually permits better visualization of central marrow on the leukocyte study).

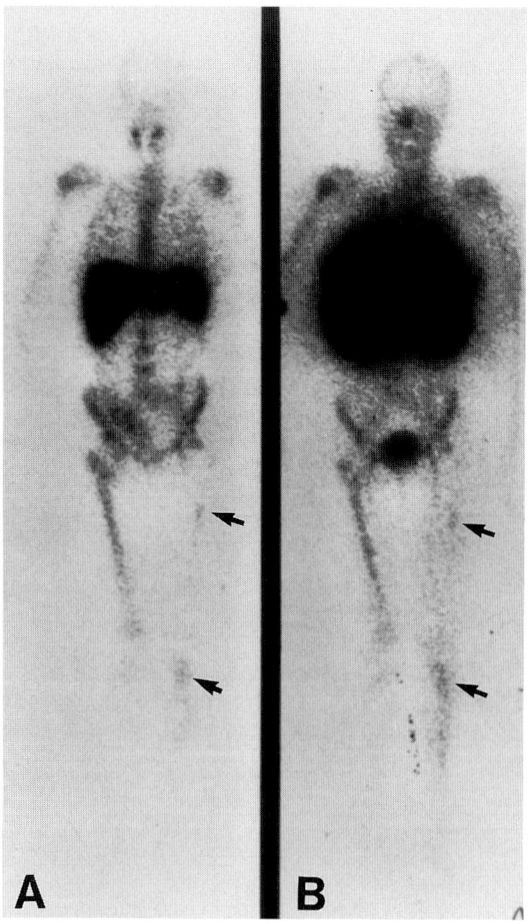


**FIGURE 2** Anterior whole-body leukocyte *(A)* and sulfur colloid marrow *(B)* images of a 43-year-old woman with a history of extensive left lower extremity trauma. Scattered foci of increased activity in the left midfemur and left tibia are present on the leukocyte images *(arrows).* However, the same foci are also seen on the marrow study *(arrows),* confirming that they are sites of (aberrant) marrow activity, not infection. Moderate marrow expansion into the distal right femur is present. (There was no explanation for the uptake in the right lower quadrant [presumably large bowel] present on the leukocyte images.)

## Technique

I recommend that the leukocyte/marrow study be performed as follows. Leukocyte imaging should be performed approximately 24 hours after injection of ~18.5 MBq (500 μCi) of mixed autologous leukocytes labeled with $^{111}$In oxine, according to the standard technique as described by Thakur. Six minute anterior and posterior images of the joint replacement(s) (hips or knees) should be performed on a large-field-of-view gamma camera equipped with a medium-energy parallel hole collimator, using 20 percent windows centered over the 174 and 247 keV photopeaks of $^{111}$In. The leukocyte images should be carefully evaluated for the presence or absence of periprosthetic activity. If no periprosthetic activity is present, the study is negative for infection and the procedure is terminated. If, however, as is generally the case, periprosthetic activity is observed, then marrow imaging with technetium-99m sulfur colloid should be performed. Immediately after completion of the leukocyte study, the patient is injected with ~370 MBq (10 mCi) of $^{99m}$Tc sulfur colloid. One to two hours later, 6 minute anterior and posterior static images of the region of interest are obtained on a large-field-of-view gamma camera (preferably the same camera used for the leukocyte images) equipped with a low-energy, high-resolution, parallel hole collimator using a 10 percent window centered on the 140 keV photopeak of $^{99m}$Tc. Although I have found that the contribution of $^{111}$In photons to the technetium image is minimal, I strongly recommend that this be verified by each individual laboratory: for at least the first few studies, before injecting the patient with sulfur colloid, a 6 minute anterior image of the region of interest, using the aforementioned parameters for marrow imaging, should be obtained to confirm that the contribution of $^{111}$In photons to the technetium image is in fact negligible.

Excellent results have also been obtained when sulfur colloid imaging is performed before the leukocyte study. My preference, however, is to perform marrow imaging after the leukocyte study, because approximately 25 percent of the patients I have studied have demonstrated no periprosthetic leukocyte activity; consequently there is no reason for these individuals to undergo marrow imaging.

Although most of the studies reported have used sulfur colloid as the marrow-imaging agent, equally satisfactory results have, not surprisingly, been described using albumin colloid for the marrow phase of the procedure.

## Study Interpretation

The interpretation of leukocyte/marrow imaging is fairly straightforward. Those studies in which the distribution of both radiotracers is spatially similar, or in which the extent of activity on sulfur colloid images exceeds the extent of activity on the leukocyte images, are classified as congruent and negative for infection (Fig. 3). Those studies in which there is periprosthetic activity on leukocyte images, without corresponding activity on marrow images, are classified as incongruent and positive for infection (Fig. 4).

## Results

To date the results obtained with leukocyte/marrow imaging have been uniformly excellent, with the overall accuracy of the study ranging between 89 and 98 percent. When the prevalence of disease in a particular patient population is low, the value of a given test is best determined by its specificity, since even a slight decrease in specificity can have a considerable (adverse) effect on the positive predictive value of the study. Even in the highly select populations that have been studied, the overall prevalence of infected joint replacements is only about 25 percent, yet the reported specificity of the procedure has ranged from 92 to 100 percent, confirming the value of leukocyte/marrow imaging for diagnosing this entity.

## Pitfalls

Despite the excellent results obtained with leukocyte/marrow imaging, the accuracy of the procedure is still less than 100 percent, and both false-positive and false-negative studies do occur.

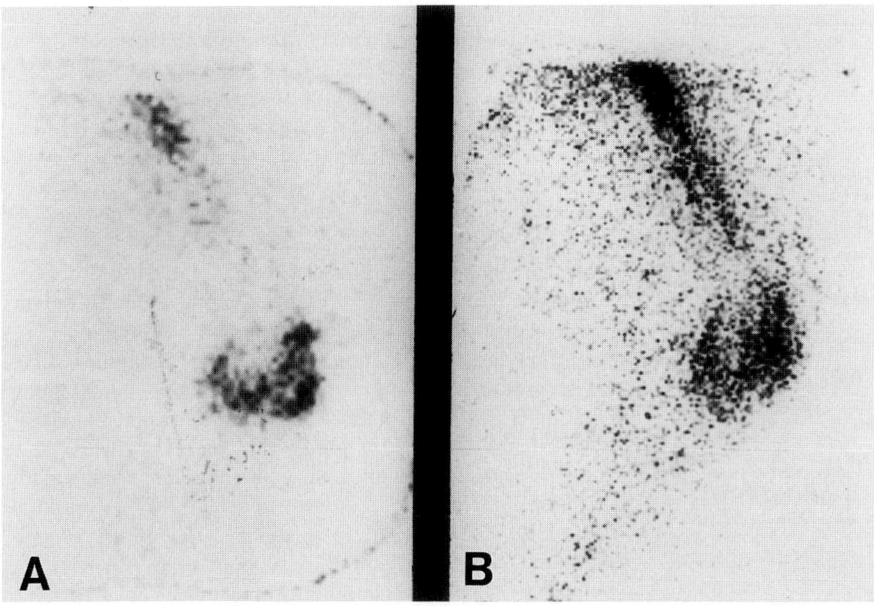


**FIGURE 3** *A,* Anterior leukocyte image of a left knee prosthesis implanted in an 80-year-old woman 8 years previously, demonstrates intense periprosthetic activity. *B,* Marrow images performed 1 hour later are congruent. (Note also the extension of marrow into the distal left femur.) A loose but uninfected prosthesis was surgically removed.

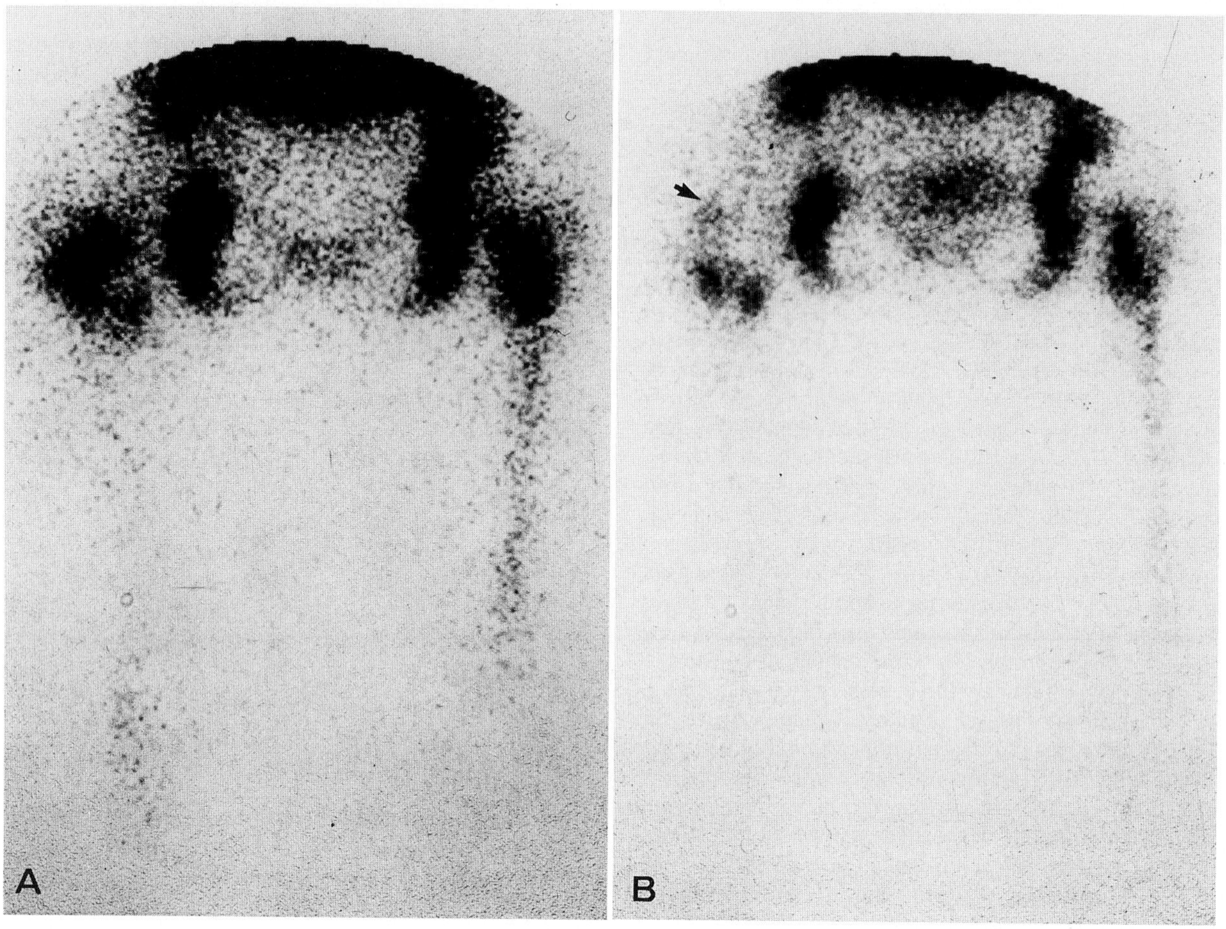


**FIGURE 4** *A,* Posterior leukocyte image of a woman with a left-sided total hip replacement implanted 3 years previously. The intensity and pattern of distribution of activity around both hips on the leukocyte image are similar. *B,* Posterior marrow image reveals incongruent distribution of activity in the proximal aspect of the left femoral component *(arrow).* Operative cultures grew *Staphylococcus aureus.*

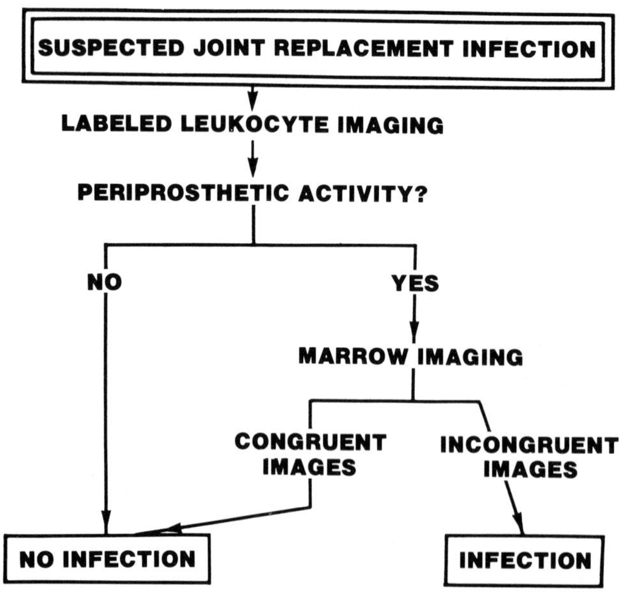


**FIGURE 5** A simple diagnostic algorithm for evaluating the patient with suspected infection of a joint replacement.

There are two conditions that can result in a false-positive leukocyte/marrow study. One potential problem is extravasation of the marrow agent at the time of injection. This problem is easily prevented by routinely viewing both the injection site and the liver and spleen before imaging the region of interest and, if necessary, reinjecting the patient with additional radiotracer. A second, more difficult, problem is the presence of extraosseous infection (i.e., cellulitis or inflammatory arthritis). Both of these conditions can result in incongruent leukocyte/marrow images, even in the absence of prosthetic infection. In the case of cellulitis, additional lateral or oblique views may help to more precisely localize the site of infection.

Inflammatory arthritis presents a more difficult problem. The success of leukocyte imaging is based on white blood cell migration and accumulation in response to a stimulus. While we generally equate such stimuli with infection, noninfectious conditions may also induce an intense white blood cell response. In the case of joints, rheumatoid arthritis, acute gouty arthritis, and pseudogout induce an intense neutrophilic response, and labeled leukocyte uptake in these conditions cannot be distinguished from uptake in a septic process. Although I know of no way to completely eliminate this potential problem, it is important for the nuclear physician to be aware of this pitfall, and in the proper clinical setting it may be reasonable to defer the study until the acute inflammatory condition has resolved.

In addition to the technical problem of dose infiltration or white blood cell damage during preparation, there are two potential causes of a false-negative study. The only one I have personally observed is not related to the dual-tracer technique itself but rather to a total absence of periprosthetic uptake of labeled leukocytes even in the presence of infection, a failure I am currently unable to explain. I have encountered this problem in 2 of 28 patients with infected joint replacements. Excluding individuals with no periprosthetic leukocyte activity, the sensitivity of leukocyte/marrow imaging in our laboratory is 100 percent.

A second potential false-negative result is related to uptake of the marrow agent in the presence of infection, since normal marrow images have been observed early in the course of osteomyelitis. I think that this is an unlikely event in patients with infected joint replacements, however, insomuch as these individuals are typically symptomatic for some time before imaging and hence not likely to be studied early in the course of their disease. In over 130 joint replacements studied to date, I have yet to observe congruent leukocyte/marrow imaging in the presence of infection.

In summary, although the diagnosis of the infected joint replacement is not an easy task, leukocyte/marrow imaging has overcome many of the limitations inherent in other scintigraphic techniques, including leukocyte imaging alone. In my opinion, among the currently available studies, it should be the procedure of choice for diagnosing this entity (Fig. 5).

## Suggested Reading

Harris WH, Sledge CB. Total hip and total knee replacement (Part I). N Engl J Med 1990; 323:725–731.

Harris WH, Sledge CB. Total hip and total knee replacement (Part II). N Engl J Med 1990; 323:801–807.

King AD, Peters AM, Stuttle AWJ, Lavender JP. Imaging of bone infection with labelled white blood cells: Role of contemporaneous bone marrow imaging. Eur J Nucl Med 1990; 17:148–151.

Maderazo EG, Judson S, Pasternak H. Late infections of total joint prostheses. A review and recommendations for prevention. Clin Orthop 1988; 229:131–142.

Mulamba L'AH, Ferrant A, Leners N, et al. Indium-111 leukocyte scanning in the evaluation of painful hip arthroplasty. Acta Orthop Scand 1983; 54:695–697.

Palestro CJ, Kim CK, Swyer AJ, et al. Total-hip arthroplasty: Periprosthetic indium-111-labeled leukocyte activity and complementary technetium-99m-sulfur colloid imaging in suspected infection. J Nucl Med 1990; 31:1950–1955.

Palestro CJ, Roumanas P, Swyer AJ, et al. Diagnosis of musculoskeletal infection using combined $^{111}$In labeled leukocyte and $^{99m}$Tc sulfur colloid marrow imaging. Clin Nucl Med 1992; 17:269–273.

Palestro CJ, Swyer AJ, Kim CK, Goldsmith SJ. Infected knee prosthesis: Diagnosis with In-111 leukocyte, Tc-99m sulfur colloid, and Tc-99m MDP imaging. Radiology 1991; 179:645–648.

Seabold JE, Nepola JV, Marsh JL, et al. Postoperative bone marrow alterations: Potential pitfalls in the diagnosis of osteomyelitis with In-111-labeled leukocyte scintigraphy. Radiology 1991; 180:741–747.

Thakur ML, Lavender JP, Arnot RN, et al. Indium-111-labeled autologous leukocytes in man. J Nucl Med 1977; 18:1014–1021.

# Scintigraphic Detection of Skeletal Metastases

*JAMES H. THRALL, M.D.*

The most common clinical application of skeletal scintigraphy is in the evaluation of patients with extraskeletal primary malignancies to detect skeletal metastatic disease. In many patients the presence and/or extent of skeletal metastases directly influences treatment decisions and prognosis. In patients with established skeletal metastatic disease, response to therapy may be assessed by skeletal scintigraphy.

## Technique

Modern gamma scintillation camera systems offer the ability to image the skeleton using either a spot view or a whole-body approach. Whole-body imaging has the advantage of providing anatomic continuity of image data (Fig. 1). Spot views provide significantly higher resolution but run the risk of missing portions of the skeleton if sufficient overlap between images is not achieved. A useful compromise is to obtain an initial whole-body survey followed by high-resolution, high-count (1,000 K), supplementary spot views of suspicious or symptomatic areas. Patients are asked to empty their bladders immediately before imaging, and care is taken to avoid contamination of the skin or misinterpretation of urinary contamination as soft-tissue or skeletal lesions.

Single-photon emission computed tomography (SPECT) is not suitable for whole-body skeletal surveys but provides high-resolution, high-contrast, regional imaging for difficult or questionable areas. Dynamic and quantitative skeletal scintigraphy have not found routine applicability in studies to detect metastatic disease.

Technetium-99m diphosphonate is the radiopharmaceutical of choice for skeletal scintigraphy; 15 to 20 mCi is used in adults, with doses reduced appropriately for children.

## Pathophysiology of Skeletal Metastases: Basis of Scintigraphic and Radiographic Detection

Nonosseous neoplasms gain access to the skeleton via three mechanisms: (1) direct extension, (2) retrograde venous flow, and (3) via the arterial circulation after venous or lymphatic access. The initial seeding of metastatic deposits via the arterial circulation is typically in the red marrow, which helps explain the predominance of metastatic lesions in the axial skeleton. In normal adults the red marrow is distributed to the bones of the axial skeleton, including the cranium, and the proximal portions of the femurs and humeri. Over 90 percent of metastatic lesions are found in this distribution, with only a small percentage outside of red marrow–bearing areas.

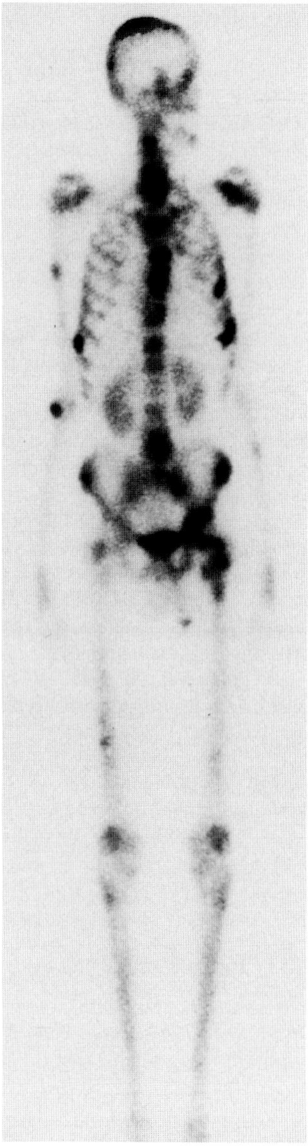

**FIGURE 1** Anterior view of whole-body scintigram in a patient with multiple skeletal metastases from cancer of the prostate. Virtually all areas of the skeleton are involved, with lesions distributed randomly. (From Thrall JH, Ellis BI. Skeletal metastases. Rad Clin North Am 1987; 25:1155–1170; with permission.)

As metastatic lesions grow in the marrow space, the surrounding bone remodels through osteoclastic (resorptive) and osteoblastic (depositional) activity. The relative degree of bone resorption and deposition elicited is highly variable between different types of tumors and sometimes even between different locations for the same tumor. The relationship between the two remodeling processes determines whether a metastatic deposit appears as predominantly lytic or sclerotic or presents a mixed pattern radiographically.

Radionuclide bone scintigrams are highly sensitive for detecting the altered local metabolism in areas of skeletal remodeling associated with metastatic deposits. On the other hand, a 30 to 50 percent change in bone density is required before small lesions can be detected radiographically.

These observations are reflected in a characteristic sequence of image findings for skeletal scintigrams and standard radiographs. Early in the natural history of the metastatic lesion, both the skeletal scintigram and standard radiograph are negative. As the metastases grow, bone remodeling results in increased skeletal metabolism and increased tracer localization; the scintigram becomes positive and the radiograph remains negative. As the process continues, net calcium content and skeletal trabecular architecture change; the scintigram remains positive and the standard radiograph also becomes abnormal. This sequence occurs over a period of weeks to months.

If healing occurs as a result of therapy, the bone scintigram may revert to negative, whereas the radiograph typically remains abnormal although there are occasional exceptions. If the cancerous process is highly indolent or diffusely lytic, the skeletal scintigram may fail to reveal an abnormality. This is due in turn to a failure to alter bone metabolism or local blood flow sufficiently to produce a focally detectable lesion. Multiple myeloma is a notorious cause of false-negative skeletal scintigrams on this basis.

It is also important to realize that the skeletal tracers do not localize mainly in the cancerous tissue per se, but in the remodeling, metabolically active bone surrounding or being invaded by the metastatic tissues. This is well illustrated in Figure 2, depicting the growth of a metastatic lesion in the calvarium. The circular rim of increased tracer uptake is in the reactive bone surrounding the cancerous tissue. As the cancer enlarges, the rim is displaced as bone is completely destroyed. The central cancerous tissue is photon deficient without tracer uptake.

Magnetic resonance imaging (MRI) has suggested a new approach to the early detection of skeletal metastases. The intense, uniform signal from marrow fat is altered by metastatic lesions. It has been demonstrated in a number of studies that early lesions in the marrow can be detected before they elicit a sufficient osteogenic response to be detected by scintigraphy. The major problems in the use of MRI for this application are the difficulty in surveying the entire skeleton and the frequent presence of incidental benign defects in marrow fat unrelated to metastatic disease, making the specificity of the observation problematic.

Although the sensitivity of the bone scan is significantly greater than standard radiography as a survey technique, the actual difference in sensitivity depends on the stage of disease being evaluated. In early disease the sensitivity of the bone scintigram is several-fold greater and the sensitivity is also significantly greater on a "per lesion" basis. However, if all patients with metastatic disease are considered, including patients with advanced disease, the relative superiority is less because both types of evaluations are positive in a higher percentage of cases. The accuracy of skeletal scintigraphy will never be precisely known because of the lack of a gold standard for comparison. The sensitivity for detecting metastatic disease is often quoted as high as 95 percent or above. The specificity is also difficult to assess but, conservatively, is probably also in the range of 90 percent.

## Scintigraphic Patterns in Metastatic Disease

The scintigraphic patterns encountered in skeletal metastatic disease are summarized in Table 1, and a decision tree or

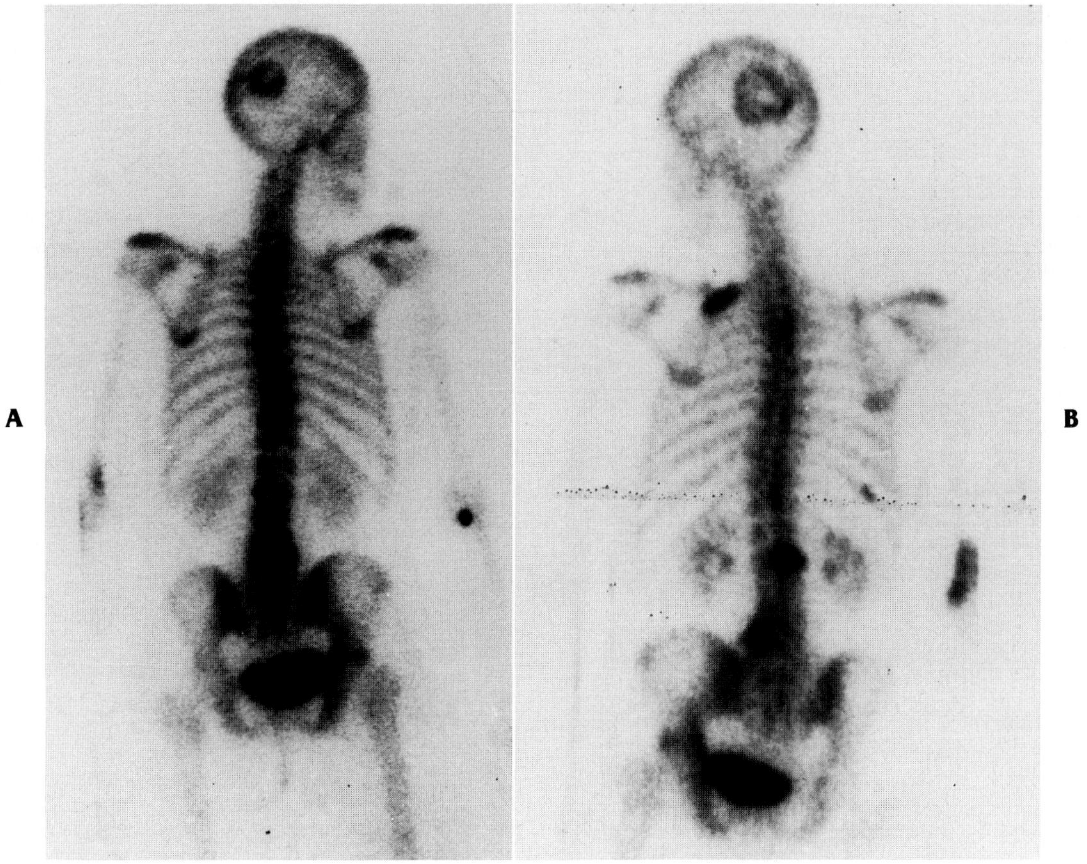

**FIGURE 2** *A,* Posterior view from Tc-99m diphosphonate skeletal scintigram. Note the doughnut configuration of tracer uptake in the skull lesion. *B,* Follow-up scintigram six months later. The skull metastasis has enlarged. Uptake of tracer is in the rim of reactive bone around the lesion.

**TABLE 1** Scintigraphic Patterns in Metastatic Disease

| |
|---|
| Multiple areas of increased tracer accumulation |
| Solitary "hot" lesions |
| Diffusely increased uptake ("superscan") |
| "Flare" phenomenon |
| Cold- or photon-deficient lesions |

algorithm for the workup of patients with proven nonosseous primary tumors is provided in Figure 3. The point of entry in the algorithm is the whole-body bone scintigram. If the evaluation is positive and characteristic for metastatic disease, the screening workup is complete. The classic "typical" pattern that provides the most diagnostic certainty is the presence of multiple randomly distributed focal lesions distributed throughout the axial skeleton (see Fig. 1).

However, there are a number of other conditions that may also result in multiple scintigraphic abnormalities (Table 2). A key feature in recognizing nonmetastatic causes for multifocal scan abnormalities is the pattern of distribution. For example, in both Cushing's syndrome and osteomalacia, there are frequently a disproportionate number of rib lesions (Fig. 4) as compared with other areas. In patients with osteoporosis, a recognition of dorsal kyphosis and patterns of associated fractures such as the H-type fracture of the sacrum provide clues to the correct diagnosis.

Trauma is a frequent cause of multiple lesions, and patients should be routinely questioned for history of trauma. In the ribs there is often a characteristic vertical alignment of fractures as a result of the mechanism of injury in falls or automobile accidents. This nonrandom pattern would not be expected in metastatic disease. Displaced fractures can be recognized by this structural deformity, but otherwise a healing fracture and a metastatic lesion may have an identical appearance scintigraphically. Persistently positive skeletal scintigrams from old trauma are a major interpretative problem, and the issue is discussed in more detail later in the chapter.

Skeletal scintigrams in older subjects almost routinely reveal evidence of osteoarthritis. This is generally recognized by its characteristic locations. The uptake can be highly intense and is not necessarily closely related in degree to current symptoms. Involvement of both sides of a joint is readily observed and is not characteristic of metastatic disease. Medial and lateral compartment arthritis in the knee, changes in the hands and wrists, especially at the base of the first metacarpal, and changes in the shoulder are extremely common scintigraphic findings. Degenerative changes in the lower lumbar spine can present a special problem, because of the high incidence of both metastatic disease and degenerative disease in this location. The pattern of scintigraphic abnormality must be assessed with caution. Degenerative changes typically involve the facet joints and vertebral end plates with hypertrophic spurring. Metastatic disease more typically involves the pedicle and body of the vertebra. The spatial resolution of bone

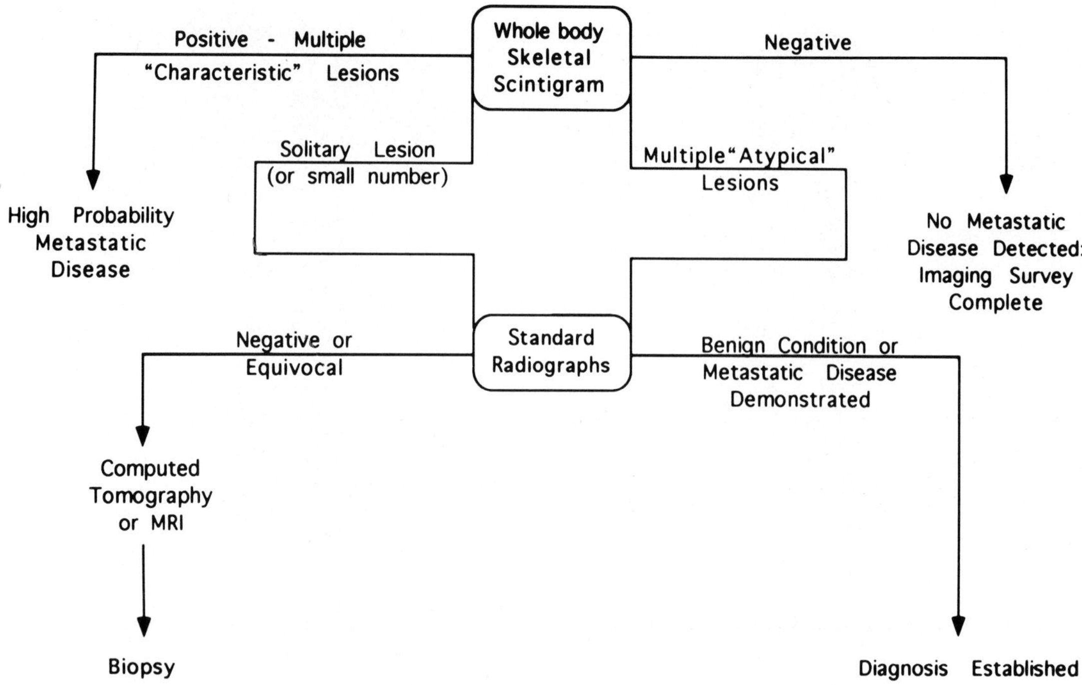


**FIGURE 3** Algorithm for workup of patients with suspected skeletal metastases. (From Thrall JH, Ellis BI. Skeletal metastases. Rad Clin North Am 1987; 25:1155–1170; with permission.)

scintigrams may not be sufficient to make these distinctions. Modern SPECT imaging may be able to make the distinction and should be considered in difficult cases.

Multifocal osteomyelitis can simulate metastatic disease, but from a practical clinical standpoint is not frequently present as an incidental and unsuspected problem in the cancer patient. Conversely Paget's disease of bone is relatively common in the cancer age group, and it may be impossible on the bone scintigram to differentiate Paget's disease from metastatic disease in specific lesions. Paget's disease can be suspected by its characteristic patterns of involvement and the extreme intensity of tracer uptake. In particular, involvement of a hemipelvis, a long portion of a long bone, and expansion of osseous structures all point to Paget's disease. Osteoporosis circumscripta causes a highly characteristic rim pattern of activity in the skull but may also be difficult to distinguish from metastasis. Radiographic correlation is frequently required when the differential diagnosis rests between Paget's disease and metastatic disease.

Multiple infarctions with reactive bone causing increased tracer uptake can also mimic skeletal metastatic disease. This pattern is most commonly observed in patients with sickle cell anemia and is rarely a practical problem. It is recognized by history and the presence of other characteristic changes on the bone scan.

Patients with either solitary scintigraphic abnormalities or a small number of detected lesions present special problems in interpretation and have been the subject of several major clinical studies (Fig. 5). The potential for diagnostic error results from the frequency with which incidental benign conditions involve the skeleton and are detected by bone scintigraphy (Table 3). When a solitary lesion is encountered, it is important to proceed in a systematic fashion using an algorithm such as the one presented in Figure 3. Frequently, standard radiographs confirm the presence of either a metastatic deposit or a benign condition, ending the diagnostic evaluation. If standard radiographs are negative or equivocal, and the presence or absence of metastatic disease is important to clinical decision making, further imaging should be carried out and, if necessary, biopsy.

**TABLE 2** Causes of Multiple Abnormalities

| | |
|---|---|
| Metastatic disease | Osteomyelitis |
| Arthritis | Metabolic bone disease |
| Fractures (osteoporosis) | Bone infarctions |

The most common cause of solitary benign abnormalities is degenerative arthritis followed by healing fracture. Other benign bone lesions including monostotic Paget's disease, enchondroma, frontal osteoma, fibrous dysplasia, and osteomyelitis can also be the cause of solitary abnormalities.

Location and pattern are important scintigraphically. Lesions in the anterior rib ends are rarely caused by metastases. This is a location subject to trauma and the costochondral junction can be highly positive scintigraphically, with no radiographic abnormality following even minor trauma. Conversely 40 to 80 percent of proven solitary lesions in the spine are shown to be metastatic in origin.

In Brown's summary of his experience with bone scintigraphy in a pediatric population combined with other large series from the literature, solitary abnormalities were due to malignancy approximately 55 percent of the time. However, rather than attempting to assign an overall probability of malignancy or a specific probability for each anatomic area, it is more important to simply recognize the potential pitfall presented by the solitary lesion and have a systematic approach.

Another scintigraphic pattern that can cause interpretative problems for the unwary is the "superscan." In some patients

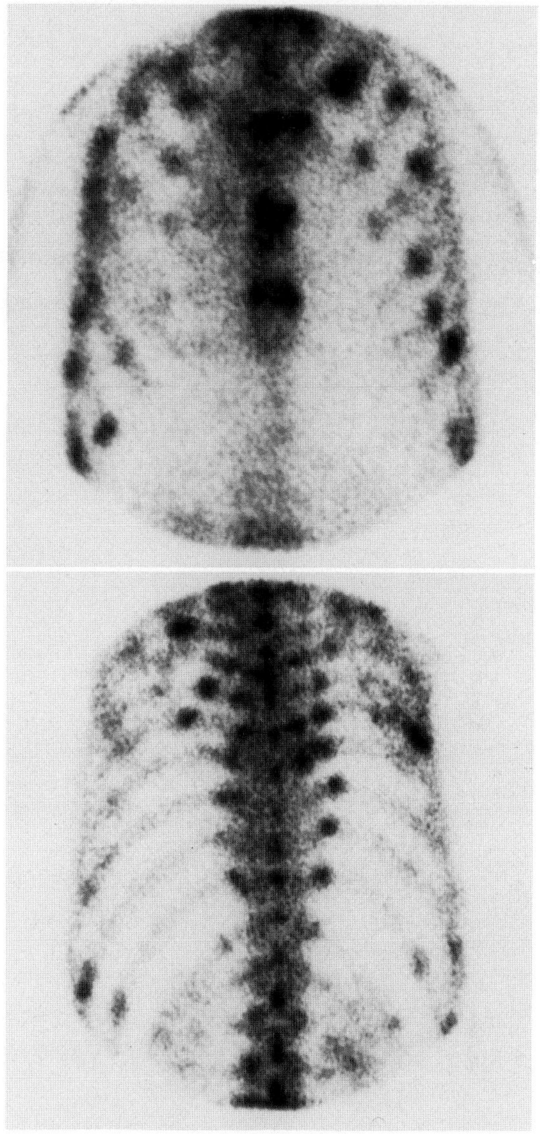

A

B

**FIGURE 4** Anterior *(A)* and posterior *(B)* spot views of the thorax in a patient with osteomalacia. The images demonstrate multiple hot areas due to pseudofractures. (From Thrall JH, Ellis BI. Skeletal metastases. Rad Clin North Am 1987; 25:1155–1170; with permission.)

with breast cancer and prostatic cancer, the entire axial skeleton becomes diffusely and rather uniformly involved with metastatic disease. If the involvement is uniform enough, the scan may appear deceptively normal (Fig. 6). There are a number of clues that provide a tipoff, including unusually good bone to soft-tissue background ratio, absent or faint visualization of the kidneys, and increase in the ratio of tracer uptake in the axial vs. appendicular skeleton. One helpful rule to avoid being fooled by uniform tracer uptake is to review at least one radiograph in every patient undergoing bone scintigraphy. Virtually all patients have had chest radiographs or other studies so that sufficient correlative information is available to avoid this uncommon diagnostic pitfall.

Another potentially perplexing pattern is observed in evaluating follow-up bone scans in patients undergoing cyclic chemotherapy. In some patients who have a good response to chemotherapy, the bone scan appears to paradoxically worsen with a "flare" of increased activity. The hypothesis to explain the flare phenomenon is that as lesions begin to heal following therapy, there is an osteoblastic response, resulting in in-

**TABLE 3** Causes of Solitary Abnormalities

| | |
|---|---|
| Solitary metastasis | Monostotic Paget's disease |
| Fracture | Fibrous dysplasia |
| Arthritis | Frontal osteoma |
| Enchondroma | Osteomyelitis |

A

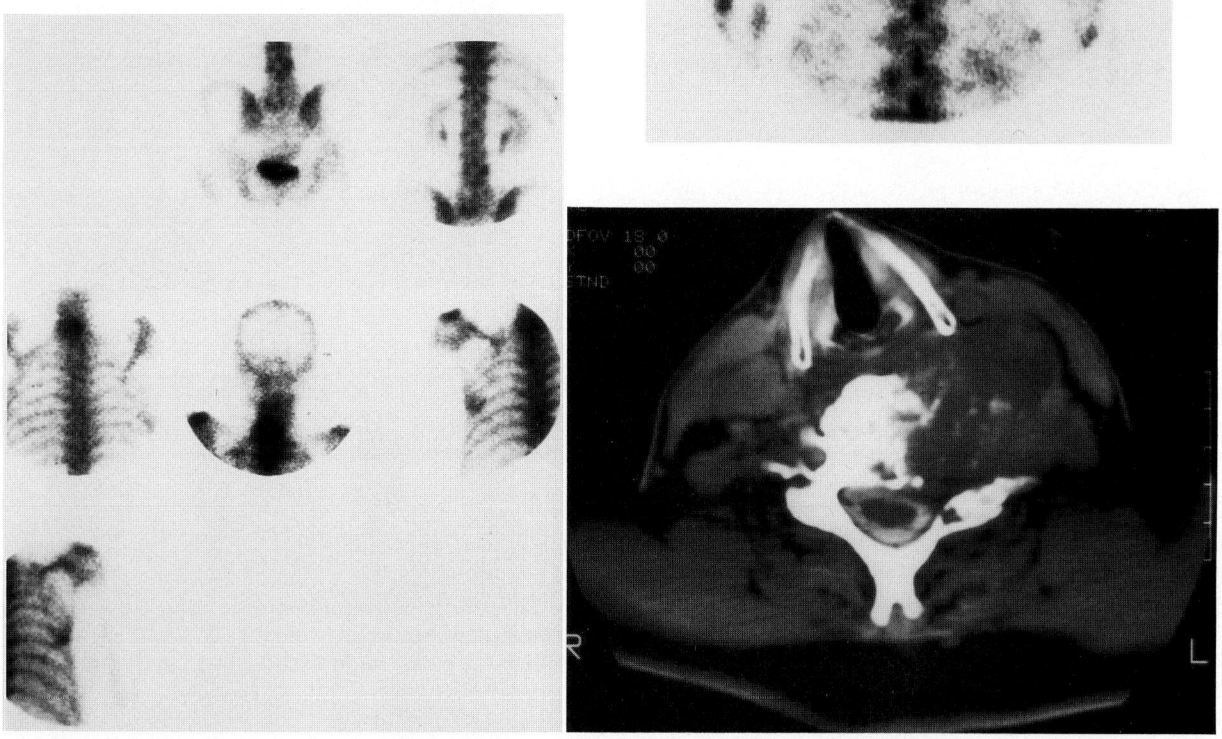


B

**FIGURE 5** *A,* Spot view scintigrams in a patient with lung cancer reveal a solitary abnormality in the lower cervical spine. *B,* Computed tomography reveals extensive bony destruction and soft-tissue mass, confirming the metastatic nature of the scintigraphic abnormality.

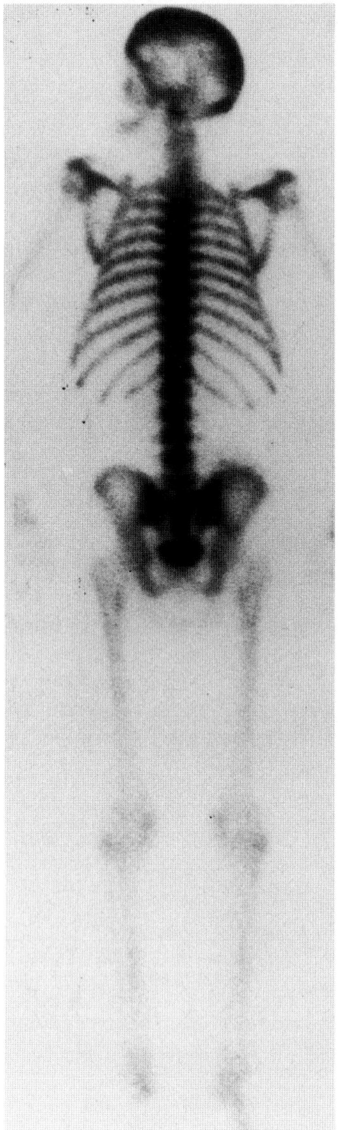

**FIGURE 6** Superscan in a patient with carcinoma of the breast. Note the increased skeleton to soft-tissue uptake ratio, the absence of renal activity, and axioappendicular disproportion in intensity.

creased activity on the scan. Some patients may experience pain in these areas following the onset of chemotherapy, further confusing the issue clinically. When these lesions are followed radiographically, healing with increased sclerosis is seen over two to six months. The flare phenomenon reinforces the fact that tracer uptake is not in tumor tissue but in the surrounding bone.

Some metastatic lesions elicit a predominantly resorptive or destructive response in bone. Areas of the skeleton that are completely replaced by metastatic tumor and/or that are purely lytic radiographically may appear as "cold" or "photon-deficient" lesions on bone scan. Therefore the focal absence of expected normal tracer uptake should be sought on bone scintigrams, as well as areas of focally increased uptake. The photon-deficient area is often bordered by a rim of increased uptake (see Fig. 2).

A more difficult problem is the scintigraphic detection of some lesions that are characterized by a permeative pattern radiographically. As noted in the discussion on pathophysiology, if the neoplastic process is indolent or causes no reactive bone formation, the scan may present as a false negative. This is a particular problem with round cell tumors and with multiple myeloma. If all sites of involvement are considered, the sensitivity of the bone scan in multiple myeloma is low, although studies in the literature suggest that the majority of patients will have some abnormality often due to pathologic fractures. The other major cause of false-negative bone scans is the quiescent or healed lesion that no longer demonstrates increased uptake. This phenomenon may be observed following successful radiation or chemotherapy.

## Primary Bone Tumors

Uptake of skeletal-seeking radiopharmaceuticals in primary bone tumors is avid and frequently striking (Fig. 7). However, skeletal scintigraphy is not commonly used in the workup of patients with osteosarcoma or other primary bone neoplasms, because the radionuclide technique does not answer the questions the orthopedic surgeon must address. The skeletal scintigram does not accurately portray the tumor margins in bone. Nor does the scintigram allow assessment of soft-tissue extent. Plain radiographs, computed tomography, and MRI are better for making these determinations.

There may be a role for skeletal scintigraphy if metastases are suspected. Skeletal scintigraphy is capable of detecting soft-tissue, pulmonary, and skeletal metastatic lesions. It must be emphasized, however, that the value of scintigraphy is for

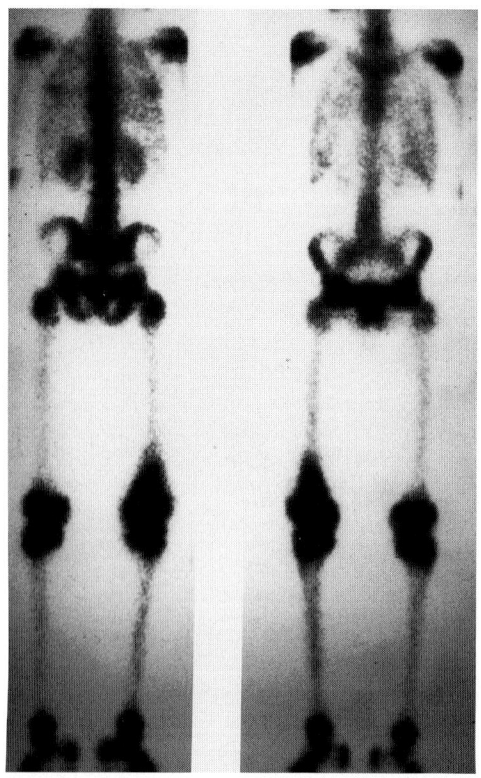

**FIGURE 7** Osteosarcoma of the distal right femur. Uptake is highly intense, equal to that in the epiphyses.

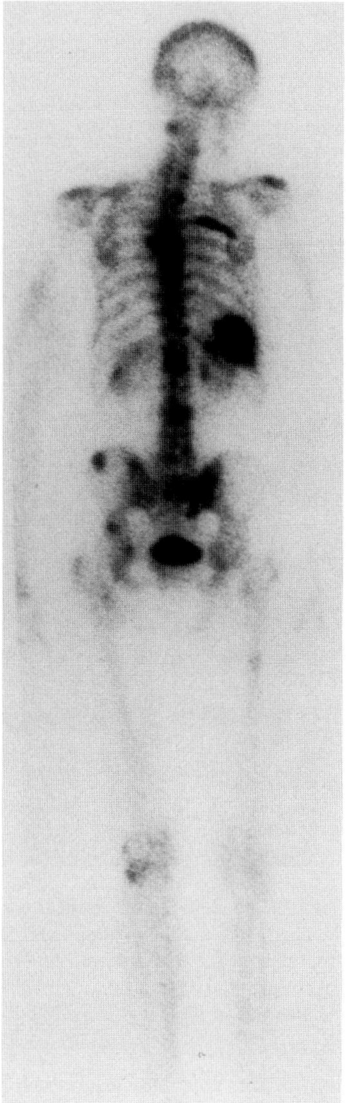

**FIGURE 8** Posterior scintigram in a patient with carcinoma of the breast reveals multiple skeletal metastases and a large area of soft-tissue uptake corresponding to an hepatic metastasis. (From Thrall JH, Ellis BI. Skeletal metastases. Rad Clin North Am 1987; 25:1155–1170; with permission.)

surveying the entire body. If metastases are suspected in a given area, a higher-resolution technique is employed. Thus pulmonary metastases are typically evaluated by computed tomography and not by scintigraphy.

Studies of primary tumors have led to at least one important observation about skeletal tracer uptake. Many tumors elicit a marked hyperemic effect. The increased blood flow is not restricted to the tumor itself, but affects the entire "watershed" distribution of regional flow, most characteristically involving an entire extremity. Thus markedly increased tracer uptake is observed in adjacent structures. The augmented or extended uptake pattern can be observed in other hyperemia-inducing lesions including fractures, osteomyelitis, and nerve injuries resulting in reflex sympathetic dystrophy syndrome.

## Extraskeletal Uptake in Soft-Tissue Neoplasms

A number of common neoplasms demonstrate variable degrees of skeletal-seeking tracer uptake in both primary tumors and soft-tissue metastases (Fig. 8). The mechanism of localization is not well understood, but felt to be a combination of tumor calcification and binding to organic macromolecules. The degree of uptake and the consistency with which it is observed are not sufficient to use the Tc-99m–labeled bone agents as primary tumor-imaging agents, although this has been explored for carcinoma of the breast.

Tumors most frequently imaged in addition to carcinoma of the breast are carcinoma of the lung, metastatic carcinoma of the colon in the liver, and melanoma and neuroblastoma.

## Discussion

Skeletal scintigraphy continues to be a highly valuable tool in the management of patients with cancer. The job of the radiologist is to exploit the exquisite sensitivity of the technique for detecting perturbations in skeletal metabolism, while adding the necessary diagnostic specificity through knowledge of lesion patterns and the natural history of metastatic disease. The strength of skeletal scintigraphy as a diagnostic test remains in the ability to survey the entire skeleton. Adjunctive techniques are used for anatomic and pathologic specificity once an abnormality is detected scintigraphically.

*Acknowledgments.* Portions of the text of this chapter are reprinted with permission from: Thrall JH, Ellis BI. Skeletal metastases. Rad Clin North Am 1987; 25:1155–1170.

## Suggested Reading

Brown ML. Significance of the solitary lesion in pediatric bone scanning. J Nucl Med 1983; 24:114–115.

Charkes ND, Young J, Sklaroff DM. The pathologic basis of the strontium bone scan. JAMA 1968; 206:2482.

Corcoran RJ, Thrall JH, Kyle RW, et al. Solitary abnormalities in bone scans of patients with extraosseous malignancies. Radiology 1976; 121:663–667.

Kaufman RA, Thrall JH, Keyes JW Jr, et al. False negative bone scans in neuroblastoma metastatic to the ends of long bones. AJR 1978; 130:131.

Kim H, Thrall JH, Keyes JW Jr. Skeletal scintigraphy following incidental trauma. Radiology 1979; 130:447–451.

McNeil BJ. Value of bone scanning in neoplastic disease. Semin Nucl Med 1984; 14:277–286.

Pollen JJ, Reznek RH, Talner LB. Lysis of osteoblastic lesions in prostatic cancer: A sign of progression. AJR 1984; 142:1175–1179.

Shirazi PH, Rayudu GVS, Fordham EW. Review of solitary $^{18}$F bone scan lesions. Radiology 1974; 112:369–372.

Shirazi PH, Rayudu GVS, Fordham EW. $^{18}$F bone scanning: Review of indications and results of 1500 scans. Radiology 1974; 122:361.

Sy WM, Patel D, Faunce H. Significance of absent or faint kidney sign on bone scan. J Nucl Med 1975; 16:454–456.

Thrall JH, Ellis BI. Skeletal metastases. Rad Clin North Am 1987; 25:1155–1170.

Thrall JH, Ghaed N, Geslein GE, et al. Pitfalls in Tc-99m polyphosphate skeletal imaging. AJR 1974; 121:739–747.

Tofe AJ, Francis MD, Harvey WJ. Correlation of neoplasms with incidence and localization of skeletal metastases: An analysis of 1355 diphosphonate bone scans. J Nucl Med 1975; 16:986.

Woolfenden JM, Pitt MJ, Durie BGM, et al. Comparison of bone scintigraphy and radiography in multiple myeloma. Radiology 1980; 134:723–728.

# Imaging Evaluation of Joint Replacements

*SUSAN V. KATTAPURAM, M.D.*

The first total joint replacement was performed in 1959 by Sir John Charnley, using a polytetrafluoroethylene acetabulum and a metallic femoral component, both embedded in methacrylate cement. Since then, advances in surgical technique and the materials and designs of prostheses have contributed remarkably to the successful creation of functional and painless joints. The majority of these procedures are hip and knee replacements. In the United States, approximately 120,000 total hips and an equal number of total knees are implanted each year.

The majority of joint replacements are performed using four materials: polyethylene, Silastic, metal, and methacrylate. These substances are biologically inert and usually provoke little if any inflammatory reaction in the adjacent tissues. Wear and tear may cause microscopic particles to be found loose in the joints.

An area of unprecedented advance from Sir Charnley's biomechanical studies was the discovery of a synthetic, biocompatible, low-friction–bearing surface, namely ultrahigh-molecular-weight polyethylene. At that time, when no plastic suitable for use in the human body was available, polyethylene along with a metal back for mechanical support was used for concave articular surfaces such as the acetabulum, tibial plateau, and glenoid fossa. The polyethylene is radiolucent and may be hidden by the metal socket at the hip and shoulder. In the knee it also prevents contact of metal against metal.

Polymeric silicone substances (Silastic) implants are used for reconstruction of small joints of the hand, wrist, and foot; carpal and radial head replacements; and preparation of a soft-tissue bed for tendon grafts and transfers. Overall results have been good; these implants are flexible and resilient and tolerated well by the body, usually eliciting only fibrous encapsulation and a mild foreign-body reaction. However, complications do occur with these implants. Severe giant cell reactive synovitis and lymphadenitis as a result of shedding of silicone particles may cause pain and limitation of motion of the joint. An erosive, destructive arthritis may manifest from fragmentation and loss of volume of the implant. Fracture and dislocation of the prostheses have also been described. Silastic is usually rendered radiopaque during manufacture.

Metal components are used where strength and stiffness are essential. Modern metals used in the fabrication of joint prostheses are super alloys of chromium-cobalt or titanium-aluminum-vanadium for maximum biocompatibility and fatigue strength.

Methylmethacrylate is an acrylic plastic, used in a putty-like form as a cement to fix metallic or polyethylene components to bone. The cement is made radiopaque by the addition of barium sulfate. Bubbles in the cement act as stress risers and are removed from the cement by either centrifugation or vacuum chamber before its use. A polyethylene plug is placed at the bottom of the prepared medullary cavity to prevent flow of cement down the shaft and also to create a closed space around the implant, so cement can be injected under high pressure.

Newer materials that may find a place in prosthetic joint replacement include ceramic and crystalline hydroxyapatite bone substitutes.

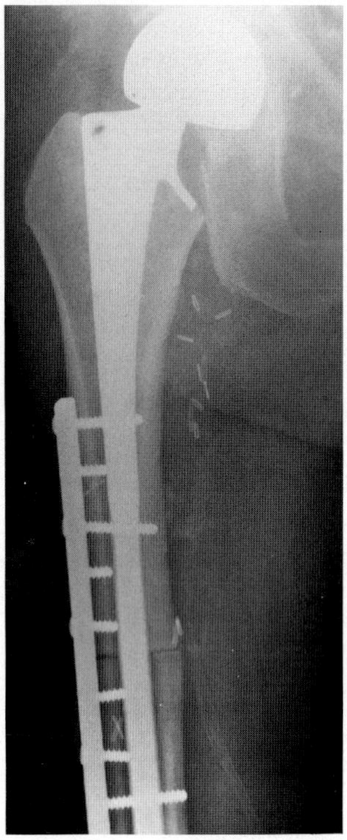

**FIGURE 1** A bipolar hip replacement used in conjunction with a proximal femoral allograft in a young patient who needed extensive bone resection for a tumor. The long femoral stem component of the prosthesis extends through the allograft into the native bone. A plate and screws fix the allograft to the native bone.

Hip prostheses can replace both acetabulum and femur or only the femoral head. Femoral head replacements may be used with an intact acetabulum, fractured femoral neck, or osteonecrosis of the head. The femoral head replacements may be of various types: simple surface replacements without moving parts or bipolar prostheses. The surface replacements articulate directly with the acetabulum and may cause accelerated acetabular wear. The bipolar prostheses have two concentric articulations: the prosthesis with the acetabulum and the femoral stem with the head. Although the acetabular component is not fixed, most of the motion occurs between the stem and the head, saving wear and tear on the acetabulum. Hip replacements may also be used in conjunction with allografts when there is major bone loss from tumor resection, major trauma, or prior surgery (Fig. 1).

In total hip replacements, both femoral and acetabular components are used. In contrast to other major hip surgeries including fusion, osteotomy, and cup arthroplasty, total hip replacement is an entirely biomechanical rather than biologic solution to arthritis of the hip.

The components are fixed either by the use of methacrylate cement or bony ingrowth. The advantages of cement fixation include adequate encasement and protection of the components from corrosion, immediate stable fixation, and elimination of incongruities between the implant and surgical bed. With methacrylate, the following histologic reactions occur in the area adjacent to the cement: (1) 0 to 3 weeks—a zone of necrotic tissue and fibrin is formed; (2) 3 weeks to 2 years—a fibrous layer from repair is formed along the cement-bone interface; and (3) 2 years onward—the histologic appearance becomes stable with a 0.1 to 1.5 mm connective tissue membrane around the cement.

The rationale for bony ingrowth implants lies in the well-established observation that bone grows into a porous surface, even in weight-bearing circumstances, if the porous surface has the proper characteristics. This is a dynamic biologic process and several parameters may influence the amount of bone ingrowth. The porous surface geometry, accuracy of initial fit, degree of rigid fixation, implant design, and weight-bearing loads are some of the key parameters. Major efforts are being made to manipulate the biologic response to enhance bony ingrowth including (1) mechanical attempts to reduce the amount of micromotion; and (2) the use of ceramic coatings containing hydroxyapatite and tricalcium phosphate, which can serve as stimuli to bone formation and the development of useful osteogenic stimuli.

Bony ingrowth occurs in an initial phase and a remodeling phase. The initial phase requires weight-bearing protection, whereas the remodeling phase progresses under weight-bearing conditions.

## Total Hip Replacement

### *Imaging*

Plain films are obtained in the operating room or immediately after surgery to document the position of the prosthesis. This portable film may suggest that the acetabular cup is in too much anteversion or retroversion, often because of the slightly flexed position that is maintained postoperatively. Subsequent films centered on the acetabulum demonstrate the true tilt of the cup. On the frontal view, the femoral stem should be in the center of the medullary cavity or in a slight valgus. When the tip of the stem is near the medial femoral cortex, the prosthesis is in valgus. On the true lateral view, the femoral head should be in 10° of anteversion or neutral position.

Subsequent plain films are the best radiographic method for follow-up. The connective tissue membrane that forms between the bone and cement is demonstrated radiologically by its relative lucency in comparison to the opaque cement on one side and the reactive zone of sclerosis that forms on the other side. In most cases these zones are established by 6 months. This zone is normally 1 to 2 mm in diameter and smooth. A stable position of the components with no change in the lucency between cement and bone on subsequent radiographs is noted in uncomplicated cases.

With cemented prostheses, a rim of sclerosis around the prosthesis corresponding to a layer of fibrous tissue may occur several months after surgery. Periosteal reaction and cortical thickening may occur near the tip of the prosthesis in response to increased stress. The location of the cortical thickening depends on the position of the stem. Heterotopic ossification occurs fairly often without much effect.

Trochanteric osteotomy may be done to facilitate surgical exposure. The trochanter is usually reattached to anatomic position or to a more distal location, depending on mechanical considerations. In over 95 percent of cases, bony union is noted at the osteotomy site by 6 to 12 weeks. If the trochanter remains unchanged in position without a bony union by 3 months, then a fibrous union has occurred. Clinical results are usually satisfactory with fibrous union. This may also progress to a bony union.

### *Complications*

Any of the systemic complications associated with major surgery may occur after total hip replacement with an increased risk of deep vein thrombosis and pulmonary embolism, because of the uniquely high incidence of femoral thrombi associated with this type of operation.

The immediate postoperative complications include dislocation of the components, fracture of the femur, and/or infection. Of these, dislocation and fracture should be visible on radiographs. Dislocation in the immediate postoperative period is usually a result of laxity of para-articular tissues combined with improper handling of the patients or improper placement of prostheses. Dislocation later than 3 months is most often from malpositioning of the components or from failure to develop adequate muscle control. Infection occurring soon after surgery usually presents with the classic clinical symptoms.

Heterotopic ossification can occasionally be a severe complication, leading to serious limitation of motion. Separation of the greater trochanter may be of clinical significance, since this is occasionally associated with pain, limp, and a tendency to develop an adduction contracture. Fracture of the trochanteric wires is of little consequence, unless it is associated with proximal migration of the trochanter. Wire breakage may occur from metal fatigue, even after a solid bony union. Occasionally symptoms may result from bursitis or irritation of the overlying soft tissues. Rarely a metal fragment can migrate into the joint.

Until recently, loosening was the dominant problem in all total hip surgery. Plain film findings of loosening and/or infection with cemented components include cement-bone interface greater than 2 mm, widening of the cement-bone or cement-metal interface, migration of the components, cement fractures, motion demonstrated on stress views, or evidence of osteomyelitis (Fig. 2). With bone-ingrowth prostheses, the only radiographic finding associated with a poor outcome was subsidence of the femoral stem component that progressed to more than 10 mm (Fig. 3). Subsidence of up to 5 mm without progression has been described by Salzer et al as a desirable response.

Femoral fractures may occur intraoperatively and may be difficult to recognize on the operative or recovery room portable anteroposterior (AP) view. Leakage of cement into the adjacent soft tissues may suggest a fracture or penetration of the femoral cortex by the tip of the prosthesis. Fractures of the medial wall of the acetabulum may occur from excessive drilling or lack of bone stock. In both cemented and noncemented prostheses, postoperative films in AP and lateral projections should be obtained before discharging the patient from the hospital. Fractures occurring later could be stress

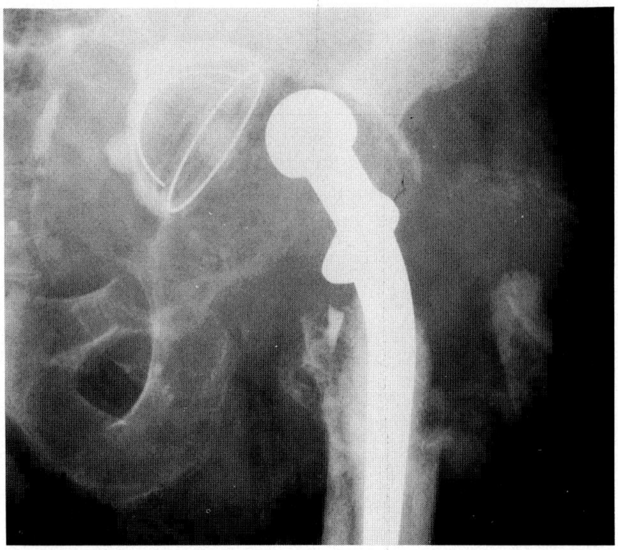

**FIGURE 2** Infected total hip replacement. There is marked destruction of the proximal femur and the acetabulum. The cemented acetabular cup is displaced supero-medially. A thin shell of periosteal new bone is noted along the destroyed acetabulum medially. The femoral head component is subluxated out of the cup. Bony fragments are also noted in the joint.

fractures, fractures caused by stress raisers in the femoral shaft or by severe trauma. The sintering process used to unite the metallic porous coating to the prosthesis, and the presence of the rough surface itself, may change the mechanical properties of the implant and make it more susceptible to fractures. The stress shielding of the proximal femur also may predispose this area to fractures.

When a complication is suspected and the plain film is unrevealing, a radionuclide scan may be appropriate. The bone scan usually remains positive for 6 months after surgery and therefore is useful only after this period. A negative bone scan speaks against loosening, infection, or fracture. However, the scan may be positive with any of these complications, and a specific diagnosis may not be possible. Scanning with indium-111–labeled leukocytes may be helpful when infection is suspected. However, joint aspiration is usually indicated to obtain fluid for culture and microscopic evaluation.

Visible motion of components on follow-up radiographs or on fluoroscopic evaluation with stress indicates loose components. Usually such evaluation is performed at the time of fluoroscopy for joint aspiration and arthrography. Radiographically visible bone destruction and/or periosteal reaction may indicate osteomyelitis.

## *Arthrography*

Hip aspiration and arthrography are usually indicated when there is continued pain after surgery and also before revision to exclude sepsis. Contrast injection confirms the intra-articular location of the needle and may show evidence of loosening and/or infection. Arthrographic findings of loosening and/or infection include (1) extension of contrast material between cement and bone or between bone and prosthesis in both cemented and noncemented components and (2) filling of irregular cavities or fistulous tracts. A joint aspiration is always

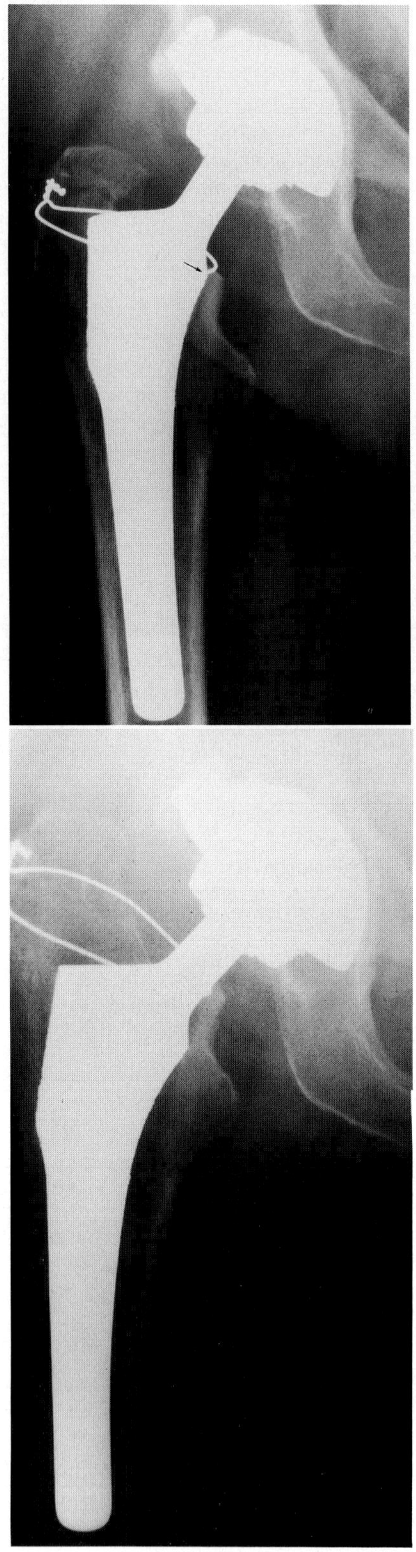

A

B

**FIGURE 3** Loosening in a porous coated anatomic total hip prosthesis. *A,* The initial postoperative radiograph shows 2 mm of subsidence of the femoral component beneath the surface of the medial cortex *(arrow)*. *B,* Two months later, the subsidence has increased to approximately 14 mm. (From Kattapuram SV, et al. Porous-coated anatomic total hip prostheses: radiographic analysis and clinical correlation. Radiology 1990; 174:861–864, with permission.)

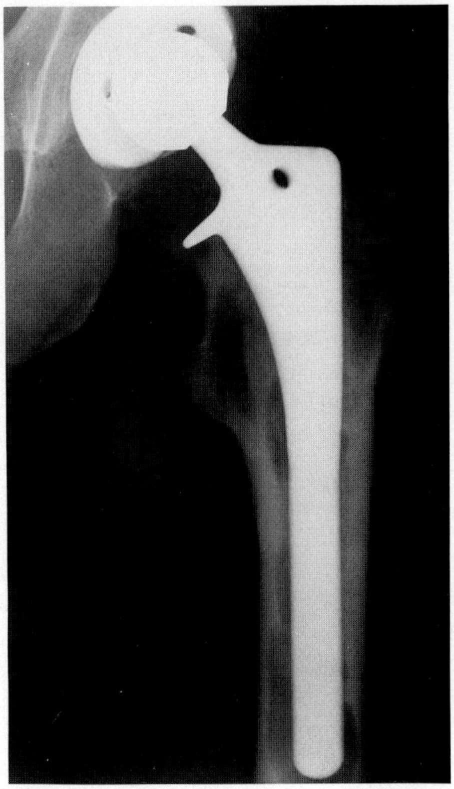

**FIGURE 4** Bone lysis in a non-cemented prosthesis. Four years after surgery. There is significant bony resorption along the femoral stem component with endosteal scalloping. This does not suggest loosening. At the time of revision, the component was not loose.

performed under extremely strict sterile precautions before arthrogram. This is done specifically to rule out infection.

Arthrography may also demonstrate lymphatic filling, a nonspecific sign of inflammation. Contrast material may also fill trochanteric bursa from trochanteric bursitis. Large quantities of fluid in the trochanteric bursa may prevent aspiration of joint fluid.

At this time in the evolution of hip replacement surgery, a major change exists in its understanding. For the first 20 years, the primary problem in THA has been loosening. Current cementing techniques have established a 97 percent solid fixation without major bone lysis. Femoral loosening, a major problem in the past, has been reduced from 30 to 40 percent in 10 years to 3 percent at 11 years using second-generation cementing techniques. Now the primary problem is particulate debris, leading to bone lysis and socket loosening (Fig. 4).

According to Harris, there are warning signs of impending failure of surgery. For the cementless implants these signs are (1) severe osteoporosis in the proximal femur, (2) "cementless disease" or bone lysis associated with cementless femoral components (Fig. 4), and (3) lack of bony ingrowth (revision operations have much smaller bony ingrowth than primary operations). For cemented components, the warning signs are (1) cement is the weak link, (2) the failure mechanism in these femoral components is initiated at the cement-metal interface, and (3) virtually 40 to 50 percent of cemented sockets will be loose at 10 years.

With the available knowledge, although the field is full of controversy, there is a certain consensus to use cementless acetabular and a cemented femoral component (hybrid total hip replacement) for most older patients who need primary replacements. Younger patients and patients requiring revisions remain a challenge.

## Knee Replacement

Replacement of the arthritic knee now has clinical results that equal or exceed those of hip replacement in terms of pain relief, satisfactory function, and survival of the implant after 10 years. The current era of knee arthroplasty began with the studies of Gunston in 1970. Since then, both the prostheses and the technique have undergone remarkable development. Total resurfacing knee arthroplasties remove the articular surfaces of all three knee compartments, including the patellofemoral, and replace them with implants. Such unconstrained arthroplasties depend on the muscular and ligamentous structures of the knee for stability. Sometimes a unicondylar prosthesis is used if only a single compartment is involved. If the soft-tissue supports of the knee are limited, occasionally a constrained or hinged prosthesis is used. The ideal alignment of the knee is parallel to the floor; standing views are necessary for documentation.

Patellar resurfacing remains a controversial issue. This is routinely done in patients with rheumatoid arthritis. In osteoarthritic knees, some authorities maintain that patellar resurfacing so improves results that it should be routine in all total knee arthroplasties. Others argue that the frequency of complications as a result of patellar resurfacing outweighs its benefits.

### *Indications and Contraindications*

The clinical results of total knee arthroplasty are reliable. Several factors must be taken into account: age, weight, level of activity, and the presence of other limitations of function. Most contraindications to knee arthroplasty are relative. A patient's youthfulness is a relative contraindication and must be considered in the context of available alternatives (further conservative treatment or tibial osteotomy). Excessive weight shortens the life of the implant. A solid bony fusion is a relative contraindication. Acute pyogenic infection is an absolute contraindication to joint implant.

### *Complications*

Most complications involve the patella. The problems include dislocation, stress fractures, avascular necrosis, progressive erosion of articular cartilage in the unresurfaced patella, and loosening of the patellar prosthesis. Virtually no modern knee replacement has failed because of loosening of the femoral component. Loosening of the tibial component is the most common mechanical failure. Infection occurs in fewer than 1 percent of knee replacements (Fig. 5). Periprosthetic fractures may also occur.

Total knee arthroplasty appears to be highly similar to total hip arthroplasty in terms of the predictability of good or excellent results, the infrequency of complications, and the ability to correct most complications to produce an eventually satisfactory result.

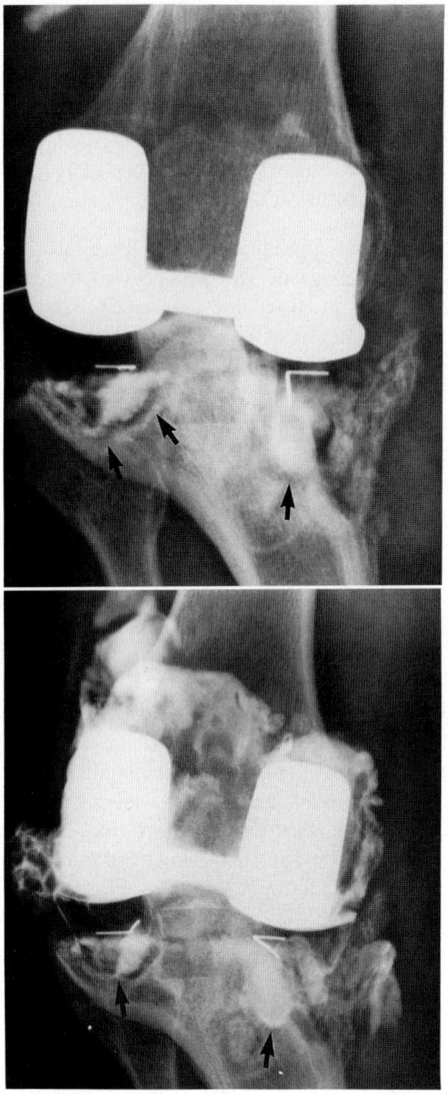


**FIGURE 5** Loose and infected total knee replacement. *A,* AP film of the knee shows marked varus angulation of the knee with destruction of the medial proximal tibia. Note the lucency between the tibial methacrylate and bone *(arrows). B,* AP view after contrast injection shows an irregular, lobulated synovium. Also, note the contrast within the lucency between tibial methacrylate and bone *(arrows),* arthrographic finding of loosening of the component.

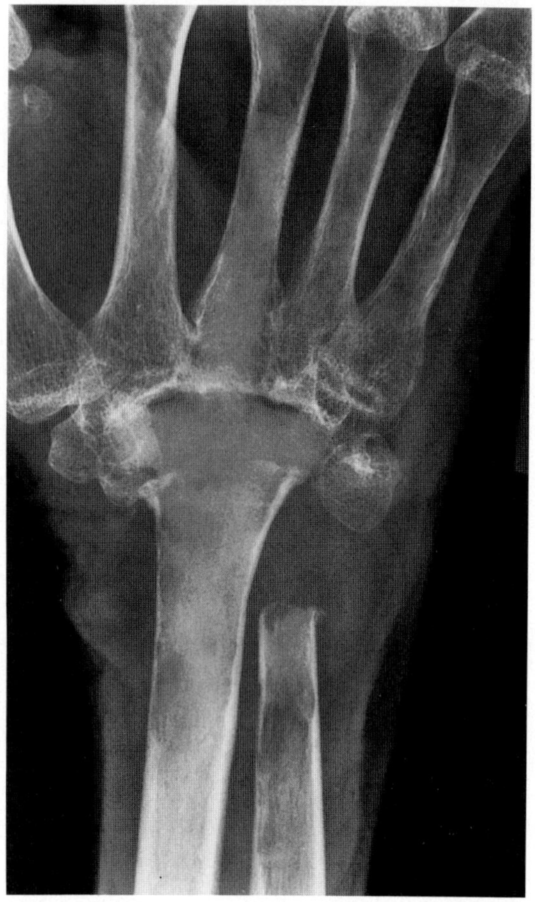

**FIGURE 6** Silastic wrist arthroplasty in a 54-year old woman with rheumatoid arthritis. (From Chew FS, ed. Skeletal Radiology: The Bare Bones. Rockville, MD: Aspen Publishers, 1989:243–254, with permission.)

## Ankle Replacement

Ankle replacements are seldom used. The tibial component is inserted perpendicular to the long axis of the tibia with the foot in neutral position. The talar component is placed parallel to the tibial component. Impingement and fracture of the lateral malleolus may occur. Arthrodesis is the usual surgical approach to severe ankle arthritis.

## Shoulder Replacement

Total shoulder replacement is primarily used in patients with incapacitating pain and secondarily for improvement in function. Normally the stability of the glenohumeral joint is provided by the joint capsule, rotator cuff, and the surrounding musculature. Depending on the stability of these structures, shoulder replacements may be unconstrained, serving only to resurface the joint, or constrained, replacing some of the stability normally provided by the soft tissues. Simple humeral head replacements may be used in conditions in which only the head is damaged.

Properly positioned postoperative radiographs should show that the inferior edge of the humeral component is aligned to the inferior edge of the glenoid component. Complications that may be detected radiographically include dislocation, superior subluxation of the humeral component, hetrotopic ossification, and widening of the cement-bone or bone-prosthesis lucency, indicative of loosening.

## Elbow Replacement

Elbow replacement is occasionally used in patients with severe sequelae of rheumatoid arthritis or post-traumatic arthritis. In the past, constrained hinged prostheses with no provision for rotational motion were used. These had a high incidence of loosening. The recent prostheses are less constrained and provide rotational motion; these are less stable and may dislocate.

## Wrist and Hand Replacements

Polymeric silicone (Silastic) implants are used primarily in the hand and wrist to replace damaged carpal, metacarpophalangeal, or interphalangeal joints. Following joint resection, the Silastic two-ended plug may be placed into the defect, with each plug seated into the medullary cavities of the involved bones (Fig. 6). Total wrist prostheses with metal components and polyethylene articular surfaces are also available, but are still considered experimental. Motion occurs at the implant because the implant itself can flex, as well as have a piston-like motion in and out of the bone. The subsequent radiographs demonstrate the degree of correction of the deformity, and the presence of complications such as dislocation of the prosthesis or silicone-induced synovitis.

## Suggested Reading

Chew FS. Joint replacements. In: Chew FS, ed. Skeletal Radiology: The Bare Bones. Rockville, MD: Aspen Publishers, 1989:243–254.

Harris WH. The first 32 years of total hip arthroplasty. Clin Orthop 1992; 274:6–11.

Harris WH, Sledge CB. Total hip and total knee replacement. N Engl J Med 1990; 323:725–731.

Kattapuram SV, Lodwick GS, Chandler H, et al. Porous-coated anatomic total hip prostheses: Radiographic analysis and clinical correlation. Radiology 1990; 174:861–864.

Phillips WC, Kattapuram SV. Prosthetic hip replacements: Plain films and arthrography for component loosening. AJR 1982; 138:677–682.

Phillips WC, Kattapuram SV. Efficacy of preoperative hip aspiration performed in the radiology department. Clin Orthop 1983; 179:141–146.

Weissman B. Total joint replacement: Fixation of prosthetic components. In: Gilula LA, Weissman BN, eds. Syllabus for the Categorical Course on Diagnostic Techniques in the Musculoskeletal System (1986). American College of Radiology, 1986:119–131.

# Imaging Evaluation of Limb Salvage Surgery

*SUSAN V. KATTAPURAM, M.D.*

Over the last two decades, there has been increasing interest in limb-salvage surgery for bone tumors as an alternative to amputation. Wide "en bloc" excision of the lesion, with an adequate margin of normal tissues, provides effective local control of many lesions including giant cell tumor, low-grade fibrosarcoma, low-grade chondrosarcoma, and parosteal osteosarcoma. The resulting skeletal defect poses major problems in functional reconstruction; if the integrity of the limb can be restored, the end result is preferable to amputation.

Various methods have been proposed and used in restoring skeletal integrity after limb salvage surgery. Filling the curettaged defect with autografting or implantation of massive autogenous bone grafts with internal fixation devices, with or without arthrodesis, remains the time-honored treatment and provides a stable, useful limb. This procedure is adequate when the defect is small and segmental rather than osteoarticular. However, if the defect is large, it may not be possible to obtain autografts of appropriate size and shape to fill the defect, and it is impossible to create a movable joint. The healing may be slow. Free vascularized fibular or rib autografts are valuable in the treatment of intercalary defects, but are not applicable to osteoarticular problems (unless the joint is sacrificed). This also has limitations in terms of length and strength of the replaced segment. Custom-made prosthetic devices have been advocated. Even when adapted to fit the defect, the currently available materials and systems are likely to fail with time.

Because of these constraints associated with the various methods, the Orthopaedic Oncology Department in our institution turned to cadaveric allografts as a solution to this problem, particularly osteoarticular defects. Allografts are easy to obtain and can be stored for long periods in the frozen state. The grafts are "sized" so that a part approximating the one removed can be substituted. If the cartilage can be preserved and ligamentous structures around the joint reconstituted, joint function that is approximately normal can be obtained. Over time, the skeleton is reconstituted and renewed to a near-normal state. The retention of ligamentous and tendinous insertions on the allograft allow the reattachment of muscles, ligaments, and capsular structures.

We have a 20 year history in allograft replacement at the Massachusetts General Hospital, the first one performed in 1971.

## Imaging Before Surgery

Before surgery, patients are staged radiographically for local extent and the presence or absence of metastatic spread including radiographs of the local site and a chest and bone scan. In most cases additional imaging procedures are involved. Tomograms of the local lesion are performed occasionally, especially if a question of pathologic fracture is entertained, or if it is thought to add more information as to what the local lesion is (i.e., stress fracture, osteonecrosis, severely comminuted fracture, Brodie's abscess). The local lesion is further evaluated using computed tomography (CT) scan and/or magnetic resonance imaging (MRI) to delineate the extent of the lesion, the size of the soft-tissue mass, and to aid in selecting appropriate surgical procedures. In most cases a CT scan provides significant information about the extent of the lesion, the integrity of the cortical bone, periosteal reaction, and the presence and extent of the soft-tissue mass. CT may also be valuable in making the diagnosis with certainty, so as to avoid further surgical intervention (e.g., calcific tendinitis, myositis ossificans, Schmorl's nodes, avulsion fracture). In addition, a tissue diagnosis can be sought using a CT-guided biopsy. In lesions such as Ewing's sarcoma and lymphoma, appropriate radiation and/or chemotherapy could be instituted. This also helps the surgeon to plan the most appropriate surgical procedure. Occasionally CT with intravenous contrast injection is needed when the margins of the soft-tissue component are not clearly defined, and to evaluate the relationship of the adjacent neurovascular bundle to the lesion. MRI clearly defines the intramedullary extent of the lesion and the presence and extent of the soft-tissue component. Occasionally the edema associated with the lesion creates a false impression of a larger soft-tissue mass on MRI.

In selected cases angiography is indicated to define the relationship and/or the vascularity of the lesion. This has also been used rarely to define the nidus of an osteoid osteoma when other imaging modalities do not demonstrate the nidus.

Arthrograms alone or in combination with CT are seldom employed in primary bone tumors. The intra-articular extent of the lesion is usually evaluated with CT and/or MRI scans. Arthrograms are employed only when a question arises as to whether a primary synovial etiology is responsible for the bony lesion.

Chest CT scans are also done preoperatively to evaluate the lungs for any possible metastases.

A

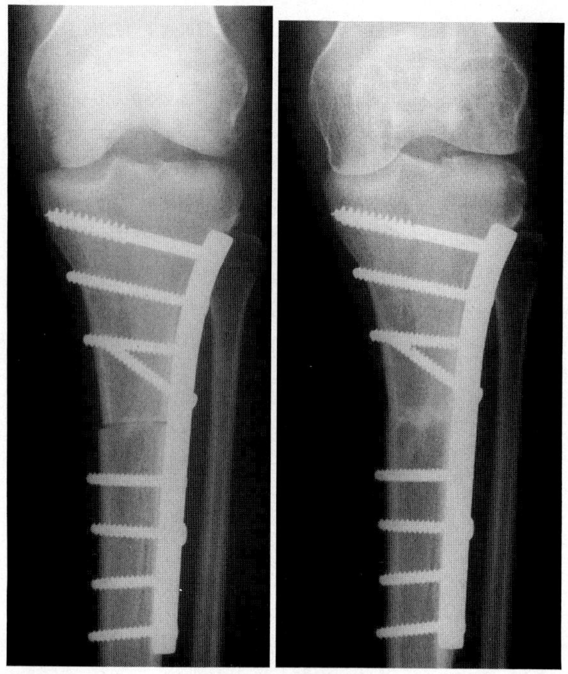

B

**FIGURE 1** *A,* Anteroposterior view of the proximal tibia and fibula 20 weeks after surgery shows an osteoarticular allograft in near anatomic alignment. *B,* Seventy-five weeks after surgery the junction site shows a healed and united allograft.

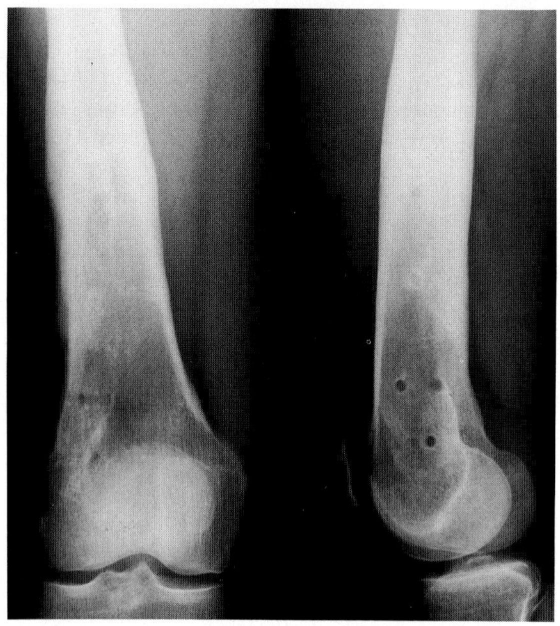

**FIGURE 2** An uncomplicated and healed hemiallograft of the distal lateral femur. This is an excellent outcome.

## Surgical Planning and Surgery

Once the preoperative imaging studies are completed, the surgeon has a fairly good idea whether to use an autograft or allograft and also what type of allograft to use. Depending on the size of the skeletal defect and adjacent muscle loss anticipated, he can choose a hemiallograft, an intercalary or segmental allograft, an osteoarticular allograft, or a combination of allograft with a prosthetic joint replacement (Figs. 1–4). If an allograft segment is to be used, an appropriate-sized allograft is chosen. The allografts are radiographed before freezing, and these radiographs are available. The patient's bone is sized by taking anteroposterior (AP) and lateral views of the involved bone, with a sizing ball, placed as close to the bone as possible. If the bone is too abnormal, the contralateral normal bone is sized instead. These films are then measured and compared with the radiographs of allografts in the bone bank until a best match is found. Particular care must be taken to ensure that films are properly marked as to "left" or "right."

After resection of the lesion, the autograft or allograft bone is trimmed to fit and fixed in place by an intramedullary rod or by compression plating. If the adjacent joint has been included in the resection, a prosthetic joint replacement may be necessary. Small tissue tags left in place during preparation of the allograft allow host muscles and ligaments to be attached anatomically. Antibiotics are administered intravenously both intraoperatively and postoperatively for at least 1 week and then orally for 5 to 6 months. Immunosuppression is not necessary.

## Postoperative Follow-up and Imaging

Intraoperative and immediate postoperative radiographs are obtained to assess the position, alignment, and apposition of the graft to the native bone. Postoperatively the patients are treated with external immobilization for approximately 3 months for lower extremities and 2 months for upper extremities. After removal of the external immobilization, the physical therapy restores a reasonable range of motion. In a patient with a graft in the lower extremity, unrestricted weight bearing is not advised until radiographic evaluation shows solid union at the graft-host site. Recently cast-type plastic braces have allowed earlier ambulation, and most patients are bearing partial weight with crutches or cane within 6 to 8 months.

We studied the radiographic changes following local excision and osteoarticular allograft placement in 40 giant cell tumors and in 20 intercalary replacements. The radiographic findings changed over time in an organized way. Both

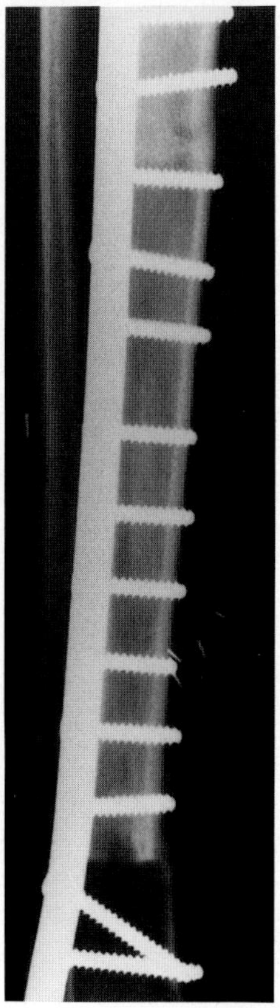

**FIGURE 3** Intercalary allograft. A normally healed segmental allograft of the midtibia 77 weeks after surgery. The allograft still remains denser than the native bone distally. (From Kattapuram SV, Phillips WC, Mankin HJ. Intercalary bone allografts: Radiographic evaluation. Radiology 1989; 170:137–141, with permission.)

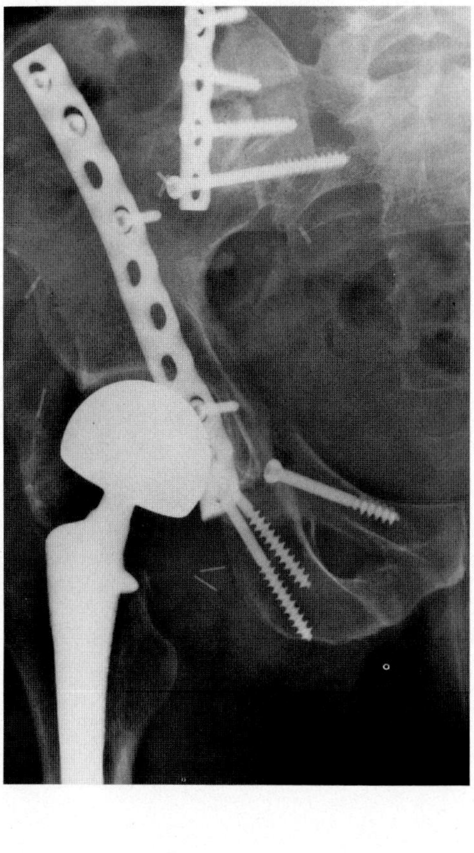

periosteal reaction and callus formation gradually increased in amount. Radiographically the healing process approaches completion some time after the first year (Figs. 1 to 3). At this time, the amount of periosteal reaction begins to decline and callus formation levels off. Mineralization of the allograft remains increased during the first 6 months (Fig. 3), then decreases gradually until stabilization is reached, approximately 2 years after surgery. Bone resorption increased quickly, leveled off 7 to 10 weeks after surgery, and thereafter remained stable. Soft-tissue swelling was present during the first 6 months, but persisted only in those cases in which complications developed (Fig. 5).

Complications with allograft surgery are early and delayed. The immediate postoperative complications of infection and hemorrhage are clinical diagnoses. The delayed complications include infection, fracture of the allograft or plate, nonunion, necrosis, recurrence of the tumor, degenerative arthritis of the adjacent joint, and prosthetic component failure. Rejection or other immunologic problems do not occur.

The overall incidence of fractures is almost 16 percent. Three types of fractures occur: type 1, rapid dissolution of the graft; type 2, fracture of the graft (Fig. 6), and type 3, fragmentation of joints. Fractures of the grafts tend to occur at stress sites where the allografts have weakened, such as through screw holes and areas adjacent to metallic plates. Fatigue fractures caused by abnormal stress secondary to malalignment at the graft-host junction did not seem to be a significant problem in our studies, presumably because of the close match between the allograft and native bone and the restoration of normal anatomic alignment at surgery. In the follow-up radiographs, changes in alignment should be noted.

Nonunion can occur following suboptimal bone contact at the host-donor junction site or inadequate immobilization. This is a complication prevented by good contact at the junction site or if needed by additional bone grafting.

Degeneration of the cartilage or fractures along the articular surface can occur as delayed complications. Although the joint space appears remarkably narrowed on plain radiographs, the majority of patients are functional. In cases in which there is functional deterioration, prosthetic joint replacements have been added.

Recurrence of tumor was found to be more common when the primary lesion was an osteosarcoma. Any evidence of soft-tissue mass or swelling or presence of matrix within the soft tissues should be viewed with suspicion, and additional studies such as CT and/or MRI or even needle biopsy may be indicated.

Infection can be a delayed complication as well. We have noticed an incidence close to 11.7 percent in our group of 283 patients. In the early years of allograft surgery, 27 infected allografts were considered failures because amputation of the limb or resection of the graft was required to control infection (Fig. 5). Recently, since 1980, in cases of infection, an attempt is made to salvage the limb by removing the graft, using a spacer or an external fixator to temporarily maintain the length of the limb, administering antibiotics orally and intravenously,

**FIGURE 4** Allograft with a prosthetic joint replacement. An iliac allograft is secured using plates and screws. The resected femoral head is replaced by a bipolar hip replacement. Some heterotopic bone formation is noted laterally along the joint.

A

B

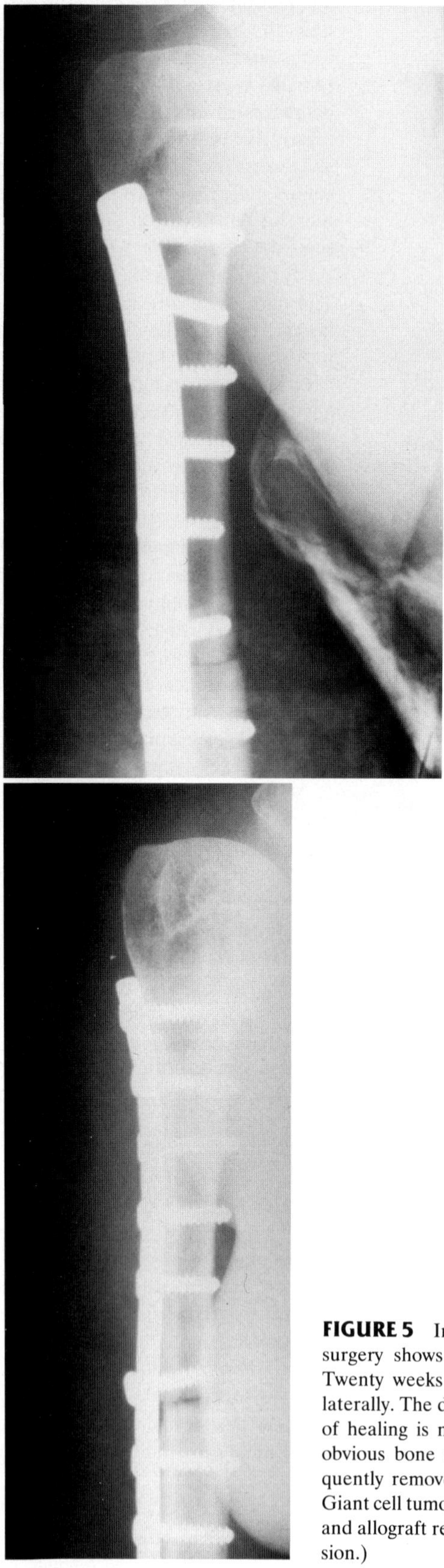

**FIGURE 5** Infection. *A,* Anteroposterior view obtained 13 days after surgery shows an anatomically aligned osteoarticular allograft. *B,* Twenty weeks after surgery, there is increased soft tissue swelling laterally. The distal screw in the allograft is getting loose. No evidence of healing is noted at the junction site. Ten weeks later there was obvious bone resorption of the allograft. The allograft was subsequently removed. (From Kattapuram SV, Phillips WC, Mankin HJ. Giant cell tumor of bone: radiographic changes following local excision and allograft replacement. Radiology 1986; 161:493–498, with permission.)

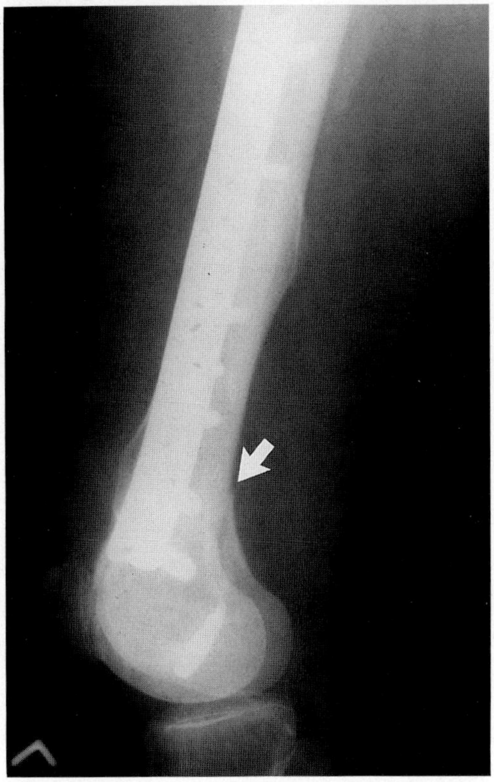

**FIGURE 6** Allograft fracture. A healed distal femoral osteoarticular allograft 190 weeks after surgery. Arrow points to an oblique fracture in the distal allograft close to the tip of the plate. (From Kattapuram SV, Phillips WC, Mankin HJ. Giant cell tumor of bone: Radiographic changes following local excision and allograft replacement. Radiology 1986; 161:493–498, with permission.)

and implanting a second allograft. This has changed the outcome significantly from failure to excellent and good.

The patients are seen at regular intervals as outpatients and are studied by radiographs for healing at the surgical site and/or development of complications. Chest radiographs are obtained at regular intervals to evaluate for metastases. If clinical symptoms warrant, bone scans are obtained. Plain radiographs of the surgical site help evaluate healing at the graft-host junction site, and detect evidence of fracture of the allograft (see Fig. 6) or plate or the junction between bone and plate (the site of stress concentration). The metallic devices used in transfixing the allograft limit other imaging modalities like tomograms, CT, and/or MRI. However, if there is any suspicion of fracture, tomograms should be obtained, although they may be somewhat limited in quality. The plain radiographs should be evaluated carefully for any bone resorption and/or soft-tissue swelling. Soft-tissue swelling may indicate an infection (Fig. 5) or recurrence of the tumor. In those cases, if possible, additional imaging using CT and/or MRI can be obtained. Bone resorption of the allograft could indicate a normal finding without any associated soft-tissue swelling. With an associated soft-tissue change, it indicates either an infection or recurrence of the tumor. Therefore, in cases with an increased incidence of recurrence, it is reasonable to have a baseline CT and/or MRI along with the postoperative plain radiographs for adequate interpretation later. The follow-up radiographs should always be compared with previous films for change. If a prosthetic replacement is used with an allograft, the radiographs should be evaluated for loosening of the components along with changes in allograft.

In summary, allograft implantation has drastically changed the surgical management of musculoskeletal tumors. The remarkable success of this procedure necessitates appropriate imaging studies in the preoperative and postoperative care. Adequate knowledge of the healing process and complications associated with the allografts enables the radiologist to participate effectively as a member of the management team.

## Suggested Reading

Kattapuram SV, Phillips WC, Mankin HJ. Giant cell tumor of bone: Radiographic changes following local excision and allograft replacement. Radiology 1986; 161:493–498.

Kattapuram SV, Phillips WC, Mankin HJ. Intercalary bone allografts: Radiographic evaluation. Radiology 1989; 170:137–141.

Mankin HJ, Gebhardt MC. Allografts in the management of bone tumors: Part 1. Surgical Rounds 1987; 48–54.

Mankin HJ, Gebhardt MC. Allografts in the management of bone tumors: Part II. Surgical Rounds 1988; 70–91.

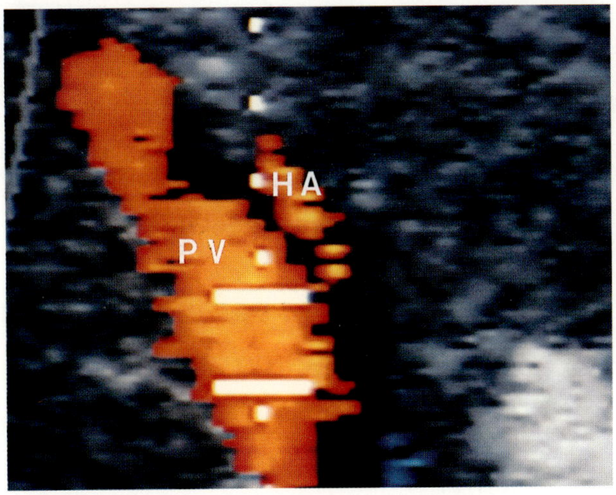


**COLOR PLATE 1** Normal hepatic artery (HA) and portal vein (PV), long-axis view. Flow in both vessels is hepatopedal.

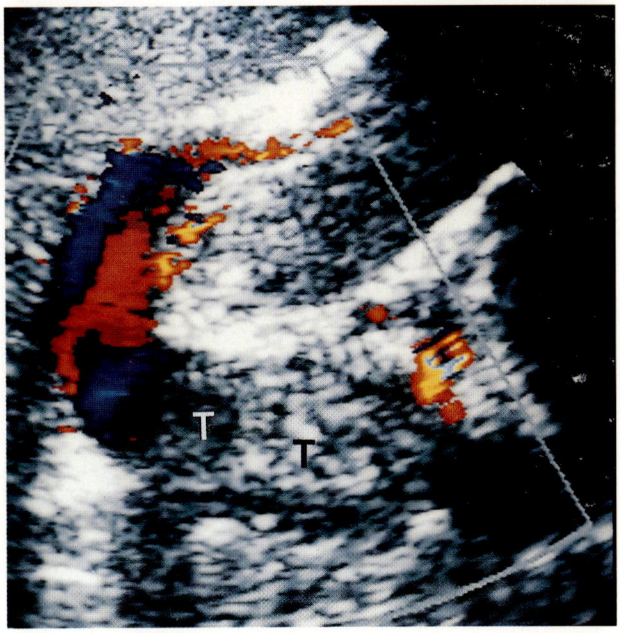


**COLOR PLATE 2** Portal vein (sagittal view). Nonoccluding thrombus (T) in patient with hepatocellular carcinoma. Color Doppler sonogram shows flow distal to thrombus. Localized regions of reversed flow *(blue)* are present, although overall flow direction is hepatopedal *(red)*. When reversed flow is detected by spectral Doppler in the portal vein, multiple regions of the vein should be examined to prevent misinterpreting a localized region of reversed flow as representative of the overall flow direction in the vein.

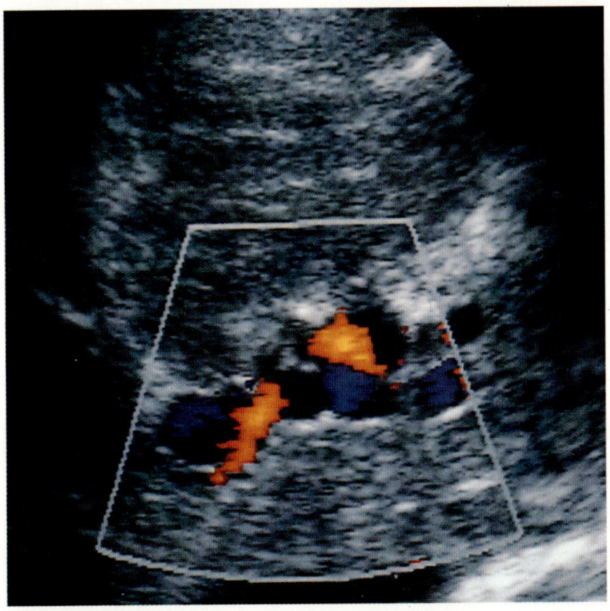

**COLOR PLATE 3** Portal vein (transverse view). Cavernous transformation. Multiple tortuous collateral venous channels adjacent to thrombosed portal vein.

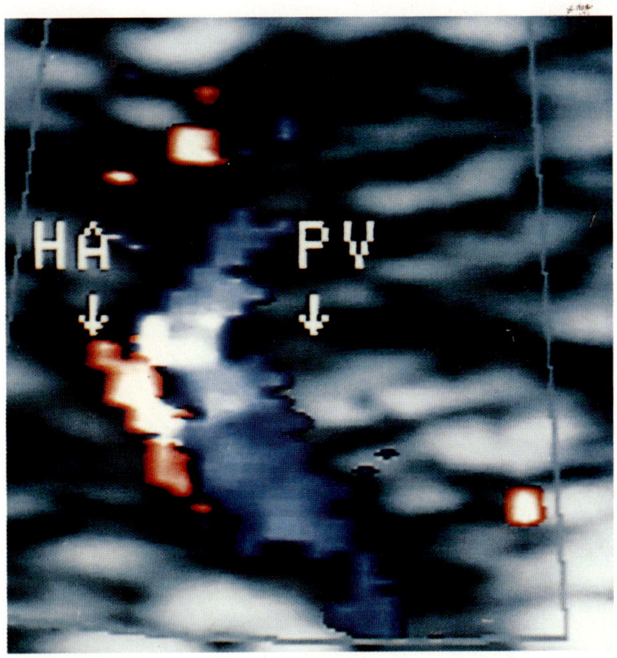


**COLOR PLATE 4** Portal vein (sagittal view). Reversed flow. Small cirrhotic end-stage liver. Color Doppler sonogram. Hepatic artery (HA) is red (hepatopedal); portal vein (PV) is blue (hepatofugal). Compare with Color Plate 1.

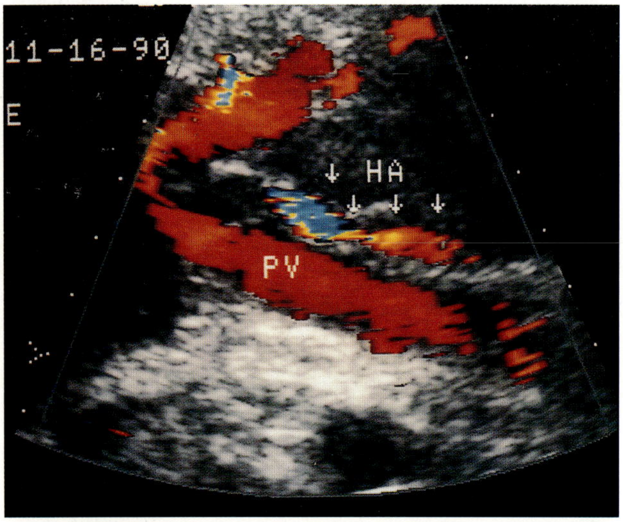


**COLOR PLATE 5** Hepatic artery stenosis. Color Doppler sonogram of the proper hepatic artery (HA) in portahepatis shows abrupt alteration in arterial flow depicted as color aliasing *(blue region)*.

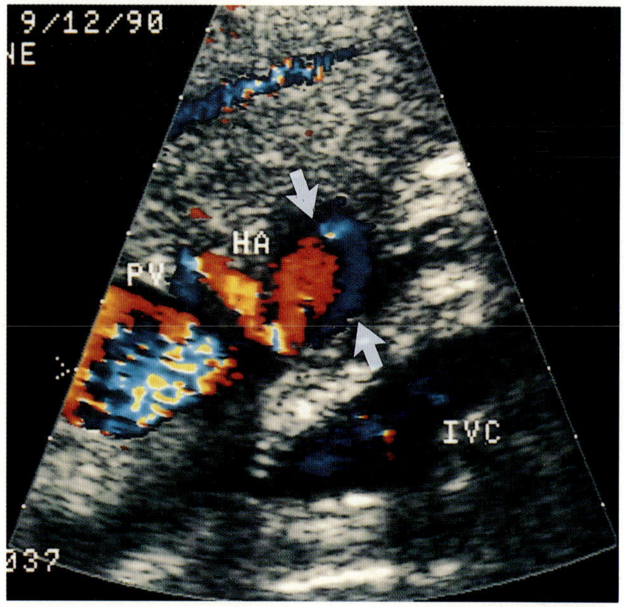


**COLOR PLATE 6** Hepatic artery pseudoaneurysm. Color Doppler sonogram shows a periportal spherical region of flow *(arrows)* adjacent to the proper hepatic artery (HA). Duplex Doppler evaluation of the spherical region demonstrated pulsatile arterial flow highly suggestive of a pseudoaneurysm.

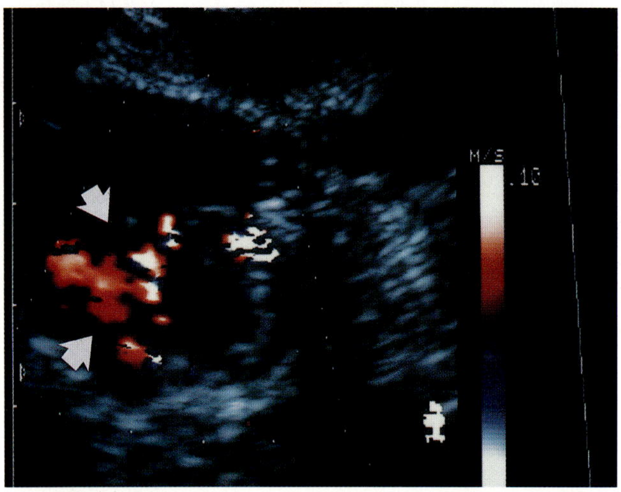

**COLOR PLATE 7** Tubal ectopic pregnancy. Color Doppler sonogram showing adnexal ring with increased blood flow at placentation site *(arrowhead)*.

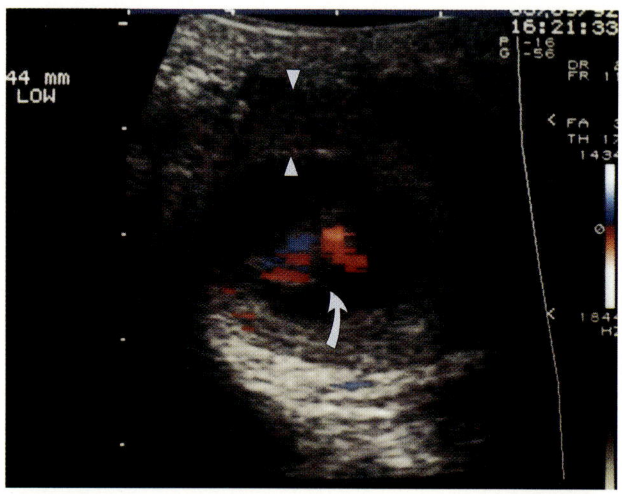


**COLOR PLATE 8** Tubal ectopic pregnancy. Color Doppler sonogram demonstrating dilated and thickened fallopian tube *(arrowheads)* and living ectopic fetus *(curved arrow)*.

**COLOR PLATE 9** Color-flow Doppler sonogram of left kidney shows large, branching renal sinus vessels, giving the appearance of hydronephrosis.

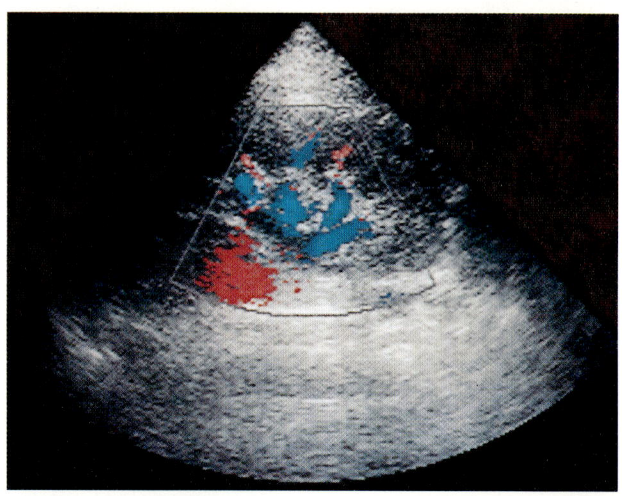

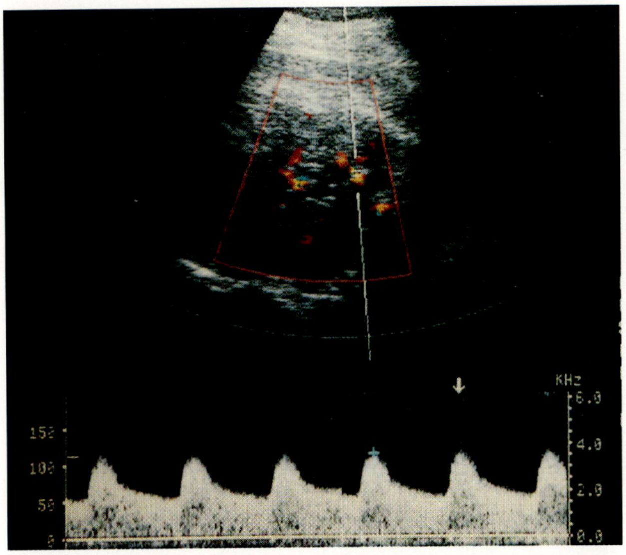


**COLOR PLATE 10** Renal cell carcinoma. Transverse view of mass on color Doppler sonogram showing chaotic neovascularity. Pulsed Doppler sonogram confirms low-impedance flow of tumor neovascularity with a Doppler shift of 4 kHz.

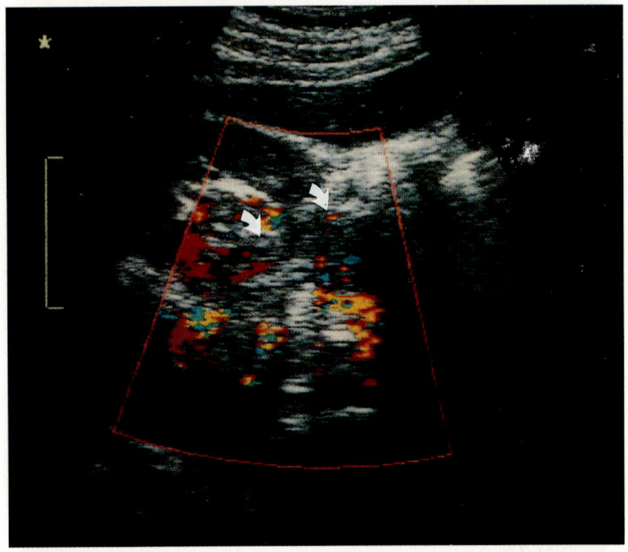

**COLOR PLATE 11** Color Doppler sonogram reveals no flow in the renal vein of this patient with a hypernephroma. Tumor thrombus can be seen within the renal vein *(arrows)*.

A

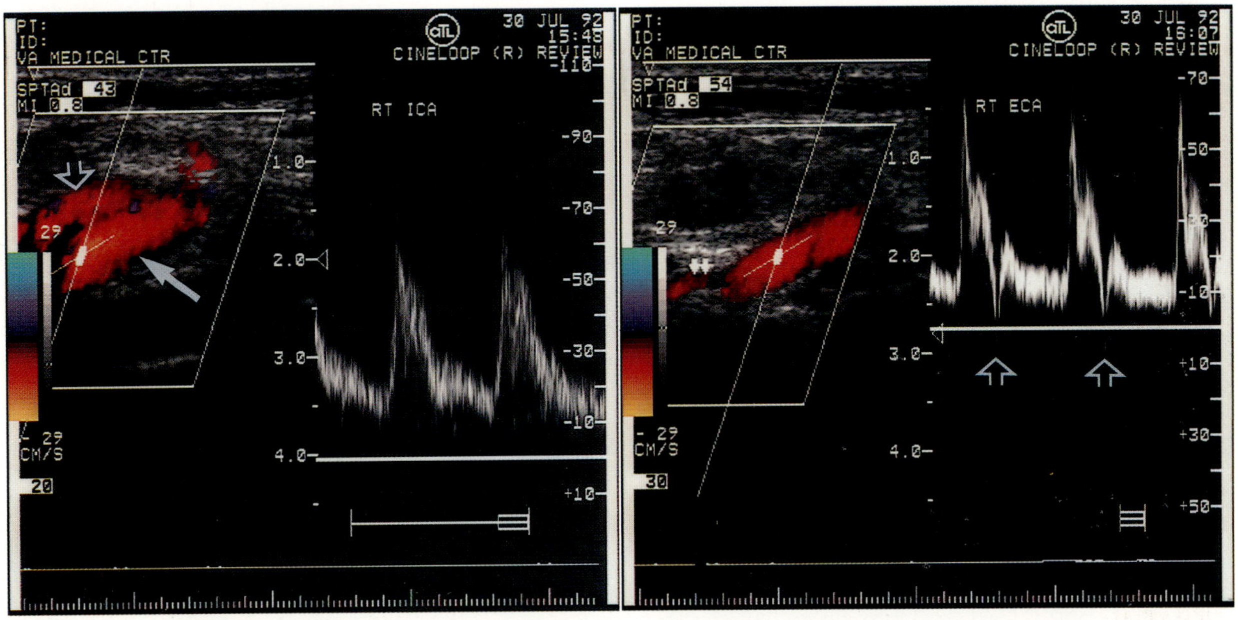


B

**COLOR PLATE 12** Normal carotid bifurcation. *A,* The internal carotid artery (ICA, *large arrow*) usually lies posterior to the external carotid artery (ECA, *open arrow*) and is typically larger. These characteristics, however, are not constant and should never be relied on to distinguish the two vessels; Doppler characteristics are far more reliable. Note the low-resistance flow pattern of the ICA. *B,* The ECA supplies the facial muscles and thus has a triphasic, high-resistance pattern characterized by minimal flow in diastole and a brief period of flow reversal *(open arrows)*. The ECA may also be distinguished by its branches *(small arrows)*; the ICA has no branches in the neck.

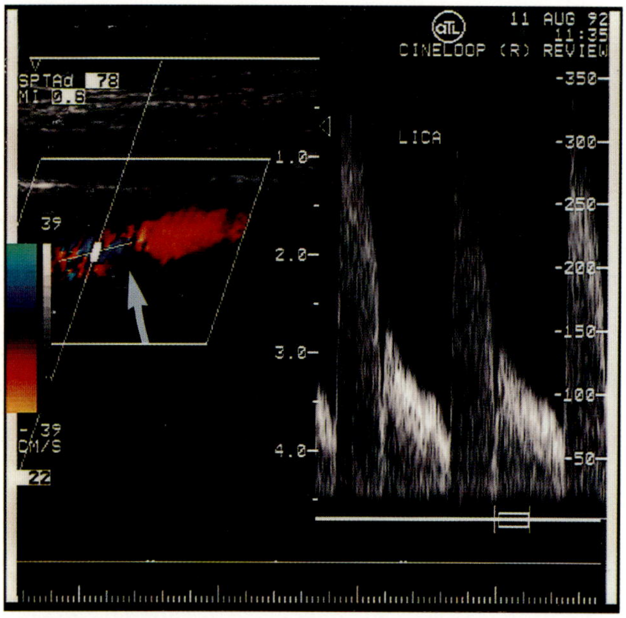


**COLOR PLATE 13** Color Doppler sonogram suggests high-grade ICA stenosis; note anechoic plaque *(arrow)* and abnormal color pattern. Spectral analysis defined lesion as narrowing lumen by 75 to 90 percent, peak systolic velocity > 350 cm/sec, VICA/VCCA > 4, end-diastolic velocity = 87.

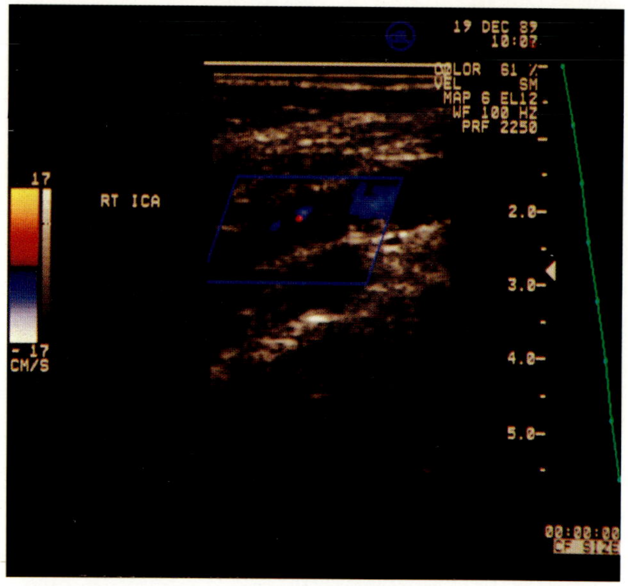


**COLOR PLATE 14** Subtotal ICA occlusion. Color Doppler image shows a minute residual lumen within an otherwise anechoic vessel *(arrow)*. Spectral tracings were difficult to obtain and demonstrated marked distortion of waveform.

A

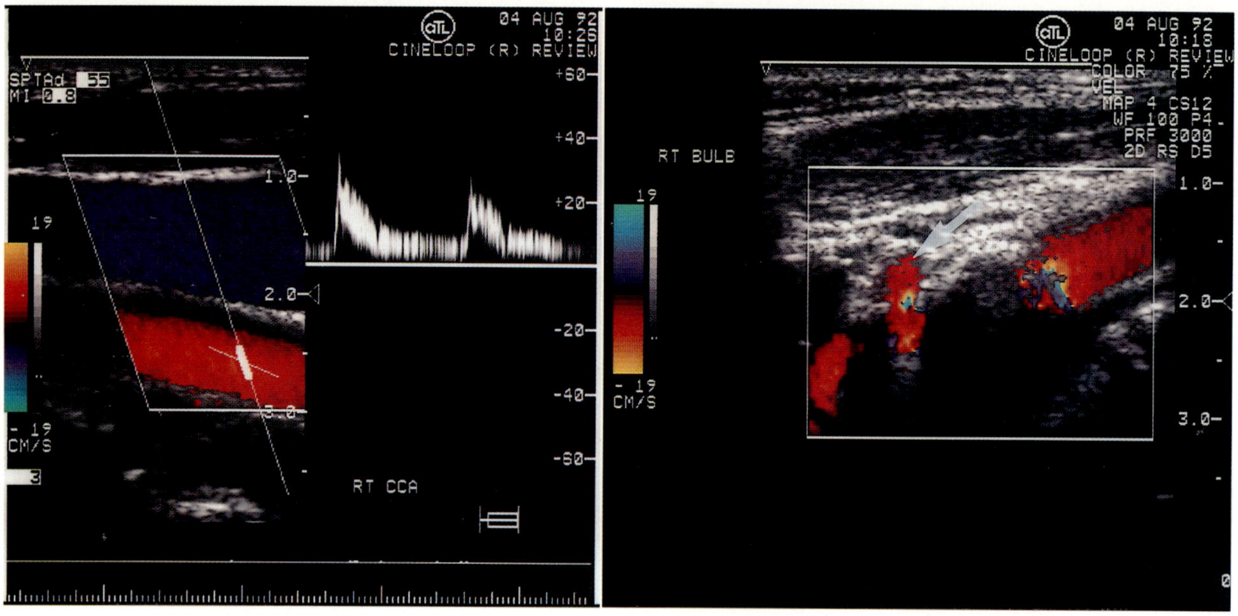


B

**COLOR PLATE 15** *A,* Scanning through common carotid artery (CCA) shows a somewhat high-resistance flow pattern. Note sharp systolic upstroke, relatively low flow in diastole, and negative component. Total ICA occlusion should be considered. *B,* Following CCA distally, the color signal is lost because of a large, densely shadowing plaque. Beyond plaque, only one vessel can be identified; branch *(arrow)* confirms patent artery is ECA.

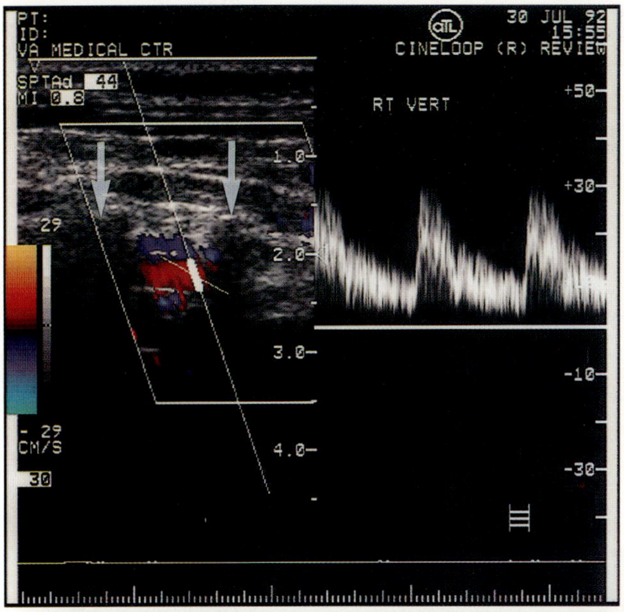


**COLOR PLATE 16** Normal vertebral artery. Two vessels with flow proceeding in different directions were identified between shadows of transverse processes of cervical spine *(arrows)*. Spectral analysis confirmed posterior vessel as the vertebral artery; note low-resistance arterial flow pattern. Anterior vessel is vertebral vein.

A 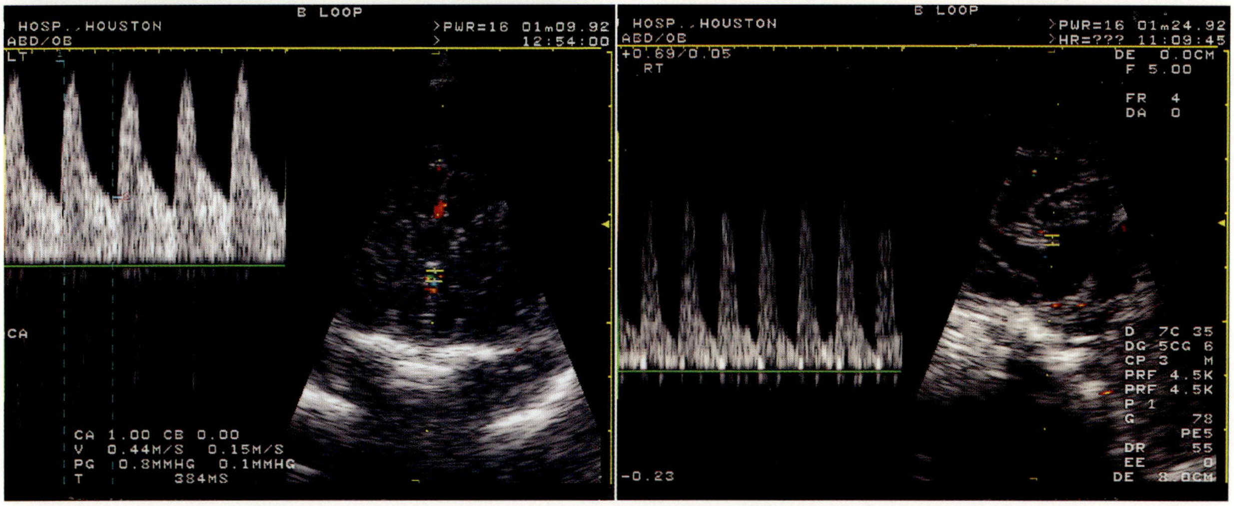 B


**COLOR PLATE 17** Doppler spectra from the anterior cerebral artery in a normal preterm neonate. *A,* Coronal projection. The configuration of the Doppler spectra is normal. Peak systolic velocity is 0.44 m/sec; end-diastolic velocity is 0.15 m/sec. Resistive index (RI) is 0.65 (within normal limits). Notice that on coronal projections no angle correction can be used and thus absolute velocities may be mildly increased. However, RI should still be within normal limits, because this measurement is angle independent. *B,* Midsagittal projection. No angle correction was used. Notice the sharp systolic upstroke and gentle diastolic downstroke. Diastolic flow should always be evident and above the baseline. In this patient peak systolic velocity is 0.4 m/sec and end-diastolic velocity is 0.08 m/sec. RI is 0.8 (within normal limits).

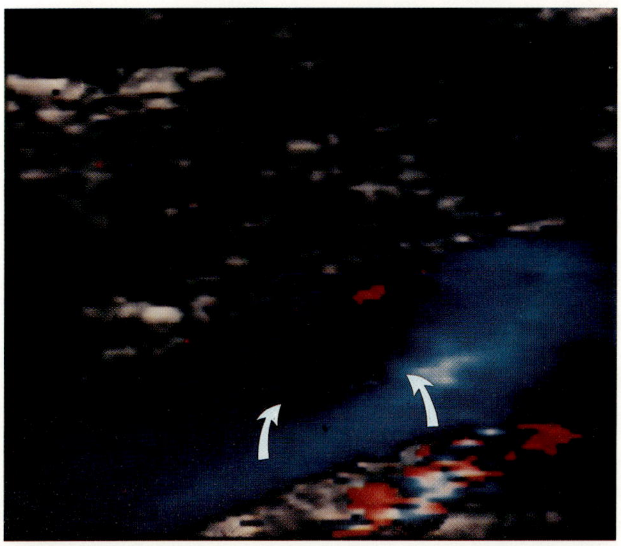

**COLOR PLATE 18** Longitudinal color Doppler image of the popliteal vein demonstrates color signal surrounding a thrombus *(curved arrows)*.

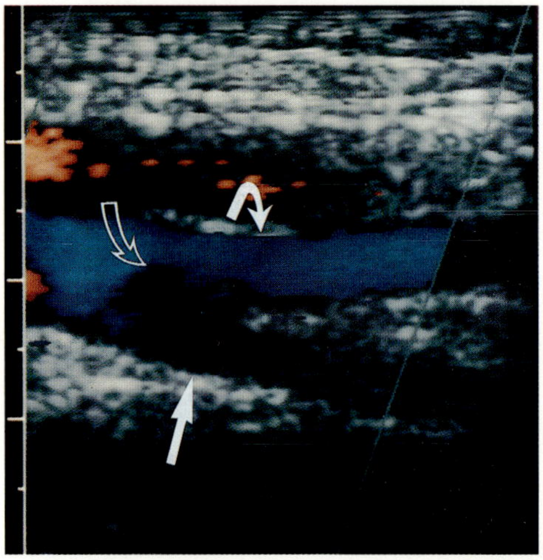

**COLOR PLATE 19** Longitudinal color Doppler image demonstrates normal flow in the superficial femoral vein *(curved arrow)*. Thrombus fills the deep femoral vein *(straight arrow)* and extends into the lumen of the common femoral vein *(open arrow)*.

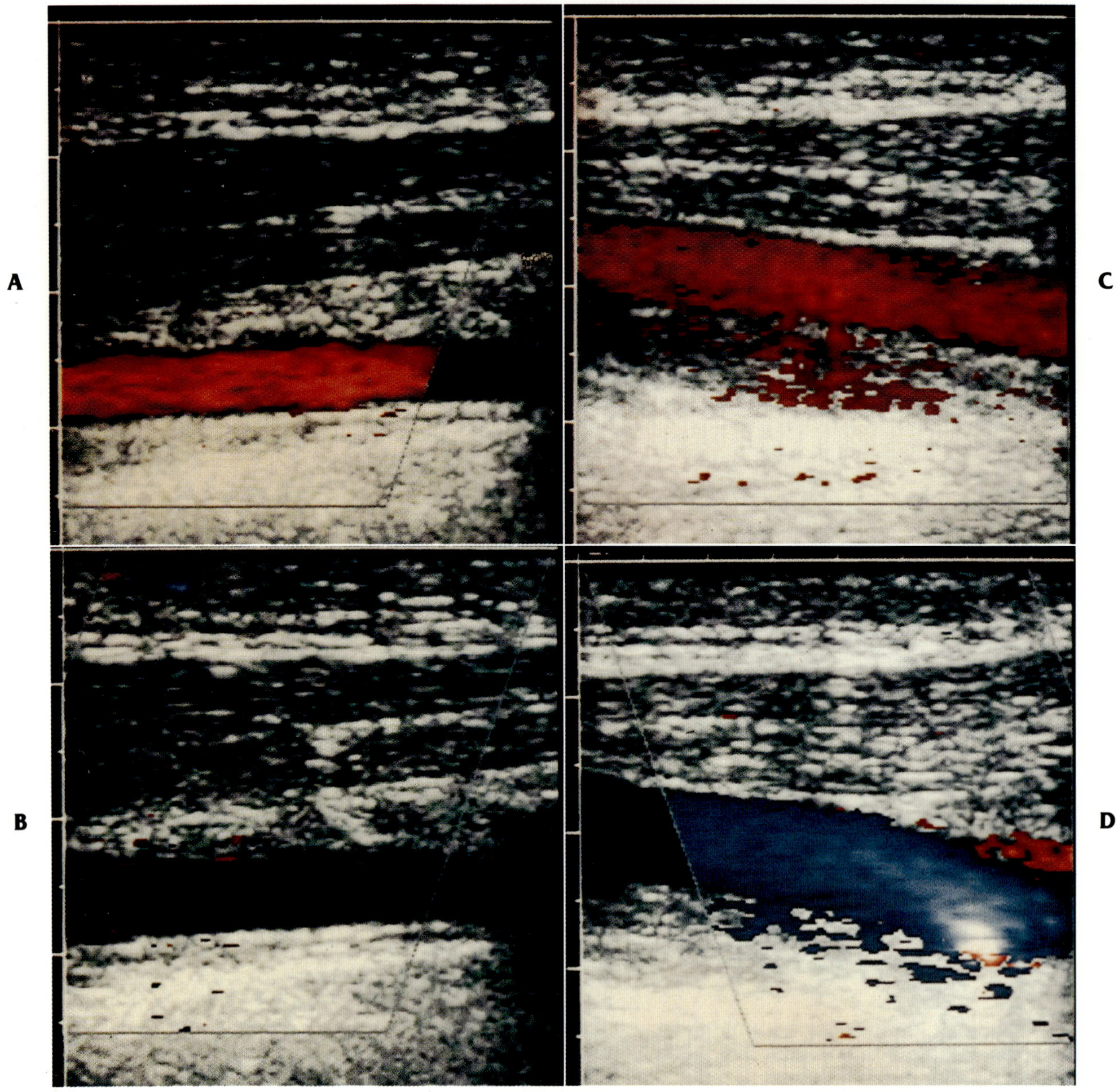

**COLOR PLATE 20** *A,* Normal femoral vein demonstrates antegrade flow in red. *B,* With Valsalva maneuver, flow in the normal femoral vein ceases completely. *C,* In this femoral vein in a patient with chronic venous ulceration, normal antegrade flow is red. *D,* With the Valsalva maneuver, retrograde flow in blue is detected, indicating venous valvular insufficiency.

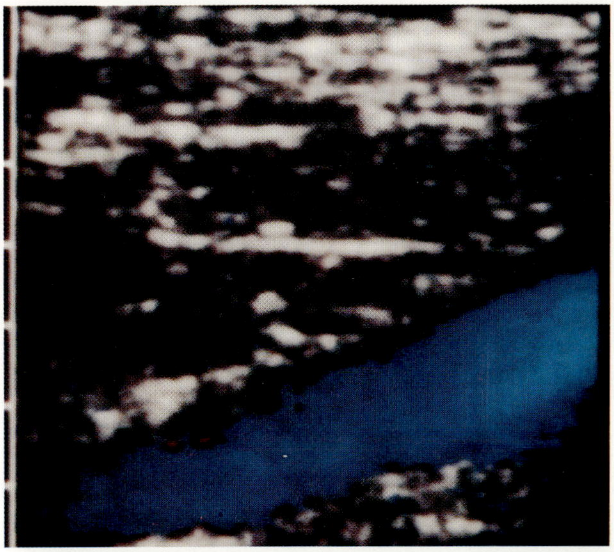

**COLOR PLATE 21** Normal flow in the subclavian vein is displayed in blue in this image taken along the long axis of the vein.

A

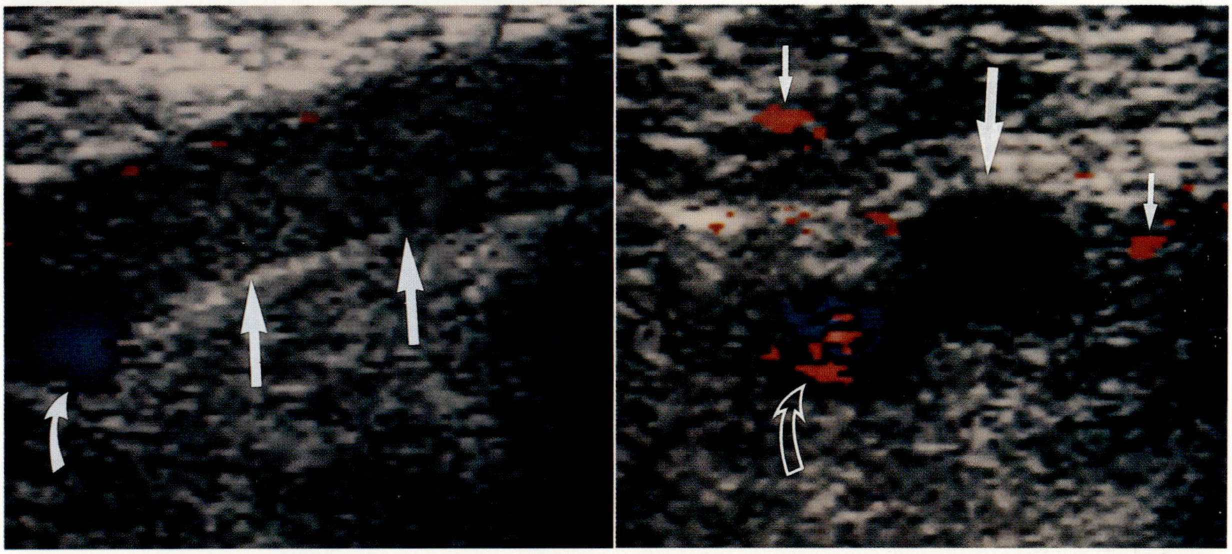

B

**COLOR PLATE 22** Long-axis *(A)* and short-axis *(B)* views of the subclavian vein *(straight arrows)*, which is filled with hypoechoic thrombus. A small area of residual flow is displayed within the vein *(curved arrow, A)*. Collateral veins *(small arrows)* and the normal subclavian artery *(open arrow)* are also displayed in *B*.

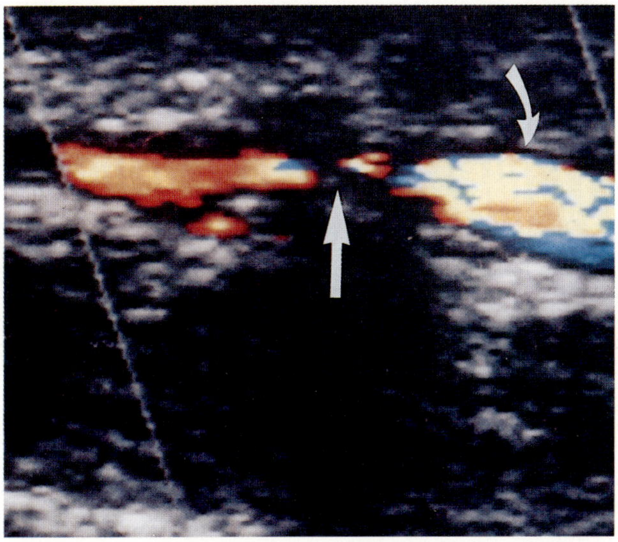

**COLOR PLATE 23** Longitudinal color Doppler image of a bypass graft demonstrates narrowing of the lumen *(straight arrow)* and marked velocity acceleration *(curved arrow)*, indicating a significant stenosis.

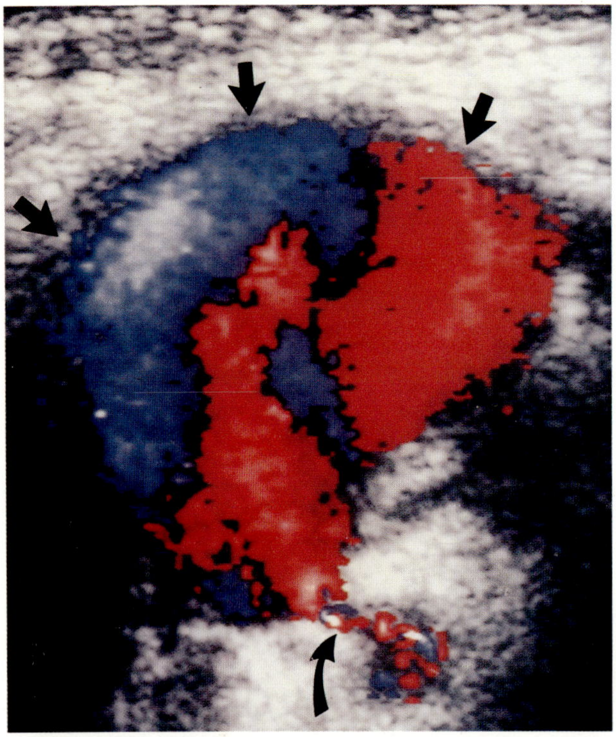

**COLOR PLATE 24** Transverse color Doppler image of a large postcatheterization pseudoaneurysm of the axillary artery *(straight arrows)*. Note the neck *(curved arrow)* connecting the pseudoaneurysm to the native vessel.

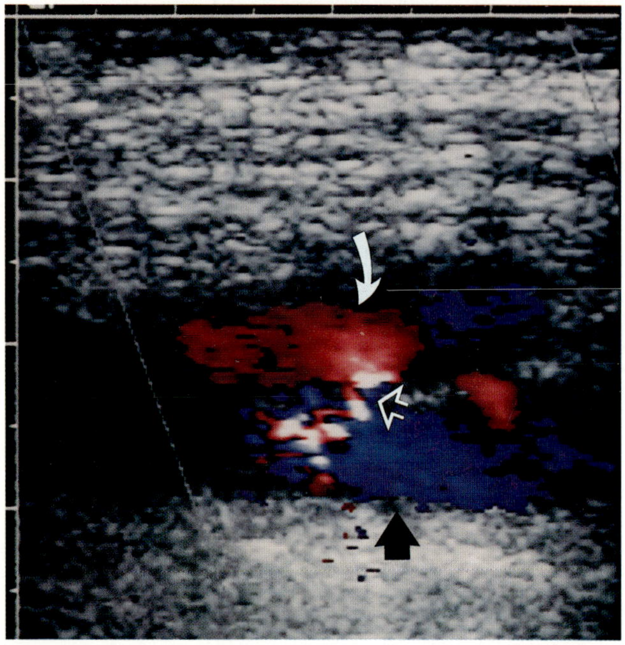

**COLOR PLATE 25** Longitudinal color Doppler image demonstrating high velocity through an arteriovenous fistula *(open white arrow)* between the superficial femoral artery *(curved white arrow)* and vein *(black arrow)*.

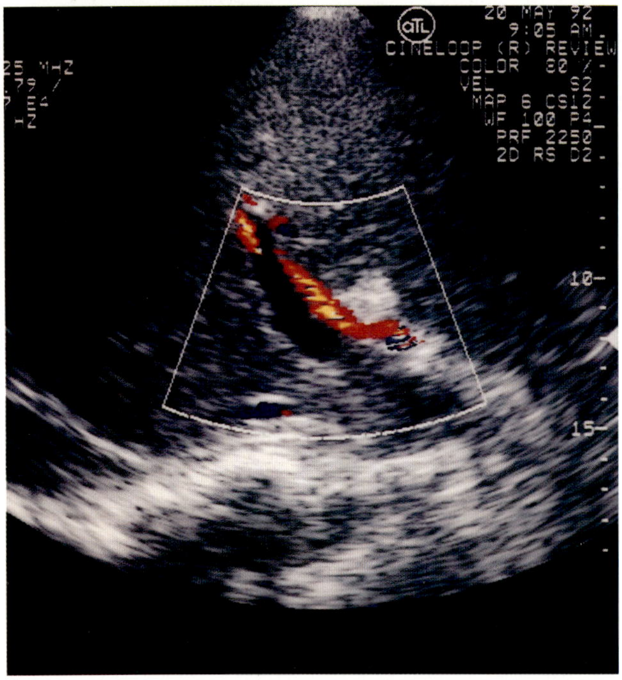


**COLOR PLATE 26** Oblique scan demonstrating dilated obstructed portal vein and prominent hepatic artery *(red)*, confirmed to represent portal vein thrombosis.

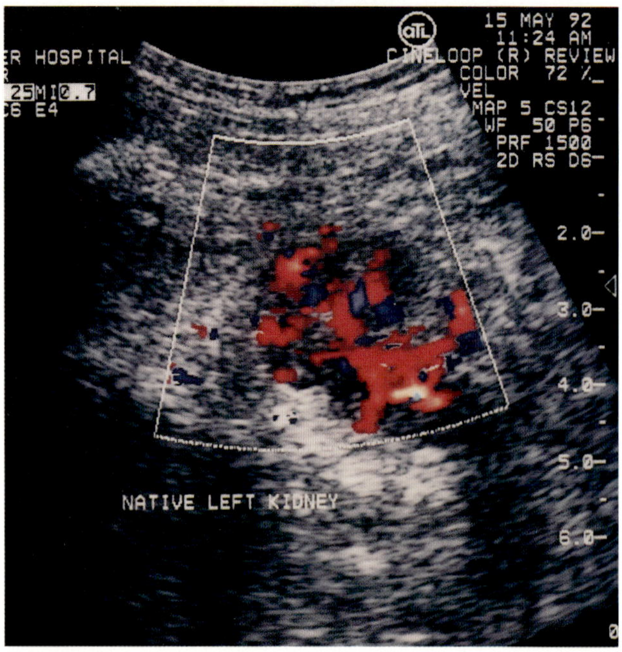


**COLOR PLATE 27** Oblique image of left kidney demonstrating hypervascular mass lesion with increased flow, surgically proven to be a hypernephroma.

# MAMMOGRAPHY

## Breast Imaging: An Organizational Approach

*DANIEL B. KOPANS, M.D.*

The primary function of mammography is the surveillance of breast tissue in the hope of detecting breast cancer at a preclinical point in its growth, and at a stage when it can be cured, or mortality delayed. Mammography is primarily a screening technique capable of detecting breast cancers in an asymptomatic population of women 2 to 4 years earlier than they might ordinarily be detected. Detecting cancers at a smaller size and earlier stage has been shown to result in diminished mortality. Mammography can be of some diagnostic use, but it cannot be relied upon, in most instances, to exclude cancer. In the symptomatic woman, its primary role is to screen the remainder of the side in question and the contralateral breast for clinically occult cancer.

It must be clearly understood by the clinician that mammography is frequently not diagnostic in the sense that it can be used to differentiate benign from malignant masses. Although there are situations in which it can be used to avoid the biopsy of a benign palpable mass, such as a lipoma, its major contribution is the ability to detect anomalous, nonpalpable structures in the breast. Many of these prove to be malignant, but others with similar morphologies prove to be benign. Since mammography and physical examination provide information based on different tissue characteristics, concerns raised by one can rarely be negated by lack of corroboration from the other. As has been often reiterated, a negative mammogram should not result in delayed intervention when a clinically suspicious lesion is present, just as a negative physical examination should not delay diagnosis in the breast containing a mammographically suspicious abnormality.

Although mammography can demonstrate most cancers when special views are used to image clinically suspicious tissues, cancers can be obscured on routine screening mammography. Since these are palpable, physical examination remains an important component of screening.

As screening programs expand, concern has been raised by the lack of consistency and standardization to ensure quality of care. Legislation has been or is being developed in many states and nationally to require appropriate equipment and the training of radiologists and technical personnel. As a consequence of the ambiguity posed by many mammogram reports, the American College of Radiology in conjunction with the Centers for Disease Control has developed the ACR Breast Imaging Lexicon, Reporting System, and Database to standardize mammographic reporting. Through the use of a standardized data collection system, the results of screening can be analyzed locally and nationally.

The marked variation in predictive value between radiology groups practicing mammography underscores the variation in interpretation, and review of reports demonstrates the failure to structure interpretation. Given the variability of the presentation of breast cancer and its frequent morphologic similarity with benign lesions, the best approach to interpretation will involve the estimation of the probability of malignancy for a given type of lesion. This will evolve as we obtain a better understanding and correlation between the morphology of breast cancers observed mammographically and their histologic characteristics. The implementation of adjunctive techniques such as fine-needle aspiration (FNA) cytology or core biopsy may prove useful to modify probabilities. Ultimately predictive values will be determined by "acceptable" false negatives, since as the false-positive rate is reduced the false-negative rate may rise. We must remember that the ultimate purpose of screening is mortality reduction, and efforts to reduce the false-positive rate should not do so at the expense of increased false negatives.

Groups involved in breast cancer detection and diagnosis

should not only try to standardize their reporting, but by monitoring their own results they can develop probabilities based not only on national data, but on their own experience, which will have greater significance in their own particular populations. Standardization will not only help the individual group compare itself with other groups in the country, but if similar data are gathered by all groups, the effect of screening can be monitored nationally. It may even be possible, by analyzing such data, to improve screening guidelines and perhaps discover new information that will affect diagnosis and therapy.

## Screening, Detection, Confirmation, Triangulation, Assessment, Diagnosis

The detection and diagnosis of breast cancer can be divided into specific tasks. These are discussed in detail in the following sections.

### *Screening*

Screening for breast cancer involves the evaluation of asymptomatic women in an effort to detect clinically occult abnormalities that have a significant probability of malignancy. The abnormality detected at screening may be of sufficient concern to instigate an immediate biopsy, or the abnormality may be borderline in appearance and require additional evaluation to resolve as inconsequential or as requiring biopsy confirmation. The latter function should be considered problem-solving breast imaging.

In an effort to reduce the expense of screening and thus make it available to all segments of the population, efficiency must be improved without sacrificing quality. The screening session is the time at which the full benefit of mammography is realized, and thus mammographic imaging at screening must be optimized. Although the psychological aspects of breast cancer detection and diagnosis are unique, the screening study is similar to a Pap smear in that the study is either negative, requires close follow-up, requires recall of the patient for additional evaluation, or is sufficiently suspicious to require a biopsy. Having a radiologist on site during the screening phase reduces the need to recall patients with questionable abnormalities, but increases the cost of screening significantly. A radiologist can read 40 to 50 mammograms in a 2 hour session, if those studies are organized on an alternator along with previous available evaluations so that film handling by the radiologist is minimized. Batch reading also permits more than one review, and double reading is facilitated at little expense with a demonstrated benefit in detection. In our practice, we found that detection of clinically occult malignancy increased by 7 percent by just having a second radiologist quickly review the batch. If a radiologist is asked to consult on each study as it is taken, the radiologist will be involved for a full 8 hour day to interpret the same number of studies. The cost will have to be increased to account for this inefficient use of radiologist time as well as the delay in patient throughput created by such a system. Double reading in an on-line system leads to increased cost. The separation of the screening component from the diagnostic or problem-solving function of breast imaging has advantages in cost-benefit as well as accuracy. The negative implications of this approach are that 5 to 10 percent of women may be asked to return for additional study, with their attendant increased anxiety and inconvenience.

The screening center need only produce high-quality contact studies. Magnification, ultrasonography, computed tomography (CT), FNA, core biopsy, localization, and excisional biopsy capabilities can be concentrated in a centralized diagnostic center fed by multiple screening sites. The diagnostic center also evaluates women with clinically evident signs or symptoms of breast cancer. Organizing breast cancer detection and diagnosis as separate functions is likely, in the long run, to be more cost-effective.

Improved efficiency is also possible by organizing the interpretive function. The radiologist should develop a reasoned approach to detection and diagnosis. Ideally guidelines will be established so that interpretation is consistent, concise, and clearly represented to the referring physician or patient. In the screening setting, the use of a computerized reporting system is highly feasible, and results in extremely consistent analysis if the approach is organized around a basic structure. Since screening in the United States is not centrally controlled, it is important for individual practitioners to do everything possible to monitor the results of their own work to ensure that they are detecting earlier-stage lesions, and in an effort to minimize the number of women who require interventional procedures and are subsequently not found to have breast cancer. The organization of mammographic interpretation is facilitated by the fact that the detection and diagnosis of breast cancer is virtually the only significant reason for evaluating the breast by imaging techniques.

### *Detection (Find It)*

Mammographic screening is only as good as the quality of the mammographic image and the skill of the radiologist interpreting the images. The imaging chain is only as strong as its weakest link. Thus equipment designed specifically to obtain high-resolution images with high contrast to enhance the separation of the inherently low-contrast structures of the breast is required. Dedicated mammographic equipment must be carefully maintained. Fortunately recent radiation risk assessments have been favorable for women of ages for whom screening is recommended, but the mammography units must be capable of producing high-quality images at as low a dose as is compatible with quality mammograms.

The technologist must be well trained to perform a rather difficult task. The amount of tissue imaged must be maximized with the breast compressed to spread the structures, reduce scatter, reduce geometric unsharpness, improve the uniformity of tissue thickness, and avoid motion without hurting the patient.

Film processing is an often neglected portion of the imaging sequence, and proper film development is required to maximize resolution, maintain high contrast, and reduce dose.

The ability to detect early cancers requires all of the foregoing to function properly and at a high level. The final link is the interpretation of the image. Radiologists must be trained to recognize the various changes on a mammogram that may indicate a malignant process. Even the most highly skilled, however, may fail to perceive a significant abnormality. Double reading has been shown to reduce this possibility.

### *Confirmation (Is It Real?)*

Before raising concern, the radiologist must be convinced that a finding at screening is truly a three-dimensional abnormality.

Lesions seen in only one projection must be confirmed as significant before suggesting any intervention. A consequence of the irregular structure of the normal breast is the superimposition of normal tissues, simulating an abnormality by forming a summation of shadows on the two-dimensional projection. Summation shadows can be differentiated from true breast lesions by various techniques. Most can be ignored on the initial screening by comparing the two standard projections. These almost orthogonal views are usually sufficient to determine whether a lesion is real or superimposed tissue. If there is any question, the radiologist should return to the projection in which the abnormality is observed and have the technologist modify that projection so as to alter the relationship of the x-ray beam to the tissues.

If the suspicious finding is distorted architecture, spot compression is used to better separate structures and eliminate confusing overlap. Alteration of the angle of the incident x-ray beam relative to the tissues may accomplish the same thing. Angling the gantry and reimaging produces a different projection of the various tissue elements on the detector. This can also be accomplished by rolling the breast and recompressing to reorient the tissue relationships relative to the beam. The absolute increase in resolution through direct mammographic magnification can be used to determine the true nature of an abnormality, as well as improve the visualization of its morphologic characteristics. The latter is important for lesion analysis.

## *Triangulation (Where Is It?)*

Once it has been confirmed that an abnormality is real, and potentially significant, its location in the breast must be determined. Certainly any recommendation for intervention should not be made unless the radiologist has an accurate idea of the three-dimensional location of a lesion within the breast. Abnormalities suggested in only one projection must be corroborated by other views or other imaging techniques such as ultrasonography or CT. Maneuvers used to establish the reality of a lesion can also be used to establish its location within the breast so that a needle can be accurately introduced into it.

The radiologist must be certain that the lesion is in fact within the breast. Since the majority of the skin surface projects over the breast on two-view imaging, skin lesions and calcifications can be mistaken for intramammary abnormalities. The radiologist and mammography technologist should be familiar with methods for excluding these benign possibilities. Raised skin lesions, or skin lesions with irregular surfaces that trap radiopaque powders and ointments, can project onto a mammogram and be mistaken as being within the breast (flat pigmented lesions usually are not visible). Any question is easily resolved by placing a marker on the skin lesion and imaging the marker en face and in tangent to the x-ray beam. Skin calcifications may be proven by placing a marker on the surface in which the calcifications are likely to be located and then imaging the marker in tangent. This confirms their dermal location.

If an intramammary lesion is seen on only the craniocaudal projection, rolled views can determine within which third of the breast the lesion lies. Simple fluoroscopic principles are applied. If the lesion moves in the direction that the top of the breast is rolled, the lesion is in the top of the breast. If it moves with the bottom, that is its location. If it remains relatively stable, it is likely in the center. Orthogonal views can then be obtained concentrating on the third of the breast in which a lesion lies to confirm its location.

If a lesion is seen only on the oblique view, a straight lateral projection should be obtained. The shift of the lesion relative to the projection of the breast tissues can be used to determine its location in the breast. We have also used ultrasonography and CT for the accurate triangulation and localization of true intramammary lesions when modified projections are inconclusive.

## *Assessment (What Is It?)*

Once the lesion has been confirmed as real, and its location in the breast has been confirmed (skin lesions excluded), lesion analysis should proceed. The first decision to be made is whether the lesion is morphologically benign. Mammographic interpretation should not be an intuitive process. The interpreter should have specific reasons for deciding that a lesion is benign. Magnification views for improved morphologic characterization and lesion definition, and ultrasonography for cyst or solid differentiation, are the primary noninvasive methods of lesion analysis.

Morphologic analysis can be used to avoid arousing concern over benign lesions. The location of a round or lobulated, circumscribed, reniform-shaped lesion in the outer periphery of the breast virtually guarantees that it represents a benign intramammary lymph node and requires no additional concern. Lucent-centered spherical calcifications are almost always a result of benign processes including the calcification of accumulated debris in and around the ducts, fat necrosis, and skin calcifications. Rod-shaped calcifications that are larger than 0.5 mm in diameter and are continuous are the result of the calcification of debris within the duct that is unrelated to a malignant process.

Magnification in conjunction with a horizontal-beam lateral projection can demonstrate the crescentic, "concave up," dependent collection of precipitated "milk of calcium" in benign cysts. Densely calcified fibroadenomas need not arouse alarm, and radiolucent encapsulated masses such as lipomas, oil cysts, galactoceles, and the mixed-density hamartoma are always benign.

An apparent focal cluster of calcifications on contact imaging may be shown on magnification imaging to merely represent a more prominent group in tissues that actually contain numerous, similar, round, amorphous, scattered calcifications reducing the likelihood of malignancy. Lucent centers may also be revealed by the higher resolution of magnification, and biopsy can be avoided.

If a circumscribed lesion is to be followed and open biopsy avoided, it should have sharp margins on magnification imaging. For lesions close to 1 cm or larger, ultrasonography can differentiate a cyst from a solid lesion. A cyst should have sharp anterior and posterior walls, with no internal echoes, and have enhanced through transmission of sound. The assessment of a solid lesion as observed by ultrasonography is purely a statistical probability, since benign and malignant solid lesions can have similar ultrasonographic morphology.

Thresholds for biopsy differ, but the radiologist should keep in mind that the best opportunity for cure is to discover breast cancers when they are under 1 cm in diameter. Any spiculated lesion that is not from previous surgery, even one that is stable over time, is highly suspicious and is only rarely benign. Any suggestion of an ill-defined "infiltrative" margin should prompt intervention. Calcifications that do not have the benign morphologies described earlier warrant careful evaluation. Those that are typical of intraductal cancer forming in necrotic cancer cells in the duct irregularly narrowed by breast cancer should be biopsied. Indeterminate irregularly shaped calcifications less than 0.5 mm in diameter should be viewed with a high degree of suspicion.

### *Diagnosis (What Should Be Done About It?)*

Ultimately, when a lesion is confirmed, but its histology is uncertain and its morphology is of concern, a recommendation for further analysis should be made according to established guidelines, such as those described earlier, and the consequences of the recommendation should be monitored so that modifications in the guidelines can be based on solid data. In general, if the lesion is circumscribed and meets the size criterion for investigation, ultrasonography or imaging-guided aspiration is recommended to establish the cystic or solid composition of the lesion. Until the accuracy of FNA is established for each radiology group, it should not be relied on to exclude cancer. If open biopsy is not used to diagnose solid lesions that have reached the threshold, these women must be followed carefully to ensure that false negatives are corrected expeditiously.

There are no absolute criteria for prompting biopsy, since imaging probabilities must be assessed in the light of individual patient factors such as age, quality of life, and risk from intervention. However, because of the true uncertainties of lesion analysis, the referring physician, whenever possible, should be given probabilities so that he or she can present these to the patient and together they can make an educated decision concerning the desirability of intervention or close follow-up. For example, some women might wish to avoid surgery and select short-interval follow-up for a lesion with a 2 to 5 percent probability of malignancy, whereas another woman might elect surgery for a 1 percent chance of cancer. If open biopsy is elected, the radiologist and surgeon must be able to offer the patient a safe accurate procedure that has a high likelihood of removing the lesion with little cosmetic damage or morbidity. The most accurate localization method involves holding the breast in the compression system of the mammographic unit and inserting a needle or wire guide through or alongside the lesion parallel to the chest wall. This permits a small amount of tissue to be removed to accurately determine the histology of the lesion in question. Specimen radiography with compression should be performed on all such lesions. If the lesion proves to be malignant, post-surgical mammography with magnification may be helpful to assess the possibility of residual cancer by defining residual calcifications. Conservation of the breast requires the removal of all the cancer to clear margins if recurrence following radiation is to be minimized.

The issue of short-interval follow-up (a period less than the recommended annual screening interval) is still debated. Many would argue that if the lesion is of insufficient concern to prompt immediate biopsy, there is little or no yield in short-interval follow-up, and unnecessary concerns are raised. There are few prospective, objective data, and most schemes rely on analysis of the expected doubling times of breast cancer. Our own experience suggests that whatever the interval, it should not interfere with the annual screening. We have adopted a 6 month "short interval," and recommend monitoring at this interval for a total of 2 years. Moskowitz suggests that in women under 50 this interval should be shortened to 3 months, because of the apparent more rapid growth of tumors in this age group. A spiculated or ill-defined lesion of any size and stability is suspect and should not be followed. Prospective studies are needed to develop policies based on data rather than supposition, but until these are available it is likely that a lesion that is stable over 2 years, and has "probably benign" characteristics to begin with, is not malignant.

## Discussion

The ability to find breast cancer earlier requires optimized imaging using dedicated mammographic equipment, highly skilled technologists to properly position the breast to maximize the visualized tissue, the proper processing of the image to enhance soft-tissue contrast and preserve high resolution, and a quality assurance program to guarantee that these elements remain constant. Once the images are obtained, interpretation requires systematic review by a trained radiologist with comparison to previous studies whenever possible, and the appropriate communication of a finding to the referring physician, or a structure to provide follow-up for the self-referred patient. Review of the images should be done in an orderly fashion. Each radiologist might wish to have his or her own approach, but it should be consistent so that the ability to recognize patterns is not compromised by haphazard review of the films.

An individual practitioner or group of radiologists should assess the various situations that arise in image production and interpretation and develop some uniform and substantiated guidelines. By maintaining these guidelines, the results of recommendations can more accurately be assessed. If, for example, a particular approach results in the diagnosis of mammographically detected breast cancers at stages that are little better than the historic ability of clinical and self-examination, the guidelines may be set at too high a threshold, and significant mortality reduction would be unlikely. If, on the other hand, there is a significant reduction in later-stage cancers by adoption of a more aggressive policy, perhaps a low threshold is reasonable. At least by having specific guidelines, one can evaluate the advantages and disadvantages and understand the effects of the program in an orderly fashion. Thus it is strongly urged that each group adopt guidelines that define thresholds for intervention. Imaging analysis should not be haphazard, but should be based on rules that can be substantiated by data, or when uncertain, tested by prospective study.

The ACR reporting system has been carefully thought through and should be adopted by those performing mammography. Final assessment should categorize all studies in the following manner according to the ACR system:

1. *Negative*—There is nothing to even comment on. The breasts are symmetrical and no masses, architectural disturbances, or suspicious calcifications are present.
2. *Benign Finding*—This is also a negative mammogram, but the interpreter may wish to describe a finding. Involuting, calcified fibroadenomas, multiple secretory calcifications, lucent (fat-containing lesions) intramammary lymph nodes,

post-surgical scars, post-radiation therapy changes, implants, and so forth fall into this category.

3. *Probably Benign Finding: Short-Interval Follow-Up Suggested*—This category will likely undergo future modification as more data accrue as to the validity of the approach, the interval required, and the type of findings that should be followed. Presently we include in this category solitary circumscribed densities under 8 mm in size, multiple round densities, multiple vague densities, and multiple groups of calcifications (assuming that none of the individual findings is of greater concern than the others).
4. *Suspicious Abnormality: Biopsy Should Be Considered*—There may be several subcategories within this general heading, but in general these are relatively low probability lesions. We include those solid lesions with a circumscribed border that have a 2 to 5 percent probability of cancer up to those ill-defined lesions that have a 50 percent or higher probability. Intermediate probability lesions are also included, such as most of the heterogeneous, clustered calcifications that lack the classic "casting" appearance. The ultimate goal is to more accurately subcategorize these lesions by morphologic as well as age criteria to provide the patient and her physician with more accurate information and probabilities to use in their decision to follow a particular abnormality or to excise it.
5. *Likely Malignant*—This category includes highly dense ill-defined lesions, or those with microlobulated margins, as well as areas of architectural distortion. These lesions have a greater than 80 percent certainty of being cancer and include the spiculated mass as well as the classic segmentally distributed casting calcifications of a comedocarcinoma.

By developing a reasoned consistent policy, a Breast-Imaging group can provide concise accurate reports based on interpretations that are not haphazard but carefully thought out. By monitoring the results of their activities accuracy will be improved.

## Suggested Reading


Brenner RJ, Sickles EA. Acceptability of periodic follow-up as an alternative to biopsy for mammographically detected lesions interpreted as probably benign. Radiology 1989; 171:645–646.

Gallagher WJ, Cardenosa G, Rubens JR, et al. Minimal-volume excision of nonpalpable breast lesions. AJR 1989; 153:957–961.

Kopans DB. Fine-needle aspiration of clinically occult breast lesions. Radiology 1989; 170:313–314.

Kopans DB. Breast Imaging. Philadelphia: JB Lippincott, 1989:331.

Kopans DB. The positive predictive value of mammography. AJR 1992; 158:521–526.

Kopans DB. Standardized mammography reporting. Radiol Clin North Am 1992; 30:257–264.

Kopans DB, Meyer JE. Computed tomography guided localization of clinically occult breast carcinoma—The "N" skin guide. Radiology 1982; 145:211–212.

Kopans DB, Meyer JE, Cohen AM, Wood WC. Palpable breast masses: The importance of preoperative mammography. JAMA 1981; 246:2819–2822.

Kopans DB, Meyer JE, Lindfors KK, Bucchianeri SS. Breast sonography to guide aspiration of cysts and preoperative localization of occult breast lesions. AJR 1984; 143:489–492.

Kopans DB, Meyer JE, Lindfors KK, McCarthy KA. Spring-hookwire breast lesion localizer: Use with rigid compression mammographic systems. Radiology 1985; 157:505–507.

Meyer JE, Kopans DB. Breast physical examination by the mammographer: An aid to improved diagnostic accuracy. Appl Radiol 1983; 103–106.

Moskowitz M. Breast cancer: Age-specific growth rates and screening strategies. Radiology 1986; 161:37–41.

Rosen PP, Groshen S, Saigo PE, et al. A long-term follow-up study of survival in stage I (T1 N0 M0) and stage II (T1 N1 M0) breast carcinoma. J Clin Oncol 1989; 7:355–366.

Sickles EA. Periodic mammographic follow-up of probably benign lesions: Results of 3184 consecutive cases. Radiology 1981; 179:463–468.

Sickles EA. Practical solutions to common mammographic problems: Tailoring the examination. AJR 1988; 151:31–39.

Swann CA, Kopans DB, McCarthy KA, et al. Localization of occult breast lesions: Practical solutions to problems of triangulation. Radiology 1987; 163:577–579.

Swann CA, Kopans DB, McCarthy KA, et al. Mammographic density and physical assessment of the breast. AJR 1987; 148:525–526.

Tabar L, Duffy SW, Krusemo UB. Detection method, tumor size and node metastases in breast cancers diagnosed during a trial of breast cancer screening. Eur J Cancer Clin Oncol 1987; 23:959–962.

Tabar L, Fagerberg G, Day N, et al. Breast cancer treatment and natural history: New insights from results of screening. Lancet 1992; 339:412–414.

Tabar L, Fagerberg G, Day NE, Holmberg L. What is the optimum interval between mammographic screening examinations?—An analysis based on the latest results of the Swedish two-county breast screening trial. Br J Cancer 1989; 55:547–551.

Tabar L, Fagerberg G, Duffy SW, et al. Update of the Swedish two-county program of mammographic screening for breast cancer. Radiol Clin North Am 1992; 30:187–210.


# Tailoring the Mammogram: Problem Solving and Special Views

*EDWARD A. SICKLES, M.D.*

The standard mammographic evaluation consists of craniocaudal (CC) and mediolateral oblique (MLO) projection exposures of each breast. However, standard imaging protocol often does not permit definitive mammographic interpretation of a visualized lesion. This situation requires additional views for further characterization, and a full understanding of how to conduct such problem-solving evaluations. All mammographers must become expert in deciding which extra views to obtain and when to use them.

This chapter presents the imaging approaches that I have developed for many clinical situations that require additional mammographic workup. Because of the great diversity of problems that are encountered, the chapter is not comprehensive in scope; however, it does cover the major issues. Further, the reader should understand that almost all mammographic problems can be solved by a variety of acceptable methods, and that I have discussed only my own personal preferences rather than a full listing of alternative imaging approaches.

## Lesion Seen on Only One Standard View

This is the most common mammographic problem, especially in interpreting screening evaluations. Usually one sees what looks like a mass or asymmetric density, although the same situation occasionally may arise with grouped microcalcifications. The finding is observed on either the CC or MLO projection, but not on the other view. The major decision to make is whether an abnormality indeed exists, or whether the "lesion" represents a fortuitous superimposition of otherwise innocuous overlapping shadows.

### *Is Additional Mammographic Workup Necessary?*

Most radiologists who monitor their mammographic evaluations before each patient is dismissed simply obtain at least one additional view, perhaps using the protocol that I describe in the next section. However, in many practices real-time interpretation of screening evaluations is impossible, impractical, or judged to be inconsistent with the rapid-throughput high-volume method that has been devised to reduce the cost of screening evaluations. These situations encourage the mammographer to develop the experience with which (in some cases) he or she may confidently make the diagnosis of summation shadow simply by analyzing the standard mammographic views, thereby eliminating the need to recall such patients for problem-solving mammography.

This latter approach, illustrated in Figure 1, is based on two cardinal principles: (1) the "lesion" as seen on one view is sufficiently close to the nipple so that it surely has been included on the second view, and (2) there is no area on the second view within which the "lesion" could be obscured by surrounding dense fibroglandular tissue. Note that in using this approach, the simplest way to estimate the depth of a finding on the second view is to make a straight-line measurement of the distance from the nipple to the finding on the first view, and then to trace an arc of this measured length, centered at the nipple, on the second view.

There are many advantages to identifying summation shadows directly from standard mammographic views. It takes less time to decide a priori that extra views are unnecessary than it does to actually expose, process, and interpret these views, especially if the patient must be recalled for problem-solving imaging. This saves time for the radiologist and technologist, thereby reducing operating costs; for the patient, it eliminates the inconvenience of a prolonged or recall visit. Such an approach also eliminates the morbidity (worry, fear, panic) that most patients experience when additional views are requested to evaluate for a possible breast abnormality. Again this applies primarily but not entirely to women who must be

A

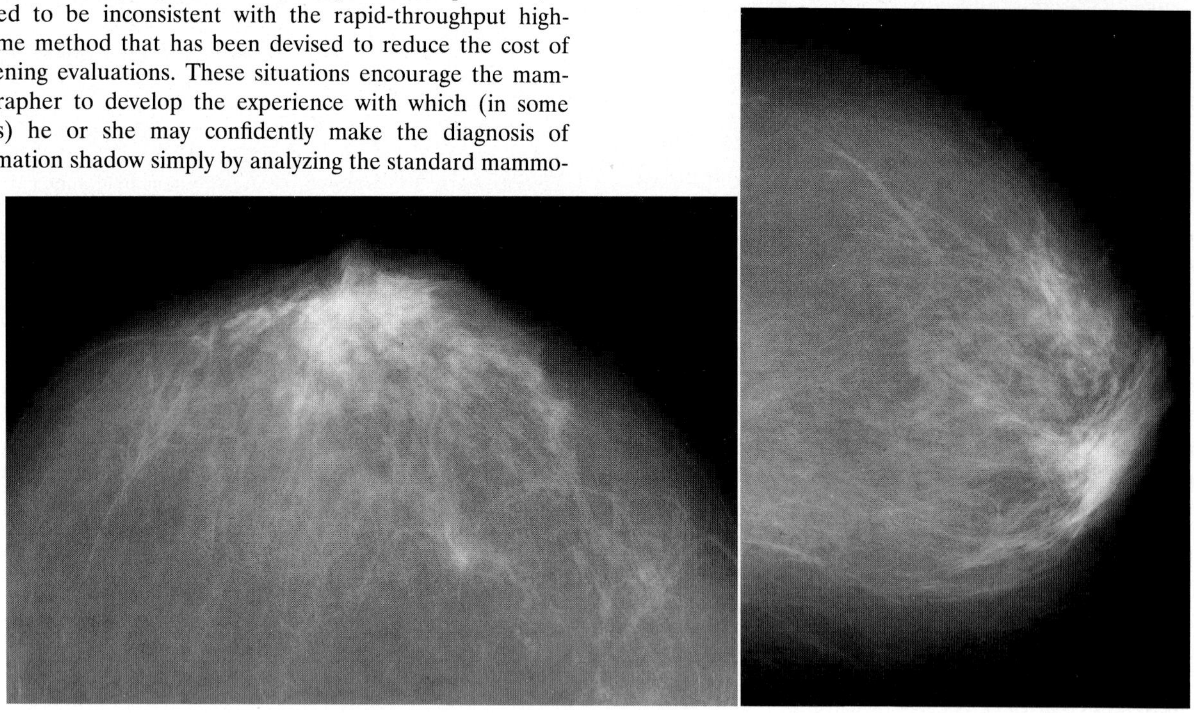

B

**FIGURE 1** Making the diagnosis of summation shadow on standard CC and MLO views only. *A,* Baseline CC projection mammogram of a 61-year-old asymptomatic woman demonstrated a 6 mm irregular, possibly spiculated density in the retroareolar region of the right breast slightly lateral to nipple level. The measured straight-line distance from the nipple to this finding was 7.5 cm. *B,* The standard MLO view mammogram from this evaluation did not show a similar finding. Note that the measured distance from the nipple to the back edge of the MLO film was 13.2 cm, indicating that the CC finding surely had been included within the MLO image. At a depth approximately 7.5 cm from the nipple on the MLO view, there were no areas of dense fibroglandular tissue that were large and dense enough to potentially have obscured visualization of the CC finding. This combination of findings is sufficient to establish the mammographic diagnosis of summation shadow, but in this case there is even more convincing evidence to support the diagnosis: on the MLO view at approximately 7.5 cm depth from the nipple (somewhat superior to nipple level) there is a much larger, less dense, and more vaguely defined area of benign-appearing fibroglandular tissue, which easily could have superimposed to create the shadow seen on the CC view. No further workup was recommended for this patient, a normal interpretation was made, and she was advised to have routine mammography screening in 1 year. Repeat evaluation done at that time also was interpreted as normal; the summation shadow seen previously on the CC view was no longer present.

recalled for additional imaging. Reduction in the number of unneeded mammographic exposures also increases the useful life of the mammography x-ray tube and reduces the radiation dose to the patient. Finally, for mammography practices that must recall screening patients for problem-solving evaluation, the number of false-positive interpretations is reduced (recall evaluations are considered "positive" interpretations), thereby increasing the positive predictive value statistic calculated as part of a basic medical audit.

### *How to Establish or Exclude the Diagnosis of Summation Shadow*

If the "lesion" as seen on one view is so far from the nipple that it may have been cut off the second view, then an additional image or images are needed for clarification. This occurs most commonly in women with small breasts and for findings located in the axillary tail or elsewhere close to the chest wall. For such cases, I direct the reader to the section entitled "Abnormality Not Included on Standard Views;" this provides a discussion of how the location of the finding as seen on the first view governs which of the many additional projections should be obtained next.

The other situation requiring extra view(s) occurs when the second standard view demonstrates a sufficient amount of potentially obscuring dense fibroglandular tissue in a location consistent with the expected depth of the finding as seen on the first view. In this circumstance, because the great majority of cases prove to be summation shadows, I believe that additional imaging should be directed toward demonstrating with confidence that the problem indeed has been caused by superimposition of normal structures. This is best done by taking an additional view in a projection only slightly different from the one in which the finding was first seen. Such a "shallow oblique" projection produces an image in which true abnormalities are readily seen again (in almost the same location and displaying virtually the same appearance), but in which summation shadows either are no longer visible or spread out into much more vague areas of benign-appearing fibroglandular density. The angle of offset for shallow oblique projection images should be approximately 5°; this is sufficient to cause substantial changes in the appearance of summation shadows, while restricting visual search to the small area immediately adjacent to that in which the finding was observed initially. In my opinion two methods are equally successful in producing 5° shallow oblique views: changing the obliquity of the x-ray beam by rotating the C-arm of the mammography unit, and changing the obliquity of the breast by obtaining a "roll" view as illustrated in Figure 2. I usually allow the technologist to decide which method works best for a given patient, but ask that she record the direction of changed obliquity so that if a true abnormality is present I will be able to make a rough estimate of the three-dimensional location of the lesion (e.g., for the case illustrated in Fig. 2, with the superior aspect of the breast rolled toward the axilla on a CC view, demonstration that the lesion shifted slightly laterally would indicate that it was located in the upper half of the breast, whereas a medial shift of the lesion would localize it to the lower breast).

Two other techniques also are helpful in differentiating between true abnormality and summation shadow. The first technique, spot compression, more effectively spreads apart overlapping islands of fibroglandular tissue than does whole-breast compression. This has the additional advantage of slightly improved resolution, since geometric unsharpness is reduced by bringing the area of interest somewhat closer to the film. Of course the spot compression device should not cover so small an area that the mammographic finding might be cut off. The second technique, magnification, produces images that are substantially higher in resolution and lower in system noise, thereby aiding interpretation. Moreover, because magnification imaging uses a more divergent x-ray beam than conventional mammography, it inherently produces a shallow oblique exposure unless the mammographic finding is exactly in the plane of the central ray.

In most circumstances an additional shallow oblique, spot compression, or magnification image is sufficient in and of itself to establish or exclude the diagnosis of summation shadow. However, in my own practice I combine all three into a single shallow oblique, spot compression, magnification exposure, because I have found that the imaging advantages of these techniques are additive, and that I get more mammographic information on this one extra view than I do on a view using only one or two of the techniques. Figure 3 illustrates how one may confidently establish the diagnosis of summation shadow with a single additional mammographic view.

Finally, one important issue must be considered concerning the workup of the lesion seen on only one standard view. If such a screening evaluation must be formally interpreted to recall the patient for problem-solving evaluation, then this interpretation should indicate that the finding is "incompletely evaluated" rather than suggesting that it is potentially suspicious for malignancy. Use of terminology that raises any concern about breast cancer is likely to prompt surgical referral, and in the absence of a palpable correlate to the mammographic finding, a needle localization inevitably is requested. Remember that most such findings are discovered to be summation shadows, which of course require no further evaluation of any kind. Should the mammographic diagnosis of summation shadow be deferred until the time of needle localization, cancellation of surgery at the last minute places unnecessary stress on the radiologist, the surgeon, and especially on the patient. Furthermore, costly radiologic and surgical resources are wasted in the process.

## Triangulating the Location of an Abnormality Using the MLO Projection

Localizing an abnormality in three dimensions by using orthogonal (i.e., CC and 90° lateral) projections is accomplished readily by radiologists, surgeons, and referring physicians. However, standard practice has substituted the MLO view for the 90° lateral view, resulting in the need to triangulate the location of an abnormality by using two films taken at an angle less than 90° apart. This situation confuses most physicians, including many radiologists.

A simple solution to the problem is to obtain an additional 90° lateral view whenever a significant abnormality is detected, but this often is not as easy as it might seem. (1) Many mammography screening practices follow the cost-efficient procedure of interpreting their evaluations in batches, after most if not all of the patients have been dismissed. Therefore there is no opportunity to obtain 90° lateral views before image interpretation, forcing the radiologist to describe the location of detected lesions based only on standard CC and MLO views.

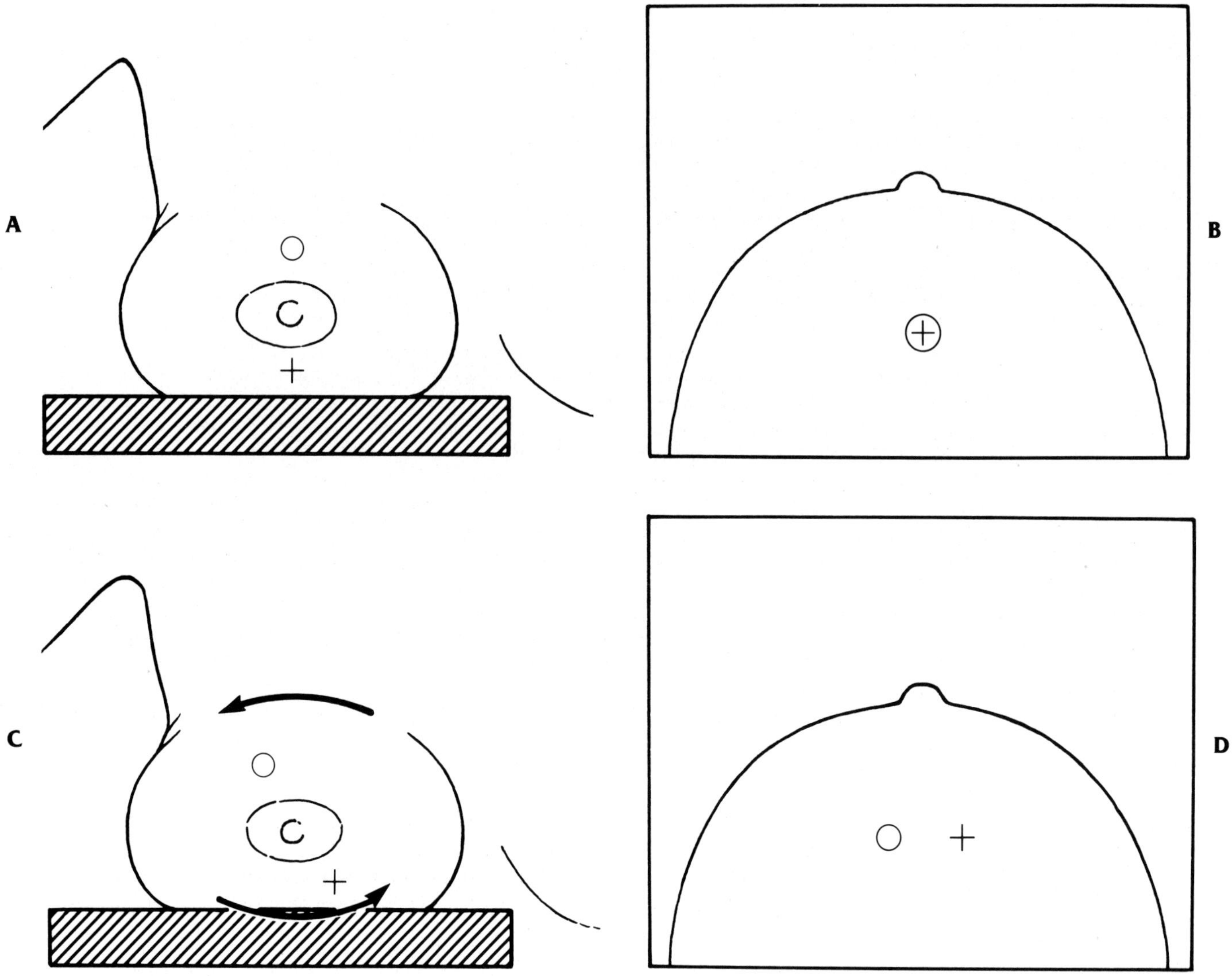


**FIGURE 2** Varying the obliquity of mammographic projection by changing the orientation of the breast ("roll" view). *A,* This breast has an area of benign fibroglandular tissue at the 12 o'clock position *(circle),* and another at the 6 o'clock position *(cross). B,* These two areas may superimpose on a standard CC view mammogram to create a summation shadow with mass-like features. *C,* The upper aspect of the breast has been "rolled" laterally, so that the two areas of benign fibroglandular tissue no longer project over each other on the CC projection. A similar effect would be produced by "rolling" the upper aspect of the breast medially. Note that the illustration indicates a much greater degree of "rolling" than the 5° that is necessary in clinical practice. *D,* A repeat CC view mammogram shows disappearance of the summation shadow. (From Sickles EA. Practical solutions to common mammographic problems: Tailoring the examination. AJR 1988; 151:31–39; with permission.)

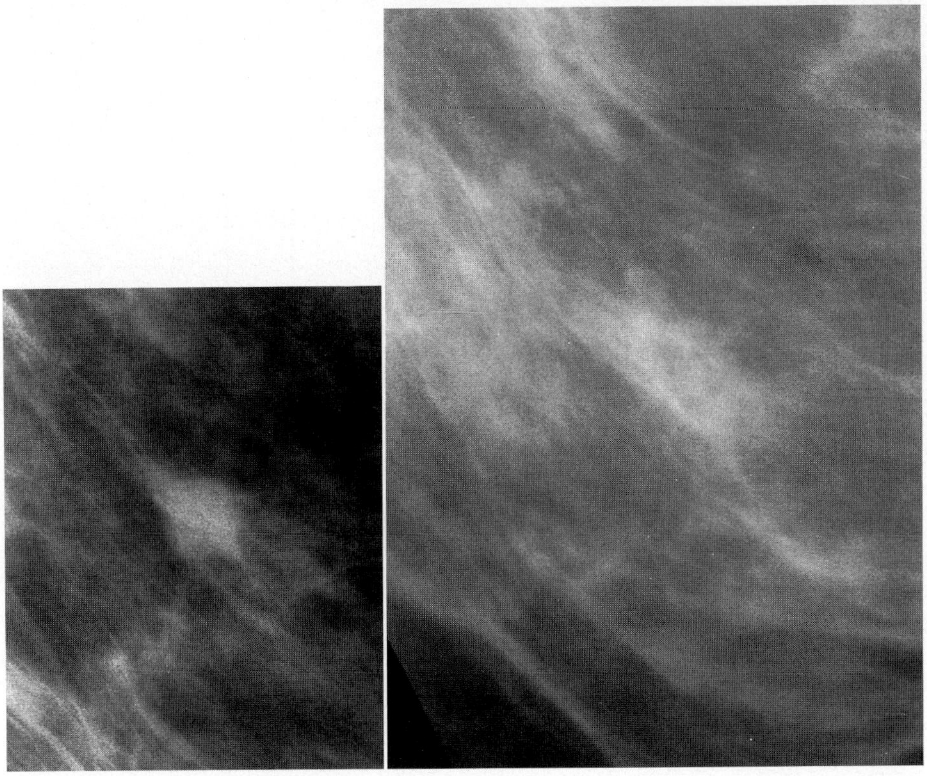

A B

**FIGURE 3** Making the diagnosis of summation shadow with a single additional mammographic view. *A,* Baseline mammography of a 52-year-old asymptomatic woman demonstrated a somewhat ill-defined and irregularly contoured 8 mm density in the lower aspect of the left breast, seen only on 45° MLO projection. The measured straight-line distance from the nipple to this finding was 8.4 cm. On the CC view (not shown), the measured distance from the nipple to the back edge of the film was 11.2 cm, indicating that the MLO finding surely had been included within the CC image. At a depth approximately 8.5 cm from the nipple on the CC view, there was one area of fibroglandular tissue that was sufficiently large and dense to potentially have obscured visualization of the MLO finding. Therefore the patient was recalled for problem-solving mammography. *B,* Shallow oblique (50° MLO) spot compression magnification mammogram, centered at the area of interest. What initially seemed to be a mass-like lesion has spread out into a much more vague area of benign-appearing fibroglandular density, thereby confidently establishing the mammographic diagnosis of summation shadow. No further workup was done, a normal interpretation was made, and the patient was advised to have routine mammography screening in 1 year. Repeat evaluation done at that time also was interpreted as normal, as were subsequent screening evaluations done over the next several years.

(2) In some cases, even though an abnormality is identified on both CC and MLO views, adjacent dense fibroglandular tissue may obscure it on the 90° lateral view. As discussed previously, this situation also may arise occasionally with either the CC or MLO view. Clearly it would be helpful to triangulate the location of abnormalities by using the (nonorthogonal) MLO projection. Unfortunately the ability to "think oblique" is not intuitively obvious.

Among the various visual aids available to teach how to make three-dimensional spatial estimates using the combination of CC and MLO views, I prefer the line drawings reproduced in Figure 4. One way to use them is to note the location of the abnormality on the CC view and then consult the appropriate set of drawings for this location. Thus, for an abnormality in the lateral aspect of the breast on CC view, one would refer to Figure 4, *A*. It should be readily apparent that if this abnormality projects approximately at the nipple level on the MLO view that it would be found in the lower part of the breast on the 90° lateral view. Similarly a lesion in the central part of the breast on the CC view (Fig. 4, *B*) that projects in the upper portion of the MLO view would be located superiorly on 90° lateral view, at the 12 o'clock position.

An even more effective way to use these line drawings is to learn the concept on which they are based, so that the drawings themselves are no longer necessary. In each set of illustrations, note that a straight line drawn between the location of an abnormality on CC and MLO views can be extended to its expected location on the 90° lateral view. Thus a radiologist viewing CC, MLO, and 90° lateral view mammograms also can expect to observe the same linear arrangement, provided that the three films are mounted on a viewbox in the same manner (oriented with the breast facing in the same direction, with the projection marker at the top of the image, with the nipple at the same vertical level, and with the MLO view in between the other two). Therefore, to use this concept without actually referring to the line drawings, the radiologist should appropriately mount on a viewbox the CC and MLO mammograms of a breast, draw an imaginary line from the abnormality seen on the CC view to its location on the MLO view, and then extend this imaginary line to estimate lesion location on the (not yet obtained) 90° lateral view.

One should not expect this approach to locate abnormalities with absolute precision, because breast positioning is usually not so exact as to place the central ray uniformly at the

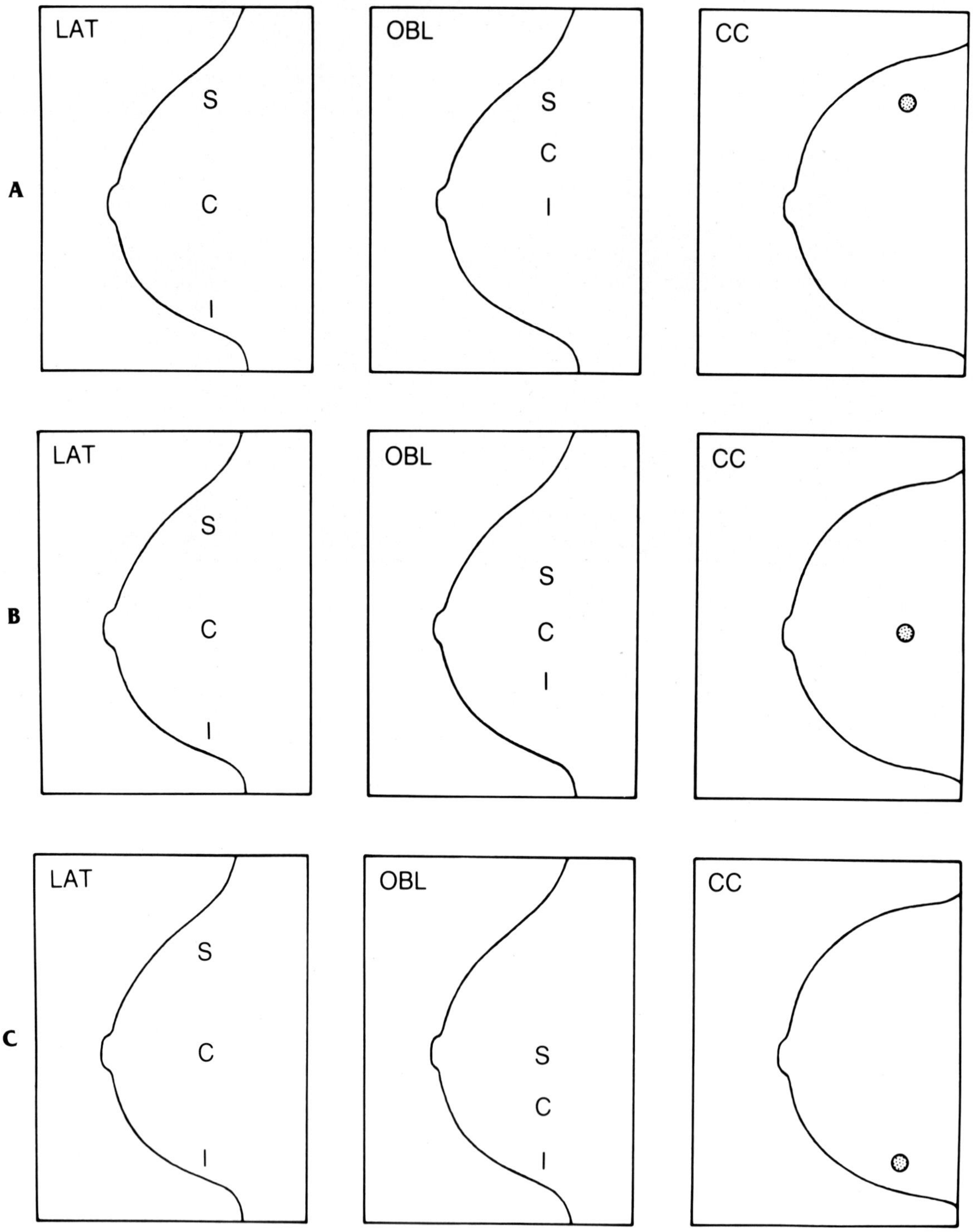


**FIGURE 4** Standard CC, MLO (OBL), and 90° lateral projections of a breast show the expected locations of abnormalities on a 90° lateral view if they were observed initially only on CC and MLO views. The abnormality is shown in the lateral *(A)*, central *(B)*, and medial *(C)* aspect of the breast on the CC views. Note the three possible locations of each abnormality on the corresponding MLO view (S = superior, C = central, I = inferior), and then find the appropriate location of the abnormality on the 90° lateral view. The illustrated mammograms have been placed equidistant from each other, which is proper for the use of a 45° MLO view. However, when using a 60° MLO view, the MLO mammogram should be placed farther from the CC view than it is from the 90° lateral view. (From Sickles EA. Practical solutions to common mammographic problems: Tailoring the examination. AJR 1988; 151:31–39; with permission.)

level of the nipple, because the same degree of breast compression often is not achieved in all three projections and because some degree of "rolling" may occur inadvertently on one or more projection. However, this is a rapid, convenient, and effective method to approximate the true position of an abnormality on the 90° lateral projection when it already is seen on MLO and CC views.

The most obvious use for this approach is in the batch interpretation of screening mammograms, during which the location of an abnormality must be described before a 90° lateral view can be obtained. This permits correlation with palpable findings without first requiring the patient to return for additional imaging. A second use is in facilitating preoperative identification of an abnormality that has been obscured by surrounding dense tissues on a conventional 90° lateral view mammogram. In this situation determination of the expected location of the abnormality permits proper positioning for spot compression magnification mammography in the 90° lateral projection, which in my experience almost always succeeds in portraying the lesion.

## Additional Mammographic Views and When to Use Them

There are two main reasons for using additional mammographic views: (1) to image in full an abnormality that is only partially included or not at all included on standard views, and (2) to better characterize an abnormality that already has been detected but is not seen as clearly as possible. The following section describes many of the additional views that can be used to help solve specific mammographic problems.

### *Abnormality Not Included on Standard Views*

#### Deep Lesions Located Far Laterally or Medially

These abnormalities usually are identified initially on the MLO view but not on the CC view. The convex curve of the chest wall simply prevents the most lateral and medial aspects of the breast from being included on standard CC projection. To overcome this problem, the patient must turn her body so that additional lateral or medial portions of the breast are included on a repeat CC view, at the expense of tissues located on the opposite side of the breast. The location of the abnormality on the MLO view determines whether the repeat CC view should be "exaggerated" either laterally or medially, as shown in Figure 5. Lesions that project in the upper aspect of the breast are likely to be found far laterally, whereas lesions that project in the lower breast almost always are found far medially. The reader may gain increased understanding of this concept by referring to Figure 4, *A* and *C*, which illustrates the potential locations on the MLO view of abnormalities located in the lateral and medial aspects of the breast. Note that for lesions seen centrally on the MLO view, either a lateral or medial location is possible. In this case, unless a mass is palpated far medially, the first attempt should "exaggerate" the repeat CC

A

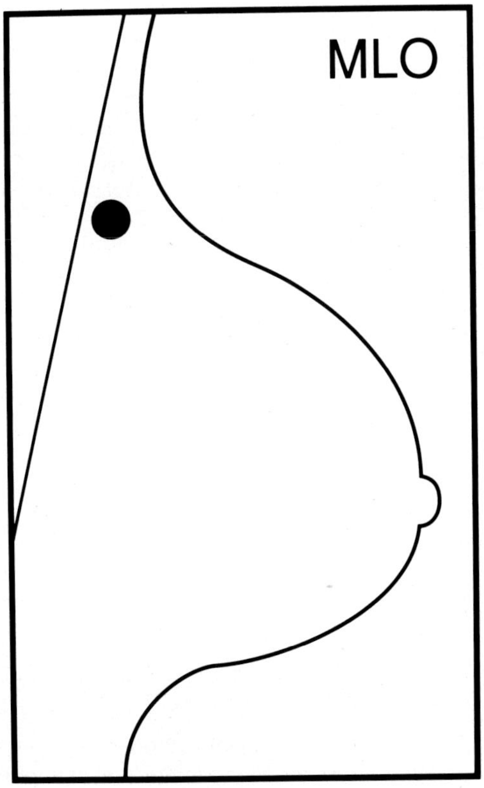


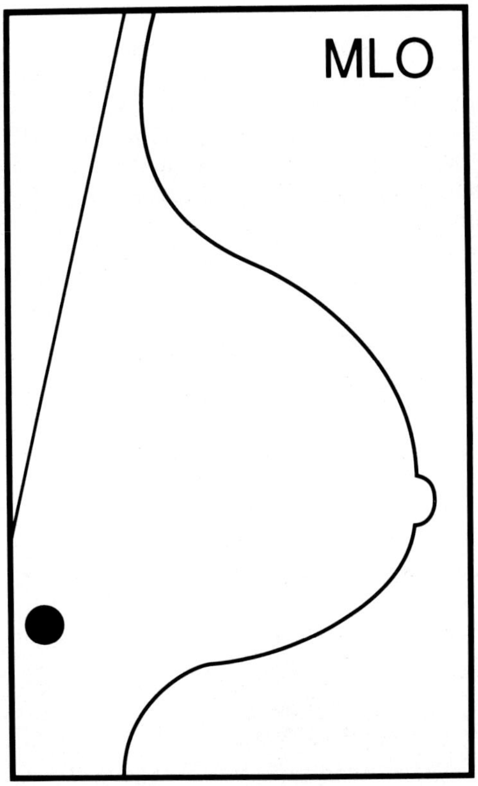


B

**FIGURE 5** The location of a mammographic abnormality seen on a standard MLO projection but not on a CC view governs the direction in which an exaggerated CC view should be taken. *A,* An abnormality that projects in the upper aspect of the breast on an MLO view should prompt a repeat CC view with the breast turned to include more lateral tissue. *B,* An abnormality that projects in the lower aspect of the breast on an MLO view should prompt a repeat CC view "exaggerated" medially. In this circumstance many technologists have even greater success by using the "cleavage" view, which also includes a substantial portion of the medial aspect of the contralateral breast.

view laterally, since most benign and malignant lesions are found there.

### Deep Lesions Located in the Upper Outer Quadrant

The projection that most effectively includes upper outer quadrant tissues is the standard MLO view, so that it is highly unusual to see a laterally located lesion on a standard CC view that has been cut off on the MLO view. However, occasionally an abnormality is partially included on an initial MLO view, for which additional imaging is required (Fig. 6). The best approach here is to show the technologist the location of the lesion on the MLO view already taken, and then request a repeat MLO view attempting to include tissues even closer to the chest wall. In my experience this almost invariably results in the imaging of at least 1 cm more of deep breast tissue, usually fully including the lesion in question.

### Deep Lesions Located in the Inner Breast, Especially in the Lower Inner Quadrant

These abnormalities may be only partially included or not included at all on either standard CC or MLO projections. An exaggerated medial CC view (or a "cleavage" view) usually includes the entire lesion, as may a lateromedial 90° lateral view. However, for the deepest of these abnormalities, the best available view is an oblique projection taken with the x-ray beam passing from superolateral to inferomedial location, the so-called SIO view.

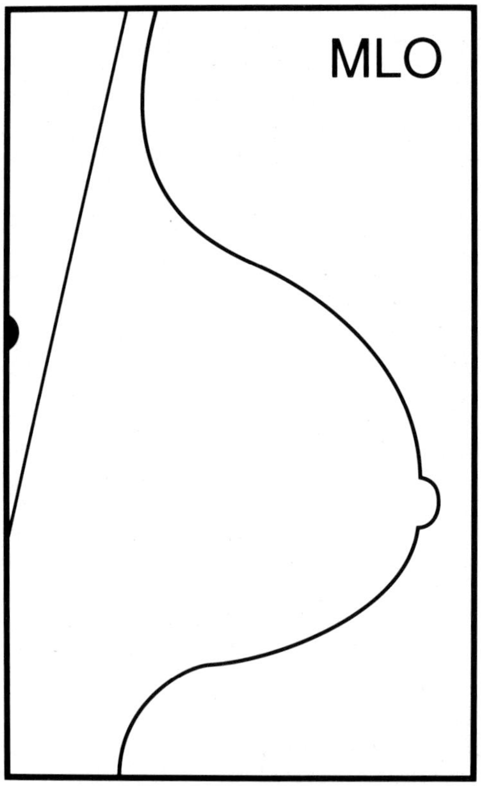


**FIGURE 6** To include the full extent of an upper outer quadrant mammographic abnormality that is only partially imaged on a standard MLO projection, simply request a repeat MLO view after emphasizing to the technologist the need to include tissues closer to the chest wall. This should encourage her to position the breast carefully, and almost always results in inclusion of deeper tissues, thereby solving the mammographic problem. Note that in this situation, a laterally "exaggerated" CC view may be necessary to visualize the abnormality with a vertical x-ray beam.

### Lesions Located High up on the Chest Wall at or Near the 12 O'clock Position

These abnormalities usually are readily seen on the standard MLO view, often are imaged successfully on the 90° lateral view, but are most difficult to include on the CC projection. Figure 7, *A* and *B,* illustrates how the firm compression needed to display breast structures with proper detail may not permit the uppermost portions of the breast to be imaged on the CC view. I prefer to overcome this problem by combining spot compression technique with positioning that includes under the compression device only the uppermost breast tissues, producing the so-called "lumpogram" that is shown in Figure 7, *C.* If there is a palpable abnormality at the same distance superior to the nipple as measured on a 90° lateral projection mammogram, then a small metal marker should be used to provide proper correlation of its location with that of the mammographic abnormality (Fig. 7, *D* and *E*). If no mass is palpable, even in retrospect, medial versus lateral positioning of the spot compression device for the CC view "lumpogram" should be deduced by triangulating the expected location of the abnormality on the CC projection from its observed location on both MLO and 90° lateral views (use the concept illustrated in Fig. 4 to work "backward" from 90° lateral to MLO to CC view).

### Lesions Located so Close to the Chest Wall That Nothing Else Works

In the hands of skilled mammography technologists who pay careful attention to proper positioning technique, it is highly unusual to encounter an abnormality that cannot be included on at least one of the mammographic views discussed previously. However, sooner or later every busy radiologist is faced with that most difficult lesion for which truly heroic efforts are required. In this situation further inventive maneuvers may well succeed. I prefer to try variants of the "lumpogram" technique in nonstandard mammographic projections, in an attempt to overcome the limitations imposed by the convex curvature of the chest wall, the concavity of the axilla, or whatever other physical constraint seems to be causing the problem. Of course one may resort to cross-sectional imaging techniques such as ultrasonography or computed tomographic (CT) scanning, but these approaches are handicapped by the fact that even if successful, they portray the abnormality with a different appearance than that seen at mammography, potentially confounding interpretation.

## *Further Characterization of an Already Detected Abnormality*

Just as there are many additional mammographic views designed to more effectively include abnormalities that have been cut off standard-projection images, so are there numerous techniques available to further characterize abnormalities that are seen with less than optimal clarity. Among this latter group, several are so obvious that they do not require discussion, including the correction of under- or over-exposure,

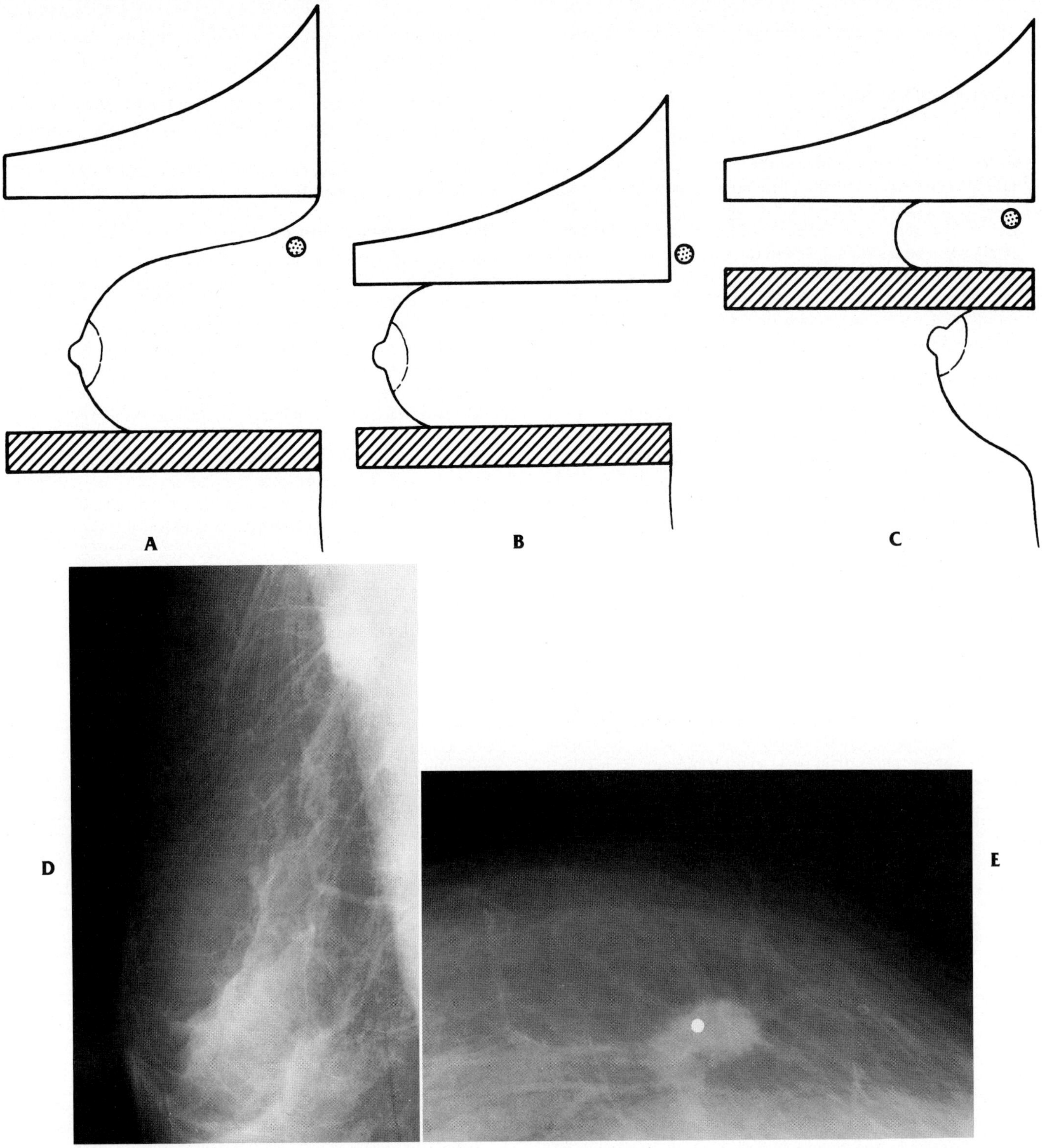


**FIGURE 7** How proper breast compression may prevent inclusion on a standard CC view of an abnormality located high up on the chest wall and how to solve the problem. *A,* A standard CC view taken without breast compression usually includes the abnormality on the film, but absence of compression so degrades the resultant image that the lesion often cannot be observed. *B,* While breast compression is applied, the compression plate may travel so far down the chest wall that the lesion is no longer included in the image. This may occur even when the breast is properly elevated by lifting the inframammary fold before application of compression. *C,* Use of the "lumpogram" technique solves this positioning problem. By imaging only the uppermost portions of the breast on the CC view, a superiorly located abnormality can still be included in the mammographic image while firm compression is applied. The only special equipment required for this view is a spot compression device. *D,* A 90° lateral view of a breast shows an ill-defined spiculated mass 14.3 cm superior to nipple level. A mass of similar size was palpated 14 cm above nipple level, approximately at the 12 o'clock position. The mammographic abnormality was imaged on a standard MLO projection, but was not included on a properly positioned CC view (both not shown). *E,* "Lumpogram" of the palpable mass in a CC projection, with a small metal marker placed over it. This additional image not only demonstrates the mammographic finding on an orthogonal view, but also indicates that the palpable and mammographic masses are one and the same, thereby eliminating the need for preoperative lesion localization. (From Sickles EA. Practical solutions to common mammographic problems: Tailoring the examination. AJR 1988; 151:31–39; with permission.)

under- or over-penetration, elimination of inadvertent patient motion, and repeat imaging after removal of overlying artifacts.

### Lateromedial versus Mediolateral 90° Lateral Views

Because most benign and malignant breast abnormalities occur in the outer half of the breast, the standard image in the 90° lateral projection is obtained with a mediolateral x-ray beam, thereby placing the outer aspect of the breast closer to the film cassette to minimize geometric unsharpness. On the other hand, when an additional 90° lateral view is needed to further evaluate an abnormality already seen to be located in the inner breast on a CC projection image, it is preferable to take the 90° lateral view with a lateromedial x-ray beam. This produces a sharper image of the abnormality.

### Full Range of Oblique Views

The standard MLO projection mammogram is taken with the plane of compression parallel to that of the pectoralis major muscle, resulting in an x-ray beam obliquity of 45° to 60° off horizontal. However, mammography units can operate in *any* plane of obliquity, permitting the mammographer to employ a much more complete range of oblique views. This capability is used most frequently in obtaining shallow oblique views to establish or exclude the diagnosis of summation shadow, as discussed previously. In addition, when a mass is partially obscured by overlying dense fibroglandular tissue on one or both standard views, it may be helpful to take another exposure using a nonconventional degree of beam obliquity. The rationale behind this approach is to project the mass so that its previously obscured margins now overlie areas of fatty tissue, where border characteristics can be analyzed more readily. Since trial and error are involved in obtaining successful results, often more than one extra exposure is needed, especially in women with dense breasts. To maximize the amount of additional mammographic information obtained, these exposures should be taken using spot compression magnification technique.

### Tangential Views

The most common clinical use of the tangential view is to establish or exclude dermal location for already detected abnormalities. This is an important distinction, since skin lesions invariably are benign. Clustered dermal calcifications not infrequently mimic the findings of malignancy, especially when they are small, when they project over the breast parenchyma on both CC and MLO views, and when the calcific particles do not show (characteristically benign) radiolucent centers. Tangential views therefore are invaluable in averting biopsy of these benign lesions.

Tangential views also can be used to further characterize selected parenchymal abnormalities, specifically those *palpable* masses that are completely obscured by surrounding dense fibroglandular tissue. Unless a mass is large, it must be fairly superficial in location to be palpable. The rationale behind using a tangential x-ray beam to image such a nonvisualized lesion is that it may project the mass sufficiently close to subcutaneous fat as to demonstrate its convex contour (or perhaps some architectural distortion), thereby permitting mammographic detection. Confirmation by mammography that a mass indeed is present may be just the stimulus needed to prompt biopsy of a palpable cancer that is not suspicious for malignancy by physical examination. As with the use of additional oblique views to visualize otherwise obscured margins of masses, these tangential-beam exposures should be taken using spot compression magnification technique.

### Spot Compression Views

The several imaging advantages of breast compression include reduced motion, decreased geometric unsharpness, increased contrast, and the spreading apart of superimposed islands of dense fibroglandular tissue. A spot compression device is especially effective in producing these improvements in image quality, because its compressive force is applied only to the area of interest, rather than being distributed over the entire breast as occurs when conventional uniform-thickness compression is provided. As a result, many mammographers obtain additional spot compression views of any abnormality that is not seen with optimal clarity on standard-projection images. However, in my practice I always combine spot compression with magnification imaging, because the theoretical advantages of these two techniques are additive, and because I get more mammographic information on a single combined view than I do on views using either technique alone.

### Magnification Views

Direct radiographic magnification produces mammographic images of superior quality, because of increased resolution and reduced system noise. Microcalcifications are portrayed with greater clarity, as are the margins of breast masses. However, to be successful, magnification technique requires the use of an x-ray tube with a tiny focal spot, usually one that is measured to be 0.2 mm or smaller. All magnification views should demonstrate noticeably finer image detail than corresponding conventional views, apart from the isolated case where motion unsharpness is encountered. As discussed previously, magnification mammography can be combined successfully with spot compression and other techniques. I routinely obtain additional spot compression magnification views for most findings not observed with sufficient detail to permit definitive interpretation; for all abnormalities that require either biopsy or periodic mammographic surveillance, I prefer to obtain these additional views in both CC and 90° lateral projections.

## Suggested Reading

Eklund GW. Problem-solving mammography. In: Sickles EA, Kopans DB, eds. Syllabus for the Categorical Course on Breast Imaging (American College of Radiology annual meeting, 1990). Reston, VA: American College of Radiology, 1990:69–75.

Homer MJ. Mammographic Interpretation: A Practical Approach. New York: McGraw-Hill, 1991.

Kopans DB. Breast Imaging. Philadelphia: JB Lippincott, 1989.

Logan WW, Janus J. Use of special mammographic views to maximize radiographic information. Radiol Clin North Am 1987; 25:953–959.

Sickles EA. Practical solutions to common mammographic problems: Tailoring the examination. Am J Roentgenol 1988; 151:31–39.

# Surveillance Mammography versus Biopsy for Probably Benign Breast Lesions

*R. JAMES BRENNER, M.D., J.D.*

A majority of breast lesions detected during routine mammography demonstrate features that are neither clearly benign nor malignant. Rather, employing appropriate imaging modalities, expertise, and experience, the mammographer attempts to correctly characterize such lesions to arrive at an appropriate recommendation for management, including routine follow-up, short-term follow-up (mammographic surveillance), surgical excision, or possibly other tissue-sampling procedures. This recommendation is subject to both a medical and legal standard of reasonableness; that is, based on experience and competent evaluation, is it reasonably foreseeable that a detected mammographic abnormality maintains a sufficient likelihood of malignancy to require surgical excision? The operational standards by which one may offer an alternative to surgical excision may be measured thusly: does a mammographically detected abnormality demonstrate sufficient characteristics for which a mammographer can reasonably presume a benign etiology? Neither the legal nor medical dictum requires a warranty of certainty with respect to the evaluation of such abnormalities. One should recall that many malignancies demonstrate no mammographic features.

This kind of analysis is supported by the recently established standard nomenclature for mammographic interpretation issued by the American College of Radiology.

This chapter discusses the management of common, probably benign, mammographic abnormalities observed during routine mammography, with an emphasis on which abnormalities may lend themselves to surveillance. Benign lesions, such as clearly defined intramammary lymph nodes or milk of calcium, are not included in this discussion. Ultimately the outcome of such management is dependent upon the particular equipment employed, diagnostic acumen, and audited experience of one's own individual practice. To the extent that suggested strategies may be successful in any particular set of circumstances, they are presented for purposes of consideration and approach.

## Well-Defined Solitary Noncalcified Masses

The most likely etiologies for a well-circumscribed solitary noncalcified mass include a benign cyst or fibroadenoma. The latter benign tumor is not uncommon in the female population and with age frequently undergoes involutionary changes often characteristically demonstrated on mammograms by the appearance of calcifications distributed circumferentially about or centrally within the tumor. Other etiologies are of course possible (such as papilloma and papillary carcinoma), but are less likely as a cause for such masses in the general population. The presentation of such masses as detected mammographic abnormalities requires diagnostic evaluation. Micro focal spot coned compression magnification views should be obtained to better define margins of lesions needing further analysis. Apparently well-circumscribed margins on conventional mammography may consequently demonstrate areas of irregularity or indistinctness. The margins most subject to mammographic evaluation occur where there is a fat and soft-tissue interface. Often, not all of the margins on the mammogram may be demonstrable, even with magnification views, because of surrounding isodense fibroglandular tissue, but may be interrogated with ultrasonography, which is not compromised by this particular problem.

The ancillary role of ultrasonography in such circumstances is twofold. Ultrasonography should be applied to prominent noncalcified solitary masses initially to establish a cystic versus solid etiology. Because ultrasonography is operator- and technically dependent, its use must be accompanied by experience and expertise insofar as time gain compensation curves may artifactually change the appearance and suspected etiology of the lesion in question. Simple cysts defined as well-circumscribed anechoic masses with acoustical enhancement may be regarded as benign and require no further evaluation or short-term follow-up.

The management of solid masses remains controversial. Many mammographers elect to employ size criteria in deciding the priority of surveillance versus surgical excision, although size in itself has little predictive diagnostic value. Consistent with the large-scale study published by Sickles, size has little significance, except when the diameter of the mass is greater than 3.0 to 3.5 cm. Because of the decrease in frequency of fibroadenomata of this size, and increased likelihood of phylloides lesions and other malignancies attaining such a size, such abnormalities are frequently referred for surgical excision.

Assuming a mass is less than 3.0 to 3.5 cm in size, any detectable irregularity of its margins by sonography invokes the same degree of suspicion as would an irregular margin mammographically detected. Although resolution capability of analog-magnified mammographic images is superior to sonographic images, appropriate imaging with high-frequency transducers can provide significant information regarding the margins of the mass. Sonographic criteria do not, however, supercede mammographic criteria in determining benign versus malignant potential. When evaluating masses sonographically, particular attention is paid to the apparent posterior margin, this margin representing different margins of the actual mass as the transducer interrogates the mass from as many directions and orientations as possible. An attempt should be made to identify a specular reflection from such a posterior margin to further increase the confidence that it is indeed smooth. An anteroposterior to transverse diameter ratio of 1:2 is a useful corroborative finding for suspected benign lesions.

I have found increased confidence employing 10 MHz transducers, but have found that the frequency of the transducers is not dispositive of high-resolution imaging. Experience with different transducers based on pathologically proven data is the best parameter of the confidence one may achieve in employing such technology. Users and transducers must be assessed on an individual basis.

Acoustical enhancement and shadowing, as well as internal echogenicity with respect to solid masses, are of indeterminate predictive value in assessing benign or malignant potential. Rather, the margins of the mass are the most useful parameter in predicting etiology, whether mammographically or sonographically. It should be noted that cysts with proteinaceous material may appear solid, but display considerable acoustic enhancement. Aspiration with disappearance of the mass (fluid may or may not be sent for cytologic and heme evaluation, depending on its appearance in conjunction with the sonogram) resolves the issue.

Simple cysts with thin septations are of little concern. Conversely, true complex sonographic masses, which by definition include both solid and cystic components, maintain a sufficiently high degree of suspicion to require a further intervention. Oftentimes clinical history may lead to the appropriate intervention, as in the case with a resolving hematoma or abscess. However, when insufficient clinical grounds exist to assign a more limited intervention to a growing or interval solid mass, or a complex sonographic mass, tissue sampling may be required.

The development of new cysts, even postmenopausally, in women not undergoing exogenous hormonal therapy, has been observed frequently. The phenomenon is difficult to explain and many sonographically guided cyst aspirations have permitted the conclusion that, given the proper imaging analysis, such lesions may be treated as benign cysts. Nonetheless, the option is reserved for aspirating interval cysts in postmenopausal women who have a history of breast malignancy.

When a solitary noncalcified solid mass can be demonstrated to be well circumscribed mammographically, sonographically (echotecture and transmission may influence management), or both, such a lesion maintains a high likelihood of representing a benign lesion, such as a fibroadenoma, and may lend itself to short-term follow-up under appropriate circumstances. Lesions are followed mammographically at a 6 month interval, with the assumption that an unchanging nature in terms of size and morphology will be corroborated. The lesion is subsequently reassessed in 6 months during an annual screening mammography; if it again demonstrates no significant change, the patient is followed annually. Thus only one additional unilateral mammogram is generally required, assuming that a patient is on a yearly screening interval program. The short-term follow-up examination is an attempt to intercept growing phylloides lesions, as well as rare, rapidly growing, well-circumscribed carcinomas. Reviews in the literature of so-called well-circumscribed masses suggest that many are indeed not well circumscribed when subject to a more critical analysis. Magnification mammography is essential to document the absence of irregular margins and provide a prudent basis for assigning such lesions to a surveillance status.

Certain exceptions to the above approach are employed. First, if a solid mass in the screening age group (>40 years) grows, surgical excision is suggested regardless of its morphology. While I have seen several fibroadenomata grow in this age group, the phenomenon is unusual and thus interferes with a reasoned basis for continued follow-up. Likewise the development of new solid masses over the age of 40 is unusual, although I have seen fibroadenomata develop in this age group with uncommon frequency. Therefore new solid masses, again regardless of morphologic evaluation, should undergo tissue sampling. It should also be noted in this context that if the mass cannot be reliably measured on the mammogram, especially the craniocaudal view, it may not lend itself to surveillance.

The presence of multiple masses, especially bilaterally, lends itself particularly well to short-term follow-up examination. Multiplicity of such masses, while inferring a benign etiology, must still be treated with care. A "worst case analysis" should be entertained by the mammographer to interrogate any particularly suspicious-looking mass among the multiplicity of such masses. If no such area or mass is more worrisome than the others, and if most appear well circumscribed to the extent that they can be defined mammographically, a short-term follow-up examination in 6 months is suggested. Attempts to evaluate all such masses with ultrasonography at initial presentation may lead to considerable frustration and error, because correlation between the mammographic and sonographic masses under such circumstances is difficult. In addition, when multiple masses abut one another, their margins do not lend themselves as well to sonographic evaluation.

The short-term follow-up examination is employed as an attempt to intercept any given mass that enlarges or any new mass that develops. The analysis applied previously to a growing or interval solid mass may then be applied under such circumstances, with management directed accordingly.

## Clustered Microcalcifications

The criteria for recognizing malignant versus benign clustered microcalcifications have been reviewed extensively in other publications. Interestingly, one such study indicated that perhaps 20 percent of malignant calcifications may present atypical manifestations, or in other words, features not classic for a consideration of malignancy. A review of such discussion is beyond the scope of this analysis; classic descriptions are available in other publications.

For questionable clusters of microcalcifications that are probably benign, the following analysis is employed. The three primary criteria by which such clusters are evaluated include number of calcifications, pleomorphism, and density per unit size. Other considerations include age at appearance, interval change, and distribution.

Many workers have chosen the number of five calcifications to begin a discussion of clustered microcalcifications, but it should be emphasized that such a number is arbitrary and of least importance in considering benign versus malignant potentials. Rather it is a term of art by which communication among clinicians and mammographers may begin when employing the term "cluster." In our experience 5 to 10 particles initiates the discussion of a cluster. Pleomorphism, differing sizes and shapes of microcalcifications, is a highly important feature in determining malignant potential. Further, differing densities per unit size (similar particles of the same size and shape that maintain different mammographic attenuation) has been a particularly useful feature in our evaluation of malignant processes, although there is little guidance in the literature to document these findings, perhaps based on the difficulty in reproducing such images in journal publications. It should be noted that pleomorphism and differing densities per unit size are perhaps paramount in importance to number when evaluating a cluster of microcalcifications. The relative importance of all three features must be considered in tandem in deciding appropriate management.

For probably benign clustered microcalcifications—namely, those that are relatively few, all round and punctate in their morphology, and of similar density per unit size—I employ short-term follow-up to corroborate a benign impression. This analysis should be buttressed with other considerations. A benign etiology needs to be considered analytically before assigning such calcifications to a benign diagnosis for which surveillance mammography may be appropriate. For example, when such benign calcifications maintain a circumferential distribution such that an early involuting fibroadenoma may be suspected, follow-up mammography is predicated on the anticipated observance that these calcifications will become larger, denser, and more classically demonstrative of a benign involuting fibroadenoma. Thus, if the distribution of such calcifications extends beyond the anticipated circumference of the presumed lesion, an impression of the benignancy may be defeated.

Similarly, vascular calcification may not always be easily correlated to mammographic demonstration of a vessel and when appearing en face may provide considerable confusion for the mammographer. The same analysis therefore is employed when considering this entity.

Age is an important factor in threshold determinations as to when to biopsy clusters of microcalcifications that are not clearly benign or malignant. In my experience the presence of small clusters of microcalcifications in an older age group has a higher frequency of benign considerations. For example, fibroadenomata within the breast may not be mammographically detectable until they begin to involute and declare themselves as small clusters of benign-appearing microcalcifications, usually in the post-menopausal age group. Although this may happen in a younger age group, its likelihood is less, and therefore the differential diagnosis of clustered microcalcification in the younger age group is more limited. Studies have suggested that tumors in the younger age group may indeed grow faster. If one considers the differential diagnosis of clustered microcalcification in the younger age group to be more limited, and assumes that an incorrect presumption of benignity may have a more adverse effect on a faster-growing tumor, the threshold for suggesting surveillance mammography versus surgical excision for such clusters changes accordingly. This does not mean that all clusters (consider lobular calcifications) in younger-aged women must be removed, but only that differing thresholds may be considered in the evaluation of a similar cluster found in a younger woman versus an older woman. I am willing to accept a somewhat higher nonmalignant/malignant biopsy ratio in the younger age group for just such a reason, so long as that ratio remains reasonable and is consistent with a general analysis of clustered microcalcifications.

The analysis previously applied to bilateral diffuse masses is analogous to the evaluation of bilateral and/or diffuse microcalcifications.

## Focal Asymmetries

Focal mammographic asymmetries must be distinguished from generalized areas of fibroglandular tissue that are asymmetries with respect to one breast or the other. Generalized asymmetries of the breast associated with palpable abnormalities maintain an index of suspicion commensurate with lesions of clinical concern, regardless of the mammogram. The directed clinical correlation is therefore dispositive in deciding to biopsy such areas or dismiss them as normal mammographic variants. It is extremely unusual to recommend short-term follow-up for general asymmetries of fibroglandular tissue if the physical examination, especially when directed to the area of concern, demonstrates no palpable area of concern.

Focal mammographic asymmetries, however, remain the responsibility of the imager, because such lesions in a screening mammographic practice are by definition nonpalpable. It is this category that lends itself more than others to an interpretative range of options.

If the focal asymmetry, as defined in two orthogonal projections, appears to "almost" represent a mass, it may lend itself to mammographic workup and sonographic evaluation and be treated as a mass in a manner previously described in this chapter.

If the asymmetry appears more focal on one view and appears to distribute itself in a more diffuse manner on the orthogonal projection (a phenomenon I refer to as the "schmear" sign), it probably has no clinical significance, because the spreading of tissue virtually negates the "focal" nature of the asymmetry.

The management of lesions that do not lend themselves to either of these circumstances and remain true focal asymmetries of the breast becomes a matter for mammographic judgment. Most of these "lesions" represent simple isolated areas of fibroglandular tissue. In our experience the more focal and unchangeable the asymmetry, the more suspicious the interpretation—a determination often aided with rolled and spot compression views. This analysis defies prescriptive guidelines and must be handled on a case by case analysis.

Thus the management options for mammographically detected focal asymmetries range from doing nothing (schmear sign abnormalities), short-term follow-up to exclude interval change, to tissue sampling.

## General Principles for Surveillance Mammography

As may be inferred from the previous discussion, surveillance mammography is predicated on establishing to a reasonable degree of confidence that a detected mammographic abnormality is most likely benign and does not warrant surgical intervention on the basis of imaging features. To this extent, all significant lesions must undergo initial and complete imaging evaluation including spot magnification mammography and possible ultrasonography. Specifically, on the basis of a full diagnostic evaluation, the election for short-term follow-up or interval-screening mammography may be established. It is unusual that any further follow-up examinations employ such ancillary studies unless an interval change is suspected on the basis of conventional films. Therefore suggesting short term follow-up with diagnostic evaluation to be applied to the future examination is by definition inappropriate and ill-advised. Sufficient benign criteria must be established to the satisfaction of the mammographer to permit surveillance mammography to be conducted on the basis of conventional imaging techniques.

Auditing one's individual practice is a most important parameter in deciding whether or not the aforementioned strategies are successful. As had been described, focal asymmetries of the breast preempt a prescribed approach insofar as the asymmetries are highly variable in their appearance. Only by assessing the success of one's individual approach to such lesions and other lesions may such strategies be validated. For example, a practice that suggests a benign etiology to well-circumscribed masses and finds that eventual biopsy of such masses for clinical or mammographic reasons yields a false-negative rate of 10 percent may not be able to pursue surveillance mammography as an alternative to surgical excision, unless methodologies and criteria are re-established and subsequently validated.

## Discussion

I am often asked, "How can you be sure that the lesion you are describing is benign and lends itself to mammographic surveillance?" Certainty is a rare luxury afforded the mammographer or radiologist involved in any other imaging practice. Rather the mammographer is responsible for rendering a reasonable evaluation and recommendation based on experience and expertise. It is important to consider surveillance mammography therefore in the context of general radiologic practice in terms of both standard of care issues as well as realistic expectations. Follow-up examinations have been recommended in recent reviews for other organ systems, including incidentally detected masses of the kidney, adrenal gland, liver (consider the high-frequency hemangiomata) and chest.

Increasing public scrutiny of mammographic practices combined with the public health–oriented approach applied in screening mammography has served as a cause for concern among mammographers choosing to reduce the number of false-positive diagnoses made during routine mammography. Consequent medicolegal exposure combined with socioeconomic concerns on the part of third-party reimbursement carriers have placed mammographers in a difficult position in attempting to offer the public a successful screening program, whose main effort is to intercept breast cancer at its earliest stages while maintaining standards of diagnostic practice commensurate with other fields of radiology. A large number of continuing education courses and literature reports in this field now offer the mammographer a reasonable basis for prudent decision making that, while difficult, reflects a degree of success commensurate with any other field of imaging. Any strategy directed toward mammographic surveillance should be validated in one's own clinical practice, supported by histopathologic follow-up results when appropriate. The role of nonsurgical intervention by means of stereotactically radiographically-guided fine-needle aspiration and core biopsy is presently being investigated. Sonographically guided tissue sampling may be more readily applicable as successful techniques adapted from other organ-specific systems are applied to the breast. Initial optimism, if validated with multicenter clinical trials, may offer additional strategies in the management of lesions whose features do not necessarily require surgical excision.

## Suggested Reading


Brenner RJ. Medicolegal aspects of breast imaging: Variable standards of care relating to different types of practice. Am J Roentgenol 1991; 156:719–723.

Brenner RJ, Sickles EA. Acceptability of periodic follow-up as an alternative to biopsy for mammographically detected lesions interpreted as probably benign. Radiology 1989; 171:645–646.

Hall FM, Storella JM, Silverston DZ, Wyshak G. Nonpalpable breast lesions: Recommendations for biopsy based on suspicion of carcinoma at mammography. Radiology 1986; 168:353–358.

Helvie MA, Pennes DR, Rebner M, Adler DD. Mammographic follow-up of low suspicion lesions: Compliance rate and diagnostic yield. Radiology 1991; 178:155–158.

Hermann G, Janus C, Schwartz IS, et al. Occult malignant breast lesions in 114 patients: Relationship of age and presence of microcalcifications. Radiology 1988; 169:321–324.

Homer MJ. Imaging features and management of characteristically benign and probably benign breast lesions. Radiol Clin North Am 1987; 25:939–951.

Kopans DB, Swann LA, White G, et al. Asymmetric breast tissue. Radiology 1989; 171:639–643.

Sickles EA. Mammographic features of 300 consecutive nonpalpable breast cancers. Am J Roentgenol 1986; 146:661–663.

Sickles EA. Practical solutions to mammographic problems: Tailoring the examination to the needs of the individual patients. In: Feig S, ed. ARRS Categorized Syllabus Breast Imaging, 1988.

Sickles EA. Periodic follow-up of probably benign mammographic lesions: Results for 3184 consecutive cases. Radiology 1991; 179:463–468.


# Ductography

*A. CHRISTINE WATT, M.D.*

Galactography is a procedure involving the introduction of contrast material into the lactiferous ducts. It is a safe, simple, and underused procedure in the evaluation of spontaneous nipple discharge. Galactography is indicated for the diagnosis of spontaneous serous or bloody discharge from a single duct. It is the only method to discover, evaluate, and localize nonpalpable intraductal lesions before a biopsy, frequently obviating the need for a major surgical procedure. Standard mammography in the presence of nipple discharge is frequently nondiagnostic.

Spontaneous discharge in a nonlactating breast can occur in approximately 10 percent of women. The discharge may be clear, creamy white, greenish-black, serous, or serosanguinous. Bilateral discharge from numerous ducts, particularly if it is green or creamy, is not an indication for galactography; this is most likely from ductal ectasia, papillomatosis, fibrocystic change, or endocrine abnormalities. Fibrocystic change may cause a chronic dark green foul-smelling discharge; these secretions tend to arise from the more peripheral tissue and drain centrally. The intraductal tumors that produce clinical discharge tend to drain through a single dilated duct.

Intraductal papilloma, either single or multiple, is the most common etiology of a bloody, serous, or serosanguinous discharge. Although these lesions are generally benign, there is also some suggestion in the literature of premalignant disposition. Serous, sanguinous, or frankly bloody discharges are the most alarming; however, carcinoma as the cause of these discharges occurs in only a comparatively small percentage but must be excluded. Intraductal carcinomas that produce discharge tend to be those located near the nipple. The discharge, which may be serous or frankly bloody, draws attention to these intraductal carcinomas resulting in their diagnosis when only a few millimeters in size and there is no invasion through the duct wall; the prognosis is most favorable.

Benign intraductal lesions cannot be differentiated from malignant lesions without histological evaluation, and galactography is able to locate the intraductal tumors for excisional biopsy.

## Technique

The patient may be examined in either the supine or sitting positions. It may be easier to locate the duct and cannulate it when the patient is supine; however, this necessitates the use of either an examining table or stretcher in, or in close proximity to, the mammogram room. When the patient is examined in the sitting position, the breast may be supported either on the cassette holder draped with a sterile towel or on an instrument or similar table. I prefer the former. A gooseneck lamp is also useful for direct illumination of the nipple area without the production of shadows. A magnifying loupe may be worn to assist in cannulization of the ostium of the discharging duct, since magnification of the nipple often helps visualize the abnormal ostium.

The procedure is dependent on obtaining at least one drop of discharge; since there may be only one drop of discharge obtainable, it is essential that the operator is ready to cannulate the duct he has seen discharge and not trust to luck, or description by the patient or referring physician, for the location of the discharging duct. Although the history can give the approximate location of the duct ostium, direct visualization at the time of galactography is essential. If discharge cannot be elicited, the procedure is canceled and may be rescheduled in a week's time, with the admonition to abstain from manipulating the breast in the interval. This is to maximize the amount of discharge available for expression at the time of cannulization. Routinely, when patients are scheduled for galactography they are requested to abstain from checking if they have a discharge for a few days before the study, and most particularly they are reminded not to check before coming in for the study. This abstention from confirming discharge by the patient herself before the study cannot be overstressed, since in some cases in which we do not elicit a discharge and must cancel and reschedule the study, patients still say, "But I got a drop when I checked this morning before I came for this exam." Usually in these cases, at the time of the re-evaluation, the procedure is completed successfully.

The cannulation system consists of a 30 gauge needle that has been blunted (Fig. 1) by cutting off the sharp point, connected by a short length of intravenous tubing (extension set 20 in. for syringe attachment or any extension [Abbott Laboratories]) to a 1 ml tuberculin-type syringe. It is essential to exclude air bubbles, which may be confused with intraluminal filling defects, when filling the system with contrast material. Water-soluble contrast material such as diatrizoate sodium injection USP (Hypaque sodium 50 percent; Winthrop Pharmaceutical) is used; since the cannula is extremely fine, it is advisable to warm the bottle of contrast material to decrease its viscosity. The whole of the cannulation system is prepared before an attempt is made to express discharge from the breast.

The nipple and surrounding breast is cleansed using povidone-iodine (Betadine) and then alcohol. A magnifying loupe may be worn to better identify the discharging duct. The nipple area itself is inspected for the presence of dried discharge or scabs. The hand holding the cannula is steadied against the breast, and the other hand is used to gently compress the areolar area and express discharge. The discharging duct is then cannulated (Fig. 2); meticulous care must be exercised to avoid injection of air bubbles, which may be confused with intraluminal filling defects. Cannulation of the

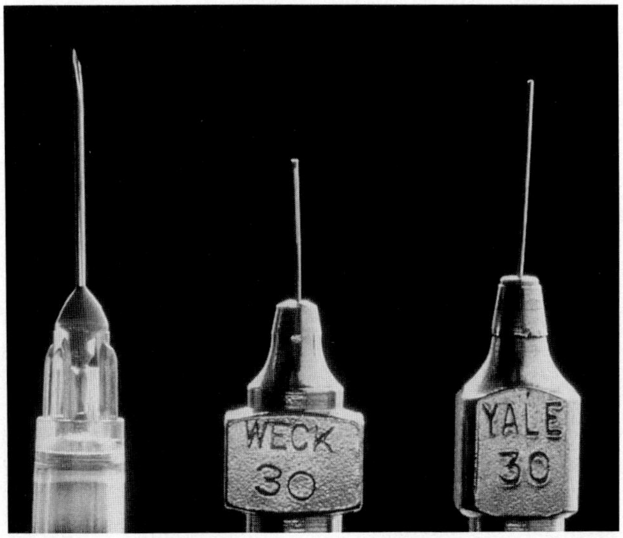


**FIGURE 1** Examples of blunted 30 gauge cannulas and a regular 30 gauge needle.

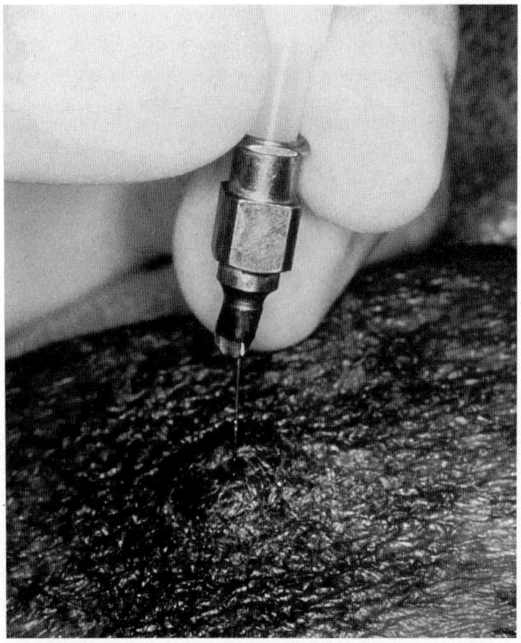

**FIGURE 2** Cannula being introduced into the duct.

duct is achieved by a gentle stroking motion over the surface of the nipple; the cannula tip drops into the ostium of the discharging duct, much as a golf ball drops into the cup. The ostium of the affected duct is usually enlarged. A delicate touch is essential to avoid rupturing the duct wall. The cannula should not be introduced more than 1 cm into the duct to avoid perforation of a duct that may angle sharply. Diatrizoate meglumine 60 percent (Hypaque 60 percent) is then injected into the duct. The end point of the injection occurs when one or more of the following conditions occurs: (1) 1 ml of the contrast agent has been injected, (2) there is backflow of contrast material around the cannula, or (3) the patient feels discomfort or burning either deep in the breast or in the nipple area. Usually the study is performed with a minimal amount of discomfort, and if the patient feels a sudden sharp pain, the injection should be terminated, because this may indicate perforation of the duct and extravasation of the contrast agent.

Craniocaudal and true lateral mammograms are obtained with limited compression to diminish discharge of the injected contrast material. Magnification views may be obtained to better identify intraluminal filling defects; the majority of lesions lie within 2 to 3 cm of the nipple surface. If there is incomplete ductal filling, a reinjection of contrast material may be performed.

## Findings

### Normal Galactogram

There is arborization of the normal mammary ducts within the breast; although there is considerable variability in appearance, usually about 15 to 20 ducts converge to open on the nipple. The proximal segment of each duct is straight and expands progressively into the subareolar portion of the ducts, which is usually 2 to 3 mm in diameter, and the ampulla is slightly wider. There is a progressive tapering of the ducts as they pass deeper into the breast. The ducts of nulliparous or postlactational women have a greater diameter. The duct walls should be smooth, without angulation or narrowing. In pathological conditions there is uneven dilatation, narrowing, and ductal displacement; reduction in number and truncation of branches of the ducts may also be observed.

### Fibrocystic Changes

The ducts are irregular in diameter; occasionally they are dilated and may even be displaced by cysts. Cysts that originate from the ducts may fill with contrast during galactography; these tend to be small, multiple, and are located in the central portion of the breast. Lack of branching is not specific for fibrocystic change, but may occasionally be observed.

### Secretory Disease, Ductal Ectasia, Ductal Hyperplasia

A normal branching pattern is observed; however, rather than the progressive tapering normally observed, the ducts widen as they pass deeper into the breast. Typically the ducts are dilated and tortuous and may contain irregular intraluminal defects produced by inspissated secretions. The ductal dilatation may be up to 7 to 8 mm in diameter, especially in the subareolar and ampullary region. The walls of the dilated ducts are usually smooth, but can occasionally be beaded with areas of narrowing. The intraluminal defects may cause difficulty in differentiating secretory disease from intraductal hyperplasia and papillomatosis. Reinjection is often useful, since secretions change position.

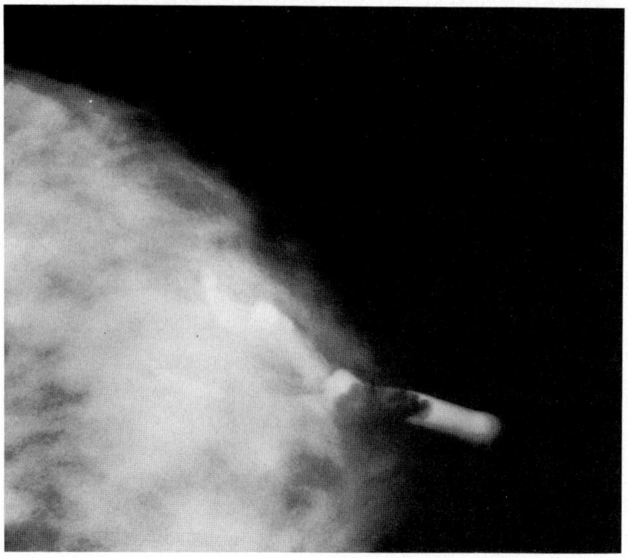

**FIGURE 3** Large lobulated intraluminal filling defect (1 cm) in a dilated duct approximately 1 cm from the nipple surface.

### Intraductal Papilloma

This entity usually presents as a single radiolucent defect within one of the major ducts in the subareolar region. The localized, smooth, rounded, or lobulated filling defect varies in size from 1 to 8 mm and is typically seen within a single dilated duct (Fig. 3). It causes obstruction to the flow of contrast and produces a meniscal effect on the contrast column, seldom causing complete ductal obstruction. Papillomas maintain a constant position if contrast material is reinjected. This is useful in differentiation from cellular debris and inspissated secretions.

### Intraductal Hyperplasia

This process has a variable appearance and may present as multiple small filling defects similar to intraductal papillomatosis, multiple blood clots, or debris.

### Intraductal Papillomatosis

Intraluminal filling defects are usually small and multiple, most commonly rounded or lobulated (Fig. 4). The duct lumen may be irregularly outlined. The ducts usually are of normal caliber or mildly dilated. When numerous irregularly shaped filling defects are observed within several branches of the duct system, each represents a discrete papilloma. Notice the marked resemblance to ductal hyperplasia.

### Intraductal Carcinoma

A malignant intraductal carcinoma most commonly presents as a diffuse lesion, but may occur early on as a single filling defect,

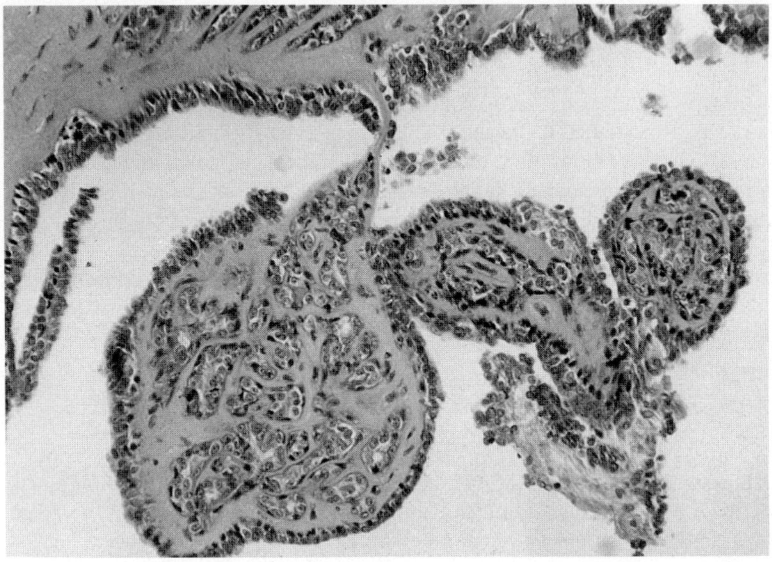

**FIGURE 4** Intraductal papilloma (in Fig. 3) that contains papillary projections with dense fibrous cores lined by benign epithelial and myoepithelial cells and displaying characteristic periductal fibrosis.

undifferentiable from benign papilloma. The distance of the lesion from the nipple is typically greater in malignant disease than in benign lesions, but is of no particular value in any one case. Numerous dilated ducts may be present, some with abrupt cutoff in a meniscus-like appearance; this represents a tumor within the duct itself. It is impossible to distinguish this from benign papillomatosis. In later stages of the carcinoma, there may be multiple intraluminal defects, ductal strictures, distortions, ductal obstruction, and wall irregularities. There may be a disordered filling of the ductal network with nonfilling and discontinuous opacification of many ducts. Malignant-appearing microcalcifications may be present.

## Discussion

Galactography is the procedure of choice in evaluating patients with serous, serosanguinous, or frankly bloody discharge from a single duct. Patients with other types of discharge may be followed clinically. In most cases ductography identifies the causative lesion and localizes the ductal system abnormality, obviating the need for a radical surgical procedure. In patients with single or multiple filling defects, reinjection of the contrast agent may be beneficial in excluding air bubbles, secretions, and cellular debris. In those patients with persistent filling defects, although a diagnosis can be suggested based on the particular features of the lesion, it is often impossible to determine if a lesion is benign or malignant, since many of the features overlap. Biopsy and resection are therefore necessary for histological diagnosis. There is some suggestion that benign lesions, such as intraductal papillomatosis and intraductal papillomas, may be premalignant.

## Suggested Reading


Diner WC. Galactography: Mammary duct contrast examination. AJR 1981; 137:853–856.

Nunnerly HB, Field S. Mammary duct injection in patients with nipple discharge. Br J Radiology 1972; 45:717–725.

Tabar L, Dean PB, Pentek Z. Galactography: The diagnostic procedure of choice for nipple discharge. Radiology 1983; 149:31–35.

Tabar L, Marton Z, Kadas I. Galactography in the examination of secretory breasts. Am J Surg 1974; 127:283.

Tabar L, Marton Z, Kadas I. Galactography and pneumocystography in the examination of breast diseases. In: Radiology. Proceedings of the Twelfth International Congress of Radiology, Madrid, 1973. Amsterdam: Excerpta Medica, 1974:133.

Threatt B. Ductography. In: Bassett LW, Gold RH, eds. Mammography, Thermography, and Ultrasound in Breast Cancer Detection. New York: Grune and Stratton, 1982:109–119.


# Fine-Needle Aspiration Cytology


*WENDE WESTINGHOUSE LOGAN-YOUNG, M.D.*
*NANCY YANES HOFFMAN, M.Sc.*


## Practical Considerations

Fine-needle aspiration cytology (FNAC) of the breast is certainly not a new procedure, but even today it is still regrettably slow in gaining acceptance. We have performed FNAC ever since our breast clinic first opened in 1975 and currently perform from 200 to 300 FNACs every month. To assess the contribution of FNAC to our patients' care, we recently reviewed our 1988 records. The same radiologist performed all the aspirations. We submit material from solid lumps only, because too many aspirates of cystic fluid are interpreted as false-positive. The University of Rochester cytology department analyzed all the aspirates. This review showed that FNAC has served us and continues to serve us (1) in verifying a probable malignancy and (2) in confirming our impression of radiographic and clinical benignity.

## Verifying a Probable Malignancy

Even when we believe a patient has a probable malignancy based on her mammogram or clinical findings, and we have advised surgical biopsy, we perform FNAC. If the cytologic evaluation verifies the presence of malignant cells, the surgeon can discuss options for treatment with the patient before her surgery. The surgeon then can bypass lumpectomy and proceed directly to wedge resection or mastectomy. Negative cytologic results never supersede a clinical or radiologic decision to advise surgical biopsy. *Because we recommend surgical biopsy for these women before we perform FNAC, we do not, in these particular instances, credit cytologic analysis with detecting any additional cancers.*

### The Symptomatic Patient

At our clinic every symptomatic patient's workup consists of a mammogram, history, physical examination, and whatever ancillary tests are necessary including supplementary radiographic views, sonography, ductography, and aspiration of any cysts. If any of these studies make us suspect cancer, we advise the patient to undergo open-surgical biopsy, and we perform FNAC if her surgeon has not already done so.

In 1988 we advised 216 such symptomatic women to undergo open-surgical biopsy because their clinical examinations or their mammograms or both were suggestive of malignancy. Open-surgical biopsy verified cancer in 134 of these symptomatic women (62 percent). Of these 134 women, 5 (4 percent) had cytologic diagnoses of "benign" aspirates, 39 (29 percent) had cytologic diagnoses of atypia suggestive of malignancy, whereas 90 (67 percent) had an explicit diagnosis of cancer. Therefore FNAC was cost-effective for these women, because its results rendered two-thirds of these patients eligible to bypass lumpectomy and proceed directly to either wedge resection or mastectomy.

### The Screening Patient

When a screening mammogram reveals a new questionable mass or area of asymmetric tissue, we perform supplementary angled radiographic views to see whether this area represents a true mass or is merely overlapped glandular tissue. If the area still appears at all questionable on these views, we assess the patient with the same supplementary tests that we perform on a symptomatic patient. If these further evaluations convince us to recommend biopsy, we perform FNAC, if possible, under clinical or sonographic guidance.

In our analysis of our 1988 FNAC results, we advised 176 women to undergo open-surgical biopsy, because their screening mammograms were suggestive of malignancy. Open-surgical biopsy confirmed cancer in 117 (67%) of these asymptomatic women. We could not obtain FNAC on 45 of these 117 women (38 percent) because their lesions were too small or located too deeply in their breasts.

Of the 72 patients whose lesions could be aspirated easily under clinical or sonographic guidance, 35 aspirates (30 percent of the original 117 patients) revealed cytologically diagnostic malignant cells, 18 revealed atypical cells suggestive of carcinoma, and another 19 were cytologically benign. Thus 30 percent of these 117 asymptomatic patients with carcinoma subsequently confirmed by open-surgical biopsy were eligible for their surgeons to proceed directly to wedge resection or mastectomy.

If we cannot clinically or sonographically localize a lesion in a screening patient, we do not resort to stereotactically guided FNAC. Dowlatshahi and his colleagues performed stereotactic 20 gauge FNAC and core biopsy on 250 mammographically detected lesions. Their cytologic evaluations revealed 11 percent more definitively diagnosed cancers than we obtained with our 23 gauge FNAC without stereotaxis in 1988. But we believe that the additional time and expense for stereotactic FNAC, just to increase the number of specific cytologic diagnoses of cancer by another 11 percent, would be unwarranted on these patients who are already scheduled to undergo biopsy.

## Confirming an Impression of Radiographic and Clinical Benignity

*In 1988 FNAC performed as a cross-check revealed a malignancy in 1 of every 225 symptomatic or screening patients whom we had considered free of breast cancer.*

### The Symptomatic Patient

If the mammogram and all the supplementary evaluations of a symptomatic woman convince us that she has no evidence of breast cancer, we still turn to FNAC for more evidence that our judgment is correct.

Certain types of palpable areas often prove to be from such benign causes as (1) relatively stable conditions such as an ancient fibroadenoma or a lipoma, physical changes associated with weight gain or weight loss; or (2) hormonally affected tissue that waxes and wanes in size.

If a patient has an area of palpable firmness so clinically and radiographically innocuous that it does not warrant a short-interval follow-up evaluation, we still perform FNAC to support our impression of benignity. In such instances the patient does not require close monitoring and returns to the routine screening schedule appropriate for her age.

If we believe the patient has hormonally influenced tissue, she still needs monitoring until the size of the palpable area recedes to normal limits. The length of the monitoring intervals depends on the nature of the patient's problem. If a patient has a palpable thickening or a mass in her breast when she calls for her appointment, but the mass disappears by the time she comes to our office, she obviously does not need FNAC and can return to her routine mammographic schedule. If the patient does have a clinically palpable thickening and we consider it hormonally induced, we do not perform FNAC at the time of her initial visit, because most cytopathologists have difficulty interpreting hormonally accentuated tissue. Instead we have her continue to abstain from caffeine, and return 7 to 10 days after the onset of her next menstrual period for another physical examination. If the thickening has disappeared or dwindled to a size that we deem within normal limits, we return her to the routine mammographic schedule appropriate for her age. If the thickening is unchanged, yet we consider it to be probably within normal limits, we perform FNAC. We introduce the needle as far into the tissue as possible in the event that a deep mass is causing the thickening. If the cytologic analysis reveals neither malignant nor atypical cells, we ask the patient to return in 4 months for a repeat FNAC. At that time we also perform a coned-down magnified radiographic view of the problematic area. If the tissue has remained stable, and the FNAC remains negative during these first 5 months of

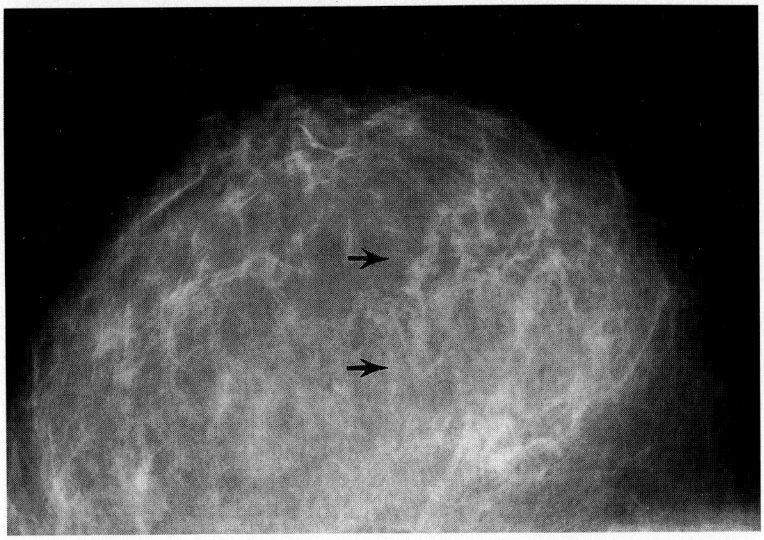

**FIGURE 1** In 1991 this 48-year-old perimenopausal woman palpated a diffusely thickened 4 cm area in the upper inner quadrant of her left breast *(arrows),* but her mammogram was normal, unchanged from her original 1988 mammogram. Cytopathologic analysis found atypical cells suggestive of cancer. Open-surgical biopsy confirmed diffuse intraductal cancer. Her lymph nodes were free of metastases.

monitoring, we have the patient return 5 months hence (10 months after her initial visit) for a complete mammographic study, physical examination, and FNAC. If the tissue is unchanged, the patient returns to her routine mammographic schedule.

In 1988 we performed FNACs on 2,248 of our symptomatic patients whose masses we had deemed benign (the remaining symptomatic patients did not have a mass). Open-surgical biopsy confirmed cancer in 8 of the 26 women whose cytologic evaluations had revealed atypical or frankly malignant cells (Fig. 1).

### The Screening Patient

If we discover either a new, benign-appearing mass or asymmetric area on a screening patient's mammogram, we perform ancillary radiographic views and whatever additional tests are necessary, just as we would in a patient scheduled for a symptomatic workup. If all the supplementary evaluations convince us that the aberration is benign, we perform FNAC to gain additional evidence of benignity and follow the patient at 3 to 6 month intervals. If we can retrospectively palpate the area, FNAC is a simple procedure. If we cannot feel the area, but can identify it sonographically, we do FNAC under sonographic guidance. We perform clinically or sonographically guided FNAC on 90 percent of our screening patients whom we follow at short intervals.

If we can readily discern the problematic area on the mammogram, but can neither palpate the area nor see it on ultrasonography, we perform FNAC under mammographic guidance and employ a variation of Novak's technique (see the following section). Although we do not perform mammographically guided FNAC on patients already advised to undergo surgical biopsy for a nonpalpable lesion, we try to obtain FNAC on those patients that we decide do not need surgical biopsy. We perform mammographically guided FNAC on only 1 out of 74 of our screening patients that we follow at short intervals.

Approximately 10 percent of our screening patients followed at short intervals have small smooth-bordered lesions located too deeply in the breast for us to reach them with mammographically guided fine-needle aspiration. Both the small size and the smooth outlines of these lesions indicate that on the rare occasions that they might be malignant, we have more time before they could metastasize, which allows us to monitor them at short intervals.

Of the 22,471 screening patients seen in 1988, we performed FNAC on 222 screening women with newly detected, benign-appearing masses or asymmetric areas. Open-surgical biopsy verified three cancers in the four women whose cytologic evaluations disclosed cancer or atypical cells suggestive of carcinoma.

## Technical Approach

Although the various techniques of FNAC all have their partisans, we prefer the simple technique outlined as follows, because the needle is in the patient's breast for only about 5 seconds. Most patients experience little discomfort, even when we aspirate a mass that is close to the nipple, the most sensitive area of the breast.

The patient undergoing FNAC is seated or supine, whichever position is best for the radiologist to palpate the density and fix it in place; most patients are in the supine position. If the density is located laterally in a large breast, we often ask the patient to roll up on her contralateral side. With this maneuver, gravity's pull stretches the breast, thereby making it easier for us to immobilize the area in question. We use no local anesthetic. Desensitizing the area necessitates introducing another needle into the breast, which would be as bothersome as the procedure itself.

To prevent the lesion from sliding when the needle is inserted, the radiologist pulls the skin tightly over the lesion, and with the index and third fingers of the nondominant hand, holds it firmly in place. If the lesion is small and slippery, the radiologist props the fourth finger of the hand grasping the needle against the far side of the lesion to keep it from slipping away.

With the nondominant hand, the radiologist wipes the skin with alcohol and inserts a disposable, 2 cm long, 23 gauge butterfly needle through the skin and into the area of palpable firmness. An assistant holds a 20 ml syringe attached to the tubing of the butterfly needle. As soon as the needle passes through the skin, the assistant pulls the plunger back almost to the end of the barrel and holds it there until the aspiration is completed. The 20 ml syringe is necessary for attaining

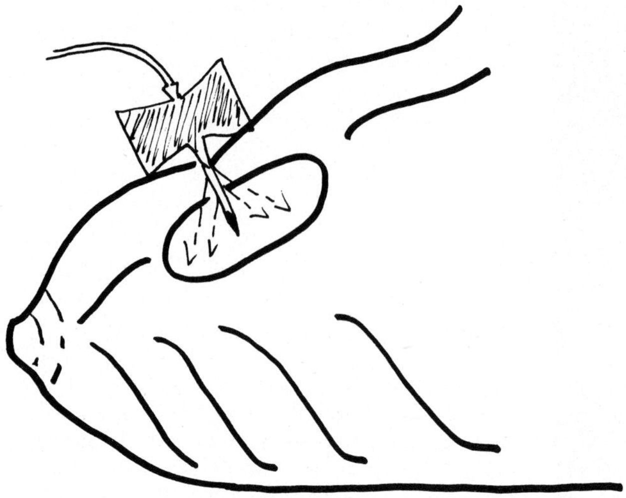

**FIGURE 2** FNAC technique.

sufficiently strong negative pressure to draw the cellular material into the lumen.

Holding the mass firmly in place, the radiologist moves the needle back and forth 10 to 20 times while angling it to sample cellular material from all areas of the mass (Fig. 2). With this maneuver, she or he usually procures enough cellular material to prepare two slides for cytologic analysis. Because the needle passes through the lesion from many different angles, it needs to enter the skin only once. If the lesion is large, the radiologist obtains cells from its periphery, because the cells in the center of a cancer tend to be more necrotic and thus more difficult for the cytopathologist to interpret. We use a small butterfly needle, because it is more maneuverable than a larger needle attached directly to a syringe. With a larger needle directly attached to the syringe, the needle's movement becomes more cumbersome and unwieldy. When the radiologist holds the small 23 gauge needle in her or his hand, the fingers can sense the needle's passage through the lesion, which reduces the chance of obtaining the sample from the wrong area.

When the radiologist finishes moving the needle back and forth (see Fig. 1), the assistant releases the syringe's negative pressure slowly and smoothly over 2 seconds. The slow release of negative pressure is important, because a sudden release of pressure might force the cells out of the needle. Only after releasing this negative pressure does the radiologist withdraw the needle from the breast. The assistant applies firm pressure with a soft folded cleansing tissue for several minutes. The firm pressure is exceedingly important to prevent a hematoma, which could obscure the border of the original lump.

In the meantime the radiologist quickly detaches the syringe from the butterfly tubing, fills the syringe with air, and expels the cells from the needle onto the clear end of a slide, which is frosted at the other end for labeling. During these maneuvers, the assistant continues to compress the tissue covering the aspirated area with one hand and with her other hand points the needle toward the slide. To smear the cellular material, the radiologist touches the cellular material on the slide to another side and then gently pulls them apart. This done, the slides are turned back-to-back, with the cellular material on the outside, and placed in a bottle of 95 percent ethanol, the same kind of bottle used for cervical Papanicolaou smears. To prevent the cells from air-drying, which could distort the nucleic parameters and impede accurate cytologic interpretation, the radiologist needs to prepare the slides swiftly.

### *FNAC on Mammographically Detected Questionable Areas*

If the mammographically detected mass is retrospectively palpable, we perform clinically guided FNAC. If the aberration is nonpalpable but sonographically identifiable as a discrete density, we locate it sonographically. Then, holding the transducer in place with the nondominant hand, we perform FNAC with the dominant hand.

If the lesion is not visible sonographically as a discrete density, we use a modified version of Novak's method to aspirate the area under standard mammographic guidance rather than stereotactic guidance. We compress the breast with a narrow fenestrated compression device at whatever angle allows the needle to traverse the shortest distance from the point of entry at the skin to the lesion. We can aspirate the majority of the lesions with the patient's breast compressed craniocaudally, although we approach inferior lesions with lateral compression.

We position the breast so that the lesion lies beneath the fenestrated plate, compress the breast, and take a check film. We then estimate the depth as a fraction of the height of the compressed breast from a previous orthogonal view. We insert a 5 to 9 cm long, 21 gauge skinny needle to the estimated depth perpendicular to the skin. Then we take a second radiograph to be sure that the needle is in the lesion.

Next, we attach a 20 ml syringe to the needle. Applying continuous negative suction, we pull the needle out of the breast with short up-and-down motions. Then we quickly remove the syringe, fill it with air, and expel the aspirate onto the slide. We prepare the slide and place it in alcohol in the same manner as we prepare the aspirate from a palpable mass. Performing this entire procedure under mammographic guidance customarily takes only about 5 to 10 minutes.

## Cellular Analysis and Monitoring Protocol

The cytologic interpretation coupled with our other findings have led us to the following recommendations for monitoring those particular patients with subsuspicious lesions:

1. If the mammogram, the physical examination, and the cytology are benign, the patient follows the routine mammographic return schedule appropriate for her age and history.
2. If the cytology reveals cancer or atypia suggestive of cancer, we advise the patient to undergo surgical biopsy.
3. If the laboratory reports that the sample is hypocellular, or that it contains insufficient cellular material for cytologic analysis, we follow the patient the same way that we monitor a patient with a negative cytologic analysis. Although the literature contains reports of false-negative findings attributable to hypocellular sampling, this problem never arose in our 1988 review of patients. In our experience repeat FNACs on these areas revealed only the same hypocellularity. For this reason, we no longer consider hypocellularity an indication to repeat the FNAC.

4. If bleeding should occur during aspiration, the cellular sample may become too diluted for accurate analysis. If the slide is only tinged with blood, accurate interpretation is usually possible. But if the amount of blood is such that the material puddles when we smear the slides, then we bring the patient back in 2 weeks for a repeat FNAC.
5. If the patient is pregnant or lactating, we also perform a control FNAC on the same quadrant of the opposite breast for comparison. This is necessary because pregnancy or lactation's heightened hormonal levels can make cytologic findings difficult to interpret.

## Pitfalls of FNAC

For FNAC to be as accurate as possible, the physician must beware of certain technical and interpretive pitfalls. Skill in placing the needle and procuring the specimen is essential. The slide requires careful preparation: if the smear is spread too thickly, the cells cannot be individually analyzed. If the smear is fixed improperly, the cells appear aberrant, resembling cytoplasmic and nuclear anomalies. The clinical aspirator and the cytotechnologist must work together to acquire better procurement and interpretation.

*Inasmuch as all cytopathologists are not equally skilled and experienced, finding a pathologist who is particularly adept at reading FNACs is essential.* Accurate cytologic analysis of breast aspirates requires training, motivation, and continuous experience with such material. One good way for cytopathologists to gain this experience is performing FNAC on lumpectomy specimens from the breast and correlating their conclusions with the final histologic diagnosis. If all else fails, slides can be sprayed with Profix and mailed in a cardboard container to a qualified cytopathologist in another city for evaluation.

### *False-Positive and False-Negative Cytologic Interpretations*

The radiologist using FNAC treads a fine line between the false-positive interpretation with its attendant unnecessary biopsy and the false-negative reading with the possibility of a delay in detecting an early cancer.

Despite FNAC's help, the radiologist should always beware of the possibility of a false-negative reading. FNAC should *never* be a substitute for biopsy. *The decision to biopsy or to monitor a patient should be made before performing FNAC.* A benign test should never supersede clinical or radiographic judgment. A 1 year follow-up of our 1988 screening and symptomatic patients who had FNAC revealed one missed cancer in a screening patient, probably resulting from the needle missing the lesion during sampling, and one missed cancer in a symptomatic patient.

The following problems arise from a false-positive interpretation:

1. A *specific* cytologic diagnosis of breast cancer. Not every physician agrees about the need for a frozen section when the cytologic evaluation demonstrates unequivocally malignant cells. Even though there were no false positives in 1988, our own experience from other years agrees with the literature's findings that even the most proficient cytopathologist may on rare occasions interpret benign cells as malignant. For this reason, even when the cytopathologist "definitely" diagnoses a cancer, we believe that a surgeon should perform mastectomy or wedge resection with lymph node dissection only if the frozen or permanent sections have irrefutably revealed a cancer.
2. Atypical cells *suggestive* of cancer. False-positive FNACs result in unnecessary biopsies. In our 1988 study, open-surgical biopsies on the 24 patients with cytologic evaluations revealing atypia suggestive of cancer found malignant cells in 6 patients and benign conditions in the remaining 18. Most of the false-positive interpretations in our experience resulted from one of the following circumstances: (1) FNAC obtained from a premenopausal woman, when the aspirate is drawn from the periareolar area; or when the woman has irregular menstrual cycling, fibrocystic disease, or a highly cellular fibroadenoma. (2) FNAC from a postmenopausal woman on estrogen replacement therapy (ERT). The higher the dose, the greater the likelihood of aspirating atypical cells. Continuous ERT without a monthly 5 to 7 day hiatus can also produce false-positive FNACs.

After determining the usual causes of false-positive interpretations, we have changed our guidelines for FNAC on patients with hormone effect. We follow these patients clinically at short intervals for 1 year, but initially do not perform FNAC. We prefer to wait on the FNAC until the patient returns after discontinuing all caffeine.

In our 1988 study, open-surgical biopsy revealed lymph node involvement in 32 percent of our symptomatic patients whose cancers were suspected clinically or mammographically. Of the screening patients with occult mammographically detected cancers, 18 percent were node-positive. The lymph node metastatic rate for subsuspicious cancers detected solely by FNAC was also 18 percent, suggesting that these patients' prognoses will be equally as promising as those with cancers discovered solely by mammography. Although these numbers are not yet statistically significant, as we continue to follow more patients over a longer period, the numbers will assume greater statistical importance. We continue to monitor these women closely. At this writing, all have remained disease-free.

Our total imaging and FNAC false-negative rates are low for patients scrutinized carefully with FNACs and interval mammograms. Screening patients who develop a palpable mass within 1 year after obtaining a screening mammogram, or who had a problem but did not tell us at the time of the screening mammogram, account for most of our 1 year interval missed cancers. Our 1988 combined 1 year interval miss rate for screening and symptomatic patients was 8 percent. If we had neglected to perform FNAC on those masses, and if open-surgical biopsy had proven that they were malignant within a year of our evaluation, our combined 1 year interval miss rate would have been 11 percent.

## Discussion

The radiologic literature repeatedly makes the point that mammography is the diagnostic gold standard for detecting cancers of the breast. In the Breast Cancer Demonstration Detection Project (BCDDP), mammography alone detected 35 percent of the cancers in asymptomatic women, but we need to remember that physical examination alone also discerned a significant number of malignancies. When clinically discovered, 1 year interval cancers are included, physical examination alone accounted for the discovery of 20 percent of the cancers.

The BCDDP data demonstrate the importance of physical

examination as a mammographic adjunct in uncovering breast cancer, but recommending surgical biopsy of every mass found by physical examination or mammographic screening would be neither feasible nor cost-effective. Many patients have radiographic or clinically palpable masses that appear or feel sufficiently innocuous for surgical biopsy not to be considered by either the surgeon or the radiologist.

In 1985, with the BCDDP data in mind, we decided to perform FNAC more frequently in patients with questionable areas that we deemed benign. Since then, we have obtained FNAC from 1 percent of our screening patients and from 62 percent of our symptomatic patients. Despite the plethora of other methods, we prefer our simple reliable method using a 23 gauge needle, because we can sample small lesions more accurately. Further, our patients find this method only minimally uncomfortable, which is crucial for gaining patient acceptance of this procedure. At our clinic in 1988, FNAC led us to the early discovery of 11 radiographically or clinically unsuspected cancers. Without FNAC, we would have had no way of knowing which of these 2,470 patients had masses that were newly surfacing carcinomas.

## Summary

For those patients with probably benign lesions, FNAC and cyst aspirations in conjunction with supplementary imaging tests and short-interval follow-ups are the crucial elements for achieving a low ratio of recommended open-surgical biopsies to surgically proven cancers. In our 1988 review, open-surgical biopsy verified cancer in 62 percent of our patients advised to undergo surgery. Thus FNAC not only detects early unsuspected cancers, but also prevents many needless biopsies, an important factor in this era of medical cost containment. Certainly the information gained from FNAC is well worth the minimal time and effort spent.

Moreover, even though these barely emerging FNAC-detected cancers are palpable, their small size and their low incidence of axillary metastases strongly suggest that the patients' survival rates will be as good as those of patients with mammographically detected nonpalpable cancers.

## Suggested Reading

Fornage BD, Faroux MJ, Simatos A. Breast masses: US-guided fine-needle aspiration biopsy. Radiology 1987; 162:409–414.

Kline TS, Kline IK. Guides to Clinical Aspiration Biopsy: Breast. New York: Igaku-Shoin, 1989.

Kopans DB. Fine-needle aspiration of clinically occult breast lesions. Radiology 1989; 170:313–314.

Layfield LJ, Glasgow BJ, Cramer H. Fine-needle aspiration in the management of breast masses. Pathol Ann 1989; 24:23–62.

Logan-Young WW, Hoffman NY, Janus J. Fine-needle aspiration-cytologic (FNAC) detection of breast cancer in nonsuspicious lesions. Radiology 1992; 184:45-48.

Novak R. Method for control of the target at aspiration biopsy of non-palpable breast lesions. Acta Radiol [Diagn] (Stockh) 1986; 27:65–70.

Parker SH, Lovin JD, Jobe WE, et al. Nonpalpable breast lesions: Stereotactic automated large-core biopsies. Radiology 1991; 180:403–407.

Seidman H, Gelb SK, Silverberg E, et al. Survival experience in the breast cancer demonstration project. CA Cancer J Clin 1987; 37:258–290.

Wilkinson EJ, Franzini DA, Masood S. Cytological needle sampling for the breast: Techniques and end results. In: Bland KI, Copeland EM, eds. The Breast: Comprehensive Management of Benign and Malignant Diseases. Philadelphia: WB Saunders, 1991:475.

Zajicek J. Aspiration biopsy cytology. In: Monographs in Clinical Cytology. New York: S. Karger, 1974.

# Mammographic Localization Techniques

*CHARLES L. ROBERTSON, M.D.*

Diagnosis of nonpalpable mammographically detected breast cancer depends on a reliable technique for directing surgical biopsy of the lesion while minimizing the excision of normal-appearing tissue. A number of techniques have been described using mammographic, ultrasonographic and computed tomographic guidance for cyst aspiration, needle biopsy, and preoperative localization.

This chapter is intended as a detailed guide to preoperative mammographic localization for nonpalpable lesions in the breast, using the hookwire localization procedure described by Kopans. Since my technique has evolved over several years, it may vary somewhat from that described by Kopans. Mammographically guided cyst aspiration, pneumocystogram, and fine-needle cytologic aspiration use the same localization principles described here.

I prefer the hookwire method for three important reasons. First, the approach is parallel to the chest wall, avoiding the risk of penetration of deeper tissues or a breast implant if augmentation has been performed. Second, this technique has been shown to be highly accurate, resulting in few missed lesions and in removal of small volumes of normal tissue. Third, the anchoring strength of the hookwire itself is superior; thus the chance of being dislodged from the lesion is minimized.

## Evaluation Before Localization

Review of available prior films and clinical history should be performed as part of any diagnostic assessment and may obviate the need for further evaluation and/or biopsy. Screening mammography is intended only to detect a potential abnormality. Prior to recommending biopsy, complete diagnostic breast-imaging evaluation is usually necessary to answer the following three questions posed by Kopans:

1. Is it real? That is, is it a single three-dimensional lesion as opposed to being superimposed nonsuspicious tissues?
2. Where is it? The location of the lesion must be clearly known. It does not have to be seen in views 90° apart, but must be visible in two views at least 30° apart for successful localization using parallax techniques. A "skin localization" procedure may be necessary to be certain that the lesion is

not in the dermis, since intradermal lesions rarely represent primary occult breast cancer.
3. What is it? Does the probability of malignancy in this lesion warrant biopsy at this time?

If biopsy is recommended, the films are reviewed with the patient by the breast-imaging radiologist at the time of diagnostic evaluation. The reasons for the biopsy, the need for localization, and the localization procedure are discussed in detail. The possibility that the lesion could be missed at biopsy is small, but that possibility is explained. Potential complications including syncope, bleeding from the localization site, and retention of a localizing wire fragment at surgery should be discussed with the patient. The report is then telephoned to the referring clinician, and the patient is asked to contact the clinician for surgical referral.

## Personnel and Scheduling

Although a breast localization often takes 30 minutes or less, we prefer to allow 1 hour for localization of one or more lesions. If the patient is late, has not had adequate diagnostic evaluation, if films done elsewhere are not available, or if the patient does not thoroughly understand what is to be done, 1 hour may not be enough, and on occasion the procedure may need to be rescheduled.

We believe that the patient must not be left alone during the procedure for fear of syncope and falling. The radiologist ideally stays with the patient while the technologist leaves the room to process films and so forth. If that is not possible, a nurse or second technologist must be available to stay in the room with the patient at all times.

## Localization in Augmented Breast

Localization in the patient with augmented breasts is expected to increase in the future because of the increasing frequency of augmentation and maturing of the augmented patients into the screening age group. These localizations require more effort and occasional ingenuity, but they can be performed safely if precautions to safeguard the implant are taken during the localization and surgery.

## Equipment

Mammography units for localization procedures must allow the tube head to rotate a full 180° to allow approaching a lesion from the inferior aspect of the breast; fenestrated paddles must be available, preferably in both standard size for most procedures and in the spot compression size for use in the periphery of the breast.

Equipment for localization is listed in Table 1. Needle-hookwire combinations ranging from 2.5 to 15 cm in length are available from several sources and should be on hand. I prefer a bevel point rather than a pencil point needle for ease of penetration of firm tissues. Film-marking pencils for annotation of the final film going to the operating room and paper tape for securing the hookwire to the skin at the end of the procedure should be available.

**TABLE 1** Equipment for Mammographic Localization

| |
|---|
| Sterile gloves (2 pairs) |
| Sterile 4 × 4 gauze pads |
| 1 ml tuberculin syringe with 27 gauge needle for anesthetic |
| 6 ml syringe for aspiration of cyst fluids, if any |
| Hookwire localization kit |
| Betadine skin preparation |
| 1% Xylocaine |

## Localization Procedure

An experienced breast-imaging technologist reviews the localization procedure with the patient and answers any remaining questions. The technologist should be certain the patient is receiving nothing by mouth, has not received sedative medications, and is able to cooperate adequately with the procedure. To minimize the risk of syncope, we may have the nurse administer atropine before localization, especially in young women who have expressed marked anxiety about the localization or who have a history of syncope. This medication should be noted and reported to operating room personnel.

The diagnostic films are then reviewed by the radiologist to select the site of entry for the localizing wire. That site is usually selected to minimize distance from skin surface to lesion (Figs. 1 and 2). If more than one lesion in a breast is to be localized, the approach to both must be planned to avoid

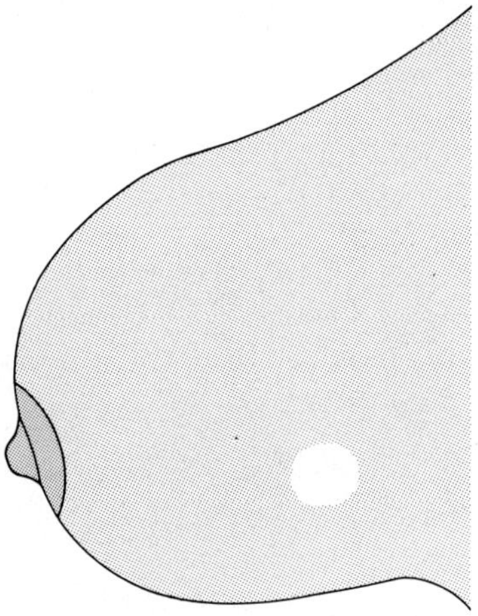

**FIGURE 1** Mediolateral view demonstrating the lesion *(open circle)* to lie in the inferior half of the breast, relatively near the inferior skin margin.

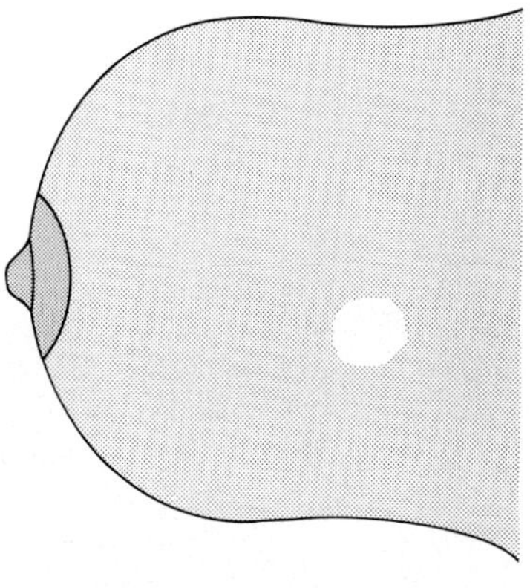

**FIGURE 2** On cephalocaudal view the lesion is relatively central and lies farther from the medial and lateral margins of the breast than from the inferior margin. Therefore the lesion is localized from the inferior aspect of the breast.

having to recompress the breast in a plane perpendicular to a previously placed needle or hookwire. Sometimes multiple localizations, or an active dermatitis at the preferred site, require approaching one or more of the lesions from a site farther from the skin surface than would ordinarily be selected.

The patient is then seated at the mammography unit, the fenestrated paddle is placed over the site selected for placement of the hookwire, compression is applied, a film is exposed, and compression is maintained while the film is processed. That film is reviewed by the radiologist to be certain the lesion is clearly visible and present within the window of the paddle. Alphanumeric coordinates derived from the film are transferred to the patient, either with shadows cast by wires built into the field light or by skin marking directly on the breast (Fig. 3).

A localizing needle is selected to allow enough length to pass through the lesion when the breast is compressed in planes both perpendicular and parallel to the needle to avoid retraction of the needle once in place.

After sterile preparation of the skin, I prefer to inject 1 percent local lidocaine (Xylocaine) intradermally and into the tissue overlying the lesion. With the localizing light on, I maintain the needle perpendicular to the skin by keeping the shadow of the needle hub superimposed over the needle shaft while the needle is advanced through the lesion. The needle may be rotated while advancing through the tissues to avoid displacement of the tip by the bevel point.

When the needle is in place, a film is obtained to confirm placement of the needle through the lesion in question (Fig. 4). Once placement of the needle has been confirmed in this plane, the radiologist should support the breast to avoid displacement while the fenestrated paddle is released, removed, and replaced with a standard compression paddle. A film perpendicular to the plane used for needle placement is then obtained, although films separated by as little as 30° work well when films at 90° cannot be obtained or when the lesion cannot be seen on those films. That film is then reviewed and needle

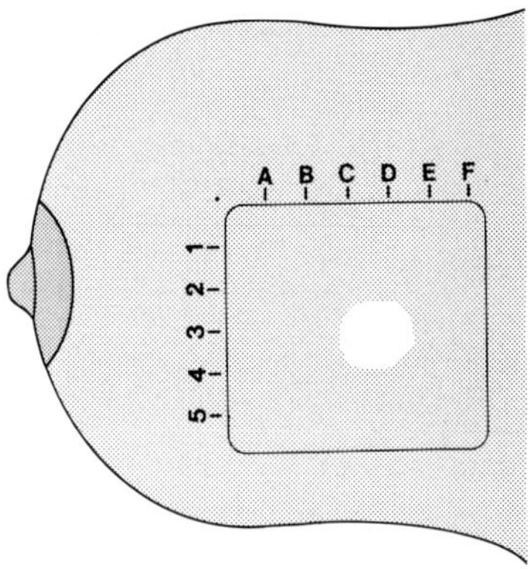


**FIGURE 3** This cephalocaudal film was obtained with the fenestrated paddle on the inferior aspect of the breast and shows the lesion to be visible at alphanumeric coordinates "3 & C-D."

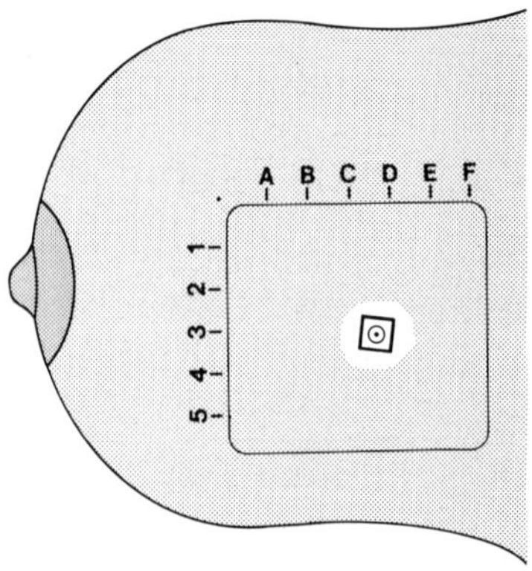


**FIGURE 4** In cephalo-caudal projection, needle has been placed with the hub superimposed on the shaft through the lesion.

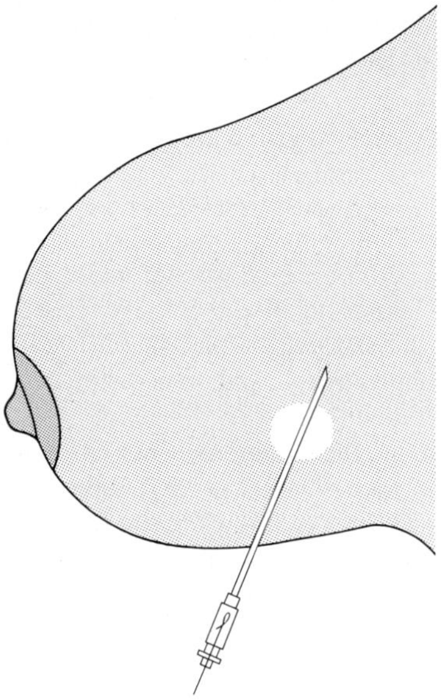

**FIGURE 5** In mediolateral projection, confirmation of placement through the lesion is obtained and depth of the needle relative to the lesion is confirmed (or adjusted) before hookwire placement.

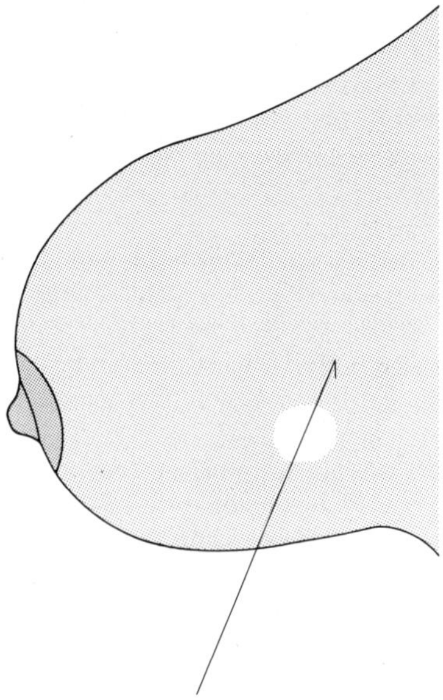

**FIGURE 6** After placement of the hookwire and removal of the needle, a final film in mediolateral projection is made to confirm the wire position. This film is annotated and sent with the patient to the operating room.

tip depth is adjusted to approximately 1 cm distal to the lesion (Fig. 5).

I prefer to slightly kink the hookwire at the burnished mark indicating needle length on the wire. This allows better visualization than the burnished mark, and if I kink the wire in the plane of the hook in the tip of the wire, I can control the point of the hook away from an implant if necessary. The hookwire is then placed in the needle to the kink or burnished mark, and the wire is fixed with one hand while the needle is withdrawn over the hookwire similar to withdrawing a vascular catheter over a guidewire.

A final film is then obtained (Fig. 6), demonstrating the position of the guidewire. I use a film-marking pencil and label the margins of the breast "top and bottom" or "medial and lateral," obviously depending on whether the plane of the final film is mediolateral or cephalocaudal. The hookwires I prefer have a palpable thick segment soldered onto the wire proximal to the hook. I circle the lesion on the film and describe the lesion and its relation to the thick segment of the wire (i.e., "calcification at the middle third of the thick segment"). That film is then sent with the patient to the operating room to assist the surgeon.

### Success and Failure in Breast Localization

The technologist, radiologist, and a mammography unit must be available for specimen radiography. That topic is dealt with in the chapter on breast biopsy specimen radiography, but several comments should be made here about accuracy of the procedure and what to do if the lesion is not observed in the specimen radiograph.

When the lesion is not observed in the specimen radiograph, a radiologist should be available to take all the films to the operating room to review with the surgeon to guide further biopsy before closing the incision. Even though the lesion is not observed in the specimen radiograph, the lesion may have been resected and not recognized. This is particularly true in biopsy of ill-defined areas of distortion or density. Films of the biopsied breast to confirm removal of a lesion may be obtained as soon as the patient is alert enough to sit up safely for additional mammograms.

### Suggested Reading

Helvie MA, Ikeda DM, Adler DD. Localization and needle aspiration of breast lesions: Complications in 370 cases. AJR 1991; 157:711–714.

Kopans DB, Meyer JE, Homer MJ, Grabbe J. Dermal deposits mistaken for breast calcifications. Radiology 1983; 149:152.

Kopans DB, Swann CA. Preoperative imaging-guided needle placement and localization of clinically occult breast lesions. AJR 1989; 152:1–9.

Robertson CL, Kopans DB, McCarthy KA, Hart NE. Nonpalpable lesions in the augmented breast: Preoperative localization. Radiology 1989; 173:873–874.

Stein MA, Karlan M. Immediate postoperative mammogram for failed surgical excision of breast lesions. Radiology 1991; 178:159–162.

Swann CA, Kopans DB, McCarthy KA, et al. Localization of occult breast lesions: Practical solutions to problems of triangulation. Radiology 1987; 163:577.

# Breast Biopsy Specimen Radiography

*EVA RUBIN, M.D.*

Specimen radiography is critical to the successful outcome of any localization procedure performed before biopsy of an occult breast lesion. A well-performed specimen radiograph is not only esthetically pleasing, but (1) assures that the appropriate tissue has been removed, (2) helps define adequacy of margins in breast cancer cases treated conservatively, and (3) provides guidance for orientation and sectioning of the specimen by the pathologist (Fig. 1). To be effective, there must be expeditious viewing of this critical radiograph by all the physicians involved in the localization and biopsy sequence: surgeons, radiologists, and pathologists.

The resected specimen, wrapped in cellophane, is transported to the mammography unit, where it is placed on the magnification stand and flattened lightly with the compression plate to produce as uniform a specimen thickness as possible. Care is taken to assure that the entire specimen is placed in the image field; if this is not possible, more than one radiograph is necessary to assure that the entire piece of resected tissue has been imaged. Exposures are performed manually at 22 kV, using the smallest focal spot size available, preferably less than 0.2 mm, and single-emulsion film with a single-sided screen (the standard mammography film in use in the department). Two identical radiographs are obtained: one remains in the radiology department, is reported separately from the localization procedure, and then filed with the remaining radiographs from the localization procedure; the other is returned along with the specimen to the operating room, the radiologist having circled the area of interest with a grease pencil. Once viewed by the physicians in the operating room, the specimen radiograph is sent to the Pathology Department along with the resected tissue.

A telephone call is placed to the operating suite as soon as the specimen radiograph has been viewed by the radiologist. The call indicates either that the specimen is satisfactory or that additional tissue should be resected. If additional tissue is requested, the surgeon is advised, whenever possible, in what direction additional tissue should be removed. In specimens that are virtually entirely adipose tissue, this may not be possible. Defining specimen margins with sutures, wire, or similar orientation aids may be helpful but does not entirely eliminate this problem. Any additional tissue obtained is radiographed, and each additional specimen is identified sequentially with leaded numbers or letters.

Routine orthogonal views of the specimen are not performed. Unless the specimen is either very large or very firm, obtaining a true orthogonal view is rarely possible, particularly when a localizing wire and stiffening cannula are still in place. However, if an abnormality is not clearly identified but is

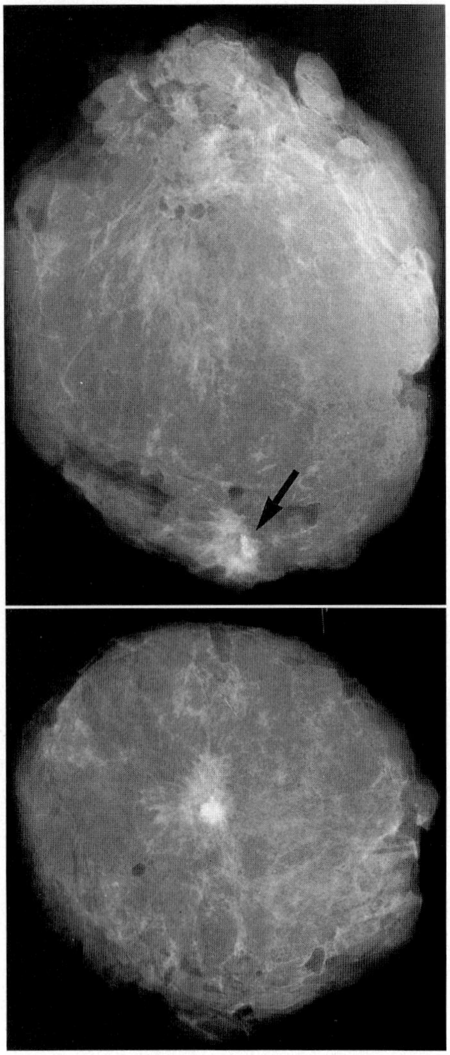

A

B

**FIGURE 1** *A,* This compressed magnified specimen radiograph shows an amorphous area of soft-tissue density containing some microcalcifications *(arrow)* at the inferior pole of the specimen. The needle localization was performed for a tiny stellate mass. *B,* Reorientation of the specimen resulted in this appearance. The stellate mass, a 1 cm invasive ductal cancer, and its associated microcalcifications, representing foci of cribriform ductal carcinoma in situ, are now readily apparent at the center of the specimen. In this case, the specimen was larger than most and the wire was extruded during surgery, allowing performance of a true orthogonal view. Had only the second specimen radiograph been obtained, the marginal location of the mass would not be perceived.

thought to be present in the specimen or if the lesion constitutes a margin of the specimen, the tissue is reoriented and an additional specimen radiograph is obtained.

I have not found it necessary to relocalize the lesion in the resected specimen other than by encircling the area of interest on the specimen radiograph. Placing needles or other sharp objects into the specimen may be hazardous (transmission of hepatitis and human immunodeficiency virus are particularly serious concerns) and makes subsequent handling of the specimen difficult. A number of devices are available that allow precise localization of an area of the specimen by radiographing it on a radiopaque grid. However, these devices are too cumbersome and costly for routine use.

Assessing margins on the routine specimen radiograph is fraught with hazard. Breadloafing the specimen and radiographing each slice provides much more accurate definition of margin involvement, but is time-consuming and hard to justify outside of a research setting. However, it is possible to predict that a margin is involved with virtually 100 percent certainty if a malignant-appearing mass or calcification extends to a margin of the specimen. In such situations, if conservative surgery is contemplated, excision of additional tissue may eliminate the need for re-excision later. Unfortunately the specimen radiograph cannot assure negative margins.

It is my practice to perform specimen radiography on *all* biopsies performed with radiographic localization of an occult breast lesion. Although some masses localized prove to be palpable at the time of resection, the specimen radiograph still can provide important information by assuring that the mammographic lesion has been excised and by defining its extent and location in the resected tissue.

## Suggested Reading

Holland R, Hendriks JHCL, Verbeek ALM, et al. Extent, distribution, and mammographic histological correlations of breast ductal carcinoma in situ. Lancet 1990; 335:519–522.

Lindfors KK, Lott SA, Abernathy MT. A new device for evaluation of biopsy specimens of occult breast lesions. Am J Roentgenol 1990; 335:519–522.

Owings DV, Hann L, Schnitt SJ. How thoroughly should needle localization breast biopsies be sampled for microscopic evaluation? A prospective mammographic/pathologic correlative study. Am J Surg Pathol 1990; 14:578–583.

Rebner M, Pennes DR, Baker DE, et al. Two-view specimen radiography in surgical biopsy of nonpalpable breast masses. Am J Roentgenol 1987; 149:283–285.

Stomper PC, Davis SP, Sonnenfeld MR, et al. Efficacy of specimen radiography of clinically occult noncalcified breast lesions. Am J Roentgenol 1988; 151:43–47.

Winchester DP and Cox JD, eds. Standards for breast-conservation treatment. CA 1992; 42:134–162.

# Large-Core Breast Biopsy

*STEVE H. PARKER, M.D.*

Interest in breast disease continues to rise, in both the medical community and the general public. As this interest increases, so does the need for a streamlined diagnostic workup of breast problems. The patient and the medical system are best served by a complete workup in the shortest time using the fewest resources. By incorporating percutaneous, automated, large-core breast biopsy into the radiologist's approach, this goal can be accomplished.

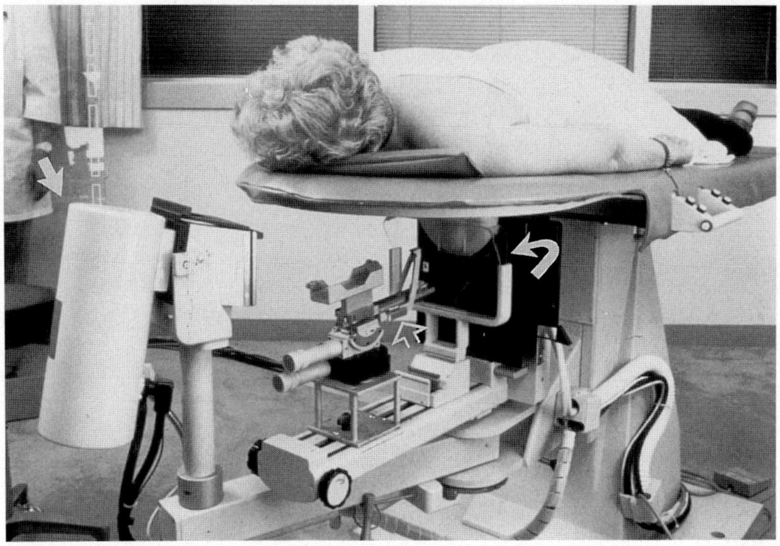

**FIGURE 1** Mammotest stereotactic system. Patient lies comfortably on the Mammotest table, shown with the x-ray tube (*arrow*) swung 15° to the right. All hardware is located beneath the table, with the compression plate (*curved arrow*) and stereotactic biopsy apparatus (*open arrow*) out of the patient's sight. (From Parker SH, Jobe WE. Large-core biopsy offers reliable diagnosis. Diagn Imaging 1990; 12:90–97; with permission.)

To appreciate the full benefit of percutaneous core biopsy, it helps to understand the drawbacks of surgical biopsy. Surgical breast biopsy has a documented "miss rate" of 3 to 6 percent and incurs substantial cost to the patient and third-party payers. Stereotactic biopsies have a similar or lower miss rate and can be performed for one-quarter to one-half the cost of surgical biopsies. In addition, the physical and psychological traumas associated with surgical breast biopsy are much greater than that with core biopsy.

Before addressing the techniques involved in large-core breast biopsy, the equipment and skills required to ensure the appropriate workup of suspicious breast lesions and to perform the biopsy itself will be reviewed. High-quality mammography is essential, as is state-of-the-art breast ultrasonography. Ideally the radiologist should have expertise in mammography, ultrasonography, and intervention.

## Mammography

In addition to standard two-view mammography, spot compression and magnification view capability is crucial for the appropriate mammographic problem solving that precedes biopsy. For biopsy guidance, the stereotactic mammography equipment must be capable of producing excellent straight craniocaudal, straight mediolateral, and stereotactic images. The stereotactic images must be able to identify any lesion detected on a conventional mammogram.

For mammographic biopsies we use Fischer Mammotest recumbent dedicated stereotactic equipment (Fig. 1) rather than the adapted standard mammography or "add-on" equipment (Fig. 2). The recumbent stereotactic table can be raised, freeing much more working room in and around the biopsy apparatus and x-ray tube than add-on systems provide. With the recumbent approach, vasovagal reactions are virtually nonexistent, and the patient is not subjected to direct observation of the biopsy itself. Lying on the table for long periods can be somewhat uncomfortable, however, and most patients find this worse than the actual biopsy. A motorized automatic-guiding device for the biopsy apparatus that can reduce procedure time approximately 20 percent has partially remedied this problem.

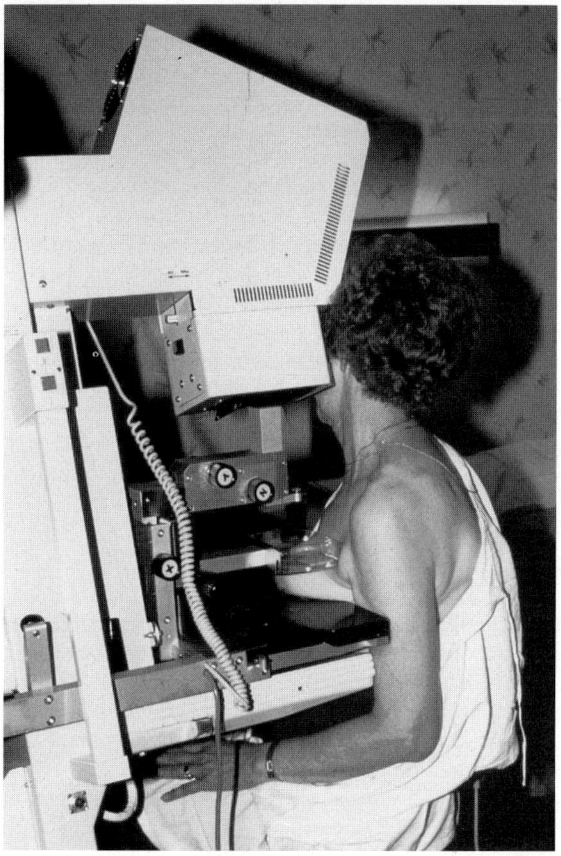

**FIGURE 2** Add-on type of stereotactic unit. Patient must hold her head back and twist it away from the tube housing to allow for stereo views, risking breast movement. (From Parker SH, Jobe WE. Large-core biopsy offers reliable diagnosis. Diagn Imaging 1990; 12:90–97; with permission.)

Unfortunately the cost differential between add-on and dedicated stereotactic equipment is considerable. Compared with other high-tech imaging equipment, however, the cost is low. One can make an argument that resources committed to the early detection of breast cancer are much better spent than the massive resources devoted to neuroradiology, a field that frequently can do little for its patients' afflictions.

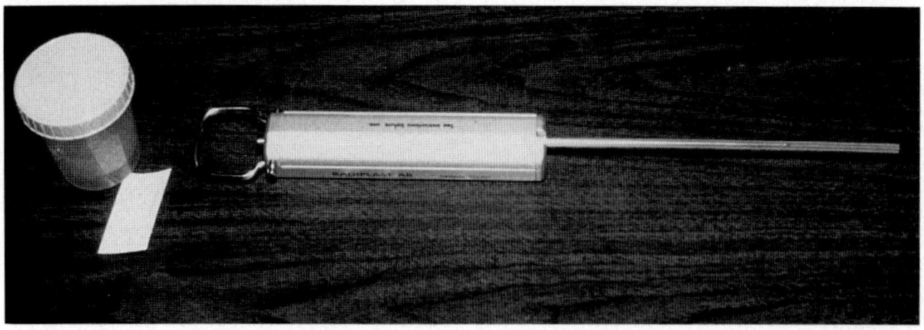

**FIGURE 3** Biopty gun with case closed.

## Ultrasonography

Conventional ultrasound equipment cannot support the kind of decision-making required for breast biopsy. It is critical to have state-of-the-art ultrasound equipment with high-frequency (7.5 to 10 MHz), electronically focused, linear array transducers. The near field resolution must be superb, with the ability to focus electronically with multiple focal zones in the first 5 to 10 mm. Older or less expensive equipment is not suitable for good breast ultrasonography. For ultrasound-guided biopsies, we use the Acoustic Imaging 5200 with 7.5 MHz linear array transducer.

## Automated Biopsy Devices

An automated large-core biopsy device is essential to realize the fruits of the efforts expended on pinpoint image guidance. Currently we use the Bard "Biopty" gun fitted with 14-gauge Bard needles (Fig. 3). This spring-loaded instrument has two separate "sleds," which accept the hubs of the trocar and cannula portions of the needle. With extensive use these springs may eventually begin to wear, causing the quality and quantity of the core specimens to decrease. To maintain original specifications, the "gun" may need to be refurbished periodically (every 1,000 to 2,000 biopsies).

## Needles

Regardless of the automated device used, it is important to select a needle carefully. The sharpness, bevel, flexibility, and sample notch of a given needle must be considered. The trocar point must be extremely sharp to pierce firm, fibrous septa and "fibrocystic changes." A duller needle will push the target out of its path while it is manually advanced to the desired point before the gun is fired. The sharpness of the cutting cannula is perhaps even more important. The sharper the cutting cannula, the less "crush" artifact results.

The trocar point should also have a bevel that slopes down from the upper distal end of the sample notch. This forces the trocar portion of the needle to dive slightly. When the stiffer outer cannula is fired straight at the lesion, this diving motion pulls the sample notch back up, gathering tissue within it the whole time. If the trocar merely projects straight ahead, one must rely on tissue passively prolapsing into the sample notch. This tends not to happen in fatty-replaced breasts. Trocar flexibility also affects this diving motion. The more flexible the distal trocar, including the sample notch, the more likely the desired diving action will occur, thus increasing specimen quantity and quality.

Likewise, the deeper and longer the specimen notch, the larger is the quantity of tissue acquired for a given needle size. Thus one should carefully compare competing needles and choose the one that provides the most of these desirable characteristics. The ultimate test is of course the quantity and quality of the tissue obtained.

## Core Biopsy Versus Fine-Needle Aspiration Biopsy

Large (14-gauge) needles obtain surgical-quality tissue rather than cytologic material obtained with fine-needle aspiration biopsy (FNAB) (Fig. 4). Since core tissue allows histologic analysis, definitive benign diagnoses can be made. Rather than the cytologic diagnosis of "no malignancy present," a definitive diagnosis such as intracanalicular fibroadenoma can be rendered (Fig. 5). Therefore it is possible to differentiate between a false negative caused by a sampling error and a true negative such as fibroadenoma. This distinction frequently is not possible with FNAB. Histologic evaluation of core tissue can also exactly classify any malignancy present. This streamlines appropriate treatment planning and implementation. With cytology, not knowing whether a cancer is invasive complicates and potentially lengthens the definitive surgical procedure.

## Training

Naturally the previously described equipment is only half the challenge. The technologists operating the equipment must be highly trained and skilled. More importantly, the radiologists should be well trained and experienced in all aspects of breast imaging. The radiologist should also have extensive experience performing image-guided needle biopsies or other interventional procedures. We initially produced this combination of skills and experience by cross-training two different radiologists: one expert in breast imaging and one expert in interventional radiology. The optimal combination of course is a radiologist skilled in mammography, ultrasonography, and interventional radiology. A radiologist who can master and blend these three areas of expertise can ensure an appropriate breast workup and ultimately perform large-core breast biopsy to its best advantage.

## Patient Selection and Workup

Once the appropriate personnel and equipment are in place, an effective breast workup can begin. The indications for large-core breast biopsy, with ultrasonographic or stereotactic

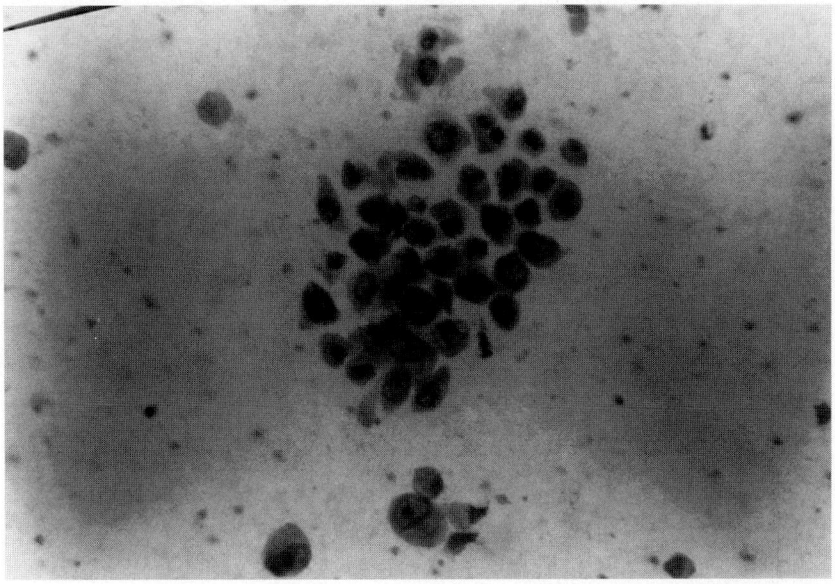

**FIGURE 4** Aspiration biopsy smear of malignant cells. It is not possible to determine whether this cancer is in situ or invasive. (From Parker SH, Jobe WE. Large-core biopsy offers reliable diagnosis. Diagn Imaging 1990; 12:90–97; with permission.)

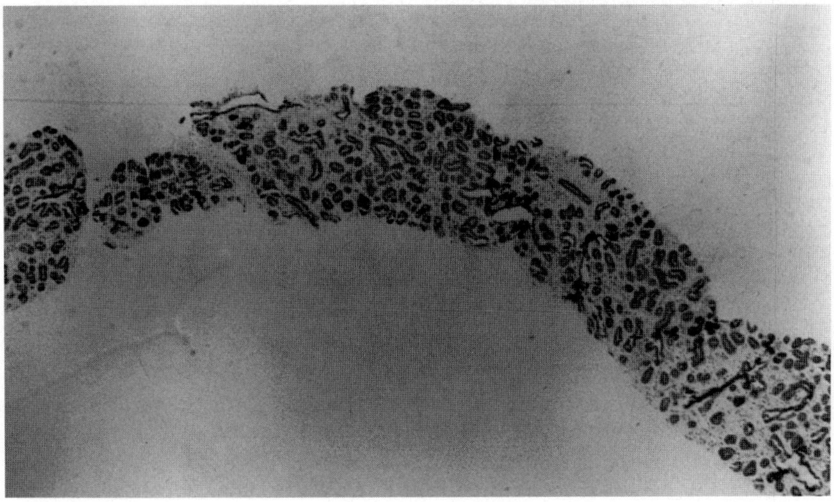

**FIGURE 5** Biopty gun core demonstrates histologic architecture diagnostic of pericanalicular fibroadenoma. This diagnosis is difficult, if not impossible, with aspiration cytology. (From Parker SH, Jobe WE. Large-core biopsy offers reliable diagnosis. Diagn Imaging 1990; 12:90–97; with permission.)

guidance, are essentially the same as that for surgical biopsy. Compared with surgical biopsy, however, stereotactic biopsy is especially useful in patients with lesions visualized well in only one projection, multiple lesions in one or both breasts, and questionable lesions in post-surgical biopsy or lumpectomy patients. In the sequence leading up to the decision to biopsy, any and all clinical or mammographic areas of suspicion must be thoroughly evaluated.

High-quality ultrasonography is especially important in evaluating mammographically dense breasts and in better characterizing mammographically detected lesions. Ultrasonographic guidance is uniquely suited for lesions visualized only on ultrasonography and for patients who are nursing. In addition, if the lesion is visualized well on both ultrasonography and mammography, we choose ultrasonographic guidance because it is quicker, less uncomfortable for the patient, and produces no ionizing radiation.

If ultrasonography verifies that a suspicious lesion is a nonpalpable, simple cyst, it can be safely left alone. If the cyst is palpable and/or symptomatic, then it can be aspirated easily using ultrasonographic guidance (Fig. 6). We aspirate cysts with a 21-gauge standard phlebotomy (vacutainer) needle with a red-top tube. In cysts with questionable mammographic findings, we take a post-aspiration mammogram to demonstrate that the mammographic lesion has resolved. There is generally no need to send the fluid from a simple cyst for analysis.

Complex cysts are aspirated for two reasons. First, there is a small but real chance that a complex cyst is associated with malignancy and the fluid obtained may contain malignant cells. Second, solid lesions are sometimes mistaken for complex cysts. Being unable to aspirate a presumed complex cyst suggests that the lesion is solid. We then proceed with ultrasound-guided core biopsy.

In questionable ultrasonographic studies, we verify that the lesion represents the suspicious mammographic lesion by placing a 25-gauge needle into the lesion under ultrasonographic guidance. We then perform a postlocalization mammogram to prove unequivocally that the lesion observed on ultrasonography is the same as that observed on mammography. We then biopsy the lesion using ultrasonographic guidance.

A

B

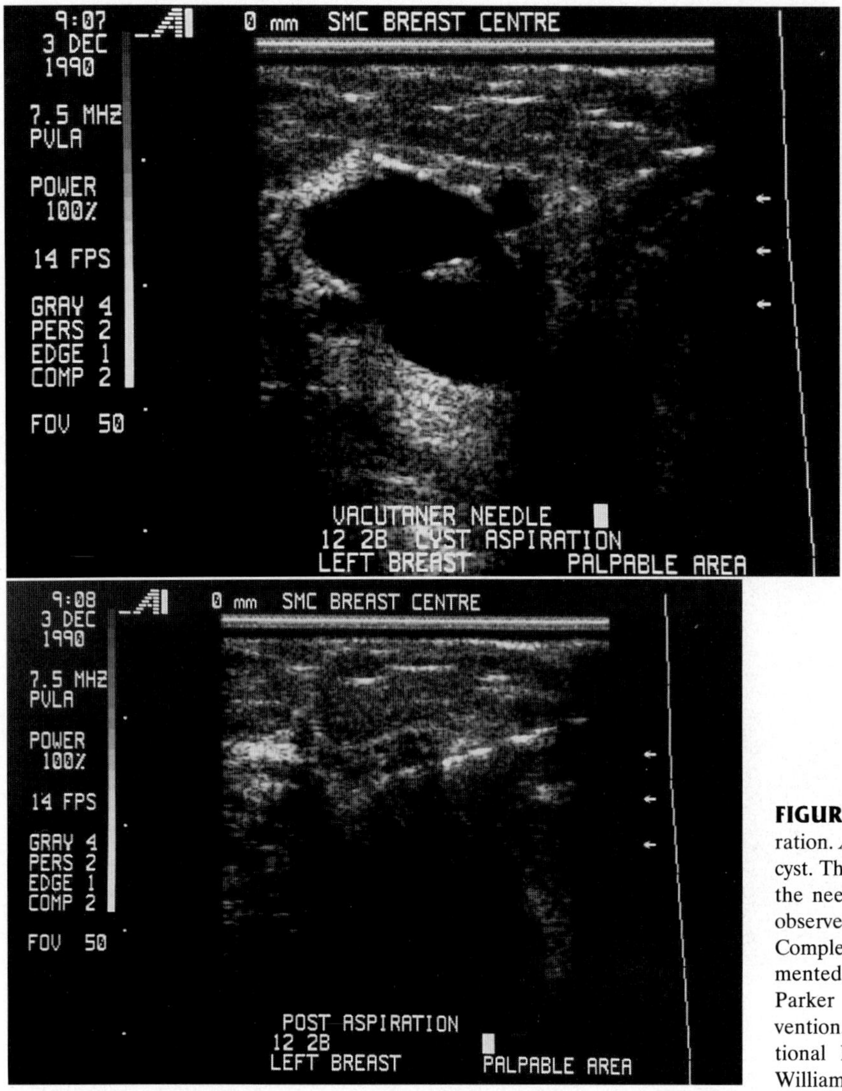


**FIGURE 6** Ultrasound-guided breast cyst aspiration. *A,* Vacutainer needle in place within the cyst. The vacuum can be activated any time after the needle pierces the skin. *B,* Needle is again observed after the cyst has been entirely drained. Complete evacuation of the cyst can be documented easily with ultrasonography. (From Parker SH, Jobe WE, Yakes WF. Breast intervention. In: Castaneda-Zuniga W, ed. Interventional Radiology. Vol 2. 2nd ed. Baltimore: Williams & Wilkins, 1992:1289; with permission.)

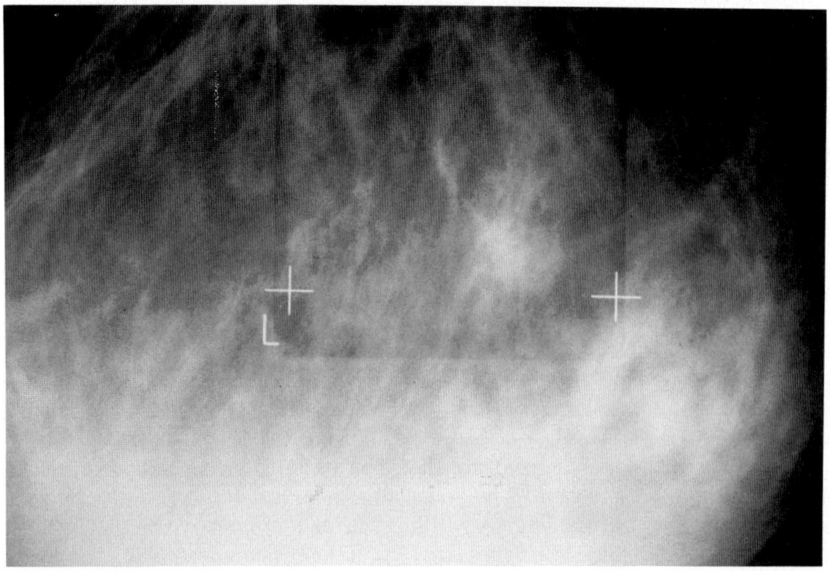

**FIGURE 7** Scout film demonstrates lesion within the compression plate aperture. (From Parker SH, Jobe WE, Yakes WF. Breast intervention. In: Castaneda-Zuniga W, ed. Interventional Radiology. Vol 2. 2nd ed. Baltimore: Williams & Wilkins, 1992:1289; with permission.)

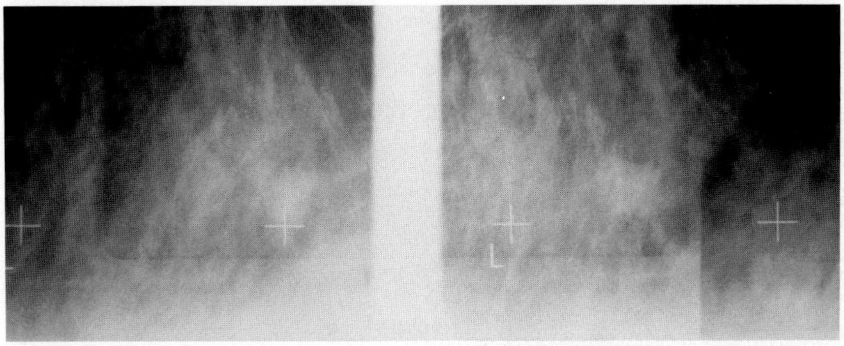

**FIGURE 8** Stereo scout films. (From Parker SH, Lovin JD, et al. Stereotactic breast biopsy with a biopsy gun. Radiology 1990; 176:741–747; with permission.)

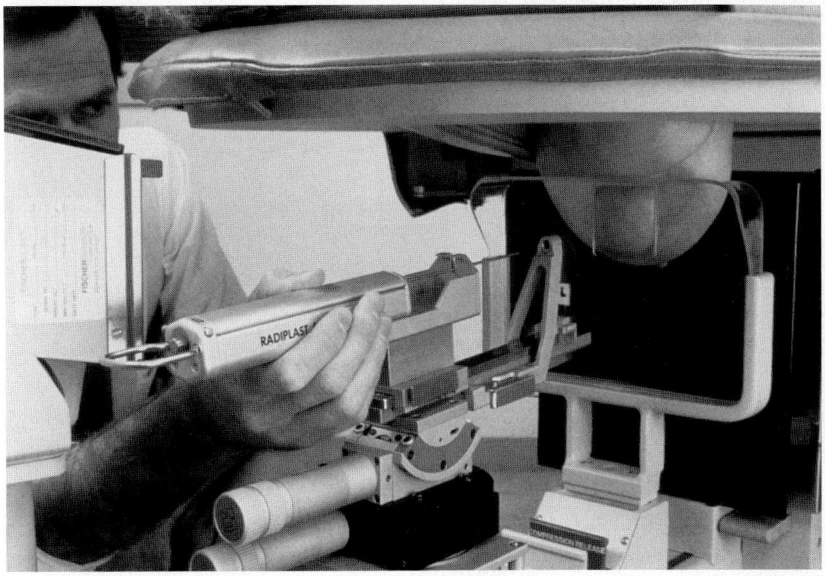


**FIGURE 9** Locking the gun in place and advancing the needle through the needle guide.

## Core Biopsy Technique

The final step is the actual biopsy. Now the interventional skills of the radiologist are especially emphasized. The first step in stereotactic biopsy is taking a craniocaudal or mediolateral scout film (Fig. 7). Using the projection that places the lesion nearest the skin increases the distance behind the lesion for maximum needle excursion. If the scout film demonstrates that the lesion is within the aperture in the compression plate, then stereotactic scout views are obtained. The two 15° off-axis stereotactic views are exposed side by side on a single film (Fig. 8). The Biopty gun is then locked into place in its dedicated housing (Fig. 9). The stereo views are placed on the adjacent digitizer and the coordinates calculated by activating a hand-held computer mouse at the center of the lesion and at reference cross hairs in each view. Older units print out the lesion coordinates, which must be manually dialed into the biopsy holder. Units with an "autoguide" place the coordinates automatically in the memory of the remote control panel attached to the main unit. The biopsy gun and needle automatically align on the proper trajectory with a push of a button.

We then administer a small amount of skin anesthetic and with a scalpel make a skin nick just big enough for easy passage of the 14 gauge needle. We advance the gun and needle to the designated depth and repeat stereo views to confirm the position of the needle (Fig. 10). After firing the gun, we obtain a final set of stereo views to document that the needle has traversed the lesion (Fig. 11). It is important to note that deep anesthetic may move or obscure lesions. Any lesion movement lengthens the procedure because the lesion must be relocalized.

We make at least five passes to obtain representative samples throughout the lesion. After the procedure, our breast center nurse manually compresses the biopsy site for 5 to 10 minutes, applies a compression bandage, and places a small ice pack between the bandage and the patient's bra. The nurse re-examines the patient the following day for any bleeding, hematoma formation, or other complications.

The same protocol described above for stereotactic biopsy is used for ultrasound-guided biopsy. Naturally ultrasonography is used instead of mammography for guidance. We prefer the freehand technique for ultrasound-guided biopsy, i.e., the radiologist holds the transducer in one hand and the biopsy needle in the other (Fig. 12). In this way we can more easily coordinate the two without the constraints of a needle guide attached to the transducer. Using the freehand technique, the needle is advanced to and fired through the lesion under real-time ultrasonographic observation. Continuous observation also ensures avoidance of the chest wall. We obtain prefire and postfire images to document the needle and sample notch passing through the lesion (Fig. 13). In over 1,000 patients biopsied with ultrasonography and stereotactic percutaneous

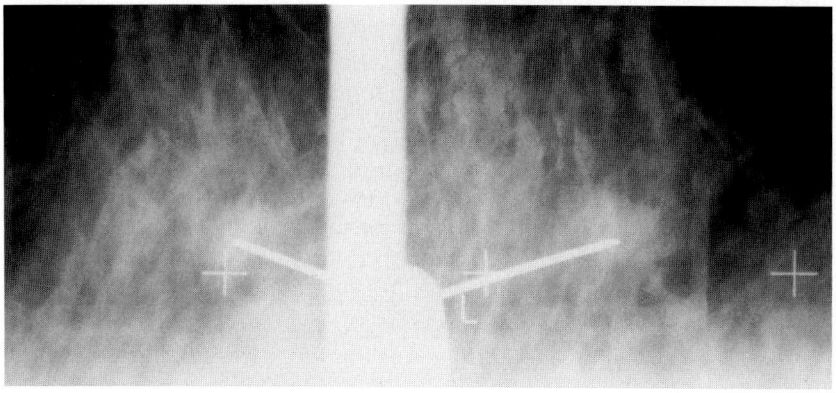

**FIGURE 10** The needle is advanced through the skin nick to the computed depth, and stereo views are obtained again to confirm that the needle tip is over the lesion in both views. (From Parker SH, et al. Stereotactic breast biopsy with a biopsy gun. Radiology 1990; 176:741–747; with permission.)

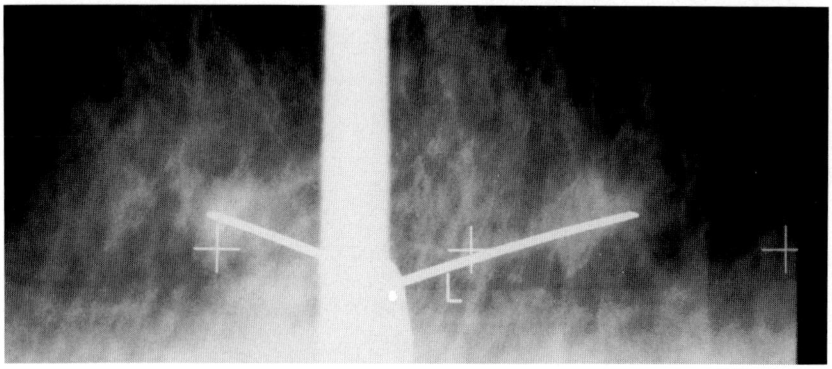

**FIGURE 11** Final set of stereo views is obtained after the gun is fired to document that the needle has traversed the lesion. (From Parker SH, Lovin JD, et al. Stereotactic breast biopsy with a biopsy gun. Radiology 1990; 176:741–747; with permission.)

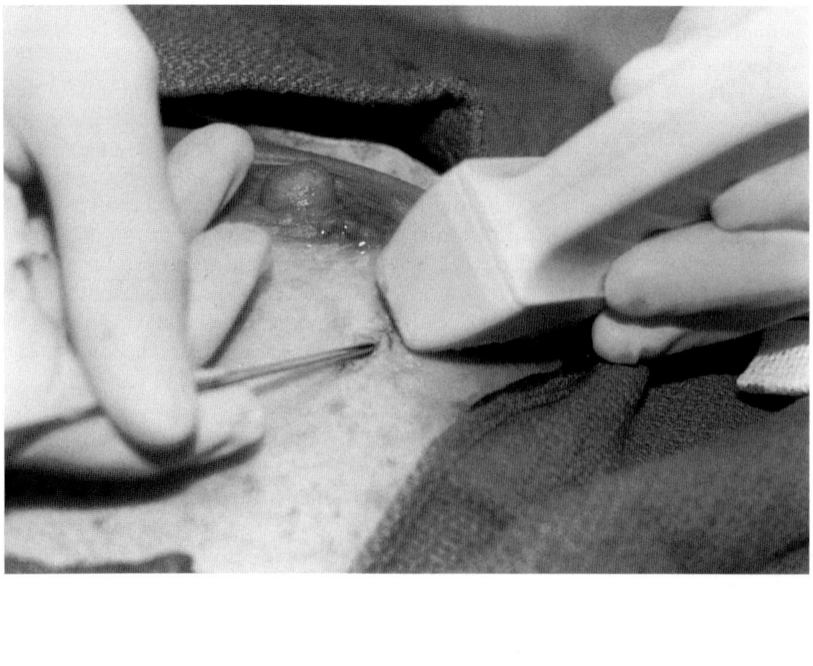

**FIGURE 12** Ultrasound-guided biopsy using the freehand technique. A 14-gauge Biopty needle is advanced with one hand while the other hand controls the transducer. A second pair of hands stabilizes the Biopty gun. (From Parker SH, Jobe WE. Large-core biopsy offers reliable diagnosis. Diagn Imaging 1990; 12:90–97; with permission.)

A

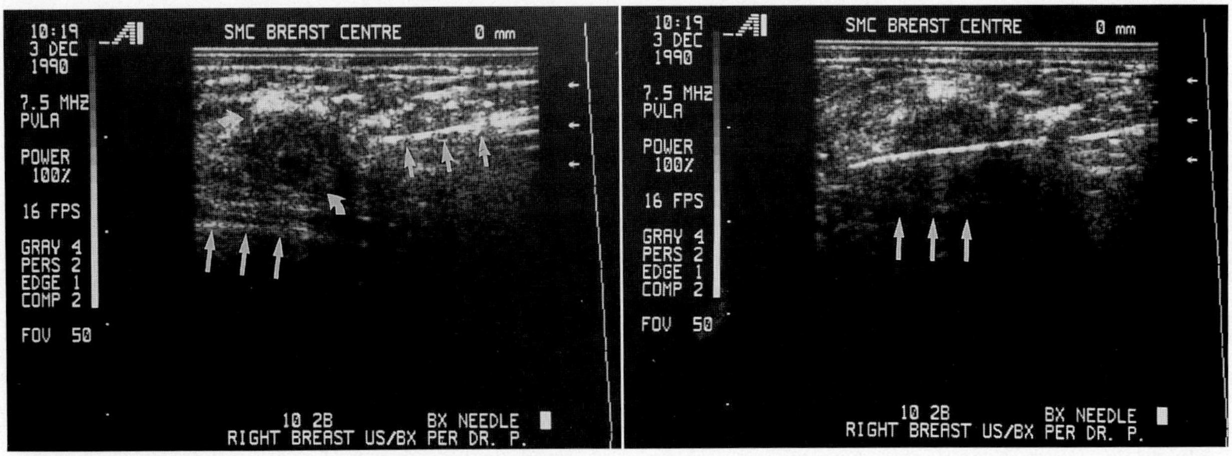


B

**FIGURE 13** Ultrasound-guided biopsy. *A,* Automated 14-gauge biopsy needle (*short arrows*) at the periphery of the lesion (*curved arrows*). Needle has been advanced such that it is nearly parallel to the chest wall (*long arrows*). *B,* Biopsy needle clearly observed traversing the lesion after firing the gun and well away from the chest wall (*long arrows*). (From Parker SH, Jobe WE, Yakes WF. Breast intervention. In: Castaneda-Zuniga W, ed. Interventional Radiology. Vol 2. 2nd ed. Baltimore: Williams & Wilkins, 1992:1289; with permission.)

large-core technique, none experienced significant hematoma or other complication.

## Discussion

The breast is one of the few areas of the body still subjected to open-surgical biopsy. In recent years improved needle and imaging techniques have allowed percutaneous needle biopsies to replace open-surgical biopsy in most other areas of the body. Excisional biopsy, however, remains the current standard in the breast. Most radiologists who have attempted to extend percutaneous biopsy to breast lesions have used FNAB. Although somewhat successful in other areas of the body, FNAB has its greatest failings in the breast. On the other hand, the combination of large-core automated biopsies and pinpoint imaging provided by stereotactic mammography and ultrasonography can provide reliable, definitive, histologic diagnosis of both benign and malignant breast lesions, thus providing a dependable alternative to surgery. Success with this procedure, however, requires a radiologist who is well trained and experienced in mammography, ultrasonography, and interventional techniques. Even so, state-of-the-art equipment and meticulous technique and protocol must be maintained to ensure successful outcomes for the patient.

*Acknowledgments.* The author gratefully acknowledges the editorial assistance of Lisa Hofsess, M.S., Radiology Imaging Associates, in the preparation of this manuscript.

## Suggested Reading

Dronkers DJ. Stereotaxic core biopsy of breast lesions. Radiology 1992; 183:631–634.

Hopper KD, Baird BJ, Reddy W, et al. Efficacy of automated biopsy guns versus conventional biopsy needles in the pigmy pig. Radiology 1990; 176:671–676.

Meyer JE. Value of large-core biopsy of occult breast lesions. AJR 1992; 158:991–992.

Norton LW, Zeligman BE, Pearlman NW. Accuracy and cost of needle localization breast biopsy. Arch Surg 1988; 123:947–950.

Parker SH, Hopper KD, Yakes WF, et al. Image-directed percutaneous biopsies with a biopsy gun. Radiology 1989; 171:663–669.

Parker SH, Jobe WE. Large core breast biopsy offers reliable diagnosis. Diagn Imaging 1990; 12:90–97.

Parker SH, Jobe WE, Yakes WF. Breast intervention. In Castaneda W, ed. Interventional Radiology. Vol 2. 2nd ed. Baltimore: Williams & Wilkins, 1992:1289.

Parker SH, Lovin JD, Jobe WE, et al. Stereotactic breast biopsy with a biopsy gun. Radiology 1990; 176:741–747.

Parker SH, Lovin JD, Jobe WE, et al. Nonpalpable breast lesions: Stereotactic automated large-core biopsies. Radiology 1991; 180:403–407.

# Imaging the Breast after Radiation Therapy and Surgery

*ELLEN B. MENDELSON, M.D.*

The breast is one of the most common sites of surgical procedures. About 180,000 new breast carcinomas will be diagnosed during the current year in the United States. If this number represents 20 to 40 percent of surgical breast biopsies, the total number of surgical procedures approximates 500,000. Radiologists should recognize postsurgical alterations and be aware that they may overlap with the radiographic features of malignancy.

Postoperative changes may be observed after benign biopsy as well as lumpectomy for carcinoma. These alterations in the breast are accentuated and prolonged by radiation therapy and include masses, scarring, edema, skin thickening, and calcifications. For analysis to be accurate, the mammograms must be placed in temporal context and correlated with the physical findings and procedures that have been performed. Many errors will be avoided, and the possibility of recurrent carcinoma can be suggested with greater confidence if mammograms are evaluated in sequence, always comparing with the earliest, not just the most recent study. Postsurgical and radiation changes are also less likely to be misinterpreted as malignant, important in avoiding unnecessary biopsy of irradiated tissues in which the healing process may be disturbed.

## Breast Conservation for Carcinoma

Radiologists have primary responsibility for breast cancer patients in making the diagnoses of nonpalpable lesions, in assessing extent of disease radiographically to determine eligibility for breast conservation, in performing precise preoperative localizations, in carefully interpreting specimen radiographs correlated with mammograms, and in analyzing sequential follow-up studies after tumor removal and radiation therapy. Radiologists are asked to make timely diagnoses of recurrent tumor, but also not to recommend unnecessary biopsies for postprocedural changes. For interpretation to be accurate, the radiographic findings must be correlated with the clinical history, the surgical procedures that have been performed, and the time intervals that have elapsed.

Although other procedures, such as segmentectomy, are performed in Europe, the *lumpectomy* or *wide excisional biopsy* is the most common operation used in the United States for breast conservation. Lumpectomy is ordinarily accomplished by means of a curvilinear incision made directly over the lesion, which is removed with a rim of tissue that is grossly free of tumor. If any skin is excised, it should only be a small ellipse.

In most lumpectomies, only the subcutaneous fat and subcuticular layers are sutured. The deeper layers of the surgical bed fill in gradually. Meticulous hemostasis decreases the likelihood that large hematomas or seromas will form. Theoretically a drain might result in a formation of a crater-like cavity, and a drain is not placed in the lumpectomy site. The contour of the breast may be better preserved if fluid resorption and filling in of the surgical bed are gradual. Axillary dissection is often performed later through a separate incision into which a drain is placed.

Radiation therapy begins as soon as the surgical site has healed adequately, ordinarily, 2 to 5 weeks after lumpectomy and axillary dissection. Forty to 50 Gy is delivered to the breast, with an optional boost to the lumpectomy site bringing the total to 60 to 66 Gy. The axilla is not irradiated after axillary dissection.

## Breast Conservation: Imaging

### *Preoperative and Perioperative Assessment*

To determine the appropriateness of lumpectomy and radiation therapy, mammography can be used to define the extent of the patient's disease, demonstrate multicentricity, and evaluate the contralateral breast. Mammographic analysis can further help to guide patient selection by suggesting the presence of certain prognostic indicators for tumor recurrence, such as an extensive intraductal component (EIC) associated with an invasive carcinoma. Pleomorphic calcifications observed within the tumor mass or stranding into the adjacent breast parenchyma are radiographic markers of EIC that should be evaluated with magnification radiography, which often shows many more calcifications and depicts morphology better than routine larger focal spot radiography (Fig. 1). Magnification in two projections can also help establish some clustered calcifications as benign, such as calcifications of cystic hyperplasia. If one of the projections is a true lateral view, the teacup-crescent configuration of milk of calcium layering in small cysts can be observed and the calcifications identified definitively as benign. A dermal origin of clustered microcalcifications can be excluded by marking the alphanumeric coordinates of the cluster using a fenestrated localization plate. A view with the x-ray beam tangential to the marker shows dermal calcifications in the skin.

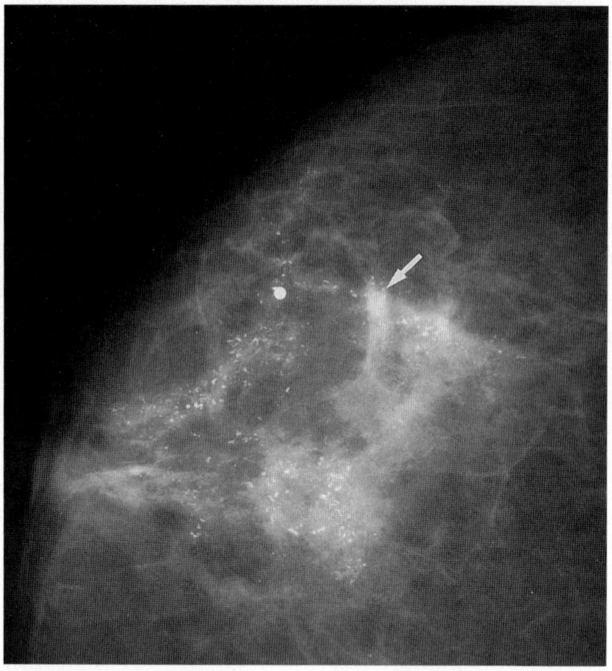

**FIGURE 1** EIC. Magnification radiography demonstrates a large number of pleomorphic, malignant-appearing calcifications suggestive of an extensive intraductal component associated with infiltrating tumor *(arrow)*. Selection of breast conservation or mastectomy is guided by careful mammographic workup.

Presurgical localization of nonpalpable masses and microcalcifications should be precise, with the tip of the hookwire or other marker usually no more than a few millimeters away from the target lesion. Specimen radiography is required to confirm removal of all presurgically localized nonpalpable and some palpable abnormalities. The specimen radiograph should be correlated with the mammogram, and an estimate made of the adequacy of the excision. Reliable assurance of a tumor-free margin cannot be obtained from specimen radiography, although if the mass or calcification is observed at the margin of resection, in any view of the specimen, the surgeon should be advised to excise additional tissue. If the specimen is generous and the abnormality small, the radiologist can assist the pathologist further by needle-localizing the abnormality within the specimen, using alphanumeric coordinates or other device. Full compression and magnification of the specimen can also increase visibility of the lesion. The specimen's findings should be communicated by the radiologist immediately to the surgeon in the operating room and then reported formally.

## *Post-Treatment Follow-up Studies*

### General Approach

For correlation with mammographic findings, such as architectural distortion or new calcifications, scars are marked with lengths of thin wire that are taped to the healed incision. The fine wires used for presurgical localization of nonpalpable lesions are suitable. These wires can be cut to the length of the scar and easily made to conform to its shape. (NOTE—A localization wire placed into the breast should not be trimmed near the skin, because the wire can retract into the breast.)

The skin marker for the scar may not always correspond to the area of tumor excision lying deeper within the breast. It is important to identify and focus on the tumor bed because more than 65 percent of recurrences are at or within a few centimeters of this site. A mammographic view tangential to the skin incision site permits differentiation of thickened skin from the tumor bed deeper in the breast.

Ultrasonography can be used as well to distinguish the cutaneous incision from the lumpectomy site. With ultrasonography, the surgical bed is a distinct hypoechoic oval area showing posterior acoustic enhancement if fluid is present or an irregularly shaped hypoechoic area with posterior acoustic shadowing after fibrosis has developed.

For radiation therapy planning and for subsequent follow-up imaging studies, the surgeon can place clips at the margins of the lumpectomy site at the time of surgery. Neither clips in the breast nor wires on the skin should compromise mammographic visualization of the breast tissue. The wires also do not interfere with gadolinium-enhanced magnetic resonance imaging, a technique under study for its applicability in differentiating mature scar tissue from recurrent tumor after lumpectomy and radiation therapy. The wires or clips may cause only small signal void artifacts.

### Findings Expected after Breast Conservation

*Fluid Collections.* During the first year after breast conservation therapy, in the area of lumpectomy, the mammogram often shows an oval mass that is fairly dense and well marginated but usually with a few spiculations or irregularities (Fig. 2). The mammographic appearance and timing are suggestive of a postoperative fluid collection; it is unlikely that a tumor will regrow to larger than its preoperative dimensions within the first year, particularly if the margins of resection have been free of tumor. If there is doubt, sonography can be used to identify the mass as fluid filled.

*Scars.* As the lumpectomy site is imaged on follow-up mammograms during the first 6 to 18 months, the discrete, dense fluid collection will be replaced by architectural distortion or spiculated soft-tissue density representing an evolving scar. Areas of radiolucency representing entrapped fat are interspersed with the soft-tissue density. The scar may elongate and develop jagged borders.

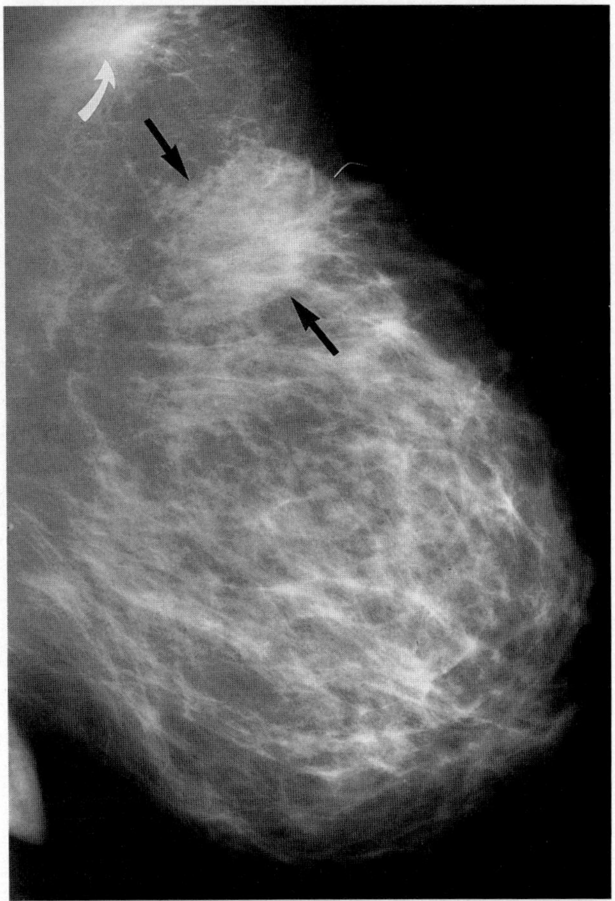

A

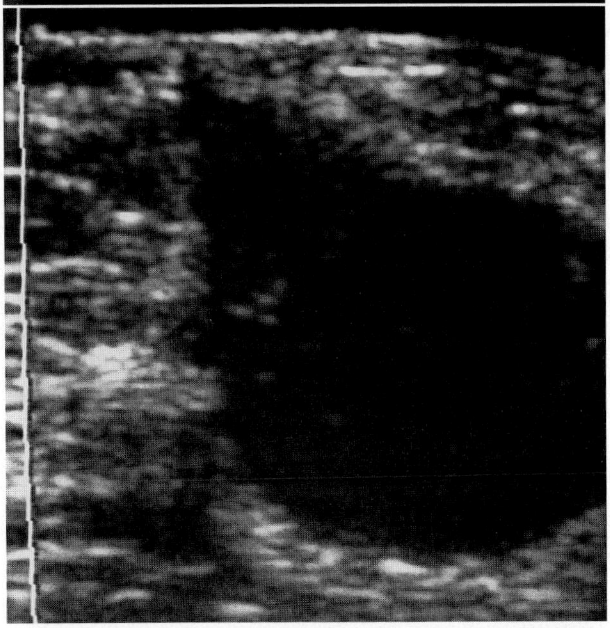

B

**FIGURE 2** Postoperative fluid collection. *A,* Mediolateral oblique view 6 months after treatment shows lumpectomy site *(arrows)* marked with a wire. Oval configuration at this time suggests fluid collection. Mild breast edema related to radiation therapy is present. Soft-tissue density in axilla *(curved arrow)* represents postsurgical changes after axillary dissection. *B,* Sonography confirms fluid collection. A tract extends to the area of incision.

A

B

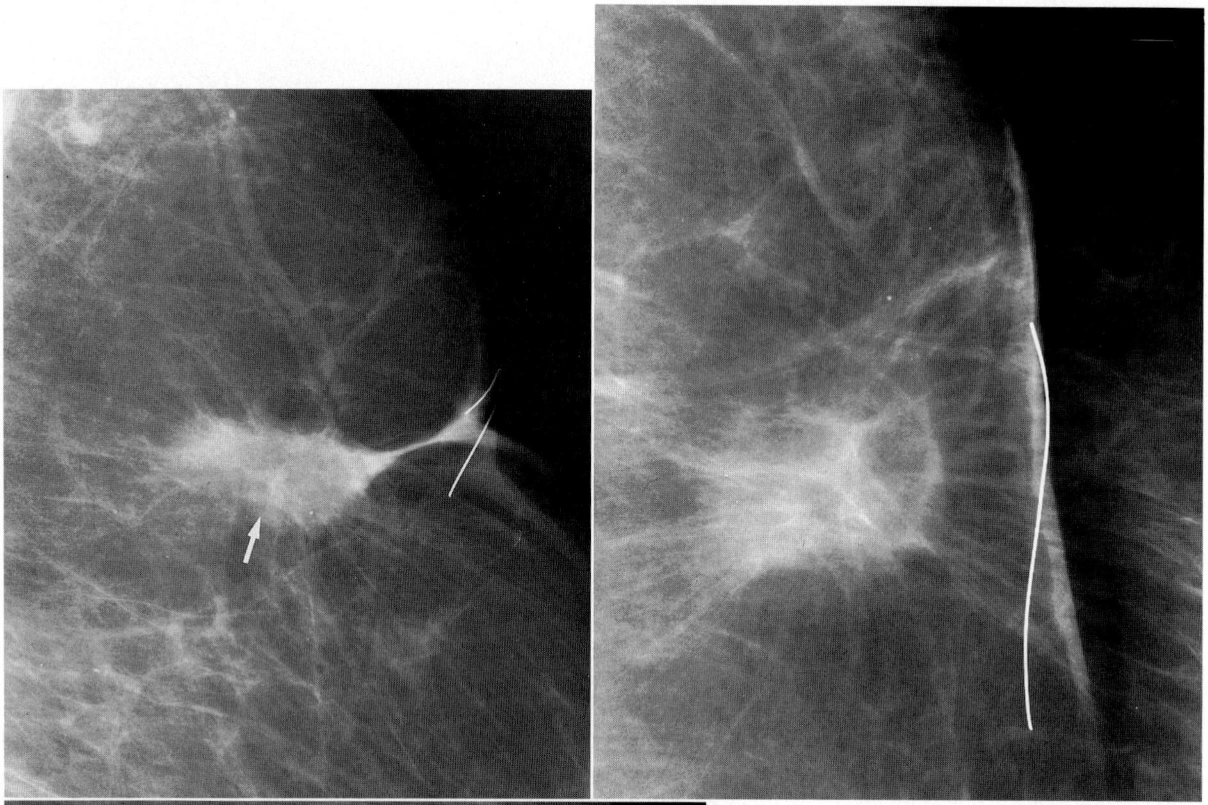

C

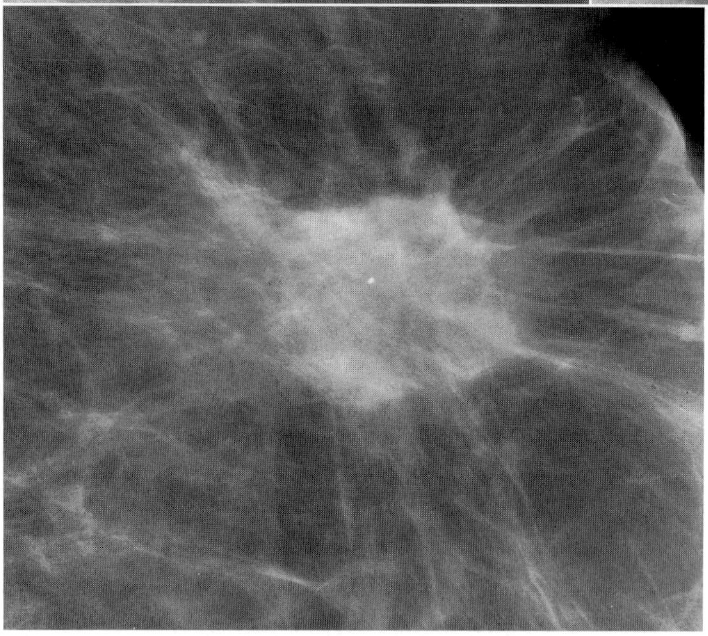

**FIGURE 3** Scar: changing shape and central radiolucencies demonstrated on three different views. *A,* Tangential view shows thin fibrous band connecting the tumor excision site *(arrow)* with the skin incision marked with a thin wire taped to the skin. *B,* Thin spiculations and benign calcifications visualized in another view of the parenchymal scar, which has a different shape in this projection. Wire at the incision is again observed. *C,* Scar looks different on this third view. Central radiolucencies are trapped within fibrous tissue. Spicule thickness and length are nonspecific. No mass is observed. Spot compression and magnification are often necessary to demonstrate radiographic features of scarring that permit differentiation from recurrent tumor.

Because both scarring and carcinoma appear as spiculated, poorly marginated soft-tissue densities on a mammogram, to distinguish them, the clinical history, physical examination, and comparison with previous studies are necessary. On physical examination, scarring uncomplicated by fat necrosis is perceived as induration rather than a mass. Radiolucencies within the central area of soft-tissue density suggest scarring.

Another finding observed in intramammary scars is a changing appearance in different projections. In one view the spiculated soft-tissue densities are masslike, but they elongate in other projections (Fig. 3).

A more reliable sign of scarring that is helpful in follow-up of the conservatively treated breast is contraction and shrinkage of the evolving scar as it matures in the first year or two. The size of the resection, volume of the postsurgical fluid collection, and whether it was drained postsurgically may affect the rate of scar formation. After two successive studies have shown no change, recurrent tumor should be suspected if the scar increases in size or becomes more nodular (Fig. 4). Fine-needle aspiration cytology, core biopsy, or surgical excision may confirm recurrent tumor as the cause of increasing soft-tissue density.

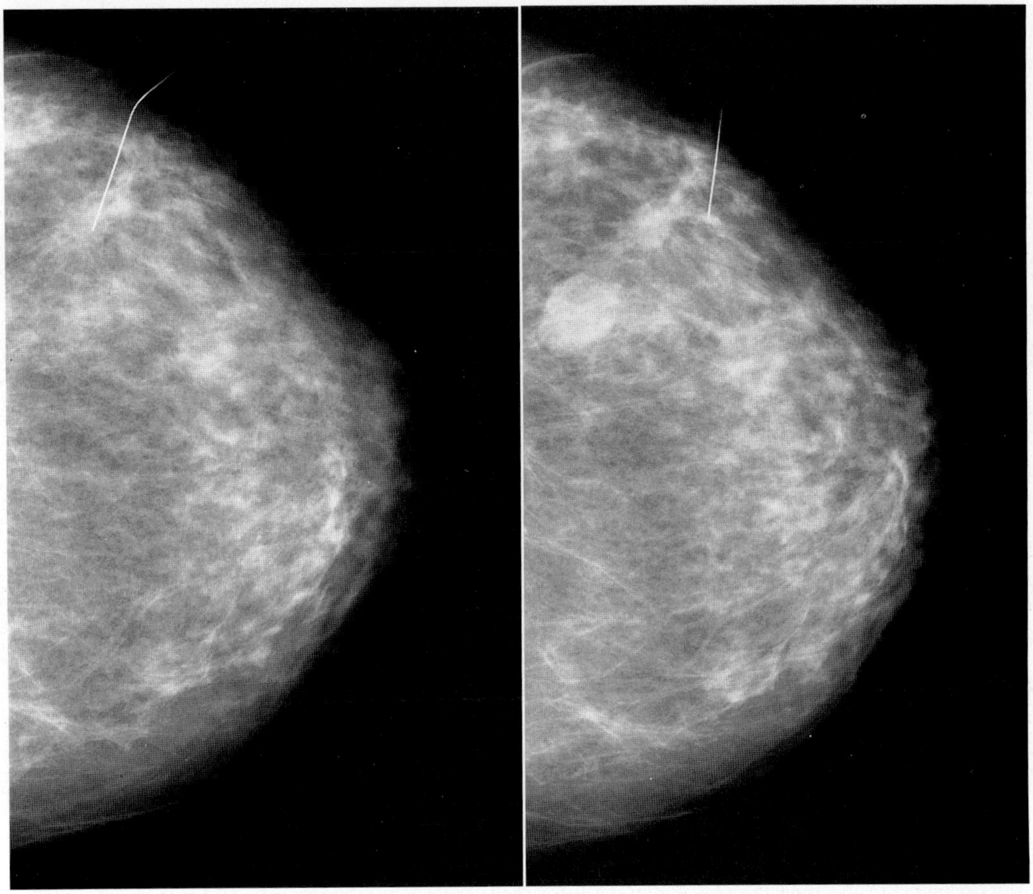


**FIGURE 4** Recurrent tumor: mass. *A,* Two years after breast conservation therapy for infiltrating ductal carcinoma, the lumpectomy site with wire taped to the incision is linear and spiculated (craniocaudal projection). *B,* One year later, a new nodule has appeared posteromedial to the scar, representing recurrence.

*Edema.* Nearly all patients who have had axillary dissection or radiation therapy have breast edema (Fig. 5). Increased breast density and thickened, stringy, linear parenchymal trabeculations are observed when edema is moderately severe. The breast enlarges and mammographic compression is more difficult as edema involves the parenchyma, subcutaneous tissues, and skin. These changes are most evident in the periareolar and dependent areas of the breast.

Breast edema gradually diminishes and resolves for many patients within 2 years. Mild edema remains in a small percentage of patients. After breast density has stabilized, recurrent edema is cause for concern.

*Skin Thickening.* Skin thickening and breast edema are companion findings that have similar time courses for maximal change and resolution after lumpectomy and breast irradiation. The skin's thickness may reach 1 cm or even greater in the periareolar region. By 2 years after breast conservation therapy, the skin has returned to near-normal thickness, although mild thickening persists in approximately 20 percent of patients.

*Calcifications.* Calcifications are a most important marker of new or recurrent breast carcinoma. The same morphologic and distributional features used preoperatively to classify calcifications are applicable to the treated breast. Postoperative preradiation magnification radiography should be performed to detect residual calcifications at the tumor excision site. Commonly the surgical bed will be re-excised if microcalcifications remain.

New calcifications occur frequently at the site of tumor excision. Several types of benign calcifications are found at the lumpectomy site. Although they coarsen later, calcifications may be fine, faint, and difficult to characterize as they begin to precipitate in scars, fibrotic tissue, or areas of fat necrosis. Once residual calcifications have been excluded, calcifications that occur soon (6 to 18 months) after surgery and radiation therapy are most often benign.

Fat necrosis is associated with all types of surgical procedures in the breast. In vague, patchy, soft-tissue densities, calcifications may be needlelike, of varied shapes, bizarre, disorganized appearing, and alarming. These dystrophic calcifications will become thick, calcified plaques. Thin arcs of calcification may form complete circles to define the rims of rounded, radiolucent oil cysts (Fig. 6).

After tumor excision and radiation therapy, small, round, and smooth dystrophic calcifications are common at the lumpectomy site. They resemble the calcifications of secretory disease or ductal ectasia and may have a similar origin, forming in areas of necrotic tissue, sloughed cells, and cellular detritus.

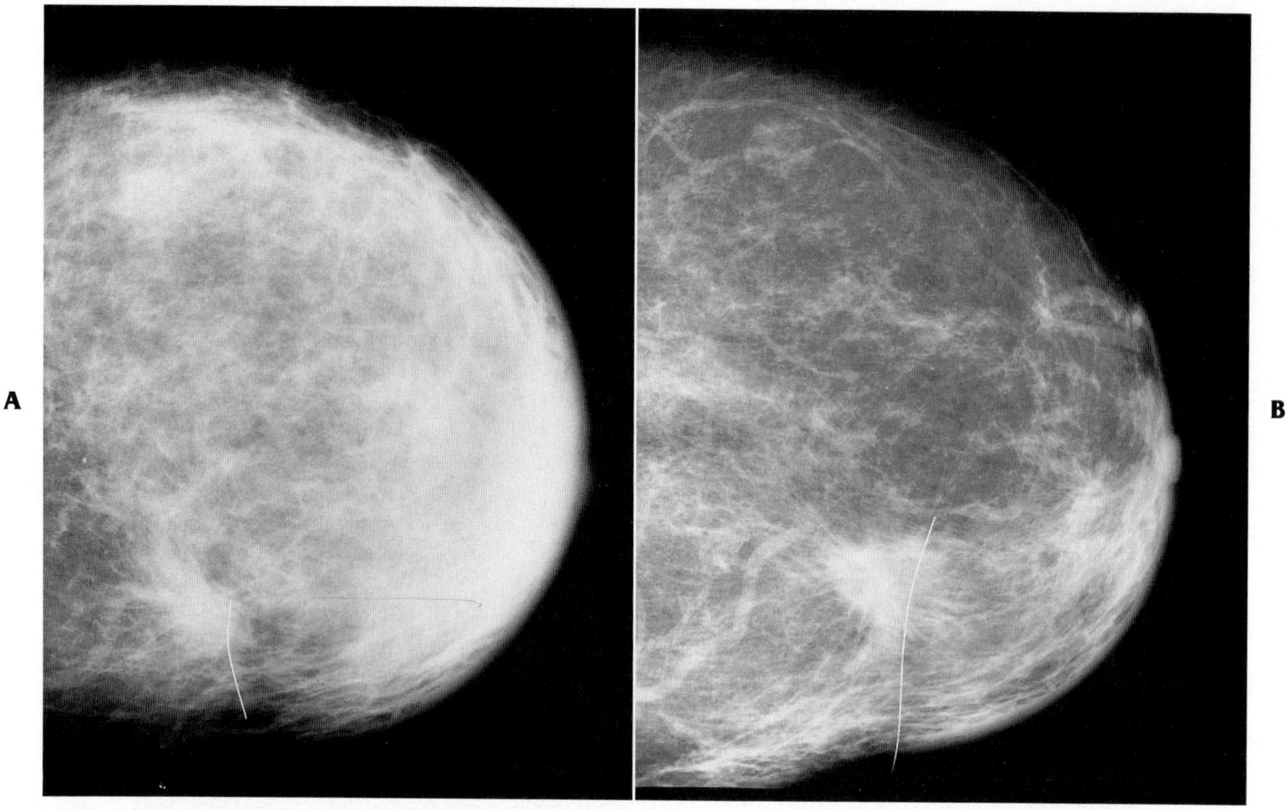

**FIGURE 5** Breast edema and skin thickening. *A,* Marked edema of the breast and skin, especially the anterior half of the breast and periareolar region. The lumpectomy site in the medial breast, marked with wire, appears masslike and is obscured by edema. Craniocaudal view, left breast, 6 months after lumpectomy and radiation therapy. *B,* Craniocaudal view, same patient, 24 months after breast conservation therapy, shows considerable resolution of edema and expected spiculation in contraction of scar without tumor recurrence observed. Mild edema and skin thickening persist.

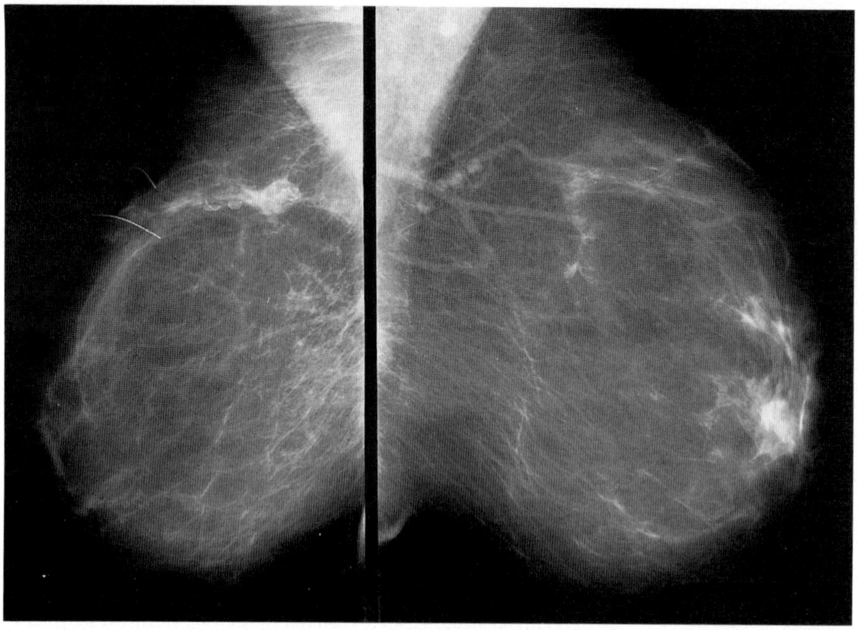

**FIGURE 6** Fat necrosis. Mediolateral oblique views of each breast show asymmetry in size, the right breast smaller because of radiation therapy and surgery. At the tumor excision site, there are oil cysts with the typical rim calcifications that may form complete circles.

Also benign appearing and somewhat less common are more coarse, plaquelike, angular calcifications. These larger calcifications are also dystrophic, developing in scars and in disturbed subcutaneous tissue.

Calcified remnants of suture material at the lumpectomy site have distinctive shapes, often containing knots (Fig. 7). Branching linear calcifications and double tracking may suggest malignancy, but these linear sutural calcifications can be wide and several millimeters long. They resemble the thick straight calcifications of ductal ectasia or secretory disease.

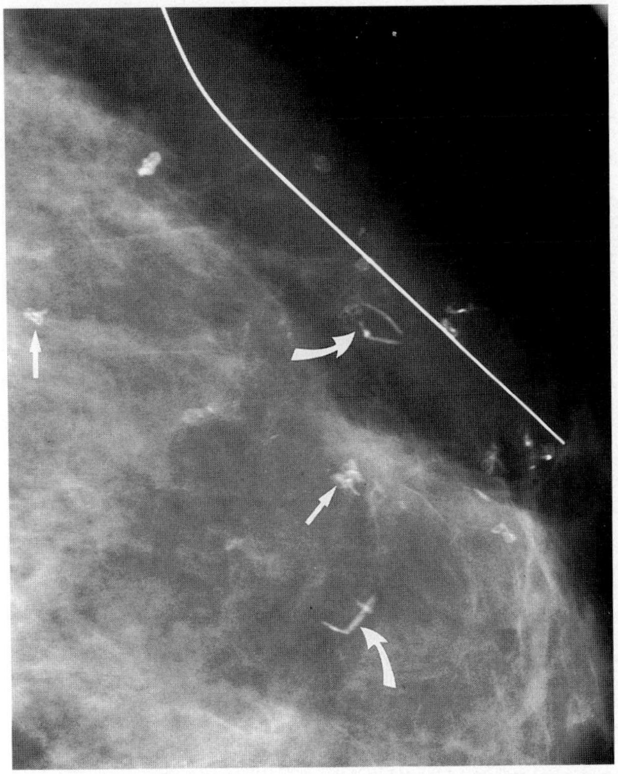

**FIGURE 7** Sutural calcifications. Magnification craniocaudal view shows angular, relatively thick, linear calcified clipped sutures *(curved arrows)* and rounded calcifications with radiolucent areas, knots, and bits of suture material *(straight arrows)*. These coarse calcifications should not be interpreted as suspicious. Magnification of the lumpectomy site is essential to accurate evaluation of calcifications.

Microcalcifications, a common radiographic sign of recurrent tumor, account for a substantial percentage of mammographically detected recurrences. An active search with magnification radiography should be made for new indeterminate or malignant-appearing calcifications at the lumpectomy site.

Unexcised calcifications may or may not disappear following radiation therapy, and their persistence does not necessarily indicate viable tumor. The expectation of recurrence will be higher after excision of invasive carcinoma with EIC or with large areas of the comedocarcinoma variant of ductal carcinoma in situ.

## Special Mammographic Views

The standard mediolateral oblique and craniocaudal views require supplementation with additional mammographic projections directed to visualization of the lumpectomy site (Table 1). The scar should be marked with wire, a small BB marker, or other radiopaque marker that does not obscure the breast tissue. The area of excision should be imaged fully in two projections. Spot compression and magnification radiography of the tumor bed should be performed in the projection in which the surgical site is visualized most completely. If the tumor has presented as microcalcifications, magnification views in two projections force the interpreter to scrutinize the surgical bed for new microcalcifications (Fig. 8). Particularly if the surgical site is near the posterior edge of the compression plate, a small spot compression device is useful both in fixing the area and in spreading apart the tissue elements.

**TABLE 1** Mammographic Evaluation After Breast Conservation

Mark scars: wires taped to scar for correlation with architectural distortion
Routine views: mediolateral oblique and craniocaudal
Additional views nearly always of value
- Tangential views to separate skin incision site from deeper tumor bed
- Spot compression: better compression in inaccessible areas
  - For posterior lesions, retroareolar area
  - With magnification for calcifications
- Particular view depends on location of lesion (place film closest to lesion): e.g., mediolateral or lateromedial, exaggerated axillary or medially rotated craniocaudal views

A view with the x-ray beam tangential to the marker shows the skin incision in profile, separate from the deeper area of tumor excision (see Fig. 3, *B*). This tangential view is of great value in analyzing changes at the operative site and should be standard in the follow-up of breast conservation patients.

## Ultrasound Evaluation

In the postoperative breast, sonography can be used to characterize a mammographic or palpable mass as fluid filled or solid. Ultrasonography is an alternate method of imaging sequential changes such as skin thickening and decreasing scar size. Sonography is useful also as a supplement to mammography in confirming resolution of fluid collections and evaluating the tumor bed for new, hypoechoic masses that might represent tumor recurrence.

## Schedule for Follow-up Imaging after Breast Conservation Therapy

There is considerable geographic variation within the United States in the treatment of breast cancer. On the two coasts, the majority of breast cancer patients may be treated with wide excision and irradiation, but in some areas up to two-thirds of women eligible for breast conservation are not being offered this option. Somewhat dependent on the prevailing surgical practices, there is also wide variation in experience with the radiologic follow-up of these patients. Currently, beyond the first year after therapy, no guidelines have been adopted for intervals between follow-up studies, although many recommendations have appeared in the literature.

Two major objectives of imaging after breast conservation therapy are (1) diagnosing recurrence early, before development of metastases; and (2) minimizing misinterpretations of postprocedural change as tumor recurrence to avoid unnecessary biopsy of radiation-treated tissue that may be slower to heal. The key to achieving these objectives is familiarity with the time course of postoperative and irradiation changes (Fig. 9). The period of greatest change occupies the first 18 months, with the most marked changes occurring around 6 months. In general, if the margins of resection have been free of tumor, recurrence will not be anticipated at the lumpectomy site until 2 to 3 years have elapsed.

Perhaps most important is recognizing stability of the breast, which we have defined as lack of change on two successive mammograms. Subsequently, a change counter to the direction of resolution suggests recurrent tumor.

There is agreement that mammography at 6 and 12 months

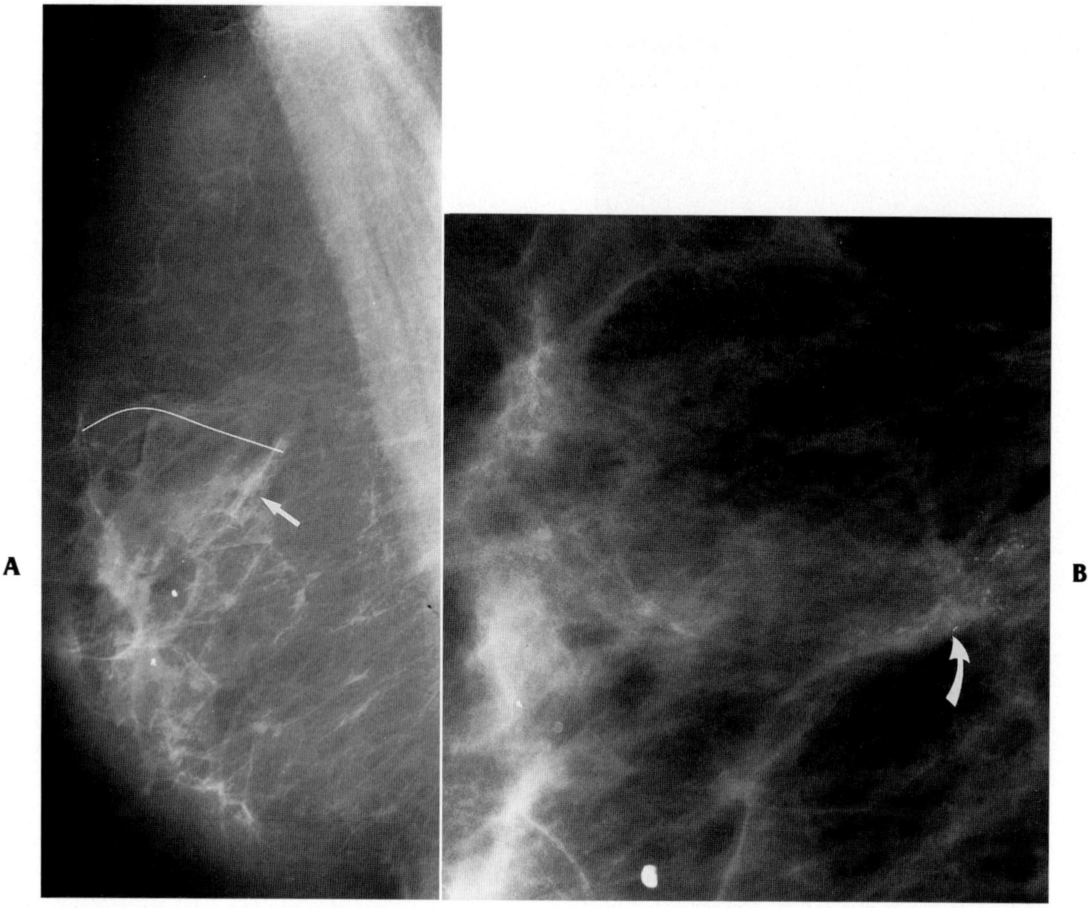

**FIGURE 8** Recurrent tumor: microcalcifications. *A,* Minimal scarring and no mass present at the lumpectomy site (wire) 5 years after breast conservation for infiltrating ductal carcinoma. New calcifications suspected *(arrow)* on this mediolateral oblique view. *B,* Lateral magnification view with spot compression shows smudge of soft-tissue density, within which are numerous pleomorphic microcalcifications *(curved arrow)*, a new area of ductal carcinoma in situ.

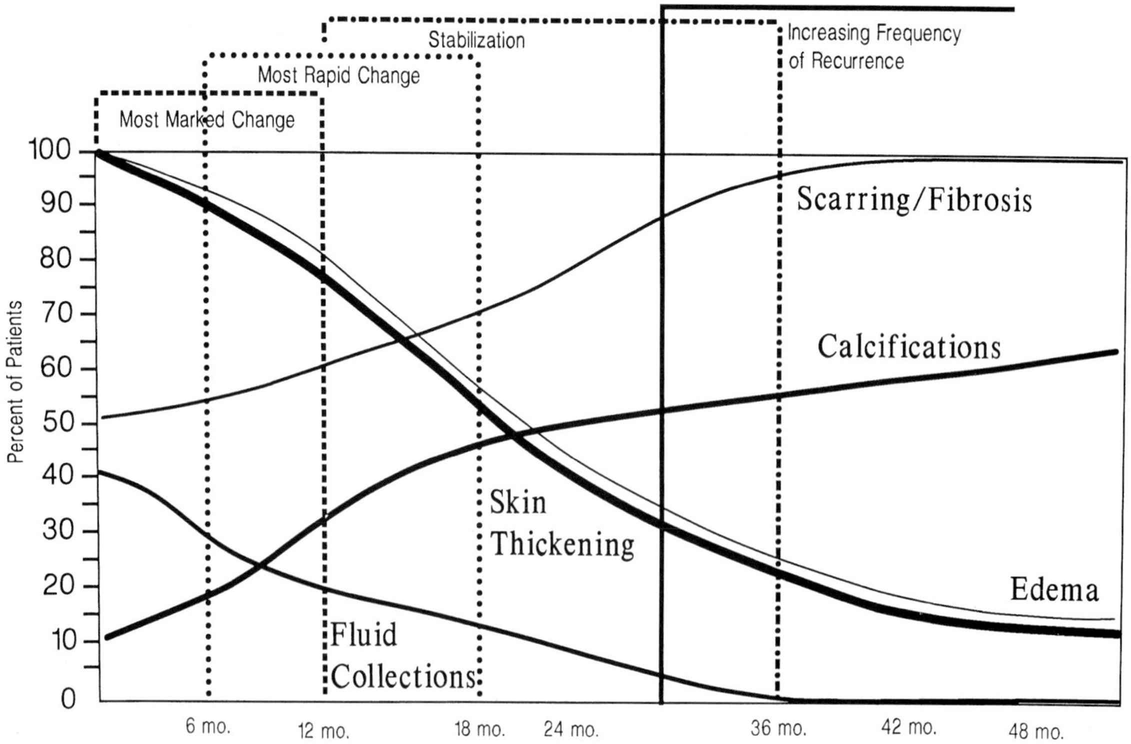


**FIGURE 9** Changing appearance of the conservatively treated breast.

**TABLE 2** Imaging After Breast Conservation Therapy

| Timing of the Study | Rationale |
|---|---|
| *Treated breast* | |
| Postoperative preradiation (2–5 weeks after lumpectomy) | Detection of residual carcinoma – important for microcalcifications |
| 6 months | Baseline study: Peak of postprocedural changes: masses, skin thickening, edema. Early calcifications form. |
| 12 months | Assess changes listed above; begin to look for mammographic stability (no change on 2 successive studies). |
| 18 months | End of time of most rapid change; confirm stability. |
| 24 months | Expect stabilization for most patients. More confident recognition of benign postprocedural changes. |
| 30 months | Mammogram should be stable for nearly all patients. |
| 36 months | Stable mammogram: Suspect recurrence if direction of change is unexpected. |
| Annual studies can be resumed after stabilization (usually by 18–36 months) | Detect recurrence: For patients at increased risk of recurrence (EIC and young patients), consider intervals of 6 months. |
| *Contralateral breast* | |
| Annually | Screening; increased risk of breast carcinoma |

after tumor excision records the greatest changes in the postprocedural breast. Beyond the 1 year study, various schedules have been proposed for follow-up mammograms. Most authors have supported studies every 6 months after the first year for some period of time. We request a postoperative preradiation mammogram of the lumpectomy site, useful for exclusion of residual microcalcifications. Studies are then performed every 6 months for 3 years to cover the 1 to 3 year period of stabilization, as much to avoid unnecessary biopsies of postprocedural benign changes as to diagnose recurrent tumor. The achievement of stability coincides with the time that recurrences begin to appear, which is 2 to 3 years after conservation therapy. After the breast appears stable mammographically, we advise annual studies of both the treated and contralateral breasts (Table 2).

Mammographic interpretation and follow-up imaging of the conservatively treated breast cancer patient can challenge the radiologist. Only with an understanding of the time course of changes can imaging evaluation of the postoperative breast be accurate.

## Suggested Reading


Fisher B, Bauer M, Margolese R, et al. Five year results of a randomized clinical trial comparing total mastectomy and segmental mastectomy with and without radiation in the treatment of breast cancer. N Engl J Med 1983; 312:665–673.

Hassell PR, Olivotto IA, Mueller HA, et al. Early breast cancer: Detection of recurrence after conservative surgery and radiation therapy. Radiology 1990; 176:731–735.

Libshitz HI, Montague ED, Paulus DD. Calcifications and the therapeutically irradiated breast. AJR 1977; 128:1021–1025.

Libshitz HI, Montague ED, Paulus DD. Skin thickness in the therapeutically irradiated breast. AJR 1978; 130:345–347.

Mendelson EB. Evaluation of the postoperative breast. Radiol Clin North Am 1992; 30:107–138.

Mitnick J, Roses DF, Harris MN. Differentiation of postsurgical changes from carcinoma of the breast. Surg Gynecol Obstet 1988; 166:549–550.

Paulus D. Conservative treatment of breast cancer: Mammography in patient selection and follow-up. AJR 1984; 143:483–487.

Sadowsky NL, Semine A, Harris JR. Breast imaging: A critical aspect of breast conserving treatment. Cancer 1990; 65:2113–2118.

Stomper PC, Recht A, Berenberg AL, et al. Mammographic detection of recurrent cancer in the irradiated breast. AJR 1987; 148:39–43.

Winchester DP, Cox JD. Standards for breast-conservation treatment. CA-A Cancer J Clin 1992; 42:135–162.

# NEUROADIOLOGY AND HEAD AND NECK RADIOLOGY

## MRI and CT Evaluation of Intra-axial Brain Tumors

*BRADLEY R. BUCHBINDER, M.D. · KENNETH R. DAVIS, M.D.*

## PART I: PRINCIPLES OF TUMOR CHARACTERIZATION

This chapter presents our current approach to computed tomography (CT) and magnetic resonance imaging (MRI) of intra-axial brain tumors. We review (1) principles of tumor characterization, (2) tumors of the cerebral hemispheres, and (3) tumors of the posterior fossa and pineal region. Essential imaging features are emphasized.

### Roles of MRI and CT

MRI is almost always the imaging modality of choice for brain tumors. Its advantages are superior intrinsic soft-tissue contrast, greater sensitivity of paramagnetic contrast agents for blood-brain barrier disruption, direct multiplanar capability, intrinsic sensitivity to blood flow, and absence of bone-related beam hardening artifact. Together, these factors result in higher tumor detection rates and more specific tumor characterization. Nevertheless, CT is helpful or necessary in several situations. It is the modality of choice to identify acute hemorrhage, calcification, and bone changes. It is often preferable in unstable, uncooperative, or claustrophobic patients. It is required when MRI is contraindicated. Once a tumor has been fully characterized by MRI, we often use CT to evaluate emergent complications such as acute hemorrhage, increasing mass effect, and hydrocephalus.

### MRI Technique

For the evaluation of a known or suspected intra-axial tumor, we use a standard imaging protocol that is modified according to individual tumor locations or imaging characteristics. Pulse sequence specifications vary with instrumentation and field strength. Our generic approach follows.

#### *Paramagnetic Contrast Material*

Gadolinium diethylene-triamine penta-acetic acid (Gd-DTPA) is indicated in virtually all cases where tumor is known or suspected. It is relatively contraindicated in pregnancy, renal failure, and hemolytic anemias. The pattern of normal MRI contrast enhancement differs from CT. Like CT, consistent enhancement occurs in the pituitary stalk and gland, choroid plexus, and cavernous sinus. Unlike CT, enhancement of the other dural sinuses, falx, tentorium, and vessels is less pronounced and more variable, while enhancement of the nasal mucosa is much more pronounced. Vascular enhancement occurs when flow is slow, as in smaller veins. We use the maximum FDA-approved clinical dose of 0.1 mmol/kg, as a slow IV bolus over approximately 1 minute.

#### *Imaging*

Although paramagnetic contrast material shortens both T1 and T2, the relative effect is much greater on T1. Therefore T1-weighted images are performed to detect contrast enhancement. Precontrast T1-weighted images are essential to differentiate between contrast enhancement and other causes of T1-weighted hyperintense signal (e.g., blood, fat, melanin). The effects of contrast material on long TR images are

**TABLE 1** MRI of Intra-axial Brain Tumors: Protocol Guidelines

Before Gd-DTPA:
- Sagittal T1
- Axial T2
- Axial T1
- Optional
  - Coronal T2 (skull base, brain stem, temporal lobes, vertex lesions)
  - Sagittal T2 (midline lesions)
  - Susceptibility-sensitive gradient-echo (blood, calcification)
  - Flow-sensitive gradient-echo

After Gd-DTPA (0.1 mmol/kg):
- Axial T1
- Coronal T1
- Optional sagittal T1 (midline lesions)

Typical Pulse Sequence Parameters for 1.5 T GE Signa:

| Parameters (Pulse Sequence) | T1-weighted (Spin-Echo) | T2-weighted (Spin-Echo)† | Susceptibility (Multislice Gradient-Echo) | Flow (3D RF-Spoiled Gradient-Echo) |
|---|---|---|---|---|
| TR (milliseconds) | 600 | 2,500 | 750 | 40 |
| TE (milliseconds) | 12 (minimum) | 30/80 | 50 | 5 |
| Flip-angle | 90/180 | 90/180 | 10 | 30 |
| Signal (NEX) | 1 | 1 | 2 | 1 |
| Slice thickness (mm) | 5 | 5 | 5 | 2–3 |
| Gap (mm) | 0 (interleaved) | 2.5 | 2.5 | 0 |
| Matrix | 256 × 192 | 256 × 192 | 256 × 192 | 256 × 192 |
| Field of view (FOV, cm) | 18–24 | 20 | 20 | 20 |
| Flow compensation | No(*) | Yes | Yes | Yes |
| Time (minutes) | 4 | 8 | 4.5 | 4.5 |

*After administration of contrast material, flow compensation sometimes reduces flow-induced artifact from enhancing veins and dural sinuses, especially in the posterior fossa. Flow compensation necessitates a longer minimum TE, resulting in fewer slices.
†Or, if available, fast spin-echo.

variable; therefore these are obtained before contrast material is administered.

Before administering contrast material, we obtain sagittal T1-weighted, axial T1-weighted, axial proton density-weighted, and axial T2-weighted images. Immediately after injection of contrast material, we obtain axial and coronal T1-weighted images. Additional imaging planes are sometimes helpful. Sagittal precontrast T2-weighted and post-contrast T1-weighted images may be useful for midline lesions. Coronal T2-weighted images may be helpful for lesions involving the skull base, brain stem, temporal lobes, and vertex. Precontrast magnetic susceptibility–sensitive long TE, low flip-angle gradient-echo images are added when hemorrhage or calcification is suspected. Flow-sensitive short TE, higher flip-angle gradient-echo images, or magnetic resonance angiography are added to evaluate abnormal vessels. The MRI protocol and typical imaging parameters are summarized in Table 1.

## CT Technique

### *Iodinated Contrast Material*

Iodinated contrast material is virtually always indicated for the initial evaluation of a known or suspected brain tumor by CT. Inclusion of an unenhanced scan depends on the likelihood of encountering calcification or hemorrhage. When a tumor is known or suspected, both unenhanced and enhanced scans are performed, because calcification and hemorrhage are relatively common. When a tumor must be excluded but is unlikely, only an enhanced scan is performed. In the few cases where it is subsequently necessary to differentiate among calcification, hemorrhage, and enhancement, an unenhanced scan is performed later. This approach is efficient, cost-effective, and spares the patient unnecessary radiation exposure. Once a tumor has been fully characterized, follow-up studies frequently require only an enhanced scan. Conversely some follow-up studies for limited indications, such as exclusion of hydrocephalus, require only an unenhanced scan.

The infusion rate, iodine concentration, total dose, and timing of image acquisition determine which features are emphasized in the contrast-enhanced scan. Dynamic scanning during rapid infusion of high iodine content contrast material emphasizes vascular opacification. Scanning during slower, sustained infusion with high total dose emphasizes parenchymal opacification at sites of blood-brain barrier disruption. The former technique is well suited to evaluation of vascular abnormalities, such as arteriovenous malformations. The latter is well suited to evaluation of processes characterized by blood-brain barrier disruption, including tumors. Our standard protocol achieves a reasonable compromise between these features, while favoring identification of blood-brain barrier disruption. In adults we administer diatrizoate meglumine 14 percent iodine (~150 mgI/ml), 300 ml by drip infusion. If low-osmolar contrast material is indicated, we use iopamidol 300 mgI/ml or iohexol 300 mgI/ml, 150 ml. In children we

**TABLE 2** CT of Intra-axial Brain Tumors: Protocol Summary

$I^+/I^-$:
  Known or suspected tumor
$I^+$ only:
  Rule out tumor (low suspicion)
  Many routine tumor follow-up cases
$I^-$ only
  Selected tumor follow-up cases (e.g., rule out hydrocephalus)
  Rule out $Ca^{2+}$ or hemorrhage

exclusively use low-osmolar contrast material, 300 mgI/ml, 1 ml/lb up to 50 ml by hand infusion. We begin the scan after infusion of one half of the total dose. Because of the higher sensitivity of MRI and higher risk of nephrotoxicity, we do not use the delayed double-dose technique.

### *Imaging*

Protocol details vary with instrumentation. With the increased speed of contemporary CT scanners and laser film printers, we favor high axial spatial resolution CT imaging. On the GE 9800 series scanners, we obtain contiguous 3 mm thick slices through the posterior fossa and contiguous 5 mm thick slices through the cerebral hemispheres on the enhanced scan or the unenhanced scan if it is the only one. When an ancillary unenhanced scan is performed, contiguous 5 mm thick slices are obtained through the whole brain. The kilovolts (peak), milliamperes, field of view (FOV), and reconstruction algorithm should be optimized for the brain. If associated bone abnormalities are anticipated, images should be reconstructed with separate brain soft-tissue and bone algorithms. Our standard CT protocol is summarized in Table 2.

## Tumor Characterization

Tumor imaging usually is not histopathologically specific. However, analysis of imaging characteristics in conjunction with clinical data can lead to a reasoned differential diagnosis that guides patient management.

MRI and CT characterize tumors by location, size, margins, mass effect, CT attenuation, MRI signal intensity, and contrast enhancement. These characteristics often reflect important underlying pathologic features, including edema, hemorrhage, necrosis, cyst formation, calcification, fat content, macroscopic vascularity, and blood-brain barrier integrity. The MRI and CT appearances of these features are briefly reviewed.

### *Localization: Intra-axial versus Extra-axial*

Localization of a mass to the intra-axial or extra-axial compartments strongly influences the differential diagnosis, anticipated vascular supply, surgical approach, and prognosis. Multiplanar MRI is superior to CT in this regard. When masses become very large, it may be difficult or impossible to definitively establish intra-axial or extra-axial location.

The cardinal features of an extra-axial mass are peripheral location, compression of the underlying parenchyma, separation from the brain surface by anatomic interfaces, and adjacent bone involvement (Fig. 1). The most frequently identified interface between an extra-axial mass and the brain parenchyma is the subarachnoid space, demarcated by cerebrospinal fluid (CSF) clefts and pial vascular flow voids. A dural boundary layer is most often observed with masses of the cavernous sinus, where the lateral dural margin separates the cavernous sinus from the medial temporal lobe. Dural thickening and enhancement are often associated with extra-axial masses ("dural tail" sign). This is characteristic of, but not pathognomonic for, meningioma. Extra-axial masses may arise from bone, invade bone, or cause bone reaction such as hyperostosis. Bone involvement is rare with intra-axial tumors in the absence of surgery.

### *CT Attenuation and MRI Signal Intensity*

Most tumors are identified because of their increased water content. High water content decreases CT attenuation and prolongs T1 and T2 relaxation times. As a result, most tumors are hypodense-to-isodense on CT, hypointense-to-isointense on T1- and hyperintense on T2-weighted images. Typical of many pathologic processes, these imaging features are nonspecific. This general pattern is frequently modified by other pathologic characteristics, resulting in greater diagnostic specificity. In all of the following discussion, the terms "hypo-/iso-/hyper-dense" and "hypo-/iso-/hyper-intense" use gray matter as a reference, unless otherwise specified.

### *Cytoarchitecture*

High cell density, high nuclear-to-cytoplasmic ratio, and high protein content increase CT attenuation and decrease T2-weighted signal intensity. Tumors that may be hyperdense on CT and iso- to hypo-intense on T2-weighted images include lymphoma (Part II, Fig. 11), germinoma, medulloblastoma, pineal cell tumors, primitive neuroectodermal (PNET) tumors, some adenocarcinoma metastases (especially colon and lung) (Part III, Fig. 1), and meningioma (see Fig. 1).

### *Hemorrhage*

The appearance of blood on MRI is principally determined by the biophysical state of iron in hemoglobin, pulse sequence, and magnetic field strength. Other factors that influence the MR image include hematocrit, clot retraction, nonparamagnetic protein content, tissue oxygen saturation, pH, and blood-brain barrier integrity. Iron affects the MRI signal by shortening T1 (T1 relaxivity effect), shortening T2* (magnetic susceptibility effect), or both. Both T1- and T2-weighted images are necessary for characterization of hemorrhage. Magnetic susceptibility effects increase with TE and field strength. They may not be evident on spin-echo images with low-midfield magnets. They are less pronounced on fast spin-echo than standard spin-echo T2-weighted images. Gradient-echo images are exquisitely sensitive to susceptibility effects. They may identify sites of hemorrhage that are not demonstrable on spin-echo images even at 1.5 T. They are especially important at low field strength. A detailed discussion of the appearances of hemorrhage on MRI is beyond the scope of this chapter. However, salient features of the stages of parenchymal hematoma evolution are summarized in Table 3.

Any tumor can bleed. Among primary brain tumors, hemorrhage is most common in glioblastoma multiforme (Part II, Fig. 5), ependymoma, and oligodendroglioma. Among metastases, hemorrhage is most common in melanoma, renal

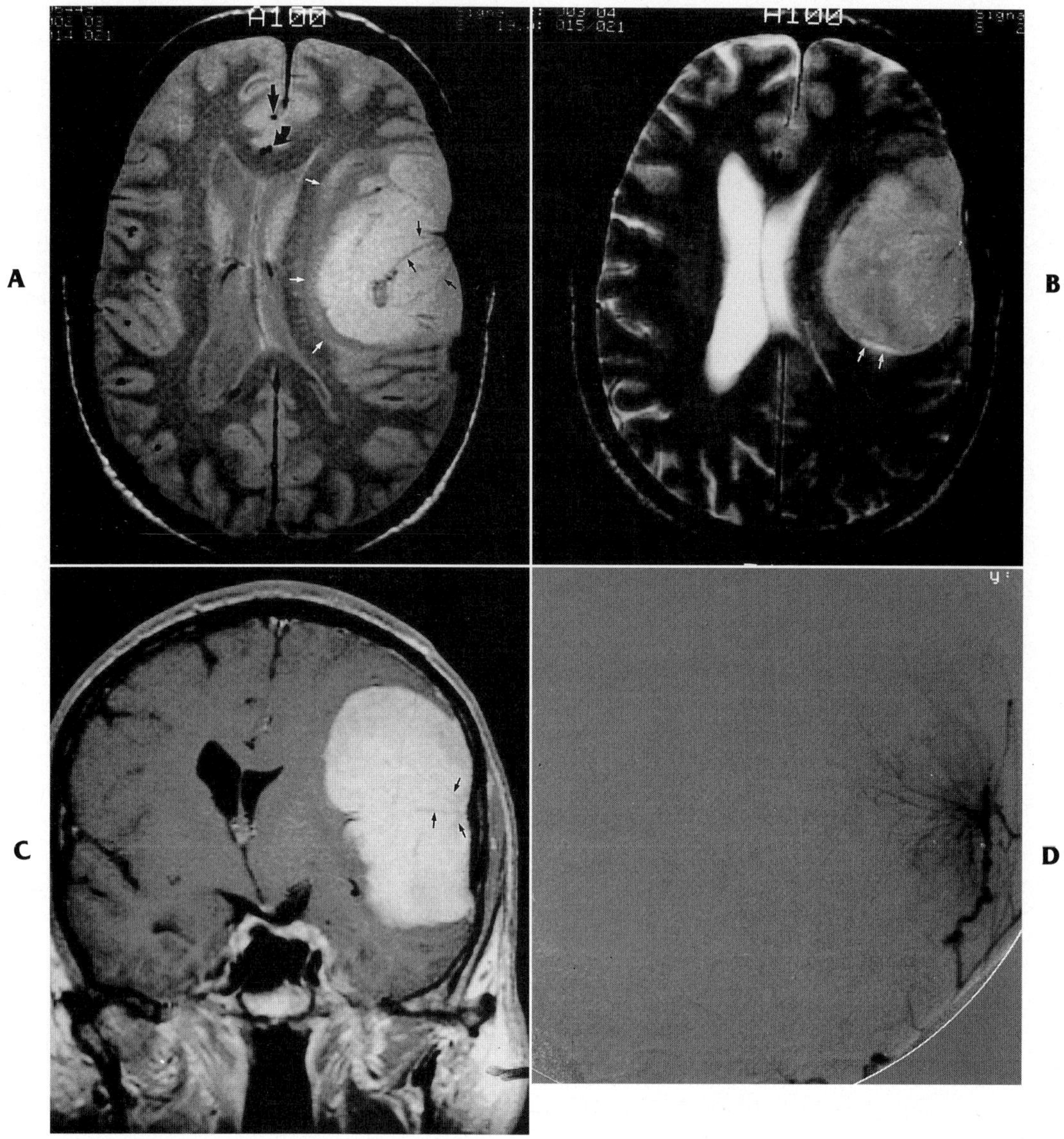

**FIGURE 1** Meningioma in a 60-year-old male, illustrating several features of an extra-axial mass. *A,* Axial fast spin-echo proton density–weighted image (effective TE18, TR2500). A sharply circumscribed mass compresses the underlying parenchyma, forming a ribbon of cortex along its medial margin *(white arrows).* Small tumor vessels radiate into the mass from the dural surface *(small straight black arrows).* Mass effect causes subfalcian herniation of the pericallosal *(curved arrow)* and callosomarginal *(large straight black arrow)* arteries. *B,* Axial fast spin-echo T2-weighted image (effective TE108, TR4000). The mass is separated from brain parenchyma by a CSF cleft *(arrows).* It is isointense to cortex, a characteristic but variable feature of meningiomas. *C,* Coronal contrast-enhanced T1-weighted image (TE12, TR800). Small dural-derived tumor vessels are outlined within the homogeneously enhancing mass. *D,* Selective left external carotid arteriogram, frontal projection. Small tumor vessels and blush radiate from a branch of the middle meningeal artery along the dural surface, well correlated with the MRI appearance.

**TABLE 3** MRI of Parenchymal Hematomas at 1.5 T

| Stage | Primary Iron State | T1 Relaxivity Effect | T2* Relaxivity Effect | T1-WI | T2-WI | Edema |
|---|---|---|---|---|---|---|
| Hyperacute (0–hours) | Oxyhemoglobin | No | No | Iso or ↓ | ↑ | No |
| Acute (hours–days) | Deoxyhemoglobin | No | Yes | Iso or ↓ | ↓ | Yes |
| Subacute | | | | | | |
| Early (days) | Intracellular methemoglobin | Yes | Yes | ↑ | ↓ | Yes |
| Late (days–months) | Extracellular methemoglobin | Yes | No | ↑ | ↑ | Decreasing |
| Chronic (days–indefinite) | Ferritin/hemosiderin | No | Yes | Iso or ↓ | ↓ | Resolved |

Adapted from Thulborn KR, Atlas SW. Intracranial hemorrhage. In: Atlas SW, ed. Magnetic Resonance Imaging of the Brain and Spine. New York: Raven Press, 1991:175.

cell carcinoma, choriocarcinoma, and lung carcinoma.

It is often difficult to distinguish between tumor and nontumor hemorrhage. Causes of nontumor hemorrhage include hypertension, infarction, vascular malformations, aneurysm rupture, amyloid angiopathy, coagulopathy, dural sinus or cortical vein thrombosis, and trauma. Characteristic features of these processes sometimes direct the differential diagnosis. Atlas has also described five features of hemorrhagic neoplasms: (1) presence of nonhemorrhage signal abnormality presumptively representing tumor (hypointense to isointense on T1-weighted images, hyperintense on T2-weighted images, contrast-enhancing); (2) markedly heterogeneous signal intensities due to combinations of various stages of blood degradation products, tumor, necrosis, cyst formation, and edema; (3) delayed hematoma evolution; (4) diminished, irregular, or absent hemosiderin ring long after hemorrhage; and (5) persistent surrounding T2-weighted hyperintense signal and mass effect, representing edema or combined tumor and edema.

## Necrosis and Cyst Formation

Tumor necrosis is important because it usually signifies an aggressive lesion. A tumor cyst is important because it can sometimes be drained to relieve mass effect. It is not always possible to distinguish between them. It is important to differentiate them from non-neoplastic cystic lesions such as arachnoid cyst, and porencephaly.

Generally, the margin of a tumor cyst is smooth and sharp, whereas the margin of a necrotic cavity is irregular. Hemorrhage may complicate either but is more common with necrosis. The presence of a fluid-blood or fluid-debris level is the only pathognomonic feature of a cystic or liquified necrotic cavity. On CT, the cavity contents are isodense to slightly hyperdense with respect to CSF; attenuation increases with protein concentration. On MRI, low protein fluid is nearly isointense to CSF on all pulse sequences. Proteinaceous fluid is hyperintense to CSF on T1-, proton density-, and T2-weighted images because protein mildly shortens T1. Hemorrhagic fluid containing methemoglobin is markedly hyperintense to CSF on T1- and proton density-weighted images and is slightly hyperintense to CSF on T2-weighted images, because methemoglobin markedly shortens T1. The contents of the cystic or necrotic cavity generally do not enhance with contrast material, although delayed imaging may demonstrate diffusion of contrast material into the cavity. The CT appearance is less specific than MRI, since solid tumor may have similar low attenuation. MRI usually identifies tumor cysts with high specificity (Part II, Figs. 3, 4, 10).

## Calcification

CT is the modality of choice for detection of calcification. While markedly high CT attenuation is characteristic, scattered microcalcification can produce mild-to-moderate high attenuation, which is less specific. Other causes of mild-to-moderate hyperdensity are hemorrhage, high cell density, and high protein content. The MRI appearances of calcification are varied and generally nonspecific. Small calcific foci ($<2$ mm) rarely alter the spin-echo MRI signal. Large dense calcifications usually attenuate the T1- and T2-weighted MRI signal, attributed to a paucity of mobile protons. Uncommonly calcification is hyperintense on T1-weighted images, hypothesized to result from associated paramagnetic cations such as Fe, Mn, Mg, Zn, and Cu, resulting in T1 relaxation enhancement. Gradient-echo imaging detects calcification with much higher sensitivity. Calcifications cause gradient-echo signal attenuation due to magnetic susceptibility effects. The magnetic susceptibility effects have been attributed to both the diamagnetic calcium salts and coexisting paramagnetic cations. Such a magnetic susceptibility effect must be differentiated from hemorrhage.

Because of its frequency, the most common primary intra-axial brain tumor to calcify is astrocytoma. Oligodendroglioma and "mixed" tumors have the highest frequency of calcification (Part II, Fig. 9). Many other primary intra-axial tumors may calcify, including neuroblastoma/PNET tumors, ganglioglioma, dermoid tumor, teratoma, lipoma, pineal cell tumors, germinoma, ependymoma, choroid plexus tumors, and medulloblastoma (uncommonly). Calcification is rare in anaplastic astrocytoma, glioblastoma multiforme (GBM), and lymphoma. Metastases that may calcify include mucinous adenocarcinomas of the gastrointestinal tract and osteosarcoma. Otherwise, calcification is uncommon in metastases before treatment. After chemotherapy or radiation, metastases may calcify.

## Fat

Fat is unusual within intra-axial brain tumors. It narrows the differential diagnosis to lipoma, dermoid, and teratoma. On CT, it is characterized by very low CT attenuation ($-50$ to $-100$ Hounsfield units). On MRI, it is characterized by short T1 and moderate T2 relaxation times, resulting in marked T1-weighted hyperintensity, and mild T2-weighted hyperintensity. The different resonant frequencies of fat and water result in slight spatial misregistration at fat-water interfaces along the frequency-encoding direction. This chemical shift artifact is pathognomonic of fat. A chemical shift–based fat-suppression pulse sequence can also be used to specifically identify fat (Part III, Fig. 5).

## Vascularity

Enlarged normal arteries feeding a tumor or macroscopic abnormal tumor vessels are frequently identified as round or serpiginous flow voids on spin-echo MR images. They may also be examined using flow-sensitive gradient-echo pulse sequences. Their observation is helpful in differential diagnosis and surgical planning. Tumors that frequently exhibit macroscopic vascularity include GBM, hemangioblastoma, and meningioma (see Fig. 1; Part II, Fig. 5).

A giant aneurysm may mimic a tumor. Standard spin-echo T1- and T2-weighted signal intensity may be increased due to slow flow or thrombus. With slow flow, a giant aneurysm may exhibit gadolinium enhancement. Flow-induced artifact through the mass along the phase-encoding direction, if present, establishes its vascular nature. Flow-sensitive gradient-echo images (including magnetic resonance angiography) can also establish vascular etiology. A completely thrombosed giant aneurysm may still be difficult to differentiate from tumor. Appropriate location and signal characteristics suggesting the presence of blood degradation products should raise suspicion of this diagnosis.

## Blood-Brain Barrier Integrity

Intra-axial tumor enhancement primarily reflects diffusion of contrast material from the vascular compartment, through the capillary blood-brain barrier, into the parenchymal interstitial space. The degree of enhancement is determined by three factors: vascular supply, capillary blood-brain barrier permeability, and volume of the extracellular space. Among these, the most important factor in brain tumors generally is the integrity of the blood-brain barrier. In intra-axial tumors, contrast enhancement identifies disruption of the normal blood-brain barrier or presence of abnormal capillaries, which lack tight junctions. Extra-axial structures do not have capillary tight junctions. Therefore extra-axial tumors readily accumulate contrast material as long as there is sufficient blood supply and volume of extracellular space. Although tumor enhancement and vascularity are related properties, they are not the same. MRI is more sensitive than CT for the detection of pathologic contrast enhancement.

## Edema

Tumors frequently incite vasogenic edema in surrounding brain. Vasogenic edema results from increased blood-brain permeability to macromolecules, resulting in transudation of water from the vascular space into the interstitial space. As the extracellular space is more abundant in white matter than in gray matter, vasogenic edema predominantly involves the white matter. Vasogenic edema appears as finger-like projections of low attenuation on CT, hypointensity on T1- and hyperintensity on T2-weighted images. T2-weighted images are most sensitive to edema (Part II, Figs. 4, 5, 6, 8, 9, 11; Part III, Fig. 1).

Associated mass effect on adjacent parenchyma and ventricles should be observed, especially herniations of brain parenchyma. These include herniations under the fixed edge of the falx (subfalcian herniation, Fig. 1; Part II, Fig. 3), under the fixed edge of the tentorium (uncal or hippocampal herniation), through the foramen magnum (tonsillar herniation), or (uncommonly) upward cerebellar herniation through the tentorial notch.

## CT Attenuation, Revisited

In summary, most tumors are hypodense or isodense to brain parenchyma. Hyperdensity narrows the differential diagnosis. Marked hyperdensity occurs with calcification. Mild-to-moderate hyperdensity occurs with hemorrhage, diffuse microcalcifications, high cell density, and high protein content. Very low attenuation is characteristic of fatty lesions.

## MR Signal Intensity, Revisited

The majority of central nervous system (CNS) pathology causes prolongation of T1 and T2 relaxation times, resulting in hypointensity on T1- and hyperintensity on T2-weighted images. Hyperintensity on T1- or iso-to-hypo-intensity on T2-weighted images narrows the differential diagnosis. The causes of high T1-weighted signal are fat, blood (methemoglobin), high protein concentration, melanin, endogenous paramagnetic cations (associated with calcification, necrosis, metabolic disorders), paramagnetic MRI contrast material (gadolinium), iophendylate (Pantopaque), and vascular flow-related enhancement. The causes of relatively low T2-weighted signal are high cell density with scant cytoplasm, blood, calcification, endogenous paramagnetic cations, dense fibrous tissue, and vascular flow voids. The mechanisms underlying T1-weighted hyperintensity and T2-weighted hypointensity are summarized in Table 4. Two other MRI effects confer

**TABLE 4** Mechanisms Underlying T1-weighted Hyperintensity and T2-weighted Hypointensity

- Causes of High T1-Weighted Signal Intensity:
  - T1 relaxation enhancement:
    - Diamagnetic:
      - Fat (lipoma, dermoid, teratoma)
      - High protein concentration
      - Pantopaque
    - Paramagnetic:
      - Blood (methemoglobin)
      - Paramagnetic cations associated with calcification, necrosis, metabolic disease
      - Melanin
      - Paramagnetic contrast agents (e.g., Gd-DTPA)
      - Free radicals (hypothesized)
  - Flow-related enhancement
- Causes of Low T2-Weighted Signal Intensity:
  - T2 relaxation enhancement:
    - Diamagnetic
      - Very high nonparamagnetic protein content
    - Paramagnetic (magnetic susceptibility effect)
      - Iron: intracellular deoxy- and met-hemoglobin; ferritin, hemosiderin
      - Paramagnetic cations associated with calcification, necrosis, metabolic disease
      - High concentration of paramagnetic contrast agents (e.g., Gd-DTPA)
      - Free radicals (hypothesized)
  - Low "mobile proton density"
    - Air, cortical bone, dense calcification, fibrous tissue, dessicated tissues
  - Flow or motion-related signal void
  - Unknown or multifactorial
    - Some pathologies with high cell density, protein content, or paramagnetic cation content (e.g., meningioma, lymphoma, sarcoid, mucinous adenocarcinoma metastases)

specificity on otherwise potentially ambiguous lesions: (1) chemical shift artifact is pathognomonic of fat; and (2) flow-induced phase-encoding artifact is pathognomonic of a vessel – for example, it may definitively distinguish between a giant aneurysm and a tumor. Its absence does not exclude a vascular lesion (e.g., thrombosed aneurysm).

In Parts II and III, these principles are used to characterize tumors of the cerebral hemispheres, posterior fossa, and pineal region.

## Suggested Reading

Atlas SW. Intraaxial brain tumors. In: Atlas SW, ed. Magnetic Resonance Imaging of the Brain and Spine. New York: Raven Press, 1991:223.

Atlas SW, Grossman RI, Gomori JM, et al. Hemorrhagic intracranial malignant neoplasms: Spin-echo MR imaging. Radiology 1987; 164:71–77.

Atlas SW, Grossman RI, Hackney DB, et al. Calcified intracranial lesions: Detection with gradient-echo-acquisition rapid MR imaging. Am J Neuroradiol 1988; 9:253–259.

Goldberg HI. Extraaxial brain tumors. In: Atlas SW, ed. Magnetic Resonance Imaging of the Brain and Spine. New York: Raven Press, 1991:327.

Holland BA, Kucharcyzk W, Brant-Zawadzki M, et al. MR imaging of calcified intracranial lesions. Radiology 1985; 157:353–356.

Kjos BO, Brant-Zawadzki M, Kucharczyk W, et al. Cystic intracranial lesions: Magnetic resonance imaging. Radiology 1985; 155: 363–369.

Latchaw RE, Johnson DW, Kanal E. Primary intracranial tumors: Neuroepithelial tumors, sarcomas, and lymphomas. In: Latchaw RE, ed. MR and CT Imaging of the Head, Neck, and Spine. 2nd ed. Vol 1. St Louis: Mosby–Year Book, 1991:449.

Russell DS, Rubinstein LJ. Pathology of Tumors of the Nervous System. 5th ed. Baltimore: Williams & Wilkins, 1989.

Sze G, Krol G, Olsen WL, et al. Hemorrhagic neoplasms: MR mimics of occult vascular malformations. Am J Neuroradiol 1987; 149:1223–1230.

Thulborn KR, Atlas SW. Intracranial hemorrhage. In: Atlas SW, ed. Magnetic Resonance Imaging of the Brain and Spine. New York: Raven Press, 1991:175.

# PART II: TUMORS OF CEREBRAL HEMISPHERES

In this chapter part a classification scheme for intra-axial brain tumors is presented, and the imaging principles that were reviewed in Part I are used to characterize tumors of the cerebral hemispheres.

## Classification of Brain Tumors

A classification system based on location and cell type of origin facilitates radiologic differential diagnosis. We follow a classification system based on the International Classification of Central Nervous System Tumors (World Health Organization, 1979), similar to Latchaw and co-workers (Table 1). For brevity, we exclude some rare tumors. Intraventricular tumors are discussed in another chapter and are not discussed as a separate category here.

Primary intra-axial brain tumors have neuroepithelial, reticuloendothelial, vascular, and maldevelopmental origins. By far, the largest group is neuroepithelial. Neuroepithelial tumors arise from glial, primitive neuroectodermal, or central ganglion cells. Of these, the glial tumors predominate. Corresponding to each glial cell type, there are four basic glial tumors: astrocytoma, oligodendroglioma, ependymoma, and choroid plexus papilloma/carcinoma. The classification of primitive neuroectodermal tumors is controversial. They constitute tumors of primitive or undifferentiated neuroepithelial cells, including medulloblastoma, primary cerebral neuroblastoma, and pineoblastoma, among other rarer tumors. The tumors of central ganglion cell origin are gangliocytoma (ganglioneuroma) and ganglioglioma. The term *glioma* is often used loosely. Some authors use it to connote the group of tumors of glial cell origin. Others use it to refer to the entire group of neuroepithelial tumors.

## Astrocytomas

### Grading Systems

Several grading systems for astrocytoma are in use. The traditional four-tiered system (Kernohan and Sayre) consists of astrocytoma grades I to IV. A more recent three-tiered system (e.g., Russell and Rubinstein, Rorke) consists of astrocytoma, anaplastic astrocytoma, and glioblastoma multiforme (GBM). Roughly, astrocytoma corresponds to Kernohan and Sayre grade I, anaplastic astrocytoma to grade II, and GBM to grades III and IV. The three-tiered system is gaining in popularity because subdivision of GBM into two grades is of questionable clinical utility. In the three-tiered classification, astrocytoma is also called benign, low-grade, or well-differentiated astrocytoma. Anaplastic astrocytoma is also called malignant astrocytoma. In practice, tumor grading is sometimes problematic because of tumor heterogeneity and temporal evolution. Tumor heterogeneity can lead to sampling errors in biopsy specimens and a low-grade lesion may evolve to high grade over time (dedifferentiation).

### Astrocytoma, Anaplastic Astrocytoma, and GBM

Astrocytomas are the most common primary brain tumors in adults. GBM is the single most common primary brain tumor in adults. The relative frequencies of the astrocytoma subtypes are low-grade astrocytoma (25 percent), anaplastic astrocytoma (25 percent), and GBM (50 percent). Low-grade astrocytoma is most common in children and younger adults, 20 to 40 years old. Anaplastic astrocytoma and GBM are most

**TABLE 1** Classification of Intra-axial Brain Tumors

Tumors of Cerebral Hemispheres:
- Neuroepithelial tumors
  - Astrocytoma
  - Oligodendroglioma
  - Ependymoma
- PNET (primary CNS neuroblastoma)
- Ganglioglioma, gangliocytoma
- Lymphoma
- Metastases

Tumors of Cerebellum:
- Neuroepithelial tumors
  - Astrocytoma
  - Ependymoma
  - Medulloblastoma (PNET)
- Hemangioblastoma
- Lymphoma
- Metastases

Tumors of Brain Stem:
- Astrocytoma
- Metastases

Tumors of Pineal Region:
- Pineal cell tumors
  - Pineocytoma
  - Pineoblastoma (PNET)
- Germ cell tumors
  - Germinoma
  - Teratoma
  - Choriocarcinoma
  - Embryonal cell carcinoma
  - Yolk sac tumor
- Parapineal tumors
  - Glioma
  - Meningioma

Intraventricular Tumors:
- Ependymoma
- Subependymoma
- Choroid plexus papilloma/carcinoma
- Astrocytoma
- Meningioma
- Colloid cyst of the third ventricle

common in older adults over 40 years of age (peak, 45 to 55 years). Males are affected more than females by a 2:1 ratio. In adults astrocytomas are most commonly located in the white matter of the cerebral hemispheres, especially the frontal and temporal lobes. They are relatively uncommon in the occipital lobes. Cortical involvement also occurs, best observed on MRI. In children and young adults, the most common locations are the cerebellum, brain stem, diencephalon, and anterior optic pathways.

Plain CT attenuation depends on cell density. Most astrocytomas are hypodense or exhibit mixed regions of hypo- and iso-density. More compact lesions may be isodense or hyperdense. Pathologically the margins of astrocytomas are poorly defined, reflecting their infiltrative nature. Low-grade lesions tend to have poorly defined margins because of their mild hypodensity, fading to isodensity with adjacent brain. Anaplastic astrocytoma and GBM tend to be better defined. On unenhanced MRI, astrocytomas exhibit nonspecific T1-weighted hypointensity and T2-weighted hyperintensity. Both low- and high-grade lesions exhibit better defined margins because of greater intrinsic soft-tissue contrast.

Cyst formation, necrosis, hemorrhage, and macroscopic tumor vessels are common in anaplastic astrocytoma and GBM; they are uncommon in low-grade lesions. As a result, low-grade lesions tend to be homogeneous, whereas high-grade lesions are often heterogeneous. Calcification occurs in about 20 percent of low-grade lesions; it is correlated with a slow rate of growth. Calcification is rare in anaplastic astrocytoma and GBM. It can be seen in high-grade lesions that have transformed over time from a low-grade tumor. Although oligodendroglioma has a higher frequency of calcification, astrocytoma is the most common calcified intra-axial tumor because of its far greater prevalence. Edema extent is variable, but tends to increase with tumor grade. Infiltrating tumor cells are frequently found pathologically at sites remote from the tumor nidus. It is not possible to define exact boundaries between tumor, edema, and normal brain by any imaging modality. Tumor cells have been found at autopsy in brain that appears normal on CT and MRI before and after contrast enhancement.

The presence and degree of contrast enhancement are only loosely correlated with tumor grade. In the cerebral hemispheres, the degree of enhancement tends to correlate with tumor grade but exceptions occur. Lack of enhancement does not exclude malignancy. Benign hemispheric astrocytomas tend to exhibit no enhancement or mild patchy enhancement. Malignant astrocytomas and GBM usually exhibit moderate or marked enhancement. The enhancement pattern is often a thick irregular ring surrounding a central nonenhancing region. The central region may represent nonenhancing solid tumor or necrosis. More homogeneous nodular enhancement also occurs. Contrast enhancement reflects the presence of an abnormal blood-brain barrier. It does not correlate well with angiographic hypervascularity. Enhancing regions identify tumor—a useful marker for MRI-guided stereotactic biopsy. However, nonenhancing regions may still harbor tumor cells.

Astrocytomas tend to spread along white matter tracts. Spread across the corpus callosum, anterior commissure, or posterior commissure into the contralateral hemisphere is common, forming the classic "butterfly glioma" appearance. GBM and anaplastic astrocytoma commonly spread to the subependymal and cortical surfaces, which may result in metastasis via the CSF pathways. GBM and anaplastic astrocytoma sometimes invade the dura. Transgression of the dura into the calvarium is rare in the absence of a surgical defect. Subependymal, subarachnoid, and dural spread are all rare in low-grade astrocytoma. Metastasis outside the CNS is rare (Figs. 1 to 6).

## *Differential Diagnosis and Imaging Pitfalls*

Differential diagnosis includes other primary gliomas, metastasis, lymphoma, abscess, cerebritis, infarction, hematoma, hemorrhagic vascular malformations, and radiation necrosis. Imaging pitfalls include the following. Small isodense astrocytomas can be missed on unenhanced CT. Nonenhancing astrocytoma with low attenuation values approximating CSF may mimic infarct, porencephaly, or arachnoid cyst. Contrast enhancement may be lessened by previous corticosteroid treatment. It may be difficult to distinguish between macrocystic (drainable) and microcystic (not drainable) components.

*Text continued on p. 447.*

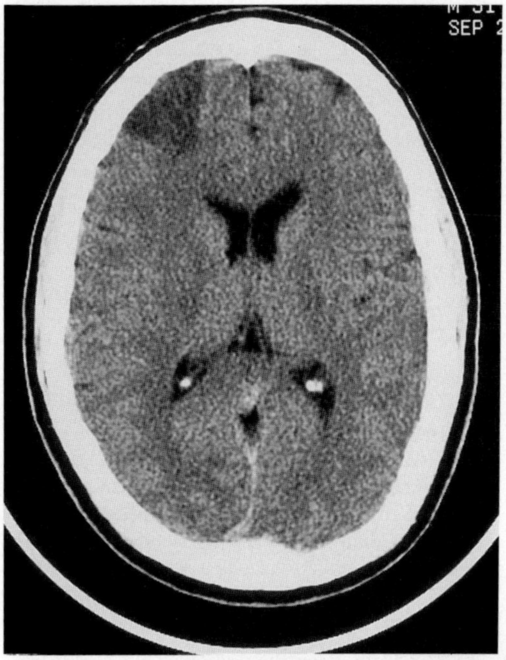

**FIGURE 1** Low-grade astrocytoma in a 31-year-old male. Contrast-enhanced CT image. Wedge-shaped peripheral low-attenuation mass in the right frontal lobe involving cortex and subcortical white matter. It is fairly well circumscribed, homogeneous, and nonenhancing. There is no evidence of edema, hemorrhage, calcification, cyst formation, or necrosis. There is minimal mass effect on the frontal horn of the right lateral ventricle. The appearance mimics infarction.

---

A

B

C

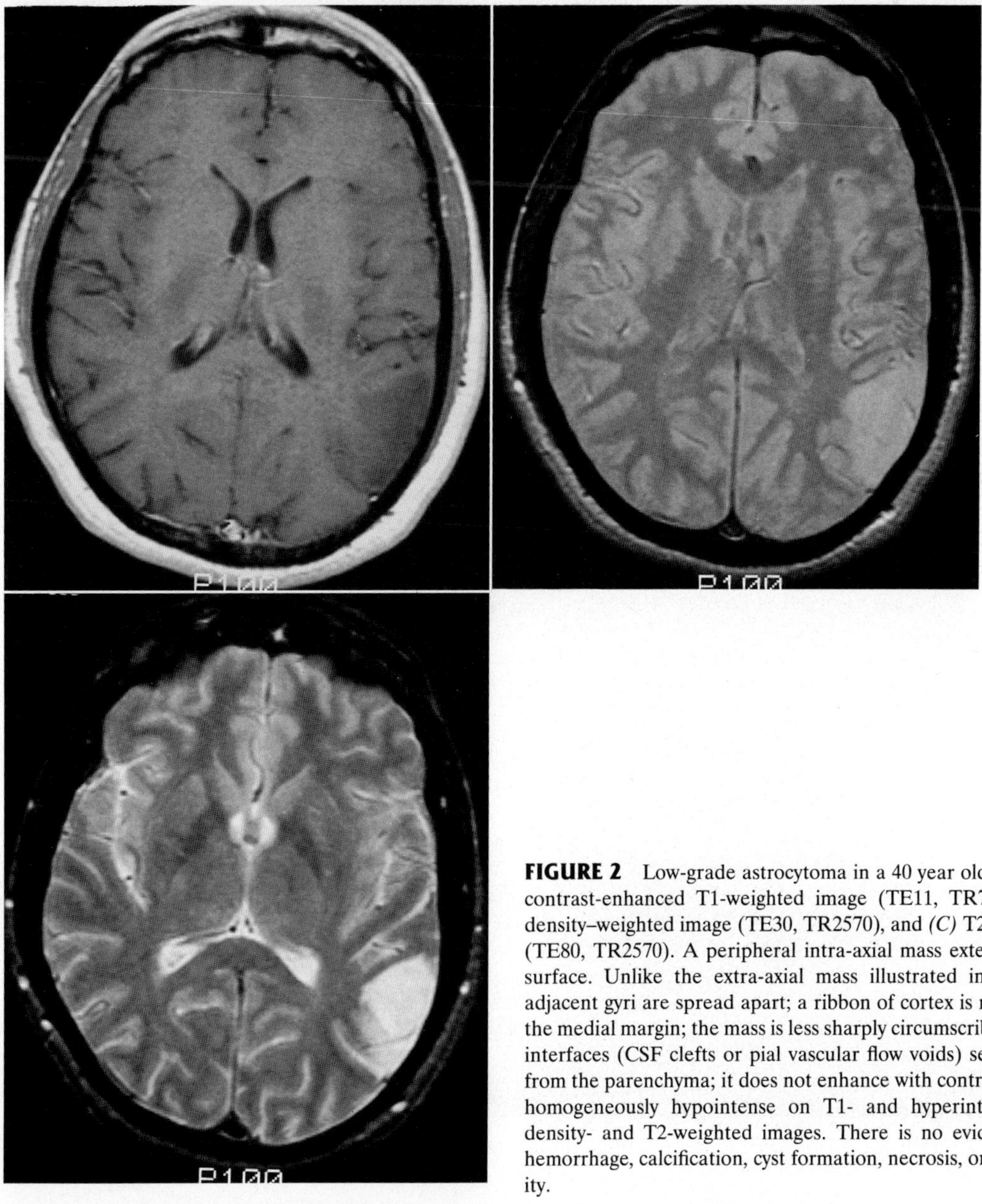

**FIGURE 2** Low-grade astrocytoma in a 40 year old male. Axial *(A)* contrast-enhanced T1-weighted image (TE11, TR700), *(B)* proton density–weighted image (TE30, TR2570), and *(C)* T2-weighted image (TE80, TR2570). A peripheral intra-axial mass extends to the brain surface. Unlike the extra-axial mass illustrated in Part I, Fig. 1, adjacent gyri are spread apart; a ribbon of cortex is not draped along the medial margin; the mass is less sharply circumscribed; no anatomic interfaces (CSF clefts or pial vascular flow voids) separate the mass from the parenchyma; it does not enhance with contrast material. It is homogeneously hypointense on T1- and hyperintense on proton density- and T2-weighted images. There is no evidence of edema, hemorrhage, calcification, cyst formation, necrosis, or tumor vascularity.

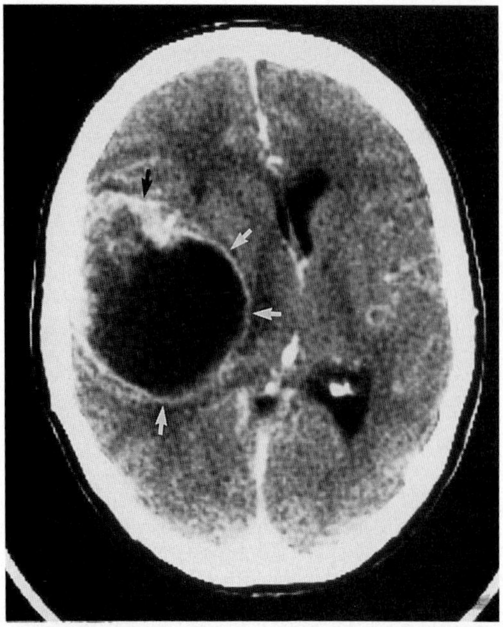

**FIGURE 3** Glioblastoma multiforme with necrosis. Axial contrast-enhanced CT image. Heterogeneous mass causing marked midline shift, ventricular effacement, and subfalcian herniation. Anterolateral aspect of tumor enhances heterogeneously, with ill-defined margin suggesting brain infiltration *(black arrow)*. Thin enhancing ring of tumor *(white arrows)* encompasses a large central region of low attenuation, consistent with necrosis.

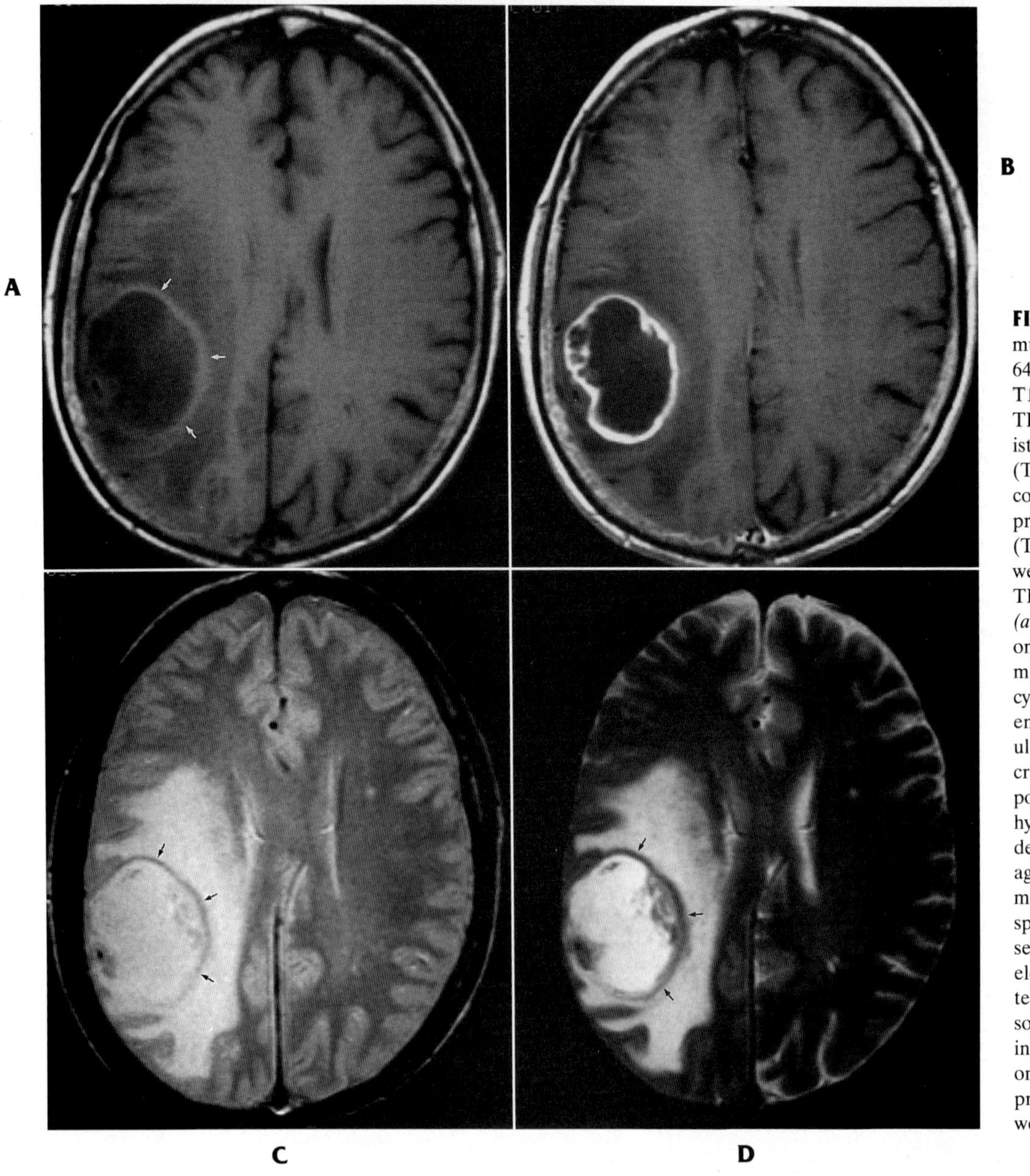

**FIGURE 4** Glioblastoma multiforme with necrosis in a 64-year-old female. Axial *(A)* T1-weighted image (TE11, TR700) before contrast administration, *(B)* T1-weighted (TE11, TR700) image after contrast administration, *(C)* proton density–weighted image (TE30, TR2500), *(D)* T2-weighted image (TE80, TR2500). The tumor margin *(arrows)* is isointense to cortex on each pulse sequence, which may reflect relatively compact cytoarchitecture. The margin enhances intensely in an irregular ring pattern. Central necrosis is nonenhancing, hypointense on T1-, and hyperintense on proton density– and T2-weighted images. The necrotic region is mildly hyperintense with respect to CSF on each pulse sequence, probably reflecting elevated nonparamagnetic protein content. Extensive vasogenic edema in the surrounding white matter is hypointense on T1- and hyperintense on proton density- and T2-weighted images.

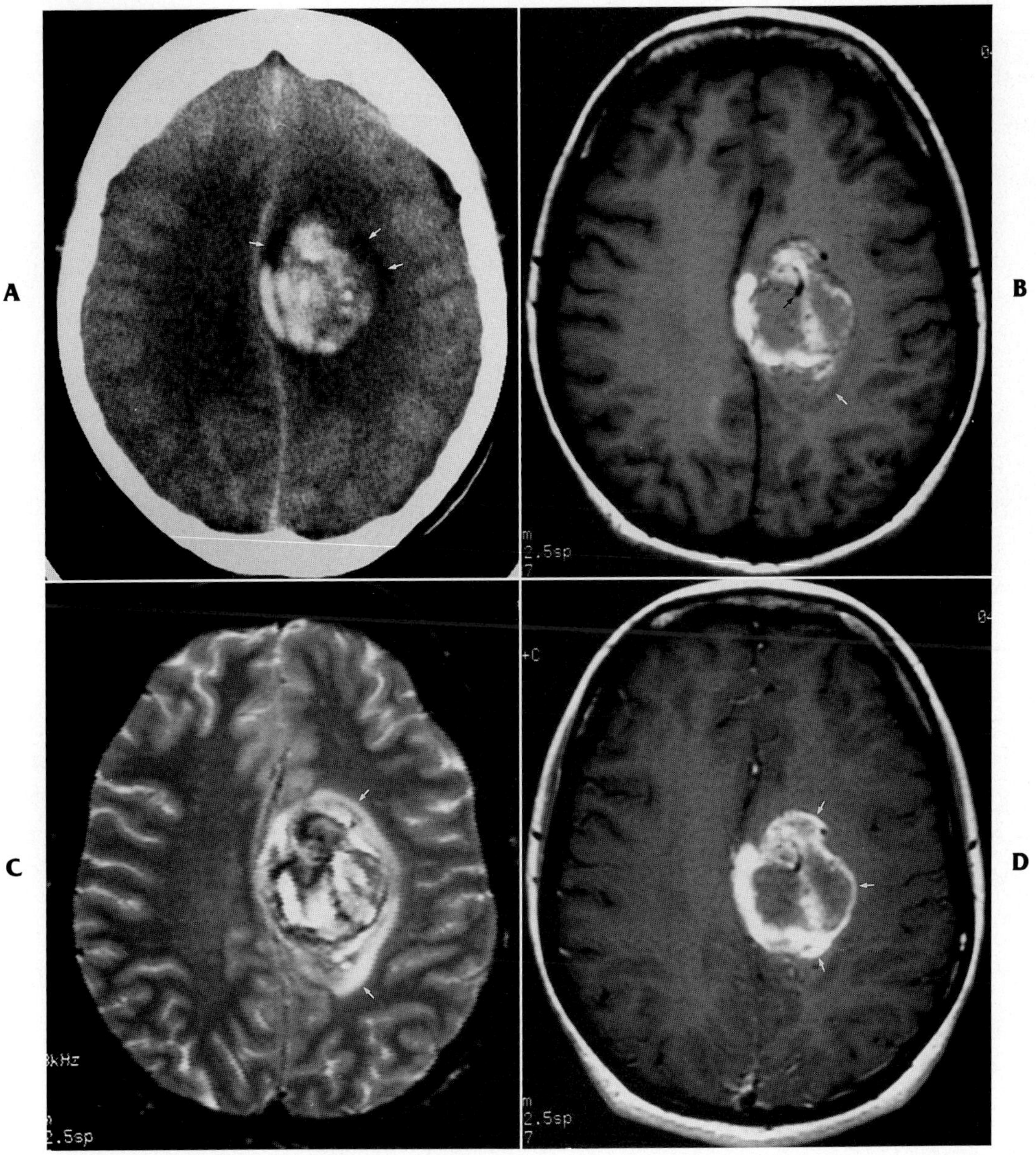


**FIGURE 5** Glioblastoma multiforme with hemorrhage. *A,* Axial CT image, without contrast enhancement, demonstrates a heterogeneous hemorrhagic left pericallosal mass with a thin rim of low-attenuation edema or nonenhancing tumor *(white arrows)*. *B,* Axial unenhanced T1-weighted (TR700, TE11) and *(C)* T2-weighted (TR3000, TE80) images, performed 10 days after CT, demonstrate markedly heterogeneous signal intensities, representing a combination of blood degradation products in various stages of evolution, macroscopic tumor vessel flow voids *(black arrow),* and tumor tissue. A surrounding zone of T1-weighted slight hypointensity and T2-weighted marked hyperintensity represents edema or infiltrating tumor *(white arrows)*. *D,* Axial contrast-enhanced T1-weighted image (TR700, TE11) demonstrates a thin perimeter of enhancement *(white arrows),* probably representing tumor tissue.

*Continued.*

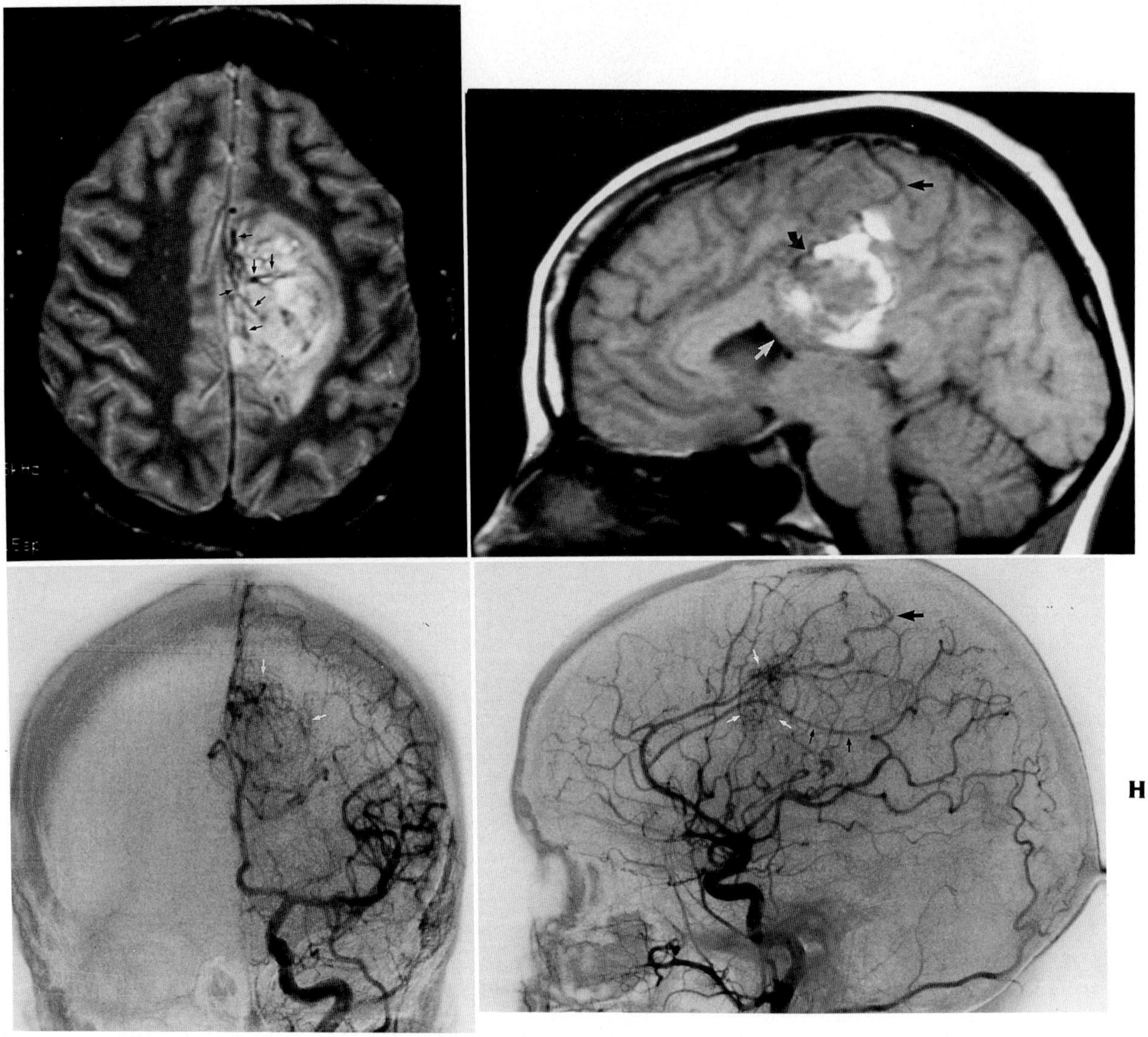


**FIGURE 5 cont'd** *E,* Axial proton density-weighted image (TR3000, TE30) demonstrates linear and round macroscopic tumor vessel flow voids arising from the left anterior cerebral artery *(black arrows). F,* Sagittal T1-weighted image (TR600, TE11), without contrast material, demonstrates invasion and marked depression of the body of the corpus callosum *(white arrow).* Serpiginous flow voids along the anterosuperior aspect of the mass *(curved black arrow)* and extending from the mass to the superior sagittal sinus *(straight black arrow)* represent an arterial feeding vessel and draining vein, respectively. Left common carotid arteriogram, frontal *(G)* and lateral *(H)* projections, confirms a tuft of tumor vessels arising from the callosomarginal and possibly pericallosal arteries *(white arrows),* marked depression of the pericallosal artery *(small black arrows),* and the early draining vein *(large black arrow).* While the hemorrhagic mass is relatively nonspecific on CT, the MRI is highly specific for an underlying vascular mass, such as a tumor or vascular malformation. Both MRI and angiography suggest tumor vascularity rather than an arteriovenous malformation. GBM was confirmed by pathologic studies.

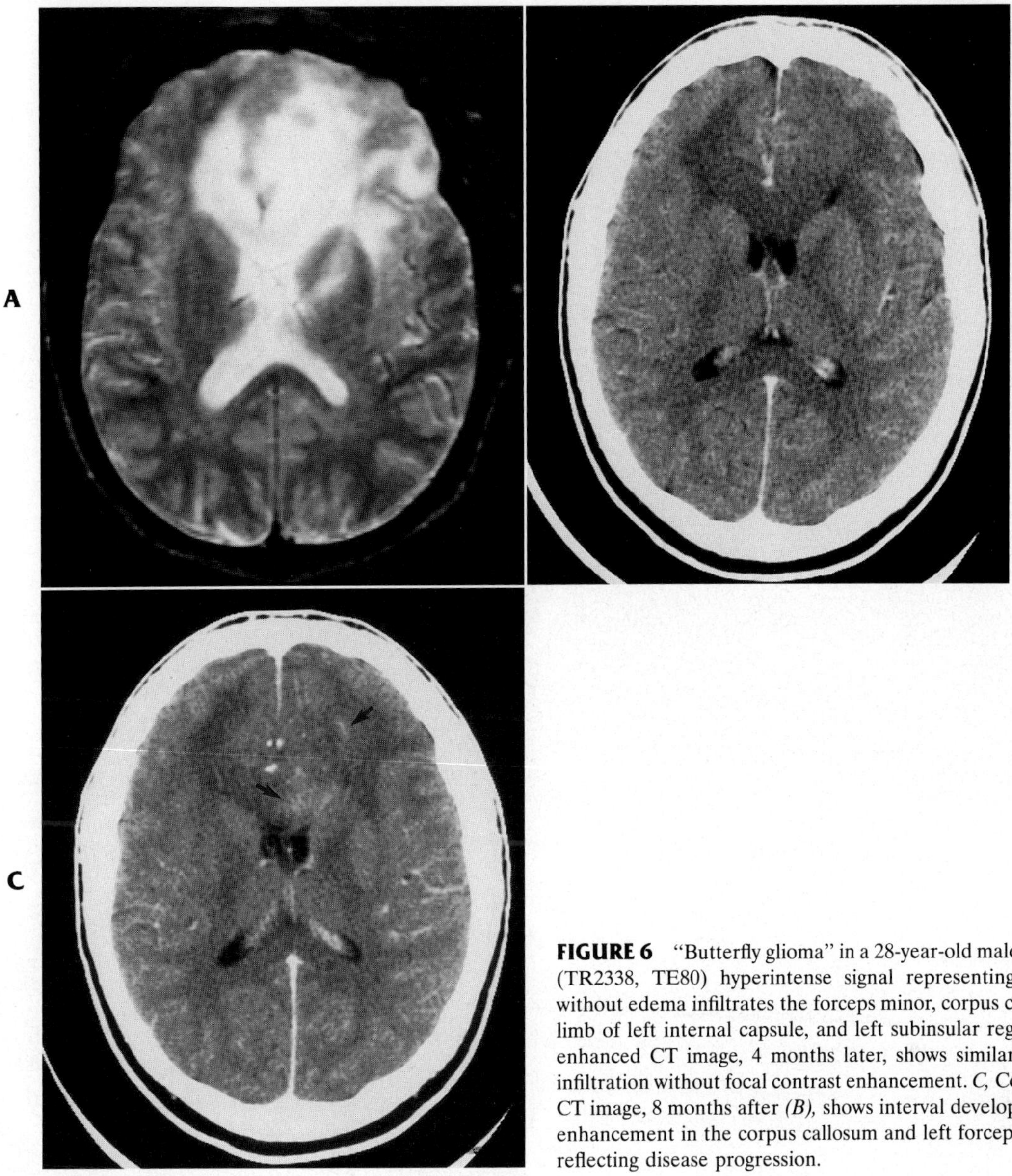


**FIGURE 6** "Butterfly glioma" in a 28-year-old male. *A,* T2-weighted (TR2338, TE80) hyperintense signal representing tumor with or without edema infiltrates the forceps minor, corpus callosum, anterior limb of left internal capsule, and left subinsular region. *B,* Contrast-enhanced CT image, 4 months later, shows similar low-attenuation infiltration without focal contrast enhancement. *C,* Contrast-enhanced CT image, 8 months after *(B),* shows interval development of contrast enhancement in the corpus callosum and left forceps minor *(arrows),* reflecting disease progression.

## *Astrocytoma Variants*

There are four astrocytoma variants which have distinct features: multicentric glioma, gliomatosis cerebri, pilocytic astrocytoma, and giant cell astrocytoma.

### Multicentric Glioma

Synchronous and metachronous multicentric gliomas are uncommon. The reported incidence varies, in the range of 2.5 to 7.5 percent based on autopsy series. The difference between multicentricity and multifocality is subtle, and can be definitively established only at autopsy. *Multicentricity* requires at least two sites of tumor without gross or microscopic connection via parenchymal or CSF pathways. *Multifocality* refers to at least two sites of tumor connected by parenchymal or CSF pathways. The pathologic basis for true multicentric glioma is still uncertain. The principal differential diagnosis is non-CNS metastatic tumor, primary CNS lymphoma, and multiple abscesses. In the absence of a known primary tumor, biopsy is important because the treatments differ. For example, a higher radiation dose is used to treat glioma than metastatic tumor.

### Gliomatosis Cerebri

Gliomatosis cerebri is rare. Peak incidence is in the second through fourth decades. It is a neoplastic process characterized by diffuse infiltration of the brain by undifferentiated and anaplastic glial cells in all stages of development, with relative preservation of the underlying neural architecture. The pathologic basis of gliomatosis cerebri remains uncertain, but Russell and Rubinstein consider it to represent the extreme end in the spectrum of infiltrating astrocytoma. The cerebral hemispheres are involved most often, but the brain stem, cerebellum, and spinal cord may also be affected. It affects white matter more than gray matter. Detection by CT may be difficult. CT abnormalities include diffuse symmetrical or asymmetrical hypodense to isodense regions with variable mass effect but without a discrete mass. Mass effect is typically manifest by

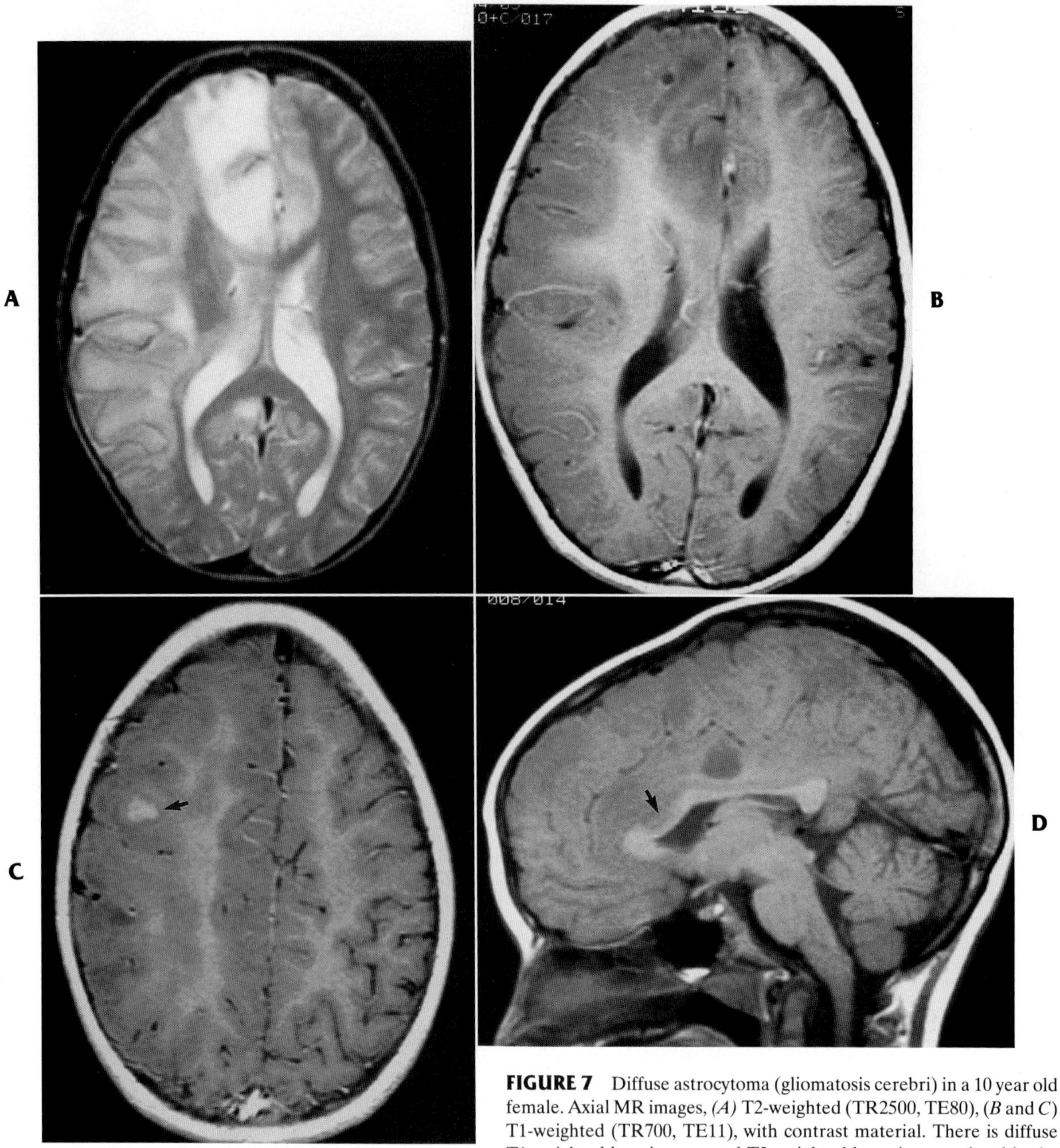


**FIGURE 7** Diffuse astrocytoma (gliomatosis cerebri) in a 10 year old female. Axial MR images, *(A)* T2-weighted (TR2500, TE80), (*B* and *C*) T1-weighted (TR700, TE11), with contrast material. There is diffuse T1-weighted hypointense and T2-weighted hyperintense signal in the right hemispheric cortex and subcortical white matter, relatively sparing the occipital lobe. There is transcallosal spread into the left forceps minor. There is marked diffuse thickening of the right hemispheric cortical mantle, with effacement of cortical sulci, reflecting tumor infiltration and generalized mass effect. Despite the widespread signal abnormalities, only one focus of contrast enhancement is present in the right frontal lobe *(arrow)*. *D,* Sagittal T1-weighted image (TR600, TE11) without contrast enhancement clearly demonstrates callosal invasion *(arrow)*. Gyral thickening and sulcal effacement are also observed.

sulcal, cisternal, or ventricular effacement and may be subtle. Complete lack of enhancement is typical, though multifocal areas of enhancement may occur. MRI has improved the diagnostic sensitivity for this disorder. It reveals large confluent regions of T2-weighted hyperintense signal in the brain. Global or regional enlargement of the brain parenchyma and associated mass effect are better defined. The process may mimic demyelinating and dysmyelinating disorders. Biopsy is essential for diagnosis (Fig. 7).

### Juvenile Pilocytic Astrocytoma

Pilocytic astrocytoma represents a histologic subtype with distinct pathologic, clinical, and imaging characteristics. Peak incidence is in the first two decades. They are most often located near the third and fourth ventricles. In order of decreasing frequency, locations include cerebellar vermis, cerebellar hemispheres, optic chiasm/nerve (optic glioma), hypothalamus, and cerebral hemispheres. Pilocytic astrocytomas are strongly associated with neurofibromatosis I, mainly optic and hypothalamic gliomas. Their biological behavior is almost always low grade. They are sharply circumscribed. They tend to be round or oval except in the optic chiasm/nerves, where they are lobulated or fusiform as they grow along the optic pathways. Macroscopic cyst formation with a vascular mural nodule is common in the cerebellum and cerebral hemispheres. Calcification is uncommon. Edema is usually absent or mild. Despite their low grade, pilocytic astrocytomas almost always enhance intensely because of a characteristic permeable blood-brain barrier. Conversely, brain stem astrocytomas are frequently biologically high grade but enhance little or none at all. These are important exceptions to the oversimplified notion that degree of enhancement correlates with biological grade. It emphasizes that blood-brain barrier permeability is only one of many physiological parameters that characterize the biological behavior of a tumor. Unlike typical fibrillary astrocytomas, pilocytic astrocytomas of the cerebellum and cerebral hemispheres are usually well defined and curable by surgical resection. Malignant degeneration almost never occurs.

### Giant Cell Astrocytoma

Giant cell astrocytoma almost only occurs in association with tuberous sclerosis, where its incidence is 10 to 15 percent. It arises from malignant transformation of a subependymal hamartoma, most often near the foramen of Monro. It is frequently densely calcified. Because of its location at the interventricular foramen, it frequently causes hydrocephalus. Although subependymal giant cell astrocytomas typically enhance, about 50 percent of benign subependymal nodules of tuberous sclerosis also enhance on MRI. Therefore enhancement does not necessarily imply malignant transformation.

## Oligodendroglioma

Oligodendroglioma is uncommon, accounting for about 5 percent of primary brain tumors. About 50 percent actually consist of mixed astrocytic and oligodendrocytic cell types, in variable ratios. Oligodendroglioma usually grows slowly. Occasionally, oligodendroglioma and mixed gliomas transform to a more aggressive lesion that behaves like GBM.

Oligodendroglioma is far more common in adults than children. Peak incidence is in the fourth and fifth decades. Eighty-five percent are supratentorial. The majority are located in the frontal lobes, near the brain surface. Rarely, they may be intraventricular. They may have well-defined or ill-defined margins. Calcification occurs in at least 70 percent, the highest frequency among intra-axial brain tumors. As mentioned previously, astrocytoma remains the most frequent calcified intra-axial tumor because of its greater prevalence. However, oligodendroglioma has a greater tendency for bulky dense calcification. Therefore a densely calcified peripheral

A 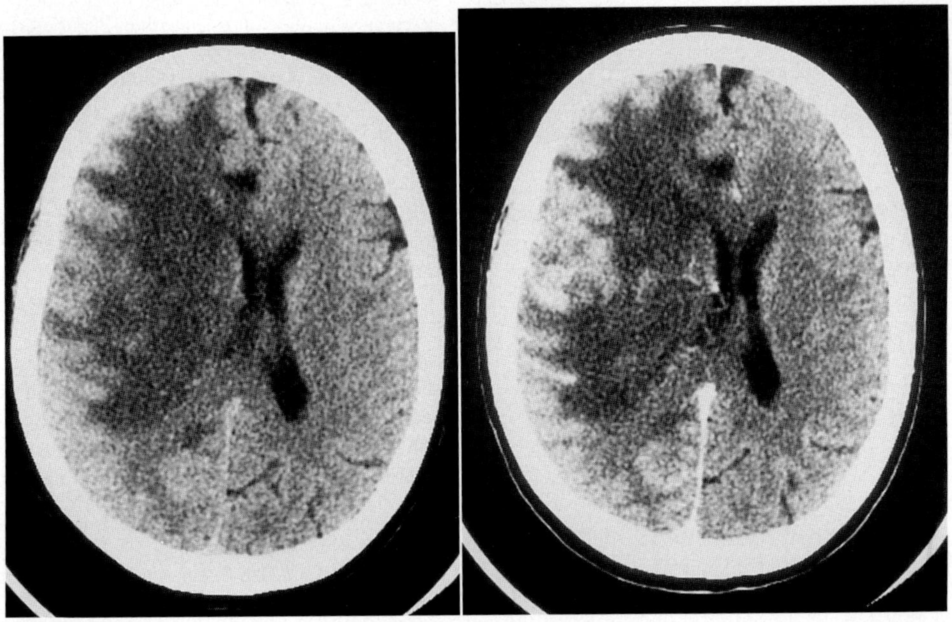 B

**FIGURE 8** Malignant oligodendroglioma. *A,* Axial CT image before contrast shows a heterogeneous hypo- to isodense right frontal mass with poorly defined margins and extensive frontoparietal low attenuation edema with or without tumor. Edema or tumor extends into the genu of the corpus callosum, favoring a neoplasm over infectious or inflammatory processes. Mass effect causes effacement of the right lateral ventricle and leftward midline shift. *B,* Axial CT image after administration of contrast material shows heterogeneous enhancement of the right frontal mass.

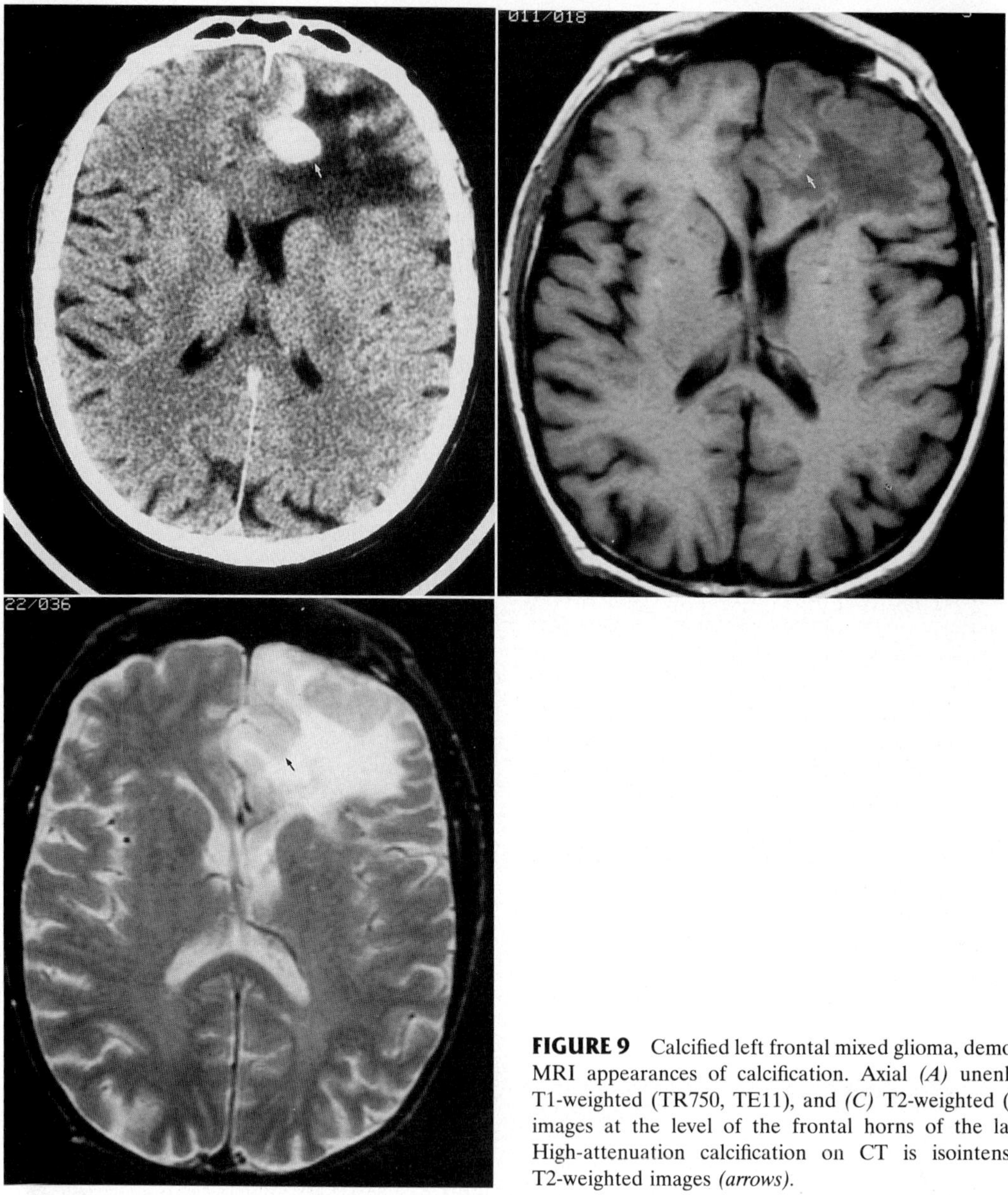


A B C

**FIGURE 9** Calcified left frontal mixed glioma, demonstrating varied MRI appearances of calcification. Axial *(A)* unenhanced CT, *(B)* T1-weighted (TR750, TE11), and *(C)* T2-weighted (TR2500, TE80) images at the level of the frontal horns of the lateral ventricles. High-attenuation calcification on CT is isointense on T1- and T2-weighted images *(arrows)*.

frontal lobe mass is suspicious for oligodendroglioma. Occasionally calcified peripheral lesions erode the calvarium. Hemorrhage and cystic necrosis are relatively common. Contrast enhancement occurs in about 50 percent and is of variable intensity. Edema is usually not prominent, except in higher-grade lesions. The CT and MRI appearances of oligodendrogliomas are similar to astrocytomas, modified by the predilection for these pathologic features (Figs. 8 and 9).

## Ependymoma

Ependymoma accounts for about 5 percent of primary intracranial tumors: 30 to 40 percent are supratentorial, distributed evenly through all age groups; 60 to 70 percent are infratentorial, primarily in children. In the cerebral hemispheres, the most common location is the body of the lateral ventricle. From there, it may invade the adjacent brain parenchyma. Less often, ependymoma originates in the hemispheric parenchyma. It has been hypothesized that in these cases it arises from ependymal cell rests. Calcification, cyst formation, and hemorrhage are common, resulting in heterogeneous attenuation and signal intensities on CT and MRI. Contrast enhancement is nearly universal, but is of variable intensity and is frequently heterogeneous. Hemispheric and lateral ventricle ependymomas are frequently large at the time of diagnosis. Metastatic seeding via CSF pathways occurs, though not as commonly as with PNET tumors. The differential diagnosis of the hemispheric ependymoma includes astrocytoma, oligodendroglioma, ganglioglioma, and PNET tumors (depending on age) (Fig. 10).

## Ganglioglioma and Gangliocytoma

Ganglioglioma and gangliocytoma are rare, accounting for less than 1 percent of primary brain tumors. They occur in children and young adults (80 percent under 30 years of age), and are often associated with seizures. Ganglioglioma consists of a mixture of differentiated but abnormal ganglion cells and glial

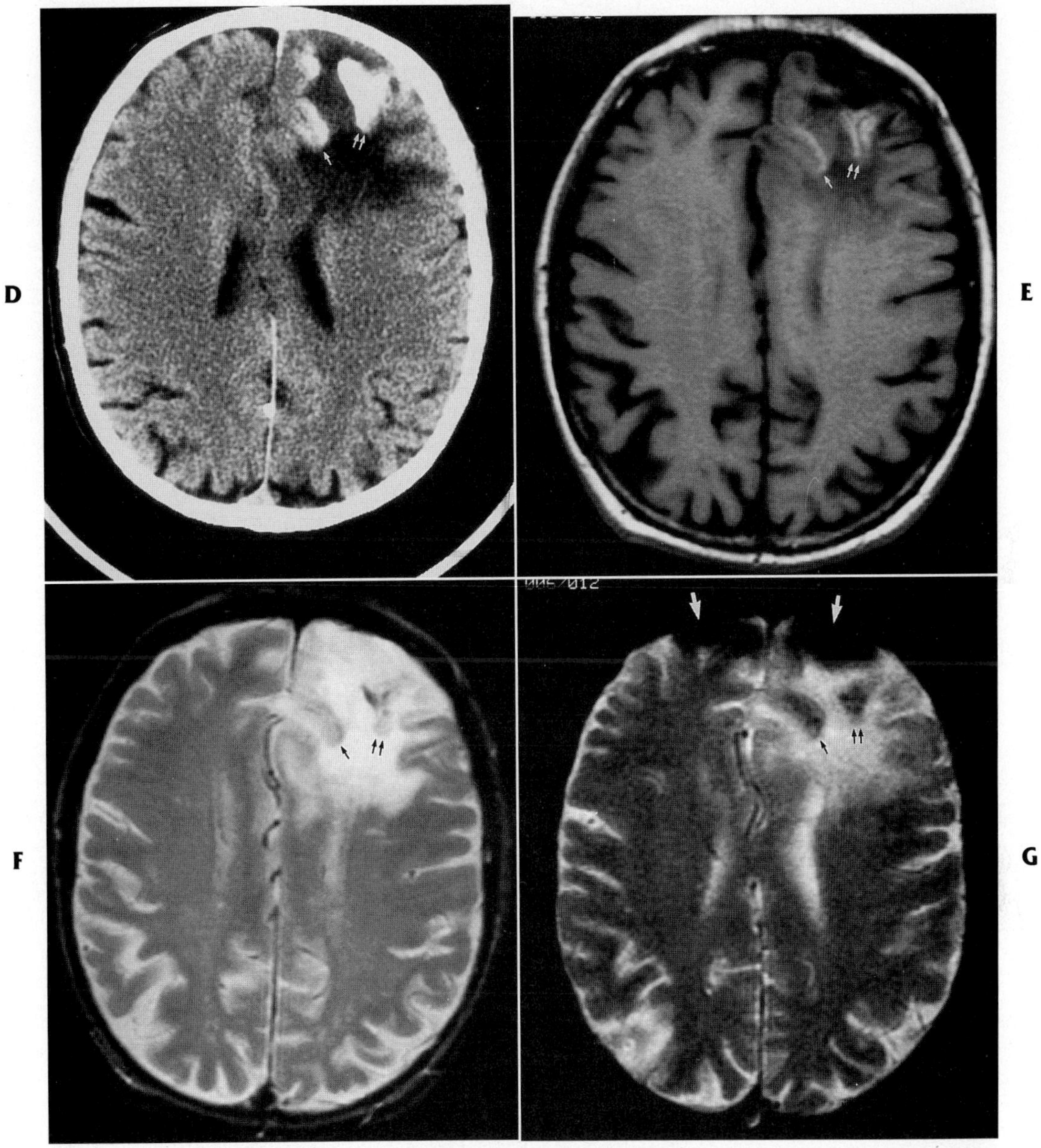

**FIGURE 9 cont'd** Axial *(D)* unenhanced CT, *(E)* T1-weighted (TR750, TE11), *(F)* T2-weighted (TR2500, TE80), and *(G)* gradient-echo T2*-weighted (TR750, TE50, flip-angle 10°) images at the level of the superior margins of the lateral ventricles, same patient. Medial calcification *(single arrow)* is hyperintense on T1- and isointense on T2-weighted images. Lateral calcification *(double arrows)* is partially hyperintense on T1- and hypointense on T2-weighted images. Both are conspicuously hypointense on the gradient-echo image, which is highly sensitive to magnetic susceptibility effects. The nearby bifrontal hypointensity *(white arrows)* is due to susceptibility effect from the frontal sinuses, and should not be mistaken for intracranial pathology. The low-attenuation, T1-weighted hypointense and T2-weighted hyperintense regions represent a combination of tumor and edema. The tumor margins are ill-defined, suggesting parenchymal infiltration.

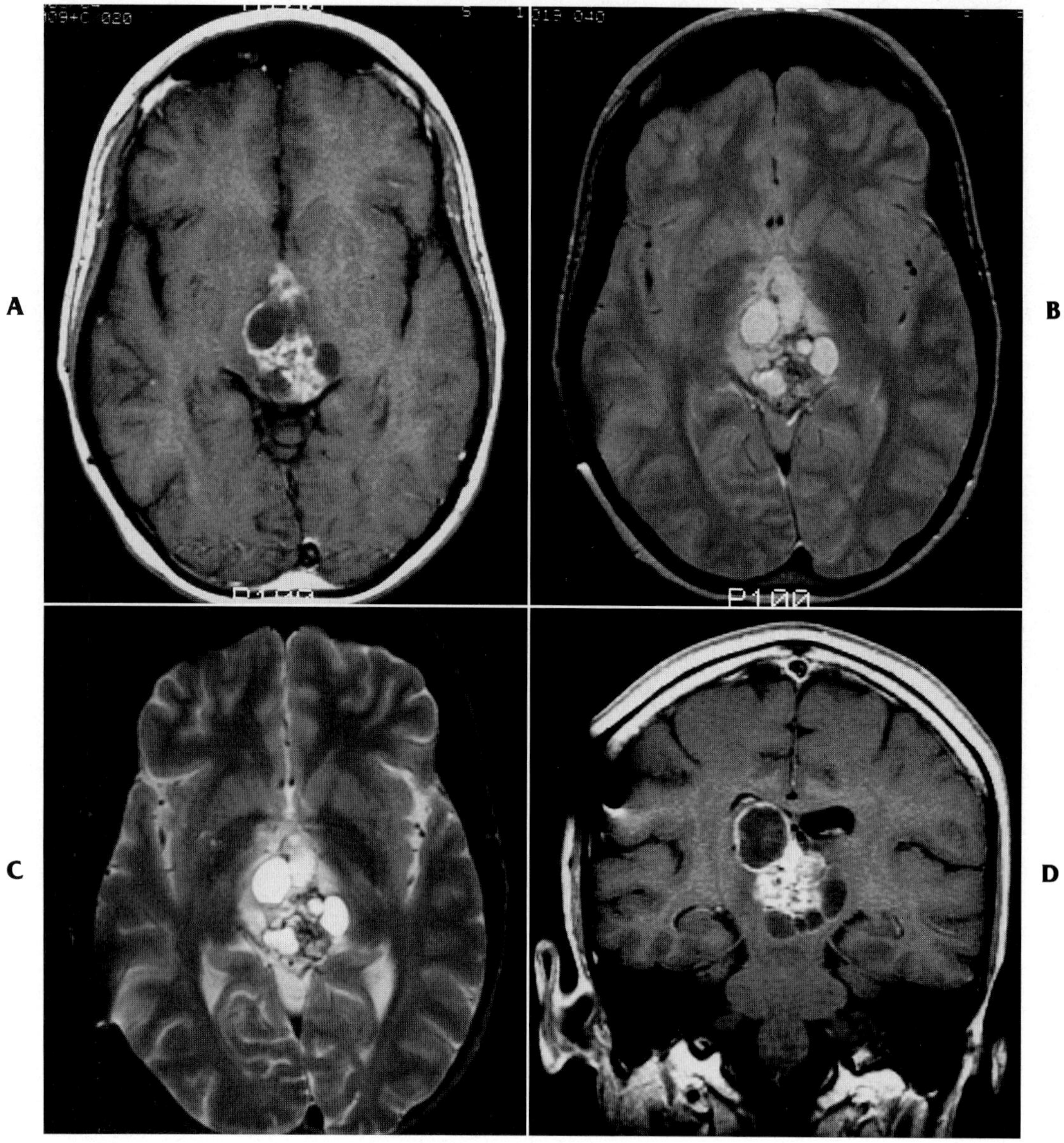


**FIGURE 10** Supratentorial ependymoma, with cyst formation, in a 25-year-old female. Axial *(A)* contrast-enhanced T1-weighted, *(B)* proton density-weighted, and *(C)* T2-weighted images. *D,* Coronal contrast-enhanced T1-weighted image. A heterogeneous partially enhancing mass fills the third ventricle and invades the diencephalon and midbrain. Several sharply circumscribed round structures are mildly hyperintense to CSF on all pulse sequences, representing cysts that probably contain proteinaceous fluid.

cells. In gangliocytoma, the glial component is absent or negligible. They favor the temporal and frontal lobes but can involve the region of the third ventricle, cerebellum, and brain stem. They are characterized by slow growth, well-defined margins, cyst formation (40 to 50 percent), calcification (30 percent), and variable (50 percent) inhomogeneous contrast enhancement. Hemorrhage and edema are not prominent features. Peripherally located lesions may erode the inner table of the calvarium.

## Primary Cerebral Neuroblastoma (PNET)

Cerebral neuroblastoma is rare, accounting for less than 1 percent of primary brain tumors. It is included by many pathologists in the class of PNET tumors. It is almost exclusively a disease of childhood (10 percent within first year, 50 percent within 5 years, 80 percent within 10 years). However, cases in adults have been reported up to 50 years of age. Cerebral neuroblastoma is most often located in the deep hemispheric white matter, with a predilection for the frontal and parietal lobes. Juxtaventricular and intraventricular locations also occur. It tends to be large at the time of diagnosis. Its margins are usually well defined. Calcification, necrosis, cyst formation, and hemorrhage are common, resulting in marked heterogeneity on imaging studies. Edema is usually mild. Contrast enhancement is almost always present but is heterogeneous. There is a high frequency of metastatic seeding along CSF pathways. Cerebral neuroblastoma may also metastasize systemically, most commonly to bone. Conversely, peripheral neuroblastoma almost never metastasizes to the brain. The most important differential diagnosis is astrocytoma. A large well-defined mass with calcification, hemorrhage, necrosis, or cyst formation in a child or adolescent should raise consideration of cerebral neuroblastoma.

## Lymphoma

In the past, primary cerebral lymphoma has also been called primary reticulum cell sarcoma, histiocytic lymphoma, and microglioma. Primary cerebral lymphoma is usually of non-Hodgkin's B-cell type. It has classically been a rare tumor, accounting for about 1 percent of primary brain tumors. However, three conditions markedly increase its risk: acquired immunodeficiency syndrome (AIDS), chronic immunosuppression after organ transplantation, and congenital immunodeficiency syndromes. In particular, AIDS is causing a marked rise in the incidence of primary CNS lymphoma. There is an additional unexplained recent rise in the incidence of CNS lymphoma in immunocompetent patients. Peak incidence is the sixth decade in immunocompetent patients and is younger in immunocompromised patients.

Primary CNS lymphoma presents as solitary or multiple (~50 percent) parenchymal masses; 75 to 85 percent are supratentorial. Favored locations are the deep gray nuclei, periventricular regions, and corpus callosum. There is a tendency for the masses to abut an ependymal or meningeal surface (75 percent). They have ill-defined margins, reflecting infiltrative growth along the Virchow-Robin perivascular spaces. Subependymal and leptomeningeal spread are common. Because of high cell density, high nuclear-to-cytoplasmic ratio, and lower free water content, lymphoma often demonstrates characteristic CT attenuation and MRI signal. On CT, it is usually hyperdense or isodense to gray matter. On T2-weighted MRI, it frequently is isointense or only mildly hyperintense to cortex. On T1-weighted images, it is nonspecifically isointense or hypointense. Calcification and hemorrhage are rare. Contrast enhancement is nearly universal. The pattern of contrast enhancement and edema appears to differ between non–AIDS-related and AIDS-related lymphoma. In non–AIDS-related cases, enhancement is usually homogeneous and edema tends to be mild. In AIDS-related cases, ring enhancement is common, reflecting central necrosis, and surrounding edema is often more prominent (Fig. 11).

Metastatic systemic lymphoma primarily involves the leptomeninges or dura. Leptomeningeal disease can extend through the perivascular spaces into the parenchyma, establishing parenchymal masses. However, parenchymal involvement is much more frequent in primary than metastatic lymphoma, and in the metastatic case parenchymal masses are rare in the absence of coexisting leptomeningeal disease. Gadolinium-enhanced MRI is much more sensitive to leptomeningeal and dural enhancement than CT.

Depending on location and multiplicity, the principal differential diagnoses are metastases, abscesses, and glioma. Occasionally meningiomas and cavernous angiomas share imaging features. In the immunocompromised host, the principal differential diagnosis is toxoplasmosis and, less often, abscesses caused by other organisms. These are often impossible to distinguish by any imaging modality. Empiric treatment for toxoplasmosis is often undertaken, and follow-up imaging is used to monitor regression. Unfortunately simultaneous lymphoma and toxoplasmosis can occur. Biopsy is sometimes required for optimal management. Progressive multifocal leukoencephalopathy also is common in AIDS patients and may appear similar to lymphoma on noncontrast MRI. However, unlike lymphoma, it does not enhance with contrast material, it is hypodense on CT, and it does not exhibit mass effect.

## Metastases

Metastases account for about 25 percent of all brain tumors. The most common sites of origin are lung, breast, skin (melanoma), gastrointestinal tract, and kidney. The incidence of brain metastasis is especially high in choriocarcinoma (80 percent) and melanoma (40 percent). Brain metastases are often multiple, but 30 to 50 percent are solitary, especially with melanoma, lung, and breast carcinomas. Brain metastases are asymptomatic in up to 25 percent of cases.

Metastases can occur anywhere in the brain, including less common sites such as pituitary gland, pineal gland, and choroid plexus. The distribution of brain metastases generally mirrors intracranial volumes: about 80 percent supratentorial and 20 percent infratentorial. For unknown reasons, renal cell carcinoma involves the posterior fossa disproportionately, in up to 50 percent of cases. Early metastases often appear at the corticomedullary junction, attributed to deposition of tumor emboli at sites of penetrating cortical arteriolar narrowing.

Metastases are usually sharply circumscribed and round. Disproportionate surrounding vasogenic edema and mass effect are characteristic but not invariable. Small metastases often exhibit little or no edema, especially when located in cortex, where the volume of interstitial space is low. Metastasis-induced edema usually does not cross the corpus

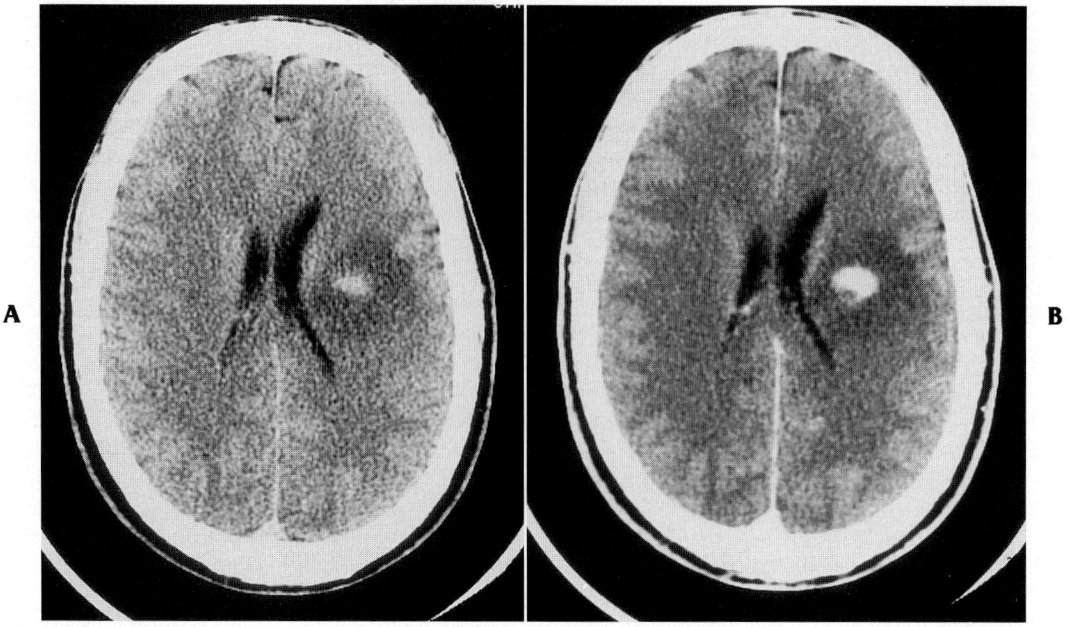

**FIGURE 11** Primary cerebral lymphoma. Axial CT images *(A)* before and *(B)* after contrast administration. A periventricular mass has central high attenuation before contrast administration. Peripheral low attenuation may represent tumor, edema, or both. The tumor margins are ill-defined, suggesting parenchymal infiltration. The central component enhances after contrast administration. High attenuation on precontrast CT image is typical of lymphoma.

callosum or infiltrate the cortex, in contrast to astrocytomas and lymphoma. Hemorrhage is most common among melanoma, lung carcinoma, choriocarcinoma, renal cell carcinoma, and thyroid carcinoma metastases. Necrosis is common in larger lesions. Calcification is rare (~5 percent). It can occur with adenocarcinomas of the gastrointestinal tract, breast carcinoma, and osteosarcoma.

On noncontrast CT, most metastases are hypo- to iso-dense. Hyperdensity may occur with high cell density, high protein content, hemorrhage, and rarely, calcification. The most common hyperdense nonhemorrhagic metastases are lung carcinoma and adenocarcinomas of the gastrointestinal tract. On MRI, most nonhemorrhagic metastases are iso- to hypointense on T1- and hyperintense on T2-weighted images. Nonhemorrhagic melanotic melanoma metastases are characteristically hyperintense on T1- and isointense on T2-weighted images. The mechanisms for T1 relaxation enhancement in nonhemorrhagic melanotic melanoma remain controversial, but may be related to intrinsic paramagnetic properties of melanin. Adenocarcinomas of the gastrointestinal tract may also be iso- or mildly hypointense on T2-weighted images, attributed to cellularity, protein content, or hemosiderin content.

Metastases almost invariably enhance after contrast administration. Homogeneous, nodular, and ring-enhancing patterns are common. Contrast-enhanced MRI is the modality of choice for detection of cerebral metastases. It is more sensitive than double-dose delayed CT. Higher doses of paramagnetic contrast material have a higher sensitivity than the standard dose (0.1 mmol/kg). Since differentiation between solitary and multiple metastases is critical to treatment planning, the use of a higher paramagnetic contrast material dose is likely to replace the standard gadolinium dose in the near future, when nonionic gadolinium-based agents become available for routine clinical use.

## Suggested Reading


Altman NR. MR and CT characteristics of gangliocytoma: A rare cause of epilepsy in children. Am J Neuroradiol 1988; 9:917–921.

Armington WG, Osborn AG, Cubberly DA, et al. Supratentorial ependymoma: CT appearance. Radiology 1985; 157:367–372.

Atlas SW. Adult supratentorial tumors. Semin Roentgenol 1990; 25:130–154.

Atlas SW. Intraaxial brain tumors. In: Atlas SW, ed. Magnetic Resonance Imaging of the Brain and Spine. New York: Raven Press, 1991:223.

Atlas SW, Braffman BH, LoBrutto R, et al. Human malignant melanomas with varying degrees of melanin content in nude mice: MR imaging, histopathology, and electron paramagnetic resonance. J Comput Assist Tomogr 1990; 14:547–554.

Atlas SW, Grossman RI, Gomori JM, et al. MR imaging of intracranial metastatic melanoma. J Comput Assist Tomogr 1987; 11:577–582.

Braffman BH, Bilaniuk LT, Naidich TP, et al. MR imaging of tuberous sclerosis: Pathogenesis of this phakomatosis, use of gadopentetate dimeglumine, and literature review. Radiology 1992; 183:227–238.

Burger PC, Vogel FS, Green SB, Strike TA. Glioblastoma multiforme and anaplastic astrocytoma. Pathologic criteria and prognostic implications. Cancer 1985; 56:1106–1111.

Castillo M, Davis PC, Takei Y, Hoffman JC Jr. Intracranial ganglioglioma: MR, CT, and clinical findings in 18 patients. Am J Neuroradiol 1990; 11:109–114.

Davis PC, Hudgins PA, Peterman SB, Hoffman JC Jr. Diagnosis of cerebral metastases: Double-dose delayed CT vs. contrast-enhanced MR imaging. Am J Neuroradiol 1991; 12:293–300.

Davis PC, Wichman RD, Takei Y, Hoffman JC Jr. Am J Neuroradiol 1990; 11:115–120.

Dean BL, Drayer BP, Bird CR, et al. Gliomas: Classification with MR imaging. Radiology 1990; 174:411–415.

Earnest F IV, Kelly PJ, Scheithauer BW, et al. Cerebral astrocytomas: Histopathologic correlation of MR and CT contrast enhancement with stereotactic biopsy. Radiology 1988; 166:823–827.

Figueroa RE, Gammal TE, Brooks BS, et al. MR findings on primitive neuroectodermal tumors. J Comput Assist Tomogr 1989; 13:773–778.

Geremia GK, Wollman R, Foust R. Computed tomography of gliomatosis cerebri. J Comput Assist Tomogr 1988; 12:698–701.

Goldstein ID, Zeifer B, Chao C, et al. CT appearance of primary CNS lymphoma in patients with acquired immunodeficiency syndrome. J Comput Assist Tomogr 1991; 15:39–44.

Hasso AN, Kortman KE, Bradley WG Jr. Supratentorial neoplasms. In: Stark DD, Bradley WG Jr, eds. Magnetic Resonance Imaging. 2nd ed. Vol 1. St Louis: Mosby-Year Book, 1992:770.

Hochberg FH, Miller DC. Primary central nervous system lymphoma. J Neurosurg 1988; 68:835–853.

Jack CR Jr, Reese DF, Scheithauer BW. Radiographic findings in 32 cases of primary CNS lymphoma. AJR 1986; 146:271–276.

Latchaw RE, Johnson DW, Kanal E. Metastases. In: Latchaw RE, ed. MR and CT Imaging of the Head, Neck, and Spine. 2nd ed. Vol 1. St Louis: Mosby-Year Book, 1991:597.

Latchaw RE, Johnson DW, Kanal E. Primary intracranial tumors: Neuroepithelial tumors, sarcomas, and lymphomas. In: Latchaw RE, ed. MR and CT Imaging of the Head, Neck, and Spine. 2nd ed. Vol 1. St Louis: Mosby-Year Book, 1991:449.

Latchaw RE, Johnson DW, Kanal E. Primary intracranial tumors: Tumors of congenital, pineal, and vascular origin and the phakomatoses. In: Latchaw RE, ed. MR and CT Imaging of the Head, Neck, and Spine. 2nd ed. Vol 1. St Louis: Mosby-Year Book, 1991:561.

Lewin JS, Estes ML, Ross JS. Magnetic resonance imaging of adult intra-axial brain tumors. Top Magn Reson Imaging 1992; 4(4):17–40.

Lee Y-Y, Van Tassel P, Bruner JM, et al. Juvenile pilocytic astrocytomas: CT and MR characteristics. Am J Neuroradiol 1989; 10:363–370.

Lee Y-Y, Van Tassel P. Intracranial oligodendrogliomas: Imaging findings in 35 untreated cases. Am J Neuroradiol 1989; 10:119–127.

Lee Y-Y, Vonofakos D, Marcu H, Hacker H. Oligodendrogliomas: CT patterns with emphasis on features indicating malignancy. J Comput Assist Tomogr 1979; 3:783–788.

Okazaki H. Fundamentals of Neuropathology: Morphologic Basis of Neurologic Disorders. 2nd ed. New York: Igaku-Shoin, 1989.

Poon T, Matoso I, Tchertkoff V, et al. CT features of primary cerebral lymphoma in AIDS and Non-AIDS patients. J Comput Assist Tomogr 1989; 13:6–9.

Russell DS, Rubinstein LJ. Pathology of Tumors of the Nervous System. 5th ed. Baltimore: Williams & Wilkins, 1989.

Sato Y. Pediatric primary brain tumors. Top Magn Reson Imaging 1992; 4(4):64–77.

Schwaighofer BW, Hesselink JR, Press GA, et al. Primary intracranial CNS lymphoma: MR manifestations. Am J Neuroradiol 1989; 10:725–729.

Spoto GP, Press GA, Hesselink JR, Solomon M. Intracranial ependymoma and subependymoma: MR manifestations. Am J Neuroradiol 1990; 11:83–91.

Sze G, Soletsky S, Bronen R, Krol G. MR imaging of the cranial meninges with emphasis on contrast enhancement and meningeal carcinomatosis. Am J Neuroradiol 1989; 10:965–975.

Van Tassel P, Lee Y-Y, Bruner JM. Synchronous and metachronous malignant gliomas: CT findings. Am J Neuroradiol 1988; 9:725–732.

Yanaka K, Kamezaki T, Kobayashi E, et al. MR imaging of diffuse glioma. Am J Neuroradiol 1992; 13:349–351.

Yousem DM, Patrone PM, Grossman RI. Leptomeningeal metastases: MR evaluation. J Comput Assist Tomogr 1990; 14:255–261.

Yuh WTC, Engelken JD, Muhonen MG, et al. Experience with high-dose gadolinium MR imaging in the evaluation of brain metastases. Am J Neuroradiol 1992; 13:335–345.

Zimmerman RA. Pediatric supratentorial tumors. Semin Roentgenol 1990; 25:225–248.

# PART III: TUMORS OF POSTERIOR FOSSA AND PINEAL REGION

## Tumors of Posterior Fossa

About 50 percent of childhood tumors and 30 percent of adult tumors are infratentorial. In the first 3 years of life supratentorial tumors predominate, while posterior fossa tumors predominate from 4 to 11 years of age. Among childhood posterior fossa tumors, about 70 percent are in the cerebellum and 30 percent are in the brain stem. In order of decreasing frequency, the most common are astrocytoma, medulloblastoma (PNET), ependymoma, and brain stem glioma. Among adult posterior fossa tumors, most are in the cerebellum. The most common are metastasis (Fig. 1) and hemangioblastoma. Less common are astrocytoma, lateral medulloblastoma (in young adults), and lymphoma.

### *Cerebellar Astrocytoma*

Astrocytomas arise in the cerebellar hemispheres (75 percent) and vermis (25 percent). Most (85 percent) are of the pilocytic subtype. They are sharply circumscribed and frequently cystic (70 percent), with a solid mural nodule. The solid portions enhance intensely. The cyst wall is composed of compressed parenchyma and does not enhance. Calcification occurs in about 20 percent. Typically, the fourth ventricle is displaced and effaced, not filled. A minority (15 percent) of cerebellar astrocytomas are of the infiltrative fibrillary type, and these usually occur in younger adults. Anaplastic astrocytoma and glioblastoma multiforme occur uncommonly in the cerebellum.

The differential diagnosis depends on age. In children a cystic tumor is most often pilocytic astrocytoma, whereas in adults it is most often metastasis or hemangioblastoma. Arachnoid cyst and trapped fourth ventricle are occasional considerations. The differential diagnosis for solid astrocytoma includes medulloblastoma, ependymoma, and metastasis.

### *Brain Stem Glioma*

Brain stem gliomas primarily occur in children and adolescents. The peak age of onset is 7 years. About 80 percent occur in patients under 20 years of age. The most common clinical presentations are cranial nerve palsies (90 percent), long tract signs, and hydrocephalus. Most brain stem gliomas (80 percent) are infiltrative fibrillary astrocytomas. A minority (20 percent) are pilocytic astrocytomas. Brain stem gliomas most commonly arise in the pons, from which they may extend rostrally into the midbrain, caudally into the medulla, and dorsally into the cerebellum. Imaging is critical to the diagnosis

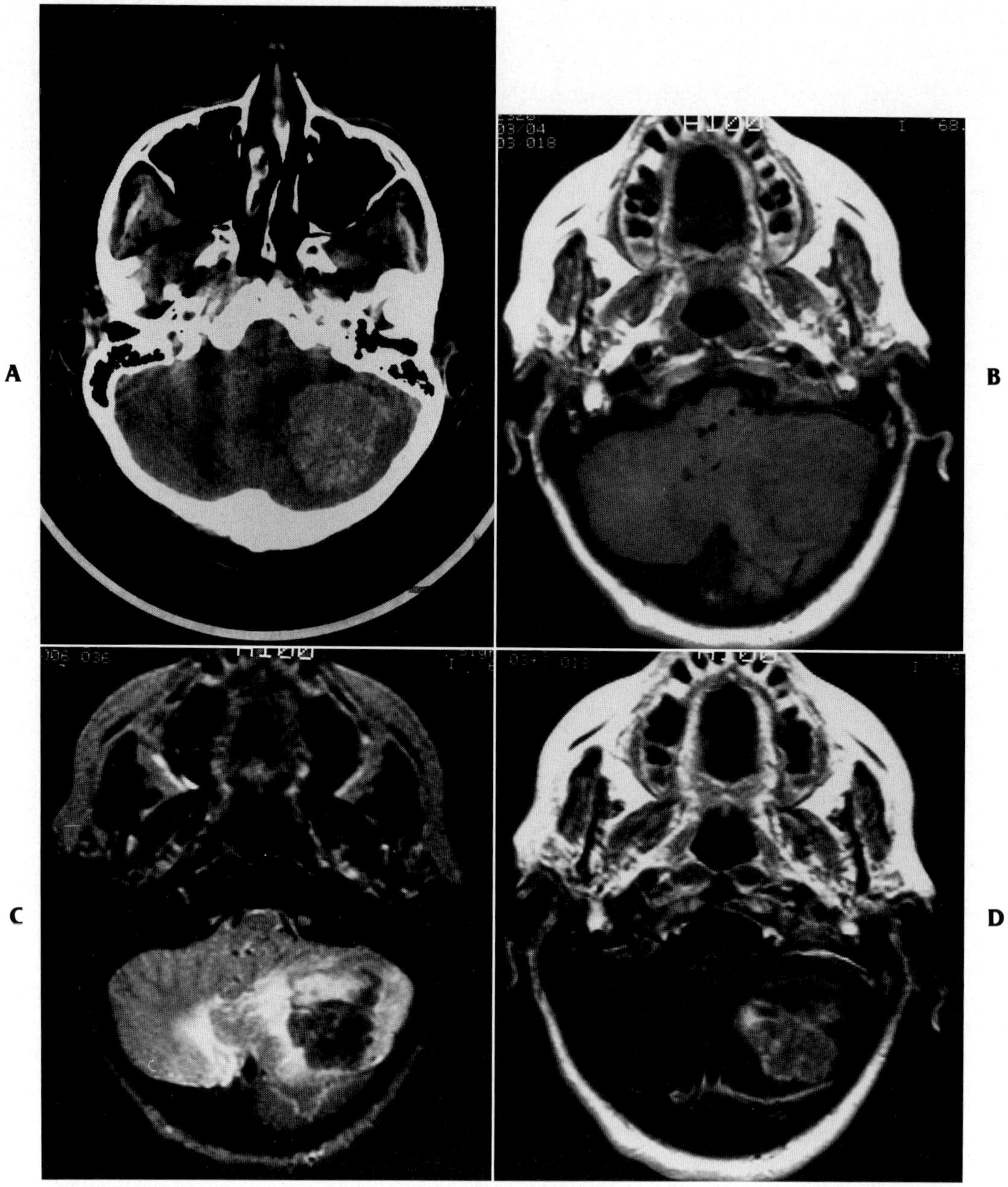

**FIGURE 1** Metastatic colon carcinoma in a 66-year-old female. Axial *(A)* unenhanced CT, *(B)* unenhanced T1-weighted, *(C)* T2-weighted, and *(D)* enhanced T1-weighted images. A large cerebellar mass is diffusely hyperdense on CT, isointense on T1-, and hypointense on T2-weighted images. These unusual signal characteristics are fairly common among mucinous adenocarcinoma metastases, especially colon and lung. They may be related to tumor cytoarchitecture, protein content, microcalcifications, or paramagnetic cations. It enhances heterogeneously. There is surrounding low attenuation, mild T1-weighted hypointensity, and marked T2-weighted hyperintensity, representing edema. There is mass effect on the midline and medulla.

A

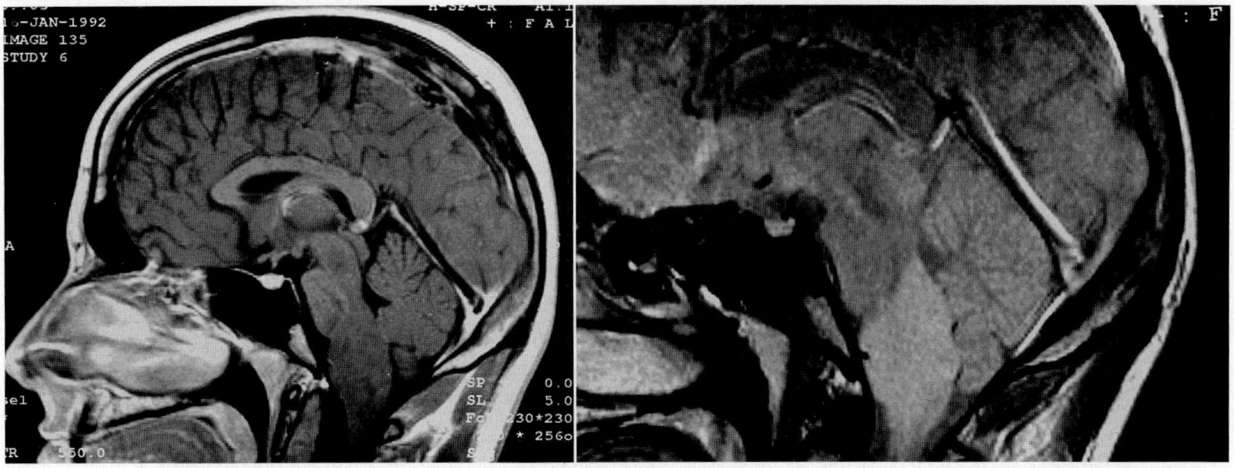

B

**FIGURE 2** Presumptive brain stem glioma. Sagittal *(A)* contrast-enhanced T1-weighted (TR550, TE15) and *(B)* proton density–weighted (TR2200, TE20) images demonstrate marked expansion of the medulla. The tumor is slightly hypointense on T1- and moderately hyperintense on T2-weighted images. There is no enhancement. It extends into the pontine tegmentum and upper cervical cord. Mass effect at the pontine level flattens the ventral pons against the clivus.

of brain stem glioma; most are diagnosed without biopsy and are treated by irradiation. Large exophytic components are sometimes debulked.

MRI is the imaging modality of choice for disease of the brain stem. On CT and MRI, brain stem gliomas may be detected by brain stem enlargement, ventral contour abnormality, effacement of the pontine cistern, encasement of the basilar artery, and posterior displacement of the fourth ventricle. They are iso- to hypo-dense on CT, iso- to mildly hypo-intense on T1- and hyper-intense on proton density- and T2-weighted images. T2-weighted images have the highest sensitivity, especially when brain stem enlargement is not present. Focal hemorrhage and necrosis may occur. Cysts are uncommon. Contrast enhancement occurs in about 50 percent of cases and is often inhomogeneous or patchy. There is no definite relationship between enhancement and prognosis. Pathologically, vasogenic edema is not found in brain stem gliomas. Therefore it is expected that MRI signal abnormality reflects tumor extent (Fig. 2).

Differential diagnosis includes demyelinating disease (multiple sclerosis, acute disseminated encephalomyelitis), encephalitis, infarction, vascular malformation, central pontine myelinolysis, and metastasis.

## Medulloblastoma

Medulloblastoma is included by many pathologists in the category of PNET tumors. It arises only in the cerebellum. Most (75 to 90 percent) occur in children, while a minority occur in adolescents and young adults. The typical childhood medulloblastoma is midline, arising from the vermis along the roof of the fourth ventricle. The inferior medullary velum is a characteristic epicenter. It frequently completely fills or compresses the fourth ventricle, almost always causing hydrocephalus (95 percent). The adolescent and young adult variant arises eccentrically from the cerebellar hemisphere.

Medulloblastoma is usually sharply circumscribed and relatively homogeneous. It is characteristically mildly to moderately hyperdense on unenhanced CT and iso- or only mildly hyperintense on T2-weighted images. These features are attributed to high cell density and high nuclear-to-cytoplasmic ratio. It is nonspecifically mildly hypo- to iso-intense on T1-weighted images. Before treatment, midline lesions usually enhance intensely and homogeneously. Eccentric hemispheric lesions tend to enhance less intensely, which has been attributed to frequent desmoplasia. Recurrent medulloblastoma sometimes fails to enhance. Edema is usually mild to moderate. Hemorrhage, calcification, cyst formation, necrosis, low CT density, lack of enhancement, and eccentric location are each uncommon (~10 percent), but up to 50 percent of medulloblastomas exhibit at least one of these "atypical" features.

Metastasis along CSF pathways to ependymal and leptomeningeal surfaces is common. Spinal drop metastases should be excluded by contrast-enhanced MRI, possibly supplemented by myelography. Medulloblastoma is the most common brain tumor to metastasize hematogenously, usually to bone. Systemic metastasis occasionally occurs via shunts. The following factors are prognostically unfavorable: young age (under 4 years old), tumor size >3 cm, necrosis, and metastasis. The most important differential diagnostic considerations are astrocytoma and ependymoma.

## Ependymoma

The majority of ependymomas are infratentorial and most of these occur in children. Although ependymoma is the third most common posterior fossa tumor in children, astrocytoma and medulloblastoma are more prevalent by factors of about 5 and 3, respectively. Ependymoma of the posterior fossa usually arises from the floor of the fourth ventricle. Less often it arises along one of the outlet foramina. It typically fills the fourth ventricle, causing hydrocephalus. It often extends through the foramina of Luschka into the cerebellopontine angle cisterns or through the foramen of Magendie into the cisterna magna. From the cisterna magna it may extrude into the cervical subarachnoid space, insinuating along the dorsal and lateral surfaces of the cord ("plastic ependymoma"). This pattern is rare in medulloblastoma. Ependymoma frequently compresses and may directly invade the brain stem. When the tumor arises

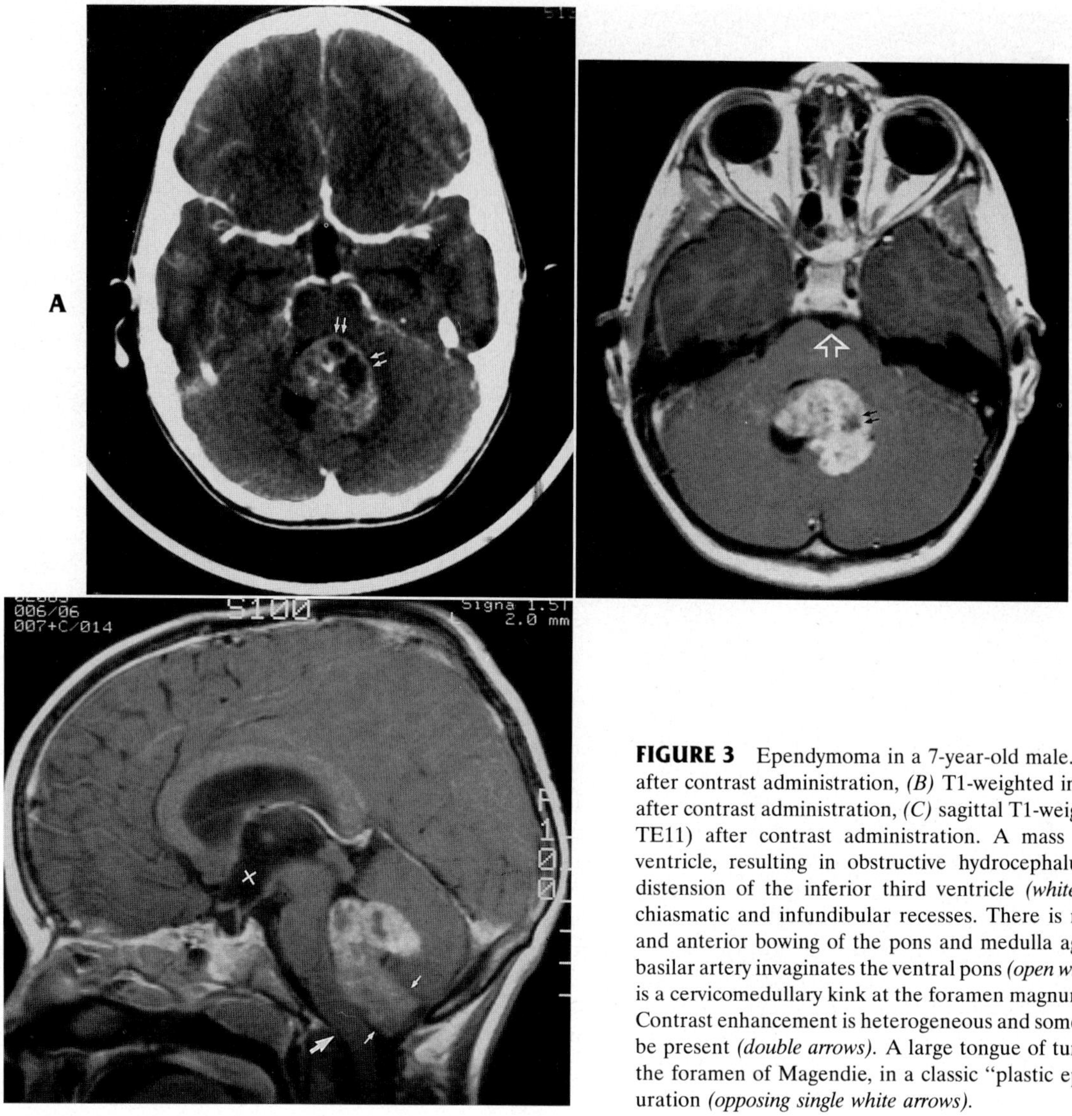

**FIGURE 3** Ependymoma in a 7-year-old male. Axial *(A)* CT image after contrast administration, *(B)* T1-weighted image (TR700, TE11) after contrast administration, *(C)* sagittal T1-weighted image (TR600, TE11) after contrast administration. A mass expands the fourth ventricle, resulting in obstructive hydrocephalus; there is marked distension of the inferior third ventricle *(white "x")* including the chiasmatic and infundibular recesses. There is marked compression and anterior bowing of the pons and medulla against the clivus; the basilar artery invaginates the ventral pons *(open white arrow),* and there is a cervicomedullary kink at the foramen magnum *(large white arrow).* Contrast enhancement is heterogeneous and some foci of necrosis may be present *(double arrows).* A large tongue of tumor extends through the foramen of Magendie, in a classic "plastic ependymoma" configuration *(opposing single white arrows).*

along the foramen of Luschka, it may present as an exophytic cerebellopontine angle cistern mass, mimicking an extra-axial tumor. Metastasis along CSF pathways is common but less so than with medulloblastoma/PNET. It usually occurs after treatment failure at the primary site rather than at initial presentation.

Ependymoma is the most common posterior fossa tumor to contain calcification (50 percent). Cyst formation is common, but less so than in supratentorial ependymoma. Necrosis and hemorrhage are less common but are more prevalent than in medulloblastoma. CT attenuation is variable. Most often it is isodense or mildly hypodense, but hyperdensity and heterogeneous density occur. Solid portions of tumor are nonspecifically hypo- to iso-intense on T1- and hyperintense on T2-weighted images. However, heterogeneous MRI signal intensity is common because of calcification, cyst formation, necrosis, or hemorrhage. Posterior fossa ependymoma usually enhances with contrast material, but it is often patchy or inhomogeneous (Fig. 3). Differential diagnosis includes medulloblastoma, astrocytoma, and choroid plexus tumors.

## *Choroid Plexus Papilloma and Carcinoma*

Choroid plexus tumors are most common in children, especially infants and young children. In children the most common location is the trigone of the lateral ventricles. In adults the most common location is the fourth ventricle. Uncommonly, it may arise in the third ventricle or foramen of Luschka. In the latter case, it presents as an exophytic cerebellopontine angle cistern mass, mimicking an extra-axial lesion. Hydrocephalus is frequent, even without evidence of mechanical obstruction to CSF flow. Although controversial, hydrocephalus is usually attributed to overproduction of CSF or impairment of reabsorption by adhesions resulting from tumor hemorrhage. The mass is sharply circumscribed with lobulated margins. Calcification, hemorrhage, cyst formation, and macroscopic tumor vessels are common, resulting in heterogeneity, especially on MRI. It is isodense to mildly hyperdense on unenhanced CT. It is isointense to mildly hypointense on T1- and heterogeneously hyperintense on T2-weighted images. Contrast enhancement is intense and homogeneous.

Choroid plexus carcinoma is uncommon ($\sim$10 percent of

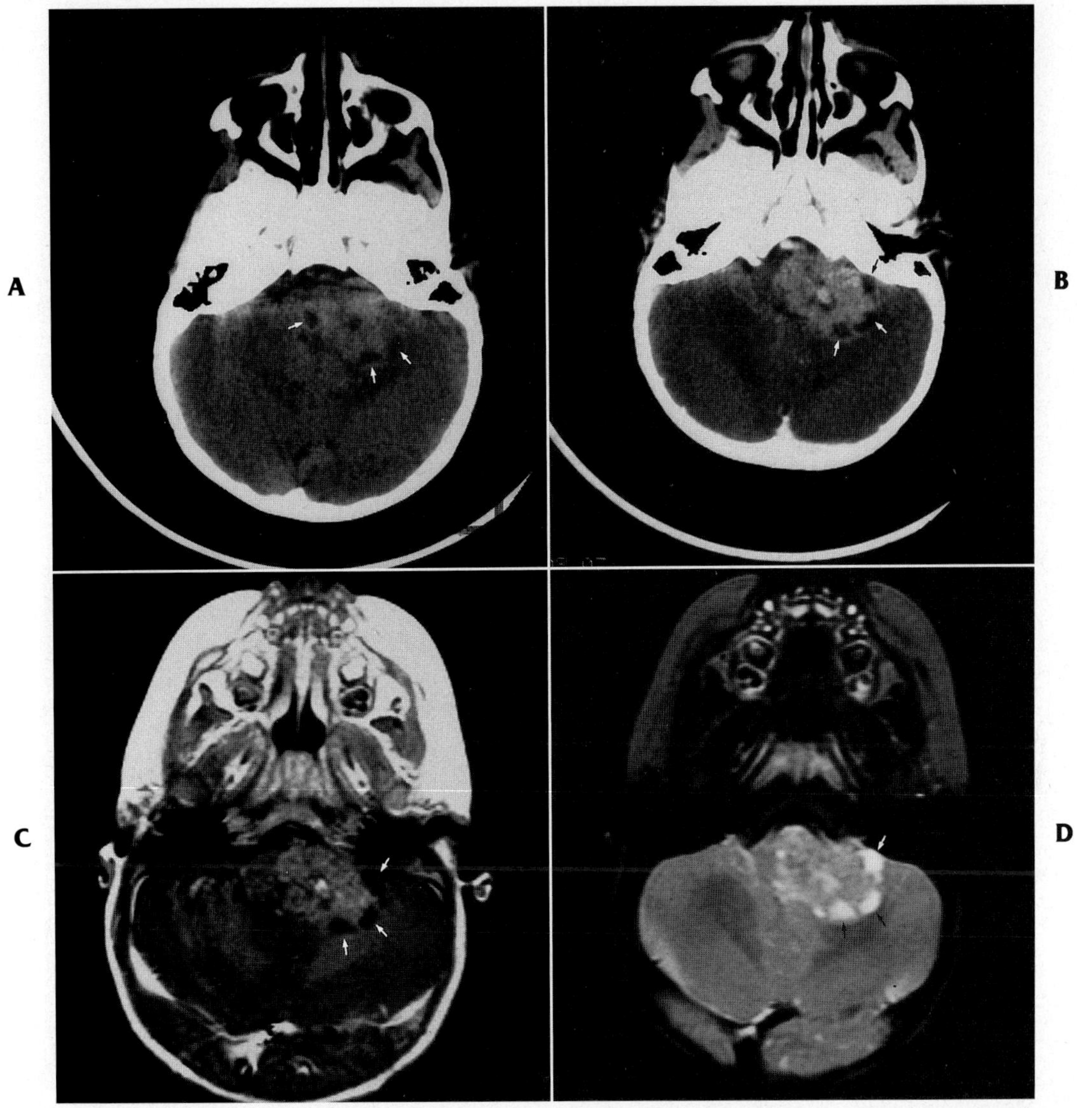

**FIGURE 4** Choroid plexus carcinoma in a 15-month-old male. Axial *(A)* CT image before contrast administration, *(B)* CT image after contrast administration, *(C)* T1-weighted image (TR500, TE11) after contrast administration, *(D)* T2-weighted image (TR2000, TE80). A large exophytic mass with lobulated margins arises from the left foramen of Luschka, extending into the cerebellopontine angle cistern. It markedly compresses the brain stem and displaces it rightward. Invasion of the brain stem is possible. It is mildly hyperdense on noncontrast CT and is slightly hyperintense on T2-weighted images. It contains multiple cysts that are isodense to CSF on CT and isointense to CSF on T1- and T2-weighted MRI *(arrows)*. There is moderate heterogeneous contrast enhancement.

choroid plexus tumors). It usually occurs in young children. There is a predisposition to parenchymal invasion and spread through CSF pathways. It is not possible to differentiate benign from malignant choroid plexus tumor on the basis of imaging (Fig. 4).

## *Hemangioblastoma*

Hemangioblastoma is the most common primary intra-axial tumor of the posterior fossa in adults. Overall, it is the second most common tumor of the posterior fossa in adults, after metastasis. Hemangioblastoma is associated with von Hippel-Lindau (vHL) disease, manifestations of which also include retinal angiomatosis, renal cell carcinoma, pheochromocytoma, and simple pancreatic cysts. Ten to twenty percent of patients with hemangioblastoma have vHL disease. Conversely 35 to 60 percent of patients with vHL disease have hemangioblastoma. The peak incidence for sporadic cases is in the fifth and sixth decades, but is younger for cases associated with vHL disease. The most common location is the cerebellum (90 percent). Other sites include the spinal cord and area postrema of the medulla. Supratentorial hemangioblastoma is extremely rare. Sporadic cases of hemangioblastoma are nearly always solitary. About 20 percent of vHL disease–associated hemangioblastomas are multiple.

Hemangioblastoma presents three radiologic patterns: (1) cystic mass with a mural nodule (most common), (2) solid mass with central cystic components, and (3) completely solid mass. Hemangioblastoma cysts are sharply circumscribed. The nodule is often relatively small compared with the cyst. The CT density and MRI signal characteristics of the cyst vary with protein concentration and paramagnetic cation content. It may

A

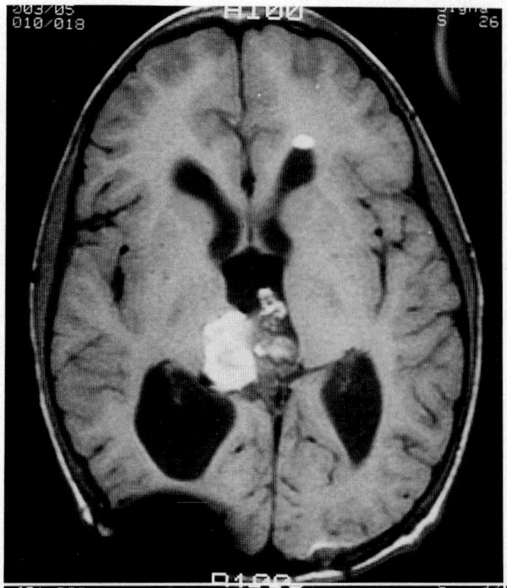

**FIGURE 5** Pineal region teratoma with intraventricular exfoliation of fat. Axial *(A)* unenhanced T1-weighted (TR750, TE11), *(B)* proton density-weighted (TR2500, TE30), and *(C)* T2-weighted (TR2500, TE80) images. A complex heterogeneous parapineal mass causes severe obstructive hydrocephalus. Exfoliated fat layers nondependently in the frontal horn of the left lateral ventricle. Chemical shift artifact is pathognomonic of fat. It is less apparent on the T1-weighted image because adjacent CSF is dark. The chemical shift artifact is amplified (by a factor of 2) on the second-echo long TE image because it is acquired at lower bandwidth (8 vs. 16 kHz).

B

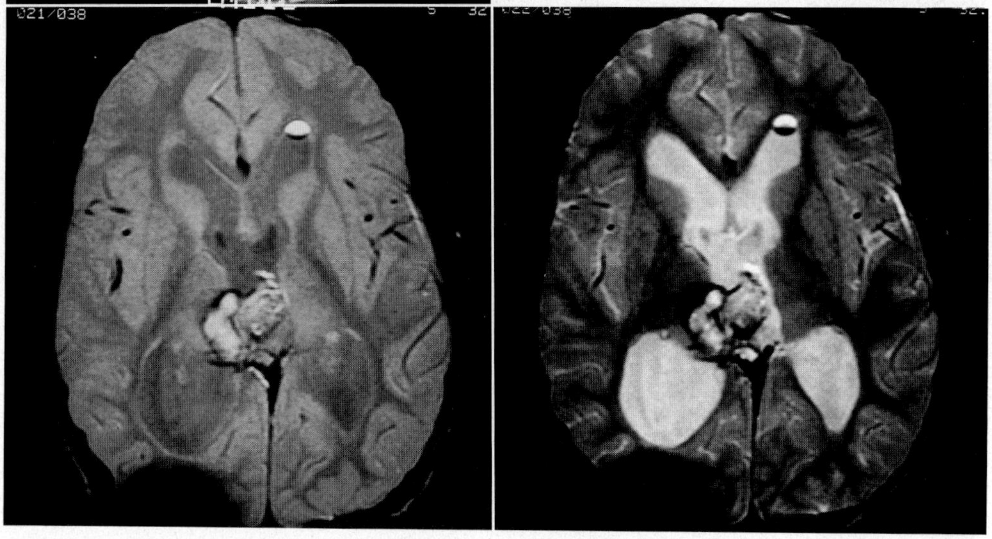

C

be isodense/isointense with CSF but more often is hyperdense/hyperintense with respect to CSF. The solid component is usually isodense on unenhanced CT, isointense on T1-, and variably hyperintense on T2-weighted images. The solid components enhance intensely. The cyst wall does not enhance and is not tumor tissue. Contrast is essential, because the mural nodule is sometimes difficult to discern without it. In each case, the mass usually abuts the pial surface. Macroscopic tumor vessels and hemorrhage are common. Calcification is rare and the surrounding edema is usually mild. The principal differential diagnosis is metastasis and astrocytoma. In adults a cystic cerebellar mass with enhancing mural nodule and macroscopic tumor vessels is virtually pathognomonic of hemangioblastoma.

## Tumors of Pineal Region

Neoplasms of the pineal region constitute less than 1 percent of all intracranial tumors and less than 4 percent of primary intracranial tumors in children. Most pineal region tumors arise from germ cell rests (~50 percent) or from pineal parenchymal cells (~20 percent). A minority arise from nearby structures, including astrocytoma, meningioma, lipoma, and metastasis. Obstruction of the cerebral aqueduct frequently causes hydrocephalus. Compression or invasion of the tectum (especially the superior colliculi) often causes Parinaud's syndrome. Compression or invasion of the hypothalamus or pituitary gland may cause endocrine dysfunction, including diabetes insipidus and precocious puberty. All germ cell tumors and pineal parenchymal tumors are malignant, except benign teratomas. The pineal region tumors have collectively been called *pinealomas* in the past; the term *pinealoma* is now outdated.

### *Germ Cell Tumors*

Germ cell tumors include germinoma, benign teratoma, malignant teratoma, embryonal cell carcinoma, endodermal sinus (yolk sac) tumor, choriocarcinoma, and mixed lesions. Germinomas and teratomas comprise the majority. Dermoid and epidermoid tumors are considered by some to represent variants of the teratoid tumors and by others to represent a separate pathologic category.

*Germinoma* is the single most common tumor of the pineal region. About 70 to 80 percent of germinomas arise in the pineal region, whereas 20 to 30 percent arise in the suprasellar region (previously called *ectopic pinealomas*). All pineal germ cell tumors are more common in males. In particular, about 90

A

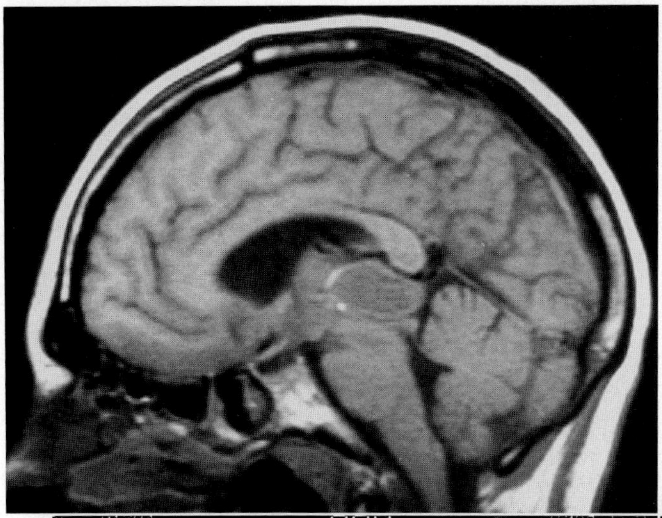

B

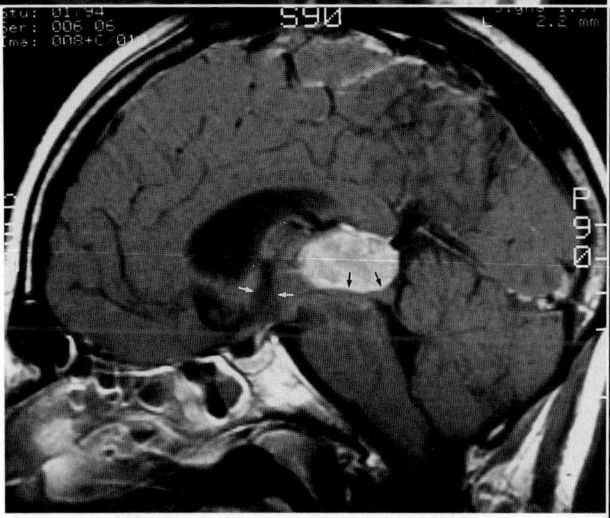

C

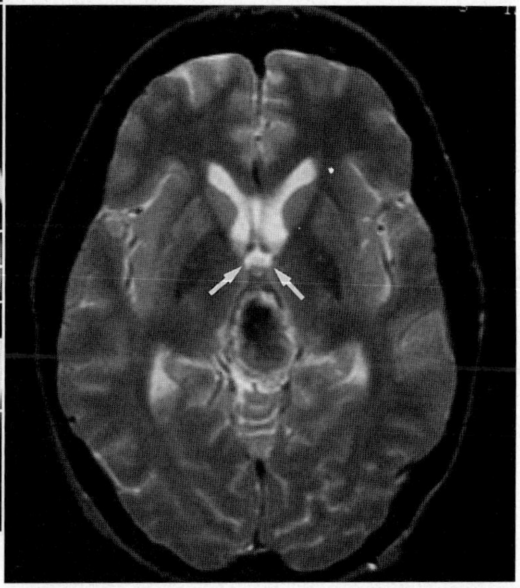

**FIGURE 6** Pineocytoma in a 41-year-old female. *A*, Sagittal T1-weighted image (TR600, TE11) before contrast administration. *B*, sagittal T1-weighted image (TR700, TE19) after contrast administration. *C*, Axial T2-weighted image (TR2500, TE80). A large pineal mass compresses the third ventricle (*white arrows*), midbrain tegmentum, and superior colliculi (*black arrows*). Primarily it is mildly hypointense on T1- and iso- to hypo-intense on T2-weighted images. There is a thin perimeter of T1- and T2-weighted hyperintense signal. The T1 hyperintense and T2 hypointense components are not typical of pineocytoma but may reflect prior hemorrhage. Nevertheless, uniform contrast enhancement is present.

percent of pineal germinomas occur in males, though suprasellar germinomas have equal sex predilection. Germinomas are most common in the first three decades of life, with peak incidence in the second decade. There is an unexplained higher incidence in Japan.

Germinomas are usually slightly hyperdense with respect to gray matter. They are iso- to hypo-intense on T1-weighted and iso- to hyper-intense on T2-weighted images. They enhance intensely with contrast administration. Hemorrhage, local invasion, edema, and spread via CSF pathways are relatively common. Cyst formation and necrosis are uncommon. Although tumor calcification does not occur, premature calcification of the pineal gland itself does. In the era of MRI, this sign is less important.

*Teratomas* contain elements of multiple germ cell layers, and as a result are usually heterogeneous. Cyst formation, fat, blood, and calcification (including bone or teeth) are common. Contrast enhancement is heterogeneous (Fig. 5). *Dermoids* are also notable for fat content and heterogeneity. *Epidermoids* tend to follow CSF in CT attenuation and MRI signal intensity; they may exhibit mural calcification. The rarer choriocarcinomas and embryonal cell carcinomas are often invasive and heterogeneous due to calcification, hemorrhage, and necrosis.

## *Pineal Cell Tumors*

The tumors of pineal cell origin are pineocytoma, pineoblastoma, and mixed lesions. *Pineocytomas* derive from relatively well-differentiated pineal parenchymal cells. They occur at all ages, with peak incidence in the later decades and a smaller peak in the first decade. Unlike germ cell neoplasms, there is no sex predilection. They tend to be well circumscribed and slow growing. They are usually slightly hyperdense on unenhanced CT, similar to germinomas. They are iso- to hypo-intense on T1-weighted and variably hyperintense on T2-weighted images. They usually enhance intensely and uniformly. Tumor calcification is common. Local invasion, CSF spread, edema, hemorrhage, cyst formation, and necrosis are relatively uncommon (Fig. 6).

*Pineoblastomas* derive from immature pineal parenchymal cells. Some pathologists include them in the family of PNET tumors. They occur predominantly in children but occasionally occur in older adults. As with pineocytoma, there is no sex predilection. They tend to be lobulated and aggressive. They are isodense or slightly hyperdense on unenhanced CT. They are iso- to hypo-intense on T1-weighted and tend to be isointense or mildly hyperintense on T2-weighted images. These imaging characteristics are similar to germinoma and are hypothesized to be related to high cell density with scant cytoplasm. They enhance intensely. Tumor calcification, local invasion, CSF spread, edema, and hemorrhage are relatively common.

There is considerable overlap among the imaging features of pineal region tumors, especially malignant germ cell neoplasms, pineocytoma, and pineoblastoma. Typically, CT and MRI are not histologically specific. Local invasion and spread along CSF spaces favor malignant germ cell neoplasms, pineoblastoma, and astrocytoma. The presence of fat is specific for teratoma, dermoid, or lipoma. Epidermoids approximate CSF in CT attenuation and MRI signal characteristics. Serum and CSF markers for β-HCG and AFP, when present, are specific for germ cell neoplasms. Contemporary approaches to treatment usually require biopsy for specific diagnosis. Therefore the most important role for imaging is to establish the presence of a pineal region mass, to characterize mass effect, hydrocephalus, local invasion, and spread along the CSF pathways.

## Suggested Reading


Atlas SW. Intraaxial brain tumors. In: Atlas SW, ed. Magnetic Resonance Imaging of the Brain and Spine. New York: Raven Press, 1991:223.

Bilaniuk LT. Adult infratentorial tumors. Semin Roentgenol 1990; 25:155–173.

Bilaniuk LT, Zimmerman RA, Littman P, et al. Computed tomography of brain stem gliomas in children. Radiology 1980; 134:89–95.

Burger PC, Vogel FS, Green SB, Strike TA. Glioblastoma multiforme and anaplastic astrocytoma. Pathologic criteria and prognostic implications. Cancer 1985; 56:1106–1111.

Coates TL, Hinshaw DB Jr, Peckman N, et al. Pediatric choroid plexus neoplasms: MR, CT, and pathologic correlation. Radiology 1989; 173:81–88.

Dean BL, Drayer BP, Bird CR, et al. Gliomas: Classification with MR imaging. Radiology 1990; 174:411–415.

Earnest F IV, Kelly PJ, Scheithauer BW, et al. Cerebral astrocytomas: Histopathologic correlation of MR and CT contrast enhancement with stereotactic biopsy. Radiology 1988; 166:823–827.

Elster AD, Arthur DW. Intracranial hemangioblastomas: CT and MR findings. J Comput Assist Tomogr 1988; 12:736–739.

Figueroa RE, Gammal TE, Brooks BS, et al. MR findings on primitive neuroectodermal tumors. J Comput Assist Tomogr 1989; 13:773–778.

Ganti SR, Hilal SK, Stein BM, et al. CT of pineal region tumors. AJR 1986; 146:451–458.

Gusnard DA. Cerebellar neoplasms in children. Semin Roentgenol 1990; 25:263–278.

Hasso AN. Posterior fossa neoplasms. In: Stark DD, Bradley WG Jr, eds. Magnetic Resonance Imaging. 2nd ed. Vol 1. St Louis: Mosby-Year Book, 1992:819.

Latchaw RE, Johnson DW, Kanal E. Metastases. In: Latchaw RE, ed. MR and CT Imaging of the Head, Neck, and Spine. 2nd ed. Vol 1. St Louis: Mosby-Year Book, 1991:597.

Latchaw RE, Johnson DW, Kanal E. Primary intracranial tumors: Neuroepithelial tumors, sarcomas, and lymphomas. In: Latchaw RE, ed. MR and CT Imaging of the Head, Neck, and Spine. 2nd ed. Vol 1. St Louis: Mosby-Year Book, 1991:449.

Latchaw RE, Johnson DW, Kanal E. Primary intracranial tumors: Tumors of congenital, pineal, and vascular origin and the phakomatoses. In: Latchaw RE, ed. MR and CT Imaging of the Head, Neck, and Spine. 2nd ed. Vol 1. St Louis: Mosby-Year Book, 1991:561.

Lee BCP, Kneeland JB, Walker RW, et al. MR imaging of brainstem tumors. Am J Neuroradiol 1985; 6:159–164.

Lee DH, Norman D, Newton TH. MR imaging of pineal cysts. J Comput Assist Tomogr 1987; 11:586–590.

Lee SR, Sanches J, Mark AS, et al. Posterior fossa hemangioblastomas: MR imaging. Radiology 1989; 171:463–468.

Lee Y-Y, Van Tassel P, Bruner JM, et al. Juvenile pilocytic astrocytomas: CT and MR characteristics. Am J Neuroradiol 1989; 10:363–370.

Lewin JS, Estes ML, Ross JS. Magnetic resonance imaging of adult intra-axial brain tumors. Top Magn Reson Imaging 1992; 4(4):17–40.

Okazaki H. Fundamentals of Neuropathology: Morphologic Basis of Neurologic Disorders. 2nd ed. New York: Igaku-Shoin, 1989.

Rollins N, Mendelsohn D, Mulne A, et al. Recurrent medulloblastoma: Frequency of tumor enhancement on Gd-DTPA MR imaging. Am J Neuroradiol 1990; 11:583–587.

Russell DS, Rubinstein LJ. Pathology of Tumors of the Nervous System. 5th ed. Baltimore: Williams & Wilkins, 1989.

Sato Y. Pediatric primary brain tumors. Top Magn Reson Imaging 1992; 4(4):64–77.

Smith RR. Brain stem tumors. Semin Roentgenol 1990; 25:249–262.

Spoto GP, Press GA, Hesselink JR, Solomon M. Intracranial ependymoma and subependymoma: MR manifestations. Am J Neuroradiol 1990; 11:83–91.

Tien RD, Barkovich AJ, Edwards MSB. MR imaging of pineal tumors. Am J Neuroradiol 1990; 11:557–565.

Zee C-S, Segall H, Apuzzo M, et al. MR imaging of pineal region neoplasms. J Comput Assist Tomogr 1991; 15:56–63.


# MRI and CT Evaluation of Intraventricular Tumors

*ANN C. PRICE, M.D. · GREGORY V. BABIGIAN, M.D.*

Intraventricular tumors comprise 10 percent of central nervous system (CNS) neoplasms. Computed tomography (CT) remains the principal modality in establishing the presence of calcifications (e.g., meningiomas, ependymomas, primitive neuroectodermal tumors [PNETs], dermoid) and acute blood. Magnetic resonance imaging (MRI) has emerged as the modality of choice in the evaluation of most CNS tumors, including those that arise within the ventricles. Lesion size, location, and extent, as well as the presence of subacute hemorrhage, are more accurately assessed by MRI. More importantly an occasional intraventricular lesion is not identified by CT (Fig. 1). This is particularly true for posterior fossa lesions, nonenhancing low-grade gliomas, and small lesions near the foramen of Monro.

Except for the CT changes of the medulloblastoma (Fig. 2) and third ventricular colloid cyst (Fig. 3), the signal intensity, attenuation, and enhancing changes of most intraventricular tumors may be nonspecific by both MRI and CT. A more accurate approach in formulating the differential diagnosis, and ultimately the correct diagnosis of intraventricular tumors, takes into consideration several factors: (1) the relative frequency of tumor occurrence, (2) its location within the

A B C D

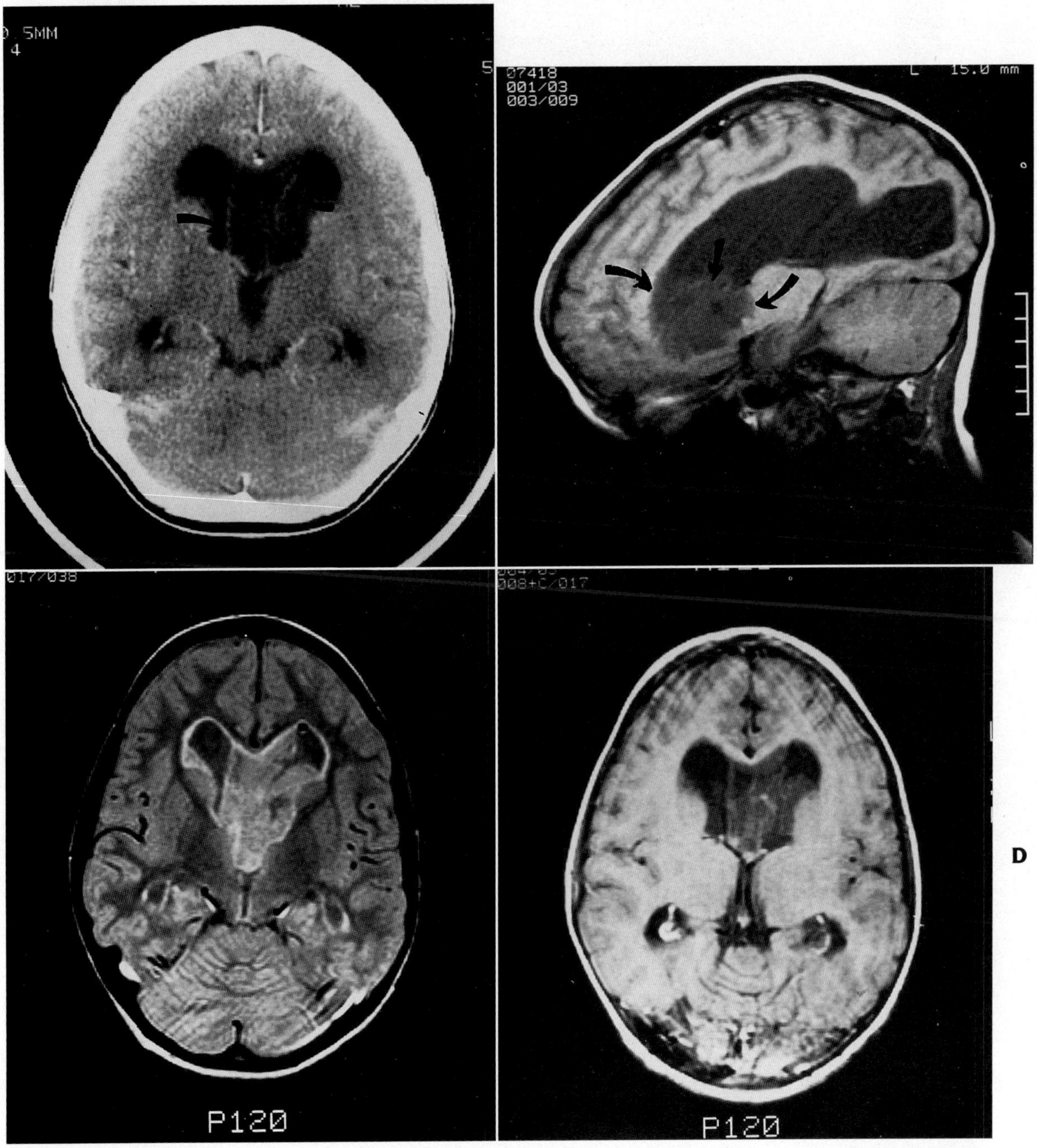


**FIGURE 1** Glioma in a 5-year-old male. *A,* Contrast-enhanced CT image shows enlargement of the lateral and anterior third ventricle. The linear densities *(arrows)* were thought to represent unusually spread leaves of the septum pellucidum. The mass was not seen. *B,* T1-weighted sagittal image (TR600, TE20) shows a large inhomogeneous mass in the left frontal horn *(arrows)*. *C,* The first echo of the T2-weighted image (TR2800, TE30) shows increase in signal intensity in the tumor and is beneficial in showing the full tumor extent into both frontal horns and into the anterior third ventricle. *D,* The low-grade glioma poorly enhances on the postcontrast T1-weighted axial image (TR600, TE20).

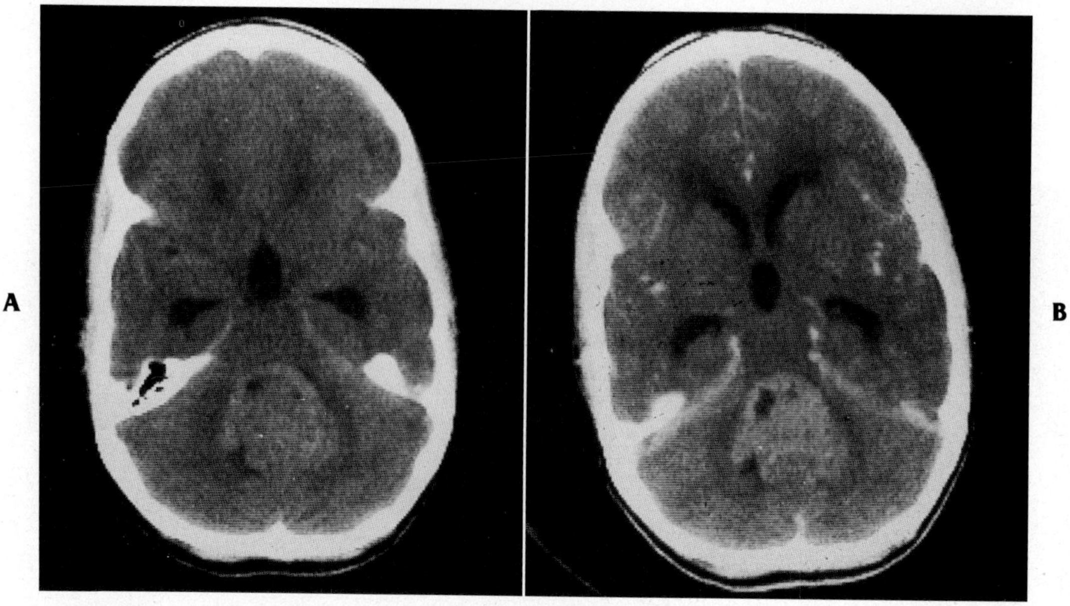


**FIGURE 2** Medulloblastoma in a 4-year-old male. *A,* A large slightly dense midline posterior fossa lesion with areas of low attenuation and heterogeneity is shown on this non–contrast-enhanced CT image. The fourth ventricle is not visualized. The dilatation of the third ventricle and temporal horns is consistent with obstructive hydrocephalus. *B,* Dense enhancement occurs on the postcontrast CT image (at a slightly higher level). The areas of heterogeneity are better defined.

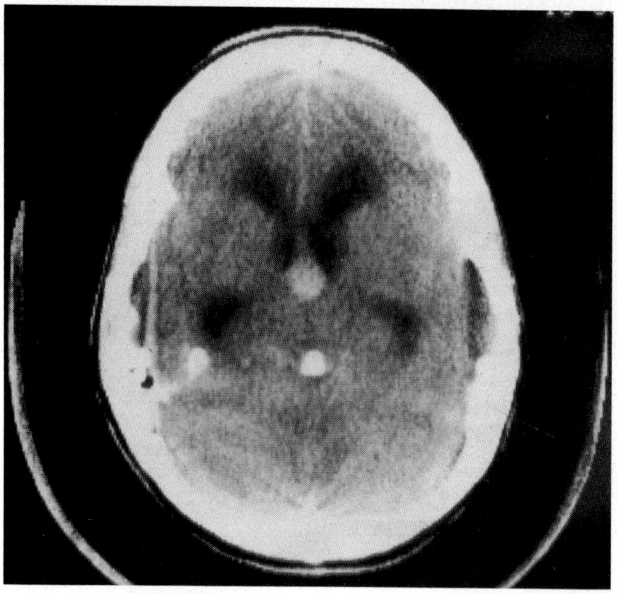

**FIGURE 3** Colloid cyst in a 25-year-old female. A 10 mm hyperdense lesion is present at the foramen of Monro. This did not enhance. There is mild-to-moderate obstructive hydrocephalus. Just posterior in the midline is a slightly prominent calcified pineal.

ventricular system, and (3) the age and sex of the patient.

To initiate this system of differential diagnosis, it is easiest to first divide the ages into broad categories: (1) childhood (0 to 15 years), (2) late childhood to early adult (15 to 30 years), and (3) adult (>30 years). The ages are not absolute but are designated as guidelines. By virtue of the variability inherent in medicine, some overlap in age groups may occur. The aim is to suggest the most likely tumor pathology that occurs in a given intraventricular location for the patient's age and sex. Only the most common diagnostic possibilities are considered in this chapter (Fig. 4), with additional differential possibilities listed in Table 1.

## Clinical Presentation

Because of their location, intraventricular tumors may obstruct the flow of cerebrospinal fluid (CSF), which almost uniformly results in headaches. When the obstruction is sufficiently severe, nausea and vomiting may occur. Other symptoms depend on the location so that posterior fossa tumors may be accompanied by ataxia. If the tumor has a stalk, as is frequent with the colloid cyst (Fig. 3), then the headache may be positional due to intermittent foraminal obstruction when the patient bends, stoops, or coughs.

Clinical detection in infancy or early childhood may be challenging as a result of the subtle clinical presentation of increasing head size, bulging fontanelle, or vomiting. Because of the deep midline position, and often associated massive hydrocephalus, surgery may be difficult. The outcome may be guarded because of these factors and because many intraventricular tumors result in drop metastases or spread via CSF pathways.

### *Fourth Ventricle*

The most common intraventricular tumors occur in the pediatric age group below the tentorium. These include the ependymoma (Fig. 5) and medulloblastoma (Fig. 6). The ependymoma arises within the ependymal lining of the ventricle, whereas the medulloblastoma arises in the cerebellar vermis or less commonly in the cerebellar hemisphere. A more lateral origin in the cerebellar hemisphere occurs in slightly older children.

Both the medulloblastoma and ependymoma are more

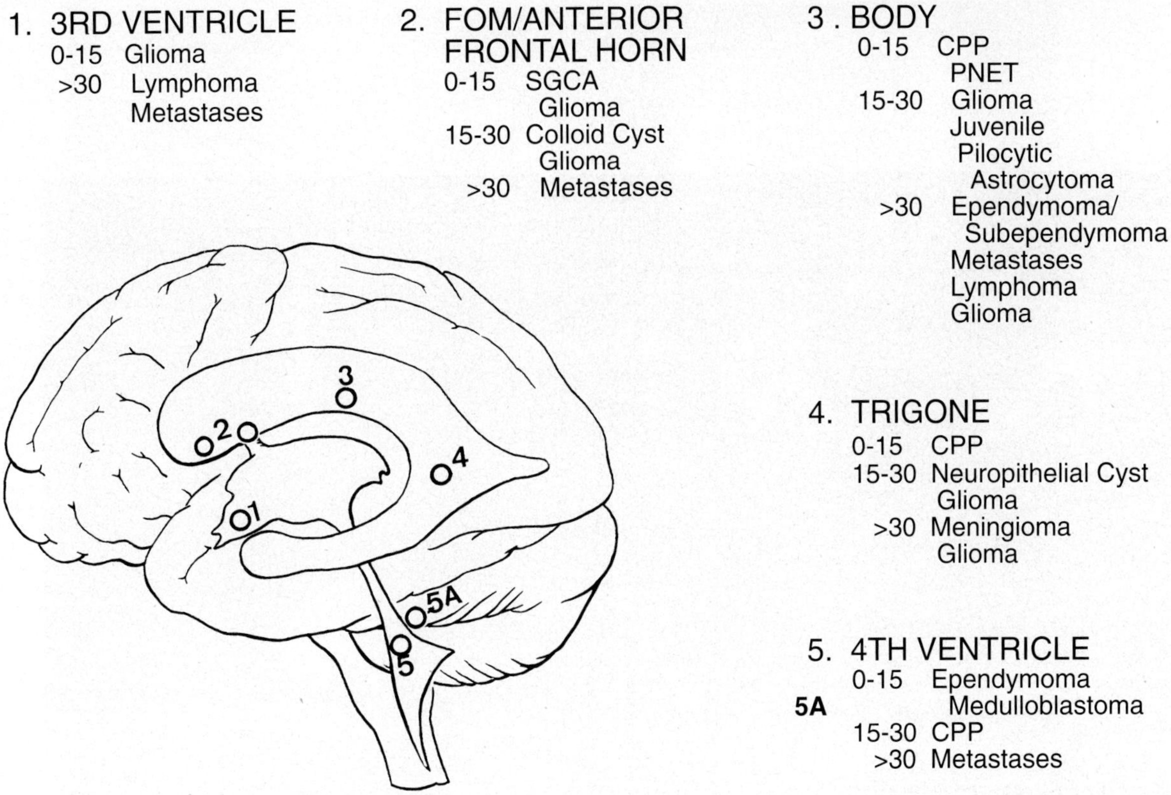


**FIGURE 4** Schematic representation of the most common tumors for age and location. CPP = choroid plexus papilloma; FOM = foramen of Monro; PNET = primitive neuroectodermal tumor; SGCA = subependymal giant cell astrocytoma. (Adapted from Jelinek J, Smirniotopoulos JG, et al. Lateral ventricular neoplasms of the brain: Differential diagnosis based on clinical CT and MR findings. AJR 1990; 155:365; with permission.)

**TABLE 1** Intraventricular Tumors

| | Age Group | | |
|---|---|---|---|
| Location | 0–15 Years | 15–30 Years | > 30 Years |
| 4th ventricle | Medulloblastoma<br>Ependymoma<br>Glioma* | CPP<br>Metastases<br>Epidermoid/dermoid* | Metastases<br>Meningioma |
| Lateral ventricle | | | |
| Trigone | CPP<br>Glioma*<br>Metastases | Glioma<br>Ependymoma*<br>Metastases* | Meningioma<br>Glioma<br>Metastases* |
| Body | PNET<br>Choroid plexus cyst<br>Glioma* | Neuroepithelial cyst<br>Ependymoma | Metastases<br>Lymphoma<br>Glioma/GBM<br>Ependymoma/<br>Subependymoma |
| Foramen of Monro–anterior frontal horn | Glioma<br>SGCA<br>CPP* | Colloid cyst<br>SGCA<br>Glioma/pilocytic<br>Astrocytoma | Metastases<br>Meningioma |

CPP = choroid plexus papilloma; GBM = glioblastoma multiforme; SGCA = subependymal giant cell astrocytoma.
*Indicates less frequent occurrence.
Adapted from Jelinek J, Smirniotopoulos JG, et al. Lateral ventricular neoplasms of the brain: Differential diagnosis based on clinical CT and MR findings. AJR 1990; 155:365–372; with permission.

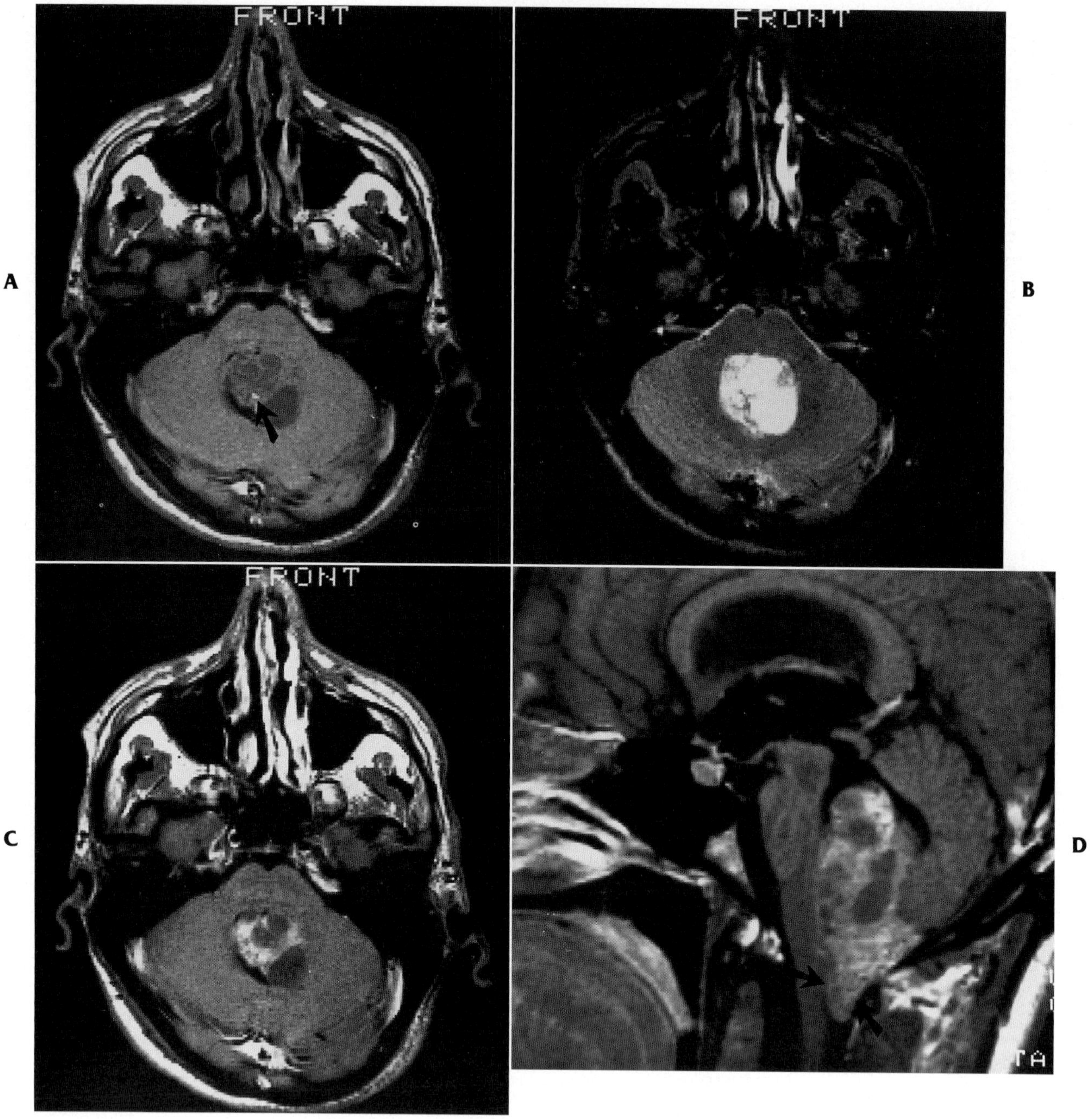


**FIGURE 5** Ependymoma in an 8-year-old male. *A,* Axial T1-weighted MR image (TR700, TE17) shows a mixed solid and cystic lesion, with a tiny dotlike area *(arrow)* of increased signal intensity that is thought to represent subacute hemorrhage. *B,* The second echo of the T2-weighted image (TR3000, TE90) shows mottled increase in signal intensity. *C,* Moderately intense mottled enhancement is demonstrated on the postcontrast axial T1-weighted image. *D,* On the sagittal postcontrast T1-weighted image, the tumor appears much larger, with extension through the foramen of Magendie into the upper cervical spine *(arrows).* (Courtesy of Fred Laine, M.D., Medical College of Virginia.)

A B

C D

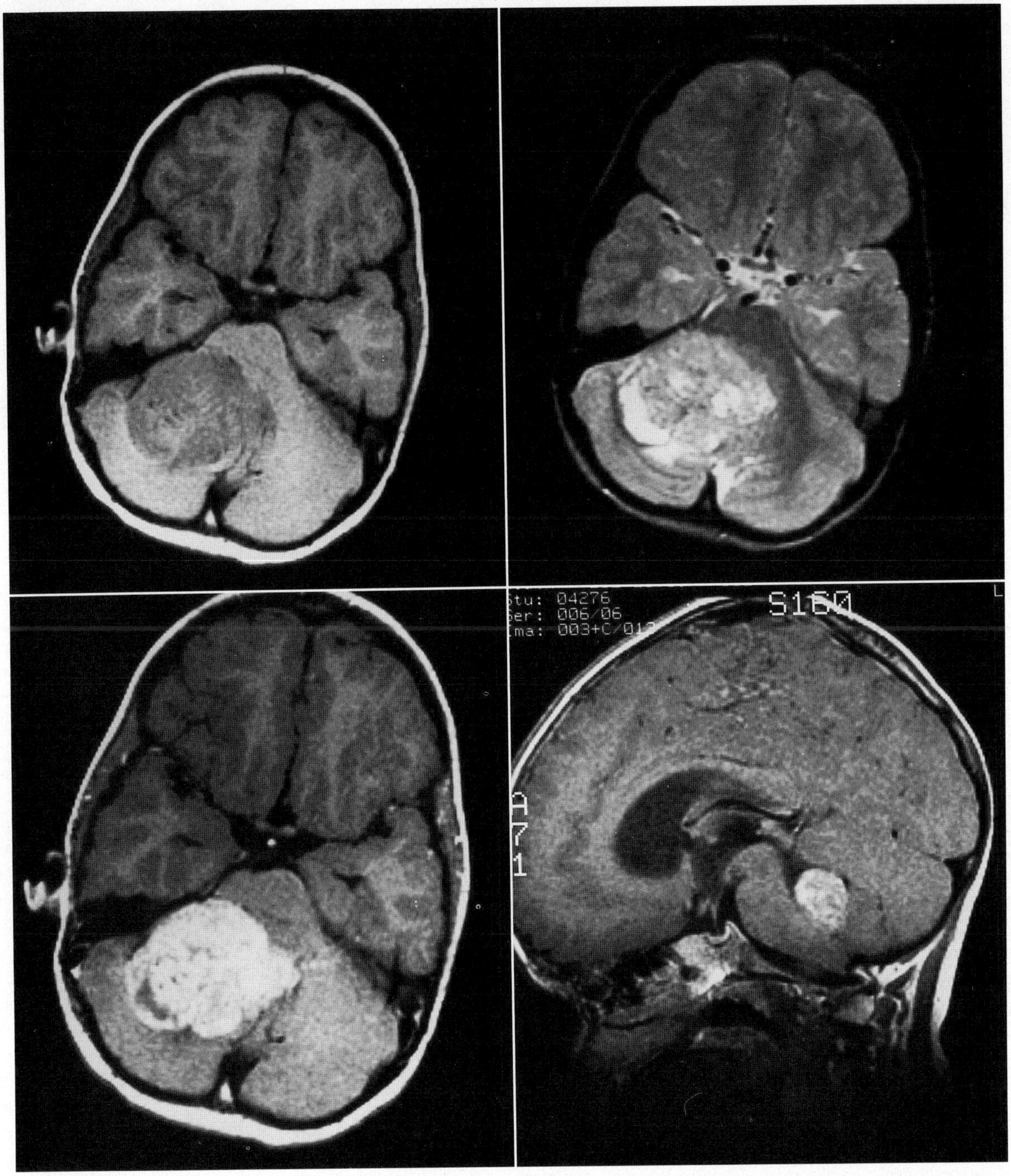

**FIGURE 6** Medulloblastoma in a 3-year-old male. *A,* T1-weighted axial images (TR600, TE20) show a mottled low signal intensity mass within the fourth ventricle, extending laterally toward the right CP angle. *B,* Mottled increase in signal intensity is noted on the second echo of the T2-weighted images (TR2800, TE80). *C,* Intense tumor enhancement occurs after contrast administration on the T1-weighted axial image (TR600, TE20). *D,* Postcontrast sagittal T1-weighted image confirms the intraventricular position of a portion of the tumor but fails to show extension through the adjacent foramina.

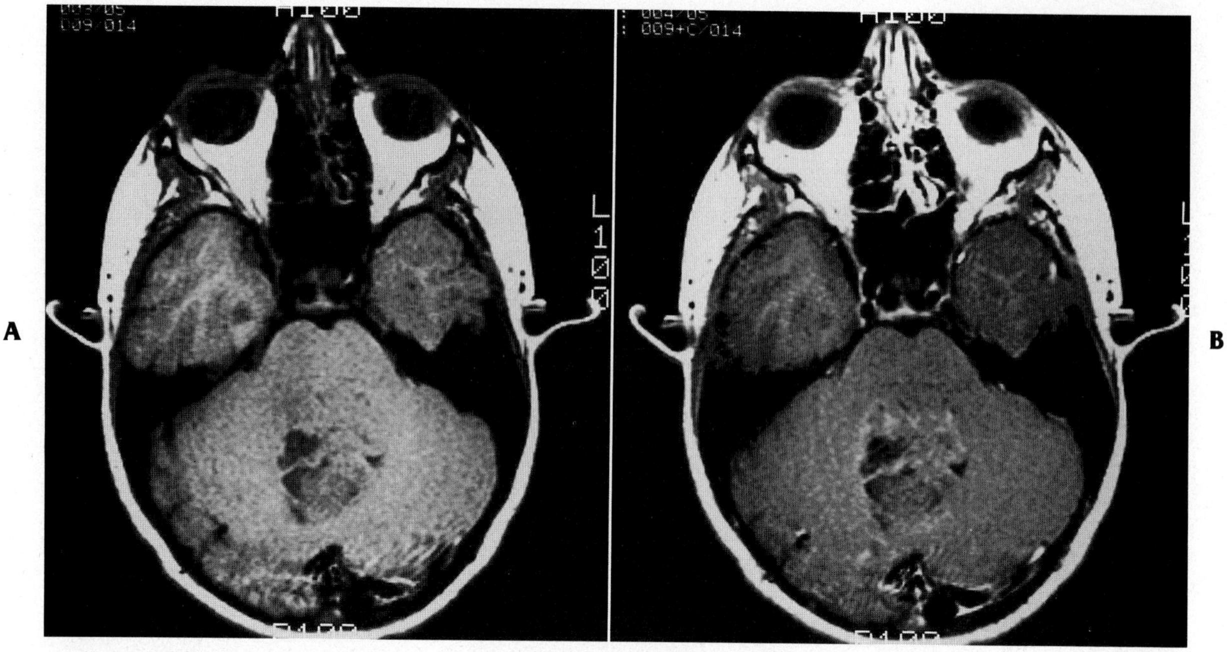

**FIGURE 7** Medulloblastoma in a 3-year-old male. *A,* On the T1-weighted axial image (TR600, TE20), the tumor has a mixed cystic and solid appearance similar to the ependymoma in Figure 5, *A. B,* Postcontrast T1-weighted axial image shows only minimal en-hancement.

common in male children. Since the medulloblastoma lies within the ventricle at the time of clinical presentation, it is included with intraventricular tumors. As previously noted, the medulloblastoma has a more characteristic appearance by CT (see Fig. 2). By MRI, the ependymoma and medulloblastoma may be indistinguishable by virtue of their signal intensity changes (Figs. 5, 6, and 7). There are several major MRI differential points between the two tumors:

1. Ependymomas tend to extend or ooze through adjacent foramina and may present in the CP angle and/or upper cervical spine (see Fig. 5, *D*).
2. Medulloblastomas show variable enhancement with up to 50 percent showing mild-to-intermediate enhancement (see Fig. 7).
3. Medulloblastomas are more common, comprising 25 percent of childhood tumors, whereas ependymomas comprise 10 percent of tumors in this same age group.
4. Calcifications occur in 50 percent of ependymomas, whereas medulloblastomas infrequently calcify (15 to 20 percent).

Therefore if a fourth ventricular mass is demonstrated in a young male patient, statistically it is more apt to be a medulloblastoma. Neither the medulloblastoma nor ependymoma has a good prognosis because of its potential for drop metastases or spread via the CSF (Fig. 8).

Since medulloblastomas arise from more primitive cells of the neuroectoderm, they are classified as PNETs. Most PNETs present in infants less than 1 year of age, and because of this have become known as "peanut" tumors. They may occur in the fourth ventricle but are usually larger and more aggressive appearing and may be calcified and hemorrhagic.

Other differential diagnoses include astrocytomas that arise from the brain stem or cerebellum and present within the ventricle. Both the astrocytomas and PNETs show no sex predilection. The origin of the astrocytoma, whether arising in the brain stem or cerebellum, is not as difficult to determine as with the medulloblastoma. Metastases are also part of the differential diagnosis, and these are discussed in the next section.

## Metastases

Intraventricular metastases are rare but may occur in any portion of the ventricular system (Figs. 8 and 9). Metastases may be direct or hematogenous. Direct spread usually occurs in tumors that arise within or adjacent to the ventricle. In young patients, these include the ependymoma, medulloblastoma, and pineal region tumors. Although spread may occur above the tentorium (see Fig. 8, *B*), they usually seed more distally into the spinal canal. Similar to the primary medulloblastoma, some drop metastases from this tumor also do not enhance densely (see Fig. 8, *B*). Therefore careful scrutiny may be required in the evaluation of these lesions regarding the necessity of myelography for spinal drop metastases. The development of gadoteridol (ProHance), a new nonionic contrast agent (E. R. Squibb & Sons, Princeton, NJ) that allows double-dose contrast injections, may prove effective in enhancing these lesions.

Most intraventricular metastatic lesions, except those previously mentioned, occur in older age groups and spread directly from primary brain tumors such as the glioblastoma multiforme (Fig. 9). Hematogenous subependymal metastases may occur in tumors of the lung and breast as well as in leukemia and lymphoma. Further subependymal growth results in spread into the ventricle followed by peripheral seeding.

MRI characteristics are nonspecific. With the exception of

A 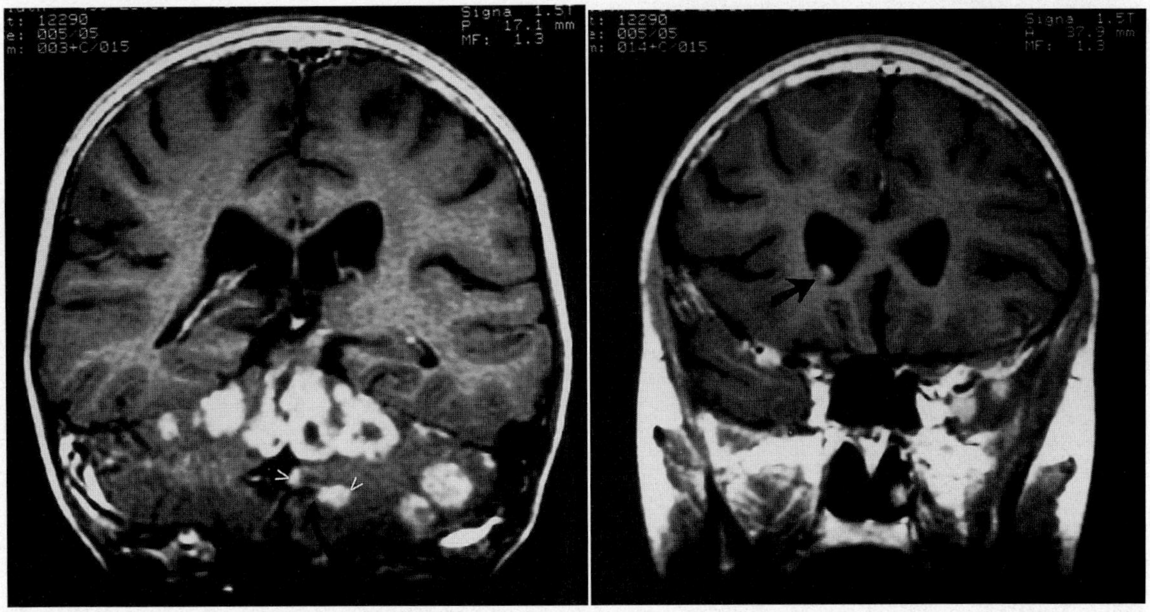 B

**FIGURE 8** Metastatic medulloblastoma in a 7-year-old male. *A,* Multiple enhancing lesions are shown on the postcontrast T1-weighted coronal image (TR600, TE20). Most of these are confluent about the tentorium and densely enhance. The intraventricular enhancement could represent either a recurrence or residual *(arrow). B,* A more anterior section from the same sequence shows a less densely enhancing intraventricular metastasis *(arrow).* A larger more densely enhancing lesion is shown in the right Sylvian fissure.

the medulloblastoma, most metastases enhance rather densely. Coronal or sagittal views may be necessary, since metastatic lesions may drop into the most dependent portions of an enlarged ventricle and simulate a parenchymal lesion (Fig. 9).

As with all posterior fossa neoplasms in the elderly, metastases should be high on the list of differential diagnostic possibilities. Regardless of age, a history of primary neoplastic disease is usually the key factor in diagnosis.

### Choroid Plexus Papilloma

Choroid plexus papillomas (CPPs) that occur below the tentorium usually present in the late teenage and early adult years. In contradistinction to the male preponderance in the childhood variety, there is no sex predilection in the infratentorial tumor (Fig. 10). The signal intensity change by MRI is nonspecific. Enhancement with a contrast agent is usually dense.

Similar to ependymomas, CPPs extend through the foramina and may appear in the CP angle or at the craniovertebral junction. It is these features and the age group that suggest the correct diagnosis. Distal seeding may occur despite the benign nature of this tumor.

Differential diagnosis includes ependymoma, which occurs in a younger male population. Meningiomas generally are more densely enhancing tumors that occur in an older age group, but less commonly in the fourth ventricle.

## *Atrium or Trigone of Lateral Ventricle*

### Choroid Plexus Papilloma

Lateral ventricular lesions that occur in childhood are usually CPPs. These are most frequently encountered in the first decade of life, especially below 2 years of age. There is a slight male and left ventricular predilection. CPPs are usually large at the time of presentation because of the patient's youth and relative lack of clinical symptoms (e.g., increasing head size, bulging fontanelles, vomiting). Massive asymmetric hydrocephalus is attributed to a combination of ventricular outlet obstruction and overproduction of CSF (Fig. 11).

Necrosis is common due to rapid tumor enlargement. Hemorrhage of varying stages and calcifications (24 percent) may be present. This highly vascular tumor has several characteristic MRI features: (1) low signal intensity vascular pedicle (Fig. 11, *D* and *E*), (2) large bulky mottled mass, (3) massive asymmetric hydrocephalus (Fig. 11, *B*), and (4) dense contrast enhancement (Fig. 11, *C*).

The prognosis is usually guarded because of the difficulty of surgical removal of such a large tumor. Therefore early diagnosis is crucial if brain damage from hydrocephalus is to be avoided.

Choroid plexus carcinomas display imaging characteristics similar to their benign counterpart. A differentiating feature is the extraventricular extension with greater white matter change. MRI is the most accurate imaging modality in the assessment of the malignant form of this tumor.

### Meningioma

Statistically a densely enhancing calcified tumor located in the atrium of the lateral ventricle of a middle-aged female is most likely a meningioma (Fig. 12). Despite the superior demonstration of calcifications by CT, MRI is preferred for tumor delineation and surgical planning. These tumors are usually large, fairly well-defined, lobulated, with a mottled internal architecture (Fig. 12). The mottling is attributed to calcifications and vascularity. Taking advantage of its greater magnetic susceptibility, gradient-echo imaging has been used to demonstrate calcifications by MRI. Although more sensitive, the changes are less specific as compared with CT.

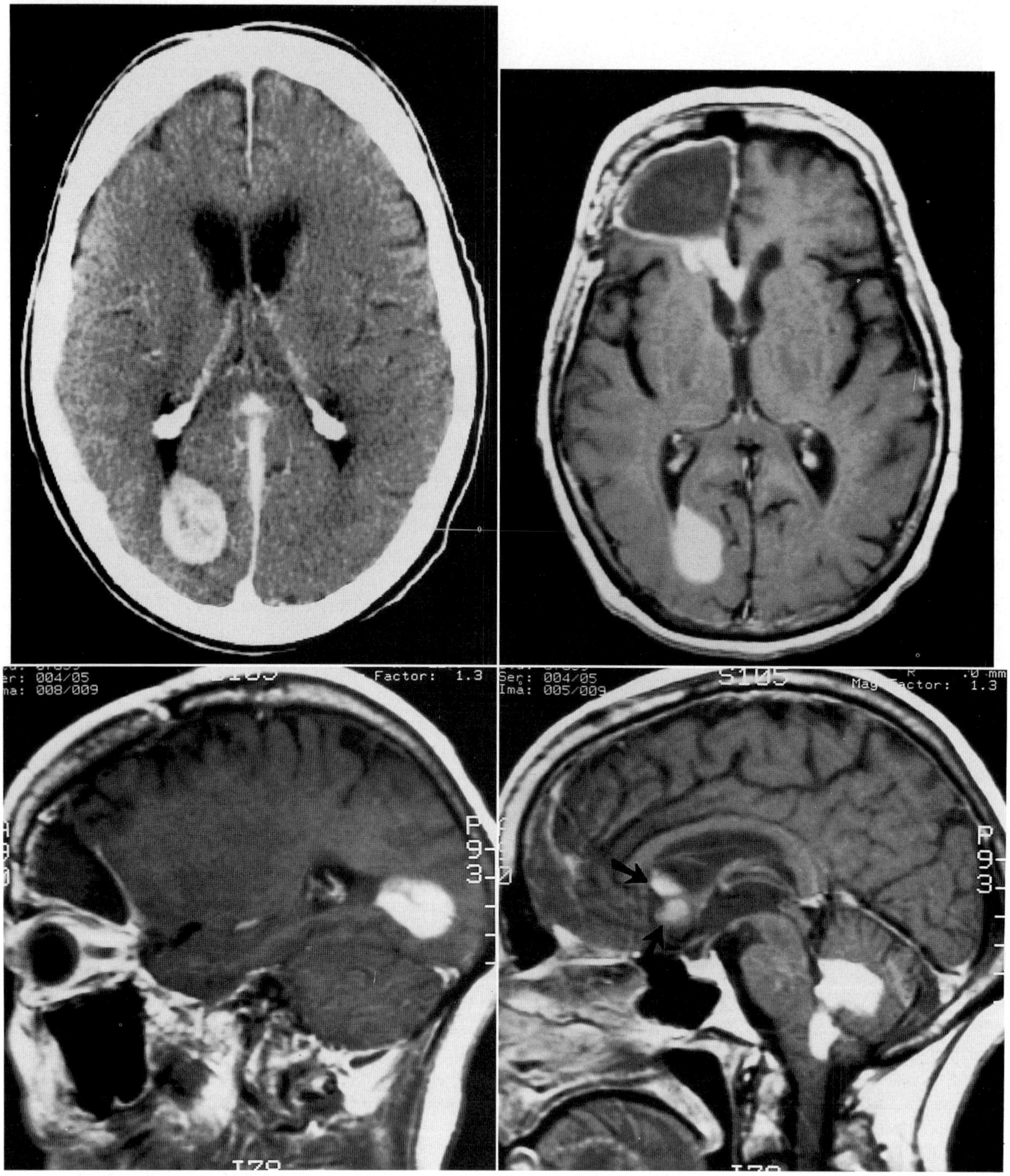


**FIGURE 9** Metastatic glioblastoma multiforme in a 60-year-old female. *A,* A rounded enhancing lesion is noted in the right occipital region on the contrast-enhanced CT image. Localizing this lesion within the ventricle is not possible. *B,* Postcontrast T1-weighted axial image (TR600, TE20) demonstrates postoperative right frontal changes with rim enhancement. The dense enhancement at the posterior surgical margin is both subependymal and extending across the corpus callosum. The position of the occipital lesion is not clearly localized. *C,* Sagittal postcontrast T1-weighted study (TR600, TE20) clearly localizes the metastasis to the occipital horn. *D,* Midline sagittal postcontrast study shows a greater extent of fourth ventricular involvement than the axial CT scan or MRI. The anterior metastases *(arrows)* are not as clearly localized as with the axial images.

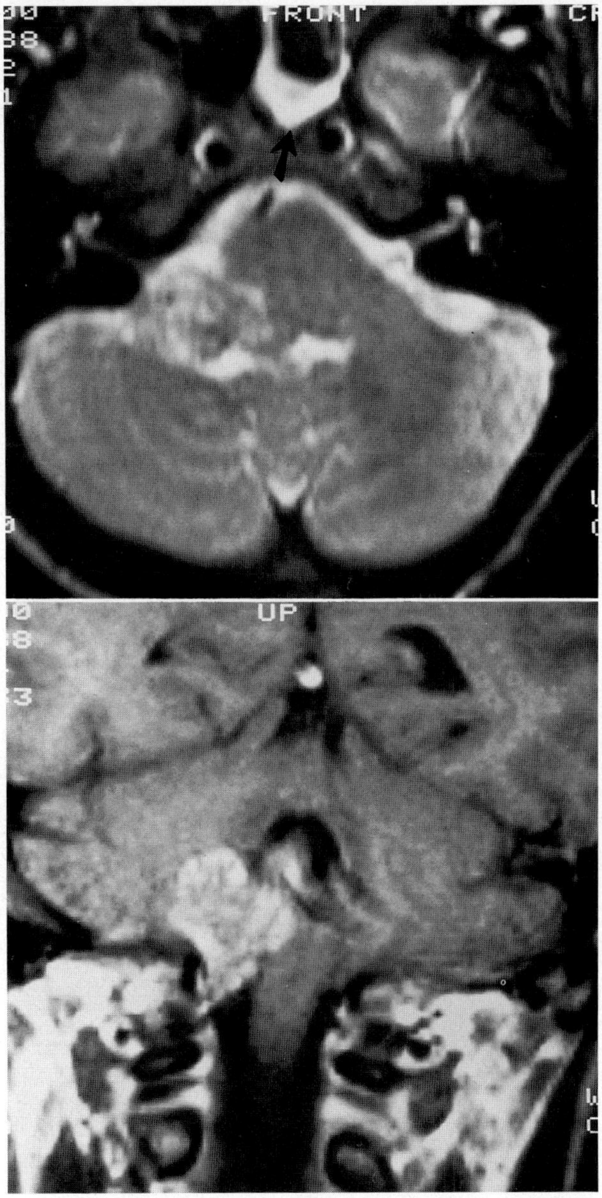


**FIGURE 10** Choroid plexus papilloma in a 19-year-old female. *A,* The second echo of the T2-weighted images (TR300, TE90) shows a heterogeneous signal intensity mass in the right CP angle, which was a heterogeneous isohypointense mass on the T1-weighted image (not shown). Note the sphenoid sinusitis *(arrow)*. *B,* Postcontrast coronal T1-weighted study (TR700, TE17) shows a moderately enhancing lesion extending from the fourth ventricle into the CP angle. The intraventricular component is more accurately demonstrated.

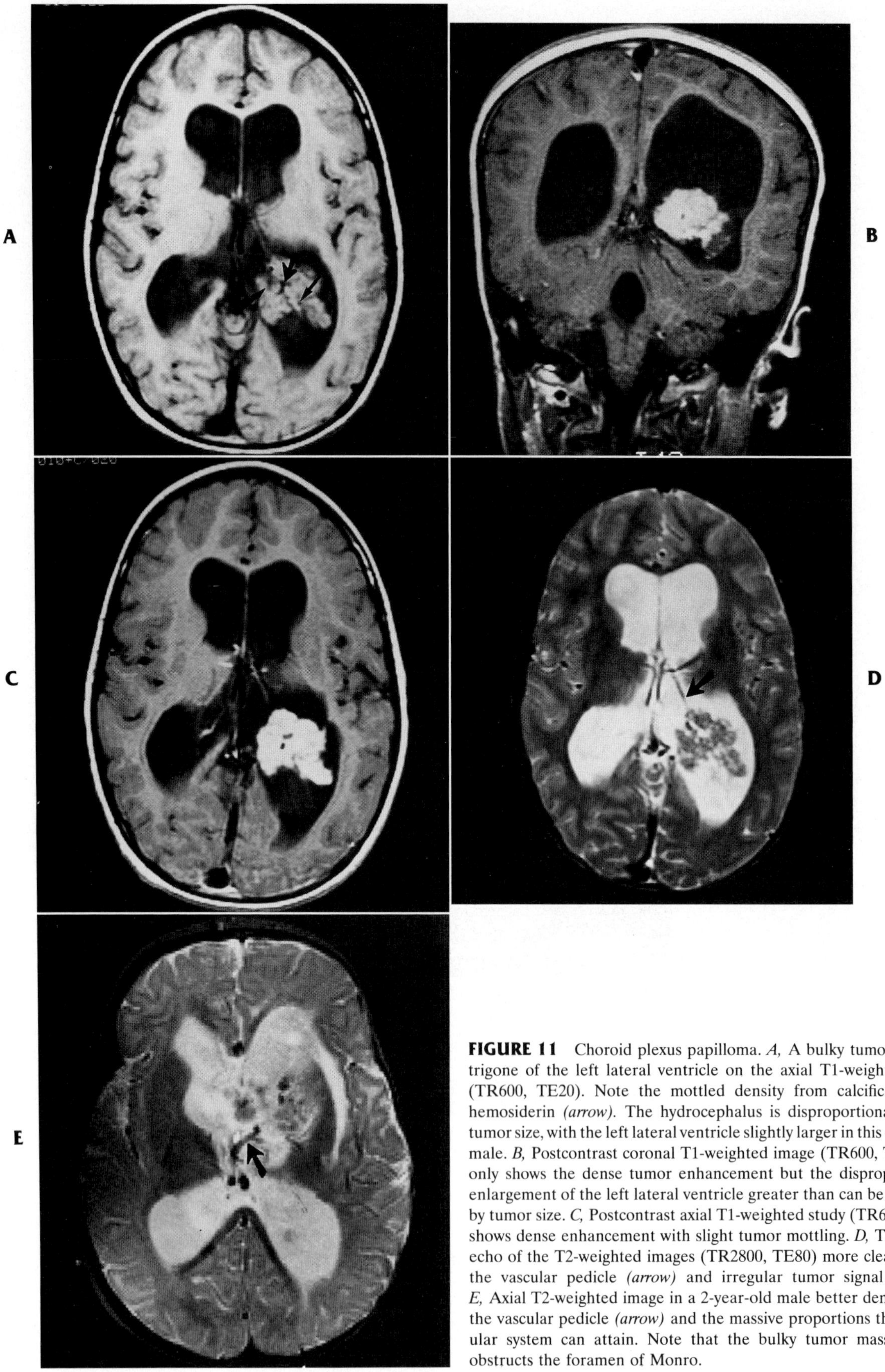

**FIGURE 11** Choroid plexus papilloma. *A,* A bulky tumor is in the trigone of the left lateral ventricle on the axial T1-weighted image (TR600, TE20). Note the mottled density from calcification and hemosiderin *(arrow).* The hydrocephalus is disproportionate to the tumor size, with the left lateral ventricle slightly larger in this 4-year-old male. *B,* Postcontrast coronal T1-weighted image (TR600, TE20) not only shows the dense tumor enhancement but the disproportionate enlargement of the left lateral ventricle greater than can be explained by tumor size. *C,* Postcontrast axial T1-weighted study (TR600, TE20) shows dense enhancement with slight tumor mottling. *D,* The second echo of the T2-weighted images (TR2800, TE80) more clearly shows the vascular pedicle *(arrow)* and irregular tumor signal intensity. *E,* Axial T2-weighted image in a 2-year-old male better demonstrates the vascular pedicle *(arrow)* and the massive proportions the ventricular system can attain. Note that the bulky tumor mass partially obstructs the foramen of Monro.

A B C

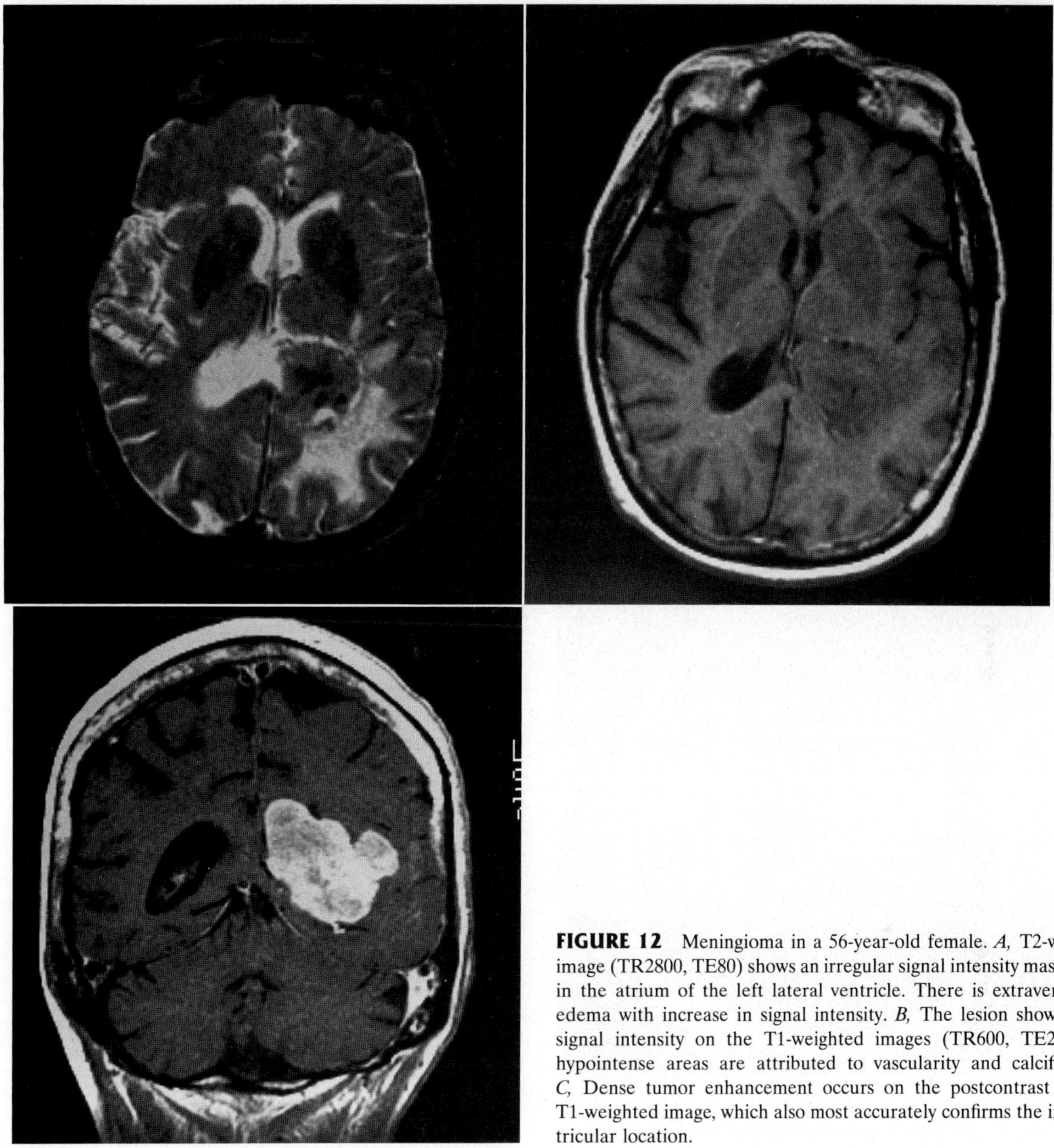

**FIGURE 12** Meningioma in a 56-year-old female. *A,* T2-weighted image (TR2800, TE80) shows an irregular signal intensity mass arising in the atrium of the left lateral ventricle. There is extraventricular edema with increase in signal intensity. *B,* The lesion shows mixed signal intensity on the T1-weighted images (TR600, TE20). The hypointense areas are attributed to vascularity and calcifications. *C,* Dense tumor enhancement occurs on the postcontrast coronal T1-weighted image, which also most accurately confirms the intraventricular location.

Meningiomas are among the most densely enhancing tumors due to the lack of a blood-brain barrier. Other than this, perhaps, its most distinctive feature is the wide spectrum of signal intensity changes on both T1- and T2-weighted images, varying from hypointense to hyperintense. Few if any other tumors show such a wide range of signal intensity change. This has been related to the tumor subtype.

In neurofibromatosis, meningiomas may be multiple, present in younger age groups, may occur in any portion of the ventricular system, and show no sex predilection (Fig. 13). The prognosis is good; however, recurrence is possible if tumor excision is incomplete.

### Other Differential Possibilities

Other lesions that can arise from the atrium of the lateral ventricle are the glioma and ependymoma. These more commonly arise in the middle-age category between the age groups affected by the more frequently occurring choroid plexus papilloma and meningioma. These are more fully discussed with tumors of the body of the lateral ventricle, since the imaging changes are the same.

## *Body of Lateral Ventricle*

### Ependymoma

Ependymomas in the supratentorial ventricular system occur in the adult years. These more commonly arise in the anterior body of the lateral ventricle. As the tumor grows, it may extend through the septum pellucidum into the contralateral ventricle. With anterior growth, the foramen of Monro is obstructed and the resulting hydrocephalus asymmetric. Similar to the infratentorial tumor, calcifications are common. The imaging features are similar to the infratentorial tumor.

Some supratentorial ependymomas may have a combina-

A B C

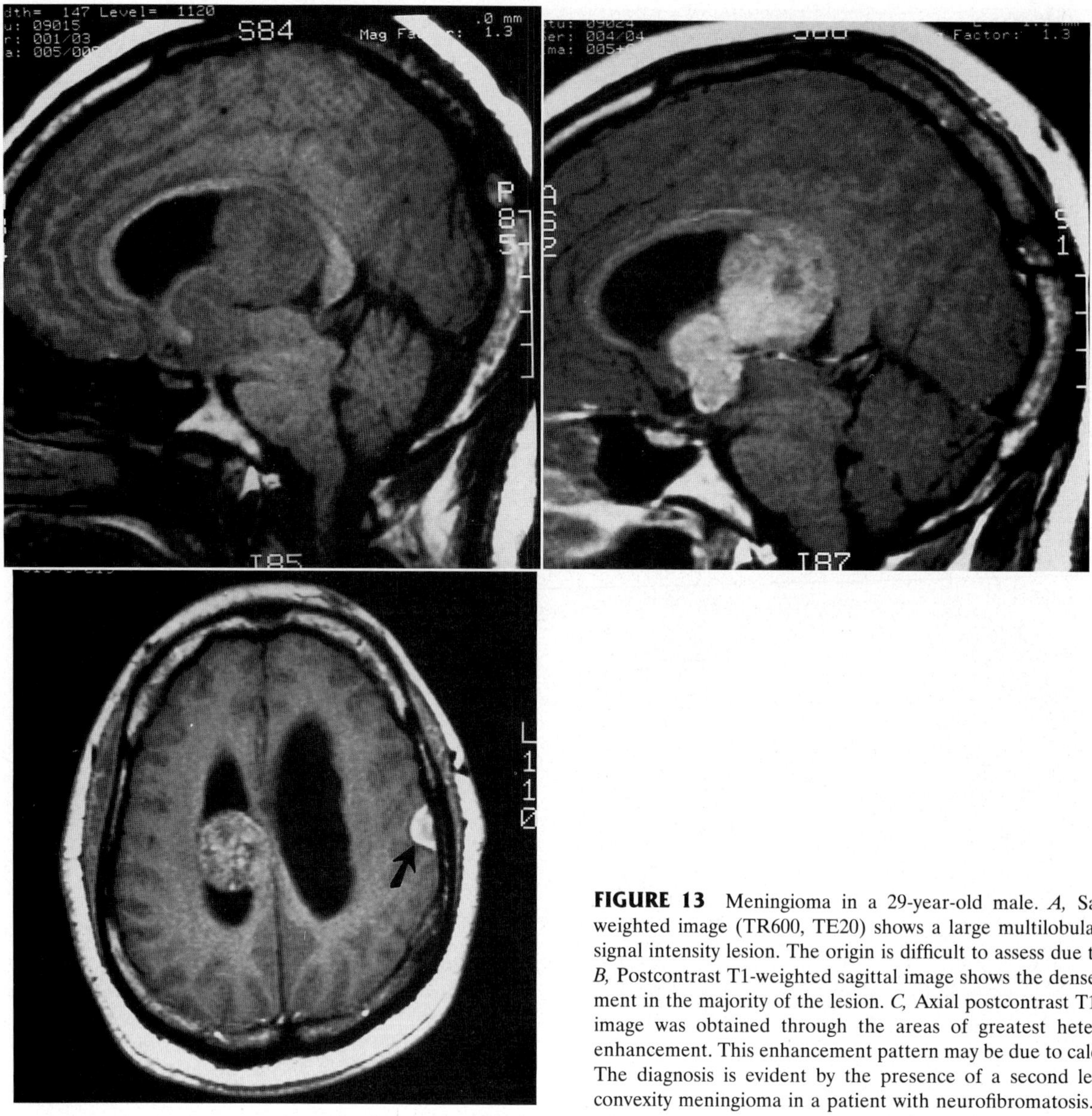

**FIGURE 13** Meningioma in a 29-year-old male. *A,* Sagittal T1-weighted image (TR600, TE20) shows a large multilobulated mixed signal intensity lesion. The origin is difficult to assess due to the size. *B,* Postcontrast T1-weighted sagittal image shows the dense enhancement in the majority of the lesion. *C,* Axial postcontrast T1-weighted image was obtained through the areas of greatest heterogeneous enhancement. This enhancement pattern may be due to calcifications. The diagnosis is evident by the presence of a second left parietal convexity meningioma in a patient with neurofibromatosis.

tion of extraventricular and intraventricular components or may be extraventricular, arising from ependymal cell rests in the white matter adjacent to the ventricles.

The subependymoma is the benign counterpart of this tumor and is a solid subependymal mass that extends into the ventricle. The age group affected and the MRI changes are such that these are distinguishable only by histological evaluation. Some subependymomas do not enhance by CT.

### Glioma

Gliomas may occur in any portion of the ventricular system and vary from low-grade lesions to glioblastoma multiforme. Whereas in the older patient gliomas tend to occur in the trigone body of the lateral ventricle, in younger patients they generally occur in the frontal horn–foramen of Monro region (see Fig. 1).

Calcifications may occur in the lower-grade tumor, resulting in tumor mottling. Otherwise the appearance is nonspecific. Enhancement is variable but is generally greater with higher-grade tumor pathologies. Enhancement, even when minimal, is more easily diagnosed by MRI.

Because of the lack of enhancement and smaller size of some of the tumors near the foramen of Monro, the only finding may be lateral ventricular enlargement (see Fig. 1). A basic and important principle is: If there is isolated symmetrical enlargement of the lateral ventricles without concomitant enlargement of the remainder of the ventricular system, a lesion at the foramen of Monro must be excluded.

## *Frontal Horns and Foramen of Monro*

### Glioma

Gliomas in this region occur in the childhood years (see Fig. 1). These are as described in the preceding section.

### Subependymal Giant Cell Astrocytoma

Subependymal giant cell astrocytomas are slow-growing tumors thought to result from degeneration of subependymal tubers or hamartomas in patients with tuberous sclerosis, a dominantly inherited genetic disorder with a variable pene-

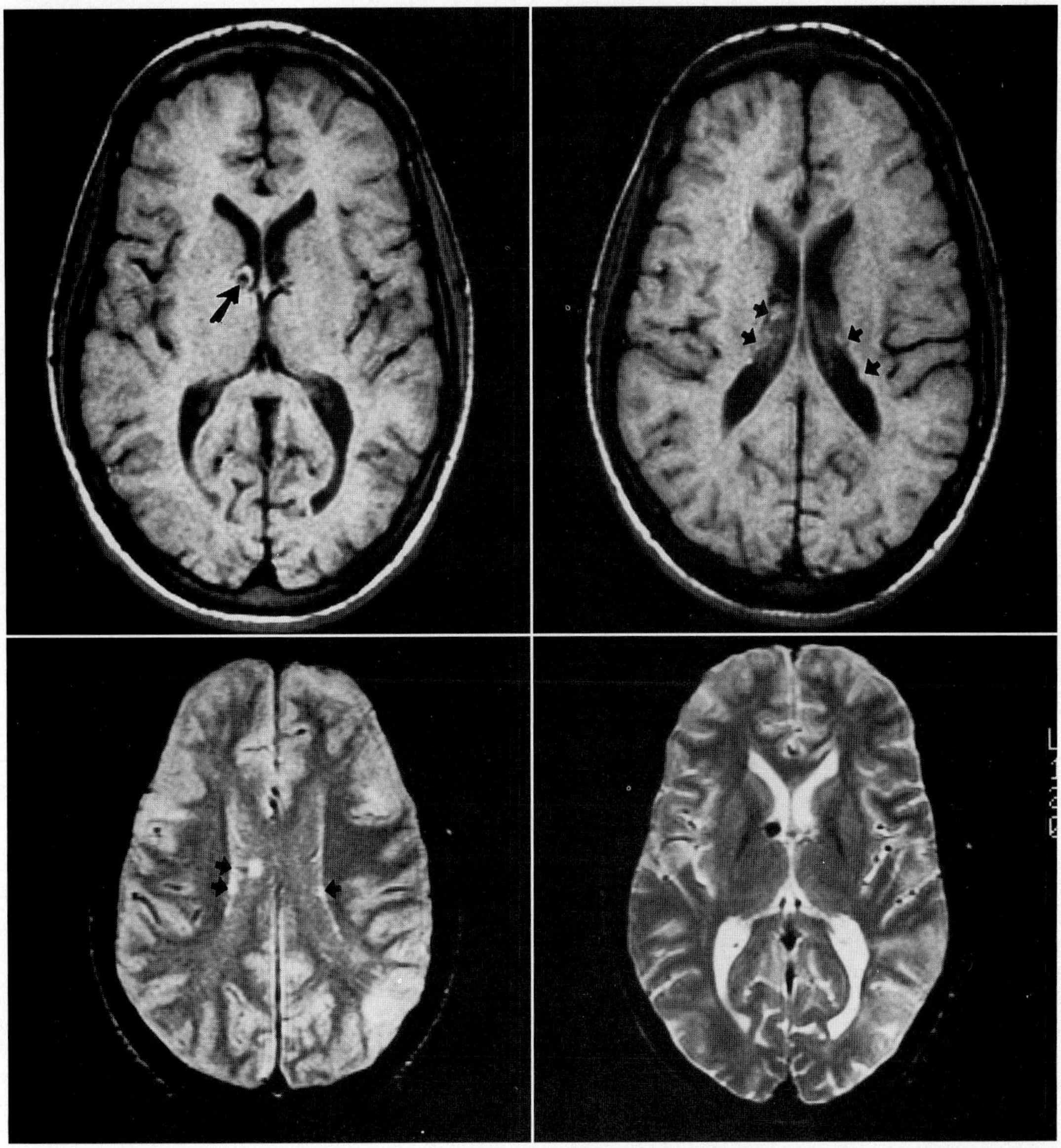

**FIGURE 14** Tuberous sclerosis in a 24-year-old male. *A,* T1-weighted axial image (TR600, TE20) shows a slightly intense subependymal hamartoma in the right frontal horn *(arrow).* The central area of diminished signal intensity is attributed to calcification. *B,* T1-weighted image from the same study at a slightly higher level shows multiple isointense to slightly hyperintense nodules *(arrows). C,* On the first echo of the T2-weighted sequence (TR2800, TE30) obtained at the same level, the nodules show increase in signal intensity *(arrows). D,* T2-weighted image at the level of *(A)* shows the right frontal calcifications as prominent areas of diminished signal intensity.

*Continued.*

trance. Since this is a genetically linked abnormality, the presentation can span the childhood and early adult years.

The calcifications that occur in the subependymal tubers are better depicted by CT; however, the subependymal location and coexistent cortical hamartomas are more readily diagnosed by MRI (Fig. 14). Because of the ease in diagnosis of the hamartomas, MRI is considered the modality of choice in screening apparently asymptomatic (forme fruste) members of families with tuberous sclerosis.

The MRI appearance of tuberous sclerosis is fairly characteristic, with small variable-density soft-tissue nodules with hypointense centers on T1-weighted images (Fig. 14, *A*). The tubers are more common in the frontal horn and anterior body of the lateral ventricles. Those that are not heavily calcified are better demonstrated on the first than the second echo of the T2-weighted images as areas of increase in signal intensity (Fig. 14, *C*). Those with heavy calcifications are visualized as areas of diminished signal intensity (Fig. 14, *D*). The cortical hamartomas are amorphous areas of increase in signal intensity on the T2-weighted images (Fig. 14, *E*).

Some tubers enhance after administration of contrast material (Fig. 14, *F* and *G*). Large or enlarging enhancing tubers in the frontal horn region are suspicious for a giant cell astrocytoma (Fig. 14, *G*).

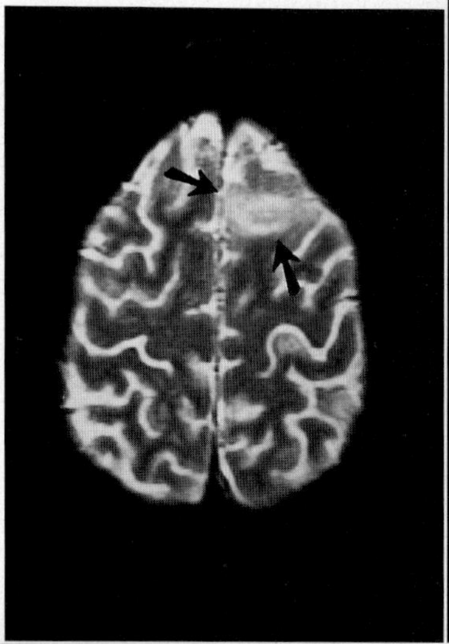

E

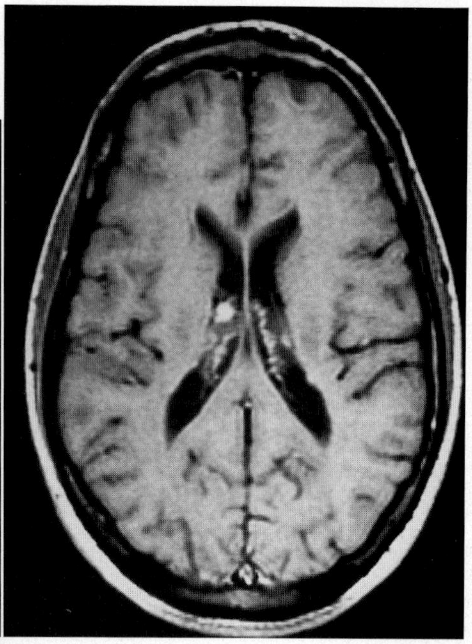

F

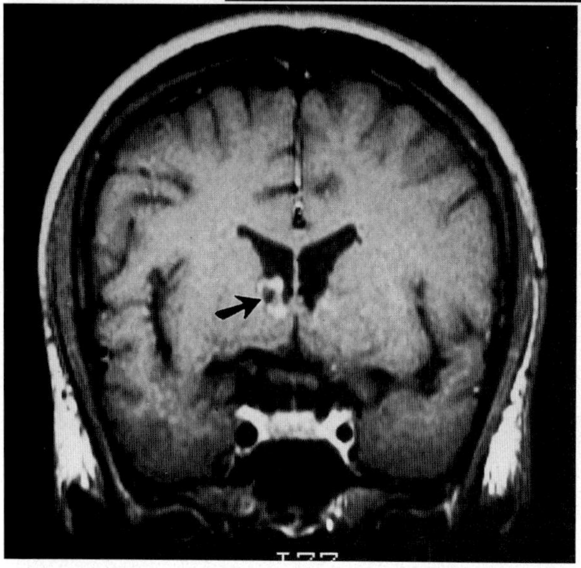

G

**FIGURE 14, cont'd** *E,* An amorphous area of increase in signal intensity is at the parietal convexity on the second echo of the T2-weighted images. This is consistent with a cortical hamartoma *(arrows). F,* Several of the nodules in the body of the lateral ventricle enhance on the postcontrast T1-weighted image. *G,* The largest nodule with the greatest enhancement is in the right frontal horn *(arrow).* This should be further observed for the occurrence of a giant cell astrocytoma.

## Colloid Cyst

The colloid cyst of the third ventricle is the most common mass to arise in this region. It is benign and congenital, arising from the neuroepithelium of the anterosuperior third ventricle. A thick fibrous capsule surrounds the epithelial lining. This lining produces a mucoid matrix and enlarges by secretory desquamation. When sufficiently large (1 cm), obstruction of the foramen of Monro occurs, resulting in symptoms as previously described.

The CT appearance is most characteristic as a smooth rounded area of increased attenuation near the foramen of Monro (see Fig. 3). The MRI appearance may be a little more variable, but it has the advantage of demonstrating smaller lesions because of the ease of multiplanar imaging. Characteristically by MRI, the colloid cyst is increased in signal intensity on T1-weighted images and diminished in signal intensity on T2-weighted images (Fig. 15). The variation in signal intensity change depends on the physical state and lipid content of the cyst. Thus a more liquid lipid tumor has the more characteristic signal intensity changes (Fig. 15). A cyst with a more solid cholesterol or protein content appears less bright on the T1-weighted images (Fig. 16) and shows variable signal intensity change on T2-weighted images. These tumors do not enhance. For time efficiency, newer fast spin-echo and fat-suppressing sequences may be used in characterizing the fatty content.

A few colloid cysts demonstrate signal intensity changes indistinguishable from those of a small low-grade glioma. A

A 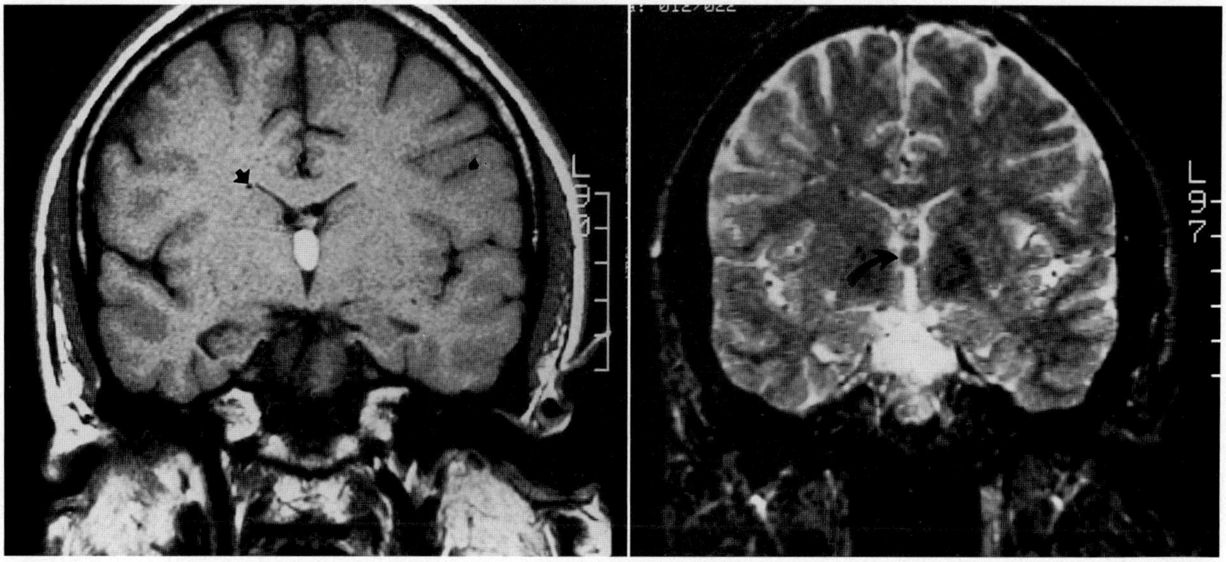 B

**FIGURE 15** Colloid cyst in a 26-year-old female. *A,* A high signal intensity lesion is shown in the anterior superior third ventricle on this T1-weighted coronal image (TR600, TE20). The ventricles have been previously shunted *(arrow),* so that there is no obstructive hydrocephalus at this time. *B,* This same area is diminished in signal intensity *(arrow)* on the second echo of the T2-weighted coronal sequence (TR2800, TE90), confirming the fatty consistency.

A 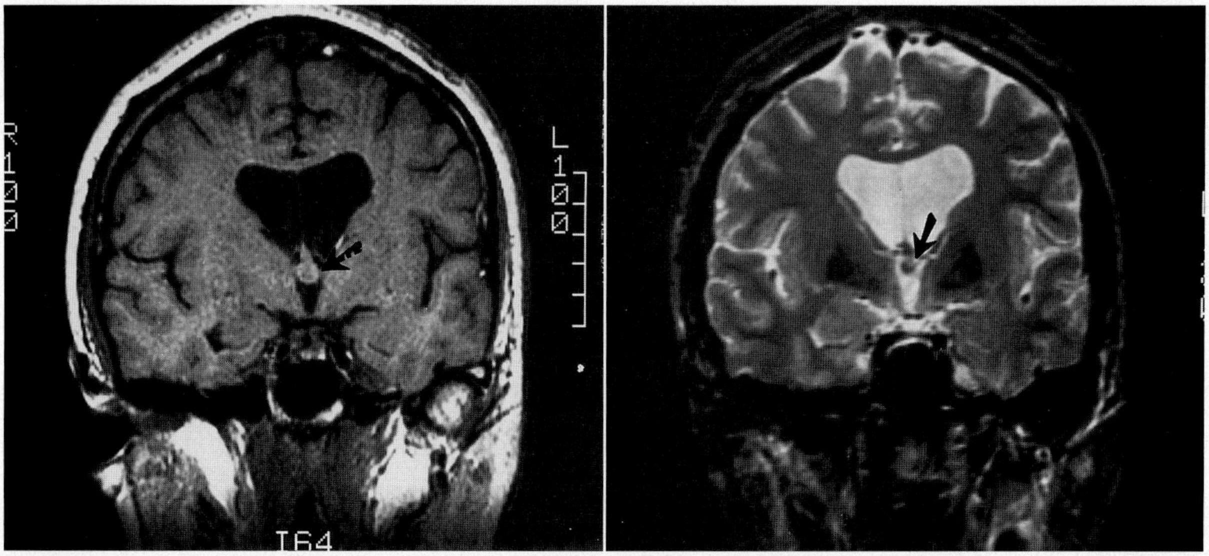 B

**FIGURE 16** Colloid cyst in a 32-year-old male. *A,* The colloid cyst *(arrow)* is not as bright as the one shown in Figure 15 on the T1-weighted coronal image (TR600, TE20). *B,* T2-weighted coronal image (TR2800, TE90) shows the area as diminished in signal intensity *(arrow)* and therefore containing fat. The difference in size might be explained as a result of a mixed component lesion.

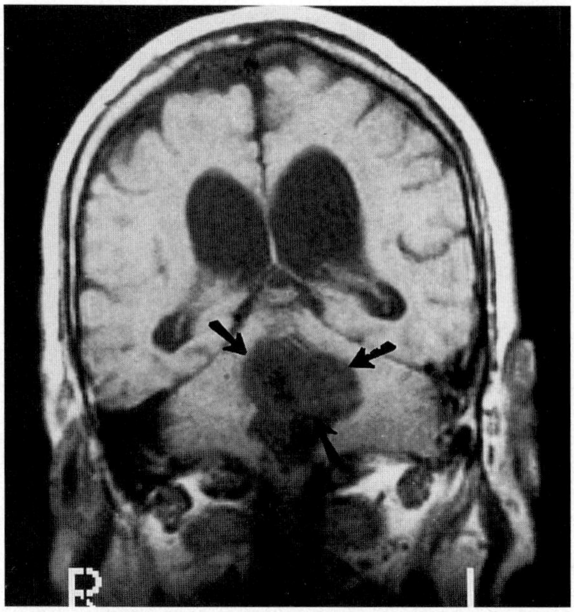


**FIGURE 17** Epidermoid in a 61-year-old male. A bulky low signal intensity mass is shown in the fourth ventricle on the T1-weighted coronal image *(arrows)*. This showed progressive increase in signal intensity on the T2-weighted images (not shown). Because of the patient's age, it is difficult to accurately assess obstructive hydrocephalus. Note how the mass conforms to the ventricular contour.

greater diagnostic dilemma is the rarer colloid cyst that has mixed solid and cystic components.

## *Other Midline Fatty Tumors*

### Fourth Ventricular Dermoid or Epidermoid

The dermoid and epidermoid are considered together, since their imaging appearance can be similar. The dermoid calcifies, whereas the epidermoid does so infrequently. Epidermoids are more commonly found in the CP angle. Like the colloid cyst, these tumors enlarge by desquamation of epithelial cells that break down into keratin and cholesterol within the tumor capsule.

Because of the soft pliable nature of the contents, the mass usually conforms to the ventricular contour, rarely reaching the size to produce obstructive hydrocephalus. Growth is slow, so that presentation usually does not occur until the early adult to adult years (Fig. 17).

The etiology of the signal intensity changes by MRI is similar to the colloid cyst. Most of these tumors, however, consist of a more complex cholesterol and thus show low signal intensity on the T1-weighted images and increased signal intensity on the T2-weighted sequences. It is the increase in signal intensity on the first echo of the T2-weighted images that distinguishes this tumor from benign cystic lesions. If there is greater fatty content, greater increase in signal intensity change can be expected on the T1-weighted images.

Cure is usually effected by surgical removal; however, recurrences are common if tumor removal is incomplete. A less common and more devastating complication is rupture of the capsule into the ventricle, producing a chemical meningitis.

## *Cystic Intraventricular Lesions*

### Choroid Plexus Cysts

The choroid plexus cyst is the most common intraventricular mass and is found in 1 percent of fetal ultrasonography. These usually arise in the lateral ventricles. There is an association with trisomy 18 and 21.

These cysts may be found in other age groups in other parts of the ventricular system. They are usually asymptomatic and can be differentiated from other masses by having MRI characteristics of CSF.

### Neuroepithelial Cysts

Patients with these benign cysts may be asymptomatic or, if the cysts are large, may present with headaches, usually occurring in young adults or adults. The cysts are lined by epithelial cells similar to those of normal choroid.

Although the true incidence of this abnormality is unknown, neuroepithelial cysts are often found at autopsy, usually in the lateral ventricle. MRI is the modality of choice in the evaluation of these masses. These follow the signal intensity characteristics of CSF, being hypointense on T1-weighted images and equal in signal intensity to the CSF on the T2-weighted images (Fig. 18). The importance in the recognition of these benign cystic lesions is their distinction from more significant pathologies such as a cystic glioma.

*Acknowledgment.* A special thank you goes to Lana Barrett, Associate Professor of Computer Sciences at Owensboro Community College, Owensboro, Kentucky. Her assistance in manuscript preparation was invaluable.

A B C D

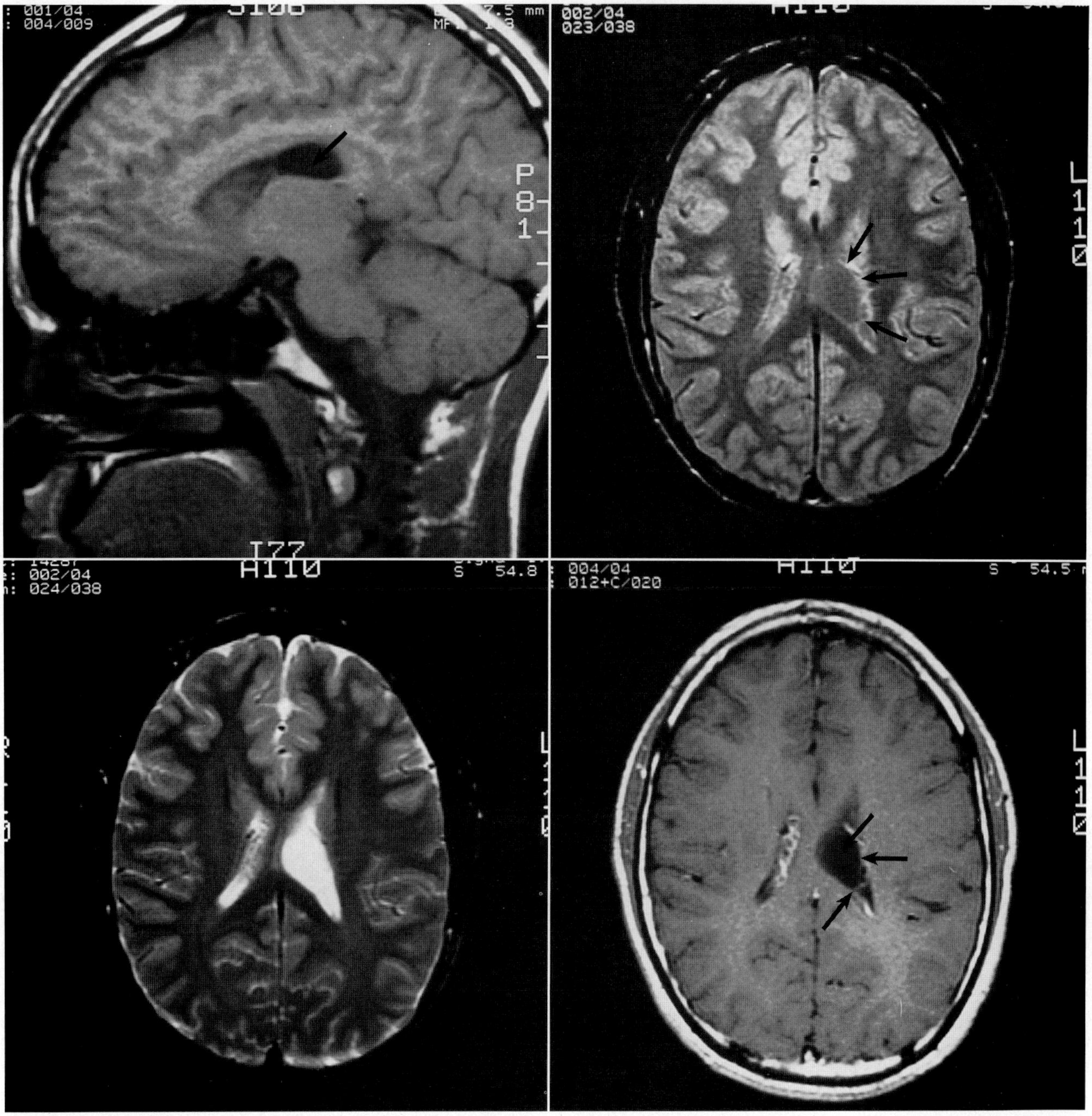


**FIGURE 18** Neuroepithelial cyst in a 24-year-old male. *A,* The thin wall of the cyst *(arrow)* is shown on the sagittal T1-weighted image (TR400, TE11). Just posterior to this is an area of hypointense cystic dilatation. *B,* The signal intensity change is the same as CSF on the first echo *(arrows)* of the T2-weighted images (TR2500, TE30). *C,* Increase in signal intensity is noted on the second echo of the T2-weighted image. The intensity is still similar to CSF, so that the lesion is not clearly outlined. *D,* No enhancement is noted after administration of contrast material *(arrows)* on the axial T1-weighted images (TR500, TE16).

## Suggested Reading

Byrd SE: Central nervous system manifestations of inherited syndromes. In Atlas SW, ed. Clinical Magnetic Resonance Imaging of the Brain and Spine. New York: Raven Press, 1991:539.

Coates TL, Hinshaw DB, Peckman N, et al. Pediatric choroid plexus neoplasms: MR, CT, and pathologic correlation. Radiology 1989; 173:81–88.

Jelinek J, Smirniotopoulos JG, Parisi JE, et al. Lateral ventricular neoplasms of the brain: Differential diagnosis based on clinical CT and MR findings. AJR 1990; 155:365–372.

Meyers SP, Kemp SS, Tarr RW. MR imaging features of medulloblastomas. AJR 1992; 158:859–865.

Russell DS, Rubenstein LS. Tumors and tumor-like lesions of mal-development origin. In Russell DS, Rubenstein LS, eds. Pathology of Tumors of the Nervous System. Baltimore: Williams & Wilkins, 1989:690.

Spoto GP, Press GA, Hesselink JF, et al. Intracranial ependymoma and subependymoma: MR manifestations. AJR 1990; 154:837–845.

# MRI Evaluation of Meningiomas

*ALLEN D. ELSTER, M.D.*

Whenever I encounter an intracranial lesion that I suspect is a meningioma, I probe the issue more deeply, asking the following questions:

1. Is it really a meningioma or could it be something else?
2. What is the exact location and extent of the tumor?
3. What is the relationship of the tumor to the adjacent arteries and veins?
4. Can I suggest any histopathologic features of the tumor that may have a bearing on its treatment or prognosis?

The magnetic resonance (MR) protocol I use for meningiomas is the conventional one I use for routine cranial imaging. Before administering contrast medium, I acquire sagittal and transaxial T1-weighted images, as well as spin-density and T2-weighted transaxial images. In all patients over age 50, and especially those with a suspected meningioma, I give gadolinium contrast agent and then acquire postcontrast transaxial and coronal T1-weighted images. MR angiography is then performed if a meningioma is encountered that potentially occludes a dural sinus or encases an artery. If the juxtasellar region or orbital apex is involved, I may also perform high-resolution (3 mm) coronal T1-weighted images with fat suppression.

## Is It Really a Meningioma?

Meningiomas are the most common benign intracranial tumors in adults. Grossly they present as globular masses or as flat, plaque-like lesions. Regardless of their shape, they are usually well demarcated and firm. Meningiomas have a propensity to invade the adjacent dura, bones, vessels, and nerves. The brain parenchyma is usually compressed but not invaded. The tumors are usually highly vascular, with a blood supply predominantly or totally of dural origin. Larger lesions may also acquire a pial blood supply at their periphery, while maintaining a dural supply centrally. Invasion or occlusion of dural sinuses is common as is arterial encasement.

Most meningiomas are found in the parasagittal regions, over the cerebral convexities, along the falx, or subfrontally. Rarely they may be found within the ventricles or even extradurally. Multiple meningiomas occur in approximately 2 percent of patients and may be associated with type 2 neurofibromatosis.

The histological subtyping of meningiomas is under constant revision, and the reader is referred to the classic textbook of Russell and Rubinstein, as well as the excellent review by Scheithauer. Regardless of the precise scheme of classification, it is generally agreed that meningiomas contain in varying proportions mixtures of the following elements: fibroblastic stroma, psammomatous calcifications, syncytial (meningothelial) cells, and vascular or hemangiopericytic components. As I subsequently discuss, the MR signal characteristics one observes largely depend on the relative amounts of each of these components within a given tumor.

A classic (but nevertheless incorrect) MR dictum has been the characterization of meningiomas as isointense to brain on both T1- and T2-weighted pulse sequences (Fig. 1, *A*). Unfortunately this incomplete (and hence erroneous) description continues to permeate modern textbooks and review articles. An equally incorrect corollary to this statement, which also may be found widely dispersed throughout the imaging literature, is that meningiomas are rather poorly documented by magnetic resonance imaging (MRI) and hence are generally better diagnosed using computed tomography (CT).

I first challenged these "classic teachings" concerning MRI of meningiomas in 1989, showing that approximately 65 percent of meningiomas are noticeably hyper- or hypo-intense compared with brain on T2-weighted images (Fig. 1, *B* and *C*). Armed with this knowledge, as well as with improvements in MRI technology and the availability of gadolinium-based contrast agents, one should now have great confidence using MRI alone to diagnose and characterize meningiomas.

Given that we can now easily detect meningiomas using MRI, other disease processes can be considered when encountering a lesion that may be a meningioma. An abbreviated differential diagnosis list is presented in Table 1.

Over the cerebral convexities or along the tentorium, benign calcified dural plaques may simulate meningiomas. Although CT is frequently indeterminate in distinguishing these two lesions, MRI with gadolinium should reveal no enhancement in a dural plaque, but definite enhancement within an en plaque meningioma. Similarly an inwardly projecting calvarial osteoma or osteochondroma should not brilliantly enhance with gadolinium, though the other features may mimic those of a meningioma.

At the skull base, the most difficult differential diagnosis for meningioma is with a schwannoma. There are no hard and fast rules to make such a distinction easy, other than careful observation concerning the exact epicenter of the tumor and its pattern of growth. Schwannomas are intimately related to the distal coverings of the cranial nerves; schwannomas therefore tend to be centered upon and grow along the course of these nerves. Conversely meningiomas prefer to spread along dural surfaces, creeping between intracranial compartments and even along the tentorium. Enhancement of the dura adjacent to the tumor, sometimes called the "dural tail sign," strongly suggests the lesion is a meningioma, but this sign can also be observed occasionally with other peripheral and extra-axial tumors, including schwannomas.

Metastatic disease in the dura constitutes an important but sometimes difficult differential diagnosis with meningioma. Although such lesions often arise as dural extensions of osseous metastases, the bony involvement may be minimal and undetectable by either CT or MRI. Breast and lung carcinoma account for most of these cases, although prostate cancer and leukemic infiltrates may also commonly produce dural-based masses resembling meningiomas. Perineural metastases from nasopharyngeal tumors may present at the skull base with a pattern of enhancement and growth similar to meningiomas.

Epidermoid tumors and arachnoid cysts are extremely common extra-axial masses, but should cause little confusion with meningiomas because their appearances are so distinct.

A B C

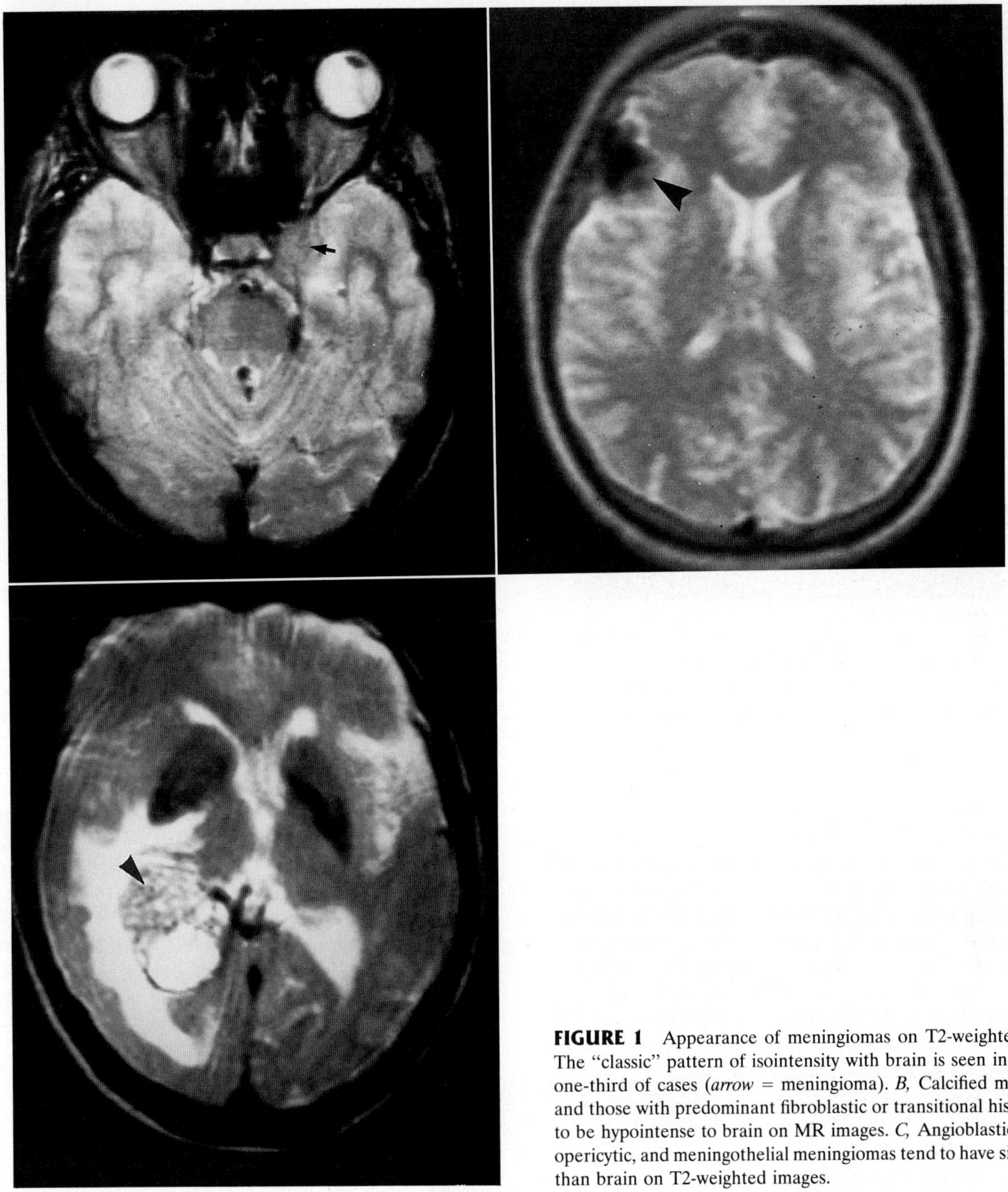

**FIGURE 1** Appearance of meningiomas on T2-weighted MRI. *A,* The "classic" pattern of isointensity with brain is seen in only about one-third of cases (*arrow* = meningioma). *B,* Calcified meningiomas and those with predominant fibroblastic or transitional histology tend to be hypointense to brain on MR images. *C,* Angioblastic, hemangiopericytic, and meningothelial meningiomas tend to have signal higher than brain on T2-weighted images.

**TABLE 1** What Is It If It Isn't a Meningioma?

| |
|---|
| Dural plaque |
| Schwannoma |
| Metastasis |
| Exophytic glioma |
| Skull lesions (e.g., chordomas, osteomas, osteochondromas) |
| Rare lesions (TB, sarcoid, germinoma, histiocytosis); additional medical history needed |

Rarely, other enhancing extra-axial masses may simulate meningiomas, such as germinomas (suprasellar and pineal regions only), ependymomas (which usually have some component within the fourth ventricle), chordomas (central skull base only), Langerhans' cell histiocytosis (perisellar region), and infectious/inflammatory processes (sarcoidosis, tuberculosis). Unless there are other clinical or radiologic findings present to suggest one of these rare diseases, the diagnosis of meningioma should be the only likely one to consider.

Although the distinction between intra-axial and extra-axial masses is fundamental and supposedly straightforward, this is not always the case. Even experienced neuroradiologists occasionally encounter lesions in which this distinction is impossible to make with certainty. In children and young adults, protoplasmic astrocytomas and other exophytic gliomas that arise within the outer cortical layers may mimic a meningioma. Here, contrast enhancement with gadolinium may be helpful to distinguish gliomas, which may not enhance or enhance weakly or irregularly, from meningiomas, which typically enhance vividly.

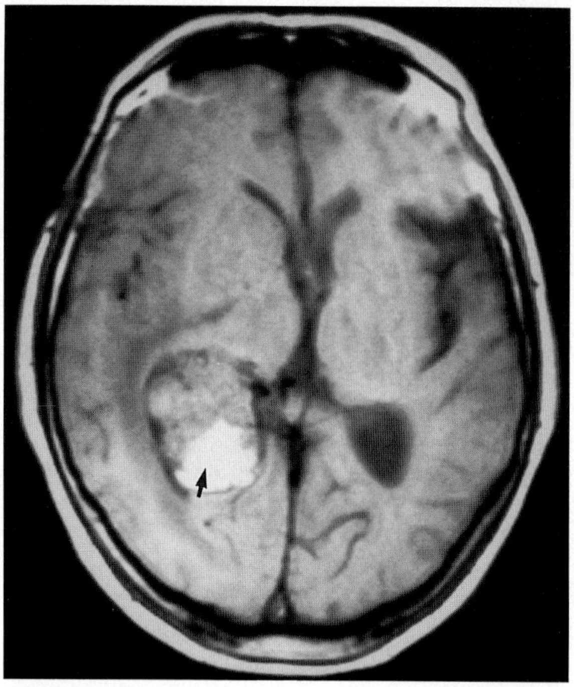

**FIGURE 2** T1-weighted image of an intravascular angioblastic meningioma shows areas of hemorrhage *(arrow).* (From Elster AD, Challa VR, Gilbert TH, et al. Meningiomas: MR and histopathologic features. Radiology 1989; 170:857–862; with permission.)

Intraventricular meningiomas (Fig. 2) present yet another diagnostic challenge and must be differentiated from choroid plexus papillomas, choroid plexus carcinomas, ependymomas, and intraventricular extension of gliomas. Because meningiomas typically involve the atria and ependymomas involve the fourth ventricle, defining the lesion location to one of these sites helps in assigning differential diagnostic probabilities. The distinction between atrial meningiomas and choroid plexus tumors can be difficult unless one observes coexistent hydrocephalus, in which the diagnosis of choroid plexus papilloma should be preferred over meningioma.

Finally, one should recognize that a small fraction of meningiomas may have bizarre or atypical appearances, which should nevertheless not dissuade one from the proper diagnosis. Meningiomas containing melanin, bone, cartilage, and fat have all been reported, and the presence of one of these elements with its characteristic attenuation on CT or signal on MRI may prove confusing. Occasionally meningiomas may be predominantly cystic, but virtually always retain an enhancing nodular component on the dural surface, which should suggest the proper diagnosis (Fig. 3).

## What Is the Exact Location and Extent of the Tumor?

Precise delineation of tumor boundaries is critical both for diagnosis and surgical therapy. Of particular surgical importance is not only the epicenter of the lesion, but also to what extent the tumor has grown away from its site of origin. Has the tumor passed from the middle fossa into the anterior or posterior compartments? Has extension through the superior orbital fissure or a skull base foramen occurred? Have the skull or brain been invaded?

The diagnosis of brain invasion by meningiomas is not as easy or as straightforward as one might imagine, even considering the vast array of sophisticated imaging tests now available. The classic radiologic sign of meningiomas, "cortical buckling," is merely a response of the adjacent brain to the extraneous mass effect and is observed with any large extra-axial tumor. About two-thirds of meningiomas have a hypointense rim at the tumor periphery, believed to represent a cerebrospinal fluid (CSF)-cleft, dural capsule, or displaced vascular structures. Whatever the explanation for this sign, if it is observed around the entire periphery of the tumor, one can presume brain invasion has not occurred. A sine qua non of brain invasion is the presence of vasogenic edema. However, it should be recognized that a great many meningiomas can excite brain edema as a result of venous obstruction or release of local vasogenic factors without invading the brain. This is

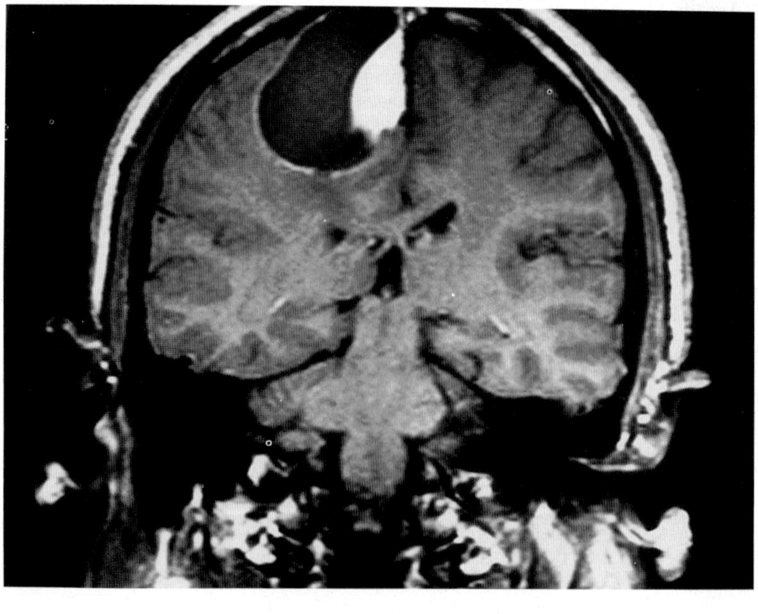

**FIGURE 3** Cystic meningioma. Note nodular enhancing component adjacent to falx.

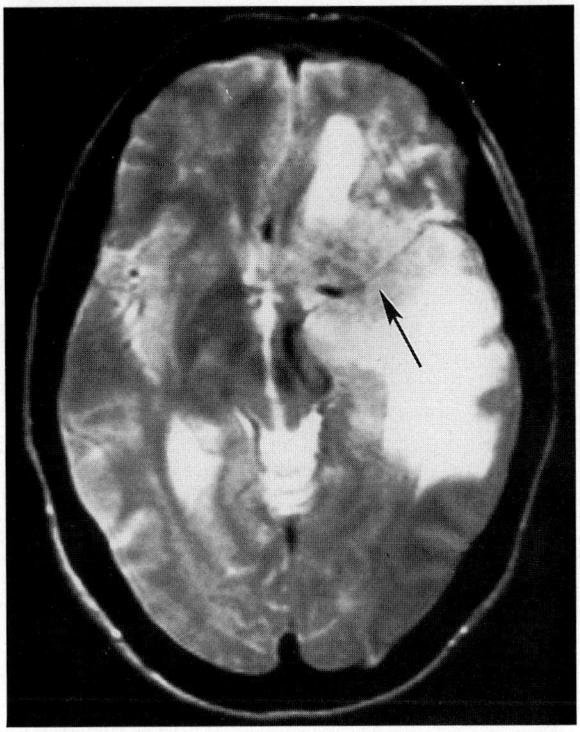

**FIGURE 4** Vascular encasement of the left middle cerebral artery *(arrow)* is well illustrated by MRI. (From Elster AD, Challa VR, Gilbert TH, et al. Meningiomas: MR and histopathologic features. Radiology 1989; 170:857-862; with permission.)

especially true for meningiomas of the sphenoid wing. Brain edema, therefore, is a necessary but not sufficient sign for diagnosing brain invasion.

## What Are the Vascular Relationships?

The presence or absence of vascular encasement and invasion is a critical feature of planned surgical resection. The diagnosis of arterial encasement is especially critical for meningiomas of the skull base (Fig. 4). The diagnosis of dural sinus invasion is important for the surgeon in deciding whether the sinus may be sacrificed.

Yeakley and co-workers have shown that arterial encasement is frequently better shown by MRI than even arteriography. MRI coronal and sagittal views can show this encasement to good advantage. If necessary, MRA may be performed in conjunction with the routine study to delineate the course of the vessels in form more familiar to surgeons.

Venous sinus invasion can best be demonstrated by MR arteriography. We use a 45 second sequence on our scanner (2D phase-contrast MRA, sagittal plane, VENC = 15, TR = 23, TE = 6, theta = 20°, slice thickness = 4 mm). This provides a superb venogram of the superior sagittal sinus, aiding in the evaluation of its occlusion by meningiomas.

## Histopathologic Features by MRI

The signal intensity of the meningioma on T2-weighted MRI pulse sequences can serve as a crude predictor of tumor histology. Tumors that are hypointense to brain tend to be calcified or fibrous and correspond somewhat to surgically "hard" lesions. Tumors that are hyperintense to brain tend to be composed of meningothelial, angioblastic, or hemangiopericytic elements; they thus tend to be somewhat "softer" and more vascular. I therefore alert the surgeon to the possibility of preoperative arteriography and therapeutic embolization when I see a hyperintense meningioma with large feeding vessels and exuberant contrast enhancement.

Presently there are no clear-cut radiologic signs that predict malignancy other than rapid growth, extensive brain or bone invasion, and postoperative recurrence. Malignant meningiomas to tend to be of high signal on T2-weighted images, but the overlap with benign forms is so great that this sign is not useful in an individual case. DiChiro and co-workers have shown that positron emission tomography (PET) may prove helpful in predicting meningioma prognosis.

## Conclusions

What appears to be a meningioma at first glance usually is a meningioma, but this is not always the case. The role of the radiologist is to define accurately the margins of the tumor, evaluate the status of nearby blood vessels, and suggest to the surgeon that the lesion may be highly vascular or malignant preoperatively.

## Suggested Reading

DiChiro G, Hatazawa J, Katz DA, et al. Glucose utilization by intracranial meningiomas as an index of tumor aggressivity and probability of recurrence: A PET study. Radiology 1987; 164:521–526.

Elster AD, Challa VR, Gilbert TH, et al. Meningiomas: MR and histopathologic features. Radiology 1989; 170:857–862.

Russell DS, Rubinstein LJ. Tumors of the meninges and related tissues. In: Pathology of tumors of the nervous system. 5th ed. Baltimore: Williams & Wilkins, 1989:449.

Scheithauer BW. Tumors of the meninges: Proposed modifications of the World Health Organization classification. Acta Neuropathol 1990; 80:343–354.

Spagnoli MV, Goldberg HI, Grossman RI, et al. Intracranial meningiomas: High-field MR imaging. Radiology 1986; 161:369–375.

Yeakley JW, Kulkarni MV, McArdle CB, et al. High-resolution MR imaging of juxtasellar meningiomas with CT and angiographic correlation. Am J Neuroradiol 1988; 9:779–785.

# MRI and Classification of Neurofibromatosis Types 1 and 2

*THOMAS R. DAMIANO, M.D. · CHARLES L. TRUWIT, M.D.*

Neurofibromatosis (NF) is the most common of the phakomatoses or neurocutaneous syndromes and has been further divided into two distinct disorders: NF type 1 (NF-1) and NF type 2 (NF-2). NF-1, or classic von Recklinghausen's disease, is more common and is characterized by café au lait spots, iris hamartomas (Lisch nodules), neurofibromas, bony and soft-tissue dysplasias, and a propensity for tumors in many organ systems. NF-2 consists of bilateral acoustic schwannomas, schwannomas of other cranial and spinal nerves, and meningiomas. Café au lait spots and neurofibromas may also occur in NF-2, but are less prominent features in comparison with NF-1. NF-1 is frequently diagnosed in childhood and tends to involve the brain parenchyma, whereas NF-2 is often not diagnosed until early adulthood and involves the coverings of the brain and nerves. NF-1 is linked to chromosome 17, and NF-2 is associated with an abnormality on chromosome 22. Some patients demonstrate features of both disorders, and this has led to the proposal of a third category: NF-3.

Magnetic resonance imaging (MRI) is the preferred means of imaging the brain of patients with NF. MRI has superior soft-tissue contrast in comparison with computed tomography (CT) and is thus able to demonstrate some parenchymal lesions not visualized with CT. Beam hardening artifacts, commonly a problem with CT, do not occur with MRI. This provides an added advantage to MRI in imaging the posterior fossa and internal auditory canals (IACs).

In this chapter we discuss our approach to imaging the brain in patients with NF. The features of NF-1 and NF-2 are described, with emphasis on the findings observed with MRI.

## NF-1

### *Indications for Neuroimaging*

#### Clinically Suspected NF-1

The findings of multiple café au lait spots or skin neurofibromas raise the possibility of NF, with or without a family history of this disorder. Clinical suspicion may also be raised by signs and symptoms suggesting an optic glioma or an appropriate skeletal deformity, such as bowing and pseudoarthrosis of the tibia. In this setting MRI is highly useful to confirm the diagnosis of NF-1. Additionally, an early MRI scan serves as a baseline for future comparison. Although a normal MRI evaluation does not exclude NF-1, it adds an additional piece of information that the clinician can use to draw a conclusion about the presence or absence of this disorder.

#### Follow-up Evaluations in Established NF-1

Any change in a patient's neurologic status clearly should prompt a neuroimaging study, preferably using MRI. Decreasing visual acuity in a young patient may herald the development or enlargement of an optic pathway glioma. Headaches or seizures may indicate the growth of an intraparenchymal neoplasm in patients of any age.

Appropriate intervals for routine follow-up scanning in clinically stable or asymptomatic patients are more difficult to define. The severity of this disorder varies greatly from patient to patient. Those who are relatively asymptomatic and have little or no abnormality by MRI require less frequent follow-up than those who are more severely affected. Serial scans are useful to monitor a known lesion for which immediate intervention is not thought to be needed. For example, mild enlargement of an optic nerve does not necessarily require immediate treatment. However, if enlargement of the lesion is documented on follow-up MRI evaluations, surgery may prevent more extensive spread of tumor and unnecessary loss of function.

#### Relatives of NF-1 Patients

NF-1 is transmitted as an autosomal dominant disorder, although approximately half of the cases occur as spontaneous mutations. Screening of asymptomatic first-degree relatives with MRI may therefore detect additional affected individuals, although the yield would be small for the resources invested. We do not routinely screen asymptomatic relatives of NF-1 patients unless there is some clinical indication or great concern on the part of the family member.

### *MRI Technique*

MRI of the brain should include intermediate and T2-weighted images in the axial plane and T1-weighted images in at least one plane. T1-weighted images with intravenous gadolinium should also be performed to improve tumor detection and characterization.

Evaluation of the orbit is best accomplished with thin-section (~3 mm) T1-weighted images without and with fat suppression and gadolinium in the coronal and axial planes. The coronal images should extend posteriorly to include the optic chiasm and tracts. The T2-weighted images of the brain evaluate the optic radiations and also demonstrate the T2 characteristics of any orbital lesions.

### *Specific Lesions*

#### Optic Pathway Gliomas

Optic pathway gliomas are said to occur in 5 to 15 percent of patients with NF-1, and of all patients with optic gliomas, at least 10 percent (probably more) will prove to have NF-1. Optic gliomas associated with NF-1 tend to occur at a younger age than those not associated with NF-1. Most of these lesions present in the first decade of life, and the majority of the remainder are found in the second decade.

Gliomas may occur anywhere along the optic pathways from the optic nerves to the optic radiations. Purely intraorbital lesions occur more commonly in association with NF-1, particularly if bilateral. Isolated chiasmal gliomas are said to be uncommon in NF-1 patients. Extensive involvement of the

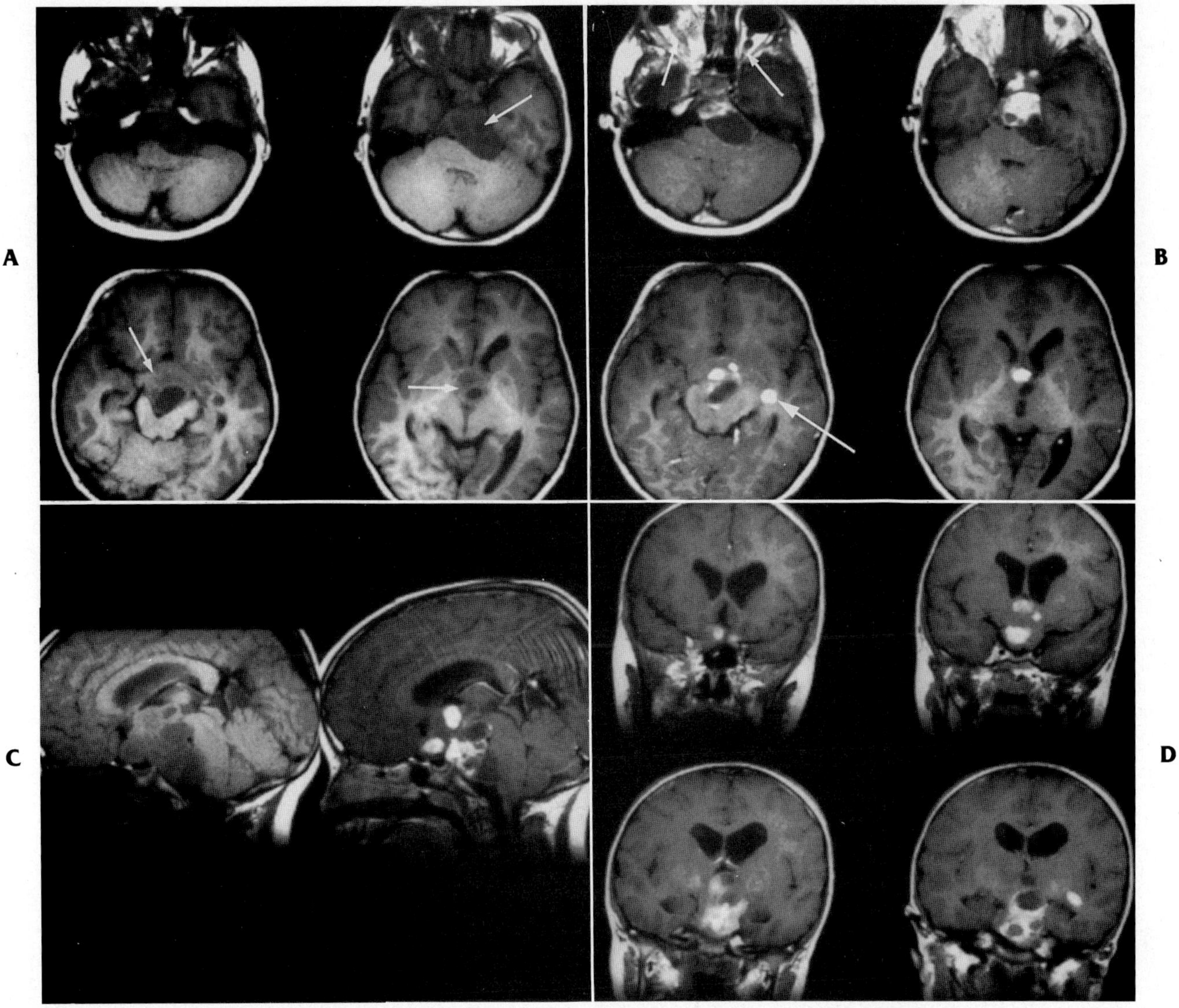


**FIGURE 1** A 6-year-old boy with NF-1 and a suprasellar mass; pathologically proven pilocytic astrocytoma. *A,* T1-weighted axial images demonstrate a heterogeneous mass in the suprasellar and prepontine cisterns and extending superiorly into the third ventricle (*arrows*). *B,* T1-weighted contrast-enhanced axial images show heterogeneous enhancement of the tumor. There is also extension of tumor into the optic nerves (*small arrows*) and left optic radiation (*large arrow*). *C,* Sagittal, and *D,* coronal T1-weighted images with gadolinium further demonstrate the extent of the tumor.

optic pathways may be observed with or without NF-1.

With the use of screening MRI, many asymptomatic optic pathway lesions are detected, particularly in the optic nerves. It is likely that many of these lesions have highly limited growth potential or actually represent hamartomas or gliosis rather than true neoplasms. This creates a difficult management decision, because surgery produces a high cure rate with lesions anterior to the optic chiasm, but at the expense of a sighted eye. Radiation therapy may also be considered, but carries the risk of cataract when delivered to the orbit, and even greater long-term risks when given to the chiasm. A reasonable alternative is to follow these lesions with MRI, clinical examination, and visual-evoked responses to determine if progression is occurring.

MRI typically demonstrates fusiform enlargement of an optic nerve and/or a mass involving the optic chiasm (Fig. 1). Extension into the adjacent diencephalon, if present, also is demonstrated with the T1- and T2-weighted images. Involvement of the optic nerve often produces elongation and kinking of the nerve (Fig. 2, *D* and *E*). Tumor extension into the optic radiations or adjacent frontal and temporal lobes is usually best observed with T2-weighted images.

Enhancement of optic gliomas is highly variable. Some lesions do not enhance at all, whereas others enhance intensely, at least in some areas. Hamartomas or gliosis would not be expected to enhance and this may be a useful finding, although at this time pathologic correlation is lacking.

Plexiform neurofibromas may mimic an optic nerve glioma, particularly if the optic nerve is surrounded by the tumor. Careful evaluation of the course and margins of the tumor usually leads to the correct diagnosis. Neurofibromas generally enhance to a greater degree than gliomas as well. Meningiomas

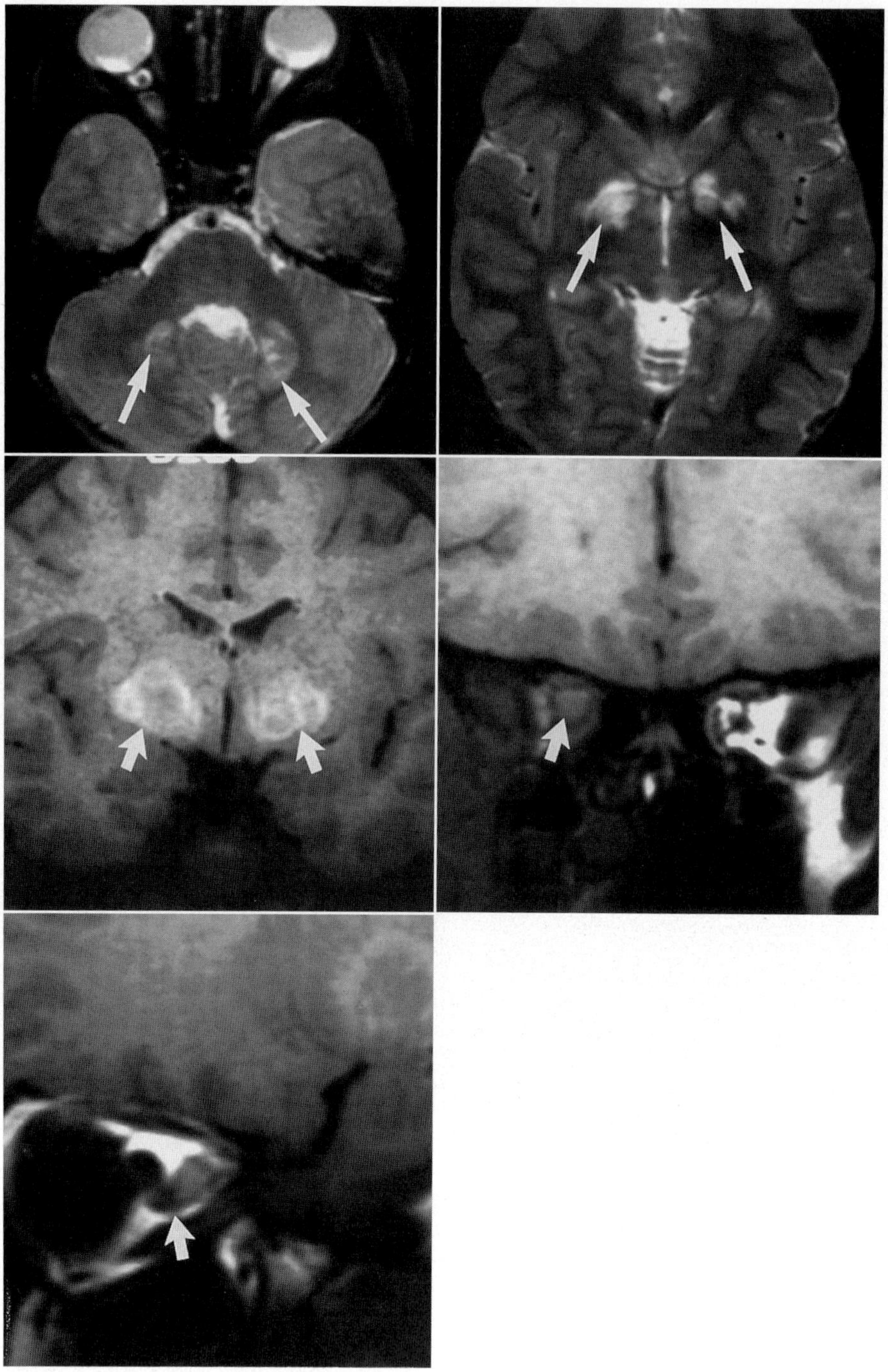

A B C D E

**FIGURE 2** A 6-year-old female with multiple abnormalities related to NF-1. *A* and *B,* Axial T2-weighted images demonstrate hyperintense foci in the cerebellar white matter (*arrows, A*) and lentiform nuclei (*arrows, B*). *C,* Coronal T1-weighted image without gadolinium demonstrates hyperintensity and mild mass effect of the lentiform lesions (*arrows*). *D,* T1-weighted coronal image of the posterior orbits shows enlargement of the right optic nerve (*arrow*), representing an optic nerve glioma or hamartoma. Note asymmetric fat suppression. *E,* T1-weighted sagittal image of the right orbit demonstrates enlargement and tortuosity of the optic nerve (*arrow*).

of the optic nerve sheath classically demonstrate enhancement of the periphery of the nerve and are not found in patients with NF-1.

### Other Tumors

NF-1 patients, particularly those with more severe forms of the disease, carry an increased risk of neoplasms compared with the general population. In the brain these consist mostly of gliomas, especially astrocytomas. High-grade astrocytomas and glioblastoma multiforme may also occur. These tumors can be located in any part of the brain and have the same imaging features as those occurring in the absence of NF.

### Multifocal Abnormalities

Many NF-1 patients demonstrate multifocal T2 signal abnormalities on cranial MRI. These are observed most commonly in the cerebellar white matter, basal ganglia, thalami, brain stem, internal capsule, and less commonly in the cerebral white matter (Fig. 2, *A* and *B*). Direct histologic correlation is still lacking, but the brains of NF-1 patients are known to harbor hamartomatous malformations and areas of glial proliferation. These likely account for some of the lesions visualized by MRI. It has also been noted that these lesions are observed with greater frequency in young patients, suggesting that they resolve over time. In some cases serial scanning reveals a decrease in the size of individual lesions.

Most of these lesions are isointense on T1-weighted images and show little or no mass effect. Occasionally, however, lesions in the lentiform nuclei will be hyperintense on T1-weighted images and show mild mass effect (Fig. 2, *C*). These lesions are different from those observed elsewhere in the brain, and the cause of the T1 shortening has not been proven. Most likely they represent a unique form of hamartomatous maldevelopment.

The significance of these abnormalities lies in the potential confusion with tumors, and the possibility that they may give rise to true neoplasms. In general, a lack of mass effect or contrast enhancement provides reassurance that an actual neoplasm is not present. Additional studies are needed to determine the neoplastic potential of these lesions.

### Miscellaneous Lesions

Hypoplasia of the sphenoid wing may occur and result in herniation of the temporal lobe into the orbit. This produces the characteristic clinical finding of pulsatile exophthalmos. Widening of the IACs may be observed as a result of dural ectasia, and this could lead to the erroneous diagnosis of an acoustic neuroma if CT is used. Gadolinium-enhanced MRI easily excludes an acoustic neuroma and confirms the correct diagnosis.

Macrocrania may be observed in NF-1, occasionally secondary to megalencephaly. A small percentage of patients with macrocrania prove to have aqueductal stenosis. Careful evaluation of the midbrain and aqueduct with contrast-enhanced MRI is necessary to exclude a small neoplasm in these patients. Ischemic disease secondary to vascular dysplasia may also occur.

# NF-2

## *Indications for Neuroimaging*

### Clinically Suspected NF-2

The indications for neuroimaging in NF-2 are similar to those stated for NF-1. Clinical suspicion may be raised by the finding of hearing loss in a patient under 30 years of age, or by the finding of multiple skin neurofibromas with few café au lait spots. MRI performed to search for schwannomas and meningiomas helps to confirm or exclude the diagnosis of NF-2. The finding of bilateral acoustic neurinomas, particularly in a young adult, is virtually diagnostic of this disorder.

### Follow-up Evaluations in Established NF-2

Once the diagnosis has been established, follow-up evaluations are necessary to monitor growth of known tumors, identify new tumors, and evaluate for recurrence following surgery. Further material on strategies for follow-up is contained in the following discussion.

### Relatives of NF-2 Patients

NF-2 is also transmitted as an autosomal dominant disorder with a high rate of penetrance. However, spontaneous mutations occur less commonly than in NF-1. Therefore most NF-2 patients have a family history of this disorder. Since intervention is unlikely to be taken in asymptomatic patients, screening relatives using MRI is probably not cost-effective. First-degree relatives should receive frequent clinical evaluation, with MRI performed at the first sign of abnormality.

## *MRI Technique*

Imaging of the IACs is best accomplished with thin-section ($\leq$3 mm) T1-weighted images using intravenous gadolinium. Occasionally focal areas of fatty marrow are present in the temporal bone surrounding the IAC and can mimic an acoustic neurinoma (Fig. 3). A precontrast T1-weighted image, or the use of fat suppression, helps avoid this diagnostic error. Focal areas of fatty marrow show high signal on precontrast images, whereas an acoustic neurinoma is bright on only the postcontrast images. Alternatively, the use of fat suppression eliminates the high signal from fat altogether.

T2-weighted images should be performed through the brain as well, particularly to evaluate the brain stem. T1-weighted images with gadolinium should also be performed through the entire brain to search for meningiomas.

## *Specific Lesions*

### Schwannomas

Schwannomas occur on multiple cranial and spinal nerves in NF-2. In particular, bilateral acoustic neurinomas are most characteristic. Most of these actually arise from the vestibular nerve, making it possible to resect some tumors without

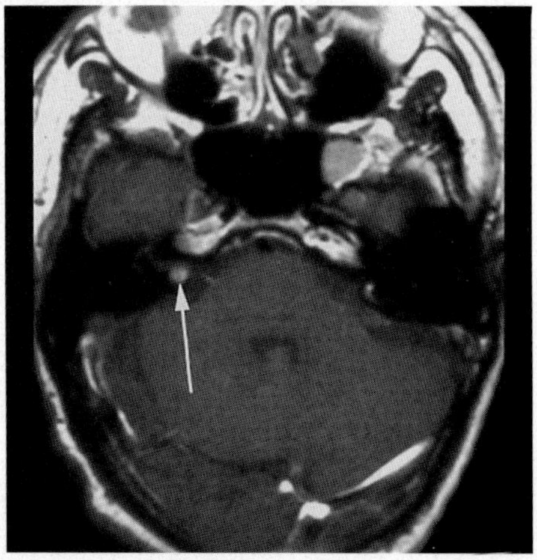

**FIGURE 3** A 54-year-old male with asymmetric hearing loss. T1-weighted axial image with gadolinium of the IACs demonstrates a small area of increased signal near the entrance of the right IAC (*arrow*). T1-weighted scan without gadolinium (not shown) also demonstrated increased signal in this location. This represents focal fatty marrow in the temporal bone and not an acoustic neuroma.

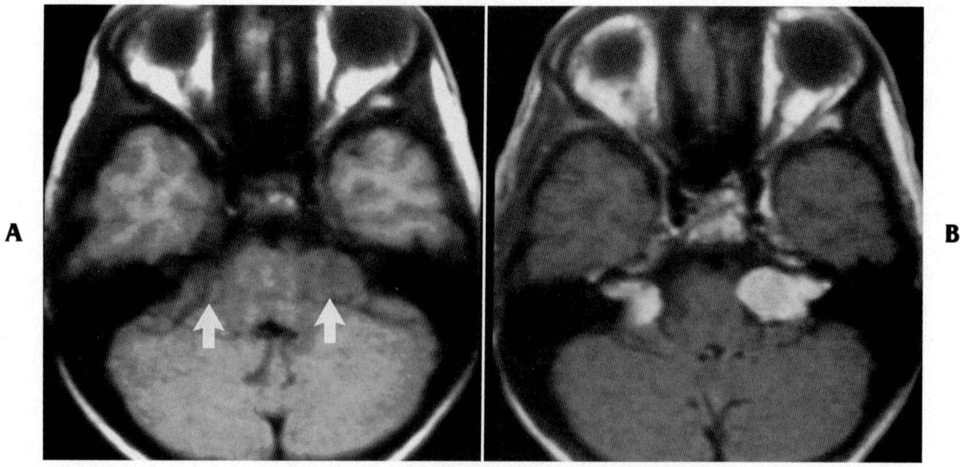


**FIGURE 4** An 11-year-old female with NF-2. *A,* T1-weighted axial image demonstrates bilateral CP angle masses nearly isointense to the adjacent brain (*arrows*). *B,* T1-weighted axial image with gadolinium at the same level shows enhancement of the schwannomas in the CP angles and internal auditory canals.

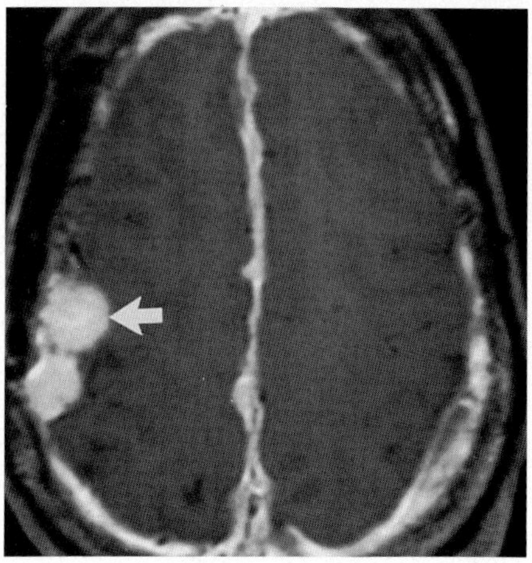

**FIGURE 5** A 29-year-old male with NF-2. T1-weighted axial image with gadolinium through the cerebral hemispheres demonstrates diffuse thickening and enhancement of the meninges. This represents diffuse meningiomatosis, confirmed at surgery. A more focal meningioma is seen on the right (*arrow*). Prior surgeries for meningioma resection had been performed.

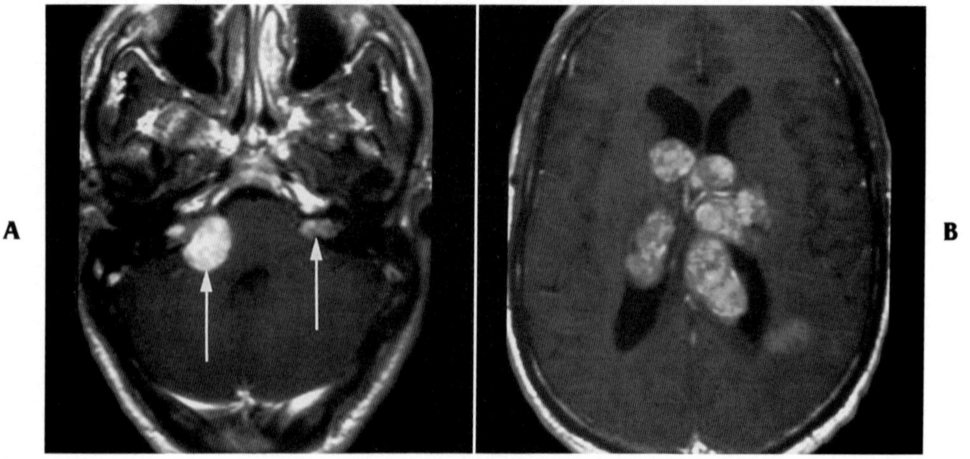


**FIGURE 6** A 32-year-old male with NF-2. *A,* T1-weighted axial image with gadolinium shows bilateral acoustic schwannomas (*arrows*). *B,* T1-weighted axial image with gadolinium through the lateral ventricles demonstrates multiple, bilateral intraventricular meningiomas. (Case courtesy of G. Momii, El Paso, TX.)

sacrificing the cochlear nerve, thus preserving hearing in that ear.

Management of acoustic schwannomas in these patients is difficult, because they are bilateral and there is the potential for total deafness. The goal should be to control the adverse effects of the tumor while preserving hearing in at least one ear. MRI can help with these decisions by providing information on the size and rate of growth of the tumors and the degree of compression of the adjacent brain stem.

By MRI, acoustic schwannomas range from small intracanalicular tumors to large masses filling the cerebellopontine (CP) angle and compressing the brain stem (Fig. 4). Small tumors usually enhance homogeneously, whereas larger tumors may show multiple areas of nonenhancement. Meningiomas also occur in the CP angle and may even extend into the IAC. The presence of a dural tail and hyperostosis of the adjacent bone often allow the correct diagnosis of meningioma to be made.

### Meningiomas

Aside from multiplicity, meningiomas in NF-2 patients appear similar to those in patients without NF. Some patients develop a diffuse meningeal proliferation referred to as meningiomatosis (Fig. 5). Intraventricular meningiomas are probably more common in NF-2 patients as well (Fig. 6).

### Miscellaneous

It has been suggested that glial tumors may occur in association with NF-2 as well. However, some of these patients may have actually had NF-1, since the differentiation of these two entities is a relatively recent development. Further studies are needed to reach a firm conclusion on this issue.

NOTE—The views expressed in this chapter are those of the authors and do not reflect the official policy or position of the Department of the Army, the Department of Defense, or the United States Government.

## Suggested Reading


Aoki S, Barkovich AJ, Nishimura K, et al. Neurofibromatosis types 1 and 2: Cranial MR findings. Radiology 1989; 172:527–534.

Bognanno JR, Edwards MK, Lee TA, et al. Cranial MR imaging in neurofibromatosis. AJR 1988; 151:381–388.

Hurst RW, Newman SA, Cail WS. Multifocal intracranial MR abnormalities in neurofibromatosis. Am J Neuroradiol 1988; 9:293–296.

Martuza RL, Eldridge R. Neurofibromatosis 2 (bilateral acoustic neurofibromatosis). N Engl J Med 1988; 318:684–688.

Meeting Report. National Institutes of Health Consensus Development Conference statement: Neurofibromatosis. Neurofibromatosis 1988; 1:172–178.

Mirowitz SA, Sartor K, Gado M. High-intensity basal ganglia lesions on T1-weighted MR images in neurofibromatosis. Am J Neuroradiol 1989; 10:1159–1163.

Packer RJ, Bilaniuk LT, Cohen BH, et al. Intracranial visual pathway gliomas in children with neurofibromatosis. Neurofibromatosis 1988; 1:212–222.

Riccardi VM. Routine cranial neuroimaging of patients with or at risk for neurofibromatosis. Neurofibromatosis 1988; 1:65–68.

Rubinstein LJ. Pathological features of optic nerve and chiasmatic gliomas. Neurofibromatosis 1988; 1:152–158.


# Detection of Cerebral Metastases with MRI and CT

*ERIC J. RUSSELL, M.D. · JAMES OSKIN, D.O.*

The early detection of cerebral metastases represents a challenge to the sensitivity of current imaging techniques. Magnetic resonance imaging (MRI) is the most sensitive test available and is therefore the procedure of choice.

It has been estimated that at the time of death, 25 percent of patients succumbing to systemic cancer have intracranial metastases. This frequency predicts that the staging of cancer, and consequently treatment planning, often depend on the presence or absence of cerebral metastatic disease. Early detection of multiple metastases can be rapidly followed by palliative radiation therapy or operative resection of solitary lesions. In patients with controlled primary tumors, this may result in significant improvement in quality of life, and survival.

Certain primary tumors produce brain metastases with relatively specific imaging findings. Adenocarcinomas of the lung and colon and primary melanomas bleed with relatively high frequency. Prostate metastases have a predilection for calvarium and dura. Lymphomatous tumors primarily metastasize to dura and leptomeninges. The pattern of involvement and structural lesional characteristics may provide specificity in patients with unknown primary tumors, thereby directing a more limited and effective initial search for the primary tumor.

## Clinical Indications

The most common indication for imaging for the detection of cerebral metastatic disease is staging of patients with known primary tumors outside the central nervous system (CNS). Although some of these patients have symptoms referable to the CNS, up to 25 percent are asymptomatic at the time of initial presentation. In this circumstance MRI, the imaging study with the highest sensitivity, is the clear choice. Advantages of MRI include a lack of interfering bone artifact near soft-tissue and bone interfaces and improved sensitivity of T2-weighted MR images to differences in tissue water content when compared with computed tomography (CT). Since small metastases may produce no detectable edema, contrast enhancement is an essential part of the screening MRI evaluation.

Patients presenting with neurologic symptoms and no known primary tumor may be initially evaluated with MRI or CT. Although it is clear that MRI is more sensitive than CT for the detection of parenchymal metastases, CT is cheaper and more easily available in many locations. In our practice CT is frequently employed as a first step for the workup of acutely symptomatic individuals, particularly those presenting emergently with seizures or hemorrhage. If multiple cerebral metastases are detected on this evaluation, there may be no need for follow-up MRI, depending on the site of the primary tumor and possible therapeutic protocols. If in these circumstances a solitary parenchymal nodule is detected, MRI is indicated to distinguish a solitary metastasis from a primary cerebral neoplasm and from other similar lesions (i.e., abscess). MRI may detect a second lesion missed by CT, permitting the certain diagnosis of metastatic disease.

Patients presenting with focal neurologic findings suggestive of leptomeningeal spread of tumor should first be studied with MRI with and without contrast infusion. CT is relatively insensitive to leptomeningeal and cranial nerve involvement with metastatic carcinoma.

Calvarial metastatic disease is not generally the primary reason for imaging in cancer patients. However, CT and MRI evaluations done for brain metastases do include the skull. Unless photographed to optimize calvarial contrast, skull lesions not extending beyond the boundaries of the inner and outer tables are easily missed.

## Technical Considerations

Most current-generation CT scanners are equally effective at demonstrating cerebral metastases. The usefulness of CT, however, is limited for small lesions in the low posterior fossa, and cortically oriented lesions involving the inferior aspects of the frontal and temporal lobes. Metastases are missed most often because of a combination of the presence of interfering bone artifact and the relative lack of sensitivity of CT to peritumoral edema (brain water distribution).

If CT is to be employed for the workup of patients suspected of harboring metastatic disease, a high-resolution protocol must be observed. Scans should be done at no greater than 5 mm section thickness, after the injection of a robust dose of contrast agent. Thinner sections reduce bone artifact. Newer fast "spiral"-type scanners may allow the acquisition of even thinner sections (1 to 3 mm), and the acquired data may be summated to produce 3 to 5 mm thick images. This technique further reduces interfering artifact. Gantry angulation may be reversed to improve lesional conspicuity in the middle cranial fossa, reducing bone artifact generated by the petrous bone. The head is positioned so that cuts are obtained through the long axis of the temporal lobe. Reduced artifact results in improved sensitivity for low temporal lobe lesions.

We routinely employ double-dose contrast infusion for lesion detection. A short delay after infusion permits optimal uptake of contrast material within poorly enhancing metastatic nodules. There is, however, a potential pitfall of double-dose infusion CT. Cortical veins enhance so dramatically that small peripherally oriented cortical metastases may be difficult to distinguish in cross section from normal veins (see Fig. 2, *D*). Enhanced MR images, performed with a T1-weighted sequence without flow compensation, are more effective at differentiating poorly enhancing venous structures from dramatically enhancing cortical metastases.

Dense bone may obscure small convexity metastases when CT images are photographed at a typical brain window (ranging from 80 to 100 Hounsfield units). For this reason, we routinely obtain additional sets of postinfusion CT photographs: one at a routine brain window, one at a window width of 150 Hounsfield units (and a relatively high window level) so that peripheral lesions are not hidden by adjacent bone, and an additional set of photographs obtained at a bone window for detection of calvarial and skull base destruction.

MR images are acquired in the transverse axial plane, employing a dual spin echo technique with a long TR ranging from 2,500 to 3,000 msec. Some current scanners permit the use of fast spin-echo (FSE) techniques, which provide T2 contrast with reduced scan time. Limited experience is currently available with FSE for detection of metastasis. Other specific sequence characteristics depend on scanner field strength and quality factors, which vary from site to site. Relatively thin sections should be obtained (5 mm) with minimal interslice gap. T1-weighted images should be acquired before and after infusion, so that direct comparison may be made between similar regions of interest. Additional postinfusion T1-weighted images may be obtained in an alternate diagnostic plane (sagittal or coronal) to improve localization.

Thin contiguous scans may be acquired using 3DFT volume techniques. The conspicuity of small metastases may improve, since these scans are heavily T1 weighted and are less subject to partial volume artifact. Also, volume data acquisition allows the performance of multiplanar reconstruction for lesion localization without the need for direct scanning in other planes.

When a high index of suspicion exists for leptomeningeal disease, postinfusion images are routinely obtained in the coronal plane for optimal cross-sectional visualization of cranial nerves. It is best to obtain preinfusion T1-weighted scans in the same plane, to allow direct comparison with postinfusion scans and aid in visualization of skull base osseous metastases that may be masked by enhancement on postinfusion scans alone.

The use of double-dose (and possibly triple-dose) contrast infusion with MRI has recently been investigated with two nonionic gadolinium-based MRI contrast agents. Clinical trials have demonstrated improved lesional conspicuity in many cases of metastatic disease, particularly in those cases with more than one lesion. When multiple metastases are present, a higher concentration of circulating contrast material makes it more likely that all lesions take up sufficient contrast material to be detectable. High-dose contrast agents may improve conspicuity, overcoming partial volume effects that might serve to hide minimally enhancing lesions poorly visualized with lower doses.

We have seen several cases of poor contrast uptake in metastatic lesions, and we believe that a slight delay following the infusion of gadolinium-based contrast agents also provides increased lesional conspicuity (in the absence of the availability of double-dose infusion). One can provide a natural postinjection delay by performing the dual-echo long TR (proton density and T2-weighted) sequence following the administration of contrast material. T1-weighted postinfusion images, done for optimal sensitivity to contrast enhancement, can therefore be performed afterward (10 to 15 minutes postinfusion). The postinfusion short TE long TR (proton density–weighted) images provide both T1- and T2-weighted information. We have observed small poorly enhanced metastases that are more readily detectable on postinfusion proton density–weighted scans than on T1-weighted contrasted images. When gadolinium-based contrast agents are approved for use at higher dose, the need for this technique will likely be reduced. Imaging strategies are reviewed in Table 1.

A

B

C

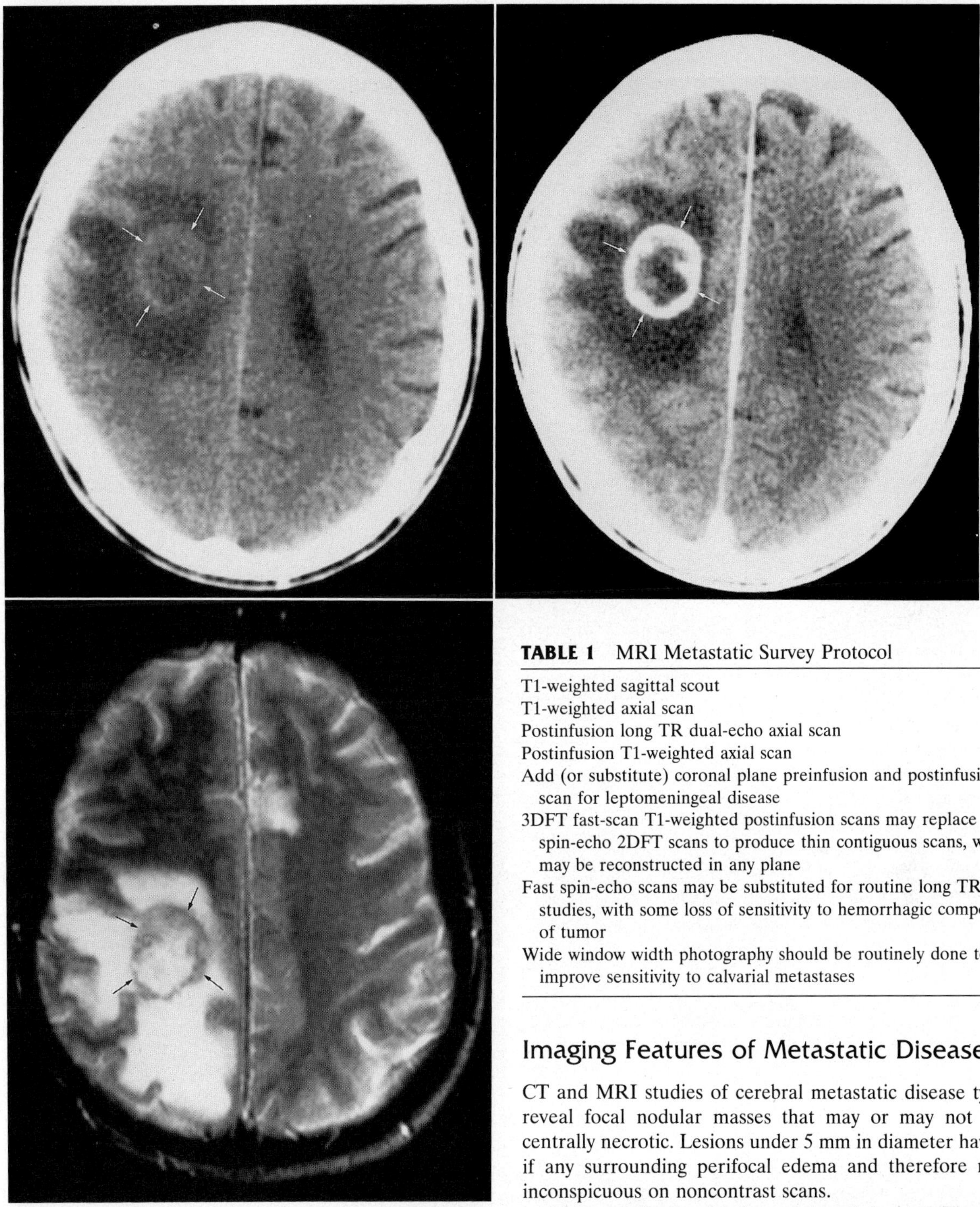

**FIGURE 1** A 65-year-old man with typical necrotic solitary lung carcinoma metastasis. *A* and *B,* Preinfusion (*A*) and postinfusion (*B*) CT scans show ring-enhanced solitary right frontal lobe metastasis, surrounded by low-density perifocal edema. Note the presence of a complete dense rim on the preinfusion scan (*arrows, A*), representing the solid tumor capsule. *C,* Axial MRI scan (SE 2000/100/2) at the same level as (*A*) and (*B*). The relatively low-intensity tumor capsule (*arrows*) is more intense than white matter, but contrasts nicely with high-intensity central necrosis and peripheral edema.

**TABLE 1** MRI Metastatic Survey Protocol

T1-weighted sagittal scout
T1-weighted axial scan
Postinfusion long TR dual-echo axial scan
Postinfusion T1-weighted axial scan
Add (or substitute) coronal plane preinfusion and postinfusion scan for leptomeningeal disease
3DFT fast-scan T1-weighted postinfusion scans may replace spin-echo 2DFT scans to produce thin contiguous scans, which may be reconstructed in any plane
Fast spin-echo scans may be substituted for routine long TR studies, with some loss of sensitivity to hemorrhagic components of tumor
Wide window width photography should be routinely done to improve sensitivity to calvarial metastases

## Imaging Features of Metastatic Disease

CT and MRI studies of cerebral metastatic disease typically reveal focal nodular masses that may or may not appear centrally necrotic. Lesions under 5 mm in diameter have little if any surrounding perifocal edema and therefore may be inconspicuous on noncontrast scans.

Metastatic foci tend to be peripherally located. The cortical and subcortical distribution is likely related to hematogenous dissemination. Although metastases are often subcortical, tumor location may not be readily apparent by gross inspection of the brain surface. Therefore operative resection of a solitary metastasis may be aided by ultrasonographic localization done in the operating room.

Large solitary metastases may be difficult to distinguish from primary brain neoplasms (Fig. 1). Ring enhancement, commonly observed with necrotic metastatic foci, is a nonspecific finding. Detection of a complete ring on noncontrast CT scans indicates the presence of a defined capsule and excludes other causes of "ring blush," such as infarction and resolving hemorrhage.

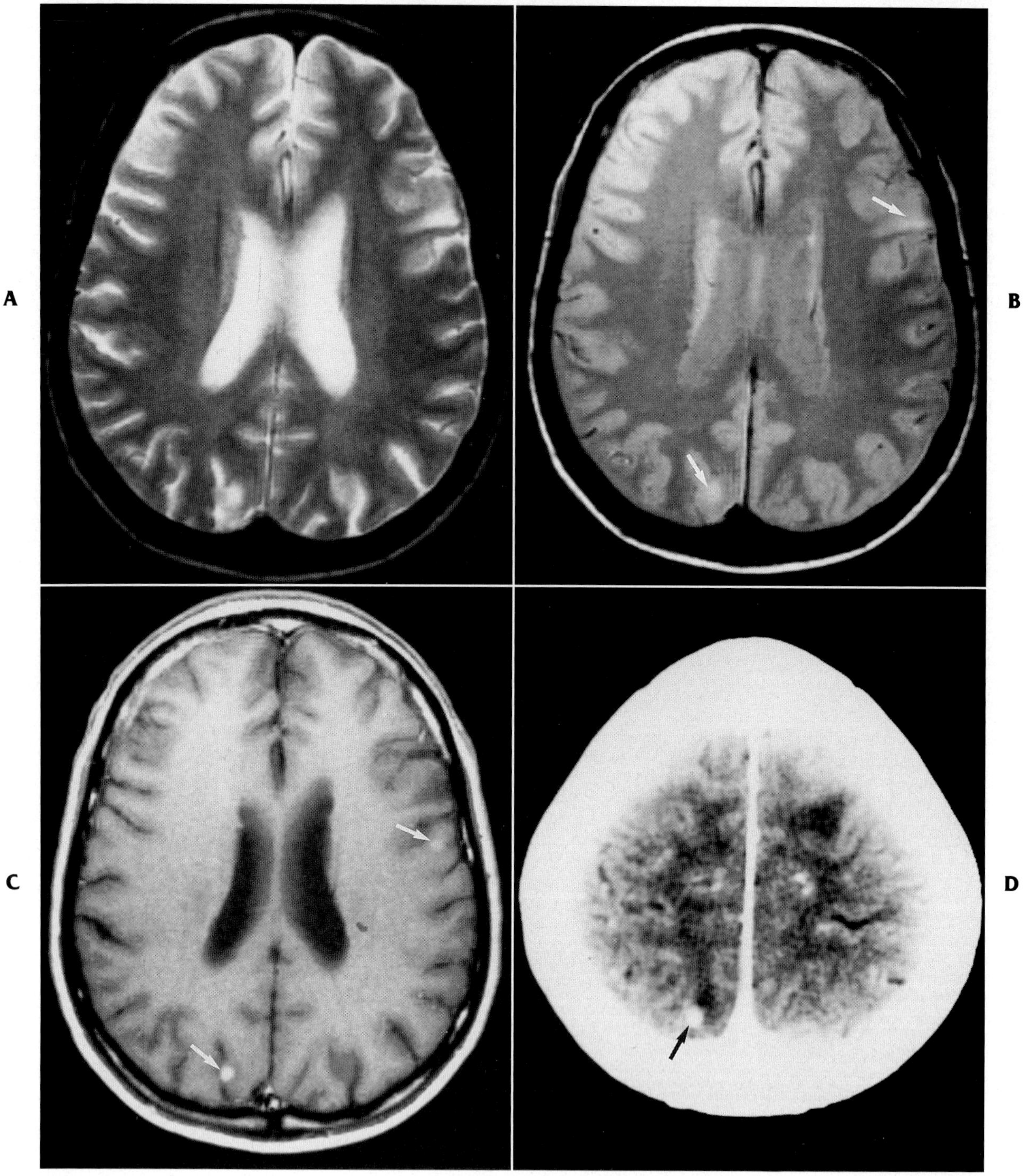

**FIGURE 2** Contrast-enhanced MRI for detection of metastasis. A 44-year-old HIV-positive male with metastatic melanoma. *A* and *B*, Noncontrast double-echo MRI scans (SE 2600/20,70/1) reveal two subtle areas of high intensity at the corticomedullary junction on proton density–weighted scan (*arrows, B*). Lesions are hidden by adjacent high-intensity CSF on the long TE (T2-weighted) scan (*A*). *C*, Contrast-enhanced MRI (SE 600/20/1) at the same levels as (*A*) and (*B*). Note the improved conspicuity of small tumor nodules (*arrows*). *D*, Contrast-enhanced CT scan through right-sided parietal metastases (*arrow*) observed on MRI scans (*A*) through (*C*). The lesion is difficult to distinguish from adjacent enhancing cortical veins. Contrast-enhanced MRI done without flow compensation provides a higher level of confidence, and can better differentiate normal cortical veins from small metastases.

The T2-weighted MRI correlate of the CT finding of ring enhancement is an area of relative T2 shortening (often ringlike) between higher-intensity areas of central necrosis and peripheral edema (see Fig. 1, *C*). Smaller non-necrotic nodules typically appear as more uniform areas of relative hyperintensity (on T2-weighted images) when compared with adjacent normal white matter. Small peripherally located metastatic deposits may not be readily distinguishable from normal cortical gray matter based on MRI intensity patterns alone (see Fig. 3). This is particularly true on heavily T2-weighted studies (Figs. 2, *A*, and 3). Careful evaluation of the first-echo (proton density) scan (Fig. 2, *B*) is essential for detecting small cortical metastases on noncontrast MR images. Postinfusion T1-weighted scans are generally more sensitive (Figs. 2, *C*, and 3). Small nodules typically enhance homogeneously.

Postinfusion T1-weighted MRI scans should be obtained without the use of flow compensation, which may produce high signal in cortical veins enhanced with a gadolinium-based contrast agent. High signal veins may then resemble parenchymal nodules and confuse the search for metastases, in a fashion similar to that observed with double-dose infusion CT (Fig. 2, *D*).

Enhancement of parenchymal metastasis is well detected with MRI in most cases, but when multiple lesions are present, unpredictably poor uptake of contrast material may occur (see Fig. 2). I believe that the use of higher-dose contrast infusion (0.2 to 0.3 mmol/kg) will significantly increase lesion detection and evaluation sensitivity in selected cases. Our own experience in this respect is supported by recent studies.

Aside from contrast dose considerations, lesional contrast uptake tends to increase over time for at least 30 minutes after infusion (Fig. 4). Delayed T1-weighted scans may therefore increase lesion detection. This observation stimulated us to begin to acquire the long TR (proton density and T2-weighted) sequence after infusion (Fig. 5). The T1 postinfusion scan is done immediately afterward, resulting in a delayed study without decreased patient throughput. We have found this technique advantageous, although a very small percentage of metastases may instead decrease in conspicuity with time. An interesting benefit of the acquisition of postinfusion proton density scans is the additive effect of T1 and T2 contrast on the proton density image (Figs. 5 and 6). Tumoral T1 shortening (very high signal) due to contrast enhancement is typically detected within an area of more intermediate high signal perifocal edema (T2 effect). Although this may be nothing more than an interesting phenomenon in most cases, on occasion the combined increase in signal afforded by the addition of T1 and T2 effects may improve evaluation sensitivity (see Fig. 6).

## *Hemorrhagic Metastases*

Metastatic foci that appear relatively hyperdense compared with normal brain on noncontrast CT studies may histologically contain areas of focal hemorrhage or mineralization. Lesions more apt to be hemorrhagic arise from primary tumors in several locations including lung (adenocarcinoma), skin (melanoma), and kidney. Areas of hemorrhage exhibit characteristic MR intensity patterns. In the acute phase, blood is hypointense on T2-weighted images, because of the accumulation of intracellular deoxyhemoglobin and clot retraction. The susceptibility effect may be more poorly detected with images obtained with FSE techniques. In the subacute phase, hyperintensity is observed on T1-weighted images, because of

A

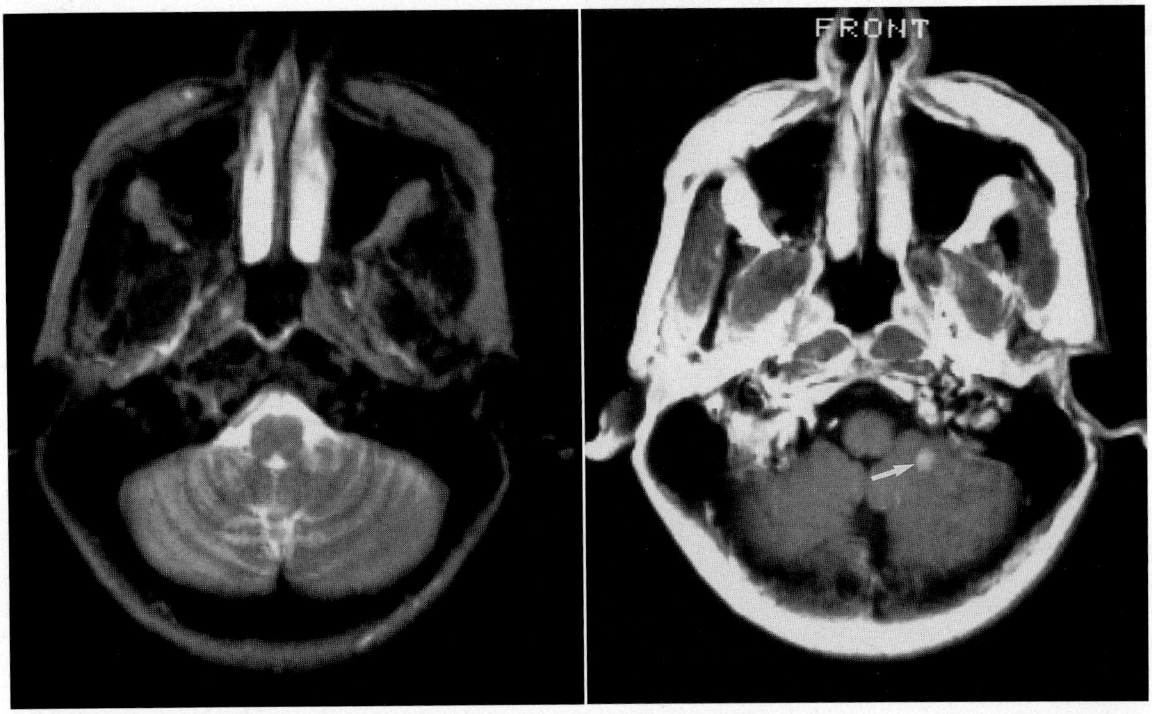


B

**FIGURE 3** A 36-year-old woman with breast carcinoma. (Small cerebellar metastases required contrast enhancement for detection.) *A* and *B*, MR images through the low posterior fossa, obtained before infusion (SE 2300/90/2, *A*) and after infusion (SE 600/15/1, *B*). The tumor nodule, less than 5 mm diameter, produces no appreciable edema (T2-weighted scan is negative, *A*). Despite the absence of bone artifact (vs. CT), the lesion required contrast enhancement for detection (*arrow*, *B*).

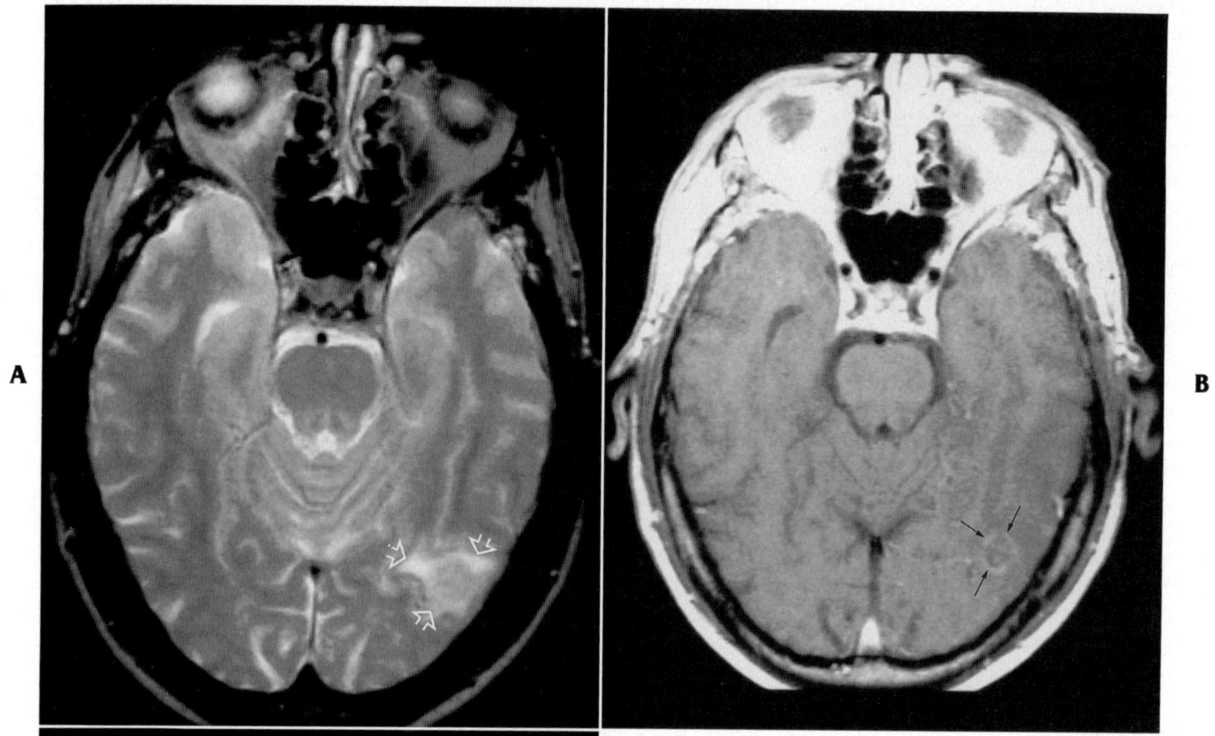

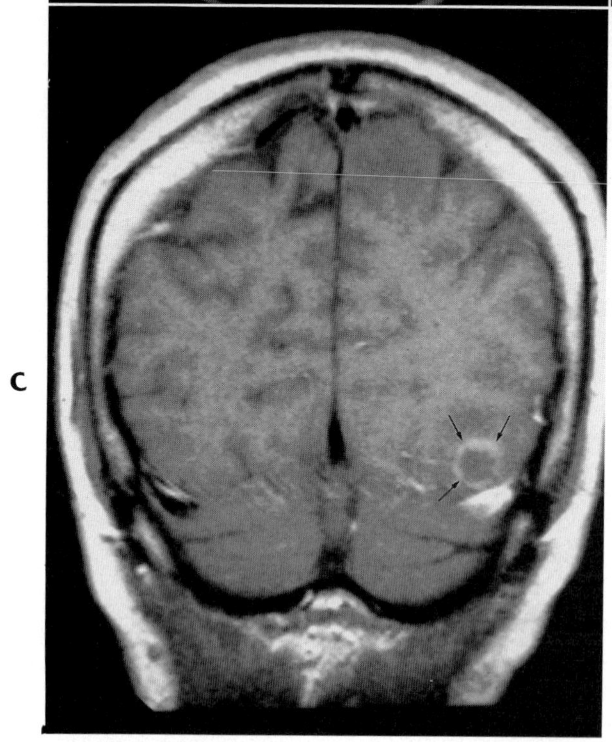

**FIGURE 4** Delayed enhancement with time after contrast infusion. A 63-year-old man with lung carcinoma metastasis. *A,* Axial scan (SE 2200/70/1) shows small solid mass in the left occipital lobe, with faint peripheral edema (*open arrows*). *B,* Immediate postinfusion scan (SE 616/19/1) reveals sharp and faint rim enhancement (*arrows*). *C,* Delayed coronal scan (SE 516/19/1), obtained 15 minutes after infusion. Note the slight improvement in degree of enhancement and lesional conspicuity (*arrows*) due to relatively slow accumulation of contrast agent. Higher doses of contrast material than employed here tend to improve enhancement of small metastases on scans obtained immediately after infusion.

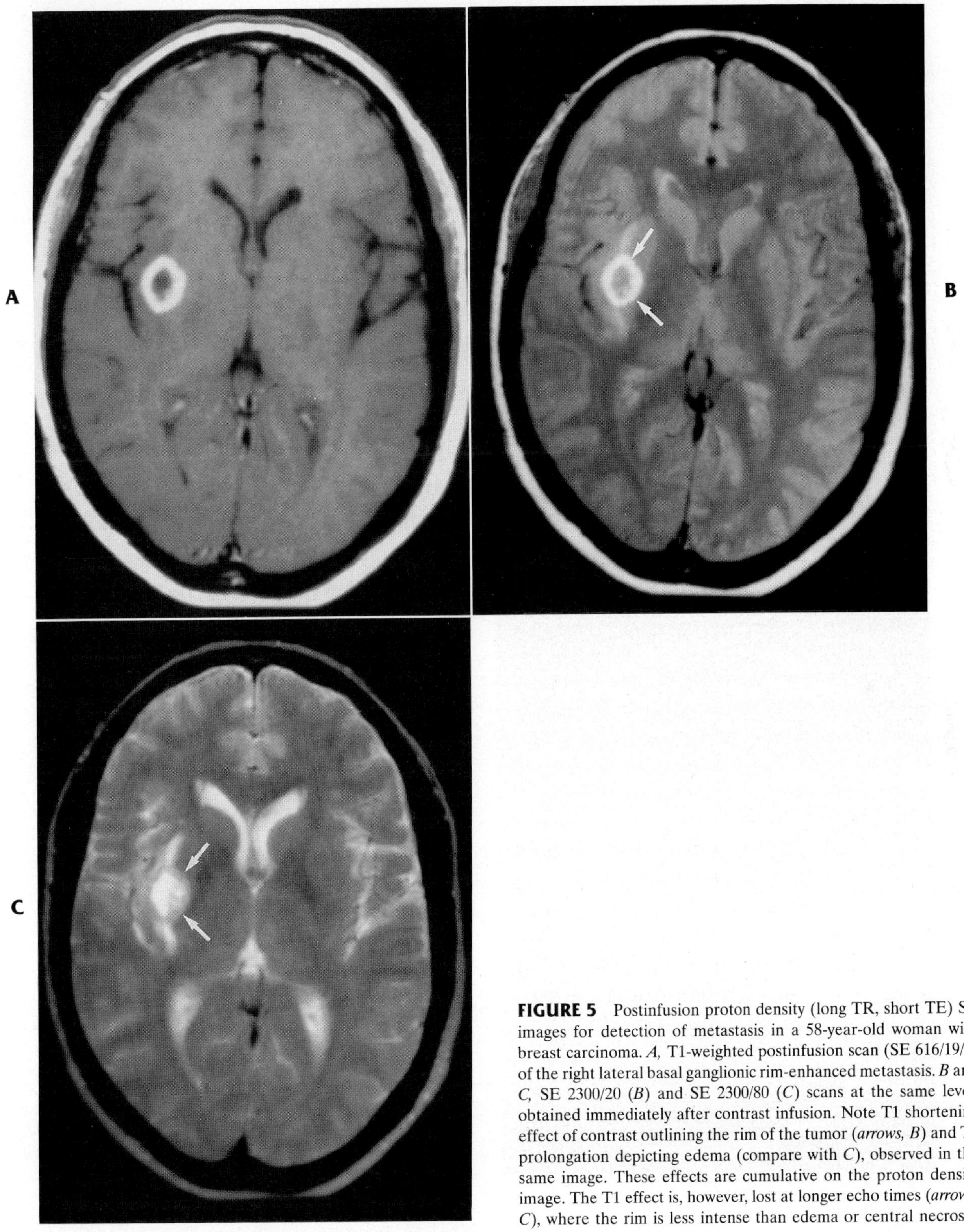

**FIGURE 5** Postinfusion proton density (long TR, short TE) SE images for detection of metastasis in a 58-year-old woman with breast carcinoma. *A,* T1-weighted postinfusion scan (SE 616/19/1) of the right lateral basal ganglionic rim-enhanced metastasis. *B* and *C,* SE 2300/20 (*B*) and SE 2300/80 (*C*) scans at the same level, obtained immediately after contrast infusion. Note T1 shortening effect of contrast outlining the rim of the tumor (*arrows, B*) and T2 prolongation depicting edema (compare with *C*), observed in the same image. These effects are cumulative on the proton density image. The T1 effect is, however, lost at longer echo times (*arrows, C*), where the rim is less intense than edema or central necrosis.

A

B

C

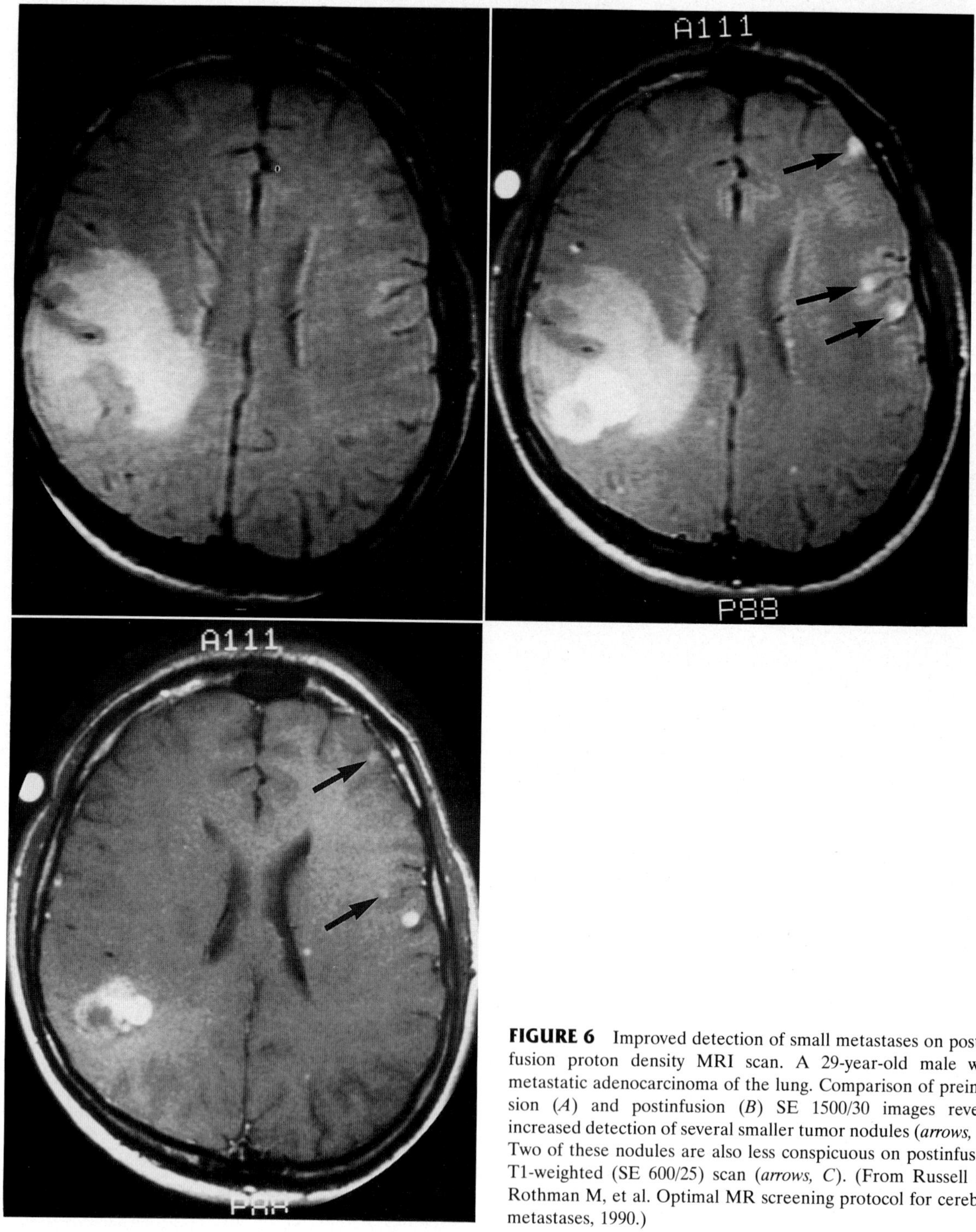


**FIGURE 6** Improved detection of small metastases on postinfusion proton density MRI scan. A 29-year-old male with metastatic adenocarcinoma of the lung. Comparison of preinfusion (*A*) and postinfusion (*B*) SE 1500/30 images reveals increased detection of several smaller tumor nodules (*arrows, B*). Two of these nodules are also less conspicuous on postinfusion T1-weighted (SE 600/25) scan (*arrows, C*). (From Russell EJ, Rothman M, et al. Optimal MR screening protocol for cerebral metastases, 1990.)

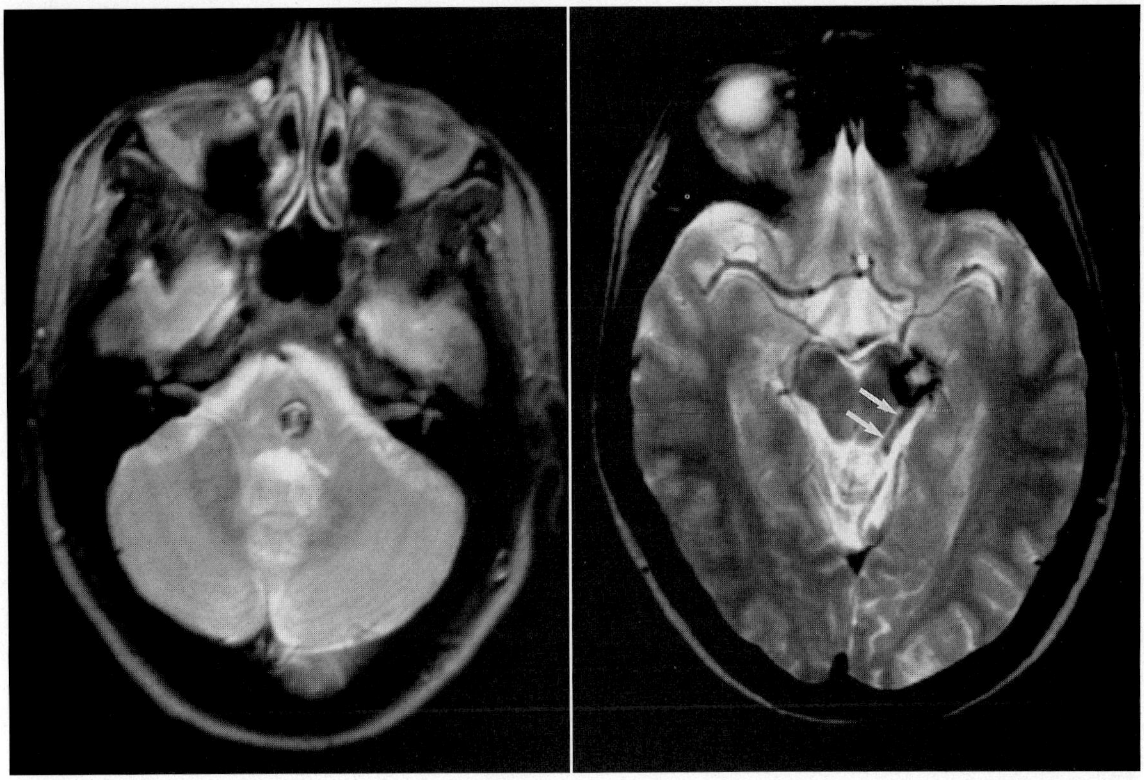


**FIGURE 7** Differential diagnosis of hemorrhagic metastases: multiple cavernous angiomata. *A* and *B,* A 36-year-old woman with intermittent brain stem symptoms over many years. Absence of mass effect and perifocal edema suggest the correct diagnosis of angioma. SE 2200/70/1 scans at two levels show the rim of low intensity representing hemosiderin and ferritin in the central pons (*A*) and medial temporal lobe (*B*). The left basilar vein of Rosenthal is dilated (*arrows, B*) (associated venous malformation).

the accumulation of methemoglobin. In the late subacute and chronic phases, hemorrhagic lesions are surrounded by a rim of hypointensity related to accumulation of ferritin and hemosiderin within macrophages. Hemorrhagic metastases may therefore contain areas of significant signal inhomogeneity. In addition, other hemorrhagic lesions, such as cavernous angioma, may present with similar MRI characteristics. Concerning differential diagnosis, cavernous angioma less frequently exhibits surrounding perifocal edema. However, it is important to note that small hemorrhagic metastases may also present without edema, and differentiation of metastasis from hemorrhage or angioma may depend on follow-up evaluation. Several authors have suggested MRI signs that might predict the presence or absence of neoplasm underlying parenchymal hemorrhage. Signs suggestive of neoplasm include a delay in evolution between the MRI stages of hemorrhage, the absence of a complete black rim, and the presence of significant perilesional edema. Regional vascular dilatation may also suggest the diagnosis of vascular malformation as opposed to neoplasm (Fig. 7).

## *Leptomeningeal Metastases*

Leptomeningeal metastases are present in up to 10 percent of patients with systemic carcinoma at autopsy. Since almost half of all patients with clinical symptoms suggestive of leptomeningeal metastases have no history of primary carcinoma, imaging plays a key role in making the initial diagnosis. Cerebrospinal fluid (CSF) cytology is a sensitive test for leptomeningeal carcinoma; however, imaging studies may be positive when CSF sampling is repeatedly normal.

Adenocarcinoma of the breast or lung frequently metastasizes to leptomeninges and subarachnoid space. Lymphoma and melanoma also have a dural predilection. Cranial neuropathy occurs in over 90 percent of patients with leptomeningeal metastases at some time during the course of the disease. The seventh and third nerves are most affected, followed by fifth and sixth nerves. Cranial and spinal metastatic disease may be present simultaneously. Patients therefore may present with radicular symptoms and back pain.

CT of the leptomeninges and dura is relatively insensitive, because of the difficulties imposed by interfering high-density bone artifact near the brain surface. CT, however, easily detects severe diffuse leptomeningeal neoplasia (Fig. 8). Subtle findings may be present on preinfusion CT studies, including an absence of normal low-density CSF in locations in which it is expected to appear. Communicating obstructive hydrocephalus in a cancer patient should be considered to be from leptomeningeal cancer until proven otherwise. Postinfusion scans more sensitively demonstrate tumor within cisterns, by demonstrating enhancement along the surface of the brain. Routine brain window images fail to detect dural enhancement unless the dura is significantly thickened. Slightly higher window widths and levels (150 to 200 WW) should be routinely employed for photography, so that the density of the overlying inner table of calvarium may be distinguished from the slightly

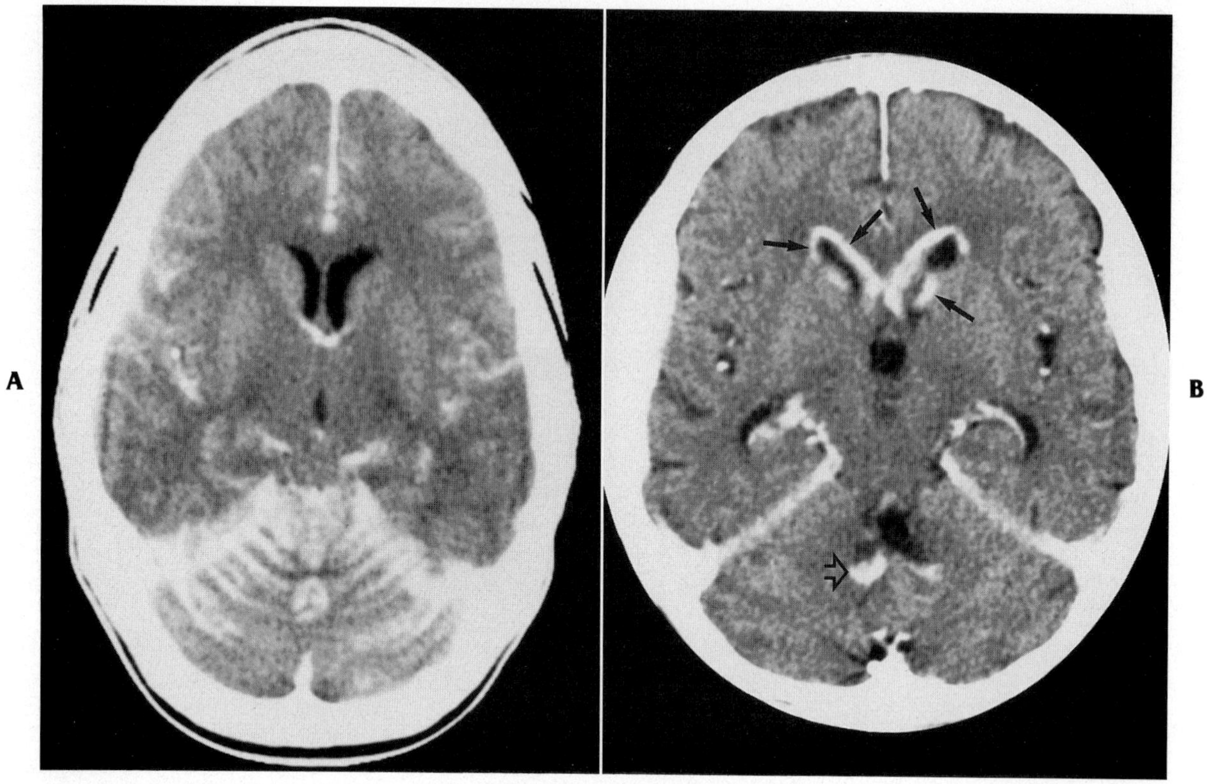

**FIGURE 8** Leptomeningeal metastatic carcinoma in two patients, shown by contrast-enhanced CT. *A,* A 35-year-old woman with breast carcinoma metastatic to pericerebellar cisterns. Note the dense enhancement of normally black cerebellar sulci. *B,* A 55-year-old man with oat cell carcinoma of the lung metastatic to the ependymal lining of the frontal horns of the lateral ventricles (*arrows*) and fourth ventricle (*open arrow*).

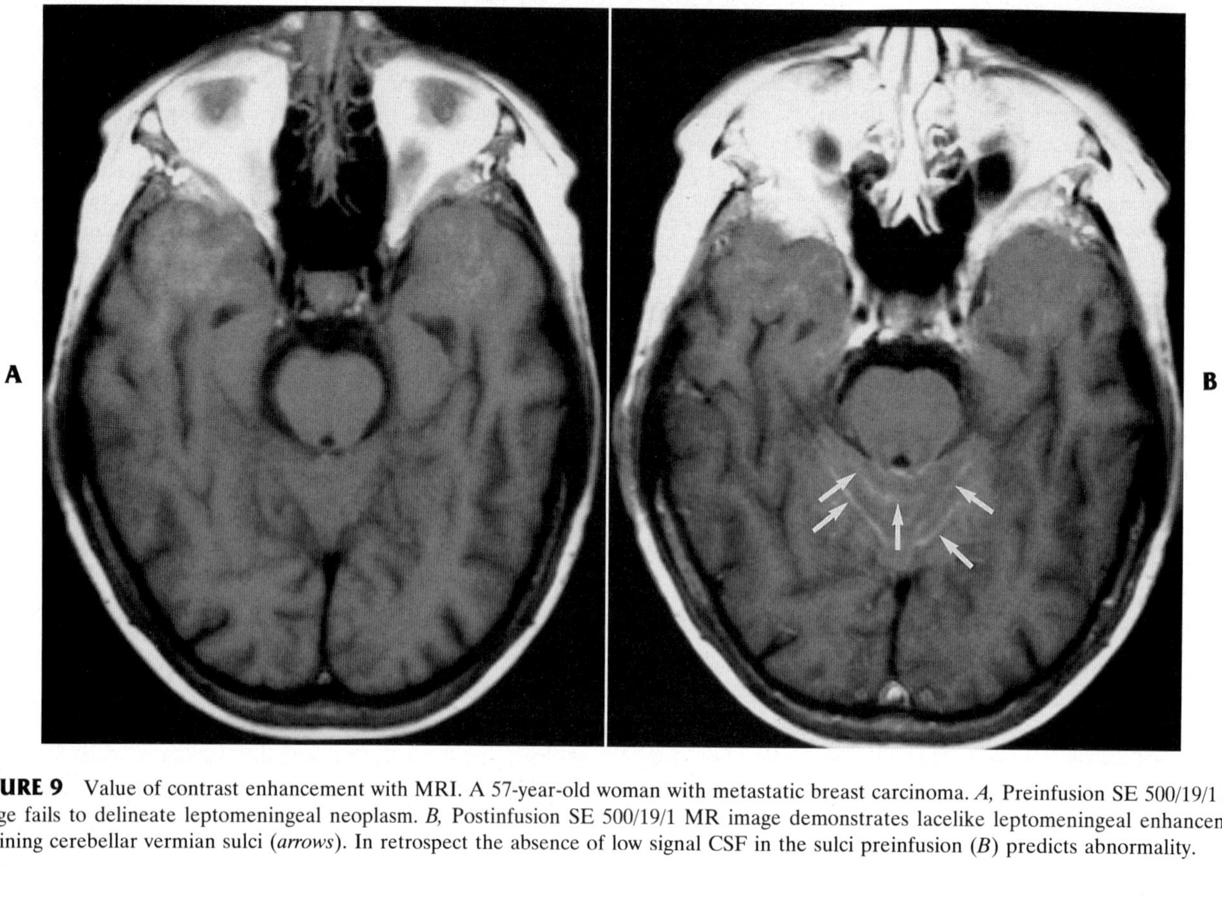

**FIGURE 9** Value of contrast enhancement with MRI. A 57-year-old woman with metastatic breast carcinoma. *A,* Preinfusion SE 500/19/1 MR image fails to delineate leptomeningeal neoplasm. *B,* Postinfusion SE 500/19/1 MR image demonstrates lacelike leptomeningeal enhancement outlining cerebellar vermian sulci (*arrows*). In retrospect the absence of low signal CSF in the sulci preinfusion (*B*) predicts abnormality.

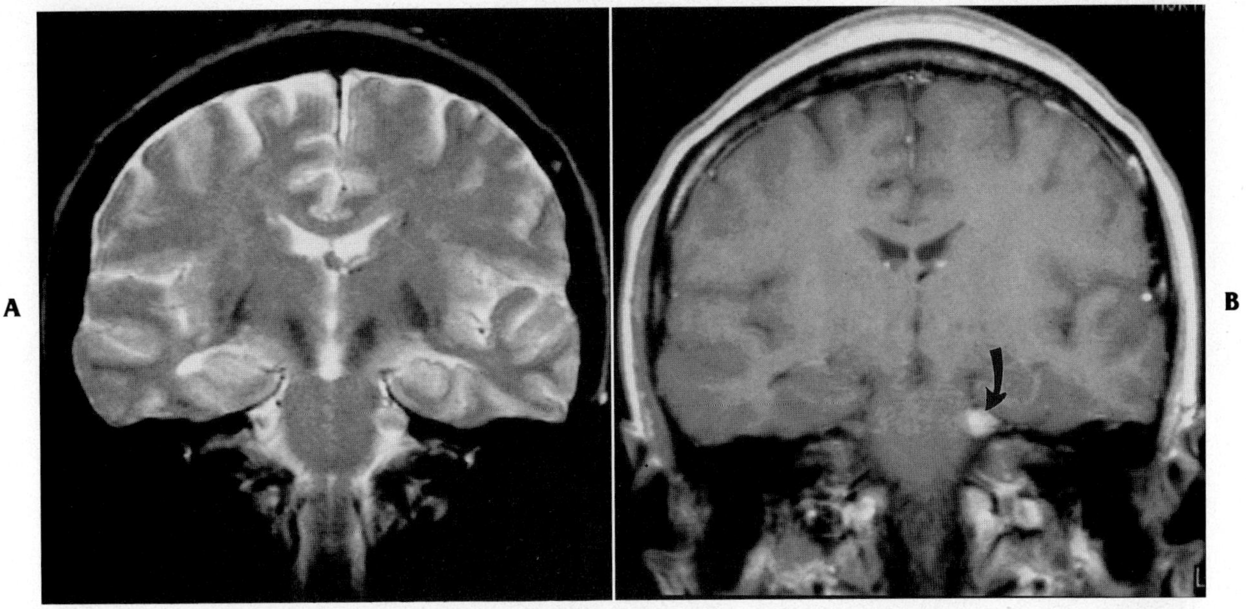


**FIGURE 10** Perineural leptomeningeal tumor in a 43-year-old woman with breast carcinoma and left fifth nerve symptoms (facial numbness). *A* and *B*, Preinfusion SE 2400/70/1 coronal image (*A*) through the midpons shows asymmetric enlargement of the preganglionic segment of the left fifth nerve. This metastatic deposit is more conspicuous on T1-weighted postinfusion image (SE 516/19/1) (*curved arrow, B*).

lower density of enhanced thickened dura.

MRI may show absence of normal CSF within basal cisterns and sulci (Fig. 9, *A*). Tumor-infiltrated leptomeninges usually appear isointense with adjacent cortical gray matter. Contrast enhancement should be routinely employed for maximal sensitivity (Fig. 9, *B*). The coronal scanning plane should be used for acquiring T1-weighted postgadolinium scans when cranial nerve involvement is suspected clinically (Fig. 10). Significant enhancement of the intracranial segments of cranial nerves is pathologic, and focal nerve thickening is a supportive finding. When neural enhancement is found, the differential diagnosis must also include primary neoplasms (schwannoma) and inflammatory disease. Abnormal enhancement in regions away from the abnormally enhanced nerve support the diagnosis of a diffuse carcinomatous process.

Benign meningeal enhancement, particularly dural enhancement, may be difficult to distinguish from dural carcinomatosis. Areas of smooth linear meningeal thickening often represent a benign reaction to an adjacent process and may be observed for several days to weeks after a simple lumbar puncture. The finding of focal nodularity, however, is strongly supportive of the diagnosis of metastatic tumor (Fig. 11, *B*). Additionally, involvement of the adjacent calvarium and the underlying leptomeninges is characteristic of neoplastic etiology (Fig. 11, *A*). The isolated finding of dural enhancement is not independently pathognomonic of leptomeningeal cancer.

## *Calvarial and Skull Base Metastases*

The detection of skull base and calvarial metastatic disease requires close comparison of precontrast- and postcontrast-enhanced T1-weighted MRI scans. Long TR MRI images are relatively insensitive, unless obtained with bone marrow–sensitive techniques such as short tau inversion recovery (STIR). Preinfusion T1-weighted images show abnormally decreased intensity replacing the normally high signal fatty marrow. Sagittal T1-weighted scout images are particularly effective at detecting tumor infiltration of clival marrow (Fig. 12). The intensity of bone marrow is age dependent, with high signal intensity progressively increasing with age. In the pediatric age group, low-intensity hematopoietic marrow is normal. Patients with severe anemia, and immunocompromised patients with marrow-suppressive disorders (acquired immunodeficiency syndrome [AIDS]), also demonstrate diffusely abnormal low-intensity marrow, because of reconversion of fatty marrow to hematopoietic elements. Such vascular marrow compartments may enhance with gadolinium and resemble diffuse marrow space metastases. Preinfusion studies are essential for complete evaluation of the skull base, since enhancing intradiploic tumor may resemble normal diploic fat, if postinfusion images are considered alone (Fig. 13). Fat-suppressed contrast-enhanced scan techniques may increase the conspicuity of calvarial and skull base tumor.

Skull metastases that invade the low-intensity inner and outer calvarial tables are readily detected on almost any MRI pulse sequence and of course are readily detected as areas of bone erosion on CT images. The detection of more subtle intradiploic metastases requires a separate set of MR photographs, with window and level settings set to optimize calvarial contrast. Even so, smaller lesions may blend with hyperintense marrow on T2-weighted images. Careful review of preinfusion T1-weighted sequences is essential for detection of intradiploic metastases. Calvarial diploic high-intensity marrow is normally symmetric from side to side. Asymmetric focal low intensity is highly suspicious for marrow replacement by tumor, in the absence of a history of trauma or surgery. Contrast-enhanced scans, which are routinely done for the detection of brain metastases, may show intradiploic metastases as focal areas of increased intensity (enhancement). Enhancement corresponds to focal areas of diploic fat replacement observed as low intensity on preinfusion scans (Fig. 14).

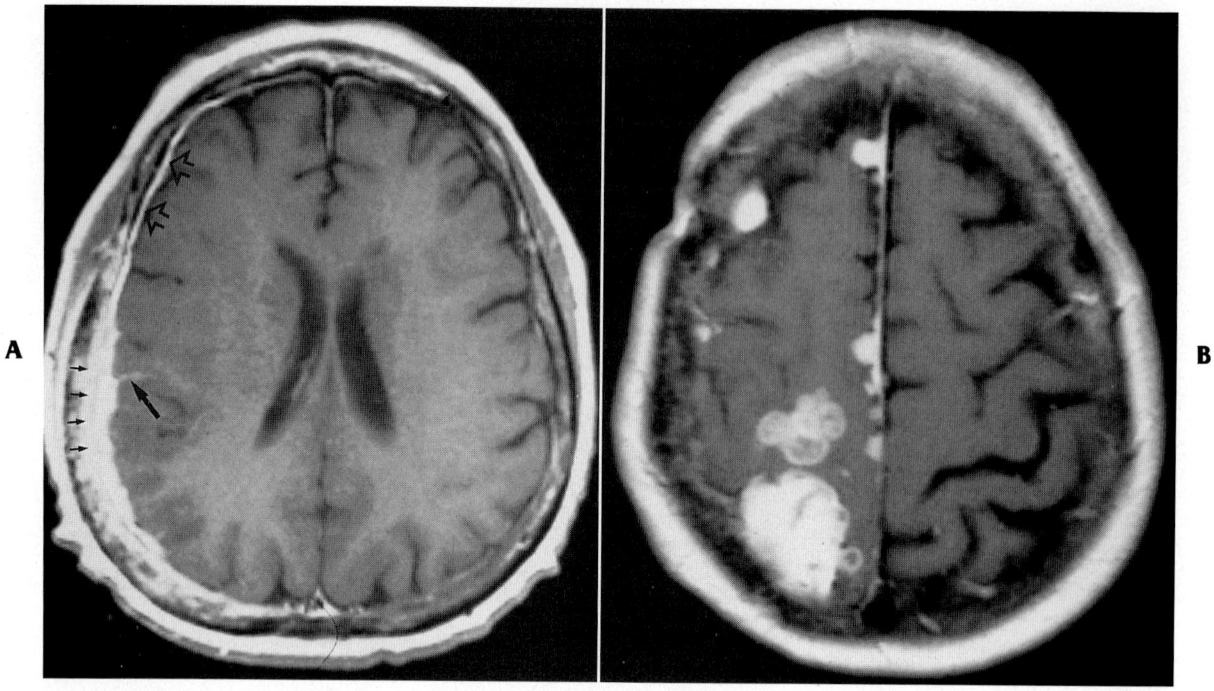


**FIGURE 11** Two patients with dural enhancement from metastatic disease, visualized by contrast-enhanced T1-weighted MRI. *A,* A 69-year-old woman with metastatic breast cancer in the right calvarium, with linear spread to dura (*bright white line, small arrows*) and leptomeninges (*large black arrow*). Linear enhancement observed more anteriorly (*open arrows*) may represent non-neoplastic reactive dural enhancement. *B,* A 77-year-old-woman with loculated nodular leptomeningeal metastasis from adenoid cystic carcinoma (postinfusion SE 500/19/1 scan). Nodularity predicts malignancy, although meningiomatosis may have a similar appearance on MRI.

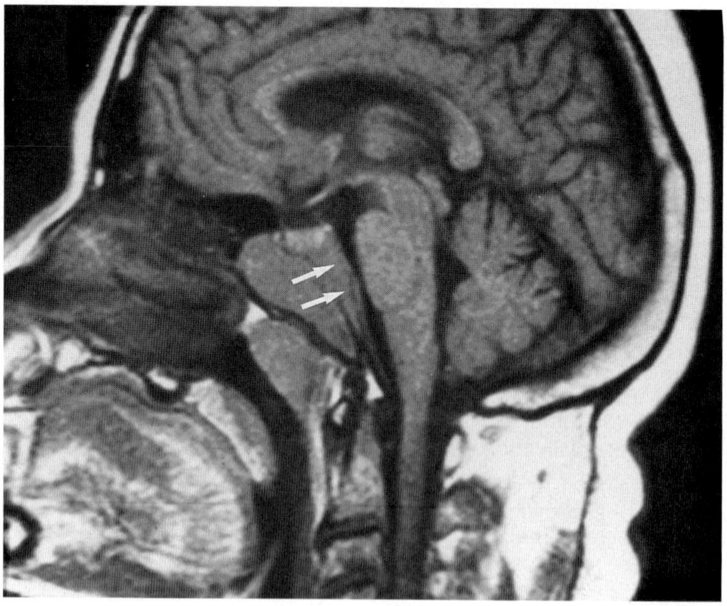

**FIGURE 12** A 78-year-old woman with left sixth cranial nerve palsy. Metastases to clivus constricting nerve in Dorello's canal. Sagittal T1-weighted SE 350/30/1 image shows a mass opacifying the sphenoid sinus. Infiltration (hypointensity) of normally white clival bone marrow (*arrows*) indicated malignancy (biopsy-proven B-cell lymphoma). Cranial neuropathy resolved after radiotherapy.

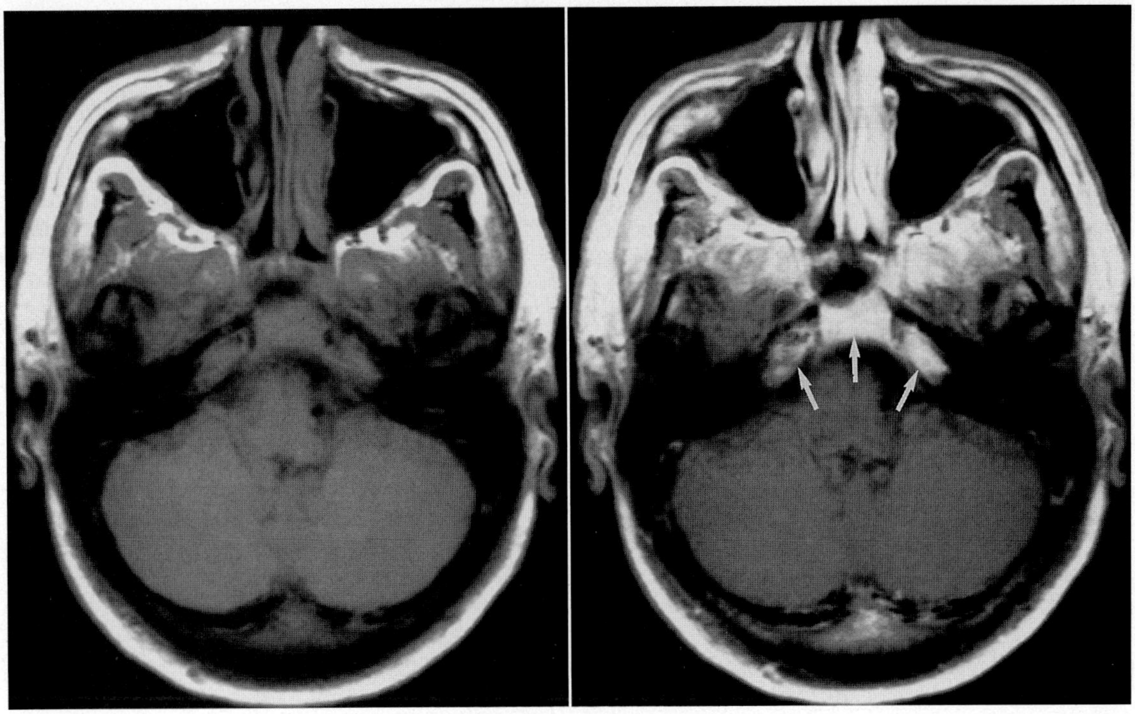


**FIGURE 13** Pitfall of employing postinfusion-only MRI for metastasis affecting skull base. Preinfusion (*A*) and postinfusion (*B*) SE 616/19/1 MR images in a 37-year-old man with Burkitt's lymphoma. Postinfusion scan appears normal, showing enhancement mimicking normal high-intensity fatty marrow in clivus and petrous apices (*arrows, B*). Comparison preinfusion scan (*A*) proves diffuse diploic marrow replacement or reconversion (intensity of marrow lower than normal).

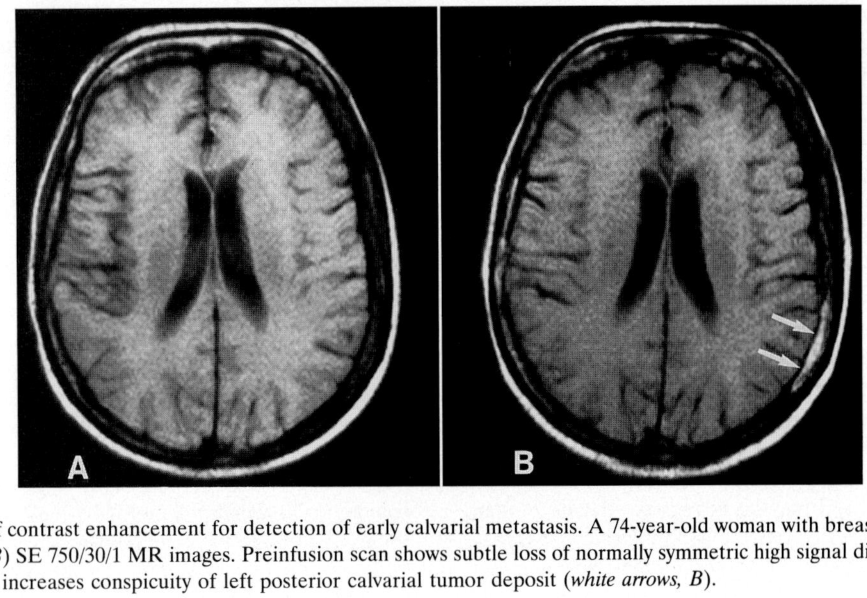


**FIGURE 14** Value of contrast enhancement for detection of early calvarial metastasis. A 74-year-old woman with breast carcinoma. Preinfusion (*A*) and postinfusion (*B*) SE 750/30/1 MR images. Preinfusion scan shows subtle loss of normally symmetric high signal diploic marrow on the left. Contrast enhancement increases conspicuity of left posterior calvarial tumor deposit (*white arrows, B*).

## Suggested Reading

Davis PC, Friedman NC, Fry SM, et al. Leptomeningeal metastasis: MR imaging. Radiology 1987; 163:449–454.

Destian S, Sze G, Krol G, et al. MR imaging of hemorrhagic intracranial neoplasms. Am J Neuroradiol 1988; 9:1115–1122.

Healy ME, Hesselink JR, Press GA, et al. Increased detection of intracranial metastases with intravenous Gd-DTPA. Radiology 1987; 165:619–624.

Hinshaw DB, Inouye CT. Metastatic brain neoplasms. Top Magn Reson Imaging 1989; 1:69–78.

Lee YY, Tien RD, Bruner JM, et al. Loculated intracranial metastases. CT and MR characteristics. Am J Neuroradiol 1989; 10:1171–1179; AJR 1990; 154:351–359.

Niendorf HP, Laniado M, Semmler W, et al. Dose administration of gadolinium-DTPA in MR imaging of intracranial tumors. Am J Neuroradiol 1987; 8:803–815.

Russell EJ, Geremia GK, Johnson CE, et al. Multiple cerebral metastases: Detectability with Gd-DTPA enhanced MR imaging. Radiology 1987; 165:609–617.

Russell EJ, Rothman M, Hesselink J, et al. Optimal MR screening protocol for cerebral metastases: The utility of post-infusion proton-density weighted scans. Presented at the 76th Annual Meeting of the RSNA, Chicago, Ill, 1990 (Cum Laude Award).

Sze G, Milano E, Johnson C, et al. Detection of brain metastases: Comparison of contrast-enhanced MR with unenhanced MR and enhanced CT. Am J Neuroradiol 1990; 11:785–791.

Sze G, Soletsky S, Bronen R, et al. MR imaging of the cranial meninges with emphasis on contrast enhancement and meningeal carcinomatosis. Am J Neuroradiol 1989; 10:965–975; AJR 1989; 153:1039–1049.

West MS, Russell EJ, Breit R, et al. Calvarial and skull base metastases: Comparison of nonenhanced and Gd-DTPA enhanced MR images. Radiology 1990; 174:85–91.

Yuh WTC, Engelken JD, Muhonen MG, et al. Experience with high-dose gadolinium MR imaging in the evaluation of brain metastases. Am J Neuroradiol 1992; 13:335–345.

# MRI and CT in Multiple Sclerosis

*TINA I. YOUNG, M.D.*

Multiple sclerosis (MS) is a chronic central nervous system (CNS) disease in which normal myelin is destroyed. Although it is the most common of the demyelinating diseases affecting the CNS, it is of unknown origin. The loss of myelin in MS results from an inflammatory reaction mediated by cells derived from the peripheral circulation, primarily macrophages and T lymphocytes that migrate across blood vessel walls into the parenchyma of the brain. The stimulus for the inflammatory reaction, assumed to be a component of myelin, may be an autoimmune response triggered by a virus.

## Indications and Clinical Utility

The diagnosis of MS is made from the clinical history, neurological findings, cerebrospinal fluid (CSF) analyses, evoked electrical potential responses, and imaging evaluations. For the patient in whom MS is a suspected diagnosis, magnetic resonance imaging (MRI) is the modality of choice. MRI, with over 90 percent sensitivity for lesion detection in the CNS white matter, is superior to conventional computed tomography (CT) (Fig. 1). CT of the brain is less than half as sensitive as MRI for white matter lesion detection. In addition, visualization of plaques in the posterior fossa and spinal cord is decreased with CT, because of bone artifact and the limitation to the cross-sectional plane. MRI has the advantage of multiplanar capability, which aids in lesion detection in the brain and spinal cord. MRI with gadolinium diethylenetriamine penta-acetic acid (Gd-DTPA), a paramagnetic contrast agent, has proved to be sensitive in distinguishing active from inactive MS lesions.

## Technical Approach

At my institution a 1.5 T magnet is used for MRI evaluation of the brain in a patient with known or suspected MS. Spin-echo T1-weighted sagittal and axial images (TR = 600 to 700, TE = 11 to 17) are initially obtained, followed by spin-echo T2-weighted axial images (TR = 2500, TE = 30/80). Gd-DTPA 0.1 mmol per kilogram is given IV and followed within 3 minutes by T1-weighted axial and coronal images through the brain. Slice thickness of 5 mm with a 2.5 mm gap, a 20 cm field of view (FOV) and a 256 x 192 matrix with 2 NEX is used for all sequences except the T2-weighted axial series in which 1 NEX is used. For the T1-weighted coronal series, a slice thickness of 4 mm with a 1 mm gap is used. T2-weighted sagittal images are an optional sequence for evaluation of the corpus callosum for MS lesions. Short tau inversion recovery (STIR) sequences have been helpful in detecting optic neuritis.

T1-weighted imaging without gadolinium is mainly for demonstrating anatomic detail. In the T2-weighted series, the first echo pulse sequence (proton density images) in which the TR is long and the TE is short is used to distinguish CSF from MS plaques, especially in the periventricular regions. In the T2-weighted series, the second echo pulse sequence in which the TR and TE are long is used to distinguish MS plaques from normal brain parenchyma (Fig. 2). The T1-weighted images with gadolinium are used to evaluate the integrity of the blood-brain barrier.

For evaluation of known or suspected spinal cord MS, spin-echo T1-weighted and T2-weighted sagittal images are obtained through the cord followed by intravenous Gd-DTPA, and spin-echo T1-weighted sagittal and axial images through the same areas. Patients in whom spinal cord MS is a diagnostic possibility should have MRI of the brain as well.

## Diagnostic Approach

Before discussing the key MRI signs in MS, it is important to have an understanding of the pathology of MS. In an acute

A

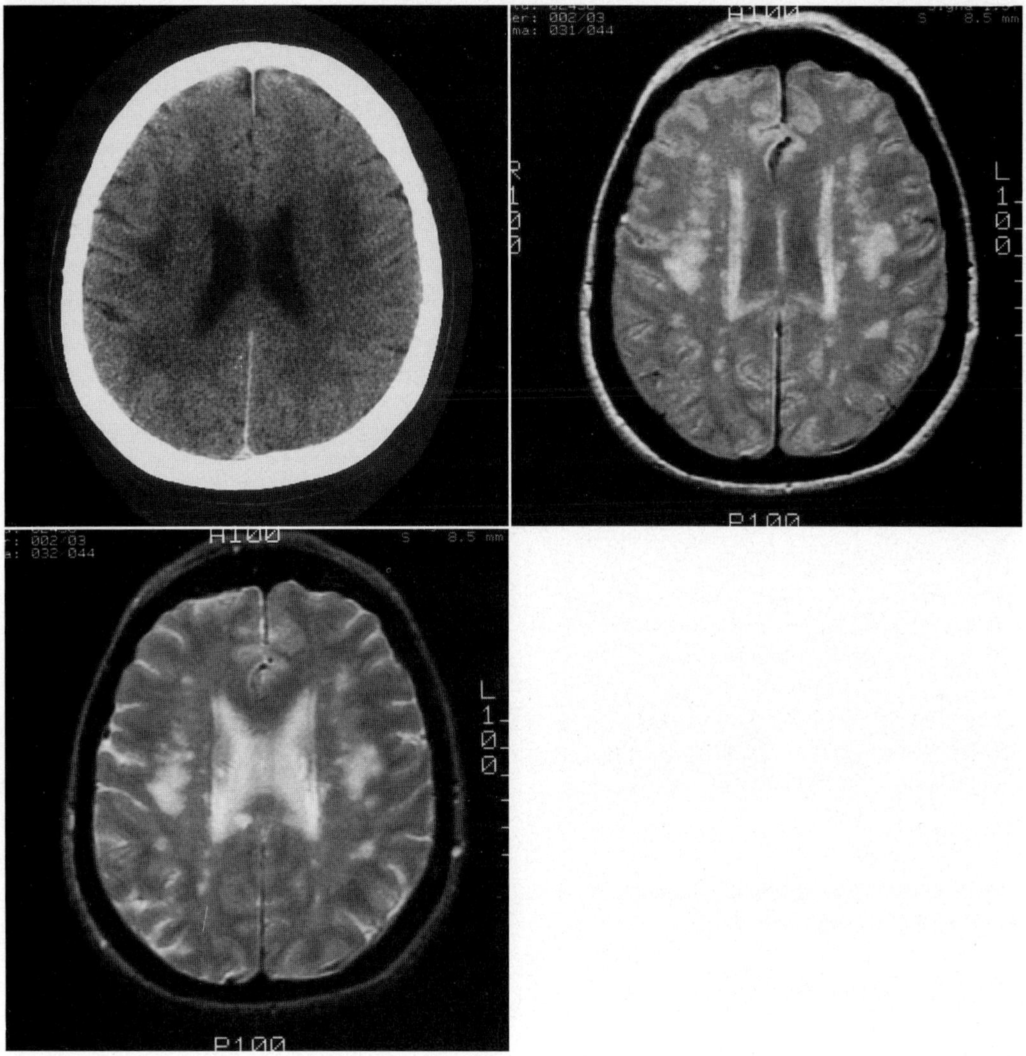


B

C

**FIGURE 1** Multiple sclerosis: CT findings vs. MRI. *A,* CT scan shows hypodensity within the periventricular white matter of the corona radiata. *B* and *C,* Axial T2-weighted proton density (first echo) and second echo images show periventricular bright T2 signal and multiple T2 hyperintense lesions within the white matter.

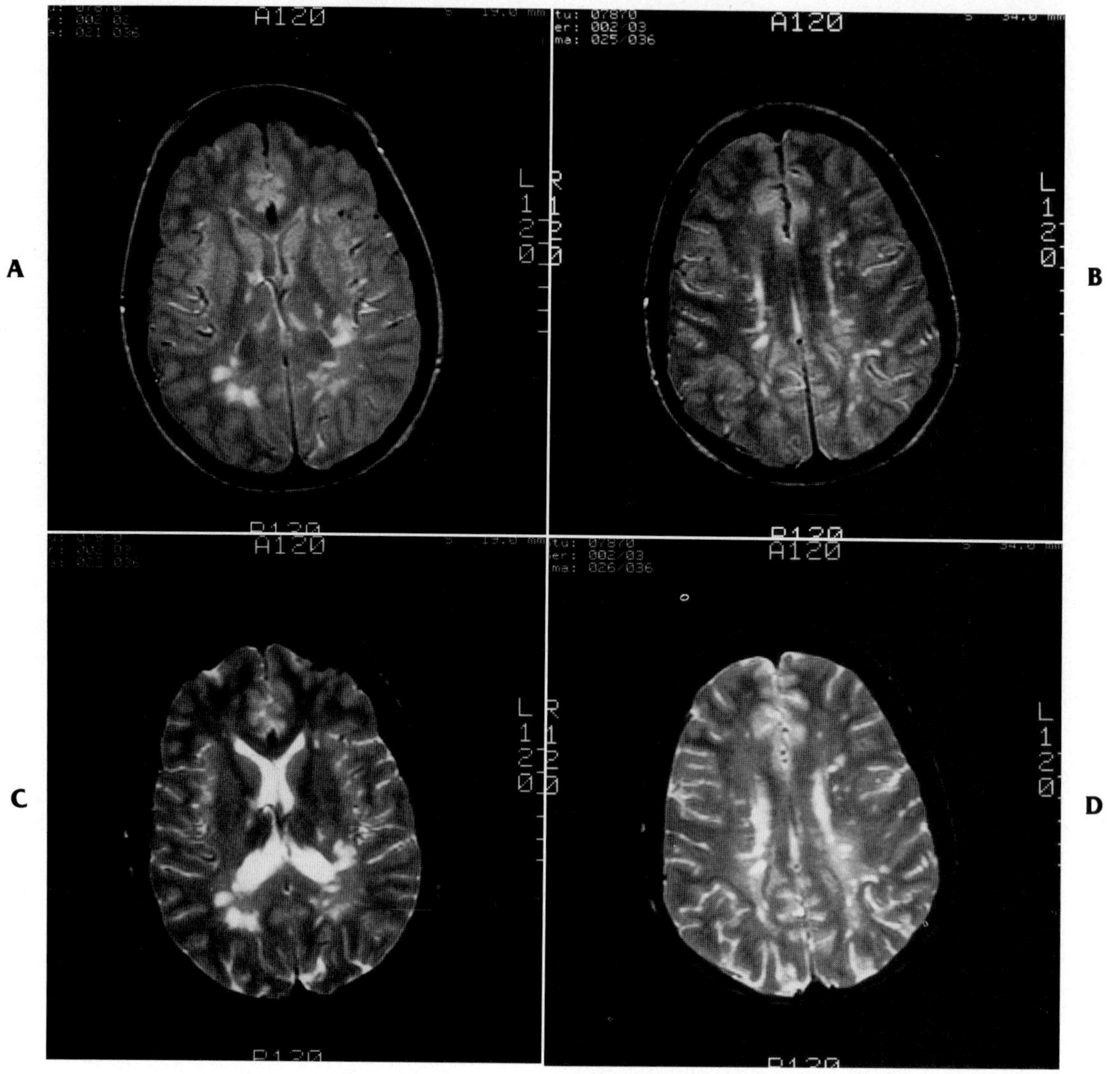

**FIGURE 2** MS patient showing usefulness of T2-weighted series in lesion detection. *A* and *B,* Proton density images of T2 series used to distinguish MS plaques from normal brain parenchyma. *C* and *D,* Second echo images of T2 series used to distinguish MS plaques from normal brain parenchyma.

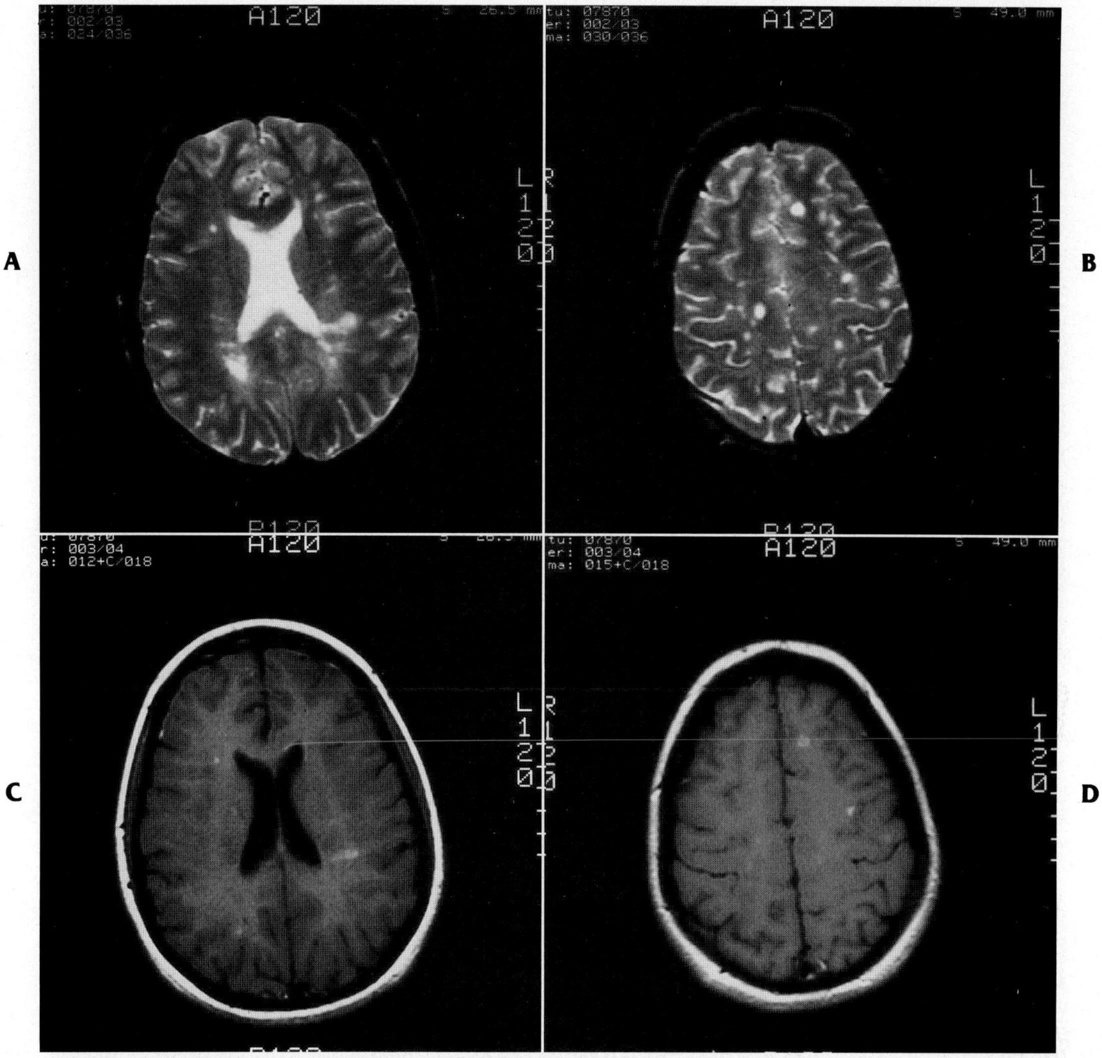

**FIGURE 3** MS plaques with gadolinium enhancement. *A* and *B,* Multiple hyperintense lesions are present in the white matter on T2-weighted series. *C* and *D,* Gadolinium-enhanced T1-weighted MRI shows enhancement in active MS plaques.

attack of MS, the blood-brain barrier is apparently disrupted. In an acute plaque, pathological studies show demyelination in a perivenous distribution with products from myelin breakdown, edema, and perivenular inflammatory cells consisting of macrophages, lymphocytes, and plasma cells. Astrocytic gliosis and hyperplasia occur in chronic plaques with decreased numbers of oligodendroglia, the myelin-producing cells. After the initial event, usually 1 month, atrophy and cavitation occur. Not all MS lesions are alike. Pathologically, there may be demyelination with axonal sparing, partial axonal interruption, or widespread necrosis of all cellular elements with cavity formation.

MS plaques occur in the periventricular white matter, subcortical U fibers, corpus callosum, corona radiata, internal capsule, centra semiovale regions, brain stem, cerebellum, spinal cord, and in any other structure in which myelin is contained. Rarely plaques may be seen in the gray matter of the cerebrum.

Although CT is not the modality of choice for imaging MS in the brain or spine for reasons elucidated previously, it may show findings of isodense or hypodense white matter foci of MS. With gadolinium-contrasted MRI, plaques with recent demyelination can be enhanced (Fig. 3). Double-dose intravenous gadolinium contrast medium provides increased sensitivity to lesion detection.

Signal intensity of MS plaques is related to water content. Plaques may be isointense to hypointense on the MRI T1-weighted series. On the T2-weighted series, the lesions are hyperintense (increased water content). The proton density image, the first echo of the T2 series, is helpful in distinguishing CSF from plaque. The plaque is hyperintense or bright and is distinguished from CSF, which is hypointense or gray. The second echo is important in distinguishing plaque from normal brain parenchyma. The regions of bright T2 signal may correspond to areas of demyelination, edema, and/or gliosis. Gd-DTPA, as a paramagnetic contrast agent, has the capability to cross an abnormal blood-brain barrier. Gadolinium enhancement has been found to occur in histologically active lesions. These may be fresh plaques with acute inflammation or in chronic plaques with reactivation at the margins. Therefore

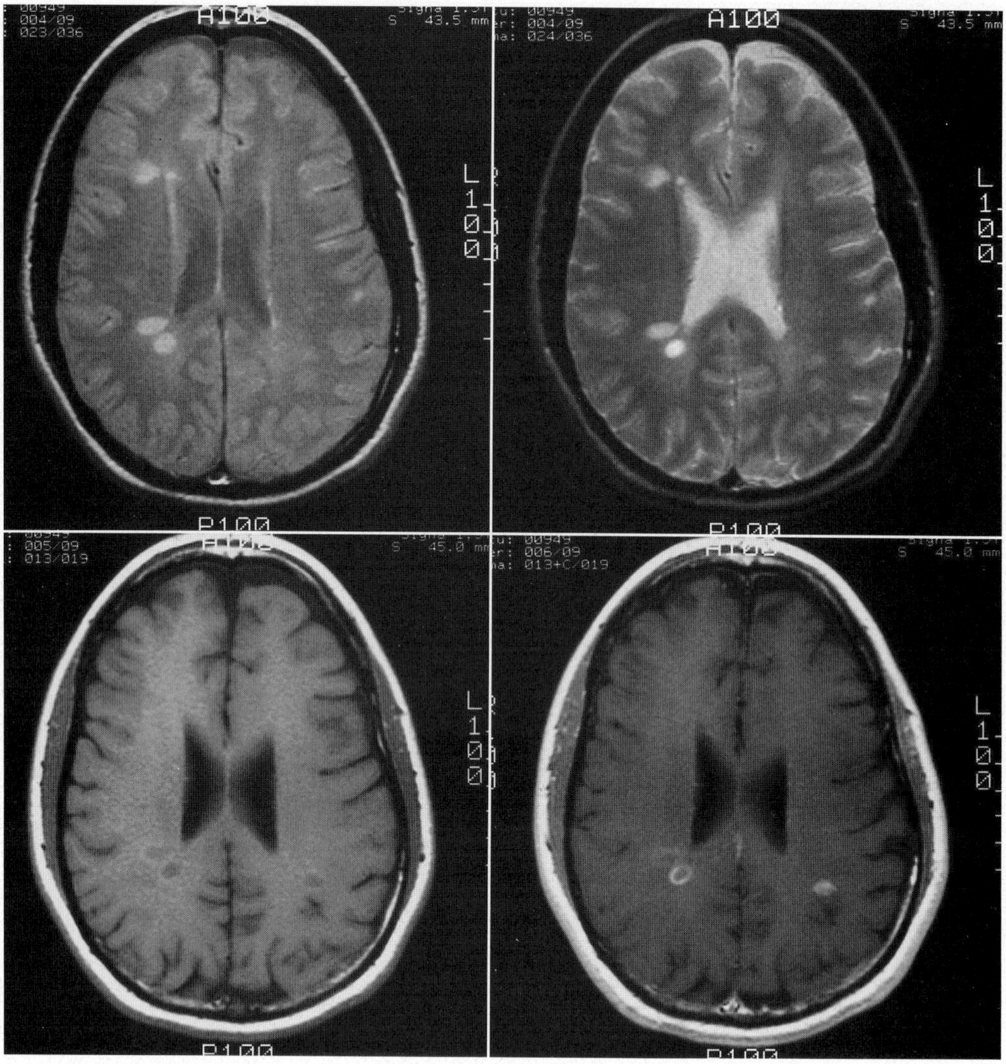


**FIGURE 4** Ovoid, elliptical MS plaque in which major axis of lesion is perpendicular to anteroposterior axis of head. *A* and *B,* T2 dual-echo series through brain. *C* and *D,* T1 axial images before and after gadolinium administration showing enhancement in the active lesion.

gadolinium is useful in distinguishing histologically active MS lesions from histologically inactive MS lesions and for determining the integrity of the blood-brain barrier. The enhancement pattern may be used to follow disease activity, outcome, and possible improvement with treatment. However, clinical course and disability do not always correlate with MRI findings. Further study in these areas is needed.

Plaques in the white matter may range in size from 1 to 2.5 mm. They can be round, punctate, or ovoid usually with little mass effect. In the periventricular white matter, they are commonly seen near the atria and occipital horns of the lateral ventricles and create a "lumpy-bumpy" pattern. The plaques can be ovoid or elliptical hyperintense lesions, in which the major axis of the lesion is perpendicular to the anteroposterior axis of the head (Fig. 4). They have been proposed to correspond to the pathologic finding of perivascular demyelination referred to as "Dawson's fingers." Rarely a plaque can simulate a mass lesion and in those cases may have mass effect, often being confused with a primary brain tumor such as a glioma (Fig. 5). Chronic plaques can cavitate or become confluent in a periventricular distribution.

MS plaques often involve the corpus callosum and are oriented in a horizontal direction (Fig. 6). MS lesions involving the callosal-septal interface, the border of the corpus callosum with septum pellucidum, have been described in a large number of MS patients. MS lesions can involve the inferior aspect of the corpus callosum with radiations to the superior aspect of the ventricular surface. In addition, in long-standing MS, the corpus callosum can be atrophied in about 40 percent of patients. Central and cortical atrophy of chronic MS is characterized by ventricular and sulcal enlargement, respectively (Fig. 7).

Decreased T2 signal intensity has been described in the thalamus and in the putamen of patients with MS. This finding may be secondary to ferritin accumulation, but its cause is unknown.

Spinal cord lesions in MS (Figs. 8, 9) may present with motor or sensory long tract signs in one or more limbs. As it can be for the brain, the clinical neurologic presentation is variable. Three patterns have been described in spinal cord lesions in MS: (1) bright T2 intraparenchymal signal abnormality in the cord without cord deformity, (2) swelling in the acute phase

*Text continued on p. 511.*

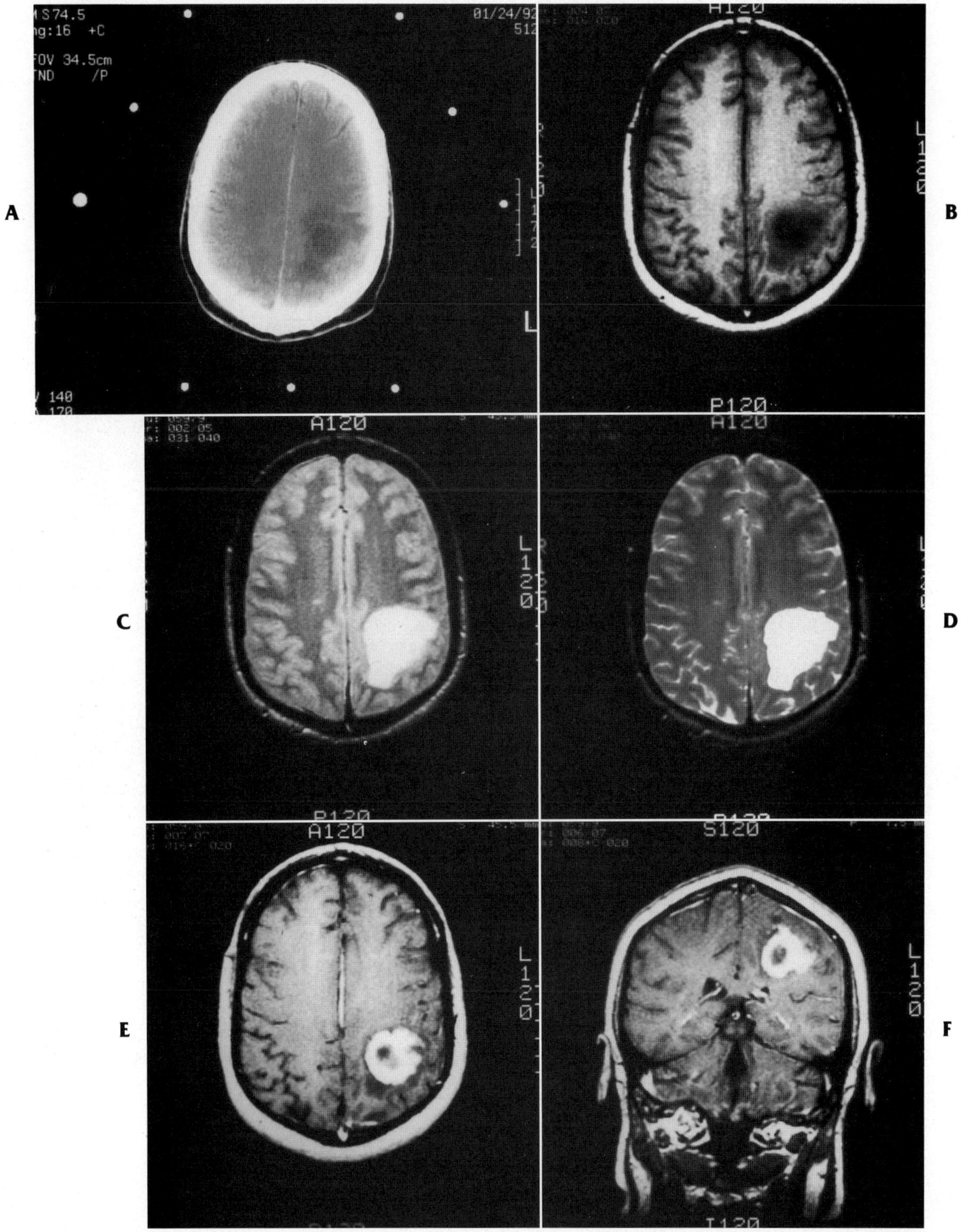

**FIGURE 5** Patient with acute MS with appearance as mass lesion. *A,* CT scan with contrast shows a mildly enhancing low-attenuation mass in the left frontoparietal lobe. *B,* T1 axial image shows hypointense T1 signal in the lesion in the left frontoparietal region. *C* and *D,* First and second echo axial T2 images show hyperintense T2 signal within the lesion. *E* and *F,* T1-weighted axial and coronal gadolinium-enhanced images show marked gadolinium enhancement.

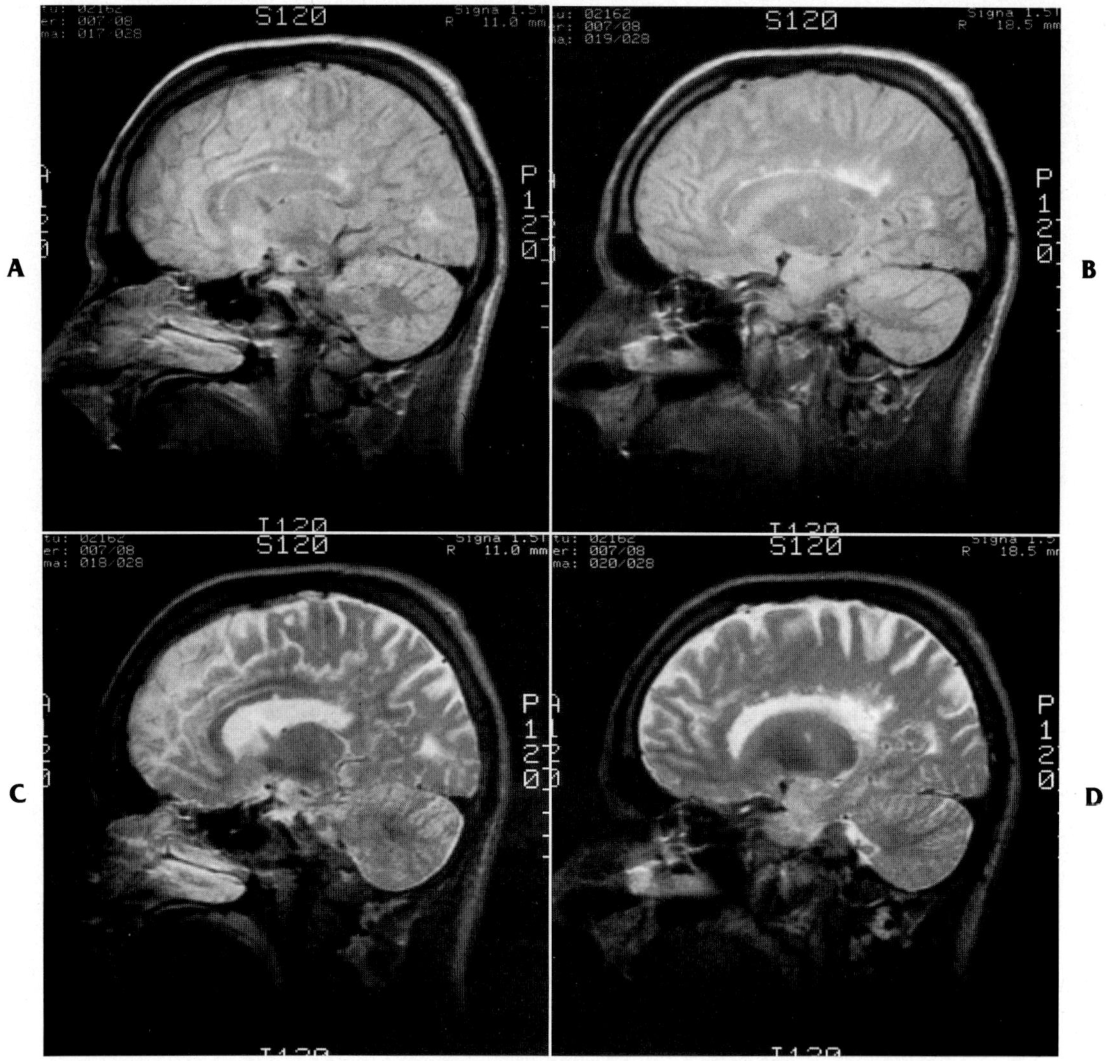


**FIGURE 6** MS lesions involving corpus callosum. Sagittal T2 first echo (*A* and *B*) and second echo (*C* and (*D*) weighted images through the corpus callosum demonstrate hyperintense MS lesions.

A

B

C

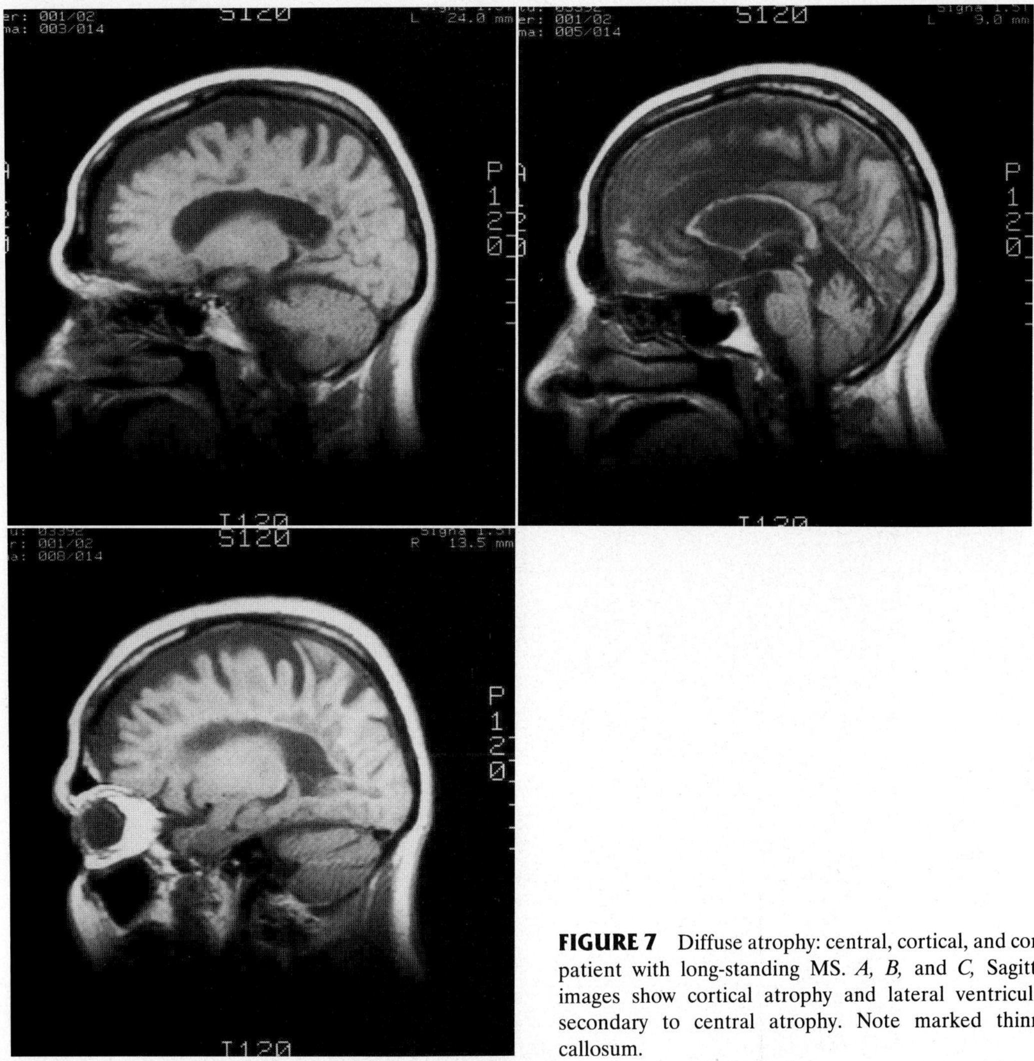

**FIGURE 7** Diffuse atrophy: central, cortical, and corpus callosum in patient with long-standing MS. *A, B,* and *C,* Sagittal T1-weighted images show cortical atrophy and lateral ventricular enlargement secondary to central atrophy. Note marked thinning of corpus callosum.

A

B

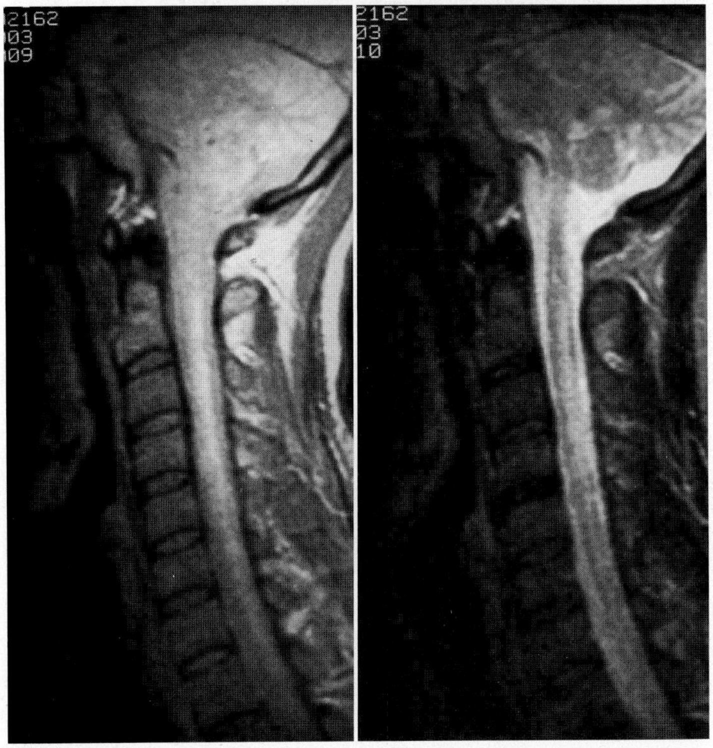

**FIGURE 8** Spinal cord MS. *A,* Sagittal T2 proton density image of the cervical spine with hyperintense intraparenchymal signal abnormality within the spinal cord. *B,* Hyperintense T2 signal within the cord on second echo of T2-weighted series corresponds to MS lesions.

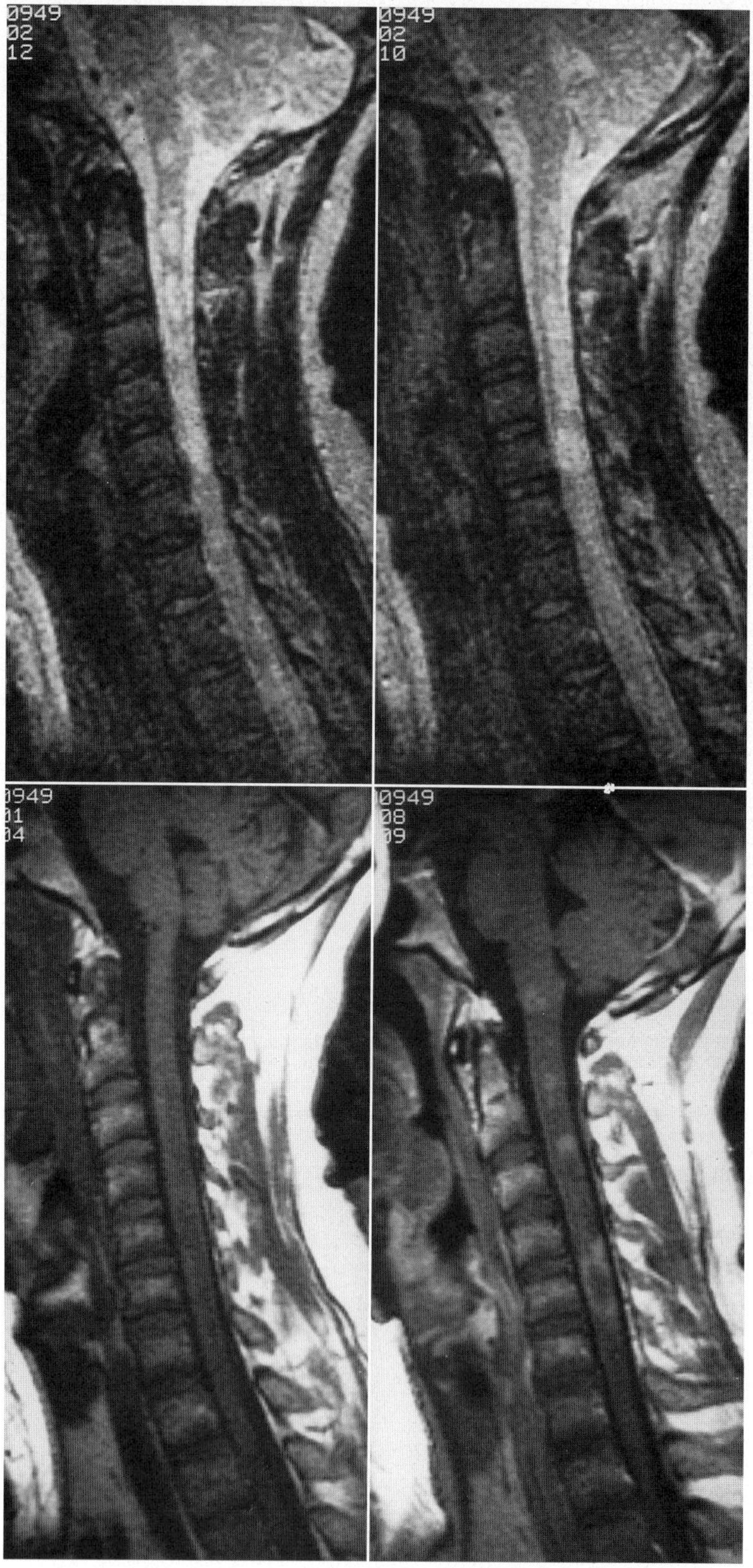


A B C D

**FIGURE 9** Spinal cord MS with active lesions. *A* and *B,* Multiple hyperintense T2 signal abnormalities within the cervical spinal cord are present. *C* and *D,* Sagittal T1 images through the cervical spine before and after administration of gadolinium demonstrate multiple enhancing lesions within the spinal cord are consistent with active MS lesions.

with spinal cord enlargement, and (3) atrophy of the spinal cord. Patients with spinal cord lesions in MS may present with or without lesions within the brain. Active lesions in the spinal cord usually enhance with gadolinium.

The differential diagnosis for bright T2 foci in the white matter is broad. Pathologic entities included are microvascular disease with white matter ischemia, lacunar infarcts, encephalitides, vasculitis, trauma, radiation and chemotherapy effects, migraine, neurofibromatosis, sarcoid, syphilis, multifocal glioma, lymphoma, neoplastic metastases, electroconvulsive therapy effect, and white matter leukodystrophies. Correlation with clinical history and the neurological evaluation are of ultimate importance in making a diagnosis, since the imaging findings are not pathognomonic.

MS is a disease affecting individuals from 20 to 50 years old, but the majority of patients are young adults in the range of 20 to 40 years of age. MS affects females more than males in a ratio of 2:1. There is an incidence of 30 to 80 cases per 100,000. In distinguishing MS from white matter ischemia, age is an important factor, because white matter ischemia is commonly observed in patients over 60 years old. There is high specificity of MRI for MS when age and sex are considered.

As described previously, MS involves the periventricular white matter near the atria and occipital horns of the lateral ventricles, and commonly involves the corpus callosum and subcortical U fibers. In white matter ischemia, there is a history of hypertension, stroke, diabetes, and cardiovascular disease. The corpus callosum and subcortical U fibers are more often spared in microangiopathic disease, because of the collateralization of blood supply to the corpus callosum and U fibers. Therefore involvement of the U fibers and corpus callosum favors the diagnosis of MS. History, including viral infections, vaccinations, acquired immunodeficiency syndrome (AIDS), headaches, trauma, radiation or chemotherapy, and immune status, can be helpful in narrowing the differential diagnosis. Many of the leukodystrophies of the white matter occur in children. Enhancement can be observed in many entities; however, it is not usually observed in white matter ischemia.

Nonpathologic entities such as Virchow-Robin spaces are usually isointense to CSF on proton density T2-weighted images, in contrast to pathologic entities that are usually hyperintense on dual-echo T2-weighted images. Virchow-Robin spaces, 1 to 2 mm in size, are small subarachnoid spaces that follow the pia around penetrating nutrient vessels of the brain. They are commonly found in the superficial white matter of the cerebral hemispheres and at the level of the lower basal ganglia and the anterior commissure. This is where the lenticulostriate arteries enter the anterior perforated substance.

## Discussion

There are many challenges ahead in understanding the pathophysiology of demyelination in MS. Further work must be done to correlate clinical course of the disease with imaging findings, grade of disability, and patient outcome. There is the challenge of distinguishing between different pathologic types of MS lesions. There is often poor correlation between the pathological plaque burden and clinical disease severity, or even between specific CNS lesions and clinical symptoms referable to that particular site. The capability of MRI to separate gliosis, edema, or demyelination is not specific. Proton MRI spectroscopy may be employed in evaluation of a variety of types of MS lesions. New imaging techniques, such as magnetic transfer imaging, may increase characterization of MS lesions by employing sequences that emphasize magnetization transfer contrast. Magnetization contrast is determined by the exchange of magnetization between water protons and protons from molecules such as myelin. Further in vivo studies of the pathophysiology of MS lesions are needed to clarify the heterogeneous pathologic clinical picture of MS.

## Suggested Reading


Drusset V, Grossman RI, Ramer KN, et al. Experimental allergic encephalomyelitis and MS: Lesion characterization with magnetization transfer imaging. Radiology 1992; 182:483–491.

Edwards MK, Bonnin JM. White matter disease. In: Atlas SW, ed. Magnetic Resonance Imaging of the Brain and Spine. New York: Raven Press, 1991:467.

Gean-Marton AD, Vezina LG, Marton KI, et al. Abnormal corpus callosum: A sensitive and specific indicator of MS. Radiology 1991; 180:215–221.

Gonzalez-Scarano F, Grossman RI, Galetta S, et al. Multiple sclerosis disease activity correlates with gadolinium enhanced magnetic resonance imaging. Ann Neurol 1987; 21:300–306.

Grossman RI, Braffman BH, Brorson JR, et al. Multiple sclerosis: Serial study of gadolinium enhanced MR imaging. Radiology 1988; 169:117–122.

Harris JO, Frank JA, Patronas N, et al.: Serial gadolinium enhanced MRI scans in patients with early relapsing-remitting MS: Implications for clinical trials and natural history. Ann Neurol 1991; 29:549–555.

Hesselink JR, Hicks RJ. Brain: Periventricular white matter abnormalities. In: Edelman R, Hesselink JR, eds. Clinical Magnetic Resonance Imaging. Philadelphia: WB Saunders, 1990:545.

Honig LS, Sheremata WA. Magnetic resonance imaging of spinal cord lesions in MS. J Neurol Neurosurg Psych 1989; 52:459–466.

Mikulis D, Kuhn M. Multiple sclerosis. In: Taveras JM, Ferrucci JT, eds. Radiology: Diagnosis, Imaging, Intervention. Vol. 3(40A). Philadelphia: JB Lippincott, 1991:1.

Nesbit GM, Forbes GS, Scheithauer BW, et al. Multiple sclerosis: Histopathologic and MR and/or CT correlation in 37 cases at biopsy and 3 cases at autopsy. Radiology 1991; 180:467–474.

Wallace CJ, Seland TP, Fong TC. Multiple sclerosis: The impact of MR imaging. AJR 1992; 158:849–857.

Yetkin FZ, Haughton VM, Papke RA, et al. Multiple sclerosis: Specificity of MR for diagnosis. Radiology 1991; 178:447–451.

# MRI Perfusion Studies of the Brain

*BRUCE R. ROSEN, M.D., Ph.D. · HANNU J. ARONEN, M.D., Ph.D.*

Over the last several years, the usefulness of magnetic resonance imaging (MRI) in neuroimaging has been significantly strengthened by developments in imaging techniques, paramagnetic contrast agents, and the exploitation of intrinsic MRI tissue contrast. Initial efforts at developing imaging techniques for the study of human neuropathology were hampered by the limitations of conventional MRI because T1 and T2, the image contrast parameters used in conventional imaging, are not always sensitive or specific in characterizing tissue or differentiating healthy from pathological states. To address these limitations, significant progress recently has been made in extending the anatomical capabilities of conventional MRI to include the acquisition of tissue function maps with high spatial and temporal resolution. These functional imaging techniques include measurements of water diffusion, temperature, and motion.

Perhaps the most significant functional imaging techniques have been those developed for hemodynamic imaging with MRI. Progress in the imaging of tissue blood flow, blood volume, and blood oxygenation has been spurred by two parallel developments. First, ultrafast techniques now have been implemented on commercially available products that can greatly increase MRI's efficiency in data collection. Ultrafast MRI, for instance, whether high-speed gradient-echo or echo-planar imaging (EPI), allows us to acquire complete, two-dimensional images in less than 1 second ($<50$ msec in the case of EPI). The second important development has involved the coupling of these rapid imaging techniques with improvements in, and a greater understanding of, exogenous and endogenous contrast agents. In neuroimaging, these achievements primarily were accomplished by exploiting high magnetic susceptibility contrast agents that are either exogenously administered (e.g., Gd-DTPA) or intrinsic (e.g., deoxyhemoglobin). Because of the intimate link between tissue function, metabolism, and blood supply, functional MRI of tissue hemodynamics can increase the specificity and sensitivity of information obtained with MRI. By using this combination of magnetic susceptibility contrast and high-speed imaging, we can measure cerebral blood volume (CBV) in tumors and stroke, as well as estimate changes in cerebral blood flow (CBF) and blood oxygenation to visualize human brain activity in real time.

## Indications and Clinical Utility

Dynamic susceptibility contrast imaging has been particularly suited to investigations of hemodynamic perturbations in the central nervous system (CNS). Gd-DTPA–enhanced, T1-weighted contrast material (the so-called relaxivity effect) is useful when the blood-brain barrier (BBB) is grossly disrupted. When the BBB is intact, however, it has little impact on most brain regions, since the intravascular space is small and T1 effects occur locally. Image enhancement for a "conventional" short-range, relaxivity (T1) study depends on the contrast agent's access to water. When the BBB is intact and the agent is intravascularly confined, enhancement is limited. Because acute infarcts, some tumors, and most neurodegenerative diseases occur in the presence of an intact BBB, conventional relaxivity-based contrast imaging often is inadequate to fully characterize these disease states. Unlike relaxivity (T1) contrast studies, magnetic susceptibility (T2 or T2*) contrast results from microscopic variations that are produced by the heterogeneous distribution of high magnetic susceptibility contrast agents within a tissue's magnetic field. Unlike that of conventional T1 contrast studies, image enhancement in susceptibility contrast (T2 or T2*) studies depends on the longer-range magnetic field perturbations that paramagnetic agents produce when they are compartmentalized within the vascular bed.

When compartmentalized within the vascular space, these magnetic field distortions ("susceptibility effects") produced by high magnetic susceptibility materials can act at a distance roughly equal to the radius of the blood vessel to relax the transverse magnetization of surrounding tissue protons. The necessary compartmentalization of contrast agent in the brain is provided by the BBB. The injection of any high magnetic susceptibility contrast agent, such as Gd-DTPA$^{2-}$ or Dy-DTPA$^{2-}$, thus produces a significant decrease in brain signal intensity for both spin-echo T2- and gradient-echo T2*-weighted images during their first pass through the microvascular bed. The magnitude of the T2 or T2* change is influenced by vascular geometry and vessel size, water diffusion, and the size of the susceptibility-induced magnetic field gradient.

To provide indices of CBF and CBV, magnetic susceptibility contrast studies can be coupled with rapid imaging to resolve the first-pass tissue transit of intravenously administered contrast materials. To measure CBV or CBF quantitatively, however, regional changes in MRI signal intensity with respect to time must be converted into contrast agent tissue concentration-time curves. Recent empirical work has shown that the degree of the signal drop depends on two factors: the concentration of an injected contrast agent within the plasma and the fractional volume of intravascular space within the tissue (CBV). After injection, the contrast agent's concentration varies with time, whereas blood volume may vary region by region. Both contrast agent concentration and blood volume reflect an approximately linear relationship to the change observed in the T2 rate, $\Delta(1/T2) \equiv \Delta R2$. This can be determined easily by measuring the percent-signal change from baseline. Within some limiting range, therefore, we are able to measure the contrast agent's concentration in tissue as a function of time (the so-called concentration-time curve) by mapping tissue signal loss dynamically over time.

Although the importance of macrovascular imaging is considerable (witness the recent activity in magnetic resonance angiography [MRA] research), the mechanism by which the brain regulates and meets its needs for metabolic substrates operates at a microvascular level. For this reason, ultrafast techniques that are able directly or indirectly to image the microvascular hemodynamics provide important information on brain function in both the normal and pathophysiological states that are characterized by altered metabolic needs. Susceptibility contrast techniques provide this opportunity in a unique way. An interesting result of the influence of the physics behind susceptibility-induced brain signal loss is that certain MRI pulse sequence techniques are better suited for the visualization of particular vascular regions of interest than others. Specifically we can obtain selective sensitivity to the microvasculature through the use of spin-echo, rather than gradient-echo, imaging. In gradient-echo images all vessels are weighted approximately equally. Thus gradient-echo–derived CBV maps represent effects from the total blood volume, including the supplying arteries and draining veins. The images produced by spin-echo techniques, however, more heavily weight contrast within the capillary bed, that is, the *microvascular* blood volume. At our center we obtain optimum tissue sensitivity, immunity to artifacts, and clinical utility by using rapid, EPI spin-echo imaging techniques to characterize lesions based on their microvascular structure.

## Technical Approach

In our work we use echo-planar spin-echo imaging and magnetic susceptibility contrast imaging to study brain microvascular perfusion after the bolus administration of paramagnetic chelates. Much of our effort has focused on the application of dynamic susceptibility contrast imaging to the study of patients with intracranial neoplasms in order to assess the effectiveness of MRI CBV blood mapping in characterizing tumor grade and assessing treatment response. Our studies of patients with brain tumors are performed on a GE Signa 1.5 T imager, retrofitted with Instascan echo-planar technology from Advanced NMR Systems Inc. (Wilmington, Mass.). Before an examination, a medical history is obtained to ensure that no contraindications to MRI exist. Patients are then positioned on the scanning table and, if they wish, provided with music to reduce discomfort. Next, an 18 gauge catheter is inserted into a large vein, usually the antecubital vein, and is secured with Tegrederm. A saline drip is used to maintain patency of the vein. Conventional noncontrast T1- and T2-weighted studies are acquired, along with other forms of high-speed imaging, such as diffusion imaging. Before dynamic MRI scanning commences, patient vital signs are acquired and monitored by an attending nurse, and venous patency is again verified. At the end of the examination, the intravenous line is removed, the patient is thanked for participating, and comments concerning the experience of the scan are invited.

After the precontrast T1- and T2-weighted images, single or multiple slices are selected for functional blood volume mapping studies. We typically perform a two-injection protocol. We use a Medrad power injector to deliver a rapid and uniform contrast agent bolus through the antecubital vein at an injection rate of 5 ml/sec. The first injection (we now use 0.05 mmol/kg Gd-DTPA) is monitored with a dynamic series of T1-weighted inversion recovery (IR) echo-planar images (TR = 3000 ms, TI = 800 ms, TE = 25 ms), acquired every 3 seconds for 5 minutes. This allows us to determine whether a BBB breakdown has occurred and permits a quantitative assessment of capillary permeability. Next, a second, larger bolus (0.15 mmol/kg) is injected at the same flow rate. During this injection, patients are typically imaged using a 1 minute series of T2-weighted, spin-echo, echo-planar sequences acquired each second (TR = 1000 ms, TE = 100 ms). A voxel size of $1.5 \times 1.5 \times 7$ mm is used for our EPI sequences. Although T1 enhancement from leaky tumors can confound the susceptibility-induced signal loss, the initial contrast agent bolus acts to "presaturate" the tissue from such regions, minimizing these errors.

Our CBV mapping protocol, developed and evaluated in over 80 brain tumor studies, has been quite safe. No major side effects have been observed from the rapid, IV, bolus injection (5 ml/sec) of either $Gd\text{-}DTPA^{2-}$ (Magnevist, Berlex) or Gd-DTPA-BMA (gadodiamide, Sterling-Winthrop). Moreover, the effects of contrast agent dose on the image quality of MRI blood volume maps and patient safety have been assessed by the use of a protocol involving 0.1 and 0.2 mmol/kg injections of gadodiamide in the same patient. CBV maps produced by the higher doses of contrast material showed better signal-to-noise ratios and depicted more detailed anatomical and pathological structures than the lower-dose maps. By simultaneously injecting contrast material and acquiring functional images, we obtain CBV tumor mapping studies during the time of a conventional MRI examination. This may help control costs, and it adds only the time needed to set up the contrast injector to the conventional study.

## Findings

The data from our investigations have demonstrated a number of important features. First, the MRI CBV maps produced by magnetic susceptibility contrast techniques are closely correlated to tumor grade (Fig. 1). The low-grade lesions show low CBV, with a typically homogeneous appearance on MRI CBV maps. Although we have seen remarkable heterogeneity in tumors originally deemed to be low grade, these were later determined to have features consistent with high-grade malignancies (Fig. 2). These focal, high CBV regions often were not seen in conventional precontrast or postcontrast T1- and T2-weighted images. More aggressive lesions demonstrate elevations of CBV at or above the level of normal brain. Additionally, in some lesions, a significant regional heterogeneity of CBV could be determined, particularly in high-grade lesions (Fig. 3). These findings concur with those of previous angiographic and positron emission tomography (PET) studies. High-grade gliomas appear more heterogeneous in blood volume maps and often contain areas of both increased and decreased blood volume. Our data support the hypothesis that MRI blood volume mapping studies will significantly aid in the grading of primary gliomas.

The heterogeneity of primary gliomas creates a significant obstacle to their characterization, since diagnosis based on stereotaxic biopsies depends a great deal on the site selected for this procedure. Selecting the most appropriate site for a biopsy can be difficult, even with $Gd\text{-}DTPA^{2-}$ enhancement or CT guidance. PET FDG studies have previously been shown to aid in the identification of optimal biopsy sites, since these can show the most active regions of the tumor. Based on our finding that MRI blood volume maps and PET FDG studies are correlated in most glioma cases, we expect MRI blood volume mapping techniques to be useful in indicating optimal sites for stereotaxic biopsies in brain tumor patients (e.g., see Fig. 2).

The local failure of external-beam radiotherapy treatment is the most common cause of poor prognosis for glioma

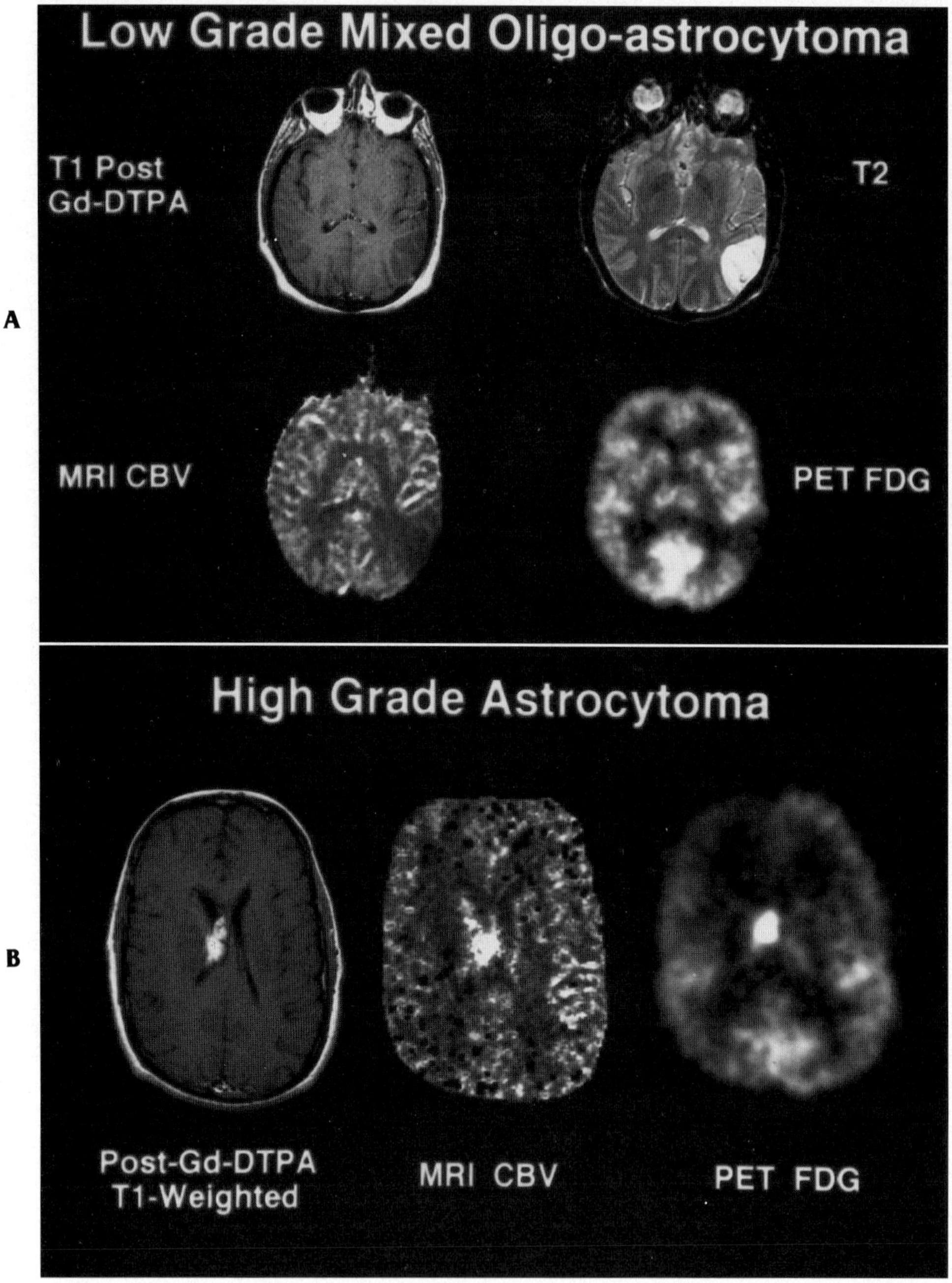


**FIGURE 1** Conventional MR images, MRI CBV maps, and PET FDG images in two patients with primary intracranial tumors. *A,* The low-grade lesion (of mixed type) demonstrates low microvascularity within the lesion, corresponding to decreased glucose metabolism. *B,* The high-grade lesion demonstrates increased microvascularity within the tumor, along with increased glucose uptake.

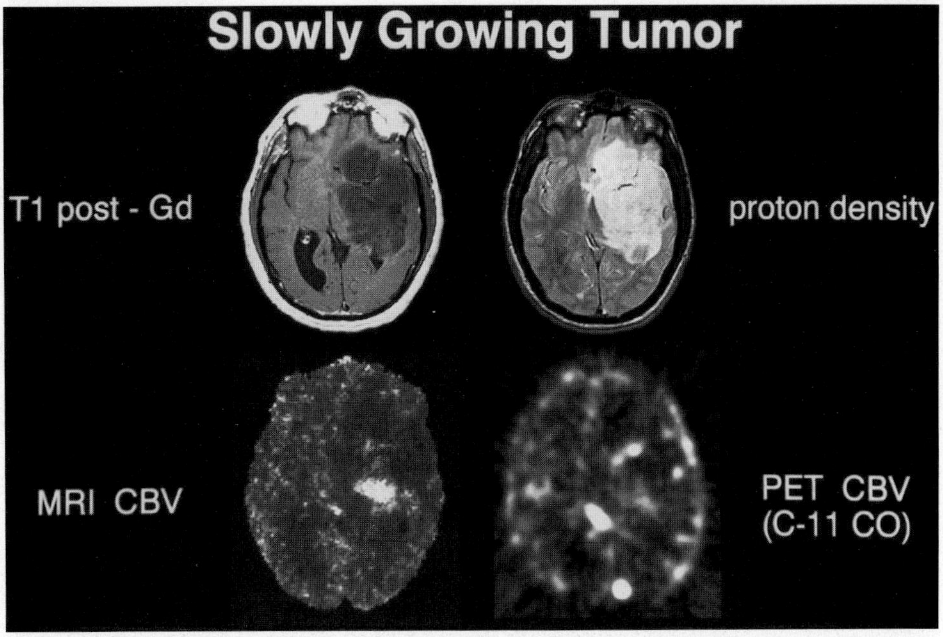


**FIGURE 2** Conventional MR images, MRI CBV map, and PET blood volume map of a patient with a large glioma. Postcontrast images reveal no significant enhancement, suggesting a low-grade lesion. However, the MR CBV image demonstrates a focal area of intense microvascularity within the tumor, verified on PET blood pool images. This lesion was subsequently debulked and found to have high-grade (3/4) components.

patients. Thus it is extremely important to determine the exact extent of the tumor and the tumor cell-free zone when planning radiotherapy. Conventional MRI, even with IV contrast material injection, is not always able to delineate the tumor zone border, because the area enhanced after contrast material injection does not always correspond to the outer edge of tumor invasion. MRI blood volume mapping may help to define the border between tumor and normal brain tissue and to delineate the border between most active and necrotic tumor areas. Also, the border between the tumor area and the edema zone is usually visible in blood volume maps. These features may be useful in planning radiotherapy.

A particularly challenging problem in neuro-oncological imaging results from the aftermath of radiation treatment, the diagnosis of radiation necrosis, and its distinction from tumor regrowth. Because of the different therapeutic approaches entailed, an accurate differential diagnosis between the two states is extremely important. Since both radiation damage and tumor regrowth may be enhanced on CT and conventional MRI studies, it has been impossible to achieve a clear differential diagnosis with these methods. PET FDG studies have proven useful in differentiating suspected radiation necrosis from tumor regrowth and dual-isotope single-photon emission computed tomography (SPECT) with $^{201}$Tl and $^{99m}$Tc-HMPAO may help to differentiate sites of viable tumor tissue from sites of radiation changes. Our preliminary results suggest that MRI CBV mapping may also be useful when evaluating patients for whom radiation necrosis is suspected. An example is shown in Figure 4, in which a left temporal glioma status after proton beam treatment demonstrates a large region of conventional contrast enhancement. CBV imaging clearly shows diminished CBV, consistent with radiation necrosis demonstrated by biopsy.

The relationship between function, metabolism, and blood supply (perfusion) has long been reported, and although it is difficult to confirm a sequential chain of increases in functional activity, metabolic activity, microvascular flow, and CBV in toto, numerous experiments have demonstrated a close relationship between these parameters. Although some of the most interesting techniques currently under investigation in perfusion imaging involve measurements of intrinsic tissue contrast, susceptibility-contrast techniques now exist that provide highly useful, functional maps of pathological states associated with CNS insult. In our studies a significantly reduced calculated blood volume has been noted in regions corresponding to known infarcts. Similar data were obtained by Warach et al. using a rapid TurboFLASH imaging technique that is combined with MRA. In a study of 34 patients with suspected cerebral ischemia, data showed a good correlation between lesions seen with MRA and those seen with dynamic contrast imaging. Furthermore, data from that study demonstrated lesions earlier than those seen with conventional T1- and T2-weighted studies, as would be expected.

Much of what we have learned about normal brain function has come from the study of deficits elicited from focal brain lesions, such as those observed in stroke patients. Paralleling recent PET imaging results, it may now be possible to study brain function safely in normal subjects using susceptibility contrast MRI. We have used quantitative imaging of cerebral hemodynamics with high-speed, susceptibility contrast MRI techniques to generate the first functional MRI maps of human brain activity. These maps are of particular interest in our laboratory for the insight they are likely to provide concerning specifically human activities, such as language, as well as the comparative information they may provide on brain pathophysiology. In our initial work, we used a visual stimulus

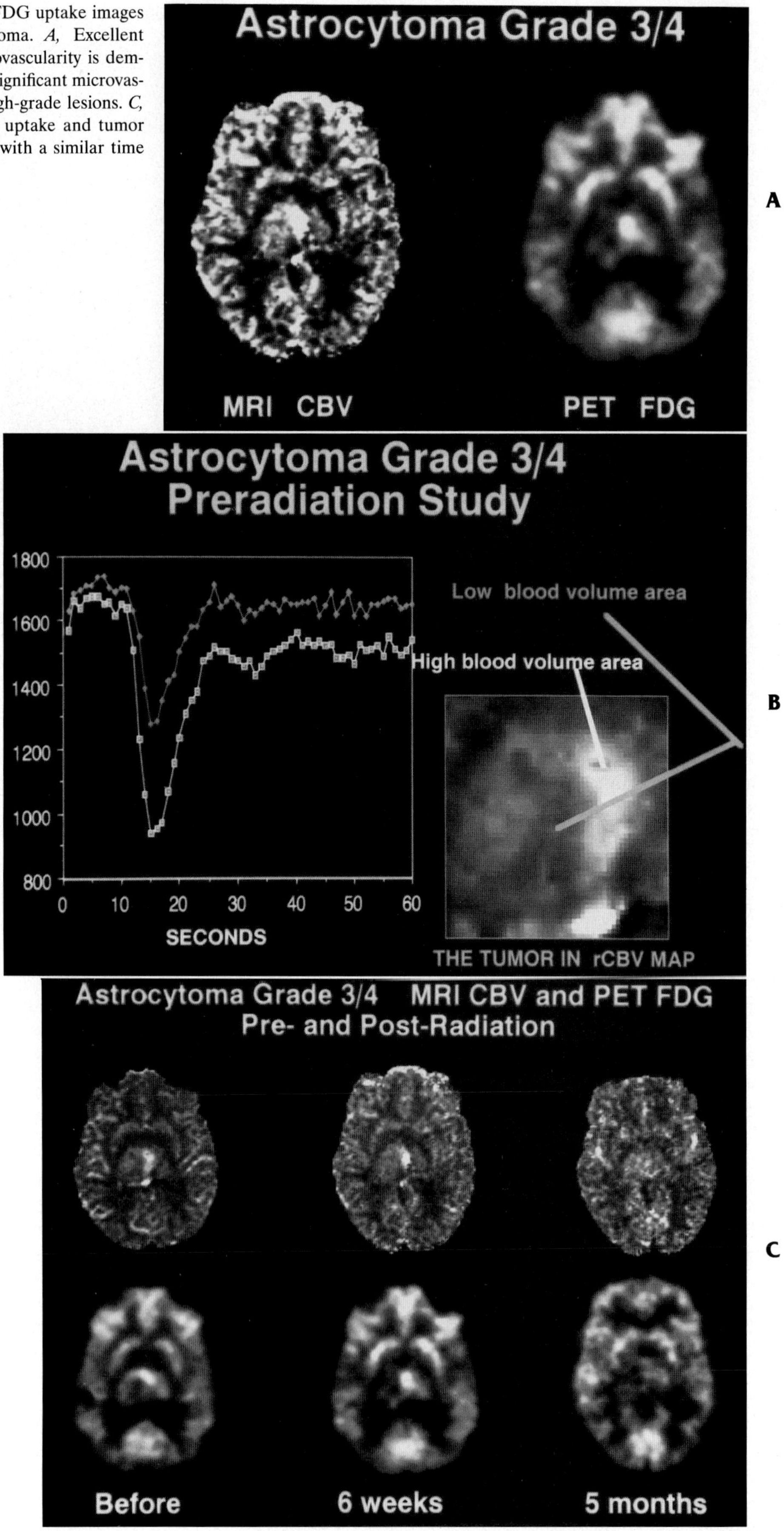


**FIGURE 3** MRI CBV images and PET FDG uptake images in a patient with a grade 3/4 astrocytoma. *A,* Excellent correlation between glucose use and microvascularity is demonstrated. *B,* These images also reveal the significant microvascular heterogeneity present within most high-grade lesions. *C,* Following radiation treatment, both FDG uptake and tumor microvascularity are observed to decrease with a similar time course.

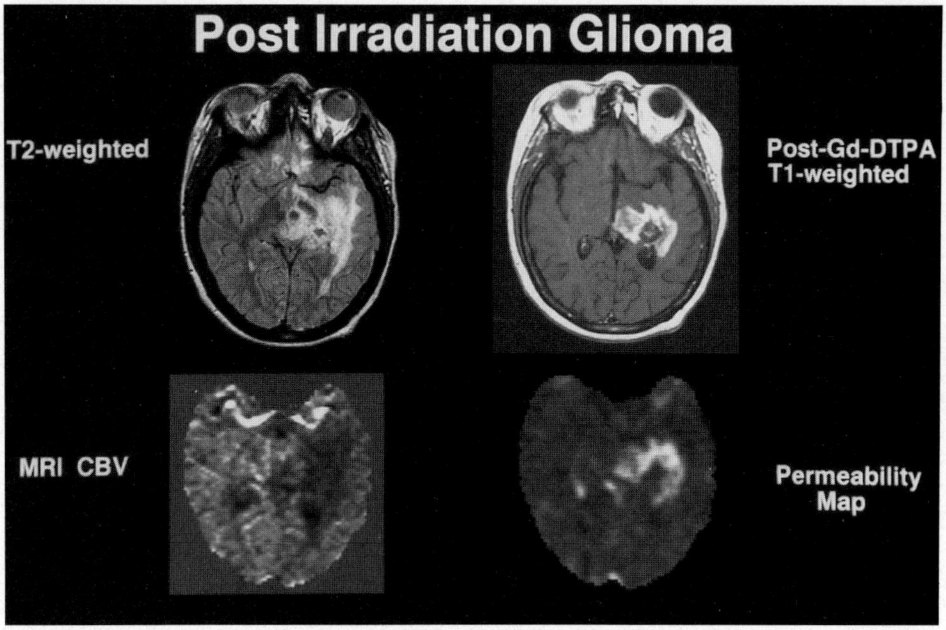


**FIGURE 4** Left temporal glioma status after proton beam treatment. Conventional MR images reveal blood-brain barrier disruption on post-contrast images, consistent with either radiation necrosis or recurrent tumor. MRI CBV map demonstrates decreased vascularity in the lesion, consistent with known radiation effects. Biopsy revealed radiation necrosis. Dynamic data can also be used to quantitatively calculate blood-brain barrier permeability, as demonstrated in the lower right.

paradigm to provide photic stimulation and measured local increases in blood volume that occurred in the primary visual cortex. Since changes in neuronal activity are accompanied by changes in CBF, CBV, blood oxygenation, and metabolism, we expect magnetic susceptibility contrast techniques to allow us to map, with increasingly high spatial and temporal resolution, both mental activity and the effects of CNS pathology by the measurement of changes subsequent to stimulation in these parameters.

Magnetic susceptibility contrast can be observed from intrinsic, as well as exogenous, paramagnetic materials. Linus Pauling established the correlation between the oxygenation state of hemoglobin and its magnetic susceptibility in 1936. In 1982, Thulborn et al. observed that the magnetic susceptibility effect of paramagnetic deoxygenated hemoglobin led to a T2 shortening in blood, thus establishing the first link between the NMR signal intensity and the oxygenation state of blood. Ogawa et al. used this intrinsic contrast effect of deoxygenated paramagnetic hemoglobin with a gradient-echo technique to study the influence of intravascular susceptibility perturbations on signal arising from large blood vessels. More recently, several groups have demonstrated that MRI signal changes occur on T2-, T2*-, and T2′-weighted images, depending on the oxygenation state of the blood. These studies have used techniques that do not measure tissue perfusion directly, but that may contribute significantly to our understanding of organ metabolism by their sensitivity to oxygen use. Because more than 70 percent of the brain's blood lies within the capillaries and venules, the measurement of magnetic susceptibility T2* signal loss predominantly reflects the regional deoxygenation state of the venous system.

Under physiological conditions where oxygen delivery to tissue is not limited by diffusion, measurement of venous oxygenation is critically linked to tissue oxygenation. Since arterial oxygen content is uniform among tissues and is easily and noninvasively measured, determinations of regional venous oxygen saturation can be used to yield regional oxygen consumption by Fick's principle. When the brain is imaged using a susceptibility contrast-sensitive technique, such as gradient-echo EPI, any decrease in blood oxygenation (i.e., hypoxia) results in a loss of signal in the surrounding tissue. Conversely, an excess of blood oxygen supply, such as that observed with increased brain activity or hypercapnia, leads to an increase in tissue signal on T2*-weighted images. The coupling of oxygenation-sensitive pulse sequences with high-speed imaging ultimately may become a powerful tool in assessing regional blood, and hence tissue, oxygenation.

In recent studies we used MRI methods sensitive to changes in CBF and oxygenation to generate functional maps of human visual and motor cortex activation. Our patients undergo dynamic MRI using an EPI technique. Changes in blood oxygenation are detected using a gradient-echo sequence sensitive to T2* (TR = 250 to 3000 ms, TE = 50 ms). Changes in tissue perfusion are evaluated using a spin-echo inversion recovery, T1-sensitive sequence (T1 = 1100 ms, TR = 3500 ms, TE = 42 ms). A series of 80 to 160 images is acquired in under 5 minutes. Neuronal activity is altered in the primary visual cortex using 8 Hz pattern-flash visual stimulation goggles as well as checkerboard stimuli. Activity within the primary motor and somatosensory cortex is induced by active finger movements and passive tactile stimulation. Changes in MRI signal intensity correspond to behaviorally induced changes in neuronal activity (Fig. 5) and match well with previous PET studies. For example, a significant increase in signal intensity was observed in the primary visual cortex of normal volunteers during visual stimulation. Similar signal changes were observed

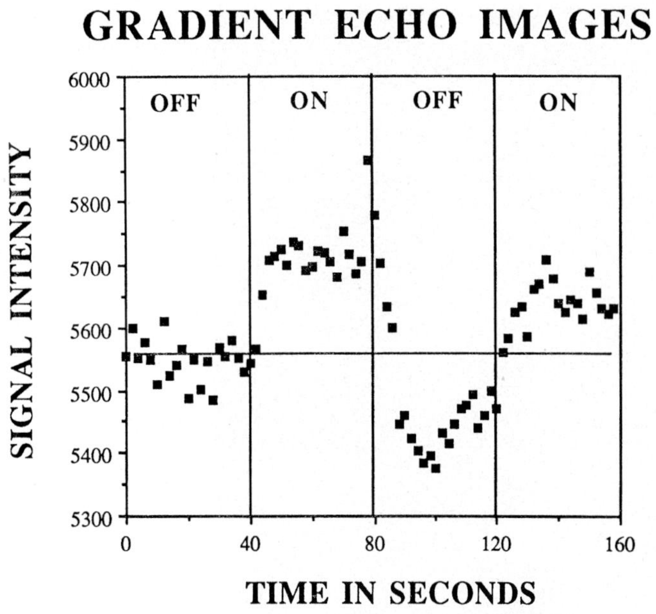


**FIGURE 5** T2*-weighted signal changes induced by visual activation within the primary visual cortex. Signal intensity increased with brain activation reflects decreased intraextravascular magnetic susceptibility differences, arising from increased venous oxygenation. The time course of these MRI signal changes precisely matches the time course of neuronal stimulation.

within the human primary motor cortex during a hand-squeezing task.

## Discussion

Functional MRI techniques that are able to image tissue hemodynamics can provide important information concerning normal and pathophysiological brain states that are characterized by altered metabolic needs. These MRI techniques are important to the study of brain activation during cognitive stimulus and the response of brain tissue to cerebrovascular, neoplastic, and neurodegenerative diseases. Although some of the biophysical principles behind susceptibility contrast techniques are becoming clearer, our understanding of the ultimate potential of these techniques in neuroimaging is in its infancy. Nevertheless, our ability to focus on the microvasculature by the use of spin-echo MRI techniques is unique among all other nuclear and x-ray modalities. High-speed, susceptibility contrast MRI, sensitive to both endogenous and exogenous contrast material, is a technology within the reach of many institutions that can provide functional studies of human neuroanatomy of unprecedented spatial and temporal resolution with which to diagnose and manage disease and to further our understanding of the human brain.

## Suggested Reading


Aronen HJ, Belliveau JW, Kennedy DN, et al. Use of functional MR imaging studies for patients with a primary brain tumor. Radiology 1992; 182:611.

Belliveau JW, Cohen MS, Weisskoff RM, et al. Functional studies of the human brain using high-speed magnetic resonance imaging. J Neuroimag 1991; 1:36–41.

Belliveau JW, Kennedy DN, McKinstry RC, et al. Functional mapping of the human visual cortex using magnetic resonance imaging. Science 1991; 254:621–768.

Belliveau JW, Kennedy DN, McKinstry RC, et al. Functional mapping of the human visual cortex with susceptibility-contrast MR imaging. J Magn Reson Imaging 1991; 1:202.

Belliveau JW, Rosen BR, Kantor HL, et al. Functional cerebral imaging by susceptibility-contrast NMR. Magn Reson Med 1990; 14:538–546.

Bleier A, Jolesz F, Cohen M, et al. Real-time magnetic resonance imaging of laser-tissue interactions. Magn Res Med 1991; 21:132–138.

Bleier AR, Panych L, Cohen MS, et al. Visualization of Laser Heat Propagation with Instant Imaging. New York: Society of Magnetic Resonance in Medicine, 1990: No. 416.

Bradbury MWB. The Concept of a Blood-Brain Barrier. New York: Wiley, 1979.

Chien D, Kwong KK, Gress DR, et al. MR diffusion imaging of cerebral infarction in humans. Am J Neuroradiol 1992; 13:1097–1102.

Cohen MS, Weisskoff RM. Ultra-fast imaging. Magn Reson Imaging 1991; 9:1–37.

Detre JA, Leigh JS, Williams DS, Koretsky AP. Perfusion imaging. Magn Reson Med 1992; 23:37–45.

Di Chiro G, Oldfield E, Wright DC, et al. Cerebral necrosis after radiotherapy and/or intraarterial chemotherapy for brain tumors: PET and neuropathologic studies. AJR 1988; 150:189–197.

Doyle WK, Budinger TF, Valk PE, et al. Differentiation of cerebral radiation necrosis from tumor recurrence by [$^{18}$F]FDG and $^{82}$Rb positron emission tomography. J Comput Assist Tomogr 1987; 11:563–570.

Fisel CR, Ackerman JL, Buxton RB, et al. MR contrast due to microscopically heterogeneous magnetic susceptibility: Numerical simulations and applications to cerebral physiology. Magn Reson Med 1991; 17:336–347.

Frahm J, Haase A, Matthaei D. Rapid three-dimensional MR imaging using the FLASH technique. J Comput Assist Tomogr 1986; 10:363–368.

Hanson M, Glantz M, Hoffman J, et al. FDG-PET in the selection of brain lesions for biopsy. J Comput Assist Tomogr 1991; 15:796–801.

Iannotti F, Fieschi C, Alfano B, et al. Simplified, noninvasive PET measurement of blood-brain barrier permeability. J Comput Assist Tomogr 1987; 11:390–397.

Kwong KK, Belliveau JW, Chesler DA, et al. Dynamic magnetic resonance imaging of human brain activity during primary sensory stimulation. PNAS 1992; 89:5675–5679.

Majumdar S, Gore JC. Studies of diffusion in random fields produced by variations in susceptibility. J Magn Reson 1988; 78:41–55.

McKinstry RC, Weisskoff RM, Belliveau JW, et al. Ultrafast NMR imaging of water mobility: Animal models of altered cerebral perfusion. J Magn Reson Imaging 1992; 2:377–384.

Moseley M, Cohen Y, Mintorovitch J, et al. Early detection of regional cerebral ischemia in cats: Comparison of diffusion and T2 weighted MRI and spectroscopy. Magn Reson Med 1990; 14:330–346.

Moseley ME, Kucharczyk J, Mintorovitch J, et al. Diffusion-weighted MR imaging of acute stroke: Correlation with T2-weighted and magnetic susceptibility-enhanced MR imaging in cats. Am J Neuroradiol 1990; 11:423–429.

Ogawa S, Lee T, Nayak A, Glynn P. Oxygenation-sensitive contrast in magnetic resonance image of rodent brain at high magnetic fields. Magn Reson Med 1990; 14:68–78.

Pauling L, Coryell CD. The magnetic properties and structure of hemoglobin, oxyhemoglobin and carbonmonoxyhemoglobin. Proc Natl Acad Sci U S A 1936; 22:210–216.

Poncelet B, Wedeen V, Weisskoff R, Cohen M. Measurement of brain parenchyme motion with cine echo-planar MRI. Radiology 1992; in press.

Rapoport SI. Blood-Brain Barrier in Physiology and Medicine. New York: Raven Press, 1976.

Rosen BR, Belliveau JW, Buchbinder BR, et al. Contrast agents and cerebral hemodynamics. Magn Reson Med 1991; 19:285–292.

Rosen BR, Belliveau JW, Vevea JM, Brady TJ. Perfusion imaging with NMR contrast agents. Magn Reson Med 1990; 14:249–265.

Rzedzian RR, Pykett IL. An instant technique for real-time MR imaging. Radiology 1986; 161(P):333.

Schwartz R, Carvalho P, Alexander E, et al. Radiation necrosis vs high-grade recurrent glioma: Differentiation by using dual-isotope SPECT with $^{201}$T1 and $^{99m}$Tc-HMPAO. AJR 1992; 158:399–404.

Thulborn K, Waterton JC, Matthews PM, Radda GK. Oxygenation dependence of the transverse relaxation time of water protons in whole blood at high field. Biochim Biophys Acta 1982; 714:265–270.

Thulborn K, Waterton J, Radda G. Proton imaging for in vivo blood flow and oxygen consumption measurements. J Magn Reson 1981; 45:188–191.

Thulborn K, Waterton J, Styles P, Radda G. Rapid measurement of blood oxygenation and flow by high-field 1H NMR. Biochem Soc Trans 1981; 9:233–234.

Turner R, LeBihan D, Moonen CTW, et al. Echo-planar time course MRI of cat brain oxygenation changes. Magn Reson Med 1991; 22:159–166.

Turner R, Le Bihan D, Moonen CTW, Frank J. Echo-planar imaging of deoxygenation episodes in cat brain at 2 T. J Magn Reson Imaging 1991; 1:227.

Tyler JL, Diksic M, Villemure J-G, et al. Metabolic and hemodynamic evaluation of gliomas using positron emission tomography. J Nucl Med 1987; 28:1123–1133.

Villringer A, Rosen BR, Belliveau JW, et al. Dynamic imaging with lanthanide chelates in normal brain: Contrast due to magnetic susceptibility effects. Magn Reson Med 1988; 6:164–174.

Warach S, Wei L, Ronthal M, Edelman RR. Acute cerebral ischemia: Evaluation with dynamic contrast-enhanced MR imaging and MR angiography. Radiology 1992; 182:41–47.

Weisskoff RM, Belliveau JW, Kwong KK, Rosen BR. Functional MR imaging of capillary hemodynamics. In: Potchen EJ, Haacke EM, Gotschalk A, Siebert JE, eds. Magnetic Resonance Angiography: Concepts and Applications. St. Louis: Mosby–Year Book, 1993.

# MR Angiography of the Extracranial and Intracranial Cerebral Circulation

*JONATHAN KRAMER, M.D. · ROBERT R. EDELMAN, M.D.*

Considering that cerebrovascular disease is the third most common cause of death in the United States, the development of noninvasive techniques to evaluate the extra- and intracranial cerebral circulation is a relevant priority. Most deaths result from massive cerebral infarctions, usually secondary to arterial embolism. Although emboli may originate from the heart and from atheromatous disease of the proximal great vessels, the source in the overwhelming majority of patients is from carotid bifurcation disease. Patients with signs and symptoms of cerebrovascular insufficiency, transient ischemic attacks (TIAs), or stroke are candidates for medical antiplatelet or anticoagulant therapy and/or surgical intervention. Carotid endarterectomy is an effective procedure, well recognized for reducing the risk of subsequent emboli and stroke in the group of patients with carotid diameter stenosis of 70 percent or more. Currently under way are studies evaluating the benefit of carotid endarterectomy in those patients with less than 70 percent stenosis. Patients with signs and symptoms of cerebrovascular insufficiency must undergo evaluation of the vascular supply to the brain to properly plan therapy. Since its inception, intra-arterial contrast angiography has been the gold standard for the evaluation of cerebrovascular disease. Complications are well recognized and include vascular injury (at the puncture site or in selective vessels from catheter and guidewire trauma), reaction to iodinated contrast material (allergic response or nephrotoxicity), and those related to procedure-induced embolism (TIA or stroke). With current technology, magnetic resonance angiography (MRA) promises to replace intra-arterial contrast angiography in the evaluation of extracranial carotid disease. With further development, it also might become the primary diagnostic tool for the evaluation of intracranial vascular disease.

## Techniques

Quite a few MRA techniques have been described to date. Of these, only a few have proved robust enough to be useful in clinical practice. These techniques all use gradient-echo pulse sequences, which have a single radiofrequency pulse and a reduced flip-angle less than 90°. In addition, a modification of the sequence structure, called *flow compensation* or *gradient motion rephasing,* is typically applied. Blood flowing along a magnetic field gradient causes a shift in the phase of the magnetic resonance (MR) signal (this is the basis of phase-contrast MRA, described later). Blood protons at different locations within a voxel have a velocity distribution that causes a spread in phase shifts; this spread in phase shifts, called *dephasing,* causes intraluminal signal loss and, in the case of pulsatile flow, objectionable ghost artifacts. The flow compensation method incorporates an additional gradient pulse into the sequence that eliminates phase shifts related to constant velocity flow and thus maximizes the intraluminal signal intensity.

Time-of-flight (TOF) MRA methods rely on the inflow of fresh unsaturated blood protons into the plane of section to cause a relatively high signal intensity of the vessel lumen compared with stationary background tissue; this phenomenon is called *flow-related enhancement.* By using a flow-compensated gradient-echo pulse sequence, short TR (e.g., 30 ms), and intermediate radiofrequency flip-angle (e.g., 40°), one can maximize contrast between flowing blood and stationary tissue. A stack of axial two-dimensional (2D) TOF gradient-echo images can be postprocessed using a maximal intensity projection (MIP) algorithm to create an angiogram-like picture. The MIP algorithm extracts the signal intensities from the brightest pixels in a set of images as viewed along a user-defined orientation, and then distributes them into a so-called *projection angiogram.* Three-dimensional TOF methods are also widely used. In this method a thick volume of tissue is excited; thin sections are created by phase encoding the data along the slice-selection direction, in addition to the usual in-plane phase-encoding direction. Two-dimensional TOF MRA is best for imaging of slow flow, because the thin sections lend themselves to flow-related enhancement. On the other hand, three-dimensional (3D) TOF MRA gives a more accurate portrayal of vessel stenoses because of the shorter echo time and smaller voxel, which reduce the amount of signal loss from flow-related dephasing.

Phase-contrast MRA makes use of phase shifts caused by a flow-sensitizing magnetic field gradient. The strength of the sensitizing gradient can be calibrated to produce a desired flow-related phase shift. Subtraction of a pair of images having flow sensitivities of equal magnitude, but opposite sign, yields a display of blood vessels with minimal signal contributions from stationary tissues. The velocity-encoded flow sensitivity (called *VENC* on some MR systems) is chosen to determine the maximum velocity of blood flow that will be correctly depicted. Compared with TOF MRA, phase-contrast MRA has the advantages that it directly gives the direction of flow and can be made sensitive to very slow flow. Its major drawbacks are the longer scan times and substantial computer requirements for image processing. Also, blood flowing faster than the selected limit for velocity sensitivity causes an artifact called *aliasing,* so that blood falsely appears to flow at a reduced velocity in the wrong direction.

## Clinical Applications

### *Extracranial Cerebrovascular Disease*

Although the promise of intravenous digital subtraction angiography has remained largely unfulfilled, over the last decade intra-arterial digital subtraction angiography has essentially replaced cut-film angiography in the evaluation of extracranial cerebrovascular disease. With smaller catheters, less contrast material required per injection, and a shorter evaluation time, there has been a concomitant reduction in the associated morbidity and mortality of intra-arterial angiographic studies. Conventional cut-film angiography continues to be heavily relied on for the evaluation of intracranial vascular pathology, including arteriovenous malformations (AVMs) and aneurysms.

B-mode, real-time, duplex Doppler, and color-flow Doppler represent a progressive spectrum of noninvasive ultrasonographic technologies that have proven effective and safe methods for carotid artery evaluation. Unfortunately Doppler ultrasonography of the cervical carotid artery is largely restricted to the region of the bifurcation. Preoperative evaluation of the entire carotid system is necessary, however, since tandem lesions involving the carotid siphon may preclude carotid endarterectomy. This information is provided only indirectly by techniques such as ocular plethysmography, and these additional indirect studies can substantially boost the overall cost of the study when used in addition to the color duplex sonogram. Duplex ultrasonography is also prone to errors in the estimation of all degrees of carotid stenosis, particularly mild-to-moderate disease. The inability to reliably make the vital distinction between extreme degrees of stenosis and occlusion is perhaps its greatest limitation. Occluded internal carotid arteries are generally regarded as inoperable, whereas restoration of normal flow in a stenotic carotid artery usually prevents further ischemic episodes.

MRA is the most recent and the most promising development in the field of noninvasive cerebrovascular evaluation. Unlike ultrasonography, MRA can image the entire vascular tree including the aorta, carotid bifurcation, and circle of Willis. As with Doppler ultrasonography, the direction and velocity of blood flow can be determined. Moreover, flow in the external carotid, ophthalmic, and vertebral arteries as well as the circle of Willis may be evaluated. The greatest clinical use for MRA has been in the evaluation of extracranial carotid disease.

Compared with the bright signal intensity of flowing blood, mural plaque appears dark in MRA, causing a narrowing of the vessel on projection images similar to a conventional angiogram (Figs. 1 and 2). Ulcerations are depicted as focal outpouchings containing bright signal (Fig. 3). It should be noted that MRA, like contrast angiography, has not proved particularly sensitive for the presence of ulcerations. Evaluation of the normal vessel, and those with moderate degrees of stenosis, is relatively straightforward. With severe stenoses, the actual site of narrowing may be rendered invisible. This is a result of the complex patterns of flow across and immediately beyond the lesion, so that continuity of the proximal and distal portions must be inferred. The stenosis is also exaggerated, more so with 2D than 3D techniques. Occlusion of a vessel may be suspected if no signal is observed along its course on 2D MRA images. Viewing the individual sections is invaluable in detecting slow flow, which might be missed in the projection images (Figs. 4 and 5).

Multimodality comparative studies involving MRA, duplex Doppler ultrasonography, and intra-arterial contrast angiography demonstrate good agreement among them and attest to the accuracy of MRA in the evaluation of carotid stenosis. Some reports have suggested that MRA imaging fails to reliably distinguish between extreme carotid stenoses and carotid occlusion. However, a recent large study comparing duplex sonography and intra-arterial contrast angiography with MRA using 2D and 3D TOF techniques showed MRA to be accurate for all degrees of stenosis. Significantly there were no cases of critical stenosis mistaken for occlusion.

As MRA is proving to be a definitive means for evaluating extracranial carotid stenosis, surgeons are beginning to perform endarterectomy without subjecting patients to the risks of conventional angiography. However, the accuracy of MRA depends on a number of factors including the type of MR system, pulse sequence, specific imaging parameters, and the experience of the radiologist performing and interpreting the studies. The merits of MRA versus contrast angiography cannot be ascertained with certainty until large multicenter trials are performed and the MRA techniques become standardized.

### *Intracranial Vascular Abnormalities*

Several reports describe a high sensitivity of MRA for intracranial aneurysms. Typically aneurysms greater than 3 mm in size can be reliably imaged (Figs. 6 and 7). Although we accept MRA as a screening method for aneurysms at our institution, some other investigators do not yet accept MRA as

*Text continued on p. 525.*

A 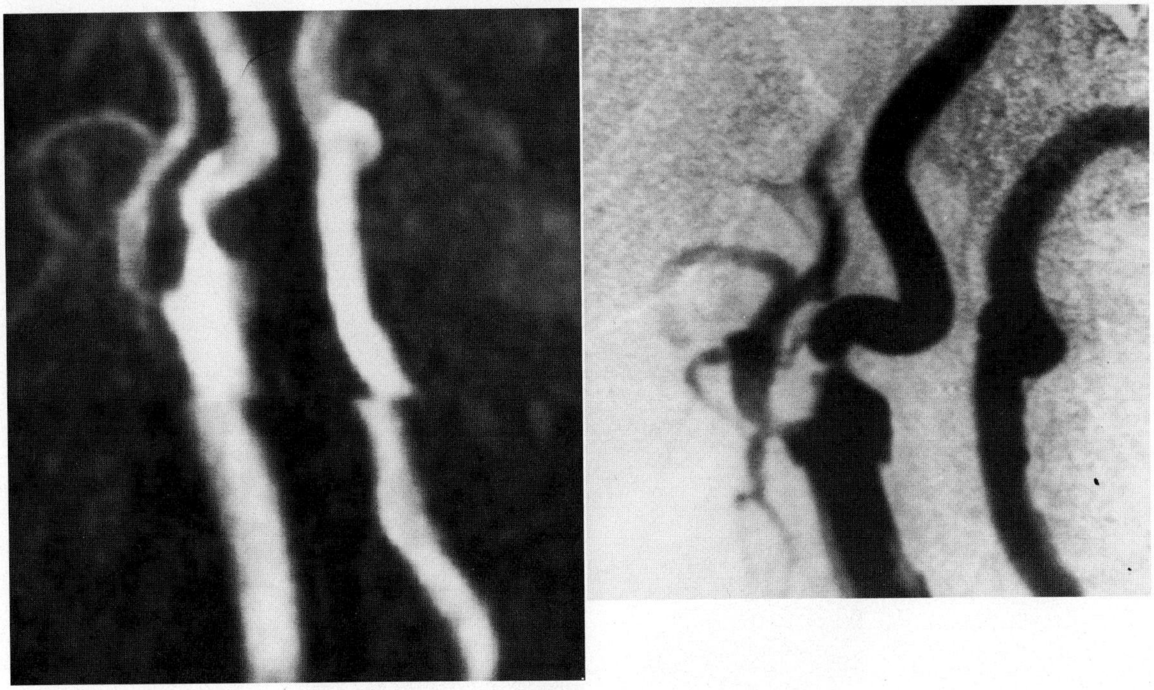 B

**FIGURE 1** Moderate stenoses of the proximal internal and external carotid arteries. *A,* Oblique lateral projection created using a MIP algorithm from a series of thin 3D sections. Two overlapping 3D acquisitions were performed using TR/TE/flip angle of 29/6/20°, 0.8 mm sections, 64 sections per 3D acquisition, field of view 20 x 17 cm, with a 256 x 192 matrix. *B,* Intra-arterial DSA shows similar findings to MRA, although the MRA did not show a small ulcer at the site of the stenosis.

A 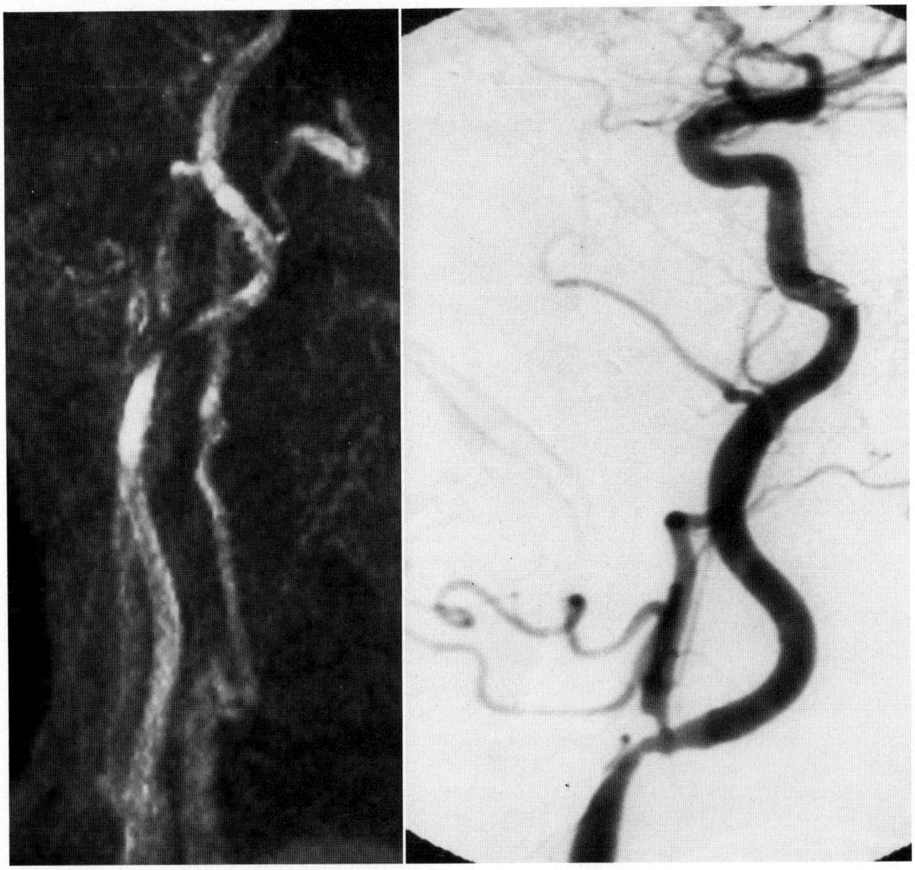 B

**FIGURE 2** Severe stenoses of the proximal internal and external carotid arteries and the distal common carotid artery. Both the sagittal 3D MRA *(A)* and the DSA *(B)* show severe pathology, but the lesion extent is slightly exaggerated by MRA.

A

B

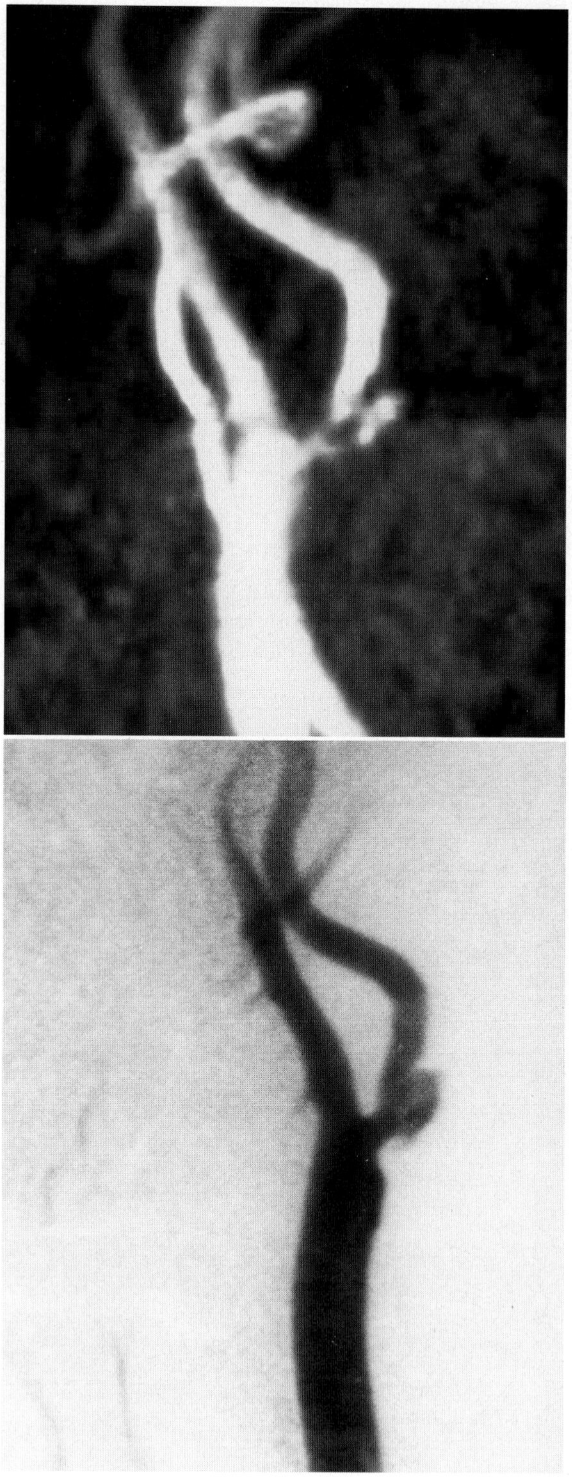

**FIGURE 3** Moderate stenosis of the proximal internal carotid artery with ulceration. The stenosis and ulcer are similarly depicted by MRA *(A)* and DSA *(B)*.

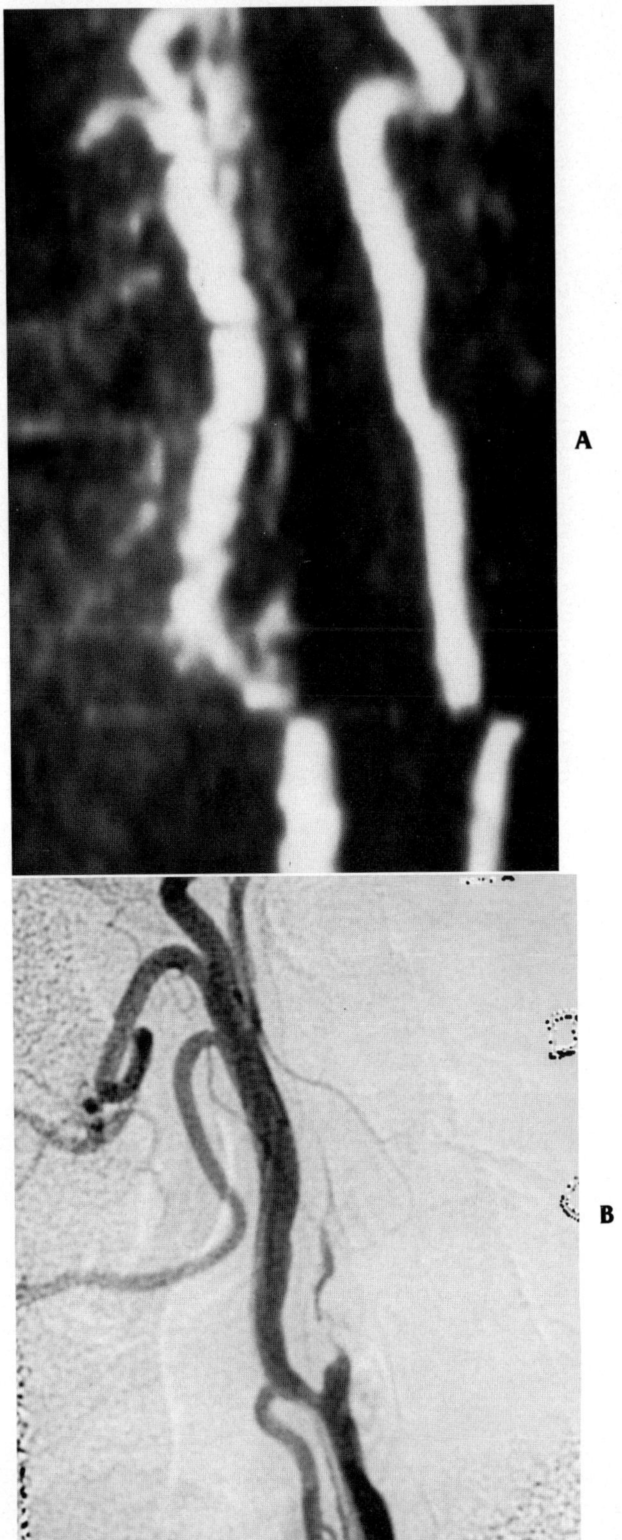


**FIGURE 4** Severe internal carotid artery stenosis with "string sign." *A,* Sagittal MIP from a sequential axial 2D MRA (30/9/30°, 3 mm section, 23 x 23 cm FOV, 256 x 192 matrix) shows the slow flow in the residual internal carotid artery lumen, as seen also by DSA *(B).* A 3D MRA (not shown) did not depict the patent lumen because of saturation effects.

A

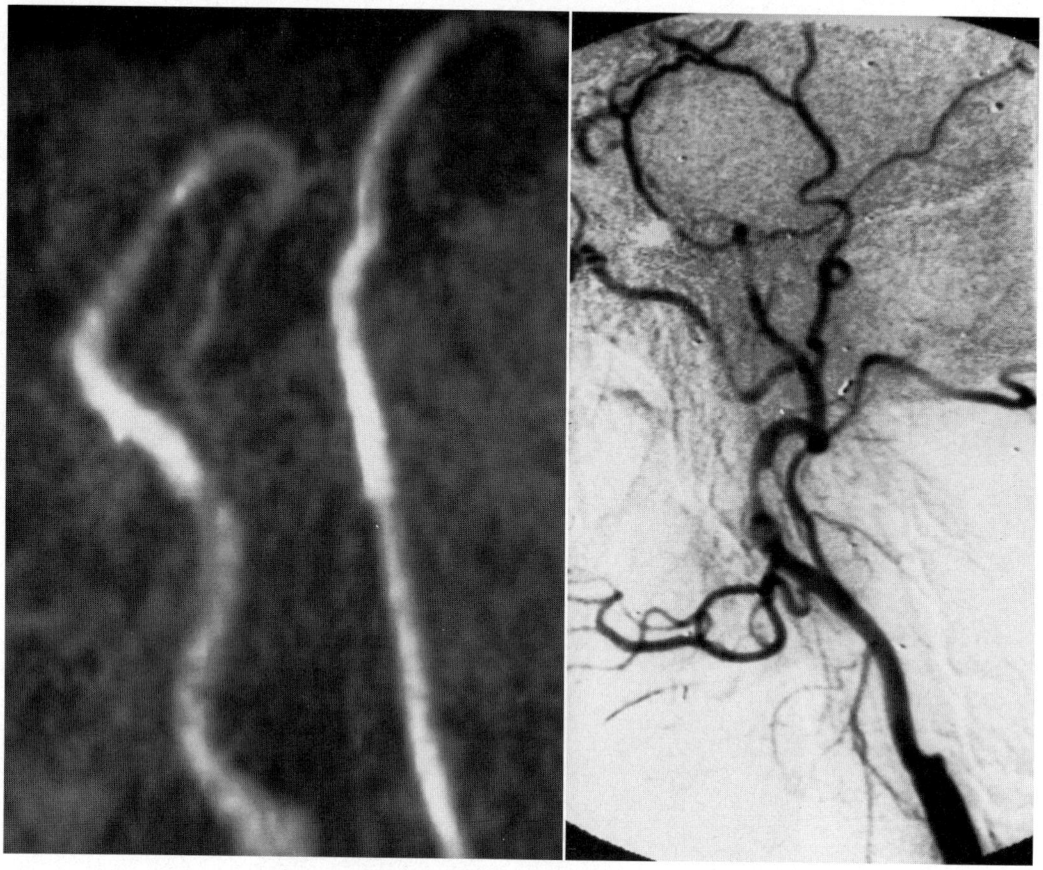

B

**FIGURE 5** Internal carotid artery occlusion. *A,* Three-dimensional MRA. *B,* DSA.

A

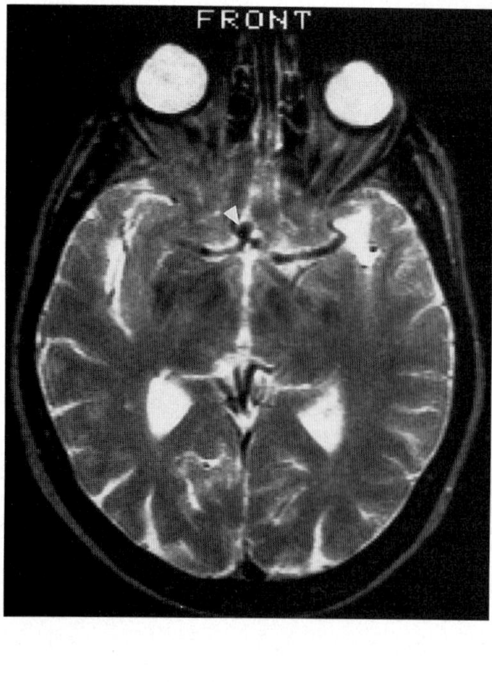


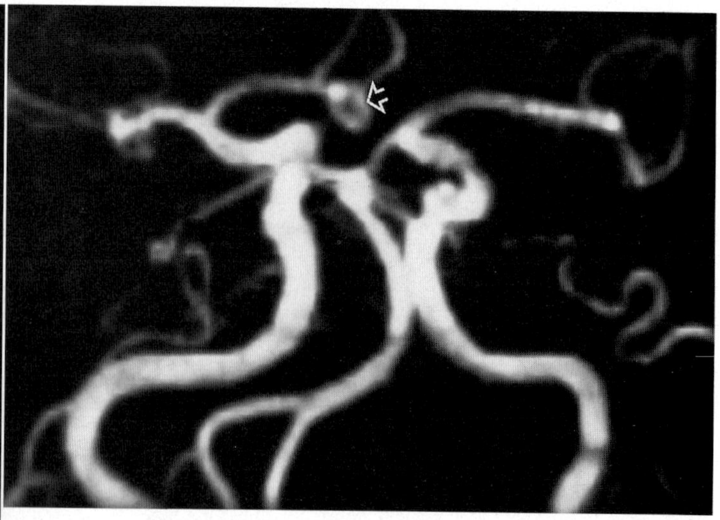

B

**FIGURE 6** Anterior communicating artery aneurysm. *A,* Axial T2-weighted SE image (TR/TE = 2500/80) shows the flow void of the aneurysm (*arrowhead*). *B,* The aneurysm (*open arrow*) appears bright on a coronal MIP created from overlapping axial 3D acquisitions.

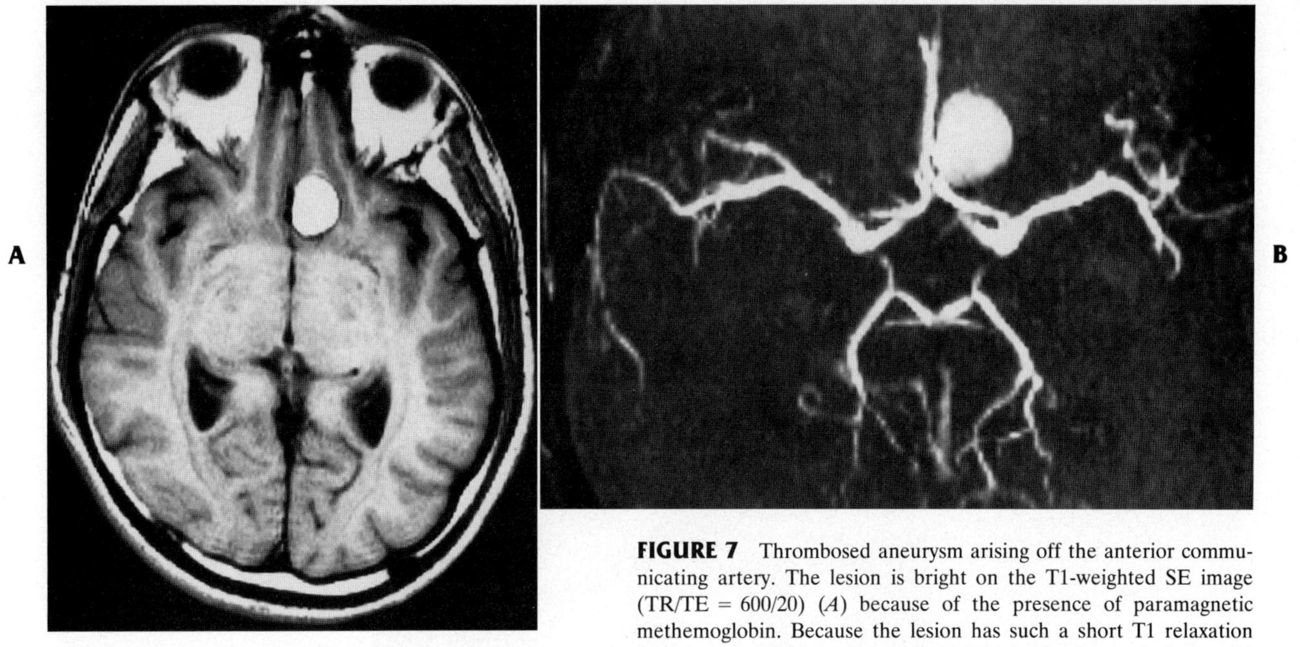


**FIGURE 7** Thrombosed aneurysm arising off the anterior communicating artery. The lesion is bright on the T1-weighted SE image (TR/TE = 600/20) (*A*) because of the presence of paramagnetic methemoglobin. Because the lesion has such a short T1 relaxation time, it appears bright also on the 3D MRA (*B*). This confusion would not occur with phase-contrast MRA, which is sensitive only to flow; even using a time-of-flight technique, the images can be properly interpreted when the SE and MRA studies are viewed together.

being sufficiently accurate to justify this approach. Presently aneurysms diagnosed by MRA require confirmation with contrast angiography. MRA is usually not appropriate for the evaluation of patients who have suffered an acute subarachnoid hemorrhage; these patients should be referred directly for contrast angiography.

MRA can show stenoses and occlusions involving the larger intracranial vessels. It is somewhat limited in its accuracy for atheromatous disease of the carotid siphon (Fig. 8); the extreme curvature of the internal carotid artery at this location causes a distortion of signal from flowing blood as a result of the time delay between radiofrequency excitation and position encoding, so that the vessel may appear falsely narrowed. Basilar stenosis is not surgically correctable, but may be treated with anticoagulant therapy. MRA can be useful for determining the severity of a basilar stenosis and thereby guiding the use of anticoagulant therapy.

Collateral flow patterns are determined by the use of saturation tagging techniques. For instance, if there is flow from the right internal carotid artery across the circle of Willis to the left middle cerebral artery, then application of a radiofrequency presaturation pulse over the right internal carotid artery will eliminate signal in the contralateral middle cerebral artery. This occurs because the dark saturated blood in the right internal carotid artery flows into and fills the left middle cerebral artery. Reversed flow in an ophthalmic artery in the setting of carotid occlusion or in a vertebral artery in the setting of subclavian steal syndrome can also be depicted.

Intracranial arteriovenous malformations are diagnosed on conventional spin-echo T1- and dual-echo T2-weighted sequences. They may also be imaged with MRA. Feeding arteries, draining veins, or vessels within the nidus are seen. The extent of the malformation may be better seen after administration of a contrast agent. In a recent study of pre- and postcontrast MRA of intracranial vascular pathology using a dose of 0.3 mmol/kg of a nonionic gadolinium chelate, we found an improvement in the depiction of small vascular structures postcontrast (Fig. 9). However, routine use of contrast-enhanced MRA is not recommended. Normally enhancing tissues, such as the pituitary gland and cavernous sinus, as well as a plethora of enhancing veins tend to overlap normal and pathological vascular anatomy. Conventional angiography is still required to completely evaluate vascular malformations when surgical or embolotherapy is contemplated.

Venous thrombosis may be reliably imaged with a combination of conventional spin-echo T1- and dual-echo T2-weighted images as well as MR venography sequences. In this instance, coronal and sagittal 2D TOF MRA distinguishes slowly flowing blood from thrombus (Figs. 10 and 11). MR venography for preoperative evaluation of meningiomas located near a major dural sinus may obviate conventional angiography.

## Pitfalls in Technique and Interpretation

As previously mentioned, in the setting of high-grade stenoses there is often signal loss at the critical segment with apparent discontinuity of the vessel between the proximal and distal portions. This problem can be reduced by use of 3D sequences with short echo time and minimal voxel size. On TOF MRA, methemoglobin in subacute hemorrhage can manifest high signal intensity because of its short T1 relaxation time. Thus mural hemorrhage in a carotid dissection could be mistaken for flow. Thrombosed berry aneurysms may falsely appear to have a patent lumen on TOF MRA (see Fig. 7). This is because of the high signal intensity of methemoglobin "bleeding" through into the MIP image. Thrombosed aneurysms can be recognized if their signal intensities are evaluated on both the T1- and dual-echo T2-weighted sequences. Distinction between hemorrhage and flow can also be made using phase-contrast MRA.

A

B

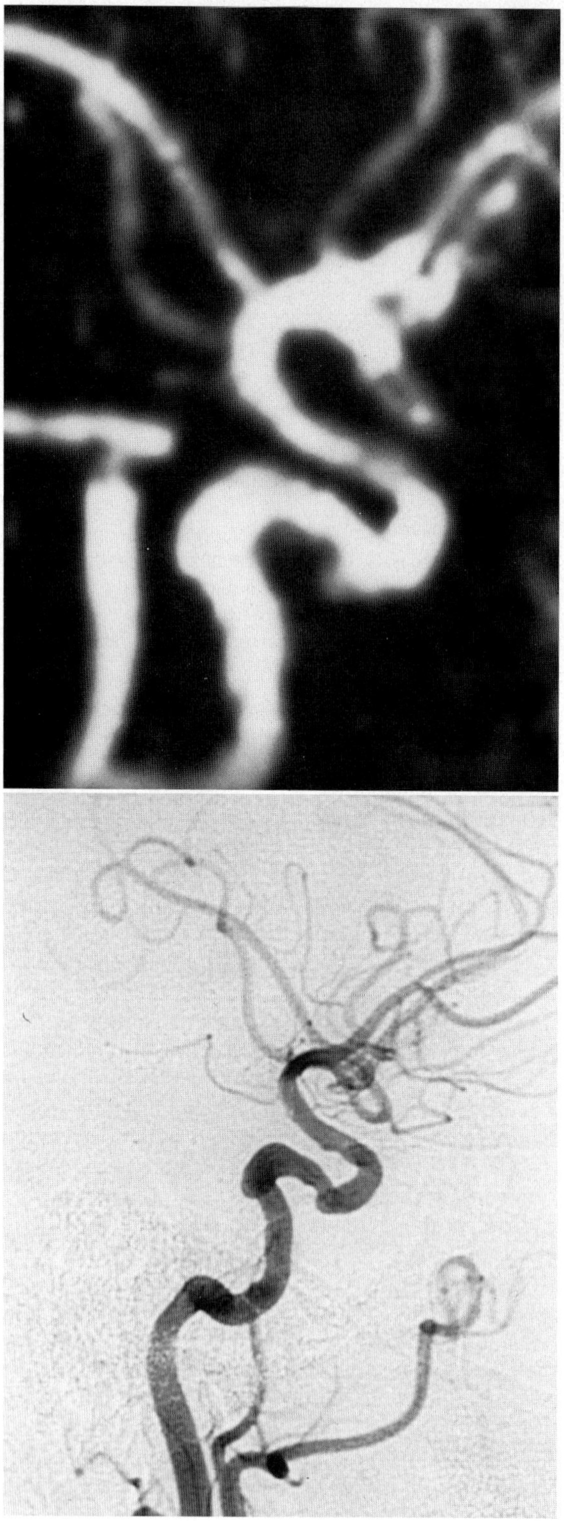

**FIGURE 8** Moderate stenosis of the carotid siphon. *A,* 3D MRA. *B,* DSA. Although the lesion is correctly shown here by MRA, the siphon is an area where flow artifacts may falsely create the appearance of a stenosis.

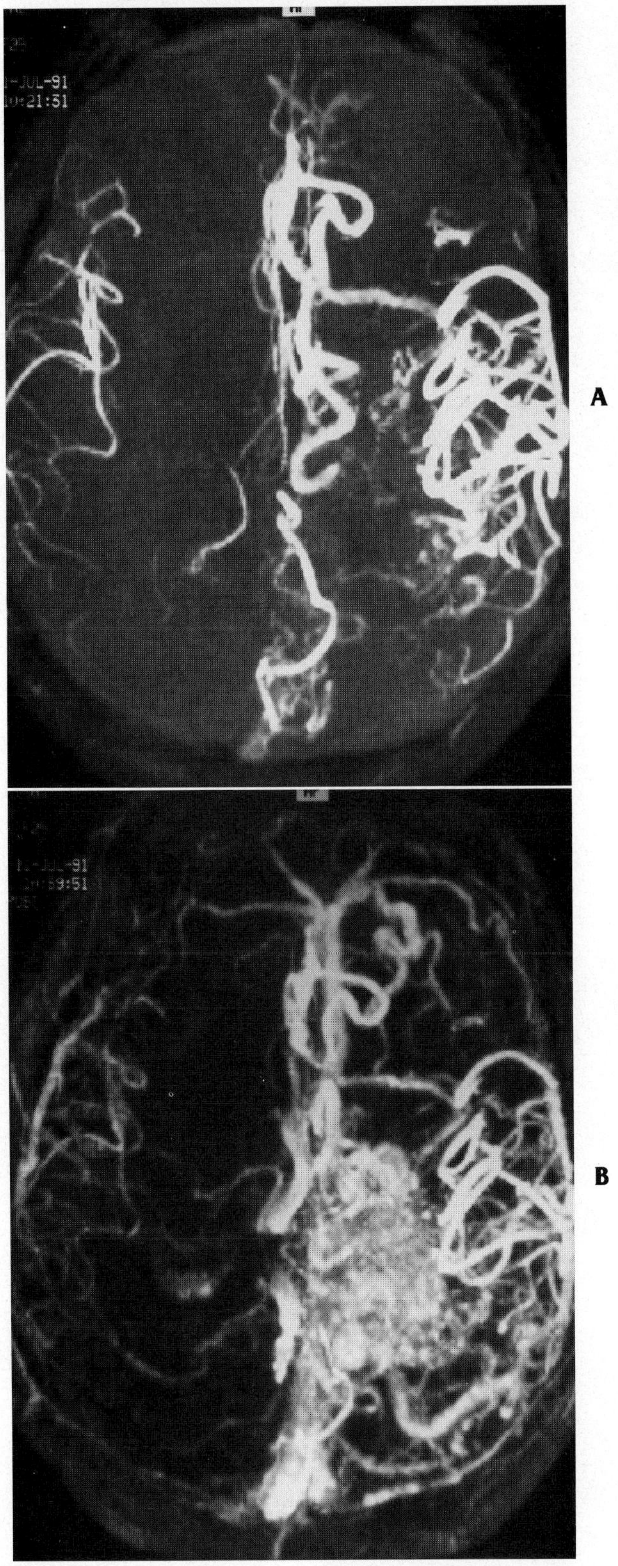


**FIGURE 9** Left temporal arteriovenous malformation. Three-dimensional MRA was acquired before (*A*) and after (*B*) intravenous infusion of gadolinium DTPA. The nidus and smaller feeder and draining vessels are best seen post-contrast.

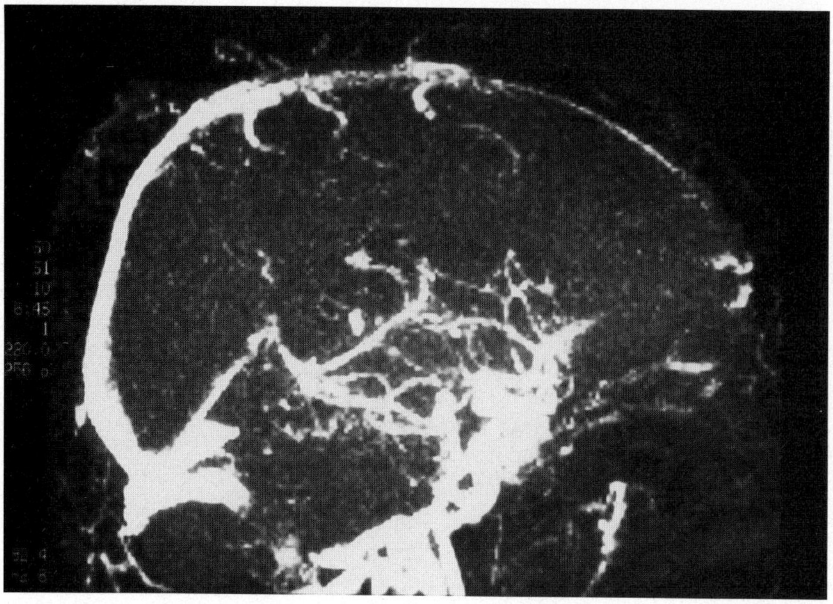

**FIGURE 10** Normal sagittal head MR venogram. A series of overlapping sagittal 2D gradient-echo images were acquired using a presaturation band placed transversely over the neck to eliminate signal from arterial inflow, and then a MIP image was created in a lateral view. The major venous sinuses are well depicted.

A

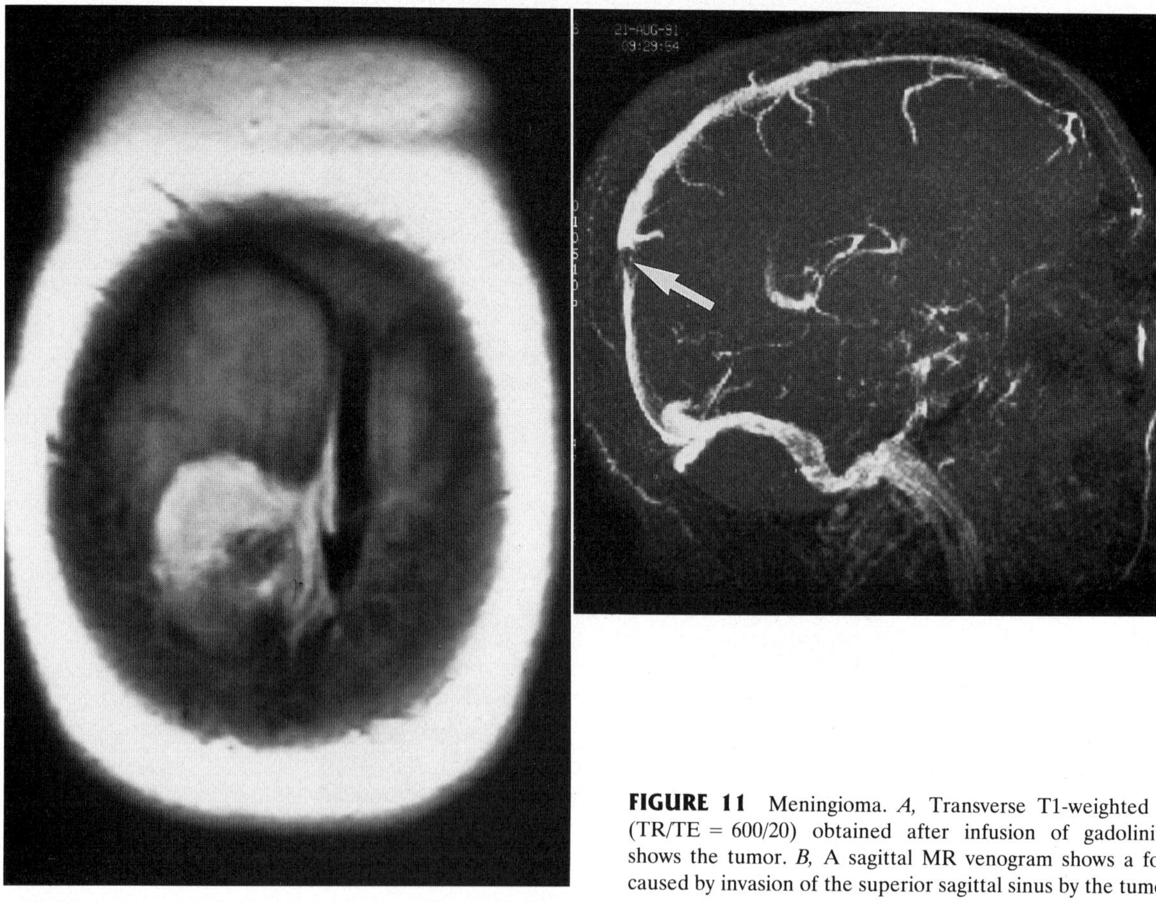

B

**FIGURE 11** Meningioma. *A,* Transverse T1-weighted SE image (TR/TE = 600/20) obtained after infusion of gadolinium-DTPA shows the tumor. *B,* A sagittal MR venogram shows a focal defect caused by invasion of the superior sagittal sinus by the tumor (*arrow*).

## Discussion

Given the relatively low cost and good accuracy of ultrasonography and its direct availability to neurologists and vascular surgeons, it will continue to be used as a screening technique for extracranial carotid disease. MRA has developed to the point that it may soon replace conventional angiography as the definitive preoperative imaging technique before carotid endarterectomy. MRA is a reliable evaluation for conditions such as intracranial dural sinus thrombosis and subclavian steal, and is useful as a screening evaluation for intracranial aneurysms and atheromatous disease involving the major branches of the circle of Willis. Certain other applications (e.g., the use of MRA to diagnose vasculitis involving small peripherally situated vessels) await further technical development to improve spatial resolution.

## Suggested Reading

Anderson CM, Saloner D, Lee RE, et al. Assessment of carotid artery stenosis by MR angiography: Comparison with x-ray angiography and color-coded Doppler ultrasound. Am J Neuroradiol 1992; 13:989–1003.

Anderson CM, Saloner D, Lee RE, Fortner A. Dedicated coil for carotid MR angiography. Radiology 1990; 176:868–872.

Blatter DD, Parker DL, Robison RO. Cerebral MR angiography with multiple thin slab acquisition. Radiology 1991; 179:805–811.

Dumoulin CL, Souza SP, Walker MF, Wagle W. Three-dimensional phase contrast angiography. Magn Reson Med 1989; 9:139–149.

Keller PJ, Drayer BP, Fram EK, et al. MR angiography with two-dimensional acquisition and three-dimensional display. Radiology 1989; 173:527–532.

Masaryk AM, Ross JS, DiCello MC, et al. 3DFT MR angiography of the carotid bifurcation: Potential and limitations as a screening examination. Radiology 1991; 179:797–804.

Masaryk TJ, Modic MT, Ruggieri PM, et al. Three-dimensional (volume) gradient-echo imaging of the carotid bifurcation: Preliminary clinical experience. Radiology 1989; 171:801–806.

Mattle HP, Kent KC, Edelman RR, et al. Evaluation of the extracranial carotid arteries: Correlation of magnetic resonance angiography, duplex ultrasound, and conventional angiography. J Vasc Surg 1991; 13:838–844.

# Artifacts in MRI of the Brain: Recognition and Avoidance

*R. GILBERTO GONZÁLEZ, M.D., Ph.D.*

Artifacts are common in magnetic resonance imaging (MRI) of the brain. The majority of artifacts encountered in clinical practice are minor, readily recognized, and do not significantly affect the diagnostic usefulness of the image. Some artifacts are serious enough to render the MR image of no diagnostic use, leading to repeated imaging studies, additional sequences, or recommendations for additional radiologic evaluations. To provide optimal care, the radiologist who reads MR images of the brain must be well acquainted with common MRI artifacts, the origin of these artifacts, ways in which they can be avoided, and how they can be rectified, if required. The purpose of the present chapter is to describe a practical approach to the recognition of artifacts and their avoidance.

My approach is to discuss artifacts in brain MRI in a different fashion from that commonly found in MRI textbooks or review articles in scientific journals. Usually the subject is systematized according to each artifact's physical cause. Here the approach is one of diagnosing artifacts. The diagnostic metaphor applies since, as in the clinic, an accurate reading of artifacts requires a "differential diagnosis" to arrive at a probable cause. The list to recall consists of signal abnormality patterns and the phenomena that give rise to them. Once the appropriate diagnosis has been ascertained, the "cure" may be either readily apparent, or textbooks or colleagues may be consulted. My purpose being explicitly practical, I do not herein discuss the science underlying the principal artifacts encountered in the practice of radiology in any detail, but instead refer the reader to a selection of other works for a more complete description of the underlying physics of artifacts in MRI.

An artifact in an MR image may be defined as an abnormal signal that is not caused by a pathological process or a normal anatomical variant. Artifacts may arise from the object imaged, from imperfections in the magnet, gradients, or radiofrequency (RF) electronics, or from improper selection of imaging parameters. Improper maintenance of an MRI system gives rise to numerous artifacts. In general, these system imperfections can be detected by quality control phantom images, which should be obtained at least once daily. When an artifact is detected on the quality control image, a system engineer must be called immediately to correct the problem. As in clinical practice, preventive care in dealing with MRI artifacts is always the best approach.

If an instrument is properly maintained and the proper parameters are selected, optimal MR images are obtained from signal produced by a motionless sample that has a simple molecule, such as water, with a single resonance in its NMR spectrum, and which magnetically is perfectly homogeneous. When these conditions are not met, artifacts arise. For example, when a sample contains substantial amounts of a second chemical, such as the fat and water mixture found in bone marrow, chemical shift artifacts arise. If the sample or a part of it moves during data acquisition, motion artifacts appear in the image. Inhomogeneities within the sample may give rise to several types of artifacts, such as those produced by magnetic susceptibility effects. All of these problems are fundamentally related and can be understood by applying the basic physical principles of MRI. Since the samples at hand in clinical imaging are to a great degree determined for us (patients who need MRI), I concentrate on artifacts that are potentially correctable and result mainly from an unwise selection of parameters and/or are directly related to the patient, such as motion.

## Blurring

Patient motion is one of the most common artifacts encountered in MRI. Blurring results from nonperiodic motion and can range in importance from minor loss of anatomical detail to a completely useless image. The problem is best avoided by discussing the effects of motion with the patient before the scan and by frequent reminders between scans to keep still. The use of foam pads and tape may also be employed to firmly hold the head in place. For patients who cannot cooperate, owing, for example, to dementing illness, I use echo-planar imaging, which has image acquisition times on the order 60 milliseconds, to "freeze" the action. This technological "fix" will be more generally available in the future.

## Abnormally Increased Signal: Ghosting Pattern

### *Pulsatile Blood or Cerebrospinal Fluid (CSF) Motion*

An abnormal increase in signal that results in a ghosting pattern is another common occurrence in MR images. Here the appearance results from an alternatingly high and low signal. The ghost artifacts are propagated in the phase-encoding direction; their intensity is related to the signal intensity of the moving tissue. In brain MRI, the CSF and blood flow are often the sources of ghosting.

I commonly see ghost artifacts within the posterior fossa of gadolinium-enhanced, T1-weighted, axial images. The ghosts arise from hyperintense flowing blood in the transverse sinuses. If phase-encoding occurs in the transverse direction, the ghosts traverse the cerebellum. This artifact can be troublesome, especially if the scan was performed to rule out metastasis. Another, more subtle manifestation that I often observe is increased signal within the brain stem on the second echo of T2-weighted axial images. This ghosting artifact arises from pulsatile CSF motion and can be problematic if there is a question of lacunar infarcts.

Fortunately the solution to each of these cases is simple. Cardiac gating can be applied and is highly effective. Gradient motion nulling (also known as flow compensation) can be applied, although it is less effective than cardiac gating. Presaturation of the blood before it enters the slice of interest is also a useful measure. These measures can all be applied at the same time to minimize these artifacts. Finally, the phase- and frequency-encoding directions can be switched, thereby rotating the direction of any ghost artifact by 90°.

### *MRI System Defects*

Abnormal ghosting patterns may be the result of a number of system defects. I emphasize here again that such abnormalities are apparent in quality control phantom images. These should be frequently obtained, and the radiologist in charge of the MR imager should regularly review them and alert service personnel to the presence of any ghost artifacts so that problems in the system may be quickly resolved.

## Abnormally Increased Signal: Normal Structure in Abnormal Location

The cause of aliasing (also known as a "wraparound" artifact) is the selection of a field of view (FOV) that is too small. Its appearance is of structures from the periphery superimposed onto the image. The obvious remedy is to increase the FOV. However, there may be important diagnostic reasons for keeping this small. At least to a certain degree, aliasing is resolved by oversampling in both the frequency- and phase-encoding directions (known as the "no phase wrap" and "no frequency wrap" methods). These oversampling methods are available in all current MRI systems. Aliasing may also occur along the slice selection axis during gradient-echo volume acquisitions. In this situation a slice of the body outside the FOV is superimposed onto a slice within it, usually toward the end of the FOV. Again the solution is to increase the FOV in the third dimension.

## Abnormally Decreased Signal

### *Magnetic Susceptibility Artifact*

Whenever I observe a region of diminished signal that is not normal, I first consider the possibility of a magnetic susceptibility artifact as its possible cause. All materials within a magnetic field interact with it in a way that either diminishes or increases the inherent magnetism of the specific material. This property is known as magnetic susceptibility. If all the material within a magnet has identical magnetic susceptibility, no magnetic susceptibility artifact can arise. This is the case, for instance, if we image a perfect sphere of water. In medical imaging, however, differences in magnetic susceptibility always exist. These frequently result in a distortion of the magnetic fields near the boundaries of differing materials and produce regional signal loss in the image near those boundaries. The greater the magnetic susceptibility differences of the materials being imaged, the greater their effect on the image obtained. This loss in signal results from spins dephasing within the imaging plane, an effect similar to signal voids that arise when spins move through magnetic field gradients (i.e., flow voids). Magnetic susceptibility artifacts are more prominent on gradient-echo than spin-echo images, and their effect is enhanced with longer echo times, a phenomenon known as "blooming." I most commonly observe magnetic susceptibility artifacts on gradient-echo images in the region of the skull base and the vicinity of the paranasal sinuses. Deep within the brain parenchyma, I commonly observe magnetic susceptibility–related hypointensity near areas of hemorrhage or calcification. This type of artifact cannot be entirely avoided, but it can be significantly reduced by the use of spin-echo imaging and short echo times.

One interesting fact is that the "blooming" phenomenon can be exploited to identify a magnetic susceptibility artifact. If a focal signal hypointensity increases in size on the second echo of a dual-echo, long TR sequence, this provides strong evidence that the effect is the result of a magnetic susceptibility difference. Immediately the possibility of the presence of blood products or some other source of the artifact should be considered. Such an effect can be used to search for tiny areas of hemorrhage that occur in, for instance, shearing injuries of the brain caused by trauma. In patients with these injuries, spin-echo images may appear normal, whereas gradient-echo images having long echo times (~50 ms) will reveal innumerable foci of low signal, thus permitting the radiologist to diagnosis the injury correctly.

### *Ferromagnetic Artifacts*

This is another type of magnetic susceptibility artifact that is observed in the vicinity of ferromagnetic objects. I am treating it separately because this artifact displays significant geometrical image distortion and focal areas of high signal. These are due to the fact that the differences in magnetic susceptibility between ferromagnetic objects and brain tissue is very high. I most commonly see this effect in patients with braces or other metallic dental equipment. Hair pins, mascara, and surgical clips are other common sources of ferromagnetic artifacts. Once again, patient education before the start of the scan is of paramount importance.

### *RF Inhomogeneity*

A perfect RF coil, such as a head coil, uniformly produces perfect 90° pulses within its volume. This is, of course, impossible to achieve. Imperfections of spin nutations within RF coils are known as RF inhomogeneity. The degree of inhomogeneity caused by the imperfections in RF coils is primarily owing to their geometric design. Bird cage head coils are usually homogeneous over a large central portion of the coil volume. Other coil designs are less satisfactory. Using volume coils, the effect of RF inhomogeneity is most marked near the edge of image, where the object comes close to the coil. In these situations I usually see an area of signal loss at the periphery of the image. An improperly maintained head coil can produce RF inhomogeneity effects significantly worse than those that commonly result. Again, I stress that evaluation of the quality control phantom image is extremely important to identify these types of problems.

The effect of RF inhomogeneity is most marked with the use of surface coils. With these, signal immediately adjacent to the coil is very high, but drops off substantially in tissue far from it. There is no true remedy for surface coil effects, although postprocessing "filters" can be employed to ameliorate the situation. Such filters use a mathematical function to decrease the signal amplitude in the immediate vicinity of the coil and to increase it in more distant tissue regions.

## Paired Increased and Decreased Signal

### *Flow Misregistration*

This is perhaps the artifact that I most commonly observe. It usually appears as a linear region of hyperintensity, paralleled by a geometrically identical linear region of hypointensity. This is usually caused by slow flow in brain venous structures that travel an oblique course through the image. The artifact is most prominent on images taken after the administration of gadolinium and arises from changes in the position of spins in flowing blood during the time required for a pulse sequence. Because of movement through magnetic field gradients, the spins undergo a "phase shift" in the period between excitation and collection of the echo signal. After Fourier transformation, the shift in phase is manifested in a change in position or misregistration on the image. There is no way, and really no need, to try to correct this artifact. It poses no diagnostic dilemma, and it is only important that one know it exists.

### *Ringing or Gibbs' Artifact*

When there is an abrupt transition from an area of high signal to an area of low signal (as between the scalp fat and calvarial bone) an artifact arises that appears as alternating lines of increased and decreased signal that parallel the high-low signal interface. This is the well-known ringing artifact, also commonly referred to as a Gibbs' artifact and a truncation artifact. It is associated with the Fourier transform and the inability to faithfully model, with the small number of data points available in MRI, what is, in effect, a step function by combinations of sine and cosine functions. I most commonly observe this artifact when employing 128 phase-encoding steps in an attempt to save time. The ringing is seen as a series of alternating bright and dark lines that concentrically parallel the calvarium. Increasing the number of phase-encoding steps does not eliminate the ringing, but it does make it much less conspicuous.

### *Chemical Shift Artifact*

Chemical shift artifacts are far more common in MR images of structures such as bone marrow and extracranial structures in general. Intracranially, in fact, a chemical shift artifact is very useful, for it allows the definitive diagnosis of a lipoma. Chemical shift artifacts arise from the fact that the resonance frequency of protons in fat is different from that of protons in water. These artifacts always appear in the frequency-encoding direction as a linear area of increased signal on one side of the fatty structure (lipoma) and as a mirror image, linear area of hypointensity on its other side.

## Straight Lines

Nothing in nature occurs in straight lines. Therefore, whenever I see one or more straight lines of increased or decreased intensity traversing an image, I immediately consider electronic or system sources for the artifact. These artifacts include central frequency line artifact, central phase line artifact, multiple oblique line artifacts, artifactual lines perpendicular to the frequency axis, mosaic patterns, and the central point artifact. These artifacts arise from a variety of sources and are observed in the quality control phantom image. The service engineer should be contacted when any of these artifacts appear.

## Discussion

In this chapter I have briefly described the most common artifacts that I encounter in the daily interpretation of MR images of the brain. The list is not exhaustive nor is meant to be. However, I believe that I have covered a substantial number of the artifacts that I observe in a busy MRI practice. An ounce of prevention is always worth a pound of cure; therefore regular preventive maintenance and daily quality control phantom imaging will prevent most system-related artifacts. The approach that I am suggesting for identification of patient-related artifacts is to keep in mind the short "differential diagnosis" lists for the appearance of the various types of artifacts herein described. With the "diagnosis" made, the cure is apparent more often than not.

*Acknowledgment.* The author would like to thank Jo Anne Fordham for her excellent suggestions during the preparation of this manuscript.

## Suggested Reading

Bellon EM, Haacke EM, Coleman PE, et al. MRI artifacts: A review. AJR 1986; 147:1271–1281.

Edelman RR, Hesselink JR, eds. Clinical Magnetic Resonance Imaging. Philadelphia: WB Saunders, 1990:74.

Partain CL, Price RR, Patton JA, et al., eds. Nuclear Magnetic Resonance Imaging. 2nd ed. Philadelphia: WB Saunders, 1988:780.

Stark DD, Bradley Jr. WG, eds. Magnetic Resonance Imaging. St. Louis: CV Mosby, 1988:138.

# CT and MRI Evaluation of Central Nervous System Complications of AIDS

*CALVIN H. FLOWERS, M.D.*

Central nervous system (CNS) disease is a major cause of mortality and morbidity in patients who are seropositive for the human immunodeficiency virus (HIV) and who meet the Centers for Disease Control (CDC) clinical criteria for acquired immunodeficiency syndrome (AIDS). Approximately 60 percent of patients with AIDS eventually develop some form of neurologic or psychiatric symptoms during the course of their illness. Even though most neurologic complaints occur in patients who have clinical AIDS, approximately 10 to 20 percent of all AIDS patients have neurologic symptoms as the initial manifestation of their disease. It is well established that a variety of neurologic manifestations exist as a result of opportunistic infections, viral and nonviral syndromes, neoplasms, cerebrovascular accidents, and central neuropathies. Neuroradiologic evaluation is frequently requested to diagnose and monitor the treatment of opportunistic and neoplastic diseases encountered in these patients. The roles of computed tomography (CT) and magnetic resonance imaging (MRI) are well established in the evaluation of AIDS patients with CNS complications. Both CT and MRI are used for screening, but today most major centers use MRI when available because of its superior contrasting between normal and abnormal tissues. With the approval of gadolinium as a contrast agent, normal and pathologic entities are more easily defined. The major neuroradiological findings in the CNS of AIDS patients are divided into four major categories: (1) atrophy, (2) white matter disease, (3) mass lesions, and (4) leptomeningeal and ependymal disease.

## Indications

The most common indications for neurologic evaluations in AIDS patients include mental status changes, focal sensory-motor deficits, seizures, headache, and cranial nerve palsies. The neurologic symptoms in AIDS patients with CNS complications may be either focal or diffuse. At our institution a review of 200 patients with AIDS who were referred for neuroradiologic evaluation showed that 65 percent were referred because of changes in their mental status. The most common neurological symptomatology in AIDS patients is the AIDS dementia complex (ADC), consisting of mental status changes, cognitive dysfunction, and recent memory loss. The ADC is a diffuse neuropathological process caused by direct HIV infection, which correlates well with the atrophy and diffuse white matter disease seen on CT and MRI. Focal neurological symptoms such as sensory-motor deficits, headaches, and seizures may also be present. Patients with opportunistic infectious mass lesions and neoplastic disease often exhibit focal neurological symptoms, although this may be superimposed with a diffuse encephalopathy. At our institution approximately 25 percent of the AIDS patients referred for neuroimaging presented with focal or diffuse sensory-motor deficits. Hemiparesis of either one or both lower extremities is most commonly observed. New-onset seizures, without documented metabolic dysfunction, are observed in approximately 10 to 15 percent of AIDS patients referred for neuroimaging. Persistent headaches without other neurologic symptoms are observed in approximately 15 percent of our referred AIDS patient population.

CT and MRI are extensively used to diagnose and follow up patients undergoing treatment for lesions such as toxoplasmosis, bacterial and fungal abscesses, and white matter disease following treatment with azidothymidine (AZT). Patients in whom focal lesions are detected on MRI or CT are empirically given a trial of pyrimethamine and sulfadiazine for the treatment of toxoplasmosis. If there are significant radiological and clinical changes after 2 to 3 weeks of treatment, maximum therapy for toxoplasmosis is given for life. Today, stereotactic biopsy is indicated only in patients who fail to respond to empiric antitoxoplasmosis therapy and in whom the cerebrospinal fluid (CSF) and neuroradiologic evaluations suggest primary CNS lymphoma.

CNS complications are rarely encountered in pediatric patients with AIDS. The onset of the disease in this population is generally observed in the first 2 years of life. Developmental milestones may be significantly delayed, and patients may demonstrate microcephaly or a chronic HIV encephalopathy. Subdural fluid collections and abscesses less frequently from toxoplasmosis may occasionally be evident. CT and MRI evaluation may show cerebral atrophy or white matter changes similar to that observed in the adult AIDS population.

## Technical Approach

CT and MRI are well established as the diagnostic imaging choice in AIDS patients with CNS complications. Although MRI is recommended as the initial screening technique for these patients, contrast-enhanced CT evaluation is still largely used at many centers throughout the United States. MRI more accurately demonstrates the extent and distribution of CNS complications in this patient population. If an acute neurologic event is suspected, the procedure of choice is a noncontrast CT or MRI evaluation. Subacute to chronic processes are imaged with either contrast-enhanced CT studies using a nonionic contrast agent or an MRI evaluation. Standard 10 mm axial CT images are obtained from the base of the skull to and including the vertex. A soft-tissue algorithm with window levels of −25 to −40 Hounsfield units (HU) and window width ranging from 300 to 80 HU is used. On visualization of the third and lateral ventricles, the window width is decreased to a range of 150 to 100 HU. Approximately 75 percent of our patients are initially screened with a standard single-dose (40 g iodine) contrast-enhanced CT evaluation, and approximately 25 percent are initially screened with an MRI evaluation because of significant patient overload. If MRI is not available, a double-dose (80 g of iodine) contrast-enhanced CT evaluation may be used as a substitute. The double-dose evaluation may be given either immediately before scanning or 1 hour before scanning on a delayed basis for adequate intracranial contrast concentration. MRI screening evaluations are performed using a spin-echo (SE) multisection acquisition technique with T1- and T2-weighted sequences. Using a head coil, 5 mm sections with 7 mm slice intervals are obtained with matrices of 192 × 192 to 256 when using a 0.5 T unit and 256 × 128 to 256 on a 1.5 T magnet. A field of view (FOV) ranging from 20 to 25 cm and two excitations are included in the protocol. Sequences include T1-weighted sagittal and axial images, with T2-weighted axial images before gadolinium infusion. Post-gadolinium studies include T1-weighted axial and coronal images. Short repetition times (TR) of 700 msec and less and short echo times (TE) of 30 msec and less provide the T1-weighted images. The T2-weighted sequences are achieved using TR of 2000 msec or greater and TE of 60 msec or greater. Intermediate proton density sequences are obtained using TR of 2000 msec or greater and TE of 45 msec or less. Post-gadolinium studies are obtained using the standard recommended intravenous dose of 0.2 ml/kg.

## Diagnostic Approach

### Atrophy

Atrophy is the most common finding on CT and MRI and is observed in approximately 30 to 60 percent of AIDS patients referred for neuroradiologic evaluation. Encephalitis from HIV and cytomegalovirus (CMV), along with aseptic and fungal meningitis, may cause significant loss of brain parenchyma, resulting in atrophy. On CT evaluation, the cerebral and cerebellar cortices are most commonly affected, although brain stem and corpus callosal atrophy may be seen. MRI may demonstrate white matter lesions in these patients, along with the cortical atrophy (Figs. 1 and 2).

### White Matter Disease

White matter disease of AIDS is most commonly caused by direct HIV infection, and demyelination is demonstrated on approximately 10 to 30 percent of CT evaluations. This frequency increases to 30 to 60 percent after MRI. On precontrast and postcontrast CT studies, HIV encephalitis is seen as focal or diffuse areas of low attenuation commonly located in the centrum semiovale and periventricular regions (Fig. 3). MRI is more sensitive than CT in demonstrating the pathological changes in the white matter because of increased tissue contrast. The T2-weighted MRI sequence is more sensitive in demonstrating the white matter disease, which may be focal, diffuse, patchy, or punctate (Figs. 4 and 5). On T2-weighted images the demyelination appears hyperintense compared with normal white matter and usually involves the periventricular and peri-insular regions (Figs. 6 to 8).

CMV involvement of the CNS is most often observed as encephalitis or retinitis, usually in patients with documented disseminated infection. On CT and MRI, the white matter disease caused by CMV or other viral syndromes may not be distinguishable from HIV encephalitis (Fig. 9). I have noticed several cases in which MRI evaluation reveals ill-defined patchy areas of high signal intensity, representing demyelination localized to the frontal or the occipital lobes (Figs. 9 and 10). Infrequently herpes virus and related viruses cause an encephalitis with documented disseminated disease. There is a

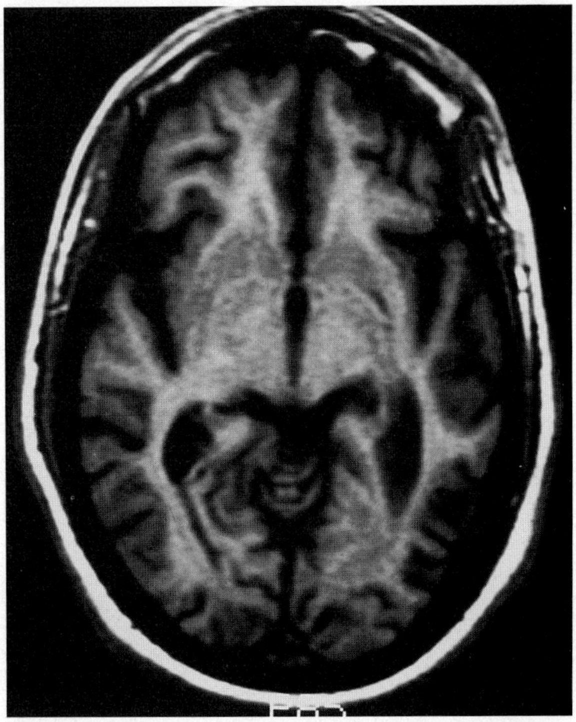

**FIGURE 1** T1-weighted axial MR image (TR417, TE20) demonstrates significant cerebral and cerebellar atrophy caused by HIV encephalopathy in this 31-year-old male. The sulci and ventricles are enlarged, with no focal lesions identified.

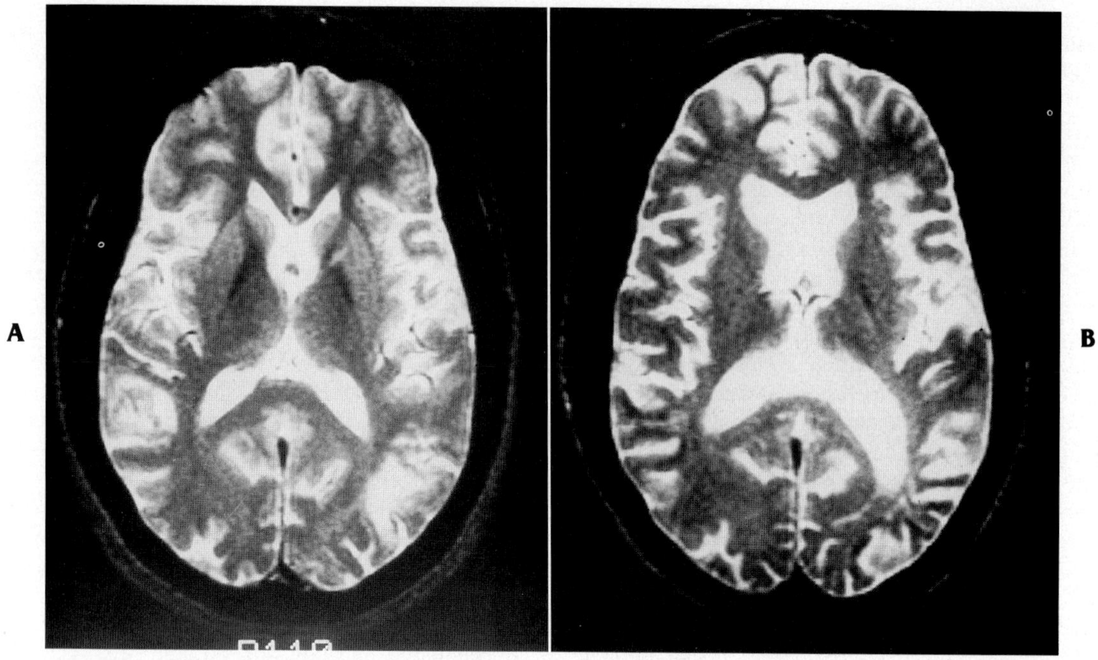

**FIGURE 2** *A* and *B,* T2-weighted axial MR images (TR2000, TE90) over six months show significant cerebral atrophy in this 39-year-old male with ADC. Notice enlargement of the sulci and ventricles as the disease progresses.

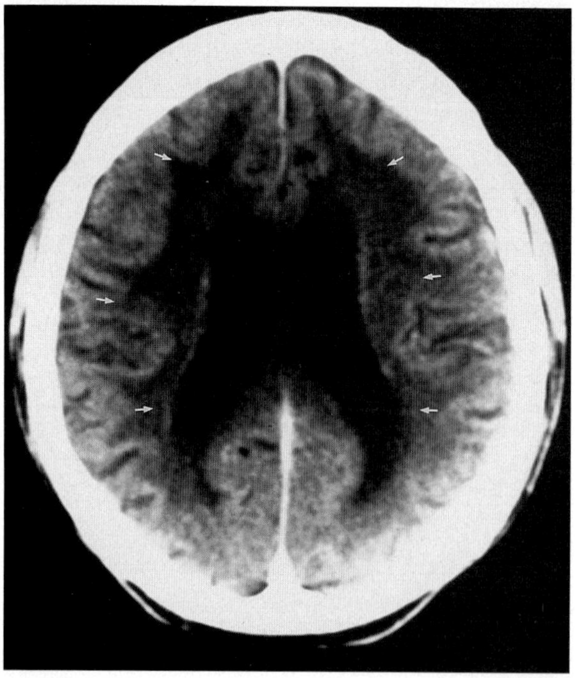

**FIGURE 3** Contrast-enhanced CT scan shows diffuse and symmetrical areas of low density in the periventricular white matter of the frontal and occipital lobes *(arrows)* consistent with HIV encephalitis. Notice the cortical atrophy in this 28-year-old man.

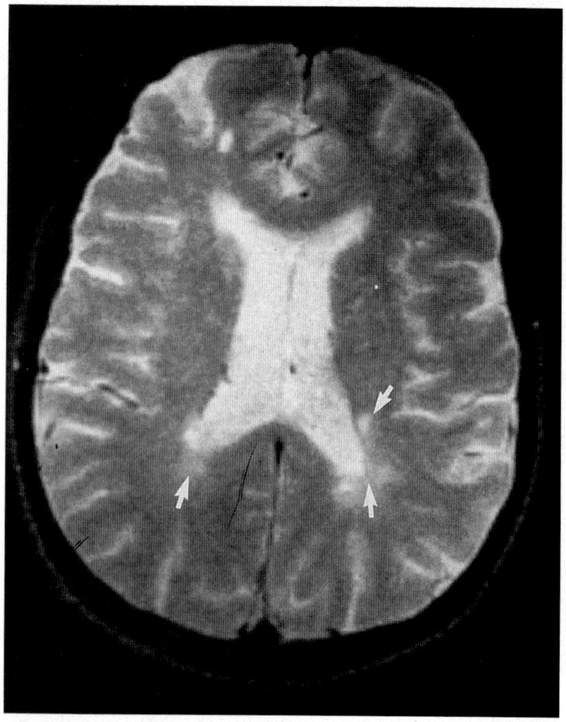

**FIGURE 4** T2-weighted axial MR image (TR2000, TE80) shows punctate areas of increased signals in the periventricular regions *(arrows),* representing HIV demyelination.

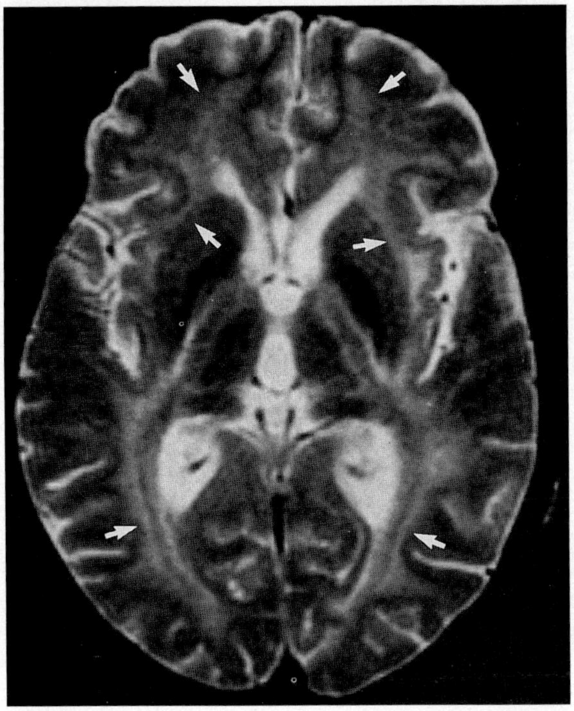

**FIGURE 5** T2-weighted axial MR image (TR2500, TE90) shows bilateral and diffuse areas of demyelination extending from the frontal white matter involving the external and extreme capsules and the optic radiation *(arrows)*.

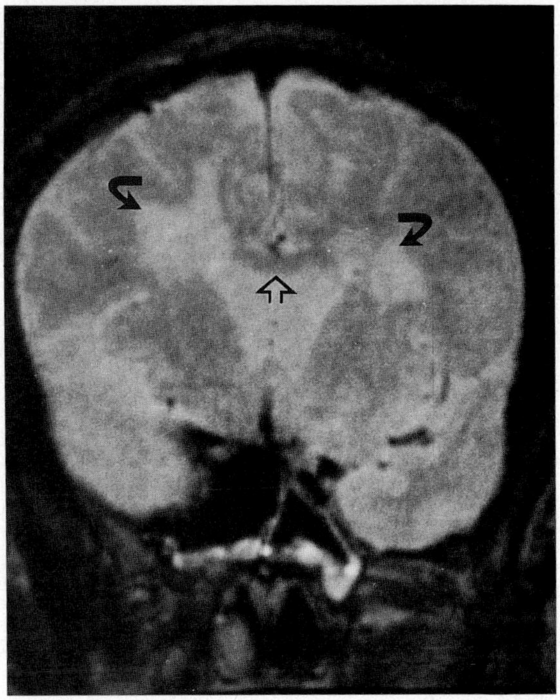

**FIGURE 6** T2-weighted coronal sequence (TR2000, TE80) shows bilateral HIV demyelination *(curved arrows)*, with sparing of the corpus callosum *(open arrowhead)*.

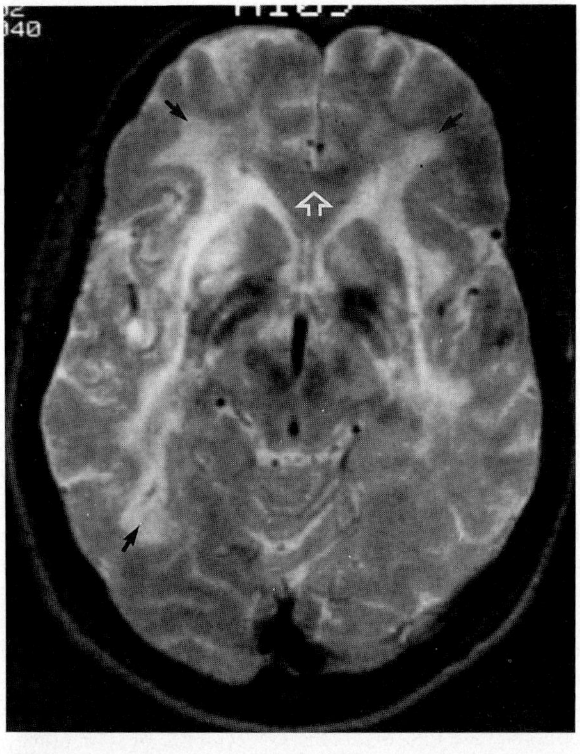

**FIGURE 7** T2-weighted axial MR image (TR2000, TE80) shows bilateral diffuse white matter disease extending along the external and extreme capsules and the optic radiation *(arrows)*. Notice no involvement of the corpus callosum *(arrowhead)*.

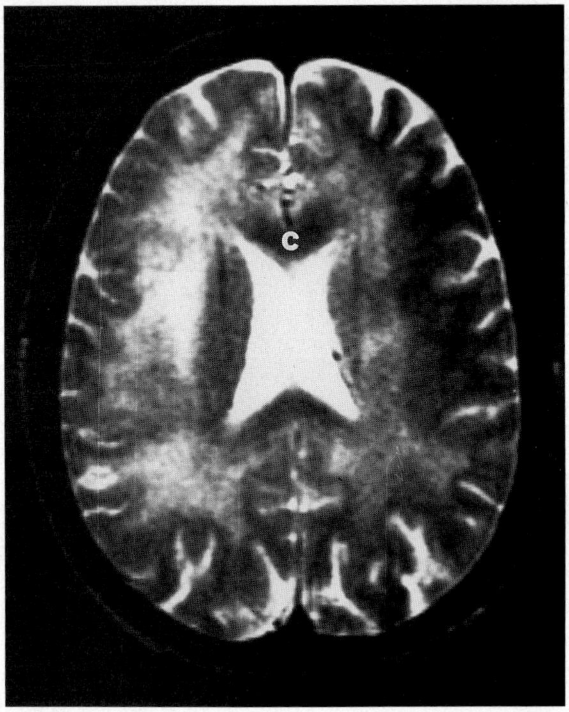


**FIGURE 8** T2-weighted axial MR images (TR2600, TE80) reveal bilateral demyelination caused by HIV with sparing of the corpus callosum (c).

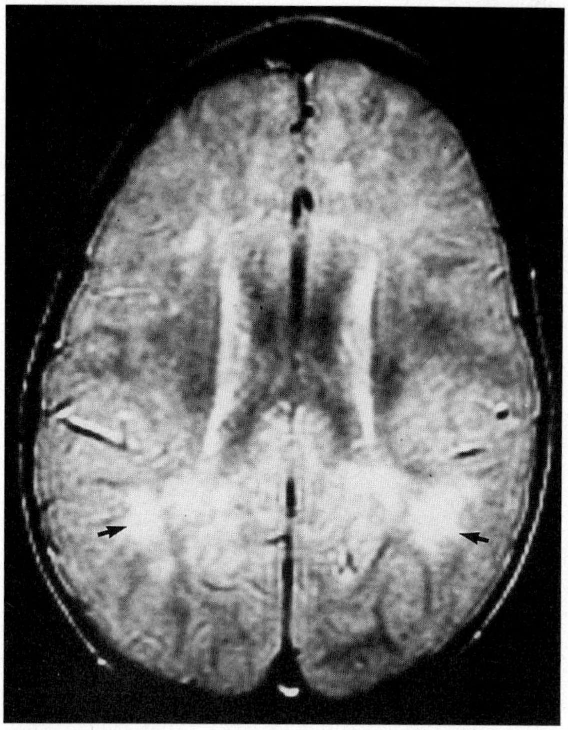

**FIGURE 9** Proton density–weighted axial MR image (TR2200, TE30) shows patchy areas of high signal intensity in the occipital lobes bilaterally due to CMV encephalitis. Contrast enhanced CT scan not shown revealed bilateral hypodense areas without enhancement.

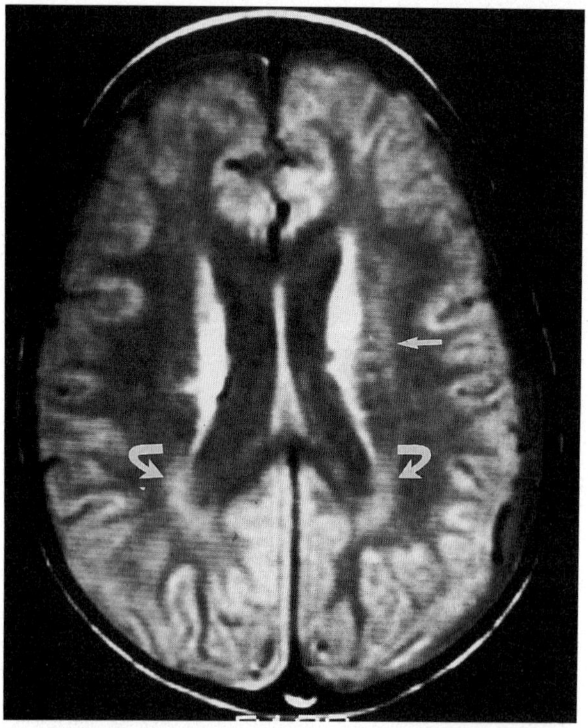

**FIGURE 10** Proton density–weighted axial MR image (TR2000, TE30) shows patchy areas of demyelination in the periventricular regions of the occipital lobes bilaterally *(curved arrows)*. Notice the area of demyelination in the left central white matter *(arrow)* and the high signals along the lateral ventricles representing CMV ependymitis.

predilection for the temporal lobes bilaterally, which appears hyperintense on T2-weighted MR images.

Progressive multifocal leukoencephalopathy (PML) is caused by a papovavirus (the JC virus) and is observed in 2 to 7 percent of AIDS patients. There is demyelination and necrosis of the white matter, with a predilection for oligodendrocytes in the subcortical areas. Precontrast and postcontrast CT studies demonstrate asymmetric and multicentric areas of low-density regions, usually seen in the parieto-occipital lobes. There is no evidence of edema or enhancement on CT and/or MRI evaluation. On T1-weighted MR images, PML demyelination may be isointense or hypointense (Fig. 11), becoming hyperintense on the T2-weighted images (Figs. 12 to 15). PML is a progressive disease and lesions may coalesce, leading to involvement of the corpus callosum (Fig. 15).

## *Mass Lesions*

### Toxoplasmosis

Toxoplasmosis is the most common intracranial mass lesion and, after HIV, is the second most common opportunistic CNS infection in AIDS patients. It may present as a space-occupying lesion or as a progressing meningoencephalitis. Most often abscesses are multiple and located in the basal ganglia but may also involve the white matter. Noncontrast CT evaluation shows the typical toxoplasmosis abscess as a hypodense mass with surrounding edema and mass effect (Fig. 16). Following contrast infusion, the abscesses exhibit ring or nodular enhancement (Figs. 16, 17 and 18). MRI often demonstrates more abscesses than CT, because of its increased sensitivity and superior tissue contrast (Figs. 17 and 18). On T1-weighted images the abscesses appear hypointense compared with the brain parenchyma. These lesions become hyperintense with surrounding edema on T2-weighted images. There is evidence of ring or nodular enhancement following gadolinium-DTPA infusion (Figs. 18 to 24). Treated toxoplasmosis is currently followed with either an MRI or contrast-enhanced CT study. Both may show a decrease in the number of abscesses, but T2-weighted MR images usually reveal a decrease in the vasogenic edema and mass effect compared with pretreated studies (Figs. 25, 26).

### CNS Lymphoma and Metastatic Disease

Primary CNS lymphoma is observed in approximately 6 percent of AIDS patients and generally presents as a focal expanding cerebral mass. Typical findings on nonenhanced CT evaluation include a solitary hypodense or inhomogeneous periventricular mass that may demonstrate homogeneous or ring enhancement on contrast-enhanced studies (Figs. 27 and 28). On T1-weighted MR images, the tumor mass may be hypointense; the mass becomes hyperintense on T2-weighted sequences (Figs. 29 to 31). On postgadolinium studies, the tumor usually exhibits homogeneous enhancement (see Figs. 28 to 31). Although neuroimaging findings are essentially consistent with specific intracranial processes, occasionally major pitfalls occur. Infrequently toxoplasmosis may present as a solitary mass that may be indistinguishable from CNS lymphoma (see Fig. 24). If there is evidence of solid homogeneous enhancement with minimal edema, the diagnosis of CNS lymphoma is highly suggested. Toxoplasmosis more often exhibits ring or nodular enhancement when present. Masses that exhibit infiltration across neuroanatomical boundaries,

*Text continued on p. 549.*

A

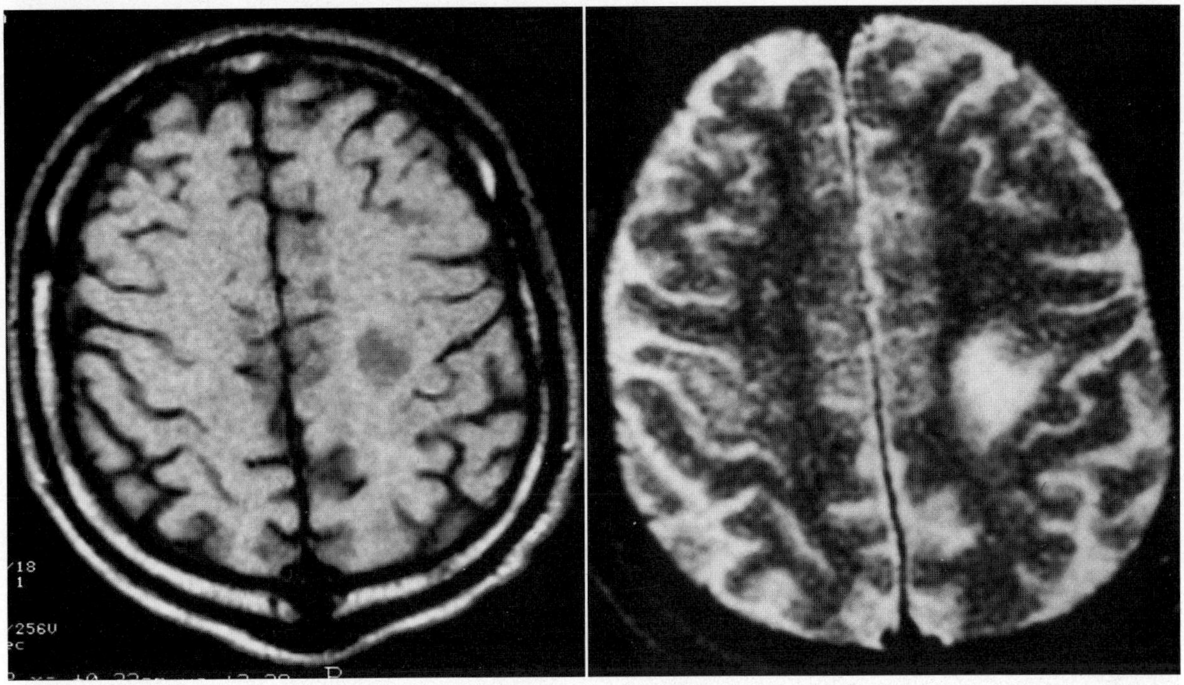

B

**FIGURE 11** *A,* T1-weighted axial MR image (TR770, TE25) shows an area of low signal in the high convexity of the left parietal region, which becomes hyperintense on *(B)* T2-weighted axial image (TR2050, TE80). This finding is typical for subcortical involvement with PML.

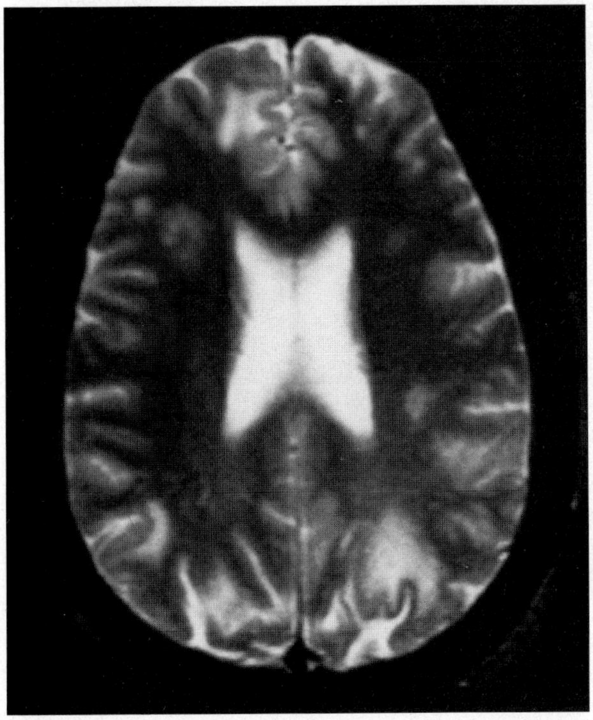

**FIGURE 12** T2-weighted axial MR image (TR2800, TE80) shows multiple areas of high signals, representing PML involvement of the peripheral white matter of the parietal, occipital, and frontal lobes.

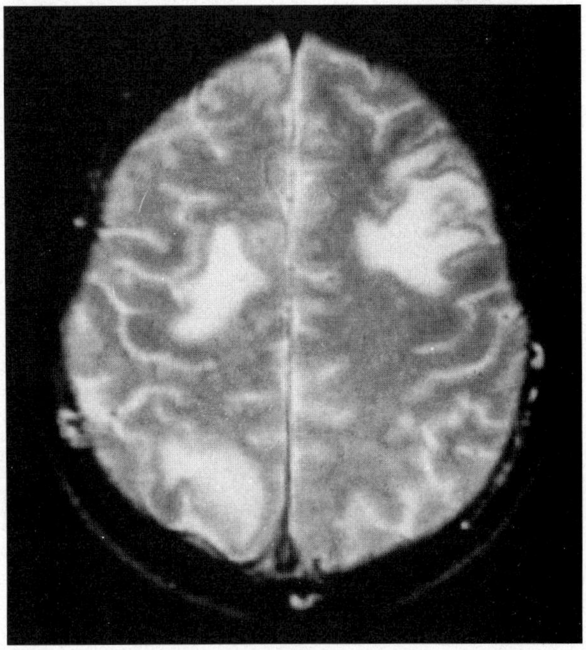

**FIGURE 13** T2-weighted axial MR image (TR2000, TE90) demonstrates multifocal areas of discrete high signals throughout the brain in this patient with PML.

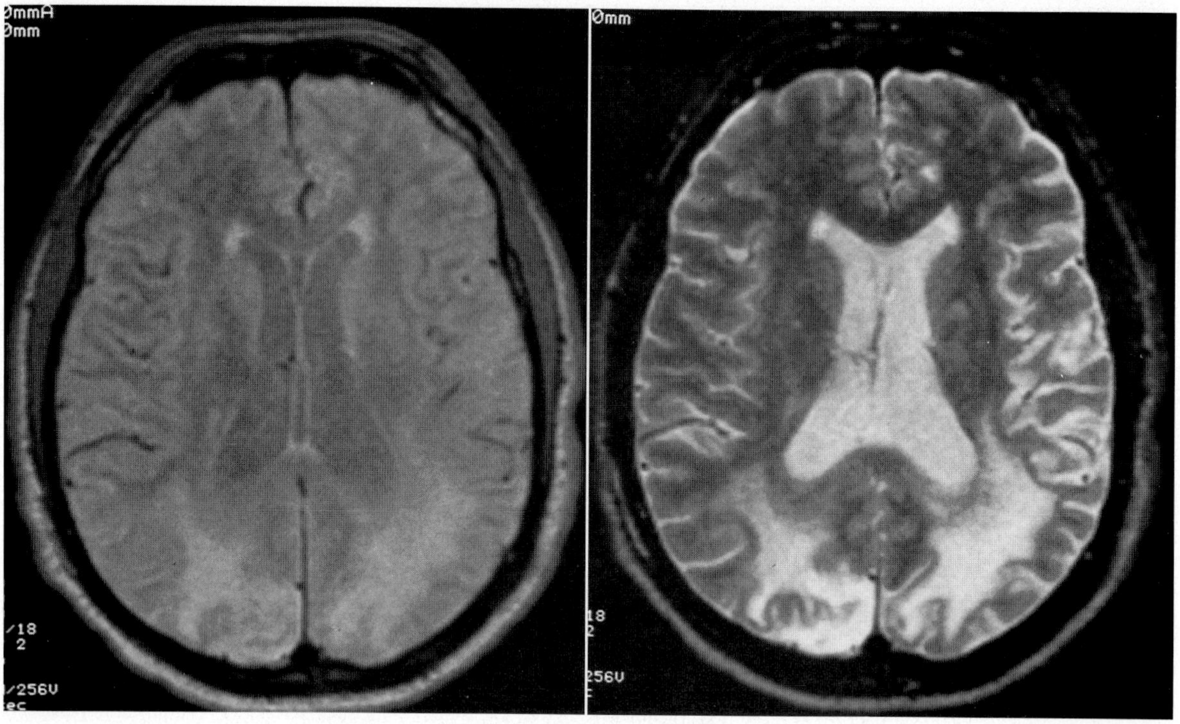

A B

**FIGURE 14** *A,* Axial proton density–weighted MR image (TR2600, TE30) shows intermediate signals in the occipital lobes bilaterally, which becomes hyperintense on *(B)* T2-weighted axial image (TR2600, TE100). These findings are typical of PML.

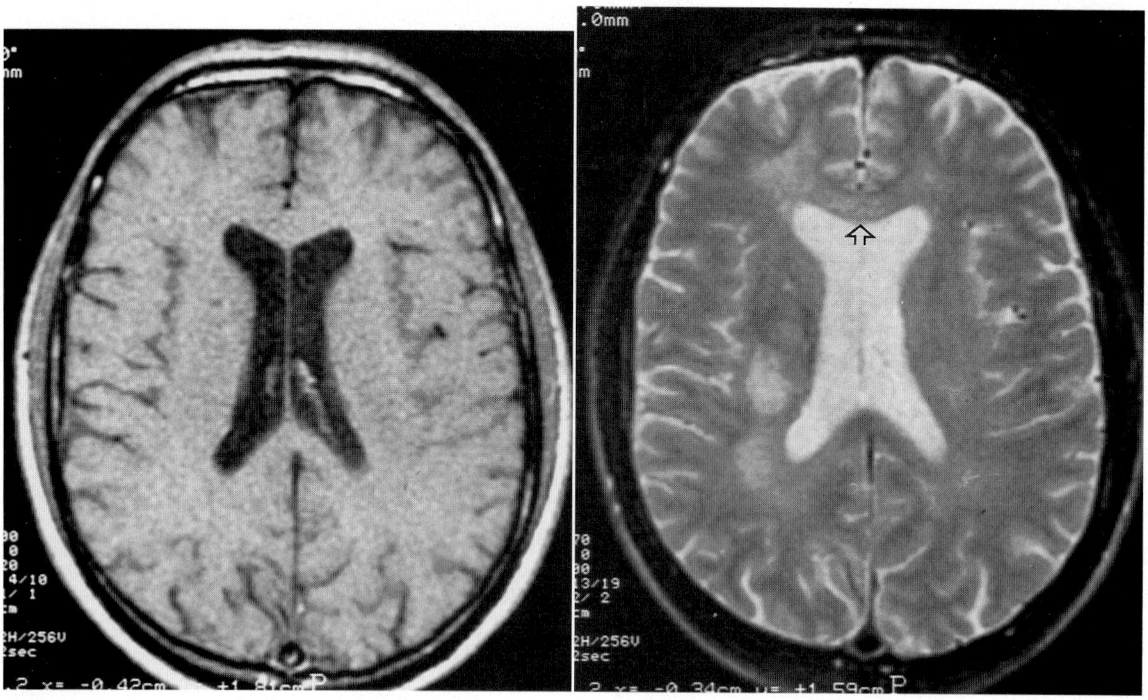

A B

**FIGURE 15** *A,* T1-weighted axial MR image (TR500, TE20) and *(B)* T2-weighted MR image (TR2670, TE100) demonstrate multiple asymmetric areas of hyperintensity throughout the frontal and periventricular regions, without significant mass effect. This finding along with involvement of the corpus callosum *(open arrowhead)* is typical of PML.

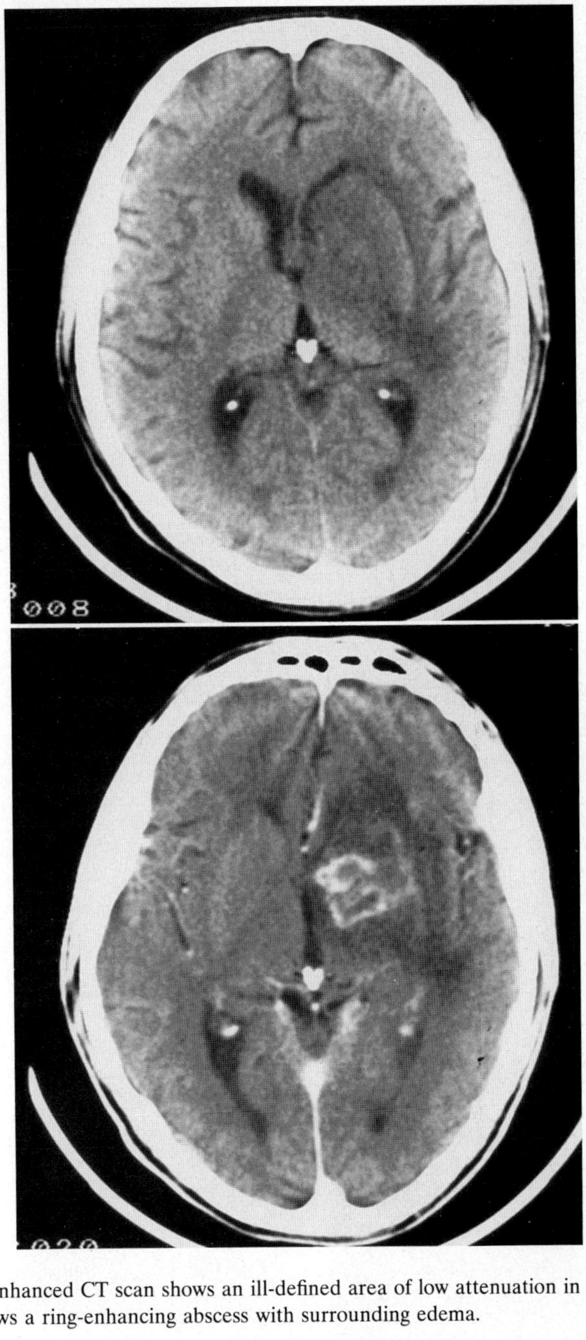


**FIGURE 16** Toxoplasmosis. *A,* Nonenhanced CT scan shows an ill-defined area of low attenuation in the left basal ganglia with minimal mass effect. *B,* Contrast-enhanced study shows a ring-enhancing abscess with surrounding edema.

A

B

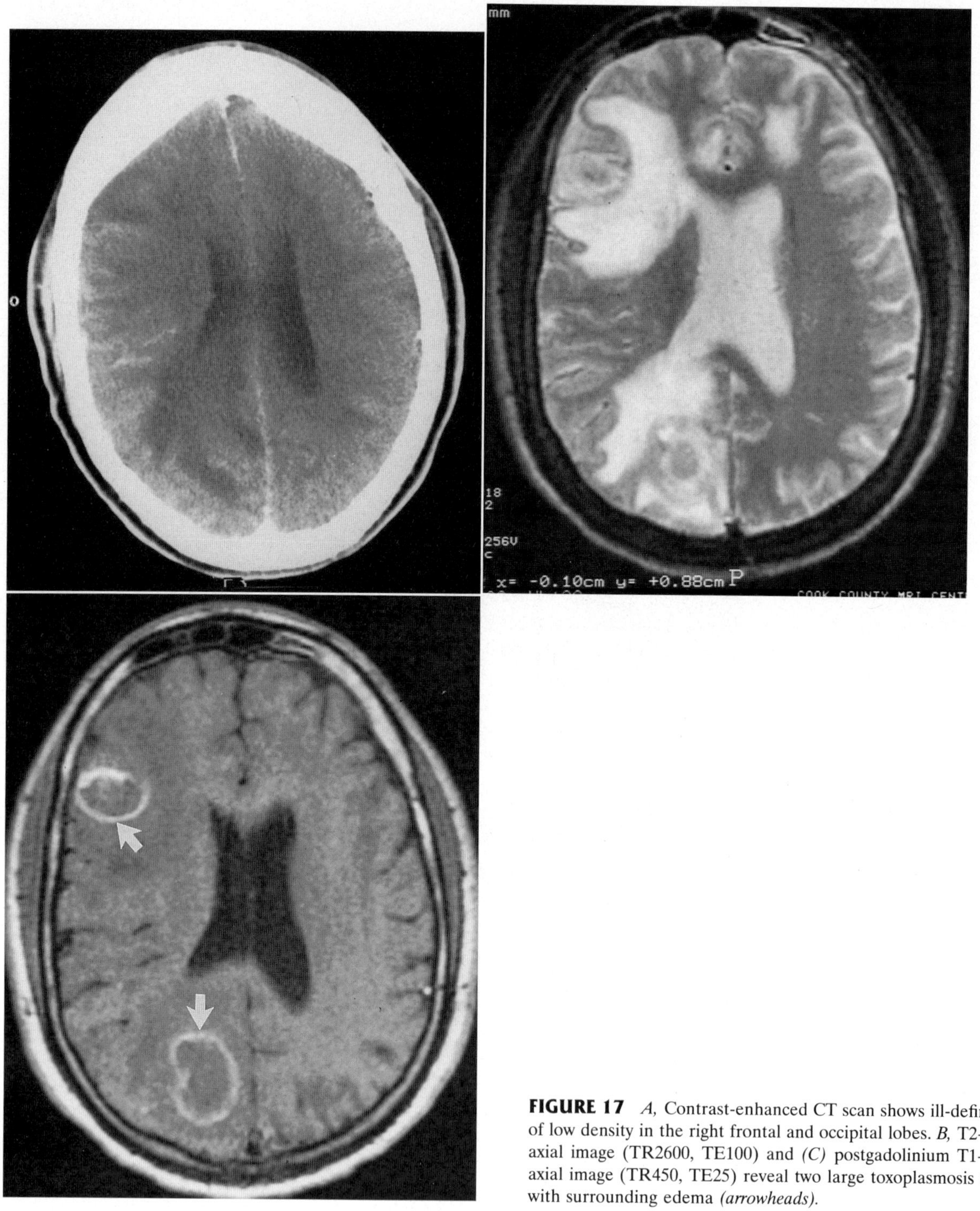


C

**FIGURE 17** *A,* Contrast-enhanced CT scan shows ill-defined areas of low density in the right frontal and occipital lobes. *B,* T2-weighted axial image (TR2600, TE100) and *(C)* postgadolinium T1-weighted axial image (TR450, TE25) reveal two large toxoplasmosis abscesses with surrounding edema *(arrowheads).*

A

B

C

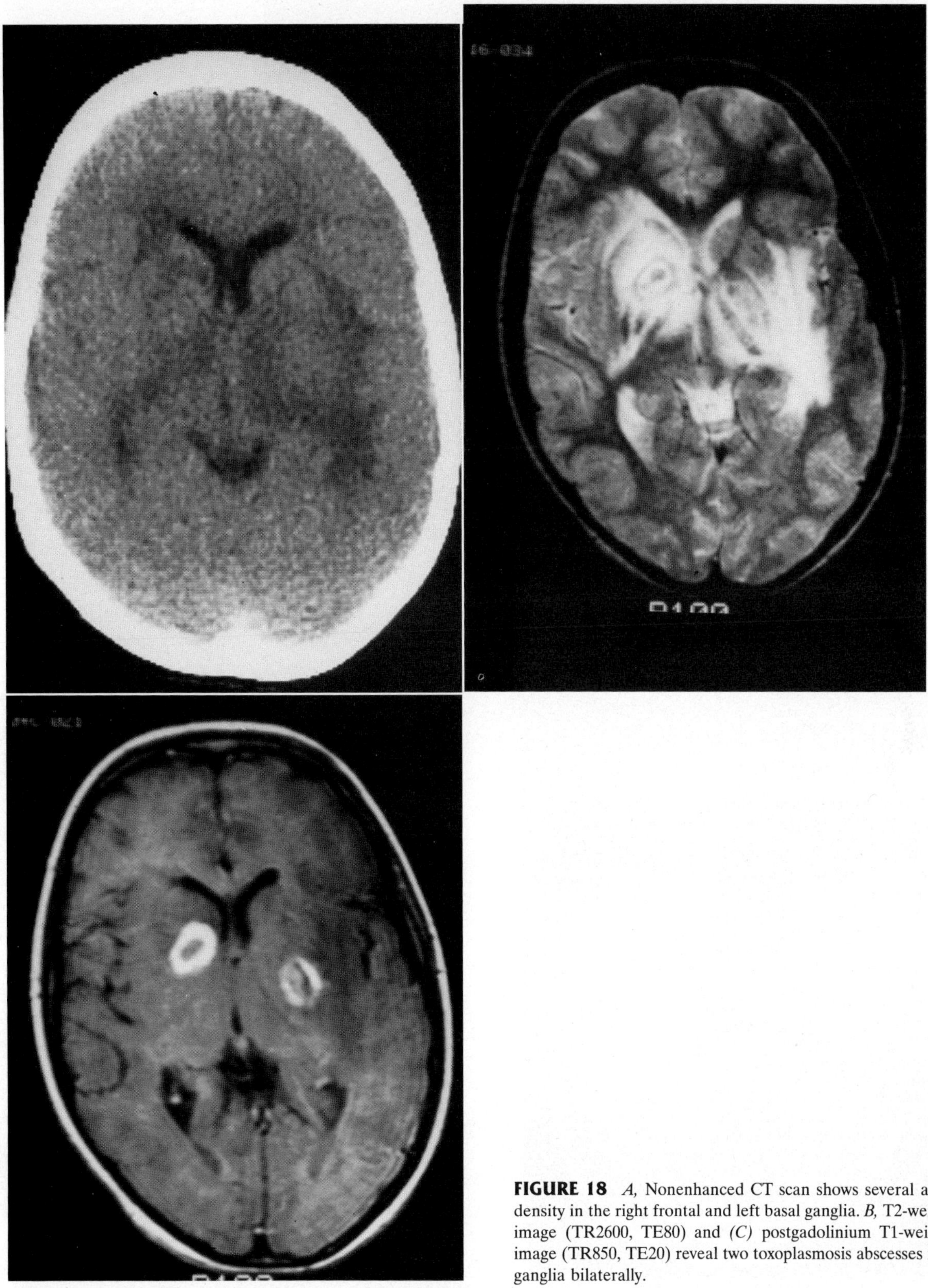

**FIGURE 18** *A,* Nonenhanced CT scan shows several areas of low density in the right frontal and left basal ganglia. *B,* T2-weighted axial image (TR2600, TE80) and *(C)* postgadolinium T1-weighted axial image (TR850, TE20) reveal two toxoplasmosis abscesses in the basal ganglia bilaterally.

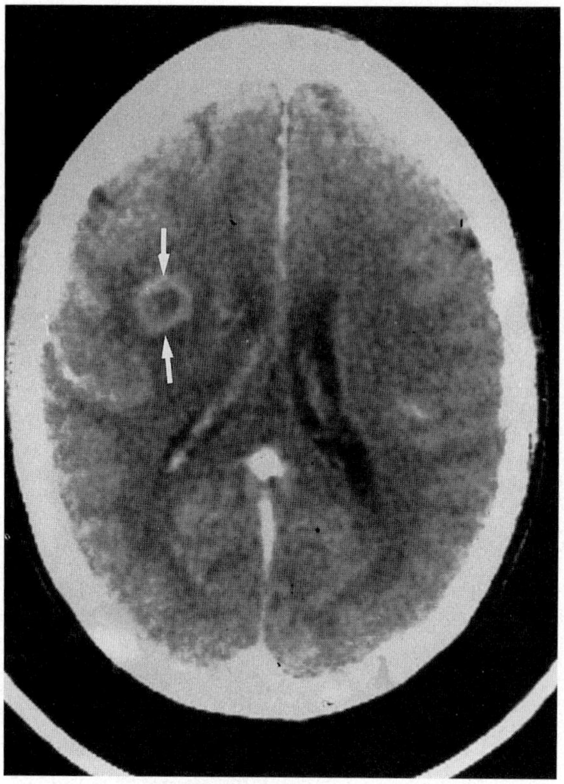

**FIGURE 19** Contrast-enhanced CT scan shows a ring-enhanced abscess in the right frontal lobe. There is evidence of vasogenic edema *(arrows)*.

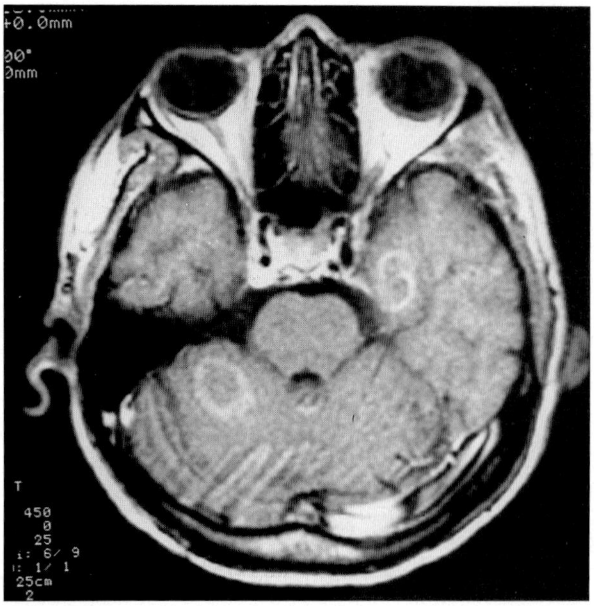


**FIGURE 20** Postgadolinium T1-weighted axial MR image (TR550, TE25) reveals several ring-enhancing abscesses in the left temporal lobe and right cerebellar hemisphere.

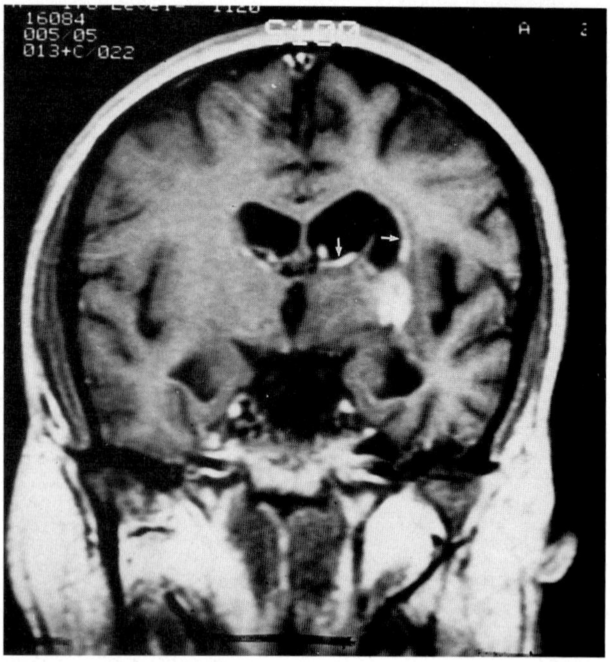


**FIGURE 21** Postgadolinium T1-weighted coronal MR image (TR550, TE30) shows a homogeneous enhancing abscess in the left basal ganglia, with slight marginal enhancement of an associated infarct and the ependymal lining of the corresponding lateral ventricle *(arrows)*. Involvement of the ependymal lining is an unusual finding with toxoplasmosis.

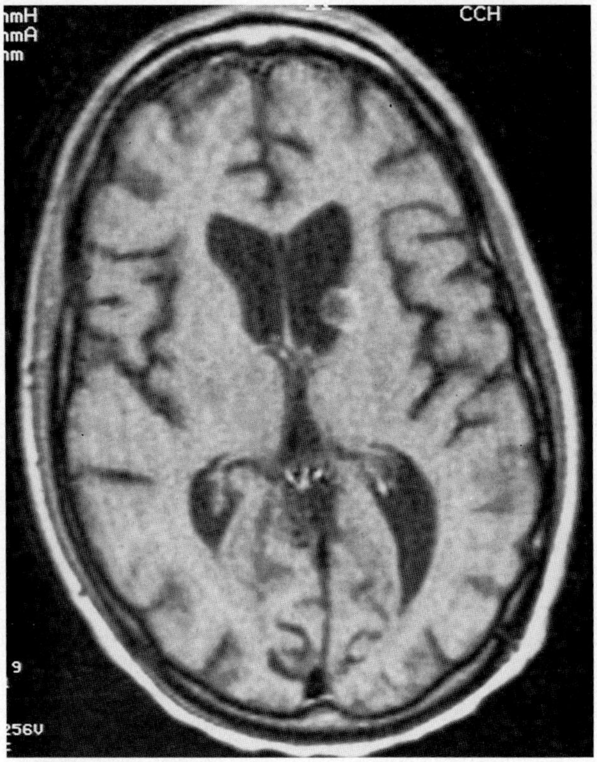

**FIGURE 22** Postgadolinium T1-weighted axial MR image (TR450, TE25) shows a small toxoplasmosis abscess along the lining of the left lateral ventricle.

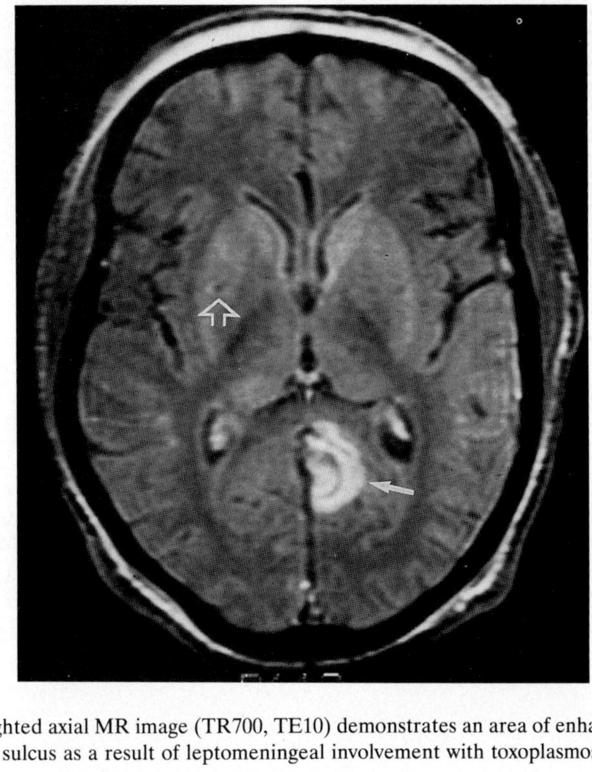

**FIGURE 23** Postgadolinium T1-weighted axial MR image (TR700, TE10) demonstrates an area of enhancement posterior to the splenum of the corpus callosum and the left calcarine sulcus as a result of leptomeningeal involvement with toxoplasmosis *(arrow)*. Notice a small abscess in the right basal ganglia *(arrowhead)*.

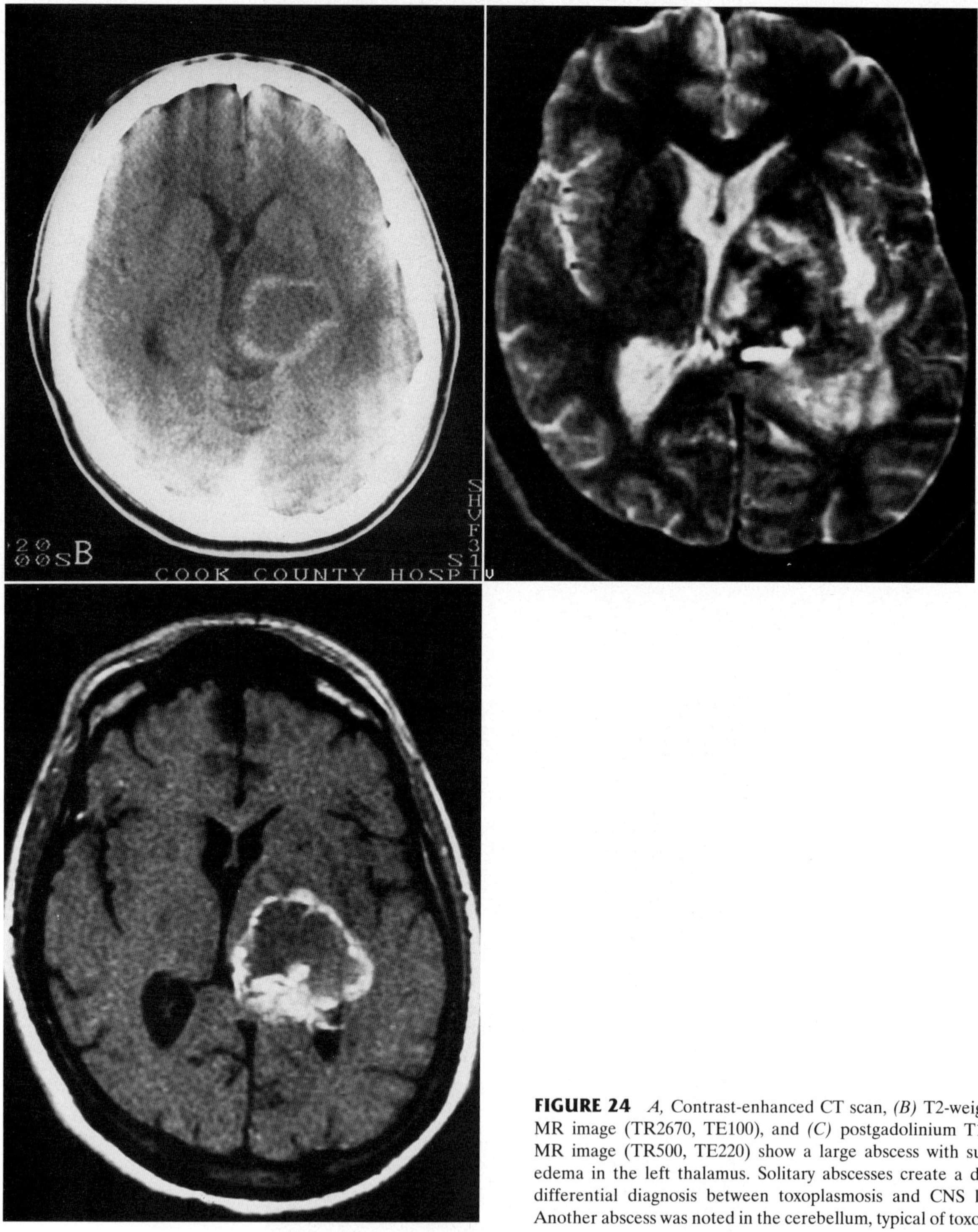


**FIGURE 24** *A,* Contrast-enhanced CT scan, *(B)* T2-weighted axial MR image (TR2670, TE100), and *(C)* postgadolinium T1-weighted MR image (TR500, TE220) show a large abscess with surrounding edema in the left thalamus. Solitary abscesses create a dilemma of differential diagnosis between toxoplasmosis and CNS lymphoma. Another abscess was noted in the cerebellum, typical of toxoplasmosis.

A

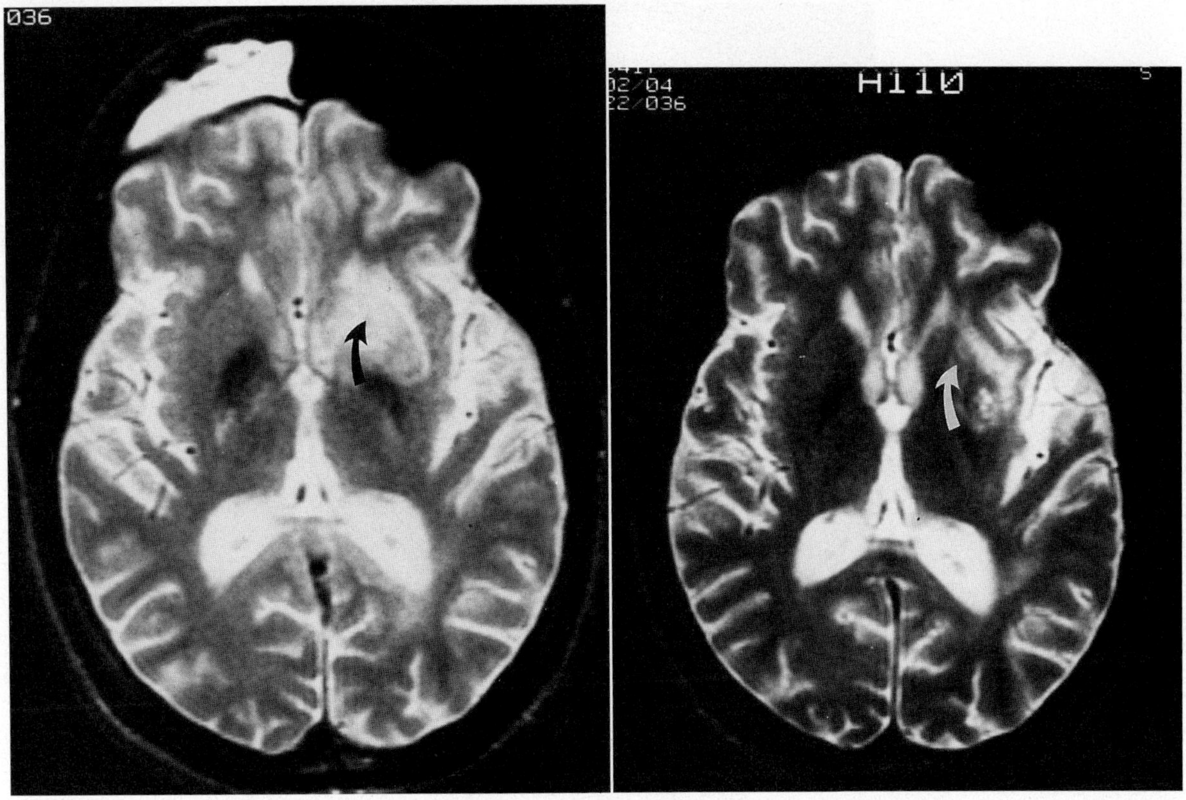


B

**FIGURE 25** *A,* T2-weighted axial MR image (TR2000, TE80) reveals an abscess with surrounding edema in the left basal ganglia and *(B)* after 3 weeks of antibiotic treatment with sulfadiazine and pyrimethamine. T2-weighted axial image shows a decrease in the size of the abscess and resolution of surrounding edema *(curved arrow).* Notice a small healing abscess in the left basal ganglia and complete resolution of the right frontal sinusitis.

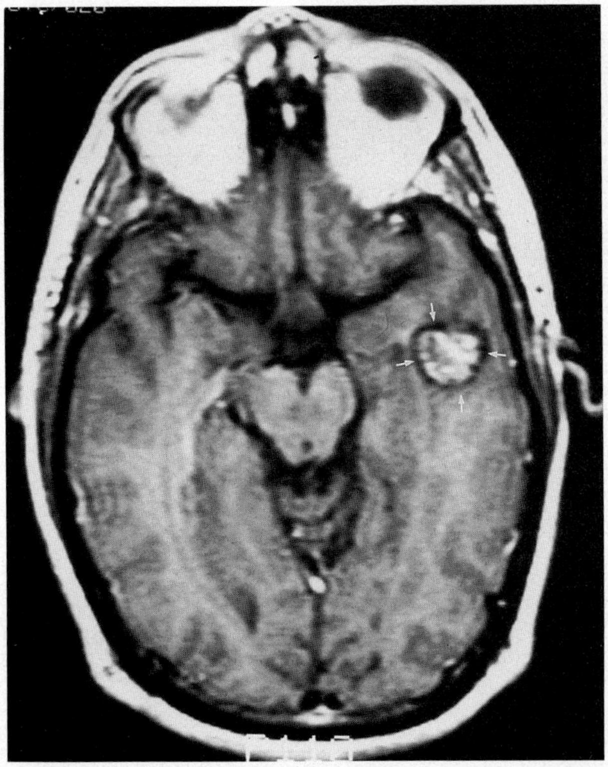

**FIGURE 26** Postgadolinium T1-weighted axial MR image (TR417, TE20) shows a healing toxoplasmosis abscess in the left temporal lobe. The low signaling capsule is clearly demonstrated without evidence of surrounding edema *(small arrows).* The inhomogeneous signals in the center of the abscess represent debris.

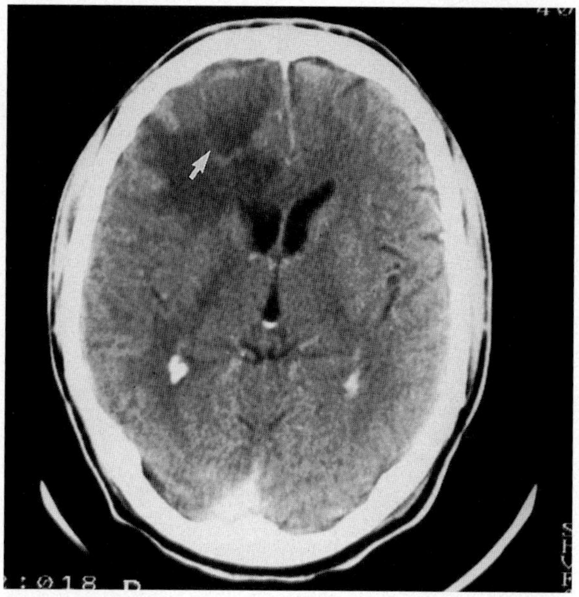

**FIGURE 27** Contrast-enhanced CT scan shows an area of minimal enhancement *(arrow)* with surrounding edema and mass effect in the right frontal lobe. Biopsy proven primary CNS lymphoma.

A

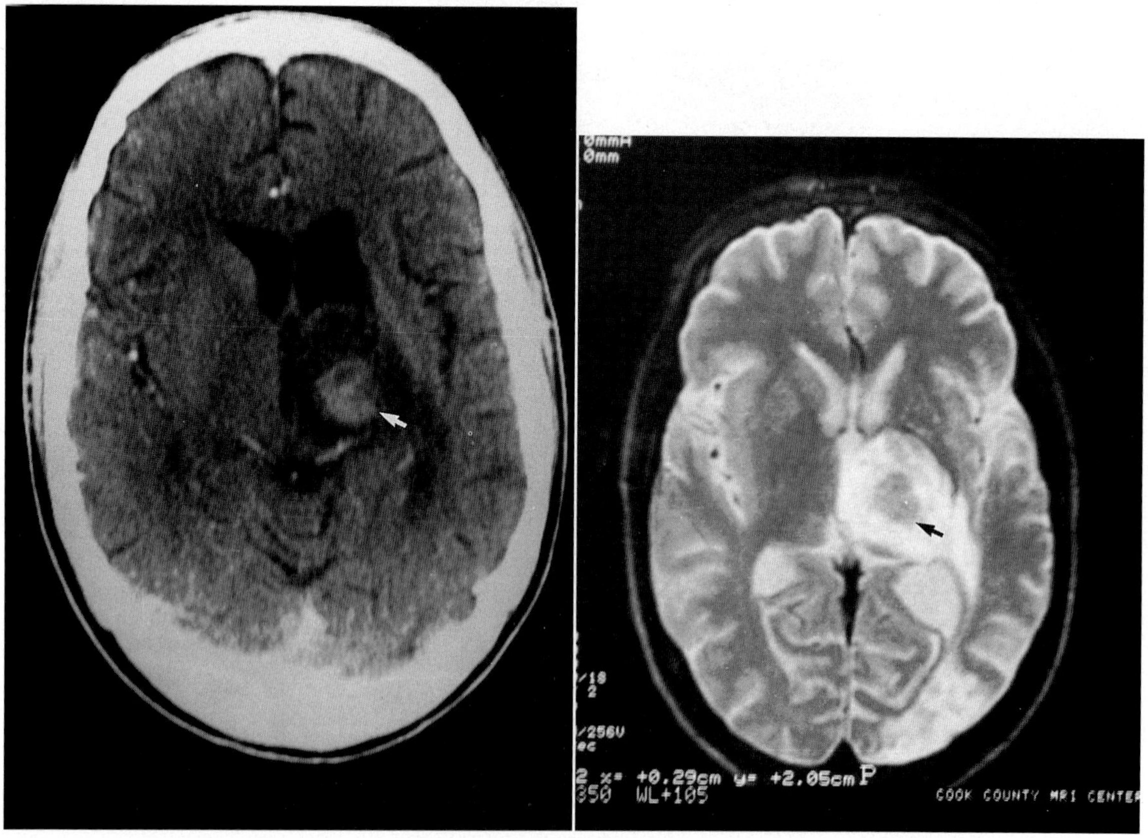


B

**FIGURE 28** *A,* Contrast-enhanced CT scan and *(B)* T2-weighted axial MR image (TR2000, TE100) show a large primary CNS lymphoma in the left brain stem *(arrow).*

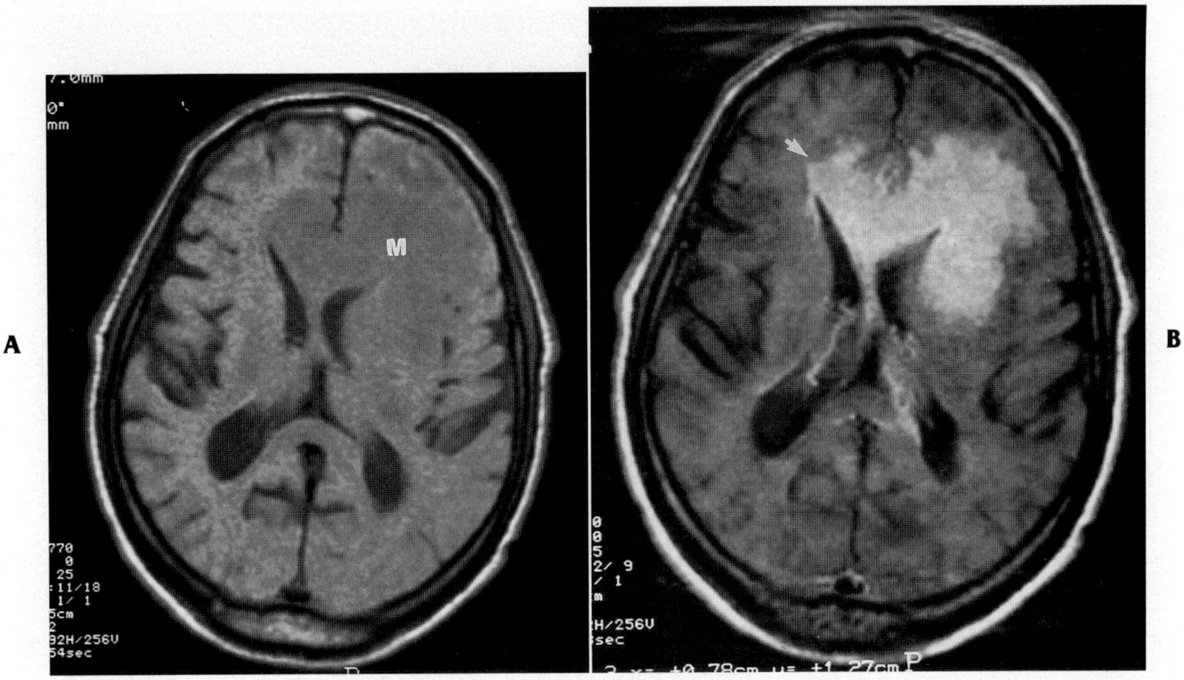


**FIGURE 29** *A,* T1-weighted axial MR image (TR770, TE25) reveals an ill-defined area of hypointense signal (M), with compression of the left frontal horn of the lateral ventricle and corpus callosum. *B,* Postgadolinium axial T1-weighted MR image (TR550, TE25) shows significant homogeneous enhancement with contralateral spread along the corpus callosum and right lateral ventricle *(arrow).* Notice involvement of the ependymal lining of the contralateral ventricle. Homogeneous enhancement with involvement of the corpus callosum is typical of CNS lymphoma.

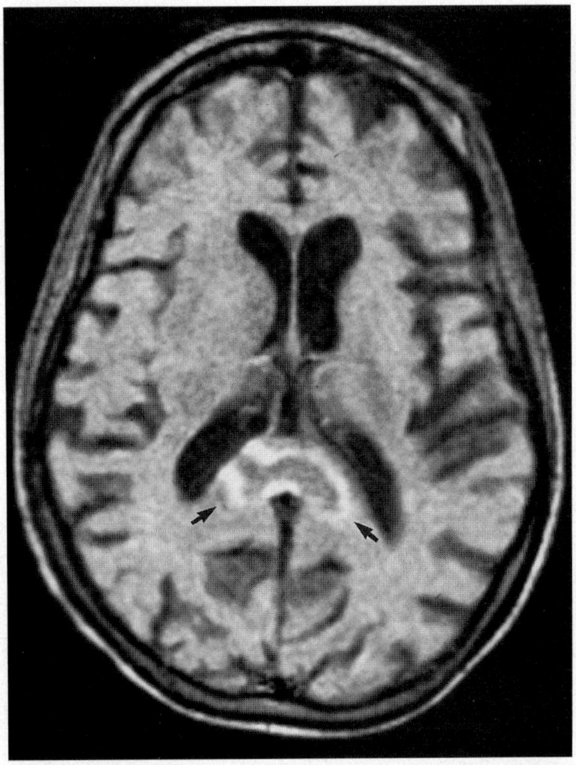

**FIGURE 30** Postgadolinium T1-weighted axial MR image (TR770, TE25) shows a nodular enhancing mass in the splenium of the corpus callosum *(arrows)* in this patient with CNS lymphoma.

A

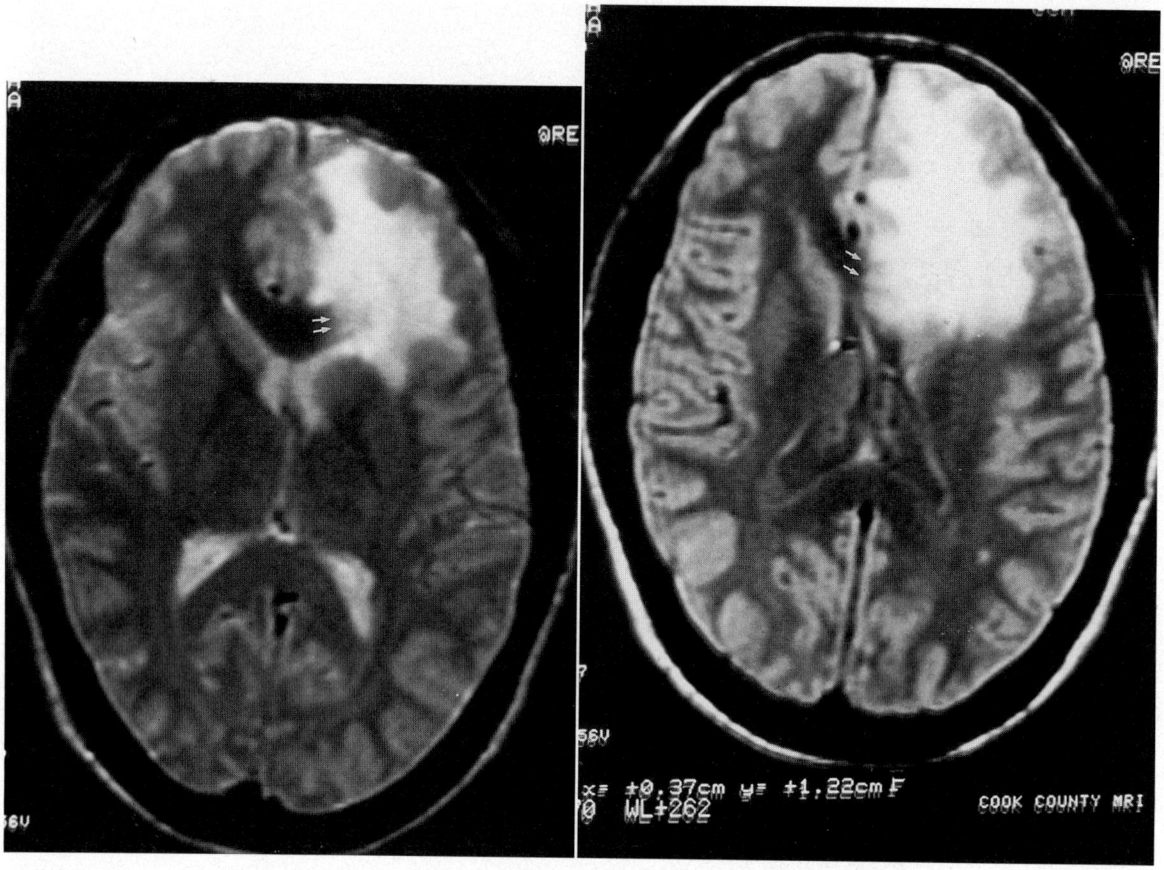


B

**FIGURE 31** *A,* T2-weighted axial MR image (TR2500, TE90) and *(B)* postgadolinium T1-weighted MR image (TR700, TE25) show a large homogeneous enhancing mass in the left frontal lobe with early involvement of the corpus callosum *(arrows).*

A

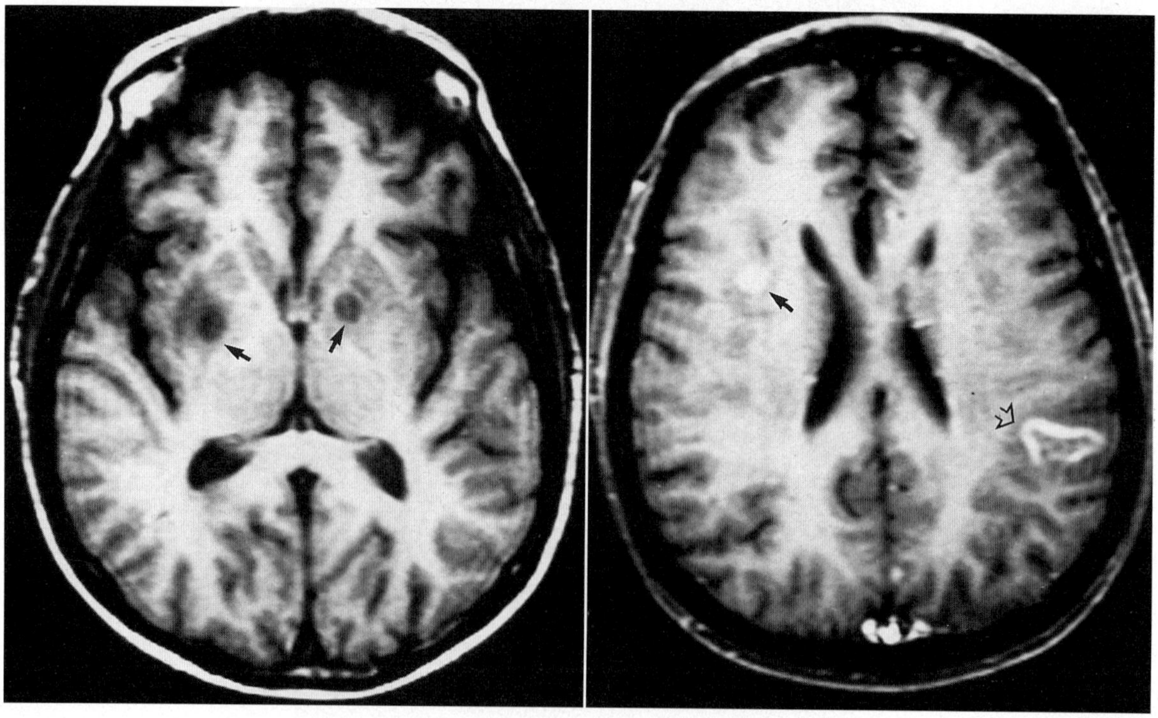

B

**FIGURE 32** *A,* T1-weighted axial MR image (TR417, TE20) shows two areas of hypointensity *(arrows)* in the basal ganglia bilaterally. *B,* Postgadolinium T1-weighted image reveals homogeneous enhancement of another lesion *(arrow)* and a linear area of enhancement *(arrowhead)* in the left parieto-occipital region in this patient with metastatic Burkitt's lymphoma.

such as the corpus callosum, are characteristic of CNS lymphoma. Occasionally CNS lymphoma may present with multiple masses, creating a diagnostic dilemma with toxoplasmosis. If there is no resolution of the masses following empiric treatment for toxoplasmosis, the diagnosis of CNS lymphoma is highly suggested if no other opportunistic infections are apparent. Intracranial mass lesions due to metastases occur infrequently in AIDS patients and are most often due to metastatic non-Hodgkin's lymphoma. Often it presents with leptomeningeal involvement, rarely with intraparenchymal involvement. Meningeal spread may cause a subacute meningitis with focal or diffuse symptoms. I have encountered two cases of metastatic Burkitt's lymphoma presenting as multiple focal lesions that appear hypointense on T1-weighted MR images (Fig. 32) and became hyperintense on T2-weighted images with homogeneous enhancement after gadolinium infusion (Figs. 32 and 33). Although an increased incidence of Kaposi's sarcoma is observed in AIDS patients, CNS metastasis is rarely documented.

## Fungal and Bacterial Abscesses

Cryptococcosis may manifest itself either as an isolated meningitis or intraparenchymal abscesses (cryptococcomas) involving both the gray and white matter. There is no specific appearance on CT evaluation, but abscesses may appear hypodense on both enhanced and nonenhanced CT studies. On T2-weighted MRI evaluation, cryptococcomas in the gray matter may appear as a cluster of small well-defined foci of high signal intensity observed in and around the basal ganglia (Figs. 34 and 35), representing microabscesses. In the presence of sufficient immune response in these patients, there may be evidence of intraparenchymal, as well as associated meningeal, enhancement following gadolinium-DTPA infusion (Fig. 34). The abscesses may extend to involve the Virchow-Robin spaces. Cryptococcal abscesses of the white matter may exhibit high signals on T2-weighted MR images without surrounding edema or mass effect. Candidal infection of the CNS is rarely

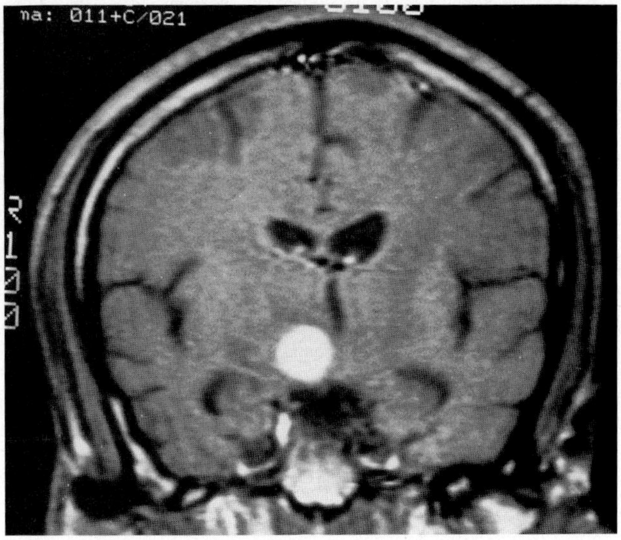


**FIGURE 33** Postgadolinium T1-weighted coronal MR image (TR550, TE20) shows a homogeneous enhancing mass in the right hypothalamic region from metastatic non-Hodgkin's lymphoma.

A

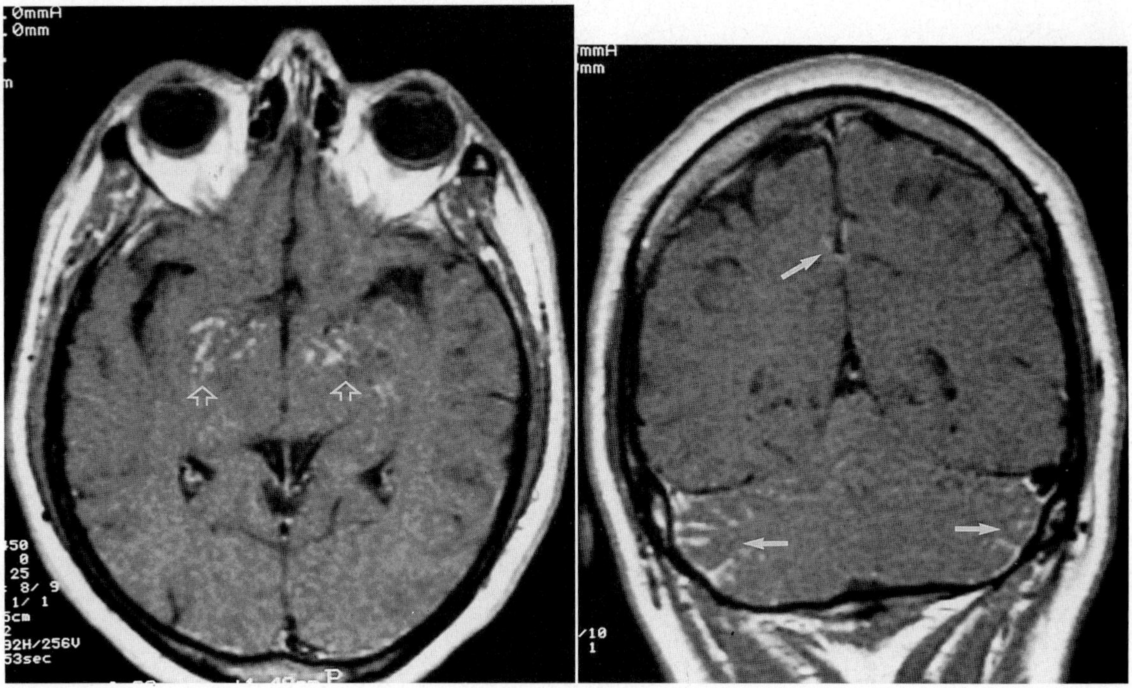

B

**FIGURE 34** *A,* Postgadolinium T1-weighted axial MR image (TR550, TE25) shows bilateral small areas of enhancement in the Virchow-Robin spaces *(open arrowheads)*. *B,* Postgadolinium coronal T1-weighted image (TR550, TE25) shows enhancement of the subarachnoid space *(arrows)* in this patient with cryptococcal meningitis. The abnormal signals in the Virchow-Robin spaces represent intraparenchymal cryptococcal pseudocysts.

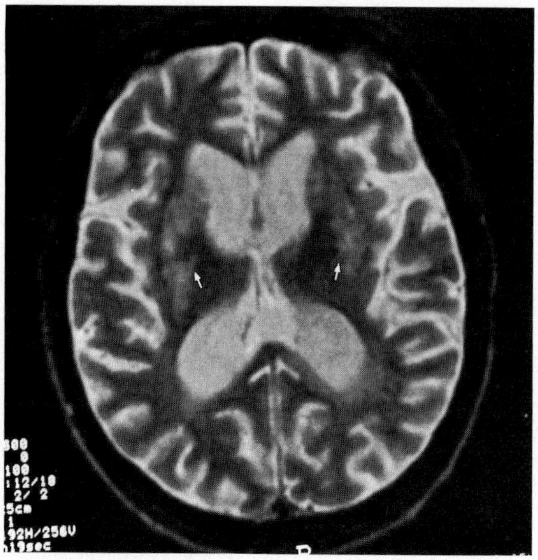

**FIGURE 35** T2-weighted axial MR image (TR2600, TE100) shows bilateral small areas of hyperintensity in the basal ganglia *(arrows)* in this patient as a result of intraparenchymal cryptococcosis.

A 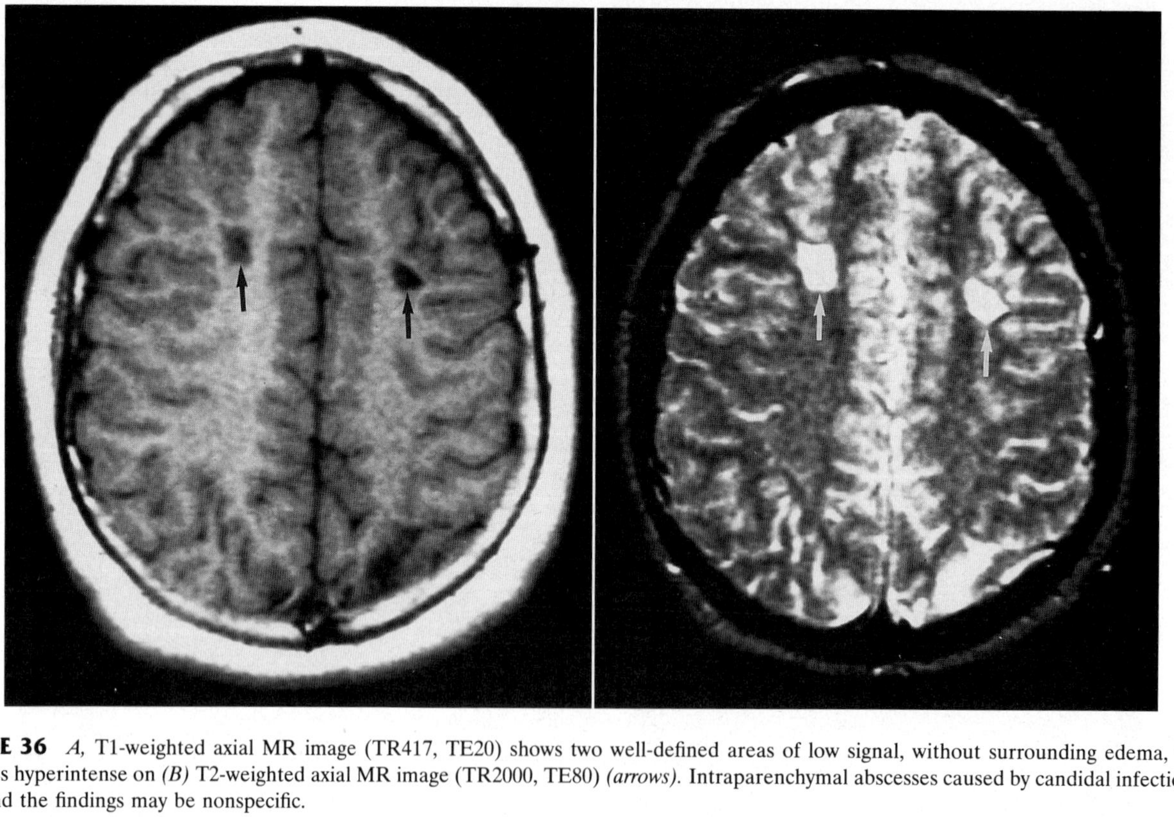 B

**FIGURE 36** *A,* T1-weighted axial MR image (TR417, TE20) shows two well-defined areas of low signal, without surrounding edema, which becomes hyperintense on *(B)* T2-weighted axial MR image (TR2000, TE80) *(arrows).* Intraparenchymal abscesses caused by candidal infection are rare, and the findings may be nonspecific.

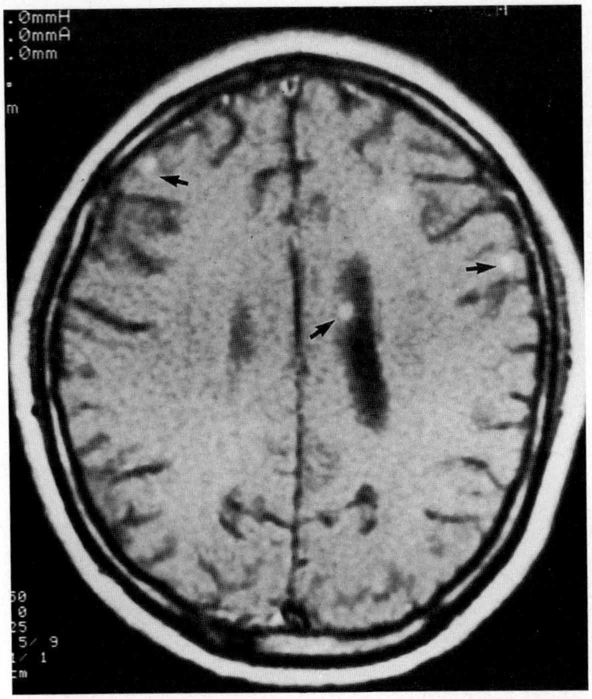

**FIGURE 37** Postgadolinium T1-weighted axial MR image (TR450, TE25) shows numerous enhancing granulomas caused by *Mycobacterium tuberculosis* infection *(arrows).*

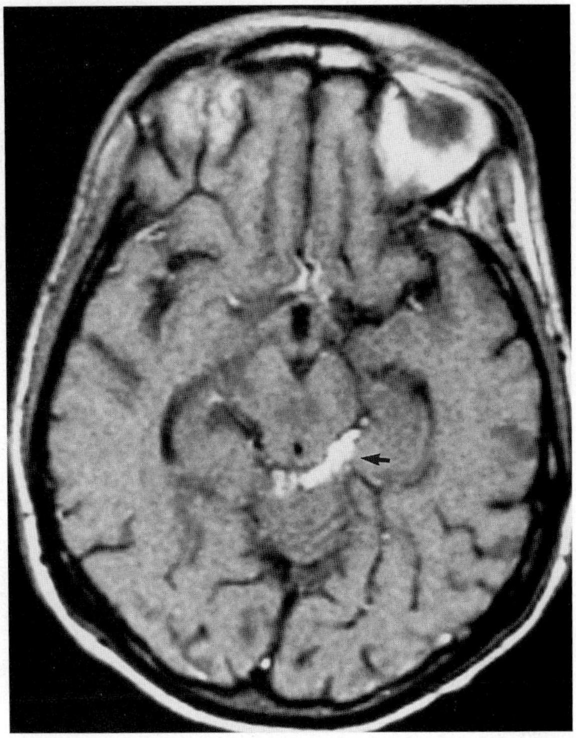

**FIGURE 39** Postgadolinium T1-weighted axial MR image (TR450, TE25) shows abnormal enhancement along the perimesencephalic cistern *(arrow)* from cryptococcal meningitis.

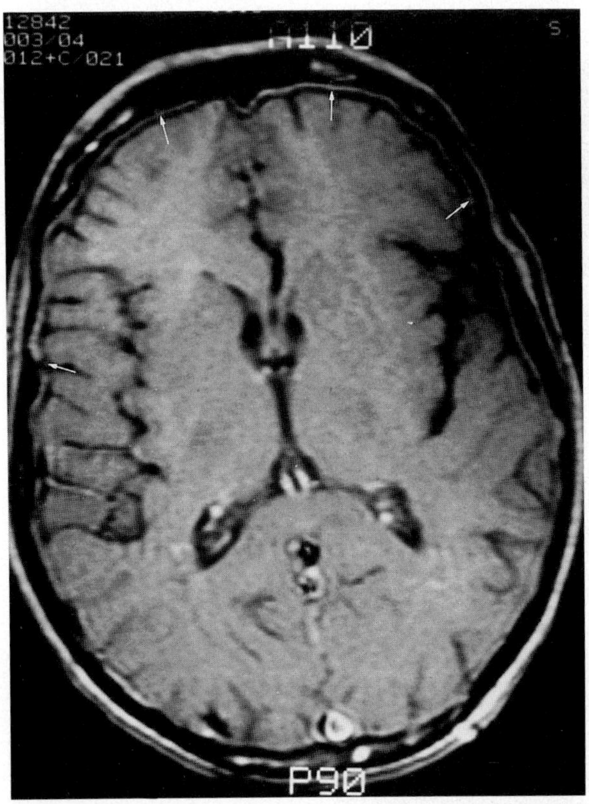


**FIGURE 38** Postgadolinium T1-weighted axial MR image (TR650, TE30) shows abnormal enhancement of the leptomeninges *(arrows)* in this patient with cryptococcal meningitis.

observed and, when present, usually is associated with disseminated candidiasis. MRI may reveal small discrete areas of low signal intensity in the white matter on T1-weighted images, which becomes hyperintense on T2-weighted sequences without surrounding edema (Fig. 36). Intraparenchymal abscesses caused by aspergillosis and mucormycosis may result from extension of disease from the nasal cavity or sphenoid sinus. Granulomatous disease caused by *Mycobacterium tuberculosis* infection (Fig. 37), histoplasmosis, and coccidioidomycosis may infrequently be observed.

## Leptomeningeal and Ependymal Disease

Today MRI is the recommended procedure of choice in diagnosing leptomeningeal infections. *Cryptococcus neoformans* is the most common cause of leptomeningitis in AIDS, and patients may present with neurological symptoms similar to those of immunocompetent patients. Both CT and MRI may be normal or show abnormal enhancement of the meninges or subarachnoid spaces following contrast infusion (Figs. 34, 38, 39). *Mycobacterium tuberculosis* infrequently produces basal leptomeningitis or intraparenchymal tuberculomas, which may be observed on contrast-enhanced CT or MRI evaluations (Figs. 37, 40, and 41). HIV and CMV may produce aseptic meningitis, observed in approximately 15 percent of AIDS patients. CMV usually involves the ependymal lining of the ventricles, causing an ependymitis or ventriculitis with subependymal necrosis. Contrast-enhanced CT and T2-weighted MRI studies may reveal an abnormal nodularity of the ependymal lining (Figs. 42 to 44), which may enhance following gadolinium (Fig. 45). Toxoplasmosis may also cause localized ependymitis or meningitis, which may be observed on postga-

*Text continued on p. 556.*

A

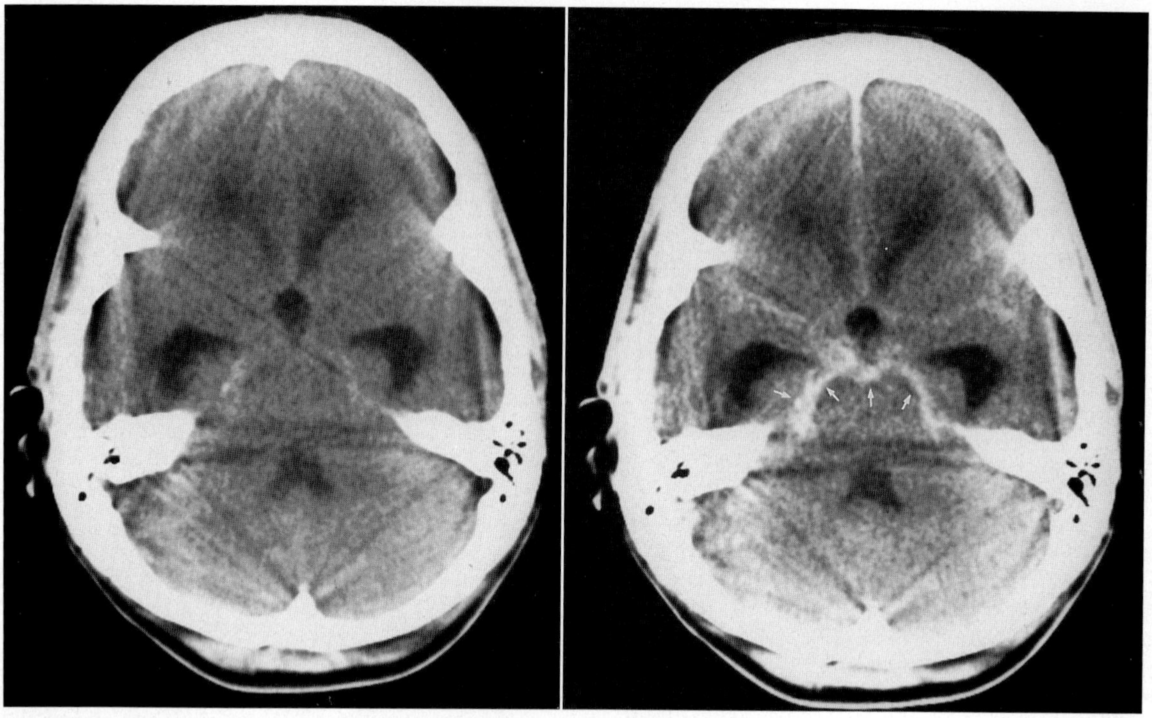

B

**FIGURE 40** *A* and *B,* Precontrast and postcontrast enhanced CT studies show diffuse nodular enhancement of the basal meninges in this AIDS patient with TB meningitis *(arrows).* Notice dilatation of the ventricles.

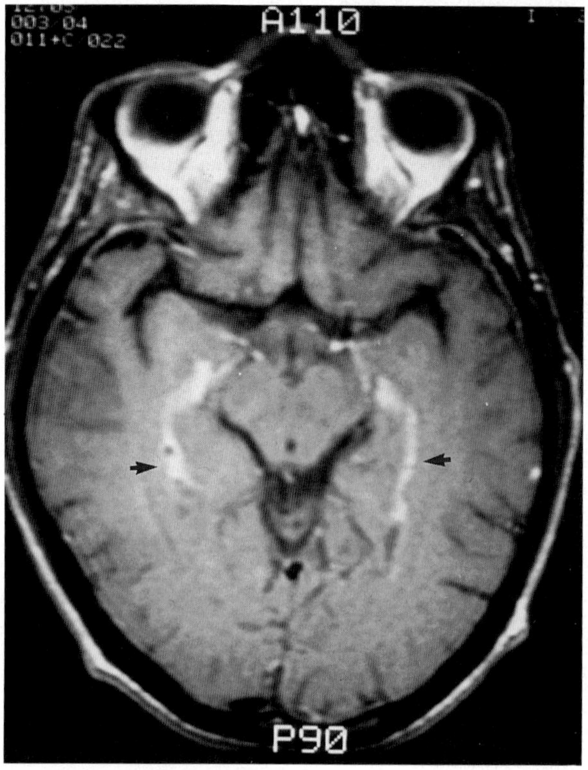


**FIGURE 41** Postgadolinium T1-weighted axial MR image (TR900, TE20) shows abnormal enhancement along the basal leptomeninges *(arrows)* in this patient with tuberculous meningitis.

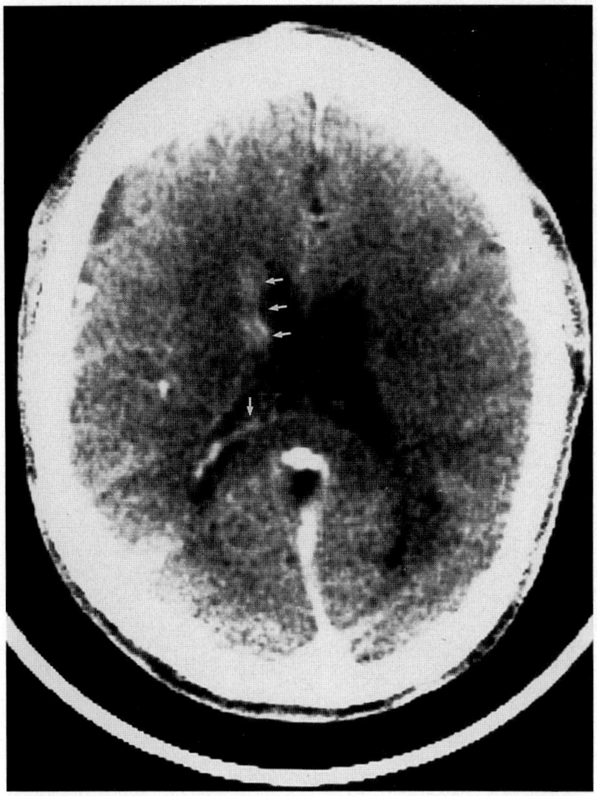

**FIGURE 42** Contrast-enhanced CT scan shows nodular enhancement along the right lateral ventricle and anterior aspect of the splenium of the corpus callosum *(arrows)* as a result of CMV ependymitis.

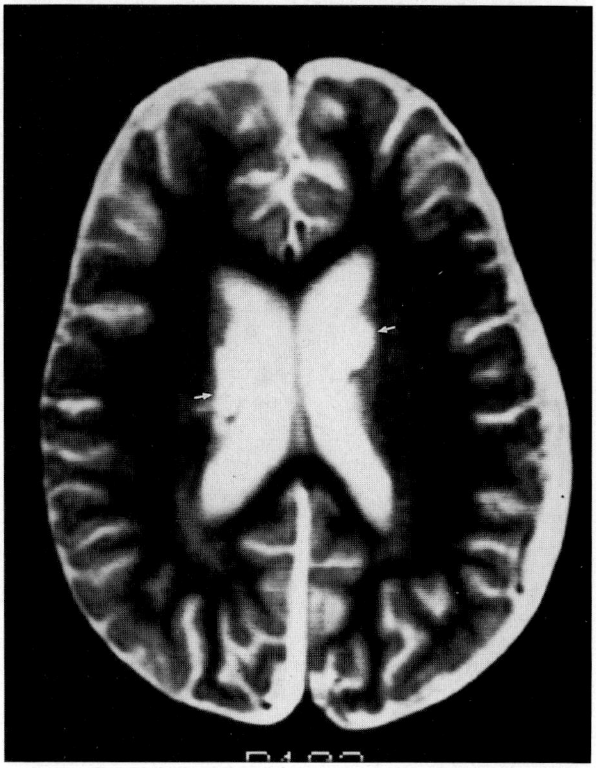

**FIGURE 44** T2-weighted axial MR image (TR2000, TE80) demonstrates bilateral subdural fluid collections along with nodularity of the ependymal lining of the ventricles *(arrows)* in this 7-year-old male child with AIDS and CMV ependymitis.

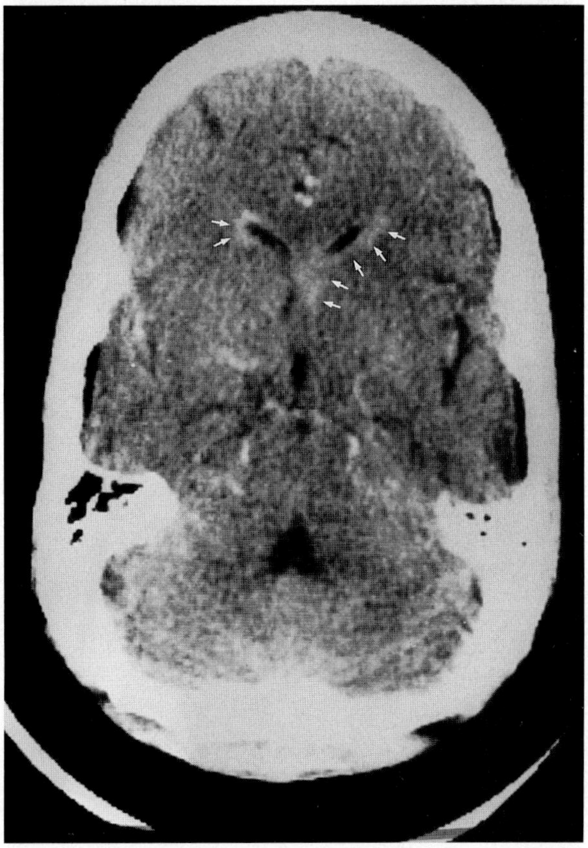

**FIGURE 43** Contrast-enhanced CT scan shows enhancement along the lining of the lateral ventricles *(arrows)* in this AIDS patient with disseminated CMV infection.

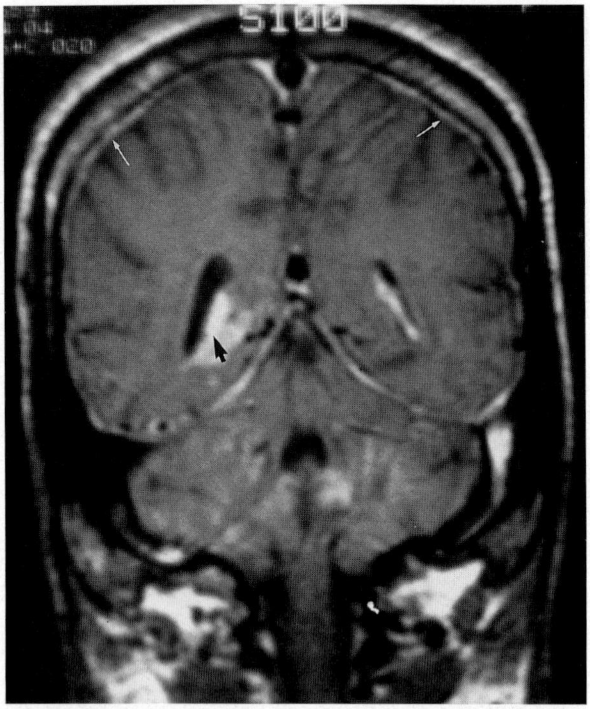

**FIGURE 45** Postgadolinium T1-weighted coronal MR image (TR850, TE20) shows abnormal enhancement along the meninges *(small arrows)* and ependymal surface of the right lateral ventricle in this patient with CMV ependymitis and aseptic meningitis.

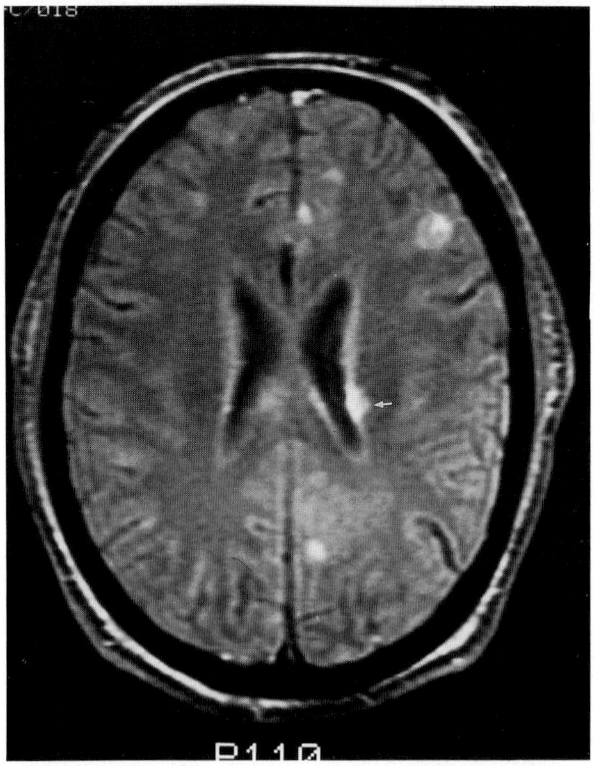

**FIGURE 46** Postgadolinium T1-weighted axial MR image (TR700, TE10) shows an abnormal focus of enhancement in the left lateral ventricle *(arrow)*. Notice several small abscesses in the left cerebral hemisphere as a result of toxoplasmosis.

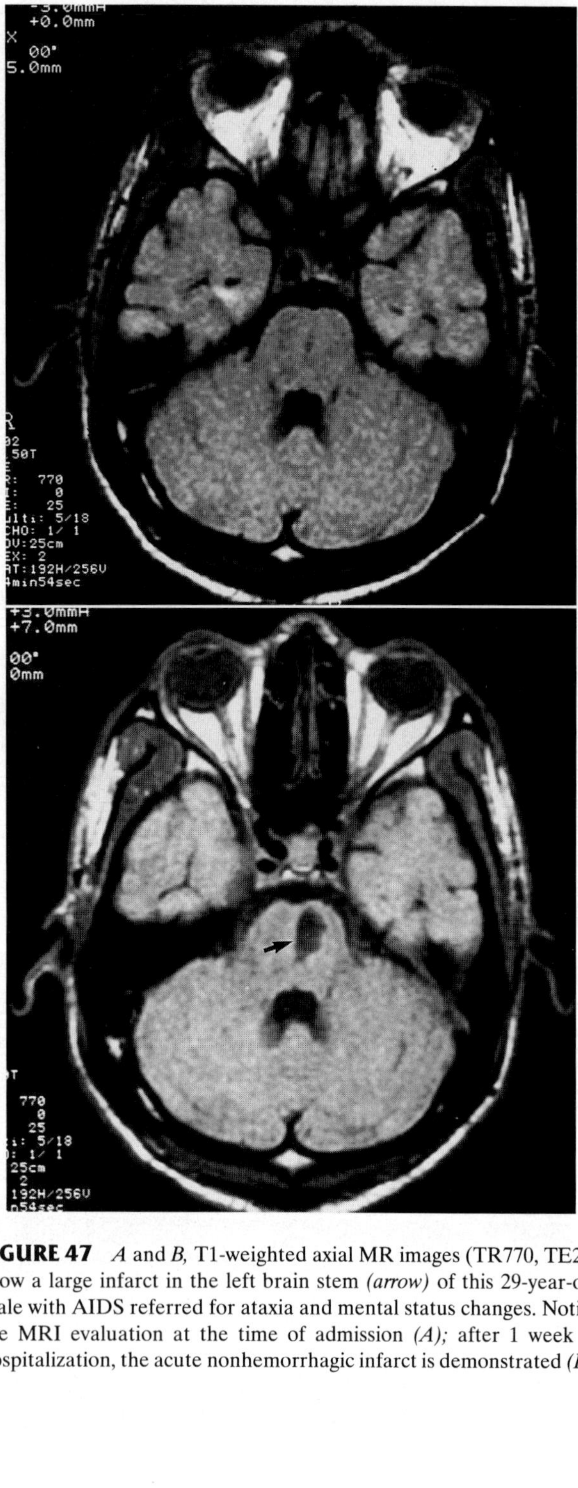

A

B

**FIGURE 47** *A* and *B*, T1-weighted axial MR images (TR770, TE25) show a large infarct in the left brain stem *(arrow)* of this 29-year-old male with AIDS referred for ataxia and mental status changes. Notice the MRI evaluation at the time of admission *(A)*; after 1 week of hospitalization, the acute nonhemorrhagic infarct is demonstrated *(B)*.

A B

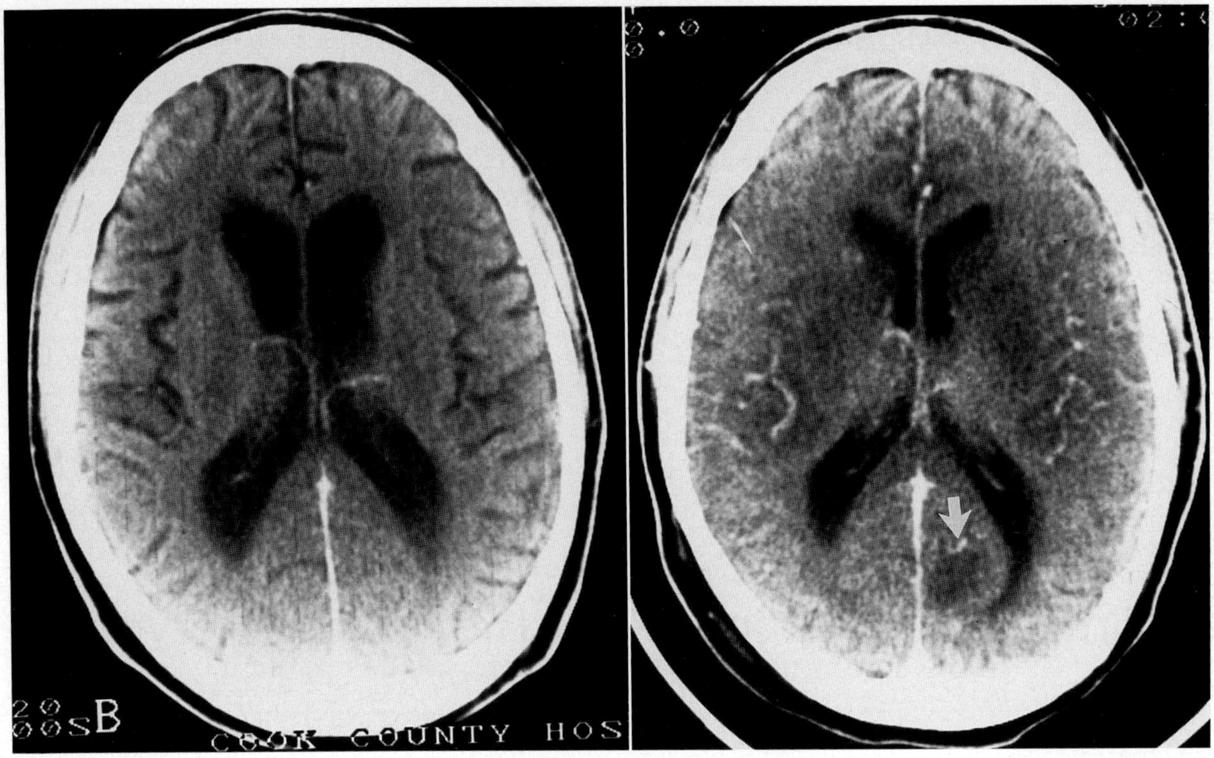


**FIGURE 48** *A* and *B,* Contrast-enhanced CT scans show evolution of an infarct in the left occipital lobe *(arrow)* after 3 days of hospitalization.

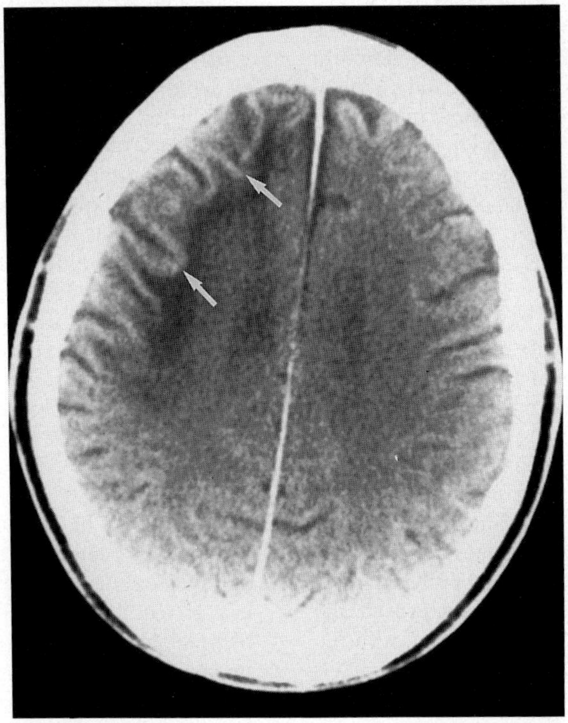

**FIGURE 49** Contrast-enhanced CT scan shows abnormal enhancement along the right frontal lobe with subcortical edema representing a hemorrhagic infarct *(arrows)* in this 27-year-old AIDS patient.

dolinium MRI sequences (Fig. 46). Usually intraparenchymal abscesses are observed in association with ependymal or leptomeningeal involvement.

### Vascular Disease

Infrequently AIDS patients are referred for neuroimaging because of cerebral infarcts and intracerebral or subarachnoid hemorrhage (Figs. 47 to 49). The imaging pattern is similar to that observed in the general population, but other findings of opportunistic infections may be present.

## Suggested Reading

Elder GA, Sever JL. Neurologic disorders associated with AIDS retroviral infection. Rev Infect Dis 1988; 10:286–302.

Flowers CH, Mafee MF, Crowell R, et al. Encephalopathy in AIDS patients: Evaluation with MR imaging. Am J Neuroradiol 1990; 11:1235–1245.

Levy RM, Bredensen DE, Rosenblum ML. Neurological manifestations of the acquired immunodeficiency syndrome (AIDS): Experience at UCSF and review of the literature. J Neurosurg 1985; 62:475–495.

Olsen WL, Longo FM, Mills CM, et al. White matter disease in AIDS: Findings at MR imaging. Radiology 1988; 169:445–448.

Petito CK, Cho ES, Lemann W, et al. Neuropathology of acquired immunodeficiency syndrome (AIDS). J Neuropath Exp Neurol 1986; 45:635–646.

Post MJD, Tate LG, Quencer RM, et al. CT, MR and pathology in HIV encephalitis and meningitis. Am J Neuroradiol 1988; 9:469–476.

Sze G, Brant-Zawadzki MN, Norman D, et al. The neuroradiology of AIDS. Semin Roentgenol 1987; 22:42–53.

# Gadolinium Chelates in MRI of the Central Nervous System

*VAL M. RUNGE, M.D.*

This chapter discusses the current clinical use of contrast media in magnetic resonance imaging (MRI) of the central nervous system (CNS), or more specifically the head and spine. Clinical indications, although almost all encompassing, are specifically addressed together with a discussion of efficacy. The use of enhanced MRI is considered relative to the major available alternative modality (in both the head and spine), enhanced radiographic computed tomography (CT). The technical approach including hardware, software, different available agents, contrast dose, rate of injection, and timing of the postcontrast scan is then discussed to the depth relevant for the clinician. This chapter concludes with a consideration of the overall diagnostic approach, in particular key signs of disease, practical differential diagnosis, and possible pitfalls in technique and image interpretation.

## Clinical Indications

In the United States today, intravenous contrast material is administered for almost half of all head MRI evaluations and nearly one-quarter of all spine evaluations. Given that U.S. Food and Drug Administration (FDA) approval came for gadopentetate dimeglumine[1] (also known as Gd-DTPA or Magnevist) only in mid-1988, the large number of studies performed with administration of contrast medium serves to underscore its clinical importance and usefulness. Lacking any unforeseen political, economic, or toxicologic problems, intravenous administration of contrast is likely to approach 100 percent of all head evaluations in the coming years, with the possible exception of infants and trauma victims. Extracellular agents such as gadopentetate dimeglumine are renally excreted and cross the placenta to the fetus; thus caution is advised with respect to administration in the young in whom renal function is not completely developed, during pregnancy, in nursing mothers (excretion of the agent in breast milk has been documented), and in patients with renal failure. The safety of contrast media in these specific patient subpopulations is as of yet not well explored. When purely structural information is sought, or when detection of damage to the brain parenchyma itself is the sole goal of the evaluation (as in most trauma patients), unenhanced evaluations may suffice. Intravenous administration of contrast is also likely to approach a high percentage of all spine evaluations in the future. Spine MRI became a clinical reality several years later than head MRI, with clinical knowledge and experience similarly lagging. Thus we are still in the relative infancy of development of spine MRI, with the usefulness of contrast media not yet well documented and communicated. Several academic institutions, including my own, perform 100 percent of all spine evaluations, aside from the relative contraindications previously noted, with intravenous contrast media as the result of clinical experience, indicating the great utility of contrast media injection. On such a basis, contrast use would be anticipated in the majority of spine MRI evaluations performed in the future across the United States.

In the head the usefulness of gadolinium chelate administration has been well documented across a vast array of pathologic states. In screening for extra-axial disease, contrast use is mandated. Small extra-axial mass lesions, such as meningiomas or acoustic neuromas (Fig. 1), can be missed on prospective interpretation of MRI studies performed without contrast injection. The size and extent of these lesions may also be grossly underestimated without intravenous contrast use. Lesions of this type, which include predominantly neoplastic and inflammatory disease states, typically display marked

[1] As of late 1992, only gadopentetate dimeglumine and gadoteridol are clinically available in the United States.

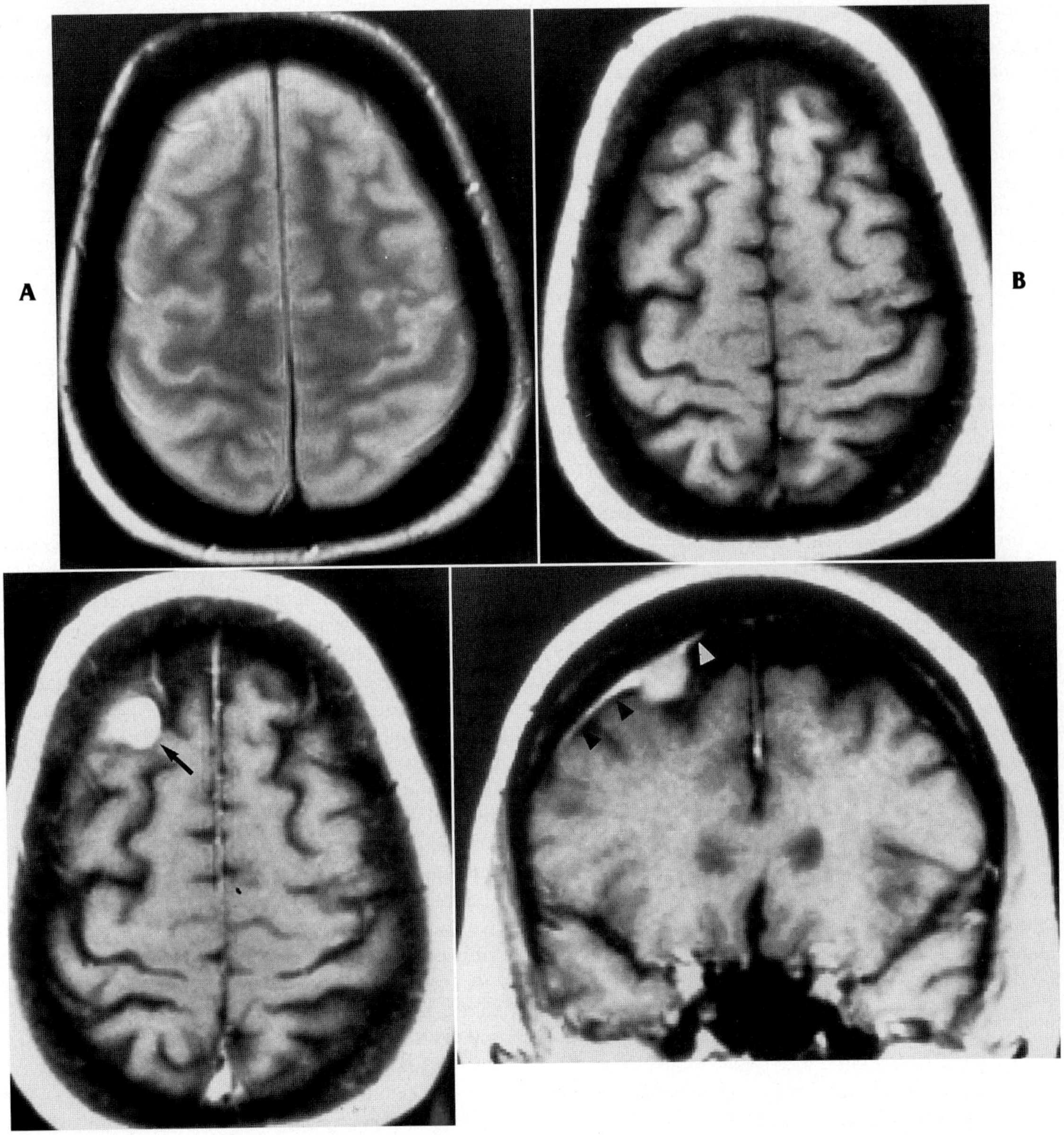


**FIGURE 1** Meningioma. Pre-contrast axial T2-weighted *(A)* and T1-weighted (*B*) spin-echo images are normal. The lesion *(arrow, C)* is well depicted on post-contrast axial *(C)* and coronal *(D)* T1-weighted images, with the prominent enhancement a result of intrinsic vascularity. The coronal image in particular well displays the extra-axial nature of the mass and a prominent enhancing dural tail *(arrowhead, D)*, the latter feature providing improved certainty with respect to pathologic diagnosis. The contrast agent used was gadopentetate dimeglumine, at a dose of 0.1 mmol/kg IV. Contrast enhancement is routinely employed on MRI for improved identification and delineation of extra-axial lesions, which are commonly isointense to brain parenchyma and thus difficult to see on unenhanced scans. (From Runge VM, Gelblum DY. The role of gadolinium diethylenetriamine penta-acetic acid in the evaluation of the central nervous system. Magn Reson Q 1990; 6:85–107; with permission.)

positive enhancement post-contrast as a result of intrinsic vascularity, which is highlighted relative to the normal brain with its intact blood-brain barrier. For intra-axial neoplastic lesions, injection of a contrast agent can result in improved (1) detection (e.g., with metastatic disease, Fig. 2), (2) delineation of lesion extent, (3) definition of necrosis (by central lesion nonenhancement), (4) grading (e.g., with glial cell tumors, where the degree of enhancement roughly correlates with lesion grade), and (5) differential diagnosis (e.g., identification of an enhancing nidus within a cystic posterior fossa mass in a young adult makes likely the diagnosis of a hemangioblastoma). In intra-axial lesions, contrast enhancement occurs from disruption of the normal blood-brain barrier. Contrast administration is particularly vital for the demonstration of tumor recurrence. Lesion recognition and characterization is also improved by contrast use with parasellar and pineal region tumors.

Intraparenchymal lesions, and specifically metastases, may be missed or underestimated with respect to size without intravenous contrast injection. In both infection and demyelinating disease (e.g., multiple sclerosis), enhanced MRI best estimates lesion activity. Lesions can also be missed by unenhanced MRI in both general disease categories. In early cerebral infarction, abnormal enhancement (or prominence) of vessels within the affected arterial territory can be demonstrated post-contrast as a result of venous engorgement and slow flow, providing a clue with respect to differential diagnosis. Gyriform enhancement is consistently observed in subacute infarction, improving differential diagnosis, and in certain cases permitting lesion detection, with some subacute cerebral infarcts appearing isointense and thus undetectable on precontrast T1- and T2-weighted MRI studies. Depiction and detection of arteriovenous malformations, in particular venous angiomas, can be improved post-contrast. Meningeal disease, whether inflammatory, neoplastic, post-traumatic, or post-surgical in origin, is also in general better detected and depicted (with respect to lesion extent) post-contrast. Administration of an intravenous bolus contrast combined with rapid sequential image acquisition holds great promise for the evaluation of brain perfusion, with quantitative evaluation of cerebral blood volume demonstrated by measurement of first-pass kinetics in recent clinical trials.

Several major clinical trials have been pursued and published addressing the efficacy of using intravenous contrast material in the head, particularly in the private clinical arena. The study by Elster and associates, who reported results in 500 consecutive patients, concluded with recommendation of routine use in all head evaluations, excluding potentially only two small subpopulations: young adults and children with a normal unenhanced evaluation and a low clinical suspicion of disease. Clearly such widespread use of contrast media is justified more on the basis of not the actual additional information provided in each clinical examination, but on the potential for failure of lesion recognition or misdiagnosis when contrast is not applied. If clinical history could only more precisely pinpoint the disease to be uncovered, then perhaps contrast use could be advocated in certain patient populations and omitted in others, permitting more selective contrast use. However, the general field is that of "diagnostic" radiology, with patients rarely if ever appropriately referred for an examination with the results, diagnosis, and staging already clearly established.

In the spine, as previously noted, clinical experience with MRI contrast media still lags considerably compared with clinical experience in the head. True efficacy studies in the general population do not exist, with reports confined to general observations in certain subpopulations of disease and to small, restricted efficacy studies. In degenerative disk disease, contrast administration can highlight disk herniation by providing enhancement of adjacent engorged venous plexus and scar, the latter of which occurs commonly even in the absence of surgery. Experience with routine contrast use in all spine evaluations has identified many individuals in whom an apparent new focal disk herniation (diagnosed simply by the presence of abnormal soft tissue on pre-contrast scans) was present, which (post-contrast and by clinical correlation) proved to represent only the result of healing, with residual granulation tissue from an older more remote event. In the post-operative lumbar spine, the efficacy of contrast enhancement for differentiation of scar, which enhances as a result of intrinsic vascularity, and recurrent or residual disk herniation, which does not enhance early post-contrast, is clearly established (Fig. 3). This application represents the single largest subpopulation for whom contrast enhancement presently is routinely employed across the United States.

For intramedullary spine lesions, contrast enhancement can improve lesion detection (e.g., with a small cord metastasis), the assessment of disease activity (e.g., by the demonstration of enhancement in a multiple sclerosis plaque), and differential diagnosis (e.g., by identification of an enhancing tumor nidus within a large syrinx). Contrast administration is particularly important in the search for intradural-extramedullary disease, with drop metastases highlighted because of their brilliant enhancement. In this application specifically, despite the typical small lesion size and greater potential resolution of CT and myelography, enhanced MRI has been accepted as the gold standard for diagnosis. Meningiomas, schwannomas, and neurofibromas all demonstrate marked enhancement post-contrast, which can be used to improve lesion depiction, delineation, and definition of extent.

Extradural disease can broadly be classified as degenerative, infectious, or neoplastic. As with degenerative disease (previously discussed), contrast administration plays a valuable role in the evaluation of suspected spinal infection, although on an altogether different basis. The typical disk space infection demonstrates prominent enhancement of adjacent involved marrow and paraspinous soft tissue, providing better definition of lesion extent and improved differential diagnosis. Compression of the thecal sac by an epidural inflammatory collection is often also better appreciated post-contrast. Neoplastic disease confined to bone is usually less well depicted post-contrast, because of the potential for enhancement to relative isointensity with normal surrounding fatty marrow. However, extent of neoplasia into surrounding soft tissue, or causing compression of the thecal sac, is often much better delineated post-contrast.

Radiographic CT today provides realistically the only true competition for MRI in the evaluation of suspected disease of the head and spine. In most academic centers, MRI is firmly established as the modality of choice, with CT still employed because of availability, lower cost, and suitability for certain patient subpopulations. When patient motion cannot be controlled, CT remains the evaluation of choice because of

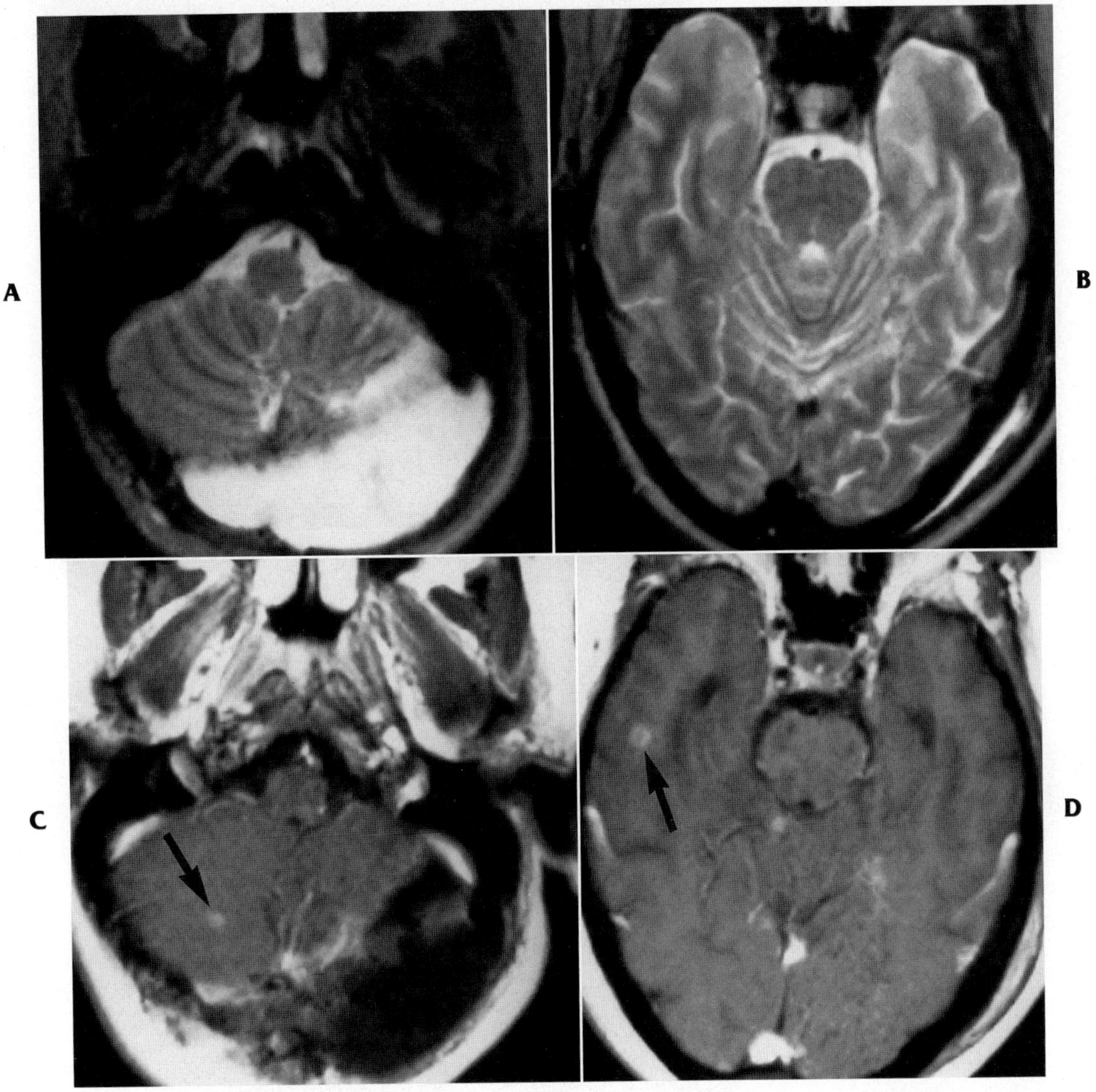


**FIGURE 2** Metastatic breast carcinoma. Pre-contrast axial T2-weighted (*A* and *B*) and T1- (not shown) weighted spin-echo images are normal, other than for identification of a postoperative pseudomeningocoel in the posterior fossa. Multiple metastatic foci *(arrows)* are identified on the post-contrast T1-weighted images (*C* and *D*), with lesion enhancement occurring as a result of disruption of the blood-brain barrier. The contrast agent used was gadoteridol, at a dose of 0.1 mmol/kg IV. In MRI of the brain, contrast enhancement is also routinely employed for identification of intra-axial lesions, which can be missed on unenhanced scans because of their small size or failure to elicit substantial reactive changes in surrounding brain. (From Runge VM, Dean B, et al. Phase III clinical evaluation of Gd HP-DO3A in head and spine disease. JMRI 1991; 1:47–56; with permission.)

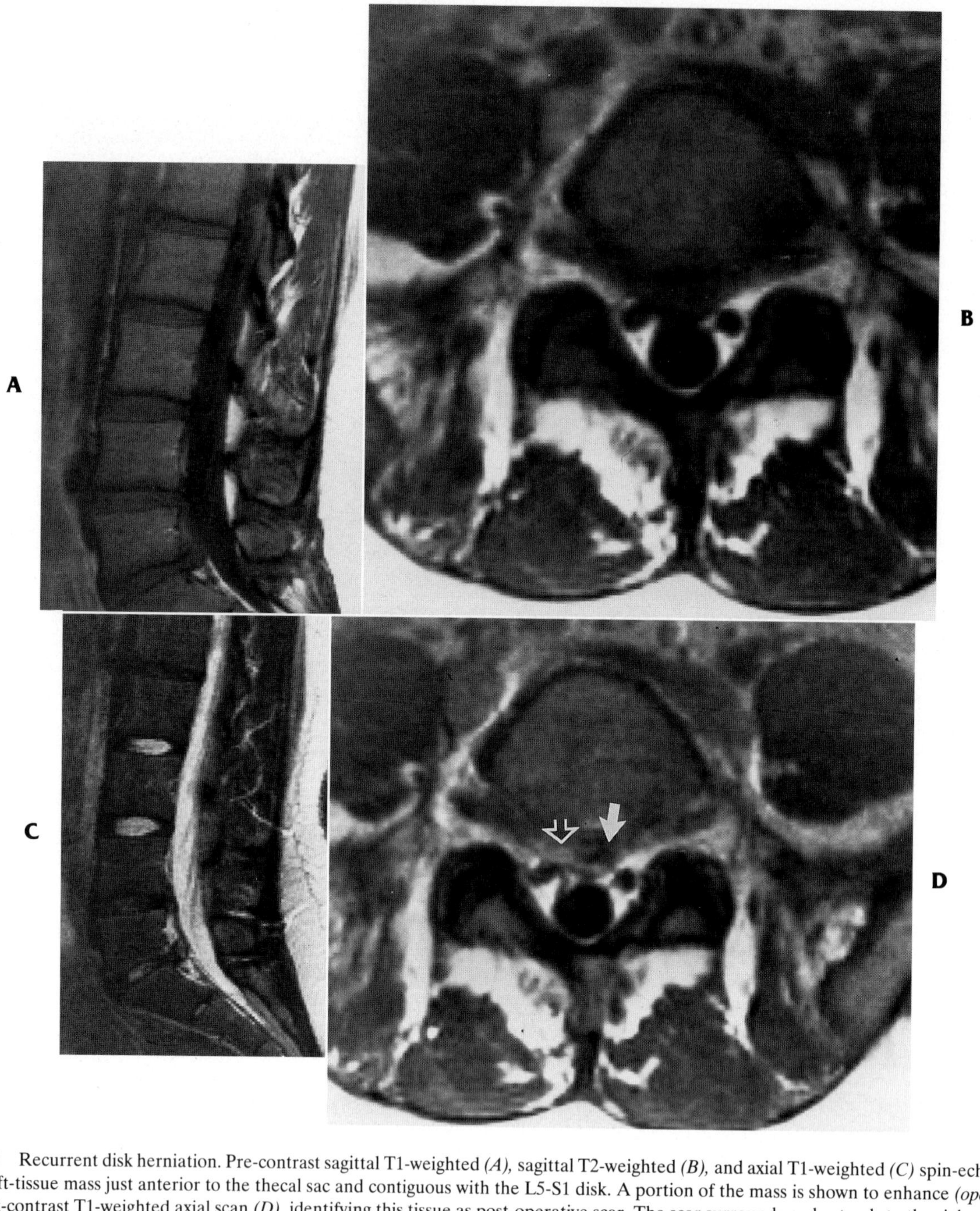


**FIGURE 3** Recurrent disk herniation. Pre-contrast sagittal T1-weighted *(A),* sagittal T2-weighted *(B),* and axial T1-weighted *(C)* spin-echo images reveal a soft-tissue mass just anterior to the thecal sac and contiguous with the L5-S1 disk. A portion of the mass is shown to enhance *(open arrow)* on the post-contrast T1-weighted axial scan *(D),* identifying this tissue as post-operative scar. The scar surrounds and extends to the right of a more centrally located nonenhancing mass *(arrow),* which can be characterized as recurrent or residual disk herniation on the basis of its appearance post-contrast. The contrast agent used was gadopentetate dimeglumine, at a dose of 0.1 mmol/kg IV. The differentiation of scar from disk material is a primary indication at present for intravenous gadolinium chelate administration in spine MRI. With appropriate clinical symptoms, identification of a disk herniation in the post-operative patient is an indication for reoperation. However, the presence of scar tissue alone, which can mimic a disk herniation on unenhanced MRI, is not an indication for surgery. (From Runge VM, ed. Clinical Magnetic Resonance Imaging. Philadelphia: JB Lippincott, 1990; with permission.)

routine availability of scan times less than 5 seconds. For claustrophobic patients and those in whom the clinical question centers on delineation of cortical bony detail, MRI can also prove less efficacious. Other competing modalities, including both nuclear medicine and myelography, have generally fallen into disuse. Enhanced MRI, however, continues to be held back, in terms of greater widespread application, because of the state of education and sophistication with regard to the modality by both radiologists and referring clinicians, which is understandable given the overwhelmingly rapid evolution of this technology. Confusion has also been caused by the broad array and price range of commercially available MRI systems, with an inherent tendency by both the commercial suppliers and the physician operators to downplay and limit dissemination of information regarding the limitation of lower-cost systems.

## Technical Approach

Hardware is the first and foremost factor to be considered in enhanced MRI of the head and spine. The use of high-field systems (1.5 T), as compared with units employing a lower primary magnetic field, translates directly to improved signal-to-noise ratio (SNR) and thus overall image quality specifically in the head and spine. This point no neuroradiologist will contest. High SNR equates to improved contrast and thus lesion detectability, combined with the potential for high resolution both in-plane and relative to slice thickness. The appearance of contrast enhancement itself is relatively unaffected by field strength, other than with regard to SNR as previously discussed. This situation thus favors the performance of enhanced evaluations on high-field systems, on the basis of overall higher diagnostic quality.

Software comes next. Spin-echo T1-weighted sequences, with relatively short TRs (400 to 600 msec) and TEs (10 to 25 msec), are favored for detection of contrast enhancement. Gradient echo sequences can, however, be employed for intravenous contrast detection, in particular spoiled FLASH (or GRASS). The latter techniques are beginning to be used on a more widespread basis, particularly in the head with three-dimensional (3D) acquisitions. Such an approach, for example, with a pulse sequence such as MP-RAGE (magnetization-prepared rapid acquisition gradient echo) can yield $1 \times 1 \times 1$ mm voxel resolution in a scan time of less than 5 minutes. Whether a spin-echo or gradient-echo sequence is employed, conventional post-contrast scanning relies on the detection of the T1 relaxivity effect of the contrast media. Gadolinium chelates enhance tissue relaxation, which means that both the T1 and T2 relaxation times that are observed decrease when a contrast agent is present. In clinical head and spine imaging, the T1 effect typically dominates, producing an increase in signal intensity on both spin-echo and gradient-echo evaluations. First-pass perfusion studies, which remain investigational to date, however, typically rely on detection of a completely different quantity, susceptibility, and influence of the contrast agent.

In the near future, physicians will likely have a considerable choice with respect to the specific gadolinium chelate used. The safety of gadolinium chelates is based principally on high in vivo stability combined with rapid excretion. DTPA (the ligand sequestering the gadolinium ion in the gadopentetate dimeglumine preparation) is a linear molecule with flexible clawlike arms binding and thus detoxifying the metal ion. The ligand in other gadolinium chelates is much more rigid as a result of the use of a cyclic or ringlike backbone structure, providing greater kinetic stability and being less susceptible to metal ion substitution. In this class lies gadoterate meglumine (Gd-DOTA or Dotarem), an agent approved for use in both Europe and South America, but unlikely to be introduced in the United States for commercial and patent reasons. Of the ringlike chelates, gadoteridol (Gd-HP-DO3A or ProHance) is likely to have the greatest impact worldwide. Approval of this agent was received in the United States during late 1992, with that in Europe and the Far East to follow. In addition to its high kinetic stability, and thus lower theoretical potential for long-term adverse effects, gadoteridol is nonionic. This agent stands as a tribute to the advance of science and technology, with the development of suitable nonionic radiographic contrast agents taking nearly 100 years, as compared with that for a nonionic MRI contrast agent, specifically gadoteridol, in less than 10 years. The high safety profile of this agent has spurred aggressive investigation of a higher-contrast dose (up to 0.3 mmol/kg) for specific clinical applications. Gadodiamide (Gd-DTPA-BMA or Omniscan), a nonionic linear chelate, has also been recently investigated in clinical trials. However, concerns have been expressed relative to this agent regarding results in animal toxicologic studies and with respect to the potential for release of gadolinium ion (as a result of a markedly lower thermodynamic stability).

With regard to dose and contrast effect, when compared on a mmol/kg basis, the four previously discussed gadolinium chelates are virtually indistinguishable. The vast majority of clinical work has been performed with a dose of 0.1 mmol/kg, with clear efficacy as previously discussed. Results have generally been poor with doses less than 0.1 mmol/kg. Large numbers of patients have only recently been studied at higher doses, and then in only restricted applications. It is, however, clearly established from even these preliminary studies (Fig. 4) that clinical evaluations in the future performed for possible metastatic disease to the brain will be obtained with a high dose (0.3 mmol/kg). FDA approval of gadoteridol, submitted with both standard and high-dose indications, was thus eagerly awaited. The high safety profile of this agent, relatively few reported adverse reactions, and extensive experience at high dose all speak well for future widespread clinical use.

The effect on enhancement due to the rate of contrast injection and the time at which (following injection) the post-contrast scan is acquired has not been closely investigated. Rates of administration for gadopentetate dimeglumine vary in clinical practice from bolus (>1 ml/sec) to slow infusion (1 ml/10 sec). Bolus injection with gadopentetate dimeglumine can elicit nausea; thus caution is advised particularly given the close confines of the typical MRI scanner. In most clinical practices, the agent is administered relatively slowly and the scan begun at a leisurely pace following completion of the injection. This coincidence is fortuitous, since maximum contrast enhancement for most intracranial pathology is not achieved until several minutes after injection. During these first few minutes, the degree of enhancement in the lesion is rapidly increasing and yet is still much below that to be anticipated at 5 to 10 minutes postinjection. Thus on a theoretical basis, early scanning could minimize the visualization of pathological enhancement. In this light, bolus injection followed by immediate rapid post-contrast imaging (with scans

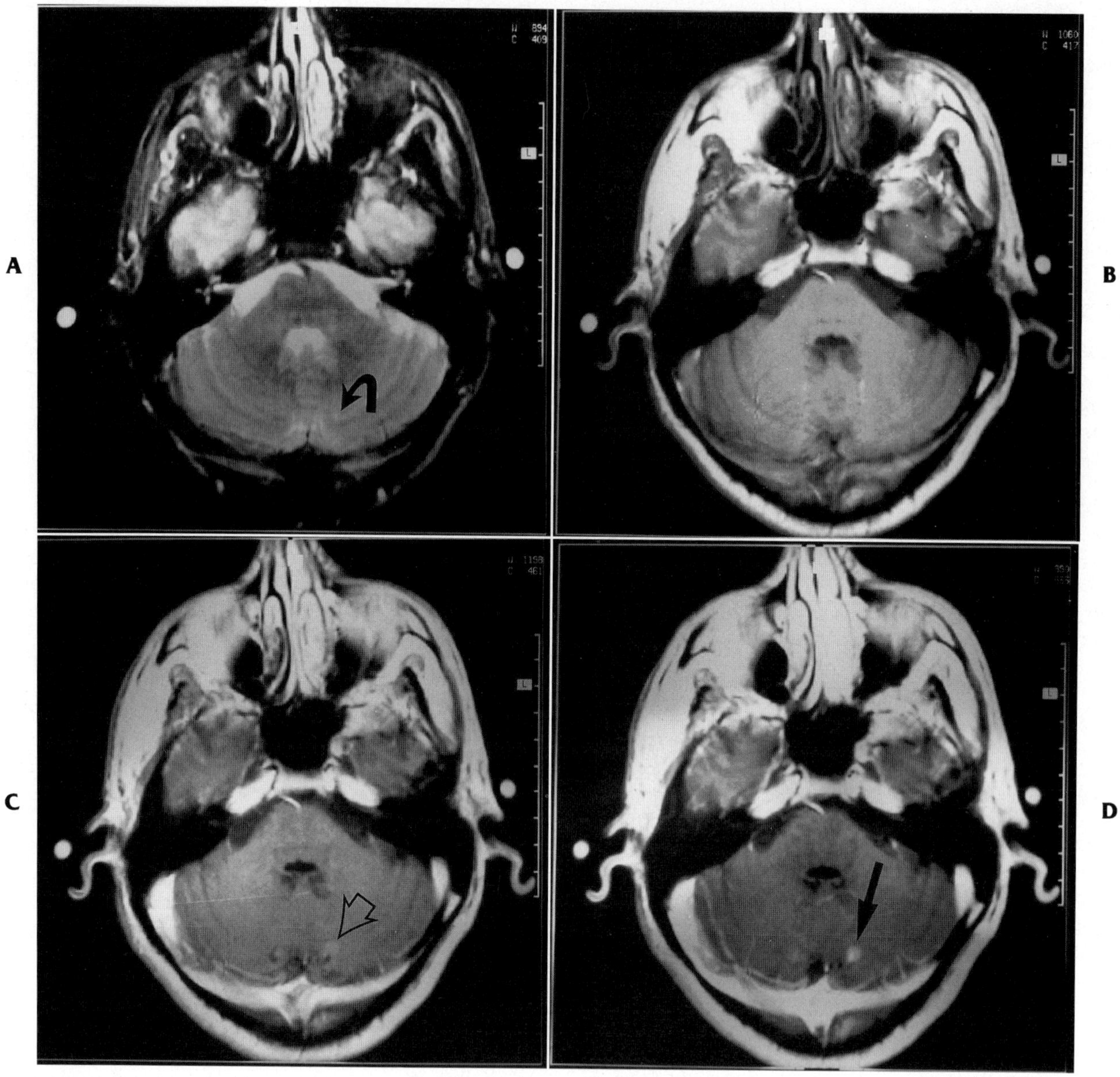

**FIGURE 4** Metastatic lung carcinoma. Pre-contrast axial T2-weighted *(A)* and T1-weighted *(B)* spin-echo images are normal. Only in retrospect might the question of an abnormality *(curved arrow, A)* be raised, on the T2-weighted evaluation, in the left side of the cerebellum. There is faint enhancement *(open arrow)* in this region on the T1-weighted image *(C)* obtained following IV contrast injection at standard dosage (0.1 mmol/kg gadoteridol). However, this small cerebellar metastasis *(arrow)* can be identified with certainty only on the *(D)* high-dose (0.3 mmol/kg gadoteridol) post-contrast T1-weighted evaluation. High-dose gadolinium chelate contrast use increases the sensitivity of MRI for the detection of intracranial metastatic disease (as compared with enhanced MRI using a dose of 0.1 mmol/kg, the current gold standard for diagnosis). Improved lesion detection has significant ramifications with respect to patient management and the appropriate choice of therapy. (From Runge VM, Kirsch JE, et al. High-dose gadoteridol in MR imaging of intracranial neoplasms. JMRI 1992; 2:9–18; with permission.)

obtained between 0 and 2 or so minutes post-injection) is to be avoided and could result in misdiagnosis. Experience with the temporal time course of enhancement relative to tissue pathology is also limited and to some extent anecdotal in nature. Enhancement in subacute cerebral infarctions does tend to progress in intensity with time up to 1 hour post-injection. Some spinal cord tumors, in particular astrocytomas, also display delayed enhancement. Most cerebral neoplastic disease peaks in enhancement at 5 to 10 minutes post-injection, with either relative constancy in signal intensity achieved for some duration (20 minutes) or a gradual loss of enhancement thereafter. Spine evaluations obtained for the differentiation of scar from disk need to be obtained early (5 to 15 minutes) post-injection, with disk material displaying enhancement on delayed scans and thus appearing indistinguishable from scar. These results with respect to the optimum time frame for imaging post-contrast are all from studies conducted with a dose of 0.1 mmol/kg. It should not be taken for granted that such results can be extended directly to higher-dose applications.

## Diagnostic Approach

### Key Signs of Disease

The key sign of disease on contrast-enhanced MRI is of course the identification of positive lesion enhancement. Recognition of abnormal enhancement, however, generally proves useful only with regard to improved lesion identification or partial characterization. Specific pathologic diagnosis on the basis of imaging findings alone is rarely possible.

Most physicians who interpret or use MRI tend to focus on the value of positive lesion enhancement. However, the lack of abnormal enhancement on a post-contrast scan also carries significant value, excluding abnormality when no lesion is observed and providing information with respect to lesion characterization and differential diagnosis when a lesion which fails to enhance is present. The importance of obtaining both pre- and post-contrast scans (with the same pulse sequence and in the same imaging plane) cannot be overstated, given that the purpose of contrast administration is to permit (with a high degree of certainty) the identification of a change between scans—what we so commonly term *enhancement.* All anatomic regions included in the field of view should be closely inspected for abnormal enhancement. In head MRI this includes the brain, extra-axial structures, the skull, and soft tissues. In spine MRI this includes two compartments commonly overlooked: the bone marrow and the intradural space. The advent of practical fat-suppression imaging sequences in the near future will also without doubt improve the depiction of abnormal enhancement within tissue containing or adjacent to fat, in particular in bone marrow and soft tissue.

### Differential Diagnosis

Unfortunately the use of contrast media in MRI only occasionally leads to a specific pathologic diagnosis. Lesion location, extent, and pattern of enhancement are all characteristics useful in differential diagnosis, with enhancement characteristics obviously playing only a partial role. Contrast enhancement is, however, typically a good indicator of disease activity. The recognition of gyriform enhancement in cerebral infarction is one of the few instances where the presence of a certain pattern can lead to a specific diagnosis. The "dural tail" was described early on to be a specific sign for meningioma and discovered later, following more extensive clinical experience, to be observed with a variety of pathological processes, including lymphoma and sarcoidosis. Ring enhancement with cerebral lesions is nonspecific on MRI, like CT, and can be observed with primary brain tumors, metastases, multiple sclerosis, and infection. In the spine contrast enhancement appears to assist more in practical differential diagnosis. Disk material can be differentiated with relative certainty from scar by the lack of enhancement on early post-contrast scans. The presence of a bulky enhancing soft-tissue mass accompanying a syrinx allows for almost certain diagnosis of tumor syrinx. It is, however, obligatory in such cases that the entire length of a syrinx be evaluated post-contrast, because a small isolated tumor nidus may otherwise be overlooked.

### Pitfalls

Possible pitfalls in technique are varied. Delayed scans can change the character and intensity of contrast enhancement. Pre- and post-contrast scans should be obtained with precisely the same technique, including both sequence type and acquisition plane. Even slight slice misregistration, which can be caused by inadvertent patient motion, can make the identification of abnormal enhancement more difficult. Slices are also not typically truly contiguous in MRI, with a slight gap maintained to prevent substantial image quality degradation as a result of "cross talk." This makes it possible to miss a small enhancing focus "between slices." Partial volume imaging may similarly lead to good detection of abnormal enhancement in one plane, with poor delineation in another, according to the orientation of the abnormal enhancing structure. In both instances the acquisition of post-contrast images in two perpendicular planes could overcome an otherwise intrinsic technique-related deficit. Attention should also be paid to the adjustment of window and center settings on the final image, with changes in these by the technologist between pre- and post-contrast scans possibly misleading the scan interpreter to describe enhancement when none is present, or the lack thereof when an enhancing abnormality is in reality present. Finally, it should not be assumed that this "technique" is totally benign, with anaphylactic reactions well described in the scientific literature. Contrast agent administration should be performed in all cases under the supervision of a physician, with adequate advance preparation for treatment of a contrast agent reaction.

A large number of potential pitfalls also exist with regard to image interpretation. Enhancement of normal structures must be recognized as such. In the head this includes the blood vessels, choroid plexus, nasal mucosa and turbinates, mucous membranes, and pituitary. In the spine this includes the dorsal root ganglion, basivertebral vein, and epidural venous plexus. Post-contrast scans should be carefully checked to confirm that the contrast agent actually reached the target organ, with "blown" veins and lack of agent delivery on post-contrast scans a real-world possibility. Contrast enhancement should not be confused with tissue, such as fat or blood, which intrinsically demonstrates high signal intensity on T1-weighted scans, again pointing to the need for comparison of pre- and post-contrast scans. Pulsation artifacts can also be accentuated by contrast agent administration and are on occasion mistaken for enhancing lesions. Such artifacts are markedly affected by the choice of TE, contrast dose, and use of motion compensation schemes such as a gradient moment refocusing (GMR). Certain relatively common disease entities, with little clinical significance, can demonstrate abnormal contrast enhancement. Such processes should not be confused with more serious disease entities. For example, type 1 end plate degenerative disease typically enhances, not to be confused with osteomyelitis in disk space infection. In addition, not all tumors or lesions display abnormal enhancement. Prominent examples include dermoids, epidermoids, and low-grade astrocytomas. Surprisingly, tumor recurrence may even not be delineated in limited instances by contrast enhancement, the best-established example being medulloblastoma. And, as always, with glial tumors (astrocytoma, glioblastoma), the correlation of blood-brain barrier disruption as demarcated by contrast enhancement with tumor extent is poor. The existence of tumor cells far beyond the limits depicted by abnormal contrast enhancement is well established pathologically.

## Suggested Reading

Carollo BR, Runge VM, Price AC, et al. The prospective evaluation of Gd-DTPA in 225 consecutive cranial cases: Adverse reactions and diagnostic value. Magn Reson Imaging 1990; 8:381–393.

Elster AD, Moody DM, Ball MR, Laster DW. Is Gd-DTPA required for routine cranial MR imaging? Radiology 1989; 173:231–238.

Hueftle MG, Modic MT, Ross JS, et al. Lumbar spine: Post-operative MR imaging with Gd-DTPA. Radiology 1988; 167:817–824.

Ross JS, Modic MT, Masaryk TJ, et al. Assessment of extradural degenerative disease with Gd-DTPA-enhanced MR imaging: Correlation with surgical and pathologic findings. AJR 1990; 154:151–157.

Runge VM, ed. Contrast Media in Magnetic Resonance Imaging: A Clinical Approach. Philadelphia: JB Lippincott, 1992.

Runge VM, Bradley WG, Brant-Zawadzki MN, et al. Clinical safety and efficacy of gadoteridol: A study in 411 patients with suspected intracranial and spinal disease. Radiology 1991; 181:701–709.

Runge VM, Gelblum DY. The role of gadolinium diethylenetriamine penta-acetic acid in the evaluation of the central nervous system. Magn Reson Q 1990; 6:85–107.

Schwaighofer BW, Klein MV, Wesbey G, Hesselink JR. Clinical experience with routine Gd-DTPA administration for MR imaging of the brain. J Comput Assist Tomogr 1990; 14:11–17.

Sze G, Abramson A, Krol G, et al. Gadolinium-DTPA in the evaluation of intradural extramedullary spinal disease. AJR 1988; 150:911–921.

Sze G, Krol G, Zimmerman RD, Deck MD. Intramedullary disease of the spine: Diagnosis using gadolinium-DTPA-enhanced MR imaging. AJR 1988; 151:1193–1204.

# Single-Photon Emission CT in Cerebrovascular Disease, Dementia, and Huntington's Disease

*B. DAVID COLLIER, Jr., M.D. · ROBERT S. HELLMAN, M.D.*
*YU LIU, M.D. · SHEKHAR C. THAKUR, M.D.*
*RONALD S. TIKOFSKY, Ph.D.*

Imaging of cerebral perfusion and metabolism with single-photon emission computed tomography (SPECT) is one of the most promising areas in nuclear medicine. Two radiopharmaceuticals for brain perfusion imaging have been approved by the U.S. Food and Drug Administration, and the introduction of additional radiopharmaceuticals for central nervous system (CNS) perfusion, metabolic, and receptor binding studies is anticipated. Both the currently available clinical radiopharmaceuticals and the agents undergoing scientific testing are suitable for SPECT imaging.

SPECT brain perfusion studies can be successfully performed using the single-detector rotating gamma camera SPECT systems that have been installed in many community hospitals and outpatient facilities. A recent development, which promises to greatly increase both the quality and number of SPECT brain studies, is the introduction of dedicated or special-purpose SPECT systems. These dedicated SPECT systems offer improved sensitivity and resolution with a corresponding dramatic improvement in image quality. In addition to superior image quality, the dedicated SPECT systems provide increased patient throughput. With radiopharmaceuticals and instrumentation for brain perfusion imaging now available, community hospitals and imaging centers throughout the United States are in a position to offer SPECT functional brain imaging for a variety of CNS pathologic conditions.

The functional information available with brain SPECT complements rather than competes with the high-resolution anatomic imaging provided by magnetic resonance imaging (MRI), computed tomography (CT), and digital angiography. The CNS distribution following intravenous injection of technetium-99m hexamethyl propylenamine oxine ($^{99m}$Tc HMPAO) and the initial CNS distribution following intravenous injection of *N*-isopropyl-*p*-(I-123) iodoamphetamine ($^{123}$I-IMP) are in proportion to regional cerebral blood flow (rCBF). Between 1 and 4 hours following intravenous injection, $^{123}$I-IMP (but not $^{99m}$Tc-HMPAO) undergoes a complex redistribution that reflects amine metabolism in multiple organs in addition to CNS perfusion and function.

The use of these two tracers to image perfusion at the CNS tissue level has been shown to be of practical clinical value for patients with cerebrovascular disease. For many other CNS pathologic conditions, such as dementia and epilepsy, the underlying primary disease process is reflected in altered brain metabolism rather than vascular occlusion or hemorrhage. Brain perfusion, however, is closely coupled to a variety of metabolic functions including glucose and oxygen metabolism. There exist some morbid states in which this close coupling may be altered. Nonetheless, for a wide variety of CNS pathologic conditions, SPECT images of brain perfusion are close proxies for the more accurate images of brain metabolism that may be obtained using positron emission tomography (PET). For this reason, SPECT brain perfusion studies often provide useful images of such principally "metabolic" diseases as senile dementia of the Alzheimer's type (SDAT) and epilepsy.

Since the first study was performed at the Medical College of Wisconsin on January 2, 1984, more than 3,000 clinical SPECT brain perfusion studies have been performed. In order of decreasing frequency, the most common clinical indications are dementia evaluation, cerebrovascular disease, epilepsy, and head trauma. Other clinical indications (although infrequent reasons for referral to Nuclear Medicine at the Medical College of Wisconsin) are much more common at other institutions (Table 1).

## Techniques for Brain SPECT

Techniques for brain SPECT using either a single-detector rotating gamma camera or the dedicated brain system currently in use at the Medical College of Wisconsin (Neurocam, General Electric Medical Systems, Milwaukee, WI) are given in Tables 2 and 3. While readers are referred to other publications for a complete account of SPECT quality control and SPECT artifacts, the more frequently encountered SPECT pitfalls should be kept in mind.

### *Pitfalls*

#### Poor Resolution Resulting from Radius of Rotation Greater than 14 cm

Proper setup for high-resolution brain SPECT requires that the detector be as close to the patient as possible. To obtain this result, the extra effort of nuclear medicine technologists and the cooperation of patients often needs to be enlisted.

**TABLE 1** Clinical Applications of SPECT Brain Perfusion Imaging at the Medical College of Wisconsin

- Common Clinical Applications:
  - Dementia evaluation
  - Cerebrovascular disease
  - Epilepsy
  - Head trauma
- Infrequent Clinical Applications:
  - Brain tumors
  - Movement disorders including Huntington's disease and Parkinson's disease
  - Schizophrenia
  - Depression
  - Brain death
  - Migraine
  - Panic disorders
  - Cocaine and other substance abuse

**TABLE 2** Single-detector Rotating Gamma Camera

- Before Acquisition:
  - Camera positioning optimal if setup allows rotation within radius of shoulders
  - Minimize effects of stimuli on rCBF:
    - Wait 5 minutes after venipuncture before IV injection
    - Minimize noise and light in injection area
  - If 1.6 camera hardware zoom is used:
    - Translate field of view to camera edge
    - New center of rotation and uniformity flood may be needed
- Acquisition:
  - 3.5–7.0 mCi $^{123}$I-IMP and image 15 minutes later:
    - Low-energy all-purpose collimator (for higher sensitivity)
    - 64 × 64 matrix (400 mm field-of-view camera with 1.6 zoom)
    - 40 second/projection, 64 projections over 360°

  *or*

  - 20–30 mCi $^{99m}$Tc-HMPAO and image 2 hours later:
    - High-resolution collimator
    - 64 × 64 matrix (400 mm field-of-view camera with 1.6 zoom)
    - 30 second/projection, 64 projections over 360°
- Processing:
  - Uniformity correction
  - Butterworth filter preprocessing (frequency cutoff of 0.41 cycles/cm for IMP or 0.44 cycles/cm for HMPAO; power factor 10; this choice of filters assumes a 12–14 cm radius of rotation)
  - Reconstruction by filtered backprojection with ramp filter
  - Attenuation correction
  - Oblique reorientation to match CT angulation (optional)
  - 8 mm thick (2 pixels) transaxial, sagittal, and coronal images
- Display:
  - Gray scale with 15 percent background subtraction preferred

**TABLE 3** Dedicated Brain SPECT System (GE Neurocam) at the Medical College of Wisconsin

- Before Acquisition:
  - Minimize effects of stimuli on rCBF
    - Wait 5 minutes after venipuncture before IV injection
    - Minimize noise and light in injection area
- Acquisition:
  - 7.0–8.0 mCi $^{123}$I-IMP and image 15 minutes later
    - Low-energy all-purpose collimator (for higher sensitivity)
    - 128 × 128 matrix in a 256 mm field of view
    - 128 projections over 360° in 42 minutes

  *or*

  - 30 mCi $^{99m}$Tc-HMPAO and image 2 hours later
    - High-resolution collimator
    - 128 × 128 matrix in a 256 mm field of view
    - 128 projections over 360° in 30 minutes
- Processing:
  - Uniformity correction on-the-fly
  - Metz filter order of 4 preprocessing
  - Reconstruction by filtered backprojection with ramp filter
  - Attenuation correction
  - Oblique reorientation to match CT angulation (optional)
  - 8 mm thick (4 pixels) transaxial, sagittal, and coronal images
- Display:
  - Gray scale with 15 percent background subtraction preferred
  - 4 mm thick images at times show more anatomic detail

### Patient Motion

This is our most frequently encountered technical problem. In addition to head holders, chin straps, and tape, it is necessary to use communication and persuasion. Patients should be told that motion will limit the value of their SPECT studies. Demented or otherwise ill subjects who move frequently will be able to follow instructions if a family member stays with them and encourages them. Pillows under the knees and firm but comfortable straps around the abdomen and arms also may be helpful. Sometimes for restless patients data acquisition times must be shortened.

### Inappropriate Data Acquisition or Processing

Even with a high-resolution dedicated SPECT system, adequate time must be allowed for image acquisition. Five to ten minute studies always will show poor resolution, and protocols similar to those suggested in Tables 2 and 3 should be followed. In addition, excessive smoothing or filtering of the data will result in unnecessary loss of spatial resolution.

## Cerebrovascular Disease

A complete quantitative analysis of the perfusion and metabolic response to cerebrovascular disease requires measurements of such parameters as cerebral blood flow, blood volume, glucose metabolism, and oxygen extraction efficiency—which currently are possible only with PET. Nonetheless, the SPECT cerebral perfusion tracers $^{99m}$Tc-HMPAO and $^{123}$I-IMP are of proven practical value for examining patients with cerebrovascular disease. Further, the promising new investigational perfusion agent $^{99m}$Tc ethyl cysteinate dimer ($^{99m}$Tc-ECD) (Fig. 1) is a stable radiopharmaceutical with favorable uptake, background clearance, and imaging characteristics.

Following initial brain uptake, which is in proportion to rCBF, $^{123}$I-IMP undergoes a later "redistribution" phase. At sites of cerebral ischemia without infarction, this redistribution is characterized by progressive filling in of perfusion defects. The decreased uptake at sites of cerebral ischemia observed with a great clarity on an initial SPECT study may be minimally

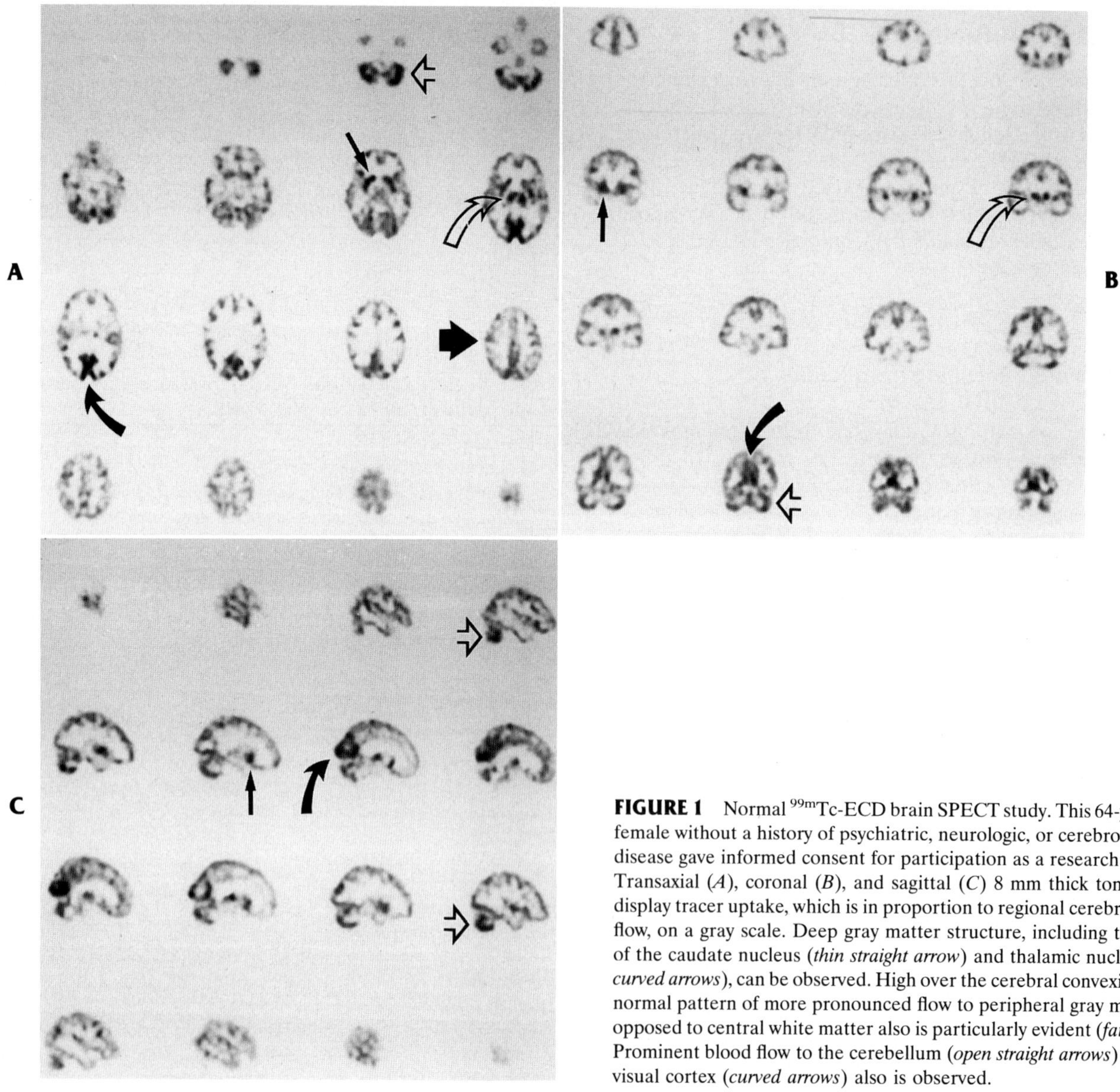


**FIGURE 1** Normal $^{99m}$Tc-ECD brain SPECT study. This 64-year-old female without a history of psychiatric, neurologic, or cerebrovascular disease gave informed consent for participation as a research subject. Transaxial (*A*), coronal (*B*), and sagittal (*C*) 8 mm thick tomograms display tracer uptake, which is in proportion to regional cerebral blood flow, on a gray scale. Deep gray matter structure, including the head of the caudate nucleus (*thin straight arrow*) and thalamic nuclei (*open curved arrows*), can be observed. High over the cerebral convexities, the normal pattern of more pronounced flow to peripheral gray matter as opposed to central white matter also is particularly evident (*fat arrow*). Prominent blood flow to the cerebellum (*open straight arrows*) and the visual cortex (*curved arrows*) also is observed.

present or appear entirely normal on SPECT images taken 3 to 6 hours after injection. Such redistribution has shown to be of value for distinguishing between infarcts and ischemia. Further, such redistribution has been shown to correlate with potential for recovery from an aphasic deficit. When asked these specific questions by referring physicians, $^{123}$I-IMP is our agent of choice. However, these questions rarely seem to arise; therefore for over 90 percent of cerebrovascular disease patients we prefer $^{99m}$Tc-HMPAO. Ready availability on a 24-hour-a-day basis in addition to superior image quality from high photon flux favor the use of $^{99m}$Tc-HMPAO.

Ischemic infarcts may be positive on clinical SPECT brain perfusion evaluations before CT, or more rarely MRI, studies show morbid changes. This is because there is decreased uptake of $^{99m}$TC-HMPAO as soon as perfusion is interrupted. In addition, the perfusion deficit seen on SPECT brain perfusion studies frequently is larger than the anatomic changes noted on CT or MRI. In particular, zones of peri-infarct ischemia in addition to brain dysfunction (so-called "deafferentation") can be imaged. Note in Figure 2, for example, the subtle reduction in uptake in the right cerebellar hemisphere when compared with the normal left hemisphere. This is secondary to and a distant effect of the left cerebral hemisphere infarction. This phenomenon, called *crossed-cerebellar diaschisis,* is a result of cerebellar deafferentation. Corticopontocerebellar tracts, which normally cross the midline as they pass from the cerebrum to the cerebellum, no longer are providing input into the right cerebellar hemisphere. The decreased input results in the decreased metabolic demands and a secondary compensatory decrease in perfusion to the right cerebellar hemisphere. Thus the full morbid results of stroke along with compensatory perfusion changes can be imaged with SPECT brain perfusion imaging.

Subarachnoid hemorrhage often produces transient vascular spasm. Severe vascular spasm may result in brain ischemia or even frank infarction. When evaluating a patient for possible aneurysm clipping, neurosurgeons may delay surgery if there is convincing evidence on SPECT of extensive and severe

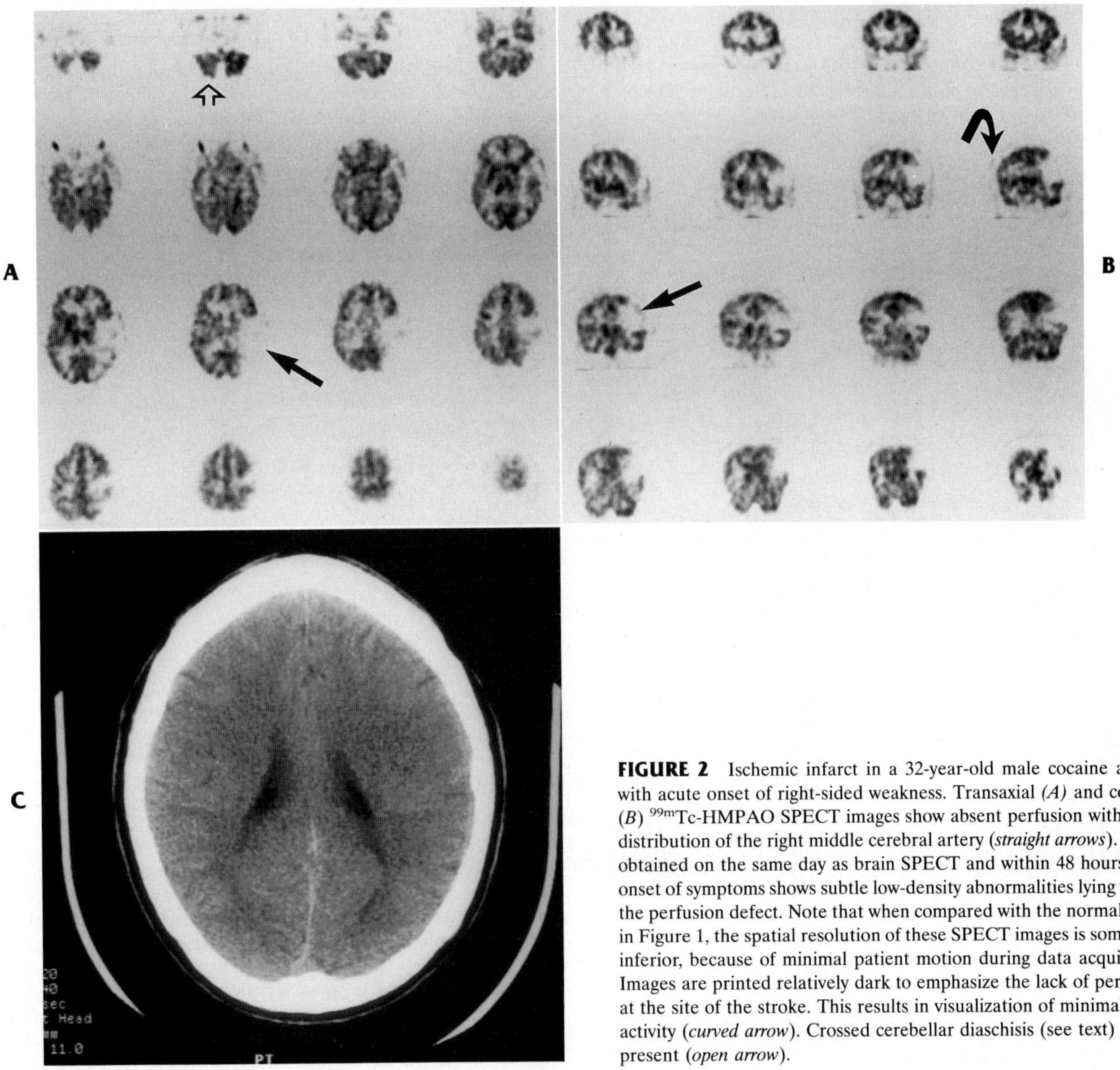

**FIGURE 2** Ischemic infarct in a 32-year-old male cocaine abuser with acute onset of right-sided weakness. Transaxial *(A)* and coronal *(B)* $^{99m}$Tc-HMPAO SPECT images show absent perfusion within the distribution of the right middle cerebral artery (*straight arrows*). *C,* CT obtained on the same day as brain SPECT and within 48 hours from onset of symptoms shows subtle low-density abnormalities lying within the perfusion defect. Note that when compared with the normal study in Figure 1, the spatial resolution of these SPECT images is somewhat inferior, because of minimal patient motion during data acquisition. Images are printed relatively dark to emphasize the lack of perfusion at the site of the stroke. This results in visualization of minimal scalp activity (*curved arrow*). Crossed cerebellar diaschisis (see text) also is present (*open arrow*).

**TABLE 4** Acetazolamide-enhanced SPECT Brain Perfusion Imaging

Indications:
- Transient ischemic attacks
- Reversible ischemic neurologic deficits
- Presurgical investigation of vascular reserve in patients with large arteriovenous malformation
- Asymptomatic patients with stenosis or occlusion of an internal carotid artery

Procedures:
- Inject 1.0 g of acetazolamide in 50 ml of normal saline IV over 10 minutes; 30 minutes after acetazolamide injection is completed, inject 20–30 mCi of $^{99m}$Tc-HMPAO.
- SPECT acquisition, processing, and displaying as described in Tables 2 and 3.
- A baseline (without acetazolamide) study is indicated and can be performed 24 hours later if the acetazolamide study shows perfusion abnormalities.

vascular spasm. Further, the decision to raise and lower blood pressure with medical therapy in patients with subarachnoid hemorrhage and loss of autoregulation can be influenced favorably by the demonstration of decreased perfusion caused by vascular spasm. For these reasons, SPECT brain perfusion studies are frequently ordered at the Medical College of Wisconsin for patients with subarachnoid hemorrhage and clinical suspicion of vasospasm.

Limited cerebral perfusion reserve frequently can be imaged in patients who have suffered transient ischemic attacks. In addition to use as a screening procedure, these studies may be used to evaluate perfusion reserve in patients with angiographically demonstrated lesions. The Medical College of Wisconsin protocol for acetazolamide-enhanced SPECT perfusion studies as a way to evaluate cerebral perfusion reserve is given in Table 4. Acetazolamide administration increases perfusion to normal vascular beds. However, hemodynamically significant lesions do not allow increased flow. Therefore, following acetazolamide administration, a flow imbalance can develop with enhanced flow to normal vascular beds but no increase in flow to regions distal to a critical stenosis or occlusion (Fig. 3). This test can be used to distinguish between patients with limited flow reserve and those with collateral flow, which fully corrects for the cerebrovascular disease. Preliminary results suggest that this test also is of value in predicting a favorable outcome following revascularization surgery.

## Dementia

When evaluating patients presenting with possible dementia, the goal of a neurologist or geriopsychiatrist is to distinguish age-associated cognitive change from organic and functional pathology such as SDAT, multi-infarct dementia, and depression (Table 5). SPECT brain perfusion imaging using either $^{99m}$Tc-HMPAO or $^{123}$I-IMP may be of value in making such distinctions. Our experience at the Medical College of Wisconsin, in addition to preliminary reports from several other institutions, suggests that the perfusion deficits associated with SDAT are more numerous and are imaged with greater contrast and clarity when $^{123}$I-IMP rather than $^{99m}$Tc-HMPAO is used (Fig. 4). For many patients with SDAT, there is bilateral decreased, but not absent, uptake in the posterior temporal lobes extending into the parietal and occipital lobes. The loca-

A

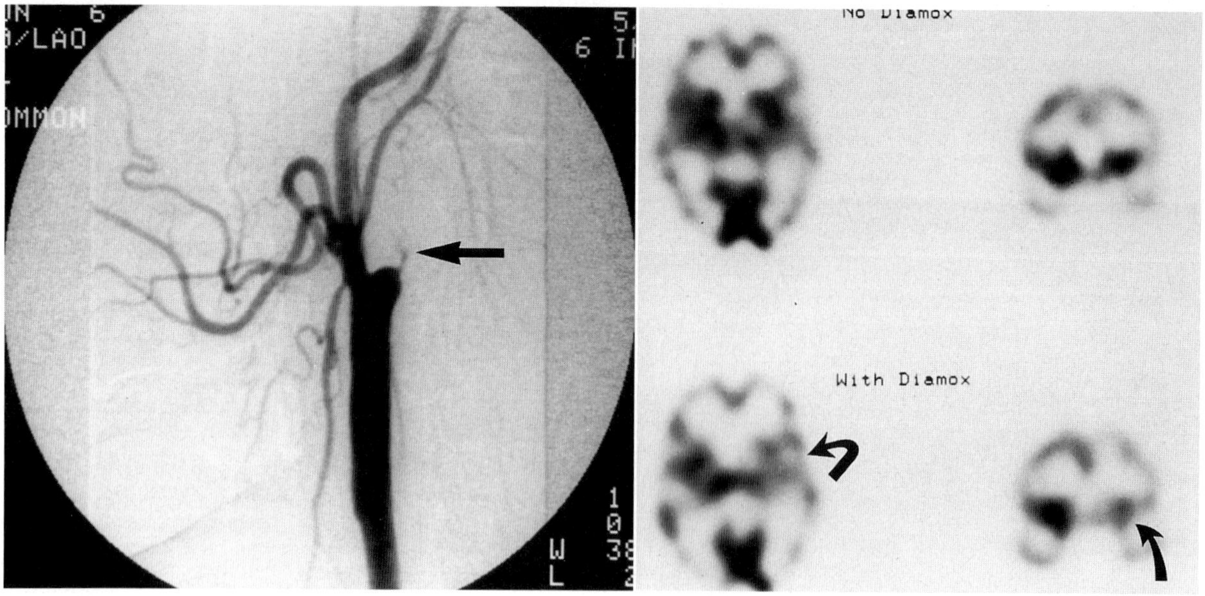


B

**FIGURE 3** Hemodynamically significant left common carotid artery occlusion in a 51-year-old male with a history of transient ischemic attacks. Patient was asymptomatic at the time of the study. *A,* Left common carotid artery arteriogram shows occlusion of the left internal carotid artery (*arrow*). *B,* Selected $^{99m}$Tc-HMPAO SPECT images with and without acetazolamide (Diamox) were obtained using a single-detector rotating camera. Note that Diamox stimulation produces a flow imbalance between the left and right cerebral hemispheres, with relatively less flow to the basal ganglia on the left (*curved arrows*). This signifies an inability to increase perfusion distal to the left internal carotid artery occlusion following Diamox stimulation. Findings indicate that there is limited flow reserve in the left cerebral hemisphere and that the internal carotid artery occlusion is hemodynamically significant.

**TABLE 5** Dementias

Senile dementia of the Alzheimer's type
Multi-infarct dementia
Extrapyramidal syndromes:
  Parkinson's disease
  Huntington's disease
AIDS dementia
Dementia syndrome of depression
Hydrocephalus
Chronic confusional states:
  Neoplasms
  Subdural hematomas
  Infections
  Toxic and metabolic

tion, size, and severity of defects correspond to the clinical presentation of SDAT. Although these findings typically are bilateral, the abnormalities may not be symmetric in both cerebral hemispheres. Frontal lobe decreased perfusion also may be observed. Usually there is normal uptake in the basal ganglia, thalamic nuclei, visual cortex, cerebellum, and sensory-motor cortical gray matter strip. Comparison with these normal areas may be of value in recognizing the characteristic perfusion changes of SDAT. Other less characteristic perfusion abnormalities may also be encountered with SDAT. Correlation with CT or MRI frequently is of great value for distinguishing SDAT perfusion changes from the perfusion deficits associated with stroke or tumor. Some investigators have reported SPECT brain perfusion imaging to be useful for evaluating patients with possible acquired immunodeficiency syndrome (AIDS) dementia.

## Huntington's Disease

Huntington's disease (HD) and other movement disorders such as Parkinson's disease have been evaluated using SPECT brain perfusion imaging. HD is a hereditary degenerative neurological disorder that is transmitted as an autosomal dominant trait. HD usually becomes symptomatic when patients are between 30 and 50 years old. First studied using PET, HD has more recently been evaluated with SPECT. Decreased uptake in the caudate nuclei usually precedes the anatomic changes that can be detected using MRI or CT. Although the results of SPECT brain perfusion imaging are highly convincing for some patients (Fig. 5), results still are preliminary. Given the great clinical significance of the HD diagnosis, caution should be used in interpreting SPECT data to predict which individuals from families with a history of HD may become symptomatic.

## Discussion

At our institution SPECT brain perfusion imaging has become a high-volume nuclear medicine examination. Using our dedicated SPECT brain system, as many as seven patients have been examined in one day. It appears that the efficiency of the system would allow one technologist to examine as many as ten patients in one day. With increasing awareness and acceptance of the indications for brain SPECT perfusion imaging, further growth of this procedure is anticipated.

A 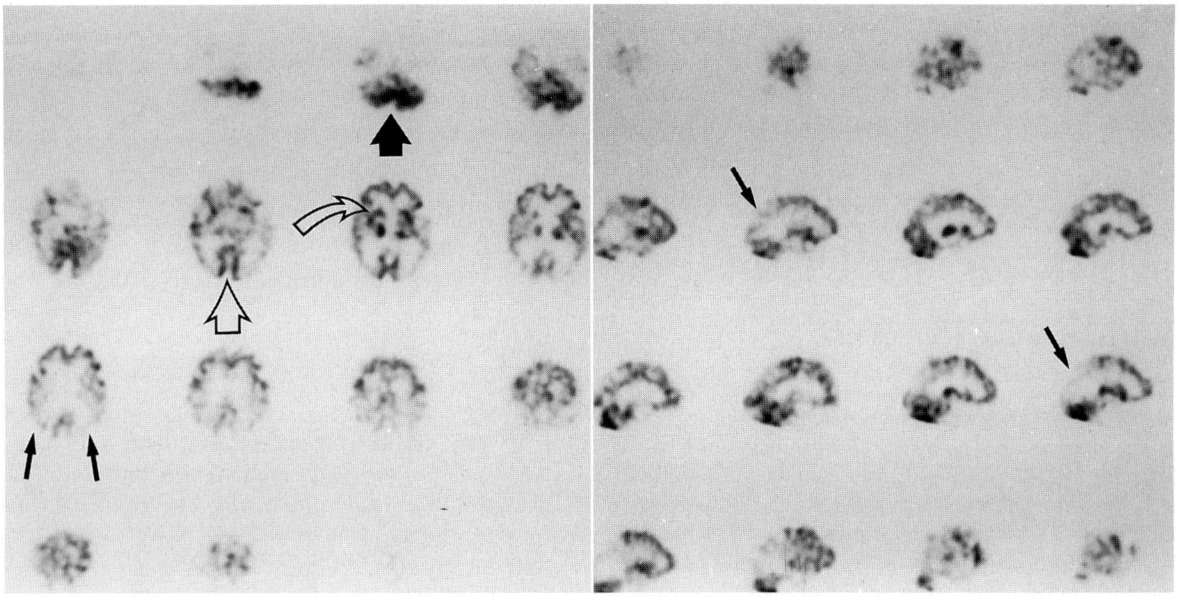 B

**FIGURE 4** Alzheimer's disease in an 87-year-old female with a five year history of progressive memory problems. CT scan was normal for age. Transaxial (*A*) and sagittal (*B*) $^{123}$I-IMP SPECT images show a generalized decrease in cortical gray matter perfusion in both cerebral hemispheres, which is most pronounced posteriorly in the parieto-occipital regions (*thin straight arrows*). Note the normal appearance of the caudate nuclei (*open curved arrow*), visual cortex (*open straight arrow*), and that portion of the cerebellum that is in the field of view (*fat arrow*).

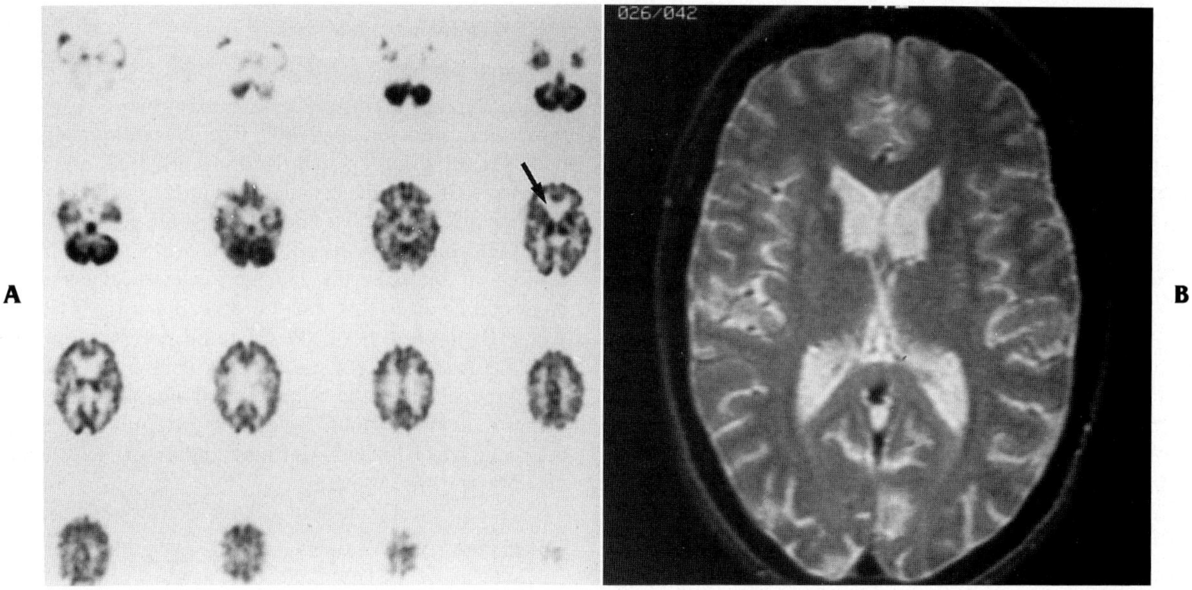

**FIGURE 5** Huntington's disease in a symptomatic 32-year-old female patient. *A,* Transaxial $^{99m}$Tc-HMPAO SPECT images show greatly reduced uptake in the head of the caudate nucleus bilaterally (*straight arrow* shows finding on right side). This abnormality is obvious only when compared with normal study in Figure 1. *B,* T2-weighted MRI in the same transaxial plane shows minimal atrophy of the caudate nuclei. Decreased flow to the head of the caudate, presumably reflecting decreased metabolic activity, is frequently observed in both preclinical and symptomatic Huntington's disease.

## Suggested Reading

Biersack HJ, Grunwald F, Kropp J. Single photon emission computed tomography imaging of brain tumors. Semin Nucl Med 1991; 21:2–10.

Bonte FJ, Hom J, Tintner R, Weiner MF. Single photon tomography in Alzheimer's disease and the dementias. Semin Nucl Med 1990; 20:342–352.

Devous MD, Leroy RF, Homan RW. Single photon emission computed tomography in epilepsy. Semin Nucl Med 1990; 20:325–341.

Hellman RS, Tikofsky RS. An overview of the contribution of Regional Cerebral Blood Flow Studies in Cerebrovascular Disease: Is there a role for single photon emission computed tomography? Semin Nucl Med 1990; 20:303–324.

Holman BL, Hellman RS, Goldsmith SJ, et al. Biodistribution, dosimetry, and clinical evaluation of technetium-99m ethyl cysteinate dimer in normal subjects and in patients with chromic cerebral infarction. J Nucl Med 1989; 30:1018–1024.

Leguin MH, Blok D, Pauwels EKJ. Radiopharmaceuticals for functional brain imaging with SPECT. Nucl Med Ann 1991; 37–65.

Van Heertum RL, O'Connell RA. Functional brain imaging in the evaluation of psychiatric illness. Semin Nucl Med 1991; 21:24–39.

# Noninvasive Diagnosis of Extracranial Cerebrovascular Disease

*EDWARD G. GRANT, M.D.*

Stroke—the most significant clinical manifestation of cerebrovascular atherosclerosis—is the third most common cause of death in the United States and a cause of major disability in at least 1 to 2 million additional people. The cost of this disease will undoubtedly continue to rise as modern medical therapy prolongs the lives of patients who previously would not have survived the initial event. Classic hemispheric stroke is heralded by the appearance of hemiparesis, aphasia, and even death. Other typical manifestations of cerebrovascular atherosclerosis include transient ischemic attacks (TIAs) and amaurosis fugax. The former is manifest by a totally reversible focal neurologic deficit originating in an appropriate portion of the brain, while the latter is the result of ischemia or, more likely, embolization to the retinal artery. The importance of TIAs and amaurosis fugax lies less in the effect of the immediate episode than in the more ominous heralding of impending stroke. The occurrence of a TIA increases the patient's likelihood of having a stroke within 5 years by threefold.

Although atherosclerosis may affect the intracranial vessels themselves, as many as 88 percent of all major hemispheric events (stroke, TIA, or amaurosis fugax) are thought to originate at the carotid bifurcation. The realization that carotid atherosclerosis was frequently responsible for hemispheric symptoms, however, took on practical meaning only after the early 1950s when it was demonstrated that atherosclerotic lesions could be removed from the bifurcation and reduce or eliminate TIAs or amaurosis fugax. Although the number of endarterectomies skyrocketed in the early and mid-1980s, the level appeared to plateau and, by the end of the decade, had fallen somewhat as the potential to affect prognosis came into question. Recently, large, cooperative studies, however, have clearly shown endarterectomy to reduce stroke in symptomatic patients with lesions that narrow the carotid lumen more than 70 percent. These studies assure endarterectomy a prominent role in the future.

With the ability to surgically correct atherosclerotic lesions at the carotid bifurcation came the requirement for a method of diagnosis. Arteriography has been the gold standard in this regard for many years. This examination, however, is an invasive procedure and even under the best of circumstances carries a small but ever-present risk. Additionally, arteriography is painful, requires contrast material, and is expensive. In an effort to minimize the number of negative examinations, noninvasive evaluations of the extracranial vasculature were developed. Originally, indirect tests such as oculoplethysmography and periorbital Doppler were used. These examinations were relatively successful and could indeed identify most patients having collateral circulation associated with a high-grade carotid stenosis. Indirect tests, however, largely have been abandoned, because they are unable to localize and quantify carotid lesions and are often negative in patients with bilateral disease. The introduction of duplex sonography significantly changed our ability to evaluate the carotid bifurcation. The combining of high-resolution real-time ultrasonography with pulse gated, directed Doppler produced a union in which each of the two components more than made up for the shortcomings of its counterpart. The real-time moiety provided a road map for the placement of the Doppler cursor, allowed for estimation of the Doppler angle, and was the first technique capable of defining the internal characteristics of plaque in vivo. High-resolution sonography, however, was not sufficiently accurate in the quantification of rate-limiting stenoses to be useful alone. In this all-important area, spectral Doppler was and still is the mainstay of diagnosis. Recently color Doppler imaging (CDI) has found increasing use in the non-invasive evaluation of extracranial cerebrovascular disease and is an integral part of the examination in many institutions. Although CDI clearly increases confidence, shortens examination time, and in specific instances may improve accuracy, a high-quality noninvasive cerebrovascular evaluation still implies a well-performed duplex examination.

## Technical Aspects of Examination

The indications and Doppler criteria for the diagnosis of rate-limiting lesions of the extracranial carotid arteries are relatively well established (Tables 1, 2). The accuracy of the examination, however, remains largely dependent on a well-performed and technically excellent scan. Even with the addition of CDI, careful attention must be given to technique and, in general, the carotid evaluation can be among the most challenging of ultrasonographic examinations. A standardized and systematic approach must be followed in every patient, and the common (CCA), internal (ICA), and external (ECA) carotids as well as the vertebral arteries should be assessed. Whether or not CDI is available, the examination should proceed along two tacks. First, a real-time evaluation of the carotid arteries should be performed to define areas of potential luminal narrowing and investigate plaque characteristics when possible. Additionally, one can obtain a good overview of essential vascular anatomy when performing the real-time scan. Specifically, the relative positions of the bifurcation and the ICA and ECA can be determined.

**TABLE 1** Indications for Color/Duplex Cerebrovascular Examination

| |
|---|
| History of TIA or possible TIA |
| Stroke |
| Amaurosis fugax |
| Asymptomatic bruit |
| S/P endarterectomy |
| Coronary artery bypass |

**TABLE 2** Spectral Criteria for Diameter Stenosis

| Percent Stenosis | Peak Systolic Velocity (cm/sec) | VICA/VCCA | End-diastolic Velocity (cm/sec) |
|---|---|---|---|
| <50 | <125 | <2.0 | <40 |
| 50–75 | 125–250 | 2.0–3.0 | 40–80 |
| 75–90 | >250 | >3.0 | >80 |
| 90–99 | Velocity criteria may not apply (see discussion in text) | | |

The real-time portion of the examination should be performed using the highest-frequency transducer available; most patients can be adequately evaluated with a 7.5 MHz transducer or greater, depending on the equipment used. Improvement in high-resolution real-time imaging has clearly allowed more routine visualization of even tightly stenosed vessels. The real-time examination is usually best performed in the transverse orientation and representative images should be taken at the proximal, mid, and distal CCA, the bulb and the immediate area of the bifurcation bilaterally. Areas of plaque should be thoroughly investigated; internal characteristics should be defined and the degree of luminal narrowing estimated.

After the B-mode assessment is completed, the transducer can be returned to the mid-CCA and the Doppler examination begun. If available, CDI may be used to obtain an overview of flow patterns and identify any potential regions of significant narrowing. Although several manufacturers claim to be capable of giving accurate estimates of peak velocity with color alone, most machines display color based on *mean* velocity readings, which are of little diagnostic value. As a rough guide, however, mean velocity is usually approximately one-half of peak. Regarding the relative importance of velocity versus kilohertz, kilohertz was successfully used for many years and was the basis of most early papers on the subject. Most authorities, however, currently recommend using angle-adjusted velocity measurements, because they are more accurate and reproducible and are interchangeable from one machine or transducer to the next.

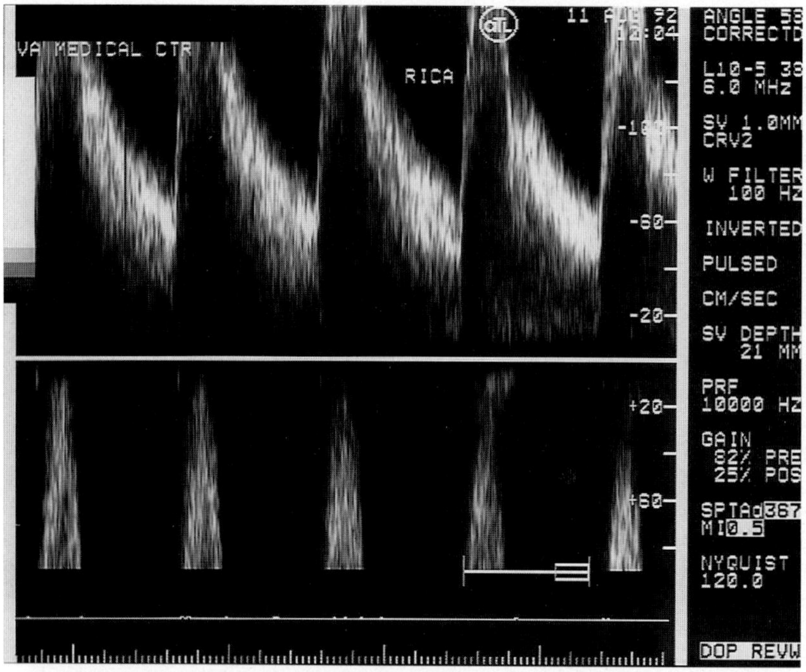


**FIGURE 1** Doppler angle is an important part of the velocity estimation, which is essential to carotid imaging. Doppler angle should be considered from two vantage points: true Doppler angle and machine-adjusted angle. True Doppler angle refers to the relationship between the actual sound beam and the direction of flow in the vessel. True Doppler angle can be changed only by changing the orientation of the transducer or Doppler beam in relation to the vessel being scanned. Machine-adjusted angle, on the other hand, automatically factors the true Doppler angle into the velocity calculation. Most units perform this function when the orientation of the small white line *(curved arrow)* is changed. This in turn tells the machine to expand or contract the velocity scale shown at the right of the image. True Doppler angle must be less than 60°; angles greater than this result in unacceptably large errors even if machine-adjusted angle has been properly adjusted.

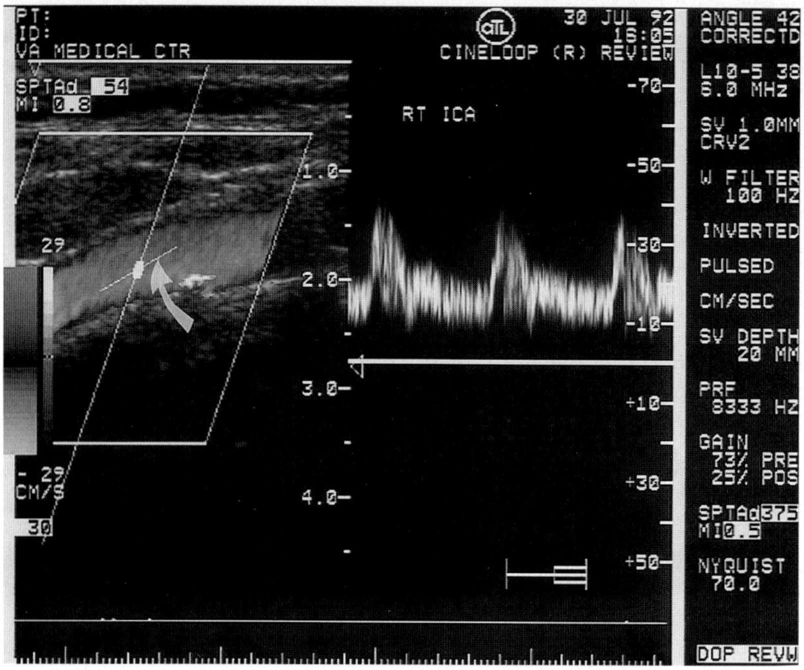


**FIGURE 2** Aliasing. Simply stated, aliasing occurs when peak velocity goes off the scale and is displayed on the opposite side of the baseline. This phenomenon is a common problem in carotid evaluations, because high-velocity jets are almost always associated with significant stenoses. Aliasing may make estimation of velocity difficult. Various maneuvers may be used to avoid this problem; the simplest include lowering the baseline and increasing the velocity scale.

The Doppler portion of the examination is best performed in the longitudinal plane, where angles can be accurately assessed. Doppler angles should always be considered when performing any form of Doppler examination, but they are of paramount importance in the carotid arteries, where estimation of flow velocity is the major diagnostic parameter. The angle between the Doppler beam and flow should be kept below 60°, and the Doppler angle itself should always be adjusted on the screen (Fig. 1). Both of these potential variables should be considered in every case. Obviously, accounting for the Doppler angle is impossible for color Doppler evaluations, and this should be taken into consideration whenever CDI information is used even as a rough guide. Changes in Doppler angle are particularly problematic in tortuous vessels and may produce bizarre color patterns that should be recognized as artifactual.

Aliasing is another technical problem frequently encountered in carotid scans because high-flow velocities at high scanning frequencies may cause Doppler shifts that exceed the Nyquist limit. In this case the spectral signal "wraps around" and is displayed on the opposite side of the scale (Fig. 2). Color Doppler aliasing is also problematic and may mimic flow reversal or severe turbulence. The complexities of the color Doppler examination should not be underestimated, and careful attention should always be given to optimizing color Doppler parameters before beginning the scan.

## The Normal Examination

Scanning is performed with the patient in the supine position; the examiner may either sit above the patient's head or adjacent to the patient in the routine position used for abdominal scanning. Both methods have their advantages, but I have found the over-the-head position to be somewhat easier on the arms and shoulders. The patient's neck should be hyperextended somewhat, but it is generally unnecessary to place towels or pillows beneath the shoulders. As was true for the B-mode examination, the Doppler scan is usually most easily begun in the midneck by locating the CCA in the transverse plane. This orientation allows the identification of several important landmarks, including the thyroid gland and jugular vein. Once the CCA is clearly depicted, the transducer should be turned longitudinally and followed as far proximal as the clavicle permits. In most patients the origin of the right CCA can be identified as it arises from the innominate artery. The origin of the left CCA, however, is from the aorta and is usually too low to be evaluated. Anomalies of the common carotid origins are not rare but, in general, have little effect on the overall performance of the examination. Scanning generally proceeds relatively rapidly through the CCA, because this vessel is large, easily visualized, and often maintains a relatively parallel course (and therefore constant Doppler angle) in relation to the skin.

The CCA eventually widens somewhat as the carotid bulb is reached. This fairly constant feature should alert the operator that the bifurcation lies immediately distal. The carotid bifurcation may be approached from either anterior or posterior to the sternocleidomastoid muscle; the posterolateral location of the ICA, however, makes the posterior approach a better method of "opening the bifurcation" in most patients. In many cases the patient's head must be turned somewhat to the contralateral side. Again, variability exists between individual patients, and any combination of these approaches may be used to lay out the bifurcation optimally. Once two vessels are identified, differentiation between ICA and ECA must be made. This seemingly simple task is one of the essential parts of the examination. Differentiation may be accomplished by means of appearance (the ICA is generally larger than the ECA, has a mildly dilated ampullary region at its origin, and is located posterolaterally), but normal variations are sufficiently common to make this inadvisable. The only infallible method of distinguishing between the two vessels anatomically is the identification of branches. The ICA has no branches in the neck, whereas the ECA has several that are often easily identified. Evaluation of Doppler spectra also offers an excellent method of differentiating between ICA and ECA. The ICA is a typical low-resistance vessel with a diphasic pattern and flow throughout diastole. The ECA supplies the muscular structures of the face and has a high-resistance, triphasic pattern (Fig. 3 and Color Plate 12). In cases in which a question exists about the two vessels, one may also tap the patient in the area of the temporomandibular joint. A large branch of the ECA traverses the area, and if one is scanning in the ECA, a reflected wave will be identified as a series of spikes in the Doppler tracing. If one is scanning in the ICA, no such reflected wave will be identified. Once the differentiation of ICA and ECA has been accomplished, the visualized portions of the ICA must be thoroughly investigated. This task is considerably simplified with the addition of color because it provides a global overview of the entire vessel. Measurement and documentation of angle-adjusted flow velocity is essential at specific areas along each carotid system, including the proximal, mid, and distal CCA; the bulb; the proximal ECA; and several sites within the ICA.

## Diagnostic Considerations

### *Plaque Characterization*

Recent articles have shown that as many as 80 percent of patients with clearly defined hemispheric events have no evidence of a significant luminal narrowing at the carotid bifurcation. Since the patients in these studies had no other obvious source for emboli (e.g., atrial fibrillation, coagulopathy), one must postulate that embolic events commonly arise from lesions at the carotid bifurcation that do not cause hemodynamically significant flow alterations. In an effort to identify those patients at risk for embolic phenomena, and possibly those who might benefit from surgical removal of non–rate-limiting lesions, high-resolution real-time ultrasonography has been used to evaluate the internal characteristics of carotid bifurcation plaque. Several studies have reported a significantly higher incidence of intraplaque hemorrhage in symptomatic patients than asymptomatic patients. Intraplaque hemorrhage may result from ischemia to the vessel wall, which causes bleeding into a pre-existing plaque from the vasa vasorum. Acute intraplaque hemorrhage may rupture through the intima, leading to distal embolization, or cause an acute increase in the size of nonsymptomatic plaque. Several groups investigated intraplaque hemorrhage and have shown that it can be identified within the vessel wall with an accuracy of as much as 90 percent, as evidenced by a heterogeneous internal echo pattern. Conversely these studies showed that homogeneous plaques never have pathologic evidence of intraplaque hemorrhage or even ulcerations.

Heterogeneous plaque typically has a mixed echo pattern. The hallmark of intraplaque hemorrhage is the identification of anechoic areas within the hemorrhage. Homogeneous plaque, on the other hand, has a relatively uniform echo texture throughout and smooth walls (Fig. 4). Although ulcerations cannot always be identified with ultrasonography, homogeneous plaques have not been found to be associated with ulceration. Calcifications have no bearing on plaque classification and may be identified in either heterogeneous or homogeneous plaques. The significance of plaque characterization remains controversial. Several recent studies, however, do show an increase in ipsilateral hemispheric symptoms in patients with heterogeneous plaque. However, longitudinal studies are needed to show conclusively whether plaque characterization is a significant prognostic indicator.

### *Doppler Evaluation*

Numerous investigations report excellent results in diagnosing internal carotid artery stenoses with duplex sonography. Accuracies of 90 percent or better are currently the norm, and the addition of CDI may improve results even further. These results are limited to the detection of lesions that compromise the luminal diameter more than 50 percent; most authorities agree that Doppler is of no value in lesions of lesser severity. Two main parameters are commonly used to diagnose stenotic

A

B

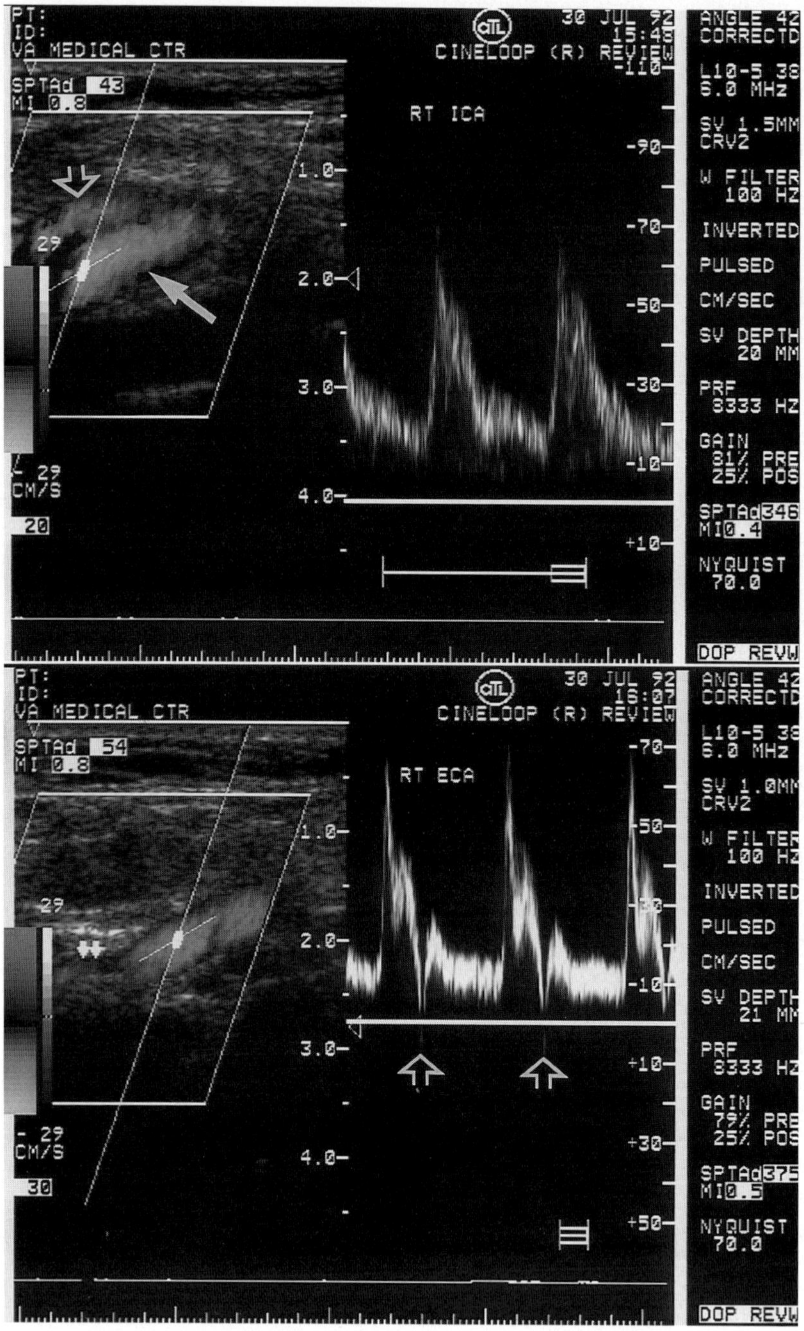


**FIGURE 3** Normal carotid bifurcation. *A,* The ICA *(large arrow)* usually lies posterior to the ECA *(open arrow)* and is typically larger. These characteristics, however, are not constant and should never be relied on to distinguish the two vessels; Doppler characteristics are far more reliable. Note the low-resistance flow pattern of the ICA. *B,* The ECA supplies the facial muscles and thus has a triphasic, high-resistance pattern characterized by minimal flow in diastole and a brief period of flow reversal *(open arrows).* The ECA may also be distinguished by its branches *(small arrows);* the ICA has no branches in the neck. See also Color Plate 12.

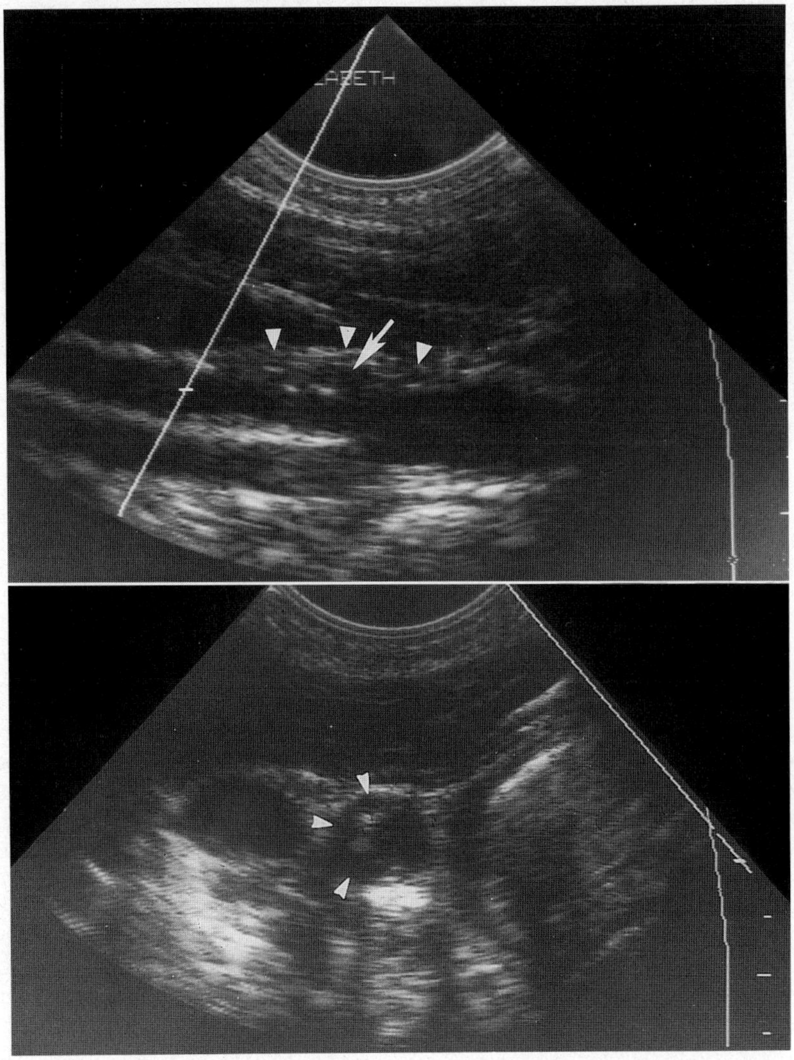

A

B

**FIGURE 4** Plaque characterization. *A,* Longitudinal section through bifurcation reveals well-defined plaque *(arrowheads)* in proximal ICA. Although plaque appeared relatively benign, several areas of decreased echogenicity *(arrow)* are present. *B,* Transverse image through right carotid bulb demonstrates plaque, which visually narrows the lumen less than 50 percent. Subintimal anechoic areas *(arrowheads),* however, suggest intraplaque hemorrhage. Patient was followed with yearly sonograms; lesion remained stable. Intraplaque hemorrhage may be difficult to differentiate from fatty deposits.

A

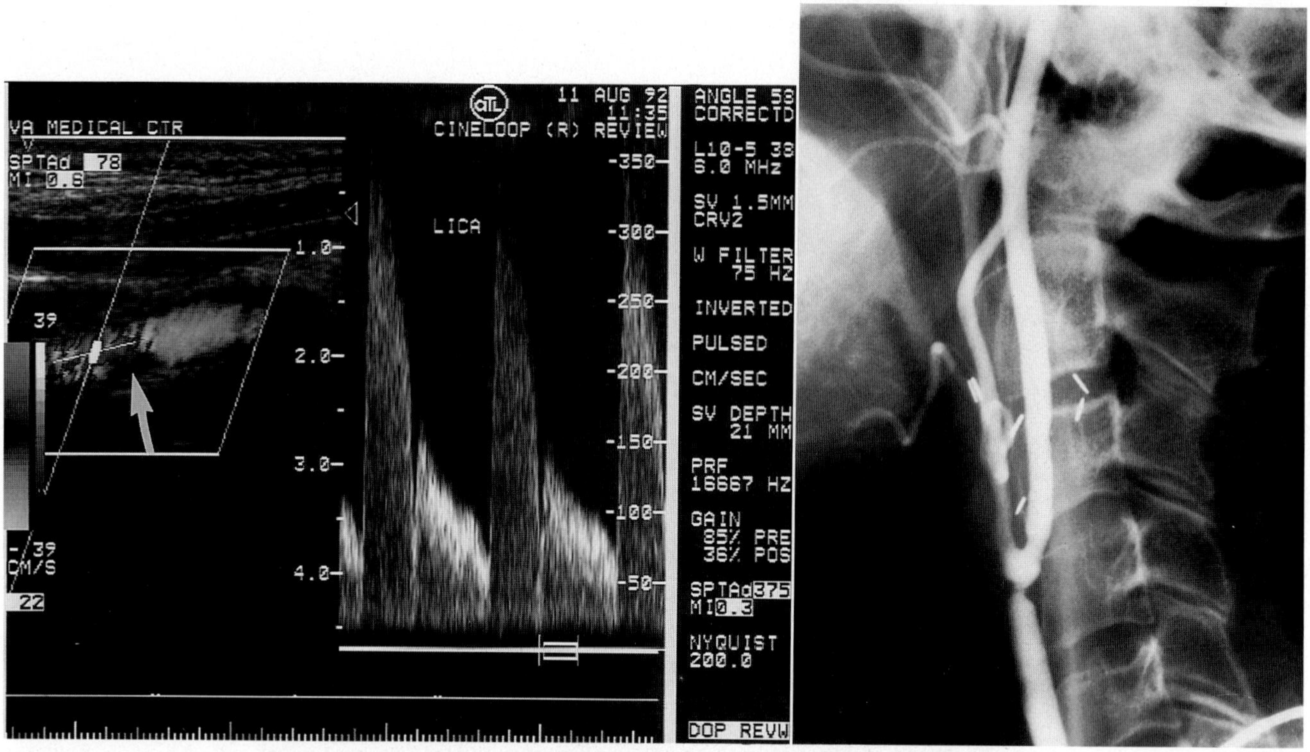


B

**FIGURE 5** High-grade ICA stenosis. Patient who had undergone carotid endarterectomy 5 years earlier presented with recent transient ischemic attacks. Real-time evaluation of left carotid bifurcation was relatively unremarkable. *A,* Color Doppler sonogram (*reproduced here in black and white*) suggests stenosis; note anechoic plaque *(arrow)* and abnormal color pattern. Spectral analysis defined lesion as narrowing lumen by 75 to 90 percent; peak systolic velocity > 350 cm/sec, VICA/VCCA > 4, end-diastolic velocity = 87. See also Color Plate 13. *B,* Angiogram confirmed 80 to 85 percent lesion.

lesions: peak systolic velocity and the ratio of peak systolic velocity in the ICA to that in the *mid/distal* CCA (VICA/VCCA). A third parameter, end-diastolic velocity, is being used increasingly as an indicator of critical stenosis (lesions that are severe enough to be considered for endarterectomy), though exactly what represents an operative lesion is changing as more experience with large, long-term studies accumulates. The most recent studies show that at this point, symptomatic patients with lesions greater than 70 percent diameter have better outcomes with surgery than medical therapy.

We have found peak systolic velocity to be the most accurate and reproducible of all Doppler parameters in the diagnosis of carotid stenosis. This relatively simple measurement is also attractive because it correlates well with increasing degrees of stenosis. Ratios are essential, however, in patients with various cardiovascular abnormalities such as hypertension, low cardiac output, arrhythmias, or tandem lesions. In this way, the patient may be used as his own gold standard, alleviating problems caused by potentially different baseline velocities. Several ratios have been described as being useful in the diagnosis of carotid disease; currently, however, only VICA/VCCA is widely applied (Fig. 5 and Color Plate 13). Specific cardiac abnormalities may also have a significant effect on the overall appearance of the Doppler pattern. In particular, a bispherious systolic waveform and occasional reversal of diastolic flow may be observed in patients with aortic regurgitation. Other cardiac lesions also likely cause alterations in the appearance of carotid spectra, but to date their effect on Doppler waveforms has not been specifically evaluated.

The Doppler diagnosis of lesions that narrow the luminal diameter between 50 and 95 percent should be relatively straightforward. One notable exception, however, is the patient with a contralateral stenosis or occlusion in whom Doppler findings in the less diseased artery may be spurious. In addition, patients with subtotal stenoses may be difficult to evaluate using the routine parameters, because peak systolic velocity may decrease into the normal range in subtotal lesions (>90 to 95 percent luminal narrowing). In such cases the duplex diagnosis must be based on the identification of a distorted spectral waveform and a relative increase in diastolic flow. Further complicating the identification of subtotal lesions using duplex technology is the difficulty one may have in finding a tiny residual lumen and the possibility of mistaking an ECA collateral for a minimally patent ICA. CDI may be of particular assistance in these lesions by being able to identify the residual lumen and assist in differentiating between the string sign of a subtotal occlusion and an ECA collateral (Fig. 6 and Color Plate 14).

The diagnosis of total ICA occlusion should be relatively straightforward with either duplex Doppler or CDI. The latter, however, has the advantage of a visual display and, with complete occlusion of the ICA, only one vessel is observed (Fig. 7 and Color Plate 15). Assuming a side branch is identified, confirming a patent ECA, the diagnosis should be made with confidence. Further adding to the ease of diagnosis is the fact that the ECA rarely occludes before the ICA. In many cases the occluded ICA lumen is visible as an anechoic or plaque-filled structure with no Doppler signals. Secondary features of

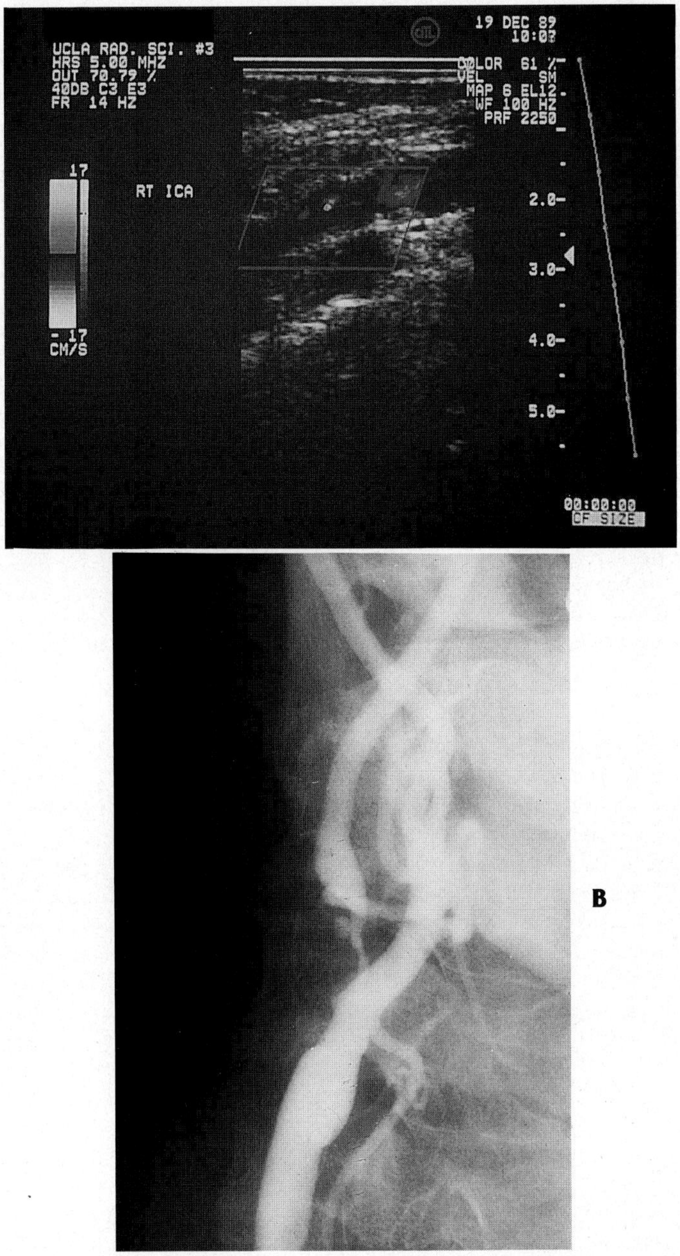


A

B

**FIGURE 6** Subtotal ICA occlusion. *A,* Color Doppler imaging (*reproduced here in black and white*) shows a minute residual lumen within an otherwise anechoic vessel *(arrow)*. Spectral tracings were difficult to obtain and demonstrated marked distortion of the waveform. See also Color Plate 14. *B,* Angiogram confirms subtotal occlusion of ICA.

A

B

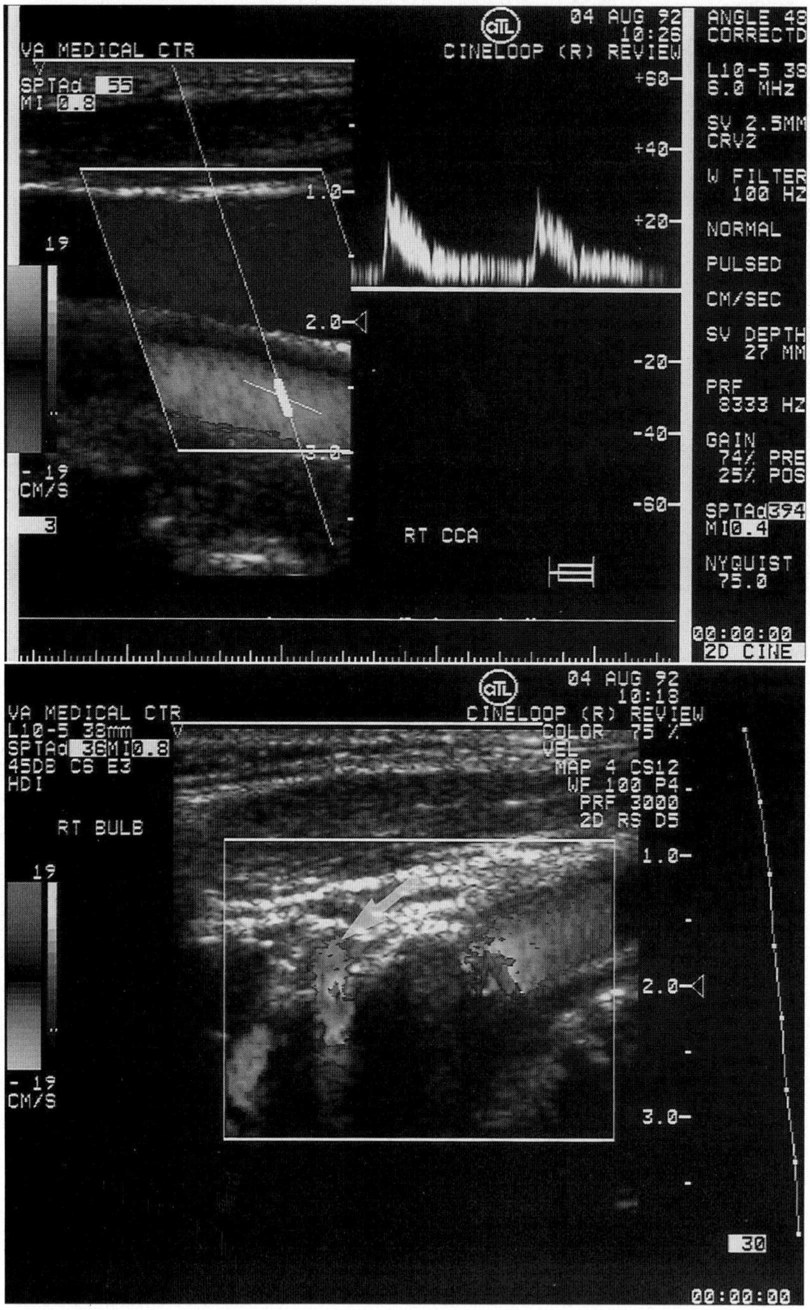


**FIGURE 7** Total ICA occlusion. *A,* Scanning through the CCA reveals a somewhat high-resistance flow pattern. Note sharp systolic upstroke, relatively low flow in diastole, and negative component. Though not specific, ICA occlusion should be considered. *B,* Following CCA distally, the color signal is lost due to presence of large, densely shadowing plaque. Beyond plaque, only one vessel could be identified; branch *(arrow)* confirms patent artery to be ECA. See also Color Plate 15.

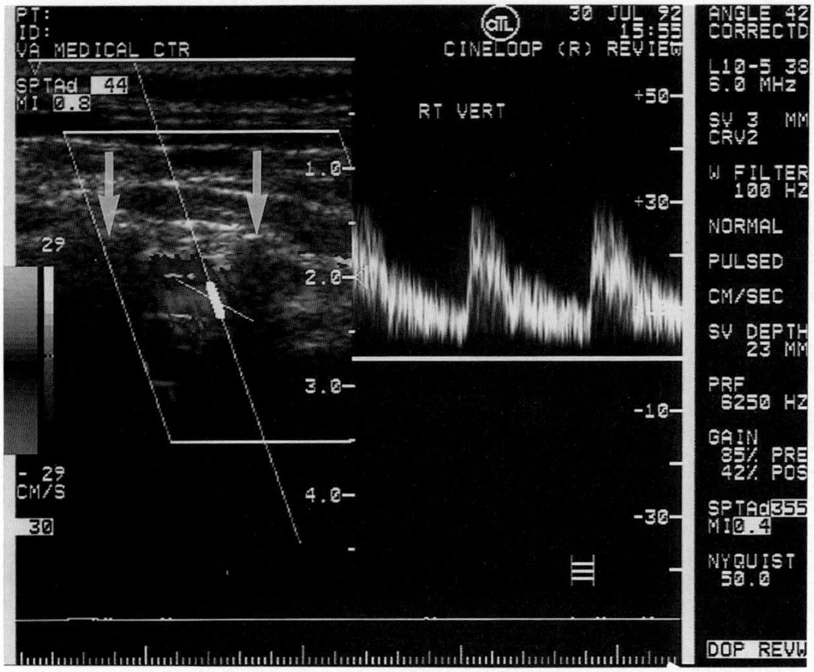


**FIGURE 8** Normal vertebral artery. Two vessels with flow proceeding in different directions were identified between shadows of transverse processes of cervical spine *(arrows)*. Spectral analysis confirms posterior vessel as the vertebral artery; note the low-resistance arterial flow pattern. Anterior vessel is vertebral vein. See also Color Plate 16.

complete occlusion may also be identified proximally. Color Doppler may reveal an area of flow reversal just distal to the occluding thrombus as a short burst of retrograde flow is reflected off the blockage. "Externalized" flow patterns may be present in the CCA as all flow is diverted to the high-resistance external vasculature. Although the latter finding is suggestive of occlusion, it may be observed in normals and should not be a cause for alarm if the ICA is clearly patent. Most total occlusions are limited to the ICA, but the CCA may occasionally be blocked completely. This is most likely the result of gradually worsening disease, because the material within the lumen tends to be fairly echogenic. Further supporting chronicity is the tendency for the bifurcation vessels to remain patent, with a reversed ECA serving as a collateral and feeding blood to the ICA. This interesting physiology should be obvious using either duplex Doppler or CDI and should be sought in any patient in whom the CCA is occluded.

## The Vertebral Arteries

The vertebral arteries should be evaluated as part of every routine duplex/CDI evaluation. These vessels are usually easily identified, but a detailed evaluation would be overly time-consuming and largely unnecessary. Although one early study suggested that a peak systolic flow greater than 2 kHz indicates a 50 to 90 percent stenosis, in practical terms the diagnosis of vertebral compromise has little clinical significance since stenosis is not a surgically correctable lesion. In addition, vertebro-basilar symptoms tend to be vague, and whether symptoms can be attributed specifically to compromise of one or the other vertebral artery is highly questionable in most patients. The anatomy of the normal vertebral arteries is also highly variable; one may be hypoplastic or completely absent and represent a normal variant. Finally, the vertebral artery origins are often difficult to visualize and much of the vessel lies within the transverse foramina of the cervical vertebral bodies.

The complete evaluation of the vertebral arteries is obviously not practical. Reversal of flow, however, should be identified in an effort to diagnose subclavian steal syndrome. The vertebral arteries are usually easily located by scanning the mid-CCA in a longitudinal plane and angling the transducer somewhat laterally. Portions of the vertebral artery appear between the shadows cast by the lateral masses of the cervical spine (Fig. 8 and Color Plate 16). A vessel thus identified can only be the vertebral artery or vein, because no other vessel in the neck courses through the transverse foramina. Once the vessel is found, spectral Doppler should be used to assess whether one is identifying flow in a vein or artery because the two often are parallel. The vein tends to be the more anteriorly located and, as is the case with many other central systemic veins, may produce a pulsatile flow pattern that should not be mistaken for the artery. The vertebral artery should exhibit typical low-resistance flow patterns with peak systolic velocity less than that of the adjacent CCA. Subclavian steal may be diagnosed when flow reversal is identified. Rarely, spectral abnormalities may be observed as well. The "bunny-rabbit" sign (vertebral waveforms having a sharp systolic peak with a bump in mid-diastole) is said to imply stenosis or impending occlusion of the proximal subclavian artery; absent diastolic flow should raise the suspicion of distal vertebral artery occlusion. Once appropriately directed flow and a normal spectral tracing have been obtained, the examination of the vertebral artery may be ended.

## Suggested Reading

Barnett HJM, Taylor DW, Haynes RB, et al. Beneficial effect of carotid endarterectomy in symptomatic patients with high-grade carotid stenosis. N Engl J Med 1991; 325:447.

Bluth EL, Kay D, Merritt CRB, et al. Sonographic characterization of carotid plaque—detection of hemorrhage. AJR 1986; 146:1061.

Bluth EL, Stavros AT, Marich KW, et al. Carotid duplex sonography: A multi-center recommendation for standardized imaging and Doppler criteria. RadioGraphics 1988; 8:487.

Cranley J. Presidential address. Stroke: A perspective. Surgery 1982; 91:537.

Erickson SJ, Mewissen MW, Foley DW, et al. Stenosis of the internal carotid artery: Assessment using color Doppler imaging compared with angiography. AJR 1989; 152:1299.

Garth K, Carroll B, Sommer G, et al. Duplex ultrasound scanning of the carotid arteries with velocity spectrum analysis. Radiology 1983; 147:823.

Jacobs N, Grant E, Schellinger D, et al. Duplex carotid sonography: Criteria for stenosis, accuracy, and pitfalls. Radiology 1985; 154:385.

O'Leary DH, Polak JF. High-resolution carotid sonography: Past, present, and future. AJR 1989; 153:699.

Polak JF, Dobkin GR, O'Leary DH, et al. Internal carotid artery stenosis: Accuracy and reproducibility of color-Doppler-assisted duplex imaging. Radiology 1989; 173:793.

Sterpetti AV, Schultz RD, Feldhaus RJ, et al. Ultrasonographic features of carotid plaque and the risk of subsequent neurologic deficits. Surgery 1988; 104:652.

# Dynamic CT Scanning in the Evaluation of Acute Cerebral Stroke

*J. RANDY JINKINS, M.D.*

Thrombotic or embolic phenomena involving the arterial and venous structures of the head and neck have been well documented using static computed tomography (CT). Occlusive disease of the major vascular structures of the head and neck produce classic findings on conventional angiography that are mirrored in the sequences obtained on intravenous dynamic CT (IVDCT). As a complement of the initial CT workup, IVDCT provides immediate, important diagnostic information, helps to direct appropriate clinicoradiologic triage with minimal delay, and may obviate more invasive studies in selected clinical settings.

## Technical Approach

Initially a noncontrast CT is obtained to evaluate for frank infarction, associated hemorrhage, or other pathologic change that might be masked by the use of a contrast agent. The level for the IVDCT is selected from this preenhanced scan and is often based on a visualized cerebral infarct. If none is seen, a section through the midcranium to include the basal ganglia is chosen. Typically a standard injection sequence for the IVDCT is used: 4 ml of Renografin-76 (or the nonionic equivalent) per second, injected through a 20 gauge antecubital venous catheter for a total of 60 ml. An appropriate dose/weight reduction in these parameters is made in pediatric patients. The scan acquisition is also standardized: one initial scan followed by an 8 second arm-to-head circulation time delay, 12 scans in rapid sequence without interscan delay (~4.5 seconds per scan), and eight subsequent scans with a 30 second interscan delay. This extends the acquisition through approximately 5 minutes.

In all patients with suspected arterial occlusive disease, a second dynamic sequence is performed at the level of the second cervical vertebrae to assess the patency of the cervical vessels. For subjects with venous occlusive disease, an additional sequence(s) is carried out in multiple axial and/or coronal planes to study the sagittal, transverse, and straight venous sinuses. This sequence acquisition spans only 60 seconds: one initial scan followed by a 6 second arm-to-neck circulation time delay, terminated by twelve scans in rapid succession without interscan delay.

## Diagnostic Approach

On IVDCT, patients with major arterial occlusion manifest a cranial picture of a delay or an absence of flow of contrast agent into major branches supplying respective regions (Figs. 1, *A*, and 2, *C* and *D*). In fact, IVDCT demonstrates this phenomenon within the first minutes or hours after the occlusive event. Such findings cannot be ascertained in these early stages by static CT alone. Even the secondary manifestations of edema and mass effect require up to 12 to 24 hours to become apparent on static imaging evaluations.

Nevertheless, it is still not possible to determine whether the observed appearance on IVDCT is due to a hemodynamically significant proximal stenosis, an embolus within a major territorial vessel, or a major proximal carotid/vertebrobasilar occlusion with collateral accounting for the delayed perfusion. Therefore at this point further radiologic evaluation is necessary.

Within 5 to 10 minutes following the initial IVDCT, the intravenous contrast agent has sufficiently equilibrated with the extracranial blood pool to allow a second successful injection. This subsequent sequence, acquired at the level of the second cervical vertebrae, may reveal a major occlusion (Fig. 1, *B*) or occlusions. In so doing, it may obviate further, more invasive, studies if an extracranial-intracranial vascular bypass procedure is not being considered. As a matter of fact, IVDCT is thought by some to be more sensitive than conventional angiographic methods in the detection of vascular patency in cervical vascular occlusive disease. In the interests of efficiency, if a vascular occlusion in the neck is a major diagnostic consideration, the cranial portion of the dynamic study may be foregone in order to focus on the cervical vessels.

However, if the cervical dynamic sequence does not reveal a delay in opacification or complete nonopacification of a major vessel(s), a proximal stenotic lesion of indeterminate severity or a more subtle abnormality, such as a vascular ulceration, cannot be excluded. A conventional arteriographic study is indicated in this setting to further evaluate the craniocervical vascular system in precise detail.

One additional finding that has implications in regard to imaging studies is that of vascular "stagnation." On static CT

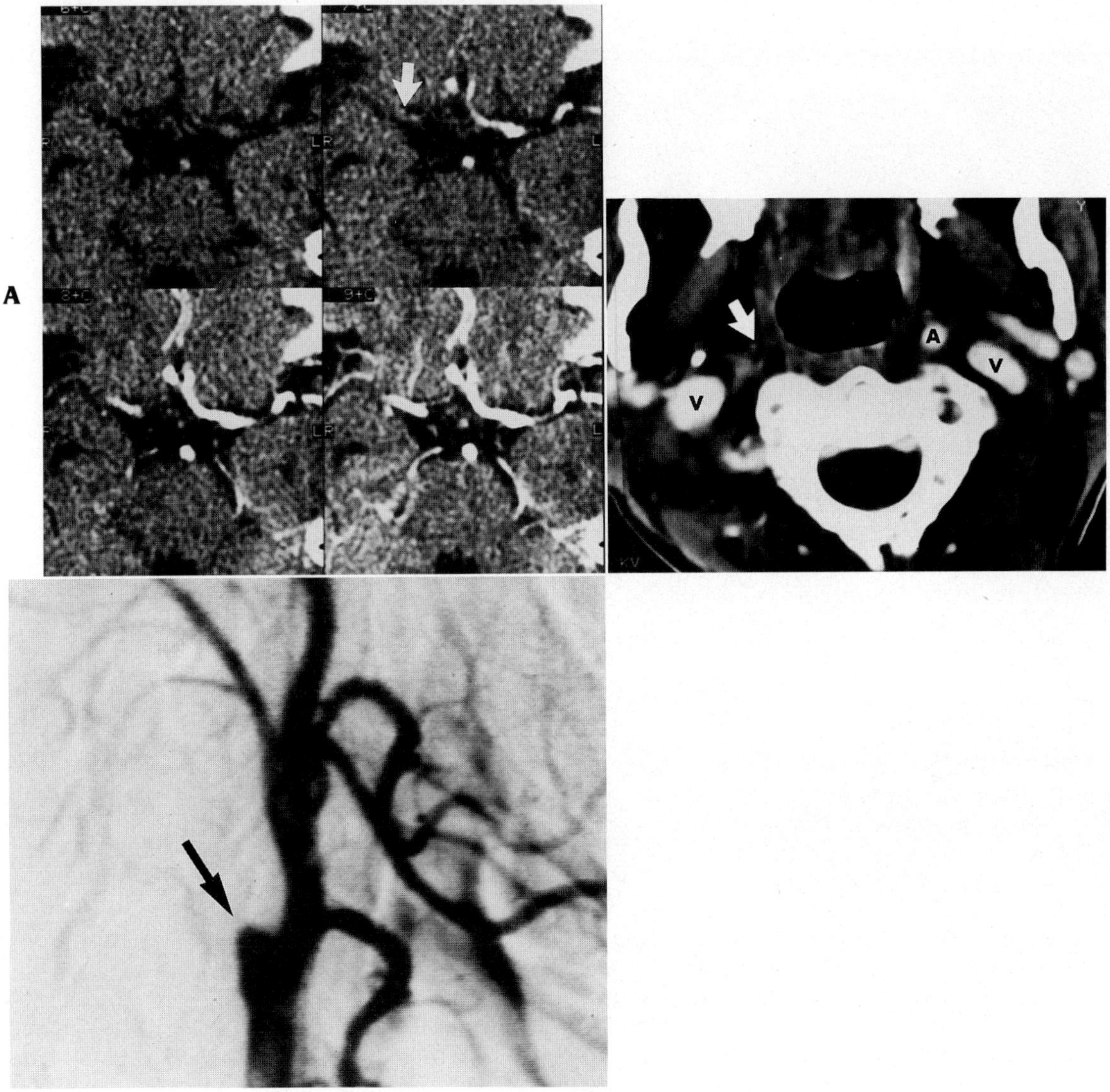


A B C

**FIGURE 1** A 92-year-old male with recent onset of left hemiparesis. *A,* Dynamic sequence centered at the level of the circle of Willis at 0, 4, 8, and 12 seconds (*left to right and top to bottom*), illustrating the delay in opacification of the right supraclinoid internal carotid artery and middle cerebral stem (*arrow*). *B,* Section from dynamic sequence recentered at the level of C2, approximately 10 to 15 minutes following the initial study in (*A*). This image obtained during peak perfusion at 12 seconds demonstrates no evidence of opacification of the right internal carotid artery (*arrow*), but normal visualization of the left internal carotid artery (A) as well as both internal jugular veins (V). *C,* Subsequent arterial digital subtraction angiogram shows complete occlusion of the right internal carotid artery at its origin (*arrow*).

A

B

C

D

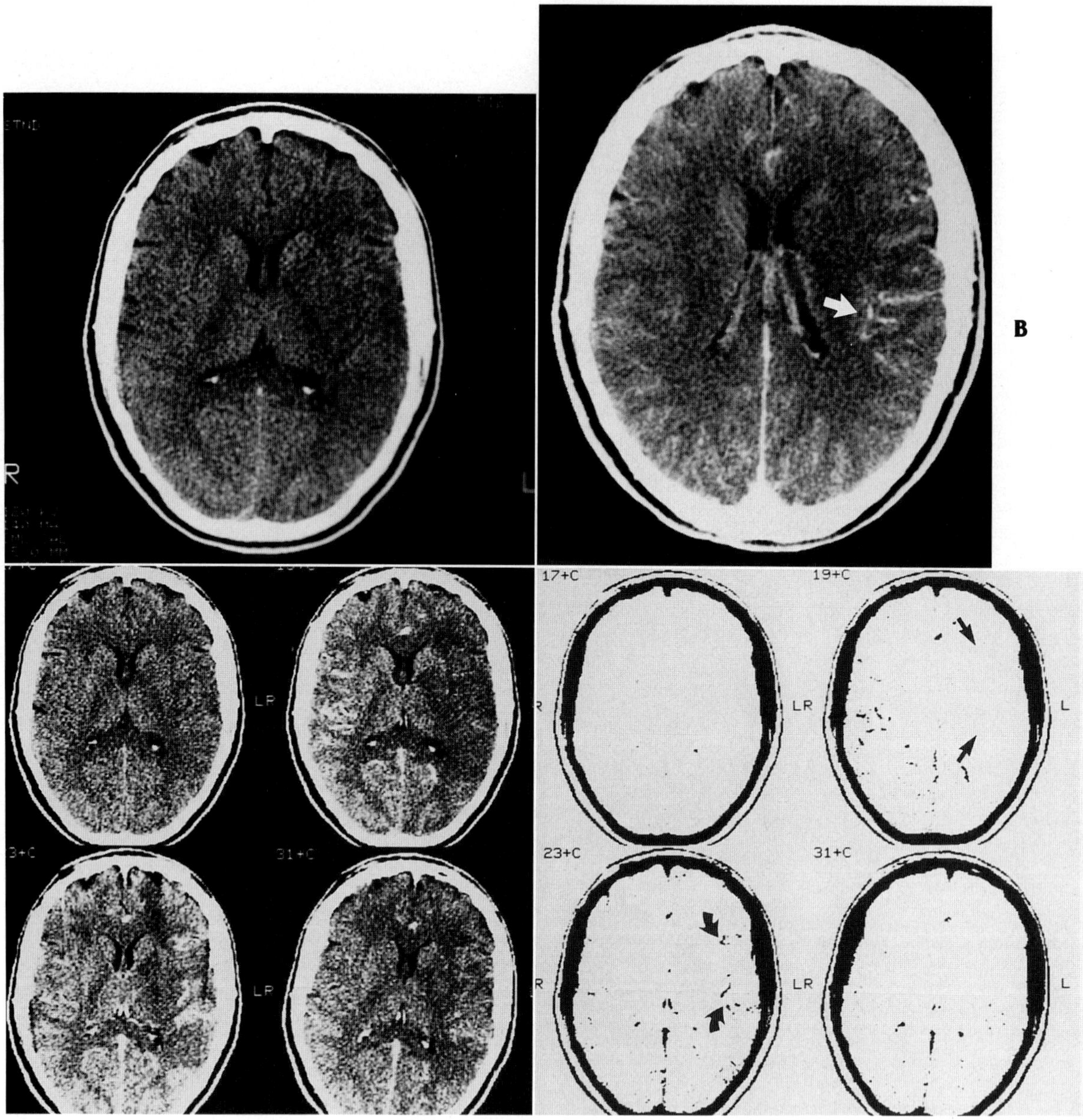

**FIGURE 2** A 39-year-old male with sudden onset of dense right-sided hemiplegia 2 hours before evaluation. *A,* Initial noncontrast cranial CT illustrates no definite abnormality, although there may be a slight diminution in sulcal prominence in the left posterior parietal region. *B,* Postcontrast CT at a slightly higher level than in (*A*) demonstrates stagnation of contrast within multiple middle cerebral vessels (*arrow*). *C,* Dynamic sequence at 4, 8, 25, and 60 seconds reveals the initially delayed opacification of the left middle cerebral region and final equilibration. *D,* Identical sequence as in (*C*) on narrow window, video-reverse imaging illustrates the early opacification absence in the middle cerebral distribution (*straight arrows*), intermediate stagnation in the same region (*curved arrows*), and final clearance.

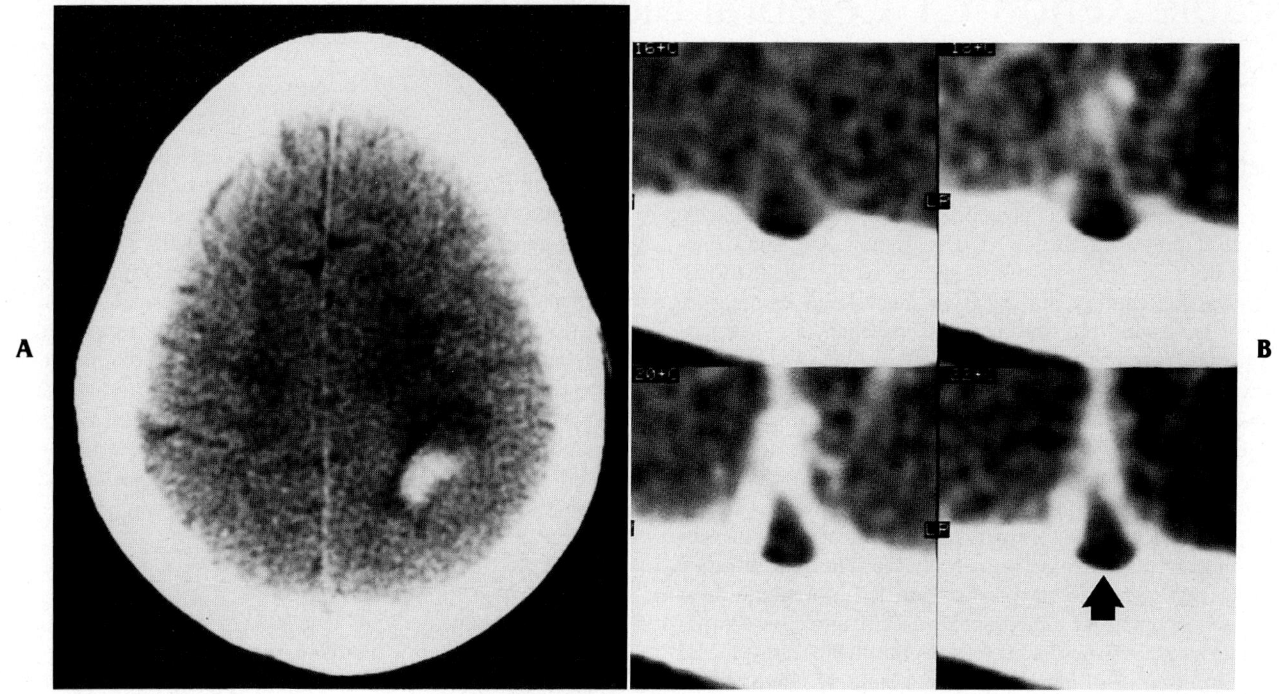

**FIGURE 3** A 32-year-old female on oral birth control medication with sudden onset of right-sided weakness. *A,* Noncontrast CT scan demonstrates the venous hemorrhage and/or infarct in the parasagittal region on the left. *B,* Magnified view of the dynamic sequence centered over the superior sagittal sinus in the occipital region at 0, 4, 8 and 12 seconds reveals the inflow of contrast material around the delta-shaped thrombus (*arrow*).

as well as on IVDCT with contrast enhancement, stagnation is manifested as intensely enhanced vessels traversing an area of infarction (Fig. 2, *B* and *D*).

Venous sinus thrombosis leading to venous infarcts and venous hemorrhages have been extensively described using static CT. In such cases IVDCT assures complete contrast opacification of the cerebral venous structures and therefore provides optimal visualization of the nonenhancing intravascular clot (Fig. 3). However, the dynamic sequence is performed at one, or at most three, fixed level(s), because contrast limitations allow only two to three injections per study. There exists therefore the possibility of missing a venous thrombus even after evaluating several cranial levels on IVDCT. In the event of a negative IVDCT of the dural venous sinuses, it may be impossible to absolutely exclude a low transverse or deep cerebral venous sinus thrombosis. In this circumstance a conventional angiographic examination is warranted.

## Discussion

IVDCT is ideally suited to the initial evaluation of subjects presenting with clinically suspected craniocervical vascular occlusive disease from any cause. Its noninvasive nature, simplicity, sensitivity, and expediency benefit patient triage and may reduce the necessity of more invasive procedures in the radiologic investigation of pathologic vascular states of the head and neck.

## Suggested Reading

Houser OW, Campbell JK, Baker HL, Sundt TS. Radiologic evaluation of ischemic cerebrovascular syndromes with emphasis on computed tomography. Radiol Clin North Am 1982; 20:123–142.

Jinkins JR. Dynamic CT of cranio-cervical vascular occlusive disease. Neuroradiology 1988; 30:105–110.

Keller HM, Valavanis A, Imhof H-G, Turina M. Patency of external and internal carotid artery in the presence of an occluded common carotid artery: Noninvasive evaluation with combined cerebrovascular Doppler examination and sequential computed tomography. Stroke 1984; 15:149–157.

Kohlmeyer K, Graser C. Comparative study of computed tomography (CT) and carotid angiography (CAG) in stroke patients. Neuroradiology 1978; 16:162–163.

Riles TS, Posner MP, Cohen WS, et al. The totally occluded internal carotid artery. Arch Surg 1982; 117:1185–1188.

Yamamoto M, Shinohara Y, Kamei T, Yoshii F. Diagnosis of internal carotid artery occlusion by dynamic computed tomography. J Comput Assist Tomogr 1981; 5:637–640.

# Stable Xenon-CT Cerebral Blood Flow Imaging

*RICHARD E. LATCHAW, M.D.*

## Methodology

A number of methods have been developed to clinically analyze cerebral blood flow (CBF). Xenon is a small lipophilic molecule that easily diffuses across the intact blood-brain barrier, thereby making it an ideal agent to measure actual perfusion into the cerebral parenchyma, not just intravascular transit time. Perfusion can be quantified by knowing the intra-arterial concentration of xenon and the time-dependent accumulation of xenon in the tissue. Xenon is inhaled and rapidly establishes an equilibrium across the alveolar-capillary membrane. The arterial concentration presenting to the cerebral parenchyma is approximated by the end-tidal concentration, which may be measured, thereby obviating the placement of an arterial line. The concentration moving into the cerebral parenchyma is sequentially measured by a computed tomographic (CT) scanner on a pixel-by-pixel basis. Scans every 60 seconds through predetermined levels are used for the production of a build-up curve of flow for every pixel scanned. The concentration of $CO_2$ in the exhalation is also measured and CBF adjusted, since CBF is affected by the $P_{CO_2}$.

This technique allows for approximately 12 percent error in reproducibility, and is quantifiable. Blood flow maps are produced, with each pixel depicting CBF in milliliters per 100 g of cerebral tissue per minute. The blood flow map is filmed next to the anatomic CT scan level from which the map is derived. A region of interest (ROI) marker of any size may be placed in an area on the map to give a direct readout of CBF.

Other techniques have been developed, including the radionuclide scanning of xenon-133. This technique uses external probes that determine the flows to the surface tissues at the expense of deeper structures. Extensive mathematical models are used to evaluate the radionuclide decay curve, along with assumptions regarding flow to two compartments (gray and white matter). Positron emission tomography (PET) scanning is a highly accurate methodology using positron-emitting isotopes attached to physiologic tracers. Many more physiological events than CBF may be measured, such as glucose metabolism, oxygen extraction, cerebral blood volume (CBV), and neurotransmitter and chemical receptor localization. Unfortunately this technology is extremely expensive (at the \$5 million level), whereas xenon-CT technology costs approximately \$60,000 to \$70,000. Single-photon emission computed tomography (SPECT) uses radionuclides attached to tracers, with derived counts reflecting both CBF and receptor population. This technique has been termed the "poor man's PET," and suffers by not being easily quantifiable. Last, a variety of magnetic resonance imaging (MRI) techniques for evaluating both intravascular transit time and actual cerebral perfusion are currently being developed but are experimental at this time.

The xenon-CT CBF procedure is most helpful in five clinical conditions. In acute stroke, the procedure demonstrates a decrease in blood flow to a region of brain tissue immediately after its occurrence. Chronic ischemia may also be evaluated using a "challenge" test to distinguish between a true low-flow state with decreased vascular reserves and decreased flow on the basis of decreased need by a previously injured tissue. Accurate measurement of blood flow following a balloon test occlusion (BTO) of a carotid artery gives a much better understanding of the risks to the brain from permanent carotid occlusion. Areas of decreased flow secondary to vasospasm following subarachnoid hemorrhage may help to determine the best timing for aneurysm clipping. Finally, our routine use of hyperventilation following head trauma to decrease CBV also decreases CBF. The xenon-CT CBF technique determines the resultant tissue perfusion and the status of altered autoregulation.

## Technique

There have been numerous articles on the xenon-CT technique including the theory, mathematics, and methodology for calculation. A number of references are given at the end of this chapter for more in-depth study. Briefly the technique involves the inhalation of a gas mixture made up of approximately 33 percent xenon and 67 percent oxygen for approximately 4.5 minutes. Because of technologic considerations, the study is limited to three or less 5 to 10 mm thick levels of cerebral parenchyma. Hence the radiologist must know the clinical problem. If the question relates to supratentorial cerebrovascular occlusive disease, I usually select the lowest level to pass through the basal ganglia so that the inferior frontal, temporal, and occipital lobes are visualized. The second level is parallel to the first, but 20 mm higher, passing through the bodies of the lateral ventricles. The third level is 20 mm above the second, passing through the supraventricular tissues. In this way all three major supratentorial vascular distributions (anterior, middle, and posterior cerebral) are visualized. If the clinical question includes posterior fossa disease, the lowest level passes through the midportion of the fourth ventricle, the second is at the level of the basal ganglia, and the third is at the level of the bodies of the lateral ventricles.

A double study may be obtained if an acetazolamide (Diamox) study is performed as a challenge test for evaluating vascular reserves in the presence of apparent chronic ischemia; both before and during balloon inflation for temporary occlusion of the internal carotid artery as part of the BTO procedure; or if there are physiological manipulations during xenon inhalation, such as hyperventilation to decrease the partial pressure of $CO_2$, or manipulation of blood pressure. Approximately 15 minutes between the two xenon studies is allowed for a decrease in the concentration of intrapulmonary and intracerebral xenon.

The difficulties with the procedure are primarily related to patient movement. Thirty-three percent xenon produces a "drunk" sensation in most people, causing them to drift into sleep, leading to movement that degrades the quality of the scan. Some people decrease their respiratory rate towards the end of the study, so that it is important to monitor them closely and coach them to continue breathing throughout the 4+ minutes of scanning. A reasonable CBF determination may be obtained in approximately 2.5 minutes, with fewer data points on the flow curves, and fewer levels require a shorter evaluation. This is not a "tech procedure," but a physician or trained physician's assistant should perform the study.

## Case Material

### *Acute Stroke*

The xenon-CT CBF technique is superb for demonstrating an acute stroke within minutes after its occurrence. A plain CT scan is obtained to exclude intracranial hemorrhage as a cause of the stroke. A two- to three-level CBF study is obtained, emphasizing the cerebrovascular distributions that might produce the clinical symptoms. If the patient is intubated, the procedure is performed by connecting the xenon inhalation apparatus to the endotracheal tube. If the patient is not intubated, cooperation is essential but difficult because of the compromised neurological status. Here one or two levels of study may be easier to perform, because of the shorter study duration and lesser need for perfect cooperation.

Figure 1 illustrates a 70-year-old male who acutely presented with symptoms of a brain stem stroke. It is well known that a CT scan is not abnormal for at least 24 hours after acute stroke. In Figure 1, *A,* obtained within hours after the onset of symptoms, the top figure (routine CT scan) demonstrates diffuse cerebral volume loss in this older individual, with the bottom portion (the blood flow map at the same level) illustrating markedly decreased flows to the brain stem and cerebellum, indicative of basilar artery thrombosis. Five days later, the routine CT scan on a repeat study demonstrates classical hypodensity of infarction (Fig. 1, *B*), along with the markedly decreased flows to the brain stem and the cerebellum. The initial CBF study immediately after the acute occlusion accurately predicted the extent of infarction.

### *Chronic Ischemia*

CBF analysis may be of help in differentiating cerebral ischemia from other neurological disorders such as Alzheimer's disease. This may help in the consideration of a flow augmentation procedure, such as carotid endarterectomy if there is cervical carotid stenosis, or the rare extracranial-to-intracranial (EC/IC) bypass procedure in selected patients with total carotid occlusion. Decreased flow may be on the basis of decreased need by a previously injured tissue, such as injury secondary to previous stroke or to other diseases such as Alzheimer's disease, or may be secondary to decreased vascular supply. This differentiation must be made by a challenge test. Before any xenon procedure, a sequential CT scan of 10 mm thick sections helps to localize the area of questionable abnormality. A three-level xenon-CT study is

A

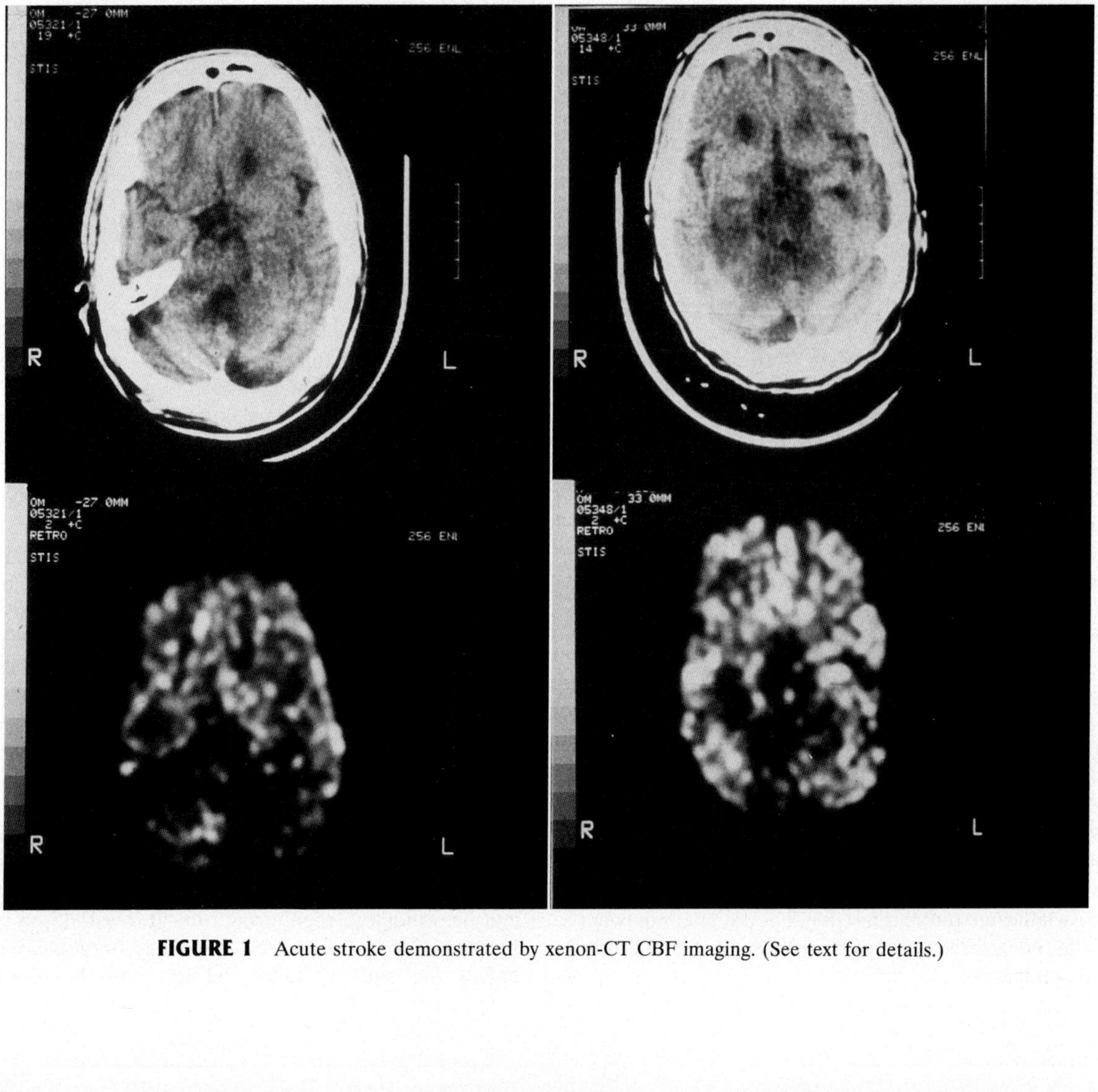


B

**FIGURE 1** Acute stroke demonstrated by xenon-CT CBF imaging. (See text for details.)

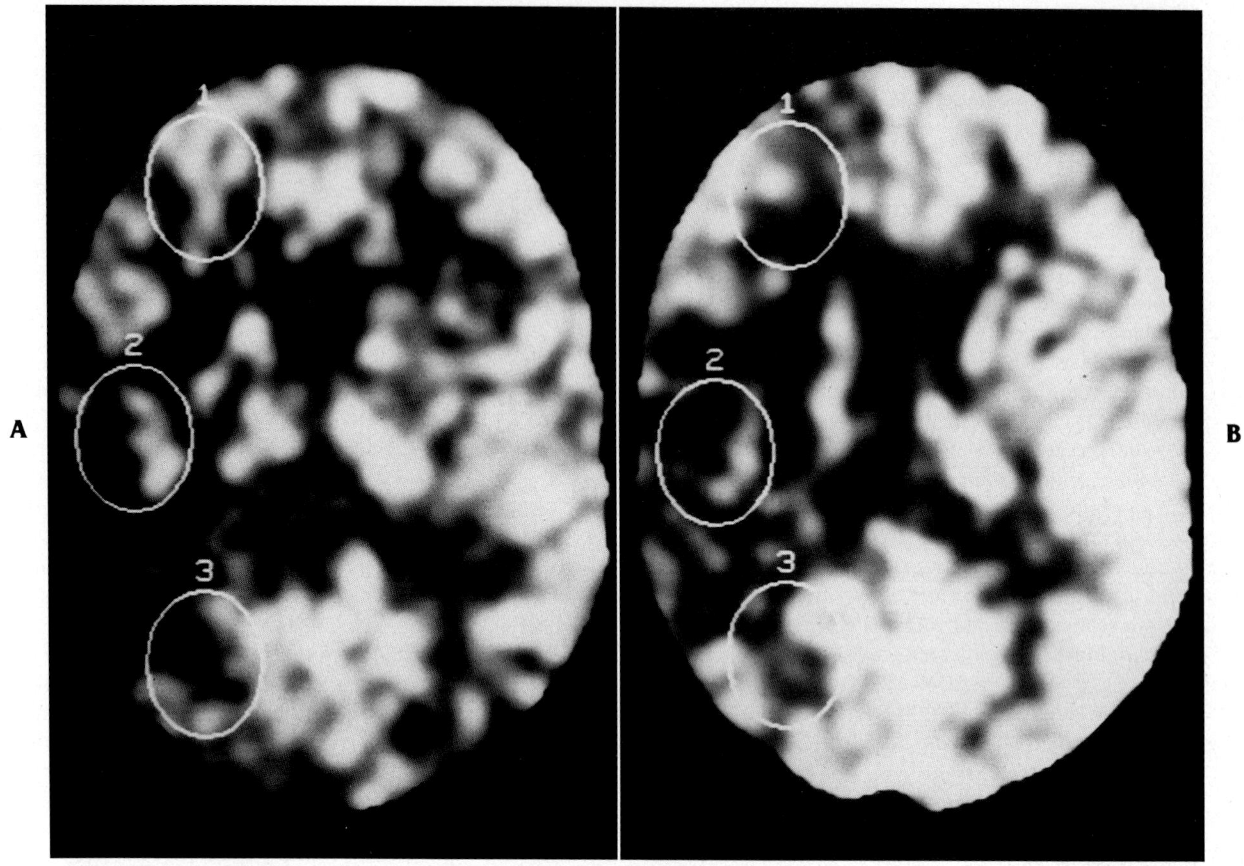


**FIGURE 2** Chronic ischemia demonstrated by xenon-CT CBF imaging. (See text for details.)

performed both on the basis of this scan and the clinical considerations. After waiting approximately 15 minutes, 1.0 g of Diamox is administered intravenously, with repeat scanning during xenon inhalation at the same three levels. Diamox acts as a vasodilator; those areas showing increased CBF on the challenge test relative to the baseline xenon study have vascular reserves that are not being used.

Figure 2 is indicative of the ability of the xenon-CT technique to determine the need for an endarterectomy. A 65-year-old male had had a previous right carotid occlusion with secondary middle cerebral distribution infarction. There was a 70 percent stenosis of the left carotid artery, and confusing symptoms of intermittent left arm and leg weakness on the side of stenosis. The pre-Diamox study (Fig. 2, *A*) shows flows in the right frontal region (ROI Box 1) of 41 ml per 100 g per minute; ROI Box 2 of 28; ROI Box 3 of 34. This scan is at the level of the bodies of the lateral ventricles. The study after Diamox injection (Fig. 2, *B*) shows ROI Box 1 measuring 30, ROI Box 2 of 23, and ROI Box 3 of 40. The increased flows in ROI Box 3 are indicative of the ability of the vessels to this region to dilate, producing increased flows. There is little change in ROI Box 2 because of the previous stroke. However, there is a paradoxical decrease in flows to the right frontal region with Diamox. In our experience such paradoxical flows have always indicated future infarction. The patient underwent left carotid endarterectomy, with reversal of the episodic left-sided hemiparesis.

## *CBF Analysis after Temporary Balloon Occlusion*

If a carotid artery is to be sacrificed, such as permanent occlusion for a giant unclippable intracranial aneurysm or as part of a skull base tumor resection, the carotid artery may be temporarily occluded by a balloon to determine if the patient can tolerate such carotid sacrifice. Although 10 percent of patients show temporary neurological deficit on the table during this test occlusion, the majority of patients do not have any symptoms. However, the degree of flow to the hemisphere in question is unknown. Since neuronal function does not decrease until flows drop as low as 18 ml per 100 g per minute, the patient could still have low flows and yet not have symptoms. Such low flow may put the patient at risk for postoperative infarction if cardiac output or blood pressure were to be transiently decreased. Hence I feel that it is essential to know the true CBF during balloon test occlusion in order to evaluate the risk to the patient of permanent occlusion. This risk may necessitate a temporary bypass during surgery, the placement of a vein graft at the time of surgery, or an EC/IC bypass.

The procedure begins in the angiographic suite, with the placement of a nonreleasable balloon in the internal carotid artery, inflation of the balloon during systemic heparinization, and neurological monitoring for at least 15 minutes. If symptoms occur, such as hemiparesis or decreased verbal ability, the patient "fails" the test and the procedure is

A

B

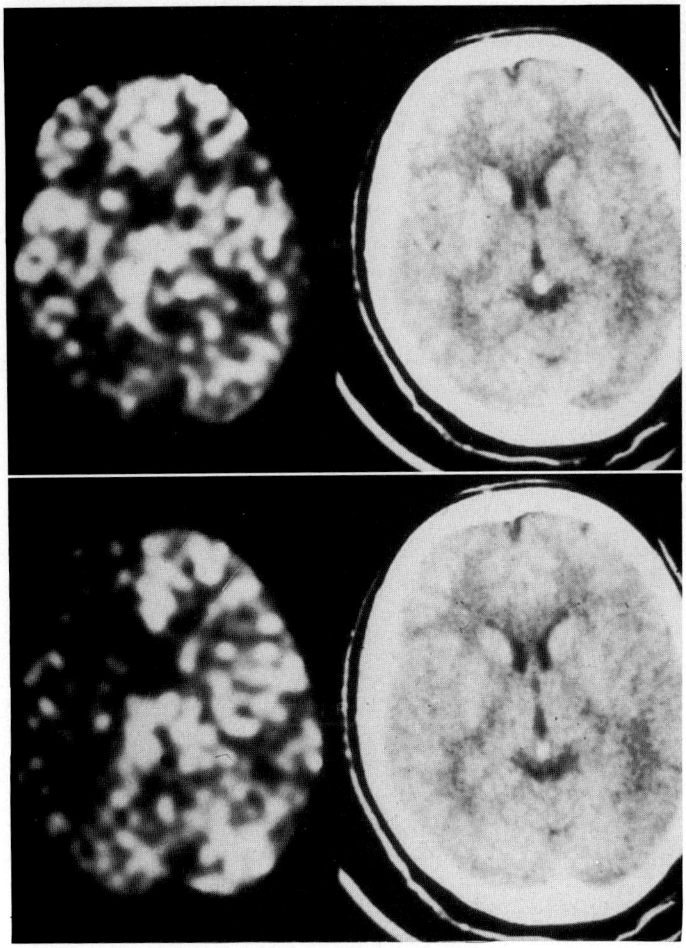

**FIGURE 3** CBF analysis after temporary balloon occlusion. (See text for details.)

terminated. If the patient passes the test, the balloon is deflated after recording the volume necessary for total occlusion as determined fluoroscopically with an injection of a contrast agent. The balloon is left in place, the patient moved to the CT scanning suite, the balloon reinflated, and a xenon-CT CBF procedure performed at two to three levels. The balloon is then deflated, the patient allowed to exhale all of the xenon over 15 minutes, and the procedure is repeated with the balloon deflated. I perform the balloon inflation portion of the procedure first in case the patient tires, since the balloon inflation portion of the procedure is the more important of the two.

In Figure 3, *A,* the CBF map at the level of the frontal horns with the balloon deflated demonstrates slight asymmetry in the parietotemporal regions, but otherwise the CBF map is unremarkable. However, after balloon inflation, there is a marked decrease in the flows to the right middle cerebral distribution (Fig. 3, *B*). These flows, however, are at the levels of 22 ml per 100 g per minute, and the patient is asymptomatic. Transient hypotension postoperatively following right carotid occlusion may have precipitated right-sided hemispheric infarction. The surgeon elected to perform a vein bypass graft at the time of skull base surgery to prevent such infarct. In our experience flows less than 30 ml per 100 g per minute during balloon inflation suggest the possiblity of complications from permanent carotid occlusion and the need for flow augmentation.

### *Cerebral Ischemia from Vasospasm after Subarachnoid Hemorrhage*

A high level of morbidity and/or mortality following subarachnoid hemorrhage is attributed to vasospasm producing cerebral infarction. This has led to earlier aneurysm clipping and the development of drugs to decrease cerebral vasospasm. However, if the patient presents a number of days after hemorrhage, when vasospasm is occurring, the surgeon may opt to wait for a later time for aneurysm clipping. The surgeon does not wish to operate in the face of vasospasm and cerebral ischemia, since manipulation of the vasculature only increases that vasospasm. Cerebral angiography has traditionally been performed to make sure vasospasm is not present perioperatively. However, the real question is whether there is decreased flow to the parenchyma. In addition, preoperative symptoms may be difficult to evaluate, with cerebral vasospasm being one of many considerations. Therefore CBF analysis may be of value in these clinical contexts.

In Figure 4 a patient presented 7 days following subarachnoid hemorrhage. On the left a low-density focus in the right frontotemporal region was indicative of cerebral ischemia, with an ROI in that region of the CBF map measuring 32 ml per 100 g per minute. The more normal appearing tissues on the routine CT scan posterior to this, however, actually had flows of 26 and 29 ml per 100 g. These flows indicated significant diffuse vasospasm, and surgery was delayed until the patient had better CBF. The right side of the illustration demonstrates

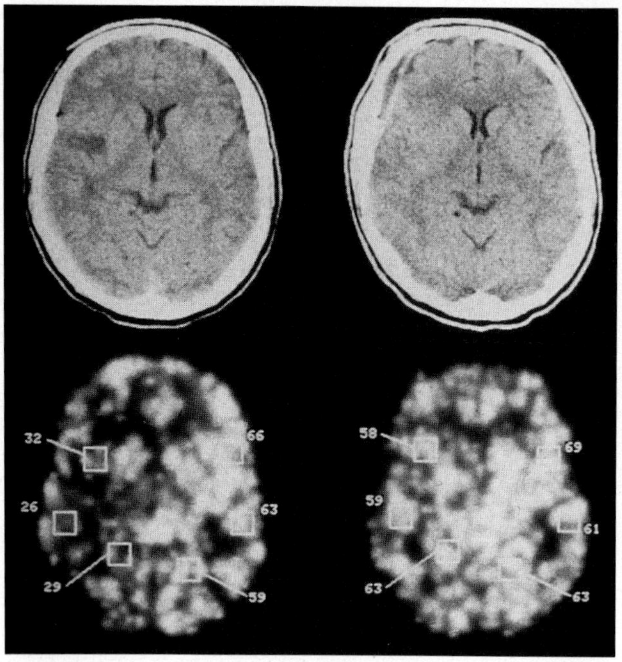


**FIGURE 4** Xenon-CT CBF imaging after subarachnoid hemorrhage. (See text for details.)

the postoperative status, with a small extra-axial collection in the right frontal region, and CBF to the right hemisphere between 58 and 63 ml per 100 g per minute. The patient was asymptomatic. The use of xenon-CT CBF analysis was thought to be helpful for determining the appropriate timing of the aneurysm clipping.

### *CBF Analysis after Trauma*

Significant closed-head injury is frequently treated by intubation and hyperventilation to decrease CBV in an attempt to decrease cerebral swelling. The decrease in the $P_{CO_2}$ with hyperventilation also leads to decreased CBF, sometimes to levels of relative ischemia. CBF analysis may therefore be of value in monitoring the effect of the hyperventilation therapy, possibly preventing the lowering of CBF to critical levels.

In addition, CBF analysis may be of help in evaluating the status of cerebrovascular autoregulation. This can be evaluated by performing the CBF study at two different carbon dioxide levels. The first is performed with the patient's respirator set at the level used for treatment, with the $P_{CO_2}$ level monitored. The respirator may then be increased in rate so that $P_{CO_2}$ is lower by 10 torr. I have seen areas of injured tissues that have lost their autoregulation paradoxically swell when the rest of the brain contracts its CBV following such $P_{CO_2}$ manipulation. This knowledge may prevent overuse of hyperventilation in a given patient.

## Discussion

The techniques described are the most important clinical applications of xenon-CT CBF imaging at this time. Validation of acute cerebrovascular occlusion and secondary ischemia as a cause of symptoms will be necessary as thrombolytic drugs are developed for treatment of acute stroke. Flow augmentation procedures may find their way back into the surgical approach as the subset of patients with true low-flow states are defined with techniques that measure CBF.

## Suggested Reading

Darby JM, Yonas H, Marion DW, Latchaw RE. Local "inverse steal" induced by hyperventilation in head injury. Neurosurgery 1988; 23:84–88.

Darby JM, Yonas H, Pentheny S, Marion D. Intracranial pressure response to stable xenon inhalation in patients with head injury. Surg Neurol 1989; 32:343–345.

Gur D, Yonas H, Jackson DL, et al. Simultaneous measurements of cerebral blood flow by the xenon/CT method and the microsphere method: A comparison. Invest Radiol 1985; 20:672–677.

Hughes RL, Yonas H, Gur D, Latchaw RE. Stable xenon-enhanced CT in the first eight hours of cerebral infarction. Stroke 1987; 18:283–287.

Latchaw RE, Yonas H, Darby JM, et al. Xenon/CT cerebral blood flow determination following cranial trauma. Acta Radiol 1986; 369(Suppl):370–373.

Latchaw RE, Yonas H, Pentheny S, Gur D. Adverse reactions to xenon-enhanced CT cerebral blood flow determination. Radiology 1987; 163:251–254.

Rogg J, Rutigliano M, Yonas H, et al. The acetazolamide challenge: Imaging techniques designed to evaluate cerebral blood flow reserve. Am J Neuroradiol 1989; 10:803–810.

Yonas H. Cerebral blood flow measurement with stable xenon-enhanced computed tomography. New York: Raven Press, 1992.

Yonas H, Good WF, Gur D, et al. Mapping cerebral blood flow by xenon-enhanced computed tomography: Clinical experience. Radiology 1984; 152:425–442.

Yonas H, Gur D, Latchaw RE, Wolfson SK. Xenon computed tomographic blood flow mapping. In: Wood J, ed. Cerebral blood flow: Physiologic and clinical aspects. New York: McGraw-Hill, 1987:220.

# CT Evaluation of Closed Head Injury

*STUART E. MIRVIS, M.D. · AIZIK L. WOLF, M.D.*
*JAMES G. SMIRNIOTOPOULOS, M.D.*

Closed head injury (CHI) resulting from blunt impact constitutes a major source of morbidity and mortality among young adults. In the United States, more than 250,000 patients a year require emergency medical attention for craniocerebral trauma, usually sustained in vehicular accidents. The appropriate management of these individuals depends on rapid and accurate triage that ascertains the significance of the injury and the most suitable clinical course of action. In our experience the evaluation of possible intracranial injury takes priority over other injuries in the multitrauma patient, once the patient's vital signs are stabilized. The initial clinical assessment of neurologic function can be measured by rapid determination of the Glasgow Coma Score, pupillary responses, oculocephalic reflex, and gross motor response to painful stimulation. Although the initial clinical assessment is important in documenting potential or probable central nervous system injury, it cannot precisely determine the nature and extent of such injury and thus guide appropriate management. In dealing with patients sustaining CHI, the foremost consideration is given to deciding between surgical intervention, medical management, or observation. Although a number of imaging studies are available to evaluate head injury, computed tomographic (CT) scanning continues to provide the most rapid, accurate, and cost-effective method upon which to base initial management decisions.

## Comparison of CT with Other Modalities

CT has a long, well-established record of diagnostic accuracy in assessing CHI, but is not the only imaging modality that can be used. In recent years many institutions have abandoned skull radiography in head trauma evaluation. Numerous studies indicate that the presence of a skull fracture does not reliably predict intracranial injury, nor does the absence of calvarial fracture exclude significant intracranial pathology. Despite these observations, many institutions continue to use skull radiography routinely in the assessment of the trauma patient. We have virtually abandoned skull radiography at the University of Maryland Shock-Trauma Center for the assessment of adult head trauma, because of its inaccuracy and limited sensitivity. On occasion skull radiographs are used to document the presence and location of foreign bodies such as ballistic fragments. In our experience skull radiography may be more sensitive than CT to the presence of linear nondepressed skull fractures, but the status of the intracranial tissues is of far greater significance than the presence or absence of a linear skull fracture. Nonetheless, the lateral digital scout radiograph of the skull that accompanies the CT study should be carefully inspected, since skull fractures crossing the temporal and parietal regions are frequently observed on this image. Use of skull radiography in patients with a high clinical likelihood of cerebral injury is in most circumstances unwarranted and should never delay more appropriate CT evaluation.

Magnetic resonance imaging (MRI) has also been shown to be valuable in diagnosing CHI. It is more accurate than CT in detection of cerebral contusions, especially those with minimal bleeding, so-called nonhemorrhagic contusions; thin extra-axial hematomas adjacent to bone; diffuse axonal shearing injuries (DAIs); and brain stem injury (Figs. 1, 2, 3). MRI, however, is not as accurate in diagnosing subtle, and more often significant, lesions such as skull base fractures; acute hemorrhage, particularly in the subarachnoid space; and minimal pneumocephalus. MRI may also be difficult to safely perform in the critically ill patient with numerous life-support systems and physiologic monitors. MRI is generally far slower than CT imaging in most centers and has not been shown to be as accurate in evaluating other injured tissues including osseous structures such as the spine, face, and pelvis, as well as the abdominal viscera. CT can rapidly assess injury to all these

A

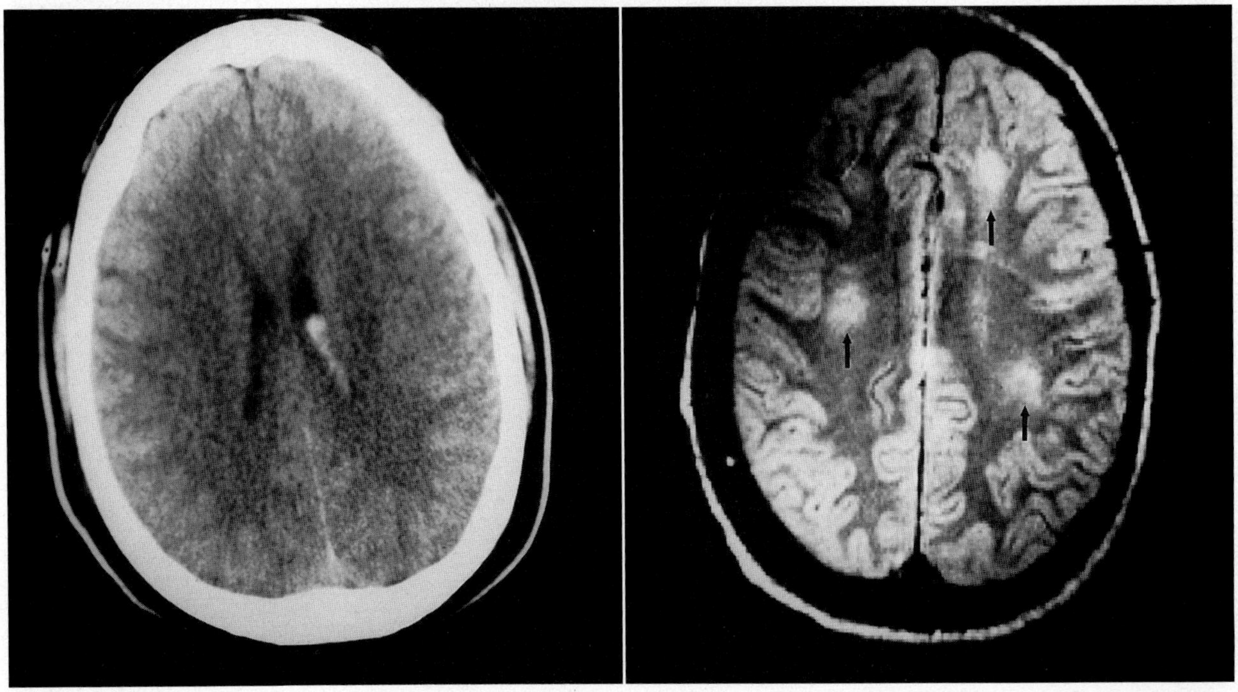

B

**FIGURE 1** White matter contusions. *A,* Axial CT image obtained in an obtunded middle-aged male after blunt head trauma reveals some blood in the left lateral ventricle, but no parenchymal contusion. *B,* Axial T2-weighted MR image acquired at a slightly more rostral level shows three foci of increased signal, representing white matter contusions *(arrows),* which were not detected by CT. (From Smirniotopoulos JG, Mirvis SE, Wolf AL. Imaging of craniocerebral trauma. In: Mirvis SE, Young JWR, eds. Imaging in Trauma and Critical Care. Baltimore: Williams & Wilkins, 1992; with permission.)

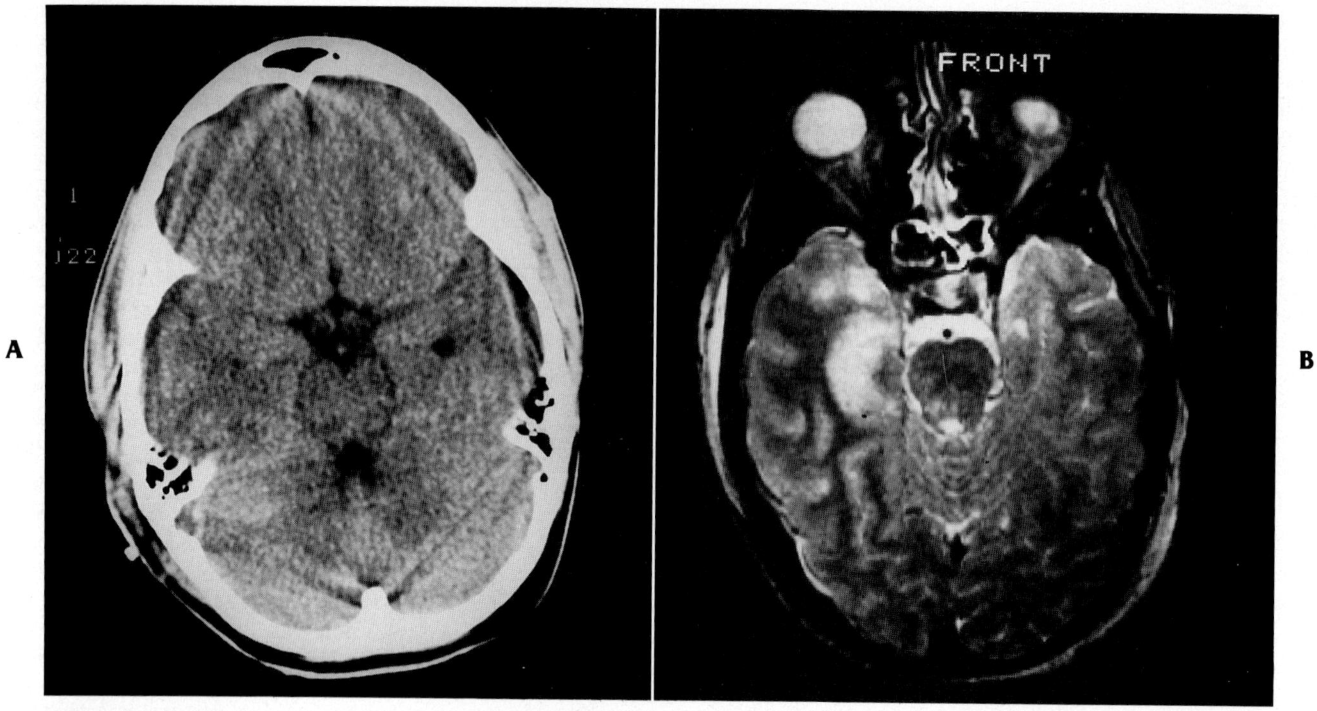


**FIGURE 2** Brain stem and temporal lobe contusion. *A,* Admission cranial CT study obtained in a 15-year-old female after a motor vehicle accident did not indicate evidence of injury, even though the patient was in coma. *B,* T2-weighted MRI study (2500/90) shows increased signal (edema) in the right medial temporal lobe and right brainstem. (From Smirniotopoulos JG, Mirvis SE, Wolf AL. Imaging of craniocerebral trauma. In: Mirvis SE, Young JWR, eds. Imaging in Trauma and Critical Care. Baltimore: Williams & Wilkins, 1992; with permission.)

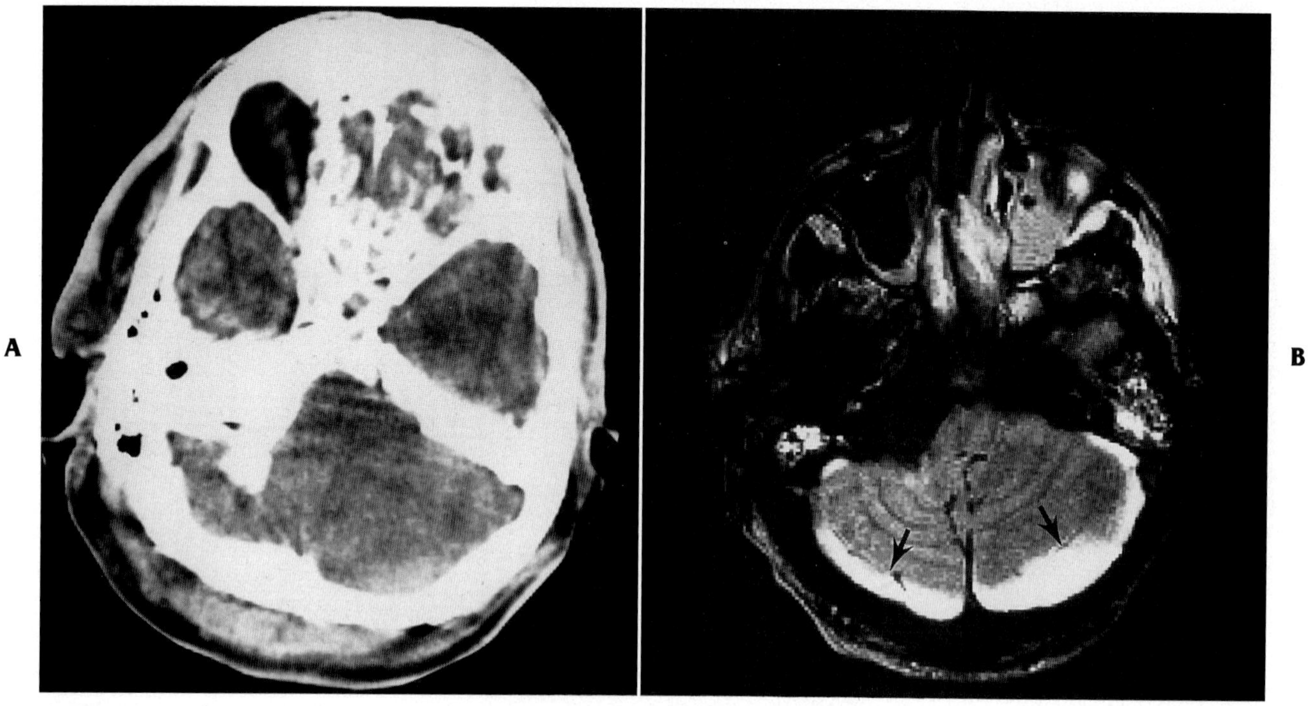

**FIGURE 3** Infratentorial subdural hematoma. *A,* Axial CT image obtained after head trauma in a 53-year-old man was initially interpreted as normal intracranially. *B,* Because of persistent neurologic symptoms, an MRI study was performed and revealed bilateral infratentorial subdural hematomas *(arrows).* Incidentally observed was left maxillary sinus fluid. (From Smirniotopoulos JG, Mirvis SE, Wolf AL. Imaging of craniocerebral trauma. In: Mirvis SE, Young JWR, eds. Imaging in Trauma and Critical Care. Baltimore: Williams & Wilkins, 1992; with permission.)

body regions that are traumatized frequently and concurrently with CHI.

In our center we selectively use cranial MRI to evaluate patients whose CT scans do not adequately explain their neurologic level of function, searching primarily for brain stem injury, DAIs, or dural sinus thrombosis (Fig. 4). On occasion we have used MRI to clarify suspected CT findings, such as thin extra-axial hematomas that lie parallel to the axial plane and are adjacent to bone (i.e., vertex or infratemporal) (Fig. 5).

Some authors have advocated routine MRI before discharge in all patients sustaining significant head injury to document all injuries. We do not concur with this suggestion and await efficacy studies of this approach relating cost and benefit to the patient.

## Technical Aspects of CT for Acute CHI

Routine CT technique for traumatized patients should include noncontrast evaluation with 8 to 10 mm slice thickness, 8 to 10 mm slice interval, and $512^2$ matrix reconstruction. Fast CT image acquisition, 2 seconds or less, is often required to diminish motion artifact. On occasion thinner CT sections can be used to clarify uncertain findings, such as to distinguish inferior frontal pole contusion from volume averaging with the orbital plates of the frontal bones. As previously noted, although CT is excellent for detecting most major intracranial pathology resulting from head trauma, some skull fractures may be underdiagnosed. It is imperative that all CT scans of the head be reviewed with "bone windows" (center 250 HU, window width 3,000 HU) to improve contrast discrimination between cancellous and cortical bone and thus optimize fracture detection. Despite ideal technique, small, linear, nondisplaced fractures can still be missed as a result of volume averaging, but in our experience such fractures are seldom of clinical significance. At the Maryland Shock-Trauma Center, we routinely obtain an additional set of CT images, termed "subdural windows" (center 60 HU, window width 120 HU). These windows increase contrast between the inner table and any adjacent thin extra-axial collections of clotted blood (Fig. 6).

In patients with suspected basilar skull fractures, i.e., cerebrospinal fluid (CSF) rhinorrhea or otorrhea or cranial nerve deficits (especially involving the optic, auditory, or facial nerves) high-resolution (bone algorithm), thin 1.5 or 2 mm contiguous sections are obtained through the optic or auditory canals in an effort to demonstrate bone impingement. Usually these high-resolution studies are performed *after* the initial baseline CT, if the patient's clinical condition permits. In the presence of posterior fossa signs or symptoms, contiguous 4 or 5 mm sections are acquired through the posterior fossa with a true horizontal orientation (parallel to Reid's baseline).

We seldom perform intravenous contrast-enhanced studies during the initial CT evaluation of the cranium. However, if the history of trauma is vague and another etiology for intracerebral hemorrhage is suspected (such as arteriovenous malformation [AVM] or aneurysm [Fig. 7]), when large quantities of subarachnoid hemorrhage are present without other cerebral injury, or when there is clinical suspicion of carotid artery injury and possible cerebral ischemia (Fig. 8), enhanced studies are performed.

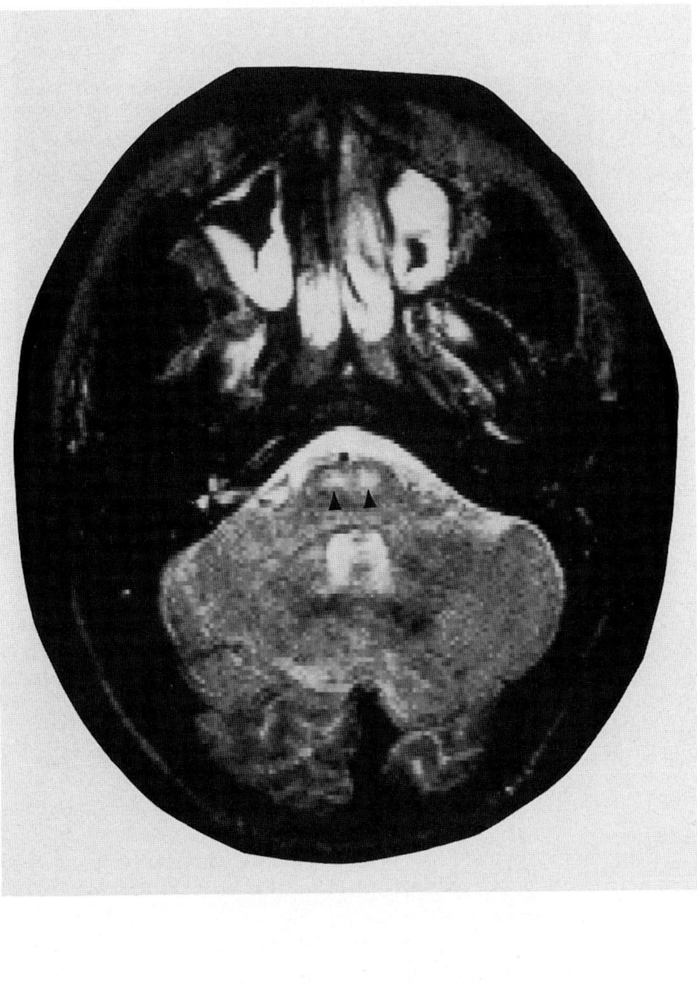

**FIGURE 4** MRI of brain stem contusion. This axial image obtained through the midpons in a young woman with complete motor paralysis reveals bilateral high signal contusions in the anterior pons *(arrowheads),* accounting for the motor deficit. Maxillary sinus fluid was incidentally noted. (From Smirniotopoulos JG, Mirvis SE, Wolf AL. Imaging of craniocerebral trauma. In: Mirvis SE, Young JWR, eds. Imaging in Trauma and Critical Care. Baltimore: Williams & Wilkins, 1992; with permission.)

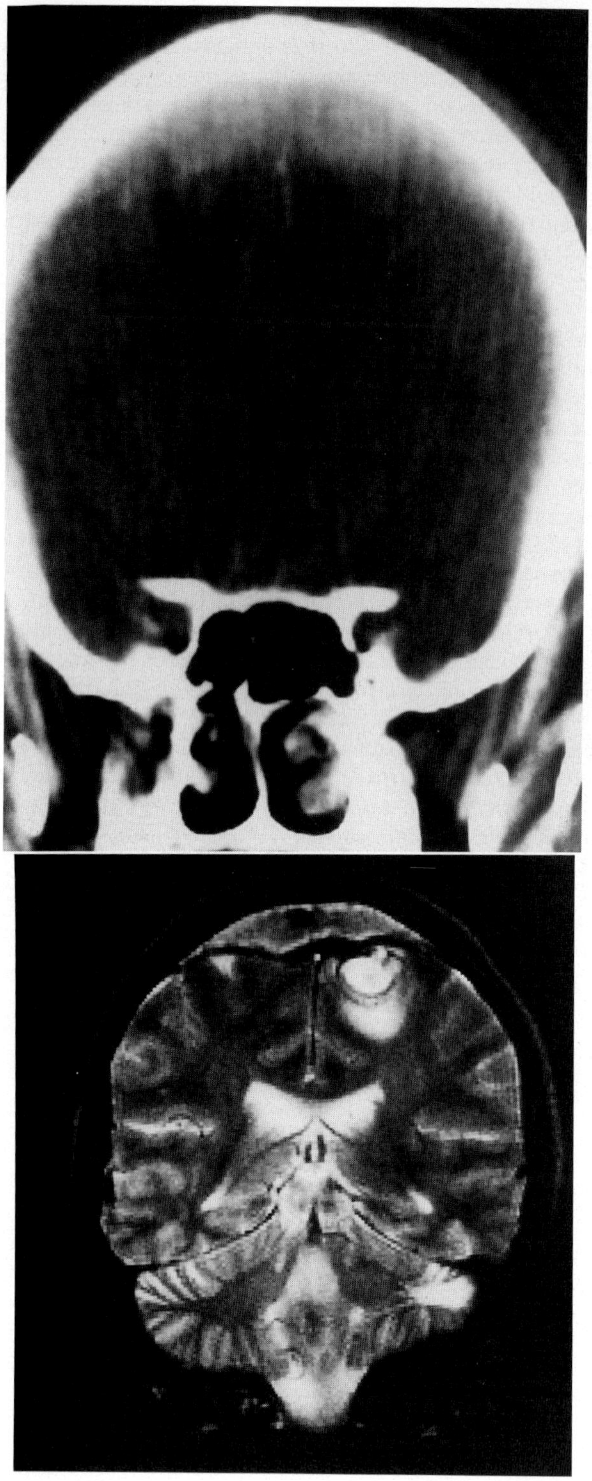

A

B

**FIGURE 5** Vertex epidural hematoma. *A,* Coronal CT image demonstrates a high-density collection at the skull vertex, but its precise localization was unclear. *B,* Coronal T2-weighted image reveals the collection of blood to be extradural. The more intense outer rim indicates the paramagnetic effect of extracellular methemoglobin, whereas the central lower signal portion represents hemoglobin in intact red cells. A hematoma surrounded by a low signal hemosiderin ring and adjacent cerebral edema was also observed in the left medial parietal lobe. (From Smirniotopoulos JG, Mirvis SE, Wolf AL. Imaging of craniocerebral trauma. In: Mirvis SE, Young JWR, eds. Imaging in Trauma and Critical Care. Baltimore: Williams & Wilkins, 1992; with permission.)

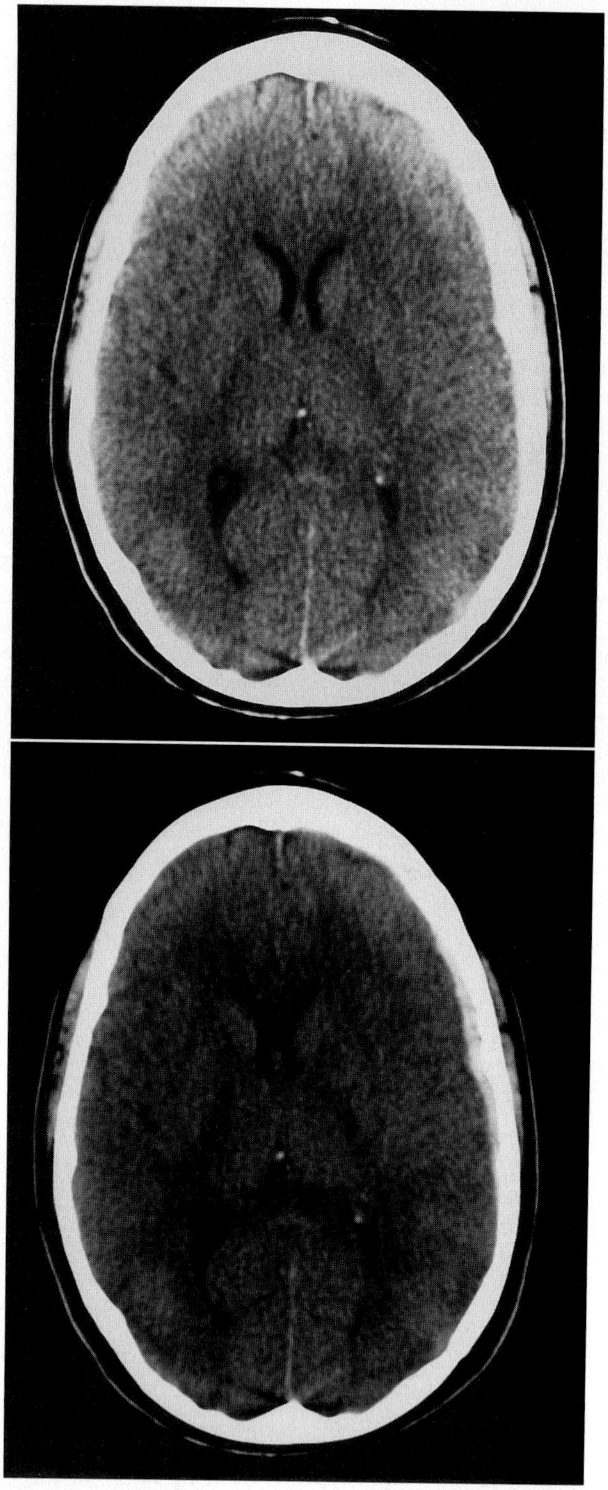

A

B

**FIGURE 6** Subdural windows. *A,* Admission CT study after blunt trauma shows no definite lesion. *B,* Photography in extended windows (center 60 HU, window width 120 HU) shows small left posterior frontoparietal SDH, which can be identified retrospectively in the routine windows for brain (center 35 HU, window width 80 HU).

A B C

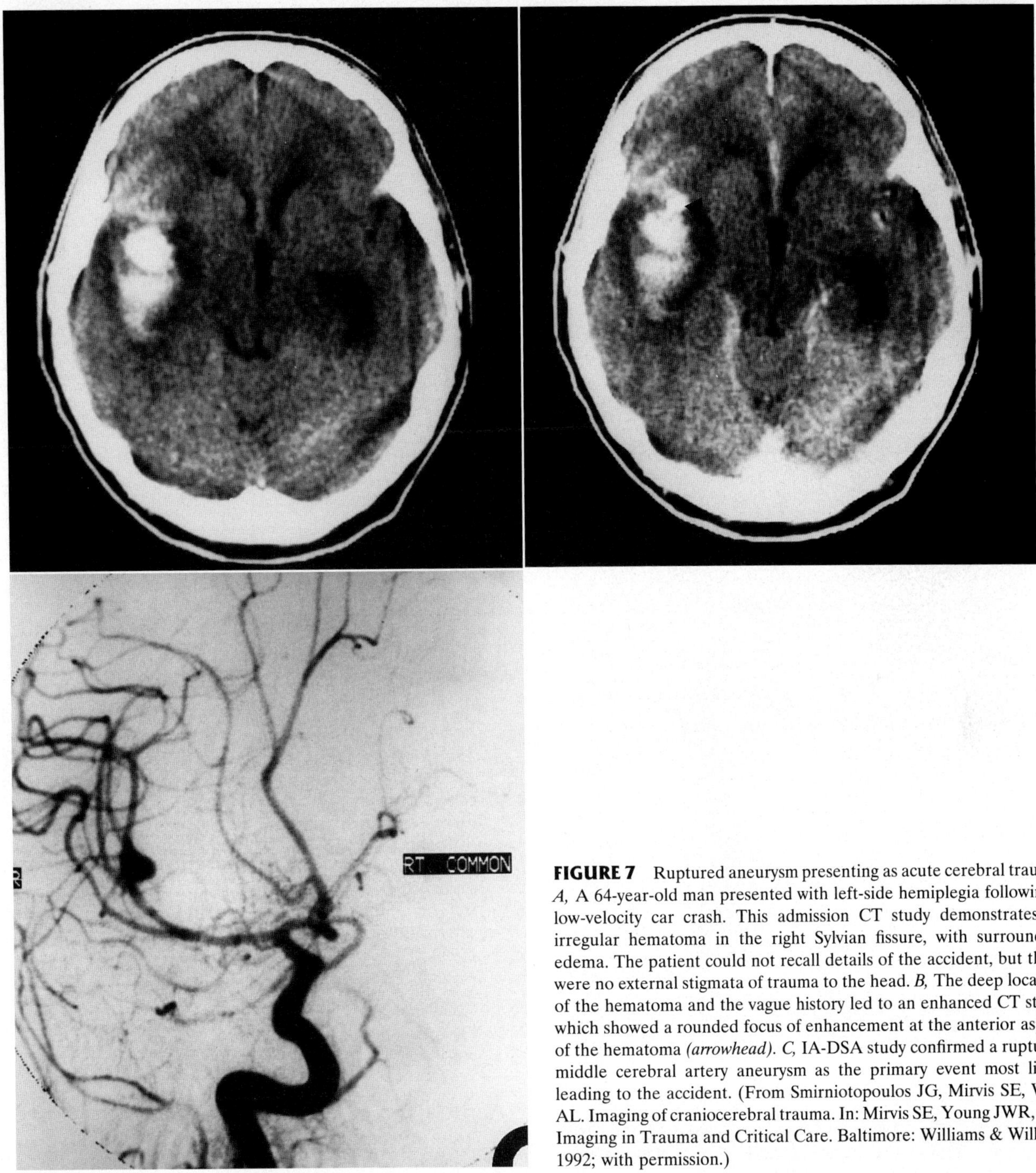


**FIGURE 7** Ruptured aneurysm presenting as acute cerebral trauma. *A,* A 64-year-old man presented with left-side hemiplegia following a low-velocity car crash. This admission CT study demonstrates an irregular hematoma in the right Sylvian fissure, with surrounding edema. The patient could not recall details of the accident, but there were no external stigmata of trauma to the head. *B,* The deep location of the hematoma and the vague history led to an enhanced CT study, which showed a rounded focus of enhancement at the anterior aspect of the hematoma *(arrowhead)*. *C,* IA-DSA study confirmed a ruptured middle cerebral artery aneurysm as the primary event most likely leading to the accident. (From Smirniotopoulos JG, Mirvis SE, Wolf AL. Imaging of craniocerebral trauma. In: Mirvis SE, Young JWR, eds. Imaging in Trauma and Critical Care. Baltimore: Williams & Wilkins, 1992; with permission.)

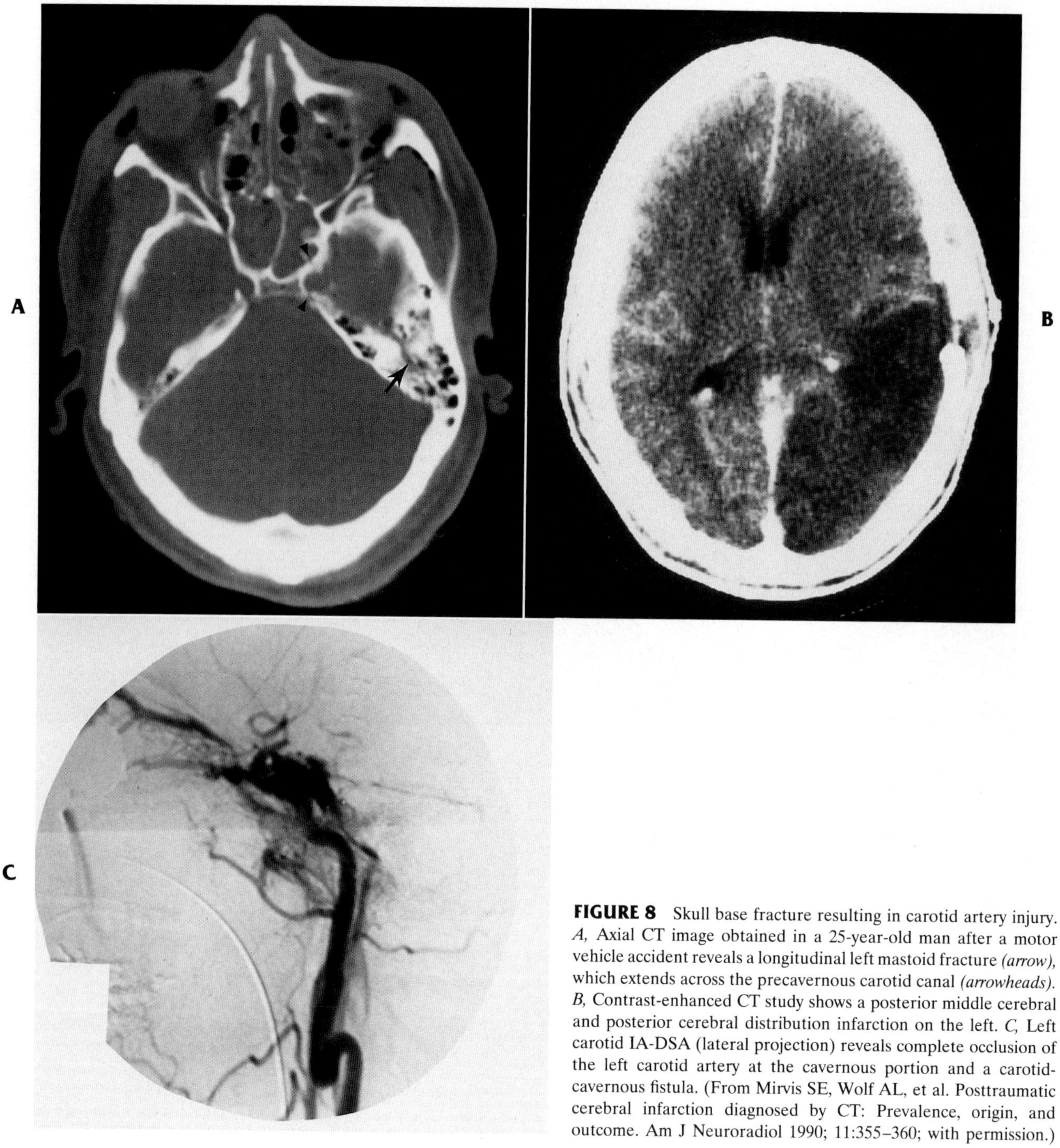


**FIGURE 8** Skull base fracture resulting in carotid artery injury. *A,* Axial CT image obtained in a 25-year-old man after a motor vehicle accident reveals a longitudinal left mastoid fracture *(arrow),* which extends across the precavernous carotid canal *(arrowheads). B,* Contrast-enhanced CT study shows a posterior middle cerebral and posterior cerebral distribution infarction on the left. *C,* Left carotid IA-DSA (lateral projection) reveals complete occlusion of the left carotid artery at the cavernous portion and a carotid-cavernous fistula. (From Mirvis SE, Wolf AL, et al. Posttraumatic cerebral infarction diagnosed by CT: Prevalence, origin, and outcome. Am J Neuroradiol 1990; 11:355–360; with permission.)

Whenever the cervical spine has not been "cleared" with plain radiography, the patient's neck is not manipulated. Rather the CT gantry is tilted to obtain the appropriate angulation for the cranial evaluation. Appropriate physiologic monitors and resuscitation equipment should always be available in the CT suite. In our center, if CT scans of several body areas are simultaneously requested, the head study is always performed first to exclude a life-threatening lesion and before administration of intravenous contrast material.

## Acute Craniocerebral Trauma

The spectrum of injuries that can occur after CHI is wide and can be organized in various manners. In this discussion we consider injuries that occur as a result of primary impact and are usually observed acutely (Table 1). Table 2 lists the frequency of primary parenchymal injuries from large series and their associated mortality.

Skull fractures can involve the cranial vault or skull base and may be described as displaced, depressed, by pattern, e.g.,

A

B

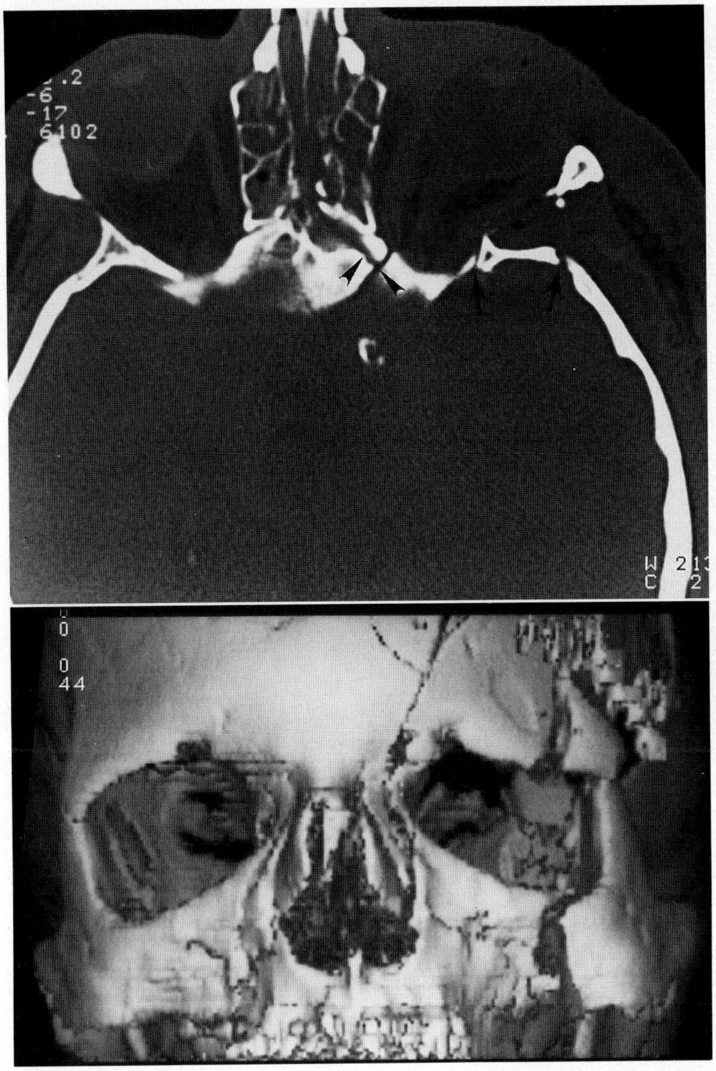

**FIGURE 9** Frontal skull base fracture secondary to lateral impact. *A,* Axial CT image obtained after left lateral impact demonstrates fractures of the left lateral orbital wall, lesser sphenoid wing *(arrowheads),* greater sphenoid wing *(arrows),* and medial orbital wall. *B,* Three-dimensional reformation depicts lateral impact disrupting zygoma (Z), medial, lateral, and superior orbit walls, and displacement of the superior orbital rim. The left frontal bone fracture is noted.

**TABLE 1** Primary Craniocerebral Injuries

| |
|---|
| Skull fractures: cranial vault/skull base |
| Extra-axial hematoma: subdural/epidural |
| Cerebral contusion |
| Cerebral hematoma |
| Diffuse axonal shearing |
| Intraventricular hemorrhage |

**TABLE 2** Incidence of Intracranial Lesions Observed by CT

| Lesion Observed | Incidence | (mortality) |
|---|---|---|
| Epidural hematoma | 5–10% | (18%) |
| Subdural hematoma | 11–18% | (30–90%) |
| Contusion | 15–25% | ... |
| Hematoma | 6–11% | (58%) |
| Intraventricular hemorrhage | 8% | ... |
| Diffuse axonal shearing | 16–68% | ... |

From Smirniotopoulos JG, Mirvis SE, Wolf AL. Imaging of craniocerebral trauma. In Mirvis SE, Young JWR, eds. Imaging in trauma and critical care. Baltimore: Williams & Wilkins, 1992: 23; with permission.

linear, stellate, or eggshell, or as open (with dural laceration) or closed. Depressed fractures do not necessarily warrant surgical reduction unless open or resulting in significant cosmetic deformity. Compound open-depressed fractures should be debrided and elevated with a watertight dural closure to minimize potential infection. The potential for injury to dural sinuses should be considered with depressed fractures overlying these structures. Although no skull fracture pattern in a child is pathognomonic of child abuse, multiple fractures, bilateral fractures, and fractures crossing suture lines should raise one's suspicion of child abuse.

Fractures of the skull base are commonly associated with severe head trauma and can lead to cranial nerve or vascular injury. The cranial nerves are tethered to the dura and bone as they exit through the neural foramina and can be directly traumatized by an adjacent fracture or a compressing hematoma. Skull base fractures typically involve the frontal base, petrous ridge, and/or clivus. Fractures involving the frontal skull base most commonly result from direct impact to the naso-orbital-ethmoid region or supraorbital frontal bone or from lateral impact to the face, producing transversely oriented fractures across the orbital roofs and both greater and lesser sphenoid wings (Fig. 9). Fragments of the orbital plate of the

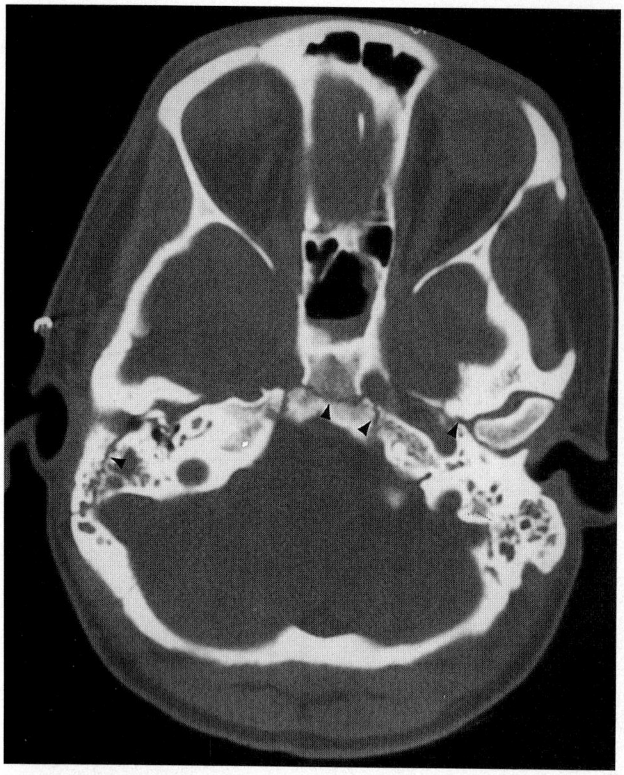

**FIGURE 10** Transverse clivus fracture. This image demonstrates a fracture extending from the right petrous ridge, transversely across the clivus and foramen lacerum, and into the left condylar fossa *(arrowheads)*. (From Smirniotopoulos JG, Mirvis SE, Wolf AL. Imaging of craniocerebral trauma. In: Mirvis SE, Young JWR, eds. Imaging in Trauma and Critical Care. Baltimore: Williams & Wilkins, 1992; with permission.)

frontal bone can be displaced into the orbit, producing damage to the globe or optic nerve (a "blow-in" fracture). Fractures through the petrous portion of the temporal bone can damage cranial nerves, the ossicular chain, otic capsule, and vestibular system. As previously noted, high-resolution, thin-section (1.5 or 2 mm) slices are required to adequately evaluate these structures. Longitudinal-oriented petrous fractures usually result from lateral impact and represent the most frequently encountered pattern (Fig. 10). These fractures have a high incidence of CSF otorrhea and rhinorrhea, and cause a conductive hearing loss, but they affect the facial nerve in only 10 to 20 percent of cases, typically transiently. Transverse petrous fractures are less commonly observed and are completed by extension through the labyrinth, leading to both sensory-neural hearing loss and vestibular dysfunction. Facial nerve injury occurs in 40 to 50 percent of cases of transverse fractures and is more likely permanent. Mixed longitudinal and transverse fracture patterns are common.

Fractures involving the deep skull base, clivus, and anterior sphenoid body have been increasingly recognized with improved CT technology. Longitudinal fractures through the clivus can result from direct occipital impact and have a high association with brain stem injury and death (Fig. 11). Horizontally oriented transclival fractures can result from high-speed lateral impact and are associated with lower mortality, but with increased incidence of cranial nerve deficits and carotid injury (Figs. 10 and 12). Oblique clival fractures can result from anterolateral impacts to the face, over the lateral orbital walls, or from posterolateral impacts to the temporal mastoid region (Fig. 13). The lateral orbital wall and petrous ridge act as buttresses, transmitting the impacting force into the region of the clivus and pituitary fossa, typically producing obliquely oriented fractures with the potential for cranial nerve and carotid-cavernous injury, especially carotid-cavernous fistulas.

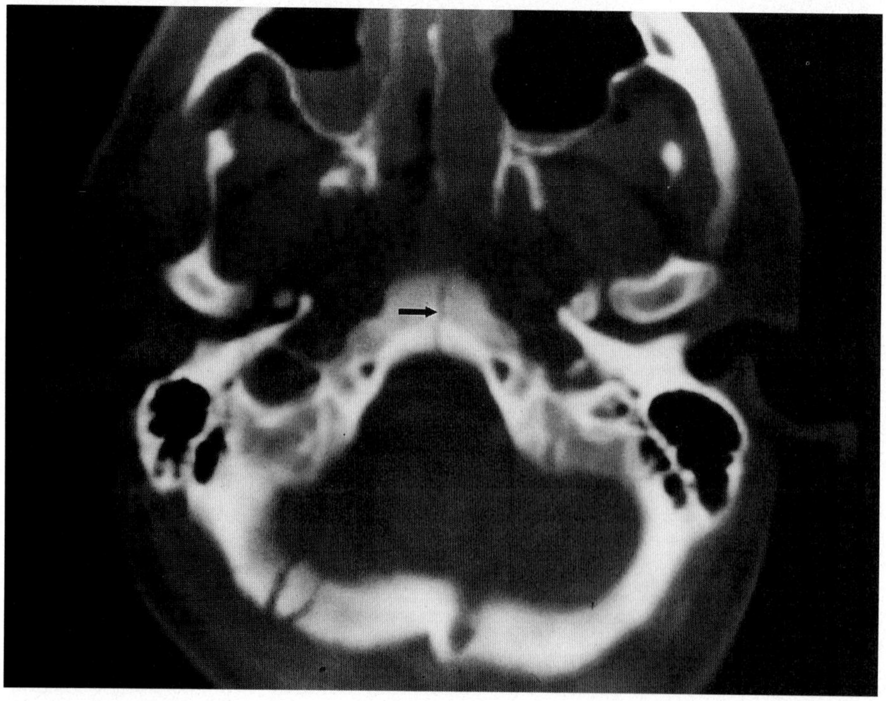

**FIGURE 11** Longitudinal fracture of the clivus. Axial CT image through the skull base was obtained in a 12-year-old child who struck his occiput on the ground after being hit by a car. Linear fractures through the right occipital bone were observed. A linear fracture line extends longitudinally through the clivus *(arrow)*. Other images showed brain stem hemorrhage, and the patient died of this injury. (From Corradino G, Wolf AL, et al. Fractures of the clivus: Classification and clinical features. Neurosurgery 1990; 27:592–596; with permission.)

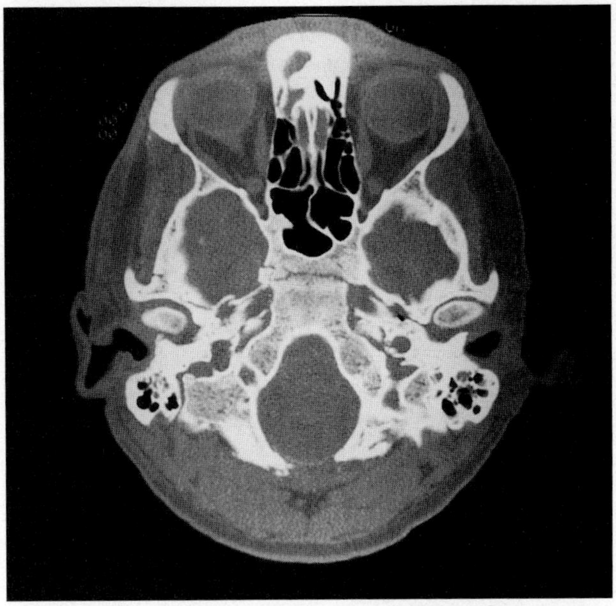

**FIGURE 12** Transverse clival fracture. This image obtained in a male patient who sustained a slow crush injury of the skull shows a deep skull base fracture that extends into the right middle cranial fossa, just anterior to the right glenoid fossa of the mandible, along the right petrous ridge, transversely across the clivus, obliquely across the left middle cranial fossa, and into the left glenoid fossa of the mandibular condyle. The patient sustained bilateral sixth and seventh cranial nerve palsies. (From Corradino G, Wolf AL, et al. Fractures of the clivus: Classification and clinical features. Neurosurgery 1990; 27:592–596; with permission.)

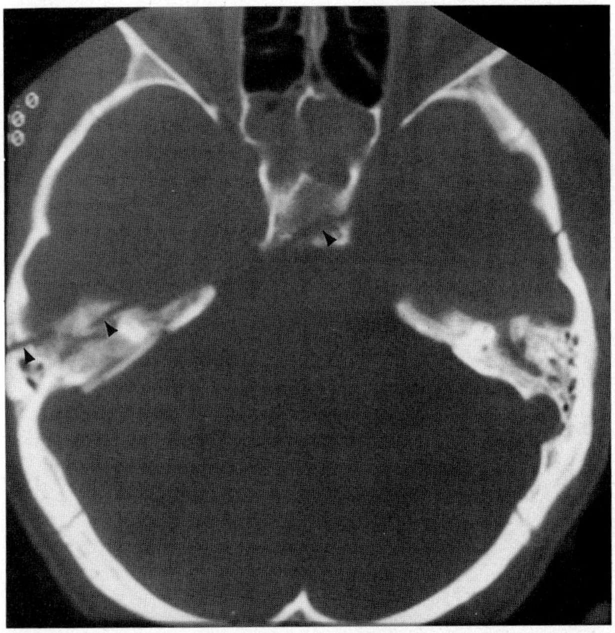

**FIGURE 13** Oblique transclival fracture. This image through the skull base demonstrates a longitudinal right-sided petrous fracture that extends obliquely across the clivus *(arrowheads)*. A left-sided temporal squamosal fracture was noted. The sphenoid sinus was opacified by hemorrhage. (From Smirniotopoulos JG, Mirvis SE, Wolf AL. Imaging of craniocerebral trauma. In: Mirvis SE, Young JWR, eds. Imaging in Trauma and Critical Care. Baltimore: Williams & Wilkins, 1992; with permission.)

## *Intracranial–Extra-axial Injury*

*Epidural hematoma* (EDH) is a relatively uncommon injury occurring in only 1 to 5 percent of major head trauma. Mortality from this injury varies from 7 to 32 percent and is less than that associated with subdural hematomas (SDHs). Patients with EDH have no significant intradural injury in 50 to 63 percent of cases, only one-third exhibit a classic "lucid" interval, and have a high association (>90 percent) with adjacent skull fractures. In children EDH is more likely to occur without an associated skull fracture than in adults, because of elasticity of the developing skull. EDH most commonly results from laceration of a meningeal artery, but can develop from laceration of a dural sinus. By CT, the EDH typically has a biconvex shape with high density (60 to 90 HU) as a result of clotted blood, most often appearing in the middle cranial fossa and lower lateral convexity (Figs. 14 to 17). The margins of the EDH are sharp, because of dissection of the dura from the inner table of the skull and are usually limited by cranial sutures. EDHs can, however, cross the falx and tentorium. Hyperacute EDH may have lower and heterogeneous density ("swirl sign") as a result of incomplete clot formation or mixing of clotted and unclotted blood. Anemia,

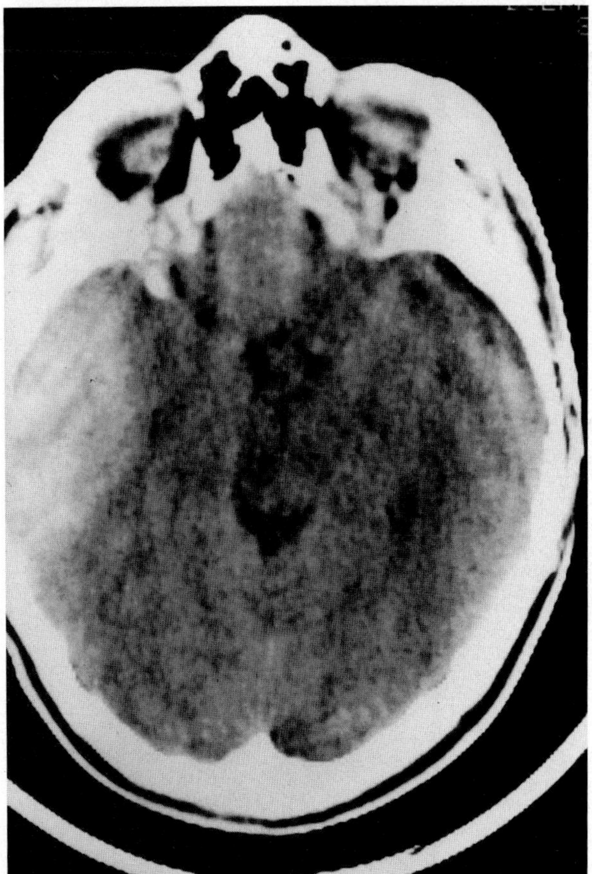

**FIGURE 14** Right-sided temporal EDH. CT image demonstrates a right-sided temporal EDH, producing local medial herniation of the ipsilateral temporal lobe. There was effacement of the ipsilateral perimesencephalic cistern and brain stem distortion. (From Smirniotopoulos JG, Mirvis SE, Wolf AL. Imaging of craniocerebral trauma. In: Mirvis SE, Young JWR, eds. Imaging in Trauma and Critical Care. Baltimore: Williams & Wilkins, 1992; with permission.)

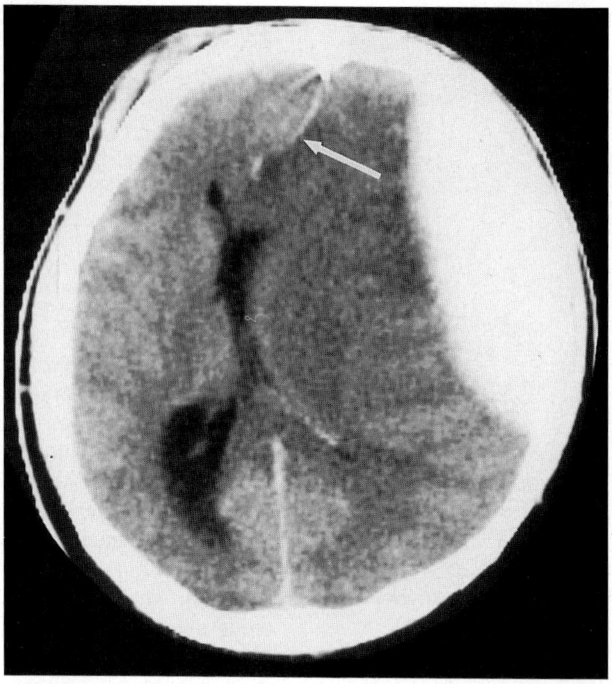

**FIGURE 15** Large left-sided EDH producing subfalcine herniation. CT image reveals an extensive EDH in the left frontoparietal area, producing bowing of the anterior falx *(white arrow)* and marked subfalcine herniation. The right lateral ventricle was obstructed because of the marked shift. (From Mirvis SE, Wolf AL, et al. Posttraumatic cerebral infarction diagnosed by CT: Prevalence, origin, and outcome. Am J Neuroradiol 1990; 11:355–360; with permission.)

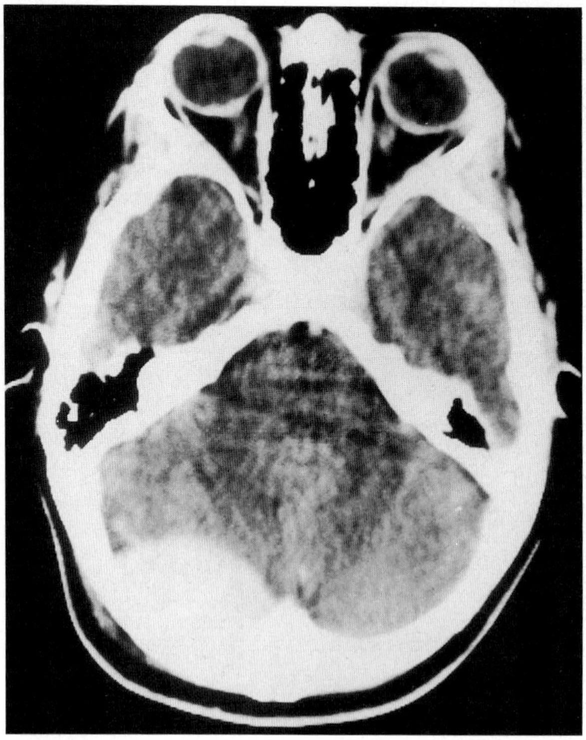

**FIGURE 16** Posterior fossa epidural hematoma. CT image acquired on an 18-year-old woman after a motor vehicle accident shows a focal right-sided posterior fossa EDH, which compresses the fourth ventricle. The patient became increasingly obtunded on the CT table and the scan was stopped after this image. The patient had complete recovery after emergency surgical drainage of the EDH. (From Smirniotopoulos JG, Mirvis SE, Wolf AL. Imaging of craniocerebral trauma. In: Mirvis SE, Young JWR, eds. Imaging in Trauma and Critical Care. Baltimore: Williams & Wilkins, 1992; with permission.)

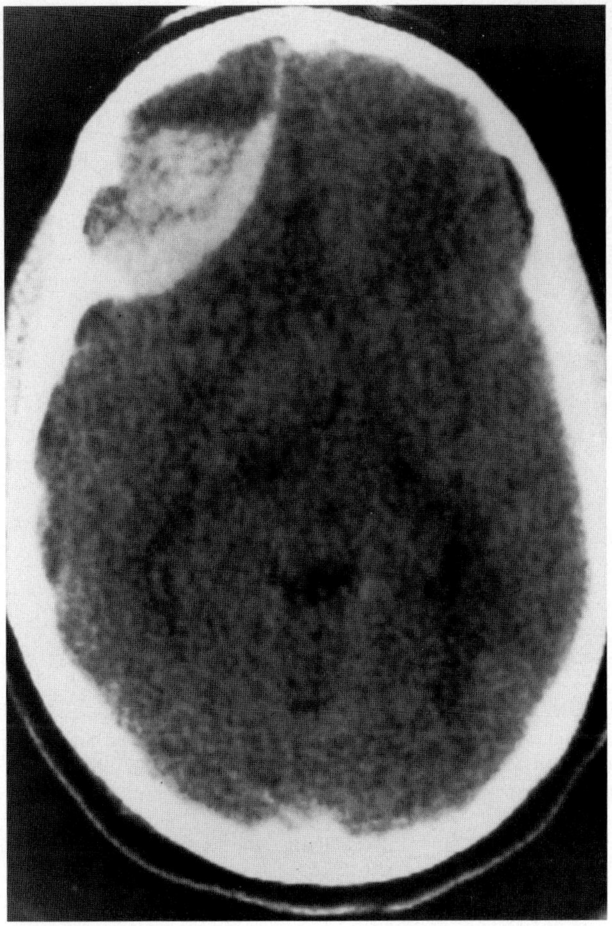

**FIGURE 17** Mixed-attenuation epidural hematoma. A right-sided frontal EDH displays a layering effect as a result of variation in clot formation with well-formed clot, highest attenuation, layering dependently, and unclotted blood on top. Diffuse cerebral edema obscures the ventricular system. (From Smirniotopoulos JG, Mirvis SE, Wolf AL. Imaging of craniocerebral trauma. In: Mirvis SE, Young JWR, eds. Imaging in Trauma and Critical Care. Baltimore: Williams & Wilkins, 1992; with permission.)

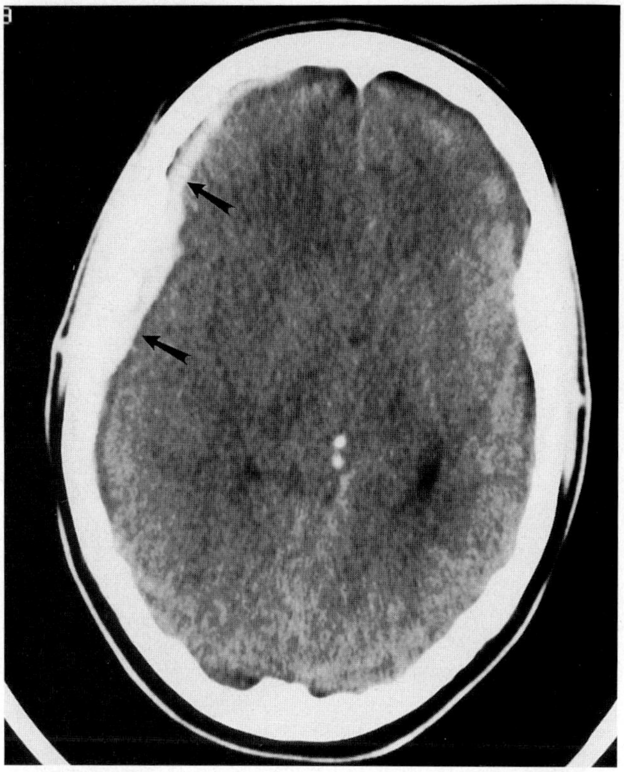

**FIGURE 18** Subdural hematoma associated with severe intraparenchymal injury. CT image reveals a thin right-sided frontoparietal SDH *(arrows)*. There is severe diffuse cerebral edema with obliteration of the lateral ventricles. The patient underwent a lifesaving right-sided deep temporal lobectomy and has had good neurologic recovery. (From Smirniotopoulos JG, Mirvis SE, Wolf AL. Imaging of craniocerebral trauma. In: Mirvis SE, Young JWR, eds. Imaging in Trauma and Critical Care. Baltimore: Williams & Wilkins, 1992; with permission.)

coagulation defects, and active bleeding can also decrease the density of EDHs. EDHs can develop in a delayed fashion in up to 9 percent of cases and can rarely decompress themselves through an adjacent skull fracture, presenting as an extracranial subgaleal hematoma.

*Subdural hematoma* (SDH) may have an acute, subacute, or chronic presentation. SDH most commonly occurs in the acute post-trauma setting and is frequently associated with concurrent cerebral injuries. Classically SDH is produced by tearing of a bridging vein (from the cortical surface to the dural sinuses) at the site of insertion into the more rigid dural sinus. In older patients with "atrophy," there is an increased risk for SDH because there is room for a greater shift of the brain after sudden acceleration/deceleration. Acute SDH occurs in 10 to 30 percent of patients after severe head trauma and carries a poorer prognosis than isolated EDH, with a mortality of 30 to 90 percent. However, this mortality is usually related to other associated parenchymal injuries such as contusion, edema, and axonal shearing rather than directly to the SDH. By CT, SDH conforms uniformly to the cerebral convexity in shape, possesses thin tapering margins, and frequently extends parallel to the falx and/or tentorium (Figs. 18 to 21). Occasionally (5 percent) the SDH displays a central convex bulge that may be related to rapid bleeding or to concurrent underlying epidural blood. SDHs are not related to skull fractures in a causal manner as are EDHs and are not limited in extent by dural sutures. Although typically hyperdense (65 to 95 HU), the acute SDH may appear less dense because of anemia, coagulation defects, admixture with CSF, or active ongoing bleeding. Acute SDH may display a "parfait" effect, with blood of differing stages of clot formation layering in a gravity-dependent fashion. On CT the density of SDH decreases linearly with time as a result of breakdown of hemoglobin and becomes isointense to brain between 10 and 21 days after injury. An isodense SDH can usually be detected by effacement of adjacent cerebral sulci, medial displacement of the gray-white interface, and mass effect on the ventricles (Fig. 22). In difficult or equivocal cases, intravenous contrast material initially increases the density of the cortex, making the SDH appear relatively hypodense. MRI is also highly sensitive to blood breakdown products in the subdural space for months following injury. These subacute and chronic collections appear as high signal on both T1- and T2-weighted sequences (Fig. 23). SDH in the interhemispheric fissure appears as a

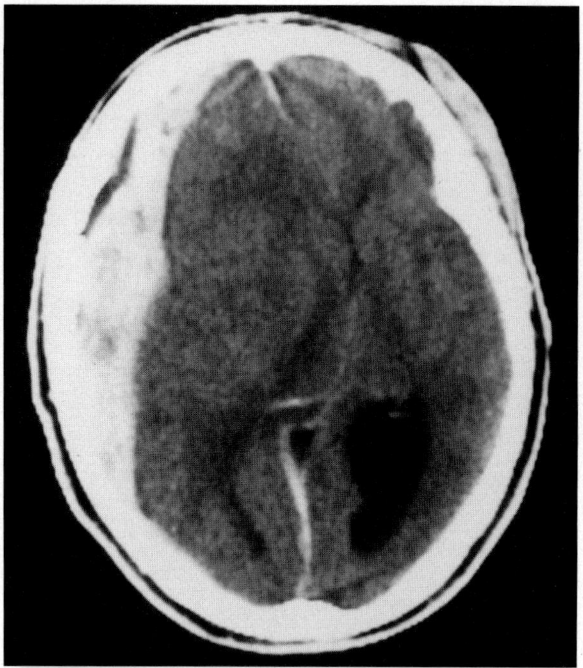

A

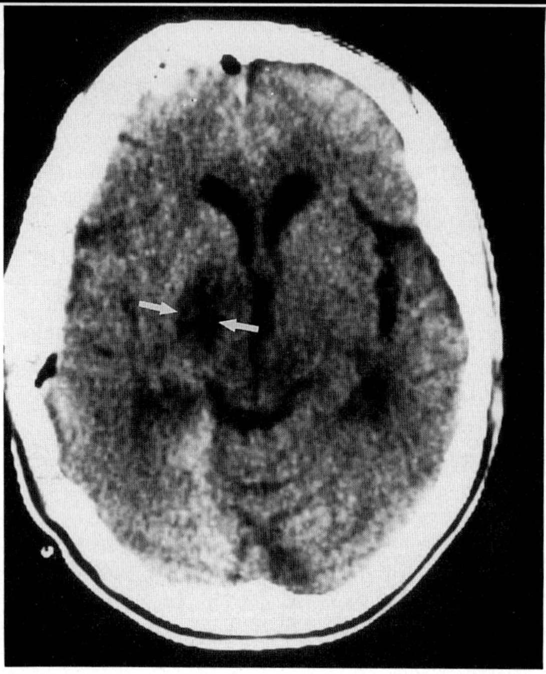

B

FIGURE 19 Anterior choroidal infarction. *A,* CT image obtained after head trauma in an elderly female demonstrates a large right-sided convexity SDH with marked subfalcine herniation. Subdural blood also tracks along the posterior and anterior falx. *B,* Follow-up CT study after surgical evacuation shows oval low density in the posterior limb of the internal capsule consistent with infarction in the distribution of the anterior choroidal artery *(arrows).* (From Mirvis SE, Wolf AL, et al. Posttraumatic cerebral infarction diagnosed by CT: Prevalence, origin, and outcome. Am J Neuroradiol 1990; 11:355–360; with permission.)

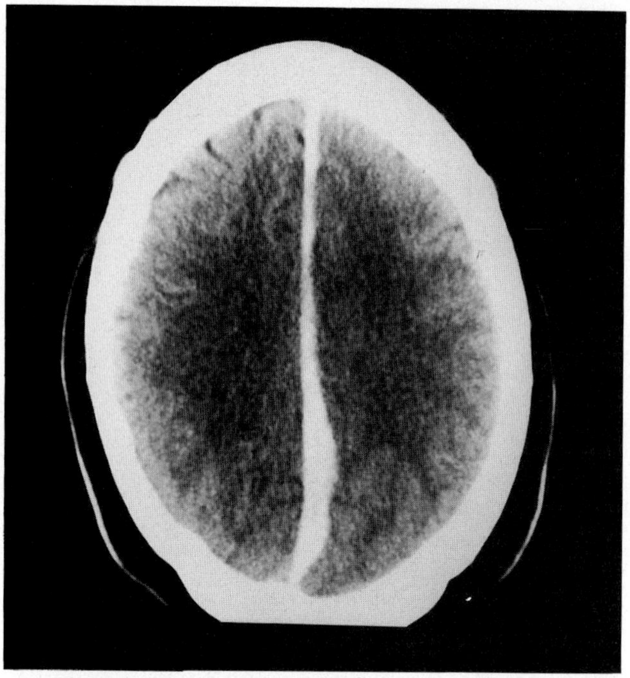

FIGURE 20 Parafalx subdural hematoma. CT image shows apparent thickening of the falx as a result of layering of subdural blood along the left side of the falx. No blood interdigitated with the adjacent sulci to suggest a subarachnoid component. (From Smirniotopoulos JG, Mirvis SE, Wolf AL. Imaging of craniocerebral trauma. In: Mirvis SE, Young JWR, eds. Imaging in Trauma and Critical Care. Baltimore: Williams & Wilkins, 1992; with permission.)

smoothly thickened falx and may be unilateral or bilateral. In contrast to subarachnoid hemorrhage (SAH), interhemispheric subdural blood does not interdigitate between adjacent medial sulci (see Fig. 20). SDH in the interhemispheric fissure in children is suggestive of child abuse. SDH tracking or extending along the tentorium appears as a V-shaped hyperdense structure that is sharply marginated medially if the blood is supratentorial in location (see Fig. 21).

## Intracerebral Parenchymal Injuries

*Cerebral contusion* is a focal area of mixed hemorrhage, edema, and ultimately necrotic tissue that arises from mechanical forces transmitted to the brain. These forces may be transmitted directly through the calvarium to the underlying superficial cortex, so-called "coup" contusion, or may appear opposite the impact site, particularly in the frontal bases and temporal tips, a "contrecoup" injury (Fig. 24). Contusions found in the deep central regions, including the corpus callosum and basal ganglia, often referred to as "intermediate," probably result from shearing stress. Contusions are usually confined to the gray matter of the cortex, involve damage to small vessels, and are self-limited. Edema associated with an acute contusion increases for several days, peaking about 3 to 5 days after injury. Serial scans may reveal progressively increasing mass effect during this time that must be carefully sought. Delayed hemorrhage may occur at sites of contusion, leading to hematoma formation with a sudden increase in mass effect (see below). Minimally hemorrhagic, predominantly edematous

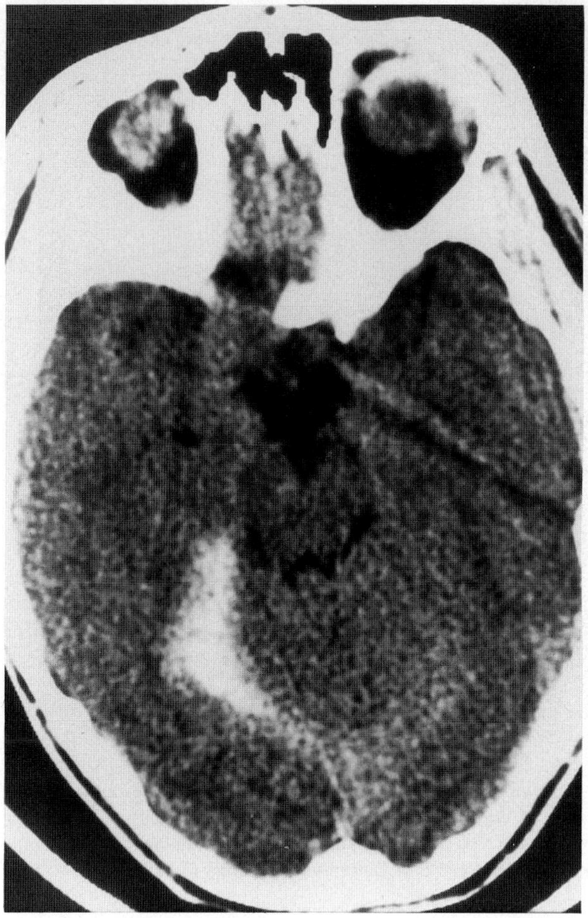

**FIGURE 21** Paratentorial subdural hematoma. CT image through the posterior fossa reveals high-density blood along the right tentorium, with a sharp medial demarcation and irregular lateral margin. This appearance suggests a supratentorial, paratentorial location of blood. (From Smirniotopoulos JG, Mirvis SE, Wolf AL. Imaging of craniocerebral trauma. In: Mirvis SE, Young JWR, eds. Imaging in Trauma and Critical Care. Baltimore: Williams & Wilkins, 1992; with permission.)

A

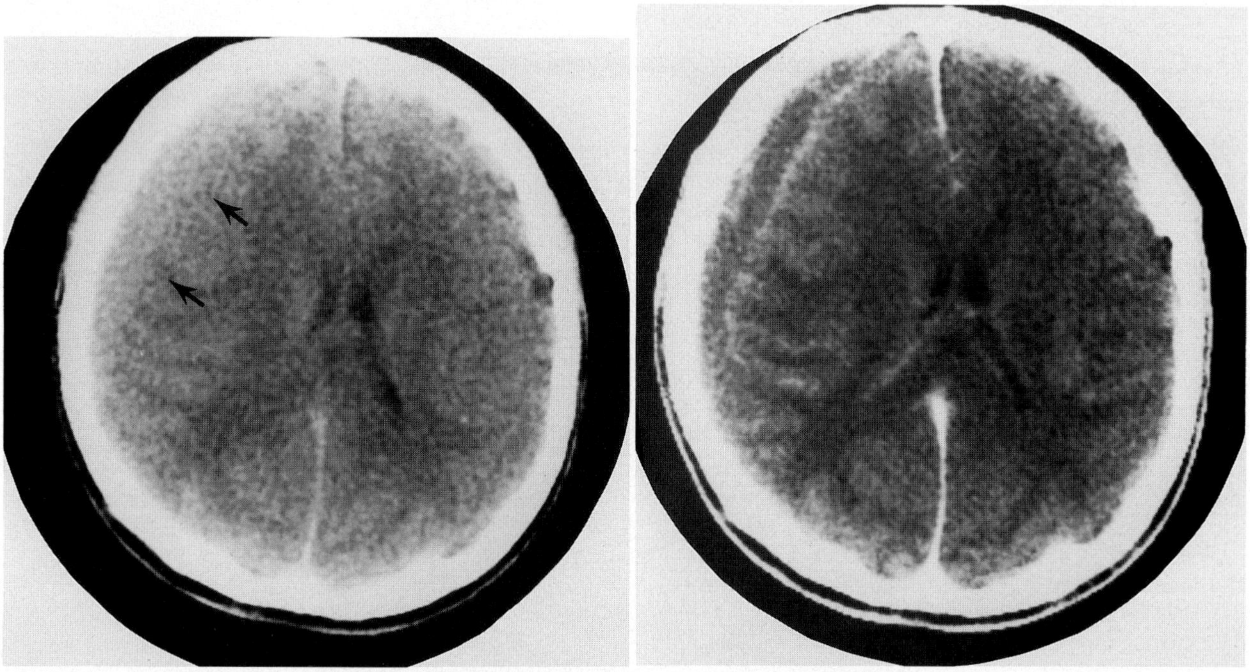

B

**FIGURE 22** Isodense subdural hematoma. *A,* Non-enhanced CT image obtained in a 33-year-old man three weeks after cranial trauma demonstrates shift of the lateral ventricles to the right and medial displacement of the right frontal gray and white matter interface *(arrows).* In addition, the cortical sulci over the right frontoparietal region are obliterated by mass effect. *B,* CT image acquired after administration of intravenous contrast material clearly demarcates the right-sided convexity SDH. (From Smirniotopoulos JG, Mirvis SE, Wolf AL. Imaging of craniocerebral trauma. In: Mirvis SE, Young JWR, eds. Imaging in Trauma and Critical Care. Baltimore: Williams & Wilkins, 1992; with permission.)

A 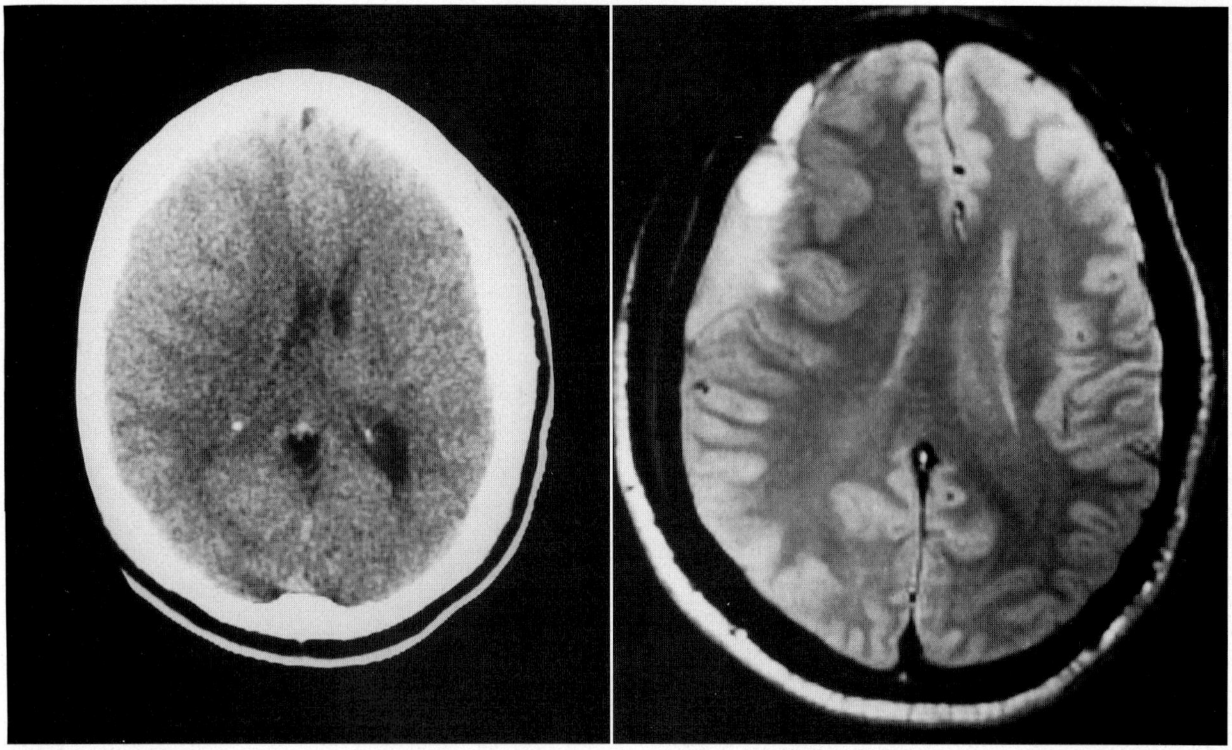 B

**FIGURE 23** Isodense subdural hematoma. *A,* CT image obtained 2 weeks after head trauma in a 31-year-old man demonstrates an isointense collection, producing mass effect and medial displacement of the gray and white matter interface. *B,* An MRI study was also performed, revealing a collection of clotted blood and proteinaceous fluid consistent with an evolving SDH. (From Smirniotopoulos JG, Mirvis SE, Wolf AL. Imaging of craniocerebral trauma. In: Mirvis SE, Young JWR, eds. Imaging in Trauma and Critical Care. Baltimore: Williams & Wilkins, 1992; with permission.)

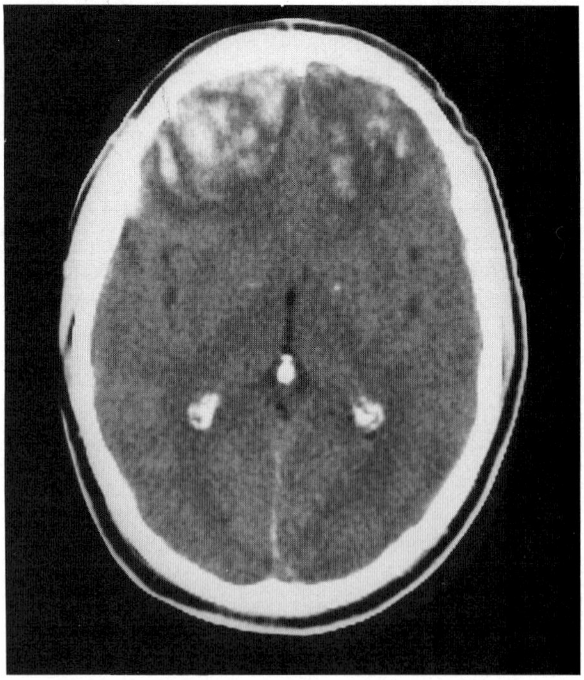

**FIGURE 24** Contrecoup cerebral contusion. CT image acquired after occipital impact reveals extensive mixed hemorrhage and edema in the frontal lobes. (From Smirniotopoulos JG, Mirvis SE, Wolf AL. Imaging of craniocerebral trauma. In: Mirvis SE, Young JWR, eds. Imaging in Trauma and Critical Care. Baltimore: Williams & Wilkins, 1992; with permission.)

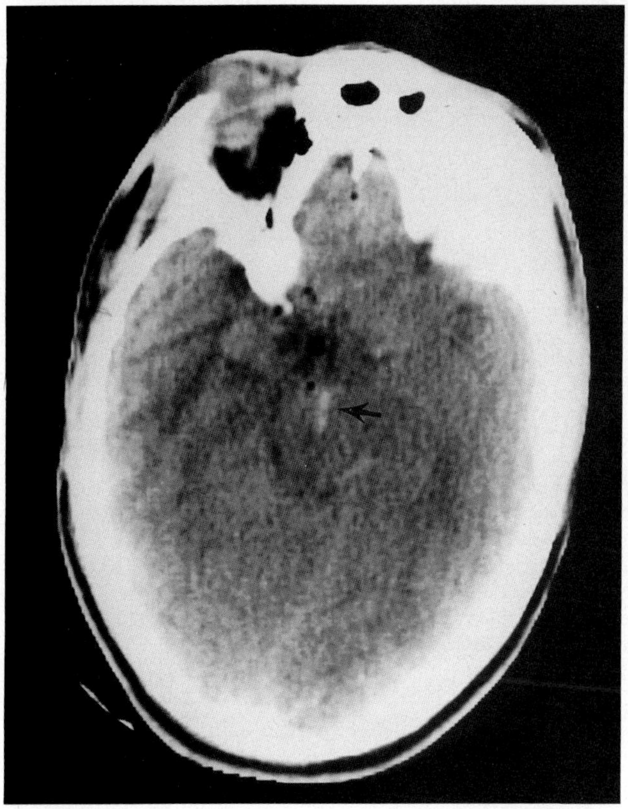

**FIGURE 25** Acute traumatic brain stem hemorrhage. CT image acquired in an obtunded man after blunt head trauma shows a focal hemorrhage in the midline of the rostral brain stem posterior to the interpeduncular cistern *(arrow)*. (From Smirniotopoulos JG, Mirvis SE, Wolf AL. Imaging of craniocerebral trauma. In: Mirvis SE, Young JWR, eds. Imaging in Trauma and Critical Care. Baltimore: Williams & Wilkins, 1992; with permission.)

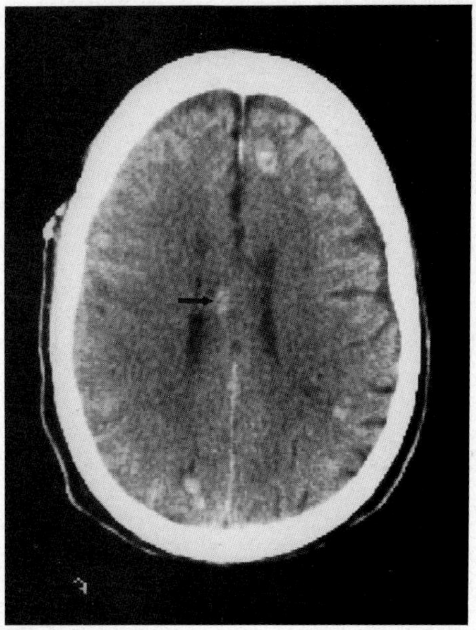

**FIGURE 26** Axonal shearing injury. CT image demonstrates numerous punctate hemorrhages predominantly at the gray and white matter interface. There is also blood in the corpus callosum *(arrow)*, indicating tearing across this structure. (From Smirniotopoulos JG, Mirvis SE, Wolf AL. Imaging of craniocerebral trauma. In: Mirvis SE, Young JWR, eds. Imaging in Trauma and Critical Care. Baltimore: Williams & Wilkins, 1992; with permission.)

contusions, particularly in the white matter, are more easily detected by MRI (see Fig. 1).

*Primary brainstem injury* after closed-head trauma is uncommon, occurring in only 0.75 to 3.6 percent of patients admitted to emergency centers. Brain stem injury is frequently associated with concurrent supratentorial injuries (31 to 45 percent) and has a high mortality rate. CT diagnosis of brain stem injury is often difficult, because of beam-hardening and other artifacts through this region. Brain stem injuries may result from impact of the brain stem against the rigid tentorium, shearing forces that typically produce dorsolateral contusions, avulsion of penetrating arteries believed to result from sudden caudal displacement of the brain, and pontomedullary tears caused by hyperextension and distraction (Fig. 25). When the CT scan does not adequately explain the level of neurologic function, MRI has proven invaluable in diagnosing brain stem injuries (see Figs. 2 and 4). MRI is not hampered by bone artifacts and has greater contrast resolution than CT, particularly for small and predominantly nonhemorrhagic lesions. Hemorrhage into the brain stem, especially the rostral pons, may appear as a delayed lesion related to cerebral herniation from any cause. These Duret's hemorrhages are associated with a poor prognosis.

*Intraventricular hemorrhage* (IVH) occurs in 3 to 8 percent of patients with closed-head trauma, either as an isolated process or in association with other lesions. Isolated IVH probably arises from tears in the choroid plexus, perhaps from inertial movements of the glomus in the open space of the trigone. IVH may also arise from a parenchymal hematoma that decompresses into the ventricular system, from intraventricular reflux of extraventricular SAH or from shearing tears in the undersurface of the corpus callosum. On CT, IVH may appear as amorphous clotted collections of blood or may layer dependently, producing blood-CSF levels. Isolated IVH after head trauma, in our opinion, is a marker of significant impact, and concurrent injuries to the brain should be carefully sought.

DAI is believed to result from shearing strains and is most likely to occur from impact-producing lateral (coronal) plane movement. Typically DAI produces multiple punctate hemorrhages in the gray-white junction, corpus callosum, deep gray nuclei, and brain stem (Fig. 26). Although MRI increases detection of nonhemorrhagic shear-induced lesions, in our experience this seldom suggests a change in likely prognosis or management.

SAH is the most common type of bleeding after craniocerebral trauma, and trauma is the most common cause of SAH (Fig. 27). In our experience, however, isolated SAH without other evidence of injury is unusual after head trauma and should prompt a search for other etiologies of SAH, such as aneurysm or AVM, unless there is a clear history of antecedent head trauma. SAH resulting from head trauma seldom produces a basilar cistern blood clot unlike SAH from aneurysm rupture. It is important to make sure the patient has not recently received intravenous contrast material for other CT evaluations that may mimic SAH on a non–contrast-enhanced head CT scan.

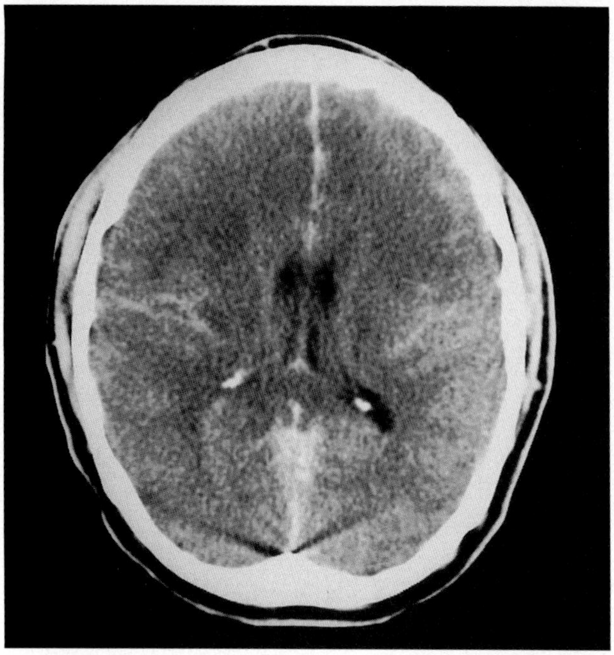

**FIGURE 27** Post-traumatic subarachnoid hemorrhage. This image reveals subarachnoid blood in the Sylvian fissures and interhemispheric fissure following blunt head trauma. Note how the interhemispheric blood interdigitates with the medial cerebral sulci. (From Smirniotopoulos JG, Mirvis SE, Wolf AL. Imaging of craniocerebral trauma. In: Mirvis SE, Young JWR, eds. Imaging in Trauma and Critical Care. Baltimore: Williams & Wilkins, 1992; with permission.)

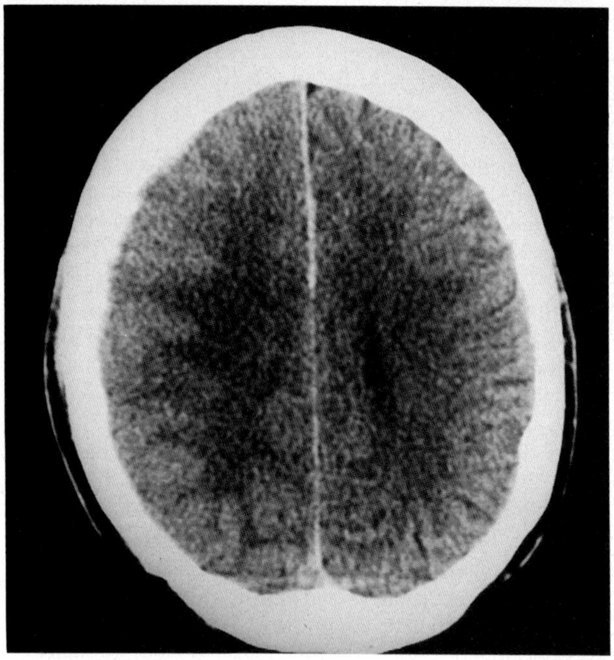

**FIGURE 28** Unilateral cerebral edema. CT image demonstrates right-sided effacement of the cerebral sulci without gross mass effect, indicating unilateral cortical edema after blunt cranial trauma. The low-density white matter extends more deeply into the subcortical region as a result of vasogenic edema. The gray and white matter interface is more sharply demarcated on the side with cerebral edema. (From Smirniotopoulos JG, Mirvis SE, Wolf AL. Imaging of craniocerebral trauma. In: Mirvis SE, Young JWR, eds. Imaging in Trauma and Critical Care. Baltimore: Williams & Wilkins, 1992; with permission.)

Cerebral edema accompanies most episodes of significant head trauma and is usually evident on the initial CT scan (Fig. 28) as decreased attenuation. Edema is multifactorial including vasogenic (loss of blood-brain barrier), cytotoxic, and vasoparalysis (loss of autoregulation). In many cases mass effects from edema are far more significant than from intra- or extra-axial hematomas. Mass effect leads to herniation across the midline (transfalcine), with truncation of the anterior and posterior horns of the lateral ventricles (see Figs. 15 and 19) and contralateral ventricular dilatation. Uncal or medial temporal herniation is associated with ipsilateral brain stem compression (see Fig. 14), downward transtentorial displacement with basal cistern effacement, distortion and compression of the brain stem with potential impaction of the contralateral brain stem against the tentorial edge (Kernohan's notch), and rarely transalar (sphenoidal) displacement, with herniation of the temporal lobe into the anterior cranial fossa. Cerebral infarction occurs in nearly 2 percent of patients with severe CHI involving all vascular territories, but particularly the posterior and anterior cerebral regions (Figs. 29 to 31). Close monitoring of intracranial pressure combined with close-interval CT scans are needed to prevent development of this complication. Severe, diffuse cerebral edema producing a "reversal sign" can mimic diffuse SAH.

*Post-traumatic pneumocephalus* indicates an abnormal communication between the intra- and extracranial spaces and typically results from a skull base or sinus fracture or less commonly an open cranial vault fracture. Fractures through the frontal sinus and anterior ethmoid region usually lead to subdural air (Fig. 32), whereas fractures involving the posterior ethmoid roof and sphenoid sinus produce subarachnoid air (Fig. 33). CT is exquisitely sensitive to pneumocephalus, but volume averaging with the mastoid or sphenoid sinuses can mimic this finding. The presence of an abnormal communication between a sinus and the intracranial contents through a dural tear is associated with an increased risk of meningitis,

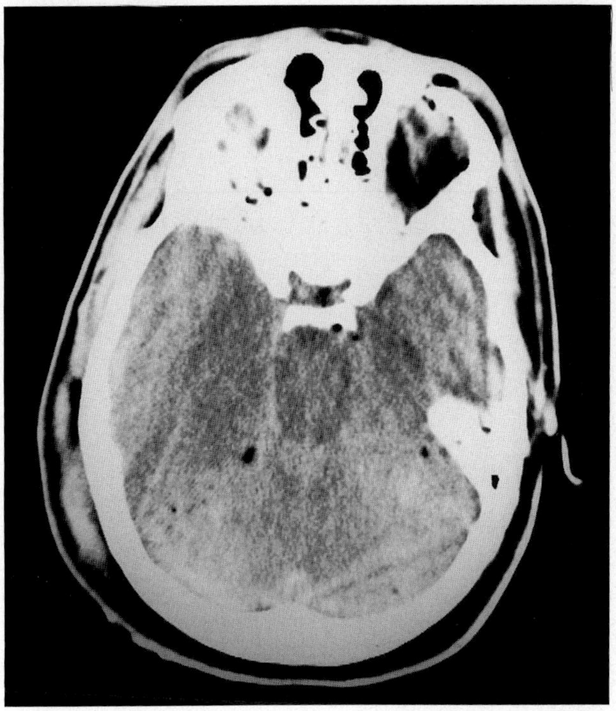

**FIGURE 29** Diffuse cerebral edema with herniation. This axial image acquired on a young male after a high-velocity car collision reveals obliteration of the basal cisterns and lateral compression of the brain stem (elongation of AP diameter) by the descending medial temporal lobes. Pneumocephalus is present. (From Smirniotopoulos JG, Mirvis SE, Wolf AL. Imaging of craniocerebral trauma. In: Mirvis SE, Young JWR, eds. Imaging in Trauma and Critical Care. Baltimore: Williams & Wilkins, 1992; with permission.)

A

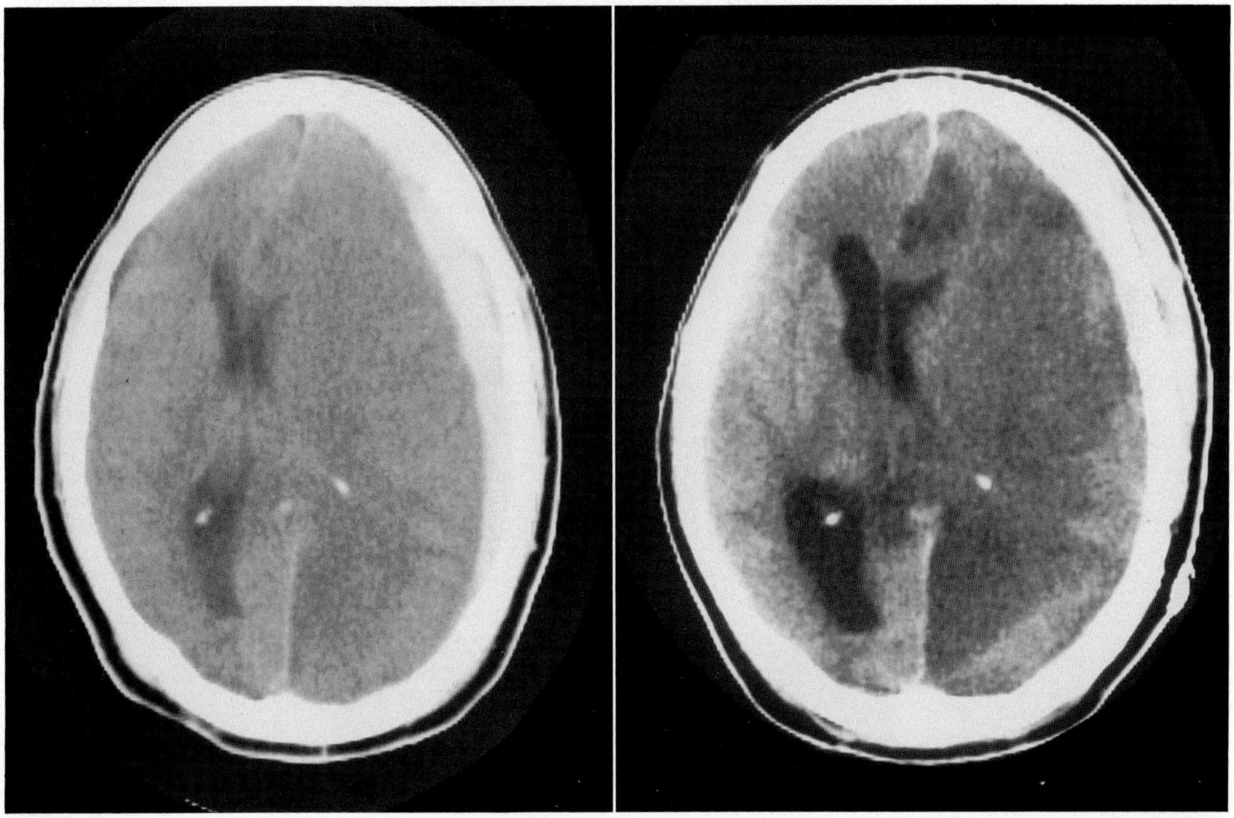

B

**FIGURE 30** Multifocal infarction following gross mass displacement. *A,* Admission CT image reveals a large left-sided convexity SDH markedly displacing the midline structures to the right. There is low density adjacent to the posterior falx, suggesting early ischemic changes. *B,* Follow-up CT at the midventricular level after evacuation of the SDH reveals infarction in the left anterior and posterior cerebral distributions, as well as in the left thalamoperforating distribution. In addition, the left anterior middle cerebral territory was of low density, suggesting infarction or edema. (From Mirvis SE, Wolf AL, et al. Posttraumatic cerebral infarction diagnosed by CT: Prevalence, origin, and outcome. Am J Neuroradiol 1990; 11:355–360; with permission.)

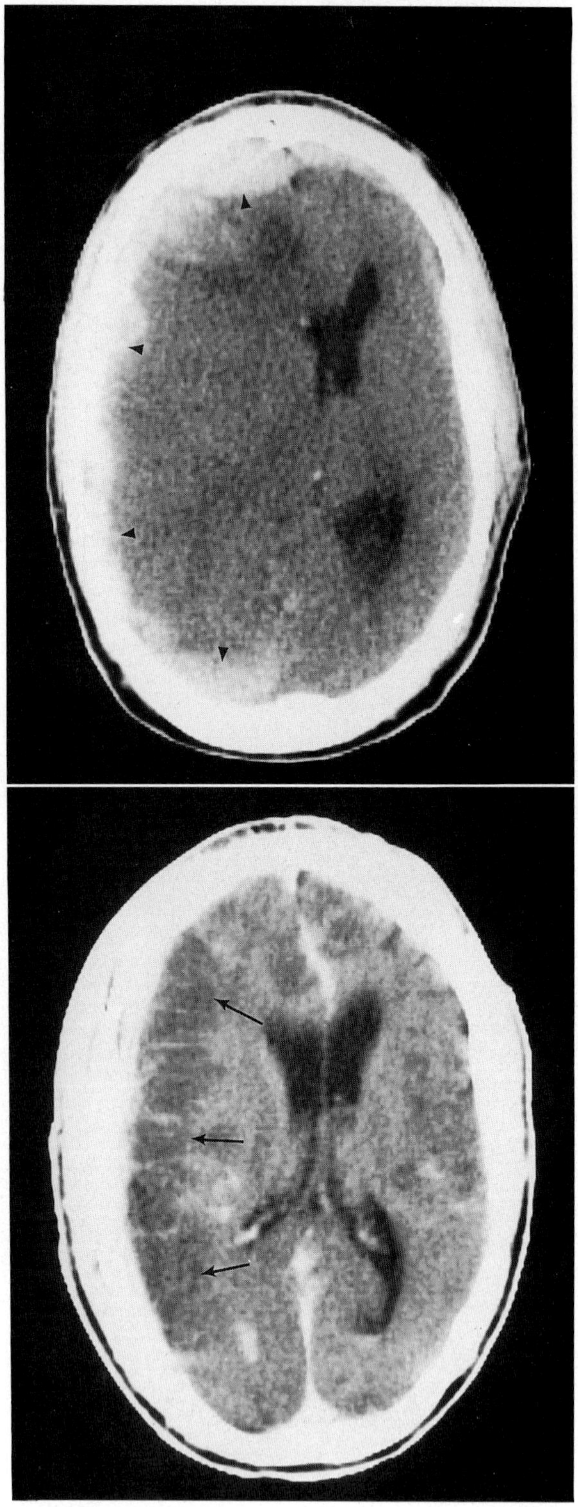

**FIGURE 31** Cortical cerebral infarction. *A,* Axial CT image obtained after head trauma in an elderly man reveals a large right-sided convexity SDH *(arrowheads),* producing marked mass effect and subfalcine herniation. *B,* Enhanced CT scan obtained after evacuation of the hematoma reveals a large band *(arrows)* of low density along the middle cerebral distribution involving the gray and subcortical white matter. The infarct is most likely a result of direct pressure effects of the overlying subdural mass, limiting arterial flow or venous outflow obstruction from the mass of hematoma. (From Mirvis SE, Wolf AL, et al. Posttraumatic cerebral infarction diagnosed by CT: Prevalence, origin, and outcome. Am J Neuroradiol 1990; 11:355–360; with permission.)

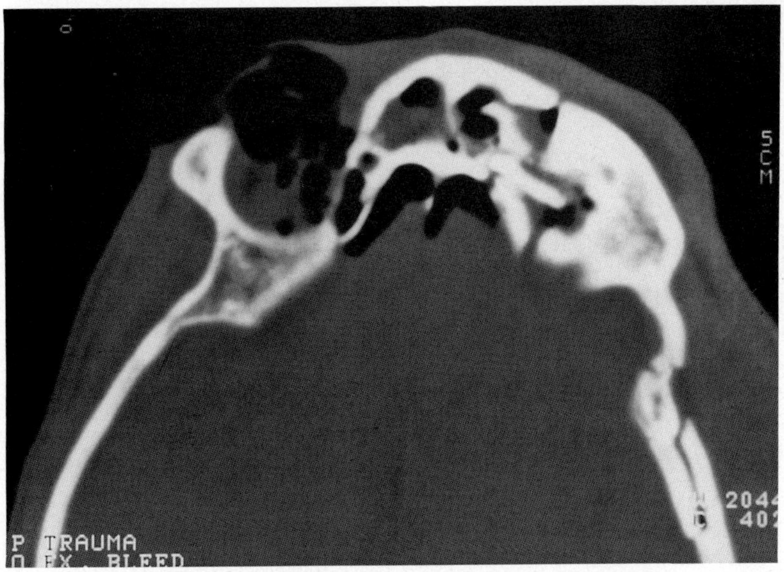


**FIGURE 32** CT of orbital roof and frontal sinus fracture. CT image demonstrates an open skull fracture, with fracture lines through the left anterior and posterior frontal sinus wall. There is blood in the base of the frontal sinus and subdural pneumocephalus. The medial left orbital roof is fractured and there is right-sided orbital emphysema. A fracture of the left temporal squamosa is also observed. (From Smirniotopoulos JG, Mirvis SE, Wolf AL. Imaging of craniocerebral trauma. In: Mirvis SE, Young JWR, eds. Imaging in Trauma and Critical Care. Baltimore: Williams & Wilkins, 1992; with permission.)

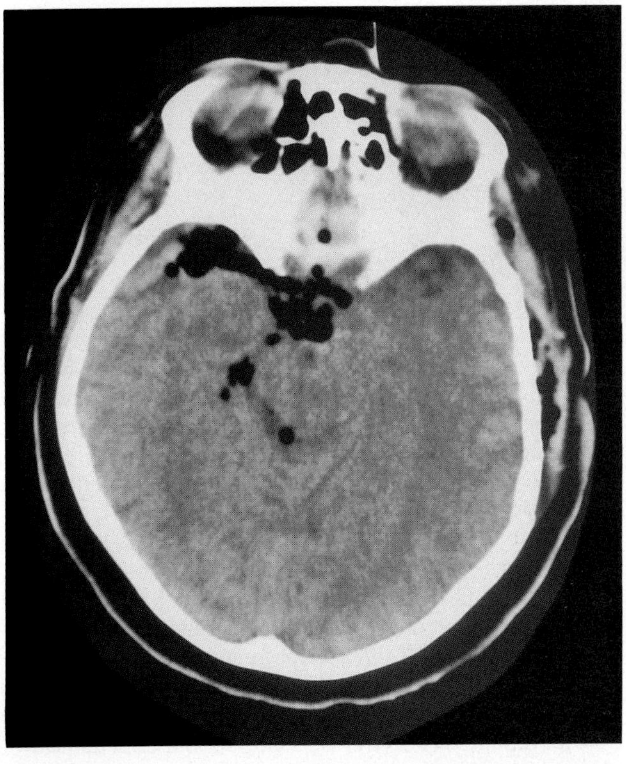

**FIGURE 33** Traumatic subarachnoid pneumocephalus. CT image through the skull base reveals pneumocephalus in the suprasellar and ambient cisterns consistent with a subarachnoid localization. A fracture of the sphenoid sinus roof (not shown) was probably the source of intracranial air.

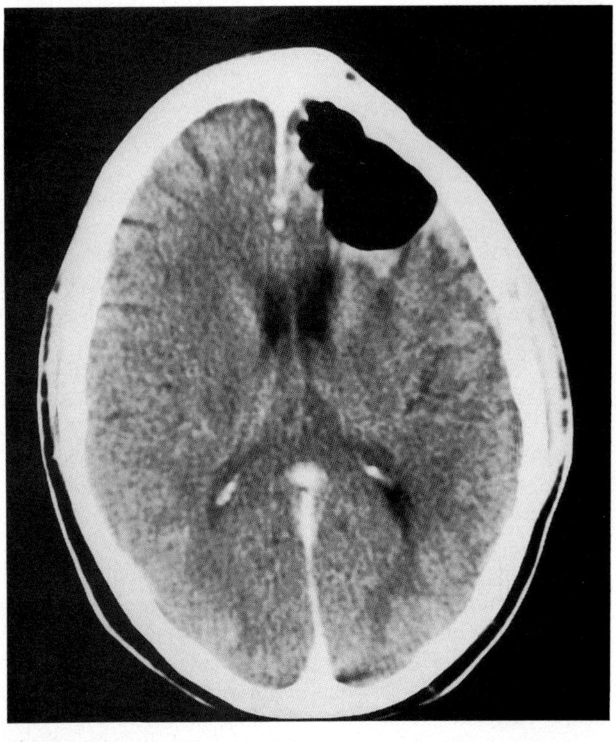

**FIGURE 34** Post-traumatic cerebral aerocele. CT image obtained two weeks after discharge of a 40-year-old man who had sustained a complex frontal bone fracture shows an air collection in the left frontal region, but no significant mass effect. The air collection results from a persistent intracranial communication with the left frontal sinus. (From Smirniotopoulos JG, Mirvis SE, Wolf AL. Imaging of craniocerebral trauma. In: Mirvis SE, Young JWR, eds. Imaging in Trauma and Critical Care. Baltimore: Williams & Wilkins, 1992; with permission.)

CSF leak, cranial nerve injury, and rarely tension aerocele (Fig. 34). Although most open skull base fractures require no direct surgical intervention, open frontal sinus fractures involving the anterior and posterior walls should, in our opinion, prompt surgical exenteration of the frontal sinus.

## Comments

Currently CT is the principal diagnostic tool used for directing initial management of patients with CHI and for detecting delayed complications of head trauma. In the future we anticipate that MRI and MR angiography will play an increasingly important complementary role, in selected patients, for both diagnosis and management.

## Suggested Reading

Cornelius RS, Gaskill MF, Lukin RR. Traumatic intracranial hemorrhage. In: Gentry LR, ed. Current Concepts in Imaging of Craniofacial Trauma. Neuroimag Clin North Am 1991; 1:435–442.

Dolan KD. Temporal bone fractures. Semin Ultrasound CT MR 1989; 10:262–267.

Frazee JG. Head trauma. Emerg Med Clin North Am 1986; 4:859–874.

Gentry LR. Primary neuronal injuries. In: Gentry LR, ed. Current Concepts in Imaging of Craniofacial Trauma. Neuroimag Clin North Am 1991; 1:411–432.

Gentry LR, Godersky JC, Thompson B. MR imaging of head trauma. Review of distribution and radiographic features of traumatic lesions. AJR 1988; 150:663–672.

Masters SJ, McClean PM, Argarese, et al. Skull x-ray examination after head trauma. N Engl J Med 1987; 316:84–91.

Murphy BP, Hicks RJ, Kirkwood JR. Neuroimaging of head trauma. Trauma Q 1992; 8:1–17.

Smirniotopoulos JG, Mirvis SE, Wolf AL. Imaging of craniocerebral trauma. In: Mirvis SE, Young JWR, eds. Imaging in Trauma and Critical Care. Baltimore: Williams & Wilkins, 1992:23.

Tsai FY, Teal JS, Heishima GB. Neuroradiology of Head Trauma. Baltimore: University Park, 1984.

Zimmerman RA, Bilaniuk LT, Gennarelli T. Computed tomography of shearing injuries of the cerebral white matter. Radiology 1978; 127:393–396.

Zimmerman RA, Bilaniuk LT, Gennarelli T, et al. Cranial computed tomography in the diagnosis and management of acute head trauma. AJR 1978; 131:27–34.

# Scintigraphic Diagnosis of Brain Death

*CONRAD E. NAGLE, M.D.*

Imagine that you and a companion are transported back in time to 1740 A.D. While visiting this time, your companion becomes critically ill and seeks medical care. After several days the doctor comes to you and says, "I'm sorry, I *think* your friend is dead." Immediately, in an agitated voice, you ask, "Don't you know for sure?" No answer is offered.

You further question, "What did the electrocardiograph show? Were heart sounds audible with the stethoscope? Was the EEG isoelectric?" Seeing the doctor's puzzled look, you then realize that the ECG was not invented until the twentieth century; that the stethoscope wasn't used until the nineteenth century; and that Hans Berger, a psychiatrist, did not invent the EEG until 1929.

Realizing your frustration over the uncertainty of your friend's death, the doctor offers several suggestions: "You might wish to bury your friend in the newly patented casket with a periscope. This will allow your friend to breathe, see, and communicate aboveground in the event I'm wrong and death hasn't occurred." Seeing your obvious displeasure with this suggestion, the doctor offers one last comment: "Well, you know what the Frenchman, Jean-Jacques Winslow, has said in his book, *The Uncertainty of the Signs of Death and the Danger of Precipitate Internments:* 'Putrefaction [is] the only sure sign of death.'"

Is the current public perception of the determination of death really different from the preceding silly scenario? Have doctors agreed on which tests are necessary? Are all doctors equally capable of determining the presence of brain death?

## Historical Background

### *Clinical Criteria*

Not until 1968 were there published criteria for "irreversible coma." The Ad Hoc Committee of the Harvard Medical School provided organized medicine with the first systematic medical approach for the determination of brain death. The committee maintained that there should be unreceptivity and unresponsivity, absence of spontaneous breathing, absence of reflexes, isoelectric electroencephalogram (EEG) pattern, and confirmation of the criteria at least twice, 24 hours apart.

No state had legally recognized brain death with somatic survival until 1970. Kansas was the first to provide an alternative to the traditional circulatory and ventilatory criteria. Other legal models were offered (California Health and Safety Code No. 7180, 1978; Capron and Kass, 1978).

Medical attention to the case of Karen Anne Quinlan raised public interest in modern death determination controversies.

The National Institute of Neurological and Communicative Disorders and Stroke proposed that a confirmatory test related to cerebral blood flow be carried out in all cases in which expeditious confirmation of cerebral death is needed. Recognition of the false-positive isoelectric EEG, in individuals with elevated barbiturate levels or significant hypothermia strengthened the need for imaging determination of brain blood flow.

In 1981 the lack of uniform medical or legal criteria from one state to another for the determination of death resulted in the publication of The Uniform Determination of Death Act.

Intending to provide a model statute for adoption by all 50 states, the President's Commission for the Study of Ethical Problems in Medicine and Biomedical and Behavioral Research had considered these issues for nearly two years.

Nearly half of the states had not adopted brain death as a criterion for death by 1982. By 1988 46 states had either adopted The Uniform Determination of Death Act, adopted it with modifications, or judicially sanctioned brain death.

Given the finality of medical decisions regarding discontinuance of extraordinary life support and the variety of legal rules regarding the medical determination of death, it is essential that physicians involved in these decisions have firsthand knowledge of the laws in their state.

## *Imaging Criteria*

As a reflection of the increasing use of imaging to prove brain death, two chapters of a recent textbook on issues of pediatric brain death were devoted to discussions of radionuclide cerebral angiography (RCA) (Goodman et al, 1989; Schwartz et al, 1989).

In 1975 Mishkin reported the use of RCA as a qualitative evaluation for cerebral blood flow. Korein and colleagues reported the use of twin probes to obtain time-activity curves at the bedside. The use of portable scintillation cameras and computers to perform RCA for evaluation of cerebral death made the studies more practical. Movement of comatose patients, who were clinically brain dead, to the imaging department for procedures had been an obstacle for use of these tests.

Four-vessel cerebral contrast angiography compared with RCA in 15 patients suspected of being brain dead showed 100 percent correlation (Schwartz et al, 1983). More importantly, in more than 40,000 patients with clinical conditions other than brain death studied by RCA at two institutions, no false-positive (absent cerebral blood flow) studies have been identified in these neurologically impaired patients (Goodman et al, 1985; Schwartz et al, 1989). Any physician interpreting RCA images should read these papers.

The absence of venous sinus tracer on static images confirms the absence of intra-arterial cerebral flow on RCA. The presence of radionuclide in the sinus can occur in the absence of intracerebral arterial flow.

In a national collaborative retrospective study in 1982, none of the 856 patients showing cerebral death by RCA survived somatically; 112 patients with absent flow by RCA had confirmation by arteriography. This same study documented five neonates with clinical and electroencephalographic brain death with normal cerebral blood flow by RCA. Cerebral blood flow was confirmed by arteriogram in two patients.

The newer lipophilic brain tracer technetium-99m hexamethylpropyleneamine oxine ($^{99m}$Tc–HM-PAO) can be used to acquire a RCA. After the flow phase, scintigraphy in a normal individual shows that the tracer has crossed the blood-brain barrier in proportion to regional blood flow and is retained by parenchymal brain receptors. Several studies have now proven that static scintigraphy with $^{99m}$Tc–HMPAO or another lipophilic brain tracer *N*-isopropyl-($^{123}$I) *p*-iodoamphetamine ($^{123}$I-IMP), together with RCA, is confirmatory in the diagnosis of brain death.

Espinola and co-workers have demonstrated the value of RCA in the diagnosis of brain death in patients being treated therapeutically with hypothermic barbiturate coma. Preliminary evidence also suggests that therapeutic phenobarbital or thiopental levels do not interfere with the cerebral penetration of lipophilic brain tracers in non–brain-dead individuals.

Four-vessel carotid and vertebral contrast angiography is more commonly used in Europe to confirm absent brain blood flow in brain-dead patients. The difficulties in transporting these supported patients to the angiographic suite; the risks of contrast compromise to potential transplant organs; the risks of compromise to blood flow in non–brain-dead, brain-damaged individuals; and the appearance of excessive procedures in a patient who is clinically brain dead are reasons that have probably minimized use of four-vessel contrast radiography.

Case reports of the use of other imaging modalities or variations on previously used modalities have appeared in the literature. Computed tomography (CT) with and without contrast enhancement, intravenous and intra-arterial digital subtraction angiography, Doppler shift ultrasonography, common carotid arterial velocity pattern with pulsed Doppler ultrasonography, xenon-CT measurements of cerebral blood flow, magnetic resonance imaging, and positron emission tomography have all been described in the clinical determinations of brain death.

## Discussion

Just as public insecurities in the 1700s led to the patented periscope casket, the public remains concerned about premature pronouncement of death and is fearful that the need for transplant organs will be a conflict of interest for physicians making pronouncements of brain death. Public concern, the fact that most states now legally define death as brain death, and the physiologic basis (as opposed to anatomic) for evaluations provided by modern scintigraphic imaging techniques are all reasons that imaging is likely to be used by clinicians.

Why not wait until a brain-dead patient undergoes somatic death? Spontaneous cessation of the heart usually occurs within 1 to 2 weeks of brain death, despite extraordinary medical life support. However, in 1982 Parisi and co-workers described a brain-dead middle-aged man who was maintained somatically for more than two months, until New York courts ordered discontinuance of extraordinary support. Somatic prolongation despite brain death will likely increase the family's medical bill, reduce the successful use of the patient's organs for transplantation, and upset the family as they agonize over the situation. The use of "living wills" may substantially reduce this problem in those states where living wills are legal.

Physicians must communicate to patients and families that there is a difference between the expeditious pronouncement of death in a patient proven to be brain dead and premature pronouncement of death. I have found that families accept brain death in a relative more readily after being shown the latter's RCA images and comparing them with normal images.

Most state laws allowing death pronouncement at the time of brain death require death of the total brain. Although no patient has survived in more than a vegetative state with a functioning brain stem in the complete absence of cerebral blood flow, documentation of absent cerebral blood flow by RCA is not evidence of total brain death, only of cerebral death. Absence of $^{99m}$Tc–HM-PAO or $^{123}$I-IMP by planar or

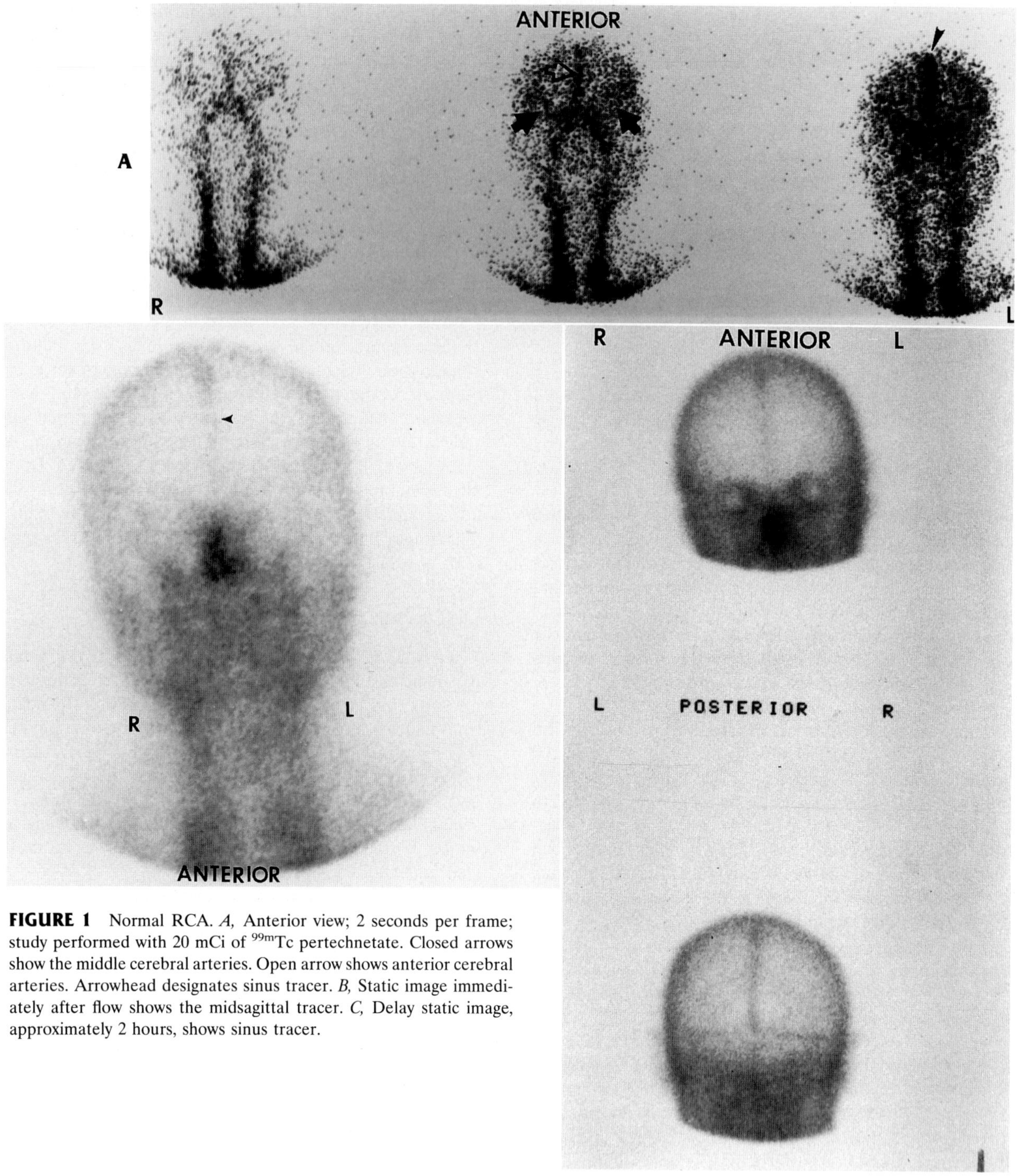


**FIGURE 1** Normal RCA. *A,* Anterior view; 2 seconds per frame; study performed with 20 mCi of $^{99m}$Tc pertechnetate. Closed arrows show the middle cerebral arteries. Open arrow shows anterior cerebral arteries. Arrowhead designates sinus tracer. *B,* Static image immediately after flow shows the midsagittal tracer. *C,* Delay static image, approximately 2 hours, shows sinus tracer.

single-photon emission computed tomography (SPECT) techniques in the cerebral cortex, cerebellum, and brain stem, however, reflects the lack of perfusion to the entire brain.

## Recommended Scintigraphic Protocol

It is recommended that the scintigraphic evaluation of a patient for brain death be performed in the nuclear medicine department, despite the complex support equipment and additional personnel necessary to care for the patient. The use of a portable scintillation camera and bedside imaging is possible but not the preferred approach. Portable scintigraphic cameras are not infrequently subject to malfunction after movement on and off elevators. In addition, critical care beds do not always allow positioning of some camera bases under the bed.

RCA is first performed using 20 mCi of $^{99m}$Tc-DTPA or $^{99m}$Tc-glucoheptonate. After the RCA is completed, a second scintigraphic study using planar or SPECT techniques is performed with 20 mCi of $^{99m}$Tc–HM-PAO, the most readily available lipophilic brain tracer. The dual study allows cross-verification of cerebral death and the diagnosis of total brain death.

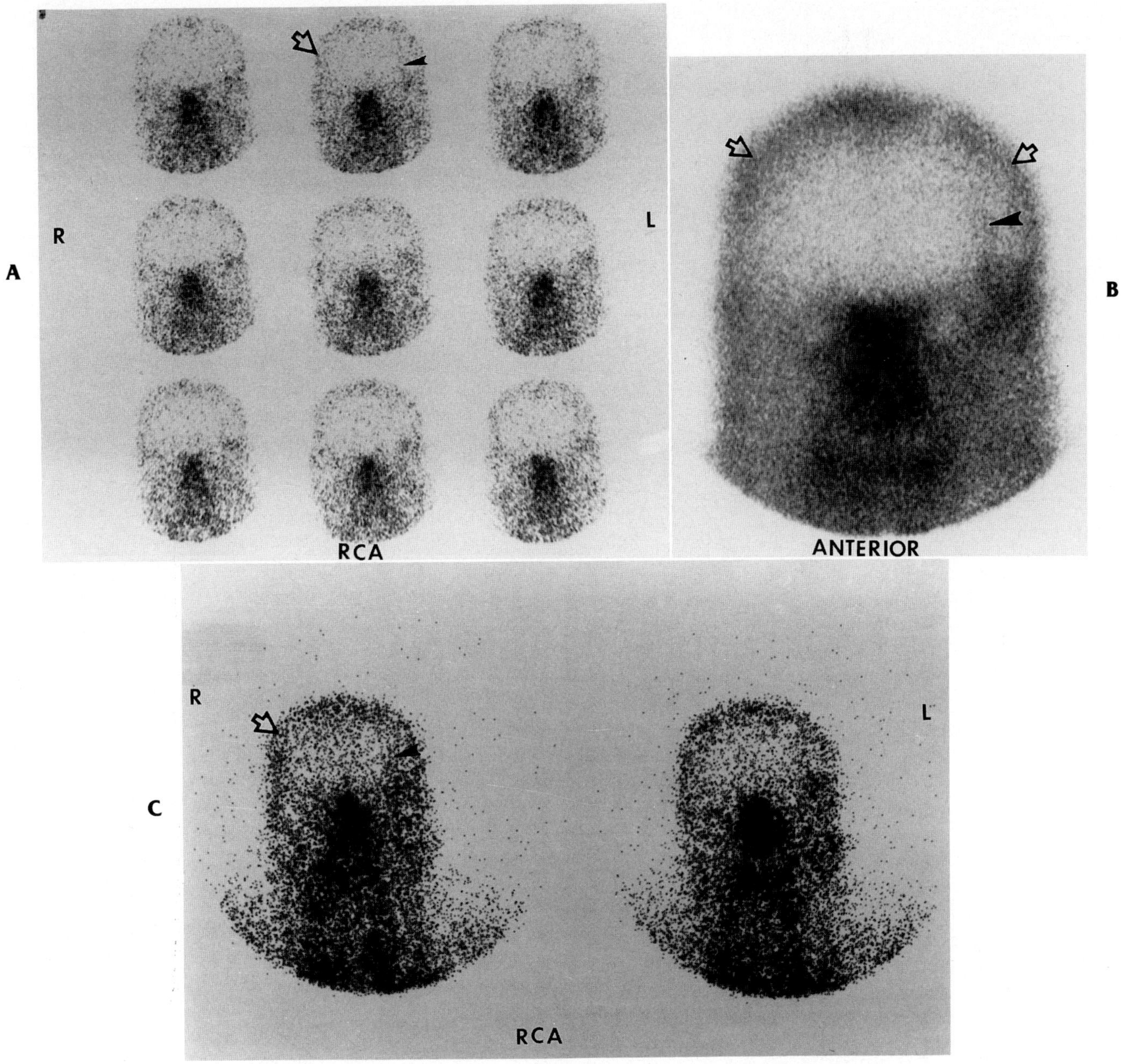


**FIGURE 2** Abnormal RCA demonstrates no cerebral flow, indicating cerebral death. This middle-aged individual had suffered head trauma related to an auto accident. An intracranial pressure-monitoring device was surgically placed into the left frontal head region. *A,* Early phase of RCA; 2 seconds per frame. *B,* Later portion of RCA. *C,* Static images showing no sinus activity. Open arrow(s) points to superficial scalp/skull tracer. Arrowhead points to site of the scalp/skull focus of tracer related to surgical placement of intracranial monitoring device.

## *Radionuclide Cerebral Angiography*

To ensure a good bolus, less than 1 ml of 20 mCi of $^{99m}$Tc-DTPA in a small syringe is coupled to a three-way stopcock and a 20 ml syringe with saline flush. Doses are fractionated for pediatric patients. Administration is performed via an established intravenous catheter. A standard- or large-field-of-view camera with a low-energy, high-sensitivity, parallel hole collimator may be used to acquire the 2 second image flow study. The camera is positioned over the anterior head with little or no separation between the head and camera. Computer acquisition is recommended for dynamic review and backup of analog images. The computer flow study is acquired in dynamic mode using a 128 × 128 matrix for 60 frames at 1 sec/frame beginning at the time of injection.

The RCA is diagnostic of cerebral death if no flow is observed in the major intracerebral arteries, including the anterior and middle cerebral arteries. Scalp/skull tracer is noted, but this is not a diagnostic problem for the experienced observer (Figs. 1 to 3).

Nuclear medicine physician training should include the

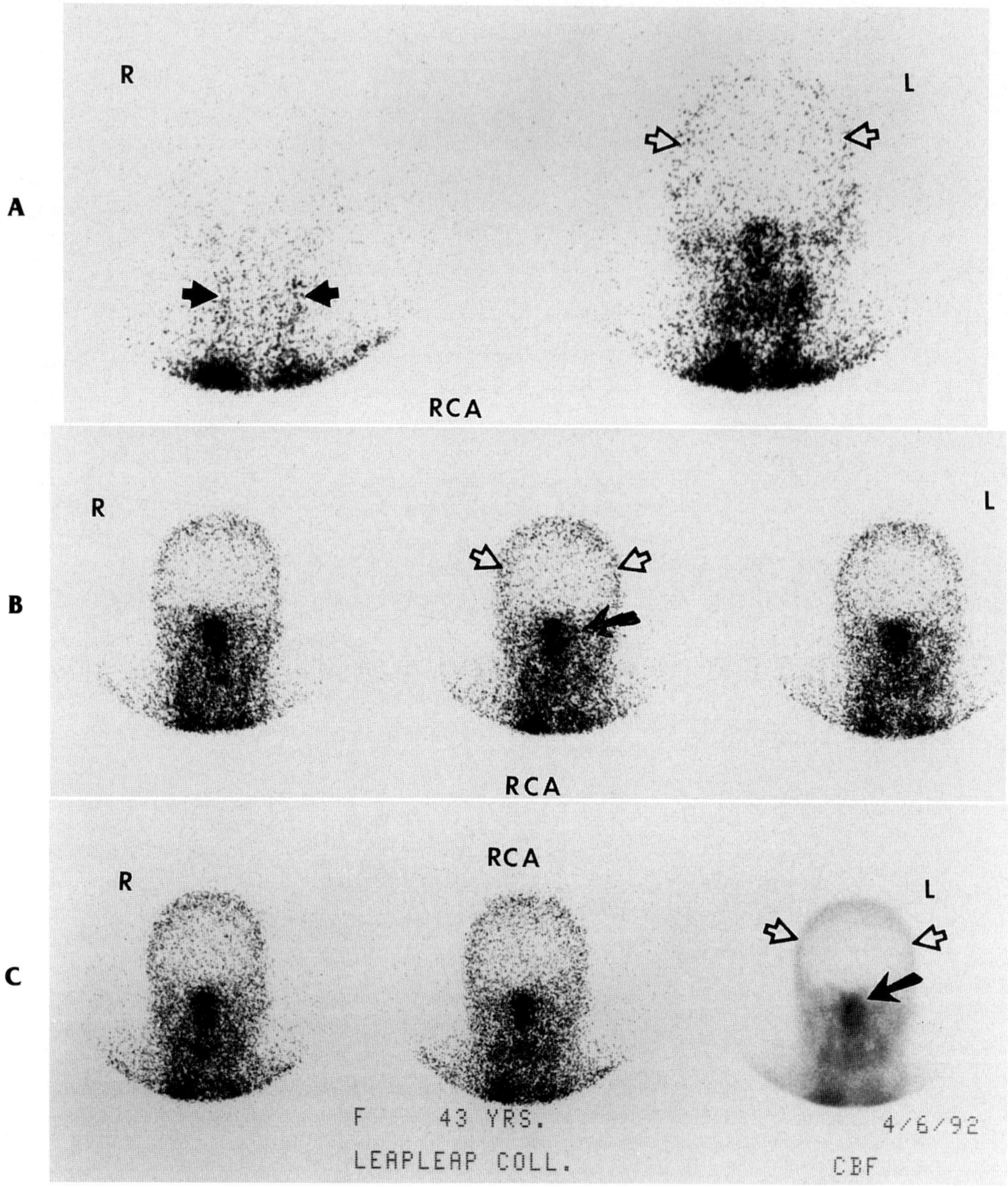


**FIGURE 3** Abnormal RCA demonstrates no cerebral flow, indicating cerebral death. This middle-aged woman overdosed on drugs and at the time of the RCA was clinically brain dead. *A,* Early phase of RCA with each image representing a 2 second acquisition. *B,* Later phase of RCA; 2 second/frame images. *C,* The left and middle images are the last of the 2 second/frame RCA images. The right image is the immediate static blood pool image. Open arrows indicate the superficial scalp/skull tracer. Solid, smaller, straight arrows point to carotid flow of tracer. Larger, slightly curved, solid arrow indicates a hot nose—a finding in cerebral death. The presence or absence of a hot nose should not affect the imaging interpretation of RCA for brain death.

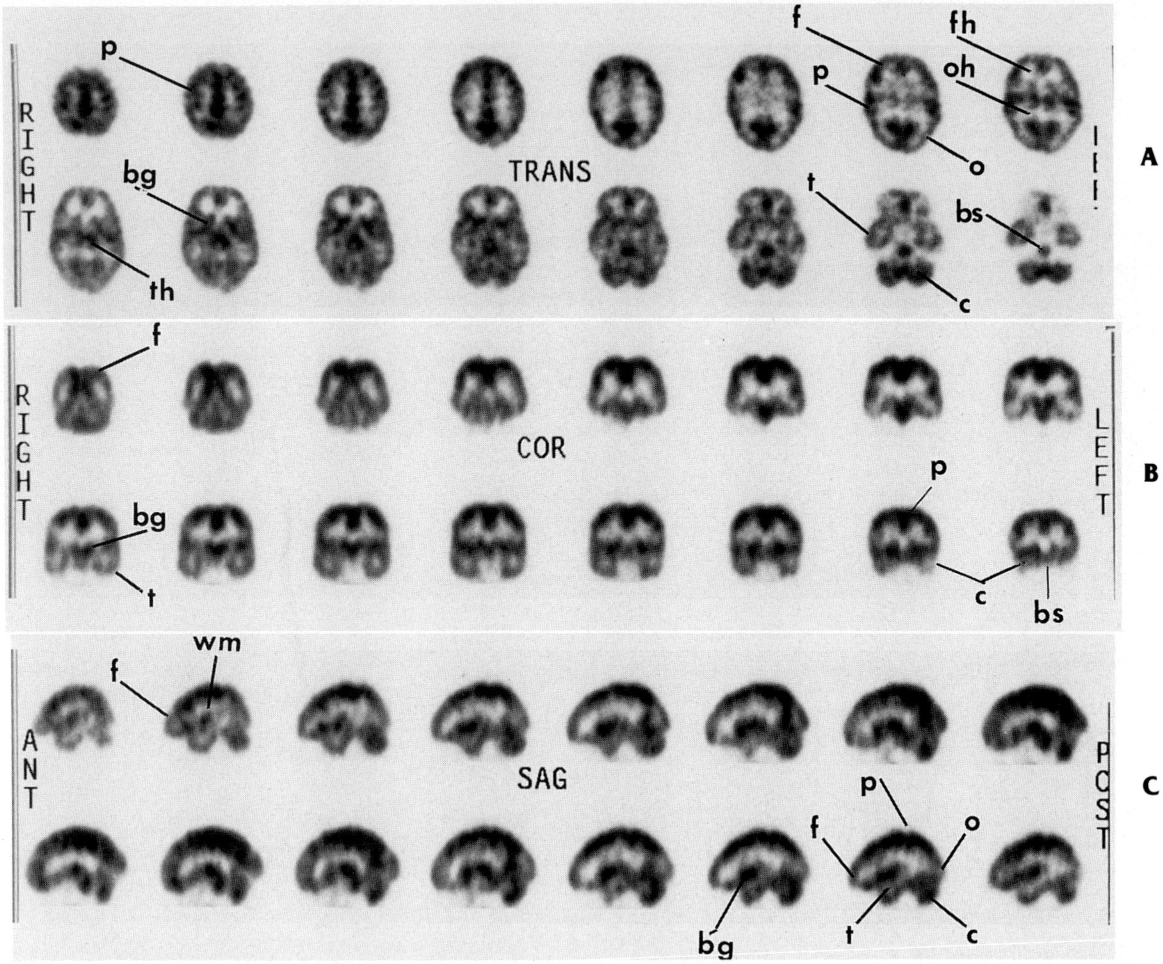


**FIGURE 4** Normal SPECT $^{123}$I-IMP study demonstrates normal tracer in the cerebral cortex, basal ganglia, cerebellum, and upper brain stem. Transaxial (*A*), coronal (*B*), and sagittal (*C*) SPECT images. f = frontal lobe; p = parietal lobe; o = occipital lobe; t = temporal lobe; c = cerebellum; th = thalamus; bg = basal ganglia; bs = brain stem; wm = white matter; fh = frontal horn; oh = occipital horn.

performance of RCA at the time of injection of radiopharmaceuticals such as $^{99m}$Tc-pertechnetate for thyroid studies. This will allow the resident physician to become familiar with the normal RCA pattern and provide a better basis for comparison with the RCA evaluation for brain death.

## *Brain Scintigraphy*

Using a fresh eluate of $^{99m}$Tc of less than 60 minutes, 20 mCi of $^{99m}$Tc–HM-PAO is injected within 30 minutes after the radiopharmaceutical reconstitution. Doses are fractionated for pediatric patients. The generator should also have been eluded at least once before in the last 24 hours. Ten to fifteen minutes after intravenous injection, SPECT images of the head are obtained. (A single-, double-, or triple-headed camera may be used.) Planar images may be obtained if SPECT capability is not available.

Radiopharmaceutical purity is essential. If labeling is improper and quality control poor, the tracer may not cross the blood-brain barrier in a living individual, leading to a false-positive diagnosis of brain death. Therefore $^{99m}$Tc–HM-PAO should be used by physicians experienced in its preparation, verifying radiochemical purity. Clinically the purity can also be validated by obtaining a scan of the liver, which should image with $^{99m}$Tc–HM-PAO. An image over the thyroid bed also verifies the absence of significant amounts of $^{99m}$Tc pertechnetate, assuming that $^{99m}$Tc pertechnetate was not used for the RCA study.

Lack of perfusion to the entire brain, which is compatible with brain death, results in no tracer in cerebral cortex, cerebellum, or brain stem. Only the superficial scalp/skull uptake of tracer is identified (Figs. 4 and 5).

## *Clinical Indication for Studies*

The two scintigraphic studies (RCA and brain scintigraphy) should be done only after direct personal communication between the nuclear physician/radiologist and the referring physician. The referring physician must indicate that clinically the patient already meets hospital policy requirements and state law requirements for brain death. Then and only then should scintigraphic studies be performed to confirm the clinical evidence of brain death.

A B C

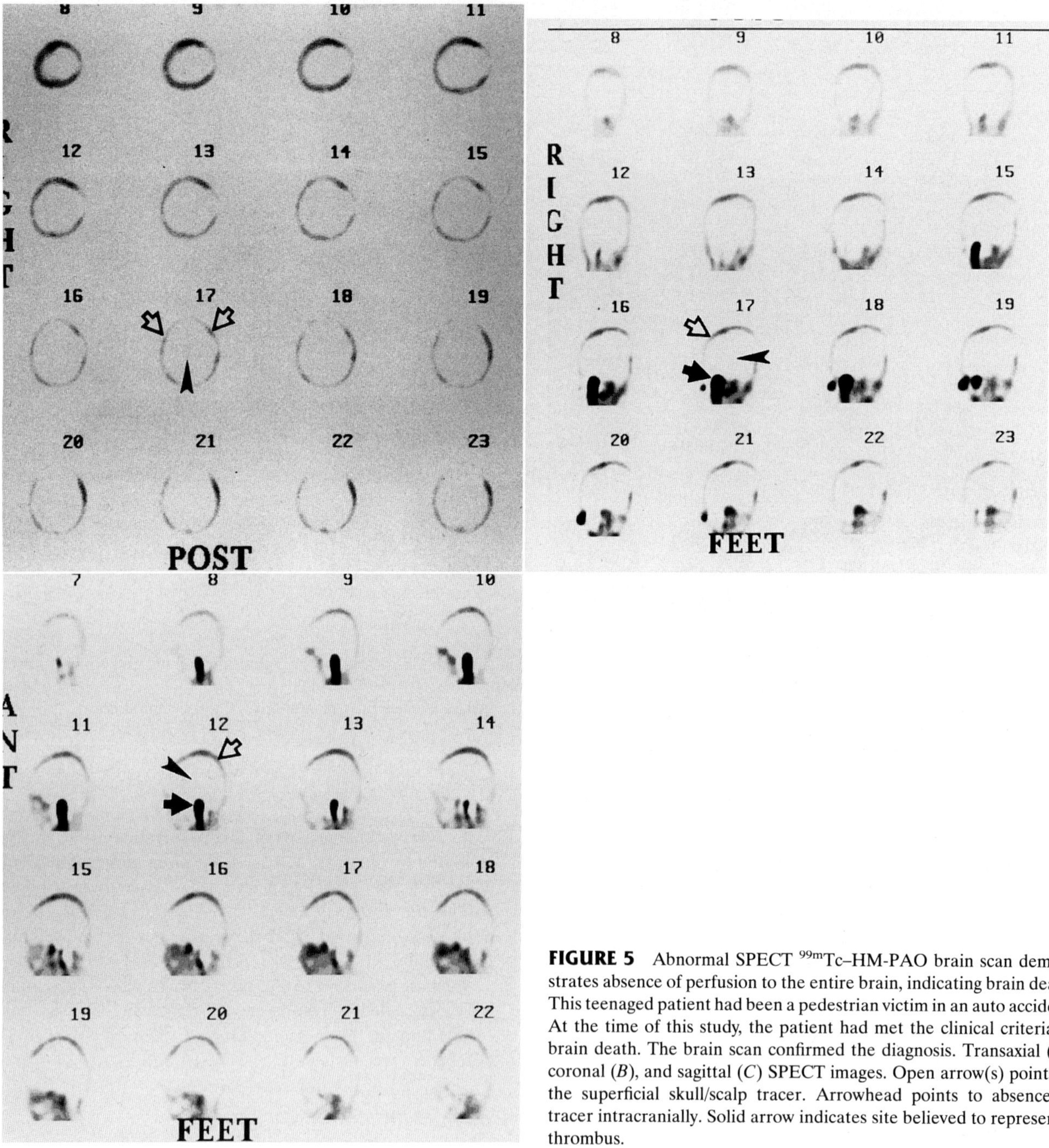


**FIGURE 5** Abnormal SPECT $^{99m}$Tc–HM-PAO brain scan demonstrates absence of perfusion to the entire brain, indicating brain death. This teenaged patient had been a pedestrian victim in an auto accident. At the time of this study, the patient had met the clinical criteria of brain death. The brain scan confirmed the diagnosis. Transaxial (*A*), coronal (*B*), and sagittal (*C*) SPECT images. Open arrow(s) points to the superficial skull/scalp tracer. Arrowhead points to absence of tracer intracranially. Solid arrow indicates site believed to represent a thrombus.

*Acknowledgments.* The author thanks Ms. Mary Mikkola for her secretarial assistance, Ms. Nancy Bulgarelli for her library research assistance, and the William Beaumont Hospital Photographic Department in the preparation of this manuscript.

## Suggested Reading

Ahmann PA, Carrigan TA, Carlton D, et al. Brain death in children: Characteristic common carotid arterial velocity patterns measured with pulsed Doppler ultrasound. J Pediatr 1987; 110:723–728.

Ad Hoc Committee of the Harvard Medical School to Examine the Definition of Brain Death. A definition of irreversible coma. JAMA 1968; 205:337–340.

Arnold H, Kuhne D, Rohr W, Heller M. Contrast bolus technique with rapid CT scanning: A reliable diagnostic tool for the determination of brain death. Neuroradiology 1981; 22:129–132.

Brandau W, Schober O, Knapp WH. Determination of brain death with technetium-99m-HMPAO. J Nucl Med 1990; 31:2075–2076.

Capron AM, Kass LR. A statutory definition of standards for determining human death. University of Pennsylvania Law Review 1978; 87–118.

Espinola D, Beyda D, Camargo EE, et al. Scintigraphic diagnosis of brain death in hypothermic barbiturate coma. J Nucl Med 1982; 23:7.

Galaske RG, Schober O, Heyer R. 99mTc-HM-PAO and $^{123}$I-amphetamine cerebral scintigraphy: A new noninvasive method in determination of brain death in children. Eur J Nucl Med 1988; 14:446–452.

Goodman JM, Heck LL, Moore BD. Confirmation of brain death with portable isotope angiography: A review of 204 consecutive cases. Neurosurgery 1985; 16:492–497.

Goodman JM, Heck L, Nugent SK, Turner MS. Validity of radionuclide cerebral angiography for diagnosing brain death in infants. In: Kaufman HH, ed. Pediatric Brain Death and Organ/Tissue Retrieval. New York: Plenum, 1989.

Guidelines for the determination of death. JAMA 1981; 246:2184–2186.

Hilfinger MF. Brain death with prolonged somatic survival. N Engl J Med 1982; 306:14–16.

Jones KM, Barnes PD. MR diagnosis of brain death. Am J Neuroradiol 1992; 13:65–66.

Korein J, Braunstein R, Kricheff I, et al. Radioisotopic bolus technique as a test to detect circulatory deficit associated with cerebral death. Circulation 1975; 51:924–939.

Laurin NR, Driedger AA, Hurwitz GA, et al. Cerebral perfusion imaging with technetium-99m HM-PAO in brain death and severe central nervous system injury. J Nucl Med 1989; 30:1627–1635.

Lewis RR, Padayachee TS, Beasley MG, et al. Investigation of brain death with Doppler-shift ultrasound. J R Soc Med 1983; 76:308–310.

The matter of Karen Anne Quinlan: The complete briefs, oral arguments and the opinion of the New Jersey Supreme Court. Vol. 2. Washington, D.C.: University Publishers of America, 1975.

Mishkin F. Determination of cerebral death by radionuclide angiography. Radiology 1975; 115:135.

Monrose T, Nishikawa J, Sasaki M, et al. 18F-FDG-PET assessment of coma and brain death. J Nucl Med 1991; 32(abstract):1077.

Morayati SJ, Nagle CE. The determination of death and the changing role of medical imaging. Radiographics 1988; 8:967–979.

Morayati SJ, Nagel [Nagle] CE. Brain death laws: 1988 update. Legal Aspects of Medical Practice, July 1989; 17:3–4.

Nagle C. Use of immediate static scans in combination with radionuclide cerebral angiography as a confirmatory test in the diagnosis of brain death. Clin Nucl Med 1980; 5:152–153.

Nagle C. Brain death with prolonged somatic survival (Letter to the Editor). N Engl J Med 1982; 306:1361.

National institute of neurological and communicative disorder and stroke: An appraisal of the criteria of cerebral death: A summary statement: A collaborative study. JAMA 1972; 237:982.

Pistoia F, Johnson DW, Darby JM, et al. The role of xenon CT measurements of cerebral blood flow in the clinical determination of brain death. Am J Neuroradiol 1991; 12:97–103.

President's commission for the study of ethical problems in medicine and biomedical and behavioral research. Defining death. U.S. Government Printing Office: 81-600150. July 1981; 13–15.

Roine R, Launes J, Lindroth L, Nikkinen P. 99m Tc-Hexamethylpropyleneamine oxime scans to confirm brain death (correspondence). Lancet 1986; 1223–1224.

Schober O, Galaske R, Heyer R. Determination of brain death with $^{123}$I-IMP and 99mTc-HM-PAO. Neurosurg Rev 1987; 10:19–22.

Schwartz JA, Baxter J, Brill D, Burns JR. Radionuclide cerebral imaging confirming brain death. JAMA 1983; 249:246–247.

Schwartz JA, Brill D, Baxter J. Detection of blood flow to the brain by radionuclide cerebral imaging. In: Kaufman HH, ed. Pediatric Brain Death and Organ/Tissue Retrieval: Medical, Ethical, and Legal Aspects. New York: Plenum, 1989.

Spieth ME, Ansari AN, Kawada TK, Siegel ME. Comparison of DTPA and HMPAO for the evaluation of brain death. J Nucl Med 1991; 32(abstract):1839.

Tan WS, Wilbur AC, Jafar JJ, et al. Brain death: Use of dynamic CT and intravenous digital subtraction angiography. Am J Neuroradiol 1987; 8:123–125.

Uematsu S, Smith TD, Walker AE. Pulsatile cerebral echo in diagnosis of brain death with Doppler-shift ultrasound. J R Soc Med 1983; 76:308–310.

Vatne K, Nakstad P, Lundar T. Digital subtraction angiography (DSA) in the evaluation of brain death: A comparison of conventional cerebral angiography with intravenous and intraarterial DSA. Neuroradiology 1985; 27:155–157.

# Imaging Approach to Spine Trauma

*ROBERT M. QUENCER, M.D.*

In the spine-injured patient, optimal use of a number of imaging techniques is necessary if the patient is to be properly diagnosed and treated. Spine trauma must be thought of in terms of (1) acute injury and (2) previous injury, and each requires a different imaging strategy. Plain radiographs, computed tomography (CT), magnetic resonance imaging (MRI), and intraoperative sonography all play a role in evaluating these patients.

## Acutely Injured Spine

### *Plain Radiographs*

Plain radiographs (Figs. 1, *A*, and 2, *A*) are obtained first when the injured patient is brought to the Emergency Room. Careful evaluation of the radiographs for fracture, subluxation, instability, and soft-tissue swelling is done in the anteroposterior (AP) and lateral projections, with an open-mouth odontoid view added in cases of cervical spine trauma. No attempt to determine spinal stability with flexion-extension views should be made on the initial evaluation. If a subluxation is present, immediate spinal reduction is performed and repeat radiographs are obtained to assure proper alignment. If the spine is nonreducible, the patient is intubated and spinal reduction is performed with the patient under anesthesia.

### *CT*

CT (Fig. 1, *B*) is routinely performed on acute spine-injured patients to confirm the presence and extent of the fractures, to disclose the presence of fractures that might not be obvious or are subtle on plain radiographs, and to determine the extent of conal compromise.

### *MRI*

MRI is performed in all spine-injured patients who are medically stable and also have abnormal neurological findings, because MRI can reveal information not available on plain radiographs or CT. If MRI shows an acute disk herniation (Fig. 2, *B* and *C*), clinical management is greatly influenced, because such information in the cervical region may influence the surgeon to perform an anterior cervical decompression and fusion (ACDF) and thus relieve cord compression. In addition, MRI can determine if there are intrinsic changes (Figs. 2, *C*, 3, *A*, and 3, *B*) within the cord (hematoma, edema, or both), findings that have some prognostic value in judging possible return of spinal cord function. Edema alone is observed as an area of high signal intensity within the cord on T2-weighted images, whereas blood yields varying signal depending on the stage of the hematoma (hyperacute, acute, subacute) and the strength of the magnet, but in general for hemorrhagic cord contusion, one expects to observe a relatively hypointense signal (Fig. 3, *A*, and *B*) within the cord parenchyma on T2-weighted spin-echo and T2-weighted gradient-echo studies. Epidural hematomas, which are an unusual sequela of

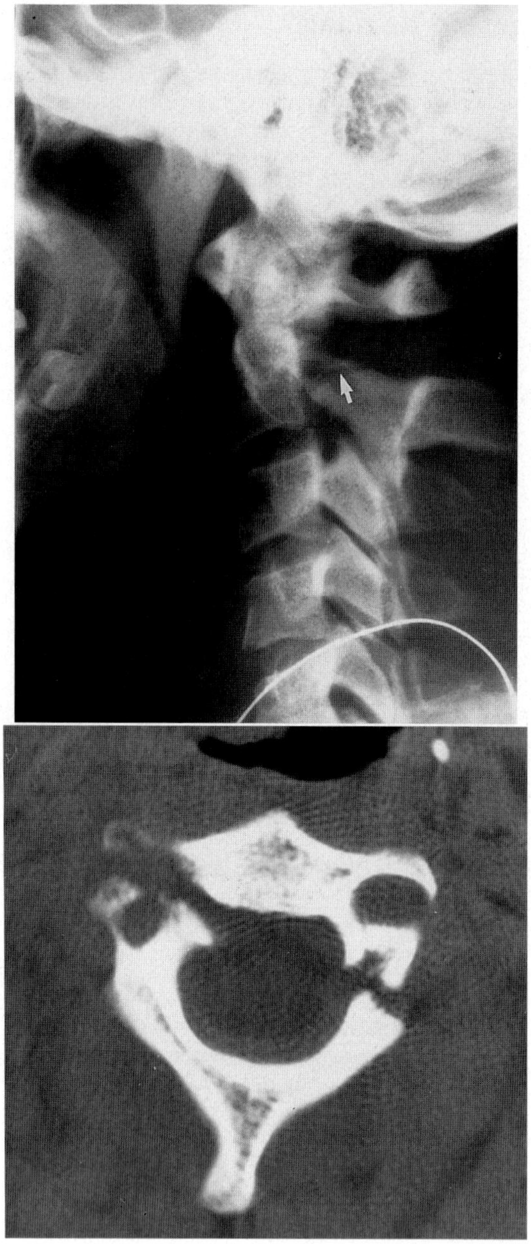

A

B

**FIGURE 1** Hangman's fracture. *A*, Lateral radiograph of the upper cervical spine shows a subtle fracture (*arrow*) with minimal anterior subluxation of C2 relative to C3. *B*, CT performed to better define the fracture and to identify other fractures, more clearly demonstrates the fractures (left lamina, right pedicle) at the C2 level. The relationship of the right-sided fracture to the foramen transverium deserves particular scrutiny because of its proximity to the vertebral artery. A limitation of this imaging sequence (CT and plain films) is the inability to clearly define associated disk herniation, epidural hematoma, and intraparenchymal abnormalities (blood and/or edema) of the spinal cord.

A B C

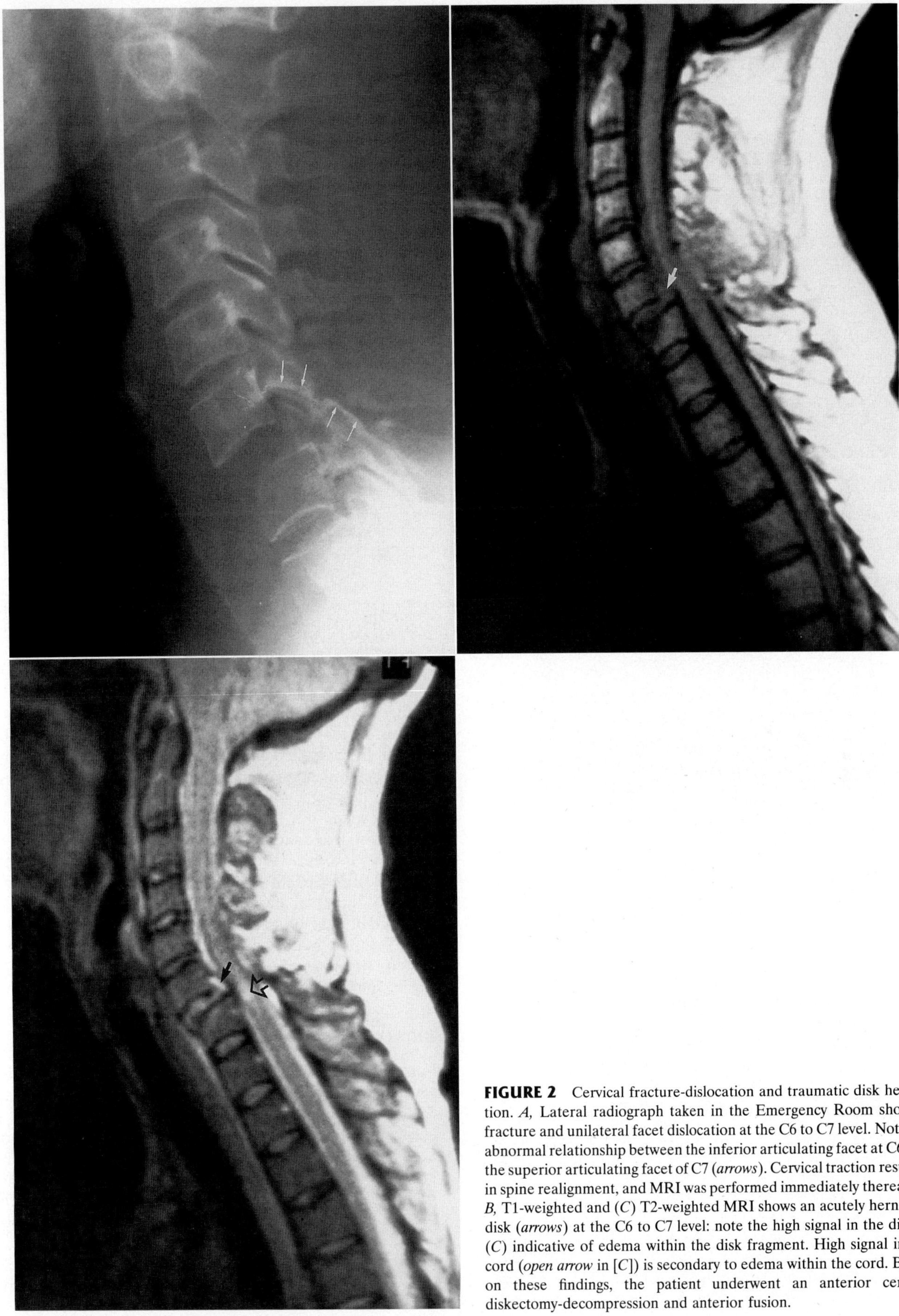

**FIGURE 2** Cervical fracture-dislocation and traumatic disk herniation. *A,* Lateral radiograph taken in the Emergency Room shows a fracture and unilateral facet dislocation at the C6 to C7 level. Note the abnormal relationship between the inferior articulating facet at C6 and the superior articulating facet of C7 (*arrows*). Cervical traction resulted in spine realignment, and MRI was performed immediately thereafter. *B,* T1-weighted and (*C*) T2-weighted MRI shows an acutely herniated disk (*arrows*) at the C6 to C7 level: note the high signal in the disk in (*C*) indicative of edema within the disk fragment. High signal in the cord (*open arrow* in [*C*]) is secondary to edema within the cord. Based on these findings, the patient underwent an anterior cervical diskectomy-decompression and anterior fusion.

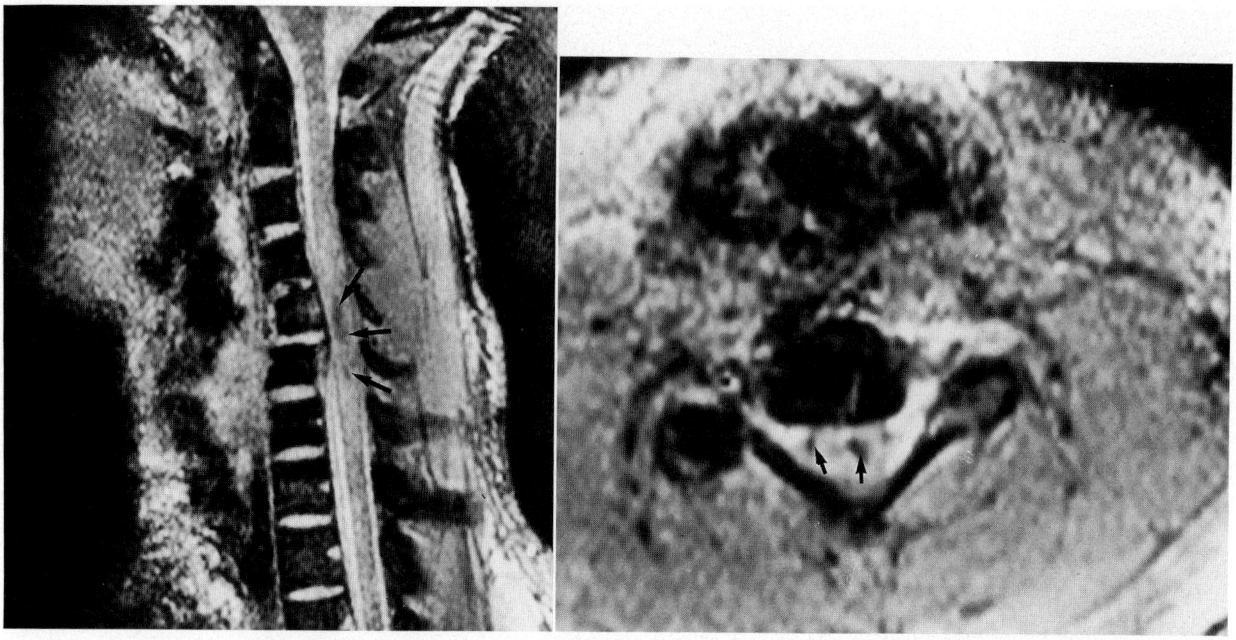


**FIGURE 3** *A* and *B*, Acute post-traumatic hemorrhagic contusion of the cord. On the day of a severe spinal injury (patient was a complete quadriplegic), sagittal and axial gradient-echo MRI images (T2* weighted) demonstrated an area of marked hypointensity *(arrows)* within the cord at the C5 and C6 levels consistent with acute blood. Note the narrowing of the canal diameter, compression of the cord, and posterior displacement of the C5 vertebral body. The presence of a hemorrhagic contusion within the cord is associated with a poor prognosis for functional recovery.

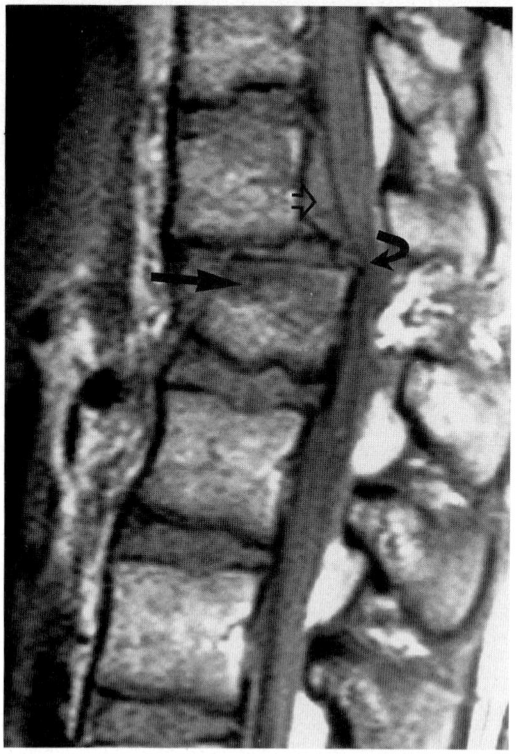

**FIGURE 4** Acute T12/L1 fracture-dislocation. Marked canal and conus compression at the T12 to L1 level is seen on this midsagittal T1-weighted image. Diminished signal in the superior portion of L1 (*arrow*) indicates post-traumatic edema within the bone. This study performed before rod stabilization shows the extent of conus compression (*curved arrow*) and a large disk fragment (*open arrow*) that has migrated superiorly from the T12-L1 level behind the T12 vertebral body. Preoperative detection of disk herniation before a posterior stabilization can influence the surgical procedure (see text).

spinal trauma, can be detected on MRI and usually are treated as surgical emergencies commonly by a multilevel laminectomy if the extra-axial hematoma is located posteriorly. MRI contrast material is not used in the evaluation of acute spine trauma, because high-quality nonenhanced MRI is adequate for the determination of spinal cord and spinal canal compression. Myelographic CT in the setting of acute spine trauma is rarely needed.

In the thoracic and lumbar spine, MRI in comparison to CT more precisely shows the degree of canal narrowing secondary to bone displacement and soft-tissue encroachment on the canal. To know that there is a herniated disk (Fig. 4) before the insertion of rods for spine stabilization is crucial information. Plans can be made preoperatively to initially perform a posterolateral or transthoracic approach for disk removal before spinal fusion.

## *Intraoperative Spinal Sonography*

Complete imaging of the spine-injured patient does not end with the preoperative studies (plain radiography, CT, and MRI), but rather the radiologist can offer the surgeon an invaluable perspective on the progress of surgery for neural decompression with the use of ultrasonography in the operating room. The vastly underused technique of intraoperative spinal sonography (IOSS), employing a real-time display of the surgical field, allows the identification of bone (Fig. 5, *A*), disk, and hematoma that may be compressing the spinal cord or thecal sac, and as importantly, shows that following spine stabilization (Fig. 5, *B*) there has been adequate decompression of neural tissue.

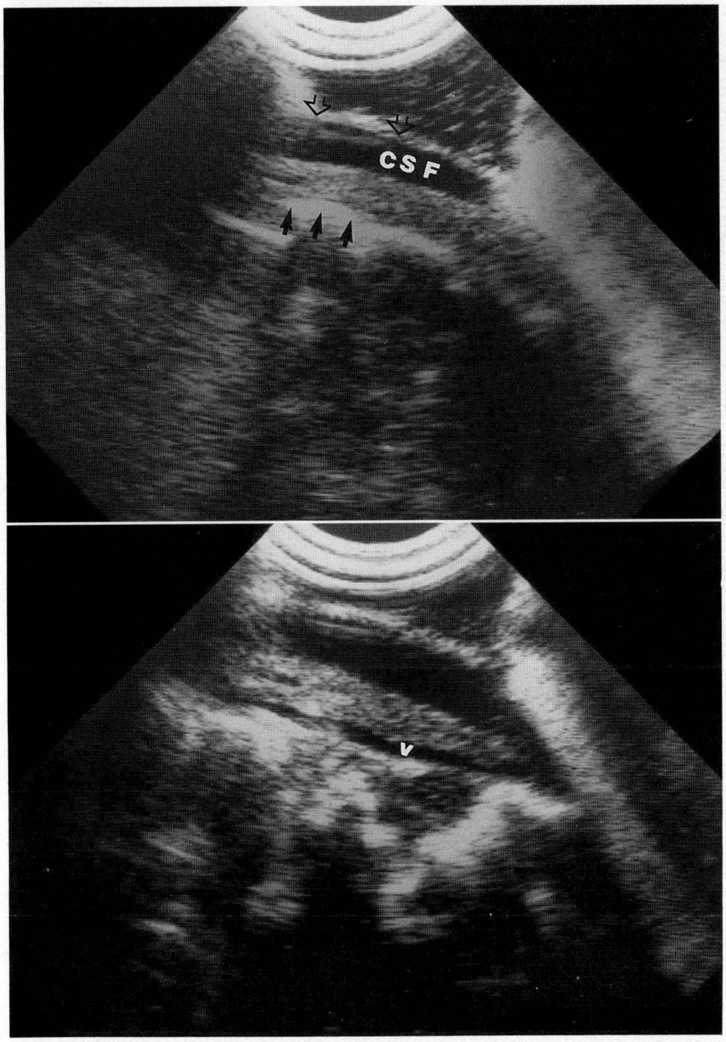


**FIGURE 5** Intraoperative sonography to monitor Harrington rod stabilization for a T12/L1 fracture-dislocation. *A,* Following a small laminotomy at T12 to allow sonographic visualization of the spinal canal, sagittal sonogram shows a large retropulsed bone fragment (*arrows*), with compression of the ventral surface of the distal cord. Note the intact dura (*arrowheads*) and the dorsal CSF. *B,* Following Harrington rod insertion, sagittal sonogram shows that there is no longer bony compression of the cord and ventral CSF (v) is now present. This study documents successful neural tissue decompression.

## The Previously Injured Spine

The clinical approach to the patient with a previously injured spine (chronic injury) has changed over the past decade. This has come about not only because MRI has the ability to show in considerable detail what other studies (CT, myelography, myelographic CT) were not able to show but because at a number of spinal cord injury centers there is a surgically more aggressive attitude towards these patients.

### *Plain Radiographs*

Assessment of gross spinal alignment, spinal stability (flexion-extension views), bony narrowing of the canal, the integrity of a prior bony fusion, and the presence of foreign bodies in the canal are all well assessed by plain radiographs. Other details often crucial to patient evaluation, particularly in patients who are deteriorating neurologically, require further studies.

### *Computed Tomography*

CT usually adds little to the information available with plain radiographs, so in the vast majority of cases one can proceed from plain radiographs to MRI. In the past, myelographic CT with delayed (4 to 6 hours) imaging had been the standard way of evaluating a previously spine-injured patient with typical progressive symptoms such as motor-sensory loss, increasing spasticity, and autonomic dysreflexia. There were misleading findings on such studies, such as a myelomalacic cord having similar appearance to an intramedullary cyst. MRI, on the other hand, can depict with a great deal of accuracy the intrinsic changes within the cord that are crucial for developing treatment strategies, so that CT is rarely employed in these circumstances.

### *Magnetic Resonance Imaging*

MRI demonstrates cord atrophy (Fig. 6), intradural adhesions (see Fig. 6), residual cord compression (Fig. 7), simple or complex spinal cord cysts (see Fig. 7), myelomalacia (Fig. 8), and the evolution over time of myelomalacia to an intramedullary cyst (Fig. 9). Each of these requires a different approach clinically and a different recommendation for follow-up imaging studies. MRI contrast agents are not needed in any of these situations.

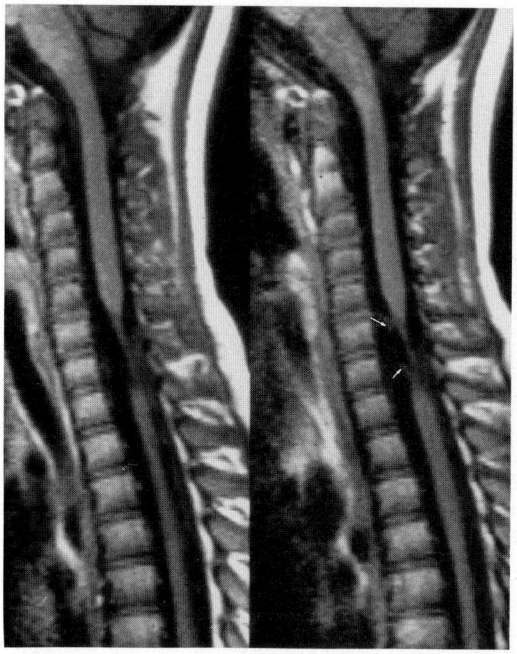

**FIGURE 6** Severe cervical cord atrophy secondary to prior stretch injury to the spine. Sagittal T1-weighted MRI shows marked atrophy of the cord from C7 to T1 in an 18-month-old child who had undergone a difficult breech delivery. Thin areas of isointense signal within the ventral CSF probably represent intradural adhesions (*arrows*). There was no evidence of spine fracture or dislocation, and the mechanism of injury was presumably a vascular one at the cervicothoracic junction.

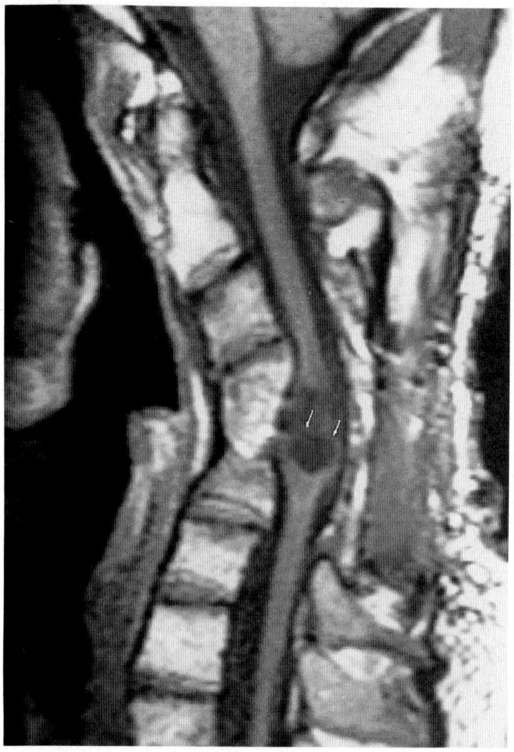

**FIGURE 7** Post-traumatic spinal cord cyst. This patient had a prior posterior cervical fusion in an attempt to stabilize a C4/C5 fracture-subluxation. Nonetheless, a gibbus deformity present at C4 is causing focal ventral cord compression. In addition, a spinal cord cyst with intracystic septations (*arrows*) is causing focal cord expansion. In a patient such as this with either progressive neurological symptoms or incomplete quadriparesis, both spinal cyst decompression via two shunt catheters (cyst to subarachnoid space and cyst to peritoneal cavity) and an anterior decompression (corpectomy) and fusion would be performed.

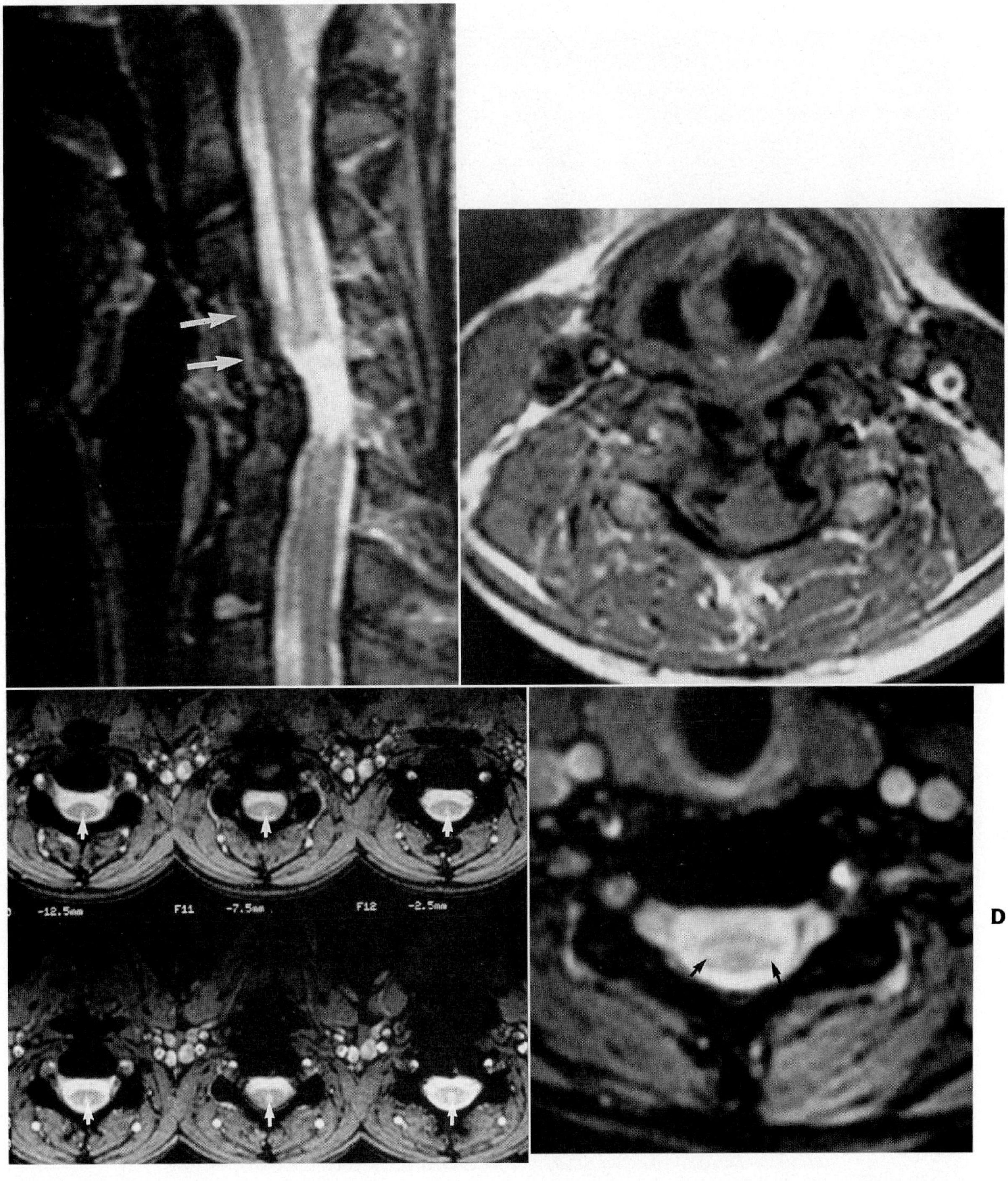


**FIGURE 8** Prior C5 cord injury with ascending dorsal column Wallerian degeneration. *A,* This patient suffered a previous C5 cord injury (high signal on T2-weighted GRE image) and had an anterior fusion (*arrows*) in an attempt to stabilize the spine. *B,* The signal within the cord on T1-weighted axial images at the injury site is hypointense to normal cord tissue, but significantly higher in signal than CSF in the adjacent SAS. These findings suggest a myelomalacia rather than a confluent shuntable cyst. *C,* Axial T2 GRE images above the injury level from C2-3 (*upper left*) to C4-5 (*lower right*) demonstrate a high signal within the dorsal columns (*arrows*), corresponding to the fascilus gracilis. Wallerian degeneration superiorly along this tract is suggested by this finding and is progressively more prominent closer to the site of injury (compare figure in upper left to figure in lower right). *D,* Below the injury level at C6-7 abnormal signal is identified in the lateral cortical spinal tracts bilaterally (*arrows*) compatible with Wallerian degeneration caudal to the injury site.

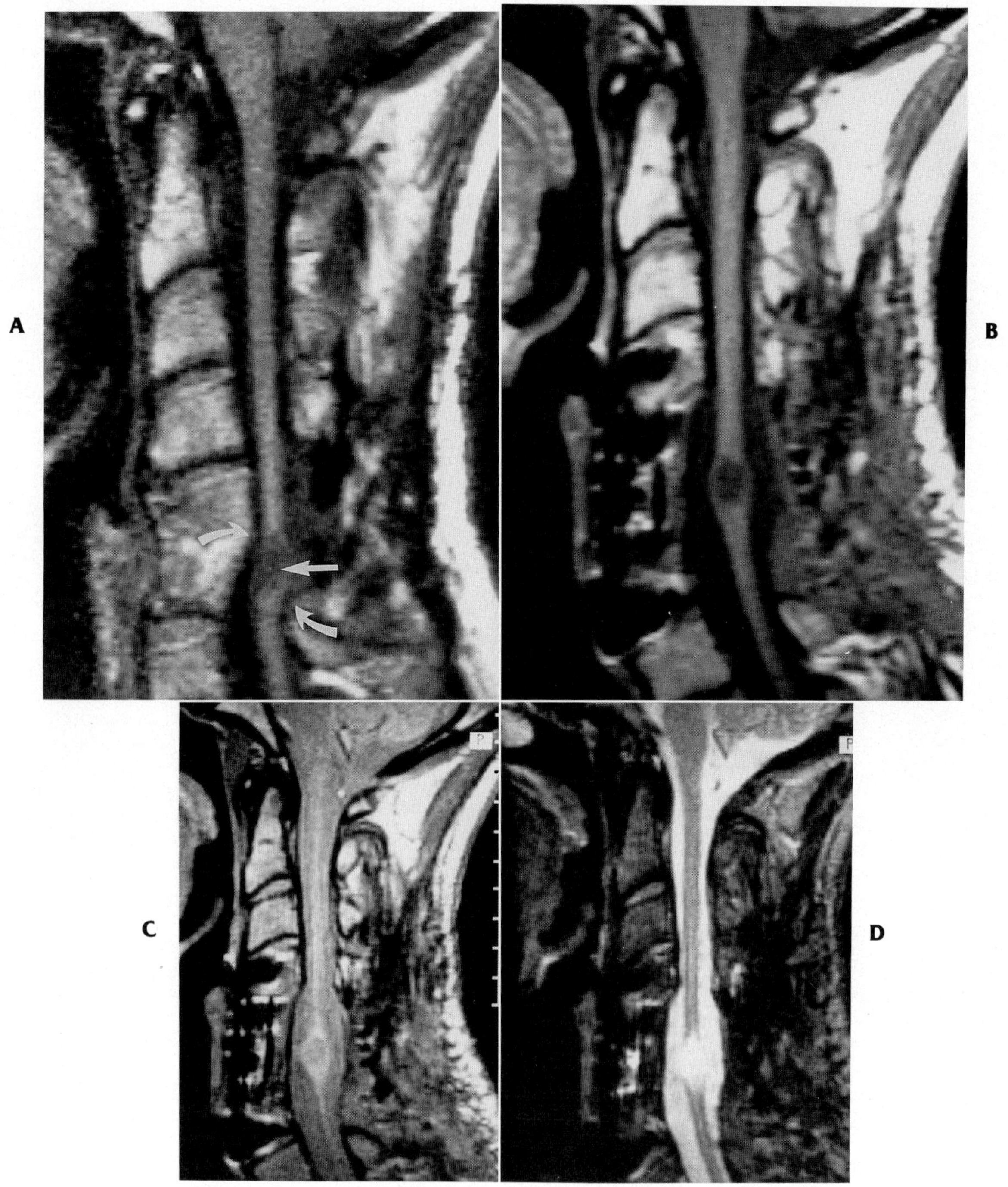


**FIGURE 9** Evolution of post-traumatic microcystic myelomalacia into a unilocular spinal cord cyst. *A,* There is an area of post-traumatic myelomalacia (*straight white arrow*) at the C6 level and narrowing of canal posteriorly at C6-C7 and anteriorly at C5-C6. *B,* An anterior and posterior decompression to widen the canal and an anterior and posterior fusion for stabilization was performed. Note that in (*B*) (performed one year after surgery), the anterior titanium plate and screws give virtually no artifact on the MRI scan. A cyst in the cord is now present; note that the signal within the cyst follows that of CSF from the T1-weighted (*B*) to the proton density (*C*) to the T2-weighted (*D*) images. Note the focal cord expansion around the cyst and a high signal of the cord's periphery in (*C*). It may be that widening the canal and the untethering of the cord was a factor in the development of a cyst from an area of myelomalacia.

In general, patients who are neurologically stable and show cord atrophy (see Fig. 6) with no other significant findings require no follow-up studies. Patients with unequivocal cord cysts (see Figs. 7 and 9, *B, C,* and *D*) are usually treated with cyst diversionary procedures, particularly if there is a deteriorating neurological situation. Two simultaneous drainage procedures are employed: cyst to subarachnoid space and cyst to peritoneal or pleural cavity. The rate of shunt malfunction and cyst recurrence is far less with this surgical approach. Cysts are distinguished from myelomalacia by the fact that the signal of a cyst follows cerebrospinal fluid (CSF) on every pulse sequence used (see Fig. 9), whereas in myelomalacia (see Fig. 8) this is not the situation. Specifically in myelomalacia, the signal from the cord tissue is more intense than CSF on T1 and proton density images. This distinction is crucial because both cord cysts and myelomalacia may present with new neurologic findings, but clearly only the former is by itself a potential surgical lesion.

Other observations on MRI are as important as analyzing the signal from within the cord. Namely, residual cord compression (see Figs. 7, 9, *A*) at, above, or below the injury level may require a bony decompression (see Fig. 9, *B*) with stabilization. Oftentimes, it is difficult to know whether new symptoms are secondary to progressive intraparenchymal changes (e.g., expanding cyst) or are caused by compressive abnormalities. It is not infrequent therefore that the surgeon might correct both situations by a decompression and fusion along with a cyst diversionary procedure.

Recent observations indicate that Wallerian degeneration (Fig. 8, *C* and *D*) along the dorsal columns and lateral columns (ascending proprioceptive pathways and descending motor pathways) occurs slowly but progressively following severe cord injuries. These changes can be seen as high signal abnormalities on T2-weighted images, and in an incompletely injured patient these findings could explain the observed clinical changes.

### *Intraoperative Spinal Sonography*

It is imperative that sonography be available whenever cases involving cord cysts, adhesions, and kinking of the cord are involved. Particularly vexing from a surgical standpoint are the complex intraparenchymal cord cysts (see Figs. 7, 10) in which fibroglial septations divide the cyst into a number of loculated components. When these cysts are shunted, the best way to know if complete collapse has occurred is by re-evaluating the cord with sonography before closing the surgical wound. Associated chronic compression of the cord or roots by bone, disk, or intradural cysts can be simultaneously evaluated and if further surgical maneuvers are performed to alleviate the compression, the consequence of such a procedure can be assessed.

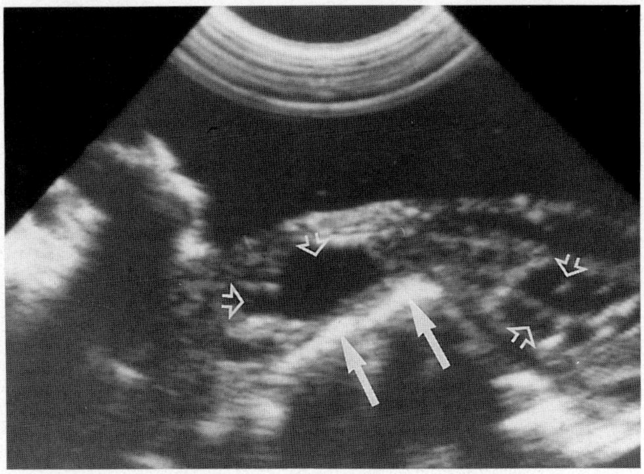

**FIGURE 10** Intraoperative sonography of a complex post-traumatic cord cyst. Sagittal sonography following a wide laminectomy at C6-7 level shows a large angulated bony fragment (*arrow*) projecting into the ventral portion of the canal. Multiple cysts within the spinal cord (*open arrows*) are seen with septations (fibroglial scarring) present within the cyst. The cysts were shunted and the bony compression was relieved.

## Suggested Reading

Kulkarni MV, McCardle CB, Kopanicky D, et al. Acute spinal cord injury: MR imaging at 1.5T. Radiology 1987; 164:837–843.

Morse BM, Quencer RM, Green BA, et al. Intraoperative sonography in spinal trauma. Radiology 1984; 153:125–134.

Quencer RM. The injured spinal cord: Evaluation with MR and intraoperative sonography. Radiol Clin North Am 1988; 26:1025–1045.

Quencer RM, Bunge R, Egnor M, et al. MR/pathological correlations in the acute post-traumatic central cervical spinal cord syndrome. Neuroradiology 1992 (in press).

Quencer RM, Montalvo BM, Eismont FJ, Green BA. Intraoperative spinal sonography in thoracic and lumbar fractures: Evaluation of Harrington rod instrumentation. Am J Neuroradiol 1985; 6:353–359; Am J Roentgenol 1985; 145:343–349.

Quencer RM, Sheldon JJ, Post MJD, et al. MRI in the chronically injured cervical spinal cord. Am J Neuroradiol 1986; 7:457–464.

Tarr RW, Drolshager LF, Kerner TC, et al. MR imaging of recent spinal trauma. J Comput Assist Tomogr 1987; 11:412–417.

# Imaging of Degenerative Disk Disease

*VICTOR M. HAUGHTON, M.D.*

Magnetic resonance imaging (MRI) effectively shows the changes in the intervertebral disk from aging and degeneration. Because back pain is so common, one of the most frequent MRI evaluations is the spine. Recognizing degenerative and normal or normally aging disks is an important responsibility of the radiologist.

The processes of aging and of degeneration of the disk are unfortunately lumped together in some reviews. For example, some journal articles imply that most of the intervertebral disks in subjects 20 years or older are degenerated. To infer that normal disks rarely occur in normal subjects makes little sense. A better understanding of disk degeneration can be obtained if progressive and age-related changes are distinguished from degeneration. It is true that both degeneration and aging of the intervertebral disk result in increasing amounts of collagen, decreasing amounts of glycosaminoglycans, and decreasing amounts of water in the intervertebral disk. However, normally aging intervertebral disks preserve their height or signal intensity to a greater extent than degenerating disks. The differentiation of age-related and degenerative changes in this chapter is based on morphological criteria derived from anatomic and MRI studies in over 150 cadavers.

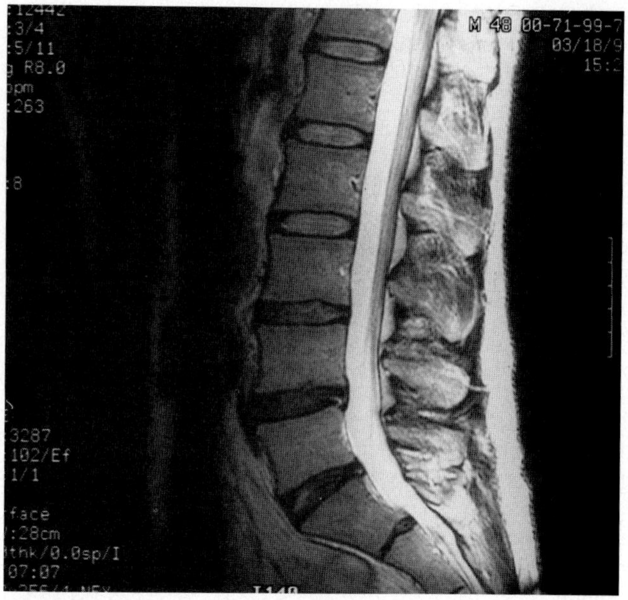

**FIGURE 1** Radial tear. A sagittal T2-weighted fast spin-echo (FSE) image shows low signal intensities in the L3-4, L4-5 and L5-S1 disks. In the lower two disks, tracts of higher signal intensity in the posterior anulus fibrosus represent radial tears.

## Age-related Disk Changes

With aging, small concentric and transverse tears develop in the peripheral portion of the anulus fibrosus. These are characterized as small spaces between the laminae in the anulus fibrosus (concentric tears) or short ruptures of one or several layers of the laminae in the anulus fibrosus (transverse tears). These concentric and transverse tears are found in the majority of the intervertebral disks of older adults and are not associated with other signs of intervertebral disk failure or degeneration. Therefore they should be considered age-related, normal, progressive, or regressive changes in the intervertebral disks. The transverse tear may be apparent in MR or CT images and, rarely, spine radiographs as a small collection of fluid or gas in the peripheral portion of the anulus. The tear is usually adjacent to the ring apophysis, either in the cervical or the lumbar spine. They may represent a stage in the development of vertebral osteophytes. The concentric tear, which is a delamination of the laminae in the anulus fibrosus, is not detected on radiographs and not usually on CT or MR images.

## Degenerative Disk Changes

The radial tear of the anulus fibrosus differs from the concentric or transverse tear in that all layers of the anulus fibrosus are involved. It has a different significance from the other tears. The radial tear in the intervertebral disk is usually associated with other degenerative changes, such as reduced signal intensity in MRI and reduced height of the disk. Although a radial tear is a necessary condition for disk herniation to occur, most radial tears exist without nuclear material herniated from its normal position. Radial tears usually are associated with decreased water content and glycosaminoglycan in the nucleus pulposus and bulging of the anulus fibrosus.

The radial tear can be recognized in MR images as a hiatus in the peripheral low signal intensity portion of the intervertebral disk (Fig. 1), where the anular fibers are torn. A radial tear can also be inferred when the disk has lost signal intensity and height. In CT imaging, bulging of the anulus and loss of disk height, which are usual findings in association with radial tears, can also be recognized. In myelography the ventral impressions on the dural sac are signs of a bulging anulus, secondary usually to a bulging anulus.

Therapeutic implications of a bulging disk or a radial tear are uncertain. Since bulging disks occur as an incidental finding, they are thought to be asymptomatic. However, some excellent clinical investigations suggest that a radial tear may produce sciatic pain or low back pain. The mechanism for back pain from a radial tear may be leakage of disk material into the epidural space, where it causes inflammatory response and/or pain, growth of granulomatous material in the disk as a part of the healing process, pain in the ligaments of the spine from destabilization of the spine by the radial tear. Whether or not the radial tear is implicated in back pain, there is no specific treatment. Therefore the radiographic detection of bulging disk or a radial tear or loss of disk height or signal intensity does not usually lead to any specific therapy.

Transverse, concentric, and radial tears must be distinguished from herniation of the nucleus pulposus. Herniation of the nucleus pulposus of course requires a radial tear of the anulus, but by definition signifies escape of disk material through the anular tear into the space that surrounds the disk. Herniation of the nucleus pulposus is not a perfectly accurate term, because often the herniated fragment of fibrocartilage is characteristic of the anulus fibrosus. Herniations of the nucleus pulposus may be asymptomatic, but are often associated with radicular pain.

Herniation of the nucleus pulposus, protrusion, extrusion, and sequestration are often used synonymously. Protrusion is usually used now to designate a small or questionable herniation, but the correct definition of protrusion is leakage of nuclear material into a radial tear in the anulus but not beyond the margin of the anulus. In that sense it is not a herniation.

Herniations of the nucleus pulposus can be divided into subligamentous, free, extruded, or sequestered fragments. A subligamentous herniation refers to nuclear material that has escaped through the anulus fibrosus and remains behind the posterior longitudinal ligament, which supplies a dense band of fibers in the midline and a somewhat thinner tough sheath of collagen along the entire posterior border of the intervertebral disk. Free fragment refers to disk material that has escaped through the posterior longitudinal ligament into the epidural space. During laminectomy, the surgeon encounters this

A 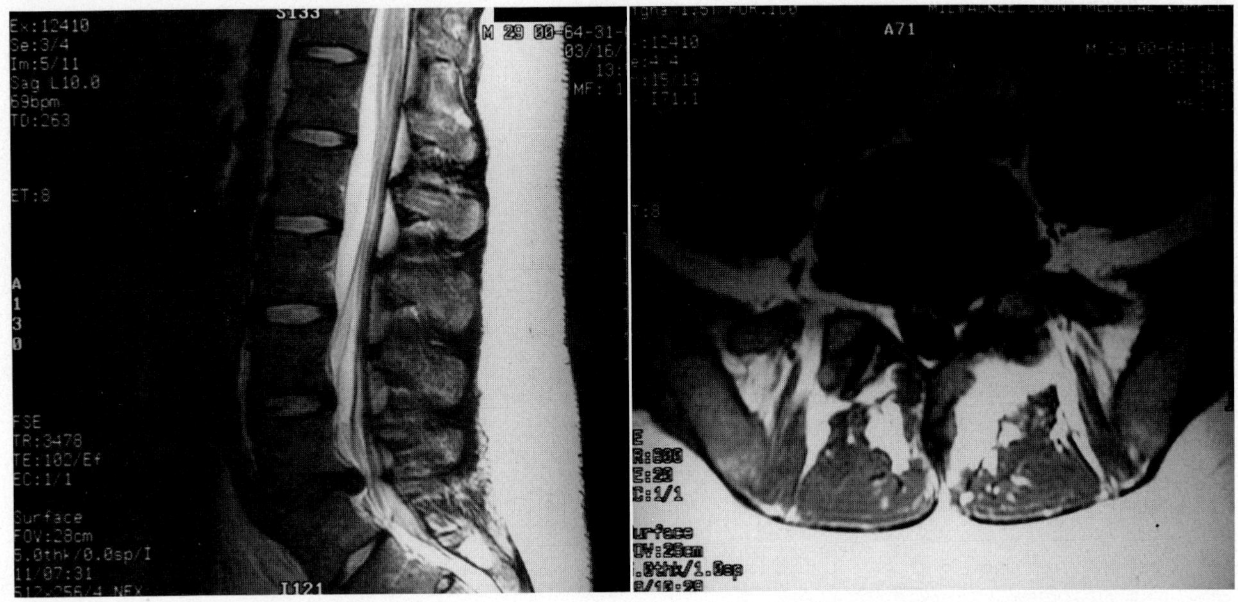 B

**FIGURE 2** Subligamentous herniation. Sagittal T2-weighted FSE (*A*) and axial T1-weighted SE images (*B*) show a herniated disk probably still retained behind the posterior longitudinal ligament at L5-S1.

fragment without the necessity of incising the posterior longitudinal ligament. In that sense this fragment is free. Extravasated disk is another term used synonymously with free fragment. Sequestration refers to a fragment that is partially free but also partially retained behind the posterior longitudinal ligament. Subligamentous herniations, free fragments, extruded fragments, and sequestrations are all examples of herniated disk. The term *prolapse* is used occasionally to signify a herniated disk without specifying its exact location.

## MRI Diagnosis of Disk Herniation

The MRI diagnosis of herniated disk is based in part on the appearance of the disk margins. Disk herniations produce a focal abnormality of the intervertebral disk margin or a focal collection of disk material in the epidural space. In the case of a subligamentous herniation, the border of the intervertebral disk is smooth and curvilinear due to the effect of the posterior longitudinal ligament on the disk fragment (Fig. 2). In extruded disks the margin of the disk may appear polypoid and irregular, because the effect of the posterior longitudinal ligament is lacking (Fig. 3). In some cases of free fragment, the disk margin may appear normal or nearly normal as a result of the migration of the fragment in the spinal canal.

### *Imaging Technique*

For effective MRI of patients with suspected disk degeneration, sagittal and axial images are required. The matrix, slice thickness, field of view, and excitations must be chosen to provide adequate spatial resolution and signal intensity. The selection of surface coil is critical. The sensitive volume of the coil must be matched as closely as possible to the region of interest. Specially designed cervical and lumbar and thoracic spine coils and phased array coils produce good results. Skips must be minimal or zero. The angulation of the axial images should be as nearly as possible perpendicular to the long axis of the spinal canal at each level. A sufficient number of sections must be obtained at each level to encompass the top and bottom of the neural foramen. Single slices through each level are not adequate.

T2-weighted sequences provide the so-called myelogram effect, with cerebrospinal fluid (CSF) achieving a high signal intensity. It also provides high signal intensity from the fibrocartilaginous portions of the intervertebral disc. Therefore radial tears in the disk and early degeneration of the intervertebral disk are readily detected in T2-weighted images. T1-weighted images provide excellent detail, especially in the lumbar region where epidural fat is plentiful. Paramagnetic contrast media are also useful in demonstrating radial tears. In the lumbar spine, T1-weighted images effectively show the tissues in the fat in the epidural space. Since CSF pulsations are minimal, good-quality T2-weighted images can be obtained of the lumbar spine with spin-echo (SE) sequences. An effective evaluation of the lumbar spine consists of a sagittal SE series with short TR and short TE, a sagittal SE sequence with long TR and long TE, and an axial short TR series (angulated appropriately for the disk levels of interest). Fast spin-echo, gradient-echo (GE), and three-dimensional (3D) techniques are a few of the effective alternatives.

In the cervical spine, epidural fat is minimal. Artifacts resulting from swallowing and CSF motion are significant problems. An effective study includes a sagittal T1-weighted SE series and a sagittal GE image with flip-angle, TE, and TR chosen to minimize artifacts and maximize contrast in the spinal cord and neural foramen (Fig. 4). Axial images with suitably thin slices ($\leq 3.0$ mm) are obtained with GE sequences at appropriate levels.

### *Indications for Surgery*

The major mission in imaging degenerative disk disease is to identify herniated disks that warrant surgical treatment. For the radiologist to diagnose such a disk herniation, three criteria

A

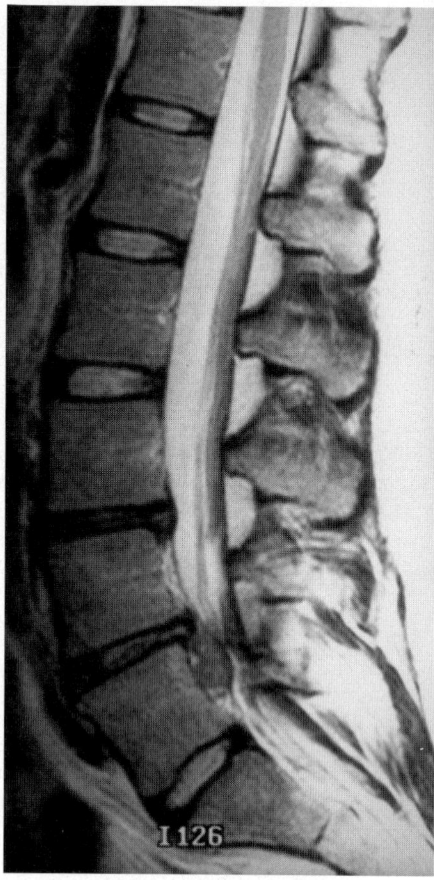


B

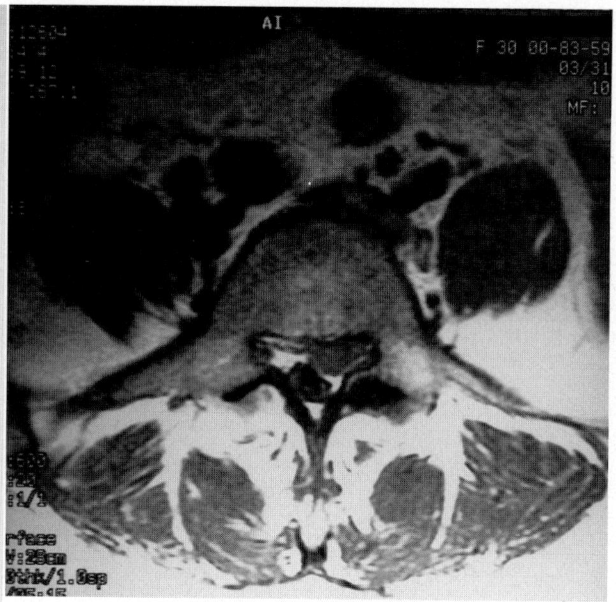


**FIGURE 3** Free fragments. Sagittal T2-weighted (*A*) and axial T1-weighted images in a free fragment at L5-S1. The fragment has migrated from the intervertebral disk to the lateral recess (*B*).

A

B

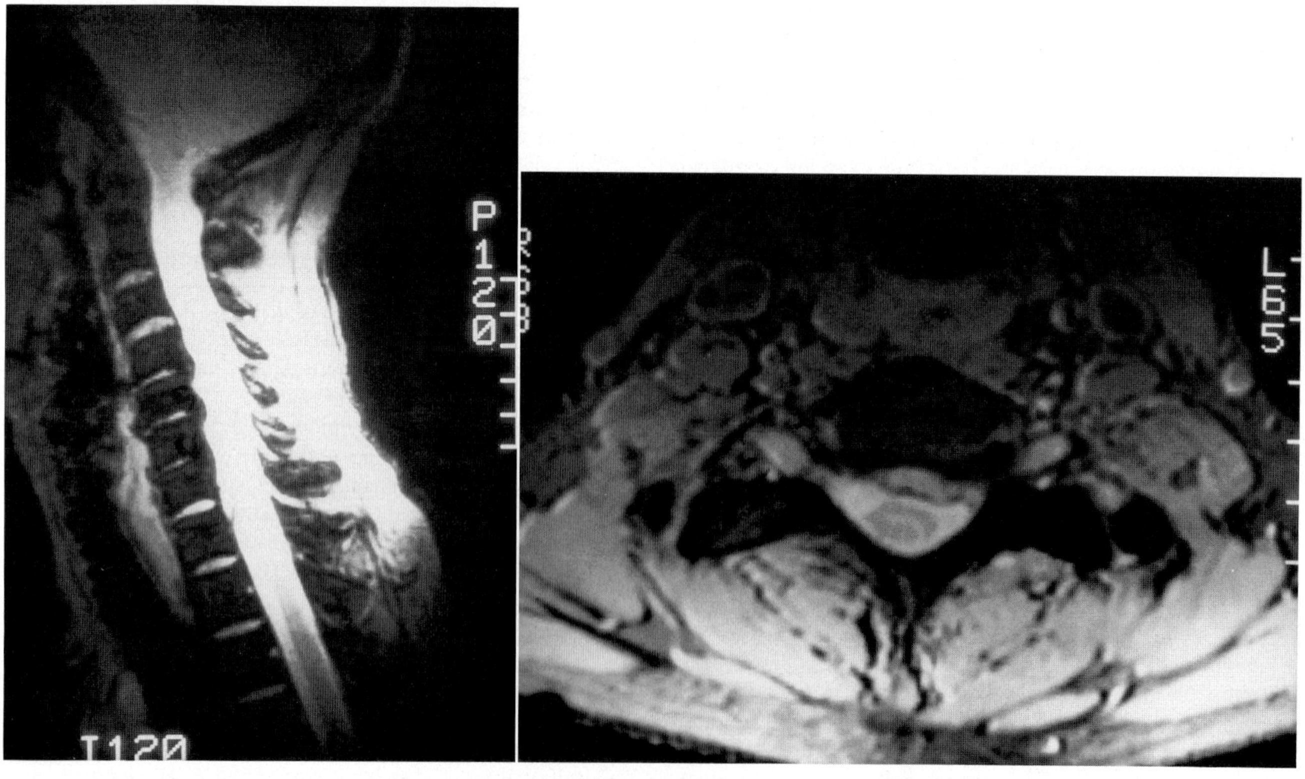


**FIGURE 4** Cervical disk herniation. Sagittal (*A*) and axial (*B*) GE T2-weighted images in a C5-6 herniated disk.

must be fulfilled. First, the appearance of the disk margin or epidural fat must suggest a disk herniation. Second, the disk herniation must compress or displace a spinal nerve. Third, the patient's pain or neurologic signs must conform to the distribution of the nerve that appears to be affected on the MRI study. Unless those three criteria are fulfilled, surgical decompression of the spinal nerve is unlikely to benefit the patient. Nerve compression or displacement of a spinal nerve is arguably the mechanism by which pain is produced. These three criteria nevertheless represent the best strategy for the MRI diagnosis of disk herniation and differentiation of symptomatic and incidental herniations. If a nerve root is not affected or if the affected nerve root is not the one that explains the patient's symptoms, then the report should convey the impression that the intervertebral disk abnormalities are of questionable clinical significance.

### *Other Findings*

Imaging in a patient with back pain provides an opportunity to detect unsuspected congenital, neoplastic, inflammatory, infectious, or traumatic conditions that may be contributing to back pain. Images need to be inspected for evidence of an unsuspected finding such as metastases or a condition such as spinal stenosis or facet joint disease that may simulate a disk herniation. The distal spinal cord should be inspected for evidence of a tumor, which may present as a disk herniation. The major indication for imaging in this group, however, is to identify a stenosis or herniated disk that may be amenable to surgical treatment. Although MRI, and to a lesser extent CT and myelography, are useful in detecting bulging of the anulus fibrosus, internal disk disruption, and postoperative changes in the disk, they are not findings that usually result in specific therapies. Therefore a herniated disk is still the object of most imaging missions.

Differentiating herniated disks from asymmetric bulging disks may challenge the radiologist; however, in these cases the radiologist can emphasize the appearance of the nerve roots. If the radiologist is able to report the presence or absence of nerve root compression and to relate the patient's clinical symptoms to a specific nerve root compression, then he has performed his job effectively, without the need to distinguish a herniation from a bulging disk.

## Suggested Reading

Blumberg ML, Ostrum BJ, Ostrum DM. Changes in MR signal intensity of the intervertebral disk. Radiology 1991; 179:584.

Jinkins JR, Whittemore AR, Bradley WG. Anatomic basis of vertebrogenic pain and the autonomic syndrome associated with lumbar disk extrusion. Am J Neuroradiol 1989; 10:219.

Resnick D, Niwayama G, eds. Diagnosis of Bone and Joint Disorders. 2nd ed. Philadelphia: WB Saunders, 1988:1494.

Ross JS, Modic MT, Masaryk TJ. Tears of the anulus fibrosus: Assessment with Gd-DTPA-enhanced MR imaging. AJR 1990; 154:159.

Ross JS, Tkach J, VanDyke C, Modic MT. Clinical MR imaging of degenerative spinal disease: Pulse sequences, gradient echo techniques, and contrast agents. J Magn Reson Imaging 1991; 1:29.

Sether LA, Yu S, Haughton VM, Fischer ME. Intervertebral disk: Normal age-related changes in MR signal intensity. Radiology 1990; 177:385.

Yu S, Haughton VM, Lynch KL, et al. Fibrous structure in the intervertebral disk: Correlation of MR appearance with anatomic sections. Am J Neuroradiol 1989; 10:1105.

Yu S, Haughton VM, Sether LA, et al. Criteria for classifying normal and degenerated lumbar intervertebral disks. Radiology 1989; 170:523.

# MRI Evaluation of Spinal Stenosis

*MARY F. GASKILL-SHIPLEY, M.D. · ROBERT R. LUKIN, M.D.*

Lumbar spinal stenosis is defined as narrowing of the central spinal canal or neural foramina secondary to bony or soft-tissue abnormalities, which produce compression of the neural and vascular structures. Neurological symptoms may be related to direct impingement of neural tissue as well as to arterial obstruction and venous hypertension.

Spinal stenosis most commonly affects men in the third to sixth decades of life. The classic presentation is neurogenic claudication, which is described as bilateral lower extremity radiculopathies and sensory-motor deficits that are exacerbated when the patient stands or walks but resolve when he lies down. The majority of patients, however, do not exhibit true claudication symptoms but may present with other neurologic complaints including low back pain, numbness, and sciatica. Often the patient's symptoms have been present for months or years; however, occasionally the onset of neurologic problems is acute.

Accurate radiologic imaging of the spine is essential in diagnosing spinal stenosis and in determining the location and cause of narrowing so appropriate surgical or medical management can be implemented.

## Radiologic Imaging

Before the development of magnetic resonance imaging (MRI), myelography and computed tomography (CT) were the primary imaging studies used to diagnose spinal stenosis. Although both evaluations provide information on the extent and degree of stenosis, each test has distinct disadvantages. Myelography is invasive, does not evaluate the entire neural foramen, and may not define the exact etiology of the stenosis (i.e., soft-tissue versus bony change). CT is restricted by the use of ionizing radiation and a limitation on the number of levels that can be scanned.

The pairing of water-soluble myelography and postmyelographic CT is a thorough and accurate method of evaluating the lumbar spine; however, because of the expense and invasiveness of these tests, this combination should be performed in select cases when other imaging modalities have not provided adequate information.

In recent years MRI has been a major development in spinal imaging, providing high resolution and noninvasive imaging of the entire spine while combining some of the best features of

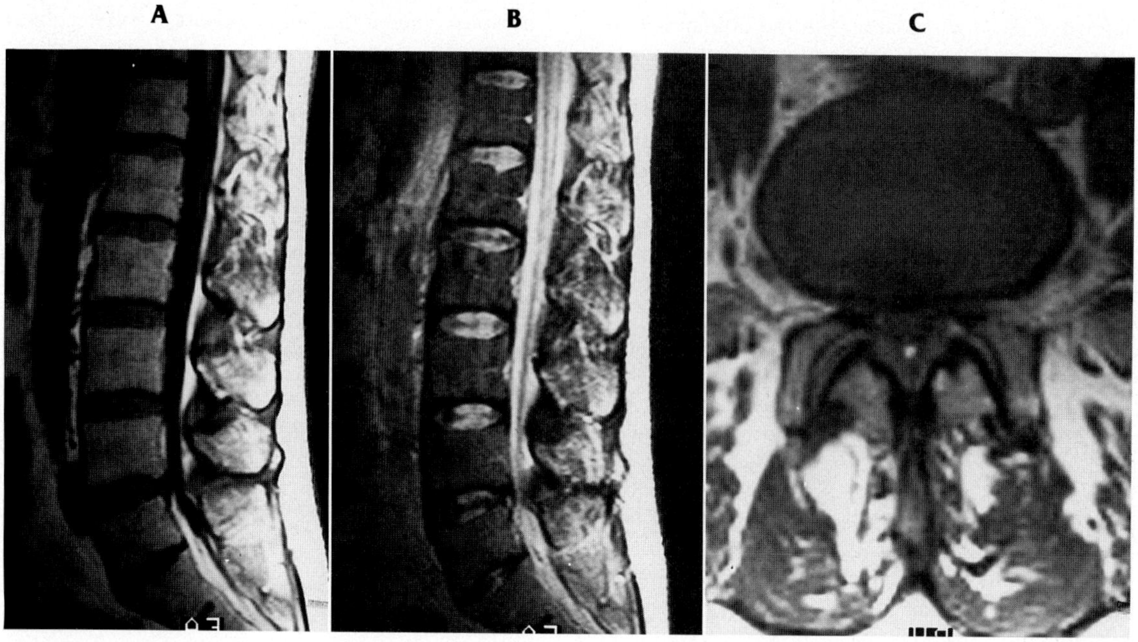

**FIGURE 1** Congenital lumbar spinal stenosis. *A* and *B*, T1- and T2-weighted sagittal images demonstrate a small central canal in the lower lumbar region measuring 10 mm in AP diameter. *C*, T1-weighted axial image at the L4-5 level reveals moderate central spinal stenosis secondary to mild disk bulging and facet arthropathy superimposed on the small canal.

myelography and CT. Advantages of MRI include the lack of radiation and the use of multiplanar imaging.

## Technical Factors

Our routine for MRI of the adult lumbar spine includes T1- and T2-weighted sagittal images of the entire region including the conus. Axial T1-weighted views are always obtained at the lower three disk spaces and are aligned parallel to the disk. Additional axial views are performed at other levels if there is suspicion of disease on the sagittal views.

Short spin-echo or T1-weighted sequences (TR = 500 to 600 msec, TE = 20 to 30 msec) provide excellent anatomic detail. The intrinsic signal characteristics of the various body tissues provide high contrast resolution between the neural structures, epidural fat, and cerebrospinal fluid (CSF) within the thecal sac (Fig. 1).

On long spin-echo or T2-weighted series (TR = 1800 to 2400 msec, TE = 80 to 100 msec), the CSF has a hyperintense signal producing a "myelographic effect." This is an excellent method to define the severity and extent of stenosis, similar to a lateral myelogram (Fig. 2).

Currently many institutions use gradient-echo T2* sequences (TR = 450 to 500 msec, TE = 20 to 25 msec, flip-angle = 15 to 20°) rather than spin-echo acquisitions. These sequences, which also give a myelographic effect, have the advantage of significantly shorter acquisition times. Despite the extra imaging time, we prefer spin-echo images since they provide additional information on disk dessication and patency of the annulus. We do use gradient-echo images during long evaluations (i.e., contrast-enhanced studies) or if the patient is in pain or unable to cooperate. Gradient-echo images may also be beneficial when using low field strength magnets where long imaging times contribute to patient motion.

Intravenous contrast material is not administered for routine lumbar spine evaluations; however, it is helpful in select cases. Gadolinium-DTPA is employed in postoperative patients to help differentiate between postsurgical fibrosis and other causes of neural impingement including recurrent disk herniations. Contrast enhancement may also aid diagnosis of other lesions such as neoplasms, synovial cysts, and vascular malformations detected on an initial noncontrast evaluation (Fig. 3).

Factors that can increase imaging resolution include obtaining thinner sections and the use of surface coils. Surface coils significantly increase the signal-to-noise ratio compared with body coils and therefore allow thinner sections with increased spatial resolution. Body coil images may be used for localization purposes or to screen large areas; however, they are inadequate to detect smaller spinal lesions.

The field of view (FOV) selected for sagittal images should be large enough to visualize the entire lumbar region including the conus. For standard surface coils, a 28 to 30 cm FOV should provide adequate coverage and maintain image quality. The recent development of phase array coils allows imaging of larger areas without degrading spatial resolution; however, these coils are not currently available on all magnets.

One of the newest advancements in spinal imaging is the development of volume acquisitions. These sequences image entire slabs of tissue in a single plane. This information can then be reconstructed at any obliquity or projected as a three-dimensional (3D) model. In the near future, volume acquisitions may increase our accuracy in defining spinal stenosis and may aid clinicians in surgical planning.

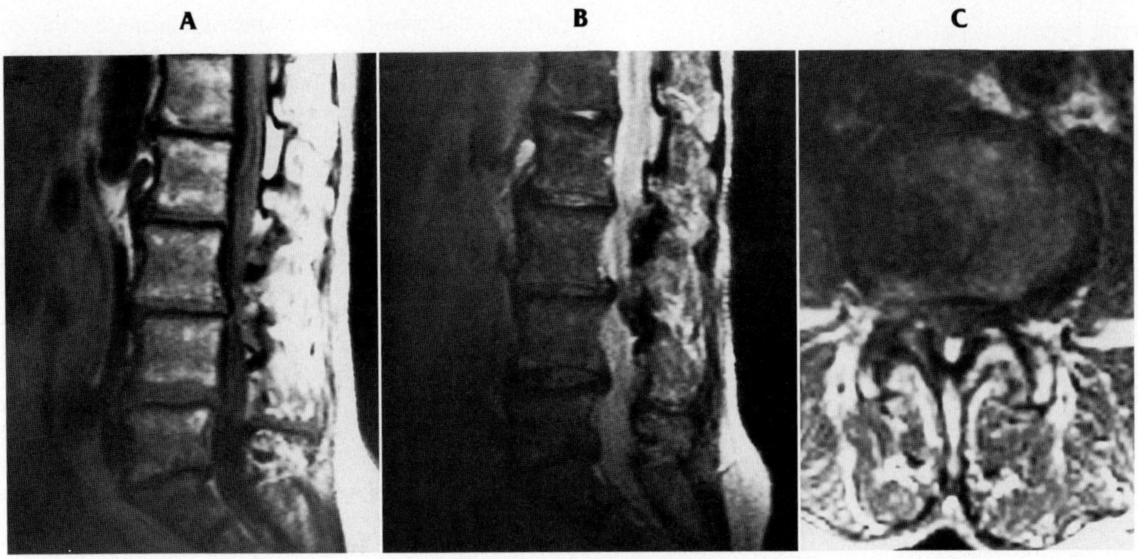


**FIGURE 2** Acquired spinal stenosis. *A* and *B,* T1- and T2-weighted sagittal images demonstrate multilevel spinal stenosis, most severe at the L3-4 level. Note how the myelographic effect of the CSF on the T2-weighted image demonstrates the degree of narrowing. *C,* T1-weighted axial image at L3-4 reveals moderate central stenosis secondary to diffuse disk protrusion and bilateral facet arthropathy.

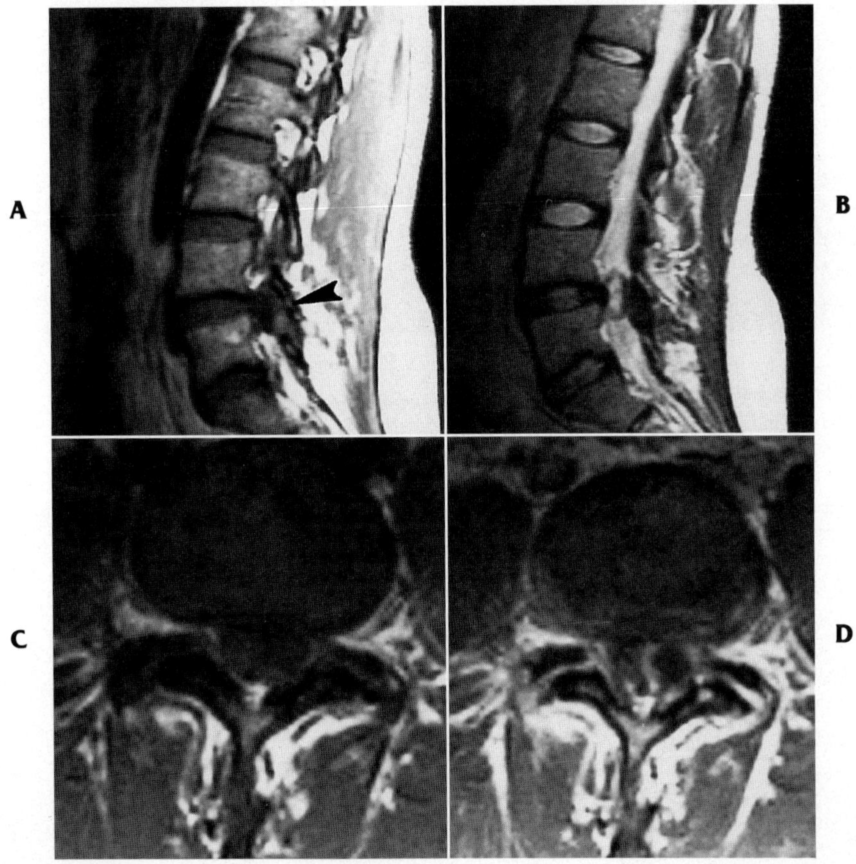


**FIGURE 3** Synovial cyst. *A,* T1-weighted parasagittal image reveals a relatively hypointense lesion in the left side of the canal at L4-5 (*arrowhead*). *B,* On the T2-weighted sagittal image, the mass becomes hyperintense consistent with a cystic lesion. *C,* On the noncontrast T1 axial image, the mass is difficult to separate from the thecal sac because of the similar signal characteristics of the lesion and CSF. *D,* Postgadolinium T1-weighted axial image demonstrates rim enhancement of the synovial cyst, which arises from the left facet joint. The contrast enhancement significantly aids detection of the lesion and helps determine the degree of thecal sac compression.

## Anatomic Considerations

Spinal stenosis lesions can be divided into three main anatomic regions including the central canal, the lateral recess, and the intervertebral foramen or nerve root canal. The lateral recess represents the section of nerve root that extends from the thecal sac to the pedicle. The intervertebral foramen refers to the bony canal beneath the pedicle.

Ullrich and co-workers established the lower limit of normal for the anteroposterior (AP) dimension of the spinal canal on CT at 11.5 cm and for the cross-sectional area at 1.45 $cm^2$. The AP diameter of the central canal should be measured at the level of the pedicle, since this region best represents the developmental diameter of the canal. Cross-sectional area measurements appear to be more sensitive in determining central spinal stenosis; however, they are seldom used and do not account for focal lesions that may cause foraminal or lateral recess narrowing. Normal measurements for the nerve root canals are 5 mm or more in width and for the lateral recesses are 3 mm or more in depth.

Sagittal images are excellent for evaluating the overall canal diameter and for detecting extradural defects produced by disk disease and degenerative changes of the posterior elements (see Fig. 2). Axial views provide additional information on the degree of neural compression. Absence of epidural fat posterior to the thecal sac at the level of the disk space is a good indication of a tight canal; however, this is a normal finding at the pedicular level. Central canal stenosis is typically graded on a scale of mild, moderate, or severe narrowing, with severe stenosis corresponding to a complete block on myelography.

The intervertebral foramina can be visualized on both sagittal and axial sequences. Foraminal compromise (Fig. 4) is indicated by loss of the normal epidural fat surrounding the nerve root or displacement of the nerve. Focal stenoses

A

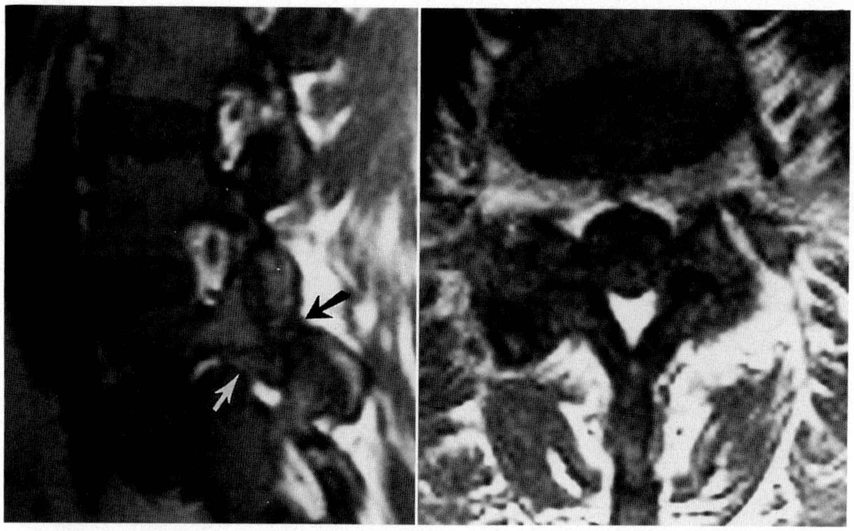

B

**FIGURE 4** Bilateral L5 spondylolysis. *A,* T1-weighted parasagittal image reveals a defect in the pars interarticularis region (*black arrow*). Note the associated deformity and narrowing of the neural foramen and compression of the L5 nerve root (*white arrow*). *B,* T1-weighted axial image confirms the presence of bilateral pars defects.

A

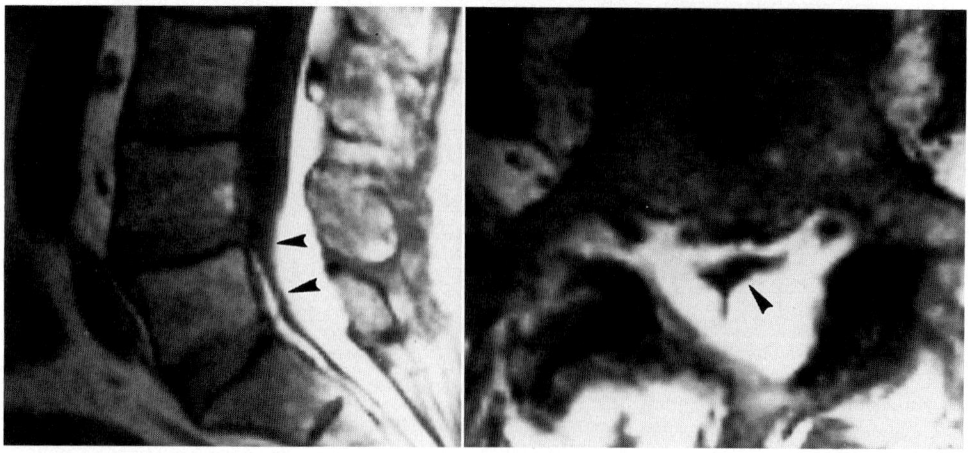

B

**FIGURE 5** Symptomatic epidural lipomatosis in a patient with long-term steroid use. *A* and *B,* T1-weighted sagittal and axial images demonstrate increased epidural fat in the lower lumbar spine. There is deformity of the posterior aspect of the thecal sac secondary to mass effect from the fat (*black arrowheads*).

involving the lateral recesses are best evaluated on axial images.

## Etiology

The numerous causes of spinal stenosis can be divided into two main categories: developmental and acquired. Developmental or idiopathic lumbar stenosis is due to underdevelopment of the central canal and/or neural foramina. These patients usually become symptomatic later in life when superimposed degenerative changes produce impingement on the neural or vascular structures (see Fig. 1). Other causes of congenital stenosis include rare disorders such as bone dysplasias, achondroplasia, Down's syndrome, and hypochondroplasia.

Acquired spinal stenosis is more common than the idiopathic form and is usually due to degenerative changes of the spine (see Fig. 2). These changes include disk disease, osteophyte formation, facet arthropathy, and ligament hypertrophy. The normal posterior ligament should not measure more than 5 mm in width.

Other causes of acquired stenosis include postsurgical changes, spondylolysis, synovial cysts (see Fig. 3), epidural lipomatosis (Fig. 5), calcification of the posterior longitudinal ligament, and bone abnormalities such as Paget's disease or acromegaly. Mass lesions such as large disk herniations or neoplasms are not usually considered in the diagnosis of spinal stenosis; however, these entities may occasionally present with stenosis symptoms.

Although simple spondylolysis does not usually produce spinal stenosis, it frequently is associated with spondylolisthesis and hypertrophic bony changes that may cause neural impingement. Pars interarticularis defects can often be detected on the sagittal and axial T1-weighted images; however, bony detail is not well visualized on MRI, and additional imaging with CT or plain films may be needed to verify the diagnosis (see Fig. 4).

## Suggested Reading


Dorwart RH, Vogler JB III, Helms CA. Spinal stenosis. Radiol Clin North Am 1983; 21:301–323.

Grenier N, Kressel HY, Schiebler ML, et al. Normal and degenerative posterior spinal structures: MR imaging. Radiology 1987; 165:517–525.

Jackson DE, Atlas SW, Mani JR, et al. Intraspinal synovial cysts: MR imaging. Radiology 1989; 170:527–530.

Johnson DW, Farnum GN, Latchaw RE, et al. MR imaging of the pars interarticularis. Am J Neuroradiol 1988; 9:1215–1220.

Modic MT, Masaryk T, Boumphrey F, et al. Lumbar herniated disk disease and canal stenosis: Prospective evaluation by surface coil MR, CT and myelography. AJR 1986; 147:757–765.

Modic MT, Masaryk T, Paushter D. Magnetic resonance imaging of the spine. Radiol Clin North Am 1986; 24:229–245.

Pleatman CW, Lukin RR. Lumbar spinal stenosis. Semin Roentgen 1988; 23:106–110.

Quint DJ, Boulos RS, Sanders WP, et al. Epidural lipomatosis. Radiology 1988; 169:485–490.

Ullrich CG, Binet EF, Sanecki MG, et al. Quantitative assessment of the lumbar spinal canal by computed tomography. Radiology 1980; 134:137–143.


# Imaging of the Salivary Glands: CT and MRI

*BARBARA L. CARTER, M.D. · COLIN KARMODY, M.D.*

There are three major and numerous minor salivary glands. The major glands are the parotid, submandibular, and sublingual glands as demonstrated in Figures 1 and 12. The minor glands are located in the mucosa of the lips, cheeks, hard and soft palate, oropharynx, floor of the mouth, and tongue. Of the major glands the parotid is most commonly involved with various diseases, the submandibular gland less often, and the sublingual glands rarely so.

In studying the salivary glands, computed tomography (CT) and magnetic resonance imaging (MRI) each have advantages and disadvantages. The considerations given for choice of imaging modality include diagnostic yield, radiation exposure, sensitivity to iodine, claustrophobia, metallic implants or foreign bodies, and cost. CT is used for identification of calculi, interstitial calcification, collections of fluid as in cysts or abscesses, and assessment of the underlying bone. MRI is more sensitive for studying tumors or inflammatory masses. There still remains a role for plain films, sialography, ultrasonography, and occasionally radionuclide scanning.

## Indications for Imaging

### *Diffuse or Generalized Enlargement*

Diffuse swelling of the salivary glands is caused by many different factors ranging from variations of normal to metabolic disorders, systemic diseases, complication of drug use, infections, and tumors. Acute bacterial and viral infections can be diagnosed clinically, but the more subtle infection, obstruction, and underlying systemic disease may require the use of imaging for determination of the causes. CT with contrast enhancement is preferable in the evaluation of bacterial infection, particularly if there is a question of abscess. Intraglandular air from infection, trauma, or mechanical derangement is more easily identified by CT than MRI.

### *Intermittent Swelling*

Partial obstruction of the submandibular or parotid duct causing intermittent swelling of the gland following a meal might be caused by a calculus or a stricture. About 80 percent of calculi occur in the submandibular duct and 80 percent of these are visible on plain film; 20 percent are nonopaque. Plain film studies are usually adequate for the identification of a calculus. For clinically suspected but nonopaque calculi, and for ductal strictures, sialography is necessary. If plain film studies and sialography are negative, CT with contrast enhancement is performed.

### Mass Lesions

A focal mass, whether single or multiple, may be adjacent to or within the gland. Although this can often be determined by ultrasonography, MRI is becoming the modality of choice for the evaluation of mass lesions within the major and minor salivary glands.

A tumor mass within the parotid gland should be localized relative to the probable position of the facial nerve and its branches. The facial nerve exiting from the stylomastoid foramen enters the parotid gland and soon divides into five major branches: temporal, zygomatic, buccal, mandibular, and cervical. The nerve and its branches are located lateral to the retromandibular vessels in a plane that artificially separates the superficial and deep portions of the gland. All branches of the facial nerve are vulnerable during partial or total parotidectomy.

A

B

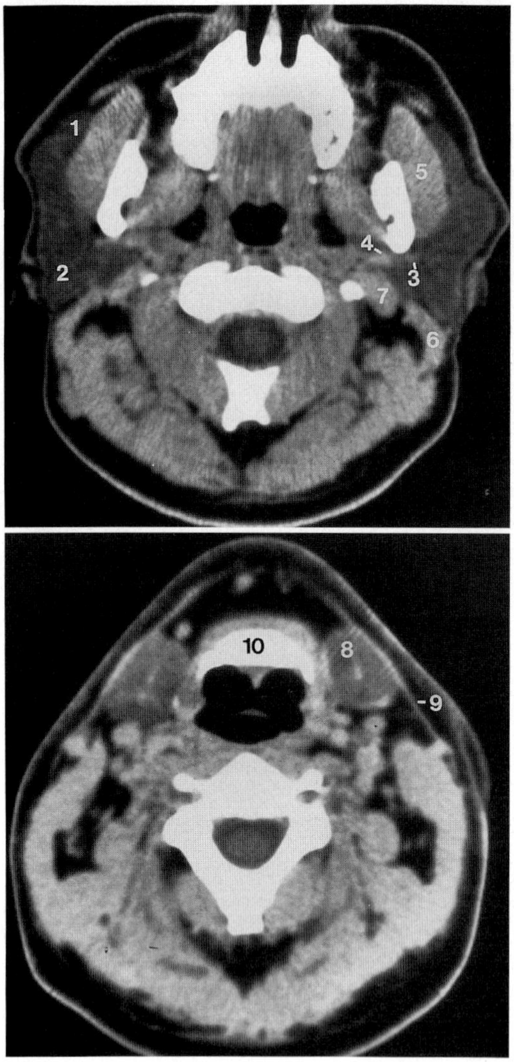


**FIGURE 1** *A,* Normal CT scan showing normal parotid gland. The accessory lobe (1) has merged with the main gland (2), resulting in a large but normal gland. The retromandibular vein (3) localizes the position of the facial nerve. The internal maxillary artery (4) is medial to the vein. The masseter muscle (5) is anteromedial to the parotid, the sternocleidomastoid muscle (6) posterior to the parotid and the posterior belly of the digastric (7) deep to the parotid. *B,* The submandibular gland (8) is deep to the platysma muscle (9) and lateral to the hyoid bone (10).

## Technique

### Plain Film Studies for Calculus

1. *Submandibular Gland and Duct*—Occlusal, lateral, lateral oblique, posteroanterior (PA). Occlusal films must be a true cephalocaudad projection to include the orifice of the duct posterior to the symphysis of the mandible. For the lateral projection, depression of the tongue with the index finger improves visualization of the hilum of the gland.
2. *Parotid Gland and Duct*—PA, lateral, tangential with cheek blown out.

### Sialography

The retrograde injection of iodinated contrast material is indicated for the identification of strictures, nonopaque stones, dilated ducts, and early parenchymal changes found in chronic infection or in autoimmune disorders such as Sjögren's syndrome. Sialography is contraindicated in the presence of an acute infection. Dilators are useful for preparing the orifice of the duct and for placement of a snugly fitted cannula, which is connected to polyethylene tubing. Water-soluble contrast material (diatrizoate meglumine [Sinografin]) is manually injected under fluoroscopic control, using 0.4 to 1.5 ml of contrast material for the parotid duct and 0.3 to 0.5 ml for the submandibular duct. Filming during and after injection permits the best visualization of the main duct and its branches.

### Computed Tomography

CT is the preferred modality for evaluation of calcifications, small calculi, acute infection including abscesses, vascular lesions such as hemangiomas and the rare aneurysm. Contiguous images 4 to 5 mm thick are obtained in the axial plane from the level of the external auditory canal or skull base to the level of or just caudad to the hyoid bone. Coronal images are occasionally a necessary supplement for better localization of some lesions, such as tumors of the minor salivary glands. A bolus injection of 100 to 175 ml of intravenous contrast material is used at a rate of 0.8 to 1.0 ml/sec. Rapid sequential imaging is started 60 to 90 seconds after the injection is begun. The slight delay in imaging permits enhancement of the area under study while the vessels are still opacified by the moderately generous volume of contrast material. The short time exposure of 1 to 2 seconds, together with suspended respiration, minimizes motion artifacts.

Dental artifacts are minimized by varying the angle of the gantry as determined by the scout image. Although most axial scans are obtained parallel to the hard palate, this is individualized according to the patient and the type of lesion, the presence of dental artifacts, and so forth. If there is a question of tumor involving the skull base, the gantry is angled 20° to the orbital-meatal line in addition to or instead of the images parallel to the hard palate. Narrow soft-tissue windows are used to maximize contrast between enhanced and nonenhanced areas, whereas wider bone windows are used for detailed study of bone, air-containing structures or air pockets in abscesses, and to further minimize dental artifacts.

### Magnetic Resonance Imaging

MRI is used primarily for studying mass lesions within or adjacent to the major salivary glands and for the assessment of tumors of minor salivary gland origin. T1- and T2-weighted images in 5 mm sections are obtained in the axial plane from the skull base to slightly below the hyoid bone. Coronal T2-weighted images are useful for evaluating malignant tumors of the major and minor salivary glands. A palpable mass is localized with a vitamin E capsule taped to the skin overlying the mass. Most benign tumors have a low signal with T1- and a bright signal with T2-weighted images. In general terms, benign tumors have sharply defined edges and malignant tumors have fuzzy ill-defined borders. Alternatively, however, some malignant tumors might have sharp edges and some benign tumors fuzzy edges from surrounding inflammatory reactions. Invasion beyond the salivary gland usually indicates a malignancy. Some highly cellular malignant tumors have low signals in both the T1- and T2-weighted images. Gadolinium enhancement is not routinely required for the demonstration of benign tumors, but it is occasionally useful for the assessment of the more aggressive neoplasms, and for tumor recurrences in areas of previous surgery and/or radiation therapy. As the salivary glands undergo fatty degeneration, a combination of gadolinium enhancement and fat-suppression techniques might be necessary to identify intraglandular masses.

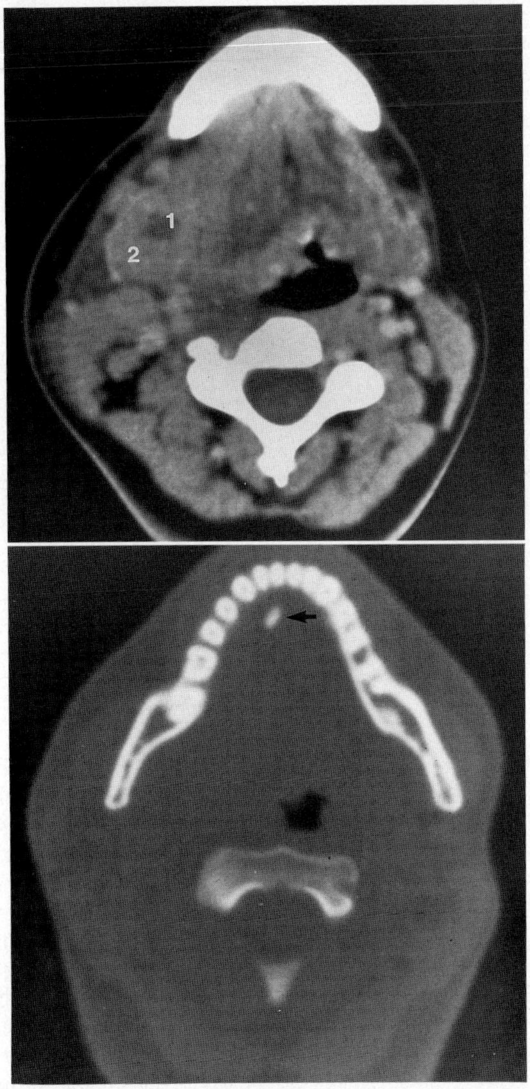


**FIGURE 2** Calculus obstructing submandibular duct. CT scans. *A,* A dilated duct (1) is observed within the enlarged submandibular gland (2). *B,* Small calculus *(arrow)* at the orifice of the left submandibular duct.

### CT-guided Needle Aspiration Biopsy

A lesion that is deep and thus difficult to palpate requires an imaging technique for guidance. A pathologist is always present during the procedure. The patient is positioned by optimal localization of the area to be biopsied. A mark placed on the skin surface is used as a reference point for determining depth and angle needed to advance the needle to the area in question. Initial scans are obtained and the patient prepared and draped in the usual fashion for a sterile procedure. The needle is then inserted and advanced in the appropriate direction. Once the needle has been positioned, and a final scan obtained to demonstrate its accuracy, a sample is aspirated and given to the pathologist. The pathologist determines immediately whether or not sufficient material has been obtained or if more tissue is needed for diagnosis. MRI is not as practical for needle-aspiration biopsy as CT scan. If MRI is to be used, special equipment is necessary that is unaffected by the magnet. With either technique the entire procedure takes 45 to 90 minutes.

## Differential Diagnosis: An Approach and Some Pitfalls

### Diffuse Enlargement

Intermittent swelling of a single gland is usually a result of calculus (Fig. 2), stricture, or infection. Involvement of both parotid and submandibular glands, however, implies some underlying systemic disease such as mumps, Sjögren's syndrome, or other autoimmune diseases. Other causes of bilateral parotid enlargement include obesity, alcoholism, diabetes, malnutrition, and drug toxicity (Table 1).

As previously mentioned, plain film studies may negate the need for further investigation. CT with intravenous contrast enhancement is the preferred imaging technique for evaluation of diffuse enlargement of the salivary gland. This reveals the presence of a small stone not detected on plain films, may show a significantly dilated duct, and reveals enhancement of an acute, subacute, or chronic inflammatory process. An abscess containing a collection of fluid surrounded by an enhancing rim is better identified by CT.

**TABLE 1** Causes of Diffuse Enlargement of the Salivary Glands

| |
|---|
| Inflammatory |
| Mumps |
| Acute suppurative sialadenitis |
| Chronic recurrent nonobstructive sialadenitis |
| Sarcoidosis |
| Sialectasis |
| Benign lymphoepithelial lesion |
| Cystic degeneration in AIDS |
| Sjögren's syndrome |
| Toxic or drug induced |
| Nutritional deficiency |
| Alcoholic cirrhosis |
| Obesity |
| Hormonal dysfunction |
| Diabetes |
| Hypothyroidism |
| Gonadal (atrophy or dysfunction) |
| Others |
| Pneumoparotitis |
| Uremia |
| Kussmaul's disease (fibromucinous plugs) |

MRI also shows altered signals in the diffusely enlarged gland that is infected or involved with some systemic disease such as Sjögren's syndrome (Fig. 3). The latter typically has multiple, small, punctate fluid collections, but this is variable. With MRI the abnormal gland has a heterogeneous low signal on T1-weighted images and a bright signal on T2-weighted images, but it might be difficult to distinguish between chronic or low-grade infection with edema, abscess, necrosis, or cystic degeneration of a tumor. For these reasons, we prefer to use contrast-enhanced CT scan to distinguish between fluid, edema, and to some extent, diffuse changes in the gland. Either modality, however, shows the diffuse fatty enlargement observed with alcoholism.

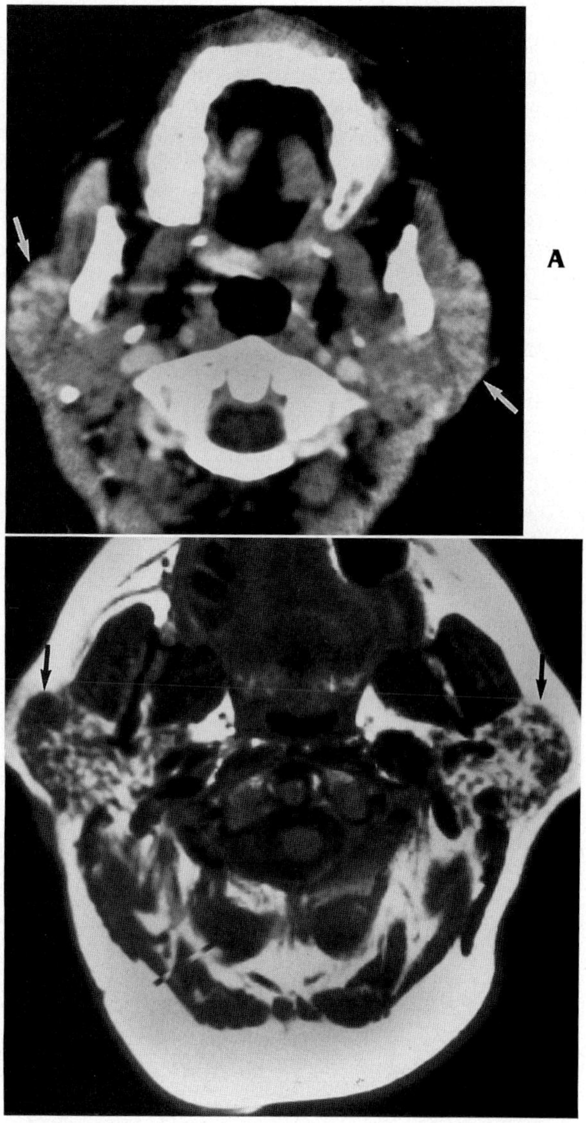


**FIGURE 3** Chronic sialadenitis. *A,* CT scan with contrast enhancement showing nodular heterogeneous enhancement of the parotid glands *(arrows)* as a result of Sjögren's syndrome. *B,* MRI T1-weighted scan (TR750, TE17). Sjögren's syndrome with areas of low attenuation consistent with punctate fluid collections.

## *Solitary Masses*

Solitary masses may be solid or cystic, benign or malignant. A solitary mass is more frequent in the parotid gland and is usually a pleomorphic adenoma (mixed tumor). Pleomorphic adenomas are also found in the submandibular gland and in the minor salivary glands. Pleomorphic adenomas are firm, almost hard, whereas Warthin's tumors are soft. The benign tumors of the salivary glands are listed in Table 2 and the malignant tumors are listed in Table 3. In the parotid gland, about 80 percent of the solitary masses are benign, whereas in the submandibular gland only about 50 to 55 percent are. About 55 percent of tumors arising from the minor salivary glands, however, are malignant. Tumors of the sublingual glands are rare. Here one usually sees a cyst or ranula that is the result of an obstructed sublingual duct.

### Evaluation of Specific Tumors

Pleomorphic adenomas tend to have heterogeneous enhancement with CT, a low signal on T1-weighted images, and a bright signal on T2-weighted images (Fig. 4). They can occasionally be homogeneous and may appear lobulated. These tumors may also have cystic degeneration.

Warthin's tumor is the second most common benign tumor of the parotid and is often multiple and/or bilateral. Although it appears solid, its cystic components may enlarge enough to simulate a cyst with a nodular border. We use either modality but prefer MRI because of its better contrast between mass and normal parenchyma. MRI is particularly useful when there has been little fatty replacement of the gland.

Solitary lesions of the deep portion of the parotid gland (Fig. 5) are less frequent than those in the superficial portion and tend to grow medially. They should therefore be differentiated from intrinsic tumors of the parapharyngeal space. A sharp line of demarcation between the tumor and the parotid gland represents fat of the parapharyngeal space that is displaced laterally with tumors of the parapharyngeal space and medially with tumors of the parotid gland. Our choice of investigating for the deep lobe tumors is MRI, although CT with a contrast agent is also valuable.

**TABLE 2** Benign Tumors of the Salivary Glands

| |
|---|
| Adenoma |
| Pleomorphic adenoma (mixed tumor) |
| Papillary cystadenoma lymphomatosum (Warthin's tumor) |
| Monomorphic adenoma |
| Sebaceous lymphadenoma |
| Myoepithelioma |
| Oncocytoma |
| Vascular tumors |
| Hemangiomas (capillary and cavernous) |
| Lymphangioma |
| Lipoma |
| Neurogenic tumors |
| Schwannoma |
| Neurofibroma |
| Tumorlike condition |
| Sialometaplasia |

**TABLE 3** Malignant Tumors of the Salivary Glands

| |
|---|
| Acinic cell carcinoma |
| Adenocarcinoma |
| Adenoid cystic carcinoma |
| Lymphoma |
| Metastatic tumors |
| Squamous cell carcinoma (skin) |
| Melanoma |
| Miscellaneous tumors |
| Malignant mixed tumor |
| Biphasic malignant tumor |
| Carcinoma arising in pleomorphic adenoma |
| Mucoepidermoid carcinoma |
| Oncocytic carcinoma |
| Squamous cell carcinoma |

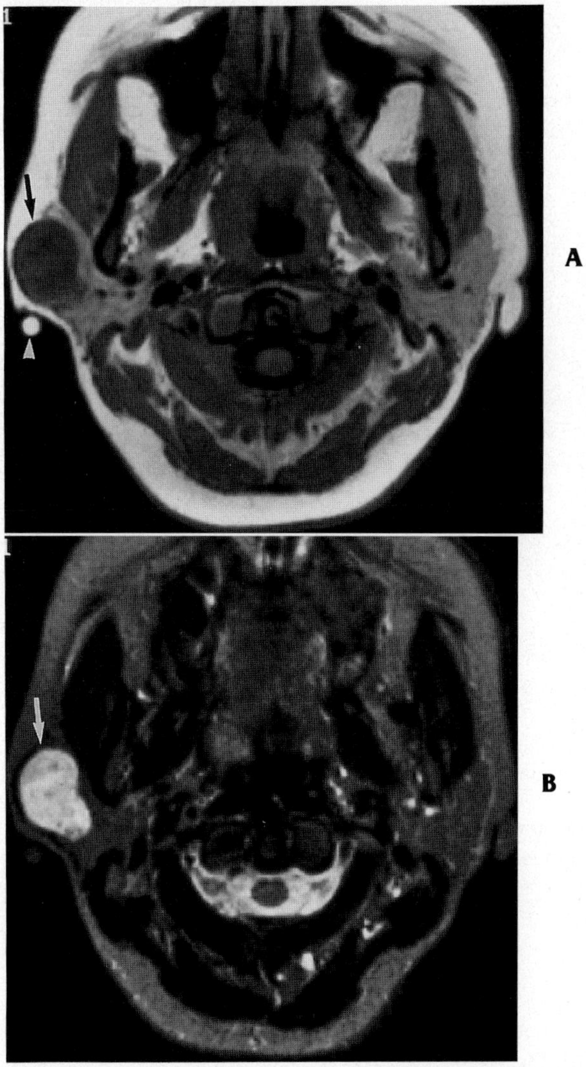


**FIGURE 4** Pleomorphic adenoma. *A,* MRI T1-weighted (TR800, TE17). Adenoma *(arrow)* is in superficial portion of the right parotid. Vitamin E capsule *(arrowhead)* placed over mass. *B,* MRI T2-weighted scan (TR3000, TE90). The heterogeneous signal of the adenoma is more readily identified *(arrow)*.

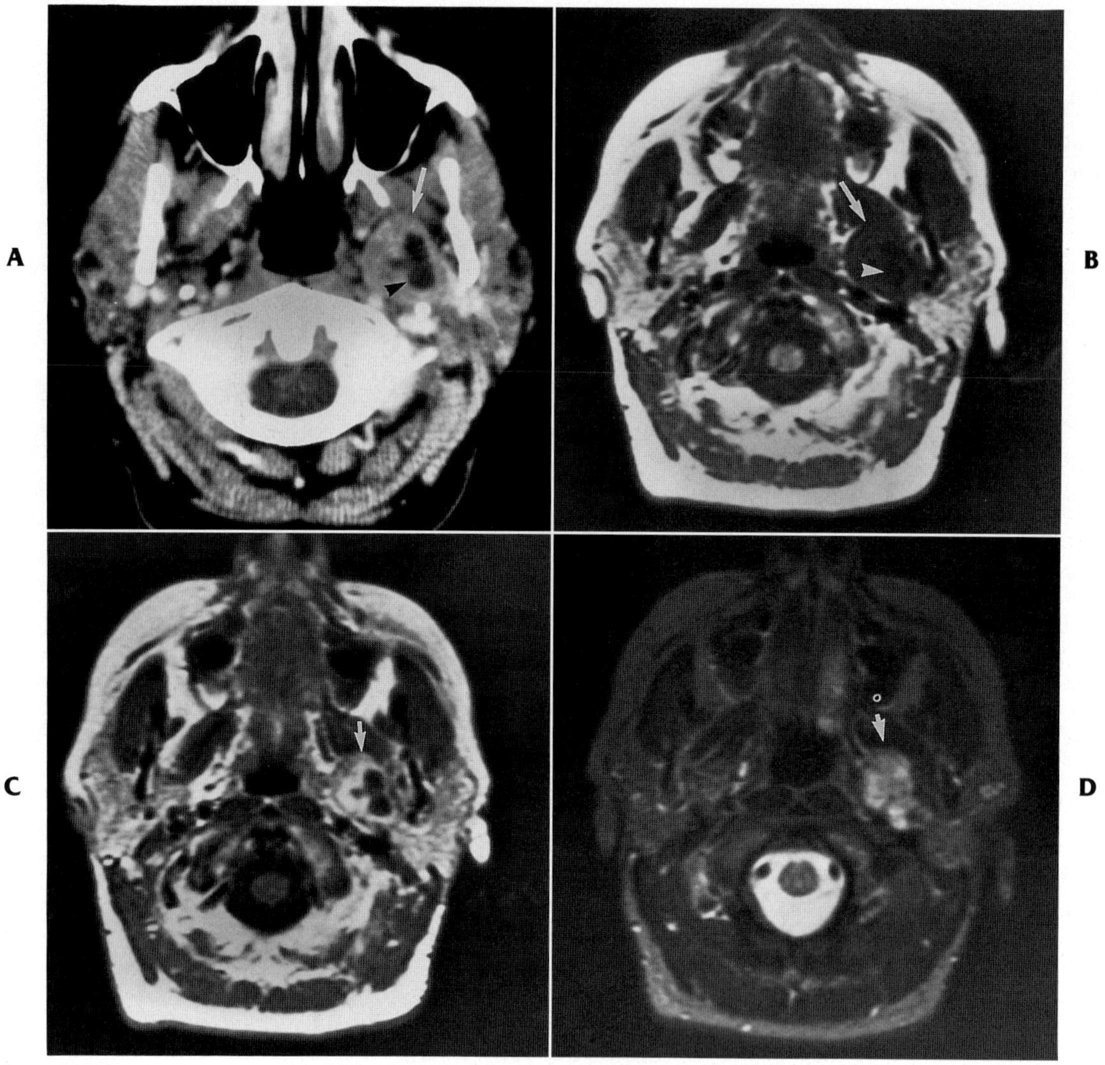


**FIGURE 5** Pleomorphic adenoma, deep portion of the parotid. *A,* CT scan with contrast enhancement. The sharply defined tumor *(arrow)* with cystic degeneration *(arrowhead)* is encroaching on the parapharyngeal space. *B,* MRI T1-weighted scan (TR600, TE20) the adenoma *(arrow)* has a low signal, making the cystic degeneration *(arrowhead)* hard to observe. *C,* MRI T1-weighted scan (TR600, TE20) with gadolinium. Note how the tumor enhances (in other cases may become isointense with the parotid), but the cystic degeneration is not affected. *D,* MRI T2-weighted (TR2500, TE80) tumor has heterogeneous bright signal.

A

B

C

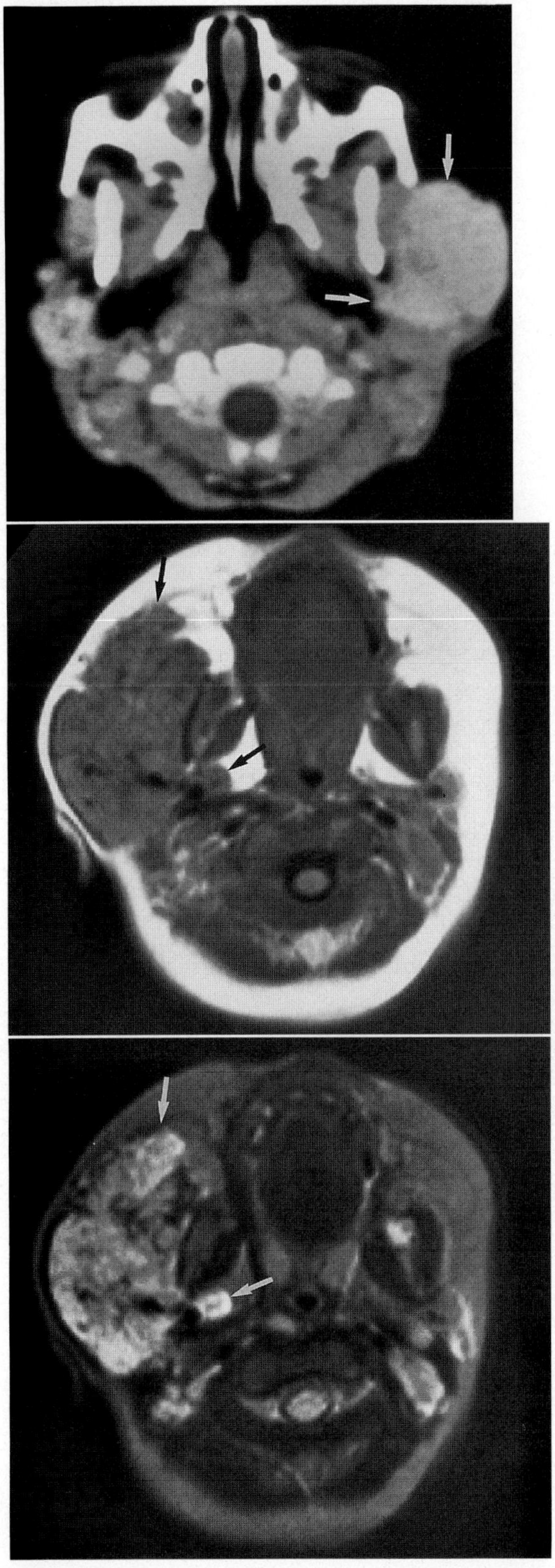

**FIGURE 6** Capillary hemangioma. *A,* CT scan with contrast enhancement. The hemangioma *(arrows)* involves the superficial and deep portions of the parotid. *B,* MRI T1-weighted scan (TR750, TE20). Diffuse enlargement of the right parotid gland in another patient shows serpiginous appearance of vessels within the tumor *(arrows). C,* MRI T2-weighted scan (TR3000, TE90). Heterogeneous bright signals are present throughout the tumor *(arrows).*

For all other lesions of the salivary glands, MRI is often preferred over CT, although either modality can be used to good advantage. Gadolinium enhancement is usually not needed for benign tumors. In fact, an adenoma which has a low signal with T1 enhances with gadolinium (see Fig. 5), making it isointense with the normal fatty parenchyma of the gland and thus invisible. Capillary hemangiomas (Fig. 6) occur most often in infants, whereas cavernous hemangiomas are observed in older children and adults. A bolus injection of contrast material with dynamic CT shows immediate enhancement with a capillary hemangioma, whereas delayed enhancement and puddling occurs with cavernous hemangiomas. A serpiginous appearance on MRI is attributed to the multiple small vessels within the lesion that may be difficult to record with slight motion artifact. Our preference is to use CT when an hemangioma is clinically a strong possibility.

## *Malignant Tumors*

The evidence for malignancy is invasiveness (Fig. 7), central necrosis, the presence of metastatic lymphadenopathy, and in the parotid gland, involvement of the facial nerve. Absence of any of these features does not rule out malignancy (Fig. 8).

If malignancy is clinically suspected, either contrast-enhanced CT or MRI can be used. We prefer gadolinium-enhanced MRI because it gives better definition of the tumor and might demonstrate perineural invasion, which is a characteristic of some salivary gland malignancies.

## *Multiple Nodules*

Although lymph nodes are normally present within the parotid gland, enlarged nodes are abnormal, usually multiple, and secondary to systemic disease. Today the most common causes of intraglandular adenopathy are acquired immunodeficiency syndrome (AIDS) (Fig. 9) and lymphoma (Fig. 10). Lymphoepithelial nodules within the parotid gland as a result of AIDS may become cystic. Multiple nodules within the parotid gland can also be from various granulomatous diseases as listed in Table 4 and from metastatic disease. With MRI these nodules have a low signal on T1-weighted images and a bright signal on T2-weighted images. These lesions are also observed with contrast-enhanced CT.

Multiple nodules in a gland with previous resection of a mixed tumor probably represents tumor recurrence (Fig. 11). The nodules are often small, close to the facial nerve, and readily identified by their bright signal on T2-weighted MRI. For the reasons as discussed here, we prefer to use MRI to investigate multiple nodules in the salivary glands. We find that, as a single modality, it gives more information.

## *Cysts of the Salivary Gland*

Ultrasonography readily identifies benign cysts, but is limited for assessment of the deep portion of the parotid gland and for evaluation of the entire neck. Cysts originating primarily from the second branchial cleft have a smooth wall, usually thin, unless there have been previous repeated infections. These cysts may occur within the parotid gland, but are more commonly observed in the neck. Cysts arising from the first branchial cleft are more closely associated with the external auditory canal with which they might communicate. CT with

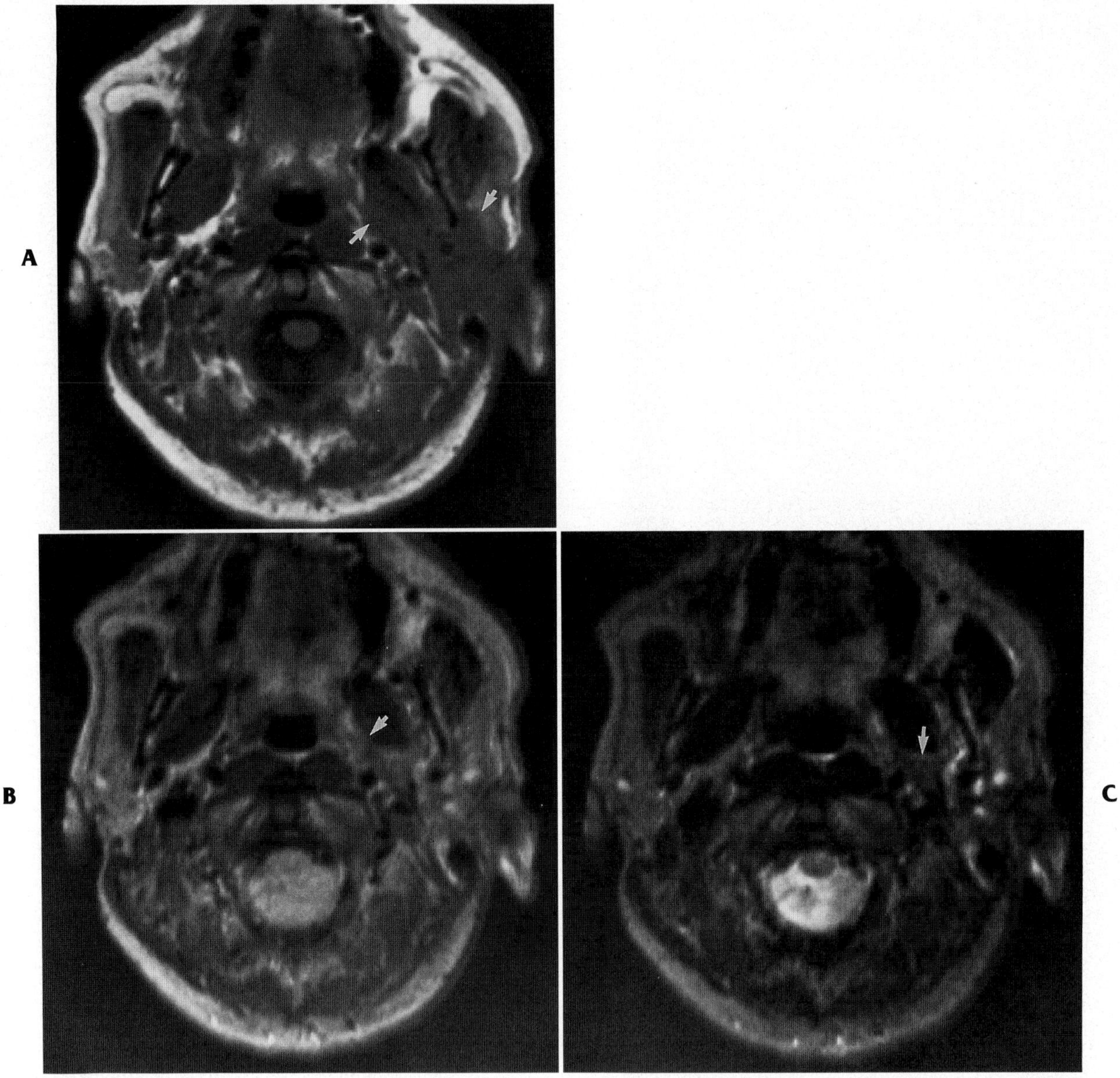

**FIGURE 7** Adenocarcinoma, recurrent. *A,* MRI T1-weighted scan (TR600, TE17). An invasive malignant tumor *(arrows)* of the left parotid gland extends to the parapharyngeal space and medial pterygoid muscle. *B,* Proton image (TR3000, TE45): the tumor *(arrow)* has low signals, making it difficult to visualize. *C,* T2-weighted scan (TR3000, TE90). The tumor is not appreciated because of the low signal *(arrow)*.

A

B

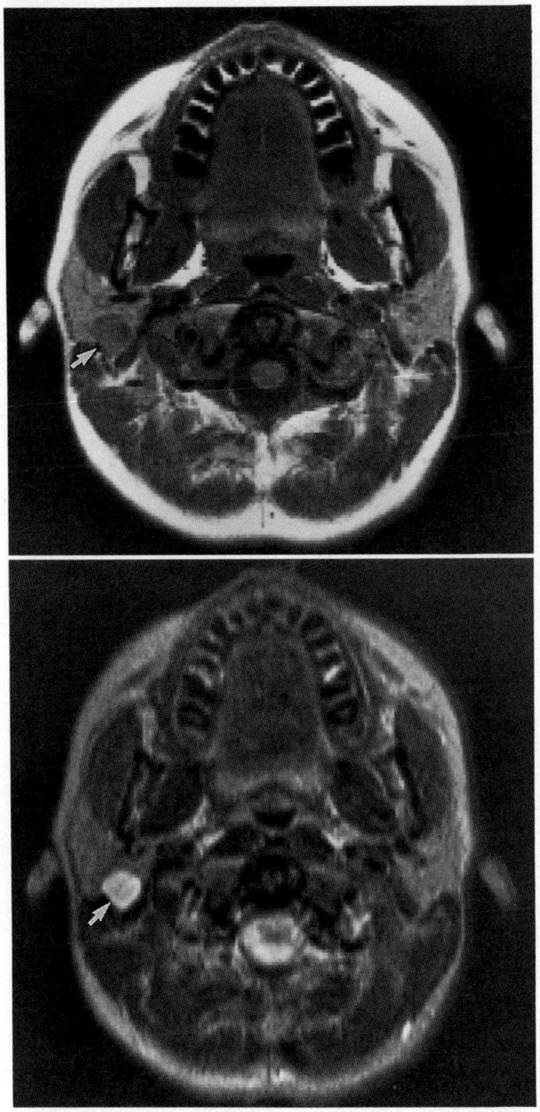

**FIGURE 8** Acinic cell carcinoma. *A,* MRI T1-weighted scan (TR600, TE17). Sharply defined tumor *(arrow)* with low signal is in the posterior superior portion of the right parotid. *B,* T2-weighted scan (TR3000, TE70). Heterogeneous signal in tumor *(arrows)* simulates a benign lesion but was proven malignant histologically.

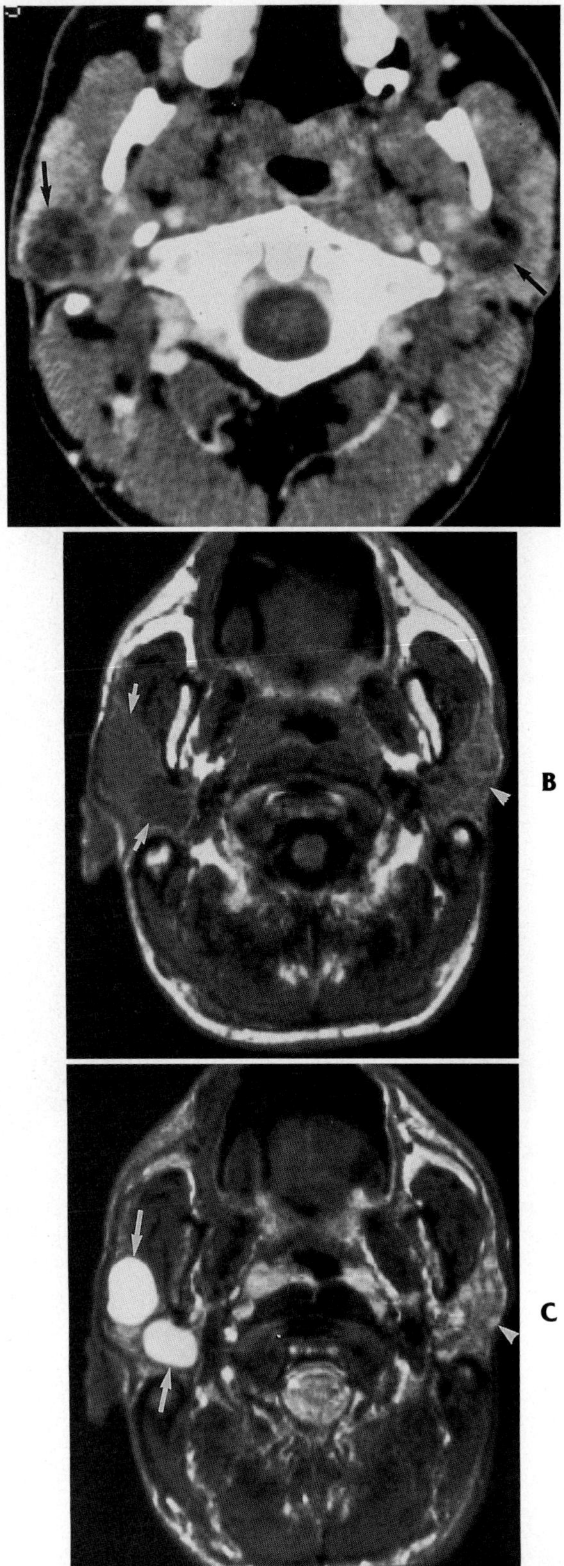

A

B

C

**FIGURE 9** AIDS. *A,* CT scan, contrast enhanced. Multiple cysts *(arrows)* are present bilaterally. The larger ones in this patient are septated. *B,* MRI T1-weighted scan (TR750, TE17). Multiple cysts (in another patient) are present *(arrows)* and have low signal. Lympho-epithelial nodules *(arrowhead)* are observed as heterogeneous signal changes within the left gland. *C,* T2-weighted scan (TR3000, TE45). The cysts on the right *(arrows)* are sharply defined with bright homogeneous signal changes. The nodules *(arrowhead)* on the left are also evident.

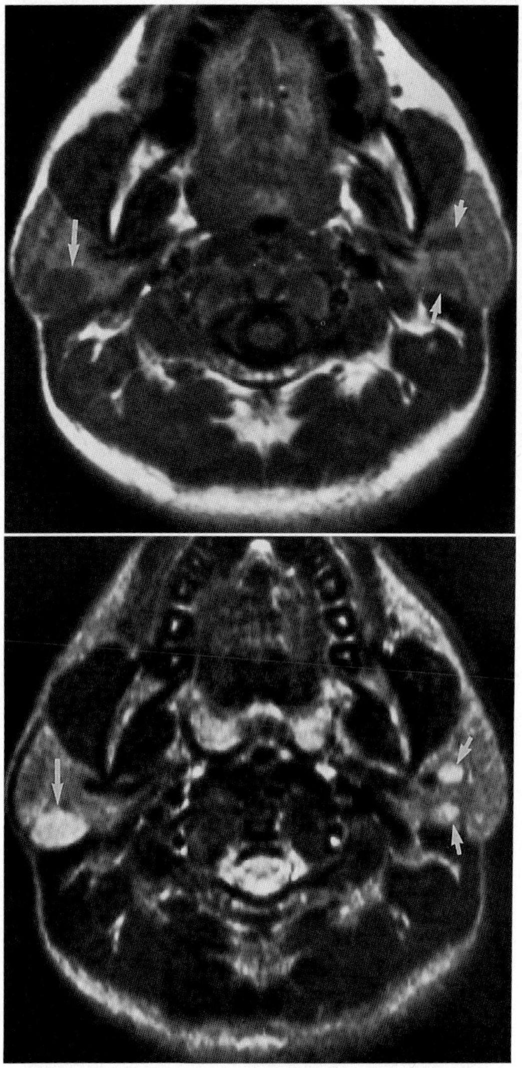

**FIGURE 10** Lymphoma. *A,* MRI T1-weighted scan (TR800, TE17). Multiple nodes *(arrows)* are present bilaterally, all sharply defined with low signal. *B,* T2-weighted scan (TR3000, TE90). Enlarged nodes *(arrows)* are now more readily identified, are sharply defined with a bright signal, some heterogeneous and some homogeneous.

**TABLE 4** Inflammatory Masses of the Salivary Glands

| |
|---|
| Focal sialadenitis, cellulitis |
| Abscess |
| Chronic autoimmune sialadenitis |
| Granulomatous disease |
|   Tuberculosis |
|   Atypical mycobacterial infection |
|   Sarcoidosis |
|   Cat-scratch fever |
|   Actinomycosis |
| Lymphoepithelial cysts (HIV positive) |
| Lymphadenopathy |

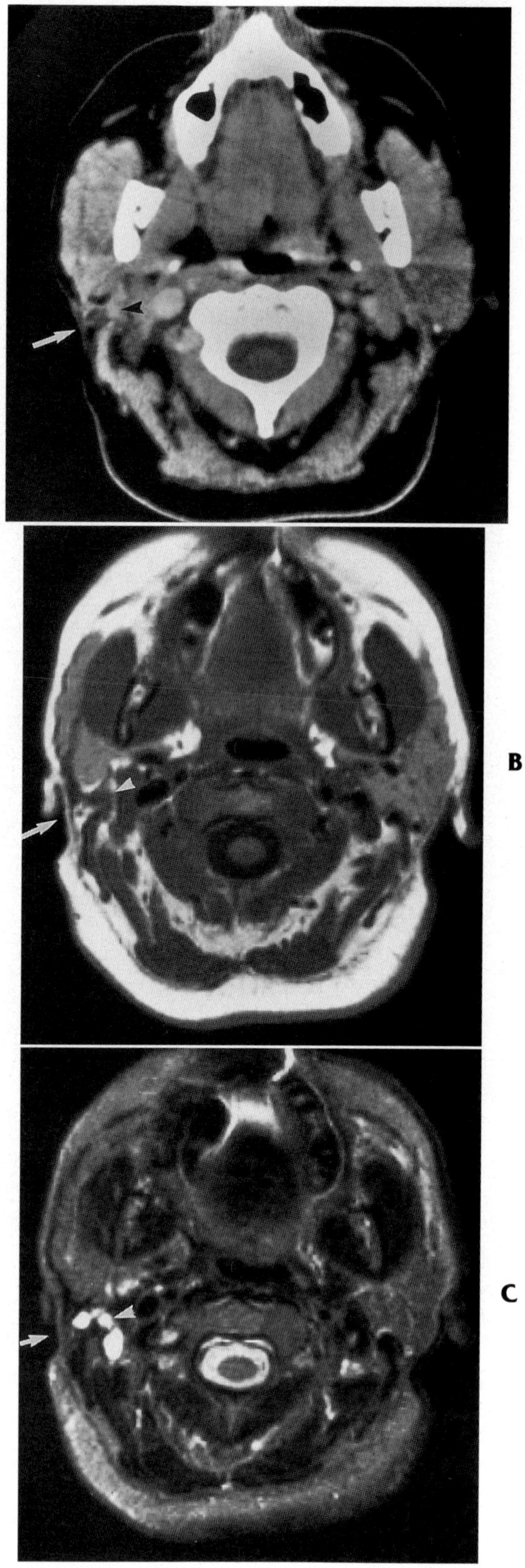

**FIGURE 11** Recurrent pleomorphic adenoma. *A,* CT scan, contrast enhanced. Postoperative changes are evident on the right *(arrows),* but the recurrent tumor *(arrowhead)* is difficult to visualize. *B,* MRI T1-weighted scan (TR650, TE17). Tumor nodules *(arrowhead)* are difficult to appreciate deep to the operative area *(arrow). C,* T2-weighted scan (TR3000, TE90). Multiple nodules *(arrowheads)* are now readily observed, all representing recurrent tumor.

**TABLE 5** Cysts of the Salivary Glands

| |
|---|
| Branchial cleft cyst |
| Postinflammatory cyst |
| Lymphoepithelial cyst (HIV positive or negative) |
| Ranula (sublingual gland) |
| Old hematoma |

contrast enhancement or an MRI study should each define the cyst, its characteristics, and other associated changes. Delineation of a fistula, if present, may require an injection of the tract. As stated previously, multiple parotid cysts are now frequently observed in HIV-positive patients (see Fig. 9). Multiple parotid cysts may be septated, are often bilateral, and are associated with diffuse lymphadenopathy. These cysts, which are actively infected with the virus, might become large enough to require aspiration for cosmesis. If necessary, ultrasound-guided needle aspiration is recommended. A ranula, a cyst of the floor of the mouth (Fig. 12), is caused by obstruction of the orifice of a sublingual gland. Recently we have seen a patient positive for HIV with an infected ranula (Table 5). Note should be made that a hematoma can simulate a thick-walled cyst (Fig. 13).

## Discussion

CT still has specific advantages for identification of ductal calculi, tumor, or parenchymal calcification and the typical findings of an abscess or an hemangioma and for assessing adjacent bone. MRI is more sensitive to soft-tissue contrast and thus preferable for the detection of subtle tumors and tumor recurrences. By using multiple pulse sequences, these different soft-tissue characteristics are enhanced. Most lesions have a low T1 signal and a bright T2 signal, but the higher protein content occasionally present is manifested with a bright T1 signal. Highly cellular malignant tumors have a low signal with both T1- and T2-weighted images, but may have some enhancement with gadolinium. The choice between CT and MRI is not necessarily clear cut. MRI does have more

A
B
C

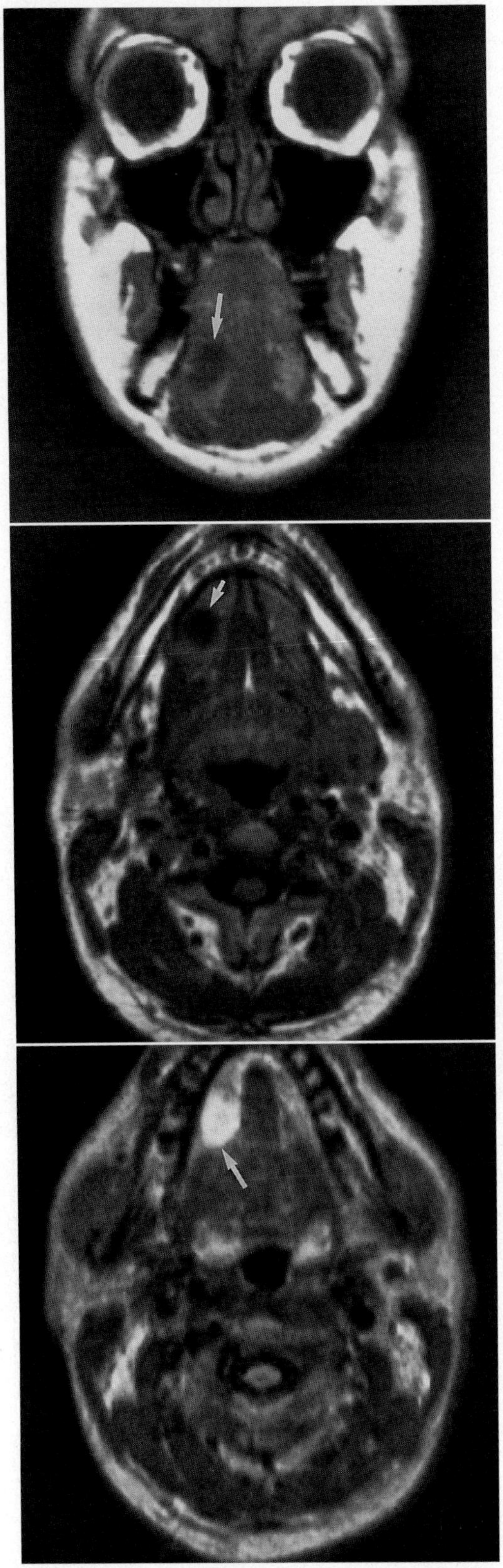

**FIGURE 12** Ranula. *A,* MRI T1-weighted scan (TR600, TE17), coronal plane. Cyst *(arrow)* in the right sublingual gland area above the myelohyoid muscle. *B,* MRI T1-weighted scan (TR600, TE17), axial plane. Cyst *(arrow)* is between the myelohyoid and geniohyoid muscles in the sublingual gland area. *C,* T2-weighted scan (TR3000, TE45). Cyst *(arrow)* has a bright, sharply defined signal.

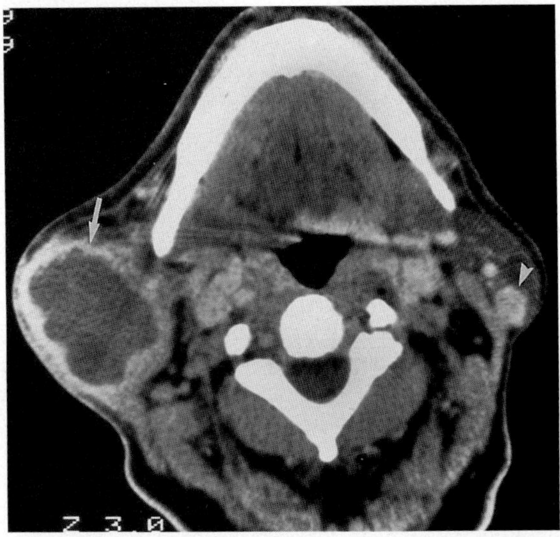

**FIGURE 13** Hematoma. CT scan with contrast enhancement. Large hematoma *(arrow)* on the right developed during biopsy of a Warthin's tumor. A small Warthin's tumor *(arrowhead)* is also evident on the left.

advantages for subtle soft-tissue differences and thus appears to be the modality of choice for evaluation of pathology of salivary glands.

## Suggested Reading


Batsakis JG. Tumors of the Head and Neck: Clinical and Pathological Considerations. Baltimore: Williams & Wilkins, 1979:1.

Byrne MN, Spector JG, Garvin CF, Gado MH. Preoperative assessment of parotid masses: A comparative evaluation of radiologic techniques to histopathologic diagnosis. Laryngoscope 1989; 99:284–292.

Cummings CW, Fredrickson JM, Harker LA, et al. Otolaryngology Head and Neck Surgery. Vol 2. Salivary Glands, Oral Cavity/Oropharynx. St Louis: CV Mosby, 1986:961.

Curtin HD. Assessment of salivary gland pathology. Otolaryngol Clin North Am 1988; 21:547–573.

Holliday R, Cohen WA, Schinella RA, et al. Benign lymphoepithelial parotid cysts and hyperplastic cervical adenopathy in AIDS-risk patients: A new CT appearance. Radiology 1988; 168:439–441.

Som PM, Bergeron RT. Head and Neck Imaging. St Louis: Mosby–Year Book, 1991:277.

Som PM, Biller HF. High-grade malignancies of the parotid gland: Identification with MR imaging. Radiology 1989; 173:823–826.

Tabor EK, Curtin HD. MR of the salivary glands. Radiol Clin North Am 1989; 27:379–392.

Takashma, Takeucni. MR Sjögren's. J Comp Assist Tom 1991; 15:393–400.

Tunkel DE, Loury MC, Fox CH, et al. Bilateral parotid enlargement in HIV seropositive patients. Laryngoscope 1989; 99:590–595.

Valvassori GE, Buckingham RA, Carter BL, et al. Head and Neck Imaging. Stuttgart, New York: George Thieme Verlag, 1988:285.

Vogel TJ, Dresel SHJ, Spath M, et al. Parotid gland: Plain and gadolinium-enhanced MR imaging. Radiology 1990; 177:667–674.


# Imaging of the Larynx: MRI and CT

*HUGH D. CURTIN, M.D.*

Imaging of the larynx must be approached within the context of modern endoscopy and modern therapeutic techniques. Excellent direct visualization of almost all the mucosa of the larynx is achieved using modern endoscopic equipment available in many otolaryngology offices. Since most lesions that come to imaging arise from the mucosa, almost all have been detected before imaging; indeed the diagnosis is seldom in question. Imaging is used to evaluate the regions of the larynx that the otolaryngologist cannot directly observe but that make a difference in therapy planning.

Most of the clinical problems that come to imaging can be put into one of three categories: mucosal carcinoma, submucosal masses, and trauma. We have different imaging strategies for each of these problems, and each is treated in a separate section. First we briefly discuss techniques for imaging the neck.

## Imaging Techniques

### *Magnetic Resonance Imaging*

Surface coils designed specifically for the neck are used to maximize signal. Currently we do a sagittal T1-weighted (short TR, short TE) localizer sequence. Axial and coronal T1-weighted sequences are then done as well as an axial long TR/variable TE sequence to obtain proton spin-density and T2-weighted information. Recently we have been using gadolinium in selected tumor cases. Fat suppression with gadolinium shows considerable promise.

The axial images are oriented parallel to the ventricle, which is often seen on the sagittal localizer (Fig. 1). The coronal images should be in a plane perpendicular to the ventricle or parallel to the posterior wall of the airway (Fig. 2).

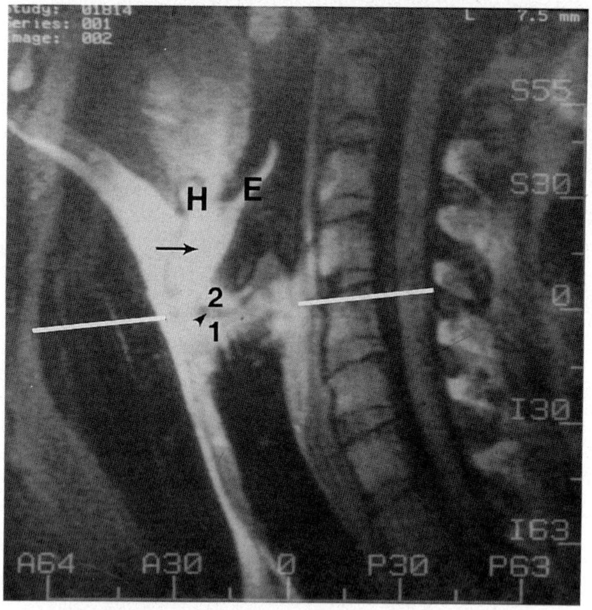


**FIGURE 1** Sagittal T1-weighted image (short TR/short TE) approximately midline shows the true cord (1), false cord (2), and the narrow air-filled ventricle (*arrowhead*) in between. The axial image(s) would be taken parallel to the ventricle as indicated by the white line. E = epiglottis; H = hyoid; pre-epiglottic fat (*arrow*).

The major problem with laryngeal magnetic resonance imaging (MRI) is motion artifact due to swallowing and respiration. To minimize the effect of respiration, the patient practices shallow breathing before imaging. The patient is told to breathe using the "belly" rather than the chest. The technologist rests a hand on the neck while the patient is

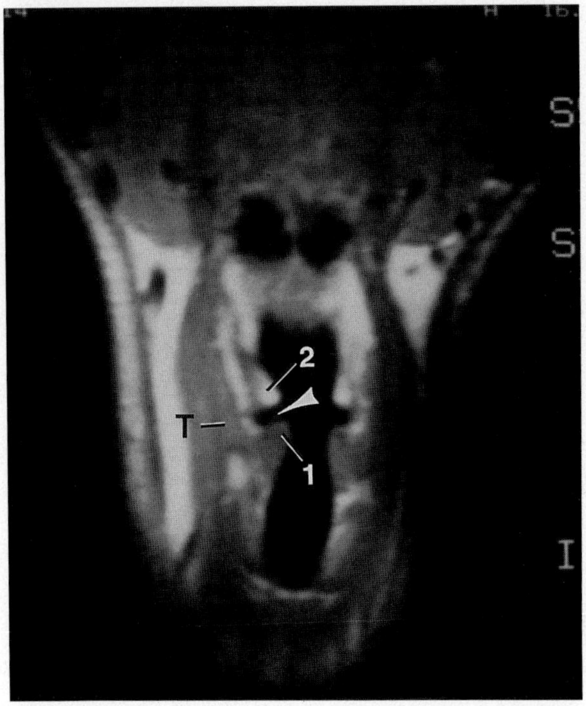


**FIGURE 2** Normal coronal short TR/short TE, T1-weighted image. Note the true cord (1), false cord (2), and ventricle (*arrowhead*) are seen in cross-section. The signal intensity of the true cord is intermediate signal representing muscle, whereas the false cord is predominantly bright signal reflecting fat. The paraglottic space represents the soft tissue deep to the mucosa, but medial to the thyroid cartilage. T = thyroid cartilage.

practicing to assure that motion is limited and to emphasize the importance of remaining still.

We also use four excitations for the axial images. Although the time of examination is longer, we feel that the images are better, because the motion artifacts caused by random events such as swallowing are averaged out.

### *Computed Tomography*

Axial images are done 1.5 mm thick at 3 mm intervals from the hyoid to the lower cricoid. The patient is instructed to breathe shallowly as with MRI. If motion is a problem, slices can be done with the breath held. The slice orientation is along the ventricle, which can often be seen on the scout view. If this landmark is not visible, the orientation is perpendicular to the axis of the spine at approximately C4 or C5.

Iodinated contrast medium is given in tumor cases, with either a bolus and drip technique or using an automatic injector. The goal is to have enough opacification of the vessels to allow easy differentiation from nodes.

## Imaging for Squamous Cell Carcinoma

### *Carcinoma*

The most frequent indication for laryngeal imaging at our institution is squamous cell carcinoma arising from the mucosa of the larynx. Virtually all have been detected by direct visualization as a mucosal lesion. In many cases, the otolaryngologist can determine all the information needed for therapy planning, and in these cases imaging is not done. Imaging is directed at answering specific questions that cannot be addressed by direct visualization. Usually these questions relate to detecting deep tumor extension, which could be a contraindication to voice-sparing surgery or radiation. The alternative to voice-sparing therapy is total laryngectomy. Imaging should be done before the biopsy, because edema and even small amounts of hemorrhage can significantly complicate the interpretation of the images.

The position of the tumor relative to precise anatomic landmarks determines the feasibility of voice-sparing partial laryngectomies, such as the supraglottic laryngectomy and vertical hemilaryngectomy. Also, determination of such factors as depth of extension and cartilage invasion can have a bearing on the likelihood that radiotherapy is successful.

### *Partial Laryngectomies*

The purpose of the partial laryngectomy is to resect the tumor but leave enough of the larynx to permit voice generation. The type of partial laryngectomy is dictated by the position of the tumor relative to the ventricle, which represents the boundary between the supraglottic larynx and the true cord.

#### Supraglottic Laryngectomy

A supraglottic laryngectomy is considered when a lesion arises above and does not cross the ventricle (Fig. 3). The resection line passes through the laryngeal ventricle, so tumor crossing this level is a contraindication to this type of surgery. A large tumor obviously crossing the ventricle is referred to as transglottic and does not necessarily require imaging. However, a smaller tumor can approach the ventricle via the paraglottic space beneath the mucosa. This region is invisible to the examining clinician.

Most of the tissue in the paraglottic space at the false cord level is fat. The thyroarytenoid muscle forms the bulk of the true cord and fills paraglottic region below the level of the ventricle. The different imaging appearances of the tissues of the true and false cords allow identification of the level of the ventricle.

We prefer to evaluate the inferior extent of supraglottic tumors with MRI. The coronal images are perpendicular to the false cord, ventricle, and true cord and thus are ideal for imaging this important region. Tumor traveling through the paraglottic space at the false cord level obliterates the fat. As the lesion crosses the ventricle, tumor infiltrates the outer edge of the thyroarytenoid muscle (Fig. 4). Tumor may have approximately the same signal intensity as the muscle on the T1-weighted images, but the increased bulk of the cord is usually easily appreciated. The fat just above the involved cord is obliterated as well. The long TR sequence or a gadolinium-enhanced sequence may be helpful, because the tumor often has a different signal than the muscle (Figs. 5 and 6).

The other point where the tumor can cross the ventricle is the anterior commissure. This is poorly seen on the coronal view, but can be evaluated with the axial or the sagittal view. Mucosal extent is difficult to assess by imaging, but if the tumor is infiltrating more deeply it may be more easily detected at imaging than at clinical examination. Tumor is seen extending

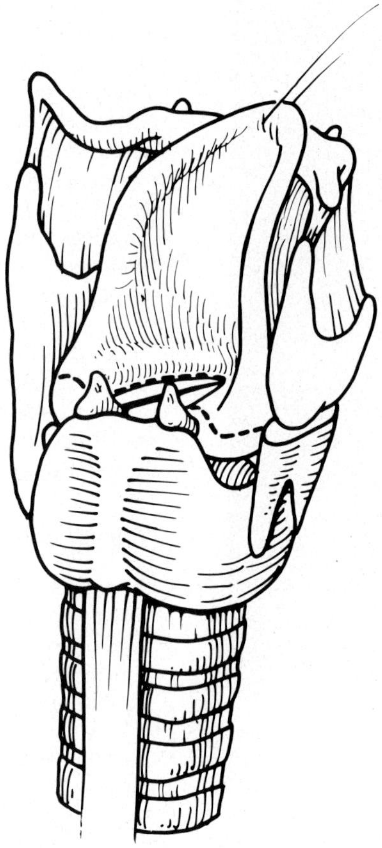

**FIGURE 3** Diagram of supraglottic laryngectomy done for lesion arising above the ventricle. The dotted line shows the line of resection. Note that the dotted line representing the incision line passes exactly along the ventricle. Tumors cannot cross this line if the patient is to be a candidate for this type of procedure.

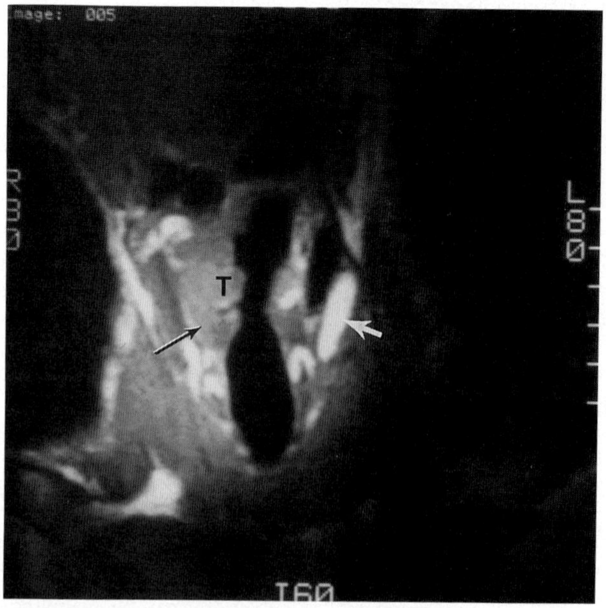


**FIGURE 4** Supraglottic carcinoma invading the true cord. The tumor (T) could easily be visualized from above. The mucosa of the true cord was normal. The tumor extended around the lateral aspect of the ventricle into the superior lateral edge (*black arrow*) of the true cord. Since the lesion extended below the level of the ventricle, a supraglottic resection was not possible. Thyroid cartilage (*white arrow*).

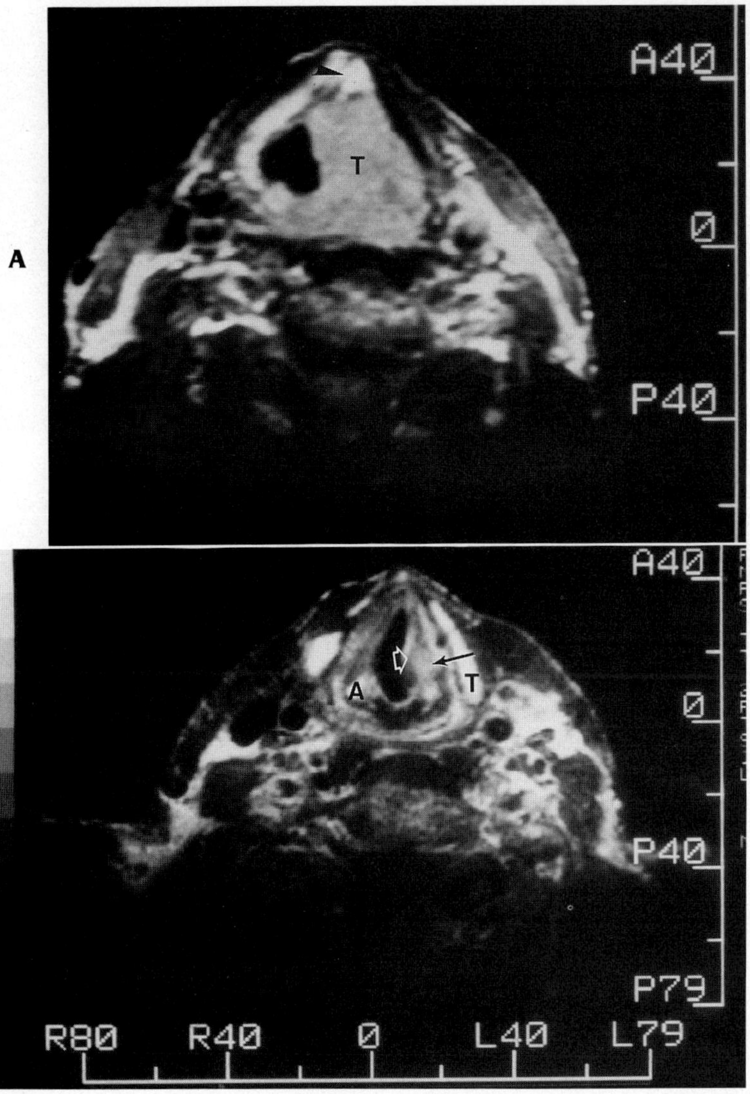


**FIGURE 5** *A,* Carcinoma. Axial T1-weighted sequence after gadolinium. The tumor (T) has an intermediate signal intensity. It can be easily differentiated from fat (*arrowhead*) in the remainder of the supraglottic larynx. *B,* Lower slice through the level close to the true cord. The tumor (*arrow*) is infiltrating into the lateral edge of the thyroarytenoid muscle (*open arrow*). A = arytenoid; T = thyroid cartilage. Compare this image with Figure 6.

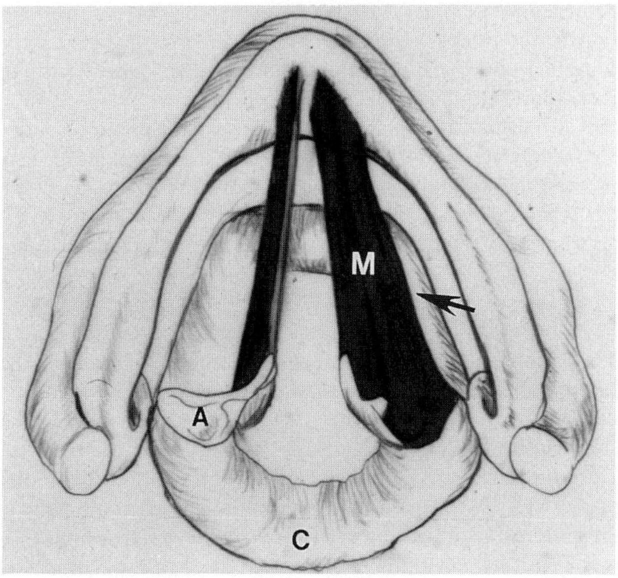


**FIGURE 6** Drawing of a view from above showing the thyroarytenoid muscle (M) stretching from the arytenoid (A) to the inner surface of the thyroid cartilage. The tumor is expected to infiltrate the lateral edge of the muscle at the approximate location of the arrow. C = cricoid.

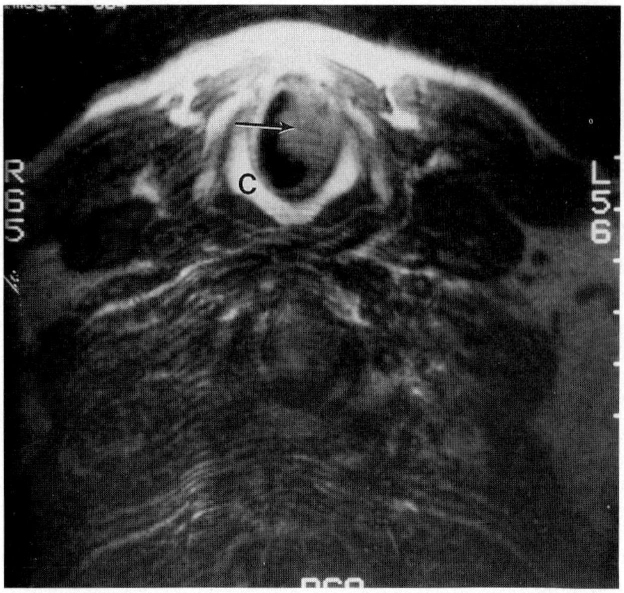


**FIGURE 7** Axial T1-weighted image. This patient had a carcinoma of the true cord. This slice is inferior to the true cord and is taken through the cricoid ring (C). The tumor (*arrow*) definitely extends within the ring and so is below the level of the upper cricoid. This patient would not be a candidate for vertical hemilaryngectomy.

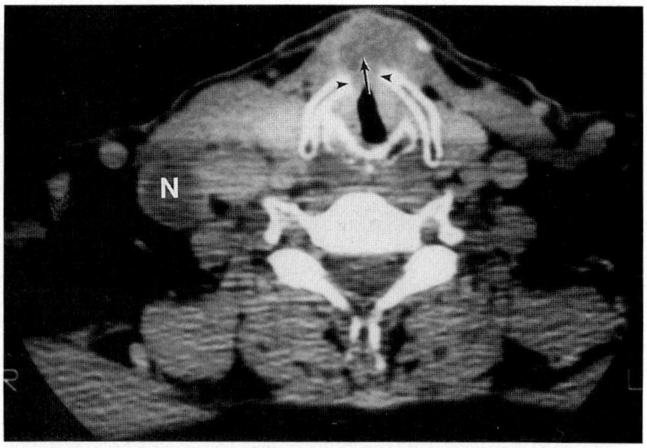


**FIGURE 8** Tumor of the anterior commissure. Most of the lesion is submucosal, but the tumor extends anteriorly through the lower thyroid cartilage (*arrowheads*) into the soft tissue (*arrow*) anterior to the larynx. N = metastatic node.

anteriorly into the tissues close to the lower margin of the thyroid cartilage.

Invasion of the thyroid or cricoid cartilage is another contraindication to supraglottic laryngectomy. This is distinctly unusual if the tumor is limited to the supraglottic larynx. Cartilage invasion is discussed in the next section.

### Vertical Hemilaryngectomy (True Cord)

Vertical hemilaryngectomy is the speech-conserving partial laryngectomy used for tumors limited to the true cord. The most important points to be addressed at imaging are the inferior extent, deep extension at the anterior commissure, and cartilage invasion. Tumor crossing the ventricle superiorly is also a relative contraindication, but this is infrequently a problem.

The cricoid cartilage is the foundation of the larynx, and most otolaryngologists consider extension reaching the upper margin of the cricoid cartilage a contraindication to vertical hemilaryngectomy. The cricoid ring has a distinctive appearance on axial imaging, and the radiologist tries to determine whether the tumor has reached the upper margin of the cartilage. For this evaluation, either axial CT or axial MRI is adequate (Fig. 7).

The axial plane is also excellent for detecting deep extension at the anterior commissure. Tumor can extend through the cricothyroid membrane into the soft tissues anterior to the larynx (Fig. 8).

Cartilage involvement is more difficult to evaluate. On either CT or MRI, the most reliable sign of cartilage involvement is identification of tumor on the extralaryngeal or outer surface of the cartilage. More subtle involvement is difficult to detect. The variability of ossification creates a problem, because the nonossified part of the cartilage can have exactly the same appearance as tumor on a CT scan. MRI has the advantage of better tissue discrimination, and early results have indicated that tumor can be differentiated from nonossified cartilage based on signal. The T1-weighted sequence is compared with either the proton spin density or the T2-weighted image of the long TR sequence. Nonossified cartilage remains relatively dark when the short and long TR sequence images are compared (Fig. 9). Tumor appears to be relatively brighter on the long TR image (Fig. 10). One cannot rely on the appearance of the cartilage on the long TR image alone, because fat may "retain" signal even on a T2-weighted image. This is commonly seen when the neck surface coil is used.

## *Radiation Therapy*

At our institution most of our referrals come from an otolaryngology group with a strong surgical bias. However, our protocols address the concerns of radiotherapists as well.

Certainly an overall assessment of the size and extent is provided with either CT or MRI. The depth of extension or the bulk of the tumor is of primary concern. How deeply into the pre-epiglottic space does the tumor extend? Does the tumor extend up into the tongue base?

Cartilage invasion is important. This is considered a relative contraindication to radiation therapy. However, MRI may provide the capability of detecting more subtle invasion than has been previously possible, and some think radiation may be appropriate treatment of cases with only minimal invasion.

## *Lymph Nodes*

The lymph nodes can be important to both the surgeon and the radiotherapist. Our CT and MRI protocols cover the principal node-bearing areas, especially when the tumor arises in the supraglottic region.

If the clinician feels that enough information about the primary tumor has been achieved by direct visualization and is only interested in the status of the nodes, we prefer CT because it is easier to do.

A 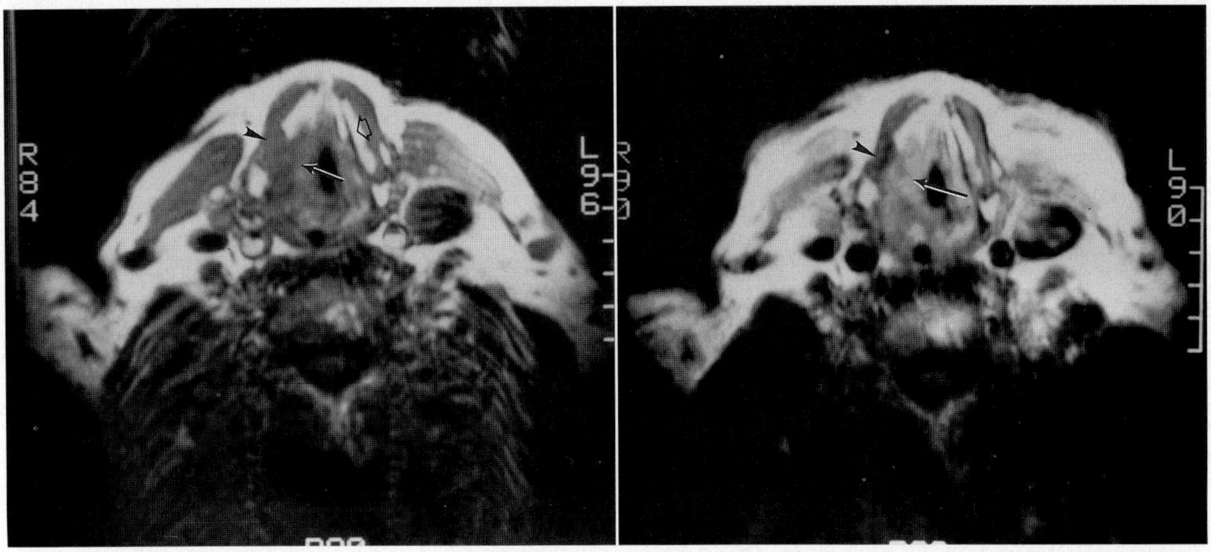 B

**FIGURE 9** *A,* T1-weighted image of tumor of the supraglottic larynx. The tumor (*arrow*) has exactly the same signal as the nonossified cartilage (*arrowhead*), and these tissues cannot be differentiated. The fat-laden medullary cavity of the thyroid cartilage on the opposite side (*open arrow*) can easily be differentiated from tumor. *B,* On a proton spin-density image (long TR/short TE) the tumor (*arrow*) is relatively brighter while the nonossified cartilage (*arrowhead*) remains dark.

A 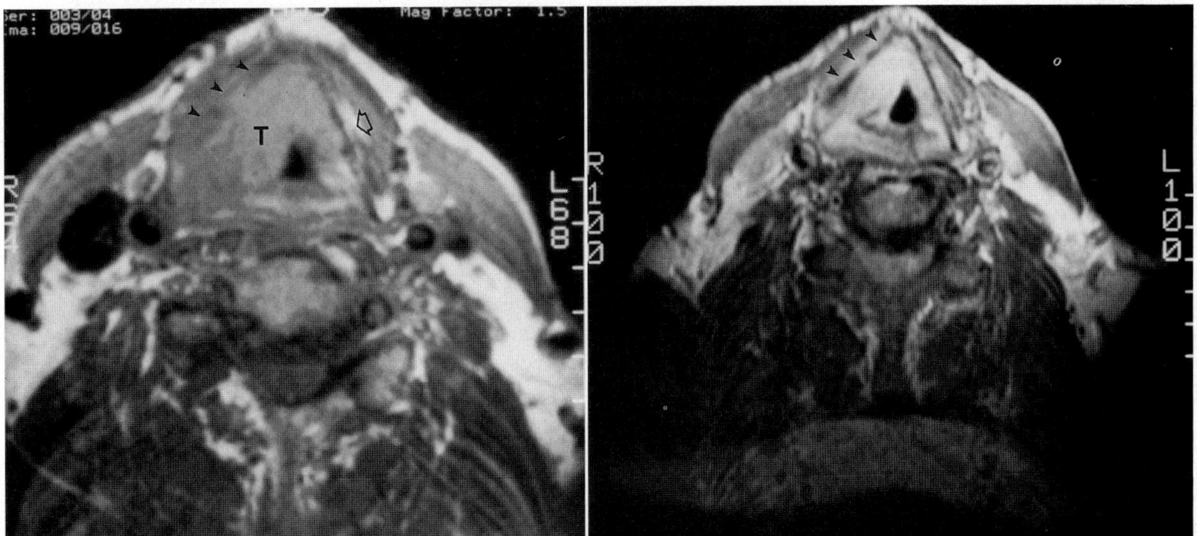 B

**FIGURE 10** Supraglottic carcinoma with cartilage invasion. *A,* Short TR/short TE, T1-weighted image shows the supraglottic tumor (T) infiltrating the fat and crossing the midline. The thyroid cartilage is of intermediate signal (*arrowheads*). Note the appearance of the thyroid cartilage on the opposite side (*open arrow*). *B,* T2-weighted image (long TR/long TE). There is "brightening" of the tissue along the outer cortex (*arrowheads*) of the involved thyroid cartilage. On this one sequence, the signal intensity of both normal and abnormal regions of the cartilage is similar. However, when this sequence is compared with the T1-weighted sequence, there is a definite difference in the appearance.

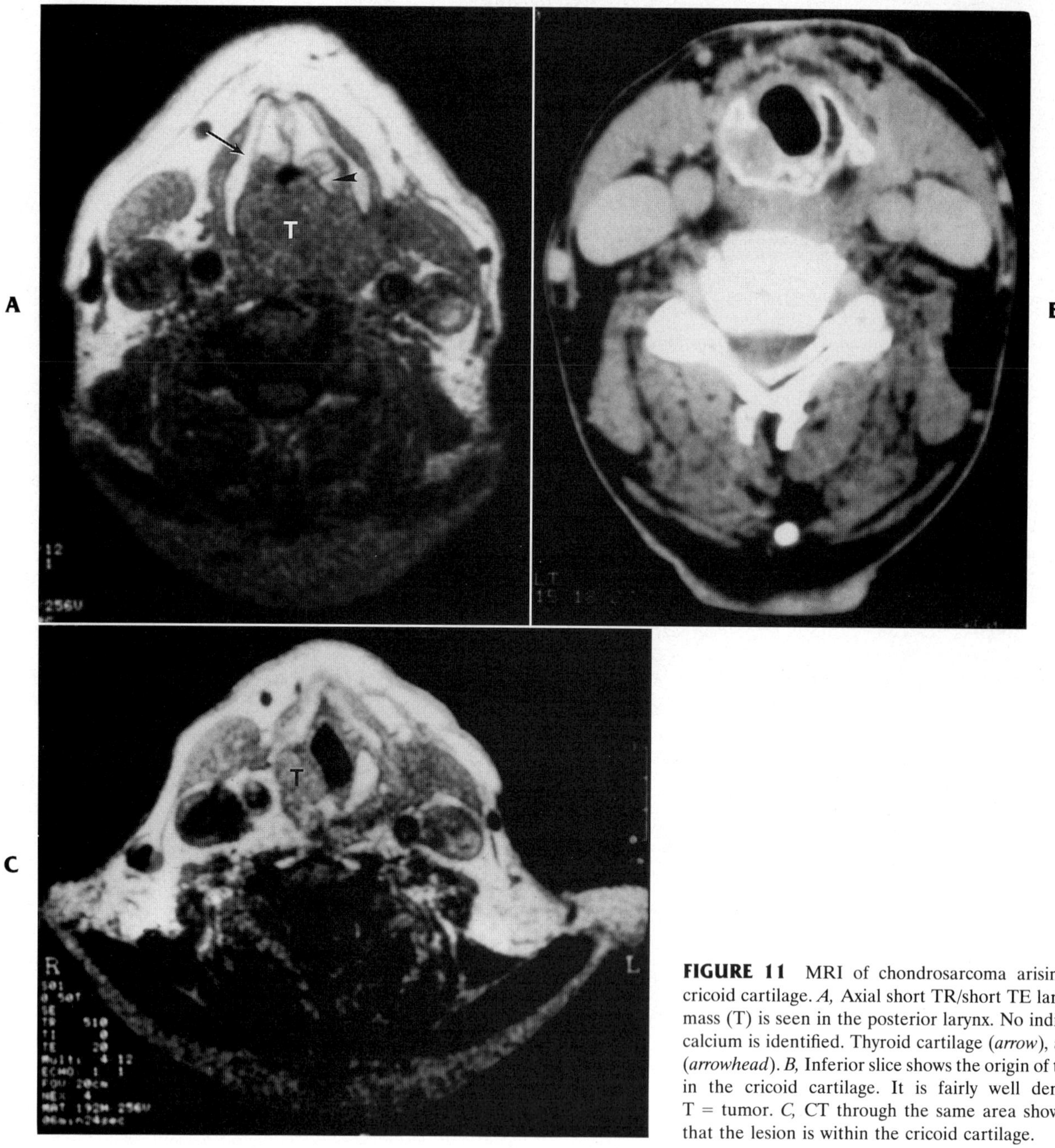


**FIGURE 11** MRI of chondrosarcoma arising in the cricoid cartilage. *A,* Axial short TR/short TE large tumor mass (T) is seen in the posterior larynx. No indication of calcium is identified. Thyroid cartilage (*arrow*), arytenoid (*arrowhead*). *B,* Inferior slice shows the origin of the lesion in the cricoid cartilage. It is fairly well demarcated. T = tumor. *C,* CT through the same area shows clearly that the lesion is within the cricoid cartilage.

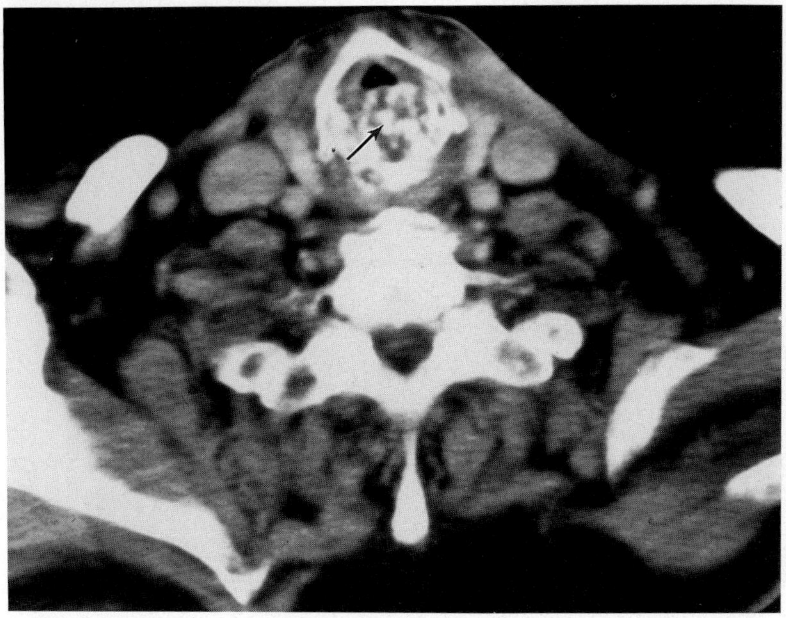

**FIGURE 12** Chondrosarcoma of the cricoid protruding into the airway. Note the obvious calcifications (*arrow*) within the lesion.

## *Pitfalls in Cancer Imaging*

Imaging of the larynx, especially using MRI, is a relatively new technique and experience is limited. Signal variations may not necessarily represent neoplasm. Inflammatory changes can mimic tumor. This is a major problem if a lesion has been biopsied before imaging. More experience is required to test the specificity of abnormal signal changes at MRI.

Another pitfall is encountered when the larynx is slightly oblique relative to the plane of the image. This is not an uncommon occurrence and can cause apparent asymmetry in the soft tissues of the larynx, which should not be misdiagnosed as tumor. Considering the narrow tolerances allowed in tumor evaluation, the radiologist must carefully evaluate the anatomic landmarks to verify that an asymmetry is due to tumor and not obliquity. Signal variations and the multiple scan orientations available on MRI can be helpful in confirming that a suspicious area indeed does represent tumor.

## Submucosal Masses

The clinician sees the submucosal mass as a bulge in an intact mucosa rather than an irregularity of the mucosa itself. In these cases, the diagnosis is not obvious and imaging can be helpful in determining the diagnosis or at least limiting the diagnostic possibilities. The extent of the lesion is also determined at imaging.

Submucosal masses include chondroid tumors, hemangiomas, and a variety of other soft-tissue neoplasms.

For evaluation of submucosal masses, we prefer CT with intravenous contrast medium. The calcifications of chondrosarcomas are much more easily detected on CT than on MRI (Figs. 11 and 12). Vascular lesions stand out clearly after intravenous enhancement. If a lesion does not enhance brightly, at least we can tell the surgeon that the lesion is not likely to be a hemangioma or a rare glomus tumor where bleeding is likely to be a more major concern.

Another submucosal "mass" that should be considered is the laryngocele or saccular cyst. This is a dilatation of the ventricular appendix, which extends superiorly from the ventricle into the paraglottic space at the level of the false cord. This cyst has a smooth wall and can be filled with air or fluid (Fig. 13). The cyst is benign, but the cause of the obstruction may be a tumor. Both the radiologist and the clinician should search for a small tumor in the region of the laryngeal ventricle.

## Trauma

We use CT, usually without contrast medium, for imaging the traumatized larynx. The cartilages are easily seen, and a fragile airway is more easily managed in the CT scanner than in the more confining MRI scanner. The thyroid and cricoid cartilages are inspected for fractures (Figs. 14 and 15). If there is a fracture, the radiologist should look carefully for any fragment that might protrude into the airway. A fragment of cartilage that breaks through the mucosa and is exposed to the airway has a high likelihood of infection, which can lead to chondronecrosis and scarring that can further restrict the airway.

Dislocations can occur at the cricoarytenoid joint or the cricothyroid joint. Often these dislocations are seen in conjunction with a laryngeal fracture. The dislocation of the cricothyroid joint is usually easy to diagnose, although one must be careful to compare images at the same level. Cricoarytenoid dislocations can be difficult to diagnose, but the radiologist should comment as to whether the cricoid and arytenoid cartilages can be identified in proper alignment.

## Discussion

Laryngeal imaging can be difficult because of various motion artifacts but can provide useful information about the deep soft tissues in selected cases.

A 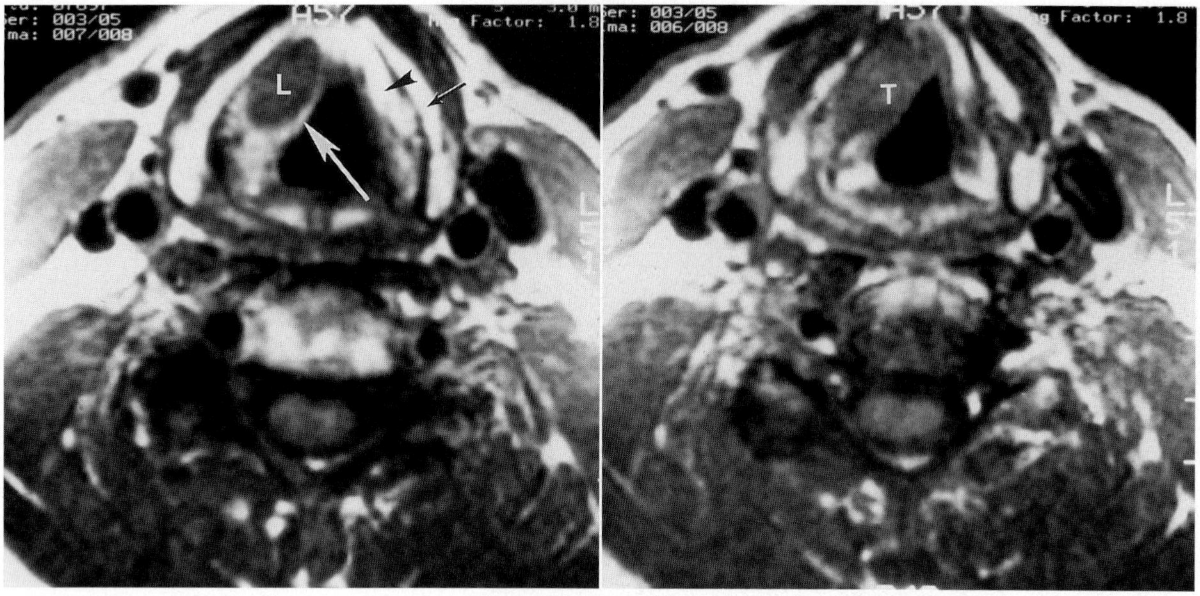 B



**FIGURE 13** Small laryngocele (saccular cyst) with carcinoma. *A,* Axial short TR/short TE (T1 weighted) through the supraglottic larynx. The fluid-filled laryngocele (L) is observed in the paraglottic fat. Note the normal mucosa (*arrow*) separating it from the airway. Paraglottic fat on the normal side (*arrowhead*), and fat in the medullary cavity of the thyroid cartilage (*black arrow*). *B,* Slightly inferior slice, same sequence, shows intermediate signal intensity of a tumor at the level of the ventricle and upper true cord tumor (T), although the laryngocele is benign and may be caused by a malignancy obstructing the appendix of the ventricle.

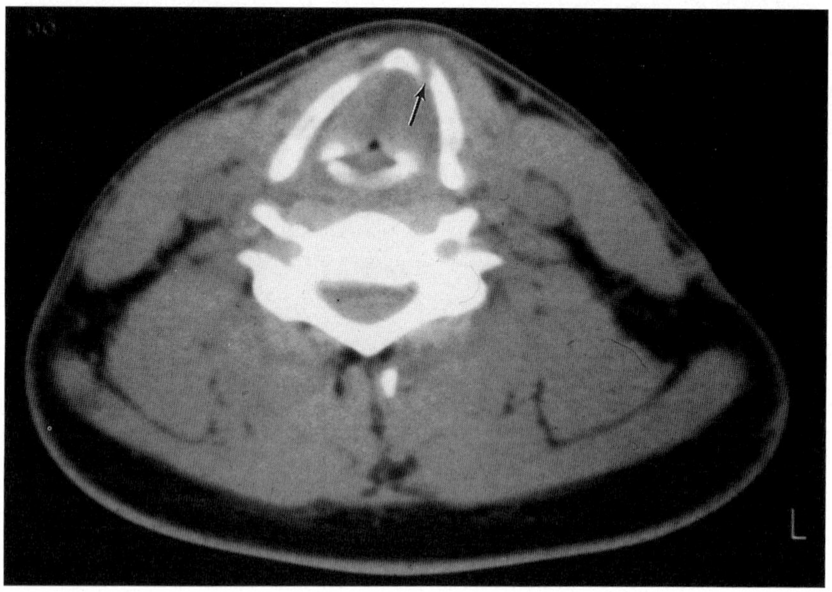



**FIGURE 14** Vertical fracture of the thyroid cartilage (*arrow*).

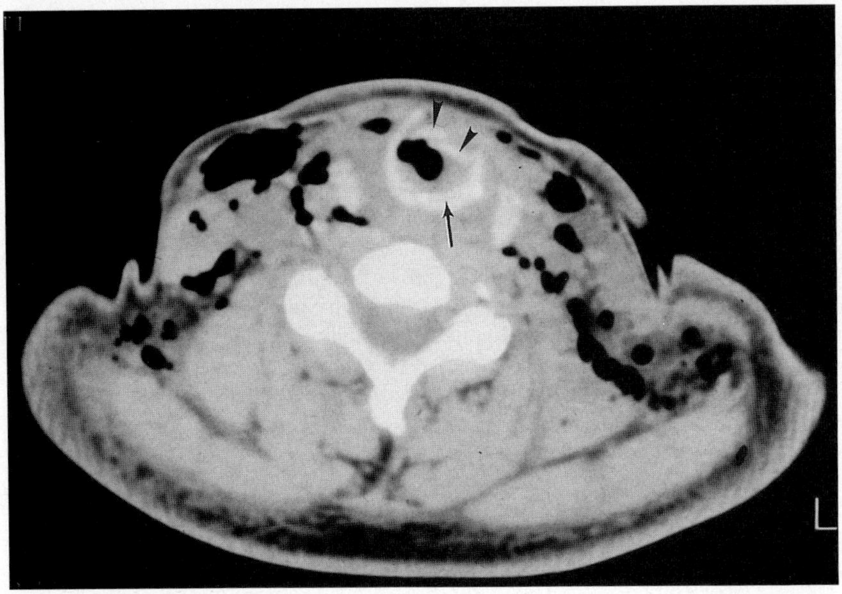

**FIGURE 15** Fracture of the cricoid. The anterior rim of the cricoid cartilage is fractured with two of the fragments (*arrowheads*) representing the anterior arch of the cricoid pushed posteriorly into the airway. Posterior cricoid (lamina) (*arrow*). Note the gas in the soft tissues.

## Suggested Reading

Castelijns JA, Gerritsen GJ, Kaiser MC, et al. MRI of normal or cancerous laryngeal cartilages: Histopathologic correlation. Laryngoscope 1987; 97:1085–1093.

Castelijns JA, Gerritsen GJ, Kaiser MC, et al. Invasion of laryngeal cartilage by cancer: Comparison of CT and MR imaging. Radiology 1987; 166:199–206.

Curtin HD. Imaging of the larynx: Current concepts. Radiology 1989; 173:1–11.

Curtin HD. The larynx. In: Som PM, Bergeron RT, eds. Head and neck imaging. St. Louis: Mosby–Year Book, 1991:593.

Giron J, Joffre P, Serres-Cousine O, et al. Magnetic resonance imaging of the larynx. Its contribution compared to x-ray computed tomography in the pre-therapeutic evaluation of cancers of the larynx. Apropos of 90 surgical cases. Ann Radiol (Paris) 1990; 33:170–184.

Kolbenstvedt A, Charania B, Natvig, Tausio J. Computed tomography in T1 carcinoma of the larynx. Acta Radiol 1989; 30:467–469.

Lawson W, Biller HF, Suen JR. Cancer of the larynx. In: Suen JY, Myers EN, eds. Cancer of the head and neck. New York: Churchill Livingstone, 1989:533.

Sakai F, Gamsu G, Dillon WP, et al. MR imaging of the larynx at 1.5 T. J Comput Assist Tomogr 1990; 14:60–71.

Teresi LM, Lufkin RB, Hanafee WN. Magnetic resonance imaging of the larynx. Radiol Clin North Am 1989; 27:393–406.

# Imaging of the Paranasal Sinuses: CT and MRI

*FRED J. LAINE, M.D. · WENDY R. K. SMOKER, M.D.*

Evaluation of the paranasal sinuses can now be performed by a number of modalities. Plain radiographs represent the most inexpensive technique, but they are insufficient for preoperative evaluation of paranasal sinus disease. With rare exception, we use plain radiographs only for (1) inpatients, too sick to travel, who require a portable procedure, or (2) as a quick screening method for facial trauma patients being stabilized or evaluated for additional life-threatening lesions. The majority of patients referred for evaluation of the paranasal sinuses at our institution are outpatients in whom we are requested to evaluate the extent of inflammatory sinus disease or a paranasal sinus tumor. Currently computed tomography (CT) and magnetic resonance imaging (MRI) are the imaging modalities of choice for evaluation of these patients.

## Computed Tomography

CT remains the primary modality for evaluation of paranasal sinus disease. CT is widely available, relatively inexpensive, and easy to perform. However, the main advantage of CT is its ability to distinguish soft-tissue structures from bone. We select from two protocols when asked to evaluate the paranasal sinuses. With either protocol, immediately before scanning, the patient is instructed to use a sympathomimetic nasal spray, in conjunction with vigorous nose blowing. The CT parameters for both are listed in Table 1.

The first protocol is a "screening" sinus technique, used primarily for preoperative planning before endoscopic paranasal sinus surgery. The majority of patients therefore are referred for evaluation of repeated acute sinusitis or chronic

**TABLE 1** CT Protocols for Paranasal Sinuses

| | Screening CT | Complete CT |
|---|---|---|
| Patient position | Prone, hyperextended head | Supine, prone |
| Scan angle | Coronal—may be of variable degree | Axial and coronal |
| Contrast medium | No | Yes; Bolus (50 ml of 60%) then drip (150 ml of 30%) |
| Slice thickness | 3–5 mm | Coronal: 3–5 mm Axial: 5 mm |
| | Contiguous | Contiguous |
| Algorithm | Bone | Soft tissue |
| Filming windows | Intermediate | Soft tissue and bone |
| First/last slice | Coronal: anterior maxillary or frontal sinus to posterior sphenoid sinus Axial: hard palate to top of frontal sinus | |

refractory disease. Radiographic evaluation is directed toward assessing the patency of the maxillary sinus ostium, infundibulum, and middle meatus—the area identified as the ostiomeatal unit (OMU) (Fig. 1). The sphenoethmoidal recess (SER), although better observed on axial images, can be indirectly assessed by evaluating the posterior ethmoid and sphenoid sinuses, areas from which it receives drainage. The screening CT scan is performed *following* treatment of an acute process. In this manner areas of residual disease that are most likely responsible for recurring problems can be fully assessed. The patient is placed in the prone hyperextended position to ensure that free fluid layers along the maxillary sinus floor and does not falsely obliterate the OMU. In general, the coronal plane provides the best demonstration of the OMU, because it simulates the plane seen by the endoscopist. The degree of CT gantry tilt for coronal imaging is variable and must be angled to maximally avoid dental amalgams.

The second scanning protocol for evaluation of the paranasal sinuses is a "complete" sinus series, used whenever noninflammatory pathology is identified on the screening sinus CT scan. This protocol is also the protocol of choice to evaluate benign or malignant tumors, complex inflammatory disease (e.g., polyposis, fungal sinusitis), and complications of sinusitis (e.g., osteomyelitis, mucoceles). Scanning is performed in both axial and coronal planes. Additional slices are obtained in any direction until the entire lesion is covered. Contrast medium is used and administered by a bolus-drip technique: 50 ml of a 60 percent nonionic medium followed by 150 ml drip infusion of a 30 percent nonionic medium. Imaging commences immediately after the bolus injection. Images are obtained using a soft-tissue algorithm and photographed with both bone and soft-tissue windows.

## MRI

Indications for MRI of the paranasal sinuses are virtually the same as for a complete sinus CT series. The decision to obtain a complete sinus CT scan or an MRI study frequently involves issues other than the information desired (i.e., patient cooperation, scanner availability). MRI is most commonly used at our institution to answer specific questions that are unanswered by CT. These specific indications are addressed subsequently. MRI offers superior soft-tissue definition compared with CT. Invasion of bone marrow spaces can be identified on MRI; however, fine bone alterations and destruction are better demonstrated on CT.

Standard spin-echo T1-weighted images are obtained in the axial and coronal planes both before and after gadolinium-DTPA administration. A sagittal plane is added if delineation of midline structures is required. Scan slices should be no larger than 5 mm thick, with a narrow interslice gap. However, sequences are somewhat variable, depending on the individual MRI unit and magnet strength, and should be optimized independently. Since distinction between inflammation and neoplasm can frequently be made by analyzing the signal characteristics on T1- and T2-weighted images, we routinely

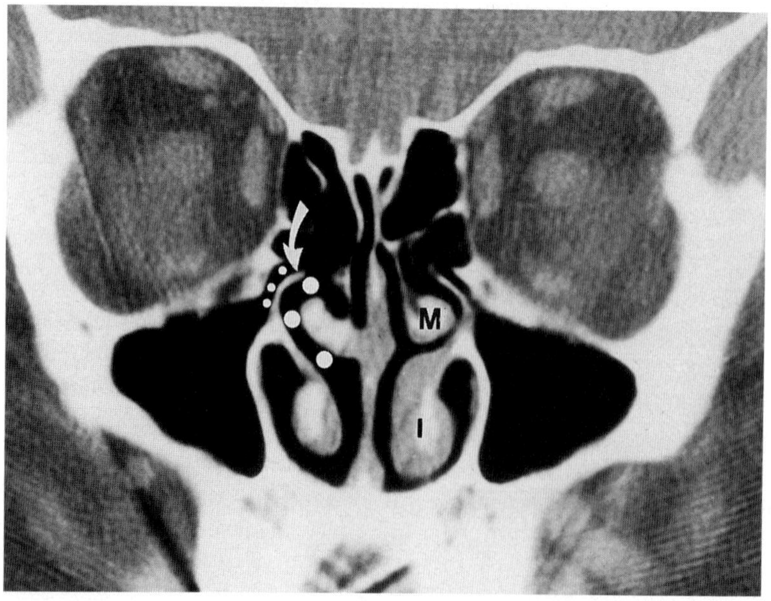


**FIGURE 1** Normal OMU. Coronal image of a screening sinus CT at the level of the OMU. This area represents the major drainage site for anterior and middle ethmoid, frontal, and maxillary sinuses and the area toward which endoscopic surgical procedures are directed. Normal anatomy of this area is well demonstrated. The uncinate process (*arrow*) separates the infundibulum (*small dots*) from the middle meatus (*large dots*). M = middle turbinate; I = inferior turbinate.

**TABLE 2** MRI Protocol for Paranasal Sinuses*

| | T1 | T2 |
|---|---|---|
| Plane | Axial and coronal (occasionally sagittal) | Axial or coronal |
| Contrast | Axial and coronal; 0.1 mmol/kg | |
| Slice thickness | 4 mm | 5 mm |
| TR | 750 ms | 2,500 ms |
| TE | 15 ms | 45/90 ms |
| NEX | 1 | 1 |
| Interslice gap | 0.1 | 0.1 |
| Matrix | 256 × 256, full matrix | 256 × 256, half-Fourier |
| FOV | 220 | 220 |
| First/last slice | Coronal: anterior maxillary and frontal sinus to posterior sphenoid sinus<br>Axial: hard palate to top of frontal sinus<br>Sagittal: lateral maxillary wall to opposite lateral maxillary wall | |

*Based on Seimens 1.5 T unit with A2.3 software.

obtain a spin-density T2-weighted sequence. The axial plane is preferred, although it may be supplemented by coronal and/or sagittal planes, depending on the information desired. The specific MRI parameters are presented in Table 2.

Recently fat-suppression techniques have proven useful in analyzing lesions adjacent to marrow spaces and within extracranial fat. If the sequence available involves a short tau inversion recovery (STIR), the sequence should precede the contrasted images, because it tends to suppress contrast enhancement. If the sequence available involves phase-dependent, chemical shift techniques (Dixon, Chopper, CHESS), the fat-suppression sequence should be performed following injection of the contrast medium. Contrast-enhanced fat-suppression techniques often provide maximal tumor-tissue differentiation in areas containing high amounts of fat.

## Specific Indications

### Trauma

Any trauma involving the head or face requires a rapid precise screening evaluation that is independent of the patient's ability to cooperate. Simple facial fractures may be adequately assessed by plain radiographs, but the more complex the injury, the more likely plain radiographs will be suboptimal. In the acute setting, if the patient is unstable or uncooperative, a rapid axial CT scan with 5 mm thick cuts is obtained. Frequently the study is performed in conjunction with an intracranial CT study. A soft-tissue algorithm is therefore used, filmed at both soft-tissue and bone windows. With this method, the site of fracture can be readily identified, as can soft-tissue abnormalities and associated complications (e.g., pneumocephalus, airway obstruction).

In the stable patient, before intraoperative fixation, a complete sinus series is performed. A more detailed evaluation can be obtained using bone window techniques with thinner slices. Three-dimensional imaging is performed only at the specific request of the referring clinician, because we believe little diagnostic information is added for the time involved.

### Acute and Chronic (or Recurrent) Inflammation

Improvements in paranasal sinus endoscopic instrumentation and the widespread availability of high-resolution CT has led to major changes in the management of sinus inflammatory conditions. Acute sinusitis is frequently treated, based on clinical examination, without the need for elaborate radiographic evaluation. However, when repeated bouts of acute sinusitis occur, or remain unresponsive to medical management, radiographic studies are frequently obtained. The screening sinus protocol is aimed at evaluation of the OMU. Disease centered at the OMU is easily identified, and the degree of ostial obstruction and extent of disease can also be determined (Fig. 2).

Differentiating acute from chronic sinus disease is often difficult unless the studies reveal the hallmarks of each. When air-fluid levels are observed in the nontraumatic patient, acute sinusitis is likely. Patients with chronic sinusitis may also present with an air-fluid level, but the chronicity is manifested by osseous thickening of the lamina dura (sinus wall), which represents remodeling and new bone formation in response to persistent inflammation (Fig. 3).

Once chronic sinusitis is identified, either clinically or radiographically, the next step is to identify its etiology. Numerous congenital variants may occur that often predispose to sinus disease by blockage of the draining ostia. These include: (1) deviation of the nasal septum, (2) concha bullosa (aeration of the middle turbinate) (Fig. 4), (3) deviation of the uncinate process, (4) the presence of Haller's cells, (5) large ethmoidal bullae, (6) pneumatization of the uncinate process, and (7) paradoxical middle turbinate (see Fig. 2). Post-traumatic bone displacement may also result in ostial blockage.

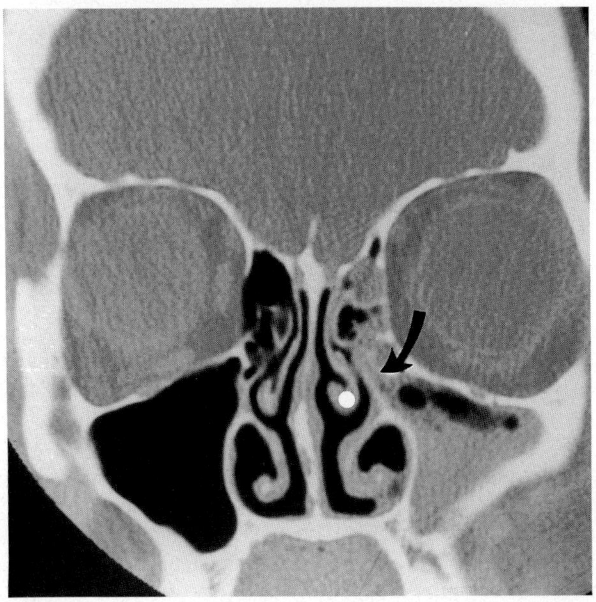

**FIGURE 2** Obstructed OMU, paradoxical left middle turbinate. Coronal CT demonstrates soft-tissue obstruction of the OMU (*arrow*), secondary to mucosal inflammation. Retained secretions are present in both the maxillary and ethmoid sinuses. The paradoxical left middle turbinate (*dot*) may have predisposed to the meatal disease. Compare the "backward" orientation of this turbinate with the normal orientation of the right middle turbinate.

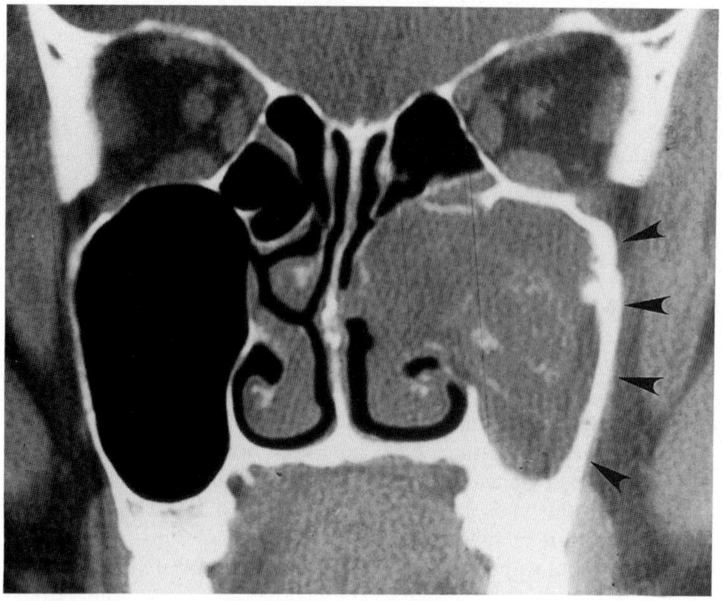

**FIGURE 3** Chronic fungal sinusitis. Coronal CT demonstrates the destructive nature of this aggressive infection, manifested by erosion of OMU structures, difficult to distinguish from tumor. An infectious etiology of this process, however, is suggested by the thickened sinus wall (*arrowheads*). Additionally, high density within the "mass" is most consistent with fungal infection.

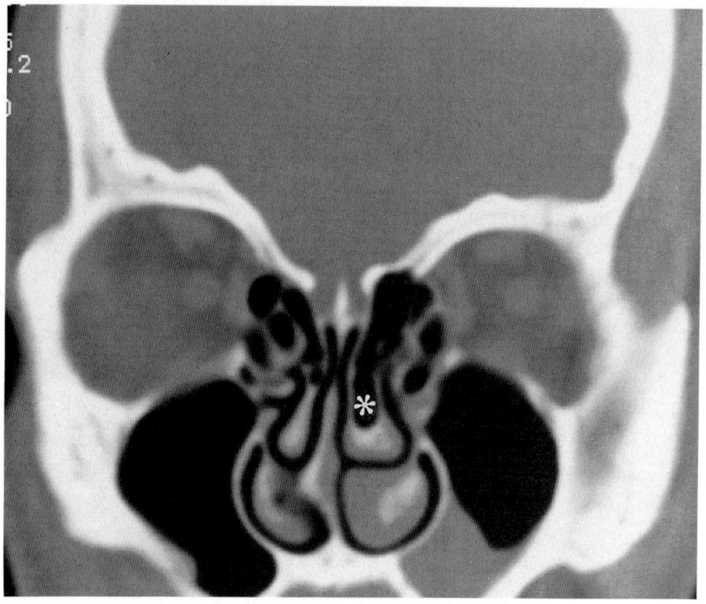

**FIGURE 4** Concha bullosa. Coronal CT demonstrates pneumatization of the left middle turbinate (concha bullosa) (*asterisk*), producing slight narrowing of the middle meatus. Inflammatory disease is seen in the floor left maxillary sinus.

In addition, mucosal thickening located at the OMU or SER can lead to persistent paranasal sinus inflammation. More importantly tumors may occasionally be responsible for repeated disease. A complete sinus CT study is required when tumor is suspected. In addition, MRI may be necessary in this regard, since most inflammatory tissue is inhomogeneous and has high signal intensity on T2-weighted images, whereas the majority of sinus tumors are homogeneous and have an intermediate signal intensity.

Fungal sinusitis is caused by a variety of fungi, all of which appear similar radiographically. Focal areas of bone destruction may mimic tumor; however, areas of bone thickening and sclerosis (evidence of chronic sinus involvement) are frequently associated with fungal lesions, but not tumors (see Fig. 3). In addition, the identification of high density within the opacified sinus on the CT scan (e.g., caused by calcification, heavy metals within the mycetoma) is highly suggestive of fungal infection. MRI may be more specific than CT in diagnosing fungal sinusitis, since the presence of these ferromagnetic metallic ions, contained within the mycetoma, produces a hypointense signal on both T1- and T2-weighted images.

Evaluation of local, regional, and intracranial complications of acute or chronic sinusitis requires a complete sinus CT study, but may be complemented by an MRI study. Local mucous retention cysts, observed as dome-shaped soft-tissue masses, usually offer no significant difficulty in their recognition. It is somewhat more difficult to differentiate among other local complications such as inflammatory polyps (membrane hyperplasia), mucoceles, and mucopyoceles. CT is useful for distinguishing between the erosive nature of inflammatory polyps (Fig. 5) and the expansile nature of mucoceles (Fig. 6).

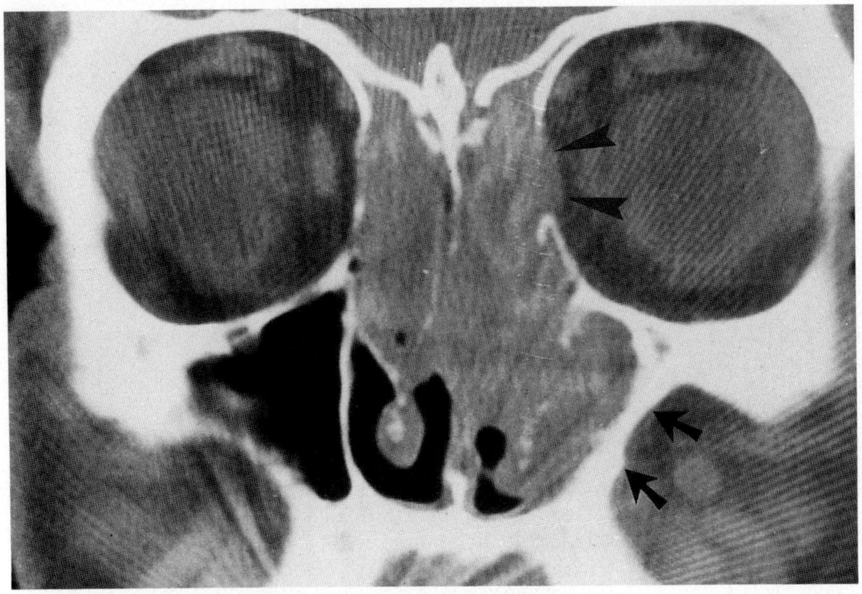

**FIGURE 5** Inflammatory polyposis. Coronal CT demonstrates the erosive changes associated with this disease. The ethmoid sinuses are expanded and the septations are virtually obliterated. The polyps have eroded through the left lamina papyracea (*arrowheads*) to enter the orbit. The thickened lamina dura of the maxillary sinus (*arrows*) suggests chronic long-standing inflammation.

A

B

C

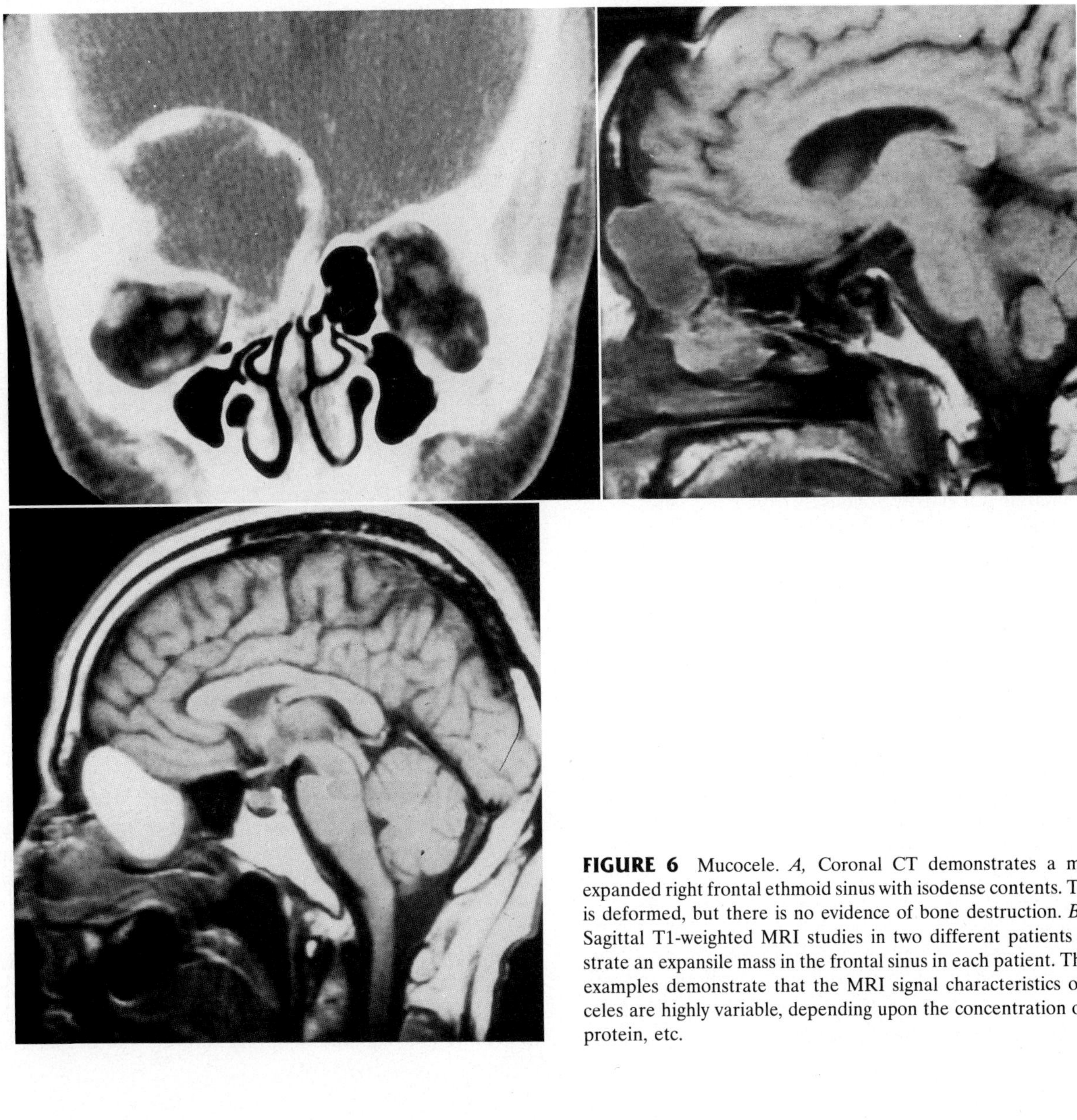

**FIGURE 6** Mucocele. *A,* Coronal CT demonstrates a markedly expanded right frontal ethmoid sinus with isodense contents. The orbit is deformed, but there is no evidence of bone destruction. *B* and *C,* Sagittal T1-weighted MRI studies in two different patients demonstrate an expansile mass in the frontal sinus in each patient. These two examples demonstrate that the MRI signal characteristics of mucoceles are highly variable, depending upon the concentration of water, protein, etc.

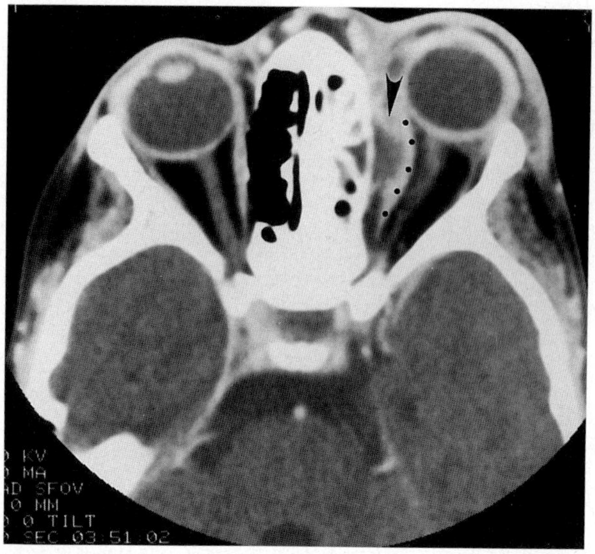

**FIGURE 7** Subperiosteal abscess. Axial contrast-enhanced CT of the orbit reveals a low-density mass along the medial aspect of the left orbital wall, laterally displacing a thickened inflamed medial rectus muscle (*black dots*). Note the marginal enhancement of the abscess (*arrowhead*). Inflammatory disease of left ethmoid sinus air cells is observed.

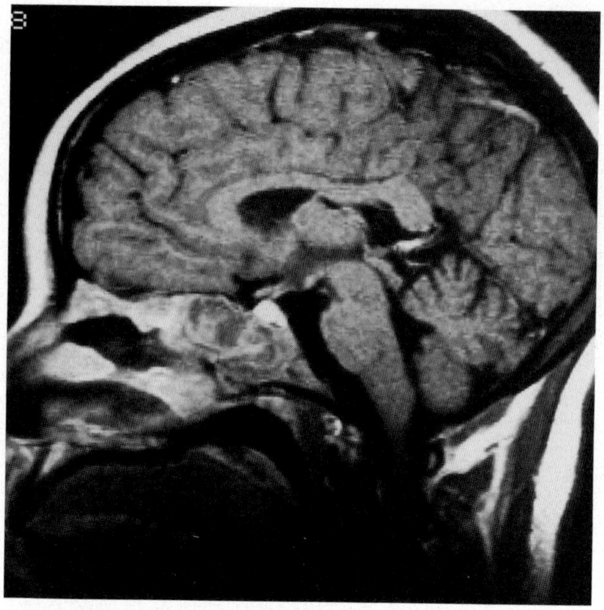

**FIGURE 8** Sphenoid sinusitis. Sagittal contrast-enhanced T1-weighted MRI demonstrates a heterogeneous-appearing mass. The darker areas probably represent desiccated secretions, whereas the areas of enhancement represent inflamed mucosa.

Among regional complications, orbital inflammation (especially subperiosteal abscesses) and osteomyelitis are the most frequently encountered. A complete sinus CT scan usually distinguishes the central low density of a subperiosteal abscess (Fig. 7) from the homogeneous increased density of orbital cellulitis. Thickened bone with patchy, lytic, erosive changes, in association with a soft-tissue mass, is evidence of osteomyelitis. Intracranial complications such as meningitis, subdural and epidural empyemas, abscesses, and venous thromboses require complete brain CT or MRI evaluations with contrast enhancement.

## *Suspected Tumor*

Differentiating inflammatory sinusitis from neoplastic disease may be difficult. If tumor is suspected on a routine screening CT scan, a complete CT study should be performed before the patient leaves the CT suite. If the patient has left the department, the clinician is notified and a follow-up complete study with MRI and/or CT is scheduled.

Contrast-enhanced MRI is the procedure of choice whenever tumor is suspected. MRI offers better differentiation between tumor and retained secretions and is more reliable in determining intracranial and intraorbital extension. Most tumors of the paranasal sinuses have intermediate signal on T1- and T2-weighted images. This distinguishes them from inflammatory processes, which have intermediate signal on T1- but a bright signal on T2-weighted images. This principle also helps distinguish granulation tissue (bright on T2-weighted images) from recurrent or residual disease (intermediate on T2-weighted images). Unfortunately overlap exists. Some tumors, especially adenoid cystic carcinomas and neuromas, have variable signal characteristics. In addition, chronic secretions become increasingly desiccated, which decreases their bright signal character on T2-weighted images, producing an intermediate signal. Contrast-enhanced MRI is beneficial in this instance, because inflamed paranasal sinuses demonstrate heterogeneous enhancement or a peripheral rim of enhancement (Fig. 8), whereas the tumor-containing sinus demonstrates a solid or relatively homogeneously enhancing mass (Fig. 9). The use of fat-suppression techniques may also be beneficial in distinguishing fat-containing marrow spaces from enhancing tumor.

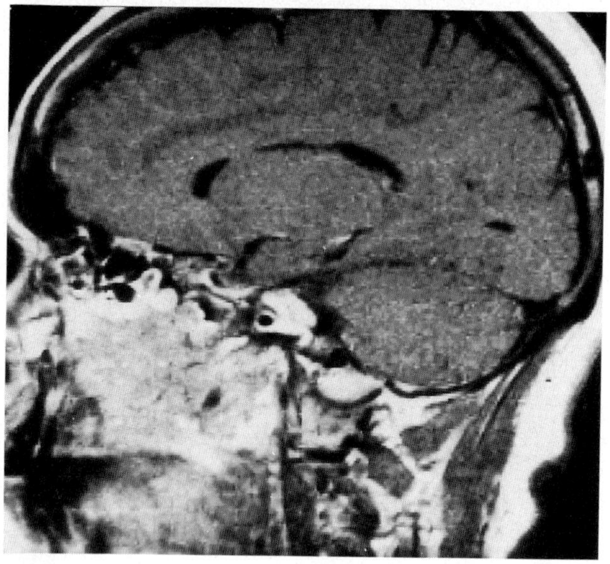

**FIGURE 9** Adenoid cystic carcinoma. Sagittal contrast-enhanced T1-weighted MRI demonstrates a fairly homogeneously enhancing mass, extending to the skull base, highly suggestive of tumor.

Tumor extension and staging is best evaluated with MRI. Tumors of the paranasal sinuses and nasopharynx have a

A

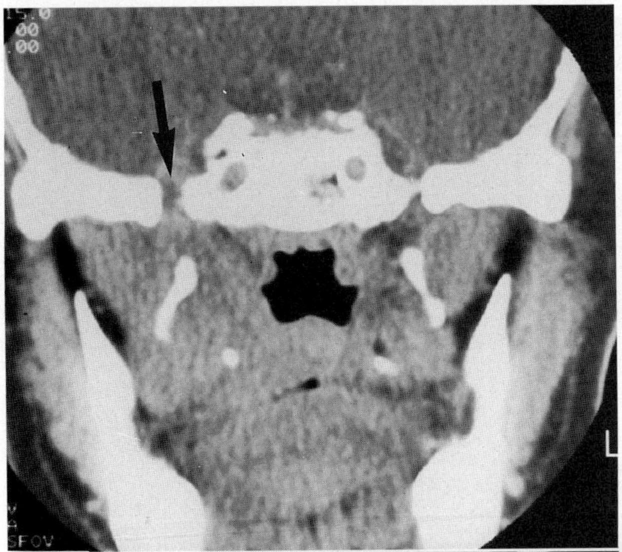

B

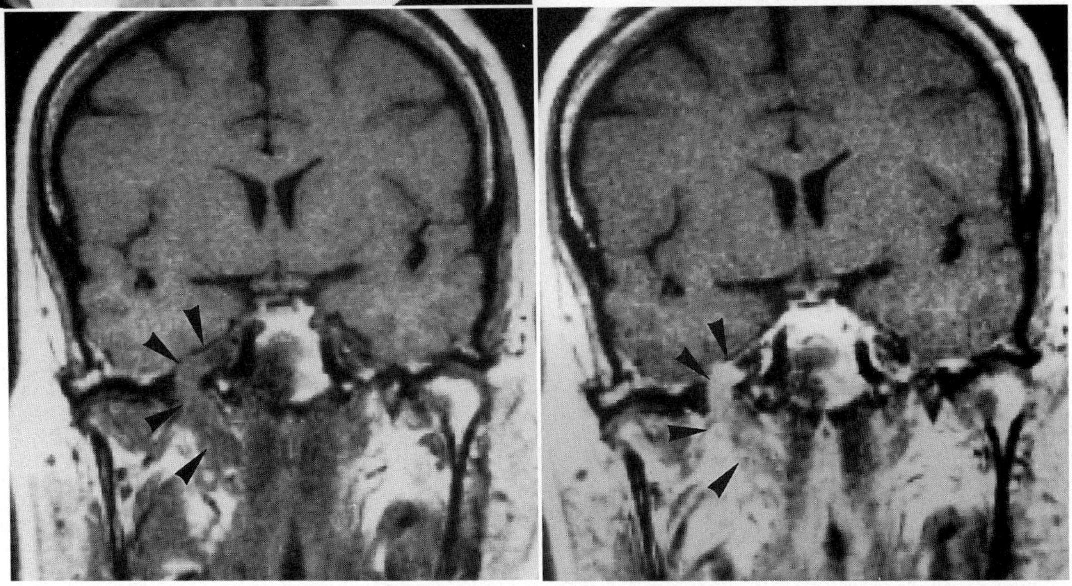

C

**FIGURE 10** Adenoid cystic carcinoma. *A,* Coronal contrast-enhanced CT shows asymmetry of the masticator spaces. The isointense tumor, impossible to distinguish from muscle, produces enlargement of the right masticator space and associated obliteration of normal fat planes. Tumor extent is not readily assessed. The foramen ovale is identified and appears normal (*arrow*). *B,* Non–contrast-enhanced and *C,* contrast-enhanced coronal T1-weighted MRI studies show perineural spread of tumor along the mandibular division of the trigeminal nerve, extending through the foramen ovale into Meckel's cave (*arrowheads*). Note how the addition of contrast helps define tumor at and above the skull base, but obscures tumor margins below the skull base, where it is adjacent to the equally bright signal from fat.

predilection for spreading along vascular and perineural spaces to enter the intracranial compartment through various foramina. MRI has made a significant improvement in detection of these forms of metastases. Non–contrast-enhanced and contrast-enhanced coronal MRI is, in particular, the preferred method of imaging (Fig. 10). MRI has also been shown to be helpful in distinguishing malignant tumor extension from benign inflammatory disease. Inflammatory disease may appear inhomogeneous due to its varying content of water and protein, whereas tumors often appear homogeneous due to their highly cellular composition (Fig. 11).

Although contrast enhancement is required to better evaluate the intracranial extension of tumor, the inherent bright signal of extracranial fat masks tumor enhancement in the extracranial region. Phase-dependent, chemical-shift, fat-suppression techniques are currently used for evaluating extracranial tumor spread. Fat suppression, coupled with contrast enhancement, can readily demonstrate extent of tumor involving the fatty compartments of the head and neck and can also aid in determining marrow involvement and tumor presence in areas adjacent to marrow.

A pitfall in the use of MRI for evaluating paranasal sinus disease is the appearance of a "signal void" within the sinus. Clear sinuses, containing only air, produce no signal and result in a "black sinus" on T1- and T2-weighted images. However, specific disease entities may result in the same appearance: desiccated secretions; fungal sinusitis; acute and/or chronic intrasinus hemorrhage; the presence of bone, calcium, or enamel-containing tumors may all appear as signal voids (black sinuses). Follow-up studies with CT may be helpful in distinguishing among these entities.

## Discussion

The availability of high-resolution CT and MRI, coupled with improvements in endoscopic instrumentation, have led to major changes in the management of sinus disease. An understanding of the normal anatomy, common variations, and specific disease processes is required of all radiologists. In addition, the imaging modalities, with their image idiosyncrasies, involved in evaluating sinus disease must be well understood. Although it is important to have routine imaging

A

B

C

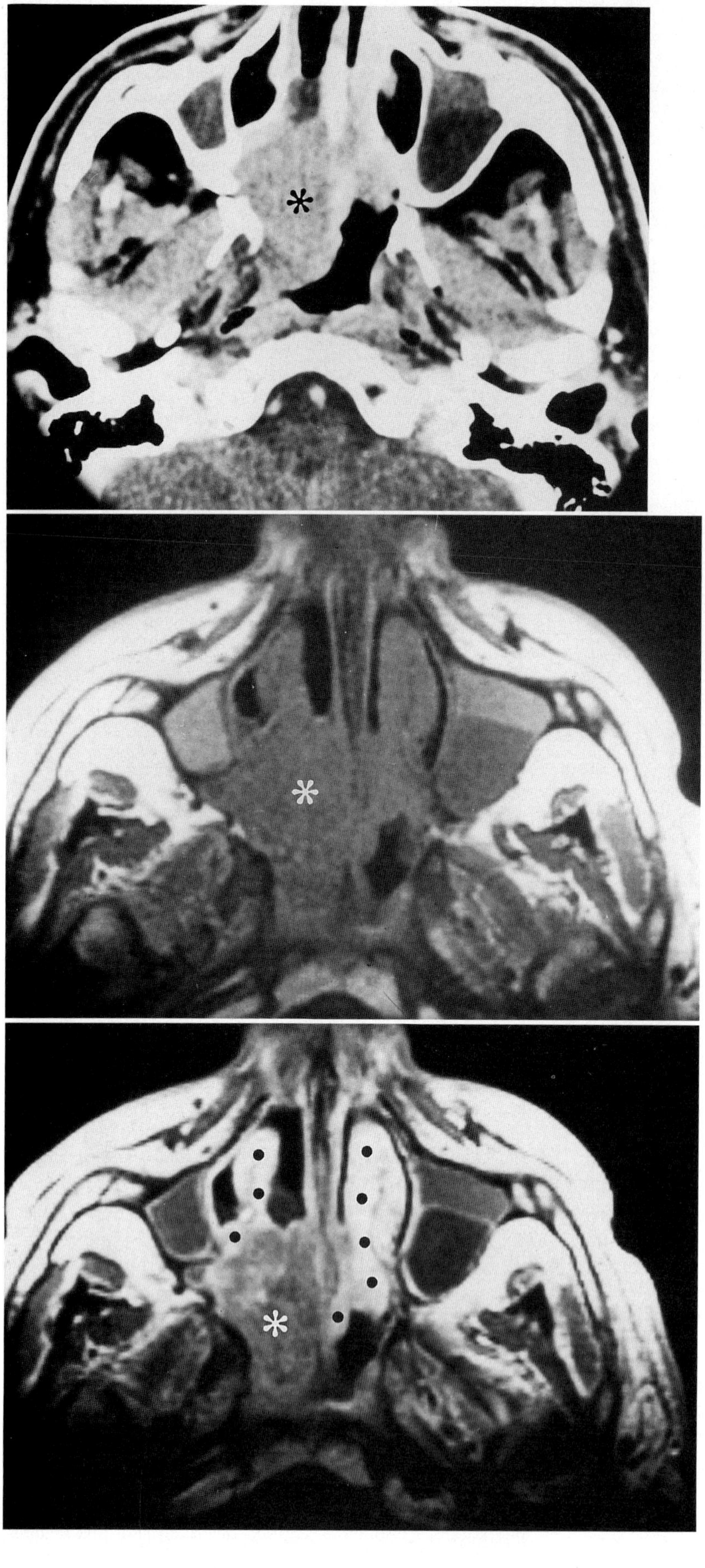

**FIGURE 11** Squamous cell carcinoma. *A,* Contrast-enhanced axial CT scan reveals a homogeneously enhancing mass (*asterisk*) in the nasal passage with destruction of the septum. The OMUs are obstructed bilaterally, and the maxillary sinuses are filled with secretions of various densities. *B,* Non–contrast-enhanced T1-weighted axial MRI demonstrates the homogeneous nature of the neoplastic tissue (*asterisk*). The obstructed sinuses contain secretions with various concentrations of water and protein. Distinction between neoplastic and inflammatory tissue is difficult. *C,* Contrast-enhanced T1-weighted axial MRI shows mild enhancement of the tumor (*asterisk*). The mucous membranes of the nasal passage (*dots*) show diffuse, extensive enhancement that helps define the true extent of the tumor.

protocols in place and understand the advantages and disadvantages of each, it is of paramount importance to maintain continuous dialogue with the referring clinician. In this way specific clinical questions can be answered by modifying protocols and by personal involvement in each case.

## Suggested Reading

Babbel R, Harnsberger HR, Nelson B, et al. Optimization of techniques in screening CT of the sinuses. Am J Neuroradiol 1991; 12:849–854.

Barakos JA, Dillon WP, Chew WM. Orbit, skull base, and pharynx: Contrast-enhanced fat suppression MR imaging. Radiology 1991; 179:191–198.

Laine FJ, Smoker WRK. The ostiomeatal unit and endoscopic sinus surgery: Anatomy, variations, and spectrum of inflammatory disease. AJR 1992; 159:849–857.

Lanzieri CF, Shah M, Krauss D, et al. Use of gadolinium-enhanced MR imaging for differentiating mucoceles from neoplasms in the paranasal sinuses. Radiology 1991; 178:425–428.

Som PM. The sinonasal cavity. In: Som PM, Bergeron RT, eds. Head and Neck Imaging. 2nd ed. St. Louis: Mosby–Year Book, 1991:57.

Som PM, Dillon WP, Curtin HD, et al. Hypointense paranasal sinus foci: Differential diagnosis with MR imaging and relation to CT findings. Radiology 1990; 176:777–781.

Som PM, Dillon WP, Sze G, et al. Benign and malignant sinonasal lesions with intracranial extension: Differentiation with MR imaging. Radiology 1989; 172:763–766.

Som PM, Shapiro MD, Biller HF, et al. Sinonasal tumors and inflammatory tissues: Differentiation with MR imaging. Radiology 1988; 167:803–808.

Tien RD. Fat-suppression MR imaging in neuroradiology: Techniques and clinical application. AJR 1992; 158:369–379.

Zinreich SJ, Kennedy DW, Rosenbaum AE, et al. Paranasal sinuses: CT imaging requirements for endoscopic surgery. Radiology 1987; 163:769–775.

# Correlative Ultrasonography, CT, and MRI of the Thyroid and Parathyroid Glands

*JOSEPH F. SIMEONE, M.D. · MICHAEL J. LEE, M.D.*

## Thyroid Imaging

The superficial location of the thyroid gland lends itself to easy scrutiny with high-resolution real-time sonography (Fig. 1). Normal thyroid anatomy and pathologic conditions can be demonstrated with remarkable clarity. High-resolution computed tomography (CT) and magnetic resonance imaging (MRI) may also be used for thyroid imaging but usually in a secondary role or to view lesions located in the mediastinum.

Sonography has come to play an increasingly prominent role in the diagnostic evaluation of thyroid disease.

### *Indications and Clinical Utility*

Thyroid disease may present either as focal nodular abnormalities or as diffuse thyroid disease. Women more commonly have thyroid nodules than men. Approximately 4 to 7 percent of the adult population in the United States has palpable thyroid nodules. In the population of patients exposed to radiation, 20 to 30 percent develop palpable nodules.

Thyroid cancer is rare and accounts for less than 1 percent of all malignant neoplasms. Therefore the overwhelming number of patients with thyroid nodules will have benign disease. In fact, much nodular disease of the thyroid is nonpalpable and is detected only by various imaging techniques.

Benign thyroid nodules include dilated follicles, dilated follicles with inspissated colloid (Fig. 2), and adenomatous nodules. These three pathologic entities probably result from cyclical changes within the thyroid gland. Hemorrhage or necrosis occurs frequently within these nodules, resulting in commonly observed cystic lesions (Fig. 3).

A true thyroid neoplasm is the benign follicular adenoma (Fig. 3). These adenomas are characterized histologically by complete fibrous encapsulation. Various histologic subtypes of benign adenomas are recognized.

There are four types of primary thyroid cancer: papillary, follicular, medullary, and anaplastic (Figs. 4 to 6). Papillary carcinoma is the most common, accounting for 75 to 90 percent of all cases. Follicular carcinoma is the second most common. Medullary carcinoma accounts for only approximately 5 percent of disease. Anaplastic carcinoma is a disease of the elderly, and is the most lethal tumor, but is rare.

All nodular entities, both benign and malignant, may be detected by palpation. However, most nodules are under 1.5 cm, and, if the morphology of the gland is not deformed, can be detected only by imaging, usually with high-resolution real-time sonography.

CT scanning of the neck is used to detect pathology deep within the neck or in the superior mediastinum. It is particularly useful in patients with scarring within the neck or multiple operations, making palpation and ultrasonographic examinations particularly difficult.

### *Technical Approach*

Almost all thyroid disease can be diagnosed solely with ultrasonography. Transducers of 7.5 to 10 MHz have theoretical resolution of 1 mm, a degree of spatial resolution unmatched by any other imaging technology. Linear array transducers are preferred to sector transducers because of the wide field of view (see Fig. 1).

The thyroid gland is evaluated with the patient's neck extended. Multiple images in both the longitudinal and transverse plane are obtained. If the inferior pole of the thyroid gland extends below the clavicles, this region may be visualized by asking the patient to swallow. The isthmus should be identified in the midline (see Fig. 1). Lymphadenopathy in the thyroid bed, and most particularly lateral to the great vessels, should be searched for (Fig. 7). A common practice in our

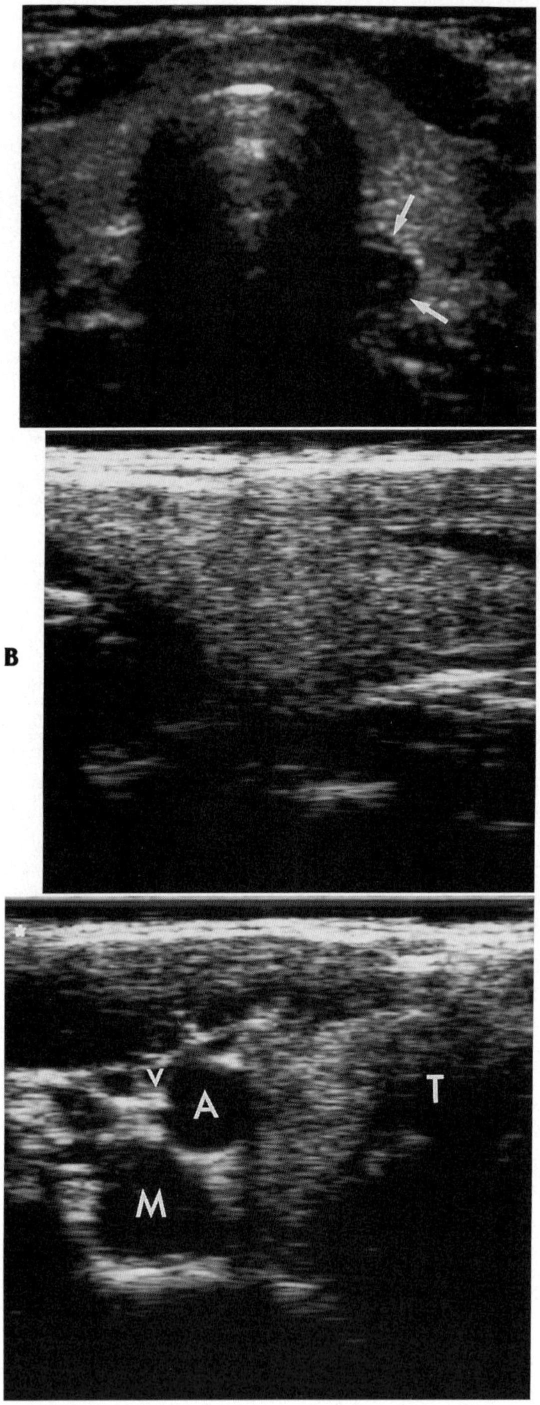


**FIGURE 1** *A,* Transverse view of the entire thyroid gland. A wide-view 5 MHz linear array transducer allows the entire thyroid gland to be visualized. Note that the anterior strap muscles are hypoechoic relative to the more echogenic thyroid tissue. The isthmus is observed just anterior to the trachea, which shows a classic reverberation artifact. Note that the esophagus *(arrows)* is just to the left of the trachea posteriorly. *B,* Sagittal view of one lobe of the thyroid demonstrates homogeneous echogenicity throughout. The muscles are only slightly more hypoechoic in this patient than the thyroid gland itself. *C,* Transverse view demonstrates the trachea (T) medially and carotid artery (A) and jugular vein (V) laterally. The longis colli muscle (M) is a posterior hypoechoic structure, and the strap muscles are anterior.

A

B

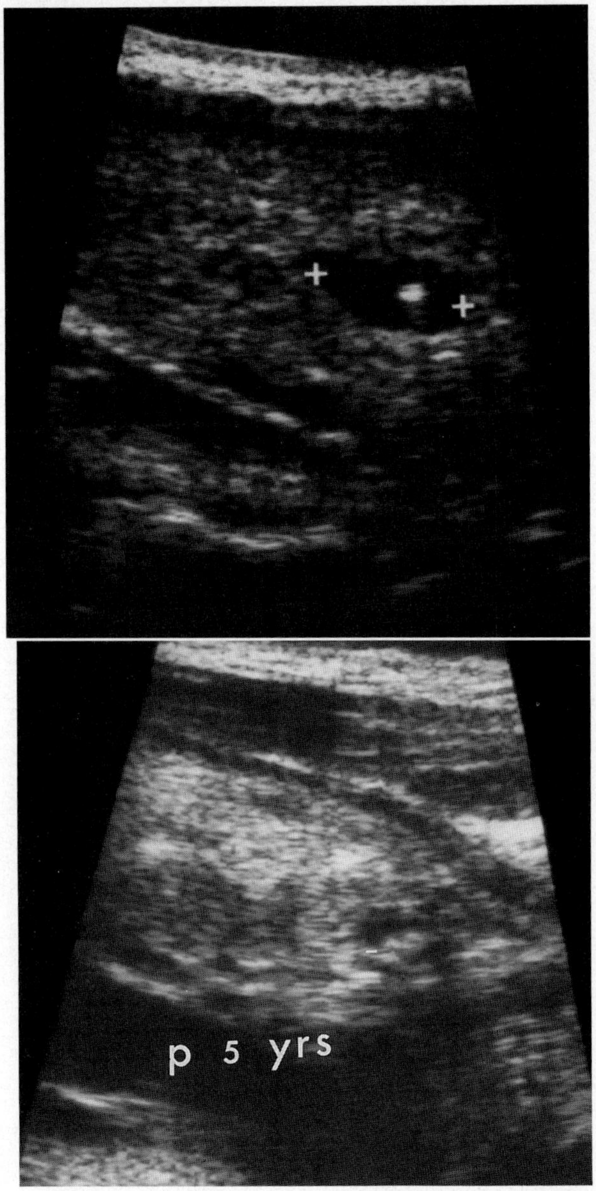


**FIGURE 2** *A,* On a routine thyroid ultrasonographic examination performed in 1987, a dilated follicle (+ +) is demonstrated as an oval-shaped, cystic, completely hypoechoic structure in an otherwise normal thyroid gland. The echogenic point with some posterior acoustical shadowing is inspissated colloid within the dilated follicle. *B,* In 1992 the patient returned for re-examination. The dilated follicle with inspissated colloid has disappeared. The gland is now inhomogeneous, probably indicating the formation of adenomatous nodules.

A

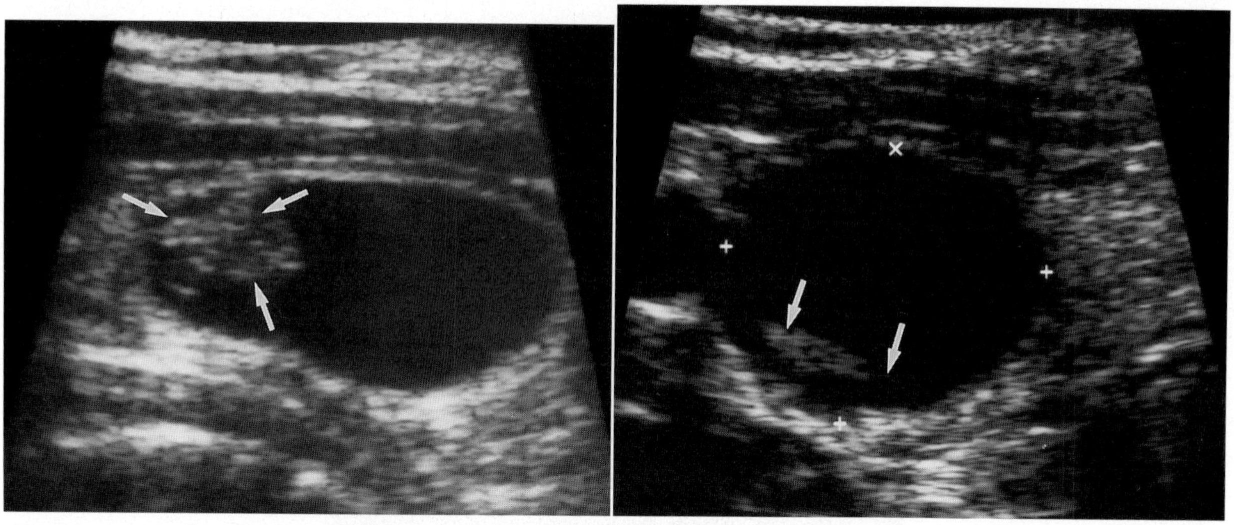

B

**FIGURE 3** *A,* In a patient with a cold nodule by radionuclide scan, ultrasonography demonstrates a 4 cm pear-shaped nodule that is mostly a cyst. The solid irregularly shaped structure in the superior aspect of the nodule is a typical follicular adenoma *(arrows).* The overall appearance is that of a follicular adenoma that has undergone cystic degeneration. *B,* Two years later the patient returned with a large neck mass. The previously observed nodule has greatly expanded and deforms the anterior tissues ( + + ). A fluid level *(arrows)* is observed in the dependent portion of the nodule, indicating recent hemorrhage within this nodule.

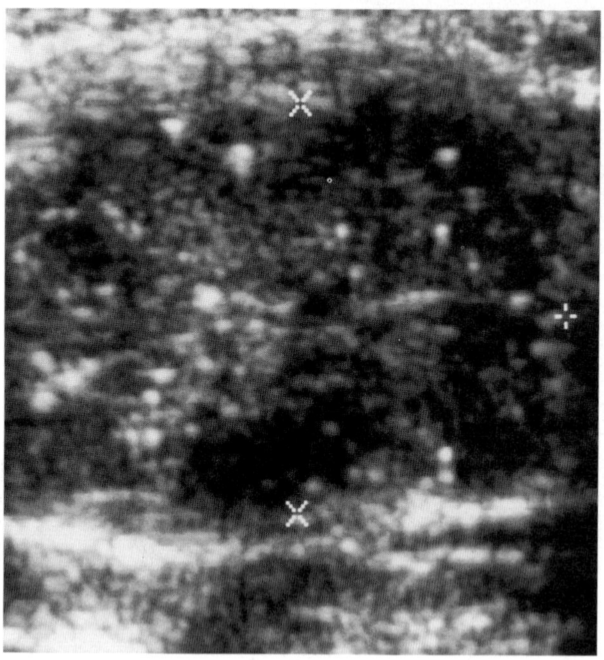

**FIGURE 4** Papillary carcinoma of the thyroid. A solid inhomogeneous mass that contains numerous calcifications proved to be psammomatous calcification at the time of surgery in a patient with papillary carcinoma of the thyroid.

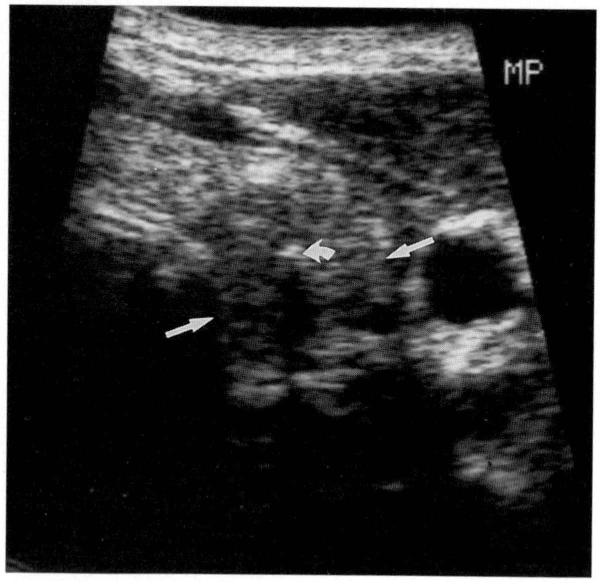


**FIGURE 5** Papillary carcinoma of the thyroid. Solid hypoechoic mass *(straight arrow)* contains a central nidus *(curved arrow)* of calcification. This lesion was stable over 4 years, without growth or change.

A

B

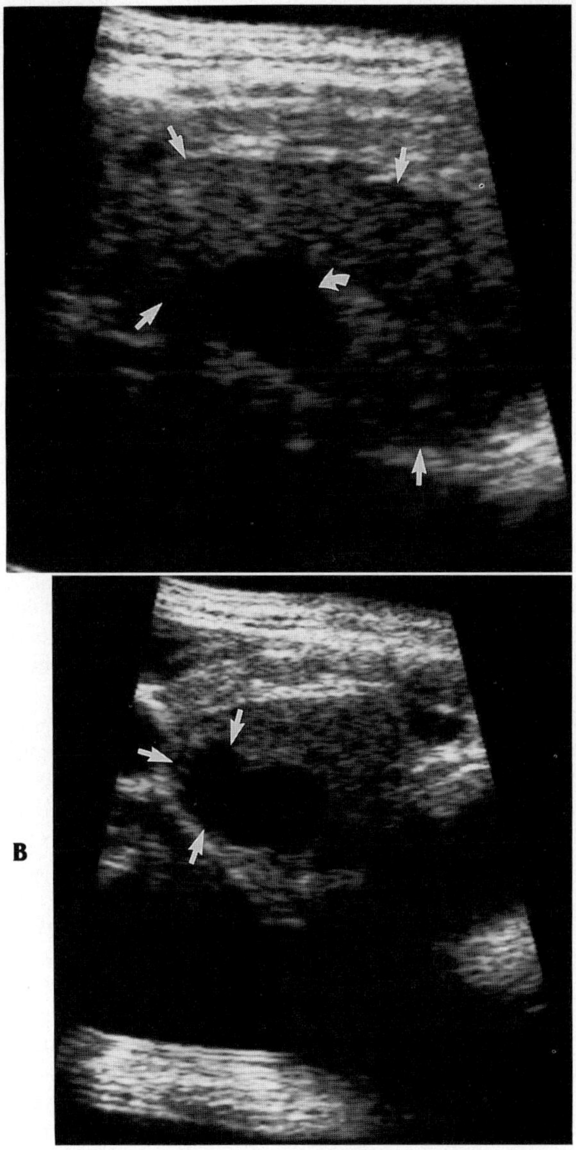

**FIGURE 6** *A,* Difficulty in detecting primary thyroid carcinoma. Longitudinal view of the gland reveals a large hypoechoic mass measuring almost 4 cm *(straight arrows).* The central portion of the mass is necrotic, with a hypoechoic center *(curved arrow). B,* At the time of surgery, only a 5 mm papillary carcinoma was observed. The rest of the thyroid mass was benign. The hypoechoic and solid area *(arrows)* was the nidus of carcinoma.

A

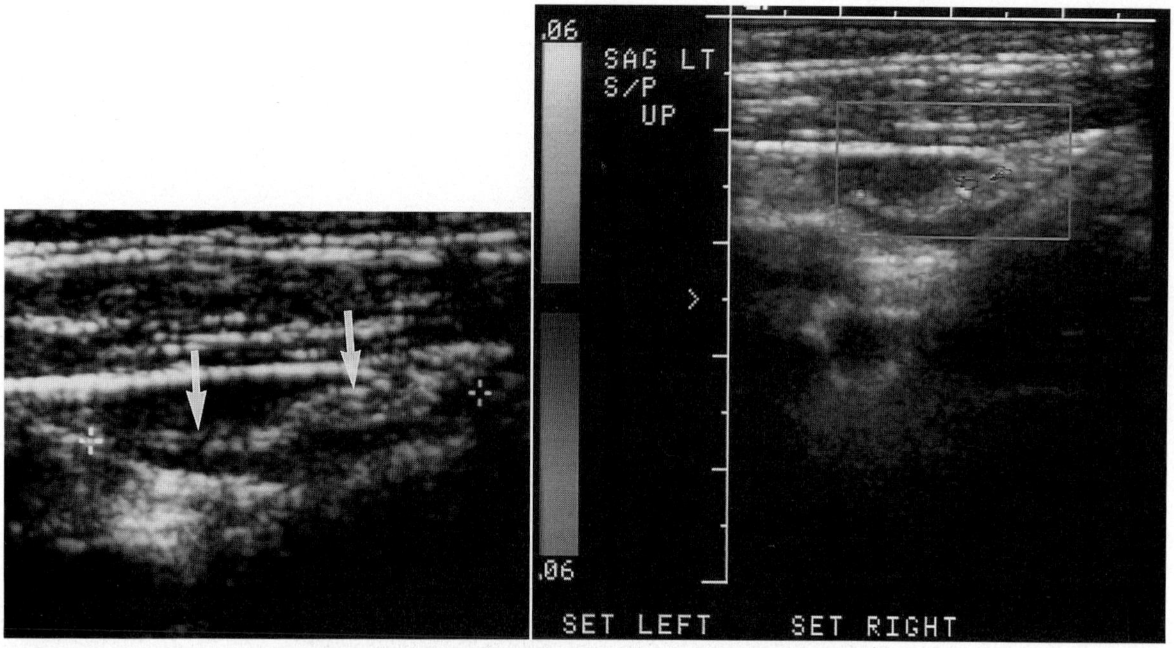


B

**FIGURE 7** *A,* Appearance of a normal lymph node. A normal lymph node is distinguished by its predominantly longitudinal (rather than spherical) shape. The linear echogenic line *(arrows)* represents the hilum of the node, which contains feeding vessels and lymph channels. *B,* Color-flow Doppler *(reproduced in black and white)* confirms the presence of a normal blood vessel in the central echogenic area. This linear structure is usually the first area to be invaded by metastatic disease within the lymph node.

institution is to construct a hand-drawn diagram of the neck including the trachea and carotid and jugular vessels, indicating where individual nodules are detected. This schematic is most helpful in the postoperative thyroid patient in clearly identifying the precise location of nodes in the thyroid bed.

Contrast agents are rarely used in ultrasonography for imaging. CT scanning can be helpful in the neck but is limited by bony artifact off the shoulder and clavicles and by lower resolution. To date MRI, although able to detect pathology in this region, provides no more additional information than ultrasonography and CT for thyroid disease.

## Diagnostic Approach

The clinical workup of the thyroid nodule hinges on close communication between the referring clinician and a subsequent effort, if desired, to determine the benignity or malignancy of a detected nodule.

Fine-needle aspiration biopsy (FNAB) is the most effective way of diagnosing malignancy in a thyroid nodule. In our practice palpable nodules are biopsied by endocrinologists as an outpatient procedure. Nonpalpable nodules are biopsied under ultrasonographic guidance. FNAB is generally the first technique used for diagnostic workup of a thyroid nodule, because of the direct information it provides about the histology of the nodule. When performed with the guidance of a physician experienced in performing needle aspiration, and a cytopathologist whose main interest is that of thyroid disease, FNAB provides a safe, inexpensive way of separating benign from malignant thyroid nodules. The patient's proper selection for surgery also is enhanced. Ultrasonographic guidance not only can help in nodules that are nonpalpable but in palpable nodules, which have a large cystic component from which only fluid is aspirated. In this situation ultrasonography can be used to obtain tissue from the solid part of a nodule, an area frequently missed by FNAB under palpation (Figs. 8 and 9).

Direct sonographic applications to thyroid disease include (1) detection of thyroid masses and adenopathy related to thyroid masses before and after neck exploration, (2) differentiation of benign from malignant masses on the basis of their sonographic appearance, and (3) guidance for aspiration. The most common use of sonography in our practice is evaluation of the postoperative neck after partial or near-total thyroidectomy. Recurrent diseases in the thyroid bed lower the patient's life expectancy, even in papillary carcinoma. Early detection of these masses leads to early diagnosis by biopsy and subsequent surgical excision. The patients in our practice are followed routinely with postoperative ultrasonography following thyroid excision for malignancy on a 6 to 12 month basis. Sonography has proved to be more sensitive than physical examination in detecting recurrent disease within the thyroid bed or metastatic disease in cervical lymph nodes.

There is no single feature or combination of sonographic features that distinguishes benign from malignant masses. A well-defined margin with a thin complete halo and hyperechogenicity are found most frequently in benign nodules. Poorly defined margins with an incomplete halo and fine internal calcification in a hypoechoic mass tend to lean toward malignancy. FNAB or close follow-up is mandatory if thyroid malignancy is suspected.

### Diffuse Thyroid Disease

Diffuse thyroid disease that results in thyroid enlargement includes Hashimoto's thyroiditis, colloid or adenomatous

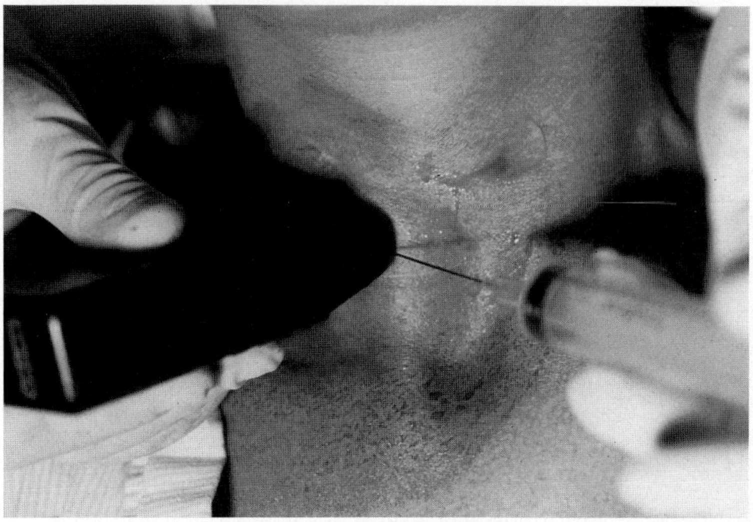

**FIGURE 8** Ultrasound-guided biopsy technique. The two-hand technique is demonstrated. One hand holds the transducer. The second hand introduces the needle. Direct visualization of needle entering the skin: subcutaneous tissue and the thyroid gland and lesion can then be visualized under real-time guidance on the ultrasound monitor.

A

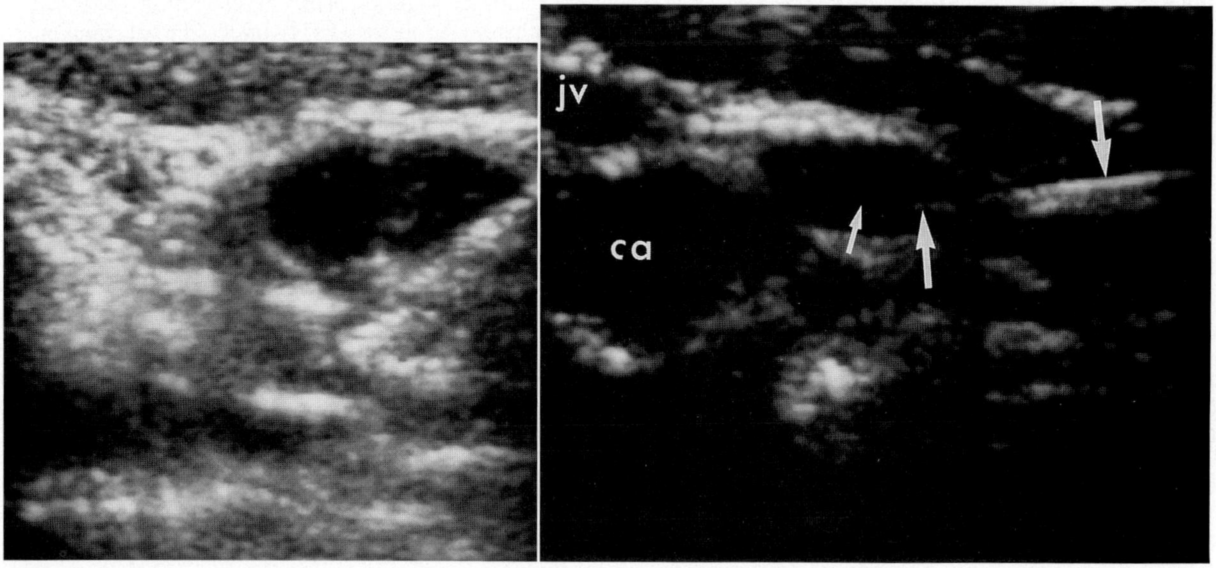


B

**FIGURE 9** *A,* Recurrent carcinoma of the thyroid. A homogeneous lymph node is found in the thyroid bed. Note the absence of the central echogenic stripe. *B,* A needle *(arrows)* was placed into the lymph node. Cytologic study revealed recurrent medullary thyroid carcinoma. (CA = carotid artery; JV = jugular vein)

goiter (Fig. 10), and Graves' disease. In these conditions sonography is usually not indicated, because diagnosis may be made by physical examination, laboratory values, and aspiration biopsy. Although an adenomatous goiter can generally be recognized clinically, diffuse non-nodular neck enlargement tends to fool inexperienced clinicians. In this category of disease, our laboratory generally makes the most useful contribution to patient care when patients are referred by an inexperienced clinician for evaluation of a neck mass. The appearance of the thyroid gland as a diffusely enlarged hypoechoic non-nodular mass is characteristic for Hashimoto's thyroiditis. These findings are generally communicated to the clinician and can lead to the proper referral to an endocrinologist for proper treatment of the thyroiditis. Our experienced endocrinologists use sonography to follow the progress of thyroiditis to ensure that (1) the thyroid gland has returned to normal size and (2) that no nonpalpable nodular densities are occurring, which may indicate an early carcinoma.

## Parathyroid Imaging

Although radionuclide scanning, sonography, CT scanning, and MRI are available in the evaluation and treatment of patients with hyperparathyroidism, in our practice ultrasonography is the first technique used to search for enlarged parathyroid glands (Table 1). Radionuclide scanning with technetium/thallium subtraction studies is used secondarily. CT scanning and MRI have a tertiary role, mostly in undiagnosed complicated patients and reoperated patients. Sonography may also be used for percutaneous biopsy, particularly when persistent or recurrent hyperparathyroidism is present. Some centers have used sonography intraopera-

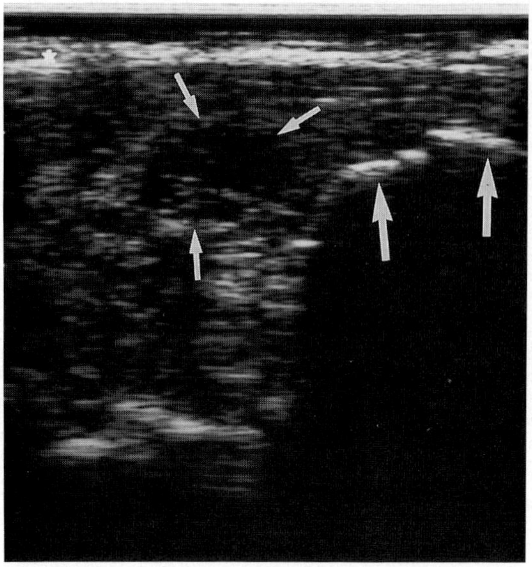

**FIGURE 10** Appearance of multinodular goiter. The thyroid gland has an increased anteroposterior diameter. Numerous calcifications are observed within the gland *(thick arrows).* Cystic and solid areas *(thin arrows)* are observed lateral to the calcification, giving an overall inhomogeneous appearance, typical appearance for a multinodular goiter.

**TABLE 1** Steps in the Detection of a Parathyroid Mass

| |
|---|
| Clinical examination (serum calcium and parathormone levels) |
| Ultrasonography |
| Technetium/thallium subtraction study |
| CT scan |
| Surgical exploration |
| Angiography |
| MRI |

tively for detection of parathyroids, but we have been asked only once to attempt to find a parathyroid in the operating room. Patients who are too sick for surgery may have parathyroid ablation with ethanol under ultrasonographic guidance.

## Indications and Clinical Utility

Technetium/thallium subtraction studies are highly accurate, easier to perform than ultrasonography, and highly sensitive and specific in detecting parathyroid neoplasms. Because they are slightly more expensive than ultrasonographic studies, and because of the high level of ultrasound experience at our institution, sonography is used first. However, if the ultrasonograph examination is equivocal or nondiagnostic, Technetium/thallium subtraction study for detection of parathyroid neoplasm is a preferred second choice. CT scanning is used if these two examinations are nondiagnostic. MRI is used only for the most complicated patients with nondiagnostic studies. Our surgeons prefer to explore the neck, rather than perform angiography in looking for parathyroid neoplasms.

## Technical Approach

Scanning of the neck is performed similar to evaluation of the thyroid gland. Because parathyroids are located at the upper and lower pole of the gland, and 70 percent of parathyroid neoplasms are found at the lower pole, these regions must be evaluated more carefully. Parathyroid glands may be found as cephalad as the submandibular gland and as caudad as near the carina. Ultrasonography may detect these lesions from the submandibular gland to the superior mediastinum. However, if bony structures interfere, CT or radionuclide scanning is recommended. High-frequency real-time linear array transducers (7.5 to 10.0 MHz) are used to examine patients with a hyperextended neck. In thick necks or in patients with a large multinodular thyroid gland, a lower-frequency transducer may be required.

## Diagnostic Approach

The diagnosis of hyperparathyroidism is made on the basis of an increased serum calcium level and an increased serum parathyroid hormone (PTH) level. Clinical symptoms most commonly associated with hyperparathyroidism are nephrolithiasis, osteopenia, muscle weakness, and dyspepsia. However, many patients with biochemical hyperparathyroidism are asymptomatic.

Primary hyperparathyroidism is caused by a single adenoma in 80 to 90 percent of patients, by parathyroid hyperplasia in 10 to 20 percent of patients, and by carcinoma in fewer than 1 percent of patients. An enlarged parathyroid gland is usually oval, hypoechoic, and homogeneous. Usually the internal architecture of the parathyroid neoplasm is solid but occasional cystic degeneration may be present. The neoplasms may vary in size from 0.6 to 5 cm and in weight from 0.5 to 10 g.

Since all parathyroid neoplasms have the same appearance, it is frequently difficult to distinguish an adenoma (Fig. 11) from hyperplasia (Fig. 12) or carcinoma. However, some signs can be helpful. The presence of more than one enlarged gland almost always indicates hyperplasia. There can be a single dominant nodule in hyperplasia, but all regions of the neck should be evaluated to see if other similar-sized or smaller glands are present bilaterally. If two or more glands are found and recognized as being enlarged, the diagnosis is almost unequivocally hyperplasia. The diagnosis of multiple adenomas has never been made in our hospital but is found in the literature.

Parathyroid carcinoma is extremely rare, but the diagnosis can be made when a single hypoechoic homogeneous nodule is present in the neck and is accompanied by an abnormal number of lymph nodes, either ipsilaterally or contralaterally. These lymph nodes do not have the typical elongated shape observed in benign nodes but are oval or round and can be located either within the thyroid bed or peripherally adjacent to the carotid vessels.

Pitfalls in technique and interpretation arise when parathyroid neoplasms occur in the mediastinum (Fig. 13) or in atypical locations. Retrotracheal adenomas are found deep in the neck posterior or posterolateral to the trachea. This is an ideal location for CT diagnosis, and we always refer patients for CT if ultrasonography is not successful in detecting parathyroid neoplasm. Frequently ultrasonography finds adenomas in the superior mediastinum, but CT may be necessary if ultrasonog-

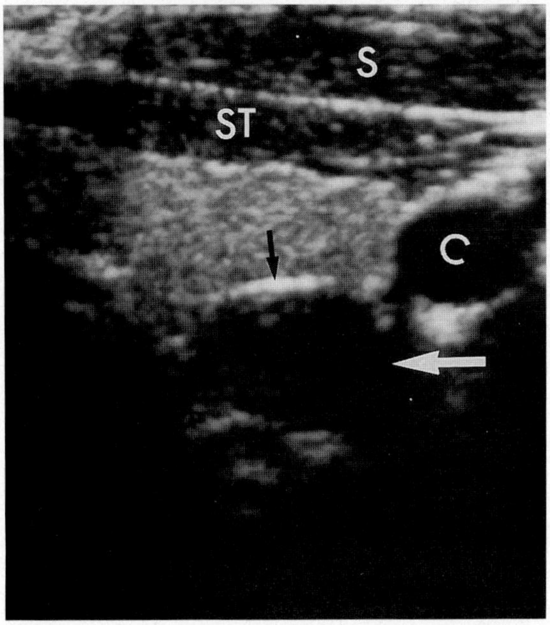


**FIGURE 11** Typical appearance of parathyroid neoplasm. On this transverse view, the carotid artery (C) and thyroid gland are normal. Posterior to the thyroid gland is a solid hypoechoic nodule in a typical location for a parathyroid neoplasm. A linear echogenic line *(black arrow)* anterior to the parathyroid gland is the aponeurotic sheath frequently observed. (S = sternocleidomastoid muscle; ST = strap muscle)

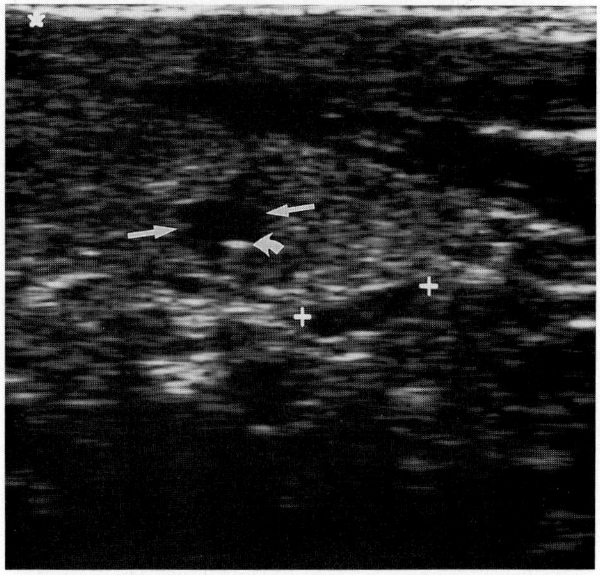

**FIGURE 12** Parathyroid hyperplasia in patient with renal transplant. The calipers denote a 7 × 2 mm hypoechoic homogeneous structure posterior to the thyroid gland, which represents a slightly enlarged parathyroid in a patient with parathyroid hyperplasia. Incidentally noted is a dilated follicle *(arrows)* containing inspissated colloid within the thyroid gland itself.

raphy cannot make a specific diagnosis. Decreased transducer frequency (5 MHz) is usually helpful in seeing deep into the mediastinum. Intrathyroidal parathyroid adenomas can frequently be missed, because they mimic thyroid nodules. They also can be missed at the time of surgery, because they are soft and therefore nonpalpable. Percutaneous biopsy may be required to differentiate an intrathyroid parathyroid adenoma from a thyroid nodule.

Careful ultrasonographic evaluation of the neck detects parathyroid neoplasms located in the carotid sheath or high within the neck. However, these areas must be evaluated carefully and meticulously when the parathyroid neoplasm is not found in a conventional location.

False-positive diagnosis of parathyroid neoplasm may be made by failure to recognize perithyroid veins, the esophagus, and longus colli muscles. Color Doppler sonography can recognize veins. Asking the patient to swallow during the examination identifies the esophagus as well as its typical location slightly left to the midline and posterior to the left thyroid lobe. The longus colli muscle can be recognized because of its characteristic anatomic appearance and location just anterior to the cervical vertebral bodies.

Thyroid nodules and cervical lymph nodes may also mimic parathyroid neoplasms. Parathyroid neoplasm can be differentiated from a thyroid nodule when the aponeurotic sheath is seen separating the parathyroid from the thyroid as a thin white echogenic line. This sheath is not present around thyroid nodules. Cervical lymph nodes have a characteristic appearance by ultrasonography manifested as a central echogenic line, which is the hilum of the node and composed of fat, vessels, and fibrous tissue. Lymph nodes also have a

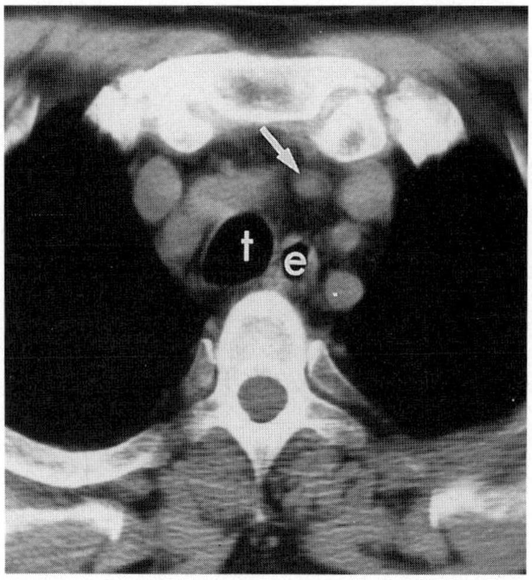


**FIGURE 13** CT scan detects parathyroid neoplasm. CT scanning is particularly helpful in finding ectopic or aberrant parathyroids within the mediastinum. This lesion was not detected by ultrasonography or radionuclide scan. CT scan shows the parathyroid *(arrow)* within the mediastinal fat anteriorly. (T = trachea; E = esophagus)

more elongated appearance, although this is not always a reliable sign.

False-negative evaluations result from ectopic adenomas, in the clinical setting of an enlarged thyroid gland, and when the parathyroid neoplasms are too small to detect.

## Suggested Reading

Hay ID. Thyroiditis: A clinical update. Mayo Clin Proc 1985; 60:836–843.

James EM, Charboneau JW. High-frequency (10 MHz) thyroid ultrasonography. Semin Ultrasound CT MR 1985; 6:294–309.

James EM, Charboneau JW, Hay ID. The thyroid. In: Rumack C, Wilson S, Charboneau JW, eds. Diagnostic Ultrasound. Vol 1. St. Louis: Mosby–Year Book, 1991:507.

Reading CC. The parathyroid. In: Rumack C, Wilson S, Charboneau JW, eds. Diagnostic Ultrasound. Vol 1. St. Louis: Mosby–Year Book, 1991:524.

Reading CC, Charboneau JW, James EM, et al. High-resolution parathyroid sonography. AJR 1982; 139:539–546.

Reading CC, Charboneau JW, James EM, et al. Postoperative parathyroid high-frequency sonography: Evaluation of persistent or recurrent hyperparathyroidism. AJR 1985; 144:399–402.

Simeone JF, Daniels GH, Hall DA, et al. Sonography in the follow-up of 100 patients with thyroid carcinoma. AJR 1987; 148:45–49.

Simeone JF, Daniels GH, Mueller PR, et al. High-resolution real-time sonography of the thyroid. Radiology 1982; 145:431–435.

Simeone JF, Mueller PR, Ferrucci JT Jr, et al. High-resolution real-time sonography of the parathyroid. Radiology 1981; 141: 745–751.

Solbiata L, Volterrani L, Rizzatto G, et al. The thyroid gland with low uptake lesions: Evaluation by ultrasound. Radiology 1985; 155: 187–191.

Sutton RT, Reading CC, Charboneau JW, et al. US-guided biopsy of neck masses in postoperative management of patients with thyroid cancer. Radiology 1988; 168:769–772.

# PEDIATRIC RADIOLOGY

## Emergency Radiology of the Pediatric Chest

*BENNETT A. ALFORD, M.D. · JOAN McILHENNY, M.D.*

Chest pathology constitutes one of the most frequent problems in infants and young children seen in an emergency department. Correct interpretation of plain chest radiographs may answer all pertinent diagnostic questions. On occasion other imaging modalities must supplement the information obtained from plain films. Rapid, accurate assessment of images may be lifesaving and requires an orderly approach based on radiographic features. Correlation of radiographic findings with age, sex, and clinical presentation allows the most accurate diagnosis to be made.

### Technique

#### *Plain Film of the Chest in Infants and Children*

Infants and children too young to cooperate for upright posteroanterior (PA) and lateral chest radiographs are filmed in the anteroposterior (AP) supine position. Lateral radiographs are obtained in the supine cross-table lateral position. Immobilization is usually needed to assure a well-positioned, motion-free film. Children are not forced to cry in an attempt to obtain "good inspiratory films"; rather they are encouraged to be calm and to stop crying in order to obtain an exposure at their basal respiratory rate, which more accurately reflects normal or pathologic lung volumes.

#### *Fluoroscopy and Decubitus Films*

Subtle findings such as focal air trapping, pneumothoraces, or pleural fluid may be verified with fluoroscopy or additional views.

To evaluate for focal air trapping as observed following aspiration of a foreign body into a bronchus, we prefer fluoroscopy over decubitus views or forced expiratory films. We find fluoroscopy extremely sensitive in demonstrating focal areas of air trapping, and the results can be recorded on videotape for review. Decubitus films or forced expiratory views are more dependent on positioning and are considered back-up techniques. When looking for a suspected pneumothorax, lateral decubitus views obtained with the side in question positioned up are preferable to cross-table lateral films. Conversely, when looking for a suspected pleural fluid collection, the lateral decubitus view is obtained, and the side in question is positioned down.

#### *Contrast Esophagography*

A contrast esophagram may be necessary to document aspiration or to suggest an etiology such as tracheoesophageal fistula. The esophagram can document tracheal compression from extrinsic causes, such as a vascular anomaly or a foreign body lodged in the esophagus. The lateral projection should be obtained first and is the most important in almost all emergency conditions that require esophagography, because the trachea and esophagus are clearly distinguished.

#### *Computed Tomography*

Computed tomography (CT) of the chest may be indicated in a few emergency situations in children. Trauma with suspected vascular injury usually occurs in older children, and dynamic, enhanced CT or aortography may be necessary. If the chest radiograph is not clearly normal, but the index of suspicion for aortic injury is low, CT is usually performed. Other cases usually require aortography, because CT may not detect a small contained aortic rupture. Mediastinal masses causing respiratory compromise may necessitate an enhanced CT scan before surgery, irradiation therapy, or chemotherapy. Great care should be taken with children who have large mediastinal masses as a cause of respiratory compromise. Sedation or supine positioning for a CT evaluation may exacerbate airway obstruction and lead to respiratory arrest.

### Ultrasonography

Ultrasonography should be performed when the chest radiograph shows an enlarged, totally opaque hemithorax to quickly detect pleural fluid, cardiac enlargement, or a mass. Decubitus films offer no help when the hemithorax is completely opaque.

### Skeletal Survey

If nonaccidental trauma or child abuse is suspected from the history or from fractures detected on the initial chest film, a complete skeletal abuse survey must be obtained. Finding rib fractures, especially in various stages of healing, strongly suggests child abuse. Rib fractures in children are unusual, except in the setting of child abuse. Posterior rib fractures are uncommon even in children with bone abnormalities, such as osteogenesis imperfecta, or in children who have received cardiopulmonary resuscitation. The complete survey includes well-exposed, high-detail AP and lateral films of the skull, spine, and thorax, and AP films of the abdomen and long bones.

## Specific Radiographic Classifications and Diseases

Reliable classification according to radiographic appearances is essential to establish a specific diagnosis in children who present with emergency chest problems. We find it helpful to divide radiographic findings into the following classes:

1. Diffuse aeration abnormalities
2. Parenchymal densities
    Focal
    Diffuse
3. Large cardiothymic silhouette
4. Asymmetry, often signifying the need for intervention
    Large opaque hemithorax
    Large lucent hemithorax
    Large cystic hemithorax

### Diffuse Aeration Abnormalities

Sometimes a disorder appears in more than one radiographic group, because it can produce more than one radiographic pattern. *Mycoplasma* infection, for example, may present several different radiographic pictures.

Diffuse obstructive airways disease is probably the most frequent nontraumatic reason for obtaining chest radiographs in children. The radiographic features of diffuse obstructive airways disease are essentially identical regardless of the underlying cause. Reactive airways disease and viral (or nonbacterial) infection are the two most likely etiologies. For this reason, clinical correlation is essential and usually establishes the correct diagnosis.

The chest radiographs in children with diffuse obstructive airways disease almost always have bilateral changes, even if there is asymmetric involvement of the two lungs. Generalized hyperinflation with low flat diaphragms is the rule, and the lungs may otherwise be clear. Bronchial wall thickening or peribronchial cuffing may present, often giving a "dirty" or indistinct appearance to the perihilar areas. Streaky or patchy densities are present in the lungs and represent areas of subsegmental atelectasis. Frank lobar or segmental atelectasis also occurs (Figs. 1 to 3).

Diffuse obstructive airways disease caused by nonbacterial infection is often from respiratory syncytial virus, but may also be a result of many other agents including other viruses, *Chlamydia,* and *Mycoplasma.* Bacterial disease, on the other hand, usually causes unilateral findings without significant generalized aeration disturbance.

A

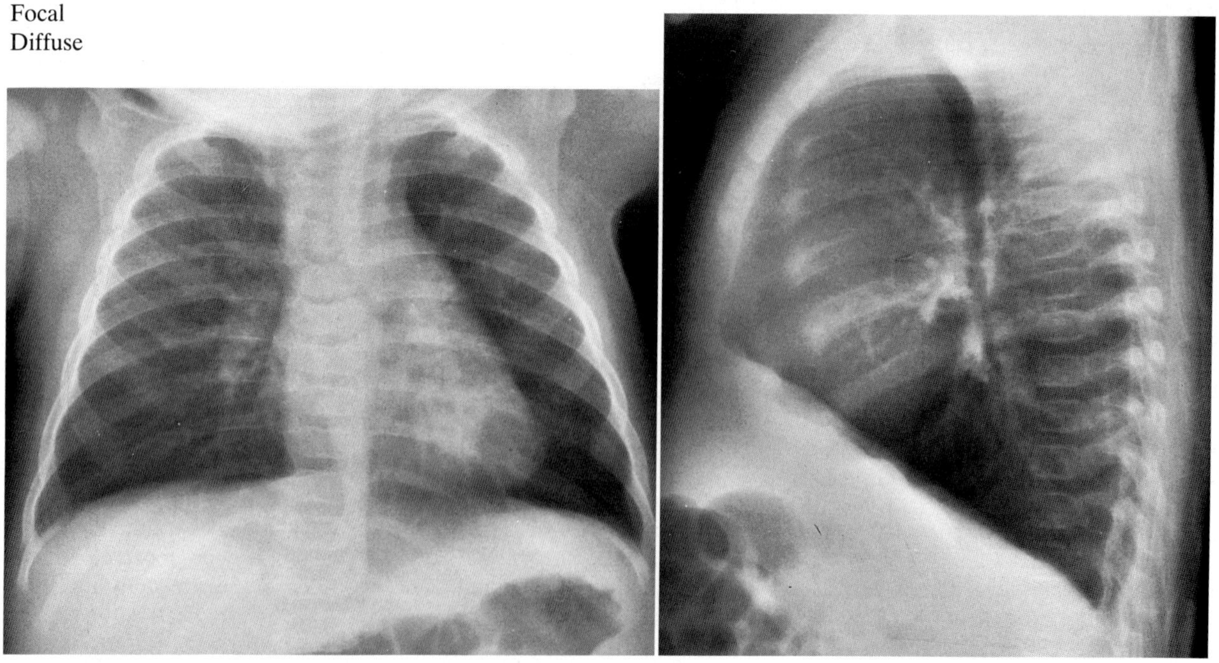

B

**FIGURE 1** *A* and *B,* Bronchiolitis. The lungs are hyperinflated, and there is subsegmental atelectasis at the left base on the frontal view.

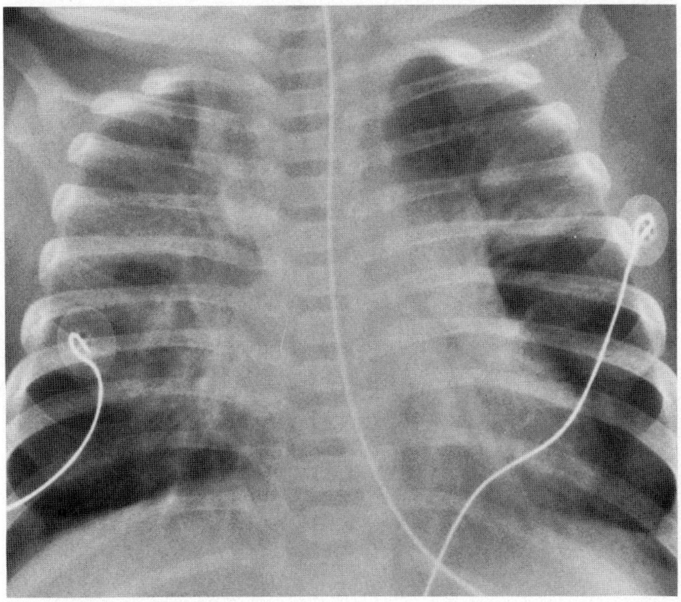

**FIGURE 2** Respiratory syncytial virus infection. The lungs are hyperinflated with patchy areas of atelectasis.

Acute problems are usually caused by nonbacterial infection or reactive airways disease. Radiographic evidence for recurrent diffuse obstructive airways disease suggests the possibility of an underlying problem, such as cystic fibrosis or an immunologic deficiency.

Occasionally it may be difficult to distinguish findings of diffuse obstructive airways disease from those observed in cardiac disease. Hilar prominence, bronchial cuffing, perihilar streaky densities, and overinflation may mimic findings observed in cardiac disease, such as significant left-to-right shunts (Fig. 4). Finding a heart of normal size on both the AP and lateral views and recognizing diffuse focal atelectatic areas in children with airways disease usually serve to differentiate the two. However, children with heart disease become infected with nonbacterial agents or may have reactive airways disease, and consequently their radiographs are difficult to interpret.

Acute or chronic aspiration may also produce radiographs similar to those observed in diffuse obstructive airways disease and should be considered in the differential diagnosis.

### Focal Aeration Abnormalities

See the section on Asymmetric Findings That Often Signify the Need for Urgent Intervention.

### Focal Parenchymal Densities

When lung volumes are otherwise normal, atelectasis of an entire lobe or lung signifies a solitary obstructing lesion. Foreign body aspiration, bronchial neoplasm, mucous plug, and a malpositioned endotracheal tube represent frequent intrabronchial causes (Fig. 5). Bronchial neoplasm is a much less common cause of lobar collapse in children. An abnormality of the bronchus itself is more likely if the right upper or right middle lobe is atelectatic. Extrinsic compression of a bronchus is a less frequent cause of complete lobar collapse, but left lower lobe or left lung collapse can occur due to compression by an enlarged left atrium in children with heart disease (Fig. 6).

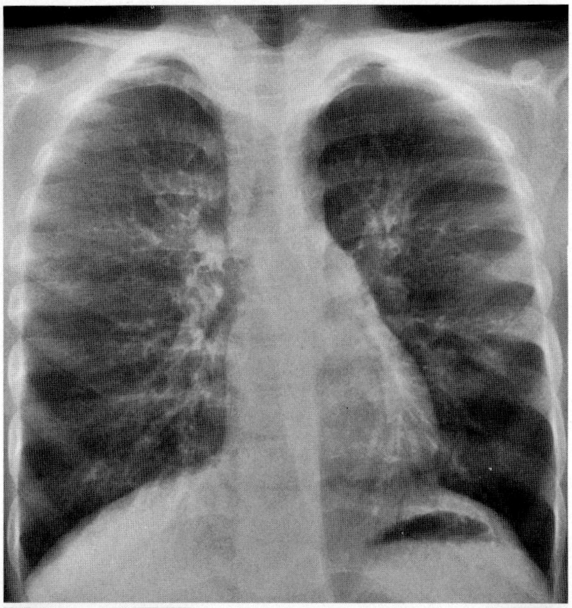

A

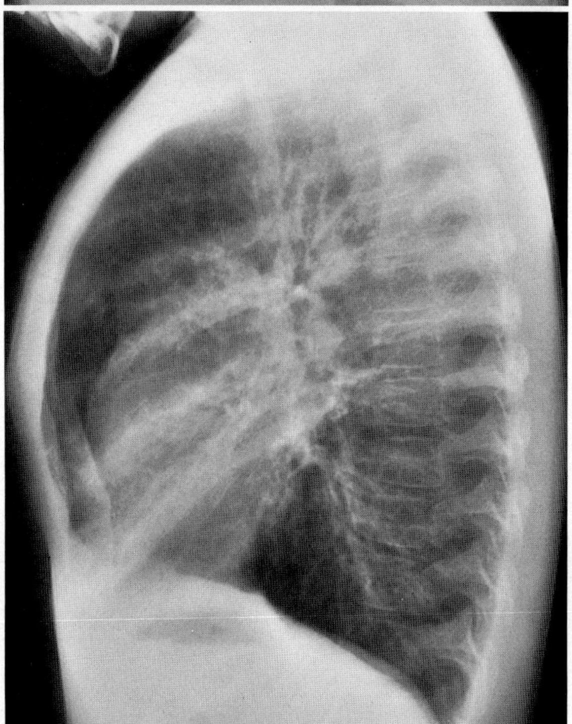

B

**FIGURE 3** *A* and *B,* Asthma. In reactive airways disease, the lungs are usually hyperinflated. There is peribronchial cuffing.

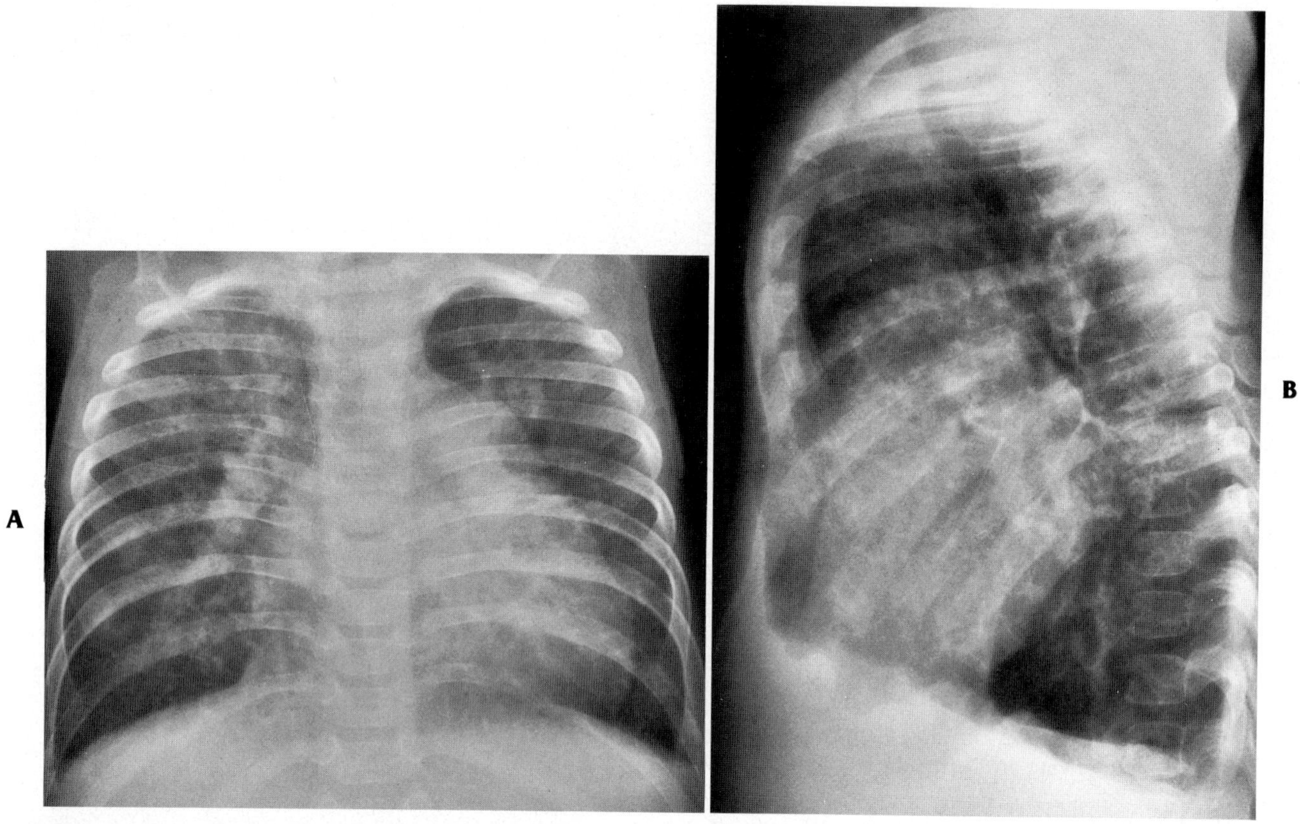

**FIGURE 4** *A* and *B*, Cardiac disease mimicking reactive airways disease. This child had a ventricular septal defect and a large left-to-right shunt. Notice that the heart is enlarged on both the frontal and lateral views.

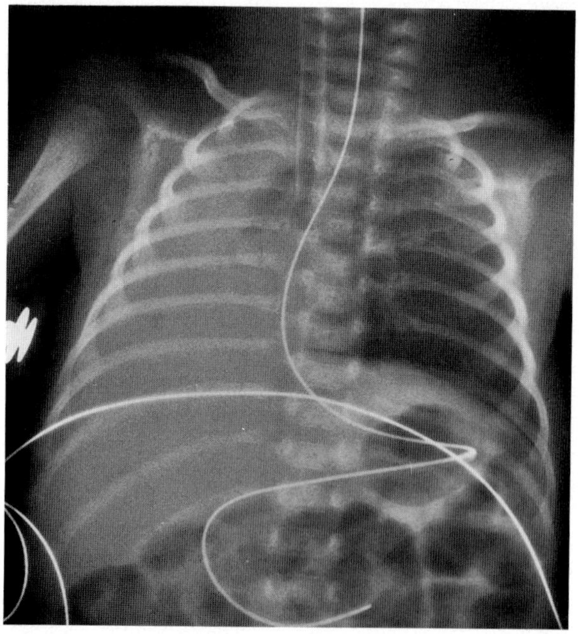

**FIGURE 5** Right lung atelectasis due to bronchial occlusion by a malpositioned endotracheal tube.

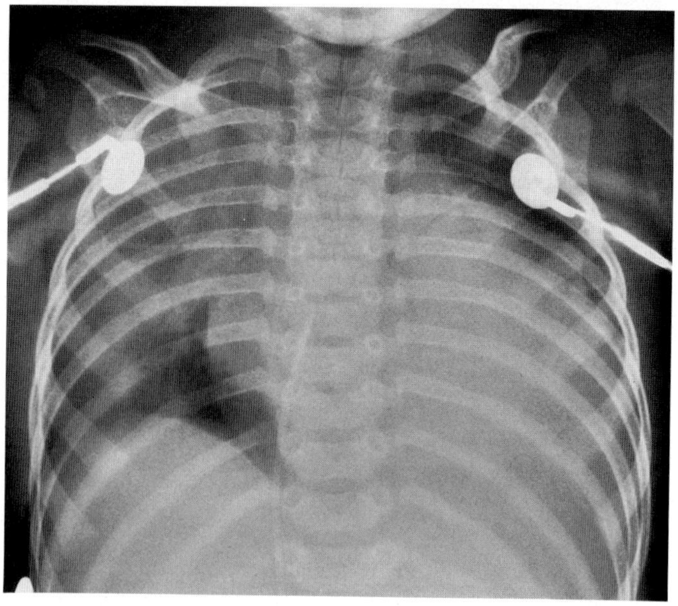

**FIGURE 6** Left lower lobe atelectasis due to cardiomegaly and compression of the left mainstem bronchus by the left atrium. The left side of the hemidiaphragm is silhouetted out by the enlarged heart and the collapsed left lower lobe. This baby had a cardiomyopathy.

**FIGURE 7** *A* and *B,* Left lower lobe bacterial pneumonia with normal lung volumes. Note the segmental distribution of the density.

A

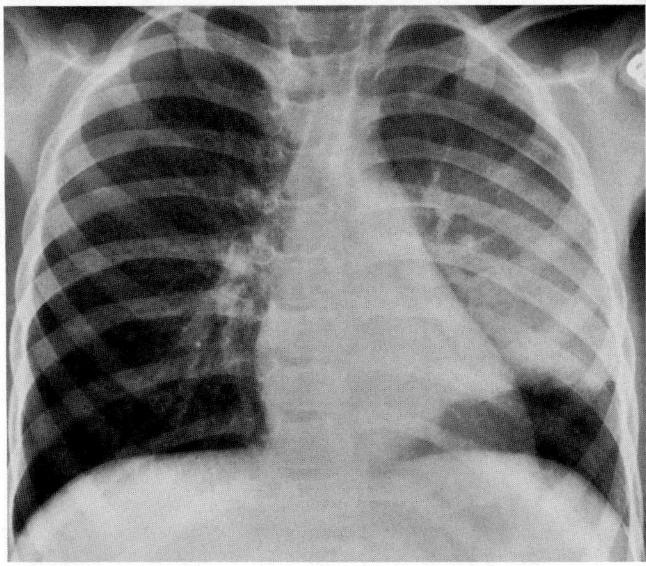

B

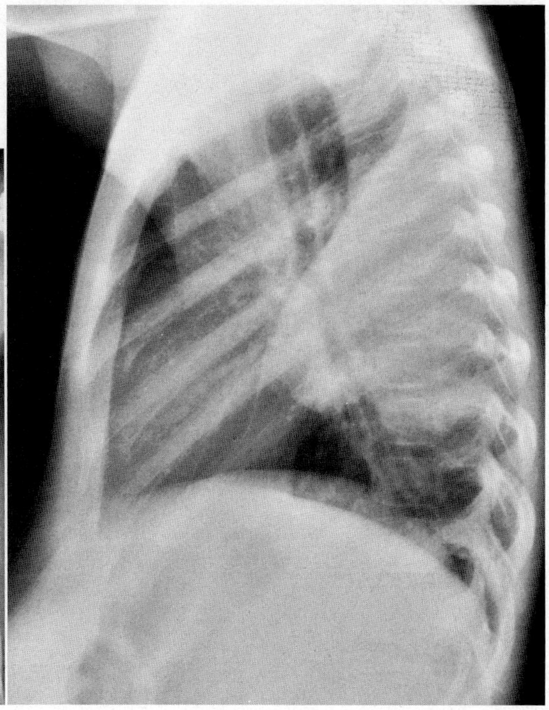

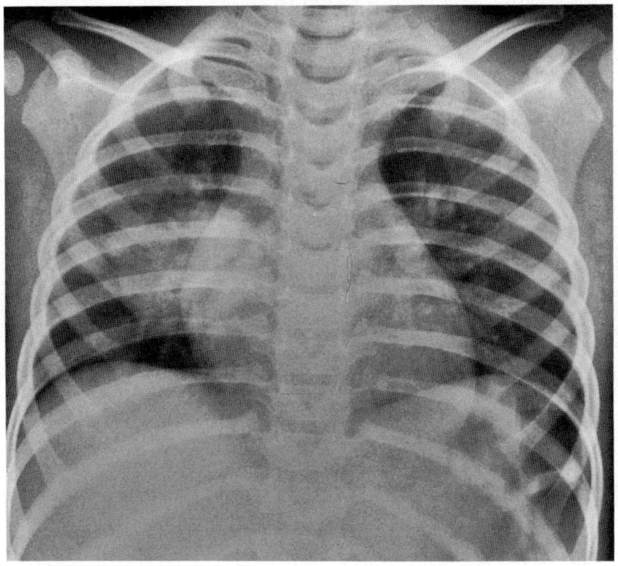

**FIGURE 8** Round masslike pneumococcal pneumonia in the right lower lobe.

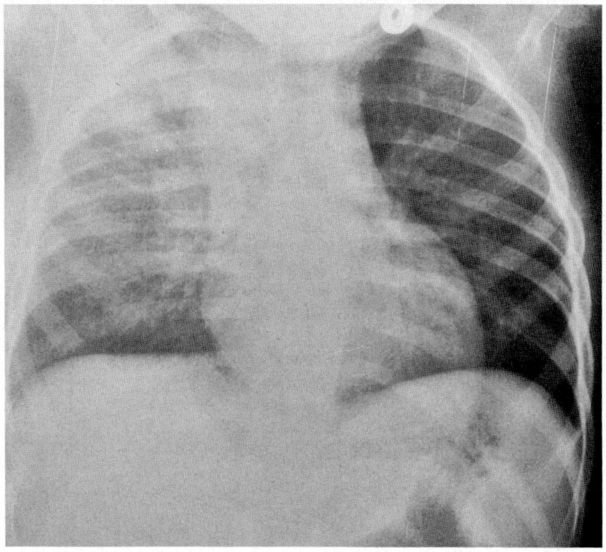

**FIGURE 9** Primary tuberculosis with right-sided paratracheal and hilar adenopathy and a right upper lobe infiltrate. There is deviation of the trachea to the left.

Lobar or segmental consolidation usually indicates infection, contusion, or infarction in children. Bacterial pneumonia usually causes focal consolidation with normal lung volumes (Fig. 7). Nonbacterial lower respiratory pathogens, except *Mycoplasma,* generally cause bilateral findings. Bacterial pneumonia usually produces radiographic density that follows lobar or segmental boundaries. The densities may be spherical, having the appearance of a pulmonary or mediastinal mass in the early stages of the disease (Fig. 8). Ipsilateral pleural fluid, occasionally in large amounts, may accompany bacterial pneumonia. A large pleural collection usually indicates staphylococcal disease in infants (see Fig. 19, *A*) or pneumococcal disease in older children, but pleural fluid occurs in other infections as well. The presence of unilateral hilar or mediastinal adenopathy, together with an area of consolidation, strongly suggests tuberculosis or a fungus such as *Histoplasma* as an etiology (Fig. 9).

Pulmonary contusion produces a focal density that may cross segmental or lobar boundaries (Fig. 10). Rib fractures may be detected in the area surrounding the contused lung. Pleural fluid representing hemorrhage may accompany contusion, as may pneumothorax. Occasionally a pneumatocele develops after trauma, but unlike postinfectious pneumatoceles, which have a delayed presentation, it appears soon after the traumatic event.

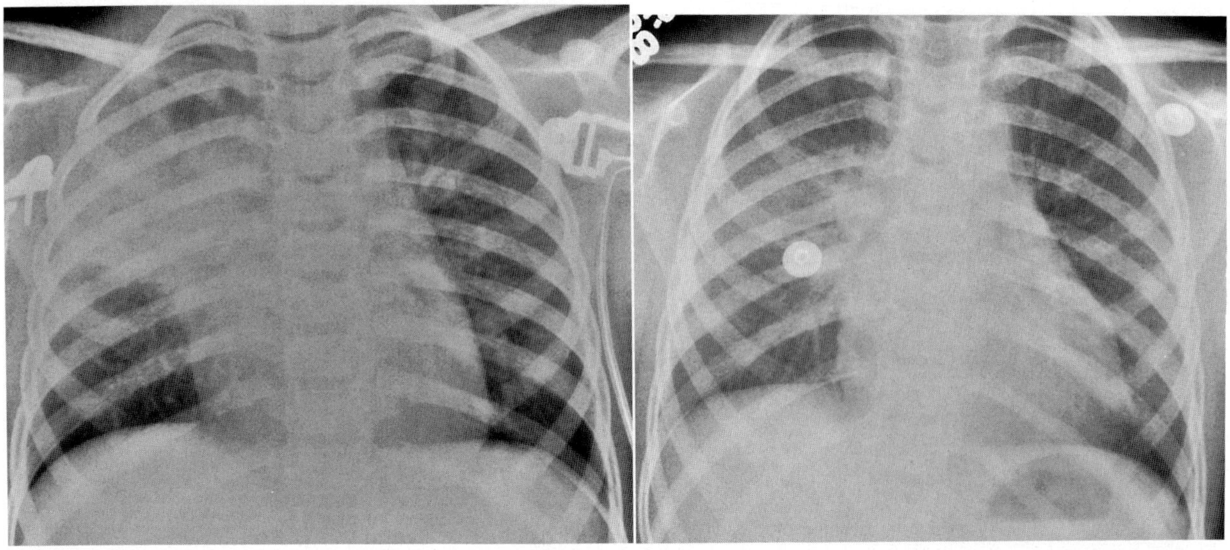


**FIGURE 10** *A* and *B*, Right lung contusion in a young child who was in a motor vehicle accident. There is significant radiographic clearing within 48 hours.

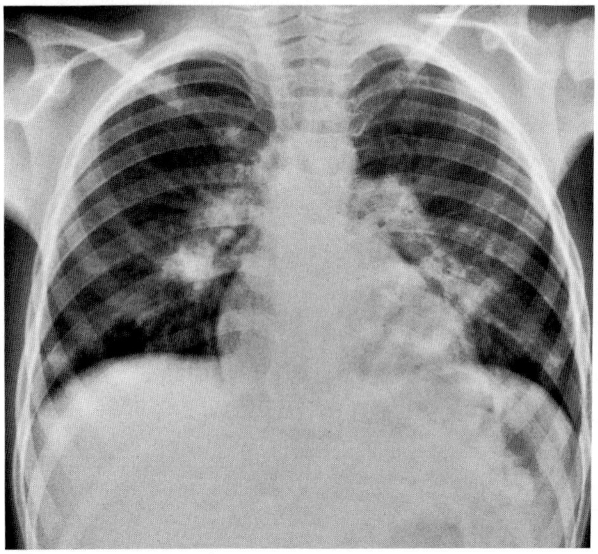

**FIGURE 11** *Mycoplasma* pneumonia with patchy airspace filling.

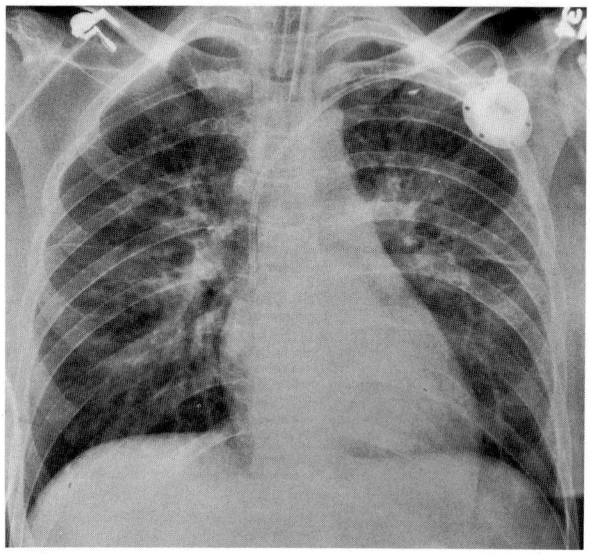

**FIGURE 12** Reticular pattern in an acutely ill immunosuppressed child with leukemia and *Pneumocystis carinii* pneumonitis.

Pulmonary infarction is unusual in children other than those with sickle cell disease.

## *Diffuse Bilateral Densities*

Patchy, irregular, or fluffy densities with normal or only slightly altered lung volumes usually indicate airspace filling. The alveoli may be filled with pus, edema, fluid, aspirated fluid, or blood. Bacterial infection with agents such as staphylococci or *Haemophilus influenzae* is a cause of an airspace filling pattern. *Mycoplasma* is the most frequent nonbacterial cause (Fig. 11). Aspiration may produce patchy bilateral densities. Other, less common, causes include fungal infections, pulmonary hemosiderosis at the time of pulmonary hemorrhage, and allergic reactions.

A reticular or reticulonodular pattern indicates interstitial disease. The list of differential considerations for interstitial disease is long, but can be shortened for practical purposes in an emergency setting. Most acutely ill children with this pattern have a lower respiratory infection caused by a virus or *Mycoplasma.* Early *Pneumocystis carinii* pneumonia may have the same appearance in an immunocompromised child (Fig. 12). Pulmonary edema is the next most likely cause of a reticular pattern, and may frequently be noncardiogenic from causes such as glomerulonephritis or fluid overload (Fig. 13). Edema and cardiomegaly in an acutely ill child suggest a cardiac cause such as myocarditis.

Diffuse hazy opacification in acutely ill children frequently indicates infection with agents such as a virus, *Mycoplasma,* or *Pneumocystis* (Fig. 14). Pulmonary edema, either cardiac or noncardiac in origin, drowning, shock lung or adult respiratory distress syndrome (Fig. 15), and lymphoid interstitial pneu-

A

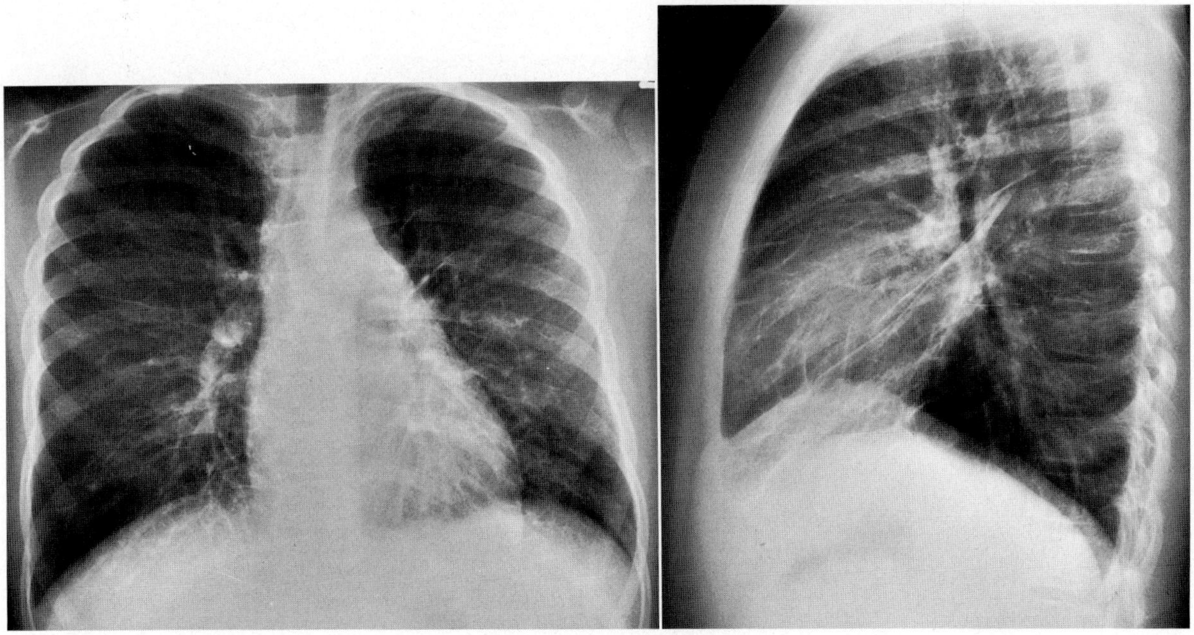

B

**FIGURE 13** *A* and *B,* Interstitial edema in a child with poststreptococcal glomerulonephritis.

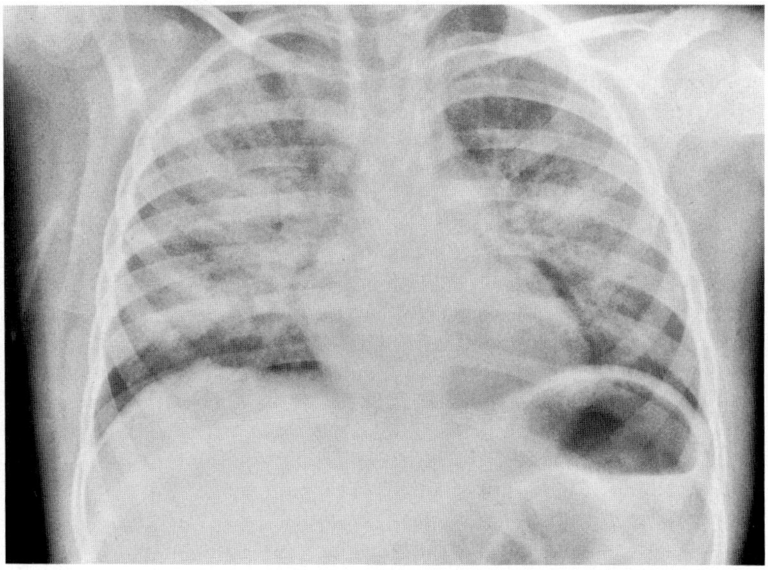

**FIGURE 14** *Pneumocystis carinii* pneumonia in an immunosuppressed child with leukemia.

A

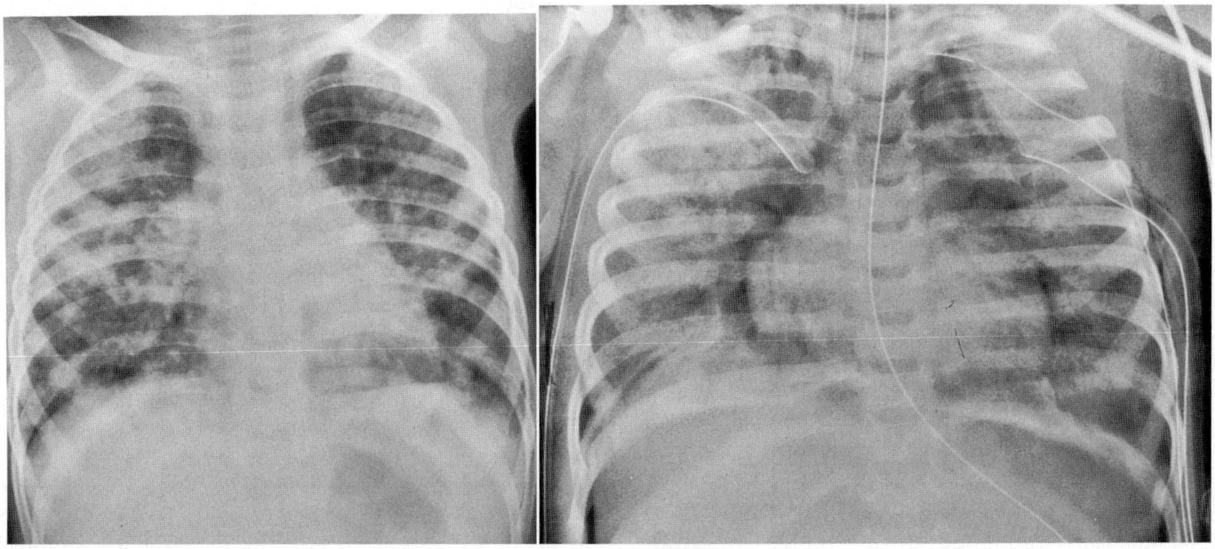

B

**FIGURE 15** *A* and *B,* Adult respiratory distress syndrome in a 3-year-old boy with pneumonia. The diffuse infiltrates rapidly progressed, and he developed a pneumomediastinum and bilateral pneumothoraces.

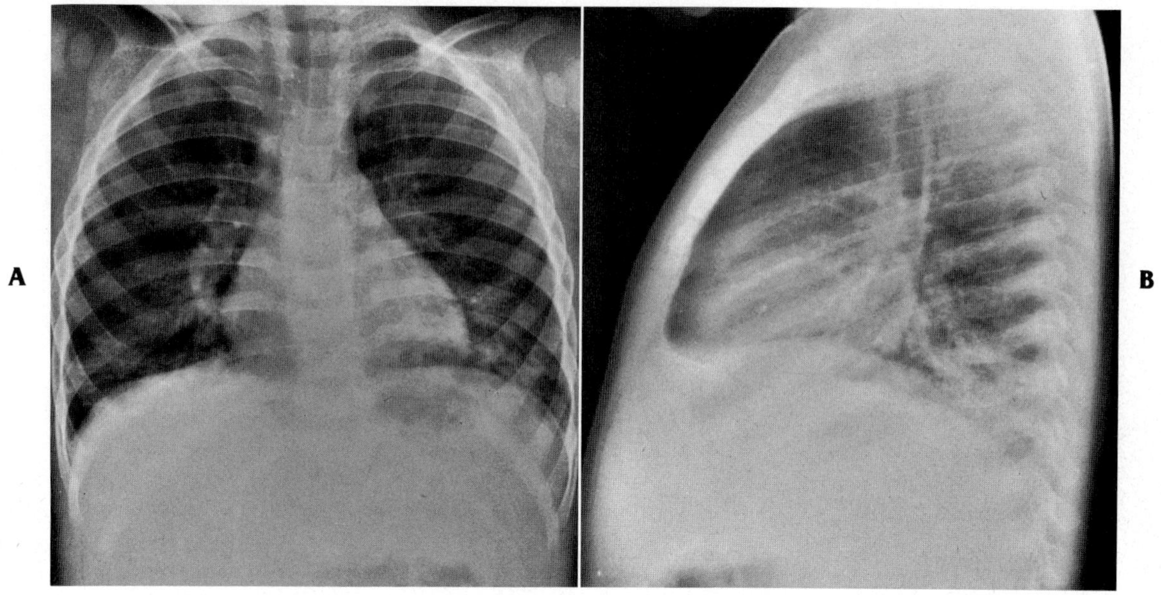

**FIGURE 16** *A* and *B*, Hydrocarbon aspiration with bibasilar infiltrates.

monitis in patients with acquired immunodeficiency syndrome (AIDS) may all have this appearance. If the hazy opacification has a basilar predominance, hydrocarbon aspiration or lipoid pneumonia is a more likely cause (Fig. 16).

Diffuse nodular opacities may be observed in infection. The size of the nodules may be miliary in miliary tuberculosis and slightly larger in histoplasmosis and varicella infections (Fig. 17). Cavitary nodules usually indicate septic emboli. Noninfectious causes for nodules, such as metastatic disease and sarcoid, are less common in acutely ill children.

## *Enlarged Cardiothymic Silhouette*

After the newborn period, the heart size should stabilize in normal children. The normal cardiothoracic ratio is 0.5 on a well-positioned inspiratory AP film. The normal thymus may increase the apparent cardiothoracic ratio on AP films, especially in children younger than four years of age. Likewise, high diaphragms caused by poor inspiration or by abdominal distention make the heart appear abnormally large. The lordotic projection frequently observed in infant chest films accentuates the cardiac silhouette. A repeat AP projection accompanied by a lateral film usually differentiates apparent from real cardiomegaly. True cardiomegaly should be present on both views. In addition, recognition of the multiple normal thymic configurations is essential to distinguish a normal, prominent thymus from an enlarged heart.

We do not discuss pediatric cardiac problems in detail. Once cardiomegaly is noted in an ill child, thorough cardiac evaluation, usually including cardiac ultrasonography, is performed.

If the cardiothymic silhouette is enlarged on both AP and lateral projections, careful attention must be paid to the vascular pattern in an acutely ill child to arrive at a pertinent differential diagnosis.

Normal or decreased vasculature may indicate a pericardial effusion or Ebstein's anomaly (Fig. 18). A large mediastinal mass may masquerade as cardiomegaly, and ultrasonography, CT, or magnetic resonance imaging (MRI) allows characterization of the mass and details the extent of mediastinal involvement.

Cardiomegaly and increased central and peripheral vascularity often indicate a left-to-right shunt or a high-output state, as in patients with anemia or peripheral vascular malformation (see Fig. 4).

Cardiomegaly and pulmonary edema are observed in children with myocarditis, myocardiopathy, or coarctation of the aorta.

## *Asymmetric Findings That Often Signify the Need for Urgent Intervention*

A number of conditions produce mass effect and may be life-threatening. Early diagnosis is essential to initiate proper interventional or surgical therapy. Plain radiographic findings in children after the neonatal period can be divided into three major categories: large cystic hemithorax, large lucent hemithorax, and large opaque hemithorax.

### Large Cystic Hemithorax

A large cystic-appearing hemithorax may be observed in children with pneumonia who develop pneumatoceles (Fig. 19). Delayed presentation of a diaphragmatic hernia, usually right sided, or a diaphragmatic eventration has a similar appearance. Ultrasonography or an upper gastrointestinal evaluation assists in diagnosing the condition. Less likely causes include lung cysts and cystic adenomatoid malformation.

### Large Lucent Hemithorax

The large lucent-appearing hemithorax is usually caused by partial bronchial occlusion, pneumothorax, or compensatory hyperinflation of the unobstructed lung. Accurate diagnosis is important to institute appropriate therapy. Tension pneumo-

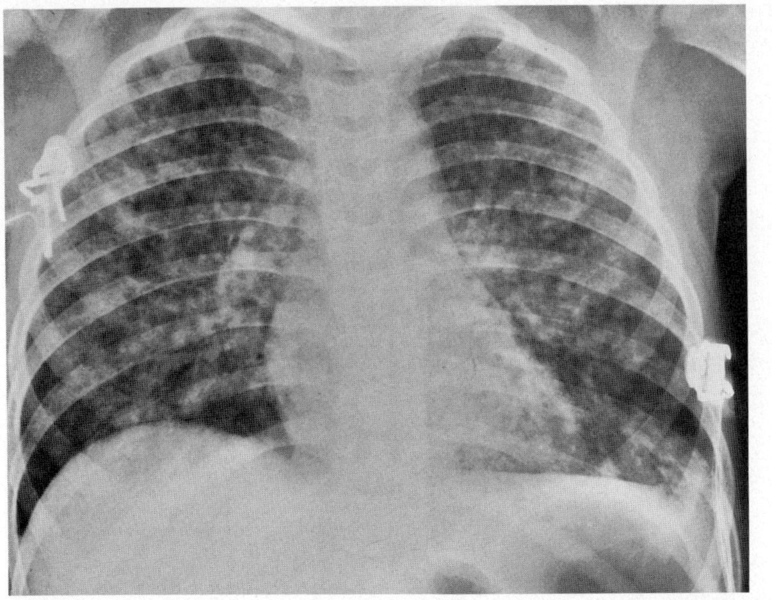

**FIGURE 17** Varicella pneumonia with a diffuse reticulonodular pattern.

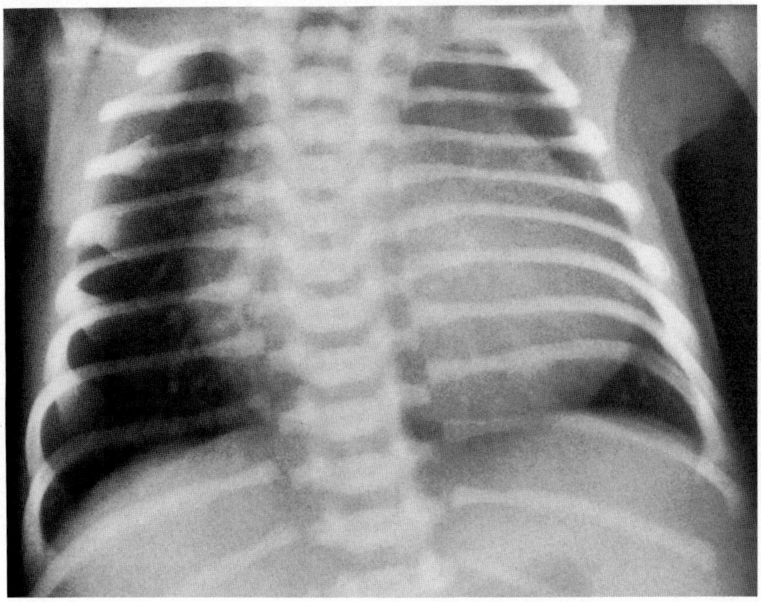

**FIGURE 18** Cardiomegaly and decreased pulmonary vascularity in an infant with Ebstein's anomaly of the tricuspid valve.

thorax requires evacuation by aspiration or a thoracostomy tube. Conditions causing bronchial obstruction, such as foreign body or mucous plug, are treated by bronchoscopic removal of the obstruction (Fig. 20). Other conditions such as congenital lobar emphysema, vascular anomalies, or bronchial adenoma require surgery.

A large tension pneumothorax may collect anterior to the lung and cause the lung to fall posteriorly. Consequently its edge may not be visible on AP supine films. A cross-table lateral or lateral decubitus film allows the lung edge to be observed and the diagnosis to be made (Fig. 21).

Partial bronchial obstruction causes overinflation of the ipsilateral lobe or lung distal to the obstruction. The increased lucency of the affected lobe or lung is accentuated because reflex pulmonary vasospasm decreases the vasculature in the affected lung. If a lobar bronchus is involved, the surrounding lobes are compressed and appear as areas of increased density. Fluoroscopy or decubitus radiographs help in doubtful cases by demonstrating selective air trapping from the "ball valve" bronchial obstruction during expiration. Foreign body aspiration accounts for most cases of acute partial bronchial obstruction after the newborn period. Nonopaque vegetable matter is the usual aspirated object, and there is a slight preponderance of right-sided aspirations.

Extrinsic bronchial compression can cause postobstructive overinflation of a lobe or lung. Tuberculosis should be suspected if there is unilateral hilar or mediastinal adenopathy. Obstruction in tuberculosis can be caused by both extrinsic nodal compression and bronchial erosion by a granuloma. An anomalous vessel may compress a bronchus to produce asymmetrical air trapping. The esophagram, especially the lateral view, identifies the position of the compressing vessel; CT or MRI delineates vascular anatomy before surgery.

Marked compensatory hyperinflation of the lung distal to an unobstructed bronchus accompanies total collapse or agenesis of the opposite lung. Vascularity may appear increased in the

A

B

C

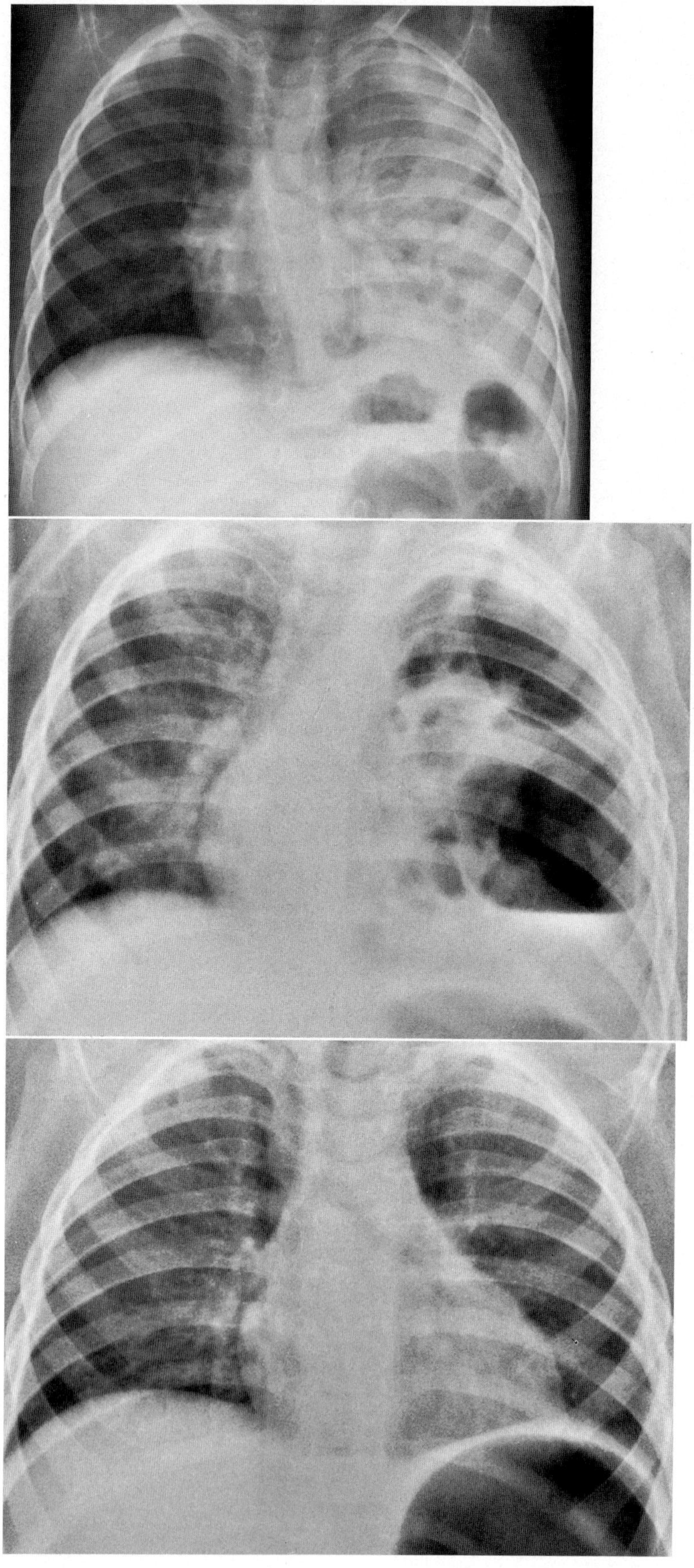

**FIGURE 19** *A,* Staphylococcal pneumonia with a left-sided pleural effusion. *B,* Pneumatoceles. *C,* Complete resolution.

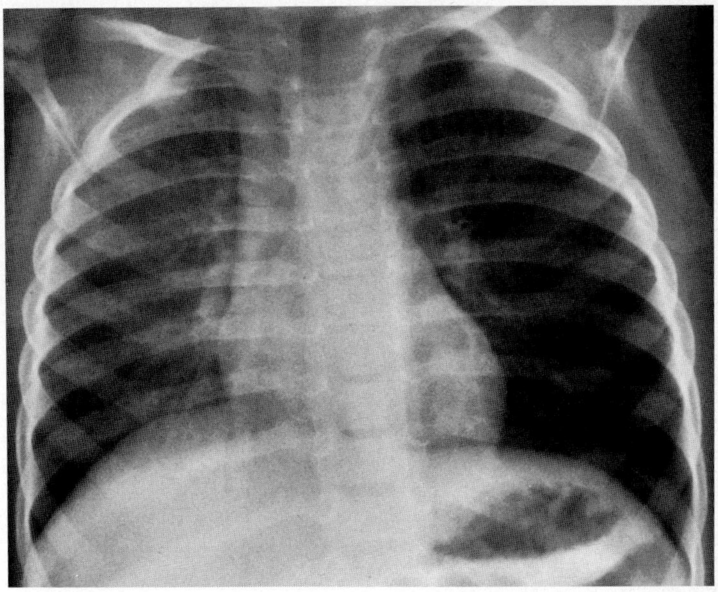

**FIGURE 20** Lucent left-sided hemithorax in a child who aspirated a nonopaque foreign body into the left main bronchus.

A

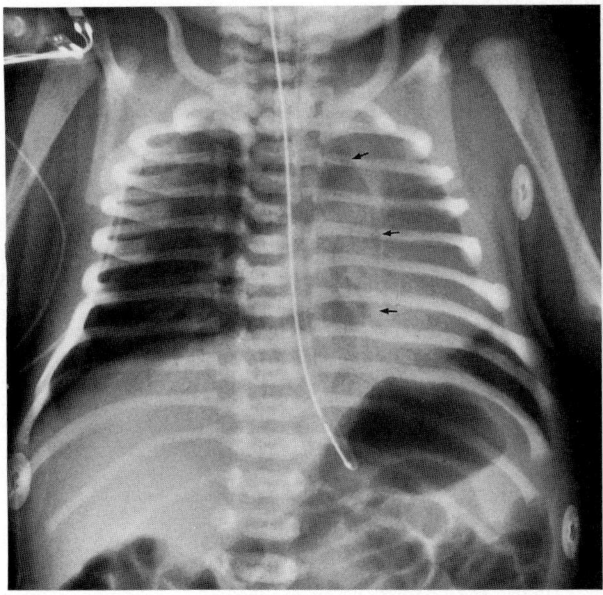

B

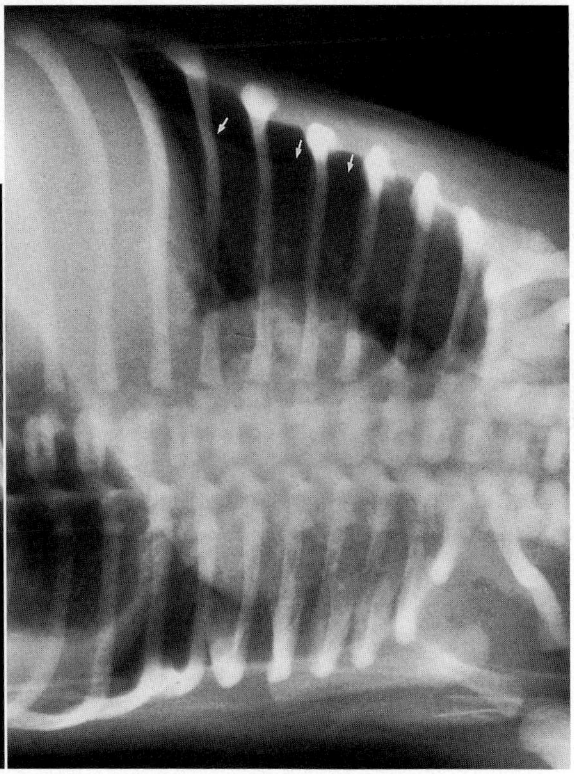

**FIGURE 21** *A,* Lucent right-sided hemithorax due to a pneumothorax. The right parietal pleura is outlined by air and herniates across the midline (*black arrows*). *B,* The left lateral decubitus film demonstrates the lung edge (*white arrows*).

large residual lung in cases of unilateral agenesis. Bronchoscopy allows differentiation of atelectasis from agenesis and facilitates extraction of a mucous plug or foreign body in the presence of atelectasis.

## Large Opaque Hemithorax

Pleural fluid collections, usually accompanying pneumonia, represent the most frequent cause of a large, totally opaque hemithorax (Fig. 22). Other types of large pleural collections include hemorrhage, chyle, lymph, or fluids infused through a catheter that has perforated a vein. Rarely a delayed diaphragmatic hernia can compromise venous and lymphatic flow in a trapped loop of bowel and produce a large pleural fluid collection.

Other causes of an enlarged opaque hemithorax include marked cardiomegaly accompanied by atelectasis of one lung, an expansile pneumonia, or a large neoplasm.

Ultrasonography allows rapid differentiation of the various

A

B

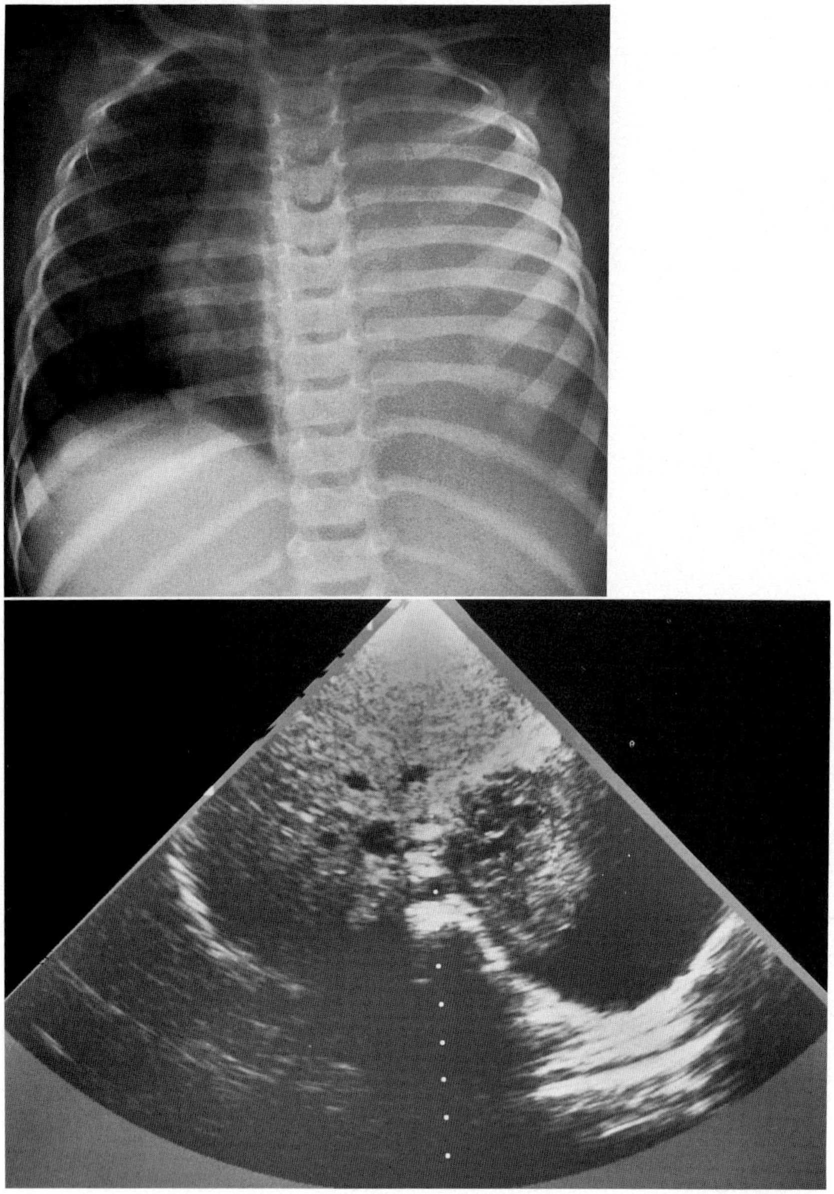

**FIGURE 22** *A,* Opaque left-sided hemithorax due to pleural fluid in a child with pneumonia. *B,* Transverse ultrasonography at the level of the diaphragm demonstrates an anechoic fluid collection surrounding the compressed left lung.

causes of the large opaque hemithorax. Ultrasonography also aids in diagnosis and classification of heart disease. CT is needed to evaluate the extent of thoracic involvement when a large mass is present.

## Discussion

The plain radiograph is key in diagnosing causes of emergency conditions involving the pediatric chest. Rapid, accurate assessment of plain films and organization of findings into basic groups are important. Careful correlation of radiographic findings with clinical information often leads to a reasonable diagnosis or a short differential list. Appropriate additional imaging is ordered if indicated by initial plain film findings.

## Suggested Reading

Alford BA, Armstrong P. Radiographic evaluation of the child who wheezes. Diagn Radiol 1983; 12(3):1–39.

Alford BA, Armstrong P. Congenital pulmonary anomalies. In: Grainger RG, Allison DJ, eds. Diagnostic Radiology. 2nd ed. London: Churchill Livingstone, 1992:373.

Alford BA, Keats TE. The infant and young child. In: Grainger RG, Allison DJ, eds. Diagnostic Radiology. 2nd ed. London: Churchill Livingstone, 1992:383.

Alford BA, McIlhenny J, et al. Asymmetric radiographic findings in the pediatric chest: An approach to early diagnosis. RadioGraphics (in press).

Armstrong P, Wilson A, Dee PA. Imaging of Diseases of the Chest. Chicago: Year Book, 1990:152.

Kirks D. Practical Pediatric Imaging. 2nd ed. Boston: Little Brown, 1991:417.

Swischuk LE. Differential Diagnosis in Pediatric Radiology. Baltimore: Williams & Wilkins, 1983:100.

# The Neonatal Chest

*BEVERLY P. WOOD, M.D.*

Chest abnormalities are the greatest cause of morbidity and mortality in the neonatal age group; however, the past 20 years have brought a remarkable improvement in survival and well-being for infants suffering from pulmonary and related chest abnormalities. The survival and improved prognosis of premature infants with pulmonary disease reflects improved understanding of the physiology of the immature lung and better methods of respiratory management and support. Unfortunately the high occurrence of preterm birth and inadequate prenatal care continues to bring immature infants to nurseries. Management of preterm infants with the pulmonary diseases of immaturity has improved remarkably. In term infants improved methods of respiratory support also have resulted in better management and prognosis and shorter hospitalization. This chapter discusses the common pulmonary and chest abnormalities of newborn infants and their management.

## Respiratory Distress Syndrome

Respiratory distress syndrome (RDS), or hyaline membrane disease, remains an important pulmonary abnormality of immature infants. RDS is well recognized as a reflection of physiologic and cellular immaturity of the lung. This immaturity presents with two important aspects of pulmonary disease.

1. The immature lung has not fully developed in the formation of terminal bronchioles and terminal air sacs, or alveolar ducts. Consequently there are a diminished number of airspaces, and the interstitium of the lung is thick. There is a less well-developed intimate relationship of the pulmonary capillaries with the alveolar epithelial lining, impeding normal gas exchange across this tissue.
2. The airspaces of the lung are lined by type 1 pneumocytes, which form the lining epithelial layer, and type 2 pneumocytes, which are more numerous but occupy the corners of airspaces and produce pulmonary surfactant. Surfactant is a phospholipid that adheres to the air/fluid hypophase of the air sacs and maintains open airspaces during inhalation and exhalation, and allows for better gas exchange and more even recruitment of alveoli. It also works to prevent pulmonary edema. Thus adequate mature surfactant results in a well-expanded and compliant lung, whereas inadequate surfactant production or immature surfactant results in poor pulmonary compliance, widespread atelectasis, and resultant hypoxemia and acidosis.

The well-known radiographic appearance of infants with RDS is of a set of small lungs of small volume and a diffuse, fine, reticular pattern that represents atelectasis, and thickened interstitium, or a diffusely opaque pattern that reflects poorly expanded pulmonary parenchyma throughout (Fig. 1).

Management of RDS is aimed toward maintenance of adequate pulmonary expansion and ventilation with adequate transepithelial gas exchange. This may be achieved by cautious mechanical ventilation adequate to maintain airspace expansion but low enough to avoid overdistention of airspaces. In the past decade, topical replacement of surfactant using surfactant obtained from exogenous sources has been successful in ameliorating the course of RDS in premature infants. Use of surfactant has resulted in improved aeration and lower oxygen and ventilatory supplementation. Although surfactant use has diminished some of the complications of RDS, it has not significantly altered the incidence of bronchopulmonary dysplasia (BPD).

## Bronchopulmonary Dysplasia

This pulmonary complication mainly occurs in infants who are premature with exposure to high levels of inspired oxygen and

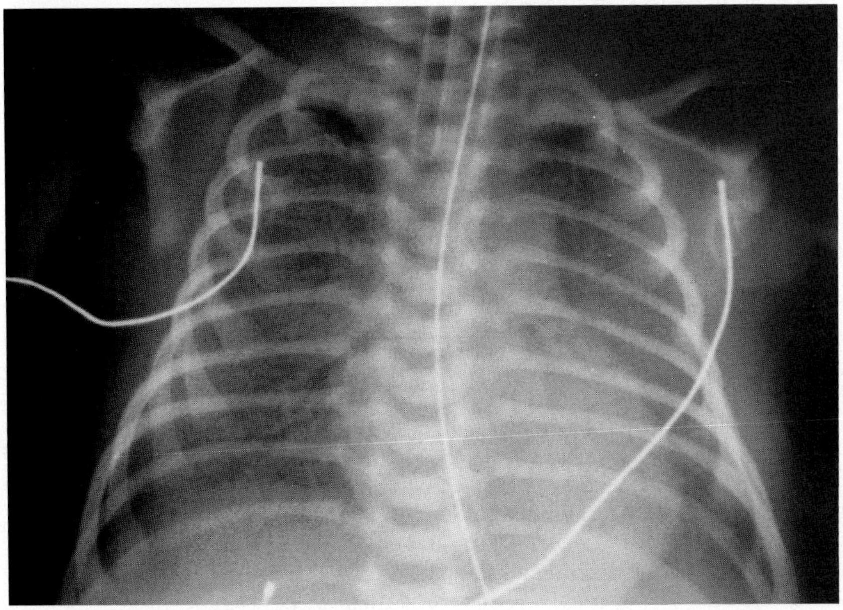

**FIGURE 1** A 30 week gestation premature infant with respiratory distress shows the presence of air bronchograms and a very fine reticular pattern throughout both lungs, which is characteristic of respiratory distress syndrome.

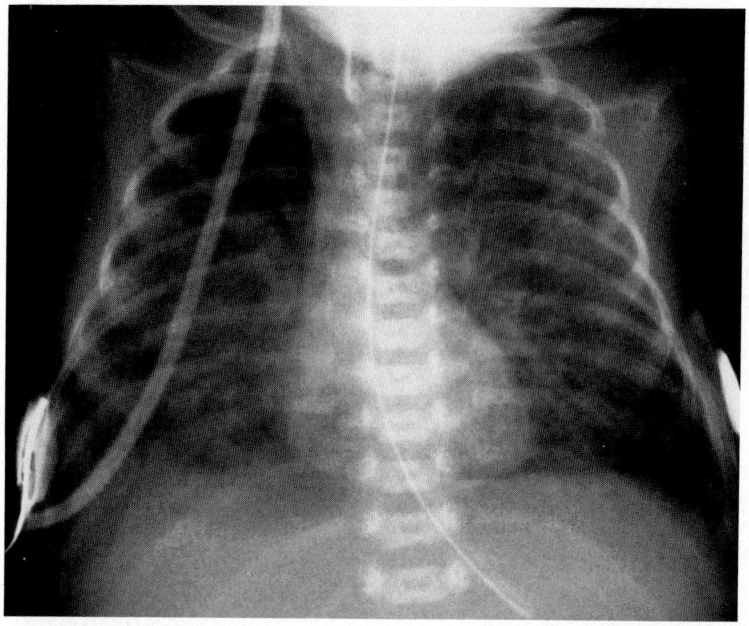

**FIGURE 2** This premature infant, with respiratory distress syndrome at birth, at 7 days of age shows diffuse vascular congestion and interstitial edema, which is an early indication of bronchopulmonary dysplasia.

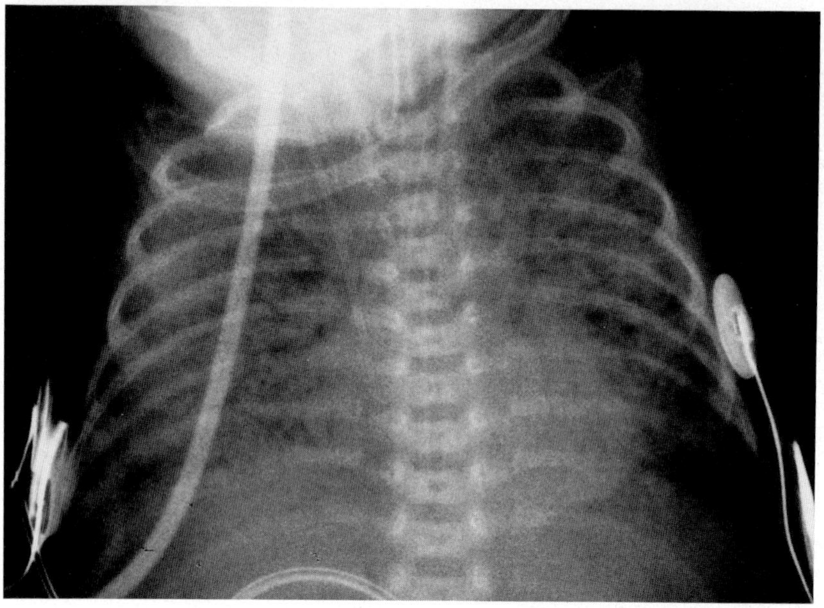

**FIGURE 3** The same infant shown in Figure 2, at 10 days of age, shows increasing interstitial and alveolar change secondary to patent ductus arteriosus, with increasing edema and microvascular leak.

positive pressure ventilation. The effects of these two insults and other factors on the immature lung are more detrimental to pulmonary integrity than the same factors would be in a more mature lung. BPD has histology that is characterized by progressive occurrence of epithelial hyperplasia and metaplasia in the small airways, with resultant partial or complete obstruction of airspaces. The peripheral airspaces become either hyperexpanded, because of air trapping and the inability of air to escape on exhalation, or they become atelectatic or scarred. Within the interstitium of the lung, the early changes of BPD are represented by progressive leaks of the pulmonary microvasculature. This damage occurs because of the effect of free radicals of oxygen on the lining airspace epithelium and on the vascular endothelium, aided by hypoxemia, acidosis, and fluctuation of intravascular volumes and pressures in premature infants. Interstitial hemorrhage occurs with interstitial edema. Later in the progress of the disease, interstitial fibroblast invasion and eventually interstitial fibrosis occur.

The early appearance of BPD radiographically is represented by interstitial edema followed by progressively uneven aeration, reflecting the areas of air trapping in airspaces in areas of hypoventilation and atelectasis (Figs. 2 and 3). Although pulmonary interstitial emphysema leads to BPD, it is not a major factor in most BPD patients. Late effects of BPD are scarring (Figs. 4 and 5) with airway hyperreactivity secondary to the hypertrophied smooth muscle in the walls of airways, pulmonary hypertension, poor lung growth, frequent pulmonary infections, and abnormal pulmonary function testing all observed in established BPD.

The most effective treatment of BPD is prevention by concentrating on use of minimal amounts of inspired oxygen and avoidance of positive pressure ventilation, the treatment of edema and infection, and, in some centers, the use of steroids to avoid scarring and cellular hyperplasia.

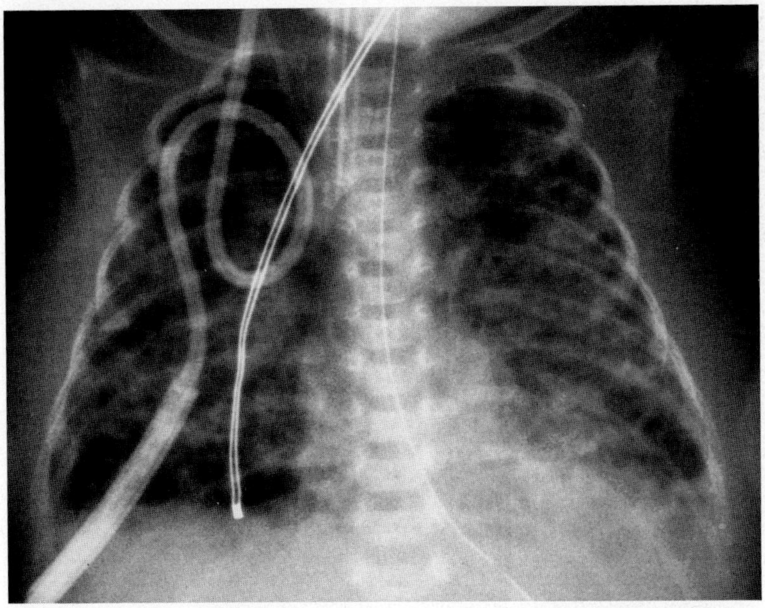

**FIGURE 4** Well-established bronchopulmonary dysplasia in the infant shown in Figures 2 and 3, now at 4 weeks of age. There is diffusely uneven aeration, with areas of hyperaeration and air trapping alternating with regions of atelectasis and scarring. Note the increased lung volume.

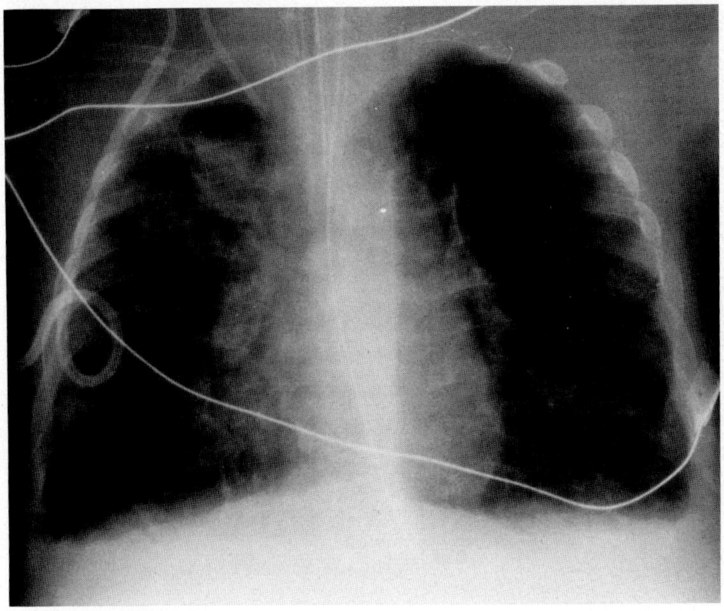

**FIGURE 5** A 2-month-old infant with long-term respiratory management shows markedly hyperaerated lungs with central scarring.

Factors that predispose to BPD are immaturity, high levels of inspired $O_2$, positive pressure ventilation, pulmonary edema (patent ductus arteriosus), infection, familial incidence of hyperreactive airways disease, and malnutrition.

## Pulmonary Infection

Neonatal pneumonia occurs more commonly in term infants than in preterm infants. The pneumonia may occur secondary to an in utero infection, an infection incurred during delivery, or a postnatal source. In utero infections may occur secondary to maternal sepsis or maternal chorioamnionitis. The organisms responsible include coxsackie virus, herpes simplex virus, cytomegalovirus, influenza virus, and *Toxoplasma.* Infections associated with passage through an infected birth canal are secondary to herpes simplex virus, streptococcus, *Escherichia* coli, and *Chlamydia trachomatis.* Postnatal infections reflect exposure in the nursery or the home and are frequently secondary to gram-negative organisms including *E. coli* and *Citrobacter* species. Neonatal pneumonia may be rapidly progressive, mainly reflecting the impaired white blood cell response of the infant; rapid identification of the infection and treatment is key to a positive outcome.

The radiographic findings of pneumonia in newborn infants are commonly those of well-expanded or hyperexpanded lungs, with dense streaky areas of consolidation and sometimes a small pleural effusion (Figs. 6 and 7). The affected infant's clinical course is one of rapid deterioration with high mortality.

Immature infants with an endotracheal tube, intravascular lines, and ventilatory support are particularly subject to pneumonia. The ventilator air bypasses the nasopharyngeal barrier of normal infant, salivary IgA is lacking, and poor host leukocyte response results in poor localization of infection and rapidly progressive septicemia. The airway abnormalities of

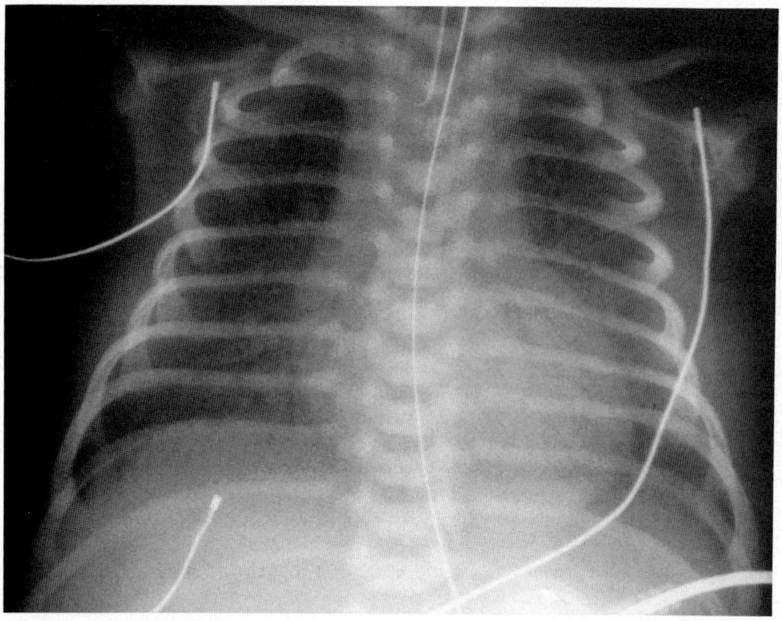

**FIGURE 6** Newborn infant with severe respiratory distress and abnormal white blood cell count. The diffuse interstitial streaky pneumonic disease is secondary to cytomegalovirus pneumonia.

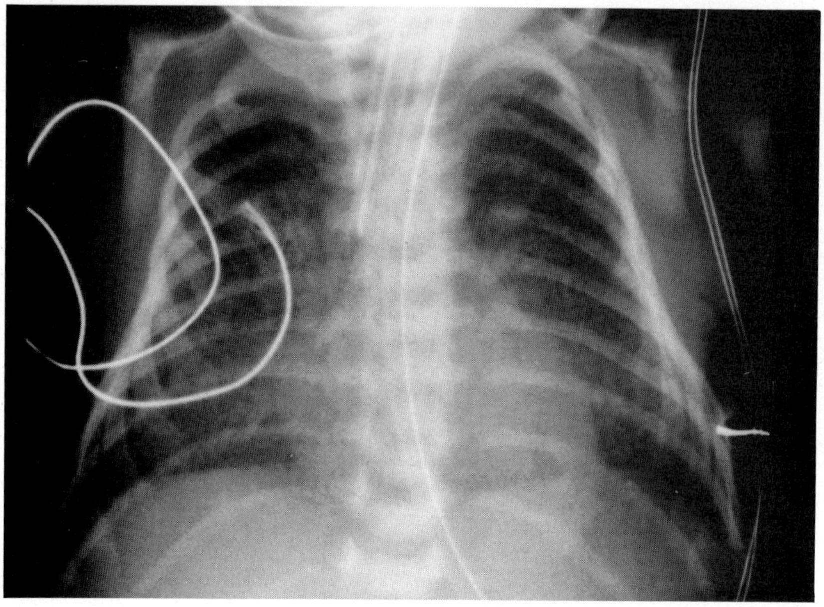

**FIGURE 7** Coarse interstitial changes with hyperaeration in a term infant with beta-hemolytic streptococcal septicemia and pneumonia.

BPD further facilitate superinfection in premature infants. Superinfecting species in premature infants are usually fungal, with *Candida albicans* being the most frequent organism. *Malassezia furfur,* which grows on indwelling lines, has proven to be a common superinfecting intracellular organism of the already ill neonate.

## Pneumothorax and Pneumomediastinum

Pneumothorax may be observed in both immature and mature infants. In immature infants a pneumothorax most commonly results from pulmonary interstitial emphysema that progresses from air within the interlobular septa into the pulmonary pleural (visceral pleural) lymphatics. These distend, rupture, and produce a pneumothorax. The most common site of air leak leading to pulmonary interstitial emphysema is from rupture at the junction of a bronchiole and its alveolar duct. The event usually occurs in poorly compliant lungs requiring high ventilatory pressures to maintain open airspaces. Once interstitial emphysema and its resultant pneumothorax are established, the leak tends to continue, and it is difficult to maintain good lung expansion, even with the use of chest tubes to drain the pleural space. The presence of a pneumothorax in a more mature infant, particularly when bilateral, reflects hypoplastic lungs and is commonly a sign of the oligohydramnios syndrome, which is observed in infants with severe renal anomalies and consequent impaired pulmonary formation and maturity.

Pneumomediastinum may occur associated with pneumothorax, reflecting rupture of air into the mediastinal spaces. It can also occur following traumatic intubation, esophageal perforation, or similar mediastinal trauma. In an infant a pneumomediastinum rarely travels upward into the subcutaneous tissues of the neck, because the thymus acts as an effective barrier against this upward migration of mediastinal air.

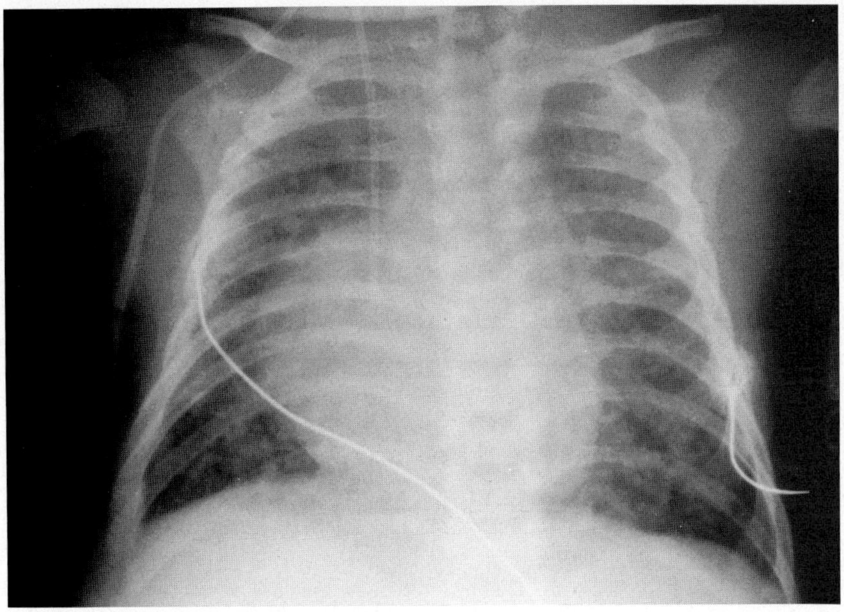

**FIGURE 8** Congestive heart failure observed in this newborn with cardiomegaly, marked dilatation of the right atrium, and marked pulmonary vascular, perivascular, and interstitial edema.

## Pulmonary Interstitial Diseases

A number of physiologic insults are reflected in interstitial abnormalities of the lung in infants. The major interstitial abnormality observed is interstitial pulmonary edema. As previously mentioned, the source of interstitial edema is a leak of the pulmonary microvasculature. This is produced by hypoxemia, acidosis, defective capillary endothelial barrier, differences in oncotic pressure between the interstitium and the intravascular space, and differences in pressure between the vascular space and the interstitium. In addition to metabolic abnormalities precipitating vascular leak, situations in which there is increased pulmonary flow or pulmonary vascular pressure (e.g., patent ductus arteriosus, intracardiac left-to-right shunts, and obstruction of pulmonary venous drainage) all result in significant pulmonary interstitial edema (Fig. 8). The pulmonary lymphatics located within the interstitium are enlarged in babies with congenital lymphangiectasia. Pulmonary infection, particularly viral pneumonia, also frequently results in interstitial prominence secondary to an inflammatory reactive response of the host.

## Aspiration Pneumonia

Perinatal or prenatal aspiration occurs at a time of severe in utero stress and hypoxemia. Amniotic aspiration is usually benign and is evidenced by an increased load of pulmonary alveolar fluid that is cleared via lymphatics in the first 24 to 48 hours of life. Meconium aspiration results from stress with passage of meconium in utero followed by gasping by the infant so that meconium is inhaled into the larger and smaller airways. In this location it results in airway obstruction with atelectasis and air trapping distal to the sites of meconium. The affected areas aerate poorly, and both a chemical and inflammatory pneumonia may ensue. Because of the severe amount of air trapping, infants are hypoxemic and develop pulmonary hypertension. Effective treatment is with extracorporeal membrane oxygenation (ECMO) to avoid the effects of pulmonary hypertension and to allow the lung to heal spontaneously without use of high levels of oxygen or positive pressure.

The other reason for aspiration is related to esophageal abnormalities, particularly esophageal atresia, in which the infant aspirates saliva and secretions as well as any feedings that are given. Because of a typical history of choking with feedings, such babies should immediately be evaluated for possible esophageal atresia. Infants with a tracheoesophageal fistula without atresia also present with aspiration of material that passes through the esophagus, and often with a severe pneumonia occurring in the early days of life.

## Small Lung

The presence of a small lung, or bilateral small lungs, is manifested by hypoxemia and severe respiratory difficulty. The etiologies of a small lung include congenital pulmonary hypoplasia, with a small main bronchus, small pulmonary artery, and small pulmonary veins. Either the artery or the veins, or both, may be systemic in origin. Pulmonary hypoplasia most commonly occurs on the right side and is associated with a small pulmonary artery and pulmonary veins that drain aberrantly into the systemic circulation below the diaphragm. The pulmonary artery may arise from the descending aorta, rather than from the main pulmonary trunk.

Bilateral pulmonary hypoplasia occurs in the oligohydramnios syndrome. There is inadequate induction of pulmonary growth and development, because of the absence of urine in the amniotic fluid and severe restriction of fetal respiratory movement in utero.

Congenital diaphragmatic hernia or other intrathoracic masses, such as cystic adenomatoid malformation of the lung, results in a small lung. The lung is proportionately hypoplastic according to the amount of compression that has occurred and the timing from early development. Thus diaphragmatic hernias present from early fetal life are associated with severe pulmonary hypoplasia compared with those that occur around the time of birth.

Infants with prune-belly syndrome have characteristically hypoplastic lungs secondary to both oligohydramnios and poor thoracic cage formation. Infants with other forms of pulmonary thoracic dysplasia, such as fatal forms of dwarfism (achondrogenesis, thanatophoric dwarfism, metatrophic dwarfism), show a small thorax and small lungs. A thoracic dysplasia is associated with giant omphaloceles.

In infants with severely hypoplastic lung secondary to congenital diaphragmatic hernia or intrathoracic mass, ECMO therapy is instituted initially before repair of the hernia to avoid pulmonary hypertension and ventilator complications.

## Large Lung

Truly large lungs are unusual, but air trapping with resultant large lung volume may occur related to an abnormality of bronchi. Best known is congenital lobar emphysema, which is associated with a large volume lobe and also with a larger lung than usual in terms of the number of airways. This is believed to occur secondary to abnormality of development of the bronchial cartilage with collapse of the bronchus on expiration and consequent air trapping. Radiographically there occurs a single large lobe that is markedly hyperexpanded and compresses adjacent portions of the lung. After removal of the abnormal lobe, the remainder of the lung expands. If the lobe is not removed, the hyperexpansion usually worsens.

## Surgical Lesions of the Chest

Intrapulmonary masses often present with severe respiratory distress at the time of birth, and once the infant is stabilized, surgery is usually necessary. Mass lesions that occur within the lung include congenital lobar emphysema, cystic adenomatoid malformation of the lung, and pulmonary blastomas. Congenital lung cysts are rare, but also compress lung in a manner similar to lobar emphysema.

Mediastinal masses in neonates are often related to cystic hygroma of the neck extending into the mediastinum, thymic lesions such as thymic cysts and germinomas, and rarely thoracic neuroblastoma of congenital origin.

## Pleural Effusion

The etiology of pleural effusion in the neonate is usually chylothorax, which occurs on the right side more commonly than the left and is considered to be related to trauma at the time of birth. Chylothorax is self-limited condition, although a large chylothorax may require drainage to alleviate respiratory distress in infants. Smaller effusions are noted in infants with beta-hemolytic streptococcal infection, congestive heart failure, or fluid overload. These effusions are also self-limited and improve as the underlying process clears.

## Therapy of Pulmonary Problems in Infants

The most common form of pulmonary therapy used in infants with respiratory distress is treatment with endotracheal intubation, supplemental inspired oxygen, and positive pressure ventilation to maintain open airspaces and allow gas exchange.

ECMO is used in cases of severe respiratory distress. This is usually reserved for term infants or near-term infants with pulmonary disease that is potentially quickly reversible. Meconium aspiration pneumonia, other pneumonias, and congenital diaphragmatic hernia are the three most common reasons for using ECMO. The principle behind this treatment is the use of venous-arterial bypass, passing the infant's blood through a membrane oxygenator and returning it to the arterial system. Bypass is obtained using the right jugular vein and the right carotid artery, which are usually ligated after management with successful outcome.

High-frequency oscillatory ventilation (HFOV) is a technique of placing infants on high rates of ventilation. The oscillatory motion of gas in the airways improves carbon dioxide exchange. Very low pressures are used, and this technique is particularly helpful in infants with air leak (pulmonary interstitial emphysema) or potential air leak.

## Suggested Reading


Auten RL, Notter RH, Kendig JW, et al. Surfactant treatment of full-term newborns with respiratory failure. Pediatrics 1991; 87:101–107.

Bancalari E. Pathophysiology of hyaline membrane disease (excluding surfactant). In: Polin RA, Fox WW, eds. Fetal and Neonatal Medicine. Philadelphia: WB Saunders, 1992:885.

Baumgart S, Hischl RB, Butler SZ, et al. Diagnosis-related criteria in the consideration of extracorporeal membrane oxygenation in neonates previously treated with high-frequency jet ventilation. Pediatrics 1992; 89:491–494.

Bonikos DS, Bensch KG, Northway WH, et al. Bronchopulmonary dysplasia: The pulmonary pathologic sequel of necrotizing bronchiolitis and pulmonary fibrosis. Hum Pathol 1976; 7:643–666.

Cotton RB. The relationship of symptomatic patent ductus arteriosus to respiratory distress in premature newborn infants. Clin Perinatol 1987; 14:621–633.

Davis JM, Veness-Meehan K, Notter R, et al. Changes in pulmonary mechanics after the administration of surfactant to infants with respiratory distress syndrome. N Engl J Med 1988; 319:476–479.

Falconer AR, Brown RA, Helms P, et al. Pulmonary sequelae in survivors of congenital diaphragmatic hernia. Thorax 1990; 45:126–129.

Greenough A. Bronchopulmonary dysplasia: Early diagnosis, prophylaxis, and treatment. Arch Dis Child 1990; 65:1082–1088.

Marchak BE, Thompson WK, Duffy P, et al. Treatment of RDS by high-frequency ventilation and tracheal injuries. Pediatrics 1986; 77:608.

Northway WH Jr. Bronchopulmonary dysplasia: Then and now. Arch Dis Child 1990; 65:1076–1081.

Northway WH Jr. Bronchopulmonary dysplasia: Twenty-five years later. Commentary. Pediatrics 1992; 89:969–973.

Northway WH Jr, Moss RB, Carlisle KB, et al. Late pulmonary sequelae of bronchopulmonary dysplasia. N Engl J Med 1990; 323:1793–1799.

Northway WH Jr, Rosan RC, Proter DY. Pulmonary disease following respiratory therapy of hyaline-membrane disease. Bronchopulmonary dysplasia. N Engl J Med 1967; 276:357–368.

Notter RH, Shapiro DL. Lung surfactants for replacement therapy: Biochemical, biophysical, and clinical aspects. Clin Perinatol 1987; 14:433–479.

Philip AGS. Oxygen plus pressure plus time: The etiology of bronchopulmonary dysplasia. Pediatrics 1975; 55:44–50.

Royall JA, Levin DL. Adult respiratory distress syndrome in pediatric patients, 1. Clinical aspects, pathophysiology, pathology, and mechanisms of lung injury. J Pediatr 1988; 112:169–180.

Short BL, Miller MK, Anderson KD. Extracorporeal membrane oxygenation in the management of respiratory failure in the newborn. Clin Perinatol 1987; 14:737–748.

Taghizadeh A, Reynolds EOR. Pathogenesis of bronchopulmonary dysplasia following hyaline membrane disease. Am J Pathol 1976; 82:241–258.

# Radiologic Manifestations of AIDS in Children

*JACK O. HALLER, M.D.*

"In this hospital, the first diagnosis you have to make is AIDS." That, unfortunately, is the statement heard most often when residents confront teaching films that show a reticular nodular pattern of the lung in children.

The World Health Organization estimates that 8 to 10 million adults and 1 million children worldwide are infected with the human immunodeficiency virus (HIV), the etiologic agent of acquired immunodeficiency syndrome (AIDS). In addition, during the 1990s, mothers or both parents of more than 10 million children will have died from HIV infection/AIDS. AIDS will remain a major public health challenge worldwide in the twenty-first century. This chapter stresses the imaging findings of children with AIDS.

## Lung

The response of the lung in children with AIDS is in some ways unique and in other ways similar to that of adults. In this disease one of the interesting features of the pediatric chest film is that it is common to observe hilar and paratracheal adenopathy. If one sees adenopathy in an adult AIDS patient, one must think of tuberculosis (TB) as a superimposed opportunistic infection. Children, however, "normally" have mediastinal adenopathy without necessarily accompanying TB. It goes without saying though that if there is a sudden growth of hilar or paratracheal nodes, one should suspect malignancy, i.e., lymphoma (Figs. 1 and 2). Apparently the pediatric chest responds to HIV by launching a lymphoid response, either as

A

B

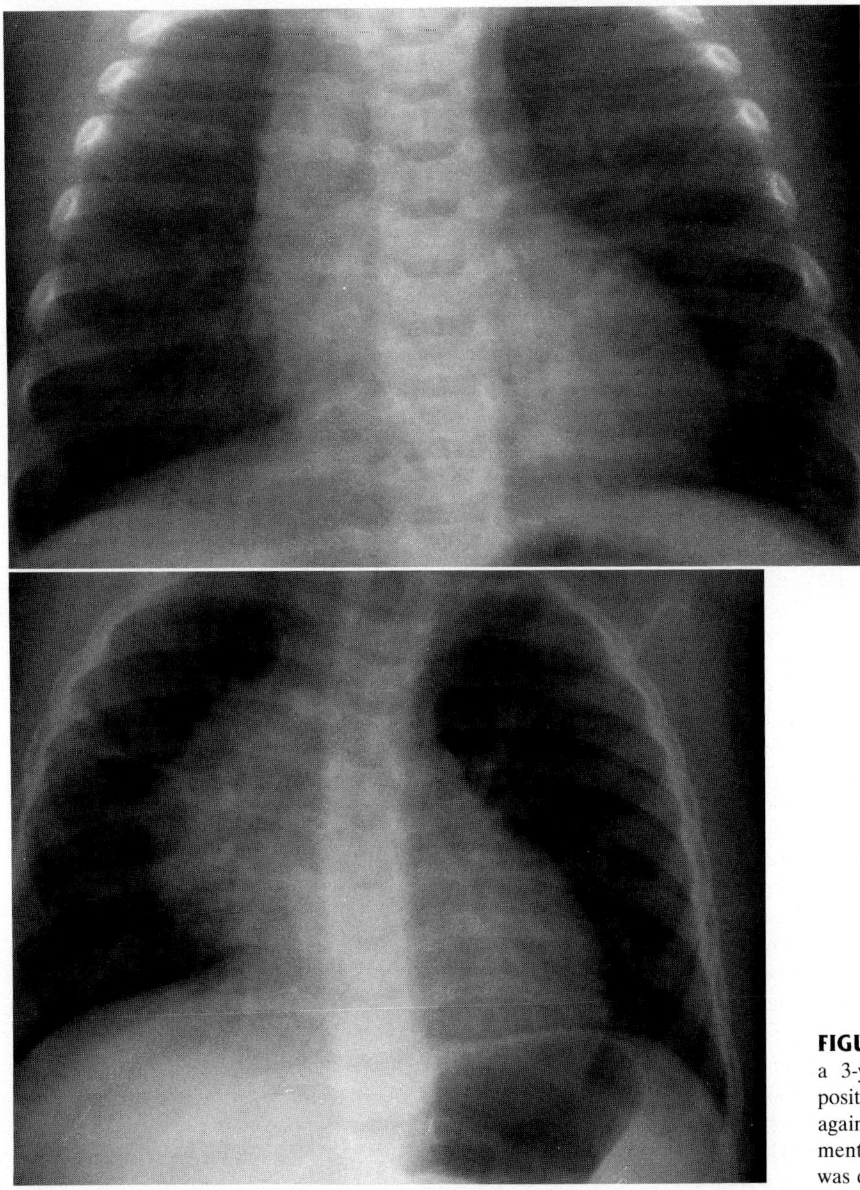

**FIGURE 1** Lymphoma. *A,* Normal chest radiograph of a 3-year-old child who was discovered to be HIV positive. *B,* Three months later the child was studied again, and the radiographs revealed marked enlargement of the right perihilar region. A biopsy of the area was diagnostic of lymphoma.

A

B

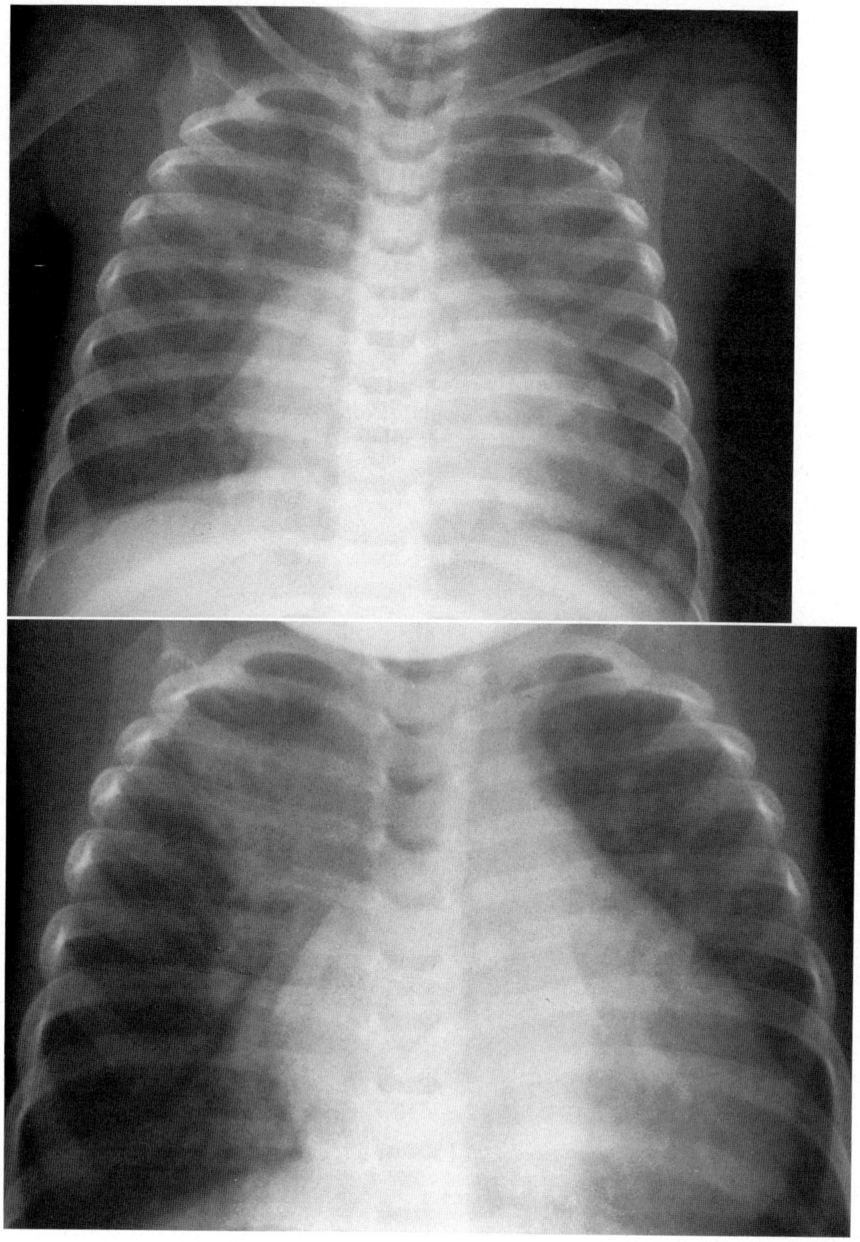

**FIGURE 2** Immunoblastic sarcoma. This 2-year-old child with known HIV disease was being followed for chronic lung disease. *A*, Frontal view of the chest shows bibasilar infiltrates and hilar and peritracheal adenopathy. *B*, Over the course of the next year, the right hilum was noted to grow at an unusual rate. Left lower lobe and right lower lobe atelectasis and infiltrates were again noted. The child subsequently died and at autopsy was found to have immunoblastic sarcoma diagnosed from the right paratracheal region.

adenopathy or as lymphocytic infiltration of the lung known as pulmonary lymphoid hyperplasia (PLH) or lymphocyte-associated disorder (LAD) or lymphocytic interstitial pneumonitis (LIP). When we reviewed our experience looking at the chest films of hundreds of these children, we found that the lung undergoes a whole spectrum of lymphoid-type changes, ranging from lymphocytic interstitial pneumonitis to bronchiolar-associated lymphoid tissue (BALT) to usual interstitial pneumonitis (UIP) to chronic interstitial pneumonitis (CIP). The corresponding chest film appears either nodular (Fig. 3, *A*), reticular nodular (Fig. 3, *B*), purely reticular, or downright fibrotic.

Other responses that the lung manifests are "reversible" bronchiectasis. This type of bronchiectasis is often manifested by a cicatrization of the lung that elongates and dilates the bronchi by traction. When the lung heals, the bronchiectasis often "reverses" (Fig. 4). This is different from the usual bronchiectasis, which these patients exhibit as well. In the typical form there is intrinsic abnormality in the bronchi. Bronchiectasis is usually seen in a middle and lower lobe distribution. These patients often have bronchial wall thickening and dilatation; cystic as well as cylindrical bronchiectasis occur and are readily detected on computed tomography (CT).

The lung is also the target for the many infections that these children contract. An organism that almost exclusively attacks immunocompromised individuals is *Pneumocystis carinii. Pneumocystis carinii* generally produces a bilateral interstitial or alveolar pattern that can evolve from a perihilar location into a more extensive and diffuse process. Pneumatoceles have been reported in association with *P. carinii* pneumonia (PCP) in AIDS patients. Both children and adults show "swiss cheese" lungs as a result of cavity formation, even without documentation of PCP. The best method for evaluating the extent of cavitary disease is CT (Figs. 5 and 6).

*Text continued on p. 693.*

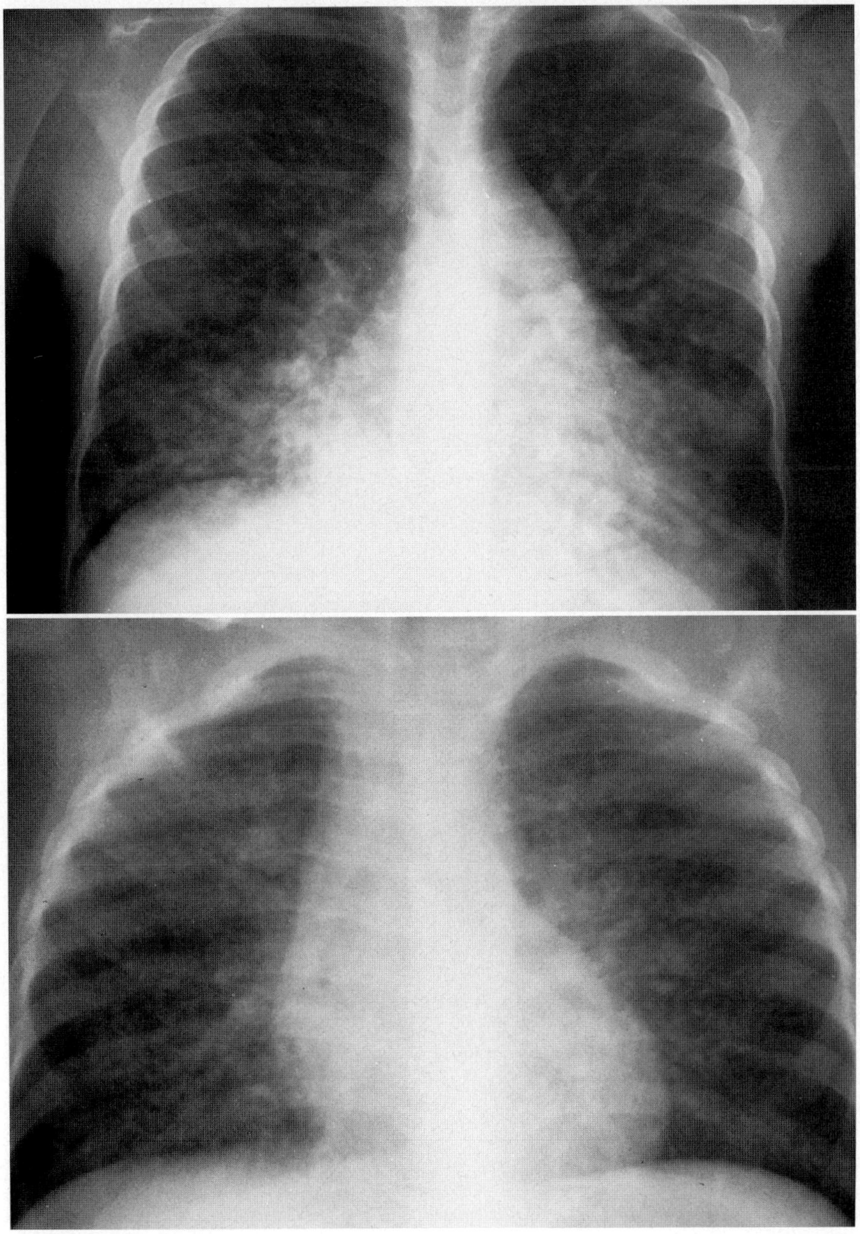

A

B

**FIGURE 3** Different forms of lymphocytic interstitial pneumonitis. *A,* This 3-year-old child displays the nodular form of LIP, predominately in the bases. *B,* This child with reticular nodular disease was more typical of the form usually associated with chronic interstitial pneumonitis, a later development in the spectrum of LIP.

A

B

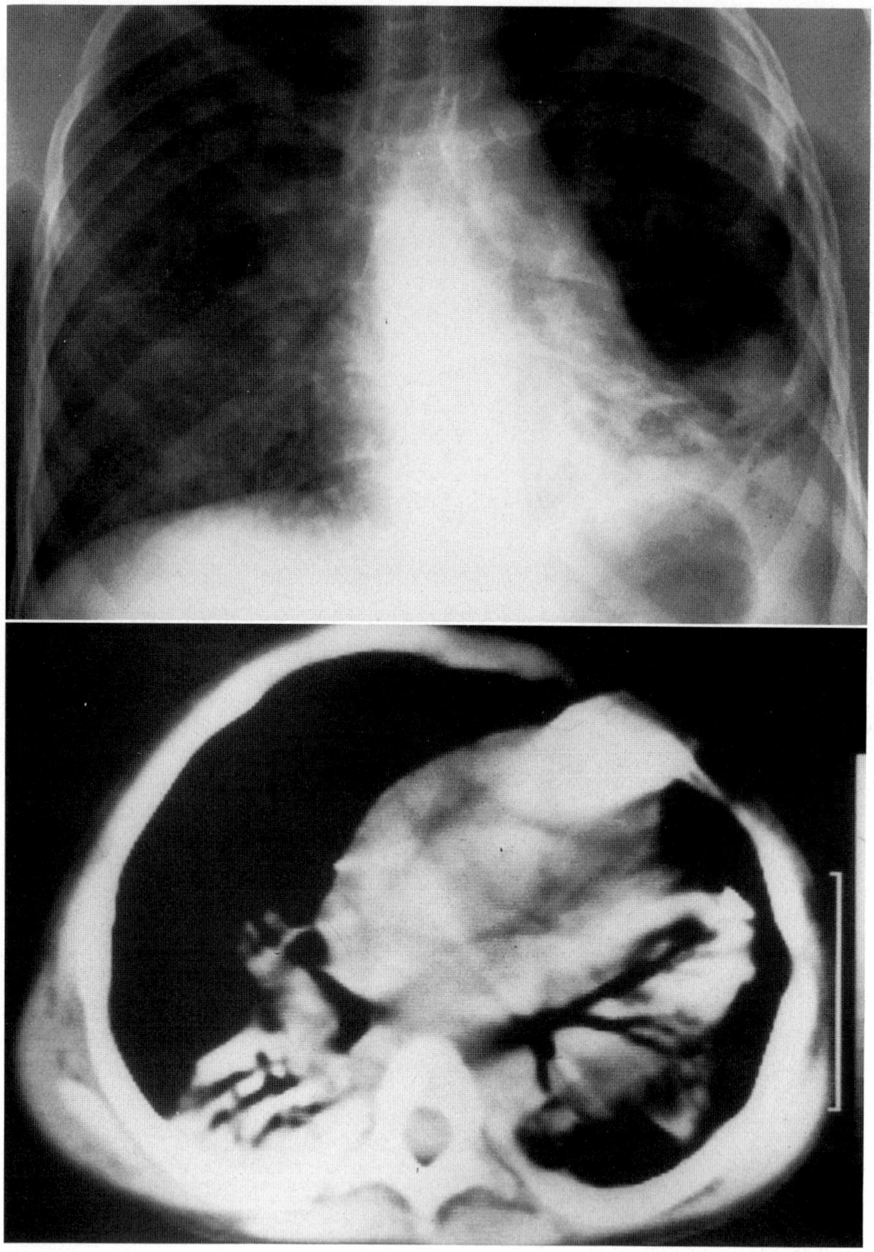

**FIGURE 4** Bronchiectasis. *A,* Frontal view of the chest of this 5-year-old child shows typical features of the left lower lobe bronchiectasis. Note the dilated bronchi coursing through the dense left lower lobe region. A pleural effusion is also noted. *B,* CT scan of the same child shows that the disease is actually bilateral and more extensive. The lung around the bronchi is consolidated and is essentially dilating the bronchi because of the fibrosis and scarring taking place within it.

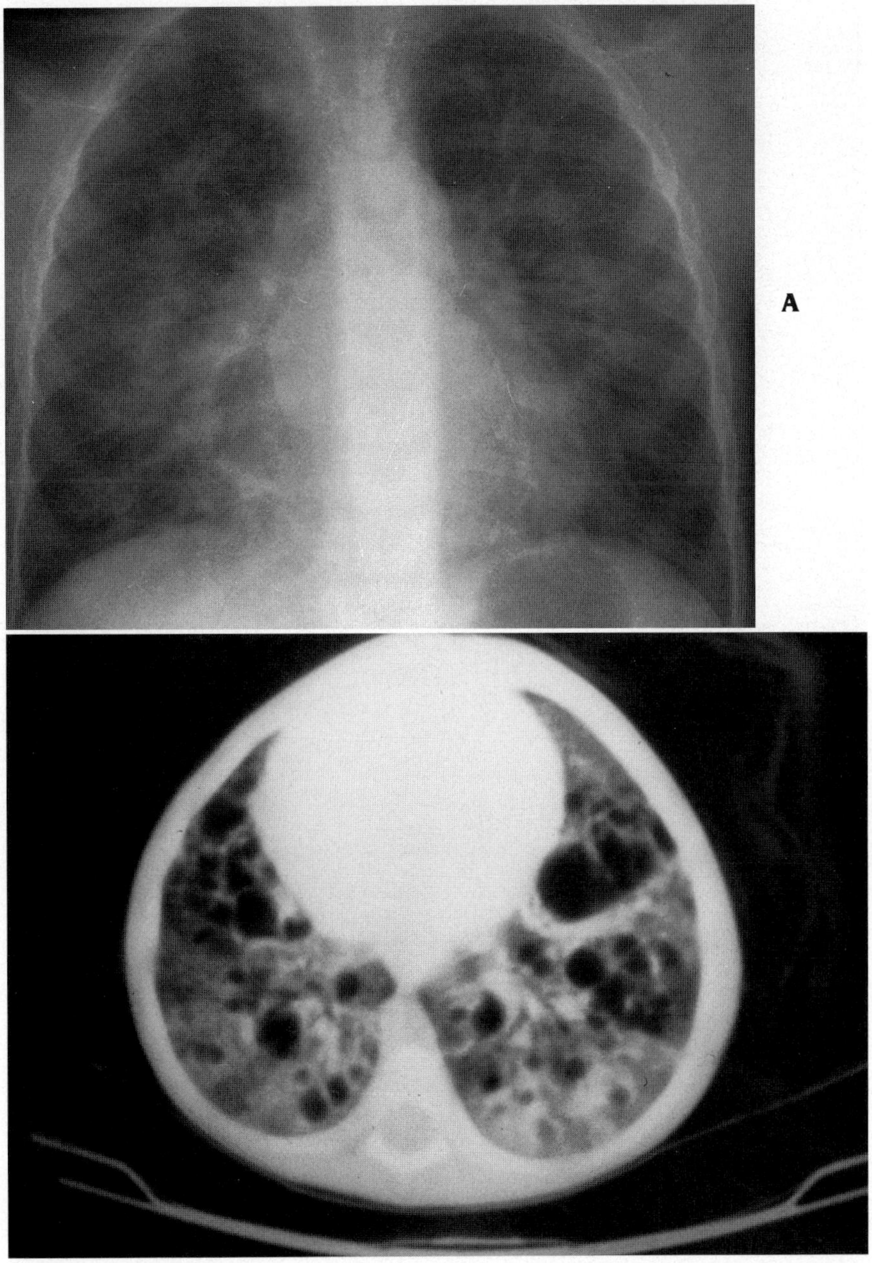

A

B

**FIGURE 5** Cavitary lung disease. This 5-year-old child presented with increasing respiratory distress. The child had had PCP diagnosed three months previously. *A,* A frontal view of the chest shows areas of cavitation, especially in the midportion of the lungs. *B,* CT scan of the same patient shows to better advantage the cavitary nature of the disease and its universal involvement throughout both lungs.

A

B

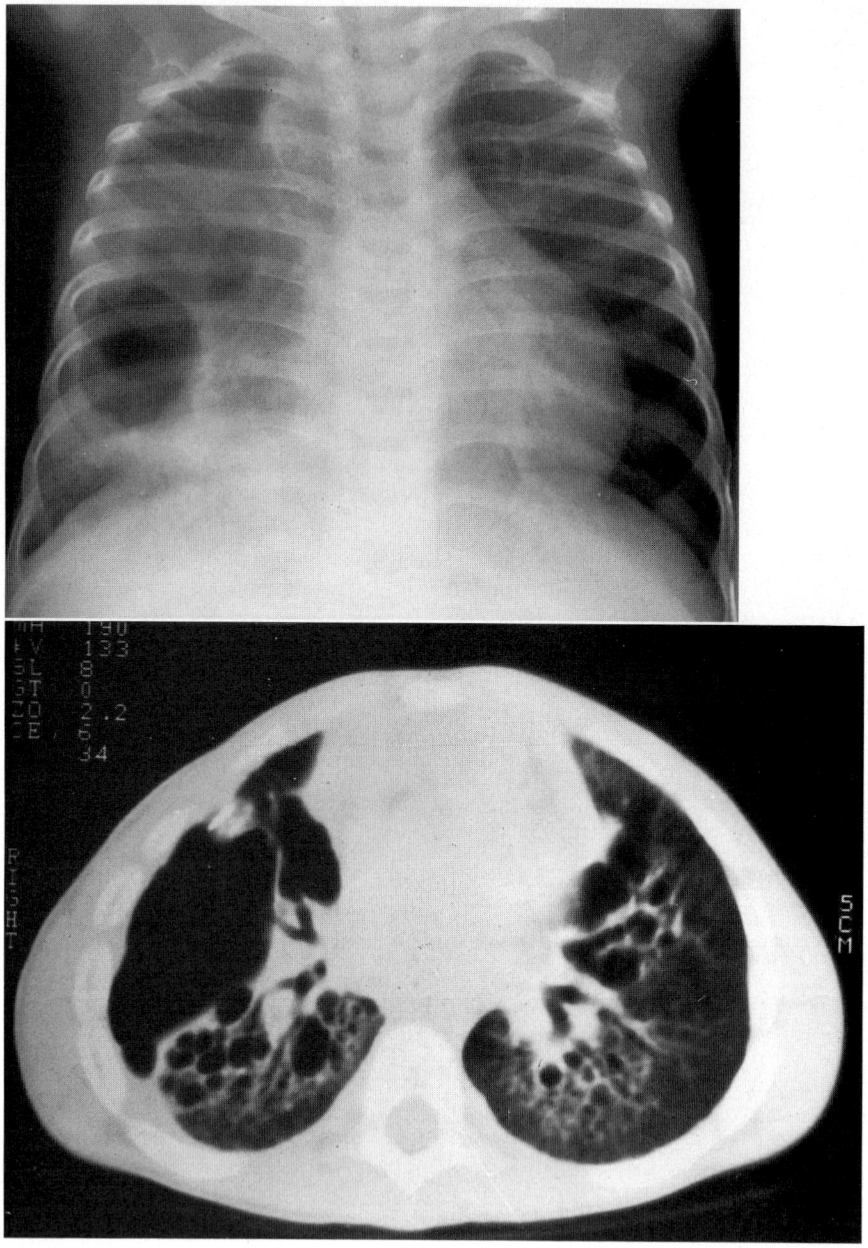

**FIGURE 6** Cavitary lung disease. This 3-year-old child presented with increasing respiratory distress. *A,* A frontal view of the chest shows right-sided cavities. *B,* CT scan of the same patient shows the bilateral nature of the disease. Note the multiple cavities in the right side of the chest with a large cavity in the periphery. This would be consistent with a loculated pneumothorax as well.

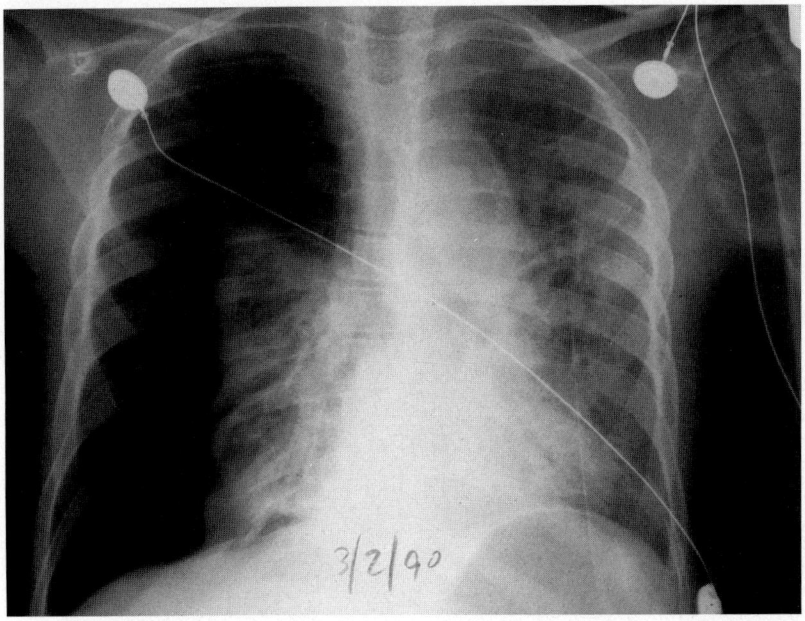


**FIGURE 7** Pneumothorax. This 6-year-old patient presented with recurrent pneumothoraces. Note the multiple cysts and cavities in the left side of the hemithorax. On the right side there is a significant pneumothorax with complete collapse of the right lung. Inside the collapsed right lung, one notices cystic cavities as well.

The precise mechanism for underlying formation of these cavities or pneumatoceles is not known. Various theories include localized pulmonary emphysema distal to a transient bronchial obstruction of a check valve type. Subpleural bleb formation, which coexists with intraparenchymal collections, results from the rupture of alveolar walls with extravasation of air into the interstitial spaces. Or, the pneumatoceles may be a result of an inflammatory process contributing to the destruction of the alveolar walls, allowing the release of air into the interstitium.

Since pneumothoraces and pneumatoceles are both the consequence of PCP, this would imply that a single pathophysiologic mechanism may underly both phenomena. Pneumothorax could result from rupture of a pneumatocele (Fig. 7). Certain characteristics of children with AIDS presenting with PCP could be predisposing factors to the development of pulmonary interstitial emphysema (PIE) and subsequent pneumatoceles or pneumothoraces. These include the relative chronicity of symptoms before admission, as well as the prevalence and severity of cough. The chronicity of the disease process allows for an increase in the number of activated macrophages known to produce elastase, which could play a role in altering the alveolar wall integrity and predispose to the rupture that is postulated with PIE. The abundant intra-alveolar *Pneumocystis* organisms and connective tissue proliferation could act as a check valve in causing an obstruction as well.

## Parotid Enlargement

Parotid enlargement in association with HIV infection has been found in both adults and children. In children with this malady sonograms reveal many small hypoechoic areas suggestive of lymphoid infiltration (Fig. 8). Large anechoic areas, suggesting lymphoepithelial cysts, may also be present. The lesions probably represent generalized lymphoid infiltration, similar to that type of infiltration seen in the lung. In fact, many of our patients had radiologic evidence of pulmonary lymphoid hyperplasia. Many of the children with parotid enlargement who had immunologic studies were sinotypically HLA-DR5, an immunophenotype associated with improved immune response occurring in less than one of four persons in the normal population. It suggests that painless enlargement may be a good prognostic sign in HIV-positive children. Parotid enlargement is found in about 10 percent of all children infected with HIV. Occasionally one observes calcifications in these parotid cysts (Fig. 9).

## Renal Disease

As many as 40 percent of children with HIV infection have been reported to have abnormal urinalyses; however, significant renal disease occurs in a much smaller number of patients. The prevalence rate of renal disease is approximately 7.7 percent. This is similar to the incidence of parenchymal renal disease complicating HIV infection in adults. Drug toxicities, fluid and electrolyte abnormalities, or septic complications also affect renal function in these patients.

The characteristic renal complication in these children is called HIV-associated nephropathy. It is characterized clinically by heavy proteinuria, mild hypertension, and often the development of nephrotic syndrome with hypoalbuminemia and edema. In both adults and children, the kidneys are typically large and highly echogenic by ultrasonographic evaluation (Fig. 10). Pathologically one sees characteristic glomerular focal sclerosis and capillary collapse. There are tubular and interstitial lesions with this disorder, suggesting that it is really a global disorder of the kidneys. These children often have a rapidly downhill course towards renal failure with end-stage renal disease developing within two years of the diagnosis of the renal disease.

The pathogenesis of renal disease in children with AIDS is not known, but circulating immune complexes that are known to occur in these patients may be involved. The HIV antigen (p24) has been demonstrated by monoclonal antibodies, and HIV nucleic acid has been demonstrated by in situ hybridiza-

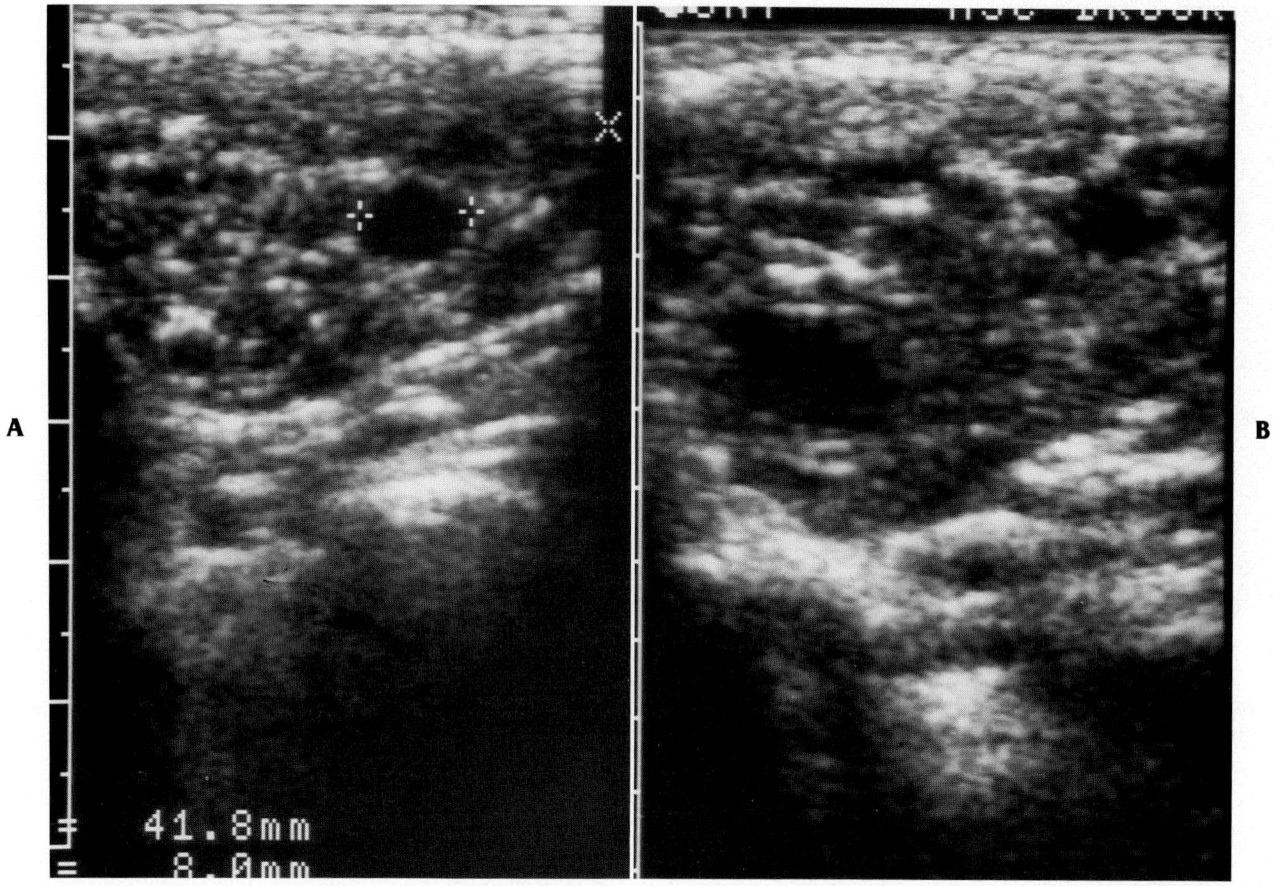


**FIGURE 8** Parotid enlargement. *A,* Enlarged right parotid gland showing multiple small hypoechoic regions in the parotid gland with one large cyst in the center. *B,* The left parotid gland showed more of the larger cysts with lots of small hypoechoic areas scattered throughout the gland.

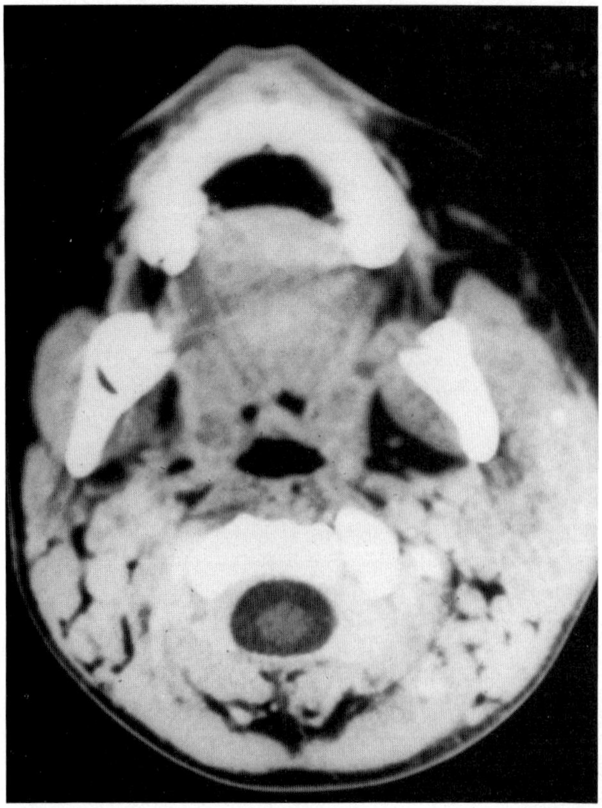

**FIGURE 9** Parotid enlargement. This child presented with left parotid enlargement. A CT scan of the face shows the left parotid enlargement with a calcific focus in the center of the left parotid gland.

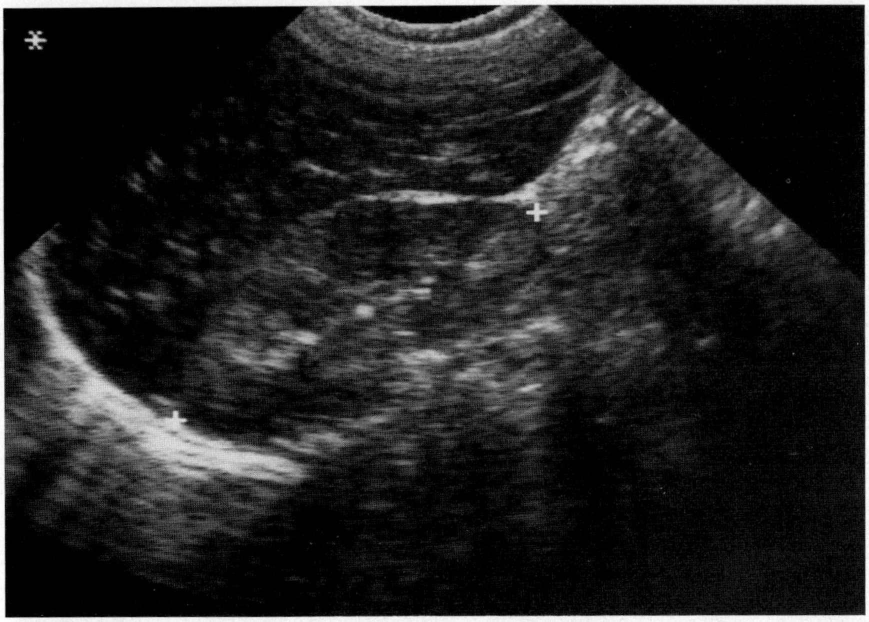

**FIGURE 10** HIV nephropathy. This 10-year-old girl was having a sonogram of her liver, and an echogenic amorphous kidney was noted in the right upper quadrant. Note the increased echogenicity of the renal cortex and note as well some foci of increased echogenicity, possibly representing a previous infection.

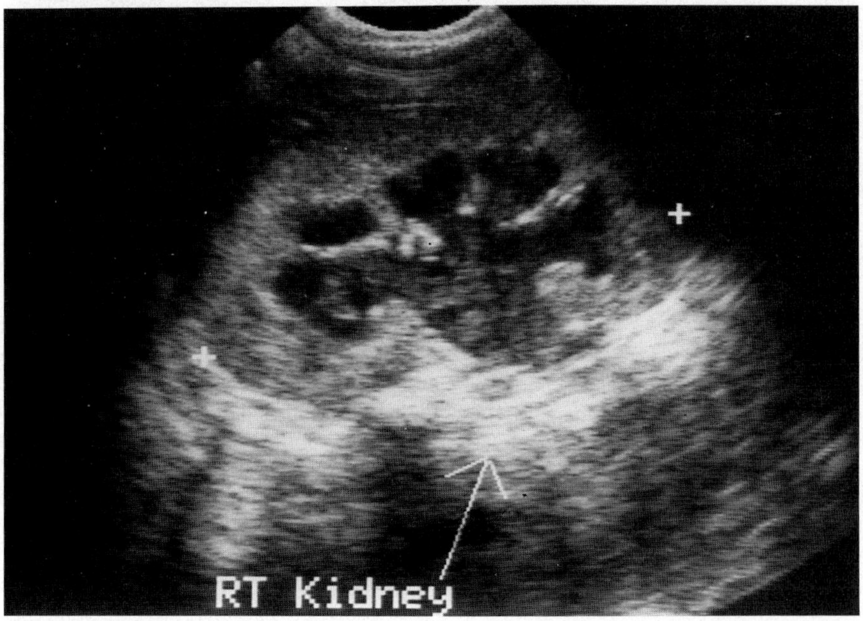


**FIGURE 11** Renal candidiasis. The echogenic kidney displays echogenic debris in the hydronephrotic pelvis and the right upper and lower pole calyx. *Candida* was cultured from the urine.

tion in the tubular glomerular epithelial cells in biopsy specimens of adults with AIDS-associated renal disease. This suggests the possibility of a direct pathogenic role of HIV.

Other imaging findings of the kidney include tiny echogenic foci that may be due to visceral calcification caused by a host of pathogenic organisms. These include extrapulmonary *P. carinii, Mycobacterium avium-intracellulare* (MAI), and other necrotizing viral infections, causing hemorrhage and subsequent calcium deposition. Finally, one sees the effects of frank infection of the kidney, causing swollen hydronephrotic kidneys, due to *Candida albicans,* with debris in the kidney or localized abscesses of the kidney parenchyma (Fig. 11). Abscesses in and around the bony pelvis, causing displacement of the bladder, have also been found.

## Central Nervous System

Complications develop in the central nervous system (CNS) in a significant number of patients with AIDS. HIV exhibits both lymphotropism and neurotropism. This dual attraction may be the result of surface antigen similarities between T lymphocytes and brain cells, particularly oligodendrocytes.

The complications include HIV encephalopathy and a variety of opportunistic infections and neoplasms. Neurologic dysfunction has been estimated to be in the range of one-third of cases. The aforementioned complications are seen much more frequently in adults than in children. The nonfocal dementing process, a result of brain infection with HIV, occurs both in adults and children and is one of the most frequent complications observed.

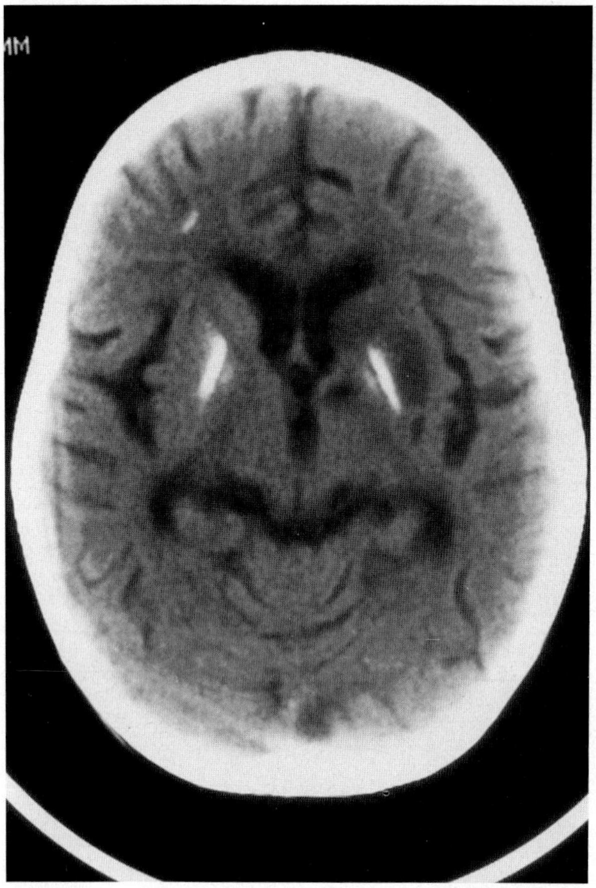


**FIGURE 12** HIV encephalopathy. This 8-year-old HIV-positive boy received a CT scan for failure to thrive. The midlevel of the brain shows the increased CSF spaces noted around the brain and Sylvian fissures. The area around the midbrain shows dilatation as well. Also of note are regions of necrosis lateral to the third ventricle in the thalamus. Calcification in the basal ganglia and brain parenchyma is seen superiorly in the right frontal lobe.

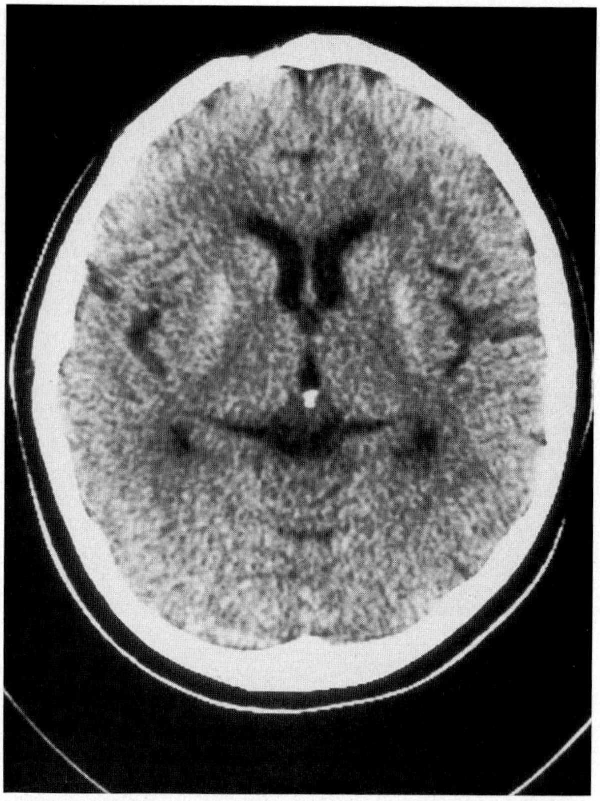

**FIGURE 13** Basal ganglia calcification. This 4-year-old boy had a CT scan for failure to thrive. Note the increased attenuation in the region of the basal ganglia. The child had calcification in the region of the pineal gland as well. The child was later discovered to be HIV positive.

Pathologically the findings of HIV encephalopathy include microglial, multinucleated giant cells and abnormalities of the white matter, most commonly diffuse myelin pallor. One finds these most frequently with magnetic resonance imaging (MRI), best appreciated on T2-weighted spin-echo images, as non–mass-producing, ill-defined, and diffuse or confluent patches of increased signal intensity in the deep white matter of the cerebral hemispheres, predominately the frontal lobes. Also, enlarged cerebrospinal fluid (CSF) spaces have been noted. These are similar to those noted in anorexia nervosa, alcoholism, and steroid therapy and are thought to be, in part, related to changes in water content (Fig. 12). The nutritional state, or state of hydration of the patient, often plays a role. Another finding is basal ganglia calcification (Fig. 13). The calcifications are found in and adjacent to blood vessel walls and may be present, in most cases, at the microscopic level.

The incidence of mass lesions from infections such as cytomegalovirus (CMV), toxoplasmosis, or TB is much lower than in similar series of adult patients. Lymphoma is the most common neoplasm associated with HIV. Lymphoma of the CNS is, however, not uncommon. It appears that in children with AIDS, systemic lymphoid lesions, including follicular hyperplasia of lymph nodes and intestinal submucosa, PLH/LIP complex, and malignant lymphoma are a spectrum. Many of these lesions may be related to Epstein-Barr virus (EBV), since the EBV genome has been demonstrated in lung tissue and in tissue derived from primary malignant lymphoma of the brain in children with AIDS. Synergism between HIV and EBV also may be involved in pathogenesis of these lymphoid lesions. (Many children with parotid enlargement are EBV positive as well.)

Infection with *Mycobacterium tuberculosis* is a common complication of HIV infection among groups with a high prevalence of TB. We have seen an increase in CNS complications as a result of TB. Approximately half of the patients have pulmonary infiltrates at the time of presentation. The clinical signs of tuberculous meningitis include fever, headache, and altered consciousness. CT findings include areas of edema and enhanced brain tissue, as well as focal tuberculomas (Fig. 14). The findings are observed even during therapy of TB. These cases are considered breakthrough TB.

## Gastrointestinal Tract

Many of the gastrointestinal (GI) complications of AIDS are related to the numerous opportunistic infections that occur in these patients and may affect the GI tract at different sites. Although these infectious agents also affect the normal population, in the AIDS population the infections tend to be more severe, difficult to irradicate, and will relapse.

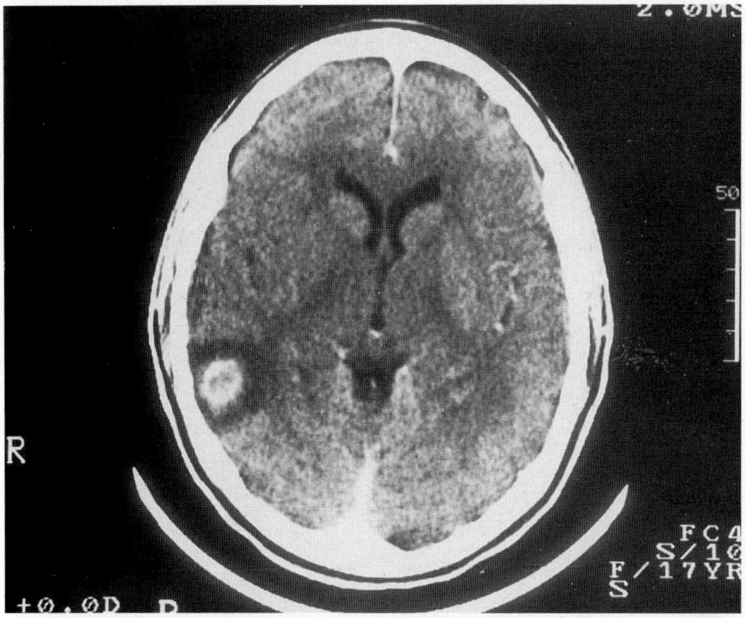


**FIGURE 14** Tuberculosis. A CT scan of the brain in this 5-year-old child showed an area of contrast enhancement in the right parieto-occipital region of the brain. An area of edema surrounds this "ring" lesion. The child had a positive spinal tap for tuberculosis.

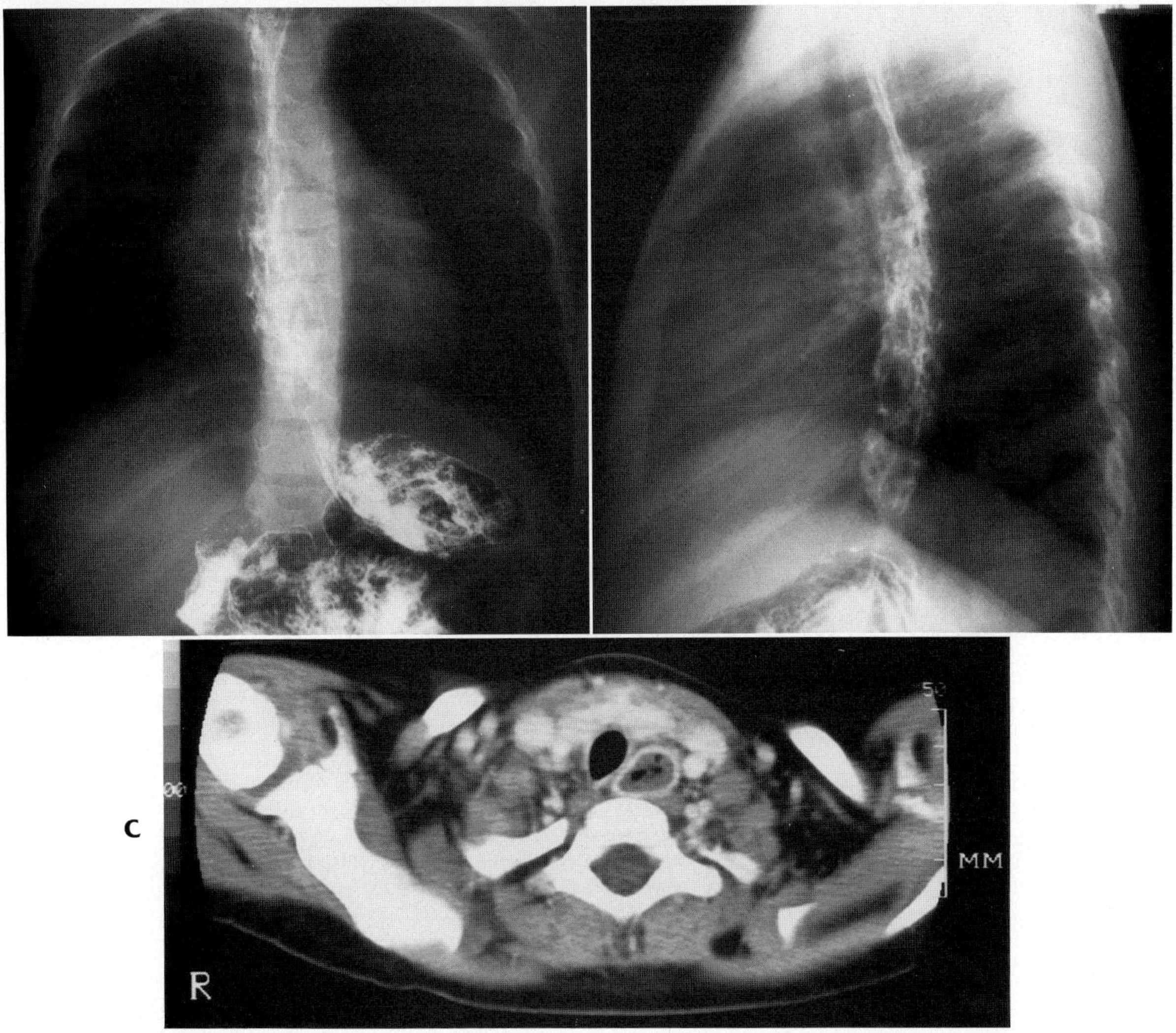


**FIGURE 15** Esophagitis. This 2-year-old child was noted to have oral herpangina and increased density behind the heart on a routine chest radiograph. Frontal *(A)* and lateral *(B)* views of barium swallow shows multiple irregularities in the esophageal lumen. There are spiculations and ulcer craters consistent with esophagitis. The offending organism was herpes simplex virus. *C,* A CT scan of the neck in this patient shows a markedly dilated esophagus with scattered air in the center and thickened mucosa surrounding the air.

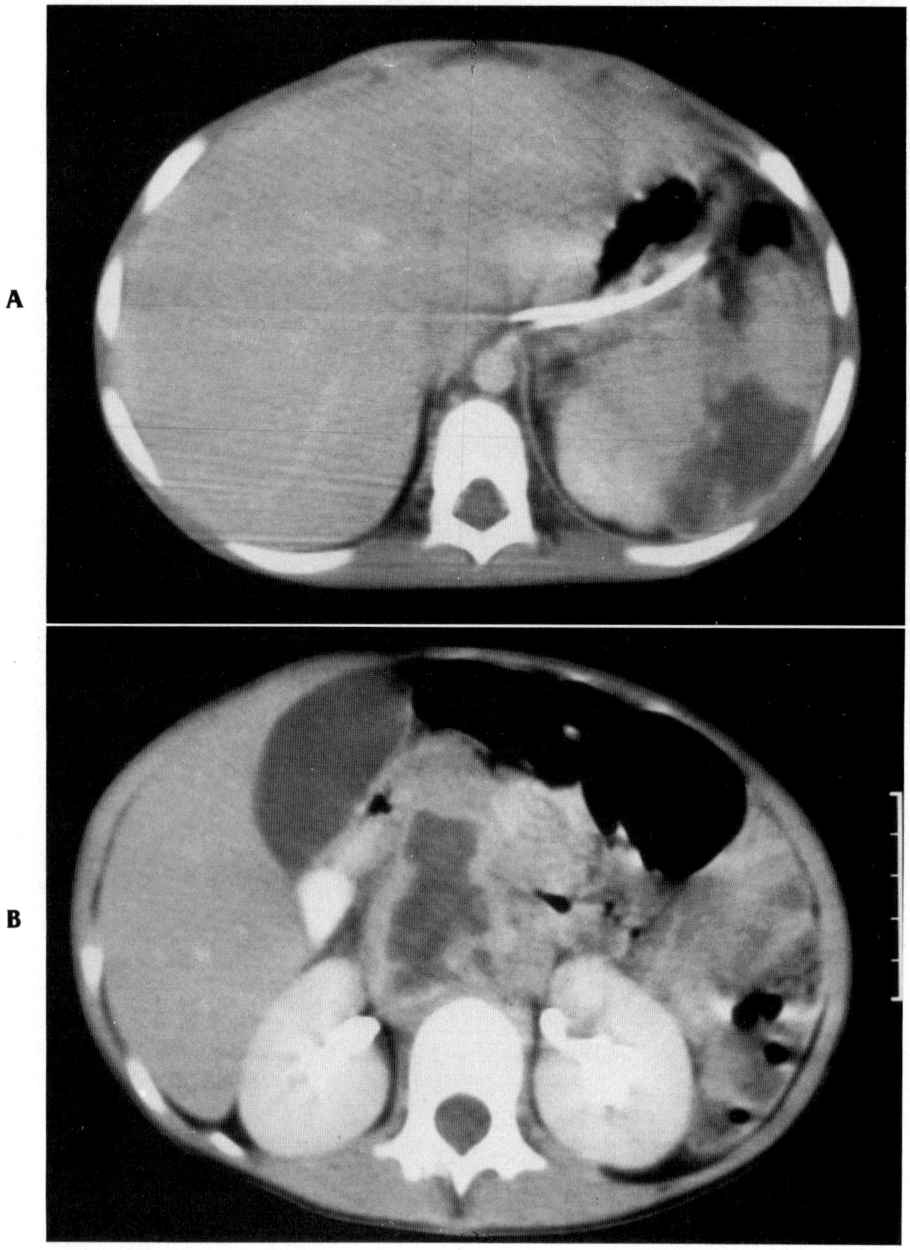


**FIGURE 16** *M. tuberculosis* infection: two cases. *A,* Splenic abscess. This child presented with left upper quadrant pain and fever and known HIV infection. A CT scan of the upper abdomen shows a large low-attenuation lesion in the spleen with a drain observed anteriorly. *M. tuberculosis* was cultured from this splenic abscess. *B,* This 6-year-old child presented with midabdominal pain and fever. A CT scan of the midabdomen shows low-attenuation lesions in the spleen, as well as a large central mass in the retroperitoneal region with low-attenuation foci observed in the center. This is consistent with splenic abscesses and necrotic low-attenuation lymph nodes centrally. *M. tuberculosis* was cultured.

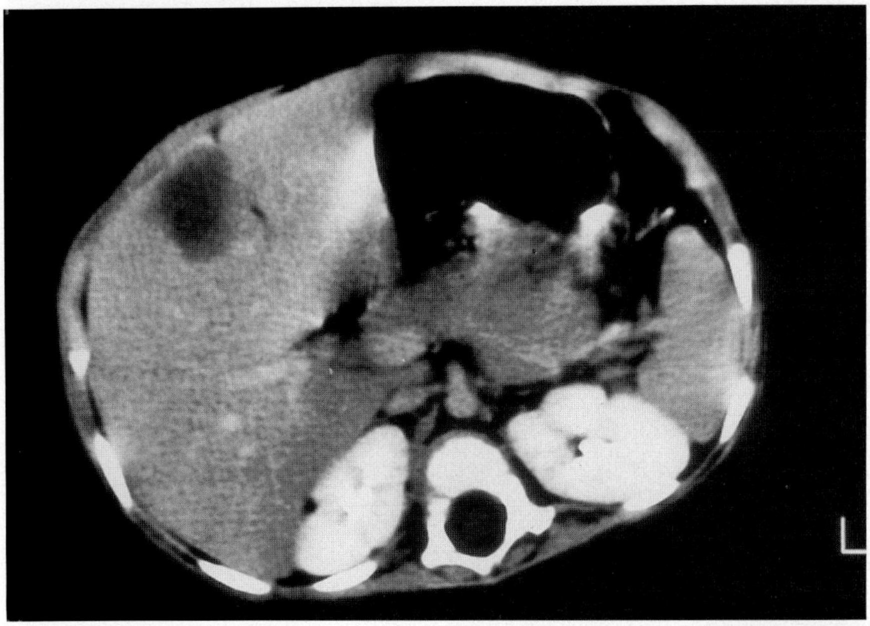

**FIGURE 17** Leiomyosarcoma. This 4-year-old child with known HIV infection was noted to have a low-attenuation lesion in the liver on a CT scan of the upper abdomen. (The child was studied for lymph nodes noted in the groin and axilla.) At biopsy, the low-attenuation lesion was determined to be a leiomyosarcoma.

The most common oral infection is candidiasis. CMV and herpes simplex virus (HSV) are also frequent infectious agents that cause esophagitis.

Esophagitis can be readily diagnosed on barium swallow by demonstration of ulcer craters, spiculation, and strictures (Fig. 15). This method, however, is not as sensitive or as specific as endoscopy with biopsy.

Diarrhea caused by common bacterial pathogens including *Salmonella, Shigella,* and *Campylobacter,* has been reported. MAI is a rare enteric pathogen in children, but it may cause enteritis in patients with AIDS. The infections seem to originate in the lungs and GI tract, and the presentation is usually with diarrhea, malabsorption of fat, and enlargement of mesenteric lymph nodes. *Mycobacterium tuberculosis* is also associated with enteritis in children as is giardiasis. The presence of focal visceral lesions and low-attenuation lymph nodes suggests disseminated *M. tuberculosis* (Fig. 16), whereas marked hepatic and splenic enlargement, diffuse jejunal wall thickening, and enlarged soft-tissue density lymph nodes suggest disseminated MAI. These are most easily recognized on CT scans. Marked hepatic and splenic enlargement is typical of MAI infection, while solid abdominal viscera involvement is more frequent in patients with MTB. Enlarged lymph nodes are typical for both groups of patients. Abnormalities observed in patients with AIDS include malignancy such as leiomyosarcoma, Kaposi's sarcoma, and lymphoma (Fig. 17). Infectious cholangitis from CMV or cryptosporidia produces morphologic changes, similar to sclerosing cholangitis. Intussusception should also be considered in patients with AIDS in the setting of acute abdominal pain. We have also noted pneumatosis, perforation of the bowel, and increased incidence of necrotizing enterocolitis in patients with HIV infection (Fig. 18).

Proctitis is unusual in children and is more likely to be observed in adolescent homosexual males.

Malignancy is rare in children, occurring in only 1 percent of patients less than 15 years of age with AIDS. Intestinal lymphoma is rare in the normal population and is similarly rare in AIDS patients. It is usually advanced at presentation and frequently of the B-cell type.

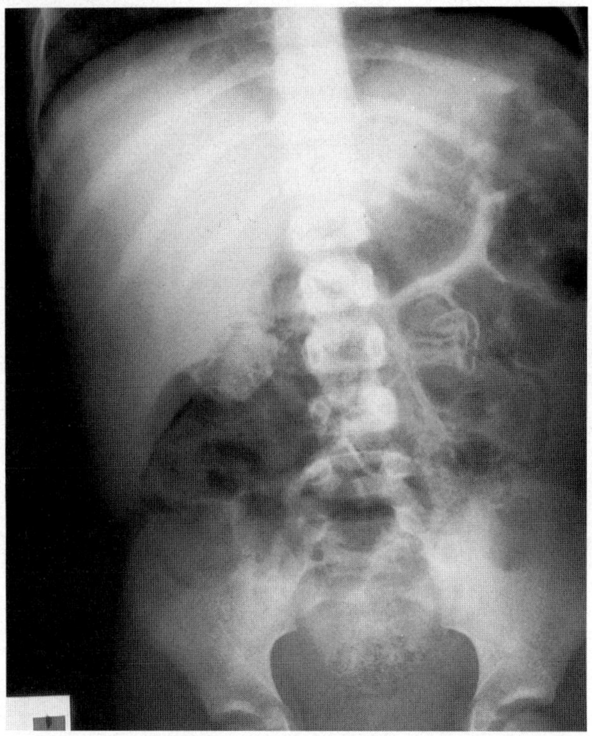

**FIGURE 18** Pneumatosis intestinalis. This child with HIV infection was noted to have abdominal abnormalities that were detected on the chest radiograph. A subsequent radiograph of the abdomen shows multiple linear lucencies scattered throughout the bowel consistent with pneumatosis intestinalis. The child was asymptomatic, referable to this, and the lucencies subsequently resolved spontaneously.

## Cardiac Disease

Cardiac involvement was initially thought to be clinically silent. Cases describing cardiac disease in adult patients infected with the AIDS virus were first reported in 1984. There have been multiple reports describing myocardial dysfunction, dilated cardiomyopathy, myocarditis, pericardial effusion, nonbacte-

A

B

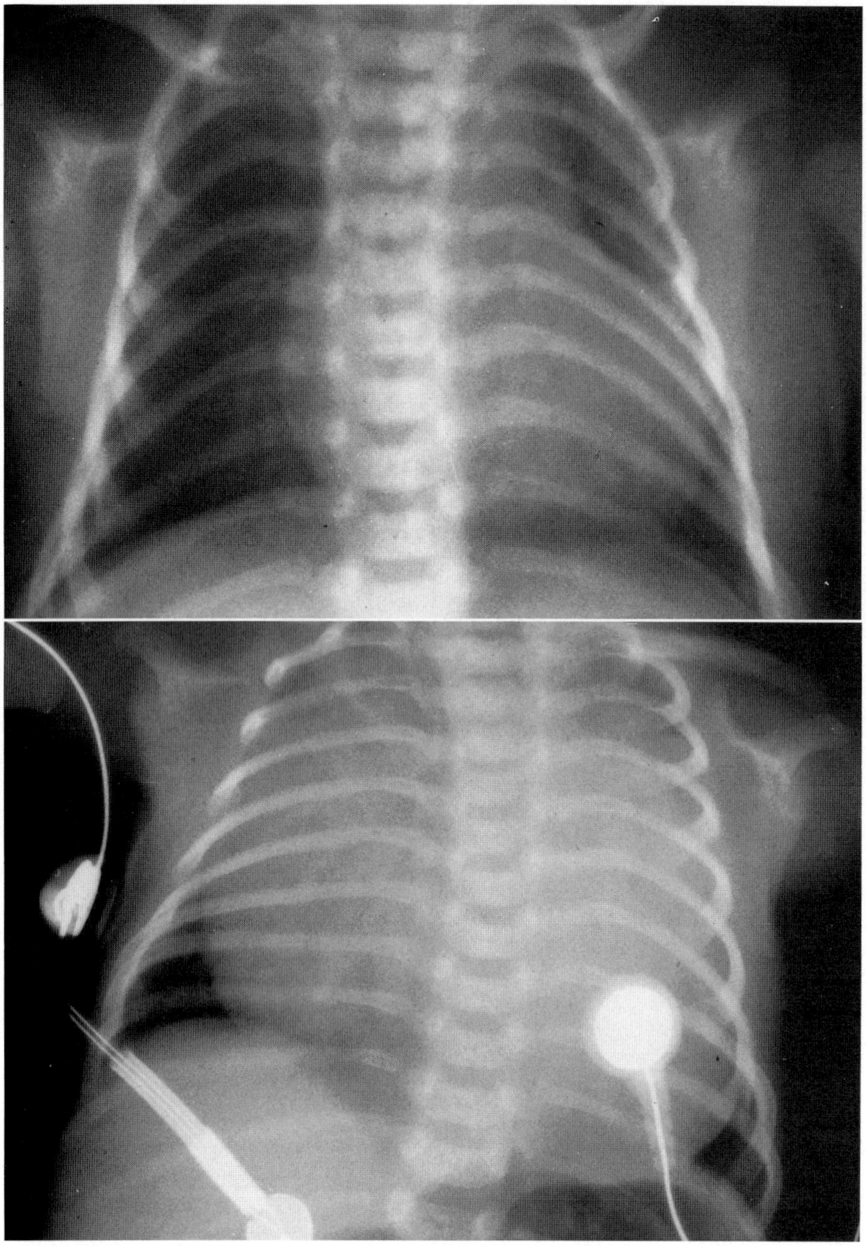

**FIGURE 19** AIDS cardiomyopathy. *A*, Frontal view of the chest of a newborn whose mother was HIV positive. The radiograph is essentially normal. *B*, Six months later, the child was noted to have increasing respiratory distress and marked cardiomegaly. A large pericardial effusion was diagnosed by echocardiography, and the AIDS virus was recovered from the aspirate.

rial endocarditis, infarction, and direct infectious and neoplastic involvement of the heart in adults with AIDS.

Recent studies suggest that cardiac dysfunction in children infected with HIV may be extensive and clinically significant. The paucity of reports dealing with this subject may be in part a result of the difficulty in identifying cardiac dysfunction in children whose signs and symptoms caused by non-cardiac causes mimic the signs of heart failure.

A retrospective evaluation was performed of all pediatric AIDS patients who had a pericardial effusion at postmortem or at echocardiography. We investigated the relationship of pericardial effusion to cardiac dysfunction in the hopes of defining a group of patients who would be at a high risk for cardiac disease.

When we evaluated children with AIDS, we found that the radiographic findings were often misleading. One-half of our patients had a normal cardiac silhouette, yet had a pericardial effusion. In two children pericardial effusion was documented by CT done for evaluation of pulmonary pathology. Our limited study suggested that in any child with AIDS and a pleural effusion and/or ascites, there may be a high risk of cardiac abnormalities and pericardial effusion. Although it is well known that a pericardial effusion can be present in a child with a normal cardiac silhouette, the frequency with which this occurs in children with AIDS should raise the radiologist's index of suspicion, especially in a child who is refractory to pulmonary therapy. Certainly when cardiac enlargement is detected on routine chest radiography in a child with AIDS (Fig. 19), or when there is a suspicion of heart disease, even with a normal cardiac silhouette, echocardiography should be recommended. A prospective study would be needed to verify (1) the association of pleural effusion and ascites with cardiac disease in these children and (2) the exact prevalence of the cardiac disease.

## Suggested Reading

Ambrosino MM, Genieser NB, Krasinski K, et al. Opportunistic infections and tumors in immunocompromised children. Radiol Clin North Am 1992; 30:639–659.

Chadwick EG, Conner EG, Guerra-Hanson JC, et al. Tumors of smooth muscle origin in pediatric HIV-infected children: An association of AIDS and cancer. J Am Med Assoc 1990; 263:3182–3185.

Jeffrey RB Jr. Abdominal imaging in the immunocompromised patient. Radiol Clin North Am 1992; 30:579–595.

Joshi VV. Pathology of childhood AIDS. Pediatr Clin North Am 1991; 38:97–120.

Mast HL, Haller JO, Schiller MS. Pericardial effusion and its relationship to cardiac disease in children with AIDS. Pediatr Radiol (in press).

New York City Department of Health AIDS Surveillance Unit. AIDS surveillance update. February 28, 1990.

Price DB, Inglese CM, Jacob J, et al. Pediatric AIDS: Neuroradiologic and neurodevelopmental findings. Pediatr Radiol 1988; 18:445–448.

Reeders JWAJ, Bartelsman JFWM, Antonides HR, Tytgat GNJ. The spectrum of gastrointestinal radiology in AIDS. Eur Radiol 1991; 1:33–45.

Zimmerman BL, Haller JO, Price AP, et al. Children with AIDS—is pathologic diagnosis possible based on chest radiographs. Pediatr Radiol 1987; 17:303–307.

# Pediatric Brain Imaging: Postinfancy

*WILLIAM S. BALL, Jr., M.D. · SPYROS S. KOLLIAS, M.D.*

The past 10 years have witnessed the evolution and transformation of pediatric neuroradiology into a complex subspecialty, encompassing a wide variety of diseases and pathologic processes that involve the central nervous system (CNS) in children. Diagnostic radiology has always required neuroradiologists to be both flexible and adaptive in their approach. The modern radiologist must be familiar with the application and practical use of the variety of modalities currently available. An individualized case-by-case approach must incorporate these modalities in an integrated fashion to obtain the appropriate diagnostic information in a concise and economically efficient manner. The term *integration,* as defined by the *American Heritage Dictionary,* means the "combining of different acts so that they cooperate towards a common end." By incorporating technically dissimilar modalities, each according to its own strengths, in a singular effort, we are practicing an integrated approach to radiologic diagnosis. Diagnostic radiology in children especially benefits from such an approach to guide and select appropriate therapy.

In the first 10 years of life, a spectrum of pathologic processes may influence the developing brain. Most common within the first decade are developmental, inflammatory, neoplastic, traumatic, and metabolic/toxic processes involving the CNS. Although these categories in no way represent the entire subject of pediatric neuroradiology, they do represent the most common entities encountered in the busy practices of today.

## Developmental Processes

Developmental delay of brain formation and/or maturation can be a result of genetic, inflammatory, metabolic/toxic, or environmental influences occurring during either prenatal or postnatal brain development. The clinical expression of such influences may vary and includes failure to thrive, mental retardation, cerebral palsy, microcephaly, isolated motor deficits, seizures, or neurocognitive delay. In children older than one year referred for evaluation, the role of imaging is to estimate the extent of injury, attempt to identify a cause, determine whether or not a congenital malformation is present that might predict the genetic expression of the disorder, indicate whether or not therapeutic intervention is warranted, and to follow the patient and document progression when present.

To accomplish these goals requires a modality that is sensitive to anatomic detail and is capable of also assessing brain maturation. Whereas computed tomography (CT) may be required to evaluate anomalies of the bony calvarium (e.g., craniosynostosis), we believe magnetic resonance imaging (MRI) is the best modality to analyze the soft-tissue structure of the brain. Since our first efforts should be in detecting the presence or absence of structural abnormalities, we initially rely on T1-weighted imaging obtained in multiple orthogonal planes. All imaging is performed in a standard send/receive head coil, preferably quadrature in design. The initial sequence should be in the sagittal projection with parameters selected to provide superior anatomic resolution (TR = 500-800 msec, TE = 10-20 msec, 256 × 192 matrix, 2-4 excitations, 5 mm thickness, 1-1.5 mm gap). The sagittal projection is useful in detecting many common congenital midline anomalies involving the corpus callosum, limbic system, hypothalamic/pituitary axis, and cerebellum. This sequence is then followed by T1-weighted imaging in either the axial or coronal projections, or both, as necessary. To assess white and gray matter development, a T2-weighted sequence in the axial projection is performed after the T1-weighted sequences. The most sensitive pulse sequence for detecting subtle abnormalities in T2 relaxation in the brain is spin echo (SE) (TR = 2,500-3,000 msec, TE = 20-40 msec and 90-110 msec, 8 kHz variable bandwidth, 256 × 192 matrix, 1-2 excitations, 5 mm thickness, 1.5 mm gap). To reduce pulsation artifact from inflowing blood with this sequence, we frequently add an inferior saturation pulse centered in the neck and/or routinely apply a refocusing gradient, such as gradient moment nulling (Flow Compensation, GE Signa). More recently, fast spin-echo (FSE) techniques have become readily available. Although these techniques are not as sensitive as conventional SE to alterations in T2 relaxation, they are useful in reducing the scan time, which is important in the sedated child. A typical FSE sequence includes: TR = 2,500 msec, effective TE's = 17 msec/119 msec, 8 echo trains (split between 17 and 119 msec), 256 × 192 matrix, 1-2 excitations. A high TR of 4,000 msec, recommended in adults, reduces the contrast differentiation between white and gray matter to such an extent that they are not recommended for use in children. Finally, gradient-echo techniques can also provide T2 weighting in the form of T2*-weighted images. To accomplish this we use TR = 400-600 msec, TE's = 15-20 msec/30-35 msec, flip angle = 20°, and 4-6 excitations. The need for gradient acquisition T2-weighted sequences has declined with the development of FSE techniques. This sequence can, however, be highly useful in detecting the susceptibility effect of calcification or hemosiderin. Contrast enhancement with gadolinium is generally not indicated in the routine evaluation of developmental abnormalities in children. However, when the child is suspected of having one of the phakomatoses as a cause of their maldevelopment, gadolinium is useful to search for the vascular and neoplastic complications of these disorders.

As with all pediatric radiology, the key to recognizing "abnormal" lies first in our complete familiarity with "normal." Alterations in development may manifest as partial or complete absence of structures such as the corpus callosum or cerebellum, anomalous formation and/or migration of gray matter in the form of heterotopic migrational defects, loss of brain substance (either gray or white matter) from a previous destructive process, delay in the normal progress of myelination, or as abnormal signal in the white matter as a result of gliosis or demyelination. A systematic approach for evaluating the images yields the best results. We begin first in assessing the size and shape of the ventricles and the surrounding extra-axial fluid spaces. Small or normal-sized temporal horns, colpocephaly, anterior point of the lateral ventricles, a small or normal third ventricle, prominence of the extra-axial fluid spaces, and/or loss of gray or white matter volume in a normo- or microcephalic child should suggest dysmorphic or atrophic ventricular enlargement rather than obstructive hydrocephalus. Ventricular dysmorphism is most frequently the result of a remote developmental defect, often beginning in utero. Loss of brain substance ("atrophy") leading to secondary ventricular enlargement, on the other hand, is usually the result of injury which can begin either prenatally or postnatally. Next should be an evaluation for the presence of major structural abnormalities (e.g., dysgenesis of the corpus callosum, prosencephaly, schizencephaly, vermian-cerebellar hypoplasia), that indicate that an adverse event did indeed occur in utero (Fig. 1). The cortex should be evaluated for normal thickness and form, carefully observing its relationship to the underlying white matter (generally, each cortical gyrus should correspond to its own finger-like projection of white matter). Often abnormalities are best detected by the asymmetries they produce from one hemisphere to the other in the same patient. Next, the white matter is carefully evaluated for thickness and signal characteristics, which may vary normally with age. Finally, the scan should be carefully reviewed for the presence of a mass or mass effect, especially in children with neurofibromatosis or tuberous sclerosis. This process of evaluation should be repeated for both the infratentorial as well as the supratentorial structures. The majority of abnormalities can be identified, and necessary observations made, by using this approach, even if the reader is not an "expert" in pediatric neuroradiology.

## Inflammatory Processes

Inflammatory conditions affecting the brain in childhood may be divided generally into either infectious (e.g., meningitis, encephalitis, brain abscess) or para-inflammatory (e.g., collagen vascular, granulomatous angiitis, hepatic encephalopathy) in origin. The clinical presentation may, however, be similar for the two groups and include fever, changes in mentation, irritability, loss of consciousness, meningeal irritation, or seizures.

A 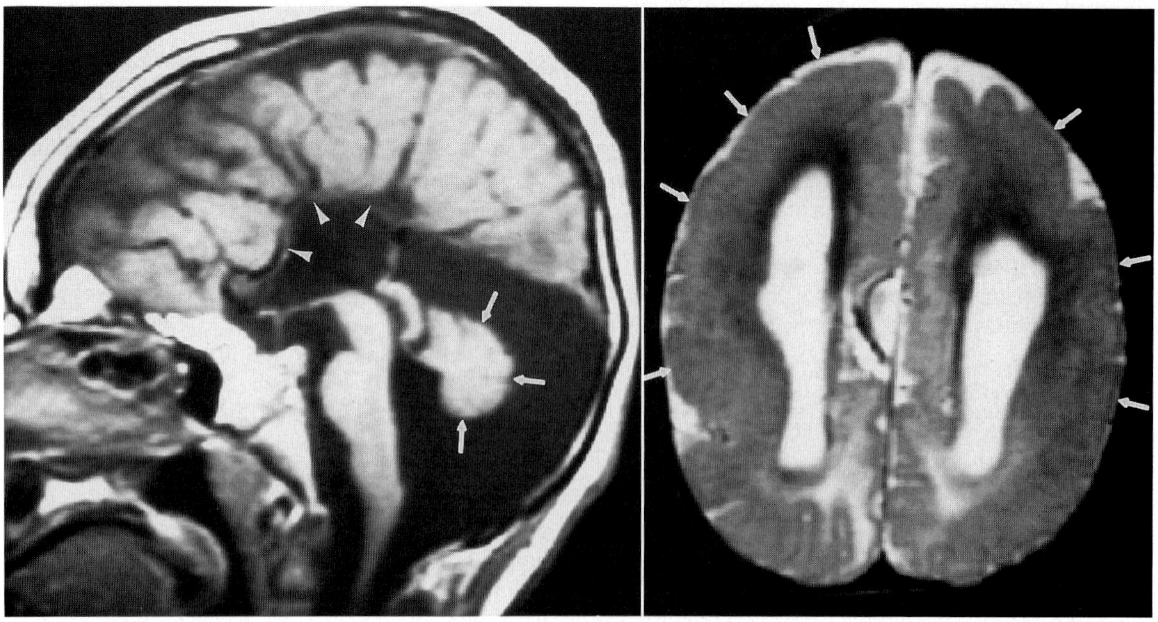 B

**FIGURE 1** A 4-year-old boy with multiple developmental abnormalities. *A,* Sagittal T1-weighted MR image shows absence of the corpus callosum with superior herniation of the third ventricle (*white arrowheads*). The posterior fossa is enlarged and the vermis is hypoplastic (*white arrows*), compatible with Dandy-Walker malformation. *B,* Axial T2-weighted MR image in the same patient reveals broad gyri in the frontoparietal regions bilaterally (*white arrows*), with thickening of the gray matter and thinning of the white matter, consistent with abnormal neuronal migration (pachygyria).

The diagnosis of meningitis is by lumbar puncture. Imaging is not routinely indicated, except to exclude a mass before lumbar puncture when there is clinical evidence of increased intracranial pressure (papilledema). For this purpose, a noncontrast CT scan often suffices. Cross-sectional imaging is indicated for the evaluation of the complications of meningitis, which may be suspected clinically by persistent fevers, seizures, focal neurologic deficits, or evidence of increased intracranial pressure. Both CT and MRI are acceptable for this purpose; however, MRI is more sensitive to the early parenchymal changes of infarction or cerebritis. Either modality requires contrast enhancement to visualize any breakdown in the blood-brain barrier from gyral infarction, cerebritis, or early abscess formation and to enhance the detection of vascular compromise in the form of venous sinus thrombosis. Cerebral abscess typically appears as a mass of low attenuation on CT or signal intensity on MRI with an enhancing peripheral rind. Subdural hygromas with or without dural enhancement are frequently encountered in uncomplicated meningitis, especially in young children. These collections represent a reactive transudate rather than an empyema. In general, reactive fluid cannot be differentiated from an empyema based on imaging findings alone. Only a subdural puncture with laboratory evaluation of the fluid is diagnostic. Nor does the presence of a subdural collection, found by imaging the patient, indicate the need for a subdural puncture, because of their frequent presence in uncomplicated meningitis.

The role of imaging in the child presenting with encephalitis is controversial. The diagnosis of encephalitis is by clinical evaluation, supported by either lumbar puncture or EEG. Imaging is useful in confirming the presence or absence of parenchymal involvement; however, rarely in children is the pattern specific for one particular etiologic agent versus another (e.g., herpes simplex virus). We believe the most sensitive means to evaluate a child suspected of having encephalitis is by contrast-enhanced MRI. T1-weighted imaging should be performed in at least two projections before and after administration of a contrast agent. For this purpose, we use SE T1-weighted imaging at TR = 600-800 msec, TE = <15 msec, and 2-4 excitations, to evaluate the entire brain from the craniocervical junction to the vertex. Routine T2-weighted imaging (TR = 2,500 msec, TE = 30-40/90-100 msec, 256 × 192 matrix, 8 kHz variable bandwidth, 1-2 excitations) is helpful for identifying alterations in brain water resulting from infarction or focal cerebritis.

Suspected parainflammatory conditions are best imaged with MRI. Routinely we employ both T1-weighted enhanced and T2-weighted SE imaging for this indication. The majority of these conditions present with focal or diffuse hyperintense signal changes in the cerebral white matter as a result of ischemia or active demyelination (Fig. 2). Rarely vasculitis appears as linear perivascular enhancement in the deep white matter. A more common pattern suggesting vasculitis consists of small multifocal brain lesions within the white matter of the centrum semiovale that indicate prominence of the perivascular spaces or lacunar infarctions. These generally do not enhance. Magnetic resonance angiography is useful in detecting associated large-vessel disease in suspected cases of vasculitis. Hyperintense signal on intermediate and T2-weighted images in the basal ganglia has been reported in association with hepatic encephalopathy. A similar appearance may be the result of hypoxia or ischemia, carbon monoxide poisoning, or Leigh's disease. There are no specific patterns that differentiate one parainflammatory process from another, and often differentiation of a parainflammatory condition from infectious encephalitis is not possible based on the findings on cross-sectional imaging.

## Neoplastic Processes

Infratentorial and supratentorial primary brain neoplasms occur with equal frequency in children of all ages; however,

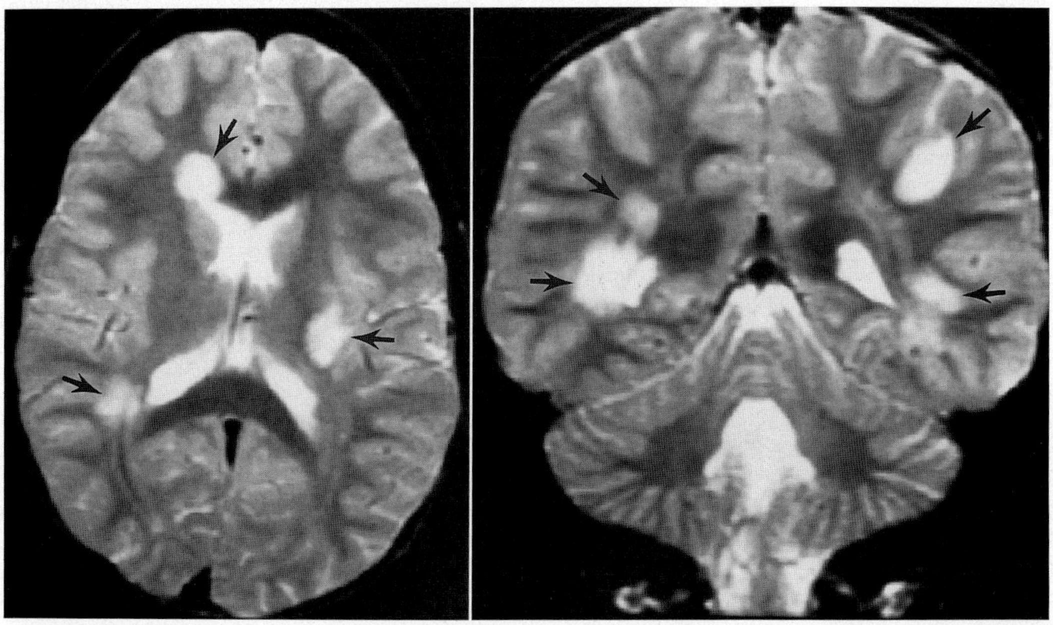


**FIGURE 2** A 6-year-old boy with parainfectious encephalitis. Axial (*A*) and coronal (*B*) T2-weighted MR images show multiple foci of increased signal intensity involving the subcortical and periventricular white matter (*black arrows*), representing focal areas of demyelination, in this patient with a clinical history of viral illness approximately 10 days before this scan.

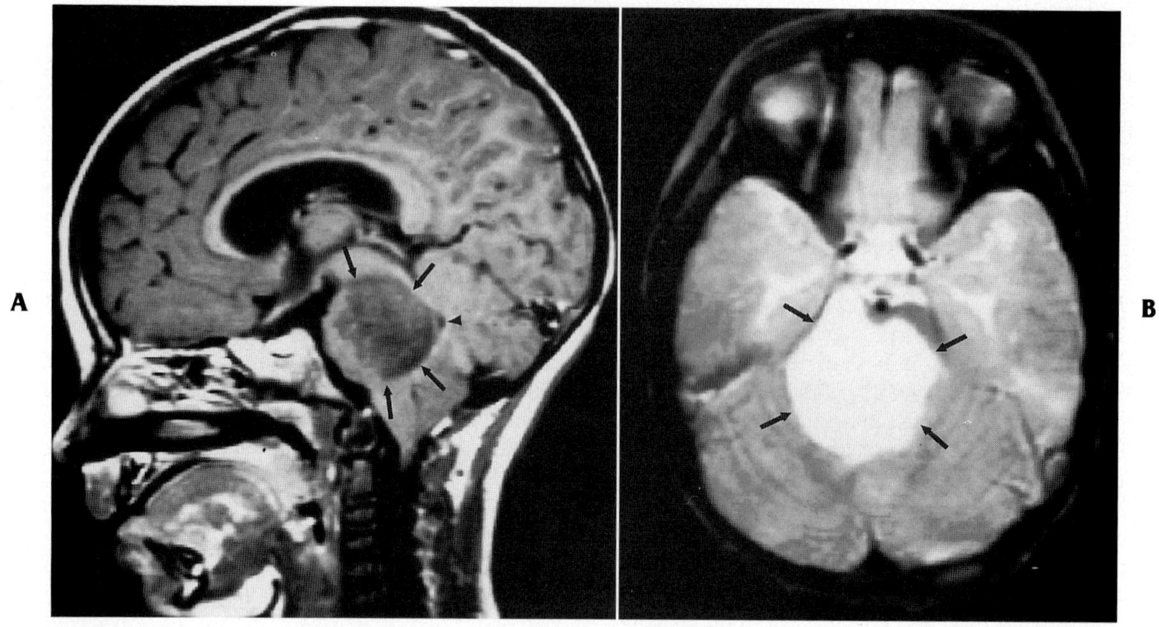

**FIGURE 3** A 2-year-old girl with brain stem glioma. *A,* Sagittal contrast-enhanced T1-weighted MR image shows a large hypointense mass, expanding the pons (*black arrows*) and compressing the fourth ventricle posteriorly (*black arrowhead*). There is no significant contrast enhancement. *B,* On axial T2-weighted MRI the mass is homogeneous, of high signal intensity, intrinsic to the pontine region (*black arrowheads*), and extends dorsally between the compressed cerebellar hemispheres without causing significant edema.

infratentorial tumors are generally more frequent between the ages of 2 to 6 years. The evidence is clear that MRI is the method of choice for the evaluation and diagnosis of tumors arising below the tentorium. A standard protocol can be adopted for the evaluation of most posterior fossa tumors involving the brain stem, cerebellum, and/or extra-axial compartment. Sagittal T1-weighted images are an essential part of the protocol, since many tumors involve midline structures. Separation of lesions in the brain stem from those involving the fourth ventricle and/or cerebellar vermis is best accomplished in this projection. Information required for the presurgical staging of tumor includes determination of the superior or inferior extent of tumor, detecting extra-axial growth of tumor (important, as for example, with detecting exophytic brain stem gliomas that may require surgical resection), and resolving the relationship of the mass to surrounding normal structures. T2-weighted images are helpful to categorize the subtype of tumor and judge the extent of involvement. Gradient acquisition imaging (TR = 30-35 msec, TE = 8-10 msec, flip angle = 10°, 4-6 excitations) can be used to detect calcification within the tumor, seen as irregular areas of signal void. The detection of calcification may be useful to differentiate one type of tumor (e.g., ependymoma) from another (e.g., medulloblastoma). Contrast enhancement with gadolinium may make the tumor more conspicuous and better separate it from normal adjacent structures, but in our experience it is not helpful in differentiating the histologic type or aggressiveness of the posterior fossa neoplasm.

Brain stem gliomas are the most common tumor involving the midbrain, pons, or medulla in children (Fig. 3). They are identified foremost by their characteristic location. Medulloblastomas arise in the midline from either the inferior (most common) or superior medullary velum in the roof of the fourth ventricle. From there, they frequently grow into and obstruct the fourth ventricle. Ependymomas, on the other hand, can arise from any ependymal surface, but most commonly they arise from the floor or lateral recesses of the fourth ventricle. Differentiation of the two based on location, extent of tumor, and signal characteristics is possible with MRI. Cerebellar astrocytomas grow from either the vermis or hemispheres of the cerebellum and therefore can be midline, posterior to the fourth ventricle, or eccentric and lateral to the fourth ventricle. The majority of these tumors are macrocystic and enhance after gadolinium administration (Fig. 4). Solid astrocytomas can arise from either the vermis of the cerebellum or from the cerebellar hemisphere.

Supratentorial neoplasms in children arise most commonly in the suprasellar/sellar and pineal regions or from the cerebral hemispheres. Each region may require a slightly different diagnostic approach. CT and MRI are equally effective in detecting the presence of a mass. CT should be performed both as a noncontrast and contrast evaluation; 5 or 10 mm thick contiguous sections are generally adequate. Evaluation of tumors in the middle cranial fossa and the sellar/suprasellar and pineal regions requires the addition of direct coronal sections through the area of interest to aid in presurgical planning. MRI, using T1- and T2-weighted imaging in multiple projections, is rapidly replacing CT for this application, as it has for infratentorial tumors. Presurgical planning is better accomplished with MRI compared with CT. Contrast enhancement with gadolinium can help define the extent of tumor, but cannot be used to differentiate tumor subtypes or determine aggressiveness. However, contrast enhancement is essential for the follow-up evaluation searching for recurrent tumor. I cannot agree with proponents who suggest that T2-weighted imaging can be replaced solely by T1-weighted imaging before and after contrast enhancement. As in adults, not all childhood brain neoplasms enhance (e.g., brain stem glioma), and many

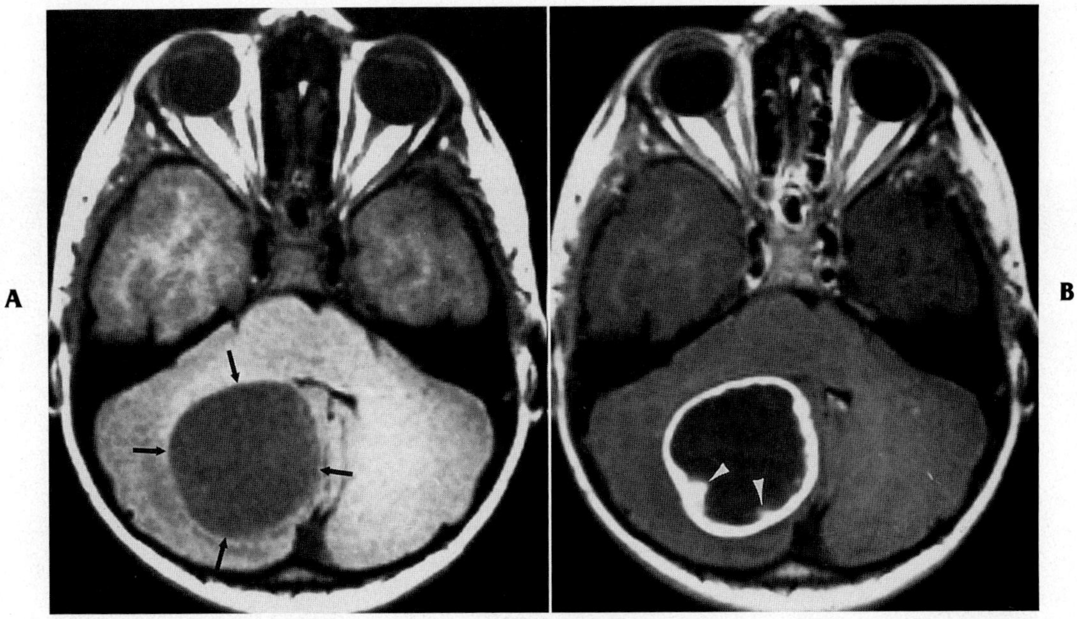


**FIGURE 4** A 4-year-old boy with cerebellar astrocytoma. *A,* Axial T1-weighted MRI through the posterior fossa shows a large cystic mass (*black arrows*) involving the right cerebellar hemisphere and compressing the fourth ventricle to the left. *B,* After contrast administration, there is intense enhancement of mural nodules within the wall of the cyst (*white arrowheads*) as well as the cyst wall itself. The location of the tumor, the macrocystic appearance, and the pattern of enhancement are consistent with a benign pilocytic astrocytoma.

may only be conspicuous on T2-weighted images because of alterations in brain water without disrupting the blood-brain barrier.

Sagittal and coronal images are most helpful to evaluate the sellar/suprasellar and pineal regions. Direct involvement of the chiasm and hypothalamus by a solid enhancing mass is most frequently from glioma. Craniopharyngiomas are more commonly suprasellar (90 percent), cystic (80 percent), and contain calcification (80 percent), either within the solid portion of the tumor or in the wall of the cyst. Detection of calcification is best accomplished with a noncontrast CT scan, which we perform whenever we encounter a cystic suprasellar/sellar mass (Fig. 5). A variety of other lesions including hamartomas, germinomas, epidermoids, metastases, adenomas, and inflammatory masses may also involve this region. Pineal region tumors common in the pediatric age group include gliomas, germ cell tumors, and primitive neuroectodermal neoplasms. Their differentiation is often not possible based on imaging, but this does not detract from imaging's primary goals of tumor detection, localization, and followup.

## Traumatic Processes

CT remains the imaging modality of choice in the evaluation of acute calvarial trauma. Its ability to detect calvarial fractures, subarachnoid hemorrhage, or the early changes of edema and hypoxic injury (Fig. 6); its ability to easily survey the upper abdomen when visceral trauma is suspected; and the ease with which unstable patients can be monitored, all make CT our first choice. We routinely begin with 5 mm thick sections through the skull base to screen for posterior fossa and basilar injury; 10 mm thick noncontrast sections are then continued to the vertex. Surgical lesions, such as large subdural or epidural hematomas, should be sought. Evidence of their presence is based on the findings of midline shift, compression of the ventricles, obliteration of the cisterns, or contralateral dilatation of the temporal horns. Obliteration of the ambient or quadrigeminal plate cisterns is an especially ominous sign, indicating significant brain swelling or transincisural herniation.

MRI is useful for the evaluation of the delayed sequelae of trauma such as headaches, seizures, or neurologic deficits not readily explained by the initial CT examination. Routine T1- and T2-weighted images are used for this purpose.

Cranial abuse in children was first described in association with long-bone fractures by John Caffey, a radiologist. The calvarial and intracranial manifestations of nonaccidental trauma (child abuse) are not dissimilar to patterns of trauma by accidental means. Severe cranial injury in the absence of an adequate clinical explanation, however, should raise the suspicion of abuse. The acute evaluation of cranial abuse is similar to that for accidental trauma. CT scanning is performed as clinically indicated. MRI should be reserved for those cases in which there is a high clinical index of suspicion in the face of a negative or equivocal CT. Small subdural hematomas high over the convexity, in the subfrontal and temporal regions, or in the posterior fossa, are best seen on MRI. MRI is also useful in explaining neurologic deficits not initially explained on the noncontrast CT scan. Caution should be exercised in attempting to stage the age of a subdural hematoma based on its MRI appearance alone, because of inconsistencies in the degradation process of intracranial hematomas.

## Metabolic-Toxic Processes

The term "metabolic" or "toxic" disease, when applied to the CNS in children, can imply a variety of different causes. Few represent inherited disease such as liposomal, peroxisomal, and mitochondrial disorders, or primary metabolic defects in

A

B

C

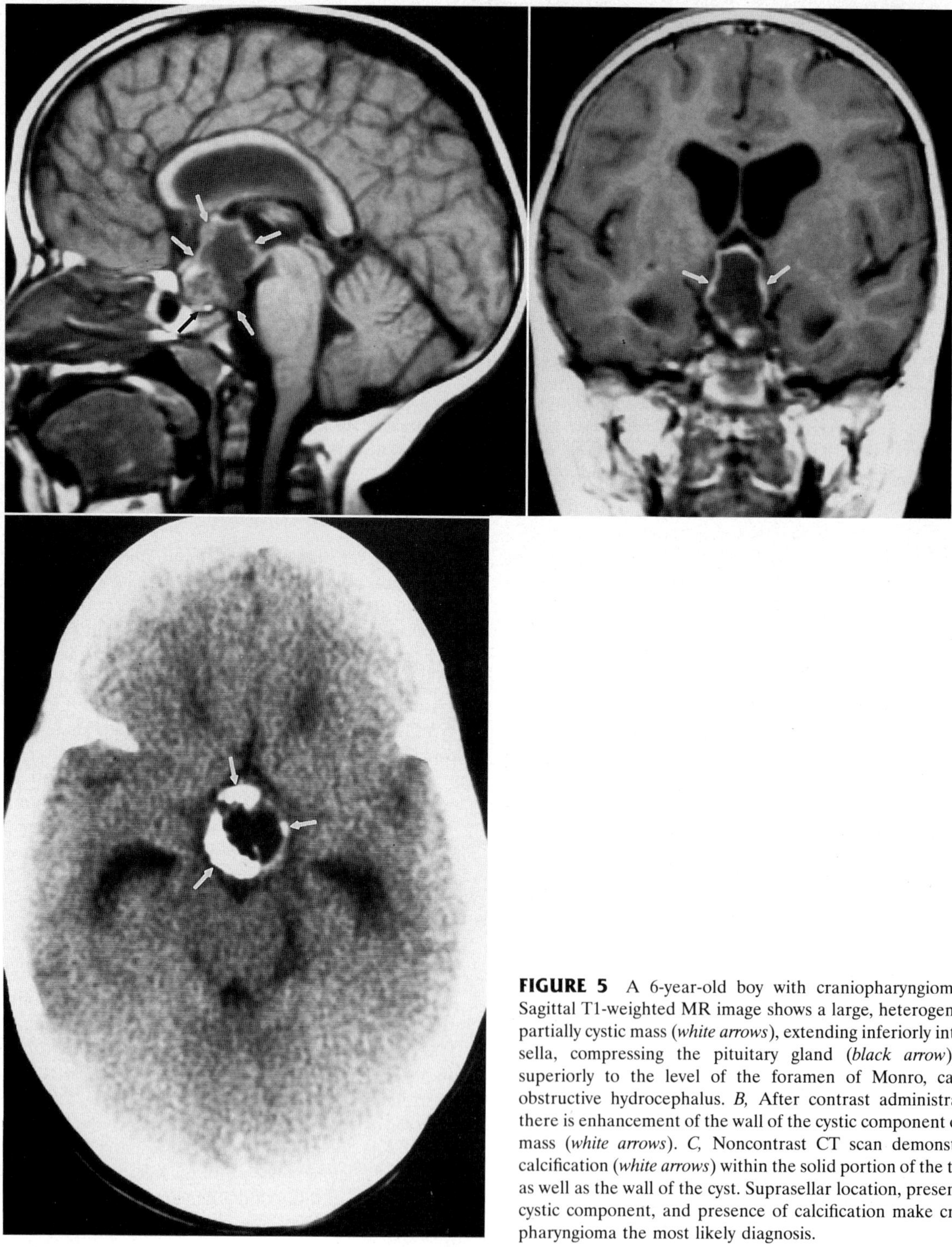

**FIGURE 5** A 6-year-old boy with craniopharyngioma. *A,* Sagittal T1-weighted MR image shows a large, heterogeneous, partially cystic mass (*white arrows*), extending inferiorly into the sella, compressing the pituitary gland (*black arrow*) and superiorly to the level of the foramen of Monro, causing obstructive hydrocephalus. *B,* After contrast administration, there is enhancement of the wall of the cystic component of the mass (*white arrows*). *C,* Noncontrast CT scan demonstrates calcification (*white arrows*) within the solid portion of the tumor as well as the wall of the cyst. Suprasellar location, presence of cystic component, and presence of calcification make craniopharyngioma the most likely diagnosis.

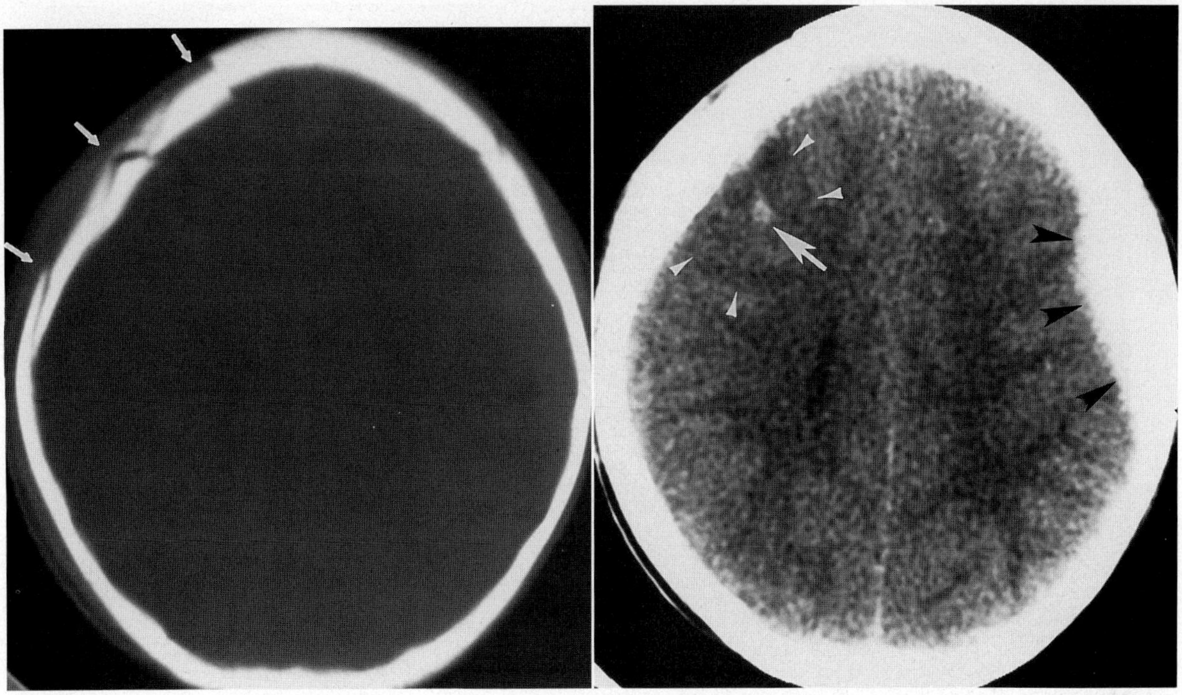


**FIGURE 6** A 2-year-old female hit in the right parietal region with a softball. Axial noncontrast CT scan. *A,* Bone windows demonstrate a comminuted depressed fracture in the right parietal region (*white arrows*). *B,* Brain windows reveal in the region of the fracture an area of hyperdensity that represents a hemorrhagic contusion (*white arrow*) surrounded by a small area of edema (*white arrowheads*). Note also the presence of a contracoup left-sided epidural hematoma (*black arrowheads*).

cerebral white matter/myelin formation. Many represent toxic or metabolic injury associated with systemic disease (e.g., hepatic encephalopathy), radiation- or chemotherapeutic-induced injury, illicit drug use, iatrogenic complication of nonchemotherapeutic medications, or reactions to immunization with demyelination.

MRI is currently the best choice to detect the changes found with metabolic disease of the brain. Yet, despite its sensitivity, changes are often not identified until late in the course of the process. Clinical neurologic findings may vary and include alterations in mental status, seizures, motor/sensory changes, progressive developmental delay or neurologic injury, and neurocognitive disorders. Not uncommonly, neurologic indicators may precede findings on MRI.

T2-weighted imaging is critical in the evaluation of metabolic or toxic encephalopathy. We rely primarily on T2-weighted SE imaging, because of its greater sensitivity in detecting subtle signal changes within the white matter. Only on occasion are T1-weighted images useful. T2-weighted images are performed in at least two projections (preferably axial and coronal) throughout the entire brain. Both FSE and gradient acquisition T2-weighted images may miss subtle alterations in white matter signal because of abnormal myelination. Rarely are the patterns of injury or signal alterations diagnostic of any one particular disorder. Patterns associated with primary white matter disease or with inherited metabolic derangements can, on occasion, suggest a specific diagnosis. For example, bilateral symmetrical involvement of the occipital and posterior parietal white matter is a typical pattern found in the peroxisomal disorder, x-linked adrenoleukodystrophy (Fig. 7), whereas anterior involvement may be more indicative of Canavan's disease. Bilateral symmetrical basal ganglia involvement may be the first sign on MRI in Leigh's disease. This finding is not, however, specific, since similar changes in the basal ganglia may be found with microvascular angiopathies, hepatic encephalopathy, or caused by hypoxic-ischemic injury. Involvement with any of the metabolic or toxic diseases can be either multifocal or diffuse. The white matter alone is most frequently involved; gray matter changes may be primary or secondary depending on the disease process.

Differentiation of a metabolic disorder from injury caused by hypoxia or ischemia may be difficult, especially in the first year of life, when normal white matter hyperintensity from hypomyelination may be confused with demyelination from injury. We have found several signs helpful in separating a demyelinating or dysmyelinating process from hypoxic-ischemic injury. With injury, white matter and gray matter volume loss often appears soon after the insult, a direct result of an encephaloclastic event, whereas, not infrequently, white and gray matter volume is often preserved until late in the course of a metabolic disease. The demonstration of progression on sequential examinations may also help differentiate an active metabolic leukoencephalopathy from a static encephalopathy caused by a previous insult. The pattern of injury from either hypoxia or ischemia is often patchy or multifocal, whereas larger coalescent areas of hyperintensity are more common in metabolic disease. Eventually, even with a severe insult (hypoxic or ischemic), the white matter that is left undergoes some degree of myelination; however, progressively increasing hyperintensity is more typical of an actively progressive leukoencephalopathy.

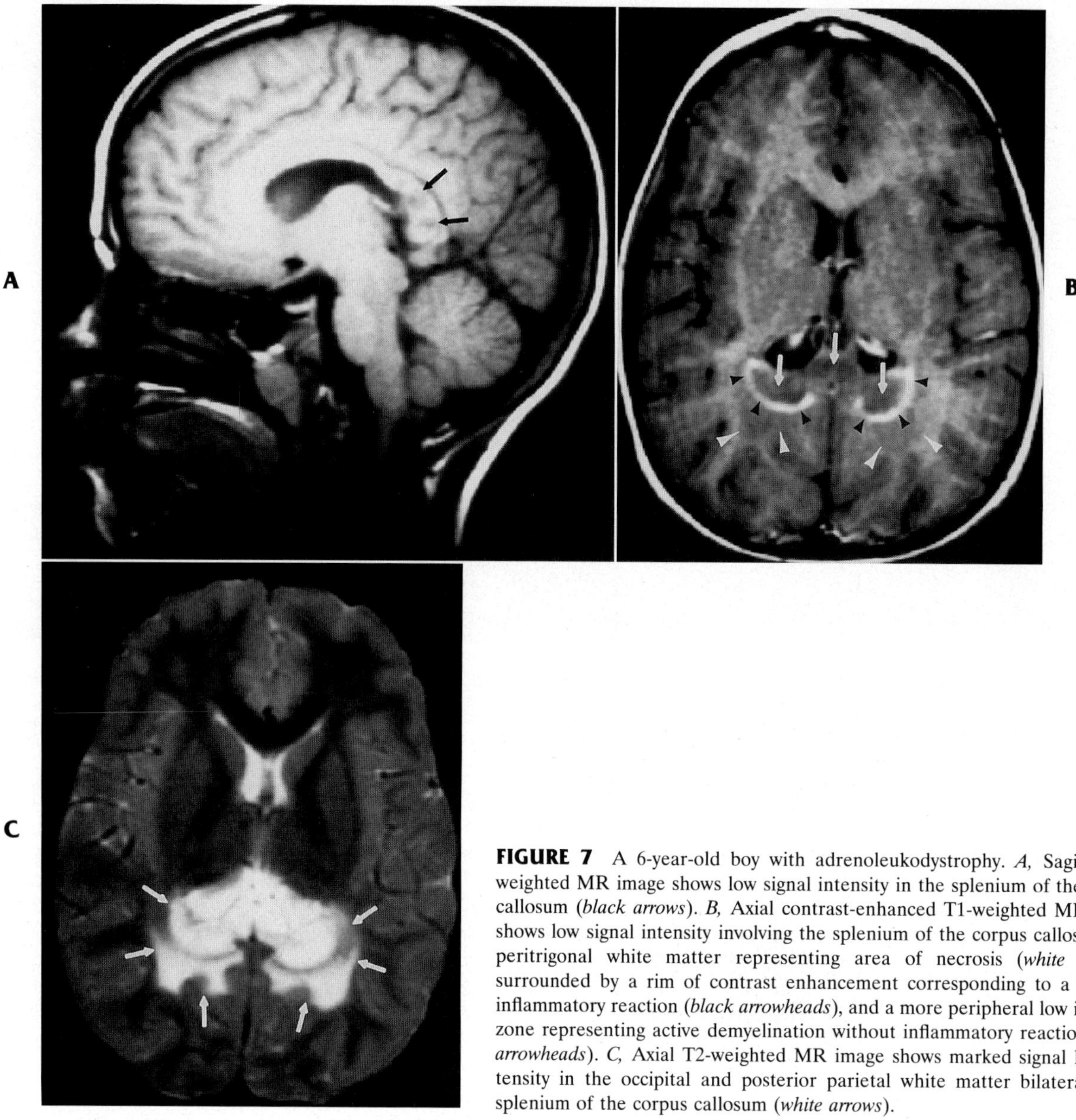

**FIGURE 7** A 6-year-old boy with adrenoleukodystrophy. *A,* Sagittal T1-weighted MR image shows low signal intensity in the splenium of the corpus callosum (*black arrows*). *B,* Axial contrast-enhanced T1-weighted MR image shows low signal intensity involving the splenium of the corpus callosum and peritrigonal white matter representing area of necrosis (*white arrows*), surrounded by a rim of contrast enhancement corresponding to a zone of inflammatory reaction (*black arrowheads*), and a more peripheral low intensity zone representing active demyelination without inflammatory reaction (*white arrowheads*). *C,* Axial T2-weighted MR image shows marked signal hyperintensity in the occipital and posterior parietal white matter bilaterally and splenium of the corpus callosum (*white arrows*).

## Discussion

In modern pediatric neuroimaging, no one modality has replaced all the rest. Radiologists practicing an integrated approach to diagnostic imaging must be familiar with multiple modalities to provide the greatest service and diagnostic sensitivity. As is often said, "Children are not just small adults." The imaging in children with CNS disease can be a challenge. However, this challenge is easily met by radiologists who are capable of matching the disease process with the appropriate modality and who have the ability to interpret their findings in relation to normal brain growth and development.

*Acknowledgments.* The authors wish to thank Ms. Juanita Hunter for her dedication to the Pediatric Neuroradiology section.

## Suggested Reading

Am J Neuroradiol 12(2), 1992.

Ball WS. Magnetic resonance imaging of the infant brain. Semin Ultrasound CT MR. 1991; 12:379–409.

Barkovich AJ. Contemporary neuroimaging, Vol 1. In: Norman D, ed. Pediatric Neuroimaging. New York: Raven Press, 1991.

Barkovich AJ, Kjos BO, Jackson DE, et al. Normal maturation of the neonatal and infant brain: MR imaging at 1.5T. Radiology 1988; 166:173–180.

Wolpert SM, Barnes P, eds. MRI in Pediatric Neuroradiology. St Louis: Mosby–Year Book, 1992.

# Head Injuries in Battered Children

*YUTAKA SATO, M.D.*

Caffey, Kempe, and Silverman, all pediatric radiologists, recognized child abuse as a medicosocial entity and established the diagnostic techniques for investigating child abuse, in which radiographs play the major role.

Child abuse is a leading killer in infancy. It is estimated that at least 1.5 million children are abused each year in the United States alone, and more than 3,000 deaths occur. Head injury is a major cause of morbidity and mortality in child abuse victims. In addition to acute life-threatening injury to the central nervous system, it has been recognized that more latent and subtle manifestations such as learning disabilities, mental retardation, and cerebral palsy can be the sequelae of child abuse.

The clinical diagnosis of a head injury in a child abuse victim may be challenging. The history of trauma may not be disclosed by the caregivers, and signs and symptoms are often vague and nonspecific. Significant intracranial injuries may be present without telltale evidence of trauma of the head and face.

The neuroradiologic examination is the key to the diagnosis of child abuse, differentiating between injuries that could be logically expected to have occurred as described and those that have resulted from other undisclosed mechanisms. Imaging procedures play an important role in the medical and legal management of abuse victims, providing objective data to document the presence and extent of head injury.

## Diagnostic Approach

### *Skull Fractures*

Skull fractures are the second most frequent skeletal injury in abused children after fractures of long bones. Plain skull radiography is the most sensitive technique for the detection of fractures. It should be noted, however, that only about 50 percent of children with intracranial injuries caused by physical abuse have skull fractures. The linear fracture is the most common fracture in both accidental and nonaccidental trauma, but complex fractures are more frequent among abused children. A casual fall does not cause depressed, diastatic, comminuted fractures; growing fractures; or fractures involving multiple cranial bones (Fig. 1). Also a fracture crossing the midline or involving the occipital bone rarely occurs in accidental trauma.

### *Extra-axial Hemorrhage*

Subdural hematoma (SDH) is the most common intracranial complication of child abuse. SDH usually results from the rupture of bridging veins extending from the cerebral cortex to the dural sinuses. Interhemispheric SDH is characteristic, although not pathognomonic, of abuse (Fig. 2). This is caused by the rupture of veins draining into the sagittal sinus, which

A

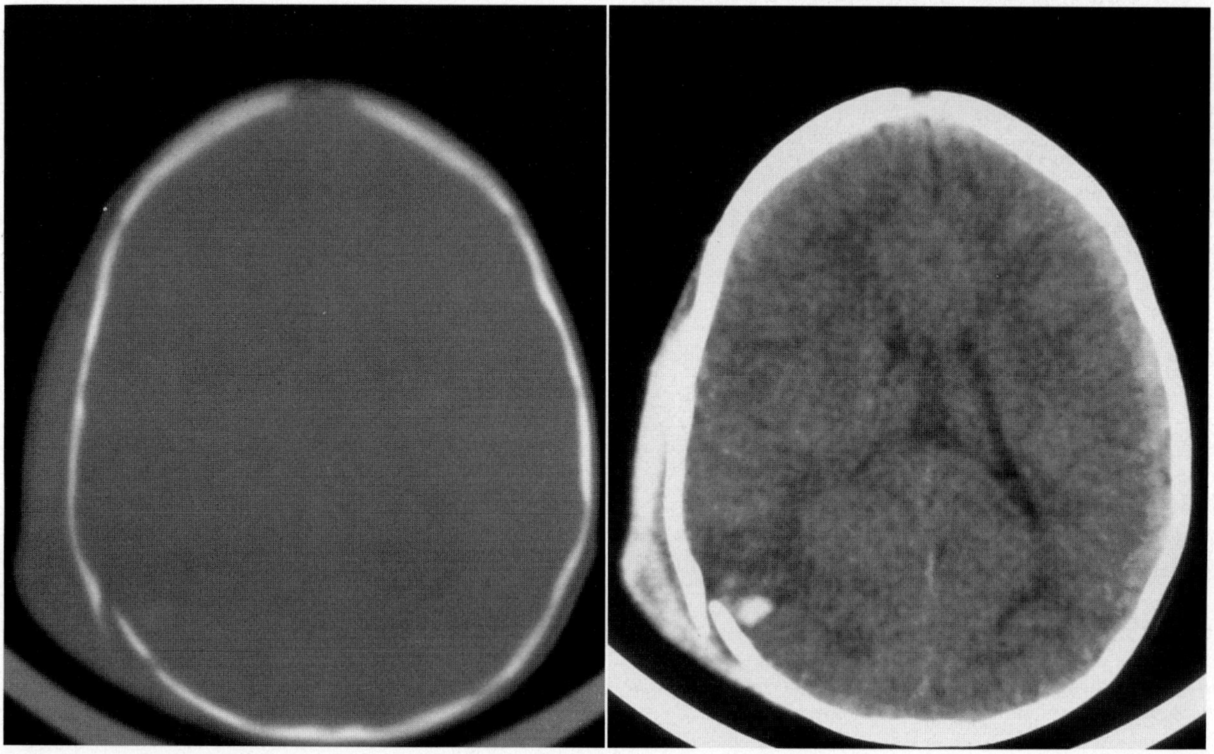

B

**FIGURE 1** Depressed skull fracture in a 4-month-old boy. *A,* CT with bone window setting shows depressed fracture and subgaleal hematoma. *B,* CT with narrower window setting demonstrates hemorrhagic cortical contusion of the underlying brain. (From Sato Y, Smith WL. Head injury in child abuse. Neuroimaging Clin North Am 1991; 1:475–493; with permission.)

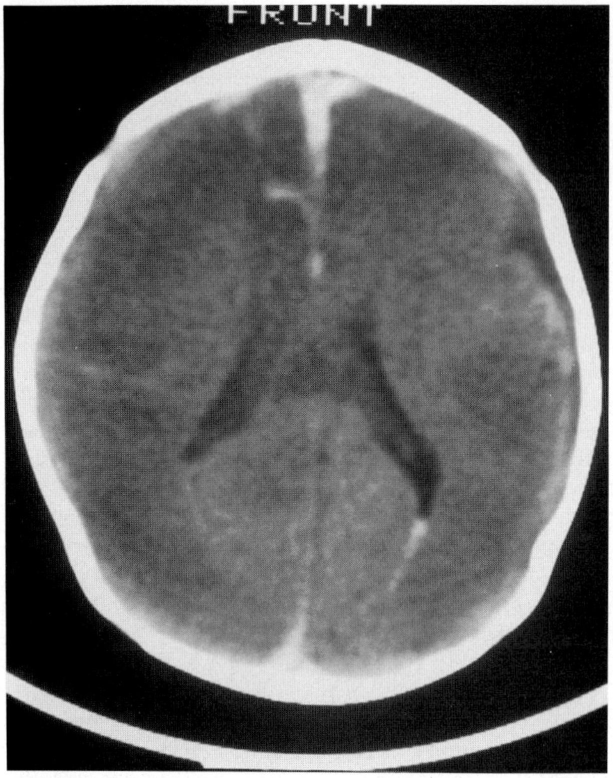


**FIGURE 2** Interhemispheric subdural hematoma. Nonenhanced CT scan shows interhemispheric subdural blood in the parafalcial location.

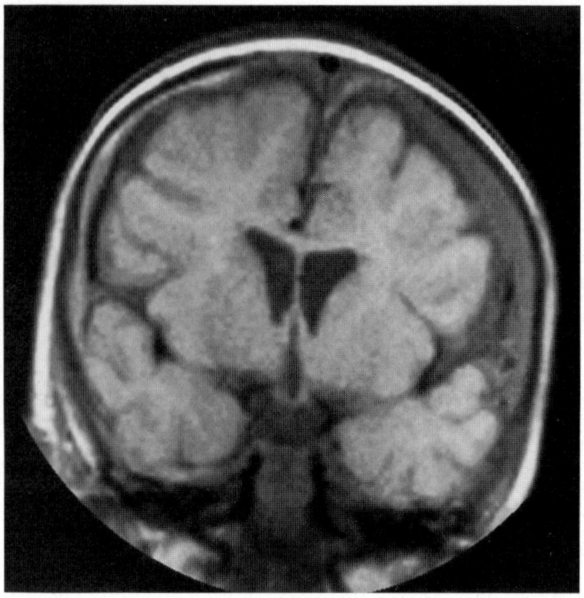

**FIGURE 4** Subdural hematomas of different ages. Coronal short TR/TE MR image shows the right-sided convexity collection with increased signal, suggesting a subacute lesion, and the left-sided convexity collection with lower signal, suggesting a more chronic lesion. This signifies the repeated nature of the insult, strongly suggesting physical abuse. (From Sato Y, Yuh WTC, et al. Head injury in child abuse: Evaluation with MR imaging. Radiology 1989; 173:653–657; with permission.)

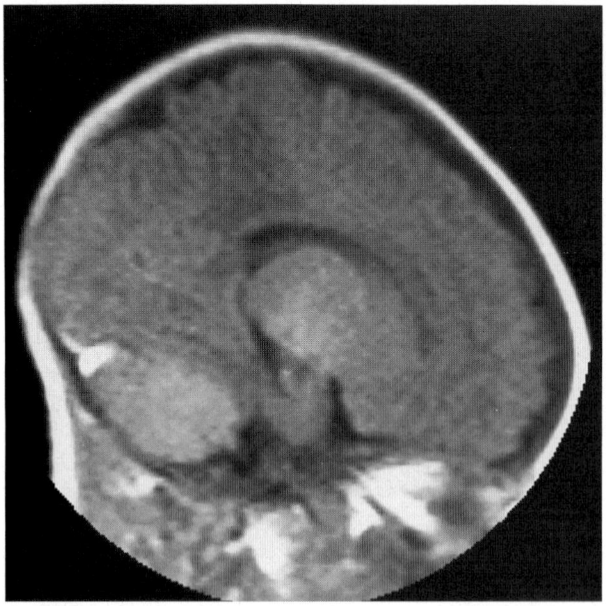

**FIGURE 3** Supratentorial and infratentorial subdural hematomas. Parasagittal short TR/TE MR image shows subacute subdural blood in the occipital, tentorial, and posterior fossa areas. Note also the edema involving the posterior portion of the centrum semiovale.

run perpendicular to the rotational force generated by acceleration/deceleration in a sagittal direction during violent shaking. SDHs are also found in the convexity, along the skull base, and in the posterior fossa. Interhemispheric SDHs and large SDHs of clinical significance are readily detected by computed tomography (CT). Intravenous contrast enhancement may be needed to demonstrate subdural "membrane" in subacute and chronic cases. The membrane may be seen as early as seven days after the trauma. Magnetic resonance imaging (MRI) is best suited to detect small SDHs, particularly those along the skull base, high in the convexity, along the tentorium, and in the posterior fossa (Fig. 3). Although the SDHs detected with MRI alone are usually clinically silent, their identification and documentation are important because they may be the only objective imaging evidence of abuse. Another advantage of MRI is the ease of identification of SDHs of various ages (Fig. 4). The existence of multiple SDHs of various ages indicates repeated insults, which, when added to the clinical evidence, suggest child abuse.

Acceleration/deceleration force may also cause infrequent but characteristic hematomas in the cerebral falx.

Subarachnoid hemorrhages are detected more reliably by CT. The cerebral falx may be prominent in the presence of cerebral edema and should not be mistaken for a subarachnoid hemorrhage.

The incidence of epidural hematomas in child abuse is lower than that of SDH or subarachnoid hemorrhage. Epidural hemorrhage is most frequently caused by the rupture of the middle meningeal artery, often associated with temporal fracture. The plasticity of the infant's skull, however, may allow avulsion of the artery from the undersurface of the skull in response to distortion and may cause an epidural hematoma without skull fracture. Epidural hematomas may also result from ruptured dural sinuses or emissary veins.

### Diffuse Brain Swelling

Diffuse brain swelling is the most common intra-axial complication associated with head injury in child abuse. In children massive, often fatal, cerebral edema may develop after accidental or nonaccidental head trauma. In children up to the age of about five years, the brain's initial response to trauma is to increase blood flow, whereas the microvascular response in adult brain is to reduce flow. This unique vascular reactivity contributes to the development of "malignant" brain edema. CT scans reveal diffuse cerebral swelling, effacement of the ventricular lumen and subarachnoid space, and obliteration of the gray-white matter interface.

### Diffuse Cerebral Infarction

Unilateral and bilateral global infarcts in the territorial distributions of the major cerebral arteries result from the compression of extracranial carotid arteries and upper airway obstruction. In the case of global ischemia, cerebral white matter may show paradoxical high attenuation relative to the gray matter ("reversal" sign), which suggests a grave prognosis.

Owing to the relatively spared circulation to the posterior fossa during acute ischemia, the relatively normal cerebellum is contrasted with the cerebrum showing decreased attenuation ("white cerebellum" sign) (Fig. 5).

Laminar cortical necrosis is a unique neuropathologic entity caused by hypoxia. Certain layers of the cerebral cortex develop necrosis in laminar fashion because of the selective vulnerability to hypoxia. Hemorrhagic infarcts confined to the cortical gray matter in laminar fashion can be observed associated with basal ganglia infarcts (Fig. 6).

### Focal Parenchymal Injuries

Constellations of focal parenchymal injuries can be observed singly or in combination. These include cortical contusions, diffuse axonal injury (DAI) involving white matter and brain stem, and subcortical gray matter injury. These lesions, especially the nonhemorrhagic ones, are best demonstrated by MRI.

Cortical contusions involve primarily gray matter and are usually hemorrhagic. The cortex directly under the region of impact and adjacent to the roughened edges of the inner table, such as along the anterior cranial fossa, sphenoid wing, and petrous ridge, is commonly involved (Fig. 7).

DAIs are caused by shear stress on the white matter by rotational force and are commonly nonhemorrhagic. The gray-white interface of the frontal and temporal lobes, brain stem, body and splenium of the corpus callosum (Fig. 8), internal capsule, and coronal radiata are commonly involved. DAI plays an important role in the development of immediate traumatic coma, subsequent cerebral atrophy, and neurologic deficits and dysfunction.

Among subcortical gray nuclei, the thalamus is the most frequently injured (Fig. 9). Disruption of multiple perforating blood vessels by shearing force is considered the mechanism of injury.

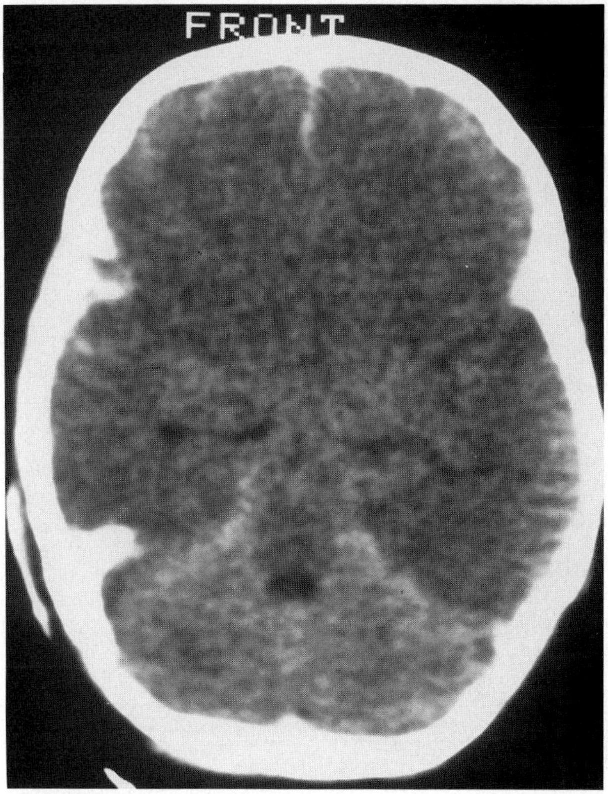


**FIGURE 5** White cerebellar sign. Axial CT scan shows relatively normal cerebellar density compared with diffusely decreased density of the edematous cerebrum in a child with global ischemia.

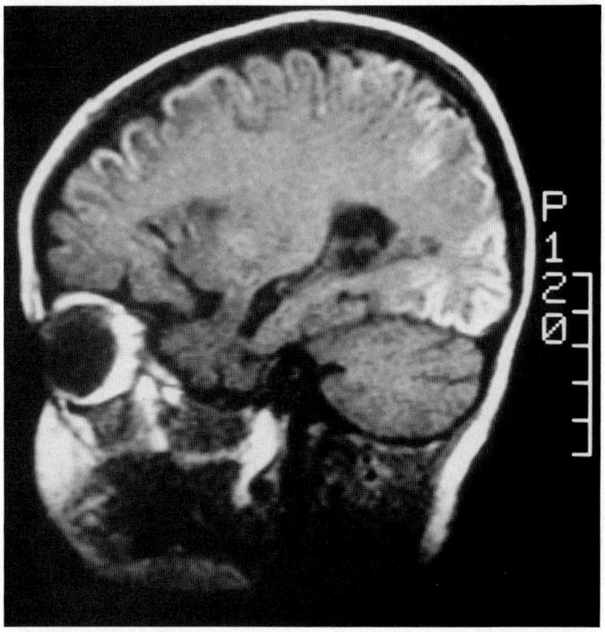


**FIGURE 6** Laminar cortical necrosis. Parasagittal short TR/TE MR image shows abnormal high intensity signal along the cerebral cortex in laminar fashion.

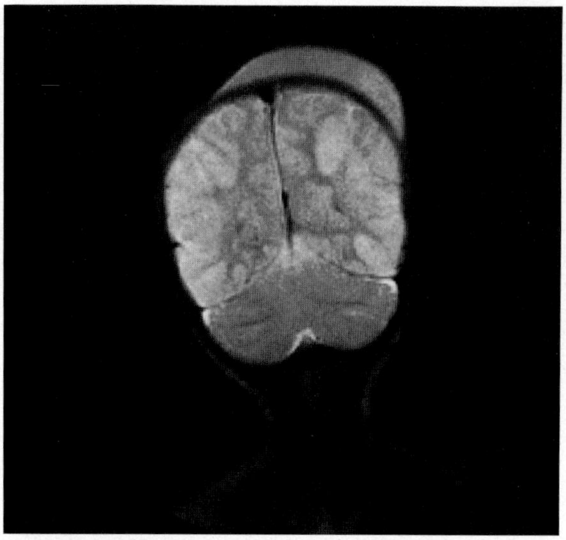

**FIGURE 7** Extensive cortical contusion in a 13-month-old girl. Coronal long TR/TE MR image shows diffuse swelling of the cerebral cortex with effacement of the underlying white matter in the left hemisphere. Note also a large subgaleal hematoma.

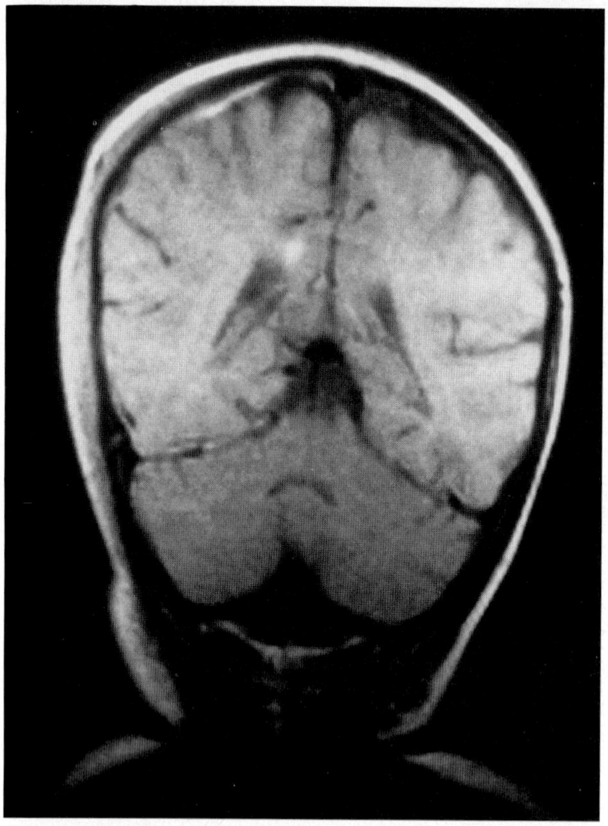

**FIGURE 8** Hemorrhagic axonal injury involving the splenium of the corpus callosum in a 5-month-old boy. Coronal short TR/TE MR image shows hemorrhagic focus in the splenium. Note also subacute subdural hematoma in the right convexity. (From Sato Y, Yuh WTC, et al. Head injury in child abuse: Evaluation with MR imaging. Radiology 1989; 173:653–657; with permission.)

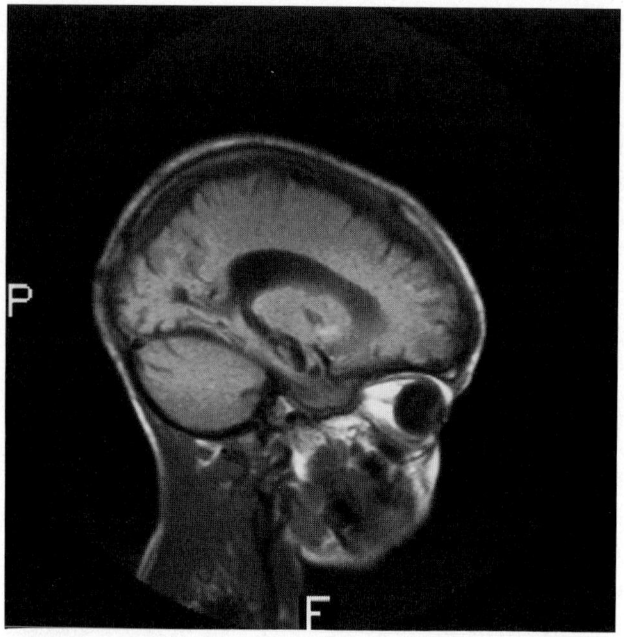


**FIGURE 9** Hemorrhagic injury to the subcortical gray matter. Parasagittal short TR/TE MR image shows injury to the striate nucleus. (From Sato Y, Yuh WTC, et al. Head injury in child abuse: Evaluation with MR imaging. Radiology 1989; 173:653–657; with permission.)

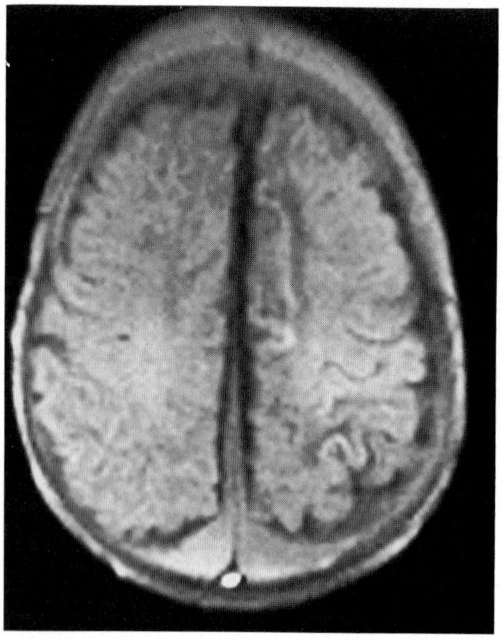

**FIGURE 10** Contusional tear in a 3-week-old girl. Axial short TR/TE MR image shows a linear cleft filled with a small amount of blood surrounded by edema in the gray-white interface of the left frontal region. Note also bilateral occipital and interhemispheric subdural hematomas. (From Sato Y, Yuh WTC, et al. Head injury in child abuse: Evaluation with MR imaging. Radiology 1989; 173:653–657; with permission.)

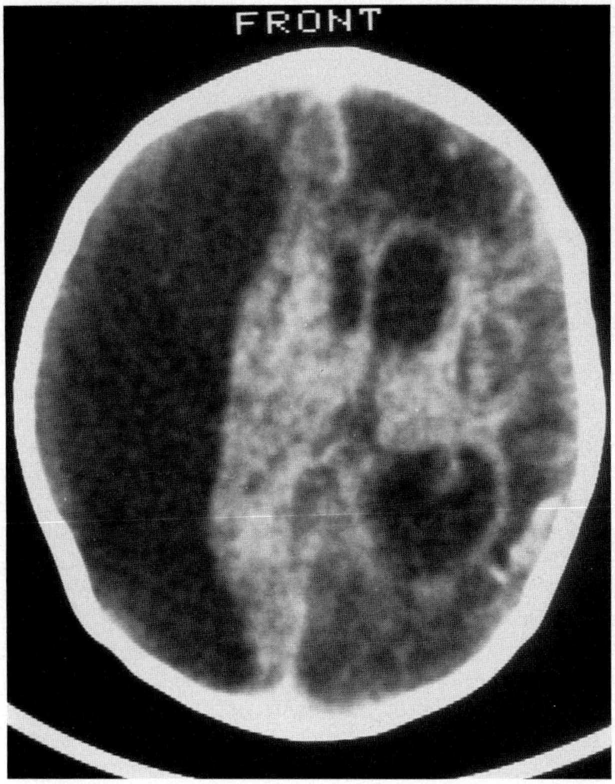


**FIGURE 11** Chronic subdural hematoma. Axial CT scan shows a large subdural collection on the right and extensive multicystic encephalomalacia of the left hemisphere.

In infants five months or younger, a unique lesion called "contusional tear" can be observed (Fig. 10). This lesion consists of grossly visible or slitlike tears in the cerebral white matter and microscopic tears in the cortex paralleling the surface of the brain. The frontal and temporal lobes are most often involved. The reason why these tears occur instead of contusions in the brains of young infants is thought to be the soft consistency of the incompletely myelinated brains and pliancy and smooth inner surface of the infant's skull.

### *Chronic Sequelae*

The immediate and delayed outcomes of head injuries caused by child abuse are, as a group, worse than that of any other head injuries in childhood. Devastation of the central nervous system can be documented by subsequent neuroimaging. Chronic subdural collections (Fig. 11), cerebral atrophy, encephalomalacia, porencephalic cyst, and dilated ventricles are often observed.

## Imaging Recommendations

Plain skull films in anteroposterior and lateral projections should be included in a radiographic skeletal survey in all patients when child abuse is suspected. Radiographic documentation of skull fractures provides objective evidence of child abuse. A discrepancy between the pattern of fractures and the alleged mechanism of injury is often instrumental in confirming child abuse.

CT is the modality of choice in the initial evaluation of acute head injury in suspected abuse victims, because of its high sensitivity in detecting acute intracranial hemorrhages, ease of patient monitoring, and rapid scanning capability. All infants with neurologic findings should be evaluated initially by CT. We use 4 mm slice thickness for evaluation of the head of an infant. Bone window image scans with wide windows should always be obtained to facilitate detection of soft-tissue and skeletal injury. Contrast enhancement is rarely needed. CT scans reliably demonstrate lesions that are amenable to surgery.

Most patients should undergo MRI evaluation to determine the full extent of the injury and prognosis, once clinical stabilization is accomplished. MRI is extremely useful to detect small subdural hematomas, nonhemorrhagic focal parenchymal injury, and hypoxic-ischemic injury. MRI, because of its high sensitivity for the detection of intracranial sequelae, may even be indicated in selected cases without neurologic findings (e.g., when other imaging modalities fail to document the evidence of physical abuse in spite of high suspicion on clinical grounds). Our routine MRI sequences for the evaluation of suspected child abuse consist of short TR/TE images in three planes and long TR/TE images in one plane using 5 mm slice thickness.

## Discussion

The key radiologic features of head injury in the abused child are:

1. Severe head injury inconsistent with the mechanism or circumstances given in the history. The presence of complex skull fractures, subdural hematomas, and/or cerebral injury with history of minor incidents such as a casual fall from a baby chair should raise suspicion.
2. Unique locations or characteristic lesions should be taken as a clue. This is analogous to the metaphyseal "corner" fractures of long bones or posterior rib fractures so uniquely seen in abused children. Examples are occipital skull fractures, fractures crossing the midline, interhemispheric subdural hematomas, intrafalcial hematomas, and "contusional tears."
3. Evidence of repeated trauma. Subdural hematomas of various ages and the presence of a fresh cerebral hemorrhage in the brain with chronic sequelae are examples.

## Suggested Reading


Caffey J. Multiple fractures in the long bones of infants suffering from chronic subdural hematoma. AJR 1946; 56:163–173.

Caffey J. The whiplash shaken infant syndrome: Manual shaking by the extremities with whiplash-induced intracranial and intraocular bleedings, linked with residual permanent brain damage and mental retardation. Pediatrics 1974; 54:396–403.

Cohen RA, Kaufman RA, Myers PA, Towbin RB. Cranial computed tomography in the abused child with head injury. AJR 1986; 146:97–102.

Harwood-Nash DC. Abuse to the pediatric central nervous system. Am J Neuroradiol 1992; 13:569–575.

Kempe CH, Silverman FN, Steele BF, et al. The battered child syndrome. JAMA 1962; 181:17–24.

Kleinman PK. Diagnostic imaging in infant abuse. AJR 1990; 155:703–712.

Merten DF, Osborne DRS, Radkowski MA, et al. Craniocerebral trauma in the child abuse syndrome: Radiological observations. Pediatr Radiol 1984; 14:272–277.

Sato Y, Smith WL. Head injury in child abuse. Neuroimaging Clin North Am 1991; 1:475–493.

Sato Y, Yuh WTC, Smith WL, et al. Head injury in child abuse: Evaluation with MR imaging. Radiology 1989; 173:653–657.

Silverman FN. Unrecognized trauma in infants, the battered child syndrome, and the syndrome of Ambroise Tardieu. Radiology 1972; 104:337–353.

Zimmerman RA, Bilaniuk LT, Bruce D, et al. Computed tomography of craniocerebral injury in the abused child. Radiology 1979; 130:687–690.

# CT and MRI in Childhood Trauma to the Central Nervous System

*ROBERT A. ZIMMERMAN, M.D.*

Head injury is the most common clinical indication for imaging the brain and its cranial vault. The clinical situation may be one in which the patient has been acutely traumatized, and by this mechanism and/or because of age (immaturity), the patient is unable to cooperate. At this moment there is a need to know whether an underlying traumatic process exists, and if so, what its nature is, so that measures can be instituted to protect the brain against still greater or irreversible damage. Within the Emergency Room, the primary care physician's responsibility is to stabilize the patient's respiratory and cardiovascular status and to make the decision that life-threatening bodily injury outside the central nervous system (CNS) either does not exist or that its evaluation and treatment can wait until the CNS damage is evaluated. Not all patients with head injuries demonstrate overt clinical signs. Some show no evidence of bone or brain damage; however, others with clinically unimpressive findings may harbor potentially fatal traumatic processes such as acute epidural hematomas. All of these head injury patients (apparent and not) need to be dealt with in a diagnostically effective and cost-efficient manner. The standard of care must conform to that of the community and should provide protection from the real or imagined threat of medical malpractice.

The resources that are available for evaluation of the skull, brain, facial bones, cervical spine and cord are radiography, computed tomography (CT), magnetic resonance imaging (MRI), myelography, and cerebral angiography. Diagnostic radiologic evaluation within the Emergency Room is usually limited to simple plain radiographic studies for the skull, facial bones, and cervical spine. Radiographs of the cervical spine are of primary importance in assessing its stability. The reason for this is to prevent injury to the cervicospinal cord with patient movement when a fracture or ligamentous injury has rendered the spine unstable. Given instability, precautions must be exercised in the form of traction or sandbags, so that the spine remains immobile. The reason for mobilizing the patient is to obtain definitive diagnostic information regarding the nature and extent of CNS trauma. This chapter covers the techniques of CT and MRI, their key image findings, and the pitfalls in both technique and interpretation.

## Indications for CT and MRI

CT or MRI evaluation of pediatric CNS head trauma is indicated when the presence or absence of intracranial, craniofacial, and upper cervicospinal and cord injury must be determined. In all instances the need for evaluation is a clinical decision. A laceration of the scalp or face, a swollen eye, or a bruise in and of itself does not constitute a need for radiographic evaluation. A decrease in the level of consciousness, the presence of a focal neurological deficit, the presence of overt fracture, or the knowledge that trauma occurred under a situation that is likely to have produced significant injury (a fall from a second- or third-story window), despite the absence of overt clinical signs, constitutes an indication for further evaluation. In the pediatric population, the pediatrician and the Emergency Room physicians also deal with another element of traumatic CNS injury, that arising from child abuse. Abused children may not be taken to the emergency department immediately after injury, but at a later point, when the etiology of their clinical manifestations (e.g., seizures, irritability, nausea, and vomiting) is not obvious. Even acute intracranial trauma, such as that arising from the shaken impact injury, may not leave physical stigmata of abuse visible on the skin, and, even here, the clinical presentation may be confused with that due to hypoxic-ischemic injury resulting from apneic episodes, seizures, sudden infant death syndrome, or it may be mistaken for disease processes such as meningitis. Thus the clinical suspicion of child abuse that may arise from the physician's interaction with parents, baby-sitter, or boyfriend may constitute a sufficient indication to proceed to an imaging study.

## Technical Approach to CT and MRI

Both CT and MRI have valuable information to contribute to one's knowledge about the brain, facial structures, and upper cervical spine. The choice between the two techniques usually depends on the nature of the problem (information desired), the urgency of the need to evaluate it, the availability of the equipment, and the ability of the patient to hold still during the period of data acquisition.

Today, CT is rapid, providing information about the bone, surrounding soft tissues, and the intracranial brain parenchyma. In general, CT is the initial imaging procedure of choice for the evaluation of the pediatric patient suffering a head injury. The diagnostic information derived is sufficient to decide whether surgical intervention is necessary to remove a blood clot that is within the brain or that compresses it from without. The information derived from the CT scan is sufficient to know whether there has been cerebral herniation, whether or not the intracranial pressure is likely to be increased, so that intracranial pressure monitoring can be instituted along with therapeutic attempts to control it. Depressed fractures of the calvarium, and even many linear fractures, can be identified. Fractures of the facial bones, cranial base, and upper cervical spine are ideally evaluated with thin-section CT, and their demonstration may be further aided by multiplanar or three-dimensional (3D) reconstruction (essential for C1 and C2 cervicospinal evaluation). Not only is performance of the CT scan quick (sections taking from 1 to 5 seconds each, total scan time 10 to 20 minutes), but the environment permits easy access to the patient within the scanner, without limiting the use of intubation devices, support or monitoring equipment, or inpatient care and support personnel involved.

On the other hand, MRI depicts the presence of intraparenchymal bleeding and nonhemorrhagic injury to an extent that is not possible with CT. The price paid with MRI is the significantly longer periods of data acquisition that require patient immobilization. There is also the difficulty of working within the magnetic field restrictions of the MRI environment. High magnetic fields require implementation of safety measures to prevent ferromagnetic objects from being pulled into the scanner, thereby acting as missiles. Selection of ventilators, intubation devices, and monitoring devices must be made so that they are safe. In addition, MRI is a poor tool for observing bone (lack of mobile protons) and does not show acute subarachnoid hemorrhage (SAH), a finding well depicted on CT.

## CT Technique

### Acute Injury (Day 1 to 3)—Routine

This study is done without contrast enhancement. Contrast injection is only performed if something nontraumatic and usually incidental is found, such as a brain tumor or an abscess.

*Slice Thickness: Axial (Transverse) Plane:*

- Infratentorial space (posterior fossa): 5 mm contiguous
- Supratentorial space:
  - Age: Birth to 2 years: 5 mm contiguous
  - Age: 3-18 years: 5-10 mm contiguous
- If a fracture of the cranial base is suspect:
  - Through base of skull: 1-2 mm contiguous
- If a fracture or dislocation of the upper cervical spine is suspect: 1 to 2 mm (C2-occiput)
- If a fracture of the orbit or facial bones is suspect (patient's clinical condition including clearance of spinal injury permits): coronal plane, 1-3 mm contiguous

*Technical Factors:*

| | |
|---|---|
| Matrix size | 512 × 512 to 1024 × 1024 |
| kV | 120-137 |
| mA | 110-250 |
| Time | 1-5 seconds/section |

Actual choices depend on scanner geometry: tube, detectors, and so on.The principle is to keep the time as short as possible to prevent sections from being ruined by patient motion but to have the time long enough and at sufficient kilovolts and milliamperes that an adequate diagnostic evaluation is obtained.

### Data (Image) Manipulation

*Windows.* The image should be photographed for hard copy display with three sets of windows:

1. *Brain window* has low window width (WW) and low window level (WL), e.g., WW = 80 Hounsfield units (HU) and WL = 40 HU.
2. *Hematoma or intermediate windows*—This set separates two relatively dense substances (bone and hematoma), which appear as the same density on the brain windows, from each other by widening the WW. The denser bone remains whiter than the less dense adjacent hematoma. NOTE—This is especially critical in demonstrating small peripheral extracerebral hematomas (subdural, epidural).
3. *Bone windows*—To see structural detail within the substance of the bone of the skull, it is necessary to increase the WW and WL until the trabecular detail of the diploic space becomes visible, e.g., WW = 2,000 to 4,000 HU and WL = 500 to 2,500+ HU.

The best settings will vary from patient to patient, depending on the thickness and density of the skull. Genetic variability (sex) and disease states (e.g., sickle cell anemia, hydrocephalus) affect the thickness of the skull.

Depending on the scanner, the method of handling the data, and the algorithms available, the data acquired may be more optimally displayed at the three window sets. For the first two, soft-tissue algorithm suffices, whereas for the third, reprocessing of the data with a bone algorithm gives sharper edge definition and permits easier identification of small fractures.

*Reformatting.* Fractures of the upper cervical spine, cranial base, orbits, or facial bones may be better visualized (e.g., they may not be visualized at all on axial section—such as fracture of the base of the odontoid) on coronal or sagittal reconstructions. NOTE—These are routinely done at our institution with the 2 mm cuts for the C2-occiput.

*Three-Dimensional Reconstruction.* Contiguous thin sections (1 to 3 mm) with or without overlap can be used as a 3D data set and then displayed over a 360° rotation with either a skin soft-tissue or bony reconstruction algorithm. NOTE—This form of display is particularly useful for correlating soft-tissue injury (laceration or swelling) with the site and nature of fracture and/or foreign body.

## MRI Technique

### Acute Injury (Day 1 to 3)—Routine

A study is rarely performed at this time because of difficulty with motion and/or support and monitoring equipment.

### Subacute Injury (Day 7 to 30)—Routine

Once the patient has become stable, MRI provides valuable information regarding the nature and extent of injury. These studies are usually done without contrast (gadolinium) injection.

#### *Types of Pulse Sequences:*

1. T1 weighted: short TR, short TE spin echo (TR = 400-600 msec; TE = 11-30 msec).

2. Proton density weighted image (PDWI)—T2WI: long TR, short and long TE spin echo (TR = 2500-3000 msec; TE = 22-35 msec and 70-90 msec). NOTE—In infants under age 2, the second echo should be longer due to the unmyelinated white matter; e.g., 120 msec.
3. Gradient-echo T2 image: This is done to look for small areas of susceptibility effect at sites of prior hemorrhage, e.g., TR = 600 msec, TE = 40 msec, Flip angle = 10°.

*Imaging Planes:*
Sagittal
Axial (Transverse)
Coronal
Number of planes: 2-3
*Slice Thickness:*
Depends on part examined
Brain: 5 mm
Orbit and optic chiasm: 3 mm
nterslice gap: 0-2 mm in brain
Number of acquisitions: 1 or 2 NEX
*Matrix Size:*
128 × 256 to 512 × 512, most often 196 × 256
*Scan Time:*
T1WI (spin echo) = 2 minutes
PDWI and T2WI (spin echo) = 7-12 minutes
Gradient echo = 4 minutes
Total scan time = 30-60 minutes.

Magnetic resonance angiography is performed if clinically indicated to evaluate intactness of intracranial blood supply. Techniques are those of 3D time-of-flight (TOF) or phase-contrast techniques.

### Chronic Injury (Day 30+)

These temporal divisions are artificial but express the concept that, once the initial event has occurred, the course is one of resolution if a process of progressive irreversible damage has not been instituted. This next period (subacute) usually extends over the remainder of the first month after injury. Beyond that, the changes are usually static or at most a slow atrophy of the brain substance (chronic).

At these points in time, MRI is often more revealing than CT, although the ability to obtain the MRI study still depends on the patient being motion-free.

With both imaging techniques, contrast agents are of little use, unless a complication such as a brain abscess, subdural empyema, or meningitis is suspect.

There is no specific formula for when or how often to obtain follow-up imaging studies after trauma. In most instances they are done to demonstrate resolution of a mass (hematoma, contusion, swelling) or to demonstrate the development of a post-traumatic complication such as hydrocephalus.

## Diagnostic Approach

### *Key Image Signs of Disease*

1. *Subarachnoid Hemorrhage* produces an increased density within the subarachnoid space. This is best observed where the full thickness of the axial CT slice is occupied by the SAH, such as adjacent to the falx cerebri.

2. *Subdural Hematoma*—The collections, whether high density or low density, usually parallel the calvarium displacing the brain inward. The potential subdural space permits hematomas in this compartment to extend around and below the hemisphere.

3. *Epidural Hematoma*—These collections are bound down by the periosteum of the calvarium. This accounts for their frequent biconvex configuration.

4. *Contusions* are usually hemorrhagic and cortical and involve the site of impact (coup) or occur opposite this site (contracoup).

5. *Diffuse Axonal Injury* is characterized by the presence of telltale small hemorrhages (CT or MRI) or focal areas of edema (MRI) at sites of axonal tearing in the corpus callosum (splenium and body), cortical gray and white matter junctures, basal ganglia, and upper brain stem.

### *Differential Diagnosis*

Hemorrhagic processes that occur in trauma can be mimicked by those found with spontaneous bleeding of many etiologies, e.g., ruptured arteriovenous malformation (AVM) and aneurysm, bleeding diathesis. The nonhemorrhagic changes of swelling, focal or generalized, found post-trauma can be observed in association with a number of disease processes including toxic, hypoxic, and metabolic. Fractures of the calvarium, of course, must be differentiated from sutures and vascular grooves.

### *Pitfalls in Technique and Interpretation*

Motion and incomplete studies preclude effective intepretation, as does failure to provide hematoma and bone windows with CT or PDWI and T2WI with MRI.

## Suggested Reading

Gentry LR, Godersky JC, Thompson B. MR imaging of head trauma: Review of the distribution and radiopathologic features of traumatic lesions. Am J Neuroradiol 1988; 9:101.

Gentry LR, Godersky JC, Thompson B. Traumatic brain stem injury: MR imaging. Radiology 1989; 171:177.

Zimmerman RA. Supratentorial trauma. In: Taveras JM, Ferrucci JT, eds. Radiology: Diagnosis/Imaging/Intervention. Philadelphia: JB Lippincott, 1985.

Zimmerman RA. Infratentorial trauma. In: Taveras JM, Ferrucci JT, eds. Radiology: Diagnosis/Imaging/Intervention. Philadelphia: JB Lippincott, 1985.

Zimmerman RA, Bilaniuk LT, Hackney DB, et al. Head injury: Early results of comparing CT and high-field MRI. Am J Neuroradiol 1986; 7:757–764.

# Color Duplex Sonography of the Neonatal Brain

*MAURICIO CASTILLO, M.D.*

Ultrasonography continues to be one of the most practical and noninvasive methods of imaging the neonatal brain. Ultrasonography not only provides morphological information but my recent experience seems to indicate that the use of Doppler ultrasonography (DU) may provide important information concerning the physiology of neonatal cerebral blood flow in specific situations. Doppler measurements obtained from the intracranial arteries (mainly the anterior cerebral arteries [ACAs]) may predict the outcome of neonates with significant brain injuries such as intracranial hemorrhage and/or cerebral edema. Neonates with hydrocephalus show altered Doppler spectra, which usually return to normal after successful ventricular shunting. Therefore DU can be used to evaluate shunt patency, even before the ventricular system has had time to return to its normal shape. I have also successfully used DU to distinguish between massive hydrocephalus and hydranencephaly. I have not found any clear use for this technique in the presence of other congenital cerebral malformations.

## Technique and Normal Anatomy

The examination is performed using 5.0 or 7.5 mHz phase array sector transducers through the anterior fontanelle as a window. If the anterior fontanelle is not accessible, the lamboid fontanelle can be used. The examination begins with the transducer in the midsagittal position. The color is turned on and flow should be evident through the ACAs (located anteriorly to the third ventricle and corpus callosum). The color gain should be set high enough for optimal visualization of the arteries but little or no background noise. At this time, the ACA is assigned red color. It is important to remember that anatomic location, rather than color assignment, determines which vessel is being imaged. For example, when the color is correctly assigned, the midsagittal image shows the posterior aspect of the pericallosal and callosal marginal arteries in blue, because the direction of the flow in these arteries is away from the transducer. The basilar artery can also be identified in the midsagittal plane. By slightly angling the transducer laterally, one is able to clearly observe the cavernous internal carotid artery. If one continues to sweep laterally, the middle cerebral artery can be followed and lastly its branches within the insula are seen. Anterior coronal views demonstrate the proximal aspect of the ACAs and the pericallosal and callosomarginal arteries in a piecemeal fashion.

Doppler spectra from the ACAs are easily obtained in the coronal or midsagittal projections (Fig. 1 and Color Plate 17). If the coronal images are used, the Doppler velocity readings may be slightly overestimated, because no angle correction can be employed. In the midsagittal plane, the angle of insonation of the ACAs is approximately 0°. The pulsed Doppler gate is then positioned at the level of the proximal ACAs (just anterior to the corpus callosum). The sample volume gate should be wide enough to obtain an adequate Doppler signal with little background noise (generally, gate = 1.5 mm). The Doppler output level should be kept at a minimal level ($\leq 94$ mW/cm$^2$) to provide adequate signal recording. The normal Doppler spectra from all intracranial arteries are characterized by sharp systolic upstrokes and gentle downslope antegrade diastolic flow (above the baseline). Absent or inverted diastolic flow is always pathological. The peak systolic and end–diastolic velocities should be measured in meters per second (m/sec) or a similar scale (cm/sec). The normal Doppler spectra reflect the presence of a low-resistance cerebrovascular system. I routinely obtain Doppler spectra from only the proximal ACAs. The ACAs are easily accessible and their Doppler measurements can be reliably reproduced. Angle correction is necessary in only some cases to correct the angle between the axis of the ACA and the Doppler sampling line. Angle correction is indispensable when sampling the middle and/or posterior cerebral arteries. I measured the velocities in the ACAs (in both sagittal and coronal planes) in approximately 50 normal premature infants (28 to 33 weeks). In all these patients, the peak systolic velocity varied between 50 and 60 cm/sec while the end diastolic velocity varied from 1 to 20 cm/sec. These velocities may increase slightly in more mature babies (normal gestational age) or in older neonates.

The resistive index (RI) from the ACA can be easily calculated from information present in its Doppler spectra and reflects the resistance of the cerebral vascular bed. The use of this ratio downplays the effect of the probe angle, that is, the RI may be considered angle independent. The presence of diastolic flow throughout the cardiac cycle and an RI of no more than 0.8 indicate normal cerebral arterial perfusion. The normal RI varies from 0.2 to 0.8. The RI is easily obtained by using the following formula: (peak systolic − end diastolic)/peak systolic. The RI may decrease slightly with progressively increasing age and maturity. The RI should be used only when one assumes normal cardiovascular status to be present. Conditions such as patent ductus arteriosus negate the utility of the RI.

Doppler spectra and velocity measurements can also be obtained in the major cerebral veins and sinuses; however, at this time I have found no clinical utility for these measurements and therefore do not use them. An examination that includes real-time evaluation of the entire brain and Doppler interrogation of at least the ACA should last no more than 3 to 5 minutes.

## Cerebral Edema

Perinatal asphyxia is the usual underlying etiology of diffuse cerebral edema in the neonate. The diagnosis of diffuse cerebral edema can be readily made if the echogenicity of the brain parenchyma is equal to or greater than that of the cerebellar vermis. In patients with diffuse cerebral edema, the normal basal ganglia cannot be separated from the surrounding structures. Other useful, but less commonly appreciated, signs include compression of the ventricular system and of the extra-axial spaces due to the swollen brain. Minimal edema can be difficult to detect but is probably of no clinical significance since the majority of these patients have a good prognosis. Ultrasonography provides better information concerning the

A

B

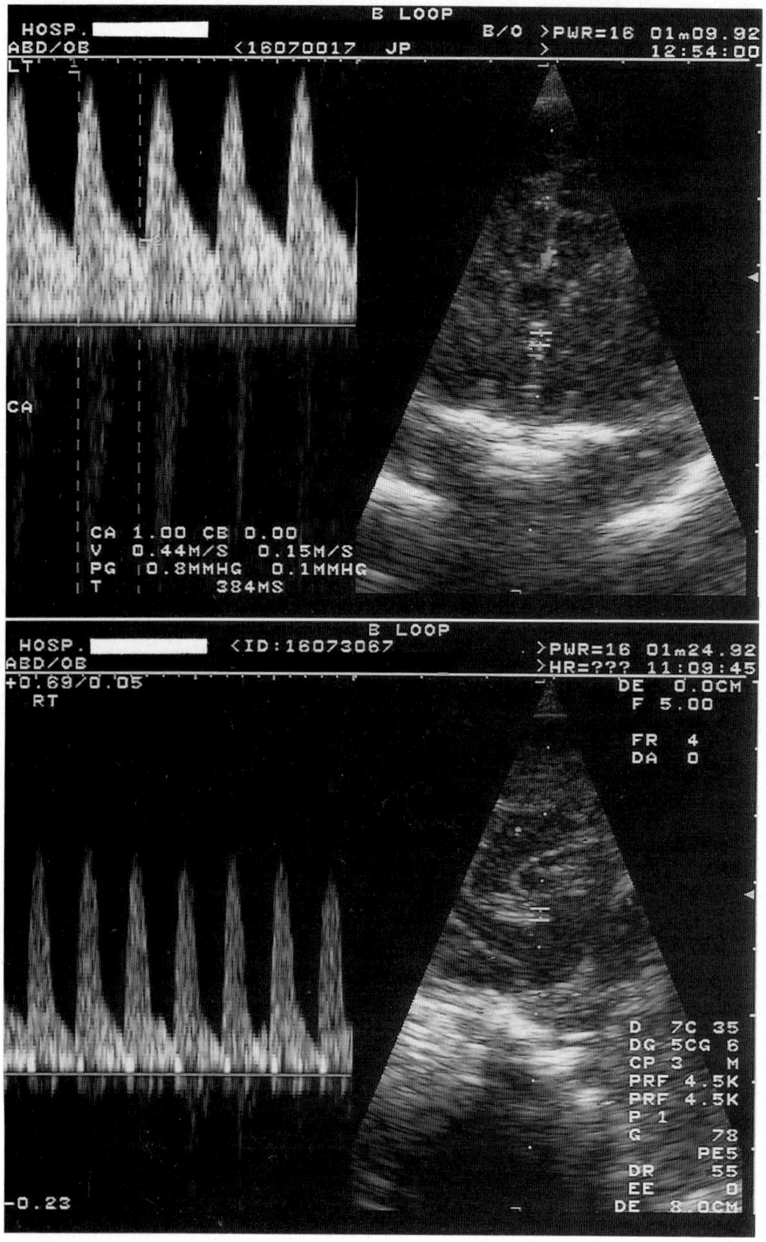


**FIGURE 1** Doppler spectra from the anterior cerebral artery in a normal preterm neonate. *A,* Coronal projection. The configuration of the Doppler spectra is normal. The peak systolic velocity is 0.44 m/sec, and the end-diastolic velocity is 0.15 m/sec. Resistive index (RI) is 0.65 and within normal limits. Notice that on coronal projections, no angle correction can be used, and therefore absolute velocities may be mildly increased. However, RI should still be within normal limits, because this measurement is considered angle independent. *B,* Midsagittal projection. No angle correction was used. Notice the sharp systolic upstroke and gentle diastolic downstroke. Diastolic flow should always be evident and above the baseline. In this patient the peak systolic velocity was 0.4 m/sec and the end-diastolic velocity was 0.08 m/sec. The RI is 0.8 (within normal limits). See also Color Plate 17.

presence of diffuse cerebral edema than either computed tomography (CT) or magnetic resonance imaging (MRI). This is because the normal neonatal brain contains a large amount of water and therefore edema may not be obvious by either CT or MRI. Using DU, neonates with diffuse cerebral edema may be classified into three different groups: those with mild, moderate, and severe diffuse edema. Neonates can be grouped within this classification according to the RI calculated from Doppler spectra measurements from the ACAs. This classification is also clinically useful, because each of these groups will have a different prognosis.

Patients within group I demonstrate normal Doppler flow profiles as well as normal systolic and diastolic velocities in the ACAs. The RI is normal in these patients; this usually indicates that the cerebral arterial blood flow mechanisms are functioning normally. In the majority of these patients, the outcome is usually good, although some of these children later exhibit minor developmental handicaps.

Patients with elevated end-diastolic velocities but normal peak systolic velocities belong in group II. These patients have moderate cerebral edema and their RI is low. Doppler spectra from the ACAs suggest that there is an increase in the total cerebral blood flow (mainly at the expense of diastolic flow), probably occurring as a compensatory and protective mechanism to the already injured brain. In the majority of these patients, follow-up real-time and DU studies show that the brain returns to normal. However, clinically these patients may later exhibit mild handicaps and/or seizures. Recently I evaluated two neonates who were initially classified as group II. Follow-up CT studies performed 2 months later demonstrated significant brain damage; therefore I recommend careful clinical and radiographic follow-up of patients in group II.

Group III patients (those with severe cerebral edema) generally show decreased diastolic velocities. The diastolic flow may be decreased, completely absent, or at times retrograde (waveforms below the baseline) (Fig. 2). Therefore in this

A

B

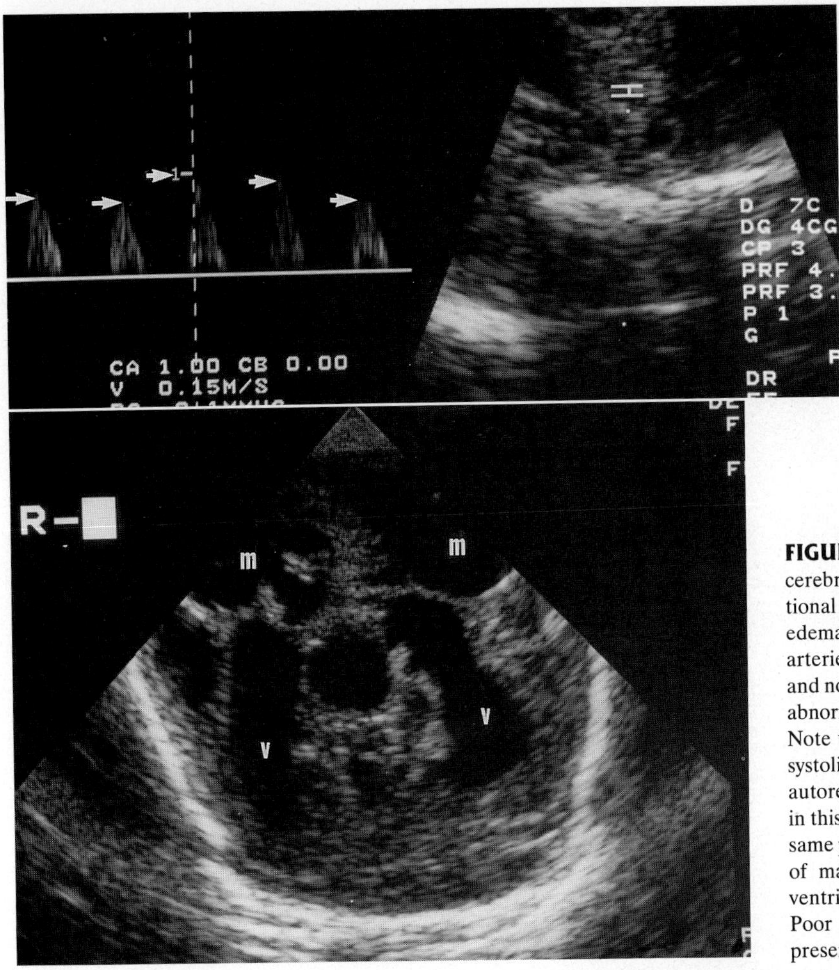


**FIGURE 2** *A,* Initial Doppler sampling of the anterior cerebral arteries in a premature infant (28 weeks' gestational age) with a history of perinatal asphyxia and cerebral edema. Doppler sampling of the proximal anterior cerebral arteries show decreased peak systolic velocity (0.15 m/sec) and no diastolic flow. The absence of diastolic flow is always abnormal. The RI is therefore markedly elevated (RI = 1). Note the unequal and varying heights *(arrows)* of the peak systolic waveforms, indicating loss of cerebral blood flow autoregulation. The prognosis can be expected to be dismal in this case. *B,* Real-time coronal sonogram obtained on the same patient at 3 weeks of age. There has been development of marked hydrocephalus with dilatation of the lateral ventricles (v) as well as multiple areas of cystic malacia (m). Poor motor development and generalized seizures were present 6 months after the initial ultrasonographic study.

group the RI is high. The Doppler profiles may also show variations in the magnitude (height) and the amplitude (width) of both the systolic and diastolic waveforms. Physiologically, these infants have only passive cerebral perfusion, an overall reduction of cerebral blood flow (secondary to severe diffuse cerebral edema and increased intracranial pressure), and lack of vascular autoregulation. Follow-up studies demonstrate major brain damage in most of these newborns, and the outcome tends to be dismal (Fig. 3). Most of these patients later exhibit signs of major mental and motor retardation, and many expire during the neonatal period.

## Intracranial Hemorrhage

It is well known that newborns with grade I and II intracranial hemorrhages have a favorable prognosis, whereas patients with grade III and IV intracranial hemorrhages later demonstrate severe mental and developmental handicaps. I have used DU to identify which patients with large intracerebral hemorrhages (grade III or IV) will not survive the neonatal period. I evaluated five premature newborns (28 to 32 weeks) with significant bleeds (at least a unilateral grade III intracranial hemorrhage) and found that in two fatal cases Doppler spectra from the ACAs showed inverted diastolic flow waves and variable magnitude of the systolic peaks (Fig. 4). In the three surviving babies, the Doppler spectra as well as the RI were normal.

## Hydrocephalus

In some newborns with hydrocephalus, the dilatation of the ventricles may be so severe that differentiating them from hydranencephaly may be impossible using only conventional real-time sonography. Obviously, the differentiation of these two entities is clinically important because the presence of hydranencephaly implies a dismal prognosis. In my opinion, MRI is the method of choice to differentiate these two entities. However, the extensive life-support system required by these neonates makes it difficult to obtain the MRI studies. I have evaluated two newborns with markedly enlarged and fluid-filled heads. In these two patients color duplex sonography failed to identify any intracranial flow and therefore the diagnosis of hydranencephaly was suggested (Fig. 5). Both of these patients expired, and autopsy confirmed the diagnosis of hydranencephaly. Although my experience is limited to these two cases, I believe that the use of duplex sonography for this purpose deserves further investigation.

In patients with less severe hydrocephalus, the dilated ventricular system behaves as a space-occupying mass, compressing the surrounding brain parenchyma. This leads to increased intracranial pressure and decreased cerebral blood flow. This abnormal blood flow physiology is reflected by an elevation of the RI (generally at the expense of reduced diastolic blood flow) (Fig. 6, *A*). After surgical decompression of the ventricular system (i.e., shunt placement), the intracranial pressure returns to normal. This is reflected by the

A

B

C

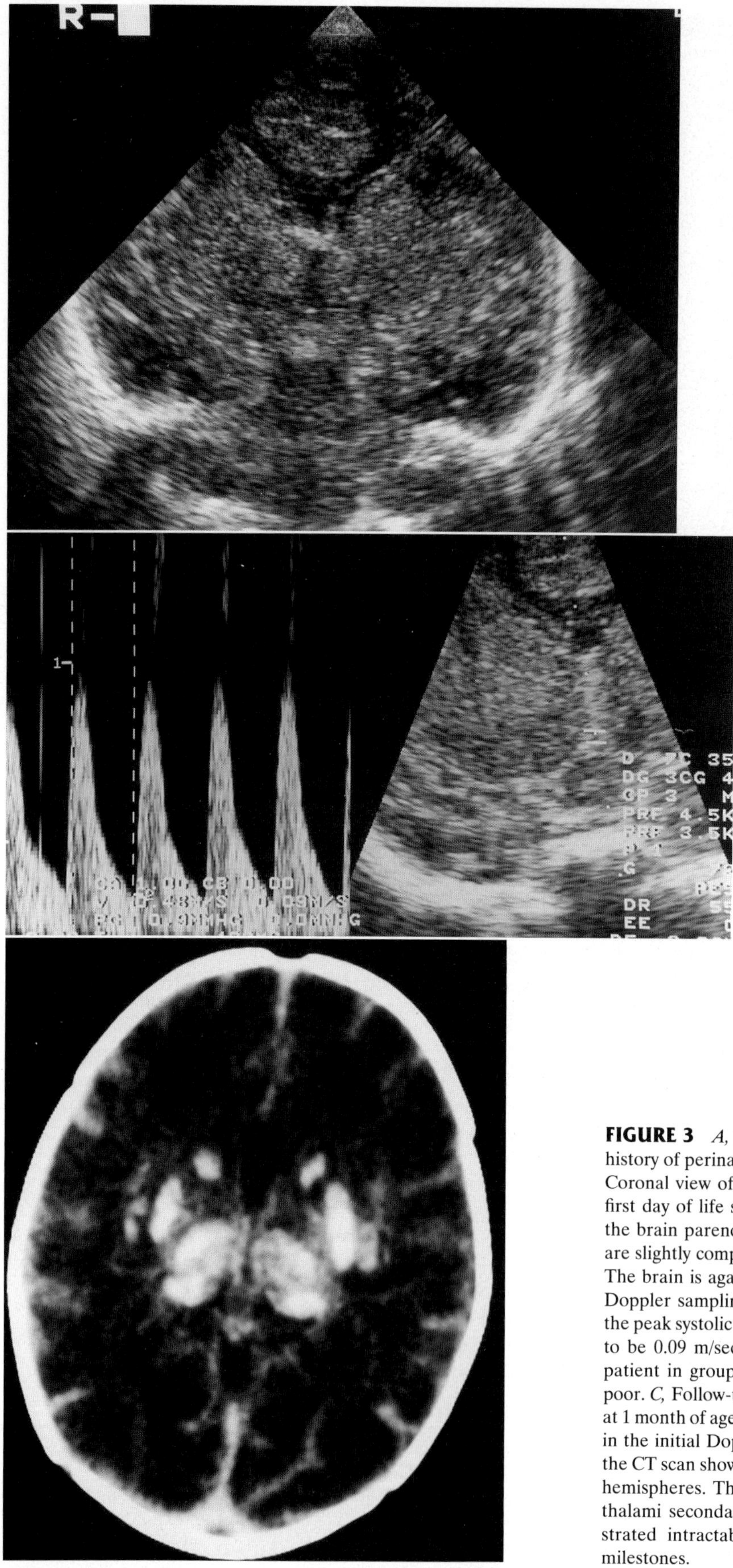

**FIGURE 3** *A,* Premature newborn (32 weeks' gestation age) with a history of perinatal asphyxia and low Apgar scores at 3 and 5 minutes. Coronal view of the initial ultrasonographic study performed on the first day of life shows increased and diffuse echogenicity throughout the brain parenchyma compatible with edema. The lateral ventricles are slightly compressed. *B,* Follow-up study obtained 3 days after *(A).* The brain is again noted to be diffusely echogenic, reflecting edema. Doppler sampling of the proximal anterior cerebral arteries showed the peak systolic velocity to be 0.48 m/sec and the end-diastolic velocity to be 0.09 m/sec. The RI is 0.82 (mildly elevated). This places this patient in group III; therefore the prognosis can be expected to be poor. *C,* Follow-up noncontrast CT scan on the same patient obtained at 1 month of age. As suspected by the hemodynamic changes observed in the initial Doppler sonogram, the poor prognosis is confirmed and the CT scan shows extensive encephalomalacia involving both cerebral hemispheres. There are calcifications in the basal ganglia and in the thalami secondary to infarctions. Subsequently, this patient demonstrated intractable seizures and a severe delay in developmental milestones.

A

B

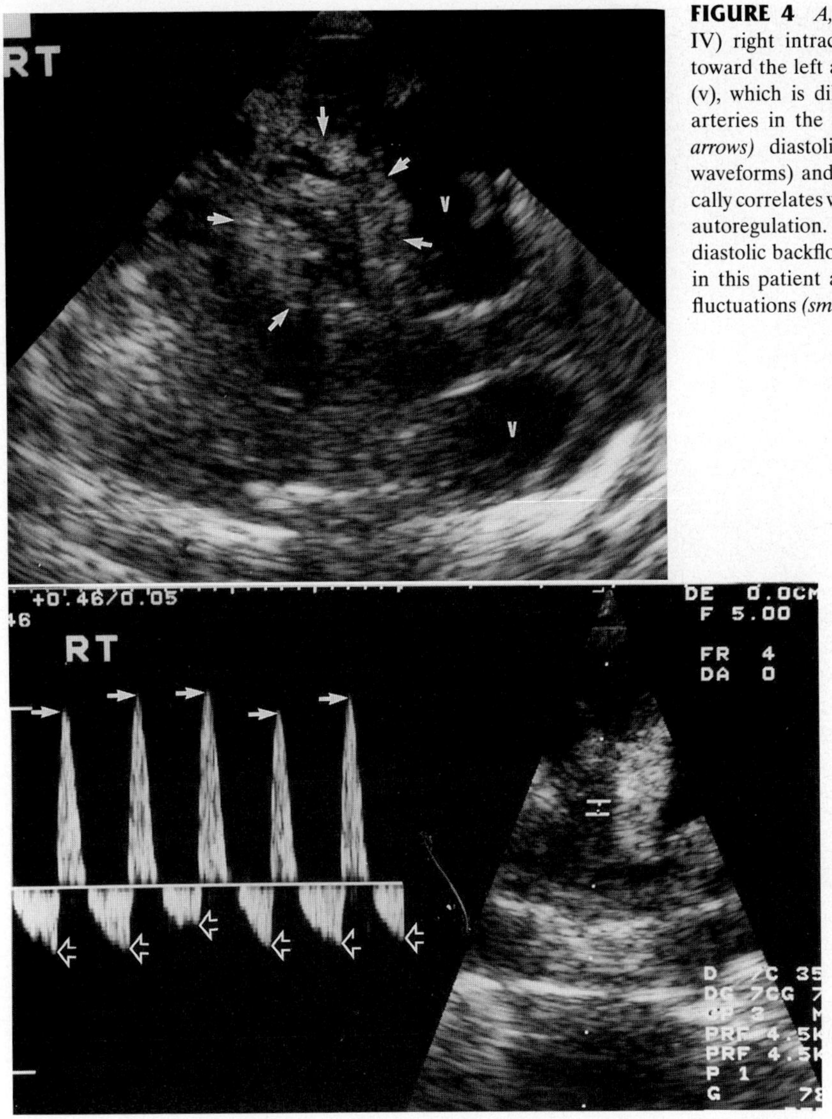


**FIGURE 4** *A,* Midcoronal real-time sonogram shows a large (grade IV) right intracranial hemorrhage *(arrows).* There is midline shift toward the left and secondary entrapment of the left lateral ventricle (v), which is dilated. *B,* Doppler sampling of the anterior cerebral arteries in the same patient. Notice the negative (backflow) *(open arrows)* diastolic flow, which fluctuates in magnitude (height of waveforms) and in amplitude (width of waveforms). This physiologically correlates with only passive cerebral perfusion and loss of vascular autoregulation. In this case, the RI is elevated. Other causes of diastolic backflow, such as patent ductus arteriosus, were not present in this patient at the time this study was performed. Also seen are fluctuations *(small solid arrows)* in the height of the systolic waveforms.

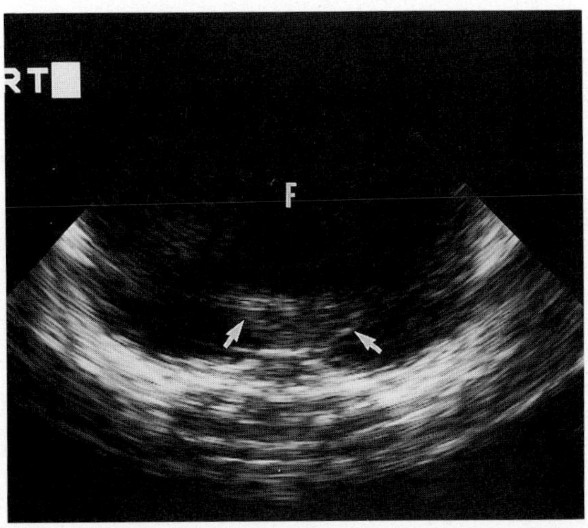


**FIGURE 5** Coronal sonogram demonstrates a large amount of fluid (F) replacing the cerebral hemispheres. The thalami *(arrows)* are preserved. Based solely on this real-time image, it is possible to determine if the findings represent hydranencephaly or massive hydrocephalus. Color duplex sonography failed to reveal any intracranial blood flow, suggesting the possibility of in utero occlusion of the internal carotid arteries and therefore hydranencephaly. Hydranencephaly was later confirmed at autopsy. The distinction between hydrocephalus and hydranencephaly is clinically significant because the latter has a dismal prognosis.

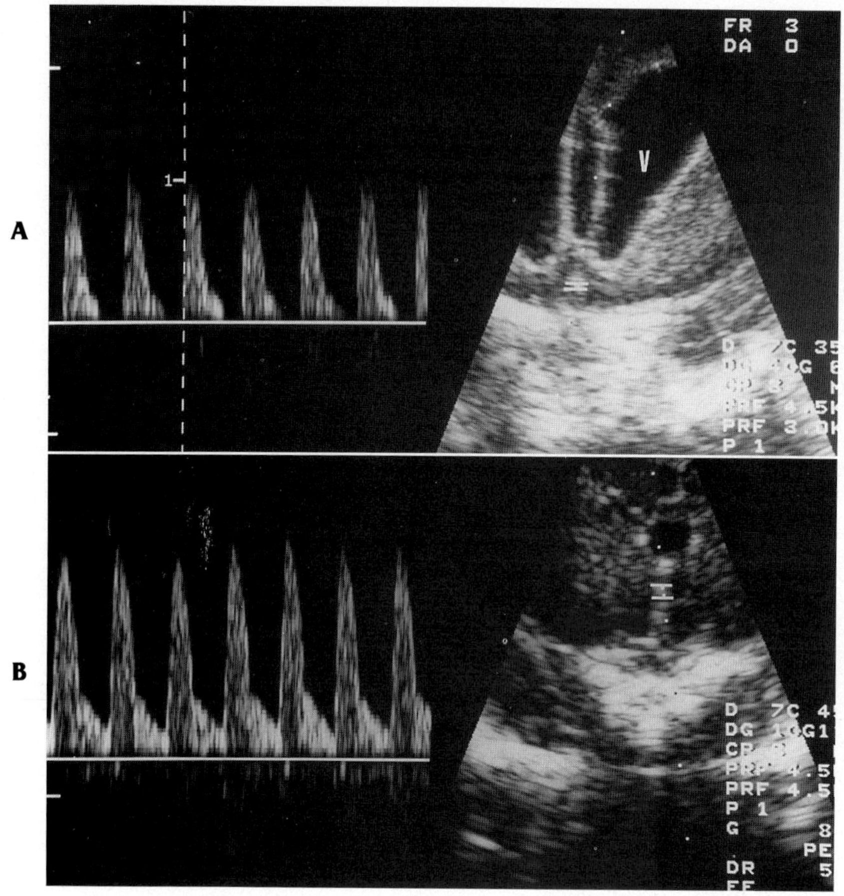

**FIGURE 6** *A,* Doppler sampling of the anterior cerebral arteries in a newborn with hydrocephalus secondary to a previous intraventricular hemorrhage (bilateral grade III bleeds). Notice the dilatation of the frontal horn of the lateral ventricles (v). Doppler spectra of the anterior cerebral arteries show a normal peak systolic velocity (0.5 m/sec) but absence of diastolic flow. The RI is therefore elevated (RI = 1). The dilated ventricular system produces mass effect on the brain, leading to increased intracranial pressure and only passive blood flow (systolic). *B,* Doppler sampling of the anterior cerebral artery in the same patient after a clinically successful ventricular shunt was placed and the head circumference had decreased. Subdural collections were not present. The size of the ventricles had also returned to normal. The Doppler spectra of the anterior cerebral arteries has returned to normal (peak systolic velocity = 0.5 m/sec; end-diastolic velocity = 0.10 m/sec; RI = 0.8).

re-establishment of normal Doppler spectra and normal RI values (Fig. 6, *B*). If large subdural collections develop after ventricular decompression, they may exert pressure on the brain parenchyma and the Doppler profiles may remain abnormal. I have successfully used this decrease in the RI to appraise the patency of recently inserted ventricular shunts. After successful shunting, the RI returns to normal almost immediately. This is especially important because re-establishment of normal ventricular size may lag somewhat. I have evaluated five neonates who received ventricular shunts for hydrocephalus secondary to intraventricular hemorrhage. In all these babies, the RI was initially elevated but returned to normal shortly after successful shunt placement.

## Discussion

DU offers a noninvasive way of determining the prognosis of patients with diffuse cerebral edema and/or intracranial hemorrhage. The patency of ventricular shunts for hydrocephalus can also be indirectly assessed. I examined five patients with severe congenital malformations of the brain (holoprosencephaly, schizencephaly, and pachygyria) and found that the blood flow through the ACA was normal in all of them. I do not presently feel that DU is useful in patients with congenital brain malformations other than hydrocephalus. There has been some suggestion, especially by European authors, that the use of DU may help predict the prognosis of neonates with meningitis. In patients with meningitis, a markedly decreased or elevated RI, as well as retrograde or absent diastolic flow, indicate that these patients will have a poor outcome. I do not presently have any personal experience in this clinical setting.

## Suggested Reading

Deeg KH. Colour flow imaging of the great intracranial arteries in infants. Neuroradiology 1989; 31:40–43.

Deeg KH, Rupprecht TH, Zeilinger G. Doppler sonography classification of brain edema in infants. Pediatr Radiol 1990; 20:509–514.

Grant EG, White EM, Schellinger D, et al. Cranial duplex sonography of the infant. Radiology 1987; 163:177–185.

Horgan JG, Rumack CM, Hay T, et al. Absolute intracranial blood-flow velocities evaluated by duplex Doppler sonography in asymptomatic preterm and term neonates. AJR 1989; 152:1059–1064.

Lopez Barrio AM. La ecografia Duplex-Doppler en las meningitis del recien nacido-lactante. Radiologia 1991; 33:567–573.

Mitchell DG, Merton D, Needleman L, et al. Neonatal brain: Color Doppler imaging. Part I—Technique and vascular anatomy. Radiology 1988; 167:303–306.

Ohlsson A, Fong K, Ryan ML, et al. Cerebral-blood-flow-velocity measurements in neonates: Technique and interobserver reliability. Pediatr Radiol 1991; 21:395–397.

Seibert JJ, McCowan TC, Chadduck WM, et al. Duplex pulsed Doppler US versus intracranial pressure in the neonate: Clinical and experimental studies. Radiology 1989; 171:155–159.

# Imaging Approach to Urinary Tract Infections in Children

*ROBERT L. LEBOWITZ, M.D.*

The two uses of imaging when an infant or a child has a urinary tract infection (UTI) are (1) to detect vesicoureteral reflux, which places the kidney at risk for ascending infection whenever she[1] has infected urine in her bladder, and (2) to detect obstructive hydronephrosis so that the obstruction can be relieved. Voiding cystourethrography (VCUG) and radionuclide cystography (RNC) are the imaging methods I use to show or exclude reflux. I usually first suspect obstruction on ultrasonography in the child in whom VCUG is negative, and then confirm and characterize the obstruction by either renal scintigraphy or excretory urography (IVP).

## Choice of Imaging Study

The imaging tests and their order depend on the age of the child,[2] the likelihood that the kidney was infected, and family history. For example, Figure 1 shows my approach to the infant or young child with a well-documented UTI. Ultrasonography and voiding cystourethrography are done in all patients. If the results of these tests are normal, no further imaging evaluations are necessary; subsequent infections, if any, are usually cystitis, not pyelonephritis. If ultrasonography is either normal or shows hydronephrosis and VCUG shows uncomplicated reflux, no further tests are done. Her therapy is then on the basis of degree and characterization of the reflux, her age, and the ability of her family to carry out prolonged medical management. If she has hydronephrosis and her VCUG shows either no reflux or reflux plus obstruction, the obstruction is confirmed and quantified by renal scintigraphy with furosemide (Lasix) provocation. If an abnormality is shown by refluxed contrast material but further depiction of anatomy is needed (e.g., the details of a duplex anomaly), IVP is the next step.

Figure 2 shows my approach in an older child who has had a UTI, and in whom, on the basis of her signs and symptoms, pyelonephritis is not likely and therefore reflux is not strongly suspected. After a normal ultrasonographic study, either nothing else is done or, if it is important to be sure about the absence of reflux, I recommend RNC. If RNC unexpectedly shows reflux, a decision is made on a case-by-case basis about whether further characterization of reflux by means of VCUG is needed. If ultrasonography shows either hydronephrosis or scarring of the kidney, the next imaging test is VCUG.

Figure 3 shows my approach to a still older child or teenager with a UTI but only lower urinary tract signs and symptoms. Reflux is highly unlikely; a negative ultrasonographic study therefore makes further imaging unnecessary. If ultrasonography unexpectedly shows hydronephrosis or scarring, however, VCUG becomes necessary.

The comparative advantage of the fluoroscopic voiding cystogram is that it characterizes reflux precisely, because of its excellent spatial resolution (Figs. 4 and 5). Its disadvantage is that, to keep radiation exposure to a minimum, fluoroscopy must be intermittent. The advantage of RNC is that since radiation exposure is determined by the amount of technetium

[1] The pronouns she/her are used throughout but the principles apply to boys as well.
[2] The likelihood that reflux will be present and the vulnerability of the kidney to infectious damage decrease with age.

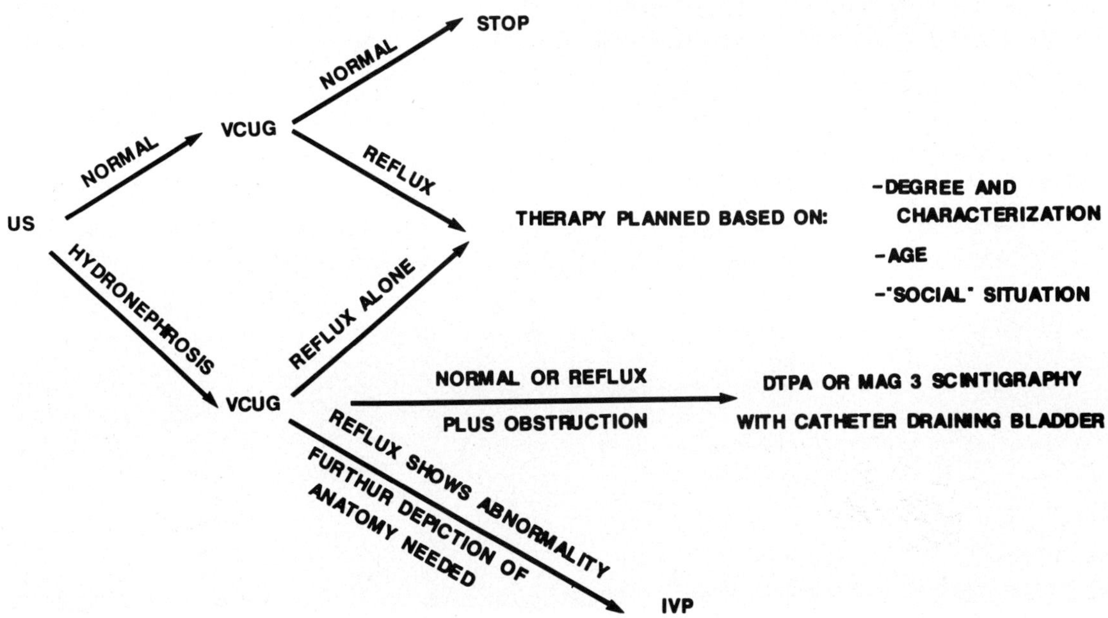


**FIGURE 1** Imaging recommendations for an infant or a young child with UTI or anyone in whom pyelonephritis is suspected (reflux is both likely and important).

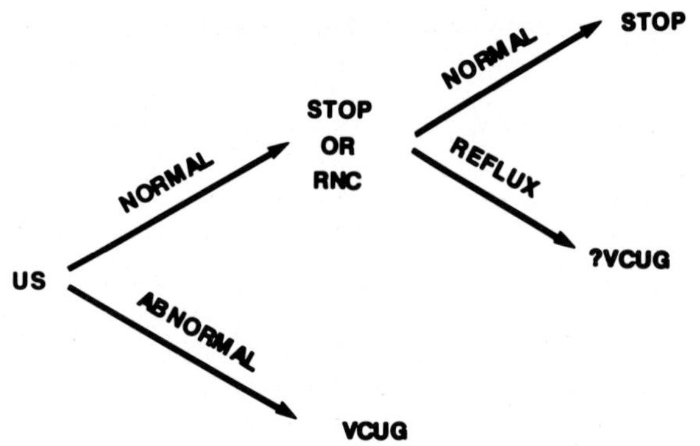


**FIGURE 2** Imaging recommendations in an older child with only lower urinary tract signs and symptoms. Pyelonephritis is not suspected (reflux is less likely and less important).

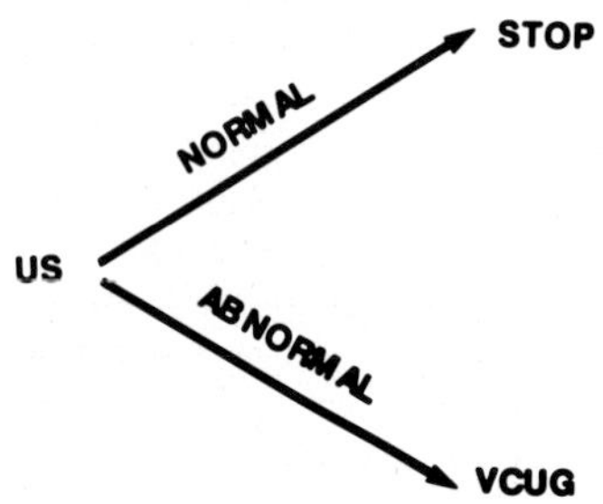


**FIGURE 3** Imaging recommendations in a still older child or teenager with lower urinary tract signs and symptoms. Pyelonephritis is not suspected (reflux is highly unlikely and much less important).

instilled into the bladder, the monitoring by the gamma camera for reflux can be continuous. The dose is exceedingly low, perhaps only 1 or 2 percent of a modern low-dose fluoroscopic study. The disadvantage is that the spatial resolution and therefore the characterization of reflux are poor (Fig. 6).

Renal imaging in the child with a UTI may be done by ultrasonography, excretory urography, renal scintigraphy using either technetium-99m diethylenetriamine penta-acetic acid ($^{99m}$Tc-DTPA), mercaptoacetyl triglycine (MAG 3), or dimercapto succinic acid (DMSA), or some combination of these. I almost always use ultrasonography first. Excretory urography adds almost nothing for the patient whose ultrasonogram is normal, whether reflux is present or not. I recommend DTPA/MAG 3 imaging when suspected obstruction needs to be confirmed or its severity quantified. DMSA scintigraphy is more sensitive to detect acute or chronic infectious injury of the kidney, but I seldom recommend it because the results do not usually affect treatment. Age, the severity and character of the reflux, the severity of the illness, and the patient's social situation, such as the stability of her family, not the presence of renal scarring, determine whether her treatment is medical (continuous antibiotic prophylaxis) or surgical (reimplantation of the ureter).

## Approach to Imaging

There is no specific time for the initial imaging studies in a child with infection. It is not necessary to wait 4 to 6 weeks after treatment. Voiding cystography and ultrasonography can be done on the same visit, and although this is convenient it is not

A

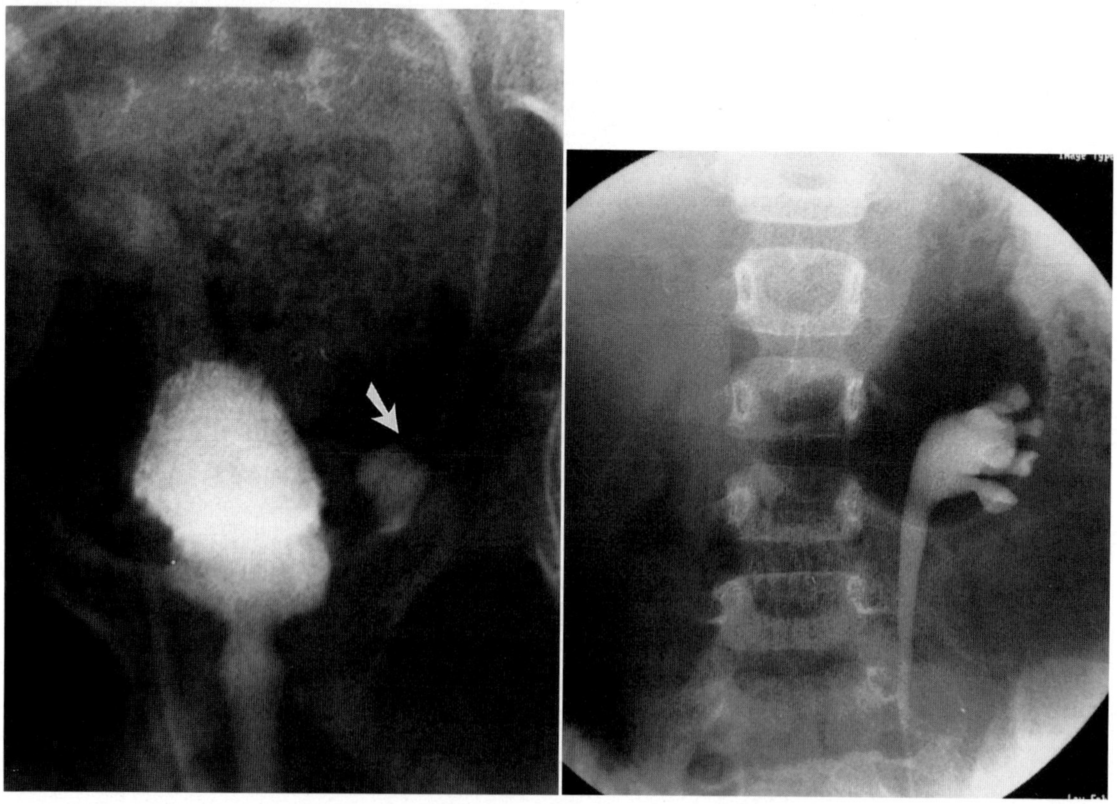

B

**FIGURE 4** Voiding cystourethrogram. *A,* Left ureter inserts into a bladder diverticulum *(arrow)*. *B,* Pelvicalyceal system shown by refluxed contrast material has the typical configuration of the lower pole of a double collecting system (same patient as *A*).

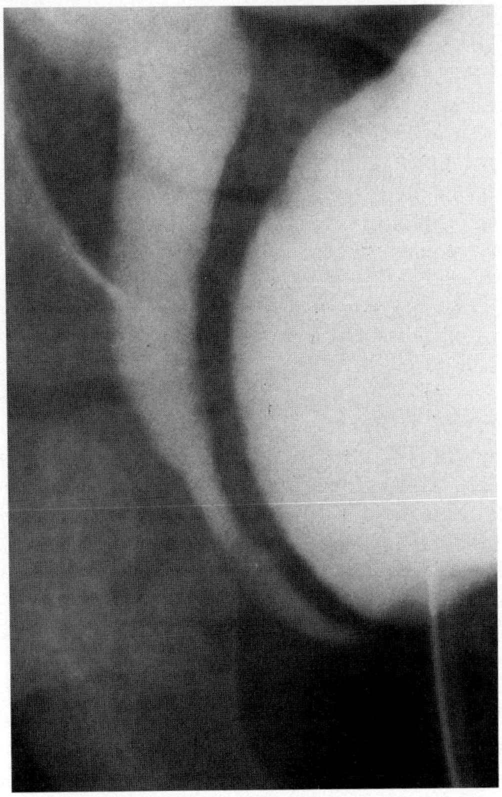

**FIGURE 5** Voiding cystourethrogram. Right ureter inserts ectopically near the neck of the bladder.

essential. Alternatively, we perform ultrasonography while the patient is in the hospital and then voiding cystography several weeks later. Timing of the studies is not crucial. It must be mentioned that a normal renal ultrasonogram does not exclude vesicoureteric reflux. Therefore the younger the child and the more likely that the episode was pyelonephritis, the more important it is to do the voiding cystogram even if ultrasonographic findings are negative.

In the rare situation where IVP is performed in a child with reflux or with some other abnormality shown on the voiding cystogram that needs further delineation, I use a nonionic contrast agent and often a catheter in the bladder to prevent artifacts that reflux can cause.

A child undergoing VCUG to verify suspected reflux should receive continuous antibiotic prophylaxis so that when the presence of reflux is confirmed, she is already being protected from further infection. (If her voiding cystogram is negative, the antibiotic can be discontinued.) I explain to her parents the rationale for the procedure, how it will be done, and what it is designed to show so that they understand the purpose and limitations of the study. I emphasize that the voiding cystogram will usually not show why their daughter got an infection in the first place, but will show conditions, such as reflux, that make infection more dangerous. I emphasize this because girls often continue to have infections even after imaging has shown no urinary tract abnormalities. These infections are usually cystitis, not pyelonephritis. I do not want the parents to think that imaging has failed when the child gets another infection.

The child should void before catheterization if she is able. I have her parent(s) sit at the head of the fluoroscopy table, and I ask what words the family uses for urination so that the child and I use the same term. I clean the area around the meatus with Hibiclens-soaked cotton balls, then I wash the Hibiclens

A

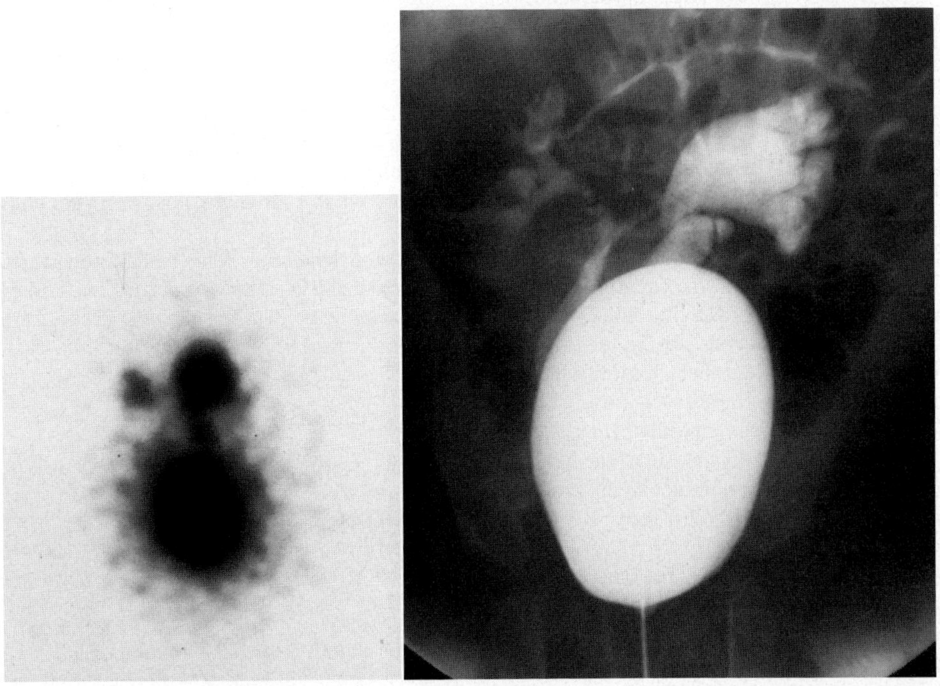

B

**FIGURE 6** *A,* Radionuclide cystogram shows bilateral reflux, greater on the left (image reversed to match VCUG). No further characterization is possible because of poor spatial resolution. *B,* Voiding cystourethrogram (same patient as *A*) reveals bilateral reflux: grade 2+ into a single (nonduplex) collecting system on the right and grade 4 into the lower pole of a double collecting system on the left.

away with sterile saline. Both solutions have been warmed. If the area around the meatus is irritated or erythematous, I apply 2 percent Xylocaine jelly to the area before cleaning to prevent stinging. In boys who are old enough to understand, I anesthetize the urethra with 2 percent Xylocaine jelly by first applying the jelly around the meatus and then injecting it through the meatus into the urethra using a fistula tip. I gently pinch the penis for 2 minutes to keep the jelly inside the lumen. After this the boy cannot feel the passage of the catheter. In boys too young to understand, it is usually more efficient simply to catheterize them without anesthetizing their urethra. In girls, if the urethral meatus is clearly identified and smoothly and gently catheterized, there will be no discomfort and Xylocaine in the urethra is not necessary.

Infant males have physiologic phimosis. The foreskin often cannot be retracted. In such a situation, I simply align the opening in the prepuce to the meatus; catheterization can then be performed without difficulty. If a tight foreskin has been retracted, I clean and catheterize quickly to avoid lengthy impedance of venous return from the glans. If such a foreskin is left retracted for too long, the glans might swell and it would not be possible to "unretract" it.

I catheterize almost all children with a no. 8 Fr infant-feeding tube lubricated with 2 percent Xylocaine jelly (in small premature infants a no. 5 Fr tube is used). If there is residual urine in the bladder, I send a specimen to be cultured. The volume of residual urine is recorded. If I have instilled Xylocaine into the urethra, that Xylocaine will temporarily occlude the lumen of the catheter. However, Xylocaine jelly is soluble; if there is any residual urine in the bladder, it will dissolve the Xylocaine in a few minutes and then flow through the catheter into the container. I instill the contrast material (17 percent wt./vol.) by gravity. It is opaque enough to be seen easily and yet is not so concentrated that it regularly causes chemical cystitis. I occasionally observe clusters of children with symptoms suggesting chemical cystitis during or after the voiding cystogram; this seems to be seasonal. Finding no relationship to the season, others have suggested that the discomfort is due to the catheterization and not the contrast material.

The filling and emptying of the bladder with contrast material should mimic the filling and emptying of the bladder by urine. Digital fluoroscopy can markedly reduce the radiation exposure. The hydration of the child should be kept constant (she should not be dehydrated), because the degree of reflux up the ureter is inversely proportional to the efflux of urine down the ureter. I compare the volume instilled to the capacity predicted for the child's weight or age. For children under 1 year of age, the weight in kilograms times seven predicts the capacity of the bladder in milliliters. For children over one year of age, the age in years plus two predicts the size of the bladder in ounces; multiply by 30 to obtain milliliters. Every voiding cystogram performed to detect reflux must have a voiding phase, since in approximately 25 percent of children with reflux, the reflux occurs only during voiding. In young children the sensitivity to detection of reflux can be improved by a cyclic study. I do this by filling the bladder and watching while the infant voids around the catheter several times. Approximately 10 percent of young children will reflux only on the second or third cycle.

Reflux must be graded. By the international grading system, grade 1 is reflux only into the ureter; grade 2 is into the ureter and pelvicalyceal system without any dilatation; grade 3 is reflux into the ureter and pelvicalyceal system with a little dilatation and tortuosity of the ureter, mild dilatation of the renal pelvis, mild rounding of the calyceal fornices, and slight effacement of the tips of the papillae; grade 4 reflux causes moderate dilatation and tortuosity of the ureter, moderate dilatation of the pelvicalyceal system, moderate blunting or rounding of the fornices, and considerable effacement of the tips of the papillae; grade 5 reflux is defined as severe dilatation and tortuosity of the ureter, severe dilatation of the pelvis and calyces, rounding or blunting of the calyces, and complete loss of the papillary impressions.

The site of insertion of the ureter should be documented carefully to make sure it does not insert into a diverticulum (see Fig. 4) or ectopically near the bladder neck (see Fig. 5) or even in the urethra. Whenever either of these situations occurs, surgery is usually needed to correct the reflux. I look carefully for intrarenal reflux: it is often fleeting and is probably under-reported. Intrarenal reflux shows which lobes are at high risk for ascending infection but does not change the grade of reflux or management.

Reflux can coexist with obstruction, and this coexistence changes management. The obstruction is usually at either the ureteropelvic or the ureterovesical junction but can be at both. Several clues suggest this coexistence. First, the refluxed contrast material hesitates at the obstruction. Second, when it passes above the obstruction it is diluted by the urine trapped there. Third, after the bladder has emptied, the contrast material above the obstruction does not drain promptly. I obtain a drainage film in every child with reflux to exclude or confirm obstruction. In young children, children who cannot void volitionally, and children in whom reflux is massive, I recatheterize their bladder to determine how well the material refluxed into the kidney subsequently drains. Recatheterization keeps me from confusing poor drainage with continuing reflux.

At the end of the examination I tell the parents the results so they can better be their child's advocate. I also telephone the referring physician with the results, especially if reflux is found, to ensure that the child will receive or continue to receive prophylactic antibiotic. I call the referring physician several days later to report any positive urine culture.

*Acknowledgments.* John A. Kirkpatrick Jr., M.D., N. Thorne Griscom, M.D., Joan Zawin, M.D., and Helen M. Lebowitz made many helpful suggestions. Elaine Donnelly and Paulette Fontaine typed the manuscript.

## Suggested Reading

Arnold AJ, Brownless SM, Carty HM, Rickwood AMK. Detection of renal scarring by DMSA scanning—an experimental study. J Ped Surg 1990; 25:391–393.

Berger RM, Maizels M, Moran GC, et al. Bladder capacity (ounces) equals age (years) plus 2 predicts normal bladder capacity and aids in diagnosis of abnormal voiding patterns. J Urol 1983; 129:347–349.

Cleveland RH, Constantinou C, Blickman JG, et al. Voiding cystourethrography in children: Value of digital fluoroscopy in reducing radiation dose. AJR 1992; 152:137–142.

Editorial. Prevention of reflux nephropathy. Lancet 1991; 338:1050.

Fairhurst JJ, Rubin CME, Hyde I, et al. Bladder capacity in infants. J Pediatr Surg 1991; 26:55–57.

Jequier S, Jequier JC. Reliability of voiding cystourethrography to detect reflux. AJR 1989; 153:807–810.

Lebowitz RL, Olbing H, Parkkulainen KV, et al. International system of radiographic grading of vesicoureteric reflux. Pediatr Radiol 1985; 15:105–109.

McDonald P, Thomas D, Burge D. Favourite words. Arch Dis Child 1985; 60:874–876.

Paltiel HJ, Rupich RC, Kiruluta HG. Enhanced detection of vesicoureteral reflux in infants and children using cyclic voiding cystourethrography. Radiology 1992; 184:753–755.

Zerin MJ, Shulkin BL. Postprocedural symptoms in children who undergo imaging studies of the urinary tract: Is it the contrast material or the catheter? Radiology 1992; 182:727–730.

# Imaging Evaluation of Ureteropelvic Junction Obstruction in Children

*JUDITH M. ASH, M.D.*

The most common upper urinary tract problem seen in the practice of pediatric urology is a dilated collecting system in a relatively asymptomatic child. The child either presents with mild complaints (abdominal discomfort, frequency, dysuria) or is completely asymptomatic, the problem having shown up on an ultrasonographic evaluation given for screening purposes.

In discussing the dilated urinary tract, traditional texts have recognized that 50 percent of all abdominal masses in infants are renal in origin and, of these, 40 percent are secondary to hydronephrosis with ureteropelvic junction (UPJ) obstruction, which is bilateral in 10 to 20 percent of cases. The causes usually cited are both intrinsic and extrinsic. An absence of smooth muscle at the UPJ may reduce the transmission of peristaltic waves, or urethral valves or polyps may be present. Extrinsic causes include aberrant vessels, adhesions, or kinking of the ureter associated with high insertion.

In the past decade, however, the advent of readily available, widely used antenatal and postnatal ultrasonography has drastically altered traditional viewpoints, particularly in the neonate, in whom the natural evolution of hydronephrosis with or without obstruction is not well established.

## Indications, Clinical Utility, and Alternative Technologies

The challenge facing clinicians and imaging consultants is to make a correct diagnosis and develop a rational plan of management. The differential diagnosis of patients with a dilated urinary tract ranges from normal through mildly obstructed to severely obstructed, and must include other causes, such as vesicoureteral reflux, primary dilatation, and duplex anomalies. Radionuclide imaging plays a prominent role in the differential diagnosis and management of these patients.

Imaging and diagnostic modalities include ultrasonography, voiding cystourethrography (VCUG), intravenous urography with and without furosemide (Lasix), retrograde pyelography, percutaneous perfusion studies (Whitaker test), and radionuclide studies with furosemide. The goals of these techniques are to evaluate (1) renal morphology, including the site of transition from dilated to nondilated urinary tract; (2) renal function; and (3) the transport function of the collecting system. No single imaging technique provides all this information; a judicious choice is necessary to achieve diagnostic accuracy.

In our institution the initial diagnosis of hydronephrosis is usually made from ultrasonography or, less frequently, intravenous pyelography. Once the diagnosis has been established, a VCUG is performed to rule out vesicoureteric reflux as a cause. Usually this test is chosen instead of radionuclide cystography as the initial procedure to assess reflux and to delineate urethral and bladder morphology. If there is vesicoureteral reflux into the renal pelvis, obstruction is not present and a furosemide renal study is unnecessary. However, if a lower grade of reflux is present, a furosemide renal scan may be done with a bladder catheter in place.

Obstructive hydronephrosis cannot be accurately differentiated from the nonobstructive type on a radionuclide renal scan without using furosemide intervention, because slow drainage from a dilated renal pelvis may be secondary to increased volume or atonicity as well as obstruction (Fig. 1). One advantage of diuretic renography is that by calculating a clearance half-time (T/2) of the radionuclide wash-out, grades of incomplete obstruction may be quantified (Fig. 2). If the patient is treated conservatively, serial renographic furosemide studies are used to follow changes both in severity of obstruction and in function. The latter is an extremely important factor in treatment decisions. In the affected kidney, renal function may be well preserved relative to the contralateral kidney. However, less than 40 percent relative renal function or incremental decreases in function of more than 10 percent on serial studies require careful monitoring and may be an indication for surgery (Fig. 3). After surgery, almost all patients have a follow-up furosemide renogram to assess improvement in drainage and possibly in function. It is usually performed 6 months following surgery.

Since the Whitaker test is invasive, it should be reserved for cases in which the diuretic renogram is equivocal or apparently normal but in which there is high clinical suspicion of significant obstruction. The test involves cannulation of the renal pelvis and catheterization of the bladder. A pressure transducer is used to measure the pressure difference between the renal pelvis and bladder during infusion of saline into the renal pelvis at a rate of 11 ml/min. In infants this rate is reduced to 5 ml/min initially and increased as tolerated. A maximum pelvis pressure of 12 cm of water or less is normal, whereas gradients greater than 20 cm indicate an obstructed system. Pressures between 12 and 20 cm are considered equivocal.

Often there is not good correlation between results of the Whitaker test and diuretic renogram, partly because each test

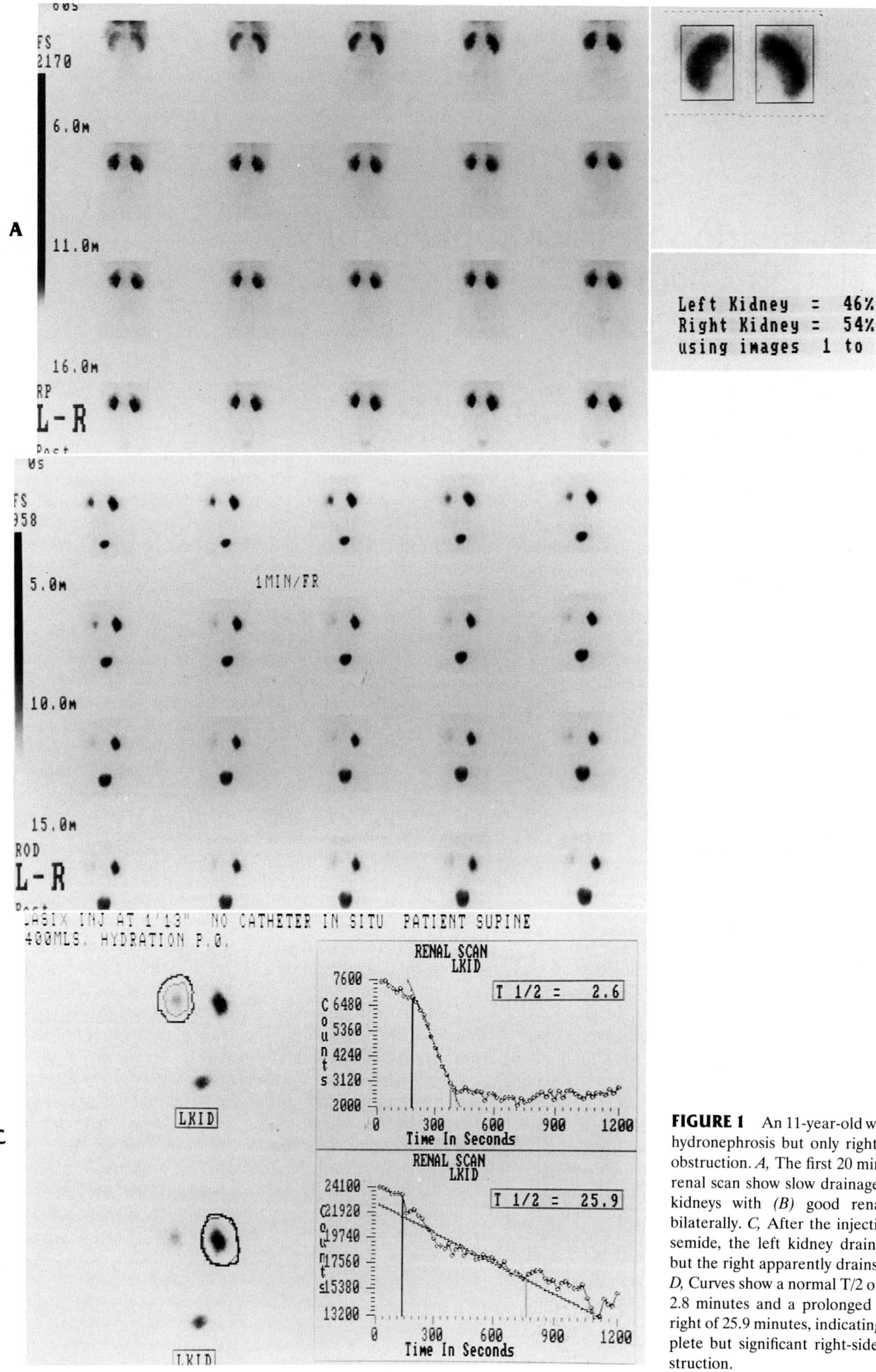


**FIGURE 1** An 11-year-old with bilateral hydronephrosis but only right-sided UPJ obstruction. *A,* The first 20 minutes of the renal scan show slow drainage from both kidneys with *(B)* good renal function bilaterally. *C,* After the injection of furosemide, the left kidney drains promptly, but the right apparently drains minimally. *D,* Curves show a normal T/2 on the left of 2.8 minutes and a prolonged T/2 on the right of 25.9 minutes, indicating an incomplete but significant right-sided UPJ obstruction.

A

B

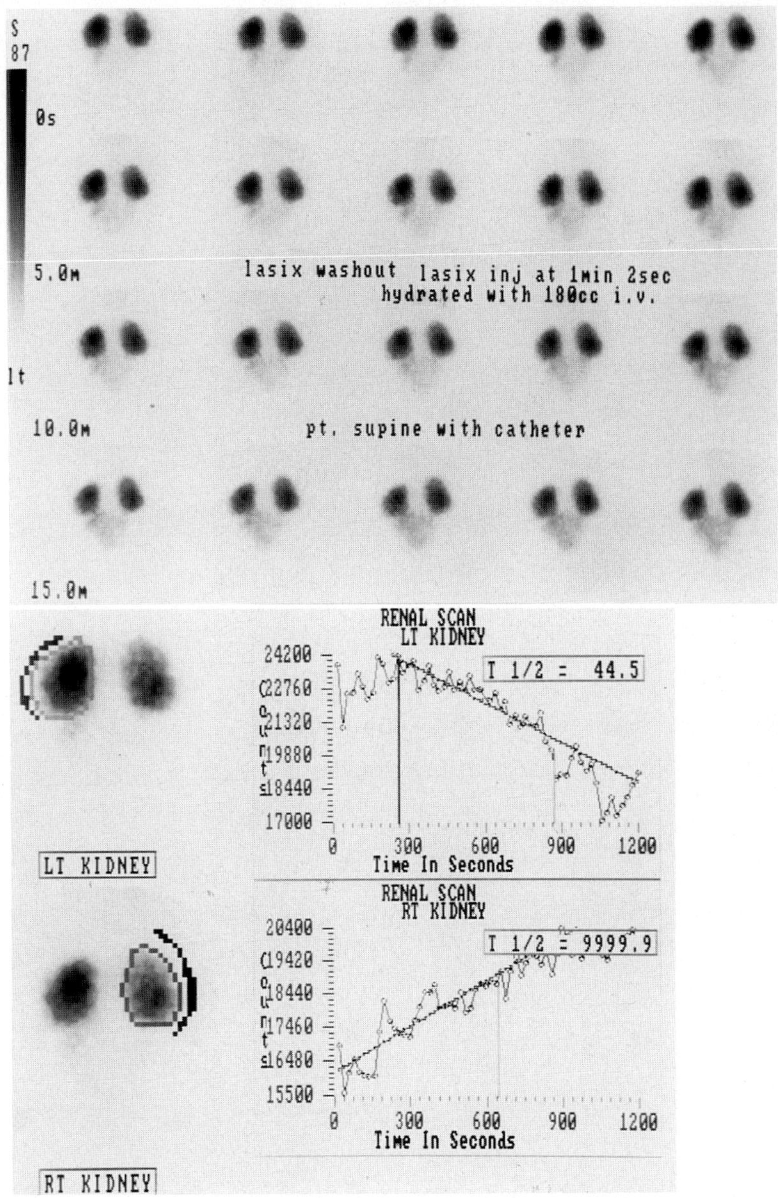


**FIGURE 2** A 2-year-old with prune-belly syndrome and bilateral UPJ obstruction, more marked on the right. *A,* There is retained activity in both renal pelves up to 20 minutes following the furosemide injection. *B,* The clearance curves show almost complete obstruction on the right side with a rising curve (therefore T/2 is calculated as 999) and incomplete obstruction on the left side. This difference in drainage between the two kidneys cannot be appreciated on the scan images alone.

**FIGURE 3** A 4-year-old with left-sided UPJ obstruction. The initial renal scan *(A)* and furosemide wash-out images *(B)* show a hydronephrotic left kidney with slow drainage. The T/2 was 32 minutes, and the left kidney had 63 percent of the total renal function. Six months later, follow-up scan *(C)* and furosemide portion of the study *(D)* show continued hydronephrosis, with delayed drainage and an unchanged T/2 of 35 minutes. However, the left renal function has decreased to 44 percent. The patient underwent pyeloplasty.

A

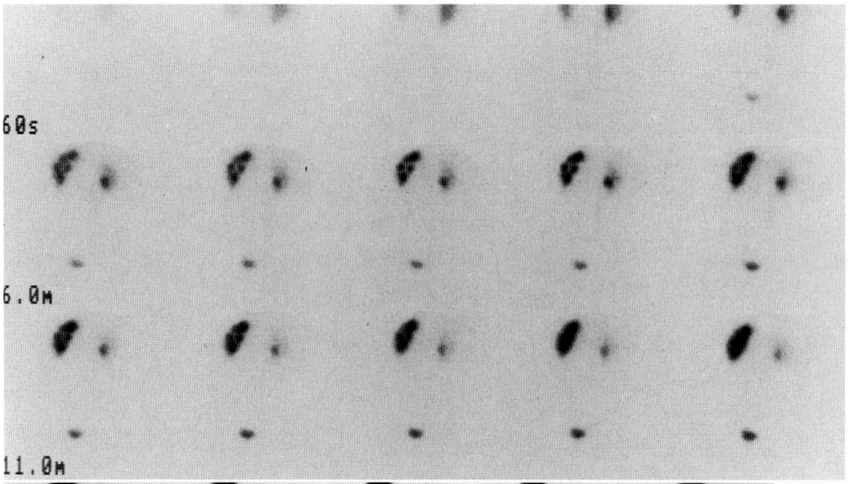


B

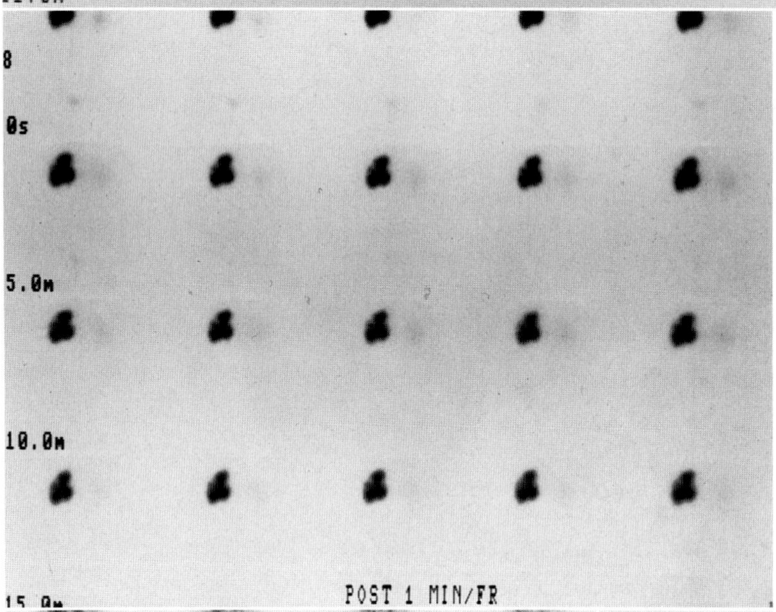


C

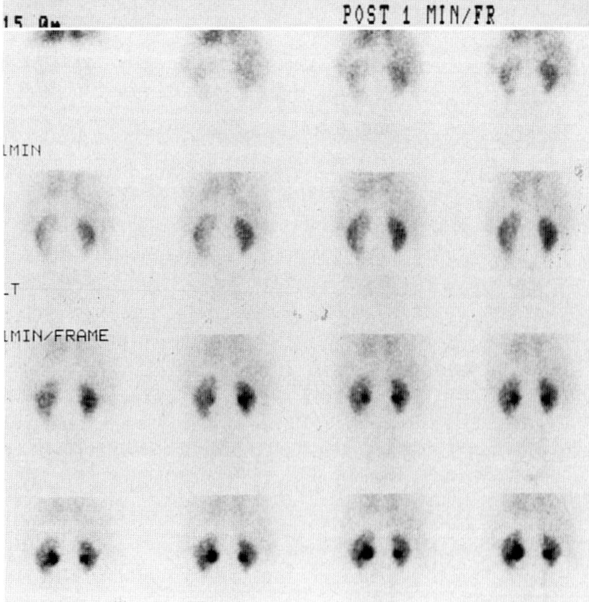


D

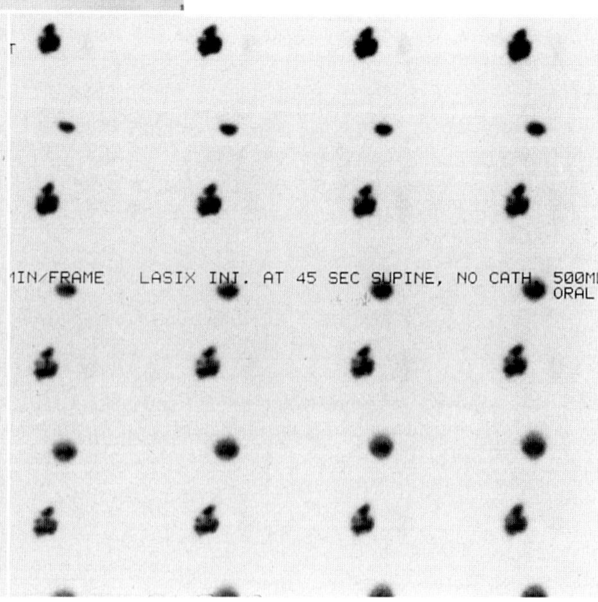

depends on different physiological factors. Diuretic wash-out is influenced by renal function, system compliance, and variable urine flow rates; perfusion pressure studies depend on measurement of a pressure gradient following fixed, nonphysiological perfusion of fluid through a needle.

Retrograde urography has the advantage of direct visualization of the urethra and bladder via catheterization of the ureteral orifice with injection of a contrast agent. It is by necessity highly invasive, requires anesthetic, and in young infants must be performed in specialized centers with small instrumentation. In our center it is used to define the morphology accurately as a prelude to complex reconstructive surgery.

## Technical Approach

### *Radiopharmaceutical*

We use technetium-99m ($^{99m}$Tc) diethylenetriamine penta-acetic acid (DTPA) for the study. The dose given ranges from 1 to 10 MCi and is based on body surface area. $^{99m}$Tc-mertiatide (MAG 3) is preferable, because its more rapid clearance from the renal parenchyma into the collecting system produces better-quality wash-out curves with fewer statistical fluctuations. At present, however, its availability is limited.

### *Patient Preparation*

We try to make the test as physiologically normal as possible by not overhydrating the patient and not using a bladder catheter.

Most children are hydrated orally 30 minutes before the study with 300 to 600 ml of liquid, either juice or water. Infants younger than 1 year or children who refuse to drink are hydrated intravenously with a solution of two-thirds dextrose and one-third saline in a dose of 15 ml/kg for 30 minutes, starting 15 minutes before the study, and continuing at a maintenance level.

Although there are many theoretical arguments for using catheter drainage in every patient, we feel that it is less invasive and traumatic for older infants and children not to have a bladder catheter inserted, particularly because most patients will void during the test. A bladder catheter is only used with children other than neonates if a full bladder is suspected of causing UPJ obstruction, thus affecting renal drainage, or if the patient is known to have vesicoureteral reflux or a neurogenic bladder.

### *Acquisition of Data*

Following the intravenous injection of $^{99m}$Tc-DTPA, 1 minute computer images are taken for the next 20 minutes. If the renal pelvis is filled by this time, a dose of 1 mg/kg of furosemide (maximum 20 mg) is given intravenously after the patient has voided. Data are then collected during the next 20 minutes at 20-second frames for 60 frames. Data acquisition in this diuretic phase is started 1 to 2 minutes before furosemide injection to obtain a baseline curve.

If the kidneys still have not drained 20 minutes after furosemide intervention, the patient is asked to void and a further image is taken.

If the renal pelvis has not filled by 20 minutes in the initial phase of the study, the administration of furosemide is delayed until radioactive filling of the renal pelvis occurs. Sometimes in a grossly dilated, poorly functioning, or completely obstructed system, there is no filling of the renal pelvis or only minimal filling by 1 hour; in this case furosemide is not given at all. Furosemide may also be withheld if the renal collecting system has drained before 20 minutes, because the resultant curves may be misleading, giving a false impression of delayed drainage.

### *Analysis*

#### Relative Function

Background-corrected regions of interest around both kidneys are used to ascertain relative (differential) renal function in the initial phase of the study. The background chosen is usually a semilunar area adjacent to the lateral margin of each kidney, extending from the upper to the lower pole. The net counts in each kidney between 1 and 2 minutes are expressed as a percentage of the total combined renal counts to derive relative function.

#### Urine Drainage

A region of interest is drawn around each renal pelvis and calices as well as a semilunar background region adjacent to the lower pole of the kidney, using data acquired during the diuretic phase of the test. After background activity is subtracted, time-activity curves of the diuretic phase beginning before furosemide injection are generated and displayed. Each curve is fitted using a least-squares fit to the steepest part of the slope to obtain a T/2 wash-out of the radioactive urine; T/2 values less than 10 minutes are normal, values between 10 and 20 minutes are equivocal, and those greater than 20 minutes are considered abnormal. A curve that is flat or slopes upward is diagnostic of almost complete obstruction, so a T/2 is not calculated. Visual inspection of the slope of the curve to assess drainage can be misleading, because the apparent steepness changes depending on the scale used for display.

Usually the curve is sigmoid (see Fig. 1). However, the response may be biphasic (Fig. 4, *A*) or delayed, particularly in kidneys with a grossly dilated renal pelvis, and it may be difficult to decide which part of the curve to use. Generally the curve is still fitted at the steepest part of the slope. If the kidney has already emptied, there will be a falsely prolonged slope because of little or no residual activity in the collecting system (Fig. 4, *B*). If these data are not interpreted in conjunction with the scan images, a false impression of obstruction will be given. Occasionally the kidney may empty initially and then refill, possibly from unsuspected reflux or intermittent obstruction (Fig. 4, *C*).

### *Factors Affecting the Results*

#### Renal Function

Renal function is not fully established in the normal child until approximately 6 months of age. This delay is even more pronounced in the face of obstruction and must be considered when evaluating the excretion of radioactivity, as well as the effects of furosemide on the kidney. During diuresis, urine output ranges from 2 to 16 ml/min in infants and children and up to 20 to 25 ml/min in adults. If the kidney has less than 10 percent of normal function, the results may not be

A

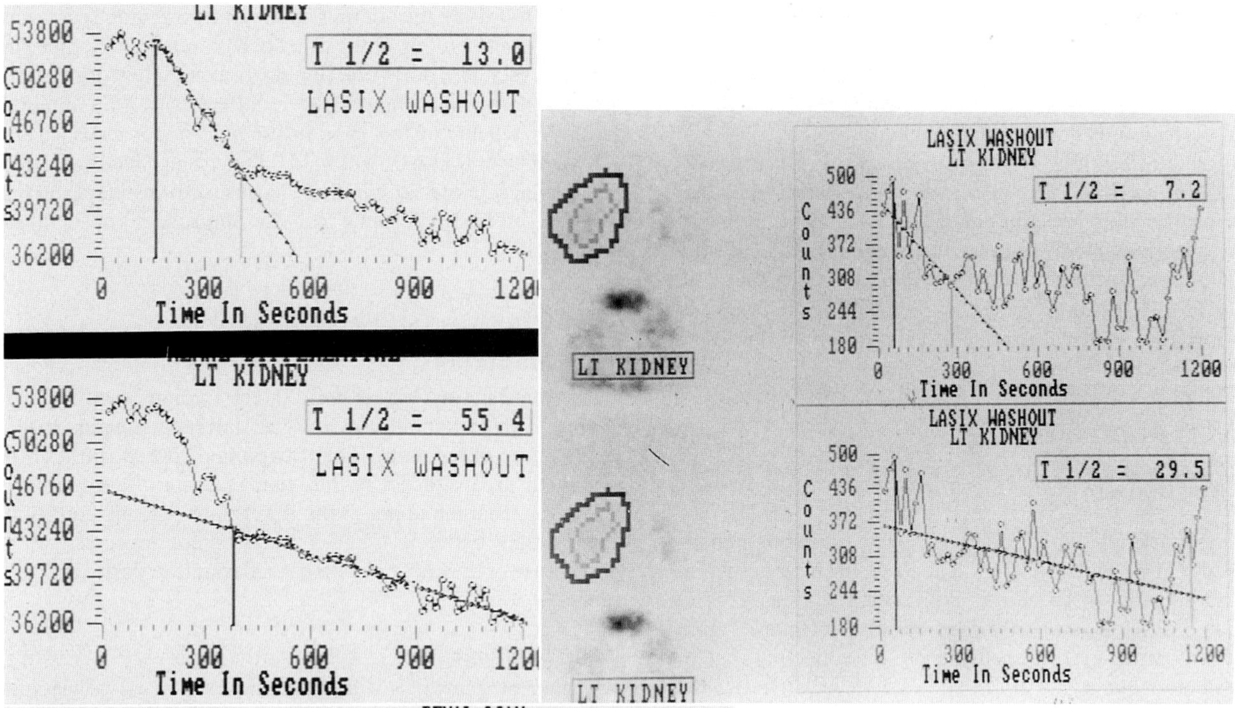


B

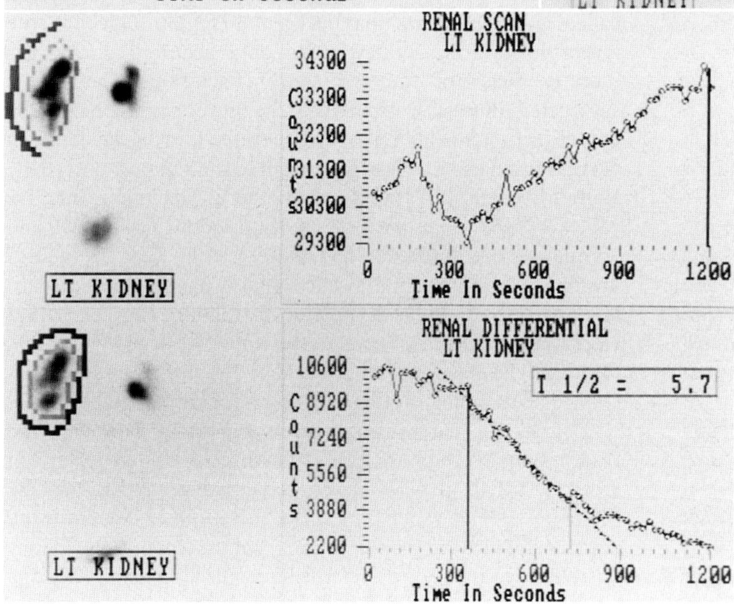


**FIGURE 4** Pitfalls in fitting curves. *A,* The curve is biphasic, and it is difficult to decide which portion to use. In this case the initial drainage gives a T/2 of 13 minutes, whereas the later portion shows drainage with a T/2 clearance of 55 minutes. Fitting to the overall slope of the curve gave a T/2 of 35 minutes. *B,* Low-count noisy curves as both kidneys have drained before furosemide administration. There is no valid fit, and assessment of the curve alone without corresponding images gives an erroneous impression of a prolonged T/2. *C,* The left kidney initially empties and then refills for no apparent reason. Reflux was not known or evident on this study. The patient was treated conservatively. Follow-up furosemide renal scan 8 months later showed good drainage with a T/2 of 5.7 minutes.

valid. A creatinine clearance in adults of at least 10 ml/min is necessary for valid results, with an achieved diuresis of 4 to 5 ml/min in these patients. However, in neonates relative function in the obstructed kidney is frequently normal or increased (see Fig. 3).

### Renal Pelvic Volume

This may be even more important than renal function in creating a false impression of obstruction. In adults pelvic volumes over 70 ml give a high number of false positive results compared with the Whitaker test, whereas those with volumes <30 ml show good correlation with Whitaker test results in 88 percent of cases. Numerical data in children are not available.

### Collecting System Compliance

A highly compliant renal pelvis may distend and not build up enough pressure to overcome an otherwise insignificant obstruction, whereas in a rigid system renal pelvic pressure may overcome the obstruction and the T/2 be normal. These factors may explain the discrepant results between the diuretic renogram and pressure perfusion studies in some cases.

### Effect of Hydration

Dehydration will cause a false prolongation of emptying. Volume expansion diuresis renography may clarify previously equivocal results, placing them in either the obstructed or nonobstructed range. However, we feel that this method is not necessary in the older child who is able to drink liquid equivalent to 15 ml/kg hydration.

### Timing of Diuretic Administration

One must wait until the renal pelvis is filled before administering furosemide. If it is not filled by the normal time of 20 minutes, wait until filling has occurred. However, as noted earlier, if the renal pelvis is not filled by 1 hour, renal function is probably not adequate for the furosemide response to be valid.

The test may be modified in ambiguous cases by giving furosemide 15 minutes before $^{99m}$Tc-DTPA to achieve maximal diuretic effect. However, we have not found this necessary in routine clinical cases. If the study result is uncertain, the patient is usually treated conservatively and followed by repeat furosemide renogram or occasionally a Whitaker test.

### Bladder Characteristics

Known ureterovesical reflux or obstruction from the bladder necessitates catheterization. If the patient is not catheterized and the upper urinary tract has not emptied, he or she is asked to void and a follow-up image is taken. In some cases this converts an apparently obstructed or equivocal picture to a nonobstructed one. We have studied a series of patients in whom poor emptying of the bladder was suspected of causing obstruction. Repeat furosemide studies on the same day, with and without catheter drainage, yielded significantly different results. A noncompliant bladder may also cause back pressure and prevent drainage.

### Regions of Interest

For relative function analysis, the entire kidney must be included in the region of interest. In a poorly functioning hydronephrotic kidney, this may be difficult to do and function may be underestimated. Appropriate background selection is extremely important, because it has a significant impact on the calculations. For these reasons, it is important to standardize the region of interest selection so that changes in results relate to differences in function and not in technique.

During the diuretic phase, the regions must be placed over the renal pelvis and calices, including as little parenchyma as possible. Residual parenchymal activity significantly changes the slope of the curve, particularly if activity in the renal pelvis is minimal. The regions, however, must be large enough to allow for patient motion. Background regions must avoid the ureter.

### Position of Patient

Ideally the patient should be positioned prone to encourage drainage. However, children are more comfortable and less anxious when supine. If drainage seems slow, the child may be moved to the prone position or placed upright to facilitate emptying.

## Special Considerations in the Neonate

### *Presentation and Differential Diagnosis*

With the advent of prenatal and postnatal ultrasonography, recognition of hydronephrosis in the neonate has increased sharply. However, many neonates with hydronephrosis have causes other than obstruction for upper urinary tract dilatation, a condition that may even be transient. The diagnosis of significant obstruction is especially difficult in the asymptomatic infant, and it is not clear when surgery should be performed. Treatment of the neonate is influenced by such factors as the effects on renal growth and development, lack of symptoms, and the resolution of a certain percentage of hydronephrosis in the postnatal period. The last factor may be related to transient fetal urinary tract obstruction or physiological diuresis in the later gestational weeks. A significant number of other infants seem to "outgrow obstruction" during the first year. Further, even if surgical intervention is deemed necessary to preserve or allow for improvement in renal function, its timing remains controversial.

Currently, in our institution any neonate with a diagnosis of hydronephrosis is given a postnatal ultrasonographic evaluation after the first week of life. If persistent dilatation is seen, the infant is referred for a VCUG to rule out reflux as a cause. Once significant reflux has been excluded, a furosemide renal scan is performed.

### *Technical Considerations*

The furosemide study is performed in a manner similar to that for older infants and children, except that it is standardized with respect to function, bladder drainage, and hydration.

1. Renal concentrating ability is not well established in the neonate, particularly in the premature neonate. Therefore all infants should be of at least 44 weeks' gestational age to ensure sufficient tubular maturation for an adequate response to furosemide, particularly in the face of obstruction. No normal values have been yet established, although the contralateral kidney may be used as a normal control. Total urine flow rates in the order of 2 to 6 ml/min may occur during diuresis, representing on average an eightfold increase in urine production.
2. All neonates are catheterized with a size 8 Fr catheter. Occasionally a size 5 feeding tube is needed. A Foley catheter is not used.
3. The infants all are hydrated intravenously with a solution of two-thirds dextrose and one-third saline. They are given 10 to 15 ml/kg of the solution over 30 minutes, beginning 15 minutes before the study, as described earlier.
4. $^{99m}$Tc-DTPA is injected and computer images are taken for 20 minutes, according to our standard protocol. If the renal pelvis is filled by this time, furosemide is given (1 mg/kg up to a maximum of 20 mg) and images are taken for another 20 minutes. At present, we continue to analyze the drainage by fitting a curve to the steepest portion of the slope. However, other portions of the curve may be included (i.e., the beginning before the furosemide starts to have an effect or the end following maximum drainage). The significance of these points of the curve and of variations in the diuretic response time is not yet clear. The normal T/2 in a neonate is assumed to be less than 10 minutes, but since this assumption remains to be validated, occasionally patients may be investigated further with a Whitaker test (Fig. 5). Because it is not uncommon to see a normal result change to an abnormal one and vice versa, serial studies are carried out at 3 to 6 month intervals for the first two years to follow changes in function and drainage. A dramatic worsening of either one of these parameters may be an indication for surgery (Fig. 6).

## Summary of Diagnostic Approach

Delayed drainage alone, without furosemide administration, does not necessarily indicate obstruction. We diagnose UPJ obstruction on the basis of the diuretic renogram, provided that the previously discussed clinical considerations have been taken into account and the technical criteria met.

Corrective surgery is generally performed if the T/2 in a

A

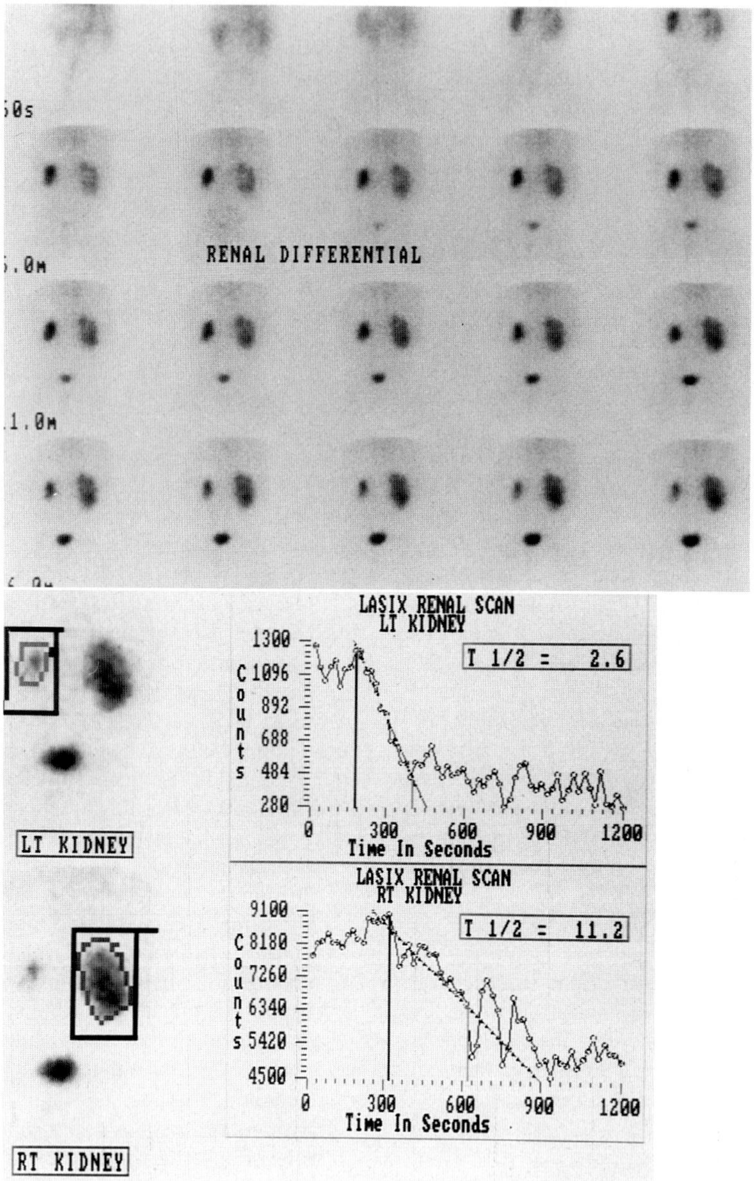


B

**FIGURE 5** Newborn with right-sided UPJ obstruction and poor function. *A,* Renal scan at 1 month of age shows right-sided hydronephrosis with virtually no drainage before furosemide administration. The right kidney has 31 percent of the total renal function. *B,* After furosemide, the left kidney drains with a T/2 of 2.6 minutes and the right with a T/2 of 11.2 minutes, which is borderline equivocal. Because of the poor function and uncertain results, the patient was given a Whitaker test. It was strongly positive with a renal pelvis pressure of 25 cm of water. The patient underwent a right-sided pyeloplasty.

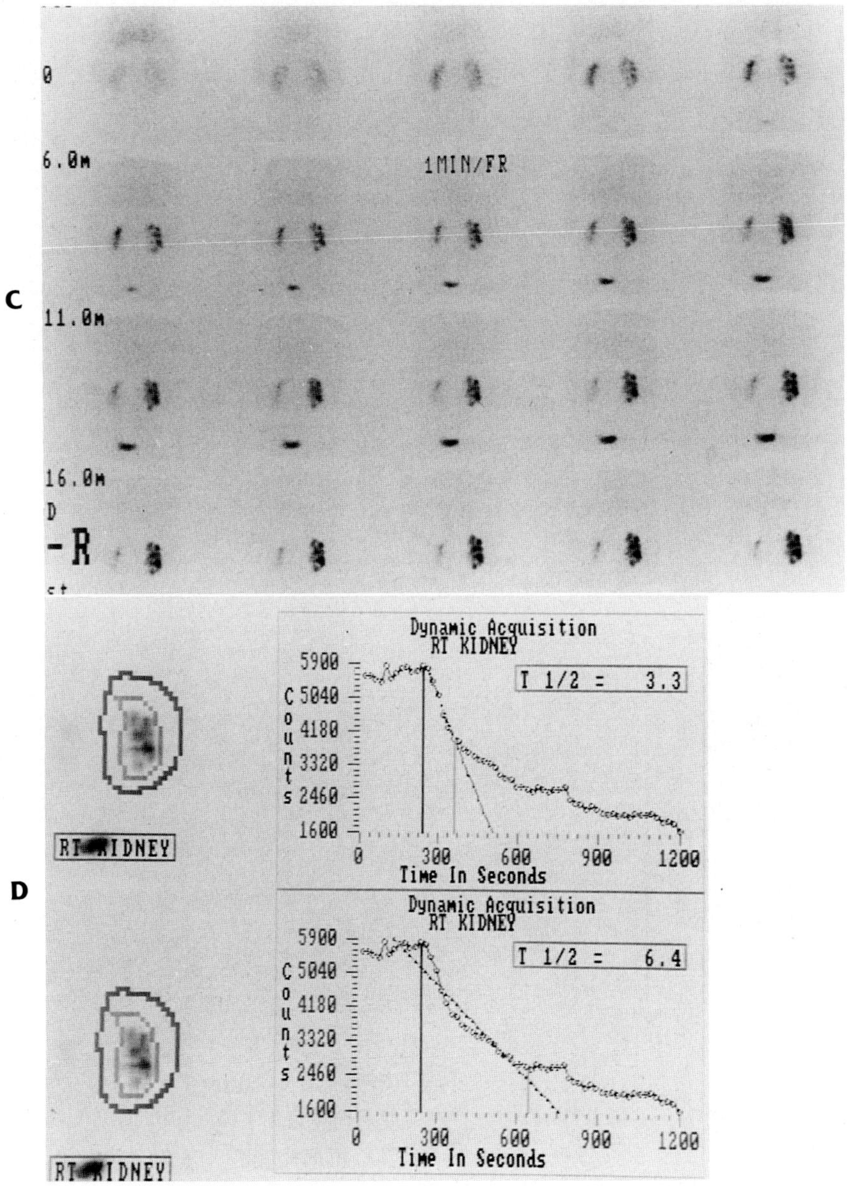


**FIGURE 5, cont'd** *C,* Postoperative renal scan at 9 months of age shows continued right-sided hydronephrosis but with improved function. The right kidney now has 54 percent of the total renal function, and *(D)* shows improved drainage following furosemide injection. Note that the curve is not sigmoid, and the T/2 is between 3 and 6 minutes, depending on how the curve is fitted.

A

B

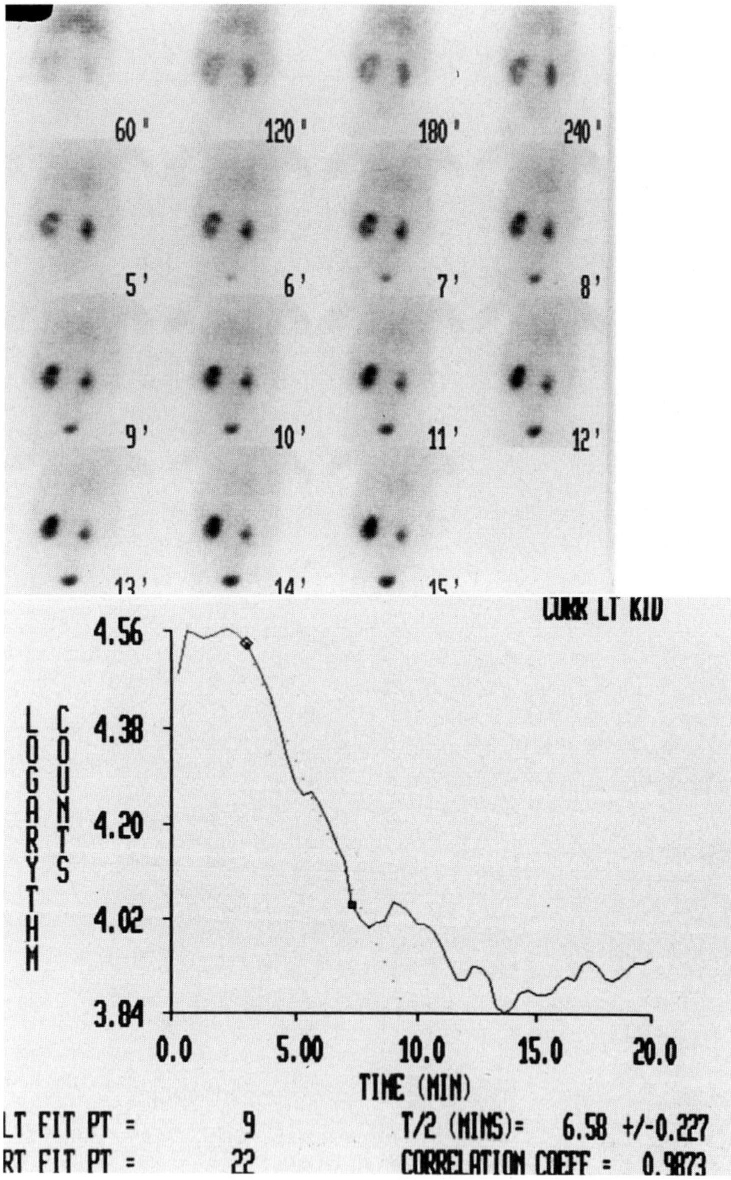


**FIGURE 6** Infant with increasing left-sided UPJ obstruction during the first year of life. *A,* The initial renal scan shows left-sided hydronephrosis with slow drainage at 15 minutes, before furosemide injection. The left kidney has 59 percent of the total renal function. *B,* After furosemide, the left kidney empties promptly with a T/2 of 6 minutes.

C

D

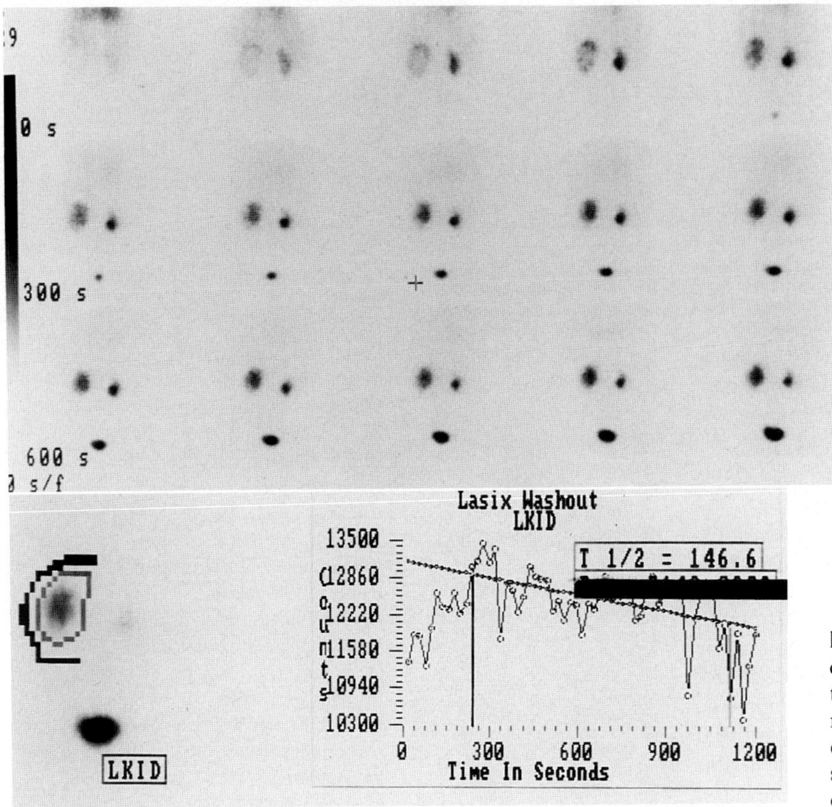


**FIGURE 6, cont'd** *C,* Repeat renal scan at 1 year of age shows continuing left-sided hydronephrosis with the left kidney contributing 62 percent of the total renal function. In spite of the unchanged function, drainage is worse, and *(D)* the left kidney now empties slowly with a T/2 of 146 minutes, indicating increasing obstruction.

child is greater than 20 minutes, particularly if associated with significant dilatation and reduction in renal function, as measured on renal scan. However, if function is poor, or if the collecting system is grossly dilated throughout, as in patients with posterior urethral valves or prune-belly syndrome, abnormal results should be interpreted with caution. To this end, both the renal images and the curves must be analyzed. We also recognize that UPJ obstruction may be intermittent and that variable results may be obtained in some cases. In these cases adjunctive studies such as the Whitaker test may be used. In the neonate it is important to assess clinical and functional changes with serial studies to follow the evolution of hydronephrosis to establish normal criteria.

## Suggested Reading

Conway JJ. "Well-tempered" diuresis renography: Its historical development, physiological and technical pitfalls, and standardized technique protocol. Semin Nucl Med 1992; 22:74–84.

English PJ, Testa HJ, Lawson RS, et al. Modified method of diuresis renography for the assessment of equivocal pelviureteric junction obstruction. Br J Urol 1987; 59:10–14.

Gillenwater JY, Grayhack JT, Howards SS, Duckett JW, eds. Adult and Pediatric Urology. Vol. 2. 2nd ed. St. Louis: Mosby-Year Book, 1991:1743.

Gordon I, Dhillon HK, Gatanash H, Peters AM. Antenatal diagnosis of pelvic hydronephrosis: Assessment of renal function and drainage as a guide to management. J Nucl Med 1991; 32:1649–1654.

Howman-Giles R, Uren R, Roy LP, Filmer RB. Volume expansion diuretic renal scan in urinary tract obstruction. J Nucl Med 1987; 28:824–828.

Kass EJ, Majd M, Belman AB. Comparison of the diuretic renogram and the pressure perfusion study in children. J Urol 1985; 134:92–96.

Kelalis PP, King LR, Belman AB, eds. Clinical Pediatric Urology. Vol. 1. 2nd ed. Philadelphia: WB Saunders, 1985:420.

Kletter K, Nurnberger N. Diagnostic potential of diuresis renography: Limitations by the severity of hydronephrosis and by impairment of renal function. Nucl Med Commun 1989; 10:51–61.

Krueger RP, Ash JM, Silver MM, et al. Primary hydronephrosis. Assessment of diuretic renography, pelvis perfusion pressure, operative findings, and renal and ureteral histology. Urol Clin North Am 1980; 7:231–242.

O'Reilly PH, Britton KE, Nimmon CC. Evaluation of urinary tract obstruction. In: Blaufax MD, ed. Evaluation of Renal Function and Disease with Radionuclides. The Upper Urinary Tract. 2nd ed. Basel: Karger, 1989:248.

Zechmann W. An experimental approach to explain some misinterpretations of diuresis renography. Nucl Med Commun 1988; 9:283–294.

# The Acute Abdomen in Infants and Children

*SIMON CHING-SHUN KAO, M.D. · EDMUND A. FRANKEN, Jr., M.D.*

An acute abdomen is a condition of sudden onset accompanied by abdominal pain for which emergency operative intervention must be considered. The role of diagnostic imaging in an infant or a child with an acute abdomen is to determine whether the patient has a medical or surgical disease and to define the nature of the process.

Differential diagnosis of the acute abdomen in the pediatric age group varies with age and gestation of the patient. Some abdominal conditions are listed in Table 1. Because of the limited space, we exclude discussion of trauma, parasitic disease (e.g., ascariasis), metabolic disease (e.g., diabetes mellitus, sickle cell crisis, and heavy metal poisoning), and referred pain from diseases in the intervertebral disk, spine, and chest (e.g., pneumonia, pleural effusion, or pericarditis).

Imaging in an infant or a child with suspected acute abdomen should include supine and horizontal-beam (upright, left lateral decubitus, or lateral cross-table) radiographs of the abdomen as well as a chest radiograph. This set of radiographs is of value to demonstrate abnormal calcification (e.g., appendicolith, renal or ureteric calculus), abnormal air-fluid levels in the gut, and to detect free intraperitoneal air. Sonography is the next line of imaging study to find the cause of an acute abdomen, especially for obstructive uropathy, acute appendicitis, biliary tract disease, and gynecologic conditions. Computed tomography (CT) is reserved for acute trauma and those patients in whom sonography is unrevealing or inappropriate. Nuclear medicine studies are used in gastrointestinal bleeding (such as Meckel's diverticulum) and acute biliary conditions. Contrast studies of the gut are used for malrotation and in the diagnosis and treatment of intussusception. Angiography is seldom needed, except occasionally in the localization and management of gastrointestinal bleeding.

In the following discussion, we cover several acute abdominal conditions in which imaging plays an important part in the workup and/or treatment. The key imaging signs of the disease, differential diagnosis, and pitfalls in technique and interpretation are included.

**TABLE 1** Some Common Abdominal Causes of Acute Abdomen According to Age

| Age | Causes |
|---|---|
| Premature neonate | Necrotizing enterocolitis (NEC) |
| Term neonate | Congenital intestinal obstruction |
| | Septicemia |
| 1 month to 2 years | Intussusception |
| | Strangulated inguinal hernia |
| | Complicated Meckel's diverticulum |
| | Malrotation with volvulus |
| | Acute appendicitis |
| | Primary peritonitis (nephrotic syndrome) |
| | Gastroenteritis |
| Postinfancy | Acute appendicitis |
| | Acute cholecystitis |
| | Inflammatory bowel disease |
| | Ruptured neoplasm |
| | Abdominal trauma |
| | Nonspecific abdominal pain |
| | Gastroenteritis |
| | Primary peritonitis |
| | Bacterial enterocolitis |
| | Viral hepatitis |
| | Pancreatitis |
| | Urinary tract infection |
| | Sacroiliitis |
| | Pyomyositis |
| | Pelvic inflammatory disease |
| | Gynecologic disorders |

## Necrotizing Enterocolitis

NEC, affecting mainly premature or low-birth-weight neonates, is one of the most common serious abdominal conditions in neonatal intensive care units. Although the exact cause of NEC is not clear, bacterial invasion of the immunologically immature gut wall is of importance. Mucosal ulceration and later transmural necrosis are often associated with pneumatosis intestinalis. The gas in pneumatosis consists of fragmentation products of bacterial action including hydrogen. Clinical manifestations of NEC are variable and may be either gastrointestinal (abdominal distention, gastric retention, and hematochezia) or systemic (apnea, acidosis, temperature instability, and lethargy).

Standard supine and horizontal-beam radiographs are indicated as the initial imaging evaluation. Although the key plain radiographic signs include evidence of pneumatosis intestinalis, portal venous gas, and perforation, some documented (including those with perforation) cases of NEC do not show pneumatosis, and interobserver variability in the diagnosis of pneumatosis is considerable. The degree of ileus and the presence of pneumatosis are most frequently overcalled, because the finding of bowel dilatation is nonspecific and frequently stool-filled bowel can simulate intramural gas. In ambiguous cases where there are discrepancies in the clinical and plain radiographic findings, we perform a contrast enema study using dilute barium or a low-osmolar contrast agent. Findings are those of colitis: mucosal irregularities or ulcerations, intramural extravasation, and persistent spasm (Fig. 1). Our experience of 126 cases shows that this procedure has been safe, despite the fact that many pediatric radiologists have been hesitant to administer enemas in an ill premature infant for fear of perforation by the enema. Although thickened bowel and portal venous gas have been identified by sonography in some neonates with suspected NEC and normal abdominal radiographs, applicability to all suspected cases is limited. The value of nuclear medicine, CT scans, and magnetic resonance imaging (MRI) is limited.

## Intussusception

Intussusception with invagination of a segment of bowel (usually the terminal ileum) into an adjacent distal bowel (usually the colon) occurs largely in the first two years of life. Although most cases are idiopathic, less than 5 percent have pathologic lead points. Classic clinical triad includes abdomi-

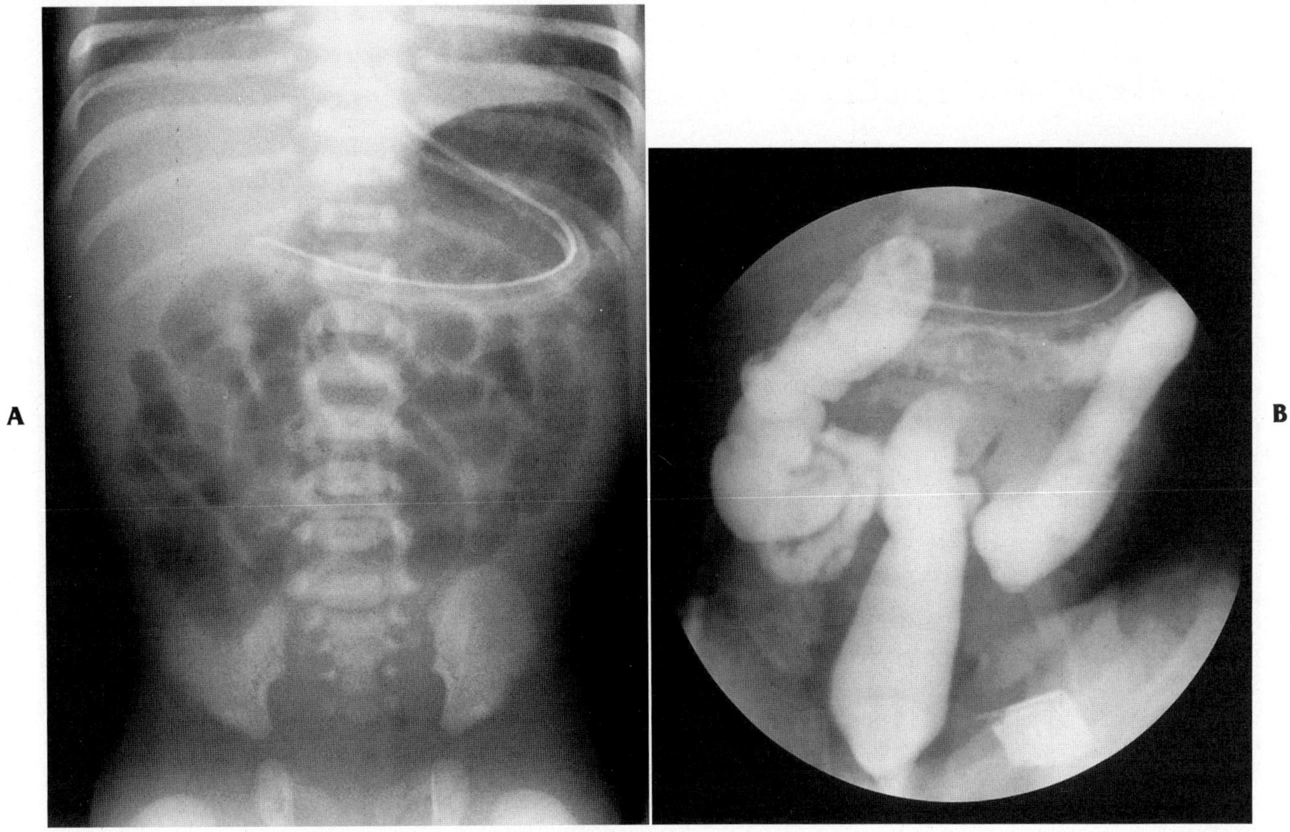

**FIGURE 1** Necrotizing enterocolitis in a 3-day-old premature newborn presenting with bloody stools. *A,* Scout abdominal radiograph shows no abnormality. *B,* Barium enema study shows abnormally spiculated mucosal outline due to ulcerations.

nal pain, vomiting, and "currant-jelly stool." Plain radiographic signs include decreased bowel gas due to vomiting, a mass lesion outlined by air (usually in the right upper quadrant of the abdomen), and abnormal air-fluid levels from mechanical small bowel obstruction. A contrast enema study is still necessary to establish or to exclude a diagnosis of intussusception and to allow nonoperative reduction if the diagnosis is confirmed and if there are no contraindications to the procedure, such as intestinal gangrene, peritonitis, and perforation. We perform therapeutic reduction with up to three attempts using limited hydrostatic pressure (3 feet above table top and up to 3 minutes per attempt) and fluoroscopic monitoring. Our double-blind study has found no value of using glucagon in the procedure.

With the increasing role of sonography in imaging abdominal diseases, intussusception can be diagnosed, appearing as a "target" on cross section and a "pseudokidney" on longitudinal section (Fig. 2). Although hydrostatic reduction can be performed successfully under sonographic monitoring, reports and experience are limited for most radiologists.

Although hydrostatic reduction of intussusception has been the standard procedure in North America for many years, there is more recent interest in the use of pneumatic reduction, a procedure that has been popular in China and Argentina for many years. From several studies, the procedure appears to be practical, safe, quick, and simple, with a higher reduction rate compared with hydrostatic reduction. There must be good control of the pressure including a pressure safety release valve, with the clinical condition of each patient taken into account. A resting maximum pressure of 120 mm Hg has been recommended. The Valsalva maneuver protects the bowel from perforation, facilitates reduction, and allows a higher maximum pressure. In case of perforation, which may be inevitable in some instances, there is less fecal contamination. If tension pneumoperitoneum occurs, one must be ready to perform urgent needle decompression.

## Acute Appendicitis

Acute appendicitis is the most common acute abdominal condition requiring operation in infants and children. Although the clinical findings of appendicitis are typical in the majority of cases, manifestations in infants may be much less specific, with rapid progression to perforation in over 80 percent of cases. The relatively low morbidity of laparotomy today and the seriousness of a missed diagnosis result in a negative laparotomy rate of about 25 percent.

Plain abdominal radiographs often show nonspecific findings and are useful in only 50 percent of cases. Calcified fecalith, a specific finding, is seen in only about 10 percent of children. Barium enema studies have been used to exclude the diagnosis of acute appendicitis if the appendix is completely filled, movable, and nontender. However, 10 to 20 percent of normal appendices may not be filled, even with good technique. Findings supportive of a diagnosis of acute appendicitis include nonfilling or incomplete filling of the appendix with cecal indentation from a phlegmon or abscess.

We use sonography with graded compression of the lower

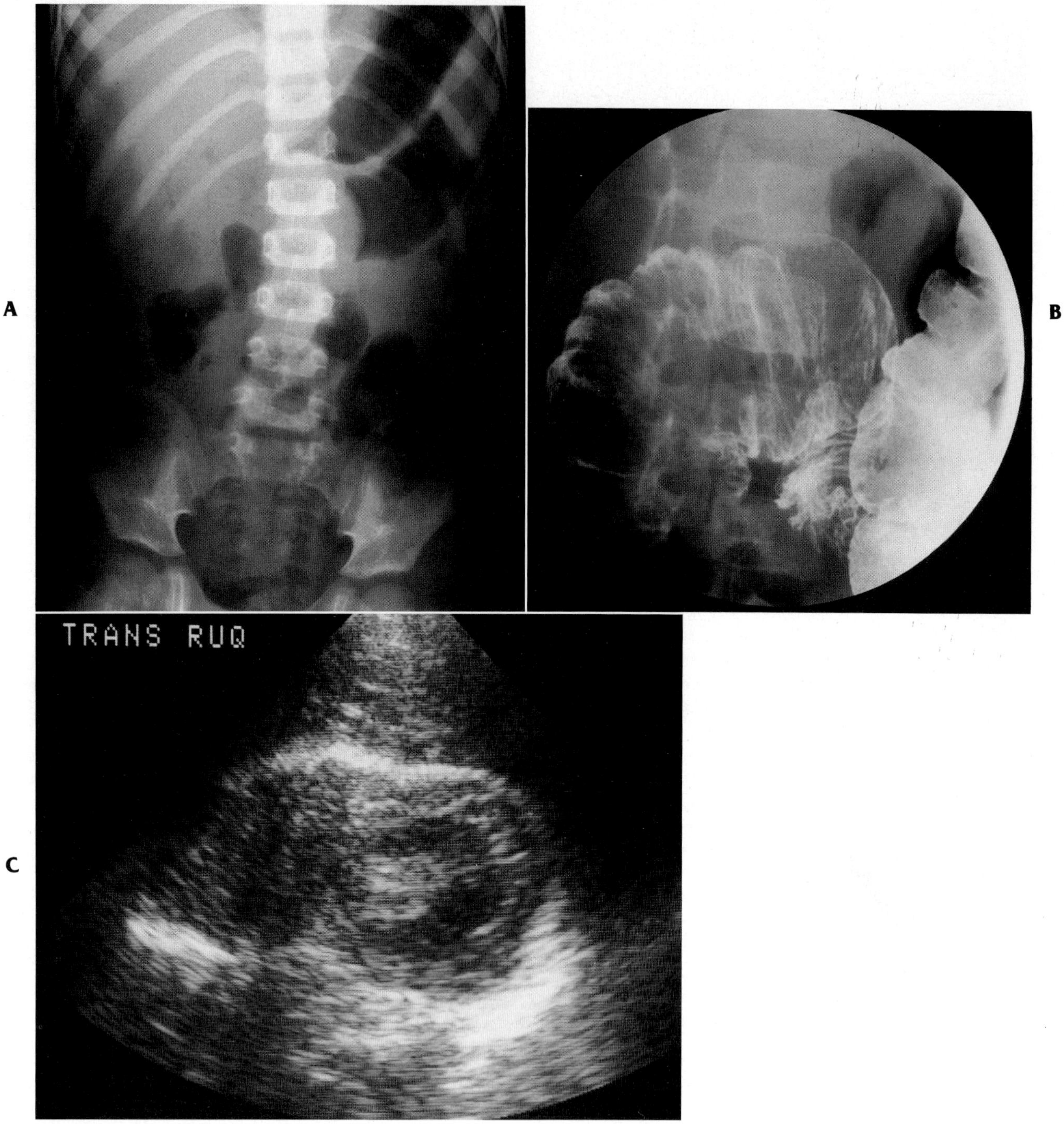


**FIGURE 2** Ileocolic intussusception in a 5-year-old boy with cystic fibrosis. *A,* Abdominal radiograph shows a soft-tissue mass outlined by adjacent gas within the transverse colon. *B,* Sonography of the upper abdomen shows a persistent mass ("pseudokidney"). *C,* Spot film during attempted hydrostatic reduction shows a large filling defect in the transverse colon with a coiled-spring appearance.

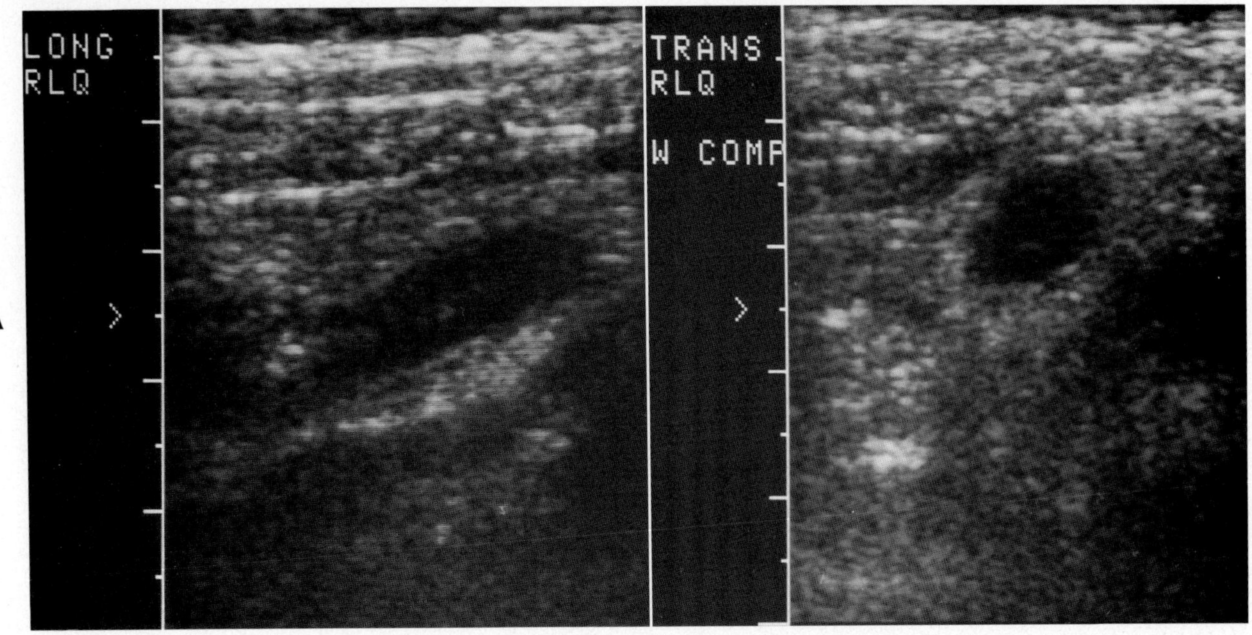


**FIGURE 3** Acute suppurative appendicitis in a 12-year-old boy. *A,* Longitudinal scan of the appendix shows a sausage-shaped structure with wall thickening and hypoechoic material due to pus distending the distal lumen. *B,* Transverse scan of the distal portion of the appendix with compression shows loss of the normal echogenic mucosa and submucosa due to transmural inflammation.

abdomen to attempt to visualize the appendix directly. The graded compression serves to displace shadowing bowel loops and to bring structures closer to the focal zone of the transducer. An inflamed appendix is recognized as a blind-ending sausage-shaped structure with no peristalsis on longitudinal section, and as a target lesion on transverse section (Fig. 3). An appendiceal wall thickness over 2 mm and a total diameter of greater than 6 mm are considered abnormal. The appendiceal lumen may be distended before perforation occurs, and appendicoliths are seen in up to 30 percent of cases. Findings in perforated appendicitis include asymmetric wall thickening, localized or free fluid, and the presence of abscess. We use CT in differentiating phlegmon from pus and in assessing the extent of the inflammatory mass to guide aspiration or operation.

We feel that the prime methods of diagnosis of acute appendicitis in children remain history, physical examination, and laboratory findings, perhaps supplemented by abdominal radiographs. In patients with considerable clinical suspicion of appendicitis, laparotomy should be the next step. However, in a select group of patients (especially younger children), in whom the clinical diagnosis is uncertain, sonography is of considerable value, provided the examination is performed properly and the limitations of the procedure, such as excess bowel gas or failure to compress adequately, are recognized. In a number of instances, an alternative diagnosis may be found. We contend that the appropriate use of sonography should increase the number of positive diagnoses without a corresponding increase in the negative laparotomy rate.

## Gallbladder Disease

With the more widespread use of sonography in abdominal imaging, concepts of biliary tract diseases in children have changed. However, there remains a substantial gap in the knowledge relating gallbladder abnormalities and specific clinical syndromes. Gallbladder dilatation occurring in a neonate due to sepsis, stress, and lack of enteral feeding may simulate a clinical picture of an acute abdomen.

Acute acalculous cholecystitis occurring in association with septicemia, dehydration, streptococcal infections, and other specific ailments such as Kawasaki disease and typhoid fever, may present as an acute abdomen with fever, vomiting, and right upper quadrant tenderness. Although an abdominal radiograph sometimes shows an enlarged gallbladder indenting on the adjacent bowel, diagnosis is usually made by sonography, showing gallbladder distention (hydrops), wall thickening due to edema, and lack of gallstone (Fig. 4).

Cholelithiasis has also been diagnosed with increasing frequency in the pediatric age groups due to an increased clinical awareness, use of therapeutic regimens predisposing to calculus formation, and better imaging techniques such as sonography. In older children cholelithiasis is often associated with hemolytic anemias and hemoglobinopathies. As only about 50 percent of gallstones are radiopaque in children, sonography is indicated if cholelithiasis is suspected.

## Gynecologic Disease

Gynecologic disorders may present as an acute abdomen, particularly in adolescent girls. Acute torsion of a normal or tumorous ovary may present with acute abdominal pain, simulating acute appendicitis or an appendiceal abscess. We would perform sonography to look for an enlarged and hypoechoic ovary associated with free fluid in the cul-de-sac, and the presence of an ovarian tumor.

Mittelschmerz, a clinical syndrome of acute pelvic pain during mid–menstrual cycle, may present as an acute abdomen. Sonography is useful to exclude other causes of pelvic pain and often just reveals transient free pelvic fluid.

Pelvic inflammatory disease and complicated ectopic pregnancy are two important considerations in female adolescents

A

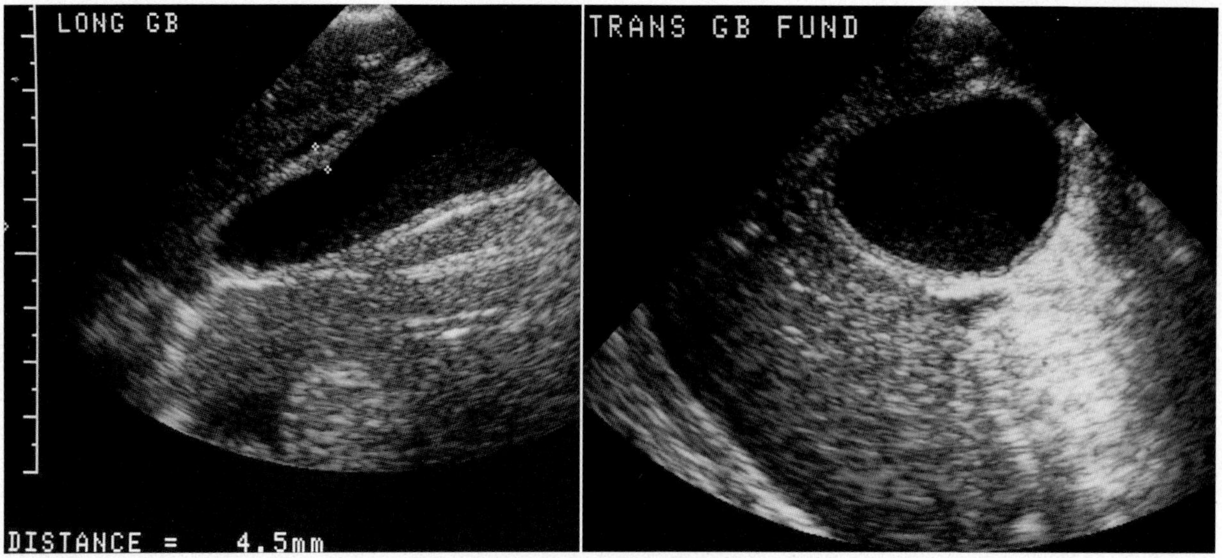


B

**FIGURE 4** Acute acalculous cholecystitis in an 11-year-old boy with prune-belly syndrome and bilateral nephrectomies, presenting with right upper quadrant pain. Longitudinal *(A)* and transverse *(B)* scans of the right upper quadrant show a distended gallbladder with wall thickening (4.5 mm) and sludge. Minimal pericholecystic fluid collection is noted. Histology of the excised gallbladder shows thickened serosa, dilated vessels, and foci of eosinophilic and lymphocytic infiltrates into the muscularis.

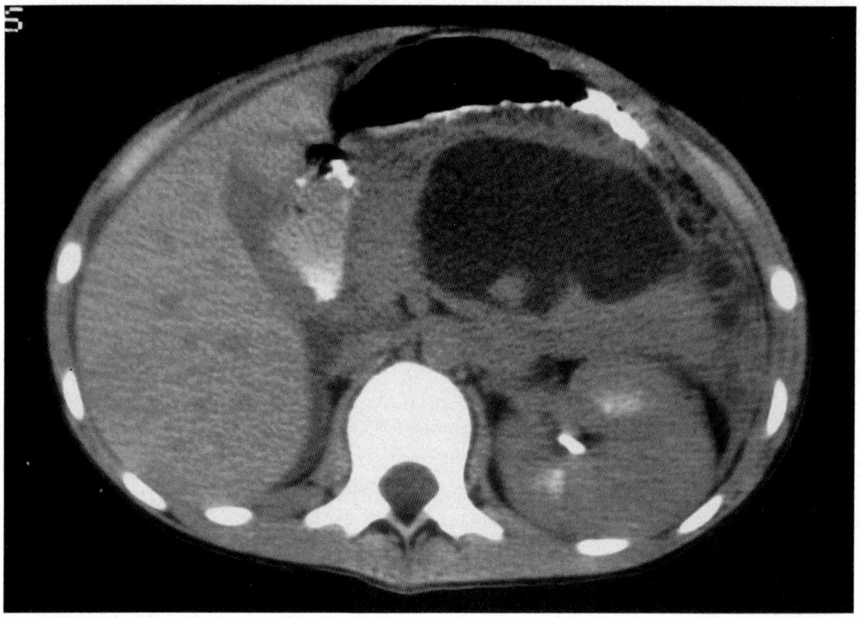

**FIGURE 5** Traumatic pancreatitis in an 11-year-old boy. Axial scan of the upper abdomen shows a large collection, with low attenuation in the lesser sac due to pancreatic rupture with pseudocyst formation.

presenting with acute lower abdominal pain. Pelvic sonography is of value to detect hydrosalpinx, tubo-ovarian abscess, and an ectopic implantation of fetus.

## Miscellaneous Causes of an Acute Abdomen

Acute dilatation of the renal pelvis (due to ureteropelvic junction obstruction or ureteric calculi) and acute pyelonephritis can produce acute abdominal pain. Sonography is useful to detect obstructive changes in the collecting system and may detect ureteric calculi.

Children with malrotation may present with an acute abdomen from volvulus, resulting in intestinal obstruction, vascular compromise, and bowel infarction. Although plain abdominal radiographs may show signs of mechanical and adynamic obstruction, a definitive upper gastrointestinal contrast evaluation is indicated to define the position of the ligament of Treitz and the site of obstruction. Although sonography to define the relationship between the superior mesenteric vessels may be useful in some cases, we do not advocate its use for exclusion of volvulus.

In abdominal trauma CT scan of the abdomen is the most efficient imaging study after plain abdominal radiographs, if clinical conditions allow (Fig. 5). If injuries to hollow viscera are suspected, a gastrointestinal contrast study may be necessary.

Acute manifestations of a syndrome of chronic recurrent functional abdominal pain may present as acute abdomen simulating appendicitis. In instances when the patient is considered for operation due to severity of pain and other clinical findings, plain radiographs and sonography may be indicated to exclude an organic cause.

## Suggested Reading

Apley J. The child with abdominal pains. 2nd ed. Oxford: Blackwell Scientific, 1975.

Franken EA Jr, Kao SCS, Smith WL, Sato Y. Imaging of the acute abdomen in infants and children. AJR 1989; 153:921–928.

Kao SCS, Smith WL, Abu-Yousef MM, et al. Acute appendicitis in children: Sonographic findings. AJR 1989; 153:375–379.

Kao SCS, Smith WL, Franken EA, et al. Contrast enema diagnosis of necrotizing enterocolitis. Pediatr Radiol 1992; 22:115–117.

Merten DF. The acute abdomen in childhood. Curr Probl Diagn Radiol 1986; 15:340–395.

O'Donnell B. Abdominal pain in children. Oxford: Blackwell Scientific, 1985:5.

Shiels WE II, Maves CK, Hedlund GL, Kirks DR. Air enema for diagnosis and reduction of intussusception: Clinical experience and pressure correlates. Radiology 1991; 181:169–172.

Siegel MJ, Carel C, Surratt S. Ultrasonography of acute abdominal pain in children. JAMA 1991; 266:1987–1989.

Stringer DA, Ein SH. Pneumatic reduction: Advantages, risks and indications. Pediatr Radiol 1990; 20:475–477.

# Diagnosis and Reduction of Intussusception in Infants and Children

*ROBERT H. CLEVELAND, M.D.*

Radiologists have played a role in the treatment of childhood intussusception since 1927, when the first successful hydrostatic reduction using a contrast enema study was recorded. Since then, the technique of reduction has changed little. More recently interest has centered on which contrast agent, if any, is superior and to the administration of drugs to aid reduction.

This chapter reviews my process in patient evaluation, preparation, and treatment of intussusception.

## Evaluation

In pediatrics, intussusception is usually observed in infants and young children, most commonly in the first year of life. Males are affected twice as often as females. Approximately 90 percent of intussusceptions are idiopathic, in which no pathologic lead point is identified, although in many instances there is concurrent or preceding gastroenteritis or respiratory infection. Presumably in these children, the intestinal lymphoid aggregates, Peyer's patches, which are normally large at this age, are further enlarged in response to the infection and act as a lead point. Much less commonly, a pathologic lead point may be encountered such as a polyp, duplication, lymphoma, lymphosarcoma, hemangioma, hematoma associated with bleeding disorders such as Henoch-Schönlein purpura, ectopic gastric mucosa, inspissated meconium in patients with cystic fibrosis, or Meckel's diverticulum. The likelihood of a pathologic lead point being present is much higher in children under 3 months or over 2.5 years of age.

Patients with intussusception present with a variety of symptoms, which can be intermittent. Some children are merely irritable or lethargic. Blood is passed in the stool in approximately 65 percent of patients, recognized as a "currant-jelly stool" or frank blood. There is abdominal pain in approximately 90 percent of patients, often recognized by the children drawing their knees to their chest, grasping their abdomen, and crying. In approximately 85 percent of patients, there is vomiting, which may be bile stained. There may be small bowel obstruction. In the most severe cases, in which bowel wall integrity is compromised, the child may present with signs and symptoms of peritonitis.

Physical examination can be normal or indistinguishable from gastroenteritis. A large intussusceptum (the invaginated portion) is palpable as a "sausage-shaped" mass in approximately 60 percent. In children with an elevated temperature and white blood cell count, it is critical to distinguish cases of peritonitis. A surgeon should evaluate each child before radiographic intervention is requested and remain immediately available in the event that a complication should arise or the intussusception not be reducible. The suspected presence of an intussusception is a pediatric emergency and should be dealt with in as expeditious a manner as possible.

The signs and symptoms are heterogeneous and often nonspecific; consequently the radiologist usually is asked to perform an emergency imaging study. This may be ultrasonography (Fig. 1) or a contrast enema study. Since an enema is the therapeutic tool, contrast enema studies are the most commonly employed imaging modality. Reduction should be attempted at the time of diagnosis; therefore the radiologist must approach all patients as if they require reduction, and decisions and policies concerning premedication and choice of contrast agent must be made before a diagnosis is known. A decision as to which patients are not candidates for attempted hydrostatic reduction also must be made.

Early in the child's evaluation, a supine radiograph of the abdomen should be performed. Occasionally the diagnosis clearly can be made from this image (Fig. 2). In many instances, however, no definite diagnosis is possible. An unequivocally normal abdominal radiograph does not exclude the presence of an intussusception. The recognized presence of an intussusception, or the lack of it, does not in fact alter the need to perform a contrast study. The most important observation to make on initial imaging is to exclude free intraperitoneal air, which is a contraindication to attempting reduction. A left lateral decubitus view of the abdomen may be of assistance in this situation, while allowing gas to rise to the cecum and possibly outline an intussusception that was not apparent on supine imaging.

The decision on whom to attempt reduction should be straightforward. Any child who is suspected of having peritonitis (or radiographically is shown to have free intraperitoneal

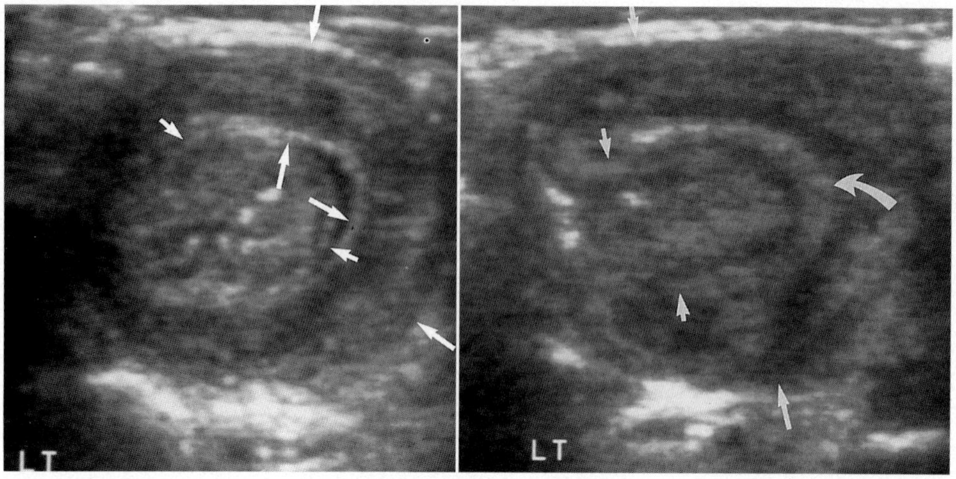


**FIGURE 1** *A,* Ultrasound image through the short axis of a colonic intussusception shows the intussusceptum, the invaginated portion *(short arrows)* surrounded by a small amount of fluid within the intussuscipiens, the portion into which the intussusceptum has invaginated *(long arrows). B,* Long-axis ultrasound image of the intussusception shows the intussusceptum *(short arrows)* and its lead point *(curved arrow)* within the intussuscipiens *(long arrows).*

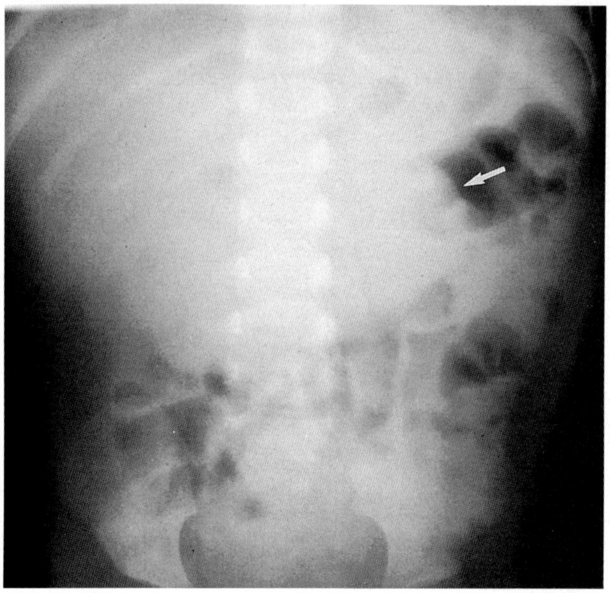

**FIGURE 2** Occasionally the lead point *(arrow)* of an intussusception is clearly observed on a supine radiograph of the abdomen. In these instances there may be a relatively small amount of air in the distribution of the distal colon. Active peristalsis makes it unlikely that large amounts of air will be observed in the colon distal to the intussusception.

air) should not undergo hydrostatic reduction. Although a diagnostic test, using water-soluble contrast material or ultrasonography, may be requested, most children are taken directly to the operating room. If peritonitis is not present, any child is a potential candidate for hydrostatic reduction.

There is approximately a 1 in 300 incidence of perforation in children with intussusception who present without evidence of peritonitis. There are no reliable predictors of which child this may be. Therefore signs or symptoms such as small bowel obstruction, presence of symptoms for longer than 24 hours, or a lead point in the left colon are not by themselves contraindications to attempted hydrostatic reduction. They do suggest a more difficult reduction, presumably because of a greater degree of edema.

There has been much interest in using contrast agents other than barium because of the known but unpredictable chance for perforation. Colonic air, insufflated via the rectum at pressures up to 80 to 120 mm Hg, monitored by manometrically controlled insufflation devices, has proven to be a safe and effective technique for intussusception reduction (Fig. 3). There is no conclusive evidence that air reduction is more successful than the use of barium or water-soluble contrast agents. Many radiologists prefer to use positive contrast material, because of the potential difficulty of differentiating insufflated air and pre-existing bowel gas, especially when there is small bowel obstruction.

Concerns about the possibility of barium peritonitis, if perforation were to occur, and the potential limitations in using air, have led some radiologists to use water-soluble contrast agents. My preference is to use iothalamate meglumine (Cysto-Conray II; Mallinckrodt; St. Louis, MO). The iodine content (81 mg/ml) offers optimal opacification, and the osmolality (404 mOsmol/L) is low enough that dehydration in smaller infants is not a problem.

## Preparation

Some individuals have advocated the use of glucagon to reduce resistance to reduction, but this has been proven ineffective. Others advocate pretreatment with antibiotics. I question the advisability of this. Theoretically antibiotic pretreatment would be of benefit to the rare child with an intussusception who perforates during or after attempted reduction. However, not all children suspected of having an intussusception actually have one. Therefore the vast majority of children would be needlessly treated with systemic antibiotics, which in itself carries a low but significant risk. In addition, the administration of antibiotics may delay performing the enema study.

Possibly the most debated question concerning premedication is over sedation or analgesia. Surgeons do not want the abdominal evaluation clouded by these agents if the child does

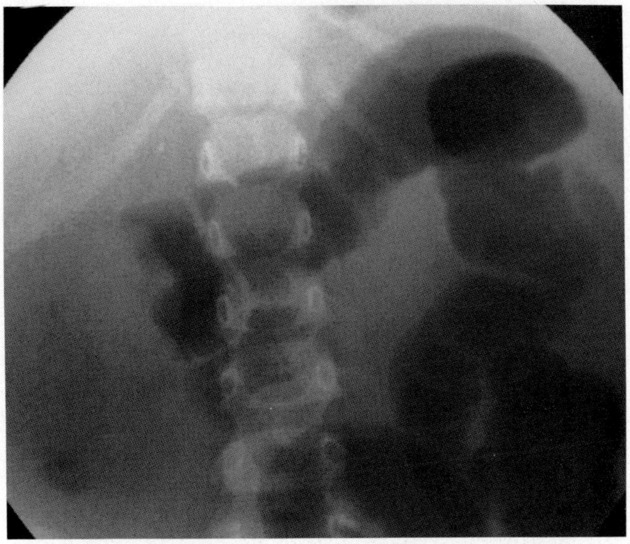

**FIGURE 3** The lead point of an intussusception is readily identified in the proximal transverse colon during attempted air reduction.

not have an intussusception. If adequately premedicated, the child will need continuous monitoring by trained medical staff, preferably with pulse oximetry and direct observation. Monitoring may require several hours of hospitalization regardless of the child's eventual diagnosis, while putting the majority of children at needless risk for cardiac/respiratory complications. Conversely, in a premedicated child who is calm and relaxed, it may be easier to successfully reduce an intussusception, if one is present.

My policy is not to premedicate with any agent. If the child is proven to have an intussusception that is initially not reducible, I may request the referring surgeon to administer appropriate analgesics. Sedation is usually less effective in children experiencing pain than analgesics with both a sedative and pain-blocking effect.

Before beginning the enema study, I always spend several minutes with the child's parents discussing the nature and possible complications of an intussusception. If both parents are present, it is important that both be a part of the discussion. Using ordinary language, avoiding the use of medical jargon, I describe what an intussusception is, how it may be treated (i.e., surgically or by hydrostatic reduction), and what the potential complications are if left untreated or if reduction is attempted. These are the same—namely, perforation and its complications, including death. If the parents agree to an attempted hydrostatic reduction, I then request that each sign a permission slip, on which the discussion is written in abbreviated form. For the child's and parents' psychological benefit, I invite one or both parents to join us in the fluoroscopy room. The presence of a parent alone is often a potent sedative for a frightened child.

I insist that a member of the surgical team be in the fluoroscopic room for the procedure. This has many benefits including smoothing communications with the referring surgeon, teaching surgical house staff, and extra help in restraining the child. Most importantly, if there were to be a perforation, there would be no delay in notifying appropriate personnel, booking an operating room, and performing surgery. It is well documented that the shorter the time from perforation to laparotomy, the better the prognosis.

## Treatment

Treatment is simply an extension of diagnosis. Techniques differ little whether using barium, water-soluble agents, or air. Some individuals prefer to insert a rectal tube with an inflatable balloon. I feel it is unsafe to inflate a balloon in a child's rectum, since the size of the rectum varies considerably according to the child's age and size. Adequate control of the contrast agent can be achieved by tightly taping and manually compressing the buttocks together. Performing the study with the child prone provides the radiologist with ready access for firmly gripping the buttocks.

I initially perform a limited rectal examination, using my fifth finger, and then insert a rectal tube. This tube should be as large as safely possible. This may be a 12 or 14 Fr caliber tube, or in slightly larger children, a special soft flexible tip designed especially for use in children. Tubes with smaller lumen size reduce the amount of hydrostatic pressure actually delivered and therefore should be avoided.

The bag of contrast material, by convention, should be 3 feet above the child (the first "rule of three's" of intussusception reduction). Although there seems to be no higher an incidence of perforation in institutions where the height of the bag is greater than 3 feet, I think it judicious not to exceed this height because this recommendation is well entrenched in the literature.

Once the contrast material is introduced, the fluoroscopist must carefully monitor the leading edge of the contrast. Total radiation exposure should be kept to a minimum. Therefore, rather than continuously monitoring the flow of contrast material, a "pulsed fluoroscopy" technique should be employed. By momentarily interrupting the fluoroscopic observation every few seconds, the total radiation exposure can be significantly reduced without compromising the imaging procedure.

There is no need to obtain images of the colon to demonstrate anatomy. The only concern is to demonstrate the intussusception and reduce it. A constant head of pressure should be maintained without slowing the flow of the contrast agent or allowing evacuation. Once the intussusception has been encountered (Figs. 4 to 6), the fluoroscopist should follow the reduction until contrast readily flows into the ileum. It is to be expected that the rate at which reduction is occurring will slow, or even stop, at the level of the ileocecal valve (Fig. 7). This should not discourage continuing the attempt at reduction. It is not advisable to palpate the abdomen in an attempt to augment reduction.

Not all intussusceptions are reducible with hydrostatic pressure. The success rate varies from approximately 55 to 90 percent. How, then, does the fluoroscopist decide when to stop? The second and third "rules of three's" are relevant at this point. It has been proposed that no single attempt should maintain pressure for more than 3 minutes and that no more than three attempts should be made before recommending surgical reduction. These are good guidelines, but judgment about the individual case should also be applied.

For me, the limiting time factor for any single attempt is my ability to maintain hydrostatic pressure by preventing evacu-

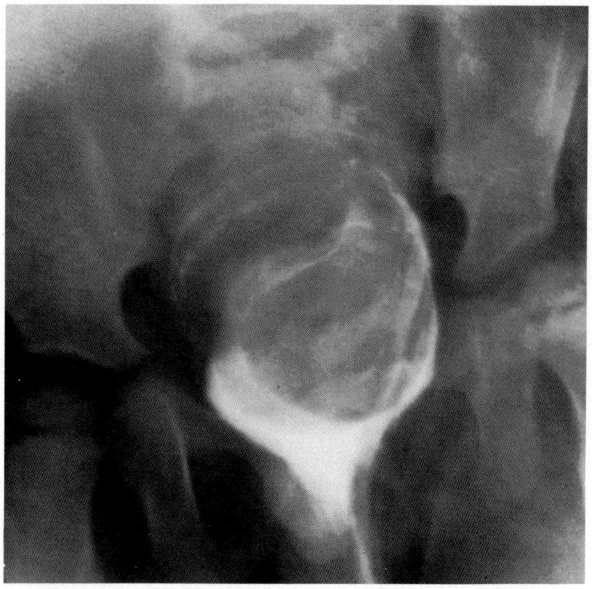

**FIGURE 4** The lead point of an intussusception was encountered just above the anus. Reduction was easily achieved without incident.

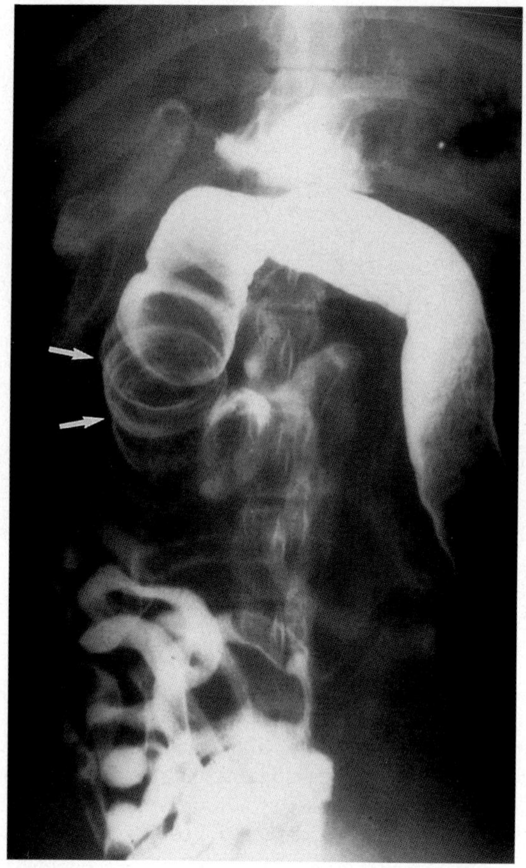

**FIGURE 6** This antegrade study (upper gastrointestinal study with small bowel follow-through) in a 2.5-year-old Irish setter demonstrates the coil spring deformity of an intussusception in the ascending colon *(arrows)*. This configuration is caused by contrast collecting between the opposing mucosal surfaces of the intussusceptum and the intussuscipiens. (This case was graciously provided by Lawrence J. Kleine, D.V.M., Department of Radiology, Tufts University School of Veterinary Medicine, Boston.)

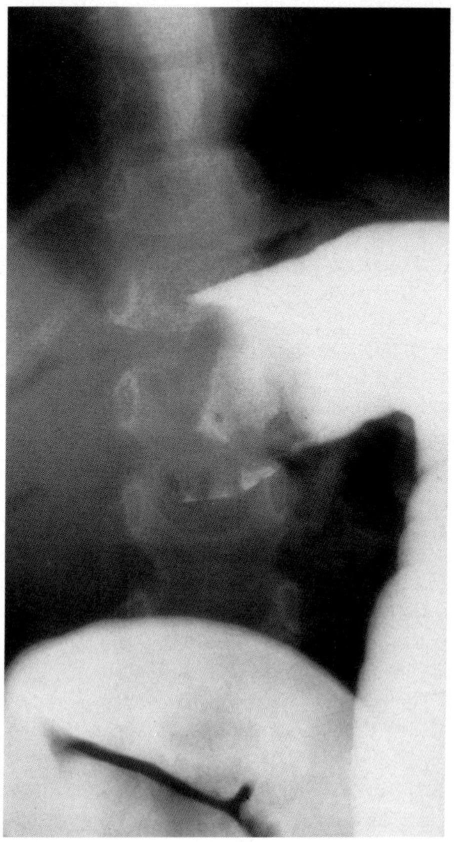

**FIGURE 5** Barium enema reduction first encountered the intussusception at the level expected from information gained from the initial supine view of the abdomen (see Fig. 2).

ation and the degree of progressive reduction of the intussusception. If I cannot prevent evacuation and/or have not shown any progressive reduction after 3 minutes, I stop that attempt. I do not promote evacuation or drainage of the colon because that may produce further intussusception. After allowing the child, and myself, to rest for a few minutes, I attempt reduction again. After three unsuccessful attempts, if there has been no progression in reduction, I recommend surgical reduction. However, if there is progressive but incomplete reduction, I may continue beyond three attempts after consulting with the referring surgeon. There have been reports that the presence of a "dissection sign" indicates nonreducibility. This phenomenon refers to the contrast material surrounding a long segment of the intussusceptum within the intussuscipiens (Fig. 8). It does seem to be an indication of a difficult, but not necessarily impossible, reduction.

A successful reduction is heralded by free reflux of contrast material into the ileum. I advocate refluxing at least 15 cm of ileum to a point above the expected location of a Meckel's diverticulum. If this degree of reflux occurs, any potential

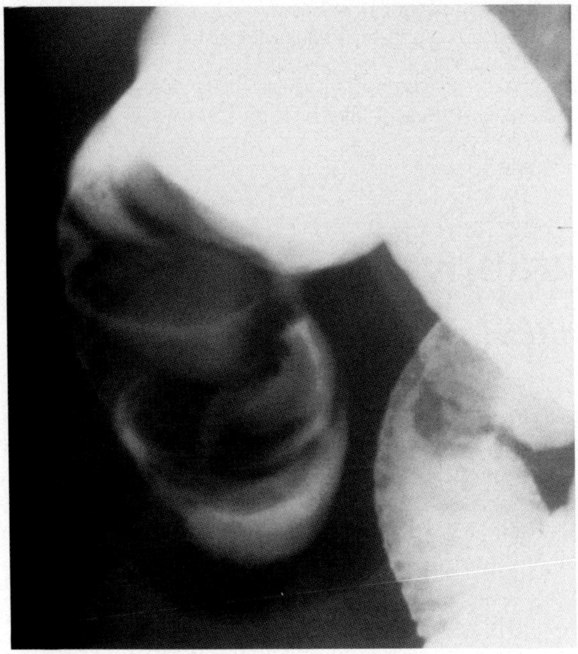

**FIGURE 7** The intussusception was successfully reduced to the level of the ileocecal valve, where further reduction was delayed for approximately two additional minutes.

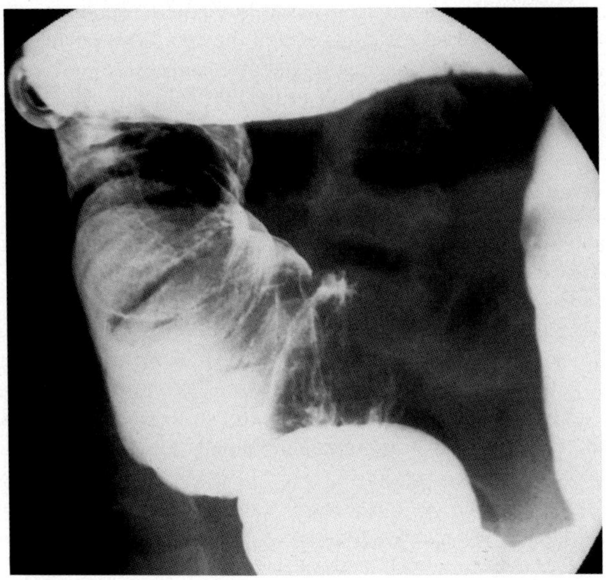

**FIGURE 8** The "dissection sign" represents a long segment of intussusceptum surrounded by contrast material. In this case the intussusceptum is shown surrounded by contrast material from the cecum to the hepatic flexure.

ileoileal intussusception that may have acted as a lead point should have been reduced.

After reduction occurs, a supine view of the abdomen should be obtained (Fig. 9). There are three important observations: (1) no free intraperitoneal contrast material, (2) contrast material in the distal ileum, and (3) no recurrent intussusception, especially after the first forceful evacuation of contrast material. The recurrence rate for hydrostatic reduction is approximately 6 to 10 percent, and half that for surgical reduction. In addition to direct visualization of a recurrent intussusception, a hallmark of recurrence on a postevacuation radiograph is complete emptying of contrast material from the small bowel. Even if no colonic component is recognized, if the previously filled small bowel is completely empty of contrast material, a repeat enema study should be performed to exclude or reduce a recurrent intussusception.

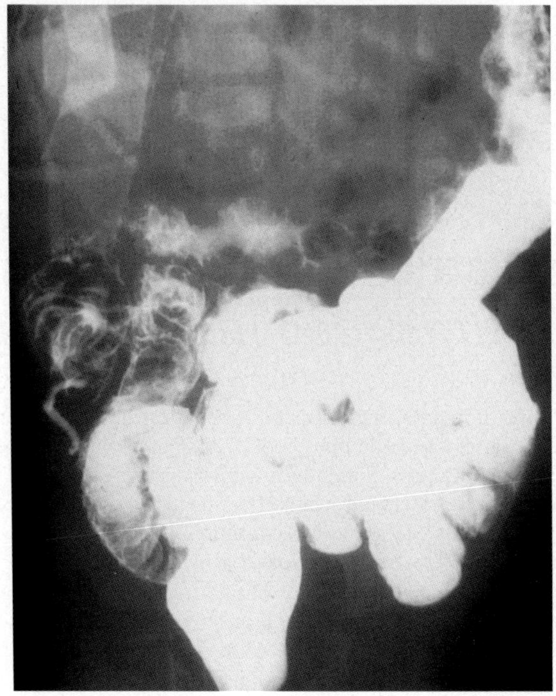

**FIGURE 9** Reflux into the ileum should occur freely and for at least 15 cm to assure reduction of a possible ileoileal intussusception and to exclude a Meckel's diverticulum, which may act as a lead point. A Meckel's diverticulum can sometimes be visualized by refluxed contrast.

No further radiographic follow-up is necessary if the child remains asymptomatic. Approximately 40 percent of recurrences occur within two days; the remaining ones may not occur for several years. If a child has more than two recurrences, a pathologic lead point becomes a serious consideration. Therefore most children with multiple recurrences are treated surgically.

## Suggested Reading


Barr LL, Stansberry SD, Swischuk LE. Significance of age, duration, obstruction and the dissection sign in intussusception. Pediatr Radiol 1990; 20:454–456.

Franken EA, Smith WL, Chernish, et al. The use of glucagon in hydrostatic reduction of intussusception: A double-blind study of 30 patients. Radiology 1983; 146:687–689.

Kirks DR, Caron KH. Gastrointestinal tract. In: Kirks DR, ed. Practical pediatric imaging: Diagnostic Radiology of Infants and Children. 2nd ed. Boston: Little Brown, 1991:708.

Ong NT, Beasley SW. The leadpoint in intussusception. J Pediatr Surg 1990; 25:640–643.

Ravitch MM. Intussusception. In: Welch KJ, Randolph JG, Ravitch MM, O'Neill JA, Rowe MI, eds. Pediatric Surgery. 4th ed. Chicago: Year Book Medical Publishers, 1986:868.

Shiels WE, Maves CK, Hedlund GL, Kirks DR. Air enema for diagnosis and reduction of intussusception: Clinical experience and pressure correlates. Radiology 1991; 181:169–172.

Stephenson CA, Seibert JJ, Strain JD, et al. Intussusception: Clinical and radiographic factors influencing reducibility. Pediatr Radiol 1989; 20:57–60.

Stringer DA, Ein SH. Pneumatic reduction: Advantages, risks and indications. Pediatr Radiol 1990; 20:475–477.

# Pediatric Abdominal Ultrasonography

*RITA LITTLEWOOD TEELE, M.D. · JANE CHRESTMAN SHARE, M.D.*

Pediatric ultrasonography functions both "inside" and "alongside" radiology and other methods of imaging. Although adults may consider ultrasonography noninvasive, an ill and frightened child considers all evaluations intrusive. Medical, psychological, and economic considerations all combine to encourage the appropriate choice of examination(s) for a particular pediatric problem. Therefore, when a clinician refers a patient to ultrasonography, it should be with the intent of having specific questions answered. We try to schedule the patient to suit the needs of the clinician, the parents, and the child. A family, worried because their baby has been identified as having an abdominal mass on a routine pediatric visit, should not have to wait long for the diagnostic ultrasonograms. On the other hand, a child who needs renal scans to check anatomy and parenchymal growth after urinary infection can have the study scheduled to coincide with the voiding cystourethrogram or radionuclide study that also needs to be done.

Before beginning an ultrasonographic examination, it is extremely helpful to have all the patient's previous radiographs and scans available to appreciate the context of the clinical situation and to know the specific concerns of the clinicians. The patient is usually in the examining room 15 to 30 minutes, depending on the complexity of the study, and that is ample time in which to conduct a brief historical review of the problem, either from the patient, the parent(s), or the medical chart.

Ultrasonography is like fluoroscopy; one has to be involved in tackling the problem, in making the images, and coming to a conclusion while the patient is being examined. There is nothing that makes one appreciate the skill of an expert pediatric ultrasonographer more than to be standing, transducer in hand, facing a 2-year-old who wants no part of any ultrasonographic study. As a rule, we do not use sedation; rarely do we have to resort to chloral hydrate or other medication for subduing a patient. Parent(s) stay in the room with young children; we try to judge the family situation when patients are older. Adolescent girls, for example, often want their parent(s) to stay outside the examining room.

Knowledge of the clinical questions determines the areas to be scanned, the sequence of scans, and the type of transducer(s) required. Scans must be systematic and labeling concise. One should account for all organs and other important structures within an area of interest. It is frequently more difficult to recognize that which is missing than to find an enlarged or abnormal structure.

If the preceding has been our philosophy of pediatric ultrasonographic practice, what follows is our practical outline for helping to solve common pediatric problems. Most children have a single disease that causes their signs and symptoms. The following material is problem-oriented by anatomic area and organ system. Each section describes preparation, technique, and typical clinical scenarios with their associated ultrasonographic findings. This description is not inclusive; only the most common situations are discussed.

## Liver, Biliary Tree, and Spleen

*Preparation* – Babies are given nothing by mouth for 4 hours preceding the study. Children and adolescents receive nothing by mouth for 6 hours preceding the study.

*Technique* – Sector scanning is done at 3.5 or 5 MHz, depending on the size of the child. Transverse scans are done from xiphoid inferiorly to include the hepatic venous confluence, left portal vein and left lobe of the liver, right portal vein and right lobe of the liver, porta hepatis, pancreas, right kidney, and gallbladder. Longitudinal and/or coronal scans include left lobe of the liver and aorta, inferior vena cava and common bile duct, gallbladder and common bile duct, right lobe of the liver, right kidney and Morrison's pouch, left kidney, and spleen.

These are the bare minimum of scans. Extra views of the gallbladder are usually needed; any area identified as abnormal on the initial screening views requires additional interrogation. Linear array scanning, using as high-frequency transducer as possible, is needed when parenchymal abnormality of the liver and/or spleen is a possibility. Scans with linear array can display the gallbladder in its entirety. Study with color/duplex Doppler is added when there is evidence for chronic liver disease, tumor, sequelae of trauma, inflammation, or vascular abnormality.

### *Jaundice in the Newborn*

An extensive medical evaluation usually precedes ultrasonographic study. After classifiable hepatitis, alpha$_1$-antitrypsin deficiency, hematologic causes, and so forth have been ruled out, ultrasonography is used to help differentiate between neonatal hepatitis of unknown etiology and biliary atresia. In general, a normal gallbladder ($>1.5$ cm in length) that contracts after feeding is not associated with biliary atresia. A small hypoplastic gallbladder may reflect disuse associated with atresia or cholestasis associated with severe hepatitis. Radionuclide scans and hepatic biopsy are other diagnostic methods for discriminating between the two problems; passage of radionuclide from biliary system to gut infers the patency of the system and rules out atresia. There are specific features on histologic evaluation of percutaneous hepatic biopsy that aid in diagnosis. Babies who have indeterminate studies may need exploratory surgery; if the gallbladder is large enough, percutaneous cholecystography under ultrasonic guidance may allow demonstration of intrahepatic ducts and obviate surgical intervention. Choledochal cyst or subhepatic cyst in the neonate may be associated with biliary atresia. Polysplenia is an associated anomaly in 10 percent of patients who have biliary atresia.

### Unexplained Jaundice in the Older Child

Diseases of the biliary tract associated with gallstones are associated with a history of hemolytic anemia, orthopedic or cardiac surgery, ileal disease, cystic fibrosis, or other metabolic liver disease. Idiopathic cholelithiasis occurs in approximately 20 percent of children (Fig. 1). If gallstones are identified, the common bile duct and pancreas should be evaluated carefully. Coronal views that show splenic enlargement (6 + ⅓ age in years = maximal length of spleen in centimeters) indicate presence of portal hypertension or splenomegaly associated with hemolytic disease. Jaundice may be the only sign of choledochal cyst. The cyst is continuous with variably dilated intrahepatic ducts; some intrahepatic systems are beaded (Caroli's disease) and some are normal in caliber. The "cyst" is identified as the dilated choledochus if the gallbladder enters it via the cystic duct.

Hepatic parenchymal disease can be identified by ultrasonography but generally not with the same sensitivity as with computed tomography (CT) or magnetic resonance imaging (MRI). Fatty infiltration (from hyperalimentation, malnutrition, obesity, chemotherapy, steroids, or metabolic liver disease) results in a hyperechogenic parenchymal pattern. Patchy increased echogenicity, predominantly periportal, results from increased fibrosis. Abscess and granuloma cause focal hypoechoic areas. Metastatic disease is rare but can result in hypo- or hyperechogenic foci. Viral hepatitis does not produce a specific ultrasonographic abnormality.

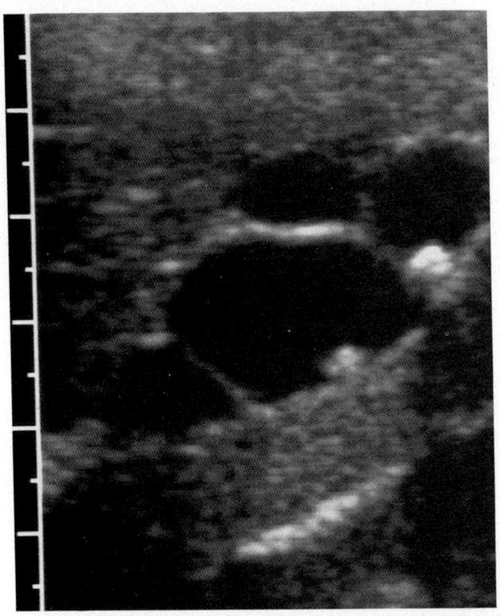

**FIGURE 1** Surprisingly this child has survived to the age of 6 years with a diagnosis of trisomy 18. She presented with abdominal pain that, because of her mental retardation, was poorly localized to the right upper quadrant. Tests of hepatic function were normal. This longitudinal scan shows not only gallstones but a septated gallbladder—a rare variant. No surgery was performed because her pain resolved spontaneously.

### Pain in Right Upper Quadrant

For the child who has this clinical presentation, we orient the study to include not only the liver and biliary tree but the right side of the hemidiaphragm, pleural space if necessary, and detailed views of the right kidney. Diagnostic considerations include those discussed in the preceding section. Other causes for pain include traumatic intrahepatic or subcapsular hematoma with hepatic laceration, right-sided pneumonia, renal disease, and high-riding inflamed appendix.

### Unexplained Hepatomegaly/Hepatic Mass

Malignant primary hepatic tumors are rare in the pediatric population. Hepatoblastoma typically occurs in infants; hepatocarcinoma occurs in two peaks: younger than 4 years of age and in midadolescence. Both hepatocarcinoma and hepatoblastoma have an abdominal mass or enlarging abdomen as their most common presenting symptom. The tumor may invade draining hepatic veins and inferior vena cava. The ultrasonographic study is directed towards identifying an intrahepatic mass, localizing it to a lobe or lobular segment, and identifying its vascular supply and vascular drainage. Benign vascular masses, such as hemangioendothelioma and vascular mesenchymal hamartoma, typically present in the newborn period either as unexplained hepatomegaly or because the child is in congestive failure. Blood supply to these lesions is dramatic.

## Kidney and Retroperitoneum

*Preparation*—No preparation is necessary unless the patient has hematuria. If hematuria is present, the bladder should be full.

*Technique*—Sector scanning is done with the highest-frequency transducer possible. We begin with transverse views of the bladder. If the bladder is large, the child is allowed to empty it before views of the upper urinary tracts are obtained. Renal scans should include transverse, sagittal, and coronal views to include the longest axis of the kidney for measurement. Evaluation includes renal position, size, parenchymal pattern, and the status of the collecting system. The upper pole of the kidney is best viewed when the patient is supine and the scanning plane is coronal. The lower pole is best displayed when the patient is prone. A linear array transducer is useful in evaluating the kidneys of small babies, evaluating the parenchymal pattern, and providing a larger view of the kidney in the near field. Color/duplex Doppler is added when vascular abnormality is suspected.

### Postnatal Follow-up of Prenatally Diagnosed Renal Abnormality

Fetal hydronephrosis, if mild, can await elective follow-up evaluation 2 to 4 weeks after the baby's birth. A baby who has severe unilateral hydronephrosis, or moderate-to-severe bilateral hydronephrosis, requires evaluation soon after delivery. Prophylactic antibiotics, begun immediately after delivery, de-

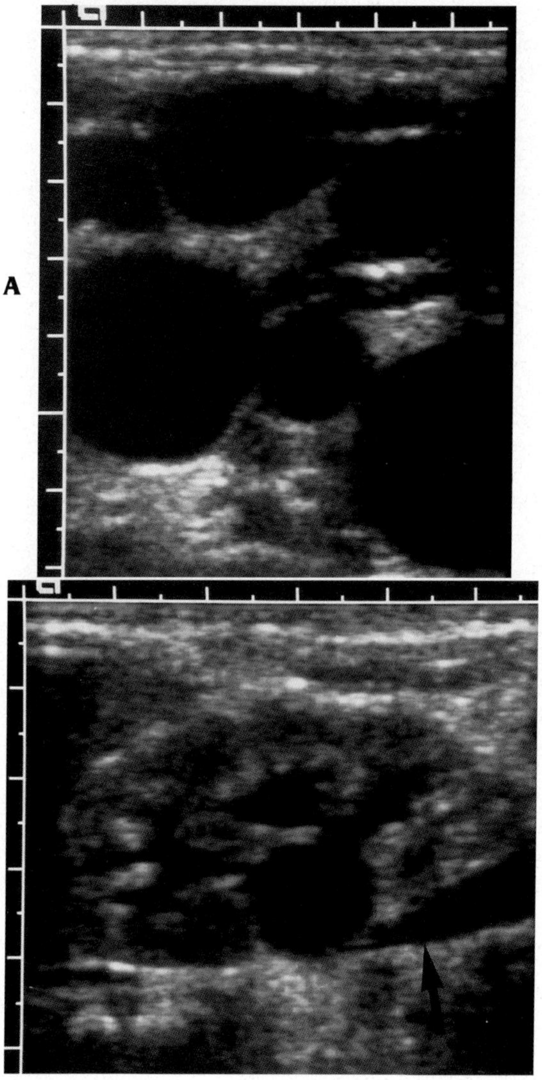

**FIGURE 2** Left multicystic dysplastic kidney (MDK) was diagnosed prenatally in this baby. Follow-up scans done at 2 days of age show typical findings of MDK *(A)* with cysts of varying sizes surrounded by echogenic stroma. There is often some degree of obstruction of the opposite kidney *(B)* in cases of MDK. The psoas muscle *(arrow, B)* is often highly lucent in babies and should not be confused with a dilated ureter.

crease the rate of urosepsis in neonates who have major structural abnormality. Ultrasonography should allow complete demonstration of the dilatation. Proximal ureteral dilatation is best shown with coronal views in the same plane as the great vessels. Careful scans of the pelvis allow identification of distal ureteral dilatation, ureterocele, or ectopic insertion. Multicystic dysplastic kidney is an irregular mass of variably sized cysts with admixed echogenic stroma. It is at the far end of the spectrum of obstructive hydronephrosis associated with proximal, pelviureteric stenosis (Fig. 2). Typically babies who have mild pelvic distention from narrowing at the ureteropelvic junction are followed with a second scan 6 to 12 months later. There is no guarantee, however, that significant dilatation will not develop at a later age. Distal ureteral obstruction occurs with primary megaureter, distal ureteral stenosis, ectopic ureterocele associated with duplex kidney, and obstruction at the outlet of the bladder such as posterior urethral valve. It is important to note that vesicoureteric reflux, unassociated with obstruction, may cause major distention of the ipsilateral upper urinary tract (Table 1).

**TABLE 1** Major Causes of Neonatal Hydronephrosis

| |
|---|
| Ureteropelvic obstruction/multicystic dysplastic kidney |
| Distal ureteral obstruction |
| Vesicoureteric reflux |
| Posterior urethral valve |
| Duplex kidney with ureterocele |

### *Urinary Tract Infection*

Ultrasonography is coordinated with voiding cystourethrography or radionuclide cystography in the evaluation of children who have had documented urinary tract infection. Scans can demonstrate structural anomalies of the kidneys, parenchymal scarring, global renal shrinkage, calculi, and abnormalities in and around the bladder. Further discussion of this topic is in the chapter on Imaging Approach to Urinary Tract Infections in Children.

### *Renal Screening*

Groups of children at risk for renal anomalies include patients with congenital scoliosis, gynecologic abnormalities, VATER association, and diverse other syndromes. Ultrasonography establishes whether two kidneys are present in their respective renal fossa. It does not give functional information and may not exclude minor anomalies (e.g., uncomplicated duplication of the renal collecting system). If questions are created by the ultrasonographic examination, urography or radionuclide studies should follow. In most cases the ultrasonographic examination is sufficient to answer the clinical questions. Common situations in which screening renal ultrasonography is employed are listed in Table 2.

## Pelvic Pain or Mass in Girls

*Preparation*—The patient should have a full bladder.

*Technique*—Sector scans are done at the highest frequency possible. Transverse views are obtained of the vagina, cervix,

**TABLE 2** Screening Renal Ultrasonography

| |
|---|
| Abnormal prenatal ultrasonographic findings |
| Myelodysplasia |
| Imperforate anus |
| Congenital scoliosis |
| Severe hypospadias* |
| Undescended testis* |
| Single umbilical artery* |
| Cardiac anomaly |
| Hemipertrophy/aniridia |
| Urinary infection |
| Hematuria |
| Hypertension |
| Familial cystic disease |
| Other syndromes |

*This is controversial. Some believe there is a higher-than-normal association with renal anomalies; others do not.

uterine body, and fundus, and each adnexa in addition to longitudinal views of the uterus and each adnexa. Screening views are done of each kidney. Color/duplex Doppler is added in cases of suspected adnexal torsion, ectopic pregnancy, and vascular abnormality. Linear array scanning rarely adds additional information.

Normal values for uterine and adnexal dimensions are available in the literature. The normal uterus in the prepubertal period is less than 3.5 cm in length. Ovaries may be small, but occasionally cysts are apparent throughout childhood. One should always be able to identify the normal uterus. All organs are easily visualized at puberty.

Solid pelvic masses in young children are rare and, when present, may be uterine rhabdomyosarcoma or ovarian teratoma. In the adolescent a solid pelvic mass is more likely to be ovarian in origin and either benign or malignant. Ovarian cysts are much more common than solid tumors; virtually all are benign.

Duplication of the genital tract with obstruction of one unit is almost always associated with renal anomalies, specifically agenesis ipsilateral to the side of obstruction. Hydronephrosis may result from any pelvic mass; thus renal scans are always included as part of a pelvic study.

## Scrotal Mass in Boys

*Preparation*—No preparation is necessary.

*Technique*—To evaluate scrotal mass in boys, 5 or 7.5 mHz linear array transducers with color Doppler capability should be used. The testicular or extratesticular site of the mass must be documented. This is characterized as cystic or solid. Solid testicular masses are generally neoplastic. Cystic extratesticular collections are usually uncomplicated hydrocele. Spermatocele and epididymal cyst are localized to the epididymis. A painful scrotal mass may be secondary to inflammation, torsion of appendix testis, trauma, epididymo-orchitis, or torsion of the testis. Absence of arterial flow in a testis, after contralateral testicular flow has been documented, is diagnostic of testicular torsion. When torsion is early and intermittent, vascular flow may be apparent in the involved testis. The clinical presentation must be appreciated when operative intervention is being considered. Inflammatory disease of the epididymis and testis results in exuberant arterial and venous flow. This pattern virtually rules out testicular torsion.

## Fever of Unknown Origin

*Preparation*—The patient receives nothing by mouth for 4 hours.

*Technique*—Sector scanning of entire abdomen is done in transverse and longitudinal axes. Linear array transducers of high frequency are then used to evaluate splenic and hepatic parenchyma for granulomas, microabscesses, or subtle changes secondary to cellular infiltration.

The search for abdominal abscess may follow surgical procedures. Patients who have Crohn disease, chronic granulomatous disease, or immunodeficiency syndromes are also at risk for formation of abscess. Localizing signs are usually evident when an intra-abdominal abscess is present. Subdiaphragmatic spaces, Morrison's pouch, and pelvis should all be carefully evaluated for loculated collections of fluid. Appendicitis as a cause of abdominal pain and/or fever may be diagnosed using the techniques pioneered by Puylaert. Gradual compression of the right lower quadrant with a small linear array transducer of high frequency allows, in most cases, demonstration of the thick-walled inflamed appendix (Fig. 3).

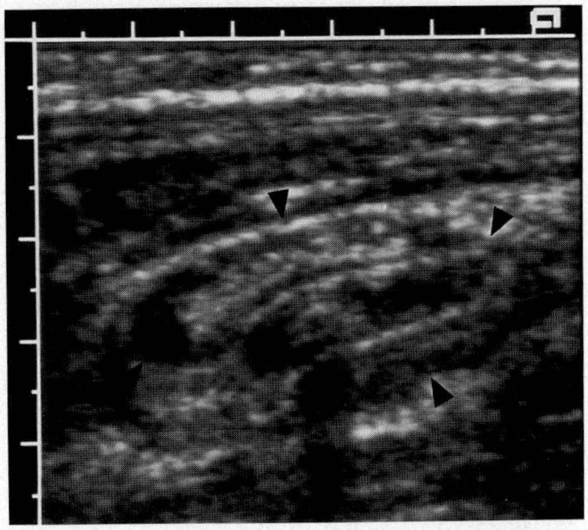

**FIGURE 3** This 14-year-old girl presented with a history of right lower abdominal pain for 30 hours, associated with fever and chills. Ultrasonography was requested to help determine if her pain was gynecologic or appendiceal in origin. Her ovaries and uterus were normal; graded compression of the right lower quadrant allowed demonstration of a noncompressible, tender, fluid-filled appendix *(between arrowheads)*. A shadowing appendicolith was present, and there was edema around the appendix. At surgery, an inflamed nonperforated retrocecal appendix was removed.

## Abdominal Mass

*Preparation*—Preferably, the patient takes nothing by mouth for 4 hours.

*Technique*—The baby or child who presents with an abdominal mass should be evaluated with ultrasonography after consultation with the clinicians and with the radiologists. Depending on the site of the mass and the age of the child, the sequence of examinations will vary. Hepatic mass and pelvic mass have been mentioned previously. The most common mass in children is one arising from the retroperitoneum. Benign disease such as hydronephrosis, multicystic dysplastic kidney (MDK), and adrenal hemorrhage may be responsible for a palpable retroperitoneal mass. If a solid tumor is identified in the adrenal gland, kidney, or other retroperitoneal structure, use ultrasonography to characterize the mass, evaluate the contralateral retroperitoneal space, establish patency or lack thereof of the inferior vena cava, and evaluate the rest of the abdomen, specifically the liver, for evidence of metastatic disease (Fig. 4). The presence of a solid mass in the retroperitoneum usually requires further evaluation with CT or MRI. Ultrasonography is relatively insensitive to the presence of nephroblastomatosis, a condition that can coexist with, and predispose a baby to, Wilms' tumor.

Anterior abdominal masses, including ovarian cyst, duplication cyst of bowel, mesenteric cyst, and mural lesions of bowel, may require only ultrasonography before surgery or confirmatory studies such as upper gastrointestinal (GI) series. With the expansion of cross-sectional imaging, urography rarely is used in the evaluation of abdominal masses in childhood.

A

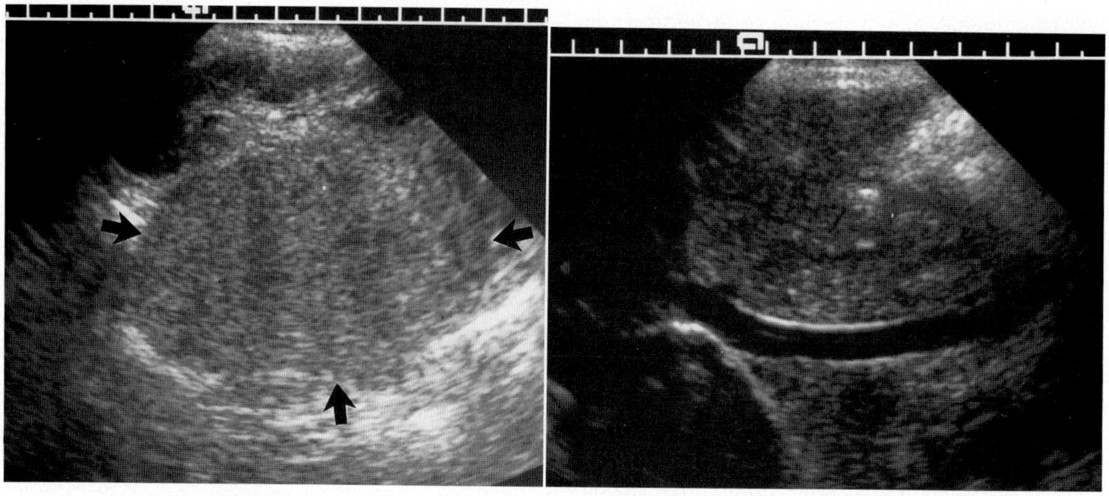

B

**FIGURE 4** This 2.5-year-old boy was referred when a left upper quadrant mass, thought to be an enlarged spleen, was palpated during a routine physical examination. His first study was ultrasonography. This showed a large mass *(arrows)* which was separate from the spleen and anterior to the left kidney on sagittal scan *(A)*. Importantly the rest of the abdominal organs were normal and the inferior vena cava was patent *(B)*. The differential diagnosis in a case such as this includes neuroblastoma and exophytic Wilms' tumor. At surgery, the mass proved to be neuroblastoma. Because the left adrenal gland is anterior and medial to the kidney, a mass involving the gland can be quite low and medial in position.

A

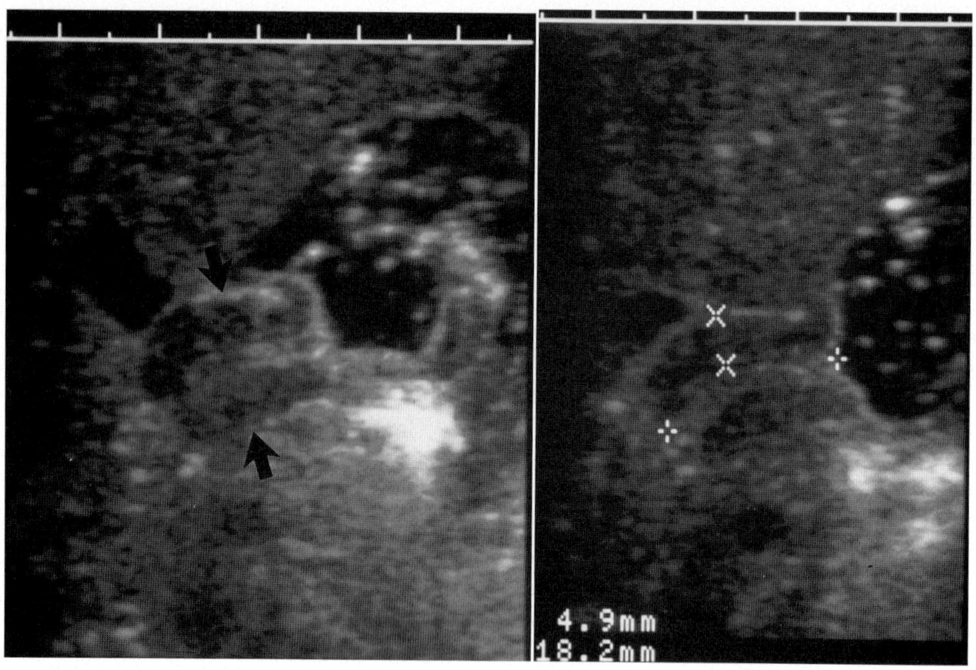


B

**FIGURE 5** *A,* Nine days of nonprojectile vomiting in this 3-week-old boy prompted a request for ultrasonography. The scans were diagnostic for pyloric stenosis. The relatively echolucent pylorus *(arrows)* is hypertrophied. The parallel lines within the muscle represent the coapted gastric mucosa. *B,* The length of the channel and the width of the hypertrophied muscle have been measured. At our institution we consider a channel length of ≥17 mm and muscle width of ≥3.5 mm as diagnostic for pyloric stenosis.

### *Pyloric Stenosis*

This highly specific abdominal mass is from hypertrophied pyloric muscle, which prevents normal gastric emptying. Babies who are affected tend to present at 4 to 6 weeks of age with projectile vomiting. Scans are performed while the baby lies supine but rolled to the right. This allows fluid to outline the gastric antrum. Fifteen to thirty milliliters of glucose water may be given to the baby in order to outline the gastric antrum. The gallbladder acts as a signpost to the pyloris. A 5 MHz linear array transducer is best for demonstrating the elongated pyloric channel, the thickened muscle, and delayed gastric emptying (Fig. 5).

## Suggested Reading

Haller JO. Review: Sonography of the biliary tract in infants and children. AJR 1991; 157:1051–1058.

Middleton WD. Scrotal ultrasonography in 1991. Ultrasound Q 1991; 9:61–87.

Miller JH, Greenspan BS. Integrated imaging of hepatic tumors in childhood. Part I: Malignant lesions (primary and metastatic). Radiology 1985; 154:83–90.

Puylaert JBCM. Ultrasound of Appendicitis and Its Differential Diagnosis. New York: Springer-Verlag, 1990.

Teele RL, Share JC. Ultrasonography of Infants and Children. Philadelphia: WB Saunders, 1991.

Teele RL, Share JC. Ultrasonography of the female pelvis in childhood and adolescence. Radiol Clin North Am 1992; 30:743–758.

Willi UV. Pediatric genitourinary imaging. Curr Opin Radiol 1991; 3:936–945.

# Visceral Injuries in Battered Children

*CARLOS J. SIVIT, M.D.*

Nonaccidental trauma is a major cause of morbidity and mortality in the pediatric population. The number of children who are victims of physical violence in the United States each year is estimated to range from 1 to 2 million. Most serious physical injury is noted in children under 5 years of age. Approximately 5,000 of these children die as a result of their injuries.

The radiologic evaluation plays an important role in the investigation and prosecution of cases involving battered children. The emphasis of the radiologic evaluation of these children has traditionally focused on the identification of skeletal and intracranial injury. Serious intra-abdominal and intrathoracic injury has been thought to be uncommon in this population.

In recent years the widespread use of abdominal computed tomography (CT) in the evaluation of blunt trauma has resulted in the identification of visceral injury in children with relatively minor or nonspecific symptoms. Thus CT reveals intrathoracic and intra-abdominal injuries in abused children that might otherwise go undetected.

Intra-abdominal and intrathoracic injuries in battered children are usually observed in an older age group than are skeletal and intracranial injuries. The median age of battered children with visceral injuries noted on CT scans at our institution has been 2 years. Most visceral injuries in this population are felt to be caused by a direct blow or to sudden deceleration after being thrown. A precise description of the mechanism of injury, however, is rarely provided.

## Technique

Proper CT technique maximizes the diagnostic value of the study. Basic principles include patient preparation, proper use of intravenous contrast material, location and spacing of CT sections, and image display.

Children should be placed on the table supine, with arms placed above the head. Restraints should be applied when necessary. Sedation is rarely required for the examination of injured children. The radius of reconstruction should be sufficiently large to include the entire abdomen and pelvis, including soft tissues. The removal of overlying metallic hardware and withdrawal of nasogastric tubes into the esophagus before scanning minimizes streak artifacts. If a Foley catheter is present, it should be occluded before the administration of intravenous contrast material to maximize bladder opacification.

Vascular enhancement is imperative to identify solid visceral injury. We use a rapid bolus injection of intravenous contrast material (3 ml/kg; 120 ml maximal dose). Approximately two-thirds of the total dose is injected before scanning. The remainder is injected continuously throughout the planned scan sequence to maximize vascular and parenchymal opacification. We do not use oral contrast opacification of the gastrointestinal tract routinely in our initial CT study of injured children. We do use oral contrast material in situations in which an injury to the intestinal tract or pancreas is strongly suspected.

Serial 1 cm thick slices are obtained at 1 cm intervals from the lower chest to the pelvis. Inclusion of the lower chest is important to identify associated parenchymal and pleural abnormalities. Imaging of the pelvis is necessary to detect intraperitoneal fluid and bony injury. We pause for approximately 5 minutes before scanning the pelvis to allow for bladder filling with intravenous contrast material.

## Indications

Children should be hemodynamically stable before CT. Our current approach to children with suspected blunt thoracoabdominal injury is as follows. If children are not hemodynamically stable after aggressive attempts at stabilization in the trauma resuscitation bay or have suspected peritonitis, they are taken directly to the operating room. Children undergo CT evaluation if they fall into one of the following categories: (1) children who are hemodynamically stable, but in whom serious abdominal injury is suspected; (2) those with multisystem injuries, especially head trauma, in whom physical examination suggests injury; and (3) children with hematuria.

Clinical suspicion of physical abuse is raised by physical examination findings, including skin bruises, burns, lacerations, and signs of skeletal trauma. Absence of radiographic abnormalities in extra-abdominal sites should not deter CT evaluation in children with physical signs of intrathoracic or intra-abdominal injury. In one-half of all children with nonskeletal thoracic or abdominal abnormalities noted on CT at our institution, no other radiographic abnormalities were observed. The most common indications for abdominal CT examination in battered children at our institution have been abdominal tenderness, abdominal bruising or ecchymoses, hematuria, and neurologic impairment such that the physical examination was considered unreliable.

## Diagnostic Approach

Battered children have constituted approximately 3 percent of all children studied following blunt trauma (33 per 1,000) at our institution over the past seven years. They constitute a high-risk group for visceral injury. Forty-eight percent of battered children studied by CT had nonskeletal injuries of the lower chest or abdomen noted at CT (Table 1), compared with a 30 percent frequency of injury in all other children with blunt trauma studied with CT. The spectrum of visceral injury noted in our battered children population has been similar to that observed in children injured by accidental blunt trauma. The most commonly injured viscera in battered children studied by CT at our institution has been the liver (Fig. 1), followed by the kidney and spleen. Thus, in contrast to many skeletal injuries that are highly specific for abuse, abdominal and thoracic visceral injuries are not pathognomonic for physical abuse. In conjunction with proper clinical findings, however, the identification of visceral injuries in this group of children is an important factor in the decision to remove the children from a high-risk setting and also may serve as evidence in clinical proceedings.

CT has proved to be highly accurate in the detection and delineation of hepatic, splenic, and renal injuries. A number of classification systems have been proposed for categorizing these injuries by CT. We classify the injuries as vascular or nonvascular. Nonvascular injuries are further characterized on the basis of percentage of abnormal parenchyma involved: minor injury (< 25 percent of organ volume), moderate (25 to 50 percent of organ volume), or severe (> 50 percent of organ volume).

**TABLE 1** Spectrum of Visceral Injury in 33 Battered Children Evaluated by CT

| | | Number (%) |
|---|---|---|
| Abdominal injury | | 13* (39) |
| Hepatic | 7 | |
| Renal | 4 | |
| Splenic | 3 | |
| Adrenal | 2 | |
| Pancreatic | 2 | |
| Bowel | 1 | |
| Thoracic injury | | 8* (24) |
| Pulmonary contusion | 5 | |
| Hemothorax | 2 | |
| Pneumothorax | 2 | |
| Total thoracic or abdominal injury | | 16* (48) |

*Some children had more than one injury.

Although the information gained by CT is useful in establishing a treatment plan, the decision to manage children with hepatic, splenic, and renal injury operatively or nonoperatively is based on the physiologic status of the child. Regardless of the extent of the injury by CT, hemorrhage stops in the majority of children, and nonoperative management is usually successful. Most intraparenchymal lacerations and hematomas undergo spontaneous absorption and healing.

We have noted post-traumatic adrenal hematoma in two battered children (Fig. 2). The characteristic CT findings are gland enlargement, oval or triangular shape, and decreased attenuation relative to enhanced liver and spleen. Thickening of the ipsilateral diaphragmatic crus may also be noted. Adjacent solid organ injury was present in both cases. Signs of adrenal insufficiency were not observed.

Bowel, mesenteric, and pancreatic injuries were not frequently observed in our group of battered children studied by CT. Prior reports had indicated that these were the most common intra-abdominal injuries observed in this population. These studies relied on findings noted after autopsy, surgery, or barium enema studies and hence are biased toward selection of patients with severe injury or injury to the gastrointestinal tract.

Pancreatic injury may be difficult to identify at CT. Delineation of the margins of the pancreas is difficult because of the small size of the organ and paucity of surrounding retroperitoneal fat in children. Minimal separation of the lacerated pancreatic fragments may be present. We have found that the presence of peripancreatic (lesser sac or anterior pararenal space) fluid is a useful marker for injury to the pancreas. On follow-up examination using CT or ultrasonography, a well-defined pseudocyst may be observed (Fig. 3).

The CT diagnosis of bowel injury also is difficult. We have noted pneumoperitoneum in only 39 percent of bowel injuries following blunt trauma. "Unexplained" fluid has been a useful indicator of bowel injury, since we have rarely observed

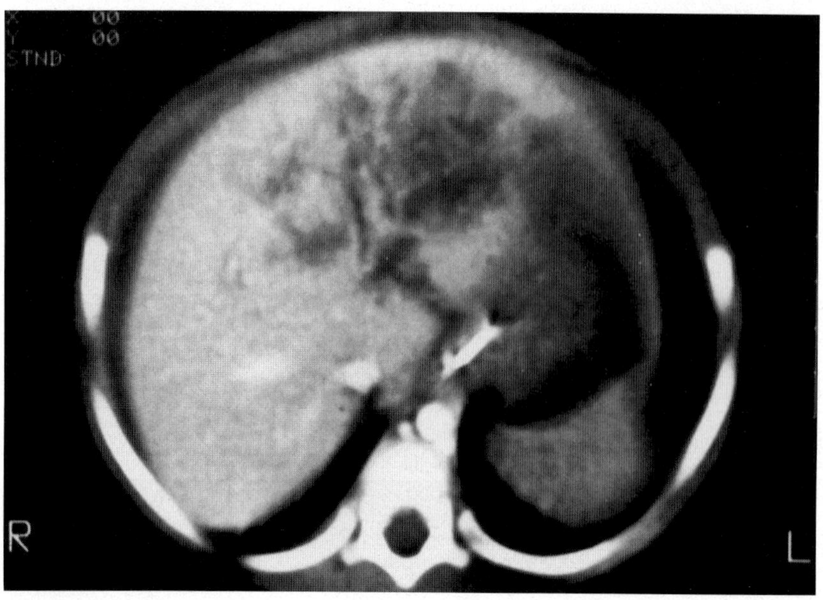


**FIGURE 1** CT scan shows complex laceration with associated hematoma in the left hepatic lobe.

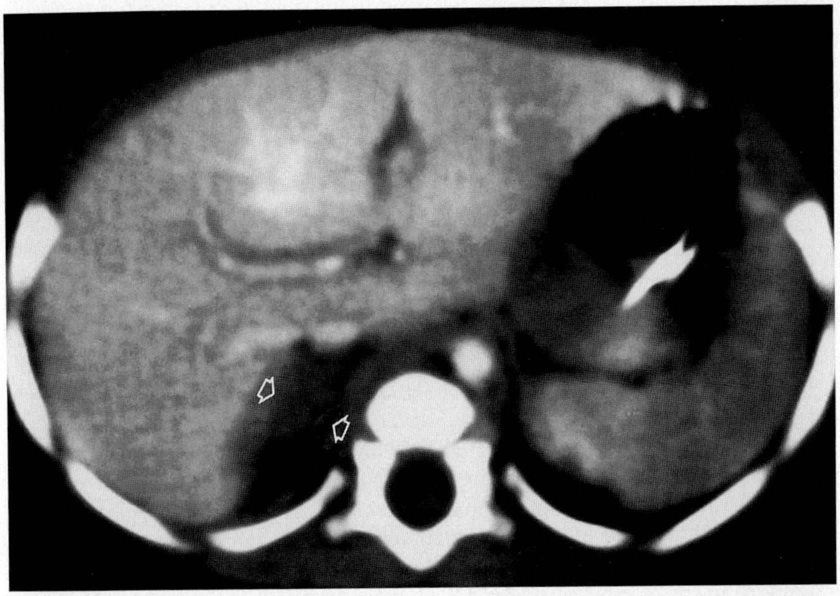

**FIGURE 2** CT scan demonstrates oval-shaped right adrenal hematoma *(arrows).*

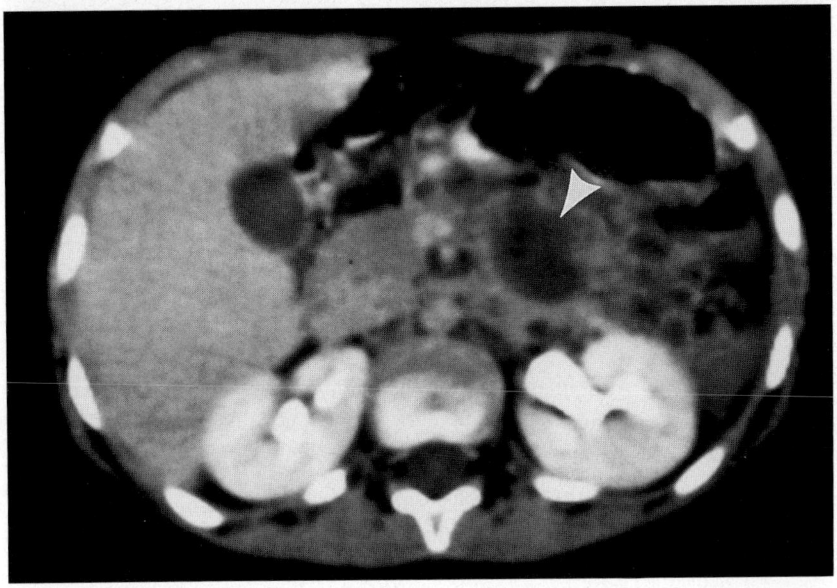

**FIGURE 3** CT scan shows an intrapancreatic pseudocyst *(arrowhead).*

peritoneal fluid as an isolated finding following blunt trauma.

The evaluation and treatment of thoracic trauma is a central feature of the early assessment and management of the injured child, because chest injury leads to hypoxia. Chest radiography remains the primary method for evaluating post-traumatic chest injury. These radiographs are usually obtained with portable equipment, with the child supine, with various monitoring devices overlying the areas of interest. As a result, even with optimal technique, the chest radiograph may underestimate or miss significant chest abnormality. Performance of a lower chest CT scan in conjunction with a CT scan of the upper abdomen is helpful in the early recognition of unsuspected chest injury. Consequently we include three or four CT slices of the chest in all children with abdominal trauma.

In conclusion, child abuse is a high-risk mechanism for abdominal visceral injury. These injuries may occur in the absence of more typical radiographic findings. Abdominal CT is a useful examination for abused children with physical signs and symptoms of abdominal trauma.

## Suggested Reading

Fontana VJ, Donovan D, Wong RJ. The "maltreatment syndrome" in children. N Engl J Med 1967; 269:1389–1394.

Heins M. The "battered child" revisited. JAMA 1984; 251:3295–3300.

Kempe CH, Silverman FN, Steele BF, et al. The battered child syndrome. JAMA 1962; 181:105–112.

Kleinman PK. Visceral trauma. In: Kleinman PK, ed. Diagnostic Imaging in Child Abuse. 1st ed. Baltimore: Williams & Wilkins, 1987:115.

Kleinman PK, Rastopoulos VD, Brill PW. Occult nonskeletal trauma in the battered-child syndrome. Radiology 1981; 141:393–396.

McCort J, Vaudagna J. Visceral injuries in battered children. Radiology 1964; 82:424–428.

O'Neill JA, Meacham WF, Griffin PP, Sawyers JL. Patterns of injury in the battered syndrome. J Trauma 1973; 13:332–339.

Sivit CJ, Taylor GA, Eichelberger MR. Visceral injury in battered children: A changing perspective. Radiology 1989; 173:659–661.

Taylor GA, Fallat ME, Potter BM, Eichelberger MR. The role of computed tomography in blunt trauma in children. J Trauma 1988; 28:1660–1664.

Touloukian RJ. Abdominal visceral injuries in battered children. Pediatrics 1968; 42:642–646.

# Dynamic Incremental Abdominal CT in Infants and Children

*ROBERT A. KAUFMAN, M.D.*

This chapter presents my personal approach to abdominal computed tomography (CT) in infants and young children. I emphasize those technical parameters that are different from CT in adults and provide helpful hints to avoid the typical pitfalls of pediatric imaging. The focus of this technique is bolus-enhanced, dynamic incremental imaging, which is applicable to most pediatric disease entities, particularly tumor, trauma, infection, and congenital anomalies.

The chapter is organized into sections on patient selection, patient preparation, and actual scanning. Incorporated into this discussion are those principles and philosophies that will allow the general radiologist to become more comfortable in understanding and proficient in examining the tiny patient, and more technically successful as well.

## General Principles

One of the disadvantages of pediatric radiology is that the patients are largely uncooperative compared with most older children and adults. To achieve technical success, I recommend the following principles:

1. The radiologist must have control of the patient, not the reverse. To make the infant or young child "cooperative," measures such as sedation and immobilization are necessary.
2. Know what your goal is and plan ahead. The ideal examination should avoid unnecessary radiation exposure and take as little time as possible while accomplishing the goal of the study. Tailor the evaluation to adhere to Sutton's law: Go for the "answer" first. A lengthy examination carries with it the risk that the patient may awaken or move out of position unexpectedly. If the diagnosis is already made, that problem is less significant.
3. Faster is better. Use the fastest scan time available. Avoid the temptation to use a longer scan time, because the image will doubtless be degraded by respiratory and abdominal wall motion, and is generally not worth the added radiation exposure or tube-cooling time.
4. Opacify everything. The lack of inherent contrast in an infant's abdomen must be compensated for by intravenous, oral, and even rectal contrast opacification.

The more meticulous the attention to the details of technique, the greater is the likelihood of success and the easier the study is to interpret.

## Candidate Selection

Not too long ago, infants less than 12 to 18 months of age were not good candidates for abdominal CT investigation; now, as a result of technical advancements, we routinely scan newborns. In the past ten years, available scan times on most CT scanners have been reduced significantly, image quality has improved, radiation dose has diminished, and reconstruction times have decreased. Most scanners sold today have a usable 1 to 2 second scan time available; a few are capable of subsecond scanning. In general, the faster the scan time available, the smaller the patient that can be accommodated. Thus abdominal CT is a viable modality for evaluation of almost all patients, yet it is neither needed nor necessarily optimal for every type of investigation.

In most pediatric radiology departments, sonography is routinely used as the initial modality of investigation for much of abdominal imaging, both to screen and to answer specific questions. CT is commonly used to characterize known lesions and to work out problems or questions. Patients are not candidates for CT if hemodynamically unstable; if there is sufficient metallic density nearby (e.g., Harrington rods) which precludes a useful investigation; or if the answer can be obtained more simply by another modality. Most hepatobiliary imaging is accomplished with scintigraphy and sonography; pancreas screening by sonography; and urinary tract investigation by combinations of sonography, scintigraphy, and cystourethrography. CT in the urinary tract often is reserved for complications of renal inflammatory disease, stones, or for problem cases. In abdominal trauma CT has displaced other modalities, except possibly for conventional radiography. For masses and tumors, conventional radiography with or without ultrasonographic evaluation is generally followed by CT and/or magnetic resonance imaging (MRI). Musculoskeletal imaging in and around the abdomen is performed by CT, MRI, or scintigraphy, depending on whether the problem is primarily soft tissue or bone in origin. Inflammatory abnormalities such as appendiceal abscesses are generally imaged first by conventional radiographs followed by sonography, but evaluation with CT either preoperatively or preintervention is useful, as well as when the sonographic diagnosis is unclear. For gastrointestinal (GI) problems, conventional radiology is still the mainstay of diagnosis.

## Patient Preparation

### *NPO Status*

Here is a simple rule for withholding food and liquid before sedation and/or injection of intravenous contrast material in infants and children: 2 hours for a newborn, 3 hours until 12 months of age, and 4 hours for patients older than 1 year. Older children and adolescents should receive nothing by mouth after midnight for morning studies.

### *Oral Contrast Medium*

For most investigations, oral contrast opacification of the GI tract is both useful and necessary. It is not necessary, however, under certain circumstances, such as in a head-injured or comatose child, when gag or cough reflex is absent or impaired, or if the patient is intubated or under general anesthesia. In

A

B

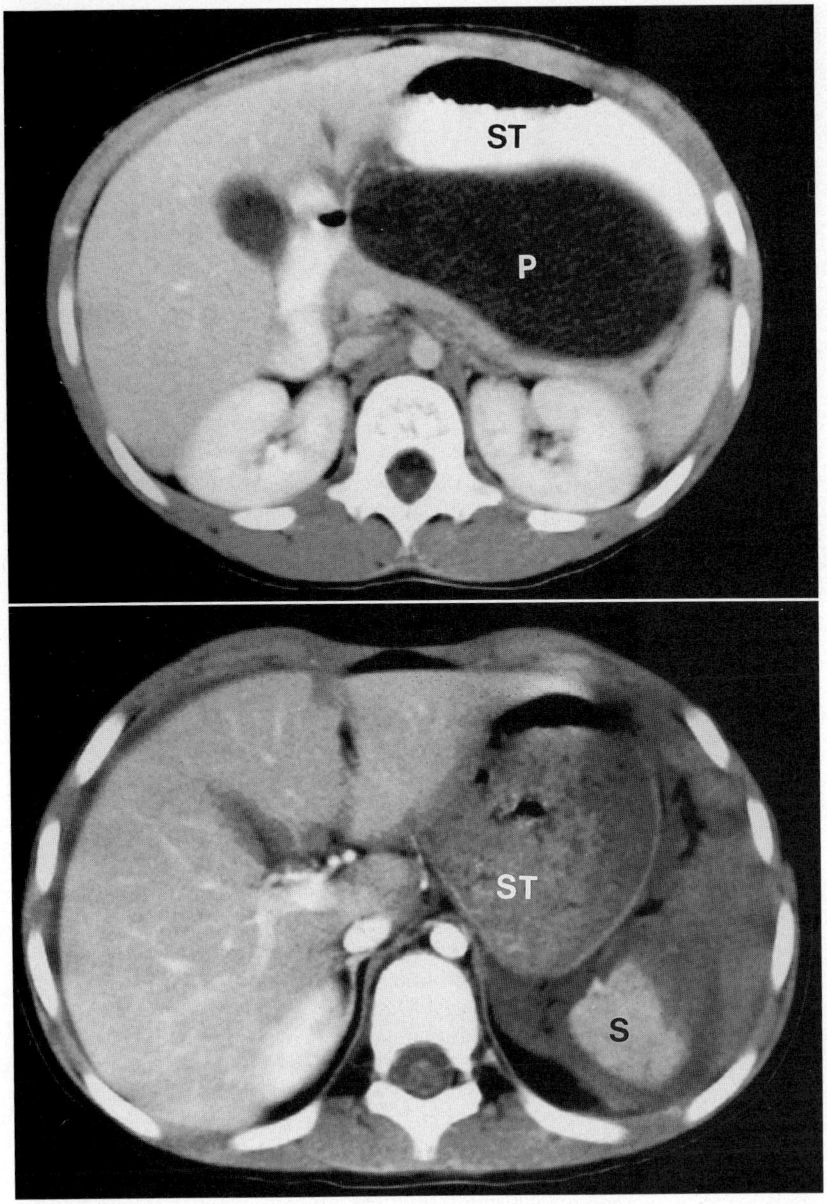


**FIGURE 1** *A,* A 7-year-old girl with post-traumatic pancreatic pseudocyst seven days after injury. Patient had elevated amylase and vomiting. Pseudocyst (P) fills the lesser sac and compresses the posterior gastric wall. Dose of the oral contrast agent was decreased by half to avoid nausea and vomiting. *B,* An 8-year-old girl with a fractured spleen. Because the gastric contents fill and distend the stomach (ST), oral contrast material was omitted. Free intraperitoneal blood and perisplenic clot were present. S = residual portion of vascularized spleen.

these circumstances we omit oral contrast material. When investigating the liver, spleen, and kidneys for fungal and/or bacterial microabscesses in the immunocompromised patient, it is omitted as well to avoid contrast-air levels in the stomach, which may cause artifact in the left lobe of the liver and anterior edge of the spleen. If the patient is nauseated, such as from pancreatitis or splenic injury, vomiting may occur during the contrast bolus or during sedation. It may be best, therefore, to decrease the volume of oral contrast material by one-third to one-half or to omit it entirely in this circumstance (Fig. 1, *A*). For trauma investigations, I have both used and not used oral contrast medium for initial emergent studies. For six years we used it routinely in most patients; for the last four years we have followed the advice of others who rarely use it unless bowel or mesenteric injury is a specific concern. I have found little disadvantage to its omission (Fig. 1, *B*). In neither case is the detection of bowel injury or perforation optimal. False-negatives are still a problem regardless of the technique used, because slit-like perforations in the small bowel are apt to seal over quickly and without detection. Using oral contrast medium in the trauma patient does delay the study slightly, and there is rarely time to opacify the distal small bowel and the large bowel in the emergent case. It can be a problem for the anesthesiologist if a general anesthetic is contemplated thereafter, such as for orthopedic or plastic surgery procedures unrelated to the abdomen. It is best to develop a protocol with your trauma surgeon.

## *Dose and Timing of Oral Contrast Medium*

The dose of oral contrast medium used to opacify the GI tract varies considerably with age: 2 to 4 oz for an infant to 16 oz for an adult-size teen. A good rule of thumb to remember is 1 oz per year over 4 years of age for a single unit dose. We use a 1.5 percent solution of sodium diatrizoate (Hypaque) oral liquid in a strong Koolaid flavor like grape or rainbow punch. Others have successfully used similar concentrations of "leftover" nonionic contrast medium kept refrigerated for same-day use.

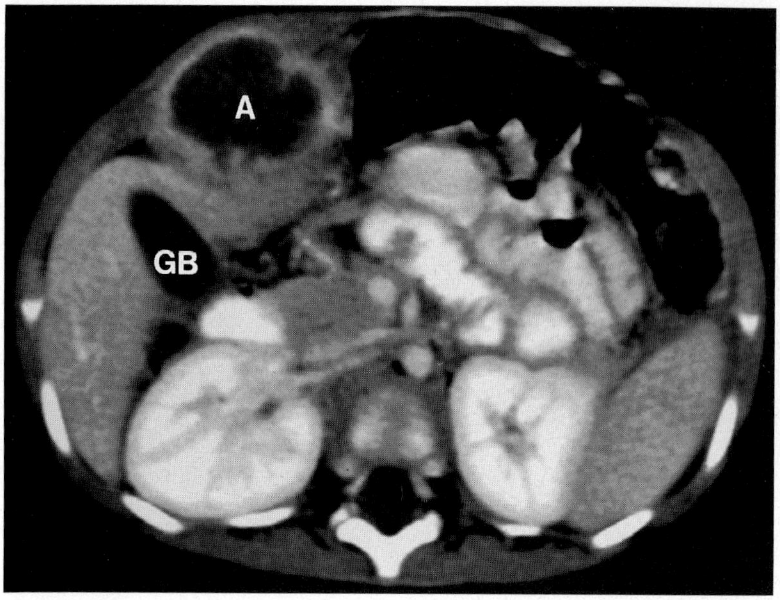


**FIGURE 2** A 6-month-old infant with liver abscess (A) arising adjacent to fissure for ligamentum teres. A single unit dose of oral contrast medium was administered 45 minutes before sedation and scanning. GB = gallbladder.

Most children and infants dislike the taste of barium preparations. The goal is to successfully persuade the child to drink; it is easier to do this if the liquid is palatable.

To opacify the bowel from stomach to terminal ileum, administer a single unit dose of oral contrast medium 45 to 60 minutes before actual scanning begins (Fig. 2). If there is ileus from appendiceal abscess, for example, wait 90 to 120 minutes. To opacify both the colon and the small bowel, give two unit doses: the first 12 hours or so before the examination (e.g., the evening before) and the second as above. In very young infants, reduce the lead time for the first dose to 4 to 6 hours.

## Intravenous Access

In general, we refrain from using lower-extremity intravenous sites to avoid vascular artifact from dense contrast medium in the inferior vena cava. Upper-extremity sites are preferred. The size of the cannula is the factor that limits the rate of bolus injection. We use the largest size practicable. We have changed from a butterfly needle to a 22 or 24 gauge intravascular catheter or larger. It provides a more secure intravenous line, and there is less chance for extravasation or dislodgement. We immobilize all intravenous access sites carefully with tape on an appropriately sized arm board. The intravenous line should remain accessible after the patient has been immobilized on the CT scan table to reduce the risk of awakening a sedated patient while unnecessarily undoing Velcro, straps, or tape.

## Psychological Preparation

In many respects it is easier to scan a sedated patient than a nonsedated one, because retaining the attention and cooperation of the sedated patient is not a problem. For those children old enough, mature enough, and well enough, breath holding for single exposures is optimal. Most 6 to 7 year olds can successfully breath hold on command, as can many 5-year-old and a few 4-year-old children. Determine the level of cooperation by practicing the breath-hold maneuver before scanning. We generally verbally prompt, "Stop breathing, . . . breathe." If breath holding appears to be reproducible and uniform, continue; if not, resort to quiet breathing or sedation.

A child who can successfully complete this maneuver will be able to "count with you" as the scans are taken. A nervous child may, in fact, perform the task better for two reasons: (1) counting the scans holds the child's attention and (2) the child automatically knows the end point of the study, and the answer to the important question, "When will I be done?" Avoid leaving a young child alone in the scan room during computer programming or scanning. A friendly face and hand holding improve cooperation and seem to be calming to most children. We make it a point to have them squeeze a finger of a parent or staff member as a focal point during the contrast injection. If the child is left unattended, he or she is more likely to move out of position while turning around to see what is going on.

## Sedation

With the exception of interventional radiology, sedation is the most risky procedure performed by a pediatric radiologist. This is an era of increasing sophistication and expectation in sedation practices, and national standards have been recommended regarding pediatric sedation for imaging procedures. (The reader is referred to recent references on this subject.) Although specifics of a sedation protocol are beyond the scope of this chapter, a few general guidelines for sedation and monitoring are important to review as follows:

1. Develop an institutional policy and procedure for sedation and follow it. It should be approved by the appropriate hospital committee(s) and be supported by the Department of Anesthesia in your hospital.
2. The patient should have routine screening for sedation and the data recorded on a form designed for such a purpose.
3. The drugs, dosages, and routes used in administration of sedatives should be recorded in the medical record.
4. Monitoring of all sedated patients is essential; at the minimum, pulse oximetry should be used.
5. Record vital signs during sedation according to your policy/procedure.

6. Postsedation evaluation is performed and recorded; a discharge scoring system is useful for decision making about safety of discharge and also for documentation.
7. Postsedation instructions should be both verbal and written and a copy given to the parent/guardian for outpatients. That instruction sheet should include a telephone number and instructions regarding whom to contact if a problem arises.

Not all patients are candidates for sedation by radiology personnel. Even the best of protocols has a small failure rate. It is better to fail once in a while than to be too aggressive and have an unwarranted complication. Consult colleagues in pediatric anesthesia when difficult cases are contemplated and for sedation failures, until your experience and comfort level increase.

### *Positioning and Immobilization*

The time spent positioning and immobilizing a patient is a good investment. It makes interpretation easier and reduces the chance that the patient will move during the study. Upper extremities are always positioned above the head and the wrists fastened by tape and/or small Velcro bracelets to the scan table. A sedated infant will move during sleep; take no chances. Most scanners come equipped with Velcro fasteners that can be used as needed for the chest, pelvis, and thighs. Do not cover the area to be scanned. We remove all electronic leads, tubing, wires, and catheters from the field of view, and we try not to scan through any material that will produce artifact.

### *Contrast Enema*

If opacification of the distal colon is needed, it is possible to administer a contrast enema to a sedated infant. We sedate first, then administer. The liquid will be retained without difficulty if you use a small volume, administer through a small tube, and give it slowly: 50 ml for infants, 100 ml for young children, and 150 ml or less for older children is usually adequate. The aim is not to cause distention and the urge to defecate, merely to opacify. The enema tip that we use is a green polyethylene, disposable catheter about 8 Fr in diameter.

### *Intravenous Contrast Medium*

We use a 2 ml/kg dose of nonionic contrast medium, to a maximum of 100 ml in most cases. For lengthy studies, 2.5 to 3.0 ml/kg of contrast medium may be used, provided that it is safe to do so. We hand-bolus all injections and have not used a mechanical injector, particularly because our patient population is largely composed of sedated babies and children. A nonionic agent causes less sensation on injection and is less apt to awaken a sleeping child or frighten one who is awake and marginally cooperative. There is also a noticeably decreased frequency of nausea and vomiting compared with ionic agents.

## Scanning

### *Prescan and Postscan Digital Radiography*

Single or biplane digital radiography for planning CT provides the opportunity to check for gastric distention in infants, to plan for withdrawal of a nasogastric tube in a patient, and to evaluate opacification of the bowel with oral contrast medium, as well as for routine programming purposes. Digital radiographs also are useful after studies, especially for problems of urinary tract distention or displacement caused by tumor, trauma, or inflammation (Fig. 3).

### *Noncontrast (Scout) Slices*

Scout slices are used sparingly in infants and children, unlike in adults. The rationale for this technique is the severe limitation that the lack of inherent contrast in the pediatric patient places on unenhanced sections. Often the radiation exposure is better spent on the bolused-enhanced work. The purpose of scout sections is to check for centering, positioning, field-of-view size, and oral contrast distribution. The number of sections taken for most abdomen studies is four to five evenly spaced sections, for trauma and inflammation, for example; one or two more if the pelvis is to be included. Exceptions to this include the evaluation of a known mass or tumor, a search for calcification or calculi, the evaluation of diffuse liver disease, or when a solitary lesion is being investigated. In such cases precontrast sections are made as needed (Fig. 4).

### *Slice Thickness and Programming*

Most "screening" is performed with 8 or 10 mm contiguous sections in infants or children. Known lesions and specific problems may require thinner sections, such as for pancreatic trauma, liver tumors, or vascular masses. When specific attention is required, 5 mm sections usually suffice. Often a combination of variably programmed 5 and 10 mm sections will be optimal, providing that tube cooling is not a problem. When a vascular lesion such as an infantile hemangioendothelioma is to be studied, one can program consecutive groups of dynamically incremented scans, temporally acquired. Such acquisitions can be planned to occur in the early bolus, late bolus, equilibrium, and delayed phases of contrast enhancement (Fig. 5).

### *Bolus-enhanced Dynamic Incremental Scanning*

For sedated infants or children, the interscan delay chosen is the shortest available to allow for table incrementation. For a breath holding patient, a 6 to 7 second interscan delay is used. The scan time chosen is always the shortest available (a 1.2 second partial arc scan on our unit). For the partial arc scan (212° to 220°), the milliampere station is intentionally increased to the next highest setting to provide high-quality images. A 1.2 second scan stops motion better than the full 360° arc 2.0 second scan. Subsecond scan times are even better.

For most studies, 50 percent of the total 2 ml/kg dose is injected as rapidly as possible, and scanning is begun while the remainder of the total dose is given. When the entire abdomen and pelvis is to be scanned, we add a "boost" of 0.5 ml/kg of contrast medium at about the level of the umbilicus to maintain excellent vascular and tissue enhancement throughout the pelvis. When only the liver is the subject of the investigation, we generally delay beginning to scan until 65 percent of the bolus has been injected, so that opacification of the hepatic veins is optimal on the first slices taken. For those scanners that allow sections to be made at a scan time of 500 msec or less,

A

B

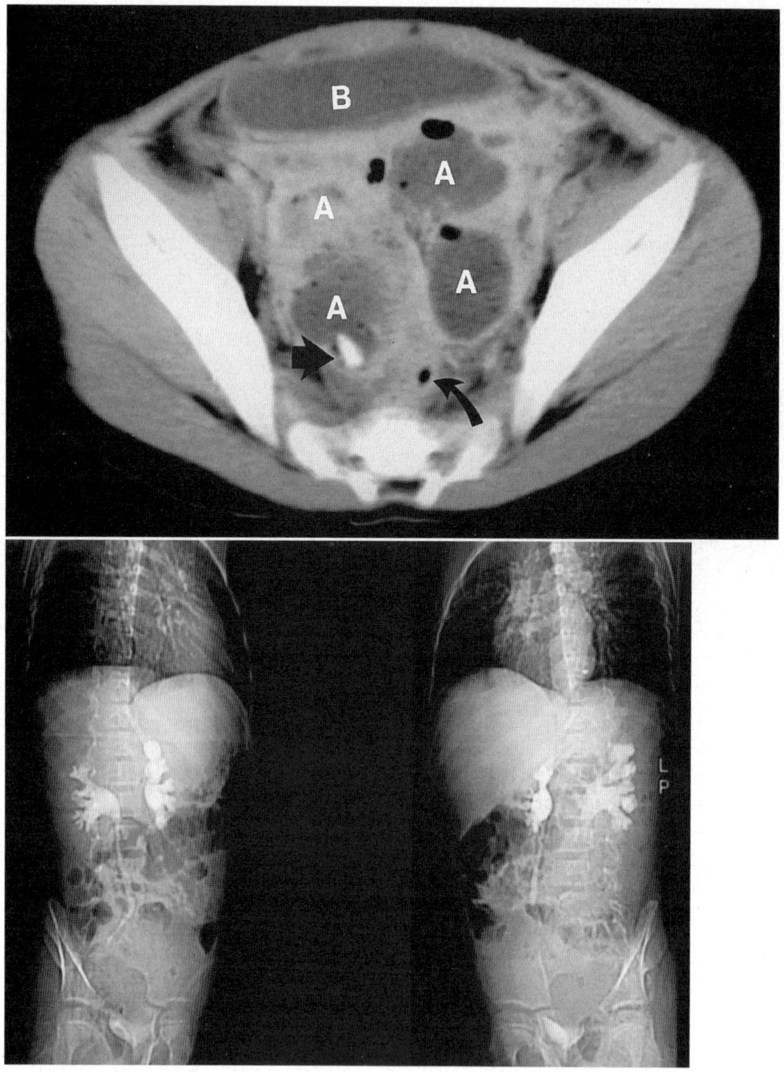


**FIGURE 3** *A,* Ruptured appendix causing multiple pelvic abscess collections (A). Note appendicolith within the right-sided collection *(arrow)*. B = bladder; curved arrow = rectum. *B,* Digital radiographs made at 45° and 135° to simulate LPO and RPO projections. Abscesses in the pelvis cause urinary tract distention and left-sided caliectasis and impress the bladder from above.

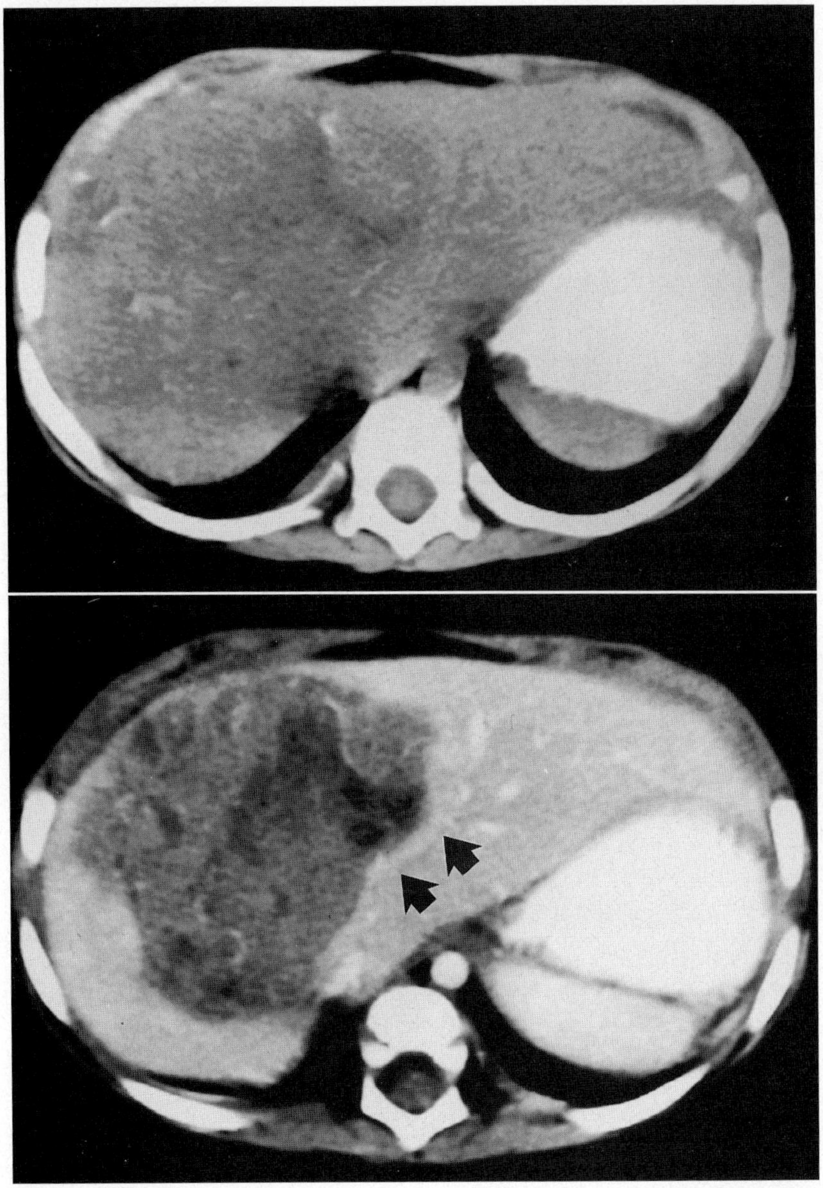

A

B

**FIGURE 4** Hepatoblastoma in a 7-month-old infant. *A,* Scout (precontrast) section shows that the liver mass is inhomogeneous and contains minute calcifications. *B,* Bolus dynamic sequential studies provide excellent liver-to-lesion contrast differentiation. Note the left portal vein displaced by the mass *(arrows).*

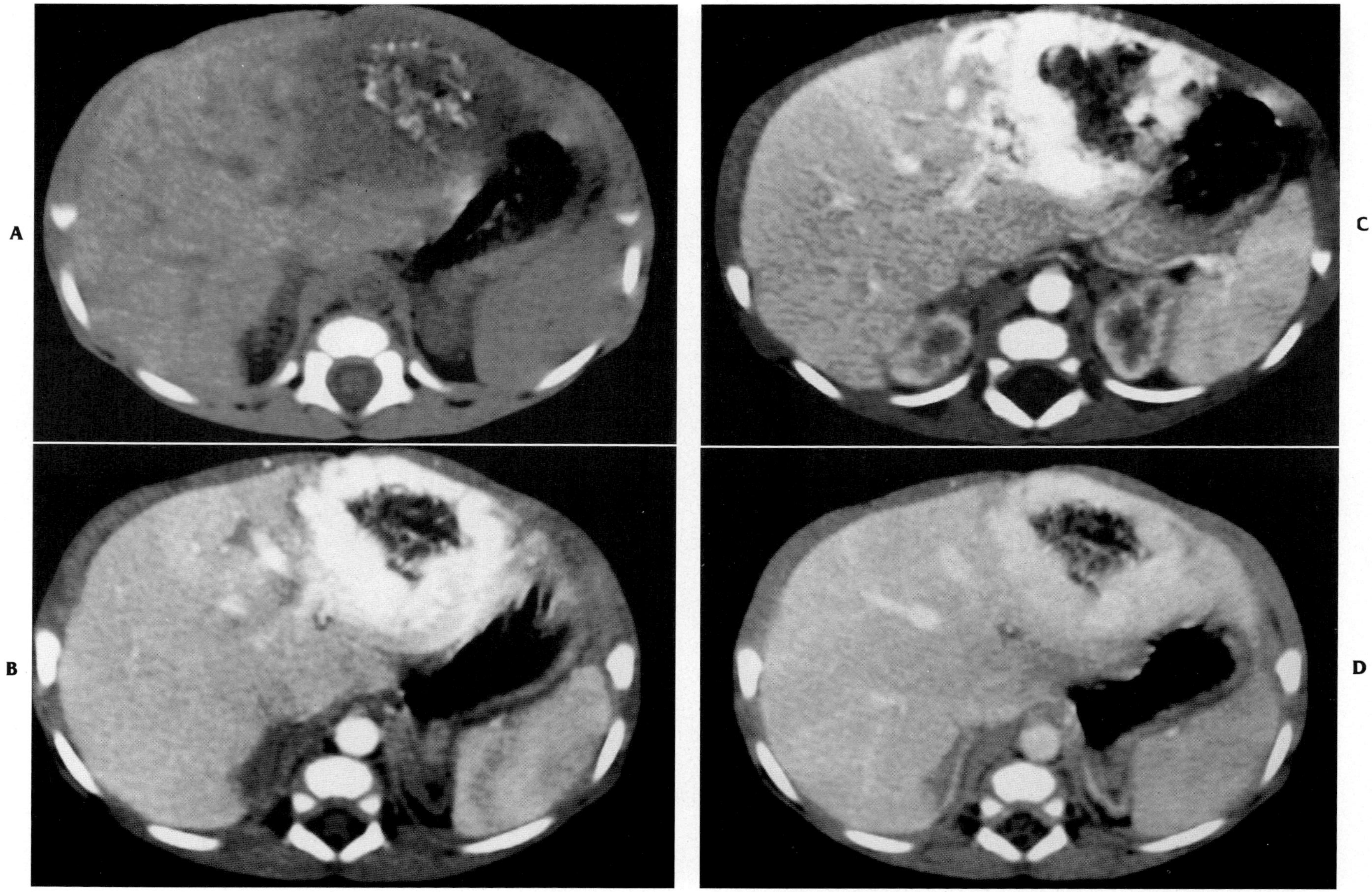


**FIGURE 5** Infantile hemangioendothelioma in a 3-week-old infant. *A,* Precontrast 5 mm section. Center of the lesion is thrombosed and contains calcification. *B* and *C,* Early bolus phase. Lesion enhances densely at the periphery. Abnormal vascularity in the liver both supplies and drains the mass. Note the large aorta caused by increased blood flow to the celiac axis and normal inhomogeneous splenic enhancement in the early arterial phase. *D,* Late bolus phase. Section taken from the second group of dynamic incremental scans immediately following the early bolus group. Same location as in *(B).* Dense peripheral blush is fading. Spleen now is uniform in homogeneity.

A

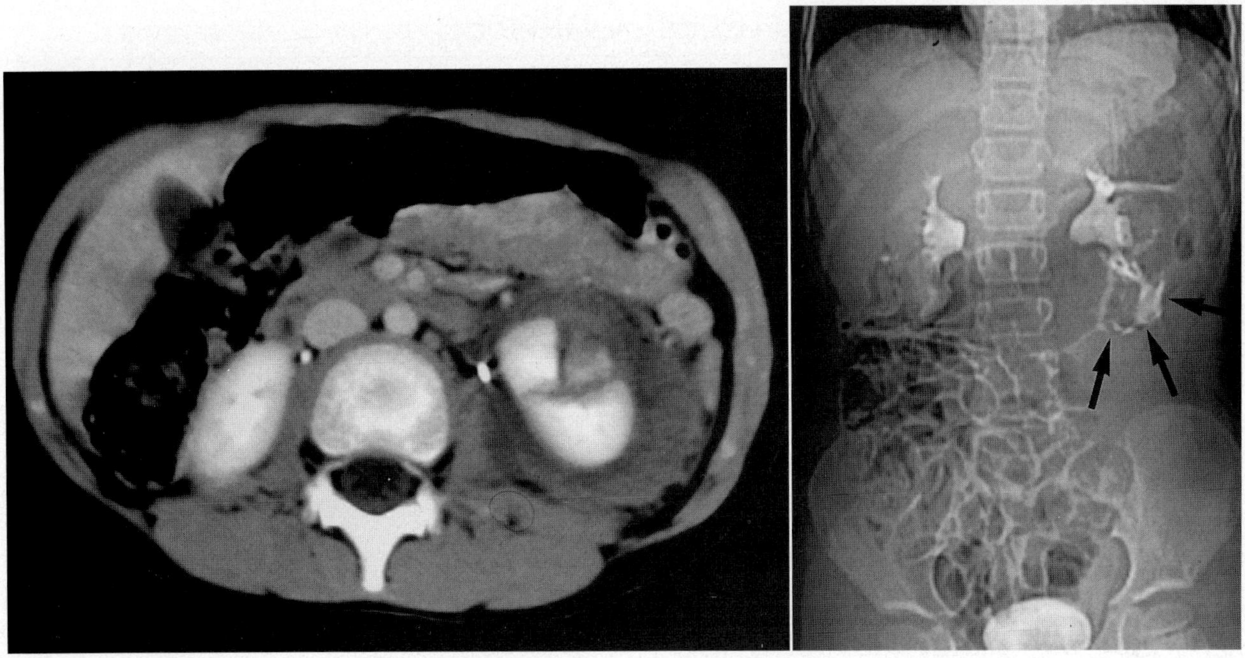

B

**FIGURE 6** Fractured left kidney with perirenal hematoma/urinoma. *A,* Dynamic sequential incrementation technique does not allow enough time for the pyelographic phase to occur. Patient can be rescanned through perirenal space to show the lacerated collecting system and contrast extravasation, or poststudy digital radiograph *(B)* can be made. Arrows indicate extravasation from left kidney.

the rapidity of the examination requires injection of all or nearly all of the contrast medium before starting the examination. Otherwise, it might be possible to complete scanning before the full dose of the contrast agent is injected.

### *Pyelographic Phase*

This technique of rapid dynamic-sequential scanning is so fast in most infants that, even on conventional scanners, kidneys are scanned in the corticomedullary differentiation phase (early arterial) or the nephrographic phase. The pyelographic phase generally is not reached until scanning is nearly completed. Thus the calyces and the ureters usually are not opacified. If this portion of the anatomy is important for the evaluation, precede the bolus injection by a tiny dose of intravenous contrast medium 3 to 4 minutes before the bolus: 1 to 2 ml in infants or young children, but not more than 5 ml in older children or teenagers. This has the advantage of slight pyelographic excretion, but without dense collection system artifact that may interfere with interpretation of the bolus phase.

In urinary tract obstruction, dilatation or laceration of the collecting system, one must remember to make additional delayed scans through the areas of interest (e.g., distended calyces, perirenal space) to opacify those structures by excreted contrast medium (Fig. 6). We find this easy to plan as one views the reconstructed scans in the bolus series.

## Suggested Reading

American Academy of Pediatrics, Committee on Drugs. Guidelines for monitoring and management of pediatric patients during and after sedation for diagnostic and therapeutic procedures. Pediatrics 1992; 89:1110–1115.

Brett CM. Sedation and monitoring for infants and children. In: Helms CA, ed. Perspectives in Radiology. St. Louis: Quality Medical Publishing, 1990; 3(2):181–204.

Cohen MD. Pediatric sedation. Radiology 1990; 175:611–612.

Fisher DM. Sedation of pediatric patients: An anesthesiologist's perspective. Radiology 1990; 175:613–615.

Kaufman RA. Technical aspects of abdominal CT in infants and children. AJR 1989; 153:549–554.

Kaufman RA. A decade of CT imaging of blunt abdominal trauma in children: Progress, pitfalls, and controversies. In: Helms CA, ed. Perspectives in Radiology. St. Louis: Quality Medical Publishing, 1990; 3(2):27–44.

Keeter S, Benator RM, Weinberg SM, Hartenberg MA. Sedation in pediatric CT: National survey of current practice. Radiology 1990; 175:745–752.

Smevik B, Westvik J. Iohexol for contrast enhancement of bowel in pediatric abdominal CT. Acta Radiol 1990; 31:601–604.

Strain JD, Campbell JB, Harvey LA, Foley LC. IV nembutal: Safe sedation for children undergoing CT. Am J Neuroradiol 1988; 9:955–959.

# Skeletal Injuries in Battered Children

*JOHN F. O'CONNOR, M.D.*

The epidemic of child abuse and neglect currently reported to be sweeping the United States and many other countries is probably not a new phenomenon. Greater awareness on the part of the public and authorities has undoubtedly resulted in better reporting of cases of child abuse and neglect. The role of the radiologist in identifying and reporting cases is central and often presents the only opportunity for society to become aware of a child at risk. For the abused child, the initial encounter with the socio-medical complex is most often a visit to the Emergency Room for soft-tissue or bony injury. Although many of these children are sexually abused or neglected, the usual final common pathway to medical care is the visit for trauma or irritability.

An accurate clinical history is the key to diagnosis of the abused or neglected child. The referral to the Radiology Department is often a requisition with a brief history, such as "rule out fracture." If the radiologist accepts the simple history of "rule out fracture," abuse will not be suspected unless multiple injuries are apparent on the part of the body that is radiographed. The key to the diagnosis for the radiologist is the simple phrase "discrepant history." The discrepancy can be related to the severity of the force alleged to have caused the injury or to age of the injury or injuries noted on the radiographs.

Knowing the actual mechanism of injury and assessing its relationship to the severity of the findings on the radiographs are keys to the diagnosis in the Radiology Department. For example, the initial injury may be as simple as a single spiral fracture of the femur in a 6-month-old infant. This type of fracture can be incurred when a child falls from a crib and the extremity in question is caught in the bars or spring mechanism. It also may be an appropriate consequence of a caretaker falling while carrying the infant in his or her arms. Such an injury is possible even in a restrained infant in an automobile accident. If, however, a fall by the infant from a bed to a carpeted or wooden floor is the tendered history, the injury should immediately arouse suspicion.

The foregoing examples demonstrate that communication between the referring physician and the radiologist is critical to the diagnosis, since the history will be accurately expanded only in that setting. In a 30 year career in diagnostic radiology of infants and children, I have yet to achieve the goal of receiving thorough, accurate histories on requests for radiographs. There is little question in my mind that we have missed numbers of cases of child abuse or neglect because of the failure of the referring physician to provide an accurate history.

Similarly, if that injury of the femur demonstrates periosteal new bone and callous formation, the date of the injury becomes critical to the suspicion of abuse. An injury that had occurred 2 weeks earlier would be expected to show evidence of healing at the time of initial imaging. Nevertheless, any fracture with extensive healing should raise some suspicion that the child, if not abused, has been neglected, since all but the most neglectful observer would note that a child with such an injury was irritable and not moving the affected extremity (Fig. 1). Because discussions of child abuse and its diagnosis by various imaging modalities often focus on the presence of multiple injuries of different ages, suspicion is raised in the minds of most physicians when this scenario is encountered.

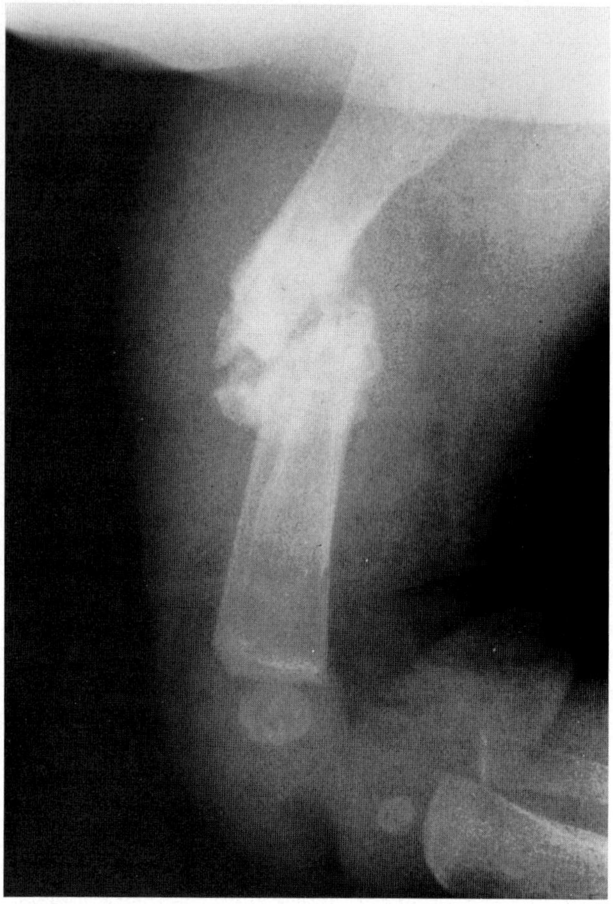

**FIGURE 1** A single lateral film of the right femur in a 2-month-old infant alleged to have fallen from a bed 48 hours before being brought to the Emergency Room. The film shows abundant callus formation with additional soft-tissue swelling, suggesting that this fracture is at least several weeks old, and that there may well have been a new superimposed injury that produced the soft-tissue swelling. This is a highly suspicious fracture, and the discrepancy with the history of injury of 24 hours' duration makes the diagnosis of abuse highly likely.

The differential diagnosis then becomes a consideration of conditions that may predispose to single or multiple injuries without history of unusual application of force. Certain forms of osteogenesis imperfecta, congenital insensitivity to pain, and abnormalities of copper and calcium metabolism may actually predispose to fractures with the minimal trauma experienced by most normal children throughout the day, and these injuries may be confused with abuse. These entities have other clinical manifestations that should make the diagnosis clear, but caregivers tend to err on the side of giving the family the benefit of the doubt.

The manifestations of child abuse and neglect are many and varied, and the skeleton is not always involved. Intracranial and visceral injuries have been covered in detail in other chapters. The shaken baby syndrome and the child with visceral hematoma or rupture may present with deliberately misleading history rather than simply discrepant history. When the responsible caretaker chooses to hide abuse or neglect, the diagnosis becomes much more difficult and the need for a high level of suspicion is increased. As in the case of skeletal trauma, communication between the referring physician and the radiologist is critical to the diagnosis. With these general thoughts in mind, let us proceed to a discussion of typical injuries observed in the appendicular skeleton of children who have been abused or neglected.

## Upper Extremities

In the newborn period and through the first month of life, the differential diagnosis must include the possibility of injury caused by obstetric trauma. Fractures of the clavicle, which can occur as a consequence of shoulder dystocia, may not be recognized by those caring for the child at the time of injury. The clinical finding most often leading to early diagnosis of these injuries is an asymmetric Moro reflex or an associated brachial plexus palsy. These are sometimes overlooked, and the child then presents with a lump over the clavicle or the mother reports pain when she moves the child's arm during routine care. The importance of dating these injuries to the approximate time of delivery is obvious. The absence of multiple injuries and of any other evidence of abuse, including axial skeletal injury such as rib fractures, intracranial injury, or retinal hemorrhage, help to exclude child abuse in the infant with simple obstetric trauma. Fractures of the femur may occur in difficult breech deliveries and occasionally are bilateral. While the injuries resulting from shoulder dystocia in vertex deliveries are often overlooked by the obstetrical team and pediatricians, the degree of difficulty in a breech extraction that results in femoral fracture is usually obvious to the attending physicians, and the obstetrician may accept these fractures as the consequence of preventing brain asphyxia. Although a clavicle fracture may be observed in child abuse as a result of a direct blow over the shoulder, it is uncommon; most fractures of the clavicle in the first month of life can be attributed to birth trauma.

Upper-extremity injuries in abused children differ depending on the age of the child. In the toddler something as simple as a pulled elbow ("nursemaid's elbow") can be evidence of child abuse, particularly if the child returns with the same injury on several occasions. This should raise suspicion and indicate the need for further clinical and perhaps imaging studies such as skeletal survey or radionuclide scan. This injury is not usually observed before the child begins to walk. Injury to the upper extremities in the pretoddler age group is more likely to involve the proximal humeral metaphyses with corner fractures and undisplaced Salter I or II fractures of the proximal humeri. These are probably the result of grasping both upper arms and shaking the child in a fit of frustration or anger (Fig. 2). Any fracture of the humerus in the first few months of life should be considered a suspicious injury in the absence of a significant fall in the caretaker's arms or other clinical history consistent with the degree of trauma (Fig. 3).

Appropriate dating of fractures is important in confirming the etiology of the injury. As previously noted, this helps in excluding obstetrical trauma as the cause. On the other hand, it should be noted that bilateral fractures of the proximal humeral metaphyses are almost never observed as a consequence of birth trauma.

Most fractures of the appendicular skeleton in infants and

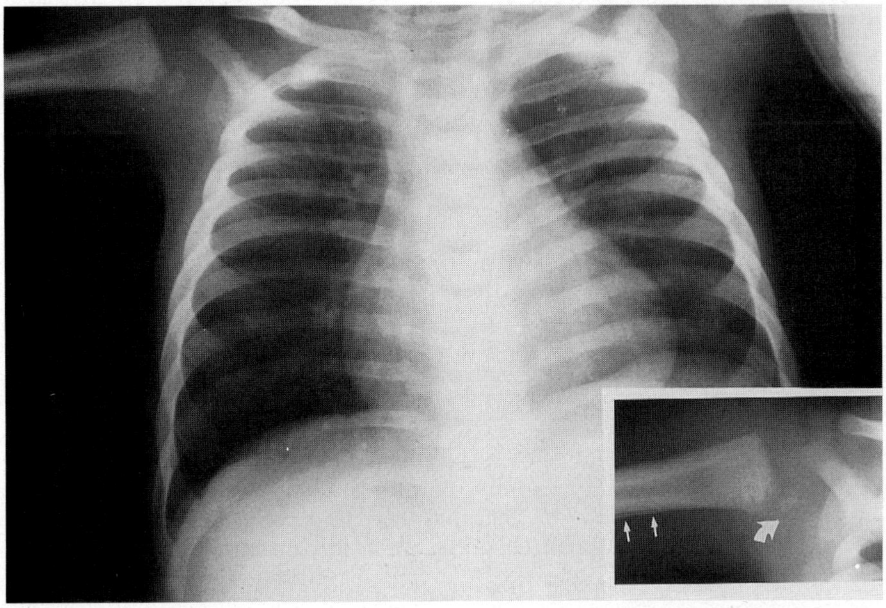

**FIGURE 2** An anteroposterior (AP) supine film of the chest and upper abdomen in a 2-month-old female referred to the Radiology Department for exclusion of pneumonia. The film shows periosteal new bone formation along both proximal humeri and corner fractures in the region of the proximal humeri. The perpetrator probably grasped the baby by both upper arms and shook her violently. The inset shows the details of the periosteal new bone formation *(small arrows)* and the corner fracture *(curved arrow)*. There were also healing fractures in the midshaft of the forearm (not shown) and in the proximal femur and tibia (see Fig. 8). Periosteal new bone such as this may be observed in this age group, but coupling this finding with the corner fractures and the fracture in the forearm makes the diagnosis of child abuse apparent.

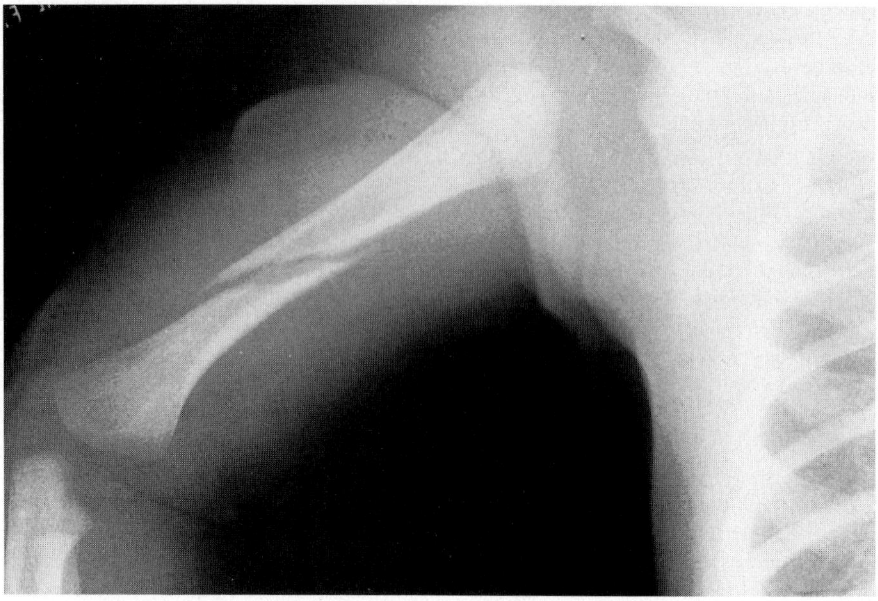

**FIGURE 3** A single AP film of the right humerus in a 1-month-old infant shows a recent spiral fracture of the humerus. This is a most unusual injury in an infant. There is no evidence of healing to suggest that this is a prenatal injury. Any such fracture in this age group should be reviewed with great suspicion.

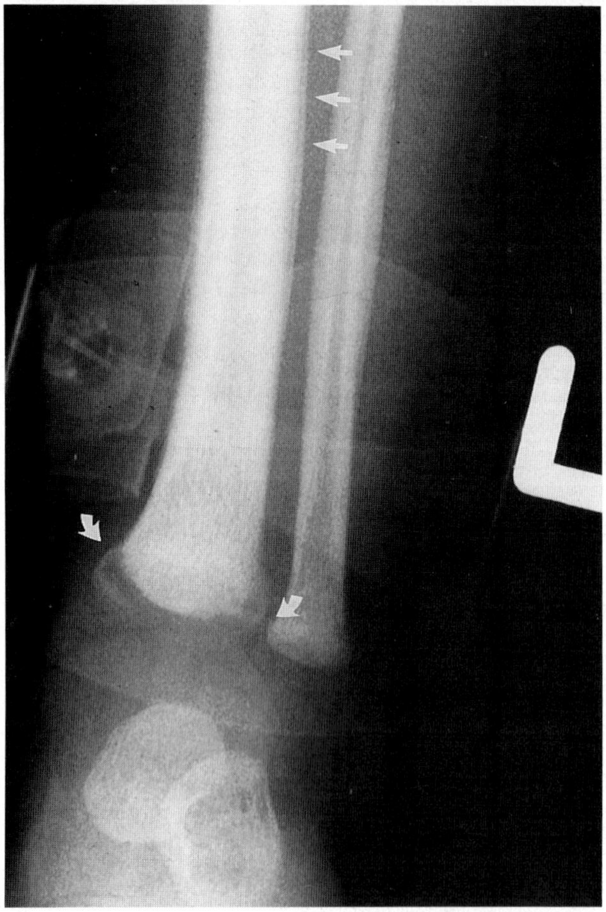

**FIGURE 4** An AP view of the ankle in a 5-month-old girl with a typical bucket-handle fracture of the distal tibia *(curved arrows)* and periosteal new bone formation along the shaft of the tibia *(straight arrows)*. These curved arcs of bone, which are similar to the Thurston Holland fragment, probably represent a combination of repetitive injury and healing.

children occur at least in part through the zone of cartilage hypertrophy in the region of the metaphysis during enchondral development of the long bones. Although fractures in the abused child may be from a single episode of trauma, they are more often the result of repetitive trauma so that there is a continuum of injury producing a distorted healing pattern. The distortion is always in the direction of prolonging the healing phase rather than shortening it. Thus, although corner fractures and "bucket-handle fractures" are probably little more than healing Salter I or II fractures, they are unusual because repetitive episodes of trauma have accentuated the unusual appearance of new bone at the corners of the metaphyses and produced the bandlike bucket handles, which represent arcs of bone similar to the Thurston Holland fragment in a simple Salter II fracture (Fig. 4).

In a significant investigation of this process, Kleinman and associates, using postmortem correlation, demonstrated that these fractures not only are somewhat different from those occurring in simple trauma, but may in fact be subtle and may require high-resolution radiography for their demonstration. Because of the present trend of using minimal radiation exposure when imaging children, the high degree of detail obtained in these postmortem studies is often not possible in the Emergency Room (Fig. 5). We are currently using an intermediate-speed system for initial imaging of all extremity trauma in children. We do not use extremely low-dose high-speed film-screen combinations, but rather a 200 to 300 speed system with detail screens for the initial assessment. We use higher-speed systems for all follow-up radiography once the diagnosis has been made and appropriate treatment instituted. The radiologist must remember that in the comatose or badly injured child who is radiographed with portable equipment in the Intensive Care Unit, *these injuries may be overlooked.* If abuse is suspected, skeletal surveys should be done with the detail system.

I am often asked about skeletal surveys versus bone scans as a means of screening children for possible abuse fractures. I have favored the use of the skeletal survey in infants up to 1

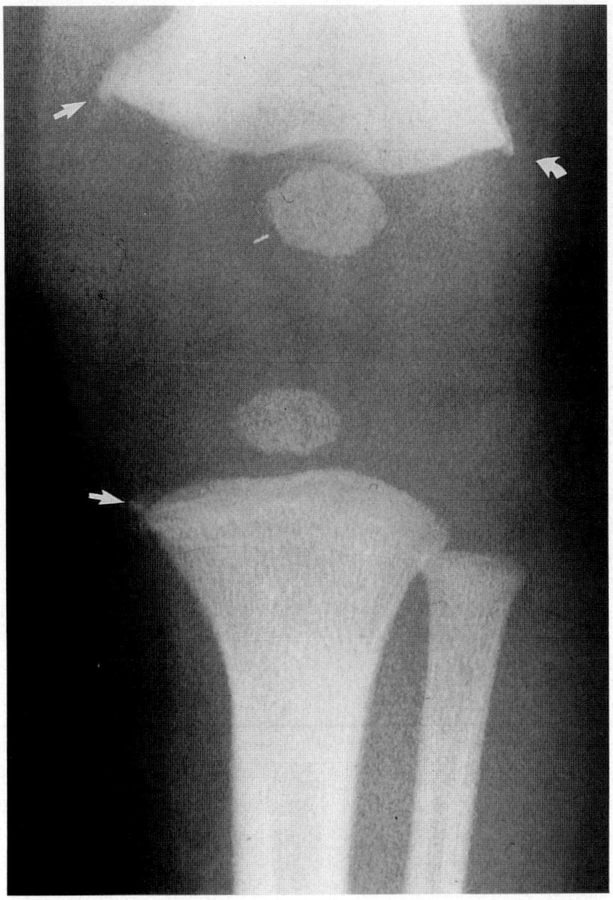

**FIGURE 5** An AP film of the knee in a 6-month-old infant shows the subtle abnormalities of the corners of the metaphyses described by Kleinman and his colleagues in postmortem studies *(straight arrows).* The tiny projection from the lateral aspect of the distal femoral metaphyses *(curved arrow)* should not be confused with an abuse fracture and may be a normal finding in some patients.

year of age, reserving bone scanning for the 1 to 4 year old age group. Radionuclide scanning may provide supplemental information, especially identifying relatively recent rib fractures, which can be difficult to identify on plain films. The usual problem with radionuclide scanning is the identification of injury that can be bilaterally symmetric and therefore difficult to distinguish from the normal avid uptake of isotope in the metaphyseal regions of the long bones. In my experience surveys are seldom useful in children older than 4 years who can communicate and who have no history of injury. If there is a history of repeated injury, selected radiographs of the allegedly affected parts are all that are necessary for either diagnosis or supporting information for court proceedings.

As previously noted, a simple pulled elbow may be a manifestation of abuse or neglect, but a sudden jerk on the arm can also produce a supracondylar fracture, a dislocated shoulder, or a fractured clavicle – so that in older children (toddlers to kindergarten age) these are sometimes observed as a manifestation of child abuse (Fig. 6). The other fracture that may be observed in this age group and the older child is the Monteggia fracture, which occurs when the child puts up the forearm to ward off a blow, resulting in a fracture of the ulna and volar dislocation of the radial head (Fig. 7).

In younger infants flail injuries may occur in the distal forearms and wrists as a result of violent shaking, usually with the child grasped around the proximal humeri or thorax. Whenever suspicious fractures are observed in the extremities, careful perusal of high-quality radiographs of the chest and spine may confirm the diagnosis by demonstrating rib fractures or vertebral injuries, including injuries to the spinous and transverse processes as well as the vertebral body itself.

## Lower Extremities

In the neonatal period transverse or spiral fractures of the femur may be a consequence of either obstetric trauma or child abuse. Because a fractured femur rarely is overlooked at the time of delivery, any fracture of the femur in this age group

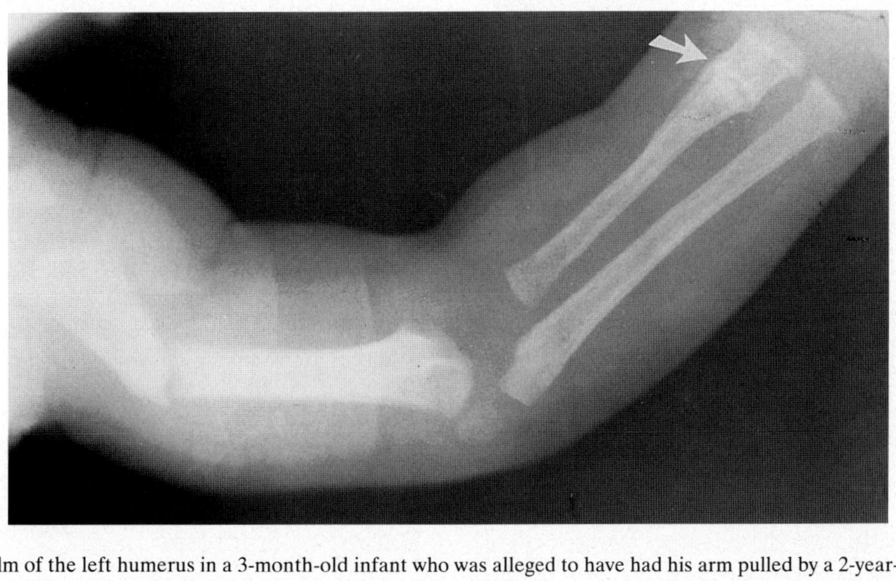

**FIGURE 6** An AP film of the left humerus in a 3-month-old infant who was alleged to have had his arm pulled by a 2-year-old sibling a few hours before. The mother noted that the arm was not moving well. There is an obvious recent transverse fracture of the proximal humerus but also a well-healed fracture of the distal radius *(arrow).* The discrepancy with the history and the absence of any other bony abnormality confirms the suspicion of abuse. This patient also had multiple fractures in various stages of healing involving both lower legs and the ribs.

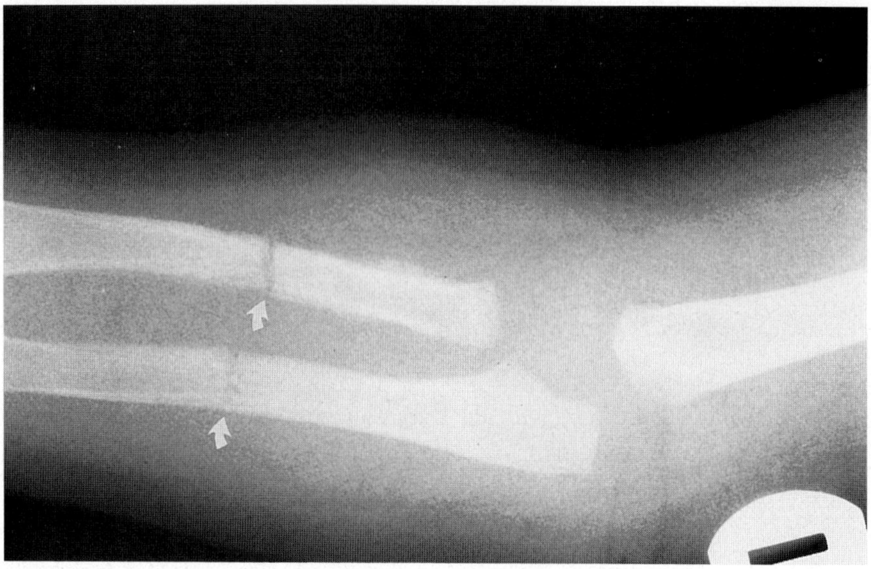

**FIGURE 7** An AP film of the right forearm in a 4-month-old infant with a history of not moving the extremity for 24 hours shows transverse fractures through the radius and ulna with some new periosteal new bone formation *(arrows)*. The injury is highly suspicious in a child of this age. While not a typical Monteggia fracture, absent the radial dislocation, the mechanism is similar.

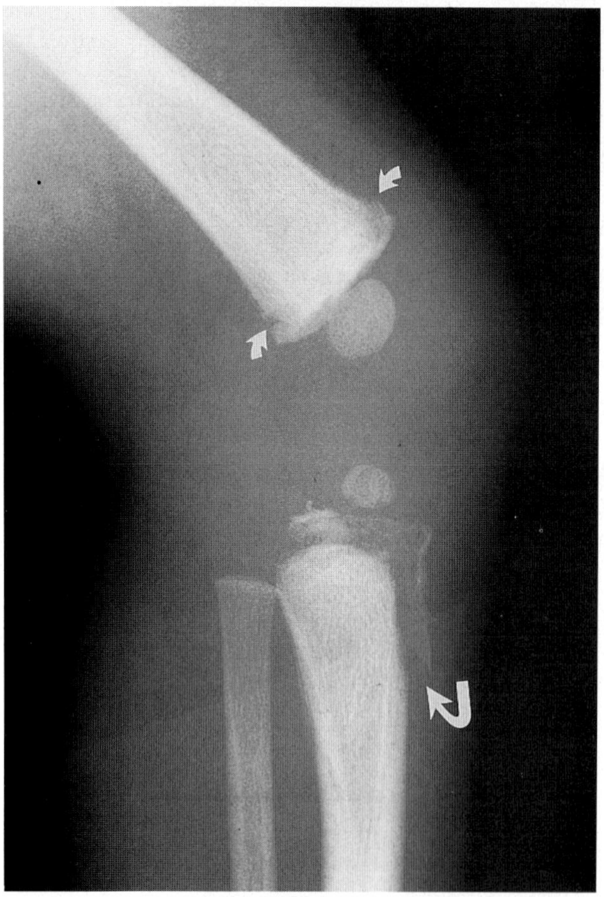

**FIGURE 8** A lateral film of the knee in the same baby whose chest x-ray was presented in Figure 2. This baby is 2 months old, and the corner fractures in the distal femur and the fracture through the tibial tubercle and proximal tibial metaphyses are of different ages and represent further evidence of abuse in this child. These fractures are highly unusual as a result of ordinary trauma in this age group.

should be viewed as suspicious unless a documented history of appropriate injury, such as a fall while being held in the caretaker's arms, is provided. Any discrepancy in the age of the fracture (see the subsequent section, Dating of Fractures) should raise suspicion of abuse. Abuse fractures resulting from repetitive injury are often observed in the lower extremities. Corner fractures, bucket-handle fractures, and abundant callous formation of periosteal new bone are all suspicious and probably occur as a consequence of flail trauma in which the child is shaken like a rag doll (see Fig. 4).

As noted earlier, common fractures in the lower extremities in abused children include simple spiral fractures of the femur. These are the injuries most likely to mislead the observer who is not alert to the discrepancy between the history and the injury. Less commonly, injuries to the proximal femoral epiphyses with fracture dislocation or a simple subcapital fracture of the femoral neck have been reported in badly abused children, but these are the exception rather than the rule. Corner fractures occur in the proximal femur but are much more common distally. It is most important to be alert to the significance of corner fractures and bucket-handle fractures of the distal femur and proximal tibia. Any such findings that are bilateral are highly suspicious of child abuse (Fig. 8).

Fractures of the distal tibia, including corner fractures and bucket-handle fractures, are also typical of child abuse and are often observed. The mechanism of these injuries is uncertain, but many authors believe that they represent flail injuries resulting from shaking the child with flailing extremities (Fig. 9).

Fractures of the foot itself are much less common manifestations of child abuse but may be the result of a direct blow or slapping or twisting of the dorsum of the foot.

## Dating of Fractures

Dating of fractures is important not only in the initial recognition of a discrepancy between the history and the

A

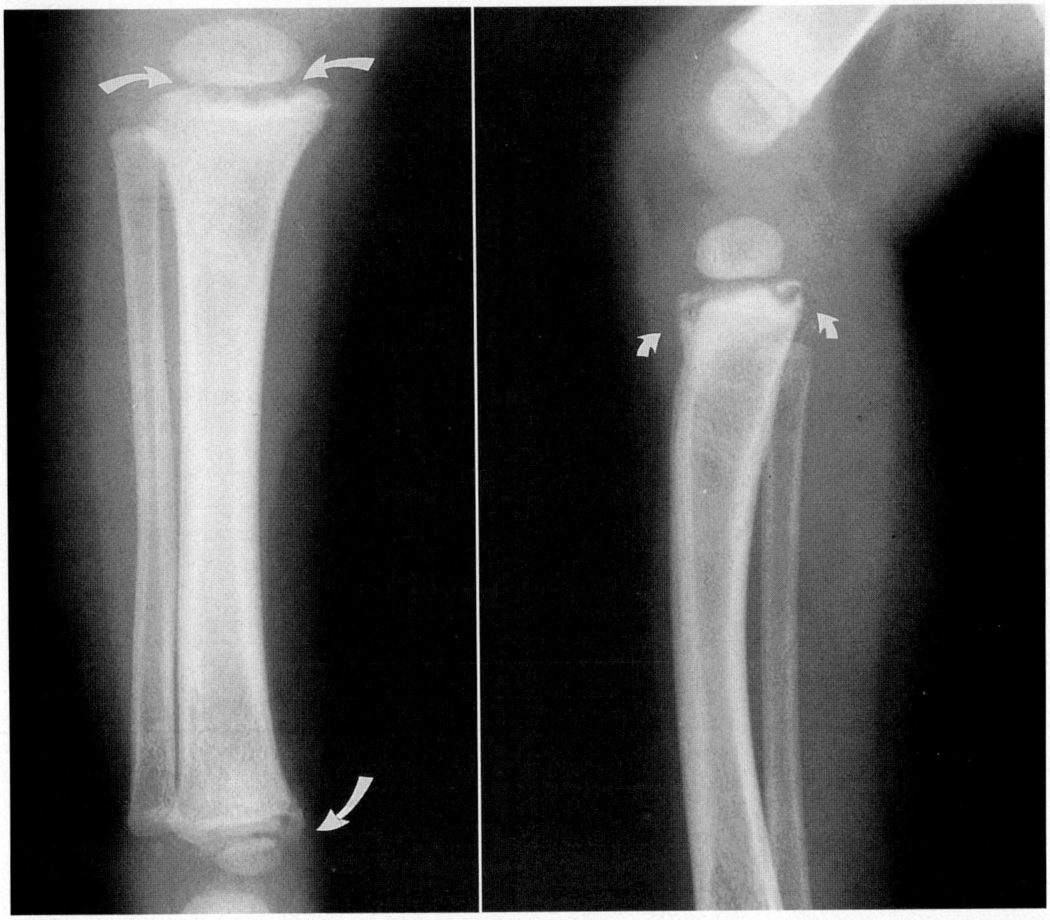

B

**FIGURE 9** *A,* An AP film of the right lower leg in an 8-month-old infant who had been living with adopting parents and scheduled to be adopted. The infant was brought to the pediatrician with a 2 day history of a swollen left arm. There was extensive evidence of abuse in this child, and the AP films of the tibia show several typical healing abuse fractures. The bucket-handle fracture in the distal tibia is indicated by a single curved arrow. Perhaps somewhat more subtle but of equal importance is the irregular widening of the metaphyses of the proximal tibia *(double curved arrows),* which probably also represents evidence of the type of injury described by Kleinman in his postmortem studies. *B,* Lateral films of the proximal tibia show the corner fractures *(arrows),* but the irregular widening of the metaphyses noted in *(A)* are sufficient evidence of injury. These abnormalities should not be overlooked and should not be confused with metaphyseal dysplasia or rickets.

**TABLE 1** Timetable of Radiographic Changes in Children's Fractures*

| Category | Early | Peak | Late |
|---|---|---|---|
| 1. Resolution of soft tissues | 2–5 days | 4–10 days | 10–21 days |
| 2. Periosteal new bone | 4–10 days | 10–14 days | 14–21 days |
| 3. Loss of fracture-line definition | 10–14 days | 14–21 days | . . . |
| 4. Soft callus | 10–14 days | 14–21 days | . . . |
| 5. Hard callus | 14–21 days | 21–42 days | 42–90 days |
| 6. Remodeling | 3 months | 1 year | 2 years to epiphyseal closure |

*Repetitive injuries may prolong categories 1, 2, 5, and 6.
From O'Connor JF, Cohen J. In: Kleinman PK, ed. Diagnostic imaging of child abuse. Baltimore: Williams & Wilkins, 1987; with permission.

severity or stage of healing of injury but also in the forensic aspects of child abuse. It should be stated at the outset that the dating of skeletal injury and its chronologic relationship with the history of injury is at best inexact. A timetable for a resolution and evolution of injury to the extremity includes several phases: the soft tissues, the periosteum, fracture-line definition, and endosteal callus formation are all helpful features of the healing process that may permit dating of fractures. Table 1 is an attempt to provide rough guidelines for the dating of skeletal injury. These criteria apply primarily to single episodes of trauma resulting in an appendicular skeletal fracture. The timetable for healing is markedly different for abuse fractures that are the result of or complicated by repetitive trauma. In particular, the fracture line and the amount of associated hard and soft callus may be greatly exaggerated in the repetitive injury associated with abuse fractures (Fig. 9). Injuries suspected of being repetitive could be expected to markedly prolong the phase of periosteal new bone formation and increase the abundance of callus and the duration of loss of fracture-line definition. It is probable that abuse fractures do not accelerate the earlier phases of this repair, so that Table 1 is helpful in dating the time of injury in the first stages.

## Discussion

I wish to stress the importance of discrepancy in the history with regard to the severity or age of the fracture in question. A high level of suspicion is important, especially in suburban communities in which pediatricians and radiologists alike are reluctant to think about the possibility of child abuse or neglect. Abuse and neglect are not exclusive to poor inner-city children; they are probably just as common in the affluent suburbs. A more important predictor than socioeconomic status is the history of abuse in the parents or caretakers. This, of course, is never available at the time of initial injury but will be sought by alert physicians. Exclusion of disease entities predisposing to trauma with discrepant history also is clearly relevant.

Children who have been abused are at great risk for continued injury and even death. Because the mortality of abused children is as high as 50 percent in some series, the importance of making the diagnosis is obvious. Although visceral and head trauma are more common antecedents of death, accompanying extremity injuries may be the only findings that alert the medical caregivers to the risk at hand.

# Differential Diagnosis of Metaphyseal Abnormalities

*DIEGO JARAMILLO, M.D. · TAL LAOR, M.D.*

The metaphysis is a funnel-shaped area located between the growth plate and the shaft. The approach to differential diagnosis of metaphyseal abnormalities requires knowledge of the anatomic and physiologic changes that occur in this area during growth. The physeal cartilage is mineralized at the junction of the zone of provisional calcification of the growth plate and the primary spongiosa of the metaphysis. The zone of provisional calcification and the primary spongiosa form a well-defined line adjacent to the growth plate, which is sclerotic on plain radiographs and hypointense on magnetic resonance imaging (MRI) (Fig. 1). This line is an indicator of endochondral ossification; interruption or lack of definition of this line suggests an abnormality of ossification or growth. On technetium-99m MDP bone scans, the primary spongiosa shows great activity, because it is an area of abundant blood flow and active deposition of osteoid.

Ossification in the periphery of the metaphysis occurs in the perichondral structures (perichondral groove of Ranvier) and is independent from the function of the growth plate. Genetic and metabolic disorders such as achondroplasia, rickets, and hypophosphatasia affect the growth plate and central metaphysis but spare the periphery. This produces the appearance of metaphyseal cupping on radiographs.

The metaphysis is a site of active remodeling of bone. The trabeculae become thinner, and the overall caliber of the bone decreases as the bone is incorporated into the diaphysis. This active rate of bone turnover probably explains why bone-forming tumors such as osteogenic sarcoma arise preferentially in the metaphysis. The metaphyseal cortex is thin throughout childhood. Most of the fractures of the long bones occur at the transition zone from the dense lamellar bone of the diaphyseal cortex to the thin metaphyseal cortex.

The vascularity of the metaphysis comes from both diaphyseal vessels and vessels that pierce the metaphyseal cortex. In the vicinity of the growth plate, the metaphyseal vessels form sinusoids. The sluggish flow in these sinusoids may explain why bactéria tend to seed the metaphysis during childhood.

The metaphyseal marrow remains hematopoietic throughout childhood. On T1-weighted MR images, the metaphyseal marrow is hypointense, while the marrow in the diaphysis and epiphysis becomes fatty (hyperintense) during early childhood. In adolescents, particularly in females, metaphyseal hematopoietic marrow is seen as patchy areas of decreased signal intensity that must be differentiated from infection and tumor (see Fig. 1). The distribution of marrow determines the location of certain tumors during childhood. For example, hematologic malignancies and round cell tumors occur in areas of hematopoietic marrow. In older children these tumors are observed more frequently in the metaphysis.

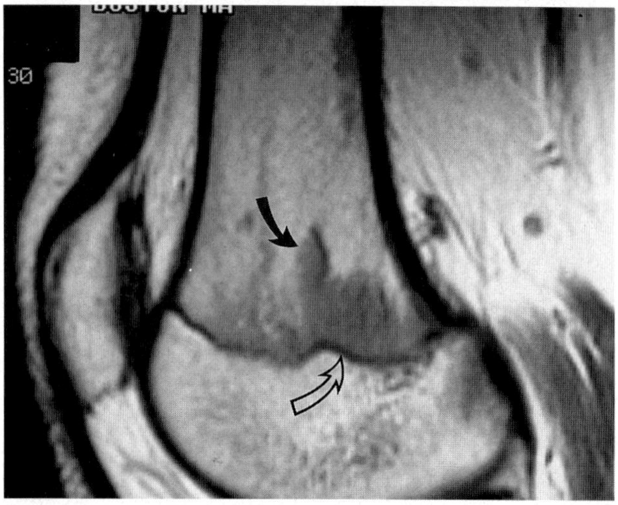


**FIGURE 1** Sagittal spin-echo (TR600/TE16) T1-weighted image of the distal femur of a 14-year-old girl. The zone of provisional calcification *(open arrow)* is observed as a band of decreased signal intensity separating the epiphysis from the metaphysis. There are patchy areas of decreased signal intensity in the metaphysis, corresponding to normal rests of hematopoietic marrow *(closed arrow)*.

In the axial skeleton, areas adjacent to apophyseal growth plates are anatomically and physiologically identical to the metaphyses at the ends of long bones. These "metaphyseal equivalents" are present in the vicinity of the synchondroses of the base of the skull, pelvis, and vertebrae and the apophyses of the pelvis, scapula, and ends of the ribs. Typical metaphyseal abnormalities, such as osteomyelitis and the fractures of child abuse, can be observed in these metaphyseal equivalents (Fig. 2).

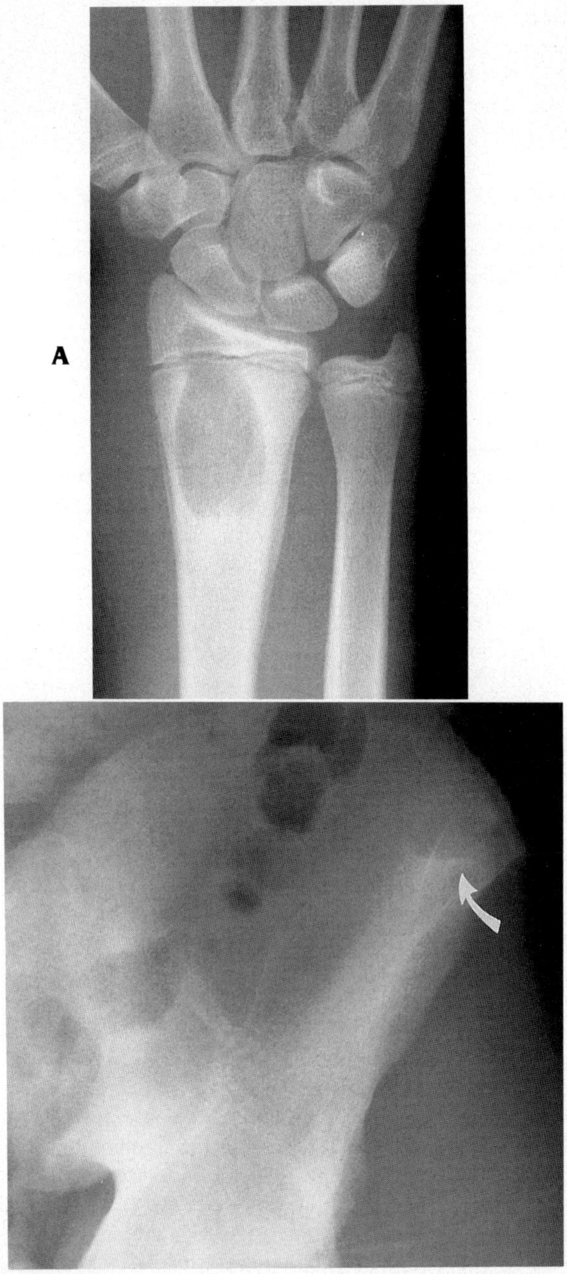

A

B

**FIGURE 2** A 15-year-old girl with multifocal osteomyelitis secondary to *Staphylococcus aureus*. *A*, Frontal radiograph of the distal radius shows a well-defined lytic lesion of the distal radial metaphysis. The lucency extends into the epiphysis. There is periosteal reaction adjacent to the lesion. *B*, Frontal radiograph of the same patient from the same time shows a lytic lesion involving the left iliac wing *(arrow)* in the proximity of the apophyseal cartilage of the iliac crest. Diagnosis was established by drainage of both areas.

## Indications and Technical Approach

The imaging evaluation of patients with suspected metaphyseal abnormalities should begin with plain radiographs. If the patient is being investigated for metabolic bone disease, such as rickets or lead toxicity, the radiographs of the knees and wrists have the greatest yield, because the abnormalities are most prominent in the areas of fastest growth. If the patient is being investigated for a possible skeletal dysplasia or child abuse, a skeletal survey should be performed. Focal metaphyseal abnormalities on radiographs can be further investigated by scintigraphy or MRI. Scintigraphy is extremely useful for detecting multifocal disease such as metastases or occult infection. MRI is more useful to detect extension of metaphyseal abnormalities into the growth plate or adjacent soft tissues. Although there is controversy surrounding the relative sensitivity of MRI and scintigraphy in detecting osteomyelitis and metastatic disease, in most diseases of childhood they are complementary rather than competing technologies. Computed tomography (CT) and sonography have a limited role in the diagnosis of metaphyseal disease. CT can help define bony abnormalities and sonography can show abnormalities in the periosteum and soft tissues.

## Diagnostic Approach

### *Key Signs of Disease*

#### Undermineralization of the Zone of Provisional Calcification and Primary Spongiosa

The junction between the growth plate and the metaphysis is a good starting point for the analysis of metaphyseal disorders, since metaphyseal abnormalities frequently reflect dysfunction of the growth plate. Diffuse lack of definition of the thin line of the zone of provisional calcification and primary spongiosa indicates abnormality of endochondral ossification.

Hypophosphatasia is an autosomal recessive disorder of the synthesis of alkaline phosphatase. Patients with hypophosphatasia do not mineralize the cartilage and osteoid of the primary spongiosa. This leads to the radiographic appearance of loss of the line of the zone of provisional calcification and irregularity of the metaphyseal border, often with a large central metaphyseal lucency (Fig. 3). The bones are bowed and osteopenic. The diagnosis can be suspected on prenatal ultrasonography because of undermineralization of the calvarium. It is confirmed by a low concentration of serum alkaline phosphatase and excessive urinary excretion of phosphonethanolamine.

Rickets is the end result of lack of mineralization of the physeal cartilage due to altered vitamin D metabolism. The columns of cells in the hypertrophic zone of the growth plate advance into the metaphysis, leading to widening of the growth plate, disappearance of the zone of provisional calcification, and fraying of the metaphyseal border (Fig. 4). The central metaphysis is more severely involved, resulting in cupping. Abnormal mineralization of the osteoid weakens the bones and causes bowing. Rickets can be secondary to dietary deficiency, malabsorption, abnormal hepatic and renal metabolism, and end-organ resistance. Rickets should be differentiated from metaphyseal chondrodysplasia in which the growth plate is wide but the zone of provisional calcification remains intact.

Diseases that block the interaction between the metaphyseal vessels and the chondrocytes of the hypertrophic zone of

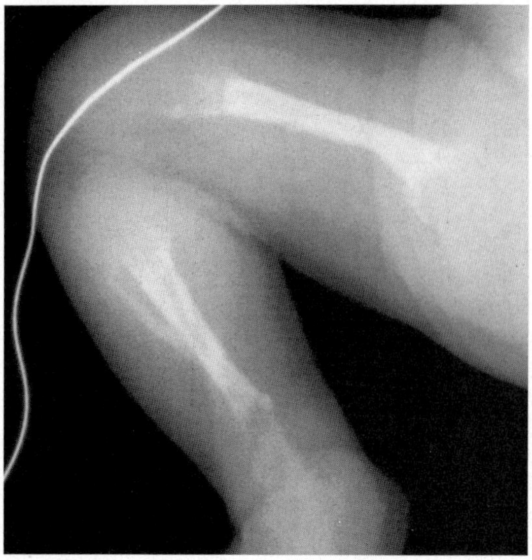

**FIGURE 3** A 1-day-old boy with hypophosphatasia. A lateral radiograph of the knee shows loss of the zone of provisional calcification of the femur, tibia, and fibula. There is diffuse osteopenia and pathologic fractures of the femur and fibula.

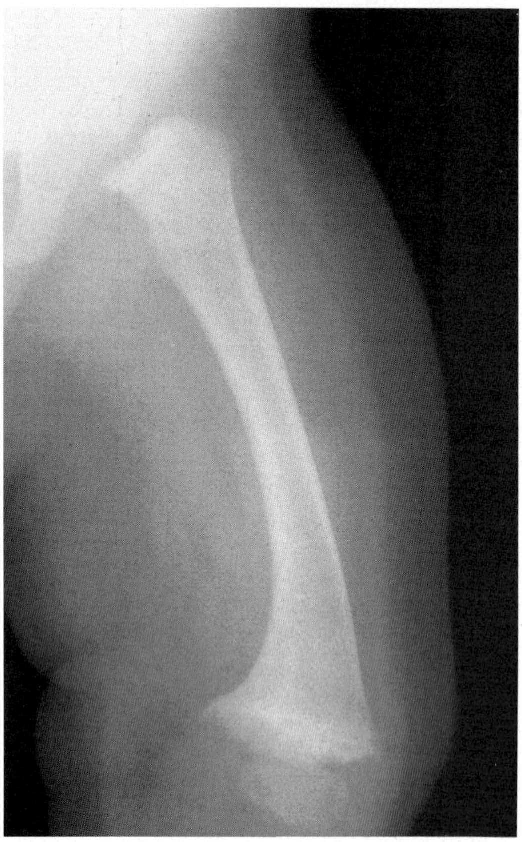

**FIGURE 4** Frontal radiograph of a 2-year-old boy with rickets. The zone of provisional calcification is lost, and there is fraying of the metaphyseal border and bowing of the femur. Notice that the changes are more noticeable in the distal metaphysis, where 70 percent of the growth of the femur occurs.

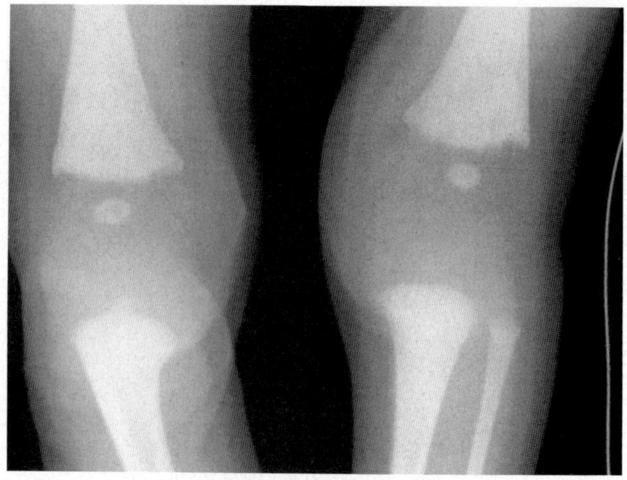

**FIGURE 5** Frontal radiograph of the knees of a 1-day-old girl with neonatal lupus. There is fraying of the metaphyseal border of the distal femora. The involvement is rather patchy, not diffuse as in rickets. The bones are not osteopenic, and there is no evidence of bowing.

the growth plate result in persistence of chondrocytes in the metaphysis. Unlike rickets, this alteration is spotty. The metaphyseal border is abnormal in scattered areas, which produces linear striations instead of diffuse fraying. This appearance can be observed with the vascular damage of perinatal infections, such as syphilis and rubella, and with other vasculitides (Fig. 5).

The blockage of endochondral ossification can be highly focal, producing a local invasion of cartilage in the metaphysis. Radiographs show a focal area of lucency extending from the growth plate. MRI shows areas of signal intensity similar to the growth plate, extending in a flamelike fashion into the metaphysis (Fig. 6). This can occur with trauma, particularly in metaphyseal injury from child abuse, embolic disease (from disseminated intravascular coagulation), and avascular necrosis (Legg-Calvé-Perthes disease).

### Increased Mineralization of the Zone of Provisional Calcification and Primary Spongiosa

The most common cause of increased density in the zone of provisional calcification is recovery following a period of arrest of growth (Fig. 7). During slow growth (as a result of disease, immobilization, deficient nutrition, or other stresses), the proliferation of the cartilage decreases, and mineralization occurs not only longitudinally, along the columns of chondrocytes, but also transversely along the metaphysis. These transverse trabeculae form a disk that persists when growth resumes. As the growth plate migrates away from this disk, there is a summation of the density from the normal zone of provisional calcification with that of the disk of transverse bony trabeculae, producing metaphyseal sclerosis. With time, the growth plate separates itself from the dense disk, and a growth recovery line becomes visible. The distance between the growth plate and the line of growth arrest indicates the amount of growth since the time of stress. If the growth recovery line and the growth plate are not parallel, focal growth arrest (usually due to a bony bridge across the physis) should be suspected.

A B

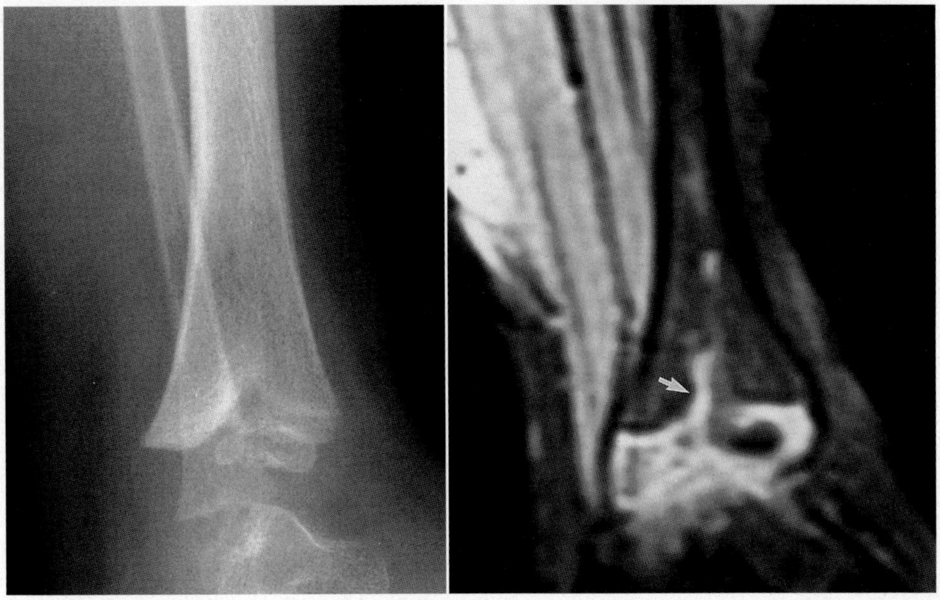

**FIGURE 6** A 3-year-old boy with a history of meningococcemia. *A,* Lateral radiograph of the distal tibia shows that the zone of provisional calcification is interrupted in its midportion. There is also cupping of the metaphysis and irregularity of the distal tibial epiphysis and of the acetabulum. *B,* Sagittal fat-suppressed spin-echo (TR2,000/TE17) balanced image of the distal tibia. There is interruption of the dark line of the zone of provisional calcification. Additionally, an area isointense with the growth plate extends into the metaphysis *(arrow).*

A B

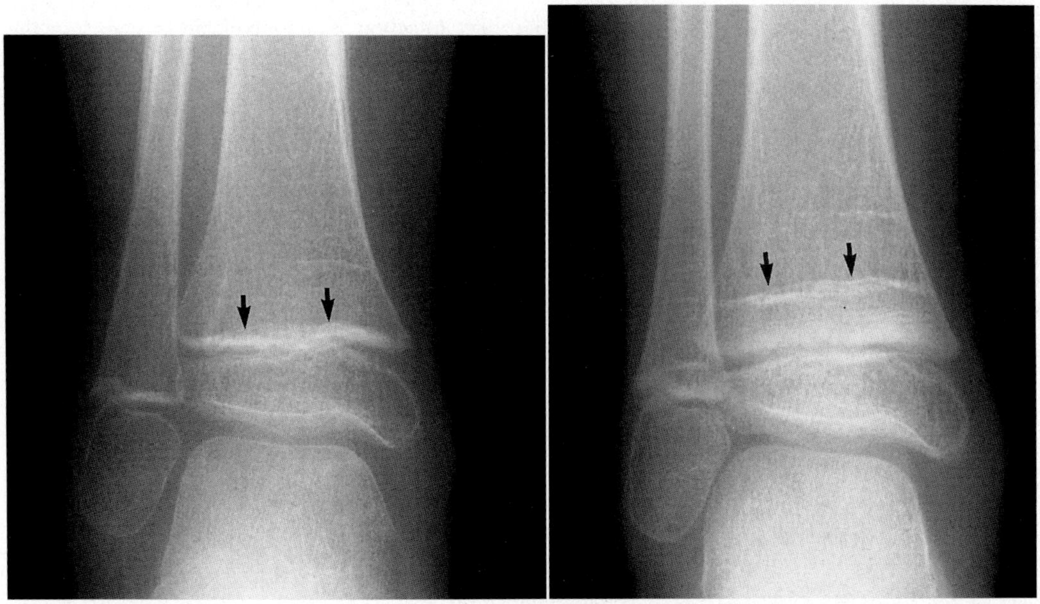

**FIGURE 7** A 5-year-old girl who fractured the midshaft of the right tibia. *A,* Frontal radiograph of the distal tibia obtained one month after the fracture. There is an area of increased density in the metaphysis, in the region of the zone of provisional calcification *(arrows). B,* Frontal radiograph of the distal tibia obtained four months later. The growth plate has migrated away from the dense line, which represents a growth recovery line *(arrows).* The growth recovery line and the growth plate are parallel to each other, indicating normal growth.

Lead toxicity interferes with the resorption of the trabeculae in the primary spongiosa of the metaphysis. This results in heavily mineralized metaphyseal bands adjacent to the growth plate that are observed both in weight-bearing and non–weight-bearing bones such as the fibula (Fig. 8). Lead lines develop with serum lead levels greater than 70 to 80 μg/ml. Sclerosis in the tibia and femur can be seen in normal children, presumably related to bearing weight. Fibular metaphyseal sclerosis is relatively specific for lead toxicity, since the fibula is a non–weight-bearing bone. It is important to note that the metaphyseal sclerosis in lead toxicity is not due to lead deposition but to the osteoclastic dysfunction that results from heavy metal poisoning. Similar changes are seen with bismuth toxicity.

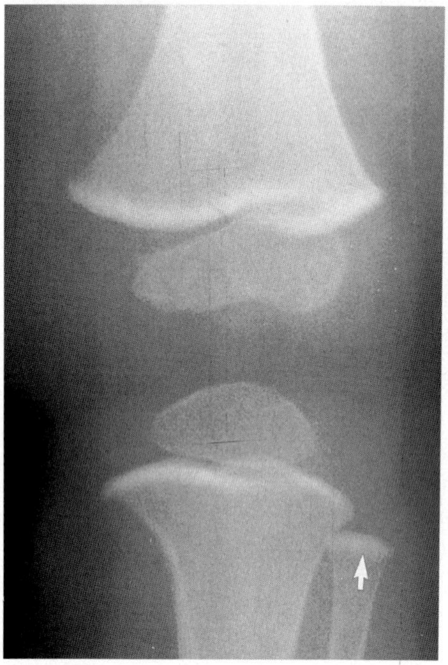

**FIGURE 8** A 19-month-old girl with a history of lead toxicity. There are dense metaphyseal bands in the metaphyses of the femur and tibia. Additionally, note the dense metaphyseal band in the fibula *(arrow)*, which is a typical osseous manifestation of lead toxicity.

Osteoclastic dysfunction also plays an important role in the metaphyseal sclerosis of osteopetrosis. The severity of osteopetrosis ranges from diffuse sclerosis to multiple parallel lines of increased density parallel to each other ("bone within a bone" appearance). The lines develop because osteopetrosis is episodic in severity. Another cause of metaphyseal sclerosis is healing of rickets, with rapid mineralization of the cores of cartilage in the metaphysis. This metaphyseal sclerosis disappears when endochondral ossification returns to normal.

## Diffuse Lucent Change in the Metaphysis

Multiple neoplasms, particularly leukemia and neuroblastoma, can decrease the mineral content of the metaphysis without affecting the growth plate. This results in a lucent line that is separate from the zone of provisional calcification. Diffuse metaphyseal lucency is normal in the neonatal period and is frequently observed with neonatal infections.

## Focal Lucent Change in the Metaphysis

The metaphysis is an area predisposed to invasion by bacteria and malignant cells. This has been attributed to sluggish flow in the metaphyseal sinusoids and decreased phagocytic activity. The infection or tumor typically spreads from the vicinity of the growth plate to the diaphysis. The growth plate is avascular and its cartilage inhibits angiogenesis. It acts as a barrier against the

A

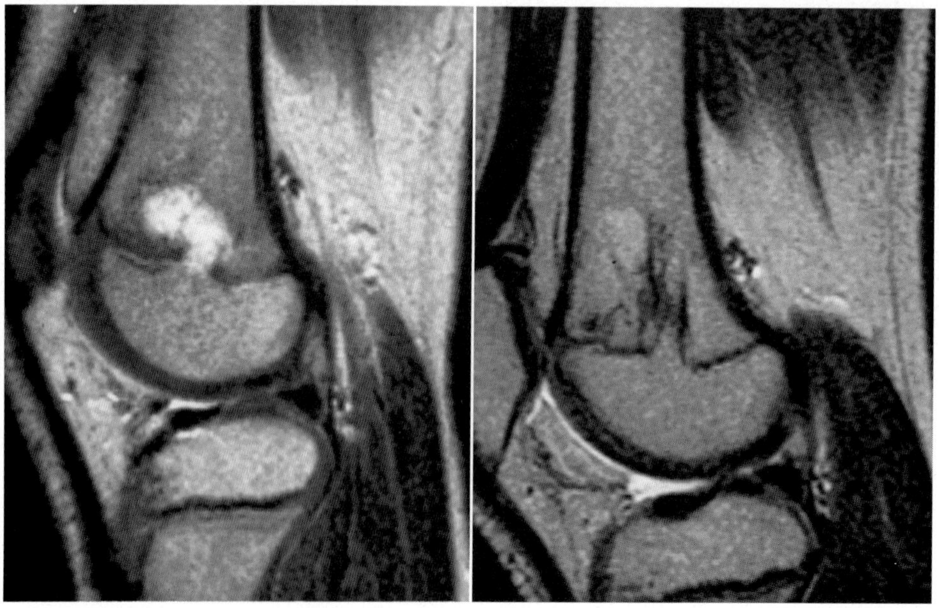

B

**FIGURE 9** A 10-year-old boy with osteomyelitis of the distal femur. *A,* Sagittal spin-echo (TR2,000/TE80) T2-weighted image of the distal femur shows an area of increased signal intensity of the metaphyses, which interrupts the bright signal from the growth plate and the dark signal from the zone of provisional calcification. *B,* Sagittal spin-echo (TR2,000/TE80) T2-weighted image of the distal femur of the same patient obtained two years later. A bridge containing fatty marrow extends from the epiphysis to the metaphysis. The inflammatory changes noted on the previous study have resolved.

spread of neoplasms and bacteria. With time, the growth plate is overwhelmed, and metaphyseal processes may spread into the epiphysis (Fig. 9).

Although systemic inhibition of endochondral ossification due to leukemia is frequently associated with metaphyseal lucent bands, direct leukemic infiltration produces focal metaphyseal destruction (Fig. 10).

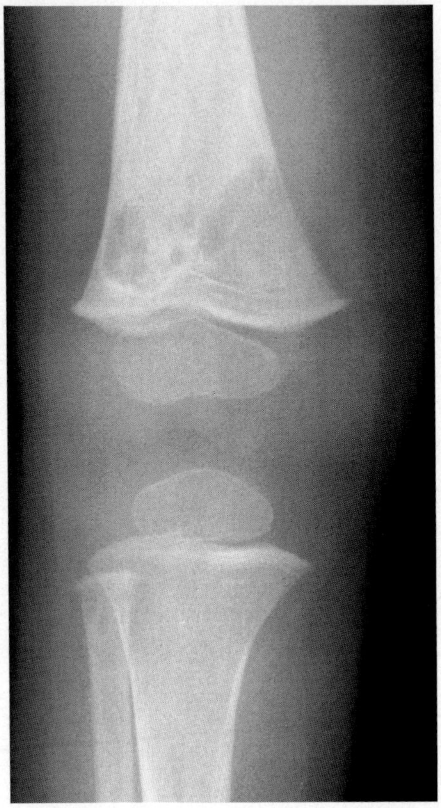

**FIGURE 10** Frontal radiograph of the knee of a 2-year-old boy with acute lymphoblastic leukemia. There is an ill-defined lytic area in the distal femoral metaphysis, indicating patchy involvement by leukemic cells. In this case the patient does not have the metaphyseal lucency typically observed with this disorder.

### Disruption of the Metaphyseal Outline

The cortex and trabeculae of the metaphysis are disrupted with trauma. In abused children a fracture through the primary spongiosa separates the epiphysis from the shaft. The metaphyseal bone attached to the epiphysis can be observed on radiographs as peripheral metaphyseal triangles ("corner fractures") (Fig. 11) or as a ring ("bucket handle fractures"). Abnormal collagen synthesis, which can be congenital (Menkes' "kinky hair syndrome") or acquired (scurvy, nutritional copper deficiency), is also associated with fragmentation of the metaphysis. Finally, destruction of the metaphyseal outline is characteristically observed with congenital syphilis.

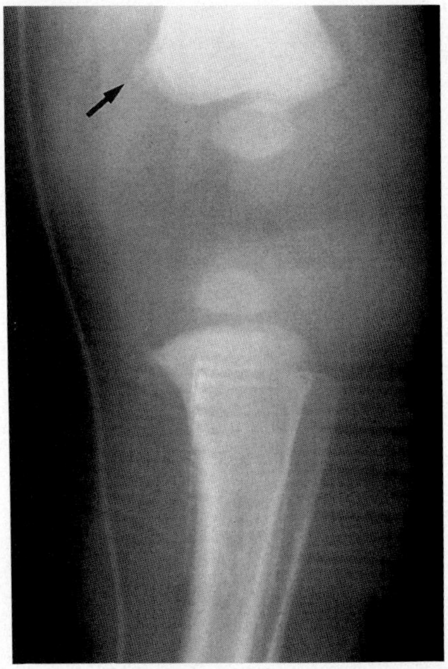

**FIGURE 11** Frontal radiograph of the knee of a 2-month-old girl who was abused. The patient had multiple fractures in the skull and the contralateral femur and tibia. Notice that the metaphyseal outline is interrupted in its medial aspect. There is a triangular fragment at the most medial aspect of the metaphysis *(arrow)*, which has the typical appearance of a corner fracture. These fractures are frequently associated with child abuse.

### Abnormal Contour of the Metaphysis

*Undertubulation.* Metaphyseal abnormalities frequently interfere with modeling. Normal modeling requires a delicate coordination between osteoclastic resorption of the outer cortex and deposition of bone along the inner cortex. A metaphysis with deficient modeling or undertubulation loses its normal "trumpet-shaped" contour, and its borders become straight ("Erlenmeyer flask" deformity). Undertubulation can result from deficient osteoclastic activity as is observed with osteopetrosis. Tubulation is also impaired by expansion of the medullary cavity by hyperplasia of the marrow, as with hemoglobinopathies, or infiltration of the marrow, as in Gaucher's disease. Finally, undertubulation may be secondary to increased vascularity in the vicinity of the metaphysis from adjacent tumors (Fig. 12), chronic arthritis (hemophilia, juvenile rheumatoid arthritis), and vascular malformation.

*Overtubulation.* Patients with neuromuscular disorders, such as cerebral palsy or myelodysplasia, lack the trophic effect of muscle traction. Their bones are gracile, with an abrupt transition from a thin diaphysis to the wider area of the growth plate (Fig. 13). Overtubulation also occurs with deficient osteoblastic activity as in osteogenesis imperfecta.

*Focal Deformity.* Osteochondromas and enchondromas represent persistence of islands of cartilage in the metaphysis. Osteochondromas result from endochondral ossification and bone formation in ectopic locations. Sessile osteochondromas deform the contour of the bone (Fig. 14). Pedunculated osteochondromas grow away from the metaphysis. Enchondromas expand the bone and are associated with growth disturbances, typically ulnar shortening.

## *Differential Diagnosis*

The differential diagnosis varies according to the age of the patient. In newborns, metaphyseal abnormalities are almost always related to perinatal stress, are metabolic (hypophosphatasia, copper deficiency), or are secondary to congenital infections. In infancy they can result from metabolic abnormalities such as rickets and lead toxicity. In this age group, metaphyseal abnormalities should always raise the suspicion of

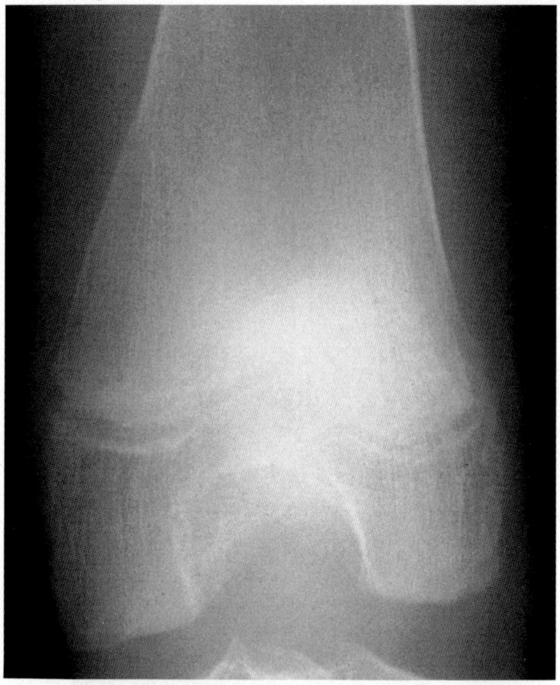

**FIGURE 12** An 11-year-old boy with neurofibromatosis. The MRI had shown multiple neurofibromata in the vicinity of the knee. Frontal radiograph of the distal femur shows lack of tubulation of the distal femoral metaphysis. Additionally, there is widening of the intercondylar notch. Both changes have been described in association with increased vascularity to the distal femur.

A

B

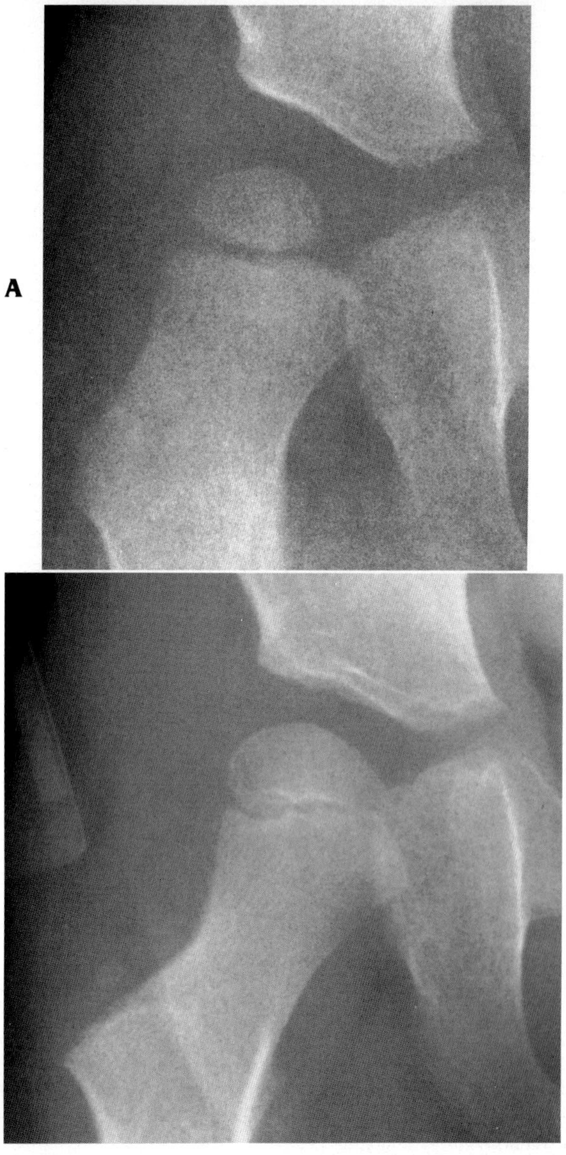

**FIGURE 13** Metaphyseal overtubulation in a boy with cerebral palsy. *A,* Frontal radiograph of the proximal femur obtained at 2 years of age shows a coxa valga deformity, which is frequently seen with cerebral palsy. The metaphyseal contour is normal. *B,* Frontal radiograph of the same patient obtained at five years of age. There is undertubulation of the proximal femoral metaphysis which expands in a bulbous-like fashion in the vicinity of the growth plate.

A

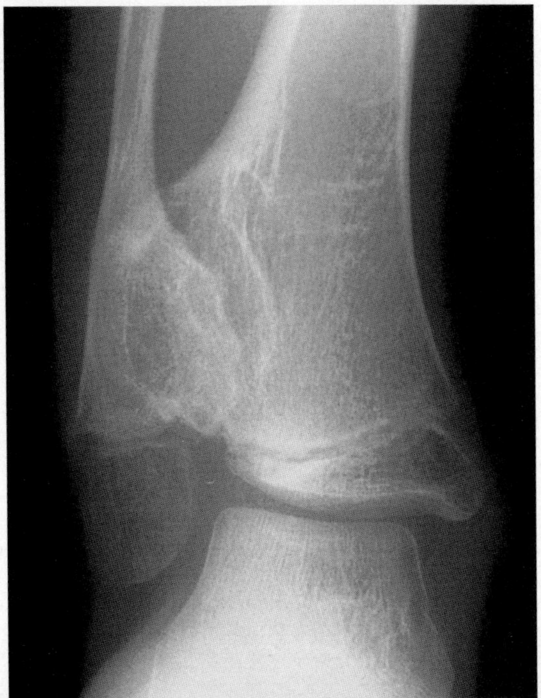

B

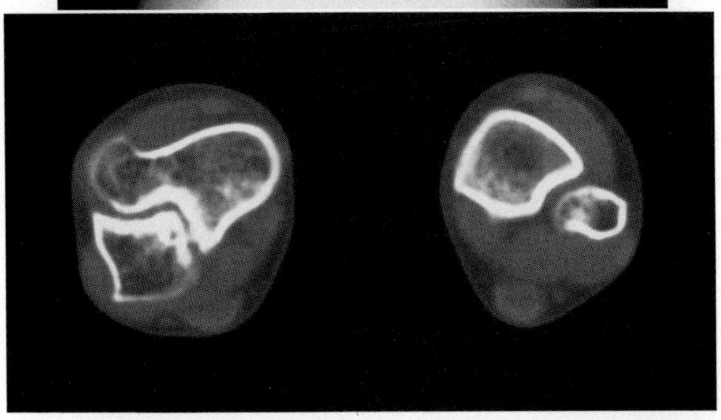

**FIGURE 14** An 8-year-old girl with multiple exostosis. *A,* Mortise view of the distal tibia and fibula show deformity of the metaphysis of both bones, secondary to osteochondromata. *B,* Axial CT scan in the region of the osteochondromata shows continuity of the marrow spaces of the native bone and the osteochondromata.

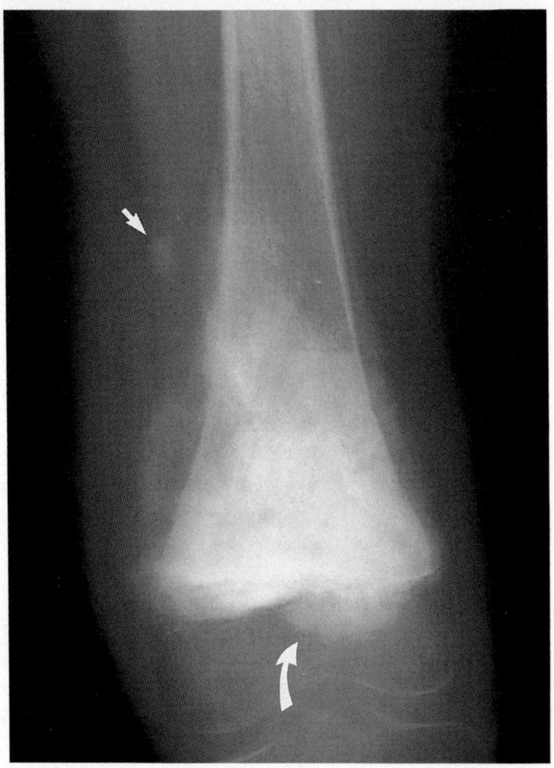

**FIGURE 15** An 11-year-old boy with osteogenic sarcoma of the distal femur. Frontal radiograph shows osteoid matrix in the metaphysis, extending into the soft tissues *(straight arrow)* and epiphysis *(curved arrow).*

child abuse. During childhood, osteomyelitis, trauma, and neoplasms are the most frequent metaphyseal abnormalities.

Metabolic diseases are more prominent where the growth is fastest, as in the distal femur. The density of the adjacent bone can help in the diagnosis of diverse conditions ranging from osteopetrosis to osteogenesis imperfecta. Signs of deficient osteoid formation, such as bowing and pathologic fractures, are often observed together with diseases that have abnormal endochondral ossification. Tumor matrix can help in the diagnosis of osteosarcomas (Fig. 15) and cartilaginous tumors.

Further imaging, such as scintigraphy and MRI, defines the pathology better, but almost never helps in the differential diagnosis.

### *Pitfalls in Technique and Interpretation*

Failure to obtain a complete skeletal survey may interfere with the diagnosis of congenital abnormalities and child abuse. When investigating metabolic disease, only the area of maximal growth, usually the knee, needs to be imaged. Imaging of multiple bones results in unnecessary exposure to radiation. In younger patients abnormalities close to the growth plate may be difficult to detect with bone scintigraphy, because this is an area of increased activity in normal patients. Knowledge of the normal distribution of the marrow for the patient's age is crucial when interpreting MR images of the metaphysis, because hematopoietic marrow can closely resemble the signal characteristics of tumor and infection.

## Suggested Reading

Brighton CT. The growth plate. Orthop Clin North Am 1984; 15:571–595.

Herman TE, McAlister WH. Inherited diseases of bone density in children. Radiol Clin North Am 1991; 29:149–164.

Kleinman PK. Diagnostic imaging in infant abuse. AJR 1990; 155:703–712.

Kricun ME. Red-yellow marrow conversion: Its effect on the location of some solitary bone lesions. Skeletal Radiol 1985; 14:10–19.

Milgram JW. Hormonal, vitamin, and metabolic imbalance affecting the bones. In: Milgram JW, ed. Radiologic and Histologic Pathology of Nontumorous Diseases of Bones and Joints. Northbrook, Ill: Northbrook Publishing, 1990:713.

Morrisy RT. Bone and joint infections. In: Morrisy RT, ed. Pediatric Orthopaedics. Philadelphia: JB Lippincott, 1990:539–544.

Park EA. The imprinting of nutritional disturbances on the growing bone. Pediatrics 1964; 33(suppl):815–863.

Pitt M. Rickets and osteomalacia are still around. Radiol Clin North Am 1991; 29:97–118.

# MRI of Musculoskeletal Tumors in Children

*BARRY D. FLETCHER, M.D.*

Approximately half of all bone tumors in children and adolescents are malignant, 90 percent of which are osteosarcomas or Ewing's sarcomas. Other bone malignancies, such as chondrosarcoma and malignant fibrous histiocytoma, occur less frequently in this age group. Rhabdomyosarcoma is by far the most common soft-tissue malignancy of the musculoskeletal system in pediatric patients, although approximately 50 percent of soft-tissue malignancies in this age group are nonrhabdomyomatous. These include fibrosarcoma, neurofibrosarcoma, synovial sarcoma, hemangiopericytoma, alveolar soft part sarcoma, leiomyosarcoma, and liposarcoma. Primitive neuroepitheliomas are soft-tissue tumors that are nearly indistinguishable from nonosseous Ewing's sarcomas on light microscopy. All of these tumors are amenable to magnetic resonance imaging (MRI), which has proven to be remarkably effective in detecting and defining musculoskeletal tumors and which provides several advantages over computed tomography (CT).

## Indications for MRI

At St. Jude Children's Research Hospital, all patients with suspected bone or soft-tissue malignancies undergo MRI examination of the primary tumor at diagnosis. We also use MRI extensively to follow our patients' responses to initial chemotherapy and to determine the results of surgical resection. Although we continue to rely heavily on plain radiographs to estimate the likelihood of malignancy of a newly presenting bone tumor and to establish a tentative diagnosis, we are increasingly confident of the capability of MRI to help determine the probable histology in specific circumstances. MRI provides higher contrast between tumor and adjacent normal tissues than does contrast-enhanced CT and produces images in a number of orientations. Our institution finds MRI an essential component of the preoperative assessment of bone and soft-tissue sarcomas when evaluating lesion resectability and extent of tumor margins and planning limb-sparing procedures.

Supported in part by the National Cancer Institute, Cancer Center Support (CORE) grant P30CA21765 and by the American Lebanese Syrian Associated Charities.

## Imaging Techniques

Our routine MRI protocol for evaluating bone and soft-tissue tumors is shown in Table 1, and representative images are shown in Figure 1. We have performed our MRI using a 1.0 T (Siemens GBS2) system and more recently at 1.5 T (Siemens Magnetom SP63).

### *General Considerations*

Most of our patients presenting with malignant musculoskeletal tumors, especially osteosarcoma, are older children or adolescents who do not require sedation. However, benign lesions, rhabdomyosarcomas, and occasionally Ewing's sarco-

**TABLE 1** MRI Protocol for Musculoskeletal Tumors*

| | Plane | TR | TE | TI | NEX | Matrix‖ |
|---|---|---|---|---|---|---|
| T1 | Longitudinal§ | 525 (600–750) | 15 (15) | | 2 | 256 × 256 |
| PD† | Longitudinal§ and/or | 2,500 (2,500) | 22 (20) | | 1 | 256 × 256 |
| T2† | Transverse | 2,500 (2,500) | 90 (80) | | 1 | 256 × 256 |
| STIR | Longitudinal§ | 2,500 (2,200) | 22 (20) | 150 (180) | 1 | 128 × 256 |
| Enhanced T1‡ | Longitudinal§ | 520 (600–750) | 15 (15) | | 2 | 256 × 256 |

*Numbers in parentheses are imaging parameters at 1.5 T; all others are for 1.0 T image sequences.
†Proton density and T2-weighted images are obtained using a double-echo sequence with a single TR of 2,500 msec.
‡Optional.
§Usually coronal.
‖Rectangular field of view on 1.5 T system.
TR = repetition time (milliseconds); TE = echo delay (milliseconds); TI = inversion time (milliseconds); NEX = number of excitations; PD = proton density; STIR = short tau inversion recovery.

mas occur in younger children who may require sedation. We carefully monitor the child's heart rate and arterial oxygen saturation with an MRI compatible pulse oximeter and expired $CO_2$ with a capnograph.

Because pain often accompanies malignant bone tumors, many unsedated patients can tolerate a long imaging procedure only if given adequate analgesia, such as meperidine (Demerol) or morphine. Claustrophobia can be reduced in patients with lower-extremity tumors by placing them feet first into the magnet.

We use the body coil to obtain bone tumor images in all but very small children. These coils provide a field of view large enough to include the bones of both the involved and the contralateral extremities or the entire pelvis, trunk, or chest. The wide variability in bone marrow signal patterns at different ages necessitates obtaining an image of the entire length of an affected long bone that includes the contralateral bone as a control. We feel these considerations outweigh both the spatial resolution and signal-to-noise limitations of body coil–obtained images. To obtain an image with improved spatial resolution, we reduce the body coil's standard 50 cm field of vision to 30 cm. Doing so, however, weakens the signal-to-noise ratio and may result in a "wrap-around" image. It is frequently acceptable to image soft-tissue tumors with a more closely coupled volume coil, such as those designed for head and knee imaging. A head coil may also be used to obtain simultaneous images of both lower extremities in very small children with nonbulky tumors. We prefer not to use surface coils, because they cause a "shading" effect with excess signal in the tissues close to the coil and gradual loss of signal in the deeper tissues (Fig. 2).

## T1-Weighted Images

Of the various sequences capable of imaging musculoskeletal tumors, T1-weighted spin-echo imaging using short repetition time/echo time (TR/TE) provides the best spatial resolution. The relatively high water content of most bone tumors makes them appear hypointense compared with the signal produced by fat-containing yellow marrow. In younger children, whose medullary cavities produce less signal because of the presence of more hematopoietic tissue and less fat, this contrast is less marked. Because the soft-tissue component of the tumor and the adjacent muscle generally are nearly isointense, T1-weighted images are not practical for imaging soft-tissue lesions. Cortical bone does not produce a signal on any type of MR image and therefore appears black; neither does fibrosis, calcification, or ossification within the tumor mass. Subacute hemorrhage, which can occur de novo or in response to chemotherapy, creates a high signal similar to that of fat.

We obtain longitudinal T1-weighted images along the long axis of the tumor and the entire affected bone. If the long axis is not parallel to the *z*-axis of the magnet, an appropriate nonorthogonal plane is selected. These longitudinal images demonstrate the distance of the margins of the tumor from the nearest joints, which influences the choice of operative procedure. These images are also evaluated for the presence of skip metastases (which occur in 5 to 10 percent of osteosarcomas), involvement of the epiphyses (which are normally intense), and invasion of the adjacent joint capsule and ligaments. Each of these features has a bearing on prognosis and subsequent therapy.

T1-weighted images enable us to detect the more remote, and therefore unsuspected, bone marrow metastases that may accompany such tumors as Ewing's sarcoma and rhabdomyosarcoma. In some cases we have also identified unsuspected marrow involvement of bones adjacent to soft-tissue sarcomas.

## T2-Weighted Images

Obtaining long TR/long TE spin-echo images is a lengthy but necessary component of the MRI procedure. These images provide excellent contrast between tumor and adjacent soft tissues, particularly muscle. Presaturation of an adjacent volume helps eliminate motion and vascular-phasing artifacts but limits the number of slices that can be produced. We routinely obtain these images through the transverse or short axis of the length of the tumor and generally find it impractical or unnecessary to image beyond the craniocaudad limits of the lesion. We may also elect to obtain longitudinal T2-weighted images.

In addition to superior tumor-tissue contrast, T2-weighted images display the "texture" of the lesion and are the most useful images for tissue characterization. For example, fluid-filled cystic portions of the lesion produce a homogeneously intense signal, whereas fibrous septa, calcifications, and ossifications within the tumor matrix remain dark on T2-weighted images. Liquefied necrotic regions of the tumor that

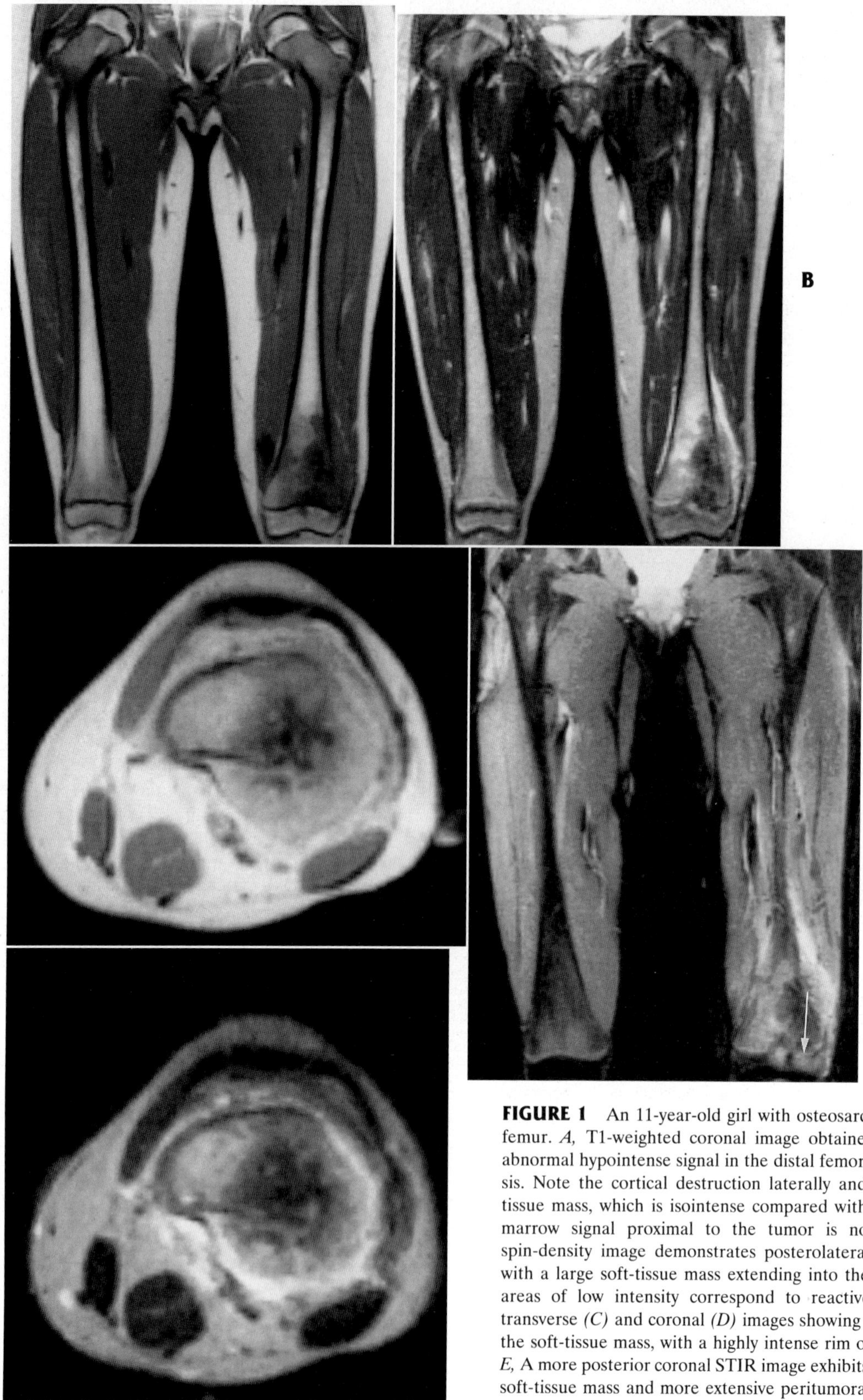


**FIGURE 1** An 11-year-old girl with osteosarcoma of the distal left femur. *A,* T1-weighted coronal image obtained at 1.5 T shows an abnormal hypointense signal in the distal femoral shaft and metaphysis. Note the cortical destruction laterally and poorly defined soft-tissue mass, which is isointense compared with normal muscle. The marrow signal proximal to the tumor is normal. *B,* Transverse spin-density image demonstrates posterolateral cortical destruction with a large soft-tissue mass extending into the soft tissues. Central areas of low intensity correspond to reactive bone. T2-weighted transverse *(C)* and coronal *(D)* images showing increased intensity of the soft-tissue mass, with a highly intense rim of peritumoral edema. *E,* A more posterior coronal STIR image exhibits hyperintensity of the soft-tissue mass and more extensive peritumoral edema. Abnormally intense signal in the lateral femoral condyle *(arrow)* indicates epiphyseal involvement, which is better visualized than on T1- or T2-weighted images.

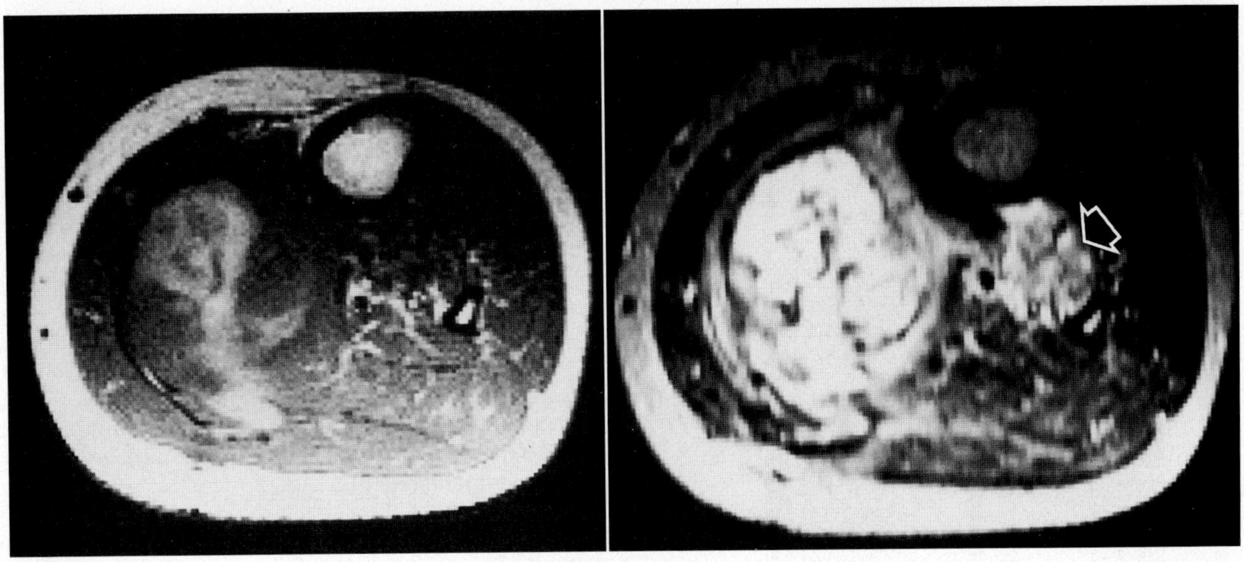


**FIGURE 2** *A,* Transverse T1-weighted image (1.0 T) of the lower leg of a 13-year-old girl with malignant fibrous histiocytoma. The gradual change in signal intensity is the result of using a posterior surface coil. The tibial and fibular marrow signal is normal and their cortices appear intact. The increase in T1-weighted signal intensity indicates hemorrhage within a soft-tissue mass that is otherwise isointense compared with muscle. *B,* T2-weighted image shows interosseous tumor extension *(arrow)* surrounding a posterior tibial vessel. This finding necessitated amputation rather than resection.

are similar in intensity to viable tumor on T1-weighted images are frequently hyperintense on T2-weighted images. Subacute hemorrhage, which is intense on T1-weighted images, remains bright on images obtained with long TR/TE. T2-weighted images also demonstrate extratumoral edema adjacent to the capsule of the mass.

We have not attempted to replace spin-echo T2-weighted images with gradient-echo sequences. Although gradient-echo images can be acquired more rapidly, their image contrast is dominated by T2* relaxation, which depends on local magnetic field homogeneity rather than molecular interactions. As a result, the images, especially of bone-forming tumors, are somewhat degraded by susceptibility artifacts, and tissue characterization is less certain.

In many MRI protocols, the heavily T2-weighted images are formed by the long TE second echoes of a double-echo sequence that are received within a single long TR. Although the "proton density," or "balanced," images formed by the shorter TE first echoes do not produce as much tumor-tissue contrast as do the second-echo images, they provide a superior signal-to-noise ratio and are less likely to contain motion artifacts, a major problem of images made with a long TE. The first-echo images are useful for assessing integrity of the cortical bone and are a reasonable substitute for transverse T1-weighted images.

## STIR Images

Short tau inversion recovery (STIR) is a fat-suppression sequence that employs a 180° radiofrequency (RF) pulse followed by a 90° to 180° spin-echo sequence. STIR images are reconstructed with a phase-insensitive magnitude algorithm, so that T1 and T2 relaxation effects are additive. An inversion time is chosen that approximates the T1 relaxation time of fat at the magnet's field strength (150 msec at 1.0 T), thereby nullifying the fat signal. Addition of the T1 and T2 signals from the remaining tissues with longer T1 relaxation times results in images with relatively high intensity and improved conspicuity of hydrated tissues, including tumors. STIR images may thus detect more tumor volume and therefore aid in the preoperative evaluation of tumor margins. We usually perform coronal STIR images to facilitate local tumor staging and to detect skip lesions (Fig. 3) and distant metastases.

The major disadvantage of using STIR imaging to evaluate musculoskeletal tumors is its lack of specificity. Peritumoral edema and bone marrow edema have high signal intensity similar to that of malignant tissues and may obscure the true tumor margins. Further, STIR images have a relatively poor signal-to-noise ratio and, with our MRI equipment, require a 50 percent interslice gap. The imaging time is minimized by the use of a rectilinear matrix.

## Contrast-enhanced Images

The paramagnetic contrast agent gadopentetate dimeglumine (Gd-DTPA) increases the signal intensity of vascularized tissue by shortening T1 relaxation time. Although administration of Gd-DTPA in the standard dosage of 0.1 mmol/kg increases the contrast between tumor and muscle on T1-weighted images, the agent is not used routinely in musculoskeletal tumor imaging primarily because the contrast it is capable of achieving is not as great as that produced by unenhanced T2-weighted images.

Contrast enhancement can help define nonvascularized portions of tumor. However, increases in intensity occur in peritumoral edema and active tumor, and well-vascularized reactive granulation tissue, common in osteosarcoma, enhances on static gadolinium-enhanced T1-weighted images.

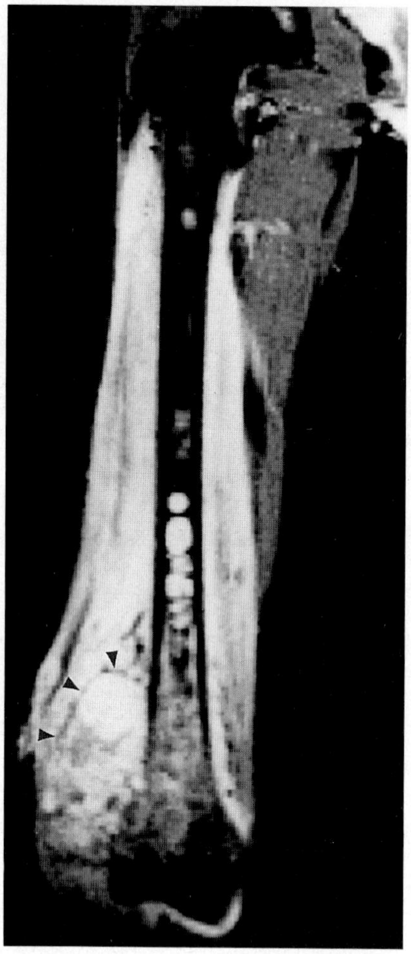

**FIGURE 3** Coronal STIR image (1.0 T) of an 18-year-old girl with osteosarcoma shows a large lesion arising from the distal femoral metaphysis, extensive edema of the vastii muscles, and multiple medullary skip lesions. High signal intensity of muscle edema nearly obscures margins of the soft-tissue component *(arrowheads)*.

Further, enhancement of the tumor reduces the contrast between the mass and the fat in adjacent marrow and soft tissues (Fig. 4). Fat-suppression sequences may alleviate this problem. We have also employed techniques using electronic subtraction to define the enhancing tissues. Static Gd-DTPA–enhanced T1-weighted imaging is an acceptable substitute for T2-weighted imaging when evaluation time is limited. It also helps assess intra-articular tumor spread in the presence of a joint effusion.

Dynamic Gd-DTPA–enhanced gradient-echo imaging has recently been introduced as a technique for measuring the rate of contrast enhancement of malignant and nonmalignant tissues. After intravenous injection of Gd-DTPA, the intensity of a representative section of the tumor is calculated on rapidly acquired fast low-angle shot (FLASH) images and plotted against time. Calculating the slopes of enhanced tissues on these time-intensity curves can help differentiate malignant disease from less rapidly enhancing necrotic tissues and edema. Dynamic Gd-DTPA–enhanced imaging is also a promising method of evaluating response to chemotherapy, because slopes of responsive tumors containing more abundant necrotic tissue become less steep. We have not found this technique successful, however, in differentiating between benign and malignant tumors.

## Key Signs of Disease and Differential Diagnosis

Although MRI excels in the local staging of musculoskeletal tumors, it less frequently provides information leading to a specific histologic diagnosis. Indeed, most tumors display low signal on T1-weighted images, homogeneously high signal exceeding that of fat on T2-weighted images, and variable enhancement on Gd-DTPA–enhanced T1-weighted images.

Low T2-weighted signal intensity of soft-tissue images suggests tumor hypocellularity and abundant collagen content. We have also observed this characteristic in Ewing's sarcoma, an extremely cellular tumor with a high nuclear-cytoplasmic ratio and little interstitial tissue.

Osteosarcomas display heterogeneous signal intensity on T2-weighted images because of their osteoid-osseous matrix; whereas cystic lesions and those containing myxoid tissue or cartilage, such as myxoid chondrosarcoma, usually have high signal intensity. Fluid-fluid levels are the hallmark of aneurysmal bone cysts that contain layers of hemorrhage. In pediatric patients these cysts are sometimes associated with telangiectatic osteosarcoma.

### *Peritumoral Edema*

Localized peri- or paratumoral edema in the soft tissues adjacent to a tumor is characterized by a zone of increased signal intensity with feathery, ill-defined margins on T2-weighted and STIR images (see Fig. 1, *C, D,* and *E*). This feature is observed in approximately two-thirds of benign and malignant tumors. Less commonly, the edema is more extensive, involving all of at least one muscle in the vicinity of the tumor (see Fig. 3). When this "massive" edema occurs in association with known musculoskeletal malignancy, it is indicative of a larger, more aggressive tumor (frequently osteosarcoma) that will likely exhibit poor response to chemotherapy.

### *Signs Associated with Tumor Therapy*

MRI frequently affords us the opportunity to observe therapeutic changes in malignant tumors. Because musculoskeletal malignancies may respond histologically to chemotherapy without significantly changing in size and because the degree of response influences subsequent therapy, efforts are being made to correlate MRI signal changes with histologic changes associated with chemotherapy, especially on T2-weighted images.

A decrease in T2-weighted signal of soft-tissue sarcomas indicates fibrosis. Treated osteosarcomas, however, are extremely heterogeneous in appearance and exhibit no consistent response pattern on MR images. The medullary portion of responsive Ewing's sarcomas increases in intensity with chemotherapy, whereas the soft-tissue component resolves. This correlates with an increase in interstitial and intracellular fluid in the affected bone marrow and may eventually be followed by fatty marrow replacement after radiation and additional chemotherapy.

Irradiation of unresected Ewing's sarcomas usually results

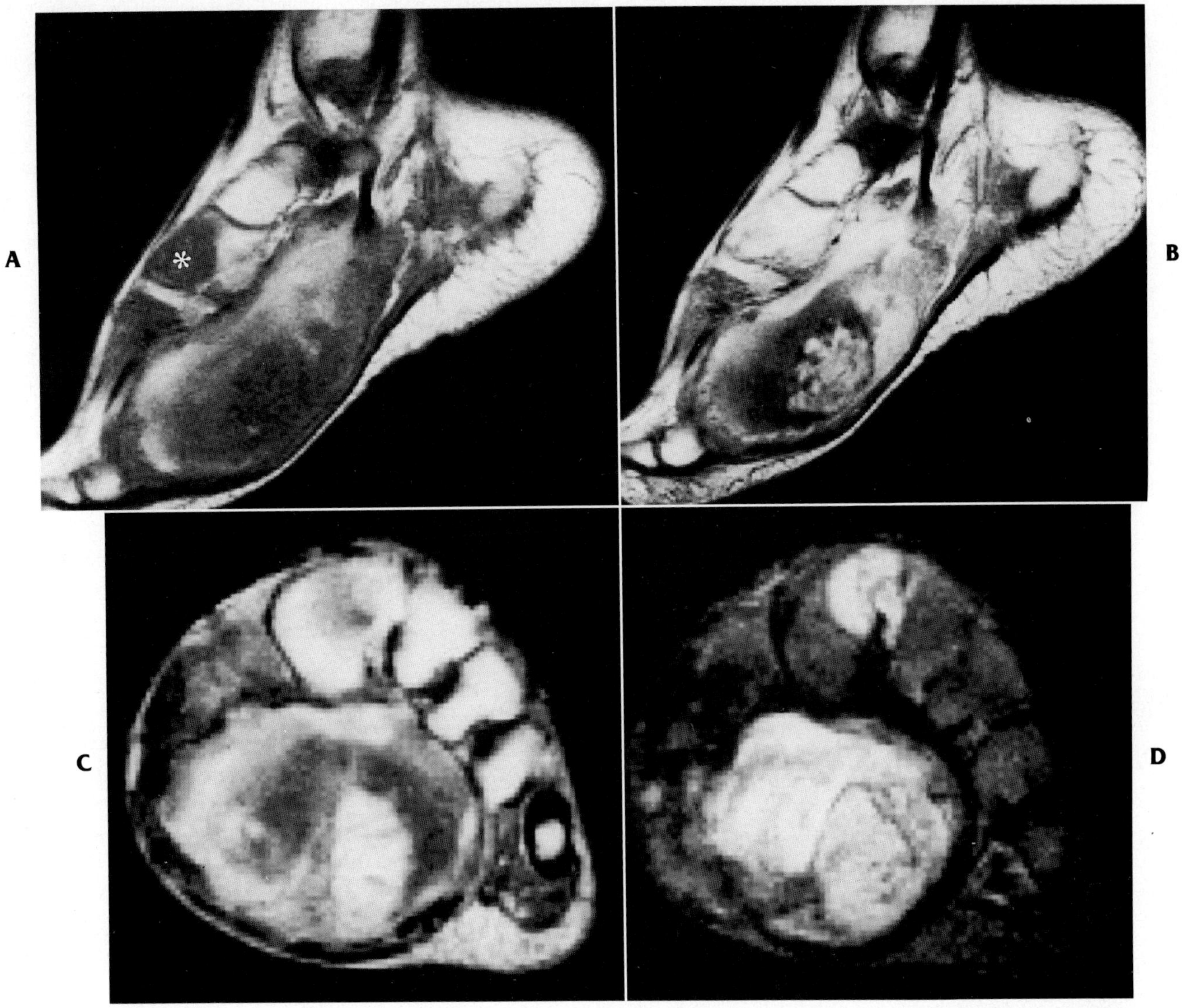


**FIGURE 4** Images (1.0 T) of the foot of a 19-year-old boy with synovial sarcoma. *A,* Noncontrast T1-weighted image shows a large plantar mass with high signal intensity from hemorrhage and a metastatic lesion of the medial cuneiform bone *(asterisk). B,* Gadolinium-enhanced T1-weighted image. Only a portion of the mass enhances, indicating extensive necrosis. Note loss of definition of the tumor margins and poor contrast between the cuneiform metastasis and the normal bone marrow with contrast enhancement. *C,* Transverse gadolinium-enhanced T1-weighted image displays less tumor/marrow contrast of primary lesion and metastasis than does the T2-weighted image *(D).* (C From Hanna SL, Langston JW, et al. Subtraction technique for contrast-enhanced MR images of musculoskeletal tumors. Magn Reson Imaging 1990; 8:213–215; with permission.)

in an increase in T2-weighted and STIR signal intensity of the normal muscles and subcutaneous soft tissues within the radiation port. The soft-tissue changes may persist for a year or more and occasionally obscure recurrent disease at the primary site.

## Discussion

MRI is capable of providing important information about pediatric bone and soft-tissue malignancies that are either more difficult to obtain or not available on CT. The ascendancy of MRI over CT is largely because of the ability of MRI to image in longitudinal and nonorthogonal planes and its improved tissue contrast and lesion characterization. CT is still valuable for initial staging and preoperative follow-up studies of bone-forming tumors, such as osteosarcoma, but MRI is the method of choice for imaging other bone tumors and for detecting and characterizing soft-tissue masses. We believe that MRI will become even more valuable in the future when the full extent of its capability to detect pathophysiologic, rather than purely anatomic, changes is realized.

*Acknowledgments.* I thank Suzanne A. Gronemeyer, Ph.D., and Soheil L. Hanna, M.D., for their advice and Kate Thomas for editorial assistance.

## Suggested Reading

Bloem JL, Taminiau AHM, Euderink F, et al. Radiologic staging of primary bone sarcoma: MR imaging, scintigraphy, angiography, and CT correlated with pathologic examination. Radiology 1988; 169:805–810.

Erlemann K, Reiser MF, Peters PE, et al. Musculoskeletal neoplasms: Static and dynamic Gd-DTPA-enhanced MR imaging. Radiology 1989; 171:767–773.

Fletcher BD. Response of osteosarcoma and Ewing sarcoma to chemotherapy: Imaging evaluation. AJR 1991; 157:825–833.

Fletcher BD, Hanna SL, Fairclough DL, Gronemeyer SA. Pediatric musculoskeletal tumors: Use of dynamic contrast-enhanced MR imaging to monitor response to chemotherapy. Radiology 1992; 184:243–248.

Fletcher BD, Hanna SL, Kun LE. Changes in MR signal intensity and contrast enhancement of therapeutically irradiated soft tissue. Magn Reson Imaging 1990; 8:771–777.

Hanna SL, Fletcher BD, Parham DM, Bugg MF. Muscle edema in musculoskeletal tumors: MR imaging characteristics and clinical significance. J Magn Reson 1991; 1:441–449.

Hanna SL, Langston JW, Gronemeyer SA, Fletcher BD. Subtraction technique for contrast-enhanced MR images of musculoskeletal tumors. Magn Reson Imaging 1990; 8:213–215.

Lemmi MA, Fletcher BD, Marina NM, et al. Use of MR imaging to assess results of chemotherapy for Ewing sarcoma. AJR 1990; 155:343–346.

Rosenthal RE, Wozney P. Diagnostic value of gadopentetate dimeglumine for 1.5-T MR imaging of musculoskeletal masses: Comparison with unenhanced T1- and T2-weighted imaging. J Magn Reson 1991; 1:547–551.

Sundaram M, McGuire MH, Schajowicz F. Soft tissue masses: Histologic basis for decreased signal (short T2) on T2-weighted images. AJR 1987; 148:1247–1250.

# Spinal Infections in Children

*JOHN R. STY, M.D. · ROBERT G. WELLS, M.D.*

This chapter discusses the inflammatory and infectious diseases of the spine in children. A range of diagnostic imaging modalities is available for the detection of spinal infections, including standard radiography, computed tomography (CT), scintigraphy, and magnetic resonance imaging (MRI). Although a child's presentation and the clinically suspected diagnosis dictate the choice and order of imaging in children with spinal infection, difficulty often arises as a result of atypical presentations, lack of temperature elevation, and inability to communicate the symptomatology. In the pediatric age group, spinal column infection can be categorized into three types: spinal diskitis, vertebral osteomyelitis, and epidural abscess. The term diskitis (or discitis) refers to a self-limited nonsuppurative disk space inflammation, while vertebral osteomyelitis indicates a pyogenic process that involves the disk and vertebral end-plate. However, a degree of overlap occurs between these two entities, in terms of both definition and pathology. Spinal epidural abscess is rare in children, but can result in devastating neurologic sequelae or death if not diagnosed early.

The vascular anatomy of the intervertebral disk and vertebral end-plate is of particular importance in the pathophysiology of diskitis. The higher incidence of diskitis in young children as compared with adolescents and adults is thought to be related to the existence of vascular pathways in the cartilaginous portions of the disk during childhood development. In adults the disk is relatively avascular, making direct hematogenous seeding unlikely. In young children organisms may gain access to the intervertebral disk through the microcirculatory subchondral vessels, which originate in the marrow space of the vertebra, enter the vertebral end-plate, and extend into the nucleus pulposus. These vessels then course between the fibers of the annulus fibrosus. This particular vascular pathway usually exists in children until about 8 years of age; however, it may persist into later years. There are other theories regarding this microvascular circulatory pattern. Some feel that the vascular supply of the disk is independent of the blood supply of the vertebral end-plate. This theory suggests that the microcirculation in the annulus fibrosus consists of terminal radial ramifications of vessels that enter the disk space from its margins. Consequently this theory suggests that childhood diskitis is actually a mild form of vertebral osteomyelitis, with the process predominantly localized to the disk because the anastomotic osseous vascular pattern in children prevents large portions of the vertebral body from being destroyed. The findings with cross-sectional imaging studies in children with diskitis tend to support this theory.

The vascular considerations in the pathophysiology of diskitis preterm hematogenous inoculation with microorganisms. However, the specific etiology of diskitis in children has not been established. Trauma, viral infection, and bacterial infection have all been incriminated. Positive cultures from blood or tissue are obtained in less than 50 percent of the patients in the early stages of disease. Cultures are not usually positive if symptoms are long-standing. The uncertain etiology of diskitis is reflected by the variety of terms that have been used for this disorder including intervertebral disk inflammation, nonspecific spondylitis, disk inflammation, and benign osteomyelitis of the spine. The disease is invariably indolent. There appear to be two peak age periods of incidence: in young children, 1 to 4 years of age and in older children, 12 to 15 years of age. Patients with diskitis may report vague pain in the buttock, thigh or knee, or backache. Symptomatic disk space narrowing in association with fever and elevated erythrocyte sedimentation rate comprise the well-known recognized triad of findings in childhood diskitis.

Vertebral osteomyelitis (infectious spondylitis) is less common than diskitis in the pediatric age group. This infection is most often a result of hematogenous spread from a focus elsewhere in the body. The most common sources are infections of the genitourinary system, skin, and respiratory tract. Direct inoculation may occur as a complication of spinal instrumentation or surgery. The most common organisms implicated in vertebral osteomyelitis are *Enterobacteriaceae* and *Staphylococcus* species.

The clinical presentation of vertebral osteomyelitis is heterogeneous and may include pain that is referred to the hip, back, or abdomen. The patient may or may not be reluctant to walk, sit, or stand, or may limp. Vertebral osteomyelitis is frequently accompanied by a systemic illness, with fever and irritability. In some cases the clinical presentation is characterized by abdominal pain, anorexia, and ileus. This triad of findings may mimic gastrointestinal disease. Because of the varied clinical presentations of vertebral osteomyelitis, the differential diagnosis can include septic arthritis of the hip, appendicitis, and meningitis, as well as diskitis and spinal epidural abscess. Hence vertebral infections present interesting and challenging diagnoses.

Fewer than 1.5 percent of cases of epidural abscess occur in the pediatric age group. Epidural abscess can arise as a primary lesion or as direct spread from infection of a disk or vertebral body. Some cases are related to surgery or a penetrating injury. The findings at presentation may include fever, back pain, and sensory-motor deficits. The early symptoms, however, are frequently mild and nonspecific, particularly in children. Without appropriate treatment, epidural abscess may lead to severe neurologic deficits and death. Acute deterioration can occur. The most common infecting organism is *S. aureus* and other gram-positive cocci.

## Imaging Strategy

As previously described, the clinical presentation of spinal column infection is highly variable, and the history and physical examination cannot accurately distinguish between spinal epidural abscess, vertebral osteomyelitis, and diskitis. At times the presentation may lead to a mistaken impression of abdominal, pelvic, or lower-extremity pathology. Standard radiographs, although typically normal during the early phases of spinal infection, are essential for excluding other etiologies of the presenting symptoms. These include diseases such as leukemia or neuroblastoma, primary bone tumor, and injury. If standard radiographs are normal and the symptoms are nonspecific, bone scintigraphy is the most reasonable imaging modality for screening the spine, pelvis, and lower extremities for bone pathology. If standard radiographs or bone scintigraphy show evidence of spinal infection or if the clinical findings are suggestive and these diagnostic modalities yield no positive information, MRI is the imaging modality that is most sensitive and specific for documenting the presence of spinal column infection and for detecting the potential complications of the disease. MRI is particularly useful in those children with neurological symptoms or signs of neural compression, epidural or intradural suppuration, arachnoiditis or myelitis. If MRI is not readily available, CT may be used. However, MRI has largely replaced CT in our diagnostic approach.

## Imaging Techniques and Findings

### Standard Radiography

The role of standard radiographs in the evaluation of spinal infections has changed over the years with the addition of new imaging modalities. Radiographs are of limited use because they are frequently normal early in the course of the process. Despite these limitations, radiographs should be obtained as part of the initial evaluation of all patients with suspected spinal infection. L2-L3 and L3-L4 are the most common sites for diskitis in young children. In teenagers the lower thoracic region is more commonly involved. The most common sites of vertebral osteomyelitis in children of all ages are the mid- and lower portion of the thoracic spine. These areas need to be scrutinized carefully for bone, disk space, and soft-tissue abnormality.

The first identifiable radiographic observation of disk infection is decreased height of the disk space (Fig. 1). This usually takes a few weeks to develop. In older children radiographic abnormalities may take as long as three or four weeks to develop. The findings are subtle and may require actual measurement. In the older age group, the initial radiographic finding of disk space narrowing is usually accompanied by irregularity and erosion of the adjacent vertebral body end plates. These are highly characteristic signs, but are not observed early. The inflammatory process may be confined to the disk space or extend to adjacent vertebrae. Most often the vertebrae adjacent to the disk have unequal involvement. A lytic lesion in a vertebral end-plate in the presence of diskitis can result either from bone destruction or extrusion of disk material into the weakened end-plate. It does not necessarily indicate the presence of true vertebral osteomyelitis.

For months to years following the infection, radiographs in cases of disk infection show persistent loss of height of the disk space. Complete resolution of disk space height sometimes occurs in young children, but older children always have some degree of permanent disk space narrowing. With healing, there is reconstitution of enchondral bone in the involved vertebrae. This may or may not be associated with reactive sclerosis.

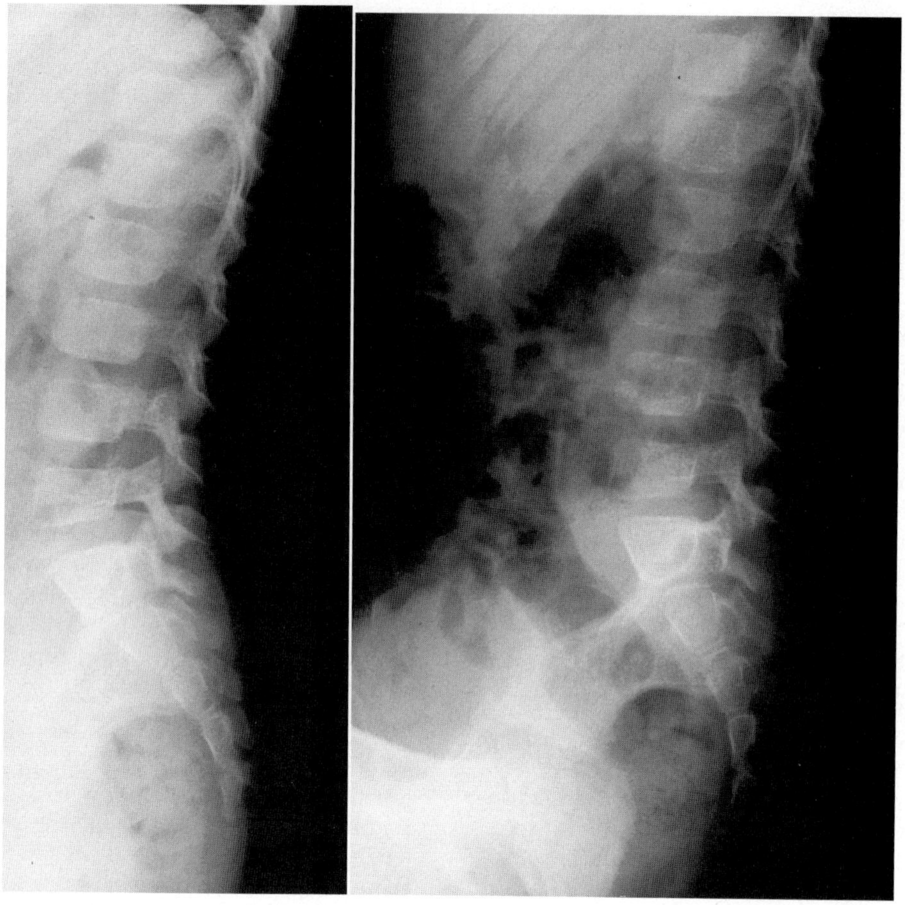


**FIGURE 1** *A,* Lateral radiograph of a 4-year-old girl with a 4 day history of low back pain is normal. *B,* Repeat evaluation 6 days later shows loss of height of the L5-S1 disk space.

Uncommon late sequelae include scoliosis, kyphosis, and, least of all, fusion. Vertebra magna (an increased anteroposterior [AP] diameter of the involved vertebra) may occur as a result of cartilage end-plate damage or from overgrowth due to a hyperemic response.

In early radiographs of vertebral osteomyelitis, one should look for localized rarefaction in the superior or inferior region of the vertebra immediately adjacent to the cartilaginous end-plate. The radiographic findings usually require 3 to 6 weeks to develop. The time of appearance depends on the virulence of the organism. The radiographic findings can include narrowing of the disk space, demineralization of adjacent vertebral end-plates, and bulging of the paraspinal lines as in diskitis. Obvious destruction of the end-plates and extension of the lytic process into the central portion of the vertebral body occur between 6 and 10 weeks. The vertebra becomes compressed and a paravertebral soft-tissue mass develops. A separate soft-tissue mass is more indicative of primary vertebral osteomyelitis than diskitis.

Both early and late in the course of epidural abscess, the radiographic findings are usually normal. At times there is reversal of the normal lordotic curve, which most likely is caused by muscle spasm and is a highly nonspecific finding.

## *Scintigraphy*

Bone scintigraphy yields positive results before the radiographic changes in both diskitis and vertebral osteomyelitis. Bone scintigraphy should be positive in all patients who have had symptoms greater than seven days. The most consistent scintigraphic pattern in diskitis is increased uptake in the disk space and in the contiguous vertebrae. Faint increased activity likewise can be seen on blood pool images. In cases of vertebral osteomyelitis, the increased tracer accumulation is usually localized to a single vertebral body (Fig. 2). Bone scintigraphy is normal in cases of epidural abscesses unless reactive bone changes occur with an indolent infection.

The increased spatial resolution provided by single-photon emission computed tomography (SPECT) imaging and pinhole collimation definitely increases the sensitivity of bone scintigraphy for the evaluation of spinal infection. SPECT imaging has been shown to increase the sensitivity by 20 percent as compared with standard bone-imaging techniques and should be employed in all suspected cases. The resultant improvement in anatomic and spatial resolution on technetium-99m bone scintigraphy may aid in the differentiation of spinal infections and inflammatory diseases. The precise localization of the focus of infection provided by SPECT imaging has virtually

A

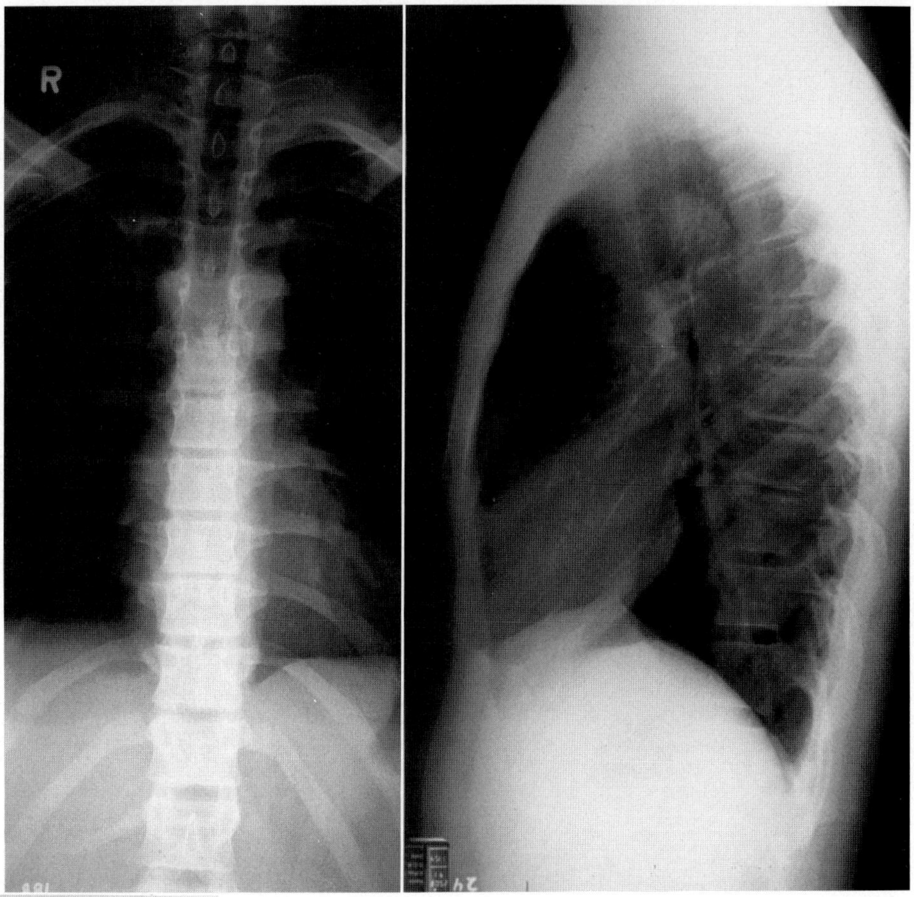


B

C

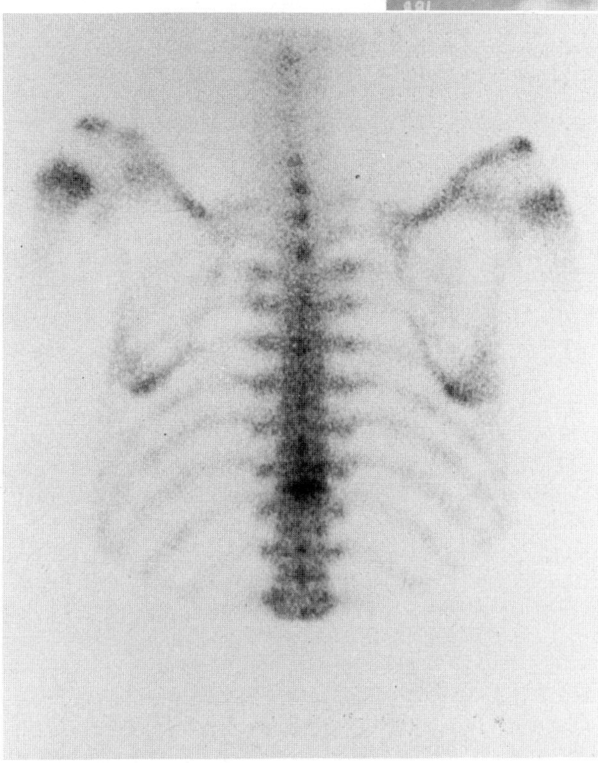

**FIGURE 2** *A* and *B,* AP and lateral radiographs of the thoracic spine in a 13-year-old boy with back pain and low-grade fever. These show narrowing of the T9-10 disc space. On the AP view there is widening of the right paraspinal soft tissues. *C,* Bone scintigraphy (posterior image) demonstrates marked increased tracer uptake in the inferior end plate of the T9 vertebral body.

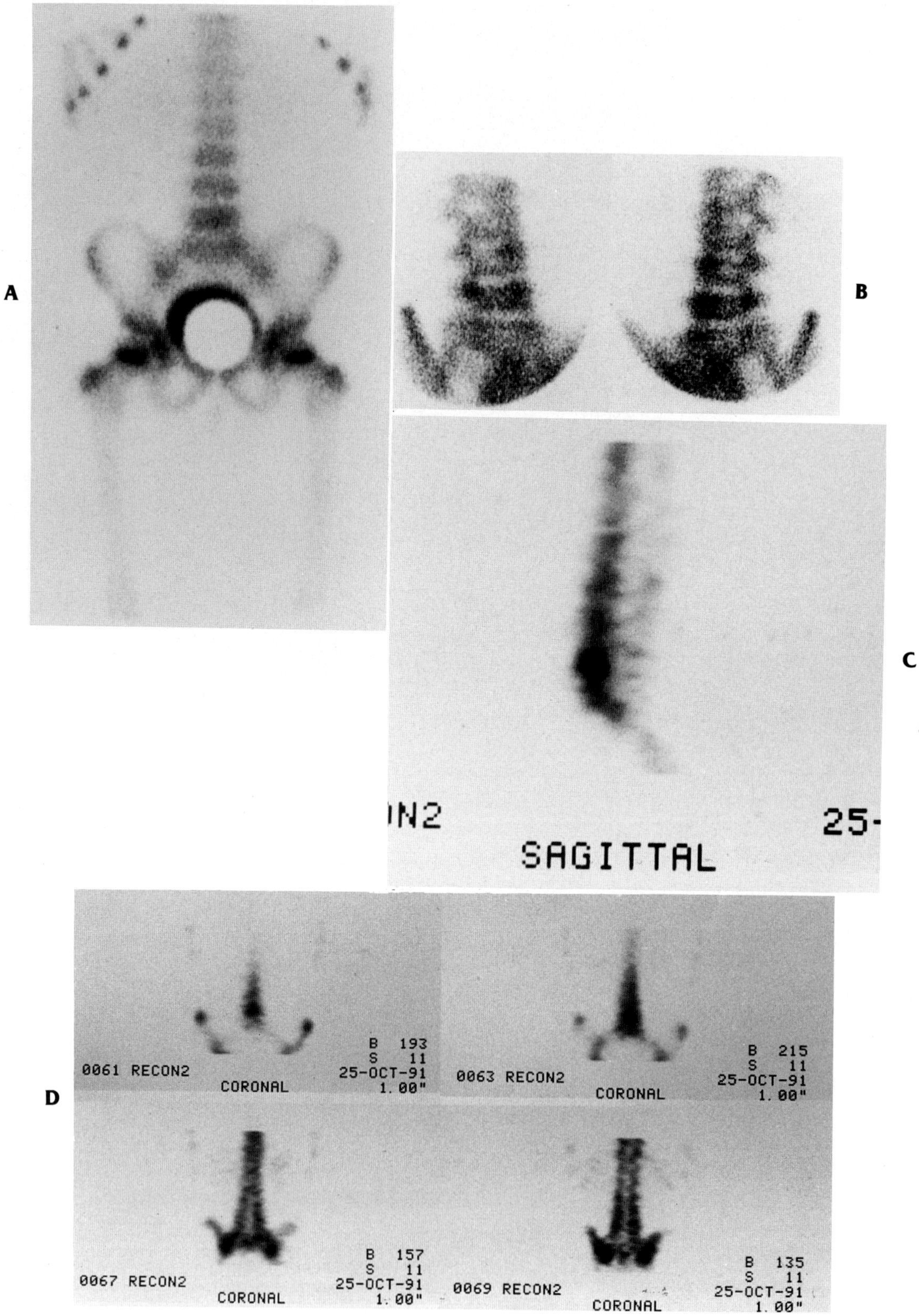


**FIGURE 3** *A* and *B*, Bone scintigraphy (anterior and oblique pinhole images) in a 2-year-old girl with fever and refusal to bear weight. These show abnormal increased uptake in the L5 vertebral body. *C* and *D*, Sagittal and coronal SPECT images confirm that the abnormal uptake is confined to the vertebral body.

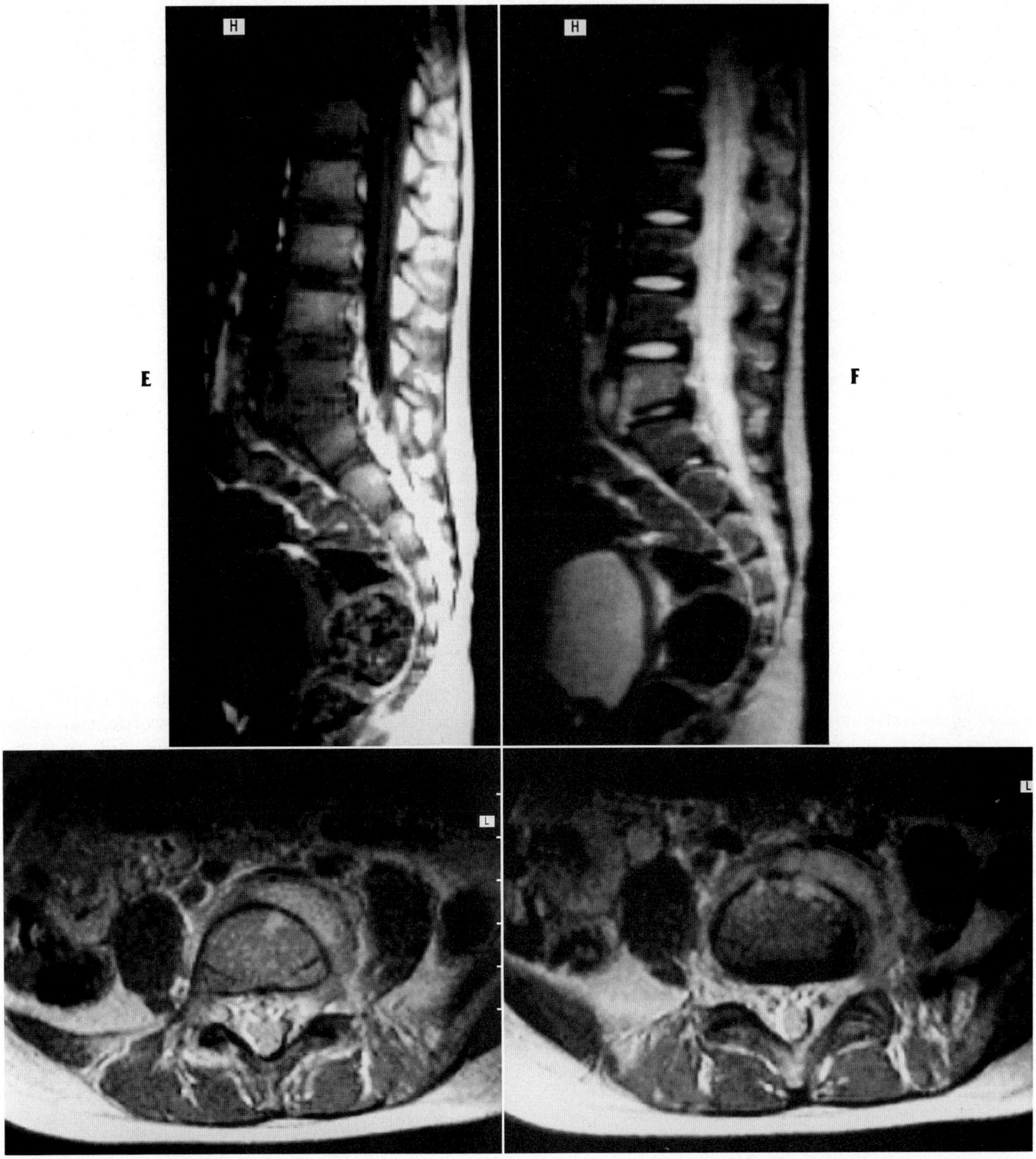

E F G H

**FIGURE 3, cont'd** *E* and *F,* T1- and T2-weighted sagittal MRI demonstrates abnormal signal throughout the L5 vertebral body. The L5-S1 disk is collapsed and there is loss of signal intensity. There is extrusion of disk material anteriorly. *G* and *H,* Axial T2-weighted MRI shows an inflammatory mass anterior and to the left of the L5 vertebral body and L5-S1 disk. This is an example of vertebral osteomyelitis, with extension into the disk and paravertebral soft tissues.

eliminated the poor distinction between the vertebral body and posterior elements that is typical with routine planar images (Fig. 3).

In general $^{99m}$Tc bone imaging should be performed before other scintigraphic studies in children with suspected spinal infection. If the scan is normal and diskitis is strongly suspected, gallium imaging can be used. In adults gallium imaging has demonstrated diskitis with nearly 85 percent accuracy. Gallium can be helpful in identifying infection when the routine bone scan is negative, because its localization is a result of affinity for polymorphonuclear cells and bacteria. When looking for diskitis, the gallium-67 evaluation should be extended to 72 hours; however, it is frequently positive within 48 hours. Since the diagnosis of this disorder is not an emergency, this time delay is not critical. A butterfly pattern of abnormal uptake on gallium scintigraphy can be seen with vertebral osteomyelitis. There is little information regarding the use of $^{67}$Ga in pediatric epidural abscesses. However, the imaging principles should be similar to those for abscesses located in soft tissues elsewhere. Time is an important consideration in the diagnosis of this process, and delay in diagnosis could result in irreversible neurologic abnormality.

There is insufficient clinical data in pediatrics regarding the use of indium-labeled white blood cells in spinal infection. Data in adults indicates that indium-111 white blood cell imaging in diskitis or vertebral osteomyelitis is neither sensitive nor specific for its detection. False-negative results can be explained by the edema and localized mass effect of the purulent debris in a nonexpansile space. Leukocyte migration is limited by vascular thrombosis and the resultant lack of blood flow to the area. However, bone scintigraphy is positive in these cases, indicating that there must be transport of the radionuclide by the vascular pathways. When positive, $^{111}$In white blood cell imaging adds specificity in combination with $^{99m}$Tc bone imaging for vertebral osteomyelitis. False-negative results are most likely to occur with chronic infection and in patients with an active bone marrow.

## *MRI*

MRI has a sensitivity and specificity of 93 and 97 percent, respectively, in early diskitis. This compares favorably with bone scintigraphy without SPECT imaging. The MRI examination is particularly sensitive to the changes in the state of disk hydration that occur early in the disease.

Ordinarily the nucleus pulposus has a higher signal than the annulus on T2-weighted MR images because of its greater water content. In disk space infection in an adult, the signal intensity on a T1-weighted image may be decreased and on a T2-weighted image may be increased. In young children the signal generated from the abnormal disk is diminished on both T1- and T2-weighted sequences. The differences in chemical structure of the developing disk in children and the adult disk are responsible for different MRI appearances in the two age groups. Additional imaging findings include loss of the intervertebral disk space height and indistinct disk margins. Signal intensity changes frequently antedate the structural disk space changes. In time the nucleus and annulus become indistinguishable, and the transition zone from the disk to the vertebral body disappears. As this process continues in adults, degeneration of the disk and loss of water occur. The T1-weighted images feature greater signal intensity than normal and lesser signal intensity on T2-weighted views.

With MRI, extension of the inflammatory process outside the osseous structures can be accurately evaluated; this is essential information for appropriate therapy. This involvement may produce a psoas abscess, or a paraspinal mass due to edema, cellulitis, or abscess (Fig. 4). Paravertebral involvement can be effectively imaged with either CT or MRI. Structures within the spinal canal are better evaluated with MRI. Disk material or osseous vertebral fragments may be displaced into the spinal canal and cause neural compression. Other potential intraspinal complications include epidural or intradural suppuration, arachnoiditis, and myelitis.

MRI is highly sensitive for the detection and characterization of osteomyelitis. Signal abnormality in the acute early stages of osteomyelitis is primarily due to intramedullary edema and exudate. These changes result in decreased marrow signal intensity on T1-weighted images; signal on T2-weighted images is isointense or hyperintense to normal marrow. Cortical destruction is imaged as interruption or increased signal in the normal black strip of cortex. Reactive bone formation is imaged as areas of low signal intensity.

Before the introduction of MRI, myelography with CT had been the primary diagnostic method for evaluating spinal epidural infection. MRI has reduced the need for myelography in most cases. The efficiency of MRI in detecting and evaluating spinal epidural abscess has been well established. An epidural abscess characteristically appears as a mass that is isointense with the spinal cord on T1-weighted images and high in signal intensity on T2-weighted images.

Despite the high sensitivity of noncontrast MRI for detecting inflammatory processes throughout the body, some epidural abscesses still can be overlooked. Contrast-enhanced MRI increases the sensitivity and specificity of MRI for spinal epidural abscesses. Two basic patterns of contrast enhancement are noted in these cases. The first pattern is that of homogeneous enhancement of the abnormal area. This may correlate with the phlegmonous stage of infection corresponding pathologically to the granulomatous thickened tissue with embedded microabscesses without a significant drainable collection. The second pattern is that of a liquid abscess core surrounded by inflammatory tissue. The core does not enhance with administration of contrast material, while varying degrees of peripheral enhancement can be detected. The area of peripheral enhancement corresponds to the edema, granulation tissue, and inflammation around a necrotic liquefied core of abscess. In addition to determining the histologic components of an abscess, administration of a contrast agent allows differentiation of epidural infection from adjoining normal cerebrospinal fluid (CSF), since epidural abscess has a similar signal to CSF on T2-weighted images. Because of the similar signal intensity, several authors have hypothesized that epidural collections may be overlooked. Because epidural abscesses may be primary or secondary to diskitis or osteomyelitis, MRI is useful in evaluating the full extent of the abnormality.

The advantages expected from the multiplanar imaging capabilities of MRI include excellent tissue contrast with improved distinction between the spinal cord and CSF, plus easier detection of paraspinal soft-tissue abnormalities and the extension and involvement of bone marrow. MRI also helps in the differential diagnosis of other entities such as disk hernia,

**FIGURE 4** *A,* Lateral radiograph of the cervical spine in a 6-month-old boy with torticollis and fever. It shows thickening of the retropharyngeal soft tissues and disk space narrowing at C2-3 with irregularity of the adjacent end plates. *B* and *C,* T1- and T2-weighted MRI demonstrates marked disk space narrowing and loss of the normal disk signal. There is an inflammatory mass in the prevertebral soft tissues that produces high signal on the T2-weighted image.

A

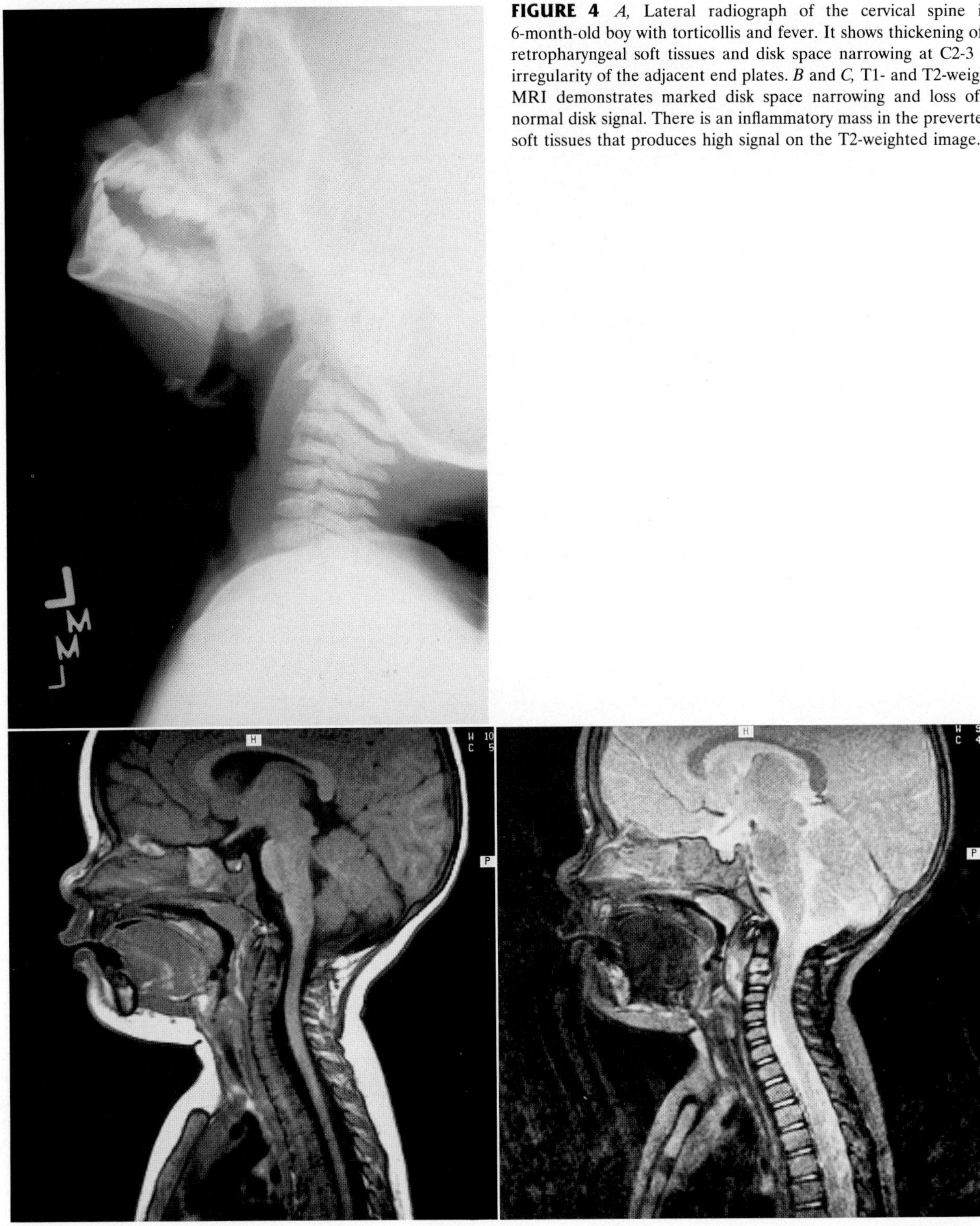


B

C

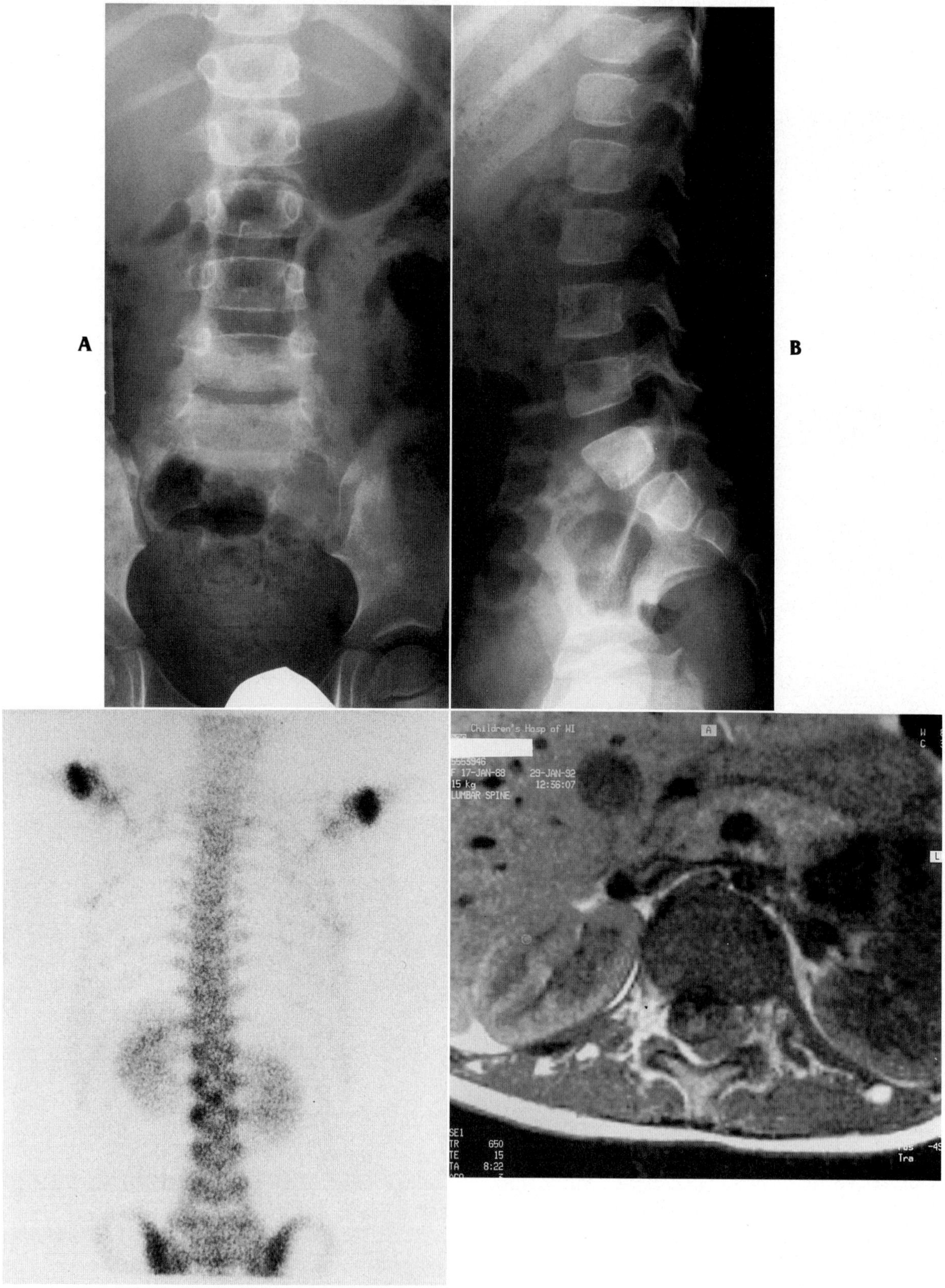


**FIGURE 5** *A* and *B,* AP and lateral radiographs of the lumbar spine in a 9-year-old girl who presented with left flank pain. These are normal except for straightening of the normal lordotic curve. *C,* Bone scintigraphy (posterior image) shows increased uptake in the posterior elements of L1,2,3 on the left. *D,* Axial T1-weighted MRI at the L2 level shows mixed signal abnormality in the left epidural space with extension into the neuroforamen. The thecal sac is displaced anteriorly and rightward.

E
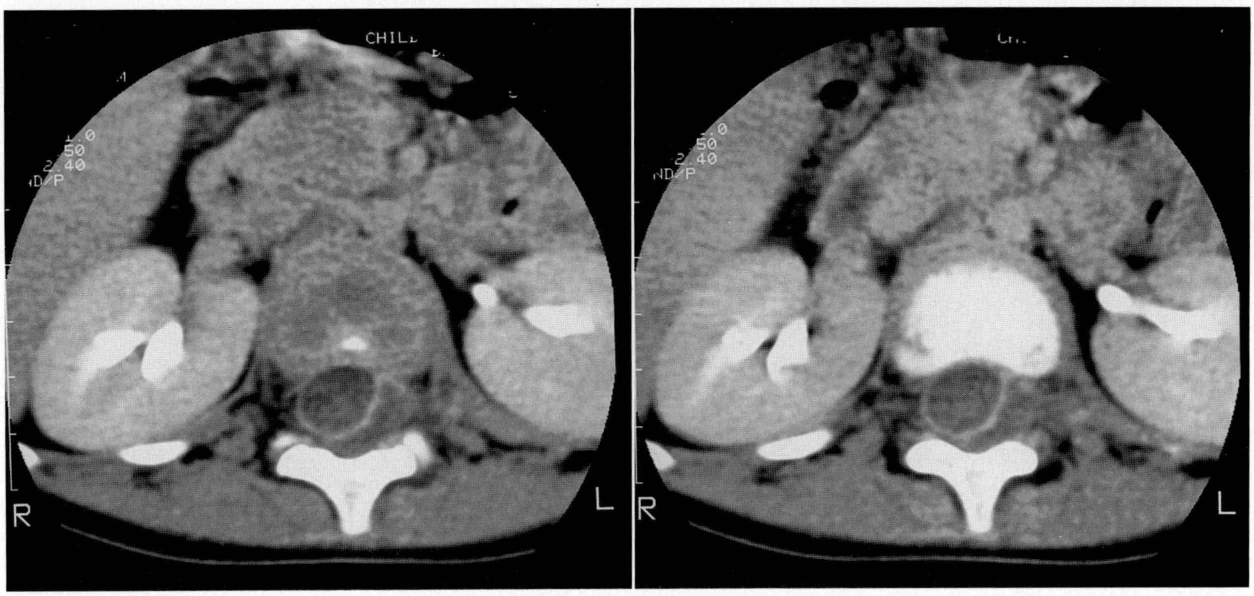

F

**FIGURE 5, cont'd** *E* and *F*, Contrast-enhanced CT scan shows the inflammatory mass in the left epidural space, with displacement of the thecal sac.

syrinx, spinal tumor, spinal hematoma, cord infarction, and some cases of myelitis.

### *CT*

CT may provide useful information in the evaluation of spinal column infections, although MRI has largely replaced this technique. CT is the best imaging modality for demonstrating areas of bone destruction. The findings typically correlate well with the abnormal sites observed with bone scintigraphy. In addition, CT often shows lytic changes not observed on standard radiographs and can identify extraosseous extension of the infection. In children with diskitis or vertebral osteomyelitis, CT can demonstrate paravertebral masses, intraspinal masses, and psoas involvement. Disk hypodensity on CT is an early sign for diskitis. CT can also demonstrate expansion of the disk with narrowing of the disk space height and irregular vertebral margins with erosions. Contrast-enhanced images sometimes show disk hyperemia. Contrast administration also aids in the detection of a paravertebral abscess. In early diskitis there is usually absence of a paravertebral soft-tissue mass. Necrotic disk space material can herniate and mimic an inflammatory mass such as an epidural abscess.

An epidural abscess is demonstrated with CT as an extradural mass within the spinal canal. With intravenous contrast, an enhancing rim may be identified at the margin of the abscess (Fig. 5). Optimal visualization of an epidural abscess with CT requires intrathecal contrast; this study, however, should not be required if MRI is available.

## Suggested Reading

Bruschwein DA, Brown ML, McLeod RA. Gallium scintigraphy in the evaluation of disc space infections: Concise communication. J Nucl Med 1980; 21:925–927.

Crawford AH, Kucharzyk DW, Ruda R, Smitherman HC Jr. Diskitis in children. Clin Orthop 1991; 266:70–79.

du Lac P, Panuel M, Devred P, et al. MRI of disc space infection in infants and children. Pediatr Radiol 1990; 20:175–178.

Fischer GW, Popich GA, Sullivan DE, et al. Discitis: A prospective diagnostic analysis. Pediatrics 1978; 62:543–548.

Förster A, Pothmann R, Winter K, Baumann-Rath CA. Magnetic resonance imaging in nonspecific discitis. Pediatr Radiol 1987; 17:162–163.

King HA. Back pain in children. Pediatr Clin North Am 1984; 31:1084–1095.

Marks WA, Bodensteiner JB. Anterior cervical epidural abscess with pneumococcus in an infant. J Child Neurol 1988; 3:25–29.

Rocco HD, Eyring EJ. Intervertebral disc infections in children. Am J Dis Child 1972; 123:448–451.

Sandhu FS, Dillon WP. Spinal epidural abscess: Evaluation with contrast-enhanced MR imaging. AJR 1992; 158:405–411.

Sartoris DJ, Maskowitz PS, Kaufman RA, et al. Childhood diskitis: Computed tomographic findings. Radiology 1983; 149:701.

Smith AS, Blaser SI. Infectious and inflammatory processes of the spine. Radiol Clin North Am 1991; 29:809–827.

Szalay EA, Green NE, Heller RM, et al. Magnetic resonance imaging in the diagnosis of childhood discitis. J Pediatr Orthop 1987; 7:164–167.

Wiley AM, Trueta J. The vascular anatomy of the spine and its relationship to pyogenic vertebral osteomyelitis. J Bone Joint Surg 1959; 41B:796–809.

# CARDIOVASCULAR RADIOLOGY

## MRI of the Heart

*ANDRÉ J. DUERINCKX, Ph.D., M.D.* · *CHARLES B. HIGGINS, M.D.*

Magnetic resonance imaging (MRI) of the heart is a noninvasive technique that is both competitive and complementary to echocardiography. Owing to the universal availability of and greater familiarity with echocardiography, MRI has been used primarily to provide diagnostic information not readily achieved by echocardiography.

MRI has several important attributes that make it advantageous for evaluation of the heart. First, there is a high natural contrast between the blood pool and the cardiovascular structures. There is lack of signal from flowing blood on spin-echo (SE) MRI pulse sequences and bright signal intensity from blood on gradient-recalled-echo (GRE) MRI pulse sequences. Contrast media are not required for discrimination of the blood pool, on either the SE or GRE images. Second, MRI is a three-dimensional (3D) imaging technique and allows precise quantification of cardiac mass and volumes without the use of any assumed formulas or geometric models. Third, cine MRI and fast GRE techniques allow the evaluation of global and regional biventricular function including measurements of wall thickening and deformation dynamics, the ejection fraction (EF), stroke volume, regurgitant fractions, and cardiac output (CO). Fourth, velocity-encoded techniques permit measurements of blood flow, which are useful for quantifying the function of both ventricles and the severity of valvular lesions.

Cardiac MRI techniques have major clinical indications in the study of vascular diseases (thoracic aorta and pulmonary arteries), acquired heart disease, and congenital heart disease.

### Techniques

Cardiac MRI requires physiological gating of the imaging sequence. MR images without gating result in poor images due to the gross motion of the cardiac structure relative to the imaging voxels during the cardiac cycle.

#### *EKG Gated Spin Echo*

For anatomic diagnosis the EKG gated multislice SE technique is used. This technique requires less than 10 minutes for the acquisition of tomograms at multiple anatomic levels (usually 8 to 12 levels). Images at adjacent levels are obtained at different phases of the cardiac cycle, with a 30 to 50 msec time difference between each adjacent level. When functional information during the cardiac cycle is needed, a multiphasic, multislice technique can be used. In this technique each anatomic section is imaged at 5 to 10 phases of the cardiac cycle. A variant of this technique is the biphasic multislice SE technique, which acquires images at multiple anatomic locations at end diastole and end systole. The biphasic multislice technique allows comparison of cardiac structures at end diastole and systole only.

#### *Cine MRI*

This is a GRE pulse sequence with EKG referencing. It allows the dynamic study of cardiac motion. Images can be laced together in a cinematic display so that ventricular contraction and blood flow patterns of the heart and great vessels can be visualized.

#### *Fast Imaging Techniques*

These GRE sequences use short TR and TE times and require a fast sampling time and rapid ramping of the magnetic field gradients. TR times as short as 4 to 8 msec and TE times on the order of 2 to 4 msec are used. One image can be acquired in less than 1 second. This approach is called by different names: Turbo-FLASH, snapshot FLASH, or magnetization-prepared rapid acquisition gradient-echo (MP-RAGE) imaging. Turbo-FLASH sequences begin with a preparation module that allows one to choose the type of contrast (T1, T2, or FATSAT). This is followed by the image acquisition module. Recent improvements in Turbo-FLASH imaging include reordering and/or segmentation of the phase-encoding acquisitions (also called the "*k*-space" acquisitions) with breath-hold imaging.

### *Spiral Scanning Techniques*

All of the preceding techniques acquire data along a rectangular grid superimposed on the image: one axis is the phase axis and the other is the frequency axis. Spiral scan imaging is part of a broad class of projection reconstruction imaging, where data are acquired in polar coordinates. Short echo times are perhaps the most important property of projection reconstructed imaging sequences. The use of radial lines minimizes flow artifacts, including flow displacement artifacts. To make projection reconstruction more efficient, spiral data acquisition has been proposed (thus "spiral scanning"). The software/hardware changes required to implement this technique presently limit its widespread use.

### *Ultrafast Techniques*

Echo-planar techniques have been available for several years and allow complete tomographic image acquisition in 30 to 50 msec. Unfortunately these techniques require special hardware not available on most commercial scanners and are available at only a few institutions.

### *Flow-sensitive Techniques*

Flow-sensitive imaging techniques now permit the measurement of flow expressed either as velocity or volume flow per unit of time. Two methods are currently being used: time-of-flight (TOF) techniques and phase-change techniques. The TOF technique is based on tracking a slab of blood in which the MRI signal has been nulled. The phase-change technique is based on the principle that the phase of flowing spins along a magnetic gradient changes in direct proportion to the velocity of flow. This technique is referred to as "phase-contrast MRI" (PC-MRI) or "velocity-encoded cine MRI" (VEC-MRI). This technique allows the quantification of blood flow at different points during the cardiac cycle within each point of a cross-sectional area through the vessel. Magnitude images provide anatomical information, whereas phase images provide the flow information.

## Thoracic Aortic and Pulmonary Artery Disease

The major clinical indications for MRI of thoracic aortic and pulmonary artery disease are shown in Table 1. Multiple imaging modalities are available to evaluate thoracic disease: contrast aortography, computed tomography (CT), MRI, and transesophageal echocardiography (TEE). Each of these modalities has advantages and disadvantages.

**TABLE 1** Major Indications for MRI of Thoracic Aortic and Pulmonary Disease

| |
|---|
| Thoracic aorta |
| Acquired diseases |
| Aortic aneurysms (Fig. 1) |
| Aortic dissection (Fig. 2) |
| Post-traumatic changes |
| Aortoannular ectasia |
| Aortitis |
| Aortic neoplasms |
| Aortic thromboembolic disease |
| Septic pseudoaneurysms |
| Periaortic abscesses |
| Congenital diseases of the aorta |
| Coarctation and interruption of the aorta (Fig. 6) |
| Aberrant subclavian artery |
| Double arch and incomplete double arch |
| Cervical arch |
| Marfan's syndrome |
| Pulmonary arteries |
| Congenital abnormalities (Fig. 7) |
| Pulmonary embolus |
| Pulmonary artery hypertension |
| Dilatation and dissection |
| Tumors |
| Branch stenosis |

The normal thoracic aortic dimensions (mean values) are 3.3 cm at the sinus of Valsalva, 3.0 cm in the midascending aorta, and 2.4 cm in the proximal descending aorta. The aorta is considered dilated when the diameter is over 4 cm (Fig. 1). In infants the diameter of the aorta at the isthmus can be as small as 40 percent of the remaining portion of the ascending aorta and still be within normal limits.

MRI is excellent for evaluating aortic dissection (Fig. 2). Both CT and MRI allow determination of the following features: intimal flap, hematoma in the aortic wall, periaortic and pericardial hematoma, the extent of the dissection, and compression of the true lumen by a thrombosed false lumen. In addition, PC-MRI allows for determination of differential flow in the true and false lumens. Pitfalls of MRI are: slow blood flow can cause intraluminal signal intensity, which could be mistaken for a false lumen; fluid in the superior pericardial recess can be mistaken for a dissection; and aneurysms with extensive mural thrombus could be confused with dissection with false lumen. Atypical patterns of aortic dissection consisting of smooth thickening of the aortic wall, and observed more frequently in acute dissection, have been described.

## Acquired Heart Disease

The major clinical indications for MRI of acquired heart disease are shown in Table 2.

### *Pericardial Disease*

MRI is highly effective for the evaluation of pericardial disease and its role is supplementary to echocardiography. The uses of MRI in pericardial disease include: evaluation of pericardial effusions, especially loculated effusions; differentiation between hemorrhagic and nonhemorrhagic pericardial effusions; detection of pericardial metastases or the extension of tumor through the pericardium; diagnosis of constrictive pericarditis;

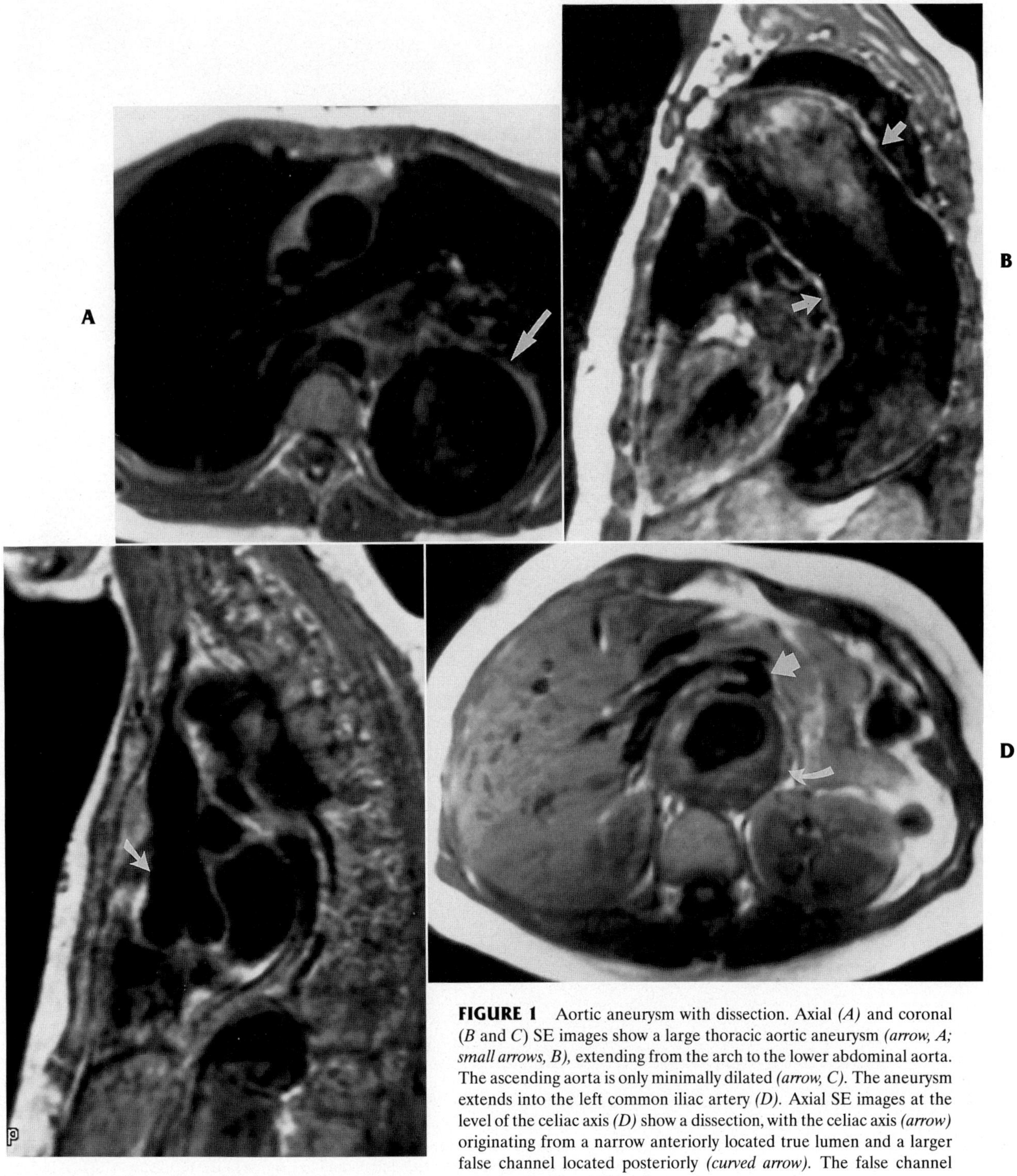

**FIGURE 1** Aortic aneurysm with dissection. Axial *(A)* and coronal (*B* and *C*) SE images show a large thoracic aortic aneurysm *(arrow, A; small arrows, B),* extending from the arch to the lower abdominal aorta. The ascending aorta is only minimally dilated *(arrow, C).* The aneurysm extends into the left common iliac artery *(D).* Axial SE images at the level of the celiac axis *(D)* show a dissection, with the celiac axis *(arrow)* originating from a narrow anteriorly located true lumen and a larger false channel located posteriorly *(curved arrow).* The false channel contains significant thrombus.

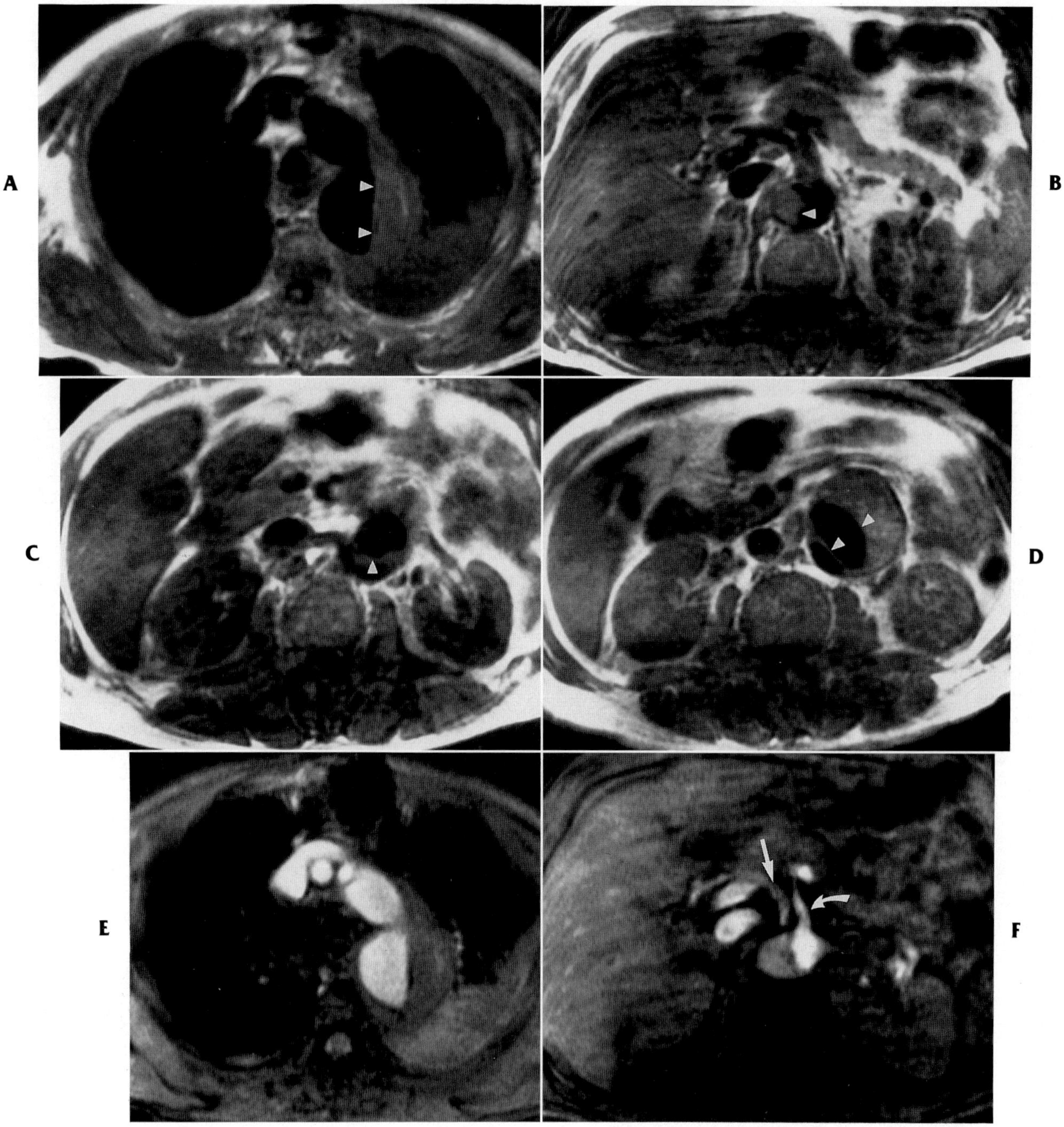


**FIGURE 2** Thoracic aortic dissection extending into an abdominal aortic aneurysm. Transverse ECG gated SE images at the level of the aortic arch *(A)* and at three levels through the midabdominal aorta *(B, C,* and *D)* are shown. The intimal flaps *(arrowheads)* are identified in the aortic arch and in the descending aorta. Signal in the false lumen is increased due to slow flow or chronic thrombus. Cine MRI images at the same levels through the aortic arch *(E)* and abdominal aorta (*F* and *G*) show high signal in the true lumen and low signal in the false lumen. Signal differences are a result of differences in blood flow. The origins of and blood flow in the celiac axis *(arrow, F),* SMA *(curved arrow, F).*

G

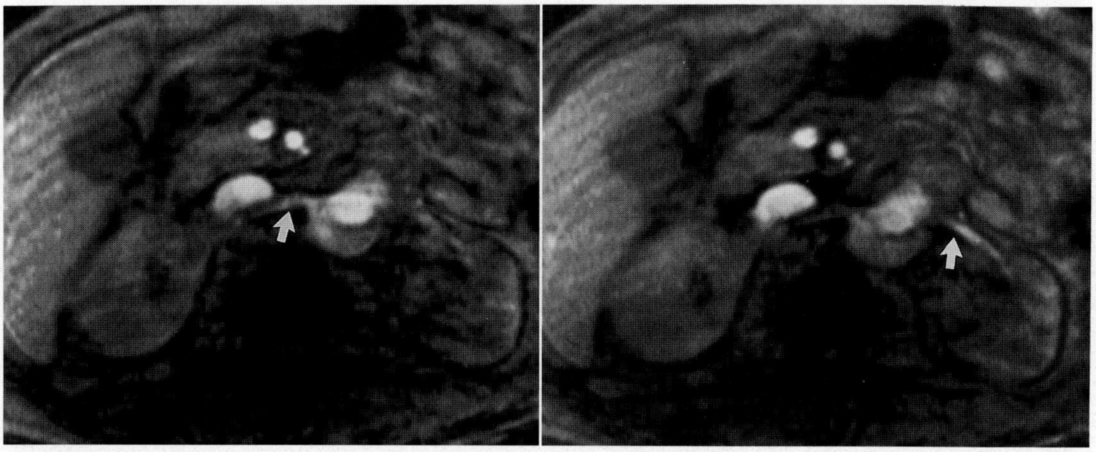

H

**FIGURE 2, cont'd** Renal arteries *(arrows, G* and *H)* are shown. (From Duerinckx AJ, Higgins CB, Pettigrew RI, eds. MRI of the Cardiovascular System: The Raven MRI Teaching File. Raven Press: New York, 1993; with permission.)

**TABLE 2** Major Indications for MRI of Acquired Heart Disease

| |
|---|
| Pericardial disease: |
| Diagnosis of constrictive pericardial disease (Fig. 3) |
| Evaluation of pericardial effusions |
| Paracardiac and intracardiac masses: |
| Evaluation of the presence, location, and extent of masses (Fig. 4) |
| Differentiation of tumor from clot |
| Myocardial disease: |
| Determination of the location and severity of myocardial hypertrophy in hypertrophic cardiomyopathy (Fig. 5) |
| Evaluation of restrictive cardiomyopathy |
| Ischemic heart disease: |
| Determination of the presence, size, and location of previous myocardial infarctions |
| Identification of complications of myocardial infarctions |
| Quantification of cardiac structures and function: |
| Ventricular volume, mass, ejection fraction |
| Quantification of blood flow within the heart and the great vessels, and identification and evaluation of valvular heart disease (Fig. 8, 9): |
| Quantification of the severity of valvular regurgitation (Fig. 8) or stenosis (Fig. 9) |
| Measurement of blood flow in pulmonary arteries |
| Evaluation of arrhythmias: |
| Right ventricular dysplasia |

evaluation of primary pericardial cysts or tumors; and diagnosis of partial or complete absence of the pericardium.

The normal pericardium is 1 to 2 mm thick. The adjacent visceral and parietal layers are bounded externally by pericardial fat and internally by subepicardial fat.

### Pericardial Effusions

A small amount of pericardial fluid is observed in most normal subjects. MRI is highly sensitive for identifying generalized or loculated pericardial effusions. It can also distinguish hemorrhagic from nonhemorrhagic effusions. Hemorrhagic effusions are characterized by high intensity on T1-weighted SE images and low intensity on cine MR images.

### Constrictive Pericarditis

Constrictive pericarditis is ideally diagnosed with MRI. A thickness of 4 mm or greater indicates pericardial thickening, and in the proper clinical setting is the diagnostic finding in constrictive pericarditis (Fig. 3). However, pericardial thickening is also observed for weeks to months after cardiac surgery, in Dressler's syndrome, and during inflammatory processes of the pericardium (acute pericarditis and uremic pericarditis). The inferior vena cava, hepatic veins, and right atrium are substantially dilated, whereas the right ventricle has normal or reduced volume in constrictive pericarditis. An elongated narrow-shaped right ventricle and a sigmoid-shaped ventricular septum are sometimes observed in this disease. Constriction can sometimes be localized to the right side of the heart, or even just the right atrioventricular groove. MRI can easily distinguish between constrictive pericarditis and restrictive cardiomyopathy. No pericardial thickening is noted in constrictive cardiomyopathy.

## *Paracardiac and Intracardiac Masses*

### Paracardiac Masses

MRI, with its wide field of view, has been highly effective in demonstrating pericardial and paracardial masses. Pericardial tumors are much more frequently secondary rather than primary tumors. Secondary pericardial tumors generally occur by extension from mediastinal lung tumors or by metastasis.

The most frequently observed paracardiac masses are (1) pericardial cysts and pseudocysts, (2) enlarged pericardial fat pad, (3) lymphoma, (4) teratoma, (5) diaphragmatic eventration and hernia, and (6) metastatic carcinoma and extension of anterior thoracic tumors.

### Intracardiac Masses

SE MRI has been highly effective at demonstrating the presence, location, extent, and in some instances also the nature of intracardiac masses. The most frequent intracardiac mass is a thrombus, which is usually located in the left atrium or left ventricle. Secondary tumors of the heart are 40 to 50 times more frequent than primary tumors. They originate from direct spread, extension, or metastasis. The significance of MRI is that it shows the extent of tumor that is attached to the cardiac wall in cases of tumor extension through the inferior vena cava from primary tumors from the abdomen.

The most frequent benign tumors are the myxoma in the left

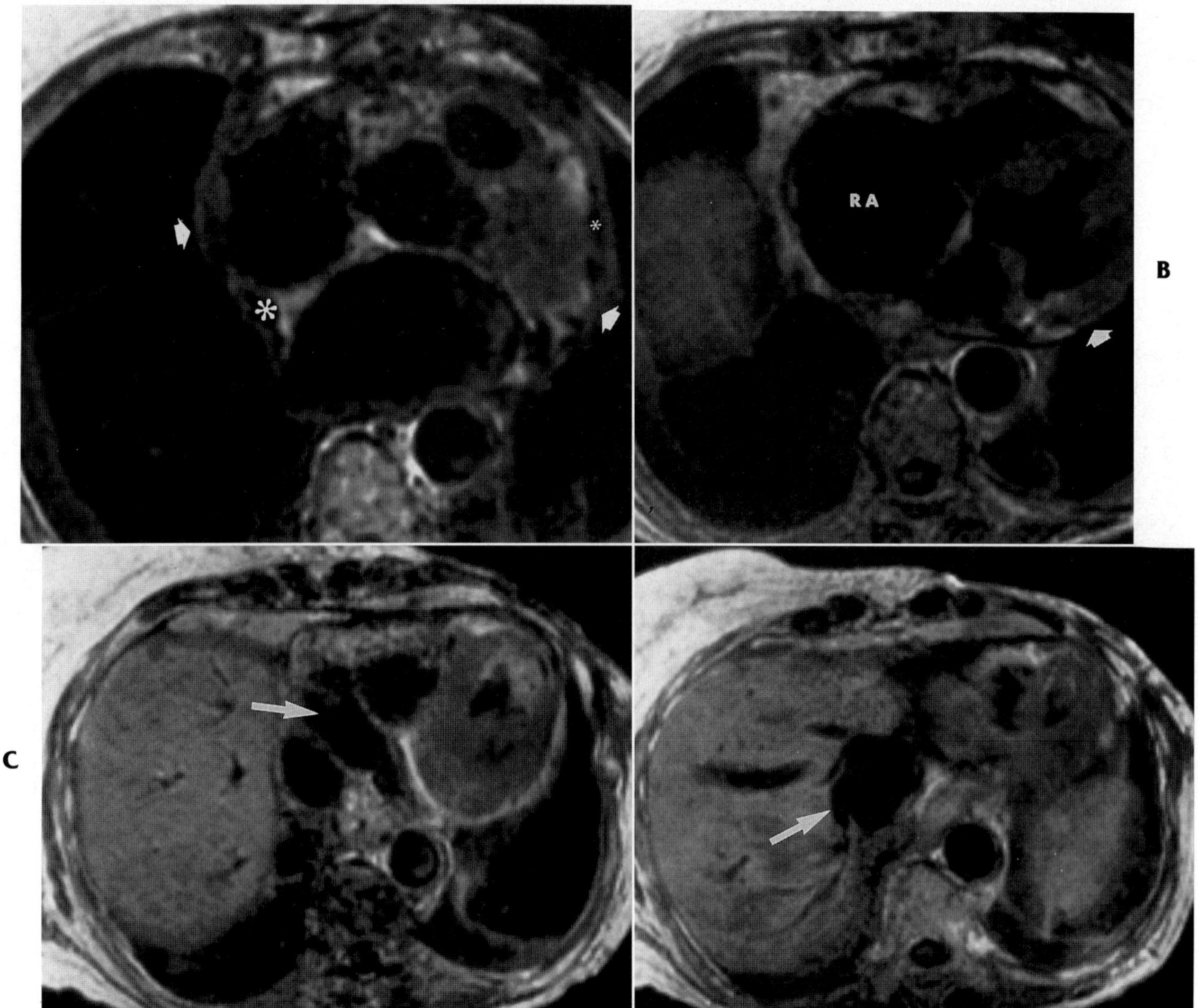


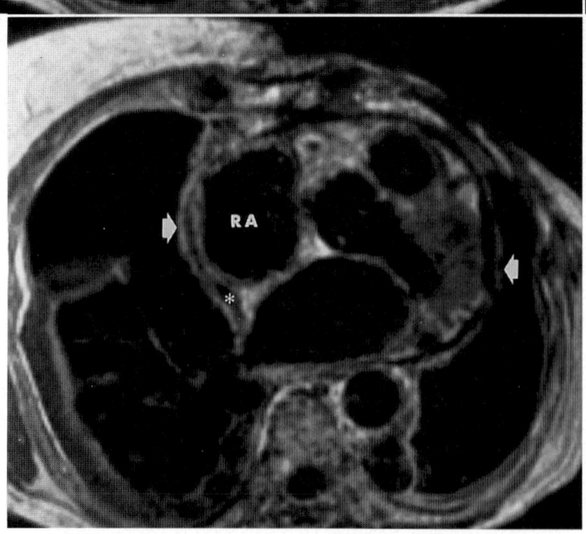


**FIGURE 3** Constrictive pericarditis in a patient with metastatic breast carcinoma. ECG-gated transaxial T1-weighted SE images at different levels through the atria and ventricles *(A* and *B)* show the thickened pericardium *(arrows)* and pericardial effusion (*). The thickened parietal pericardial line produces a low intensity and is recognized between the subepicardial and the pericardial fat layers. Pericardial effusion has low signal intensity. The coronary sinus *(arrow, C)* and inferior vena cava *(arrow, D)* are dilated. The right atrium (RA) is enlarged. Postgadolinium images show the pericardial effusion (*) and enhancement of the pericardium *(arrows, E).* Bilateral pleural effusions are present. (From Duerinckx AJ, Higgins CB, Pettigrew RI, eds. MRI of the Cardiovascular System: The Raven MRI Teaching File. Raven Press: New York, 1993; with permission.)

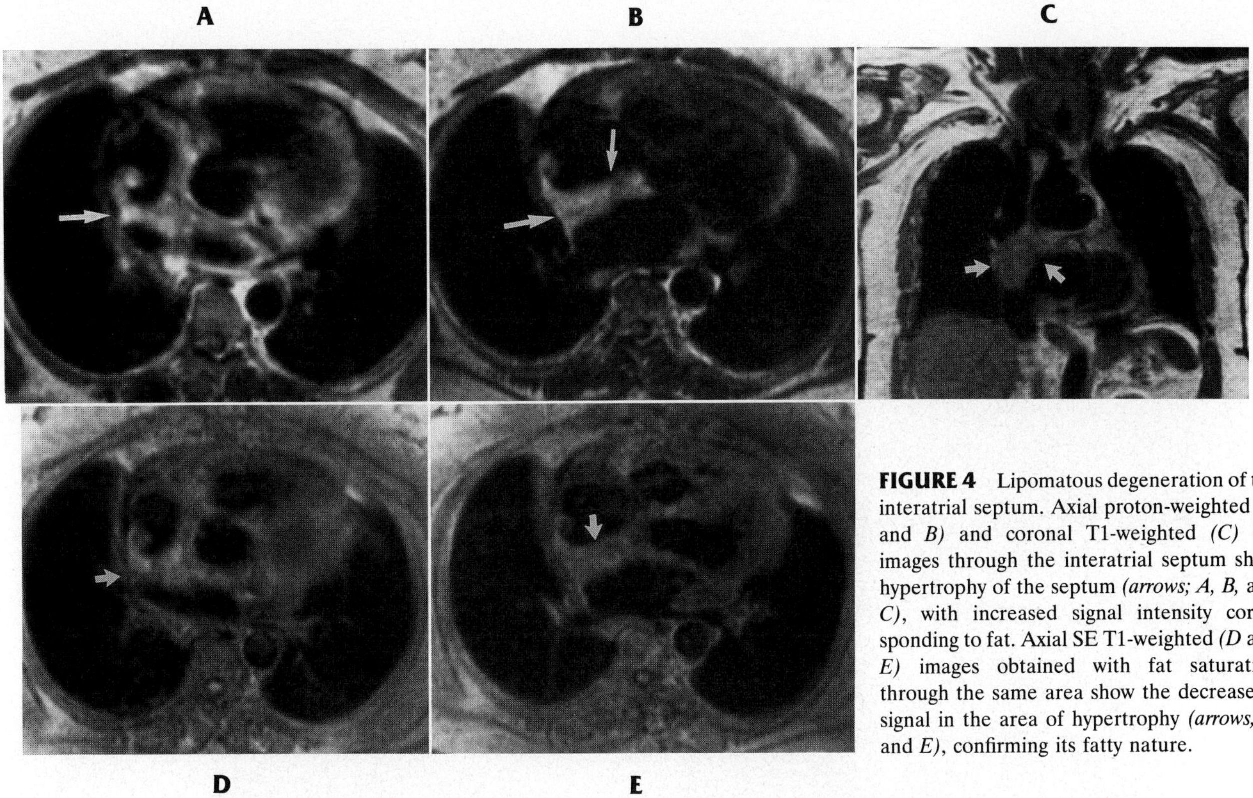


**FIGURE 4** Lipomatous degeneration of the interatrial septum. Axial proton-weighted *(A* and *B)* and coronal T1-weighted *(C)* SE images through the interatrial septum show hypertrophy of the septum *(arrows; A, B,* and *C)*, with increased signal intensity corresponding to fat. Axial SE T1-weighted *(D* and *E)* images obtained with fat saturation through the same area show the decrease in signal in the area of hypertrophy *(arrows, D* and *E)*, confirming its fatty nature.

atrium and the lipoma in the right atrium. This includes the cases of lipomatous degeneration of the atrial septum, which are best visualized by using T1-weighted and FATSAT sequences (Fig. 4). The most common malignant intracardiac tumor is the angiosarcoma, which usually involves the right atrium. In children the most common tumor is the rhabdomyoma. Some rhabdomyomas have demonstrated higher signal intensity than the myocardium. Another tumor is fibroma, which usually has low signal on the T2 images.

### Differentiation Between Clot and Tumor Thrombus

MRI can frequently differentiate between tumor thrombus and blood clot. MRI is superior to echocardiography for the visualization of clots in the atrial appendage or along the lateral left atrial wall. On SE sequences, fresh clot has bright signal intensity and an older clot has low signal intensity. Tumors have high signal intensity on SE T2-weighted images. On GRE images, clot has signal intensity lower than myocardium and solid organs, whereas tumor has medium signal intensity. Atrial myxomas may have a signal intensity indistinguishable from that of clot on cine MRI. They may have very low signal intensity because of the presence of considerable fibrosis, calcification, and iron within the tumor. Another method for differentiating tumor from thrombus is the use of gadolinium-DTPA. Contrast medium enhances tumor but does not enhance clots.

## *Myocardial Disease*

MRI has been used for the evaluation of congestive cardiomyopathy, hypertrophic cardiomyopathy, and restrictive cardiomyopathy. The SE technique is used to demonstrate the morphological abnormalities, whereas cine MRI can demonstrate functional abnormalities.

### Congestive Cardiomyopathy

In congestive cardiomyopathy SE MRI has demonstrated dilatation of the ventricles, the usually normal wall thickness, and in cases of ischemic cardiomyopathy, the extreme wall thinning in regions of prior myocardial infarct. Cine MRI can provide accurate and highly reproducible quantification of the left ventricular mass, volumes, ejection fraction, wall thickness, and wall stress.

### Hypertrophic Cardiomyopathy

The major role of MRI has been to document the presence of unusual forms of hypertrophic cardiomyopathy, since there is considerable variation in the ventricular morphology in these patients. The different focal forms of hypertrophy can involve the outflow septum (Fig. 5), entire septum, midventricle, and apex. Cine MRI has been used to demonstrate functional abnormalities and associated mitral valve abnormalities.

### Restrictive Cardiomyopathy

Imaging studies are usually done to differentiate between constrictive pericarditis and restrictive cardiomyopathy. MRI is highly useful in making this distinction, since the pericardium has normal thickness in restrictive cardiomyopathy. The wall thickness of either or both ventricles is usually increased in restrictive cardiomyopathy associated with amyloidosis. In amyloidosis the ejection fraction is decreased. There is often evidence of mitral and tricuspid regurgitation. Stasis of blood in the atria causes bright signal within the atrium on SE images.

## *Ischemic Heart Disease*

MRI has multiple applications for the evaluation of ischemic heart disease. It allows determination of the size and extent of the myocardial infarct, and the amount of residual myocardium. It also demonstrates complications of myocardial

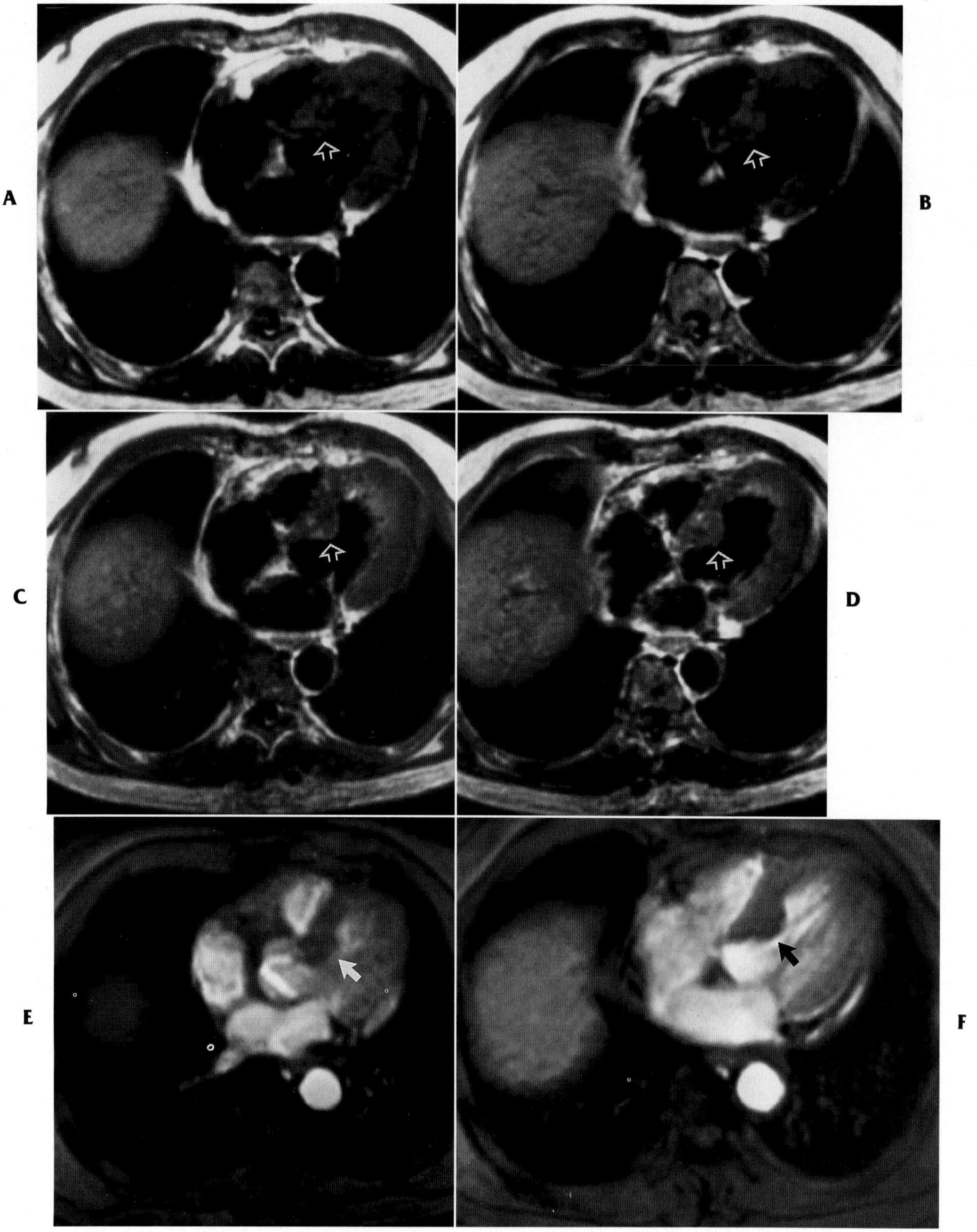


**FIGURE 5** Focal hypertrophy of the outflow septum. Axial SE T1 images *(A* and *B)* through the interventricular septum show a focal bulge *(open arrow)* in the interventricular septum. Postgadolinium axial SE images at the same level *(C* and *D)* show minimal inhomogeneous enhancement of this focal mass *(open arrow)*. Cine MRI images *(E* and *F)* confirm that this mass *(arrow)* is part of the septum. (From Duerinckx AJ, Higgins CB, Pettigrew RI, eds. MRI of the Cardiovascular System: The Raven MRI Teaching File. Raven Press: New York, 1993; with permission.)

infarcts, such as aneurysm and thrombus. True and false aneurysms can be distinguished by MRI. False aneurysms are usually larger, have a small ostium, and are typically located on the posterior or diaphragmatic wall. Thrombi are easily recognized in both subacute and chronic forms, which each have different signal characteristics. Regions of acute myocardial infarct (<3 weeks old) have increased signal on the T2-weighted SE images. In patients with chronic myocardial infarcts, there is evidence of wall thinning and disturbed left ventricular function with stasis of blood during systole.

Cine MRI can be used to quantify the regional myocardial function. Normal myocardium has up to 60 percent wall thickening and more than 2 mm absolute wall thickening. Abnormal regions are easily detected. The potential future use of gadolinium to study regional myocardial perfusion is being investigated.

**TABLE 3** Major Indications for MRI of Congenital Heart Disease

| |
|---|
| Evaluation of thoracic aortic anomalies (Fig. 6) |
| Definition of the pulmonary artery morphology (the presence, central confluence, size) in pulmonary atresia, tetralogy of Fallot, and other right-sided obstructive lesions (Fig. 7) |
| Definition of intracardiac and extracardiac morphology of complex ventricular anomalies |
| Determination of pulmonary venous connections and other pulmonary venous anomalies |
| Monitoring of the status of patients after surgical procedures for congenital heart disease |
| Determination of situs abnormalities |
| Identification of systemic venous anomalies |
| Quantification of blood flow separately in the right and left pulmonary arteries |

## Congenital Heart Disease

The major clinical indications for MRI of congenital heart disease are shown in Table 3. SE MRI is used to demonstrate the normal segmental anatomy of the heart. Axial cuts are obtained from the top of the aorta to the diaphragm. Depending on the pathology, additional oblique views can be used (i.e., LAO-equivalent to evaluate coarctation). The following structures can easily be visualized: the great vessels (relative size and position); the situs (epiarterial and hyperarterial bronchi); the pulmonary venous return; the ventricular loop (infundibulum in the right ventricle); the atrioventricular connections; the atrioventricular septa; and the systemic venous return. Cine MRI is used to determine abnormal flow across intracardiac defects and across sites of obstruction.

The following specific abnormalities have been studied effectively by MRI: coarctation of the aorta (Fig. 6), abnormal situs, transposition of the great arteries, double-outlet right ventricle, truncus arteriosus, tetralogy of Fallot, pulmonary stenosis (Fig. 7) and atresia, and atrial and ventricular septal defects. MRI has been used to evaluate patients postoperatively after surgery involving supracardiac anastomosis (Rastelli, Fontan, Damus, Norwood, and Jatene) or systemic-to-pulmonary artery shunts (Fig. 7).

## Quantification of Cardiac Function

Cine MRI and PC-MRI allow for quantification of cardiac dimensions and contractile function and blood flow in the heart and great vessels. Cine MRI provides a 3D data set with adequate temporal resolution and thereby is likely the most precise and reproductive technique for quantification of ventricular dimensions and function. PC-MRI provides a direct measurement of forward and retrograde flow across cardiac valves.

### *Global Ventricular Function*

Ventricular function can be assessed using cine MRI to acquire multiple images for each cardiac cycle. Cine MRI allows acquisition of images at a rate of 16 to 30 frames per cardiac cycle. After obtaining 10 to 12 tomographic slices encompassing the entire heart from apex to the base, the left and right ventricular volumes can be calculated using the multislice summation technique (i.e., the sum of the cavity area times the slice thickness). These calculations can be repeated at different portions of the cardiac cycle, such as end systole and the end diastole. This allows the determination of the end-diastolic and end-systolic volumes, ejection fraction, and cardiac output for the right and left ventricles.

### *Regional Myocardial Function*

The use of short-axis planes is essential for the measurements of left ventricular wall thickening during the cardiac cycle. Cine MRI defines both the endocardial and epicardial borders. Wall motion abnormalities and wall thickening can easily be determined.

### *Measurements of Blood Flow*

Both bolus tagging (TOF technique) and PC-MRI techniques allow for determination of flow velocity and vessel cross section. This flow information can then be used to determine the flow volume through the ascending aorta and main pulmonary artery, which allows determination of stroke volumes and shunt flow, and evaluation of valvular regurgitation.

Phase-contrast cine MRI has been used to measure flow separately in the right and left pulmonary arteries and to quantitate flow in pulmonary arteries after lung transplant surgery. It has been shown that in normal pulmonary arteries, there is almost no retrograde flow during diastole or systole. In the case of pulmonary arterial hypertension, the peak velocity of blood flow is achieved earlier during systole, and there is retrograde flow during portions of both systole and diastole. Moreover, it has been noted that directional blood flow in the pulmonary arteries during systole is antegrade in some regions and retrograde in other regions in patients with pulmonary arterial hypertension.

### *Valvular Heart Disease*

The combination of cine MRI and PC-MRI can be used to evaluate patients with valvular heart disease.

On cine MR images, the severity of valvular regurgitation can be estimated by measuring various dimensions or volumes of the flow void caused by the regurgitation (Fig. 8). The volume of flow void can be quantitated on adjacent images encompassing the chamber receiving the regurgitant flow. Such quantification can differentiate between mild, moderate, and

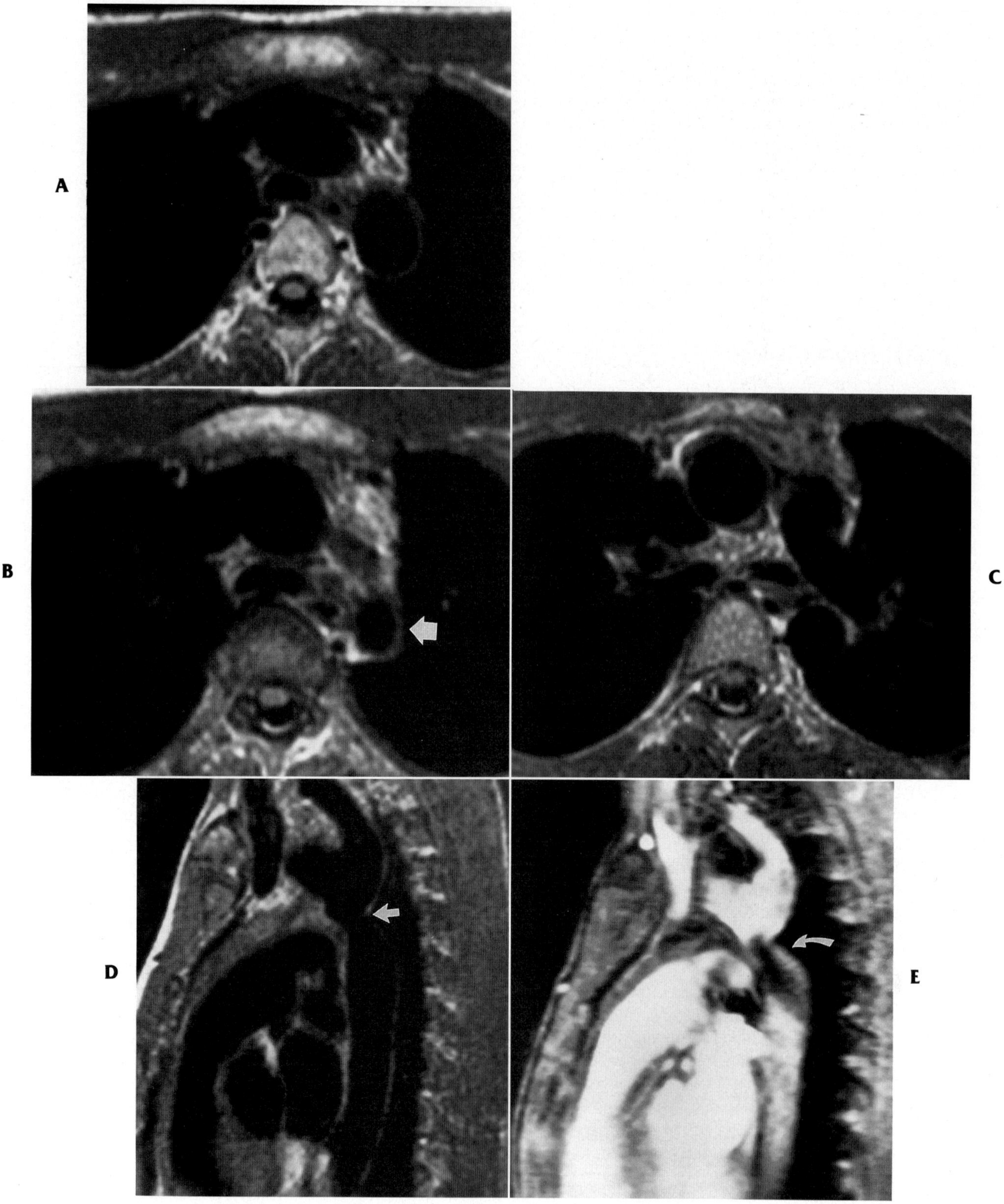


**FIGURE 6** Coarctation of the aorta. Axial SE images *(A, B,* and *C)* at three consecutive levels (5 mm thick slices) through the proximal descending aorta show the focal narrowing *(arrow, B)* of the aorta. This is confirmed on a coronal-oblique SE image *(arrow, D)*. A coronal oblique cine MR image *(E)* demonstrates the systolic flow jet *(curved arrow)* across the area of coarctation. (From Duerinckx AJ, Higgins CB, Pettigrew RI, eds. MRI of the Cardiovascular System: The Raven MRI Teaching File. Raven Press: New York, 1993; with permission.)

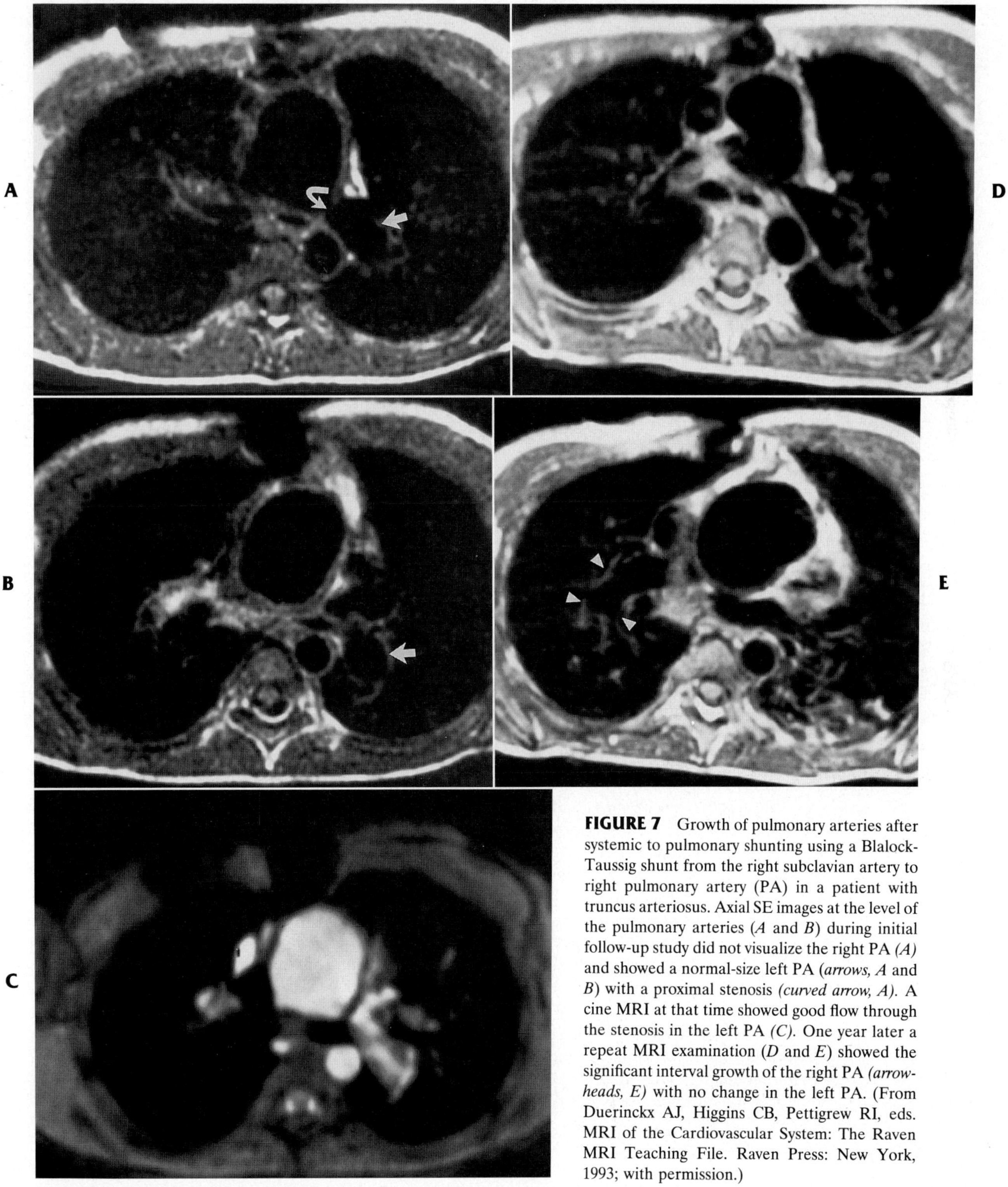


**FIGURE 7** Growth of pulmonary arteries after systemic to pulmonary shunting using a Blalock-Taussig shunt from the right subclavian artery to right pulmonary artery (PA) in a patient with truncus arteriosus. Axial SE images at the level of the pulmonary arteries (*A* and *B*) during initial follow-up study did not visualize the right PA *(A)* and showed a normal-size left PA (*arrows, A* and *B*) with a proximal stenosis *(curved arrow, A)*. A cine MRI at that time showed good flow through the stenosis in the left PA *(C)*. One year later a repeat MRI examination (*D* and *E*) showed the significant interval growth of the right PA *(arrowheads, E)* with no change in the left PA. (From Duerinckx AJ, Higgins CB, Pettigrew RI, eds. MRI of the Cardiovascular System: The Raven MRI Teaching File. Raven Press: New York, 1993; with permission.)

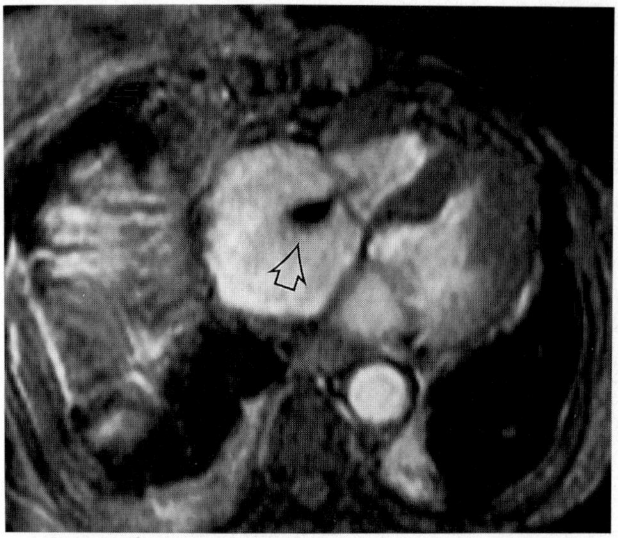

**FIGURE 8** Tricuspid regurgitation in patient with constrictive pericarditis. A cine MR axial image during systole at the level of the tricuspid valve shows the area of flow void *(arrow)* due to turbulence in the regurgitant jet. The thickened pericardium and dilated right atrium are also shown. (From Duerinckx AJ, Higgins CB, Pettigrew RI, eds. MRI of the Cardiovascular System: The Raven MRI Teaching File. Raven Press: New York, 1993; with permission.)

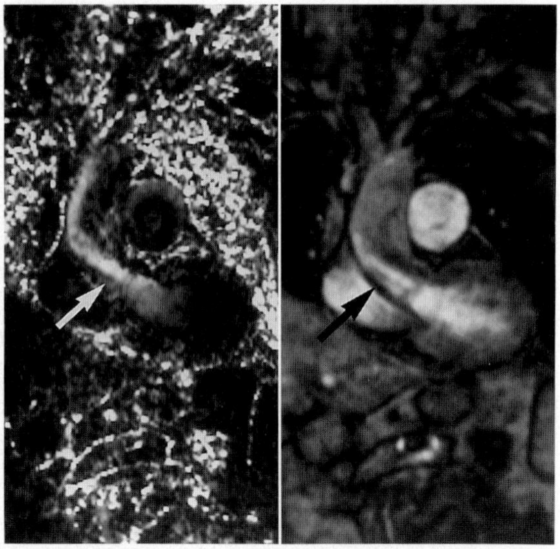


**FIGURE 9** Aortic stenosis. Coronal phase-contrast MRI *(A)* and cine MRI *(B)* images through the proximal ascending aorta and aortic valve area show the flow jet *(arrows)*. The signal intensity within areas of flow on the phase-contrast MR image is proportional to the speed of blood flow. Thus, from the phase-contrast MR image the velocity at any point within the flow jet can be determined. (From Duerinckx AJ, Higgins CB, Pettigrew RI, eds. MRI of the Cardiovascular System: The Raven MRI Teaching File. Raven Press: New York, 1993; with permission.)

severe lesions in both the aortic and mitral regurgitation and has correlated with echocardiographic and/or angiographic gradings.

Another method for quantification of aortic regurgitation is PC-MRI (Fig. 9). Usually the cardiac cycle is segmented into 15 to 30 phase-contrast images equally spaced throughout the cycle. For each image, the average velocity in a cross-sectional area of the aorta and pulmonary artery is measured. Instantaneous blood flow is calculated as the product of average flow velocity in the cross section and the area of the great artery. Integration of blood flow values from images in systole estimates stroke volume for the left and right ventricles. The technique can distinguish between antegrade and retrograde flow, so that retrograde flow in diastole can be measured to directly quantify aortic regurgitation. Aortic regurgitation can be estimated in two ways with this technique. For isolated aortic regurgitation, difference in calculated stroke volume between the two ventricles is the regurgitation volume. The retrograde flow in the aorta is a direct measurement of regurgitation and should be valid even in the presence of pulmonic regurgitation. Integration of the area under the retrograde part of the flow curve is a measure of the volume of aortic regurgitation.

The peak systolic ejection flow in cases of aortic stenosis can be measured, using PC-MRI, which then allows the estimation of the aortic valve pressure gradient using the Bernoulli equation. Mitral flow can also be quantitated using PC-MRI.

## New Frontiers

### *Coronary Artery Imaging*

Spiral scanning and *k*-space segmented TurboFLASH have provided images of portions of and even long segments of the coronary arteries (Fig. 10). Echo-planar techniques are also very promising for coronary artery imaging. This may open up a whole new area of applications for cardiac MRI.

### *Myocardial Motion and Strain*

A newer technique for regional myocardial function determination is the use of myocardial tagging to quantitate myocardial motion and local deformation (the strain). These techniques spatially encode a pattern of tags in the myocardium before imaging. In the MR images, these tags appear as a set of dark lines. Any translation or rotation motion occurring between the period of tag placement and the imaging sequence will cause these dark bands to be displaced in the image.

Another recently developed technique for myocardial motion analysis uses phase-contrast cine MRI. Phase-contrast cine MRI acquisitions provide information on the velocity as a function of position. This information is used to calculate changes in position between frames taken at different points in the cardiac cycle. This interval change in position allows for calculation of myocardial strain. The clinical utility of this approach has not been fully determined.

### *Perfusion Imaging Using Contrast Agents*

The role of MRI in ischemic heart disease has been relatively minor up to the present time and has been limited primarily to the demonstration of the complications of acute myocardial infarction. The differentiation of normal from ischemic myocardium using MRI has been accomplished by demonstrating the differential distribution of MRI contrast media. Most information has been obtained in experimental models. The jeopardy zone produced by an acute coronary occlusion is demonstrated as a region of decreased signal intensity using

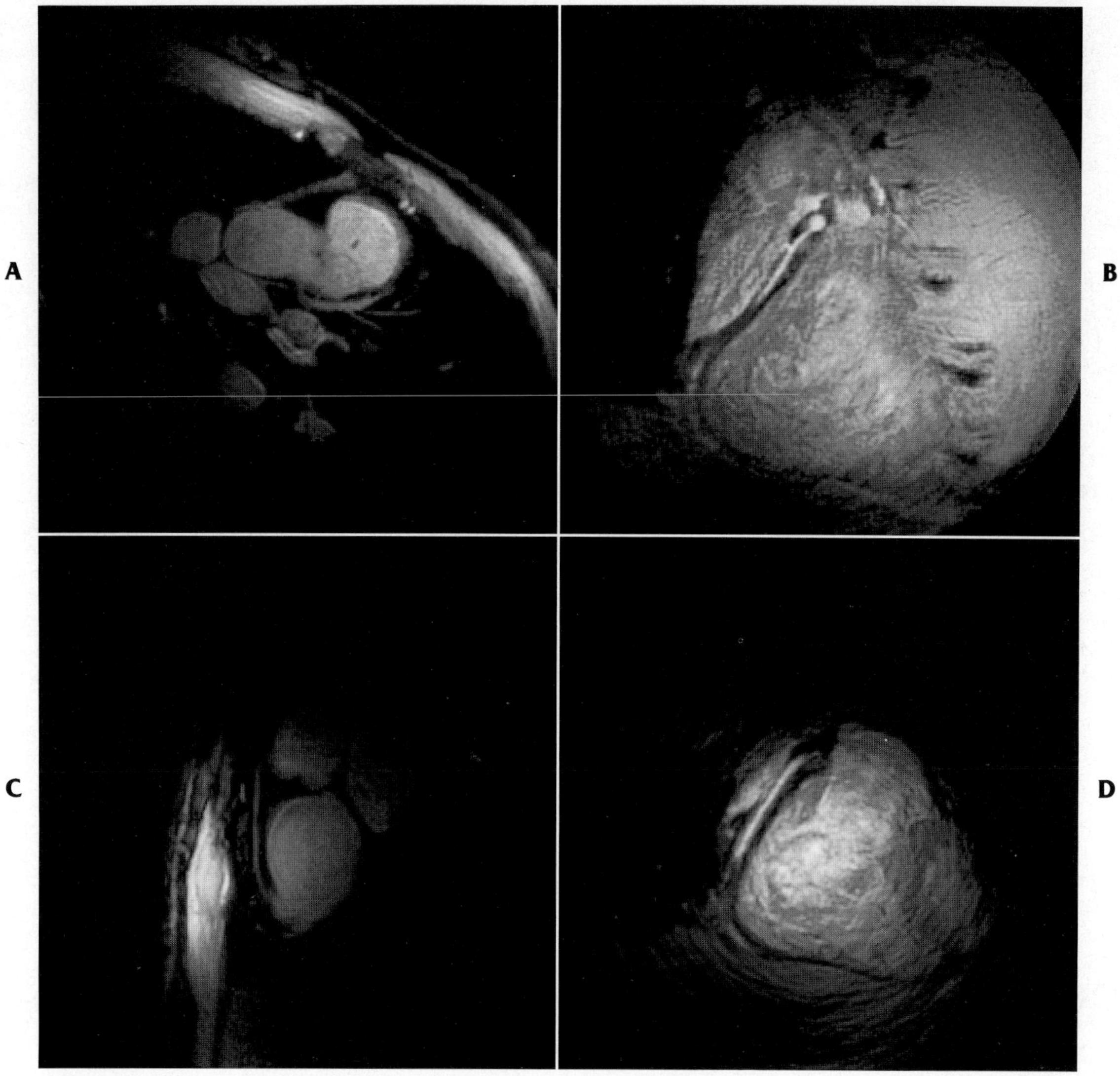


**FIGURE 10** Normal coronary arteries using MRI spiral scanning technique. *A,* Oblique axial view of the LAD and several diagonal branches. *B,* Axial view of the RCA. *C,* Double oblique image of the RCA. *D,* Coronal view of the RCA. (Courtesy Craig H. Meyer, Information Systems Laboratory, Stanford, Calif.)

T1-enhancing contrast media, and is shown as a region of increased (hot spot) signal intensity with the use of magnetic susceptibility agents. In humans paramagnetic contrast media, such as Gd-DTPA, have been shown to increase the signal intensity of the entire infarction (or the periphery of the infarction) during the acute and subacute phases.

## Discussion

Our experience agrees with a recent survey of 70 MRI sites, which revealed that cardiac MRI is most often used in the evaluation of acquired thoracic disease, congenital cardiac malformations, and para- and intracardiac masses. Cardiac MRI is most often used to delineate anatomic abnormalities. Evaluation of ventricular and valvular dysfunction is the most common functional objective.

### *Comparison of MRI and Other Cardiac-Imaging Techniques*

Both standard SE and cine MRI are inherently 3D techniques allowing for quantification of volumes and globular ventricular function. This is an advantage over techniques such as 2D echocardiography and angiography, which provide measurements based on geometrical assumptions regarding the shape of the ventricles. The advantages of MRI over other tomographic techniques such as CT are that MRI does not require ionizing radiation or injection of contrast media.

The advantages of MRI over echocardiography are (1) the better edge definition of the ventricular walls, (2) a wider field of view, and (3) independence of image quality from either operator experience or body habitus of the patients. Echocardiography has the advantages of greater functionality among clinicians in addition to portability and lower cost.

MRI is also superior to radionuclide imaging because of the greater temporal and spatial resolution. However, MRI has not currently been shown to be effective for demonstrating regional myocardial perfusion necessary for the detection of myocardial ischemia, such as is possible with thallium scintigraphy. However, recent work on the usage of MRI contrast agents with rapid imaging techniques for myocardial perfusion shows that this may become feasible in the near future.

MRI provides both anatomical and functional diagnosis of acquired and congenital heart disease. It is the most precise technique for the quantification of ventricular dimension and function. The measurements are highly reproducible between studies, indicating that MRI can be used for the assessment of response to therapeutic interventions in a variety of cardiac disease states.

## Suggested Reading

Caputo GR. Coronary arteries: Potential for MR imaging (editorial). Radiology 1991; 181:629–630.

Caputo GR, Kondo C, Masui T, et al. Right and left lung perfusion: In vitro and in vivo validation with oblique-angle, velocity-encoded cine-MR imaging. Radiology 1991; 180:693–698.

Dulce MC, Mostbeck GH, O'Sullivan M, et al. Monitoring of the severity of aortic regurgitation: Interstudy reproducibility of velocity encoded cine MR measurements of aortic regurgitation. Radiology (in press).

Higgins CB. Congenital heart disease. In: Higgins CB, Hricak H, Helms CA, eds. Magnetic Resonance Imaging of the Body. New York: Raven Press, 1992:567.

Higgins CB. The vascular system. In: Higgins CB, Hricak H, Helms CA, eds. Magnetic Resonance Imaging of the Body. New York: Raven Press, 1992:629.

Higgins CB, Caputo GR. Acquired heart disease. In: Higgins CB, Hricak H, Helms CA, eds. Magnetic Resonance Imaging of the Body. New York: Raven Press, 1992:525.

Higgins CB, Saeed MM, Wendland MF. The myocardium. In: Higgins CB, Hricak H, Helms CA, eds. Magnetic Resonance Imaging of the Body. New York: Raven Press, 1992:1289.

Higgins CB, Silverman NH, Kersting-Sommerhoff BA, Schmidt K, eds. Congenital Heart Disease: Echocardiography and Magnetic Resonance Imaging. New York: Raven Press, 1990.

Kondo C, Caputo GR, Masui T, et al. Pulmonary hypertension: Pulmonary flow quantification and flow profile analysis with velocity-encoded cine MR imaging. Radiology 1992; 183:751–759.

Masui T, Finck S, Higgins CB. Constrictive pericarditis and restrictive cardiomyopathy: Evaluation with MR imaging. Radiology 1992; 182:369–373.

Mohiuddin RH, Amanuma M, Kilner PJ, et al. MR Phase-shift velocity mapping of mitral and pulmonary venous flow. JCAT 1991; 15:237–243.

Mohiuddin RH, Paz R, Theodoropoulos S, et al. Magnetic resonance characterization of pulmonary arterial blood flow after single lung transplantation. J Thorac Cardiovasc Surg 1991; 101:1016–1023.

Petasnick JP. Radiologic evaluation of aortic dissection. State of the art. Radiology 1991; 180:297–305.

Seelos K, Caputo GR, Carrol CL, et al. Cine gradient refocused (GRE) echo imaging of intravascular masses: Differentiation between tumor and nontumorous thrombus. JCAT 1992; 16: 169–175.

Wagner S, Auffermann W, Buser P, et al. Diagnostic accuracy and estimation of the severity of valvular regurgitation from the signal void in cine MR. Am Heart J 1989; 118:760–767.

White RD, Ehman RL, Weinreb JC. Cardiovascular MR imaging: Current level of clinical activity. J Magn Reson Imaging 1992; 2:365–370.

# Echocardiography

*CONRADE CARL JAFFE, M.D.*

Echocardiography is most commonly employed to solve clinical problems in the following categories:

- Abnormal chest radiograph (cardiomegaly)
- Clinical murmur (valve disease, shunts)
- Chest pain
- Assessment of left ventricular function
- Assessment of left ventricular hypertrophy
- Endocarditis

## Indications, Clinical Utility, and Alternative Technologies

Since echocardiography has no significant biologic adverse effects and is highly diagnostic for a large spectrum of cardiac disorders, portable, readily repeatable, potentially inexpensive, and convenient, the indications for use of this technique are initiated at relatively modest diagnostic uncertainty and are primarily limited by the experience of the clinician. The main impediment to diagnosis is an adequate acoustic window into the heart free from lung interference. But much of even this limitation is obviated by the ready availability of the minimally invasive transesophageal technique, which offers superb valvar and chamber imaging. In experienced hands, echocardiography reveals considerable information of high specificity regarding the anatomic configuration within the pericardium. Echocardiography offers unchallenged usefulness for the diagnosis of pericardial effusions, valvular stenosis, insufficiency and vegetations, myocardial thickness, regional wall motion, and pragmatic clinically effective assessment of left ventricular ejection fraction.

Alternative technologies available include angiography, cine computed tomography (CT), nuclear blood pool and myocardial perfusion imaging, and magnetic resonance imaging (MRI). Despite the capacity of echocardiography to visualize the proximal coronary arteries, especially by the transesophageal technique, coronary arteriography remains unchallenged for diagnosis of coronary insufficiency. On issues of valvular stenosis and regurgitation, however, experience has proved that combined two-dimensional and Doppler echocardiography correlates so well with catheterization data that catheterization is now less of a primary diagnostic tool on those questions and is more commonly employed in these cases to assess coronary anatomy before valve surgery. Cine CT offers some ability to reveal myocardial motion and chamber sizes, but requires injection of intravenous iodinated contrast material, is generally nonrepeatable without risk of significant radiation dose, is nonportable, and expensive.

Cardiac gated MRI, particularly with high-speed acquisition, offers generally excellent anatomic definition of the heart in predictable tomographic orientations. MRI is particularly advantageous for mediastinal masses that may include the heart, and great vessel diseases such as congenital malformations, coarctations, and dissections. Its shortcomings, however, include poorer image quality in patients with arrhythmias, lack of portability, difficulty with monitoring and imaging patients on respirators, and expense. In addition, it is contraindicated for patients with pacing wires. Despite a useful ability of MRI to provide some valve and intracardiac flow definition, echocardiography has such high temporal and spatial resolution, particularly with transesophageal technique, that echocardiography is likely to remain the pre-eminent tool for diagnosis of valve disease for the foreseeable future. Nuclear cardiac imaging offers both blood pool imaging for ejection fraction estimation and myocardial perfusion imaging for localization of coronary insufficiency. Although not free of its own limitations and artifacts, quantitative ejection fraction calculation by nuclear technique can be considered to have a reproducibility superior to echocardiography. Where sequential assessment of ejection fraction is required for monitoring therapeutic progress or coronary perfusion deficit detection, nuclear imaging would be the tool of choice. But from a pragmatic clinical point of view, day-to-day assessment of normal, moderately depressed, or markedly depressed cardiac function can certainly be easily achieved by visual observation on cardiac echocardiography.

## Technical Approach

Although emphysematous elderly patients notoriously generate noisy echocardiograms, much can be done to overcome these difficulties. But even very noisy images are remarkably informative for narrow diagnostic questions (e.g., to rule out pericardial effusion, which can be done even on the noisiest of images). The key to optimal imaging is patience, a methodical approach, placing the patient in a high left-lateral decubitus position, and use of the end-expiratory and end-inspiratory positions as appropriate. Modern ultrasound equipment optimized for cardiac studies encourages the use of the highest possible scanning frequency for best resolution, and most instruments now offer adequate signal penetration and recovery.

Color Doppler imaging is used to quickly survey the four valves for regurgitation, but a thorough evaluation requires careful pulsed-wave Doppler interrogation of the atria and outflow tracts, and continuous-wave Doppler is employed to accurately measure the velocity of stenotic jets. The Bernoulli equation, which relates transvalvular pressure to that velocity, is used to estimate valve gradients. When interatrial shunts are questioned, rapid injection of bubble contrast material (saline agitated with air) intravenously safely allows swirling signals entering the right-sided atrium to be observed for any evidence of inappropriate crossing over to the left side of the circulation.

Transesophageal echocardiography has become convenient and is readily offered when endocarditis or prosthetic valve imaging is required or whenever a high-resolution image is required for diagnostic certainty (Fig. 1). Steerable transesophageal probes of high frequency (5 MHz) are now available in biplane configuration and of small diameter even for pediatric patients. Individuals can be evaluated as outpatients with minimal light sedation (1 to 3 mg of midazolam hydrochloride [Versed] given IV) and topical lidocaine viscous liquid and spray to the oropharynx. No routine antibiotic prophylaxis is required. With reassurance, the patient in the left lateral position will usually swallow the probe in a few minutes. The probe can be guided to the proper position for viewing behind the left-sided atrium. With no lung to interfere with the acoustic path, the imaging is superb and the procedure can generally be concluded within 45 minutes.

## Diagnostic Approach

### *Cardiomegaly*

Cardiomegaly or abnormal configuration of the heart on chest radiograph is readily resolved by conventional two-dimensional real-time echocardiography. Unless otherwise indicated, examination by using a methodical sequence of imaging planes should be performed to avoid errors of

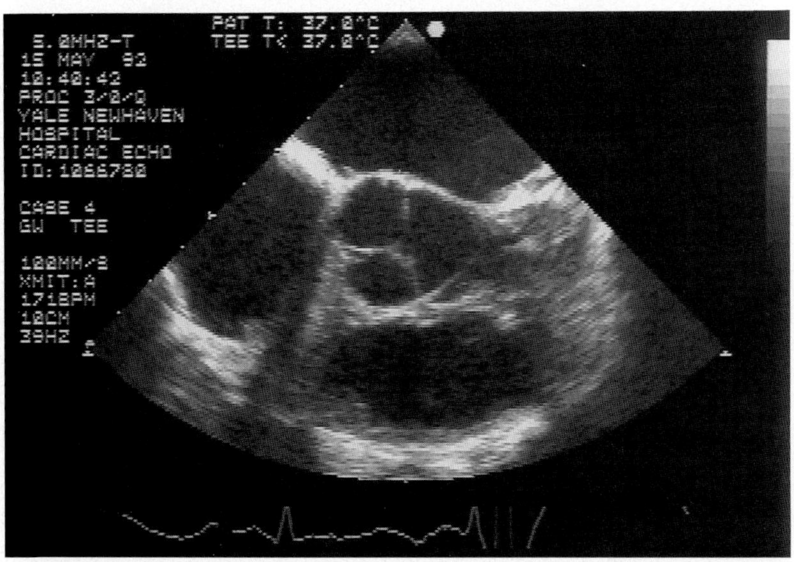


**FIGURE 1** Transesophageal short-axis view of the aortic valve shows the fine detail and resolution offered by this technique.

omission. Standard imaging sequences include parasternal long-axis and short-axis multiple views as well as apical long-axis and four-chamber views. M-mode examination is now seldom used as a primary diagnostic modality, and two-dimensional imaging is sufficient for characterizing the size and shape of the chambers. Current equipment allows freeze-framing of end diastole and end systole, as well as on-screen linear and area measurements of the various chambers and great vessels. Published tables are available for the range of normal dimensions. With experience those measurements should be reviewed qualitatively to be sure they are consistent with judgment of the relative size of each chamber to each other, such as the left-sided atrium versus the left-sided ventricle. Although the dimensions usually quoted are linear ones, it is important to observe and record qualitative shape and function abnormalities of the various regional segments of the myocardium.

Dimensional measurements of the right-sided chambers are more problematic, and it is more difficult to determine when right ventricular enlargement has truly occurred, since the shape of that chamber is in the form of a crescent. Cardiomegaly caused by pericardial fluid collections are easily recognized on the echocardiogram. Distinguishing between pleural versus pericardial fluid is generally simple and reliable. Pericardial fluid has a distinct location, being contained laterally and anteriorly, a configuration not shared by pleural effusions. Once a large pericardial fluid collection is detected, the more problematic issue is decision making concerning tamponade. Compression or collapse of the right-sided chambers is a hallmark that is not ambiguous, but the more subtle judgments required when the effusion is large but the patient not yet symptomatic stretch the bounds of clinical experience. In those circumstances conservative judgment and deferral to clinical presentation is wise. Also, tamponade can occur with small effusions when the effusion accumulates quickly such as with traumatic injury. Little doubt occurs when there is tachycardia with right atrial and ventricular compression accompanied by distention of the inferior vena cava. However, large effusions should be reported with the caution that clinical correlation is required.

### *Murmurs*

Although cardiac structure and configuration are resolvable with two-dimensional echocardiography, I still value the additional information provided by color Doppler integrated into every examination since there is little additional cost or time needed. Presence of regurgitation of a valve can help explain disproportional enlargement of a specific chamber and permits a more comprehensive evaluation of the functional components of the structural image. Murmurs are perhaps the most common motivation for obtaining an echocardiogram. Color Doppler and two-dimensionally directed spectral Doppler imaging are the most rapid and effective way of diagnosing murmurs caused by valve dysfunction or shunt such as septal defects. Although color Doppler imaging is diagnostically powerful, it is best to recognize that it has technical limitations particularly at greater distance from the transducer, or when flow is expected to be low velocity or perpendicular to the axis of the transducer beam. This is particularly the case with shunt questions where an atrial septal defect or patent foramen ovale is the clinical question. The apical four-chamber view, both imagewise and using color Doppler, may not create sufficient certainty for excluding such a diagnosis. The subxyphoid view, which looks more axially at the interatrial foramen, assists in improving certainty of a negative diagnosis. Nonetheless, there is still a value in venous injection of bubble contrast material (10 ml of agitated saline injected as a rapid bolus) to determine whether shunting might be present, despite apparently negative color and two-dimensional Doppler imaging.

Conventional valve disorders—the important ones being aortic or mitral stenosis and regurgitation—generally achieve high diagnostic accuracy by combining color Doppler and directed continuous-wave Doppler sampling. The characteristic diastolic doming of the mitral valve in mitral stenosis and its specific Doppler pattern leave little likelihood of error. Regurgitation of either the aortic or mitral valve creates such a strong color Doppler signal that, despite the distance from the transducer and the sometimes less than optimal approach angle, there is little likelihood of negative errors. The most problematic aspect is the grading of the degree of regurgitation and the attempt to provide a sharp distinction between moderate and severe mitral regurgitation. The presence of a flail leaflet automatically deserves the appellation of severe regurgitation, but moderate regurgitation will always be a somewhat judgmental call despite published claims for measured indices. Aortic stenosis is also an item needing discrimination between moderate and severe. Adult aortic stenosis is characterized by calcification, but there is frequently some evidence of slight flexibility at the central portion of the valve. Attempts to use simple Doppler velocity criteria for rigorous decision making can create false security. Using supporting evidence of the "continuity equation" is helpful, but still subject to errors from angulation differences between the interrogating beam alignment and the direction of the stenotic jet. Thus critical aortic stenosis (as opposed to moderate) will generally involve some judgment to avoid errors of underestimation. The calcific rigidity of the valve and presence or absence of hypertrophy are secondary items that help support decision making. Aortic regurgitation accompanying stenosis raises the peak Doppler velocity but rarely leads to overestimation of the stenosis.

### *Chest Pain*

Chest pain is an increasing indication for echocardiography, since the assessment of regional myocardial function can generally be made if sufficient effort is made to achieve a high-quality image from all viewing windows. Patient cooperation and persistent technical effort are essential ingredients for successful echocardiography. The high left-lateral patient position and deep expiration if necessary are important parts of the examination strategy. Combinations of views, particularly the apical long-axis, four-chamber, and short-axis views, allow an assembly of the various myocardial segments for functional assessment. Noncontractile thinning and aneurysm formation are hallmarks of past or present transmural ischemic processes. Adherence to naming conventions for the various segments is essential if diagnostic consistency is expected. The main specificity of echocardiography occurs with transmural rather than subendocardial ischemia, and therefore apparently normal contractility does not fully exclude coronary insufficiency—although a positive finding of regional noncontractility is highly specific. Recently exercise- or drug-induced echocardiography stress testing has become popular. Although there is some merit in this technique and it is occasionally helpful, I have found a high-quality nuclear perfusion image (thallium or sestamibi) to be more diagnostically valuable to the referring clinicians.

### *Assessment of Left Ventricular Function*

Left ventricular function and measurement of left ventricular myocardial wall thickness are reliably present in the echocardiogram. Estimation of left ventricular ejection fraction can be achieved, but I am not a strong believer in rigid adherence to linear measurements, or even area planimetered measurements, for numerical calculation. Although the numerical measurements have value in helping support a visual assessment of ejection fraction, clinical experience based on feedback, from nuclear medicine or angiography, allows the development of a visual expertise that permits rough categorization of the global and regional functional status of the myocardium and pumping function from simply viewing the moving two-dimensional echocardiogram. With reasonable experience, it is possible to categorize function into the categories of normal, mildly depressed, moderately depressed, and severely depressed left ventricular function. These correspond to rough categories of ejection fractions of greater than 55 percent, 55 to 45 percent, 45 to 30 percent, and lower than 30 percent ejection fraction. These categories are generally sufficient for most clinical decision making.

### *Assessment of Left Ventricular Hypertrophy*

Left ventricular myocardial thickness is available from a linear measurement either from the two-dimensional image or an M-mode line. Simple geometric equations are available for estimation of overall left ventricular mass. There is increasing evidence that the echocardiographic estimate of left ventricular mass has better sensitivity than ECG criteria and may be valuable in stratifying risk in hypertensive patients.

### *Endocarditis*

Infection of the valves, and rarely of the myocardium (abscess), are particular strengths of echocardiography. For survey purposes in a patient suspected of infection, and presuming adequate image quality, the conventional two-dimensional examination with particular narrow angle viewing of the valve structures is essential and may be sufficient. Here the value of technical persistence is critical, and rigid adherence to the specific view planes is to be discouraged. Off-angle views of all valves, and thorough mapping of the valve architecture from as many views as possible, are the hallmark of a good examination. The greatest factor creating difficulty is the presence of degenerative valve abnormalities or calcification; prosthetic valves also make discrimination of infectious processes more difficult. The friable mobility of a vegetation is usually a hallmark, but the presence of abnormal structures on a valve, even when rigid, would not exclude the possibility of infection. In these circumstances and where there is a strong clinical likelihood of infection with an indeterminate transthoracic examination, use of transesophageal technique is the method of choice. Transesophageal echocardiography is far easier and less difficult than most referring clinicians realize. Views of the myocardial structure are without peer and offer very specific diagnostic capacity as well as strikingly clear view of the anatomy.

## Discussion

Echocardiographic imaging should be considered as a first line imaging tool for most structural problems of the heart and its valves, and to a more limited extent the great vessels. Although examinations can be customized for the sake of time, a thorough and methodical series of image planes is by far the better methodology and much less likely to result in diagnostic errors. The most important issue impacting image quality is the commitment to reposition the patient and persist in acquisition despite variations caused by breathing. The ready availability of color Doppler and now transesophageal probes adds value to the examination, producing far greater accuracy and obviating the need for alternative or more elaborate imaging technologies.

## Suggested Reading

Kisslo J, Adams DB, Belkin RN. Doppler Color Flow Imaging. New York: Churchill Livingstone, 1988.

Nanda NC. Atlas of Color Doppler Echocardiography. Philadelphia: Lea & Febiger, 1989.

Salcedo E. Atlas of Echocardiography. 2nd ed. Philadelphia: WB Saunders, 1985.

Seward JB, Khandheria BK, Oh JK, et al. Transesophageal echocardiography: Technique, anatomic correlations, implementation, and clinical applications. Mayo Clin Proc 1988; 63:649–680.

# Positron Emission Tomography in Ischemic Heart Disease

*MICHAEL W. HANSON, M.D. · R. EDWARD COLEMAN, M.D.*

The multiple adverse consequences of atherosclerotic coronary artery disease continue to be a major issue of medical concern. Short of prevention, the early diagnosis of this illness provides the best opportunity to reduce the morbidity and mortality associated with ischemic heart disease. Traditionally patients with suspected atherosclerotic coronary artery disease have been evaluated with conventional treadmill or bicycle exercise in conjunction with radionuclide ventriculography or myocardial perfusion scintigraphy with thallium-201 or, more recently, technetium-99m–labeled radiopharmaceuticals. These studies have been useful in the diagnostic workup of these patients and have been used to help define which patients needed further evaluation with cardiac catheterization. With coronary angiography, the anatomy of the epicardial coronary arteries can be easily defined. However, the complexity of this disease is not determined by these anatomical findings alone. In those instances in which coronary angiography may be done as the initial investigational study, there is often a need for additional investigation with these scintigraphic techniques. Decisions regarding prognosis and the need for further therapy frequently depend upon the combination of the anatomical findings and the functional or physiological data that can be acquired by these studies.

Positron emission tomography (PET), a technology that has been available for more than 15 years, has only recently emerged as a clinical diagnostic option for the evaluation of myocardial ischemia and viability. PET offers selected advantages over either planar or tomographic imaging of Tl-201 or Tc-99m–labeled agents. The inability to correct for attenuation in either planar imaging or single-photon emission computed tomography (SPECT) can confound the accurate interpretation of myocardial perfusion studies. In contrast, PET can accurately correct for attenuation. In addition to accurately demonstrating the distribution of perfusion, PET can evaluate myocardial metabolism, which is important in evaluating myocardial viability. PET can measure the concentration of radioactivity in a given volume of tissue, and it is the only modality currently available that can provide quantitative measurements of in vivo biochemistry. The array of detectors in the PET scanner is highly sensitive in the detection and localization of the high-energy coincident photons that result from the annihilation of the positron. The combined characteristics of the radiation emitted by the positron emitters and the design of the scanner result in a high-resolution image that can be analyzed qualitatively, quantitatively, or semiquantitatively.

## Evaluation of Myocardial Ischemia

Regional myocardial blood flow can be assessed by several available positron-emitting myocardial perfusion tracers. The radionuclides incorporated into these radiopharmaceuticals are produced either by a cyclotron (nitrogen-13–labeled ammonia and oxygen-15–labeled water) or by a generator (copper-62–labeled pyruvaldehyde-bis-(*N*-4-methylthiosemicarbazone) [PTSM] and rubidium-82). The most commonly used tracers for the evaluation of myocardial ischemia are $^{82}$Rb and $^{13}$N-labeled ammonia. Facilities that have a cyclotron use $^{13}$N ammonia, whereas facilities that do not have a cyclotron use $^{82}$Rb.

$^{82}$Rb is similar to $^{201}$Tl in that it acts as a potassium analog. The main advantage of $^{82}$Rb is that it is a generator-produced radionuclide. An on-site cyclotron and radiopharmacy are not needed for its use, thus making it more readily and widely available. $^{82}$Rb is approved by the Food and Drug Administration (FDA) for myocardial perfusion imaging. $^{82}$Rb has a short physical half-life of only 76 seconds, which allows for rapid imaging and allows for serial studies to be done easily. The energy of the positron from $^{82}$Rb is 3.3 MeV, which is undesirable, since it travels farther in tissue before it annihilates with a free electron than the positrons from either $^{13}$N or $^{15}$O. This factor in part results in lower image resolution. The extraction fraction of $^{82}$Rb is approximately 65 percent at normal resting myocardial blood flow and is nonlinear at higher blood flow rates. The parent radionuclide, strontium-82, has a 25 day half-life. Thus the generator must be replaced monthly, and the cost of the monthly replacement of $^{82}$Sr is \$25,000. Several studies have reported myocardial perfusion imaging with $^{82}$Rb to have sensitivities of 90 to 95 percent and specificities of 75 to 95 percent for the detection of coronary artery disease.

$^{15}$O-labeled water (positron energy of 1.72 MeV; half-life of 2 minutes) is close to an ideal perfusion tracer; the extraction fraction is nearly 100 percent, and myocardial extraction is linear relative to blood flow without compromise at higher flow rates. However, the free transmembrane diffusion characteristics of water create technical problems for imaging. Due to rapid equilibrium of tracer in the myocardium and the blood pool, definition of the left ventricular myocardium is lost. Thus far, the proposed solution to this problem is less than desirable, and involves a cumbersome dual-isotope injection for identification and subsequent subtraction of the blood pool from the entire image, leaving the myocardium then identifiable. This process results in lower image resolution and possible errors during the subtraction process. No clinical studies have been reported that address the accuracy of $^{15}$O-labeled water in the diagnosis of coronary artery disease. $^{15}$O-labeled water has been used widely for the evaluation of cerebral blood flow, but it has not been used clinically in the evaluation of myocardial perfusion. Its ultimate use for perfusion imaging may depend on improved instrumentation and/or alternative means of image acquisition and analysis.

The primary positron-emitting agent used at our medical center for the evaluation of myocardial perfusion is $^{13}$N-labeled ammonia. Ammonia, labeled with $^{13}$N (positron energy of 1.2 MeV; half-life of 10 minutes) has an extraction fraction of approximately 90 percent at normal resting myocardial blood flow, which is not as good as $^{15}$O-labeled water, but is greater than either $^{82}$Rb or $^{201}$Tl. The extraction of $^{13}$N ammonia is not linear at higher flow rates. It clears rapidly from the blood pool, enters the extravascular space, and is converted in the myocardium to $^{13}$N glutamine. Clearance of $^{13}$N from the myocardium is slow, resulting in a high-contrast image between myocardium and blood pool activity. These properties result in overall excellent image quality for $^{13}$N ammonia myocardial perfusion images. Although pulmonary accumulation of $^{13}$N ammonia occurs in smokers and in patients with congestive heart failure, the tomographic technique of PET produces good-quality images of the myocardium in those instances. Studies have reported sensitivities and specificities for the diagnosis of coronary artery disease with $^{13}$N ammonia comparable to that with $^{82}$Rb.

Conventional myocardial perfusion imaging with $^{201}$Tl or $^{99m}$Tc-labeled agents is most often performed with treadmill or bicycle exercise. However, because of the technical requirements for PET imaging, myocardial stress by treadmill exercise is not practical. Supine bicycle exercise is feasible, but is difficult and cumbersome to perform. The recent introduction of pharmacologic stress agents for the evaluation of myocardial ischemia offers an alternative to exercise. Intravenous infusions of either adenosine or dipyridamole can cause coronary artery vasodilatation that is adequate for evaluation of stress-induced differential coronary artery blood flow. Perfusion-imaging studies with $^{13}$N ammonia and $^{82}$Rb, using intravenous dipyridamole and unilateral handgrip exercise, have been reported. After obtaining transmission images,

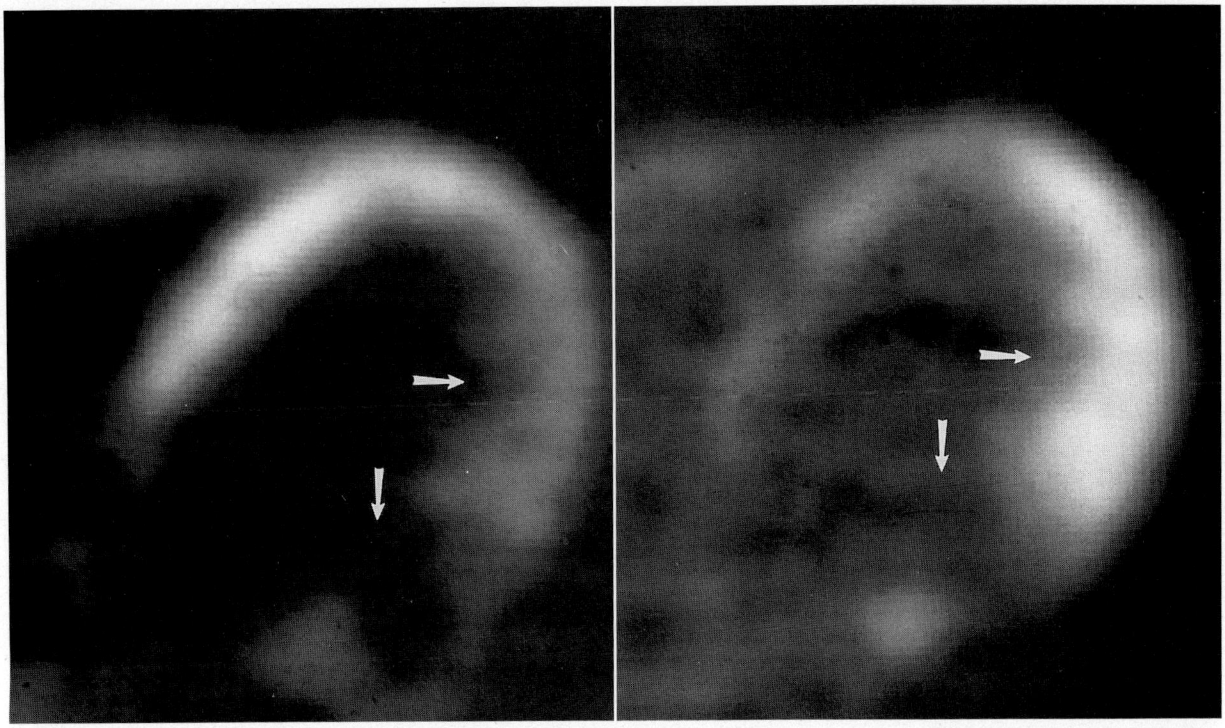


**FIGURE 1** A 59-year-old man with a prior myocardial infarction and two-vessel coronary artery bypass surgery. After presenting with recurrent chest pain, cardiac catheterization demonstrated a patent graft to the left anterior descending, an occluded graft to an obtuse marginal branch of the circumflex, and a 95 percent stenosis of the proximal circumflex. *A,* The transaxial image of $^{13}$N ammonia demonstrates decreased tracer uptake *(arrows)* in the anterolateral and posterolateral walls of the left ventricle. *B,* The transaxial image of $^{18}$F-FDG, acquired in the same plane as the ammonia image, demonstrates a corresponding increase in FDG accumulation *(horizontal arrow)* in the anterolateral wall and decreased FDG accumulation *(vertical arrow)* in the posterolateral wall, while perfusion is diminished in both of these regions. This study was performed in the fasting state. Note the normal lack of significant FDG accumulation in the normally perfused interventricular septum. The mismatch of diminished perfusion with preserved metabolism identifies the anterolateral wall as ischemic, while the matched perfusion and metabolism defect identifies the posterolateral wall as infarcted myocardium. The patient had successful angioplasty of the circumflex coronary artery.

intravenous $^{82}$Rb or $^{13}$N ammonia was injected at rest followed by 5 to 8 minute emission images for $^{82}$Rb or 15 to 20 minute emission images for $^{13}$N ammonia. At 10 minutes after the first rubidium injection (40 minutes for $^{13}$N ammonia), dipyridamole was infused in a dose of 0.142 mg/kg/min for 4 minutes. Two minutes later (6 minutes after the dipyridamole infusion was started), unilateral handgrip exercise with a dynamometer was begun and held for 4 minutes. At 4 minutes after the termination of the dipyridamole infusion, $^{82}$Rb or $^{13}$N ammonia was injected again and emission images were repeated for comparison with the rest images. Dobutamine, a beta-agonist catecholamine, can also be used as a pharmacologic stress agent. By increasing heart rate and myocardial contractility, this agent increases myocardial oxygen demand, thereby allowing for evaluation of stress-induced ischemia. These pharmacologic agents offer an alternative that is more suitable for use with PET imaging than either treadmill or bicycle exercise.

For a resting $^{13}$N ammonia study, the patient is placed in the gantry of the PET scanner and a 15 minute transmission scan is acquired for attenuation correction. When the transmission scan is completed, the patient is given 20.0 mCi of $^{13}$N ammonia by intravenous injection. After waiting 3 minutes for equilibration, an emission image of myocardial perfusion is acquired for 20 minutes.

For determination of myocardial viability, areas of diminished myocardial perfusion on the $^{13}$N ammonia study are further delineated by fluorine-18 fluorodeoxyglucose into ischemic or infarcted myocardium (Fig. 1).

## Evaluation of Myocardial Viability

With increasing resources and capabilities of performing coronary artery bypass graft surgery and percutaneous transluminal coronary angioplasty in patients with known atherosclerotic coronary artery disease, the question of tissue viability becomes increasingly important. These patients generally have a history of myocardial infarctions and have wall motion abnormalities. The ability to distinguish viable from nonviable myocardium in the distribution of the involved coronary arteries can dramatically alter the clinical decision whether to treat a patient medically or to proceed to surgery, angioplasty, or cardiac transplantation.

Wall motion analysis by contrast ventriculography, echocardiography, or multigated acquisition studies cannot accurately distinguish a region of ischemic and thus, viable, myocardium from a region of completed myocardial infarction (thus nonviable myocardium). The conventional method of distinguishing viable from nonviable myocardium has been with $^{201}$Tl scintigraphy. However, studies have shown that this modality,

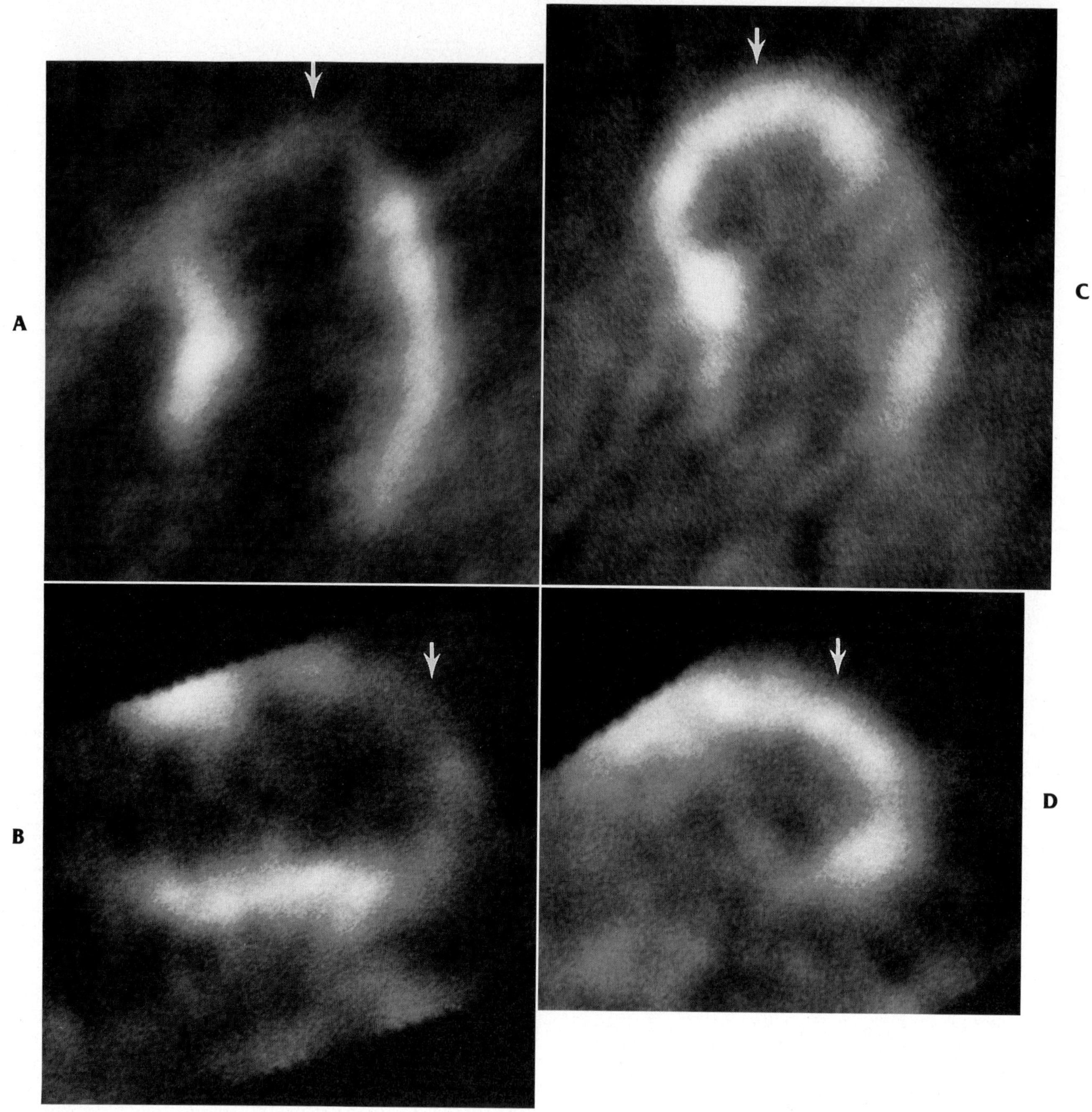

**FIGURE 2** A 56-year-old woman who had an acute anterior wall myocardial infarction treated with thrombolytic agents. Subsequent catheterization demonstrated severe proximal stenosis in the left anterior descending coronary artery with anterior wall dysfunction. An exercise $^{201}$Tl scan demonstrated a nonreversible defect in the anterior wall and apex consistent with a completed infarction in these locations. The horizontal *(A)* and vertical long-axis *(B)* $^{13}$N ammonia PET images show decreased perfusion in the apex and anterior wall of the left ventricle *(arrows)*. The corresponding horizontal *(C)* and vertical long-axis *(D)* $^{18}$F-FDG images demonstrate increased FDG uptake in these same locations *(arrows)*. This perfusion-metabolism mismatch is consistent with viable myocardium in the anterior wall and apex. The patient underwent coronary bypass graft surgery, since the lesion was not amenable to treatment with angioplasty.

A D B E C F

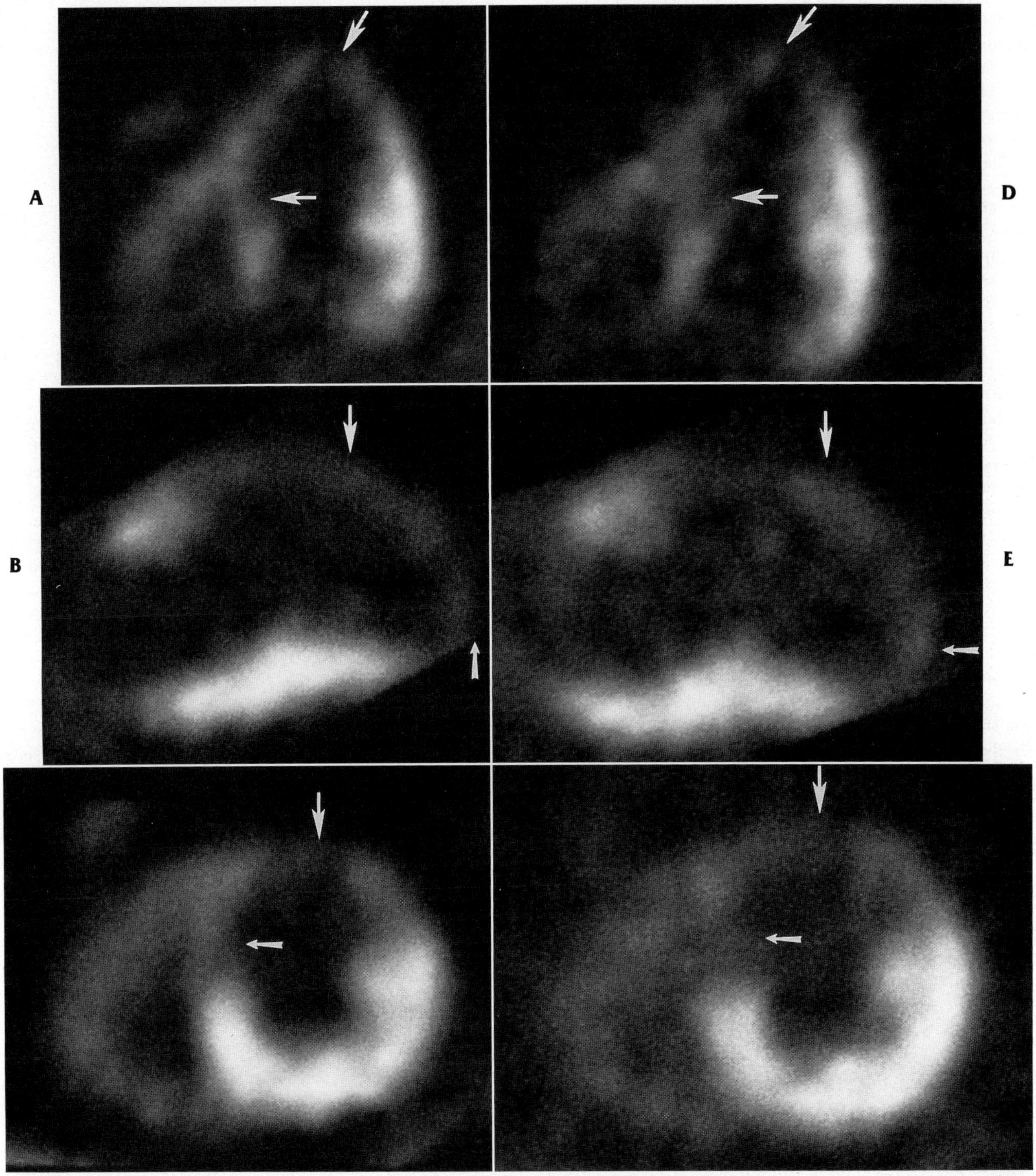

**FIGURE 3** A 60-year-old man who had an acute myocardial infarction, treated with streptokinase and later with tissue plasminogen activator on two occasions due to recurrent chest pain. Emergency cardiac catheterization demonstrated a total occlusion of the left anterior descending coronary artery, with anterior wall dysfunction. An emergency angioplasty of the left anterior descending coronary artery restored perfusion. However, at repeat catheterization 1 week later, there was restenosis of the left anterior descending vessel and persistent dysfunction of the anterior wall of the left ventricle. The horizontal long *(A)*, vertical long *(B)*, and short-axis *(C)* $^{13}$N ammonia PET images show diminished perfusion in the interventricular septum, apex, and anterior wall of the left ventricle *(arrows)*. The corresponding horizontal long *(D)*, vertical long *(E)*, and short-axis *(F)* $^{18}$F-FDG images demonstrate correlative defects in FDG accumulation in these same locations. These matched perfusion-metabolism defects confirm a completed infarct with nonviable myocardium in these regions. The patient had no further intervention and was discharged on medical therapy.

using conventional imaging techniques, overestimates nonviable myocardium in approximately 30 to 40 percent of patients. Reinjection techniques and/or 24 hour delayed redistribution imaging increases somewhat the accuracy of $^{201}$Tl scintigraphy to identify viable myocardium. However, $^{201}$Tl imaging remains less than optimal in accurately defining regions of viable myocardium. Thus there is a need to develop better noninvasive methods of identifying and distinguishing viable from nonviable myocardium.

Myocardial viability can be assessed by PET by evaluating cell membrane integrity or by evaluating myocardial metabolism. Cell membrane integrity can be assessed by the ability of the myocardial cell to extract and retain intracellular elements such as potassium or potassium analogs, such as $^{201}$Tl or $^{82}$Rb. In myocardial fibrosis there is less uptake of $^{82}$Rb than there is in regions of normal or dysfunctional, but viable, myocardium. In the setting of a recent myocardial infarction, $^{82}$Rb will be taken up into the infarcted segment, if blood flow has been restored with lytic agents and/or angioplasty. However, due to the damaged cell membrane integrity, the rubidium then leaks out of the cell, leaving a perfusion defect. Thus sequential imaging after the injection of $^{82}$Rb has been used as one method of evaluating myocardial viability.

The second PET method for assessing viability is by evaluating myocardial intermediary metabolism with $^{18}$F-FDG. This modality is the preferred method for assessing viability at Duke University Medical Center. In ischemic, but viable, myocardium, metabolism is shifted to anaerobic glycolysis, which results in a relative greater uptake of glucose (thus FDG) into those segments, relative to the surrounding normal myocardium. This characteristic allows identification of ischemic, viable myocardium, since nonviable myocardium will not take up FDG. The finding of maintained or increased FDG accumulation, relative to coronary artery blood flow, assessed with $^{13}$N ammonia, can identify regions of viable myocardial ischemia (Fig. 2) or regions of myocardial scar (Fig. 3). The combination of $^{13}$N ammonia and $^{18}$F-FDG has been reported to have a positive predictive accuracy of 78 to 85 percent in the identification of viable myocardium and a negative predictive accuracy of 78 to 92 percent.

For the $^{18}$F-FDG study, the patient is given 50 g of glucose orally 30 minutes before injecting FDG. A 15 minute transmission scan is then acquired for attenuation correction. The patient is then given 10 mCi of $^{18}$F-FDG IV. After waiting 30 minutes for adequate FDG uptake, the emission scan of the myocardium is acquired for 20 minutes. Because of the need for the accurate overlay of the transmission scan and the emission scan, the patient must stay on the gantry bed during the entire time of these image acquisitions, with as little motion as possible. For some patients, this requirement has proven difficult for performing these studies. Therefore, to shorten the length of time for these studies, variations of this technique are being evaluated. For one method under investigation, the transmission scan is acquired after the emission scan is completed, thus eliminating the need for the patient to stay on the imaging table during the uptake phase for the various tracers.

At Duke we have found that if these studies are done in the fasting state, the unpredictability of FDG uptake in that setting results in as many as 30 percent of the studies being uninterpretable. Therefore, to assist in a more reliable uptake, patients are given 50 g of oral glucose approximately 30 minutes before the injection of FDG. Even with this protocol, imaging patients with diabetes has proven difficult at times, with inconsistent patterns of uptake. Some investigators are administering insulin at the time of FDG administration in diabetic patients with high serum glucose levels, and the resultant images are interpretable. However, this is an area that needs further evaluation.

## Discussion

In spite of some of the benefits with myocardial PET imaging, a major issue continues to be the cost and the lack of reimbursement for these procedures. At Duke University Medical Center, the initial noninvasive evaluation for myocardial ischemia in the routine patient is done by standard rest and exercise perfusion imaging with $^{201}$Tl or $^{99m}$Tc-labeled Cardiolite or with rest and exercise MUGA studies. If these studies are equivocal or unhelpful for evaluating ischemia, the patient may be referred for PET scanning.

The initial study for the evaluation of myocardial viability at our medical center is still performed with an exercise/reinjection $^{201}$Tl study. However, in those instances when the $^{201}$Tl study fails to satisfactorily answer this increasingly important question, cardiac PET with $^{13}$N ammonia and $^{18}$F-FDG is used. Further, the patient with a severe compromise in left ventricular function (EF $<25$ percent) is studied initially with an FDG-PET viability study.

The costs of cardiac PET and the lack of reimbursement policies for these procedures by third-party payers remain major obstacles in the further development and widespread use of these techniques at this time. Most third-party payers are reimbursing for the studies, but only a few have policies for reimbursement. The advantages of PET must be shown to result not only in improved accuracy in the diagnosis of coronary artery disease, as compared with existing modalities, but also to be cost-effective in the management of the patient. This challenge will determine the future role of cardiac PET in the overall management of patients with ischemic heart disease.

## Suggested Reading

Berry JJ, Baker JA, Pieper KS, et al. The effect of metabolic milieu on cardiac PET imaging using fluorine-18-deoxyglucose and nitrogen-13-ammonia in normal volunteers. J Nucl Med 1991; 32:1518–1525.

Bonow RO, Berman DS, Gibbons RJ, et al. Cardiac positron emission tomography—a report for health professionals from the committee on advanced cardiac imaging and technology of the council on clinical cardiology, American Heart Association. Circulation 1991; 84:447–454.

Brunken R, Schwaiger M, Grover-McKay M, et al. Positron emission tomography detects tissue metabolic activity in myocardial segments with persistent thallium perfusion defects. J Am Coll Cardiol 1987; 10:557–567.

Cloninger KG, DePuey EG, Garcia EV, et al. Incomplete redistribution in delayed thallium-201 single photon emission computed tomographic (SPECT) images: An overestimation of myocardial scarring. J Am Coll Cardiol 1988; 12:955–963.

Council on Scientific Affairs. Report of the positron emission tomography panel; application of positron emission tomography in the heart. JAMA 1988; 259:2438–2445.

Gould KL, Yoshida K, Hess MJ, et al. Myocardial metabolism of fluorodeoxyglucose compared to cell membrane integrity for the potassium analog rubidium-82 for assessing infarct size in man by PET. J Nucl Med 1991; 32:1–9.

Kuhl DE, Wagner HN, Alavi A, et al. Positron emission tomography: Clinical status in the United States in 1987. J Nucl Med 1988; 29:1136–1143.

Schelbert HR, Buxton D. Insights into coronary disease gained from metabolic imaging. Circulation 1988; 78:496–505.

Tamaki N, Yonekura Y, Senda M, et al. Value and limitation of stress thallium-201 single photon emission computed tomography: Comparison with nitrogen-13 ammonia positron tomography. J Nucl Med 1988; 29:1181–1188.

Tillisch J, Brunken R, Marshall R, et al. Reversibility of cardiac wall motion abnormalities predicted by positron tomography. N Engl J Med 1986; 314:884–888.

# Radionuclide Ventriculography

*EDWIN L. PALMER, M.D. · JAMES A. SCOTT, M.D.*

The last decade witnessed dramatic advances in cardiac imaging. Despite rapid development of echocardiography and magnetic resonance imaging (MRI), radionuclide techniques remain the method of choice for accurate evaluation of ventricular function. Although originally used primarily to study valvular disease, ultrasonography today provides a reasonable estimate of ventricular contraction. The cross-sectional profile used to generate an ejection fraction (EF), however, may inaccurately estimate the true global value in some patients. When reliable assessment of ventricular function is important, radionuclide ventriculography is preferable.

Two general approaches have been applied to radionuclide ventriculography: first-pass angiocardiography and gated equilibrium blood pool imaging. The former is performed in a manner analogous to conventional cardiac angiography. A bolus of tracer is injected intravenously and rapid sequence images recorded as the activity transits the heart. This approach quickly assesses cardiac function, but count density and spatial resolution are limited, and the method is better suited to specialized multicrystal cameras than to the standard gamma camera.

Gated equilibrium blood pool imaging uses a tracer that remains within the blood pool during image acquisition, usually 20 mCi (740 MBq) of technetium-99m–labeled red blood cells (RBCs). The stable blood pool distribution of labeled RBCs allows imaging during a longer time than is possible with the dynamic first-pass method. The resulting images are of better quality, but show activity in all the cardiac chambers simultaneously. As a result, multiple image projections must be chosen to minimize overlap of important structures.

There are three basic ways to label RBCs with pertechnetate ($^{99m}TcO_4^-$): in vivo, in vitro, and modified in vivo methods. The in vivo technique is the simplest, but least satisfactory. Stannous chloride is injected intravenously, usually in the form of a commercially available pyrophosphate kit. Twenty minutes later, an intravenous injection of $^{99m}TcO_4^-$ follows. The pertechnetate diffuses into red cells, where it becomes reduced by the stannous ion and binds to hemoglobin. The problem with this method is that some $^{99m}Tc$ binds to plasma constituents that subsequently diffuse out of the vascular space, often resulting in poor image contrast.

The modified in vivo method also begins with an intravenous injection of stannous ion. Twenty minutes later, about 3 to 5 ml of blood is withdrawn into a heparinized syringe that contains the $^{99m}TcO_4^-$. Labeling then proceeds for 10 to 15 minutes in the syringe. This greatly reduces binding to plasma constituents and yields better image quality. The syringe can be left attached to the patient's arm during labeling, avoiding any possibility of reinjecting labeled RBCs into the wrong patient.

The best RBC label, however, results from an in vitro labeling method. The original in vitro method required painstaking technique, including centrifugation of the blood specimen. There is now a commercially available kit that allows convenient in vitro labeling of RBCs in about 30 minutes. This system chelates and oxidizes plasma stannous ion and does not require centrifugation. The in vitro method provides much better image quality than does the in vivo method, but its advantage over the modified in vivo method is less striking.

We routinely use the modified in vivo method. In a busy department with multiple RBC-labeling procedures going on simultaneously, we feel that the chance of reinjecting the wrong patient outweighs the advantages of the in vitro method. This is an individual choice, however, and in some circumstances, the potentially higher reliability of the in vitro kit may make it a better selection. Limited venous access occasionally presents a problem, since two different injection sites are needed with the in vivo RBC-labeling methods. When venous access is a problem, we sometimes use $^{99m}Tc$-labeled albumin, prepared from a commercial kit. Albumin gradually diffuses out of the vascular space, and so usually produces images inferior to those obtained with RBCs.

The photon flux available from a typical dose of $^{99m}Tc$-labeled RBCs distributed in the vascular space is insufficient to record images of the heart in "real time." Instead, the electrocardiogram (ECG) serves as a physiological gate to record and sum multiple cardiac contractions. The QRS complex identifies end-diastole and signals the beginning of image acquisition. By measuring the heart rate, it is possible for an imaging computer to calculate the length of the average cardiac cycle and to divide that time into a predetermined number (usually 16 to 32) of frames. Information from each cycle is recorded and added to the summed data from all previous cardiac contractions. In this manner gated images from about 400 to 600 beats can be recorded and viewed in an endless-loop cinematic display, showing a stylized cardiac contraction. Figure 1 shows selected frames from a normal radionuclide ventriculogram acquired in this way. This technique is called frame-mode acquisition. It is technically simple and provides good-quality images in the vast majority of patients. Changes in heart rate during acquisition degrade image quality, but fortunately the typical beat-to-beat variation in most patients does not greatly impair evaluation of systolic function. Severe arrhythmias, however, may make a standard frame-mode acquisition impossible. Some computer software

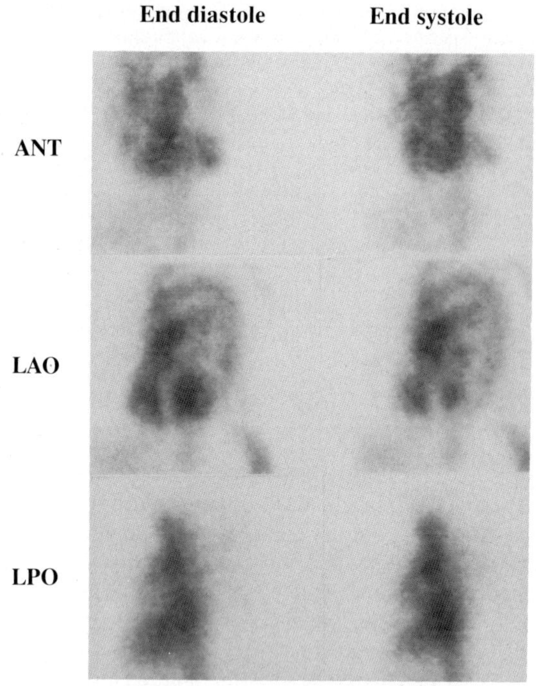


**FIGURE 1** Normal equilibrium gated cardiac blood pool scan showing selected end-diastolic and end-systolic images. Symmetric contraction of the ventricles is visible on all views.

programs provide ways to handle the problem of arrhythmias by sorting and holding images in a buffer memory so that only those beats of a specified length are processed. This variation of the standard frame-mode acquisition may be helpful, but is usually not required. Severe arrhythmias may present so few beats of desired length that imaging becomes impractical.

An alternative approach is the list-mode acquisition. Here, the computer stores data about event location during acquisition and images are later reconstructed. This provides more flexibility in the ways that images can be processed, but is rarely needed in clinical practice.

Several quantitative parameters are often used to characterize ventricular function. The most commonly used is the left ventricular EF, derived from the left ventricular time-activity curve. The EF is a measurement of systolic function; that is, the ability of the ventricle to contract. It is calculated using a fully or semiautomated computer algorithm that defines the left ventricular blood pool on the end-diastolic and end-systolic frames. The shallow (~45°) left anterior oblique (LAO) view best separates the left ventricle from other cardiac structures and is thus suited for the calculation. Most nuclear medicine computer systems yield a normal EF range between about 50 and 65 percent. The value calculated is subject to several errors, including incorrect background subtraction, improper placement of the ventricular region of interest, and excessive superimposition of atrial and ventricular activity. When carefully performed, the left ventricular EF is reproducible to about 5 percentage points in most patients. Reproducibility falls if the EF exceeds 65 percent or declines to below 25 to 30 percent. There are occasional patients in whom it is not possible to obtain a reliable EF. When this occurs, we report a range of numbers that appears to include the true value. Quantitative evaluation of the right ventricle is more difficult than the left because of its asymmetric shape and considerable superimposition of right atrial activity. We provide a qualitative description of right ventricular function and do not routinely calculate its EF. The normal right ventricular EF range is about 5 percentage points lower than that of the left ventricle.

Several types of parametric analysis can be applied to the quantitation of systolic function. Perhaps the most common of these is the Fourier transform image set. Fourier images show a map of the amplitude and timing of maximal ejection from each pixel of ventricular activity. In practice these often do not add greatly to visual inspection.

Diastolic dysfunction results when a stiff ventricle does not relax normally, impeding ventricular filling. This usually results from left ventricular hypertrophy, although it may also occur in patients with coronary artery disease (CAD). It is possible to evaluate diastolic function by analyzing the diastolic (filling) portion of the ventricular time-activity curve. Quantitative evaluation of diastolic function using parameters such as the peak filling rate requires higher temporal resolution than does EF calculation, so more frames must be acquired per cardiac cycle. Slight variation in heart rate has a much greater effect on the diastolic portion of the cardiac cycle than it does on systole. The resulting errors introduced into the gated images can cause significant inaccuracies. Reliable diastolic evaluation requires careful technique, usually with modification of the standard approach to record a higher framing rate and avoid aberrant beats. We do not routinely measure diastolic function, reserving this for specific clinical situations.

## Clinical Applications

Patients with CAD and infarction show regional wall motion abnormalities proportional to the amount of myocardium damaged. Small, nontransmural infarcts may show no detectable abnormalities of wall motion. Transmural infarctions (typically associated with an electrocardiographic Q wave) usually cause focal abnormalities. These may be characterized by either reduced contraction (hypokinesis), absent contraction (akinesis), or systolic expansion (dyskinesis). The regional wall motion abnormality is usually largest immediately after infarction, and becomes smaller in subsequent weeks. Right ventricular wall motion abnormalities are less common than those involving the left ventricle. They are usually accompanied by an inferior wall left ventricular abnormality, a territory also served by the right coronary artery. Right ventricular abnormalities tend to be global rather than focal, and often improve markedly in the weeks following infarction.

Small regional ventricular wall motion abnormalities may not affect global ventricular function, but large infarctions reduce the EF. Left ventricular aneurysm (Fig. 2), a sharply circumscribed region of akinesis or dyskinesis that may result from infarction, often occurs at the left ventricular apex. If an apical aneurysm is large, it may spuriously decrease the calculated EF.

CAD without infarction usually does not affect ventricular function at rest. It is common to see patients with severe CAD and normal ventricular contraction. With exercise, however, hemodynamically significant coronary disease becomes manifest. Under some circumstances, it may be desirable to evaluate ventricular function with exercise. Unlike myocardial perfusion testing, however, these images must be recorded while exercise continues. For practical purposes, this means using a

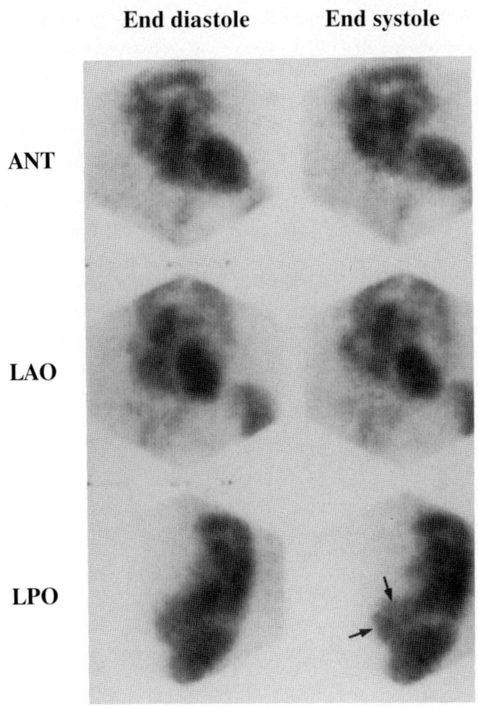


**FIGURE 2** Apical left ventricular aneurysm following left anterior descending coronary artery infarction. The aneurysm is best shown on the LPO view *(arrows)*. Note the preserved contraction in the basal portion of the ventricle, adjacent to the arrows. The left ventricle is dilated, while the right ventricle is normal.

semiupright bicycle so that the patient remains in a nearly fixed relationship to the camera. A baseline study is recorded at rest, followed by exercise images. An abnormal response to exercise may include ventricular dilation, falling EF, and development or progression of regional wall motion abnormalities. Although exercise ventriculography was commonly used in previous years as an alternative to thallium stress testing, it is now infrequently applied. The abnormal findings are not specific for CAD and the examination is technically demanding. Although exercise ventriculography has a role in selected patients, we use it infrequently in clinical practice.

Radionuclide ventriculography is often performed to detect, evaluate, and follow the clinical course of patients with cardiomyopathy. Hypertrophic cardiomyopathy usually shows a normal or small ventricular cavity accompanied by myocardial hypertrophy. Systolic function may be normal or hyperdynamic in these patients, often with an EF of above 65 percent. Diastolic abnormalities, such as reduced peak filling rate, may occur because of diminished wall compliance and are usually the most important functional pathology. Dilated cardiomyopathy, on the other hand, typically shows markedly abnormal systolic function (Fig. 3). This usually appears as global right and left ventricular hypokinesis and a reduced EF. Occasionally the right ventricle is spared or there is a focal left ventricular wall motion abnormality. The scan appearance in these patients is indistinguishable from that seen in CAD.

The common chemotherapeutic agent doxorubicin (Adriamycin) often causes myocardial toxicity when given in large cumulative dosages. The left ventricular EF provides an important indicator of developing cardiac toxicity. Patients usually undergo a baseline examination before beginning treatment. They are subsequently evaluated before each additional dose. A progressive fall in the EF indicates myocardial toxicity. Both the magnitude of the decline and the final value of the EF are important parameters to determine the feasibility of further treatment. In patients with an initially normal EF, treatment is usually withheld if the absolute decrease is 10 percentage points or more, to a final value of less than 50 percent. In patients with a baseline EF below 50 percent, therapy is usually stopped if the value falls 10 percentage points, or to a value below 30 percent. Ventricular function often stabilizes if further treatment is withheld.

Although ultrasonography is the procedure of choice for the initial characterization of valvular disease, radionuclide evaluation can assist management. Patients with chronic aortic insufficiency may remain asymptomatic for many years. Valve replacement is deferred until either increasing symptoms or declining EF occur. It is important not to delay surgery beyond this point, because the long-term survival after valve replacement falls once the ventricle begins to decompensate. Sequential ventriculography provides a reliable way to monitor asymptomatic patients and ensure that valve replacement is undertaken before left ventricular function deteriorates. Measurement of the EF has also proven prognostically important in predicting the results of mitral valve replacement.

Although not a sensitive indicator, the left-to-right ventricular stroke volume ratio derived from the gated scan can be used to estimate the degree of left ventricular volume overload in patients with valvular disease. Volume overload can often be suspected when the scan shows a dilated ventricle with a normal or increased EF, suggesting a regurgitant component to the ejected volume. The stroke volume ratio is determined

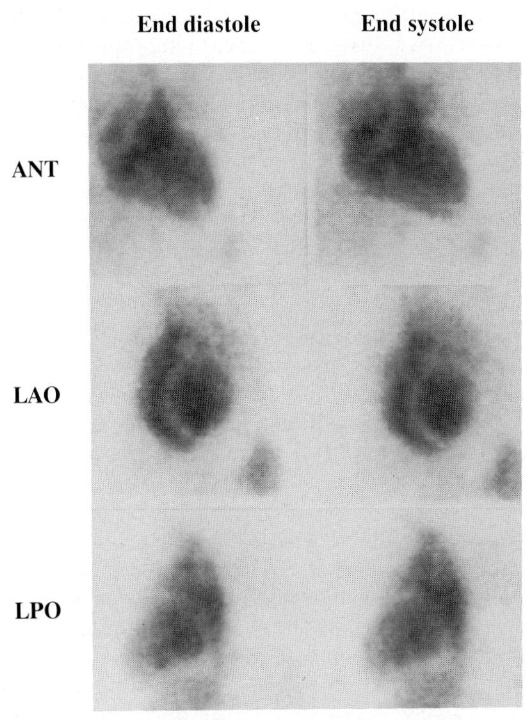


**FIGURE 3** Idiopathic dilated cardiomyopathy. Both the right and left ventricles are dilated, with severe global hypokinesis. There is almost no change between the end-diastolic and the end-systolic images. The left ventricular EF is reduced to 15 percent.

from the LAO projection by subtracting the end-systolic from the end-diastolic frame and drawing regions of interest over both ventricles. The volume of blood ejected by the ventricles is normally identical, but technical factors result in a calculated left ventricular to right ventricular ratio of up to 1.7:1. A greater value suggests left ventricular volume overload, usually from valvular regurgitation.

## Suggested Reading

Chilton HM, Callahan RJ, Thrall JH. Radiopharmaceuticals for cardiac imaging: Myocardial infarction, perfusion, metabolism, and ventricular function (blood pool). In: Swanson DP, Chilton HM, Thrall JH, eds. Pharmaceuticals in Medical Imaging. New York: Macmillan, 1990:442.

Dilsizian V, Rocco TP, Bonow RO, et al. Cardiac blood-pool imaging II: Applications in noncoronary heart disease. J Nucl Med 1990; 31:10–22.

Forman R, Firth BG, Barnard MS. Prognostic significance of preoperative left ventricular ejection fraction and valve lesion in patients with aortic valve replacement. Am J Cardiol 1980; 45:1120–1125.

Jain D, Zaret BL. Antimyosin cardiac imaging: Will it play a role in the detection of doxorubicin cardiotoxicity? J Nucl Med 1990; 31:1970–1974.

Patrick ST, Glowniak JV, Turner FE, et al. Comparison of in vitro RBC labeling with the UltraTag RBC kit versus in vivo labeling. J Nucl Med 1991; 32:242–244.

Rocco TP, Dilsizian V, Fischman AJ, Strauss HW. Evaluation of ventricular function in patients with coronary artery disease. J Nucl Med 1989; 30:1149–1165.

# Selection and Relative Safety of Iodinated Contrast Media

*MICHAEL A. BETTMANN, M.D.*

The selection of iodinated contrast agents raises two broad questions. First, the question arises as to when, specifically, iodinated contrast agents should be used. The second question is which specific agent should be used for any given procedure. The former is essentially beyond the scope of this chapter. Individual radiologists and other clinicians have developed guidelines, some personal and some broader, for the use of iodinated contrast agents in specific procedures and disease states. Such indications are clearly open to debate and form an important focus in the general discussion of the assessment of health technologies, for example, in regard to the use of mammography and of magnetic resonance imaging (MRI). The assessment of the effect of a contrast-enhanced examination on patient outcome, as compared to the use of a nonenhanced examination, is an important one in several examinations, including thoracic and cerebral computed tomography (CT). This question has not yet been satisfactorily answered, but this and similar questions must be addressed as health care costs continue to soar and careful examination of the utility of expenditure of specific health care dollars increases.

This chapter focuses on the selection of specific contrast agents, based on the understanding that a decision has been reached that the use of such agents is likely to provide useful information.

## Concentration

There are several components to the question of selection. Perhaps the easiest is the choice of concentration of contrast agent for a specific evaluation. Although this is still a matter of personal preference and debate, relatively broad guidelines have been accepted. For example, for intravenous urography, contrast agents with an iodine concentration in the range of 280 to 320 mg of iodine per milliliter are used. For cut-film angiography, contrast media with a concentration of 300 to 400 mg of iodine per milliliter are administered. In essence, the lowest iodine concentration should be used that allows satisfactory visualization of the target structures. This raises the question of a possible trade-off between concentration and dose. That is, it is possible that the use of a higher concentration of iodine may allow the use of a smaller volume of contrast material. Conversely, if a lower concentration is used, a larger total volume may be necessary. The question of the effect of volume per se has been addressed in a study by Redman and more recently confirmed in a study by Miller and colleagues. Both studies showed that there is no direct relationship between total volume of contrast material and the incidence of adverse general or renal effects. Although a dose effect has often been postulated, in general, as these studies suggest, none has been shown to be present. One exception to this, however, appears to be in patients with underlying renal failure. A recent study by Cigarroa and colleagues showed that in patients with abnormal renal function, an increased dose of contrast material does lead to an increased likelihood of further renal failure. In general, however, such renal failure is not related to obvious symptoms or to the need for treatment.

It has been shown previously that in certain settings, the incidence of complications can be lowered, without compromising the quality of the study, simply by lowering the contrast concentration. On the other hand, it has been shown in the case of cerebral CT that the quality of the study can be enhanced and the total volume decreased by increasing the concentration of the contrast material used.

## High-Osmolality Versus Low-Osmolality Contrast Media

The major question regarding the selection and relative safety of contrast agents is the relative role of high- and low-osmolality contrast media. Three points of view are possible, two of which are currently vying for primacy. One view that is rarely accepted is that high-osmolality agents should be used exclusively. The best defense for this view is the available data, which suggest that there is no difference in mortality rate between patients receiving high- and low-osmolality agents. Nonetheless, for reasons ranging from safety to comfort, this first view is rarely advocated. The selection of contrast agents, then, for all practical purposes rests on a choice between universal use and selective use in certain patients. Universal use is often advocated, and many different arguments are used to justify such an approach. The proponents of the view that low-osmolality agents should be used exclusively point to several factors. First, the incidence of mild adverse reactions, particularly those that relate to patient comfort such as pain, nausea, and vomiting, is lower with low-osmolality contrast agents (LOCAs) than with high-osmolality contrast agents (HOCAs). Second, numerous studies conclude that incidence of severe and highly severe adverse reactions is higher with HOCAs than with LOCAs. Finally, some investigators suggest that if HOCAs are used instead of LOCAs merely because of their decreased cost, and an adverse reaction occurs, the physician may be open to successful litigation. All three of these arguments represent opinions based on interpretation of available data and are supported by the data to varying degrees. The argument concerning litigation is the least valid, as both HOCAs and LOCAs are widely used, to varying degrees, throughout the world. Litigation based solely on the use of one versus the other, in the absence of events that actually fulfill the strict definition of liability, is exceedingly unlikely to be successful. In the current climate in the United States, litigation can be instituted for almost any reason, and the outcome is often unpredictable, but liability does have a strict definition, and it is unlikely that any action will ultimately be successful unless it meets the four necessary criteria: a defined duty, a clear breech of this duty, the occurrence of an adverse event, and a clear relation between the breech of duty and the adverse outcome. Given what is known about adverse reactions and contrast agents, proof of a relation between an adverse outcome and the choice of one category of contrast material over another is almost impossible.

The arguments against universal use are based on considerations of cost and cost-benefit ratio. In favor of universal use of LOCAs, as noted, the argument most often used is safety. In fact, given equal mortality between HOCAs and LOCAs, and the increased comfort with LOCAs, the most compelling argument for exclusive use of LOCAs is that such an approach is simpler. That is, the physician need not be concerned about cost-benefit issues or specific patient characteristics or settings that would suggest or dictate the use of one class versus the other. Although such an argument does clearly make life easier in a busy practice, based on the available data it is not a reasonable approach. The most rational approach remains one of selective use of LOCAs in certain patients and certain situations.

## Adverse Reactions to Contrast Media

Selection of contrast agents has been extensively examined, and various strategies have emerged for classifying risk and determining which patient should receive which class of contrast agent. Recent information has helped to define specific risk categories, and work continues in defining both the etiology of specific reactions and those patients at greatest risk. Underlying the selection of specific agents for specific settings are two questions, however, that are incompletely answered at present: (1) What is the etiology of any given reaction? and (2) What patient characteristics predispose to such reactions? Once these questions can be answered even partially, the selection of a specific contrast agent becomes relatively easy.

Certain reactions are relatively specific to certain examinations. The best defined of these is pain, which may be fairly intense on intra-arterial injection into upper- and lower-extremity arteries or into the external carotid circulation. It is perhaps surprising that discomfort in general is far less marked with all other injections, both arterial and venous, and is more often related to nausea and vomiting than to pain. The etiology of this pain or discomfort is in large part osmotic. That is, in general, the higher the osmolality of the contrast agent injected, the greater the pain. Even this particular reaction, however, is not so simply defined. It has been shown that below a certain level of osmolality, there are differences in the degree of discomfort experienced that are related specifically to the formulation. Additionally, with intravenous injection, it has long been thought that the higher the sodium content of HOCAs, the more discomfort is experienced with both peripheral arterial and intravenous injections.

It has also been thought that the incidence of adverse reactions to contrast agents is higher with venous than with arterial injections. Although this has in the past been supported by the work of Shehadi and others, more recent studies suggest that this is probably not true. It is then easiest, perhaps, to define patients at risk by examining specific kinds of reactions first, with secondary consideration of patient characteristics.

### *Systemic Complications*

In part because contrast agents, when administered intravenously or intra-arterially, have systemic effects, systemic complications are always important and are the most feared. They range widely in severity, however, from nausea and vomiting to cardiopulmonary arrest. To a large extent, these reactions are diagnosed as to cause by exclusion. That is, nausea, vomiting, laryngeal edema and bronchospasm, as well as full-blown anaphylactoid responses, have etiologies that cannot yet be clearly defined. Some such reactions, such as urticaria, are clearly histamine mediated, but despite extensive investigations, no clear and reproducible pathway has been elucidated that explains even these reactions. It is known that systemic reactions that have allergic manifestations, such as urticaria, are not classically allergic: patients who have experienced a reaction to a given contrast agent do not necessarily experience a reaction when the same agent is readministered. An additional problem is the definition of the frequency and severity of such reactions. For example, if a patient complains of pruritus and is examined and found to have urticaria immediately after the administration of contrast material, it is easy to establish that such a patient has had a systemic reaction to contrast agents, which is, in some fashion, immune mediated. Conversely many patients may experience urticaria without pruritus, and such a reaction is often not noted. In addition, pain or feeling of warmth on injection may be classified as reactions, when in fact they represent physiologic responses to the contrast agents rather than systemic reactions. This distinction becomes important only in attempting to define those patients who are likely either to have a recurrent "reaction" or to benefit from low-osmolality agents.

Patients who have had pain on a peripheral arterial injection with a HOCA clearly have less pain if a lower-osmolality agent is used in a subsequent arteriogram. This is true if a LOCA is specifically used but also if digital subtraction angiography using dilute contrast material is performed instead. If pain is considered an adverse reaction, the incidence of adverse reactions will be lower on a second examination with both approaches. If only immune-mediated systemic reactions (e.g., urticaria, laryngeal edema) are considered as true adverse reactions, however, re-examination of such a patient with a LOCA is associated with a lower likelihood of causing a recurrent reaction, whereas restudy using a dilute conventional agent, as far as is currently known, is not. A further consideration is the somewhat subjective nature of classification of adverse reactions. This continues to be a major problem in attempting to understand reactions to contrast agents in general.

Many categories of adverse reactions exist, and this makes comparison of results from one series to another difficult. In some ways this is perhaps analogous to an assessment of pain. It is well known that what may be called severe pain by one individual would be considered only moderate by another. The same holds true for various other reactions such as difficulty breathing. An additional aspect of this subjectivity is that the incidence of adverse reactions, even objective ones, varies with the expectation of the observer. In prospective, randomized, double-blinded studies, when a HOCA and a LOCA are compared, the reported incidence of complications is higher with the LOCA than the incidence observed when two LOCAs are similarly studied. Large unblinded studies, particularly ones that do not use objective definitions of adverse reactions, must be addressed critically. It is clear that adverse reactions are expected to be less frequent with low-osmolality contrast media, and available data suggest that this expectation is to some extent an explanation for the difference that is found.

There is therefore reason for uncertainty concerning conclusions about the relative incidence of systemic adverse reactions between HOCAs and LOCAs. Nonetheless, certain guidelines concerning systemic reactions are reasonable at this time. Patients with a clear history of systemic reactions are at increased risk of having a recurrent reaction compared with patients who have had a contrast evaluation and have not experienced a reaction. Interestingly, however, the likelihood of a recurrent reaction is not 100 percent. Rather, in various studies, it has ranged from 10 to 60 percent. This probably reflects in part different classifications of reactions. It has also long been thought that patients with a strong allergic diathesis are more likely to experience a reaction to contrast media than are patients without such a history. A problem arises in this regard, however, when "allergies" are defined. It is clear that almost everybody experiences at least mild seasonal rhinitis. Similarly, most patients develop contact dermatitis to certain toxins such as poison ivy or poison oak. Are all such patients in the same category in regard to the risk of an adverse reaction? It is fairly clear that they are not. It is also difficult to assess the previously widely held opinion that patients who are allergic to seafood, specifically shellfish, are at particular risk of experiencing an adverse reaction. Most recent studies, although somewhat limited in size, suggest that such an association does not exist. The most reasonable conclusion at this time therefore is that immune-mediated systemic reactions, such as urticaria and laryngeal spasm, are difficult to predict. Severe reactions of this type are rare. The incidence of such reactions appears to increase among patients with a strong allergic diathesis and severe asthma, although a definition of this risk is still unclear. The incidence of such reactions is lower overall with low-osmolality contrast media. Although there is a difference overall in incidence, the extent to which LOCAs decrease the incidence of severe reactions remains unclear.

One interesting illustration of this puzzling situation is evident when adverse reactions to sodium meglumine ioxaglate (Hexabrix) are compared to reactions to nonionic formulations. Hexabrix is a low osmolality ionic dimer. The incidence of pain with Hexabrix appears to be the same as or lower than that with low-osmolality nonionic formulations. The incidence of certain reactions, most notably nausea and vomiting, are clearly higher with Hexabrix than with nonionic agents and arguably higher than with conventional HOCAs. The incidence of severe systemic reactions, however, appears to be the same with Hexabrix as with nonionic formulations. This merely confirms that osmolality alone is not a sufficient explanation for adverse reactions, nor is the presence or absence of ions. Clearly more work needs to be done to define the incidence, nature, and etiology of systemic reactions.

### *Nephrotoxicity*

Data concerning other reactions are perhaps somewhat clearer. Nephrotoxicity is a feared complication of contrast agents, perhaps second only to the worry about sudden death. Recent studies suggest that contrast-related nephrotoxicity is rare and almost invariably inconsequential in patients with normal serum creatinine clearance. There is the possibility of worsening of renal function among patients with underlying renal disease, as manifested in elevated serum creatinine clearance. Most studies have suggested that this incidence differs little if at all between HOCAs and LOCAs, but these studies have primarily examined patients with a relatively mild elevation in serum creatinine. More recent studies have suggested that in patients with significant elevations of serum creatinine, for example, above the level of 2.0 to 3.0 mg/dl, the likelihood of worsening of serum creatinine is greater with HOCAs than with LOCAs. Data also indicate that among such patients, although not among patients with normal renal function, there is an adverse effect of increasing dosage. In regard to the risk of contrast-induced renal failure, the following conclusions are reasonable at this time. In patients with normal renal function, the risk of nephrotoxicity is low and there is no discernible difference between HOCAs and LOCAs. Among patients with mild renal dysfunction, with serum creatinine in the range of 1.5 to 2.5 mg/dl, the likelihood of worsening of renal failure is moderate, and there is again no evidence currently to suggest a clinically significant difference between HOCAs and LOCAs. In patients with more severe renal failure, as noted, evidence suggests that there is a dose-effect relationship, so that dose should be limited as much as possible. Data also suggest that the risk is lower with LOCAs than with HOCAs.

### *Cardiac Effects*

Cardiac effects of contrast agents are invariable, although in general they are not clinically manifested. Such effects may be divided into those that are reflex and those that are direct. The direct effects are relatively easy to evaluate with intracardiac injection. They are rarely of significance with other applications, such as intravenous injection, although they are noticeable with careful hemodynamic monitoring. Many of the severe systemic reactions such as hypotension, shortness of breath, or cardiac arrest may actually be manifestations of cardiac effects, rather than true immune-mediated systemic effects. Perhaps the best understood and most striking example of this concerns electromechanical dissociation. This can present as a sudden cardiac arrest. It is also related, at least in some cases, to calcium binding by the contrast agents, with sudden decrease in ionized calcium. This manifestation is easy to confuse with an anaphylactoid response. The only real difference may be that, in at least some cases, with the former the etiology is clear. Similarly vasovagal reactions, which can perhaps best be classified as reflex cardiac manifestations, are relatively common. When severe and unrecognized, they may also present with cardiac arrest. When less severe, they may present with hypotension, which can be ascribed to systemic effects or to direct cardiac effects. The only means of differentiation is that vagal reactions are accompanied by bradycardia or a lack of tachycardia. The significance of this different etiology is that the treatment is different. Vagal reactions are often in part related to anxiety, presumably on the part of both the patient and the personnel involved in the examination. The extent to which the incidence of such reactions varies between high and low osmolality contrast media is speculative. It is likely, however, that vagal reactions are less frequent with LOCAs, because both medical personnel and patients tend to be more comfortable with them.

Other direct cardiac effects are related, in large part but not exclusively, to osmolality. For example, hypotension and tachycardia invariably follow the injection of contrast agents into the coronary arteries. Such a response is far more marked with LOCAs than with HOCAs. Similarly hypotension, with reflex bradycardia related to systemic vasodilatation, follows left ventricular injections. Again, large magnitude changes, although they occur with LOCAs, are far less frequent. Therefore certain patients are particularly likely to benefit from the use of LOCAs, whether directly into the heart or systemically. These include patients with borderline cardiac compensation, such as those with congestive heart failure. Also likely to benefit are patients with limited cardiac compensatory ability such as those with significant aortic stenosis, significant pulmonary hypertension, or severe coronary artery disease, as well as those who might be likely to have adverse effects in the face of severe hypotension (e.g., severe cerebrovascular disease). It has also been shown, in one of the few studies with high-risk patients, that patients with acute cardiac instability have a lower incidence of adverse reactions when LOCAs are used.

### *Vascular Effects*

Specific vascular effects on the endothelium and endothelial cell junctions are generally of little concern, although they have been investigated to some extent. Endothelial damage leading to thrombosis is thought to occur secondary to contrast agents. The most common clinical manifestations occur during leg venography, with infusion of large volumes of contrast material into a vascular bed with slow flow. As noted previously, such reactions, by objective criteria, are more common with HOCAs. When HOCAs are diluted from 280 to 200 mg of iodine per milliliter, bringing the osmolality from approximately 1,400 mOsm per kilogram to approximately 1,000 mOsm, the incidence of such reactions decreases and is no different than that found with LOCAs at an osmolality of 600 to 800 mOsm. For such evaluations as venography, as with other evaluations, the most logical approach is to use the lowest iodine concentration consistent with achieving the necessary diagnostic accuracy.

Other vascular effects of concern are primarily related to pain as discussed previously. The question of the relative anticoagulant efficacy of the various categories of contrast agents has been raised over the last several years in a series of articles. These were precipitated by an observation that clumping of blood, and perhaps the formation of thrombi, in syringes and in catheters, was more likely to occur with a nonionic formulation than with an ionic formulation, either high or low osmolality. After several studies, it is still not entirely clear whether this is of clinical concern. One conclusion that does seem clear is that careful technique should always be used, and this in itself is likely to be sufficient to avoid thrombotic complications related to contrast agents per se. Appropriate technique includes frequent flushing of catheters, both arterial and venous. It also includes avoiding prolonged static contact of blood and contrast material, as in a syringe.

## Relative Safety of Contrast Media

The concept of relative safety of contrast agents is a difficult one, in large part because of difficulties inherent in defining reactions and establishing their incidence. There are the added difficulties of the general, if somewhat surprising, lack of understanding of the etiology of reactions on one hand, and the high level of safety of all contrast media on the other. Given the current state of knowledge, and taking into account considerations of both the cost-benefit ratio and the needs of society as a whole, limited use of low-osmolality contrast media in certain settings is the most appropriate approach. Such an approach should be adopted with the knowledge that work continues on both understanding adverse reactions and improving the safety of contrast media. That is, any conclusions must be based on the realization that this is not a static field. It is clear that the use of low-osmolality contrast media is beneficial in certain situations (Table 1). In general, LOCAs are useful in painful examinations such as upper- or lower-extremity angiography (but dilute HOCAs and digital subtraction may be substituted). Nonionic LOCAs are useful in decreasing the incidence of

**TABLE 1** Indications for the Use of LOCAs

| |
|---|
| Prior documented idiosyncratic reaction to contrast material |
| History of significant allergies or allergic diathesis |
| Active bronchial asthma |
| Acute cardiac or cardiovascular instability (e.g., acute myocardial infarction, cardiogenic shock) |
| Marked limitation of hemodynamic reserve (e.g., significant aortic stenosis, class IV congestive heart failure, severe pulmonary hypertension) |
| Painful procedures |
| Marked patient anxiety |
| Underlying process (e.g., suspected cervicospinal injury) that would make minor adverse reactions possibly harmful |

other minor adverse reactions, such as nausea or vomiting in patients who are likely to be particularly harmed by their occurrence, e.g., patients who are extremely anxious or have had recent significant central nervous system or extremity trauma or have an unstable fracture. LOCAs are also indicated in patients who are hemodynamically unstable or have limited cardiovascular compensatory ability and in those with significant prior idiosyncratic or immune-mediated reactions.

## Suggested Reading


Barrett BJ, Parfrey PS, Vavaseur HM, et al. A comparison of nonionic low-osmolality radiocontrast agents with ionic, high-osmolality agents during cardiac catheterization. N Engl J Med 1992; 326:431–436.

Bettmann MA. Clinical experience with loversol for angiography. Invest Radiol 1989; 24(Suppl 1):561–566.

Bettmann MA, Robbins A, Braun SD, et al. Contrast venography of the leg: Diagnostic efficacy, tolerance, and complication rates with ionic and nonionic contrast media. Radiology 1987; 165:113–116.

Bourdillon PD, Bettmann MA, Poole-Wilson P, et al. Effects of a new nonionic and a conventional ionic contrast agent on coronary sinus ionized calcium and left ventricular hemodynamics in dogs. J Am Coll Cardiol 1985; 6:845–853.

Campbell DR, Flemming BK, Mason WF, et al. A comparative study of the nephrotoxicity of iohexol, iopamidol and ioxaglate in peripheral angiography. J Can Assoc Radiol 1990; 41:133–137.

Cigarroa RG, Lange RA, Williams RH, Hillis LD. Dosing of contrast material to prevent contrast nephropathy in patients with renal disease. Am J Med 1989; 86:649–652.

Doust BD, Redman HC. The myth of 1 ml/kg in angiography. Radiology 1972; 104:557–560.

Fareed J, Walenga JM, Saravia GE, Moncada RM. Thrombogenic potential of nonionic contrast media? Radiology 1990; 174:321–325.

Feldman RL, Julowiec DA, Hill JA, Lambert CR. Contrast media-related complications during cardiac catheterization using Hexabrix or Renografin in high-risk patients. Am J Cardiol 1988; 61:1334–1337.

Gasperetti CM, Feldman MD, Burwell LR, et al. Influence of contrast media on thrombus formation during coronary angioplasty. J Am Coll Cardiol 1991; 18:443–450.

Kahn MJ, Baker MR. Optimization of low-osmolality contrast media for cranial CT: A dose comparison of two contrast agents. Am J Neuroradiol 1990; 11:847.

Katayama H, Yamaguchi K, Kozuka T, et al. Adverse reactions to ionic and nonionic contrast media: A report from the Japanese Committee on the Safety of Contrast Media. Radiology 1990; 175:621–628.

Miller DL, Chang R, Wells WT, et al. Intravascular contrast media: Effect of dose on renal function. Radiology 1988; 167:607–611.

Palmer FJ. The RACR survey of intravenous contrast media reactions: Final report. Australas Radiol 1988; 32:426–428.

Parfrey PS, Griffiths SM, Barrett BJ, et al. Contrast material-induced renal failure in patients with diabetes mellitus, renal insufficiency or both. N Engl J Med 1989; 320:143–149.

Shehadi WH, Toniolo G. Adverse reactions to contrast media. A report from the Committee on Safety of Contrast Media of the Interventional Society of Radiology. Radiology 1980; 137:299–302.

Smith DC, Yahiku PY, Maloney MD, et al. Three new low-osmolality contrast agents: A comparative study of patient discomfort. Am J Neuroradiol 1988; 9:137.

Wexler L, Cohen MB, Rudnick MR, et al. Multicenter trial of ionic and nonionic contrast media: Nephrotoxicity following cardiac angiography. Radiology 1991; 181(Abstr):292.


# Treatment of Contrast Media Reactions

*WILLIAM H. BUSH, Jr., M.D. · DENNIS P. SWANSON, R.Ph., M.S.*

Severe systemic reactions to conventional ionic intravascular contrast media are uncommon, even less frequent with the lower-osmolality nonionic agents, and very uncommon with magnetic resonance imaging (MRI) agents. However, clinically significant reactions do occur with all agents; fatal reactions are not eliminated by switching to nonionic media. Life-threatening situations can be minimized by early recognition of the various acute reactions to imaging agents followed by prompt and specific treatment.

## Preparation and Planning

The key to treating a contrast medium reaction effectively is being prepared to deal with the reaction should it occur.

Do not inject contrast media in an isolated setting; be able to readily summon additional assistance. Have immediately available equipment and drugs necessary to treat a reaction (Table 1). Have basic knowledge about the patient's medical history, including risk factors and allergies. If a reaction occurred with a previously administered contrast medium, a nonionic contrast medium should now be used (if contrast is necessary) and a premedication protocol used (Table 2). Know how to recognize the types of reactions. Have training in the treatment of various types of reactions, including training in cardiopulmonary resuscitation. With early treatment, lower doses of drugs can be used and drug side effects are minimized. To facilitate the rapid systemic administration of treatment drugs, IV access used for injection of the contrast medium should be maintained throughout the examination.

## Typical Reactions to Contrast Media

1. Scattered to extensive urticaria (hives) without respiratory symptoms
2. Bronchospastic reaction: asthma-like symptoms without coexisting cutaneous or vascular manifestations
3. Hypotension (isolated) with normal sinus rhythm or compensatory tachycardia. (NOTE—Compensatory tachycardia may be lacking in patients taking beta-adrenergic receptor blockers.)
4. Anaphylactoid (anaphylaxis-like) reaction: manifested by rapidly accelerating or severe bronchospasm with asthma-like wheezing, angioedema, laryngospasm, and developing profound hypotension

**TABLE 1** Acute Reactions to Contrast Media: Treatment Outline

**Urticaria:**
- Mild:
  - Observation
  - Diphenhydramine, 25–50 mg PO/IM/IV
- Severe:
  - Cimetidine, 300 mg, diluted, slow IV (pediatric: 5–10 mg/kg, diluted, slow IV
  - Ranitidine, 50 mg, diluted, slow IV (pediatric use not established)

**Bronchospasm (Isolated):**
- Oxygen (3 L/min)
- Beta$_2$-agonist metered-dose inhaler (2–3 deep inhalations):
  - Metaproterenol (Alupent)
  - Terbutaline (Brethaire)
  - Albuterol (Proventil)
- Epinephrine:
  - SC: 1:1,000, 0.1–0.2 ml (0.1–0.2 mg) (pediatric: 0.1–0.2 mg)
  - IV: 1:10,000, 1 ml (0.1 mg), slowly (pediatric: 0.01 mg/kg)

**Anaphylaxis-like Reaction (Generalized):**
- Oxygen (3 L/min)
- IV fluids: 0.9% sodium chloride for injection (normal saline); Ringer's solution
- Epinephrine:*
  - SC: 1:1,000, 0.1–0.2 ml (0.1–0.2 mg) (pediatric: 0.1–0.2 ml)
  - IV: 1:10,000, 1 ml (0.1 mg), slowly (e.g., 5–10 minutes) (pediatric: 0.01 mg/kg)
- Antihistamines:
  - H$_1$ blocker:
    - Diphenhydramine, 50 mg IV
  - H$_2$ blocker:
    - Cimetidine 300 mg, diluted, slow IV (pediatric: 5–10 mg/kg, diluted, slowly); or,
    - Ranitidine 50 mg, diluted, slow IV (pediatric use not established)
- Beta$_2$-agonist metered-dose inhaler (2–3 inhalations)
  - Metaproterenol (Alupent)
  - Terbutaline (Brethaire)
  - Albuterol (Proventil)
- Corticosteroids:
  - Hydrocortisone, 0.5–1.0 g IV; or,
  - Methylprednisolone, 500 mg IV over 30 seconds or 2,000 mg over 30 minutes

**Hypotension (Isolated):**
- Oxygen (3 L/min)
- IV fluids (primary therapy): rapidly, 0.9% sodium chloride for injection or Ringer's solution

**Vagal Reaction (Hypotension and Bradycardia):**
- Oxygen (3 L/min)
- IV fluids: rapidly, 0.9% sodium chloride for injection (normal saline) or Ringer's solution
- Atropine: 0.8–1.0 mg IV, repeat every 3–5 minutes to 2–3 mg total (pediatric: 0.02 mg/kg IV, maximum 0.6 mg, repeat to 2 mg total)

*Avoid epinephrine for patients taking noncardioselective beta-adrenergic blocking drugs. Alternative drug therapy: isoproterenol 1:5,000, IV, 0.5–1.0 ml (0.2 mg/ml) diluted to 10 ml with normal saline.

**TABLE 2** Premedication Options

Prednisone: 50 mg by mouth every 6 hours for 3 doses (e.g., 13, 7, 1 hour before contrast medium)
Diphenhydramine: 50 mg by mouth or intramuscularly 1 hour before contrast medium
Nonionic contrast agent (essential)

or

Methylprednisolone (Medrol): 32 mg by mouth 12 and 2 hours before contrast medium)
Nonionic contrast agent (essential)

5. Vagal reaction: hypotension with associated sinus bradycardia

## Treatment of Specific Reactions

Each physician or department should develop a specific plan or protocol for dealing with the various reactions that may result from administration of a contrast medium, update the plan periodically, and be ready to implement it quickly and effectively should a reaction occur.

### *Scattered to Extensive Urticaria with No Respiratory Symptoms*

If only a few scattered hives or pruritus develop, treatment likely is not necessary.

1. Observe the patient closely for other signs and symptoms and maintain IV access.
2. If scattered urticaria is the only sign and is protracted or troublesome to the patient, administration of an H$_1$ antihistamine (e.g., diphenhydramine 25 to 50 mg) is often effective.

Profound urticaria or diffuse cutaneous reactions may not respond completely to the administration of an H$_1$ antihistamine. In such situations the addition of an H$_2$ blocker (e.g., cimetidine 300 mg, diluted, slow IV; or ranitidine 50 mg, diluted, slow IV) may provide relief.

### *Bronchospastic Reaction*

Bronchospasm may be the primary manifestation of a reaction to contrast medium. For mild-to-moderate bronchospasm (i.e., without coexisting cardiovascular symptoms), an inhaled beta-agonist bronchodilator, such as albuterol, metaproterenol, and terbutaline, is recommended instead of epinephrine. These potent beta-adrenergic agonists, when inhaled, preferentially deliver medication to the airway tissue with minimal systemic effects. Epinephrine IV in low dose (e.g., 1 ml/1:10,000), given slowly, is recommended if bronchospasm does not respond to two to three metered doses of an inhaled beta-agonist drug or if laryngospasm develops. Epinephrine is an agonist (stimulator) of both alpha- and beta-adrenergic receptors. With slow subcutaneous release or slow intravenous injection, the beta-adrenergic effects of epinephrine predominate; whereas with rapid systemic administration, its alpha-adrenergic effects are more prominent. Intravenous administration of epinephrine in a slow, controlled manner is recommended, titrating the dose to the reaction response and avoiding erratic subcutaneous absorption.

In summary, the recommended treatment for a mild-to-moderate bronchospastic reaction includes the following:

1. Oxygen (nasal prongs or mask, 3 L/min)
2. Inhaled bronchodilator, 2 to 3 inhalations
3. Epinephrine, 1:10,000, IV, 1 ml (0.1 mg) slowly (e.g., 5 to 10 minutes) if patient does not respond to inhaled bronchodilator

### *Isolated Hypotension with Normal Sinus Rhythm or Tachycardia*

Some patients have reactions to contrast media that are manifested as profound hypotension with no respiratory symptoms. Isolated profound hypotension is treated most effectively and safely by the rapid infusion of a large volume of an IV fluid (0.9 percent sodium chloride for injection [normal saline] or Ringer's solution).

### *Anaphylactoid Reactions*

An anaphylactoid (anaphylaxis-like) reaction manifested as rapidly accelerating or severe bronchospasm, developing or profound hypotension (with compensatory tachycardia), laryngospasm, and angioedema requires prompt treatment, including maintenance of airway patency, supplemental oxygen, administration of adrenergic drugs, and rapid infusion of IV fluids.

For anaphylactoid reactions, epinephrine should be administered IV to provide rapid drug effect and to avoid erratic or incomplete absorption from subcutaneous sites associated with hypotensive circulatory collapse. It is recommended that a low dose (1.0 ml, 0.1 mg) of 1:10,000 epinephrine be given at a slow infusion rate (e.g., over 5 to 10 minutes) so as to maximize its beta-adrenergic effects and reduce its alpha-adrenergic activity. When administered early in the reaction course and at low doses, IV epinephrine is safe and effective in reversing a potentially life-threatening situation.

IV epinephrine must be used cautiously in elderly patients or if hypoxia is present, because the combination can cause severe cardiac arrhythmias. Additionally, patients who are receiving noncardioselective beta-blocking drugs (e.g., propranolol) may respond adversely to IV epinephrine. For these patients isoproterenol hydrochloride injection can be used. Isoproterenol is a sympathomimetic amine related to epinephrine, but acts almost exclusively on beta receptors. It can be administered IV at a dose of 0.5 to 1.0 ml (0.2 mg/ml) of the 1:5,000 concentration (diluted to 10 ml) to over-ride the beta blocker and treat bronchospasm and hypotension.

The $H_1$ histamine receptor antagonist, diphenhydramine (25 to 50 mg IV), is used commonly in addition to IV epinephrine and fluids to treat an anaphylactoid reaction. However, diphenhydramine alone should not be used in place of IV epinephrine to treat an anaphylactoid reaction.

If hypotension associated with an anaphylactoid reaction is refractory to treatment with IV fluids, consideration may be given to the administration of an $H_2$ histamine receptor blocker such as cimetidine or ranitidine. In patients with coronary artery disease, the injection of an $H_2$ receptor blocker must be accompanied by the injection of an $H_1$ receptor blocker to prevent coronary artery constriction.

High doses of IV corticosteroids are often used in the treatment of anaphylactoid reactions. However, onset of action is slow, making the administration of corticosteroids of little value in the treatment of an acute reaction to a contrast medium.

If the patient has or is progressing to a severe, anaphylactoid reaction, the following treatment plan is recommended:

1. Oxygen (nasal prongs or mask, 3 L/min)
2. IV fluids: 0.9% sodium chloride for injection (normal saline) or Ringer's solution
3. Epinephrine 1:10,000, IV, 1 ml (0.1 mg [adult]), slowly (e.g., 5 to 10 minutes)
4. Diphenhydramine, IV, 25 to 50 mg (adult)
5. Cimetidine, 300 mg (diluted), IV; or, ranitidine, 50 mg (diluted), IV
6. Corticosteroids: hydrocortisone, 0.5 to 1.0 g IV; or, methylprednisolone, 500 mg, IV

### *Vagal Reaction*

Prominent sinus bradycardia (pulse rate <60 beats per minute) and hypotension (systolic pressure <80 mm Hg) characterize the vagal reaction. Treatment is specific and different from that for a hypotensive reaction with normal sinus rhythm or tachycardia. Elevation of the patient's legs and the rapid infusion of IV fluids treat the vasodilation and hypotension; IV atropine blocks vagal stimulation of the heart and corrects the bradycardia. Atropine should be given in large doses, because small doses may accentuate cardiac arrhythmias. Therefore 0.8 to 1 mg should be injected IV initially; the patient's pulse rate determines the need for further therapy. If bradycardia persists, repeat IV doses of 0.8 to 1 mg can be given every 3 to 5 minutes to a total of 2 to 3 mg in adults. Despite resolution of the bradycardia, hypotension may continue, requiring further intravenous fluids:

1. Intravenous fluids: 0.9 percent sodium chloride for injection (normal saline) or Ringer's solution
2. Atropine, IV, 0.8 to 1 mg (adult)

## Reactions to MRI Contrast Agents

Since reactions to gadopentetate dimeglumine are similar to those caused by ionic and nonionic intravascular contrast media, albeit much less frequent, treatment of a specific reaction will be similar, irrespective of the causative agent. However, because of the strong magnetic field in the imaging room, special equipment requirements exist. Patient monitoring, such as by pulse oximeter, electrocardiogram (ECG), and noninvasive blood pressure devices should be routine during the examination. A source of oxygen should already be in place in the MRI Suite. Suction and a respiration AMBU bag are also necessary. IV fluids in plastic bags solve fluid needs. IV drugs need to be available in nonmagnetic syringes or containers. If a severe reaction occurs and full resuscitative efforts are necessary, it is our recommendation that the patient be moved quickly onto a stretcher and immediately out of the MRI Suite, so that the full array of resuscitative equipment can be used and all personnel can respond. Such an approach also avoids having to supply each MRI Suite with total resuscitative equipment.

## Suggested Reading

Barach EM, Nowak RM, Tennyson GL, Tomlanovich MC. Epinephrine for treatment of anaphylactic shock. JAMA 1984; 251:2118–2122.

Bush WH. Treatment of systemic reactions to contrast media. Urology 1990; 35:145–150.

Bush WH, Swanson DP. Acute reactions to intravascular contrast media: Types, risk factors, recognition, and specific treatment. AJR 1991; 157:1153–1161.

Cohan RH, Dunnick NR, Bashore TM. Treatment of reactions to radiographic contrast material. AJR 1988; 151:263–270.

Curry NS, Schabel SI, Reiheld CT, et al. Fatal reactions to intravenous nonionic contrast material. Radiology 1991; 178:361–362.

Goldstein HA, Kashanian FK, Blumetti RK, et al. Safety assessment of gadopentetate dimeglumine in US clinical trials. Radiology 1990; 174:17–23.

Greenberger PA, Patterson R. The prevention of immediate generalized reactions to radiocontrast media in high-risk patients. J Allergy Clin Immunol 1991; 87:867–872.

Salomen OLM. Case of anaphylaxis and four cases of allergic reaction following Gd-DTPA administration. J Comput Assist Tomogr 1990; 14:912–913.

Stanley RJ, Pfister RC. Bradycardia and hypotension following the use of intravenous contrast media. Radiology 1976; 121:5–7.

Swanson DP, Shetty PC, Kastan DJ, Rollins N. Angiographic contrast media. In: Swanson DP, Chilton HM, Thrall JH, eds. Pharmaceuticals in Medical Imaging. New York: Macmillan, 1990:13.

van Sonnenberg E, Neff CC, Pfister RC. Life-threatening hypotensive reactions to contrast media administration: Comparison of pharmacologic and fluid therapy. Radiology 1987; 162:15–19.

# Digital Angiography

*MARGARET E. HANSEN, M.D. · HELEN C. REDMAN, M.D.*

The role of digital subtraction angiography (DSA) is expanding with advances in computer and imaging technology. Although we virtually never performed intravenous DSA, we find that intra-arterial DSA has many advantages over conventional screen-film angiography. These include reduced volume of contrast medium, faster frame rates and image processing, greater contrast sensitivity, and reduced film usage. In some cases images of the desired vessel may be obtained with a nonselective contrast medium injection, or smaller catheters may be used. Other useful features such as real-time road mapping, edge enhancement and filtering techniques, zoom capability, and stenosis quantitation are unique to DSA. Portable DSA equipment has recently been introduced, which may expedite diagnostic studies on critically ill patients in the intensive care unit or the emergency suite.

Some disadvantages and potential limitations of DSA remain, despite recent improvements. Spatial resolution of screen-film angiography is still greater than that of DSA, although modern 1,024 × 1,024 digital systems produce excellent angiographic images. DSA is highly sensitive to patient motion (e.g., respiratory, cardiac, peristaltic), with resultant loss of image quality. Image quality may be limited in body areas with large variations in density, although some systems have built-in filters that can be placed in the image field to compensate for such variations. Finally, the subtraction process itself can produce artifacts. This chapter provides a brief overview of our current approach to DSA and the clinical situations in which we find it particularly helpful.

## Indications

A discussion of the indications for DSA might best begin with a review of situations for which DSA is *not* the method of choice at our institution.

The basic limitations already discussed apply to all clinical situations. In addition to these, DSA is not ideal if the region of interest contains high-density material, such as metallic foreign bodies or barium, which produces blind spots in the image. Problems that require very high resolution are better addressed with screen-film angiography. These include detection of subtle wall abnormalities (e.g., tumor encasement of a vessel, or a small intimal flap), detection of small pulmonary emboli, and distinction between a 99 percent stenosis and complete occlusion of a vessel (e.g., the carotid artery). Studies that may be nondiagnostic if even a small amount of misregistration occurs due to motion should be done with screen-film technique rather than DSA. An example of such a case is angiographic evaluation of bleeding from the lower gastrointestinal (GI) tract. Patients who are unable to hold still or to hold their breath, if needed, are not good candidates for DSA examination.

Situations in which we find DSA helpful cover the range of angiographic procedures. We frequently use DSA as an adjunct to screen-film angiography in lower-extremity disease, especially if there is poor opacification of pedal arteries due to proximal arterial occlusion(s) (Fig. 1). Rapid frame rates available with DSA are highly useful in pulmonary angiography (Fig. 2) and in the study of arteriovenous fistulas (Fig. 3). Another setting in which we often use DSA is to document normal vessel anatomy distal to the major vessel of interest after a cut-film study of that region (e.g., to show arm, forearm, and hand vessels in a patient with subclavian artery occlusion or stenosis). We also use DSA to evaluate the central venous system both diagnostically (in patients with dialysis fistulas, for example, or patients with superior vena cava syndrome) and in conjunction with caval filter placement (Fig. 4). Another common use of DSA is to assess progress in interventional procedures such as embolotherapy or angioplasty, during which multiple sets of images need to be acquired, usually with hand injection of contrast material (Fig. 5). DSA facilitates this process and also makes subsequent image development and manipulation faster and easier. We often use DSA to obtain oblique projections to demonstrate branch vessel origins if they are obscured on an initial study (Fig. 6) or to supplement a large-field-of-view screen-film study with targeted magnification views (e.g., the femoral bifurcations).

A

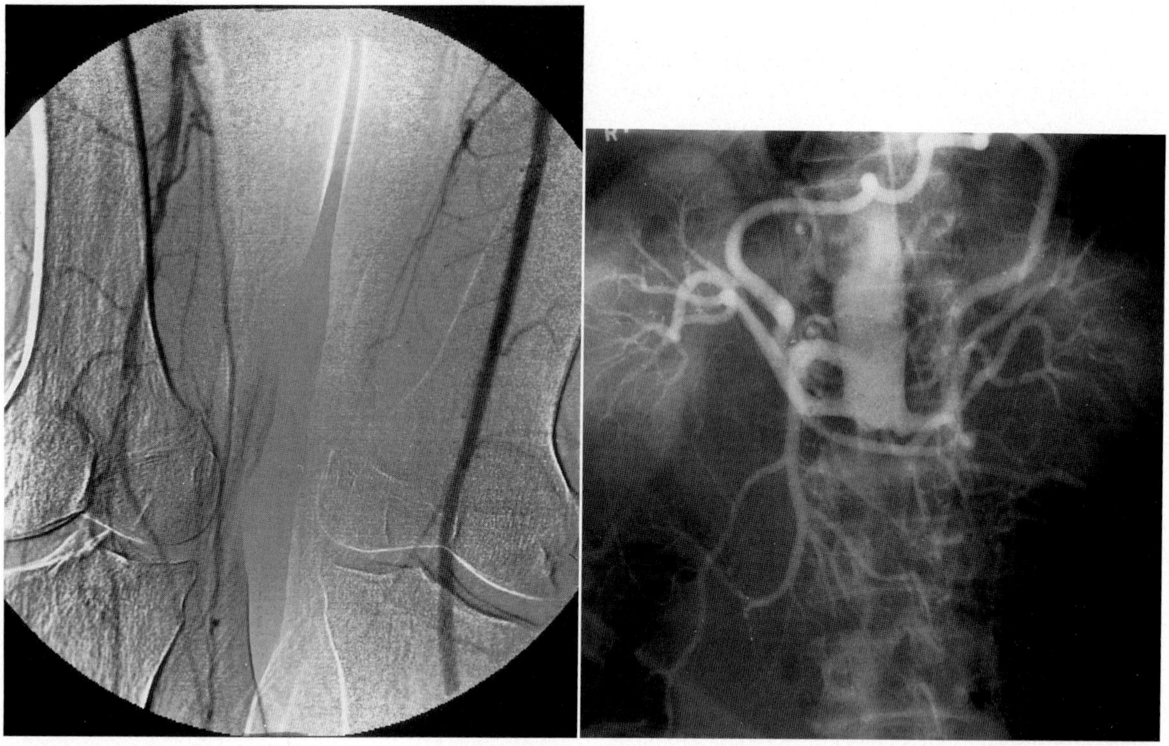

B

**FIGURE 1** Anteroposterior DSA study of legs shows good opacification of popliteal arteries (and occlusion of distal right popliteal artery) *(A)* despite infrarenal aortic occlusion shown on cut-film aortogram *(B)*.

A

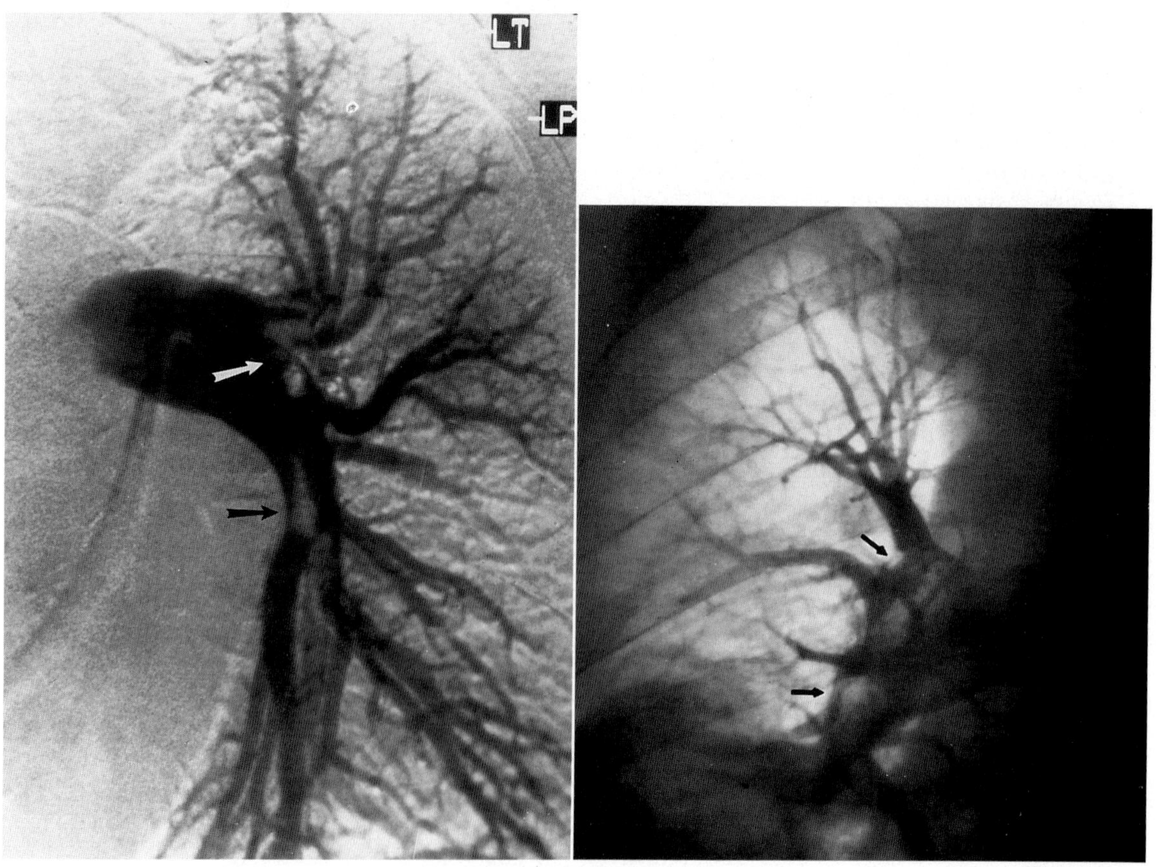


B

**FIGURE 2** Subtracted *(A)* and nonsubtracted *(B)* digital pulmonary arteriograms in two patients with multiple pulmonary emboli *(arrows)*. Images were obtained at 7.5 frames/sec. (Courtesy of Arthur C. Waltman, M.D., Massachusetts General Hospital, Boston.)

A

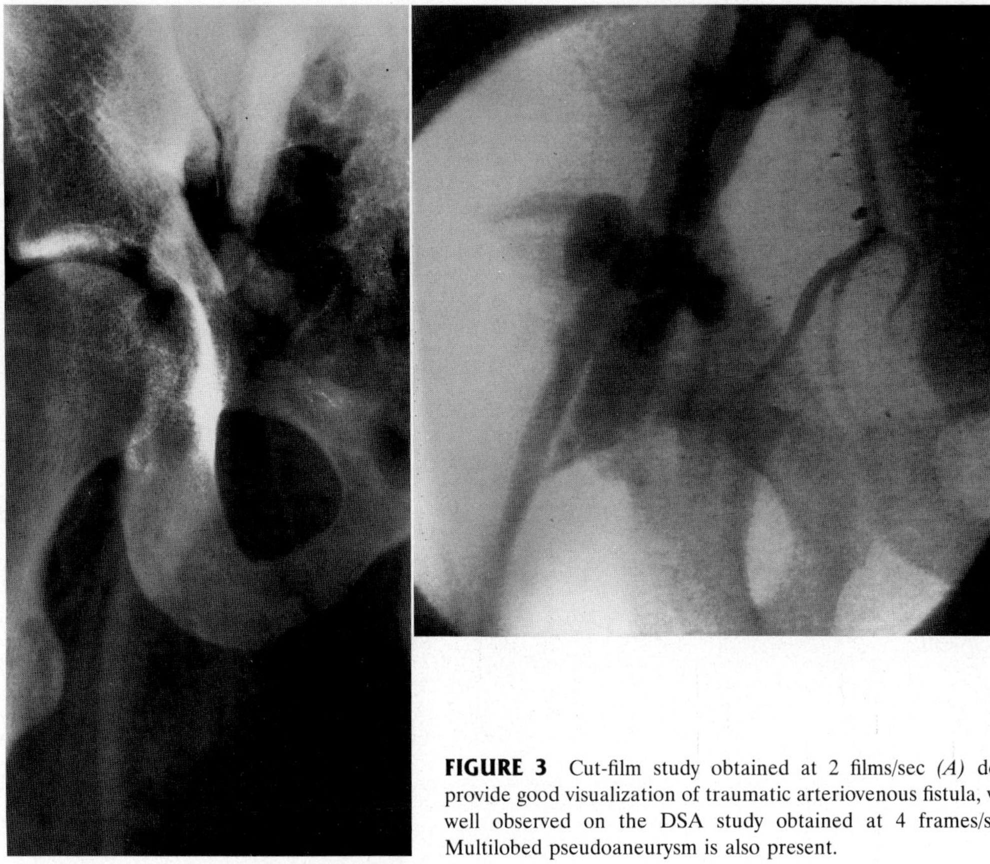

B

**FIGURE 3** Cut-film study obtained at 2 films/sec *(A)* does not provide good visualization of traumatic arteriovenous fistula, which is well observed on the DSA study obtained at 4 frames/sec *(B)*. Multilobed pseudoaneurysm is also present.

A

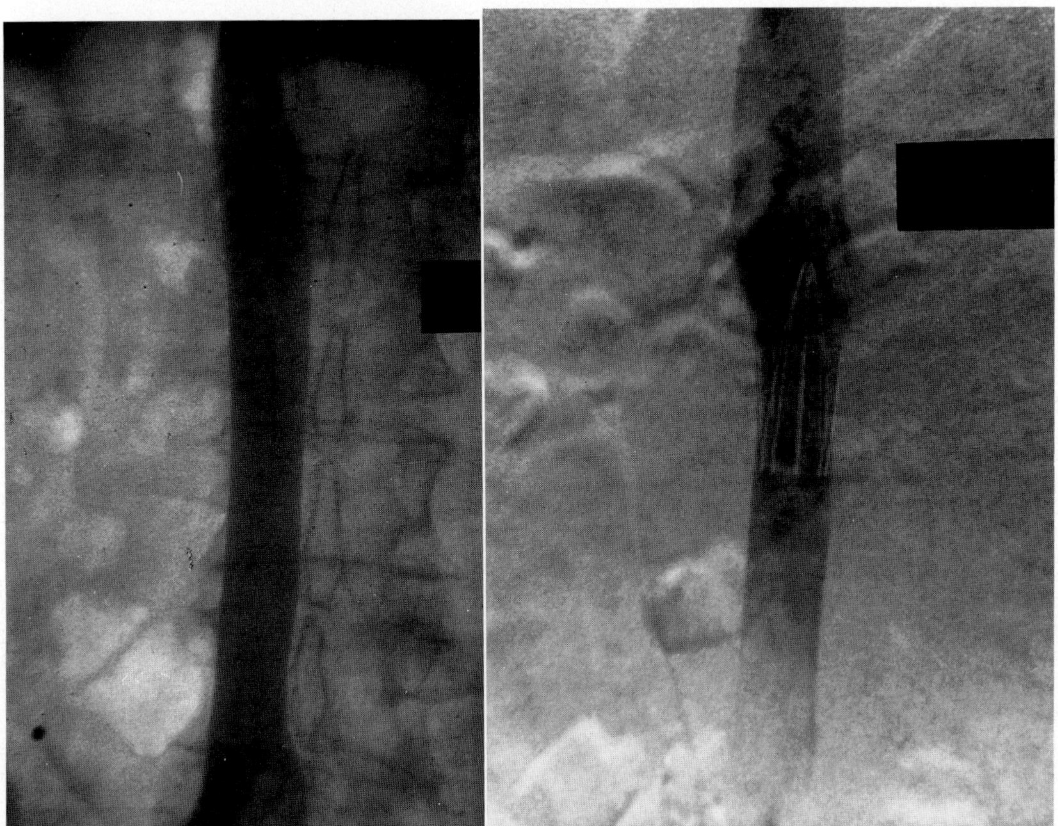

B

**FIGURE 4** DSA evaluation of inferior vena cava before *(A)* and after *(B)* placement of a Vena Tech filter. (Courtesy of Arthur C. Waltman, M.D., Massachusetts General Hospital, Boston.)

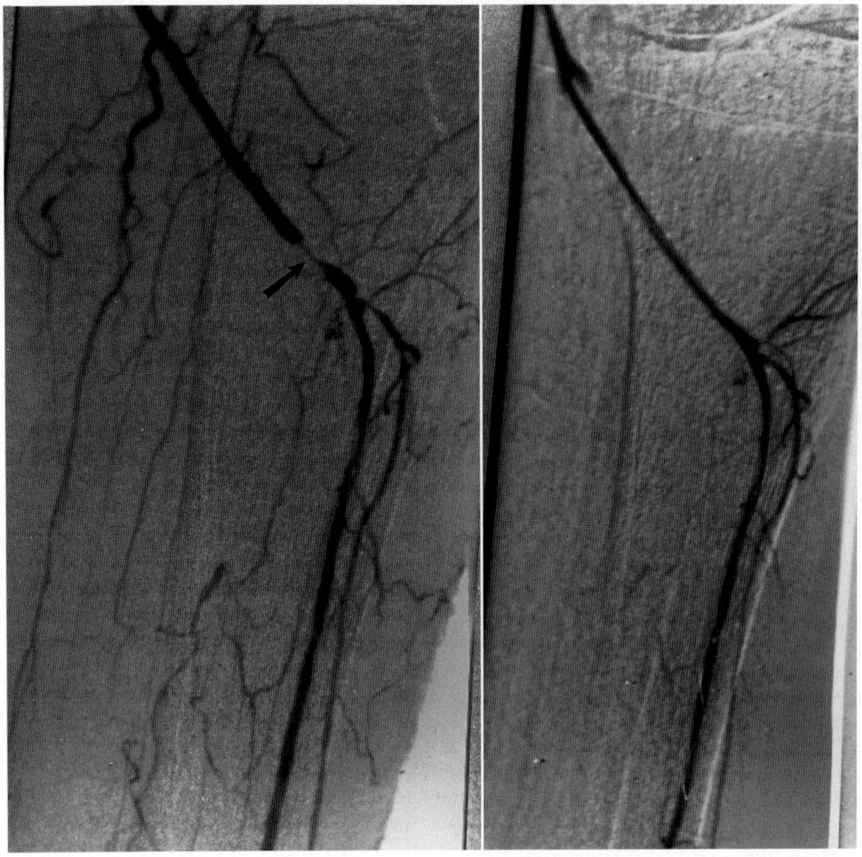

**FIGURE 5** DSA studies during hand injection of contrast material before *(A)* and after *(B)* angioplasty of stenosis in proximal anterior tibial artery *(arrow)*. (Courtesy of Arthur C. Waltman, M.D., Massachusetts General Hospital, Boston.)

## Technical Approach

Technical factors to be considered in DSA are much the same as for screen-film angiography. Although each system is slightly different, most have an automated feedback mechanism for setting exposure factors based on a test image. Some equipment, for example, allows milliamperes and time (milliseconds) to be selected by the operator and automatically sets the kilovolts (peak) to an appropriate value after test exposures are obtained. Just as in conventional angiography, the exposure time should be as short as possible, to minimize image degradation caused by motion. The chosen frame rate must be appropriate for the vessel to be imaged, considering its flow rate and the rate of any physiologic motion in the region of interest. The total duration of the run must be sufficient to include all desired information (e.g., the venous phase of an arterial injection).

Patient positioning should be done just as for conventional screen-film angiography. Magnification views can be obtained simply by selecting a small image intensifier size, rather than by using geometric magnification or an air gap as in screen-film angiography. If the region being evaluated has large density variations (e.g., the chest), placement of filters or water boluses over the less dense areas helps to equalize exposure throughout the image (Fig. 7). Areas that do not contain useful information, such as space between the legs on a run-off study, should be covered with lead strips or collimated out to reduce burnout on the image from unfiltered radiation. Patient cooperation is essential to minimize subtraction artifacts caused by motion.

Approaches to injection of contrast material in DSA are varied. In general, the duration of contrast material injection should be the same as it would be if the study were being done with conventional screen-film technique. Some angiographers prefer to use a smaller amount of full-strength contrast material, whereas others use more diluted contrast material than they would use for a screen-film study, but do not reduce the volume injected. Our practice falls somewhere between these two approaches, depending on the vessel(s) being evaluated and the indication for arteriography. Examples of average contrast media injection rates for selected studies are given in Table 1.

## Diagnostic Approach

### *Signs of Disease*

Most signs of vascular disease on DSA studies are very similar to those on conventional screen-film angiograms, and intra-arterial DSA has been shown to have diagnostic value comparable to that of conventional angiography in many clinical settings. Vessel occlusions, stenoses, filling defects (Fig. 8), abnormal arteriovenous communications, aneurysms and pseudoaneurysms (Fig. 9), vascular spasm, and neovascularity all have much the same appearance on DSA and screen-film angiograms. Intimal flaps, particularly if they are small, may appear as vessel wall irregularity on DSA studies rather than the well-defined line seen on conventional angiography. Even fairly extensive intimal flaps, as in aortic dissection, may not be readily apparent on DSA (Fig. 10). Extraluminal contrast medium collections are usually easily observed on DSA but must be distinguished from subtraction artifacts.

A

B

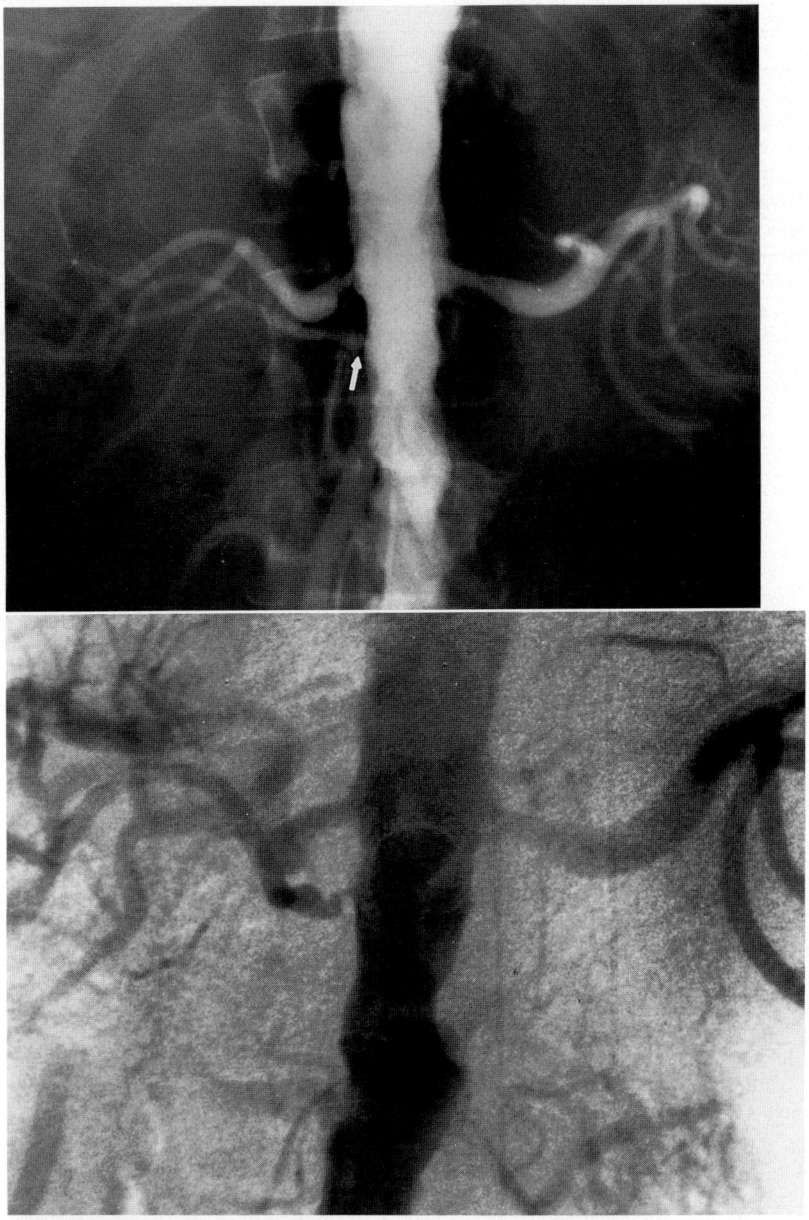

**FIGURE 6** Origin of lower right renal artery *(arrow)* is not well observed on AP cut-film study *(A)*, but is profiled on RPO DSA study *(B)*, which shows a critical stenosis. (Courtesy of Arthur C. Waltman, M.D., Massachusetts General Hospital, Boston.)

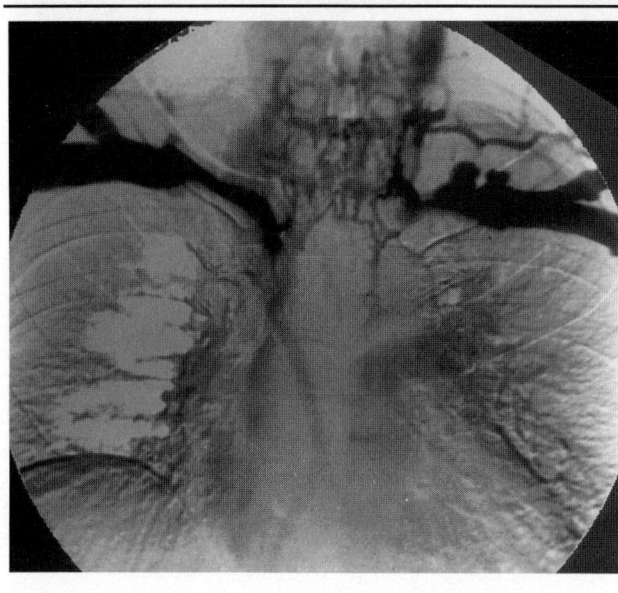

**FIGURE 7** DSA study of superior vena cava and subclavian veins shows a large area of burnout over the right lung, which could have been reduced with filters or water boluses.

**TABLE 1** Selected Average Rates for Injection of Contrast Media

| Vessel | DSA Technique | Screen-film Technique |
|---|---|---|
| Aortic arch (atherosclerosis) | 43–60% contrast; 40 ml at 25 ml/sec | 76% contrast; 70 ml at 35 ml/sec |
| Aortic arch (trauma, dissection) | 43–60% contrast; 70 ml at 35 ml/sec | 76% contrast; 70 ml at 35 ml/sec (minimum) |
| Inferior vena cava | 43–60% contrast; 30 ml at 20 ml/sec | 76% contrast; 40 ml at 20 ml/sec |
| Common carotid | 60% contrast; 8 ml at 5 ml/sec | 60% contrast; 11 ml at 7 ml/sec |
| Distal aorta/iliacs | 43–60% contrast; 16–30 ml at 8–10 ml/sec | 76% contrast; 30–40 ml at 10 ml/sec |
| Abdominal aorta | 43–60% contrast; 25-30 ml at 15–20 ml/sec | 76% contrast; 40–50 ml at 20–25 ml/sec |
| Superior mesenteric artery | 43–60% contrast; 24–42 ml at 5–6 ml/sec | 76% contrast; 50–70 ml at 5–7 ml/sec |
| Pedal arteries (catheter in ipsilateral external iliac) | 60% contrast; 24–32 ml at 4 ml/sec | 60–76% contrast; 44–48 ml at 4 ml/sec (minimum) |
| Pulmonary artery (proximal R or L PA) | 43–60% contrast; 25–30 ml at 10–15 ml/sec | 76% contrast; 40–50 ml at 20–25 ml/sec |

A

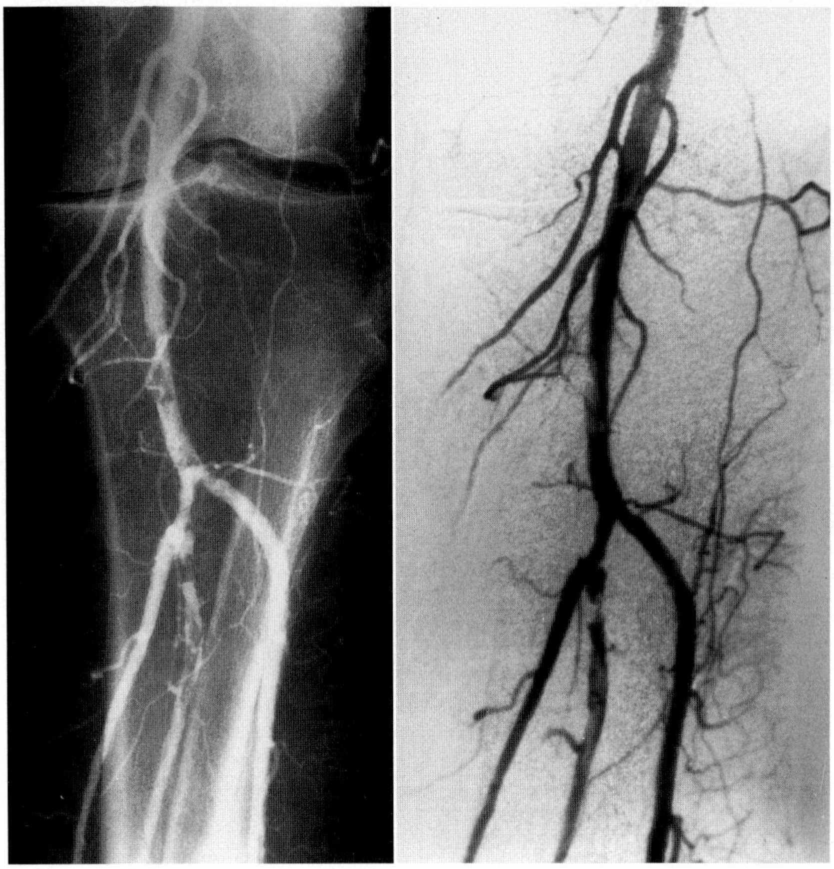

B

**FIGURE 8** Cut-film *(A)* and DSA *(B)* arteriograms show multiple emboli in distal popliteal artery and proximal peroneal artery. (Courtesy of Arthur C. Waltman, M.D., Massachusetts General Hospital, Boston.)

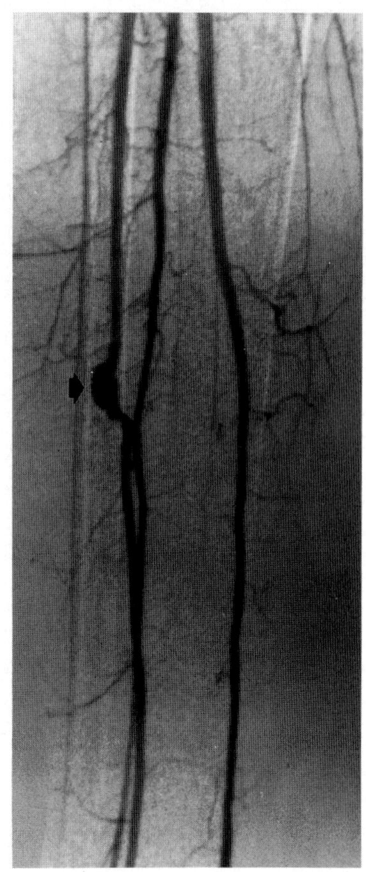

**FIGURE 9** DSA study of calf shows small pseudoaneurysm of midanterior tibial artery *(arrow)* in patient with history of blunt trauma. (Courtesy of Arthur C. Waltman, M.D., Massachusetts General Hospital, Boston.)

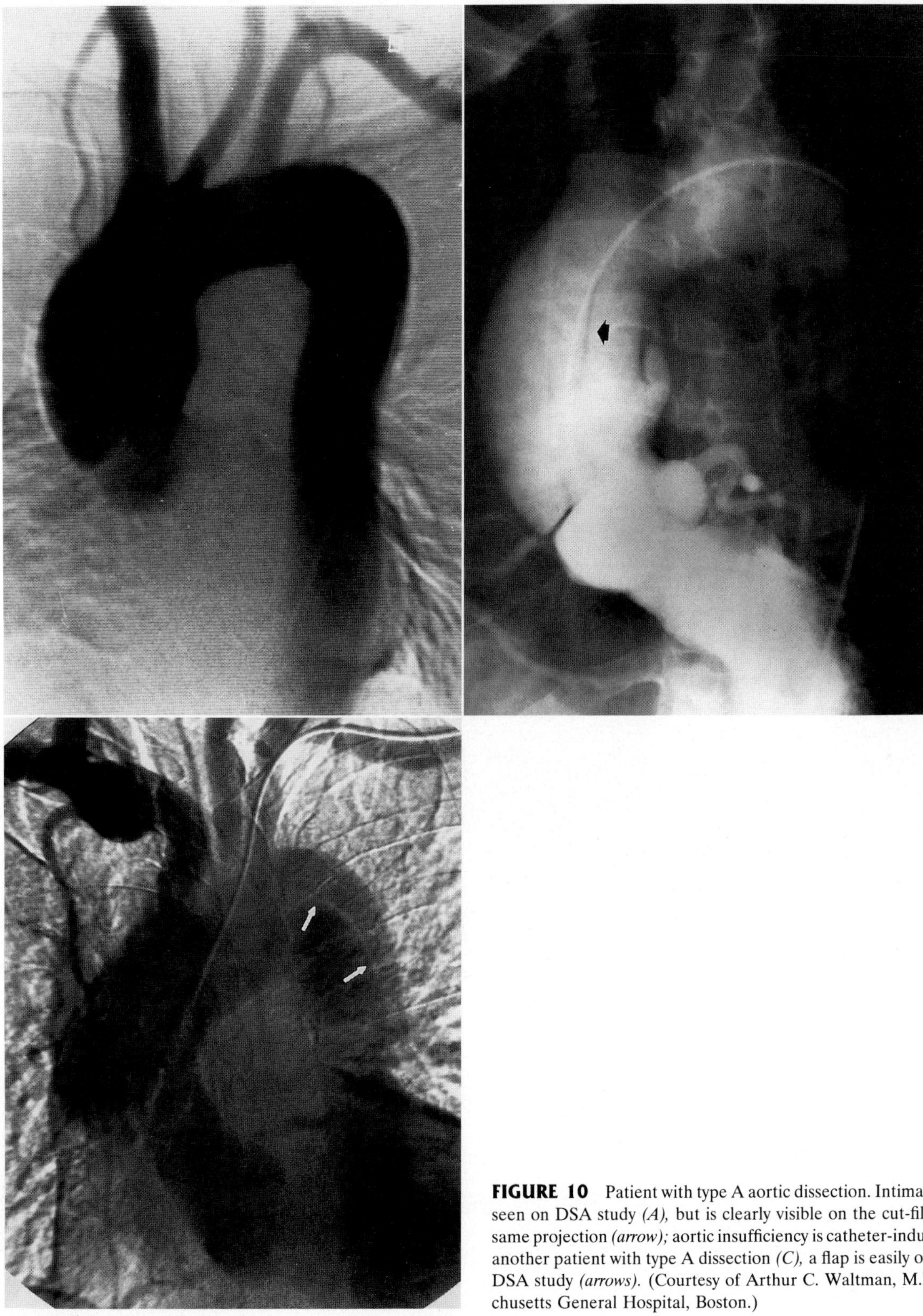

A

B

C

**FIGURE 10** Patient with type A aortic dissection. Intimal flap is not seen on DSA study *(A),* but is clearly visible on the cut-film study in same projection *(arrow);* aortic insufficiency is catheter-induced *(B).* In another patient with type A dissection *(C),* a flap is easily observed on DSA study *(arrows).* (Courtesy of Arthur C. Waltman, M.D., Massachusetts General Hospital, Boston.)

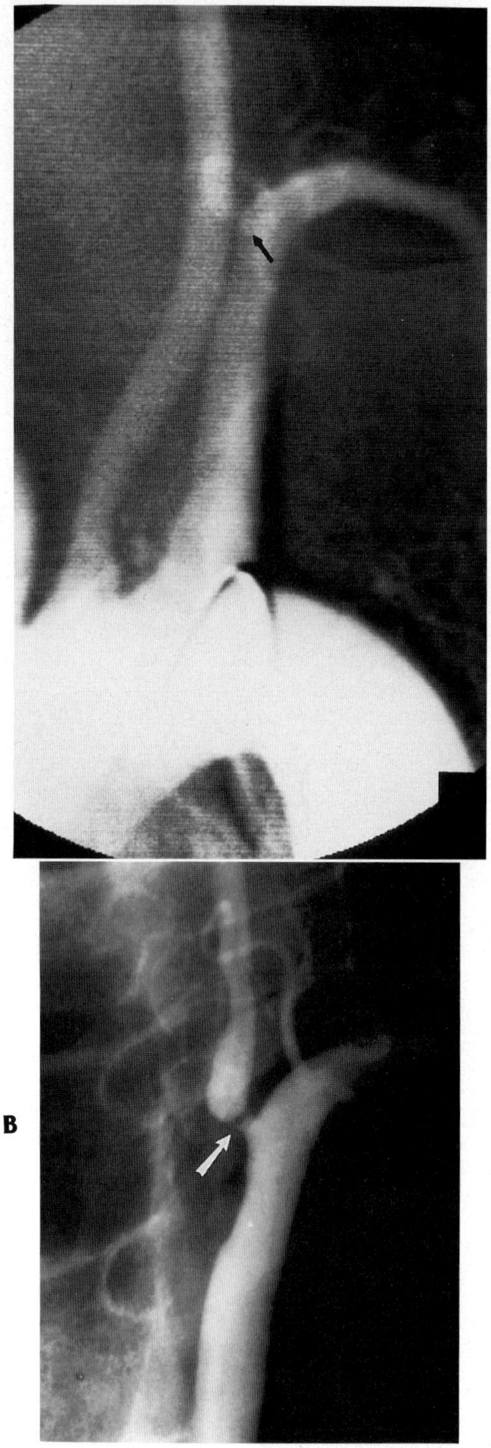

A

B

**FIGURE 11** On DSA study with nonselective injection into aortic arch *(A)*, the left vertebral artery appears occluded at its origin *(arrow)*. Cut-film study with injection into subclavian artery *(B)* shows a critical stenosis *(arrow)*, rather than occlusion. Overlap of left vertebral and left common carotid arteries and nonselective injection both contribute to error on DSA evaluation.

A 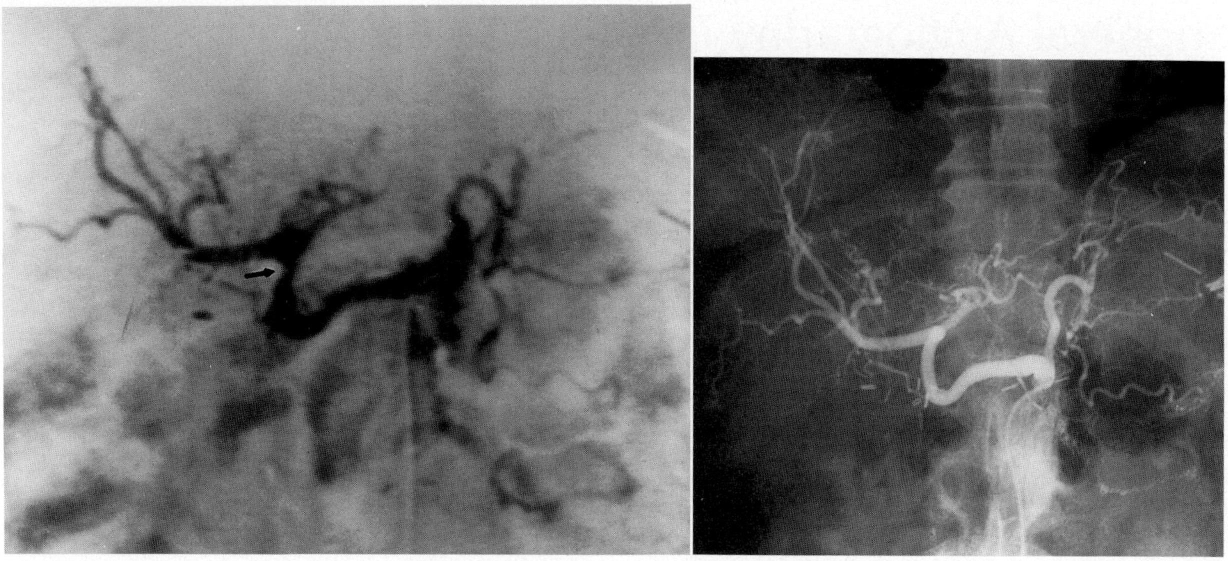 B

**FIGURE 12** Poor exposure and windowing on DSA study of hepatic artery *(A)* cause stenotic appearance in proximal portion of vessel *(arrow)*, which is completely normal on subsequent cut-film study *(B)*.

### *Diagnostic Pitfalls*

Pitfalls in DSA image interpretation are, for the most part, related to the inherent limitations of the technique and the potential artifacts it is subject to. Abnormalities of small vessels may not be as well demonstrated on DSA due to its lower resolution, but magnification views generally show even small vessels well. Perhaps the most vexing artifact in DSA is misregistration caused by motion, which can mimic extraluminal contrast material. This is especially common in the abdomen owing to peristaltic motion of bowel loops. Administration of glucagon (0.5 to 1.0 mg IV) before DSA helps to reduce bowel motion but does not eliminate it; for this reason evaluation of lower GI tract bleeding should not be done with DSA alone. Motion is not as problematic in the upper abdomen, and DSA can sometimes be highly effective in diagnosis of upper GI bleeding.

If a nonselective catheter position is used for injection, care must be taken to ensure that the vessel to be studied is not obscured by overlying vessels. This is a particular problem in evaluation of the extracranial carotid arteries and the vertebral arteries. Misinterpretation of a critical stenosis as an occlusion has obvious clinical implications, and in such cases DSA should be supplemented by a screen-film study (Fig. 11).

Technical factors can also affect the diagnostic quality of a DSA study. Improper selection of exposure technique can produce misleading appearances, as can inappropriate window and level settings on the display console or on the filmed images (Fig. 12). The angiographer should look at all the images before filming and indicate any that may be of particular diagnostic significance, rather than relying on the technologist to select the images to be filmed. Although an experienced technologist can film DSA studies adequately, we find that physician input is the only way to obtain the most correct information from the study.

## Suggested Reading

Dawson P. Digital subtraction angiography: A critical analysis. Clin Radiol 1988; 39:474–477.

Ferris EJ, Holder JC, Lim WN, et al. Angiography of pulmonary emboli: Digital studies and balloon-occlusion cineangiography. AJR 1984; 142:369–373.

Howard CA, Thal ER, Redman HC, Gibson P. Intra-arterial digital subtraction angiography in the evaluation of peripheral vascular trauma. Ann Surg 1989; 210:108–111.

Jeans WD. The development and use of digital subtraction angiography. Br J Radiol 1990; 63:161–168.

King JN, Orrison WW, Keck GM, et al. Arteriography with portable DSA equipment. Radiology 1989; 172:1023–1025.

Levin DC, Schapiro RM, Boxt LM, et al. Digital subtraction angiography: Principles and pitfalls of image improvement techniques. AJR 1984; 143:447–454.

Lipchik EO, Mewissen MW. A comparison of normal intraarterial digital subtraction angiography with standard angiography in patients with symptomatic cerebrovascular ischemia. Am J Neuroradiol 1990; 11:837–838.

Ovitt TW, Newell JD II. Digital subtraction angiography: Technology, equipment, and techniques. Radiol Clin North Am 1985; 23:177–184.

Picus D, Hicks ME, Darcy MD, Kleinhoffer MA. Comparison of nonsubtracted digital angiography and conventional screen-film angiography for the evaluation of patients with peripheral vascular disease. JVIR 1991; 2:359–364.

Rees CR, Palmaz JC, Alvarado R, et al. DSA in acute gastrointestinal hemorrhage: Clinical and in vitro studies. Radiology 1988; 169:499–503.

# Peripheral Angiography in Acute Trauma

*P. C. SHETTY, M.D. · DAVID J. KASTAN, M.D.*

Vascular injuries in the extremity can result in long-term disability, loss of limb, and occasionally even death. These may occur despite accurate diagnosis and appropriate treatment in a timely fashion. In many cases there is some delay in the management of peripheral vascular injury because of delayed patient presentation, transportation, and referral to the appropriate specialist. Evaluation and treatment of extremity vascular injury may also be delayed because of the time needed for evaluation of other associated traumatic injuries and underlying medical conditions. Injuries resulting in arterial occlusion, producing limb ischemia or active massive hemorrhage, need immediate confirmation and treatment. Injuries that may produce delayed occlusion, formation of a false aneurysm, and arteriovenous fistulas in the absence of hemorrhage and limb ischemia can be worked up in a semielective fashion. For cost-effective management of patients with suspected extremity vascular injury, we have developed a protocol agreed upon by the involved specialists—in this case, Emergency Room physicians, trauma surgeons, orthopedic surgeons, vascular surgeons, and interventional radiologists. Although there is still some controversy in the workup and management of extremity vascular injuries, this mutually agreed upon protocol, which is discussed in the section on Indications for Angiography, allows a cost-effective, safe, practical approach to these patients.

## Clinical Evaluation Before Angiography

In our setting, history and physical examination with special emphasis on underlying medical conditions, including screening for alcohol and other drugs, is performed by the Emergency Room physician. After this initial examination, the trauma surgeons are consulted and become the primary service in charge of management for these patients, who often require concurrent treatment by many specialists. Most of our trauma surgeons are credentialed to treat vascular injuries. Vascular surgery is consulted as needed. Neurology and neurosurgery are consulted when associated nerve injury is suspected. All bone injuries and joint injuries are treated by orthopedic surgeons.

We routinely obtain a complete blood cell (CBC) count, creatinine clearance, blood urea nitrogen (BUN), prothrombin time (PT), and/or partial thromboplastin time (PTT) before angiography. Before the procedure the radiologist examines the extremity with special attention to local bleeding, hematoma, distal pulses, paresthesia, and paralysis. This examination just before the angiogram is essential for two reasons: (1) we have experienced significant difference in the recording of the distal pulses by different individuals, and (2) the findings, again especially the distal pulses, may vary with time. It is also important to compare the pulses in the contralateral extremity in all patients, particularly in patients with suspected atherosclerotic disease. Some centers use noninvasive testing in the evaluation of extremity vascular injuries. However, in our practice, this is limited to the use of a portable Doppler velocity meter as an adjunct to the clinical examination.

## Indications for Angiography

We divide the indications for angiography into two categories: patients who need emergent angiography and patients who undergo angiography on a semielective basis.

1. Indications for emergency arteriography (if not explored directly)
   A. Pulse deficit with distal ischemia
   B. Arterial bleeding
   C. Expanding hematoma
   D. Suspected vascular injury because of a proximity injury in patients going to the operating room emergently for other reasons
2. Indications for semielective angiography
   A. Pulse deficit without distal ischemia
   B. Stable hematoma
   C. Penetrating wound near major vessel or signs of injury to an adjacent nerve
   D. Suspected injury to the vessels near the thoracic outlet and in the pelvis
   E. Proximity injuries in patients unlikely to allow appropriate followup

## Patient Preparation for Angiography

We make sure that there is a well-functioning large-bore IV access in all patients before starting the procedure. Informed consent for angiography, transcatheter intervention, and possible surgery is obtained before the administration of premedication. We premedicate our patients with 50 to 100 mg of IV meperidine (Demerol) injection. Demerol is given in 25 mg incremental doses. We avoid premedication in patients intoxicated with alcohol or who are suspected of using other drugs. Also, in patients with other suspected injuries, especially intracranial or intra-abdominal injuries, studies are done without sedatives to allow appropriate evaluation of those areas.

EKG, vital signs, and oxygen saturation are continuously monitored throughout the procedure.

## Angiographic Procedure

With the patient under local anesthesia, arterial puncture is performed using a single-wall puncture needle. In all cases we use a 3 mm J-guidewire and recommend using a dilator before the insertion of the pigtail catheter if this is the first catheter to be inserted. We prefer the transfemoral approach whenever possible. If there is a significant decrease in the femoral pulses bilaterally, we use a high brachial artery approach. We feel that better hemostasis can be obtained by using a high brachial artery puncture rather than an axillary artery puncture. Also, it is easier to recognize and treat local complications, such as bleeding from a high brachial artery puncture. For a majority of our lower-extremity angiograms, we use the ipsilateral common femoral arterial puncture. If the site of injury is the upper thigh, we use the contralateral common femoral artery for catheter insertion. If the contralateral pulse is compromised, we use a high left brachial artery puncture for catheter insertion. We reserve antegrade puncture of the ipsilateral common femoral artery for rare cases where we cannot fill the distal popliteal outflow tract from the retrograde puncture and injection in the ipsilateral external iliac artery. We also use antegrade common femoral artery puncture for interventional procedures, such as embolization of a bleeding vessel or occlusion of an arteriovenous fistula. In our experience only about 2 percent of patients require antegrade puncture of the common femoral artery for better visualization of the distal popliteal outflow tract or for interventional procedures such as embolization. Because of this low percentage of cases where antegrade puncture is required, we start all of our patients with a retrograde puncture and external iliac artery injection. If antegrade puncture is required, we pull the retrograde catheter, establish hemostasis, and perform antegrade puncture. We do not recommend converting retrograde puncture for antegrade catheterization. In our experience this increases local complications such as hematoma and does not permit adequate flexibility for superselective catheterization. In our practice most of the trauma victims are young patients who have a fairly acute aortic bifurcation. Selective catheterization of the femoral arteries from the contralateral approach often takes more time and requires more than one catheter exchange. Hence we do not use this routinely.

An aortogram is performed using a pigtail catheter prior to selective catheterization when subclavian artery injury or iliac artery and common femoral artery injury is suspected. Attempts to selectively catheterize the subclavian arteries or the iliac arteries may cause further damage from guidewire and catheter manipulation at unsuspected proximal sites of injury (see Fig. 6). For most of our unilateral lower-extremity angiograms, we use a 4 Fr straight catheter with ten side holes introduced over a J-guidewire from the ipsilateral common femoral artery. The injection is performed in the ipsilateral external iliac artery. This method is fast, simple, and can be performed without fluoroscopy. We are almost always able to visualize the infrapopliteal vessels by injecting the ipsilateral external iliac artery with the safer retrograde puncture. We use a Cobra or a Chung catheter to selectively catheterize the contralateral iliac artery. If selective catheterization of the femoral artery is required, we may also use a 45° angled catheter with a soft tip. We use a Headhunter-1 catheter for selective catheterization of the subclavian and brachial arteries. We almost exclusively use 5 Fr catheters for our selective catheterizations.

We use low-osmolar contrast agents (LOCAs) in all of our trauma patients. This standardized approach speeds set-up time and procedure time in patients who often cannot give accurate medical histories. Volume and flow rate vary depending on the site of injection and whether we are performing a localized cut-film study or runoff study of an entire extremity. In our experience injecting 50 ml of a LOCA (300 mg/ml iodine) in the external iliac artery at the rate of 5 ml/sec almost always visualizes the femoral, popliteal, and the popliteal outflow tract vessels.

For imaging of a localized segment of the vessel without runoff, 15 to 20 ml of contrast material at the rate of 5 to 8 ml/sec is injected several centimeters proximal to the suspected site of injury. When we perform an aortogram using conventional filming we use a LOCA with a 350 mg/ml iodine concentration, and we use a 300 mg/ml iodine concentration LOCA when imaging is performed using digital subtraction angiography (DSA). Even though the amount of contrast material used during angiography of the extremity is small, most of these patients may receive additional contrast material during other procedures such as computed tomographic scanning; therefore, hydration before, during, and after the procedure must be carefully monitored.

The extent of imaging and the rate of filming are tailored to the nature and extent of injury. In a case of localized gunshot injury (GSW) or stab wound (SW), we usually use a 14 inch field-of-view DSA or 14 × 14 inch cut-film study to demonstrate a segment of normal vessel proximal to the injury, the site of injury, and a segment of normal vessel distal to the injury. In patients with thrombosis of the vessel caused by injury and in elderly patients suspected of significant atherosclerotic disease, we try to demonstrate the entire distal runoff in the upper and lower extremities. Also, in cases of shotgun injury to the extremity, we routinely try to demonstrate the distal runoff to the level of the distalmost pellet observed on plain radiographs. It is not uncommon to see arterial and venous pellet emboli resulting from shotgun injury (see Fig. 8).

When using a cut-film study or DSA for localized injury, we generally use two exposures per second during the length of the contrast injection and then one exposure per second for at least double that length of time. When using a long film changer, one exposure is made every 2 seconds initially, with the interval between exposures lengthened depending on the clinical evaluation of the circulation in the limb and the age of the patient.

It is not uncommon to observe varying degrees of spasm of the vessel near the site of injury. In some cases it may be difficult to distinguish intimal injury from spasm. We may use vasodilators such as tolazoline (Priscoline) (25 to 50 mg) or nitroglycerin (100 μg) given intra-arterially proximal to the site of the suspected spasm. Rarely a follow-up study is obtained to confirm the diagnosis of spasm (see Fig. 1).

We usually use intra-arterial DSA (IA-DSA) for the evaluation of localized vascular injury. There is no clinically significant loss of resolution with 1,024 matrix DSA, and opacification of the distal vessels via collaterals is improved because of the increased contrast resolution with DSA. Even with patient motion and resultant artifacts, the study is diagnostic in a vast majority of patients (see Fig. 4). Availability of instant subtraction and improved visualization of veins are additional benefits. In our experience IA-DSA suffices in a majority of our trauma patients. Only in a small number of these patients is IA-DSA nondiagnostic, requiring imaging using conventional film-screen combinations.

## Pitfalls in Peripheral Angiography in Acute Trauma

In upper-extremity angiography, it is important to remember that in 20 percent of patients, there is high takeoff of the radial artery. This vessel could even originate from the axillary artery. Hence, for all brachial and distal forearm angiograms, initial injection must be performed in the proximal axillary artery before injection in the distal brachial artery. Second, a hypoplastic ulnar or radial artery is not uncommon. Although this anomaly is usually obvious, occasionally it may be necessary to image the palmar arches and their branches for

*Text continued on p. 843.*

A 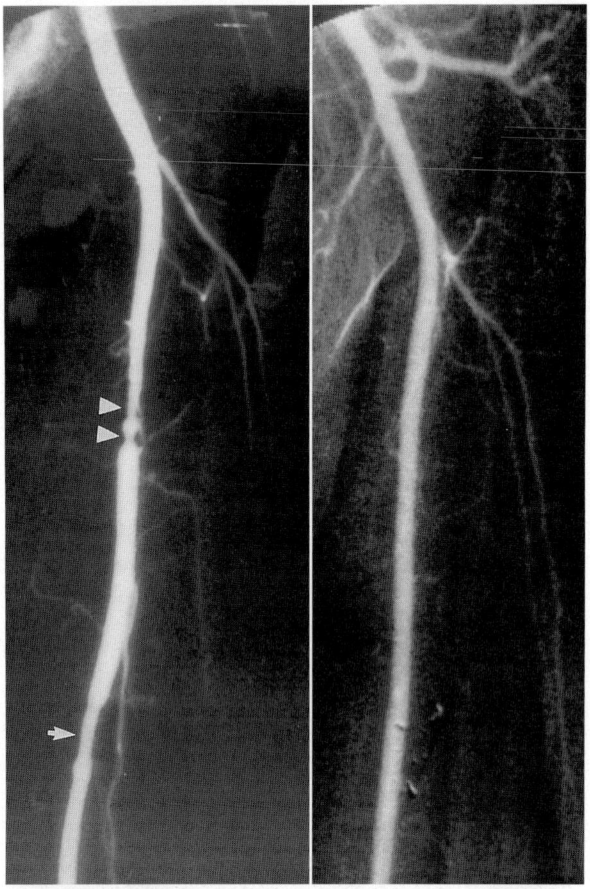 B

**FIGURE 1** Gunshot wound to proximal left upper extremity. *A,* Arteriogram performed soon after injury demonstrates segmental areas of spasm *(arrow)* and question of intimal injury *(arrowheads). B,* Follow-up IV-DSA, performed 3 days later, demonstrates resolution of the arterial spasm. No intimal injury is detected.

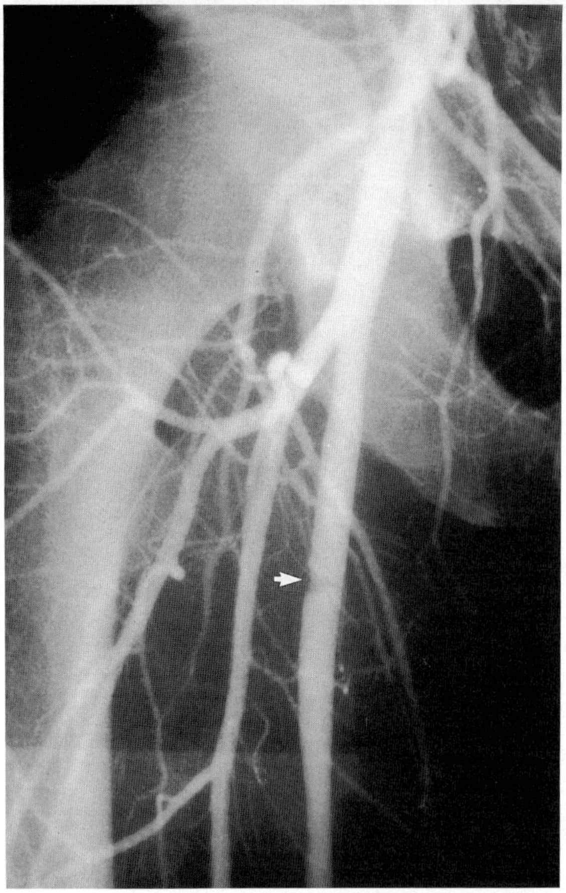

**FIGURE 2** Gunshot wound to proximal right thigh. Femoral arteriogram demonstrates intimal injury *(arrow)* of the proximal superficial femoral artery. This injury was successfully managed with conservative therapy.

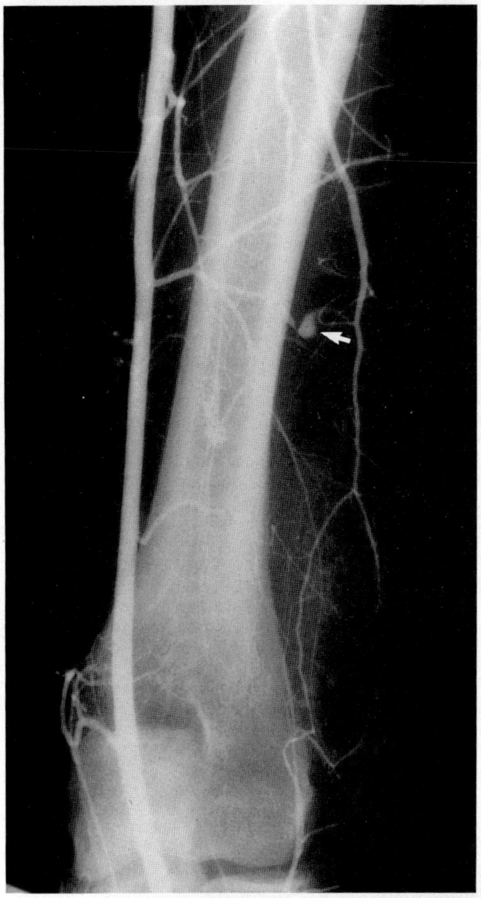

**FIGURE 3** Stab wound to left upper extremity. Pooling of contrast material *(arrow)* indicates active bleeding from a branch of the left brachial artery.

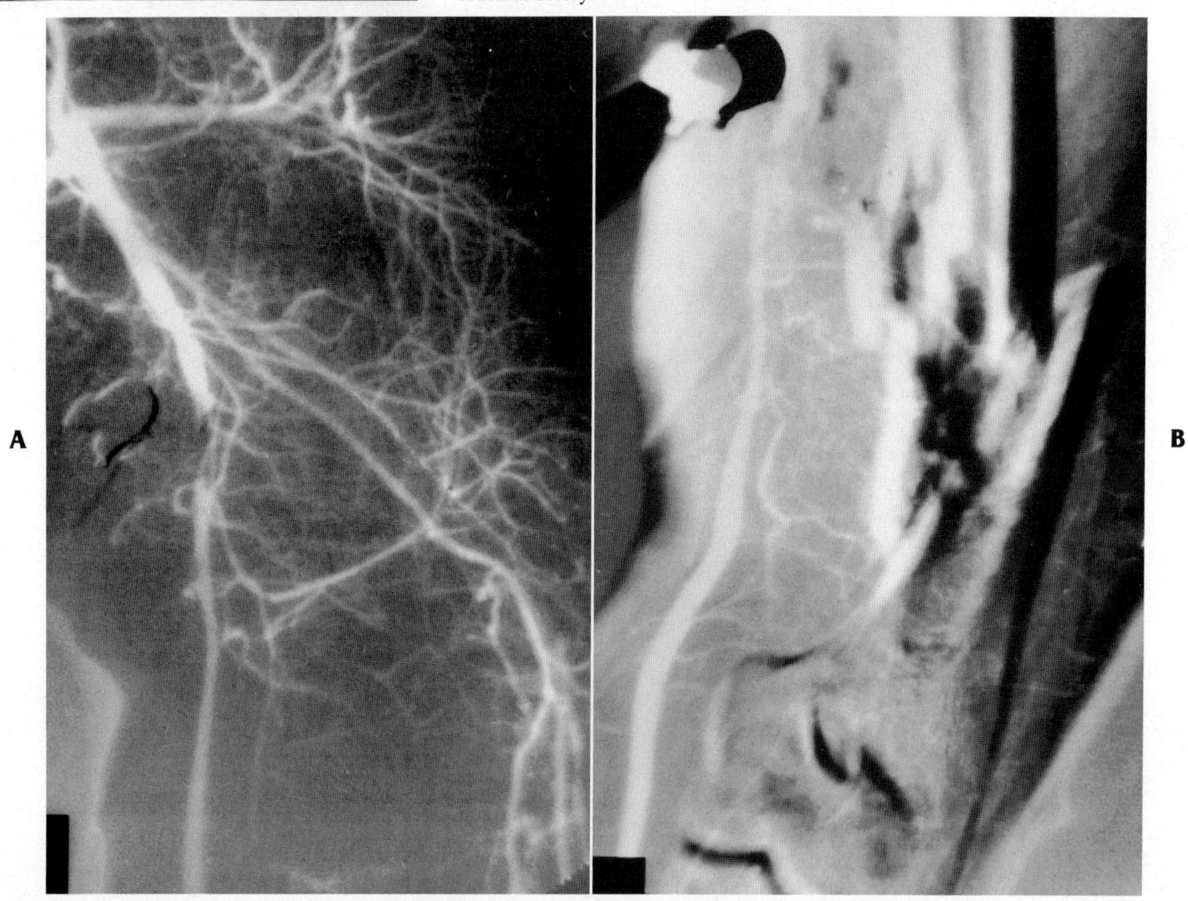

**FIGURE 4** Gunshot wound and resultant fracture of left upper extremity. *A* and *B,* DSA demonstrates partial transection and thrombosis of a short segment of the brachial artery, with collateral reconstitution. Note that distal vascular opacification is not hampered despite significant patient motion.

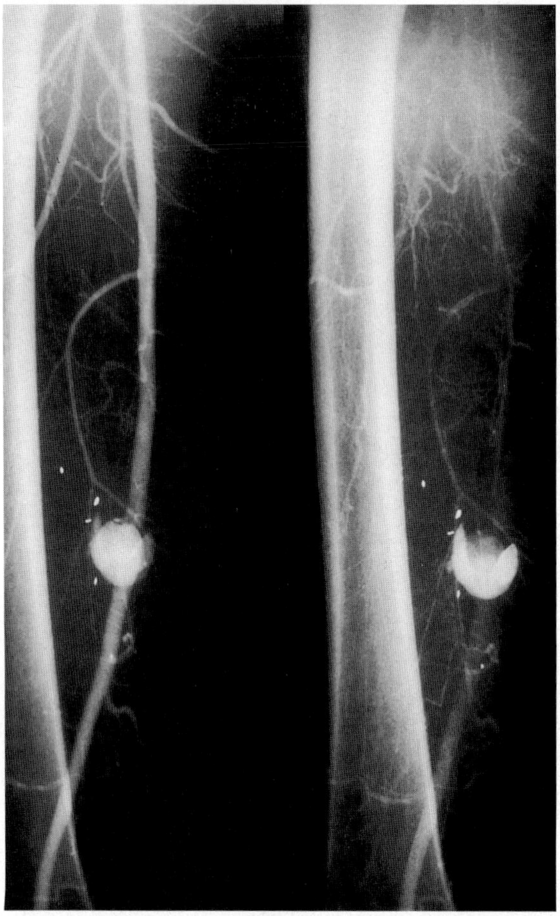

**FIGURE 5** Gunshot wound to right thigh with intact distal pulses. Moderately large pseudoaneurysm arising from the superficial femoral artery (SFA) at the approximate level of the adductor canal. There is antegrade flow in the SFA/popliteal artery.

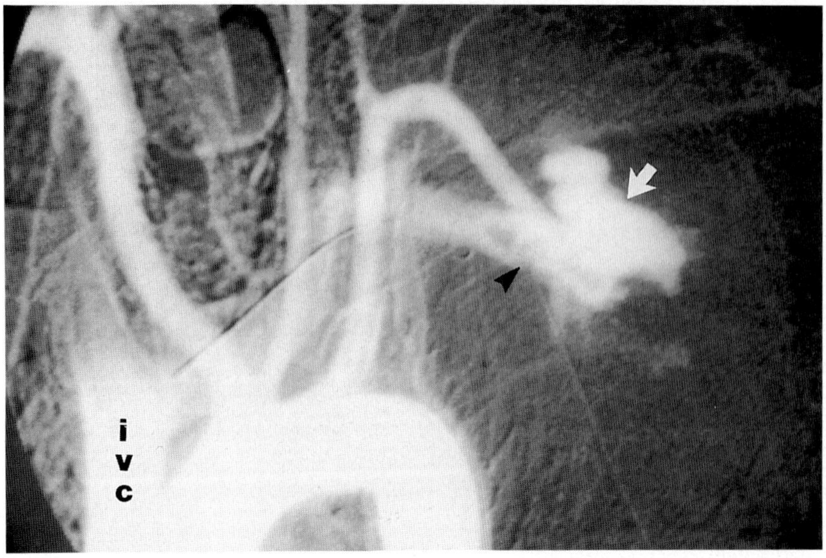


**FIGURE 6** Stab wound to left upper chest with ischemic left upper limb. Pseudoaneurysm *(arrow)* with arteriovenous fistula *(arrowhead)* involving the left subclavian artery. No distal arterial reconstitution is demonstrated despite delayed DSA filming.

A 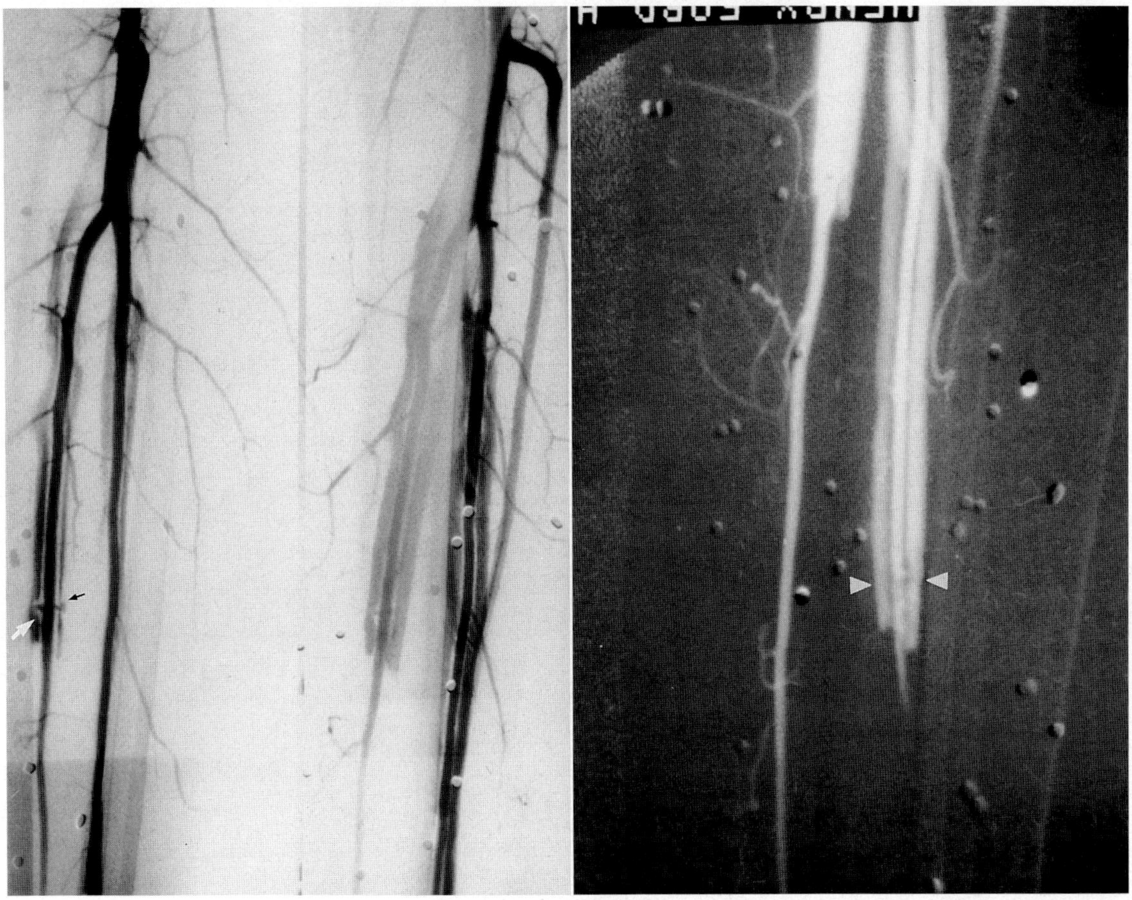 B

**FIGURE 7** Shotgun injury to lower leg. *A* and *B,* Femoral arteriogram demonstrates arteriovenous fistula *(arrows)* arising from the posterior tibial and peroneal arteries. Paired draining veins *(arrowheads)* from each of these arteries are opacified.

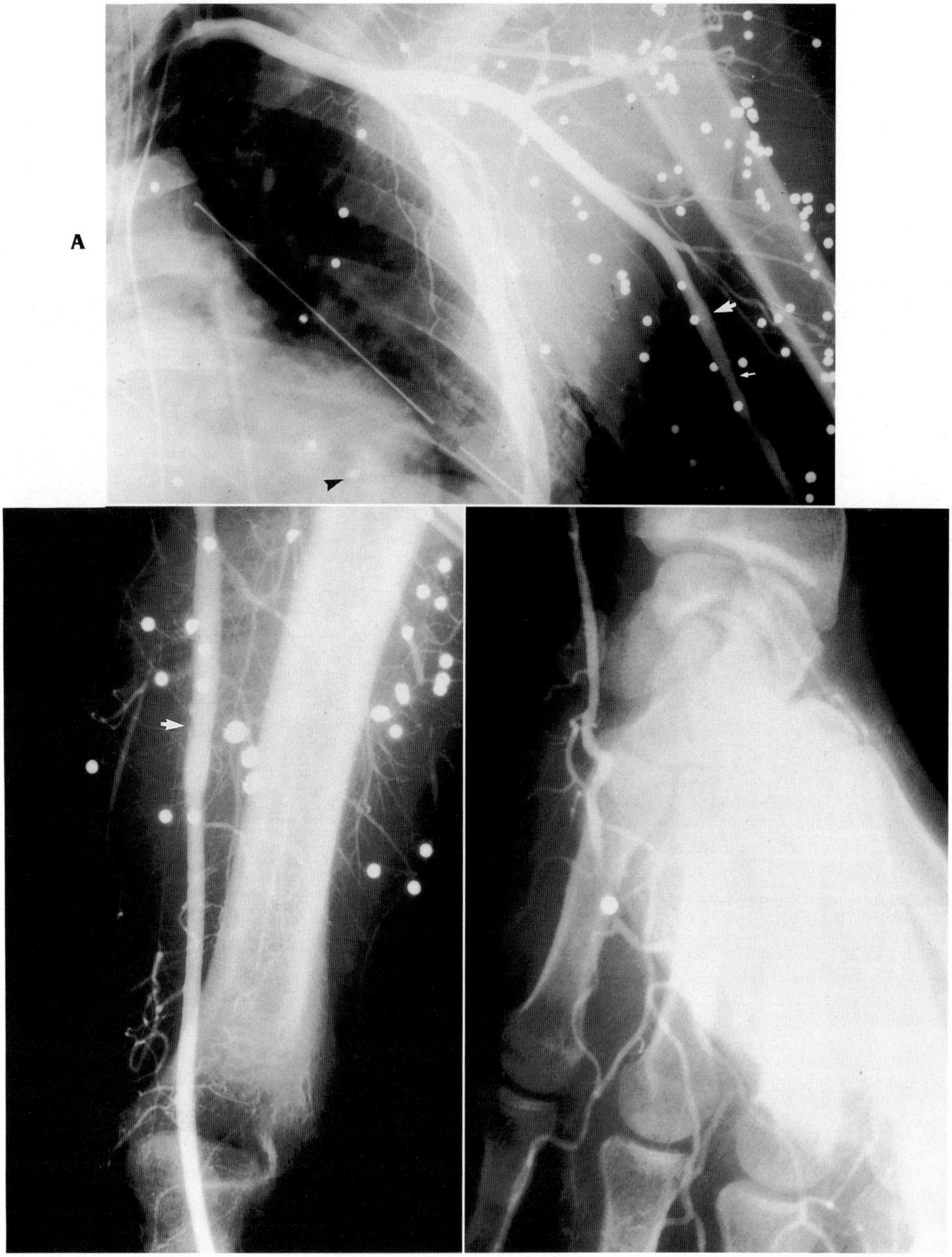


**FIGURE 8** Shotgun injury to left shoulder. *A,* Multiple buckshot pellets are distributed about the left shoulder. Multiple areas of intimal irregularity are present *(arrows).* Motion of one pellet *(arrowhead)*, confirmed to be located within the right ventricle by echocardiography. *B,* Arteriographic evidence of intimal injury *(arrow)* and spasm involving the distal left brachial artery. *C,* Distal arterial embolization of one of the shotgun pellets occluding a short segment of the distal ulnar artery.

confirmation of this anomaly. Hypoplasia of one of the popliteal outflow tract vessels is not uncommon. In most cases there is hypoplasia of either the anterior tibial or the posterior tibial artery, with peroneal artery continuing into the foot as the dorsalis pedis artery or as a posterior tibial artery. In these cases there is gradual tapering of the hypoplastic artery. The peroneal artery continues uninterrupted into the foot in these situations, rather than appearing as a collateral vessel reconstituting the anterior or posterior tibial artery. Rarely is there hypoplasia of both the anterior and posterior tibial arteries with a remaining large peroneal artery.

Spasm induced by the guidewire, especially the J-guidewire in a small artery such as the brachial artery, may be difficult to differentiate from the spasm produced by injury. For this reason, great care must be taken to avoid the passage of a guidewire, especially a J-guidewire, near the site of suspected injury.

## Radiographic Findings in Penetrating Extremity Trauma

Vascular extremity trauma may be manifested angiographically as follows:

1. Spasm (Fig. 1)
2. Intimal injury (Fig. 2)
3. Contrast extravasation (Fig. 3)
4. Transection (Fig. 4)
5. Pseudoaneurysm (Figs. 5 and 6)
6. Arteriovenous fistula (Figs. 6 and 7)
7. Occlusion, thrombosis, peripheral emboli (Fig. 8)
8. Dissection
9. Displacement

## Suggested Reading

Ben-Menachem Y, Handel SF. Angiography in Trauma: A Work Atlas. Philadelphia: WB Saunders, 1981.

Frykberg ER, Crump JM, Vines FS, et al. A reassessment of the role of arteriography in penetrating proximity extremity trauma: A prospective study. J Trauma 1989; 29:8.

Hollerman JJ, Packler ML, Coldwell DM, Ben-Menachem Y. Gunshot wounds: 2. Radiology. AJR 1990; 155:691–702.

Rutherford RB. Diagnostic evaluation of extremity vascular injuries. Surg Clin North Am 1988; 68:4.

# MRI of the Abdominal and Peripheral Vasculature

*FRED STEINBERG, M.D.*

Noninvasive vascular imaging by magnetic resonance imaging (MRI) and magnetic resonance angiography (MRA) is aiding radiologists in diagnosing diseases affecting the arteries and veins of the abdomen, pelvis, and lower extremities. Taking advantage of two fundamental effects of protons in blood flow exposed to magnetic field gradients (velocity-induced phase shifts and flow-related enhancement) MRI specialists are applying tailored pulse sequences to diagnose the spectrum of diseases from deep vein thrombosis (DVT) to aortic aneurysms. This chapter communicates some of the specifics of these tailored pulse sequences and discusses the principles and practices of customizing pulse sequences.

## Peripheral Vasculature

The earliest applications of MRA were tested in the peripheral circulation. The goal of vascular imaging is to aid in assessing the severity of peripheral vascular occlusive disease and planning interventions. This requires identification and grading of the lesion, and assessment of the inflow and outflow arteries. For the radiologist, the application of MRI to the diagnosis of blood vessel abnormalities holds the promise of complete noninvasive diagnosis of vascular diseases.

### *Atherosclerotic Peripheral Vascular Disease*

In the United States, atherosclerotic disease is the most common disease affecting the arterial side of the circulation. Atherosclerosis may lead to aneurysm formation, vessel wall rupture, dissection, arterial embolization, occlusion or stenosis, and hypertension.

### *MRA Techniques*

Since 1988, essentially two MRA techniques have been tested clinically. They are cine phase-contrast (PC) MRA and two-dimensional time-of-flight (2D TOF) MRA. There are several advantages of cine PC MRA over 2D TOF MRA. Wide fields of view (up to 40 cm) and short imaging times ($<2$ minutes per acquisition) allow an entire study of the pelvic and lower extremity arteries to be acquired in under 40 minutes. Current cine PC MRA techniques are able to freeze respiratory motion and bowel motion. Since cine PC MRA is a direct projection technique, no additional post-processing is required. By adjusting the velocity-encoding gradients, cine PC MRA is more sensitive to slow arterial flow and yields better suppression of stationary tissues as well as elimination of pulsatile artifacts. This allows visualization of arterial flow distal to high-grade stenoses (Fig. 1) and occlusions (Fig. 2). Because of the wide range of velocity sensitivities and the temporal resolution of cine PC MRA, this technique tends not to overestimate the severity or length of stenoses or occlusions.

However, there are also advantages of 2D TOF MRA compared with cine PC MRA. First, 2D TOF MRA does not require cardiac gating or MRI devices with shielded gradients.

A

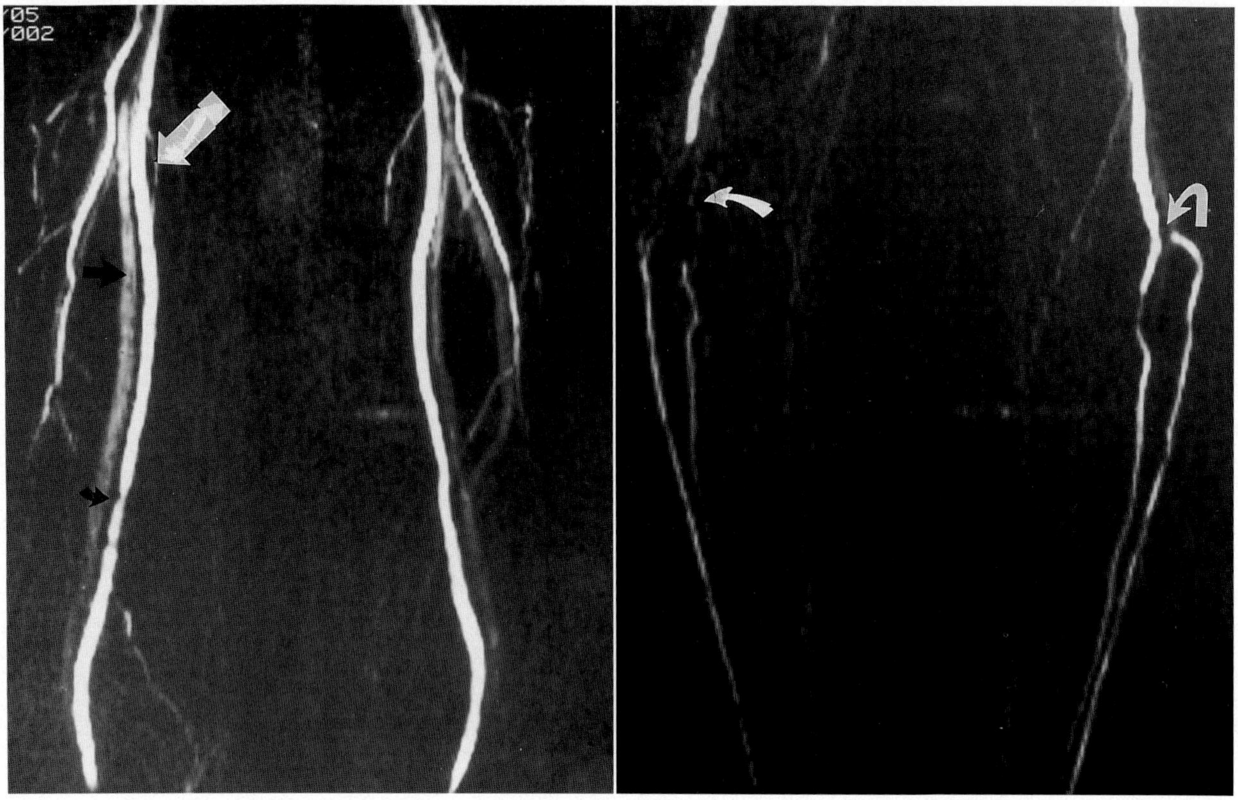

B

**FIGURE 1** Femoral and popliteal artery stenosis. Cine PC MRA (TR/TE 22/8 ms, 20° flip-angle, 60 cm/sec VENC, superoinferior flow direction, 2 NEX, NP). *A* and *B,* These images illustrate the appearance of the right SFA *(white arrow),* a right SFA stenosis *(small black arrow),* and unsuppressed flow in the femoral vein *(large black arrow)* causing an artifact. The distal right popliteal artery is occluded *(white arrow)* and reconstitutes two tibial vessels. Note the artifact in the left anterior tibial artery *(curved white arrow)* due to flow in an orthogonal direction to the flow-sensitive gradients.

A

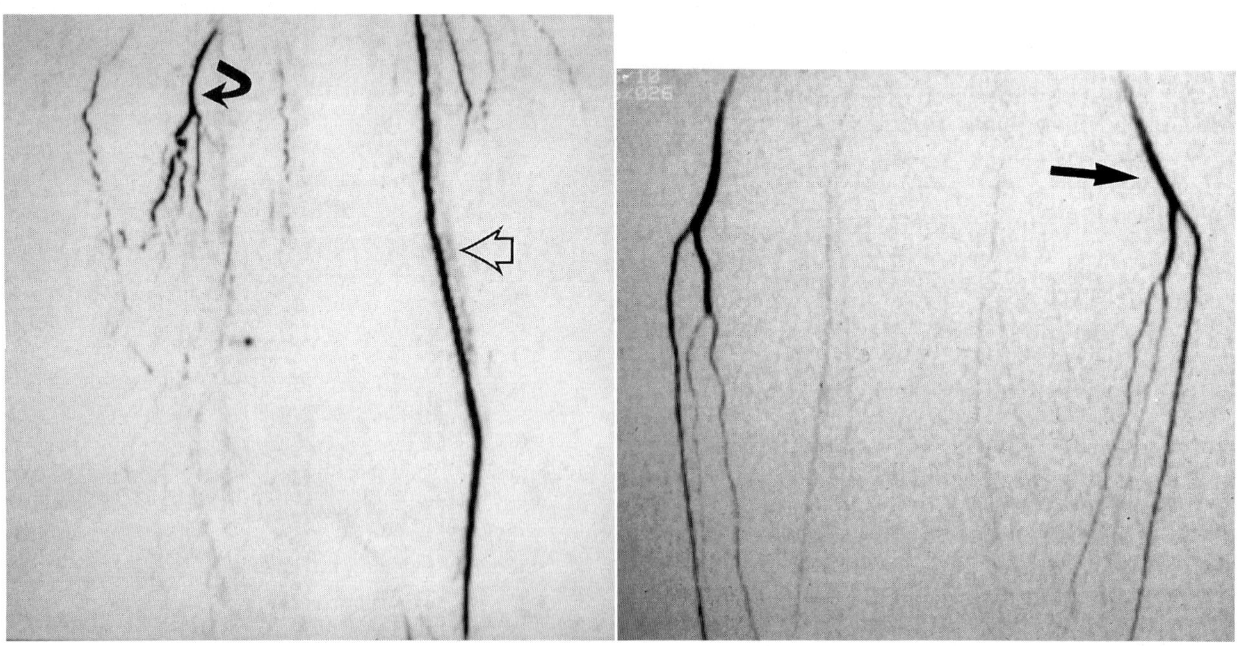

B

**FIGURE 2** Peripheral vascular occlusive disease. Cine PC MRA (TR/TE 22/8 ms, 20° flip-angle, 60 cm/sec VENC, superoinferior flow direction, 2 NEX, NP). *A* and *B,* These images show a patent left SFA *(open arrow)* with occlusion of the right SFA and enlarged right profunda femoral artery *(curved black arrow).* At the knee the popliteal arteries *(black arrow)* are patent with three tibial vessel runoff.

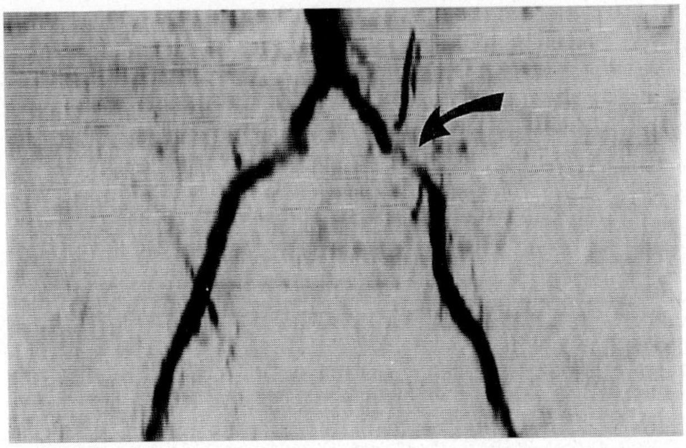

**FIGURE 3** Left iliac artery stenosis. Axial 2D TOF MRA (TR/TE 45/8 ms, 60° flip-angle, 3 mm slice thickness, SAT/i, 1 NEX, body coil). Note the moderate stenosis *(curved arrow)* in this patient with mild claudication.

Another major advantage of 2D TOF MRA is the acquisition of a three-dimensional (3D) data set from which projections at any oblique angulation can be created.

## *Results and Reliability*

In a report to the 44th Annual Meeting of the Society of Vascular Surgery in 1990, I compared cine PC MRA, 2D TOF MRA, and angiography in the lower extremity of 25 patients. The highlights of the study were the following: in 14 patients studied by cine PC MRA, the overall accuracy was 94 percent, whereas 2D TOF MRA was 85 percent accurate for the identification of arterial stenoses, occlusions, and characterization of the runoff vessels in 11 patients.

Mulligan and Lanzer at the University of Alabama have reported their results of a study comparing 2D TOF MRA with angiography. They found that this MRA technique overestimated the severity and length of a stenosis or occlusion and that the pelvic arteries were difficult to visualize. However, Yucel at Massachusetts General Hospital has been using 2D TOF MRA with increasing degrees of success in detecting target arteries distal to proximal occlusions (Fig. 3).

## *Image Interpretation Hints*

The interpretation of cine PC MRA differs slightly from angiography. However, 2D TOF MRA differs greatly. First, an area of flow signal dropout may indicate a severe stenosis, rather than an occlusion. Second, collateral vessels and arteries with flow in-plane or retrograde flow may not be visualized. Care must be taken not to overestimate severity of stenoses or occlusions. To help resolve problems, higher-resolution images with surface coils targeted to the abnormality are suggested.

## *Pitfalls and Artifacts*

Since MRA is looking at blood flow rather than the wall of the artery, all MRA techniques have a tendency to overestimate both the length and severity of arterial stenoses. High-resolution images with short TEs and motion suppression are mandatory to decrease this problem. Although MRA has been reported to be sensitive to slow flow in the peripheral arteries, large voxel size may lead to false-positive occlusions. Finally, a word of caution is in order in the evaluation of patients after vascular surgical bypasses and those patients who have had prior implantation of metallic surgical clips: MRA is sensitive to the artifacts produced by metal. These artifacts tend to overestimate lesions.

## *Clinical Applications*

### Popliteal Aneurysms

The radiographic workup of suspected popliteal artery aneurysms consists of two components: (1) confirmation of the aneurysm and distinguishing it from other masses, and (2) identification of inflow and outflow arteries for surgical planning. MRA has been applied to detect popliteal aneurysms. Together with thin-slice axial MRI, we have studied four patients with suspected popliteal aneurysms. Both cine PC MRA and 2D TOF MRA accurately identified the aneurysm and the tibial vessels and the more proximal femoral arteries. MRA was able to accurately depict the arterial anatomy with respect to distal occlusions, anatomic variants, and proximal stenoses (Fig. 4). MRI more accurately sizes aneurysms and detects the presence of intraluminal thrombus than does angiography. It may also be more accurate at detecting leaking aneurysms due to the presence of characteristic MRI signal intensities indicating the presence of hemorrhage.

### Diabetic Foot Ulcers

Severe tibial trifurcation disease, with sparing of the iliac and femoral arteries, frequently characterizes diabetic vascular disease. For the diabetic, target vessels in the distal tibial distribution or even the foot need to be identified for surgical planning. Although the velocity of blood flow in these vessels may be low, high-resolution 2D TOF MRA frequently can

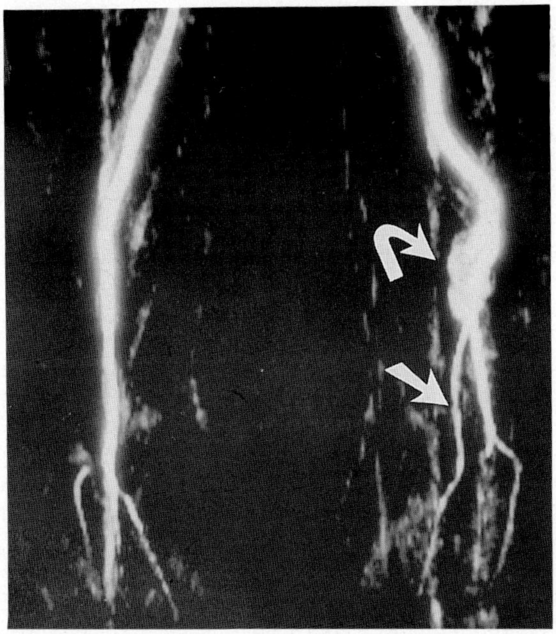

**FIGURE 4** Left popliteal artery aneurysm. Cine PC MRA (TR/TE 24/10 ms, 20° flip-angle, 40 cm/sec VENC, superoinferior flow direction, 2 NEX, NP). Note the anomalous origin of the posterior tibial artery *(straight white arrow)* directly from the aneurysm *(curved white arrow)*.

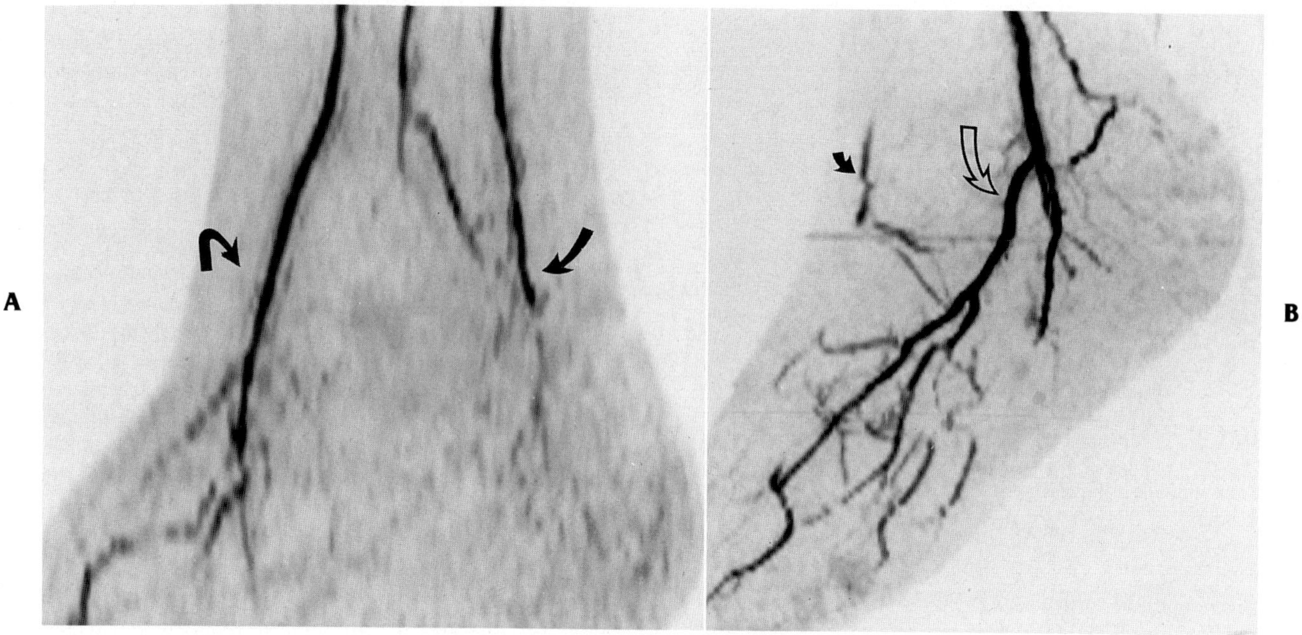

**FIGURE 5** MRA of the foot. Axial 2D TOF MRA (TR/TE 45/8 ms, 60° flip-angle, 1.5 mm slice thickness, SAT/i, 1 NEX, extremity coil). *A,* Occlusion of the posterior tibial artery *(black arrow)* and the dorsalis pedis *(curved black arrow)* in a diabetic man with foot ulcer. *B,* Traumatic occlusion of the dorsalis pedis artery *(black arrow)* with collateral flow to the metatarsals arising via the plantar arch *(curved arrow).*

detect the reconstituted dorsalis pedis artery and plantar arch vessels, but may not visualize flow more distally due to in-plane saturation (Fig. 5). Cine PC MRA, even with strong velocity encoding, may not detect some of the target vessels due to unsuppressed stationary tissue signal, but in general has a greater sensitivity to detecting small vessels in the foot.

### Venous Disease of the Lower Extremity: Superficial and Deep Vein Thrombosis

MRA has been employed in the diagnosis and staging of venous occlusions with great success. Spritzer and co-workers have reported a high accuracy finding DVT using 2D TOF MRA. In general, MRA is highly sensitive for detecting venous flow in the popliteal vein and above, but is less sensitive for flow in the tibial veins and veins of the calf. It has been our experience that flow in the tibial veins may be stagnant, or at least slower than the prescribed MRA velocity sensitivity, and that the tibial veins are frequently not visualized. In addition, patient position and external compression either at the popliteal space or the groin may cause loss of flow signal from the veins.

MRA is the only noninvasive imaging modality that can reliably identify pelvic vein DVT. In clinical practice, patients with suspected DVT are evaluated primarily by color-flow ultrasonography of the legs. If iliac vein thrombosis is still in question, MR venography (MRV) is performed. We use a combination of 2D PC projections and 2D TOF MRA to evaluate for the presence of DVT (Figs. 6 and 7). Although the slices are reformatted into venogram-equivalent images, it is important to view the raw data images to find intraluminal nonoccluding thrombi. Rarely, bright T1-weighted clot may fill the lumen of a vein and appear completely normal on TOF images. In these circumstances, a 2D PC image is invaluable in preventing a false-positive interpretation.

## Renal Artery Stenosis: Diagnostic Imaging with MRA

### *Indications and Clinical Utility*

Renal artery stenosis (RAS) is present when there is a narrowing of the main blood supply to the kidneys that can lead to decreased blood flow. If the stenosis is tight enough, it can lead to occlusion of the renal artery and loss of function from the affected kidney. However, for the majority of patients, the reduced blood flow affects mainly the renin-angiotensin system and leads to elevation of systemic blood pressure.

The gold standard in the diagnosis of RAS is conventional angiography. Since the prevalence of RAS is low, several noninvasive diagnostic procedures have been used as a screening test before angiography. Although these tests have relied on altered physiology to predict the presence of RAS, MRA is the first noninvasive test to image the renal artery itself.

### *MRA Techniques and Imaging Hints*

Because of their motion in the abdomen, the renal arteries present a technical challenge for MRA. Suppression of respiratory motion and stationary tissue, as well as elimination of overlapping venous flow, are essential to performance of successful renal artery MRA. Except for the cine PC technique which uses a thick-slab excitation, renal artery MRA methods rely on postprocessing reconstructions using the maximum intensity projection (MIP). Well-known artifacts can be produced by this technique if the input image slices do not have sufficient contrast between blood flow and stationary tissue, or contain overlapping blood vessels such as the inferior vena cava (IVC) or renal veins.

A

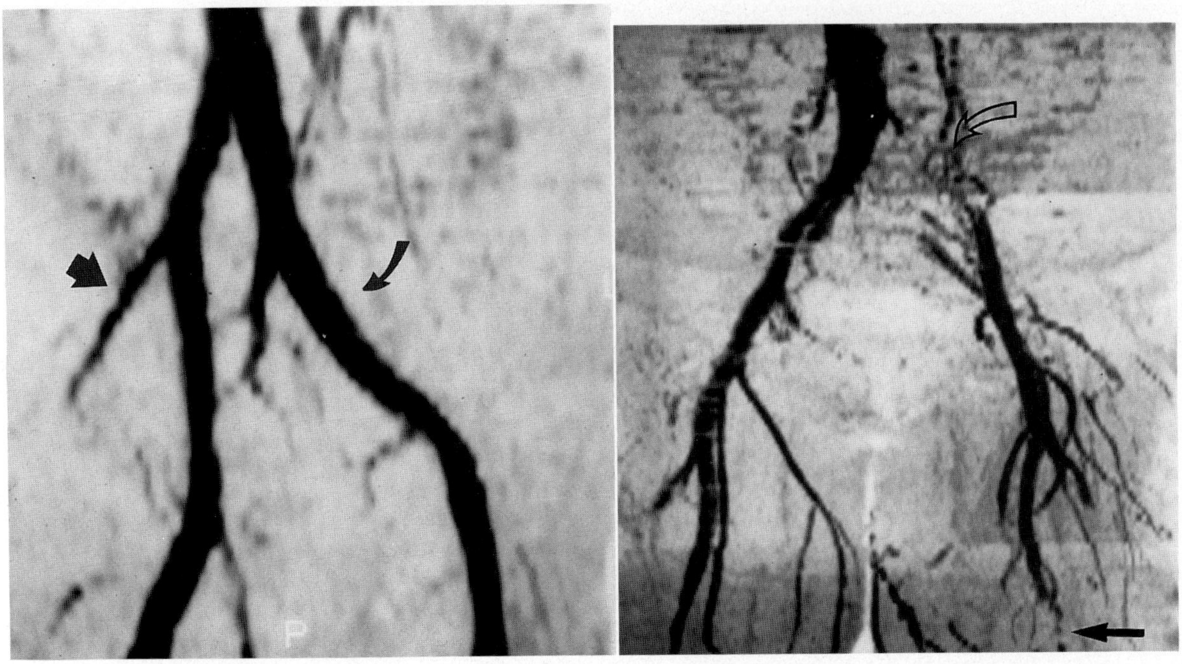

B

**FIGURE 6** 2D TOF MRA of the iliac veins (TR/TE 45/7 ms, 60° flip-angle, 3 mm slice thickness, SAT/s, 1 NEX). The acquisition time for 100 slices was under 10 minutes. The common iliac, external iliac *(curved arrow),* and internal iliac veins *(straight arrow)* are patent and well visualized in *(A)*. *B,* The left common iliac vein *(curved open arrow)* and the left femoral vein *(black arrow)* in the thigh are both occluded due to a chronic deep vein thrombosis.

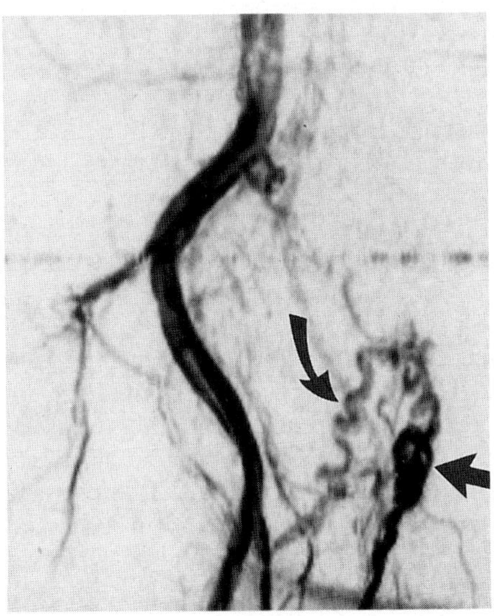

**FIGURE 7** Left iliac vein occlusion. Thick-slab coronal 2D PC MRA (TR/TE 25/10 ms, 20° flip-angle, 30 cm/sec VENC, all flow-encoding directions, SAT/s, 8 NEX). The left femoral vein in the groin is dilated *(straight arrow),* and venous return from the left leg is via transabdominal collaterals *(curved black arrow)* to the right femoral vein.

The first report describing aortorenal MRA in patients used a 2D TOF MRA technique, with acquisition of overlapping axial and coronal images obtained during breath holding. These images were postprocessed using MIP to produce projection MRAs. Additional reports testing MRA have used 3D TOF MRA, 3D PC MRA, 2D PC MRA, and cine PC MRA.

## Strategies to Suppress the Renal Veins and IVC

There are two main methods of venous flow signal suppression: venous presaturation and postprocessing phase information. In the first method, presaturation bands are placed upstream of the area of interest to eliminate signal in flowing blood. This eliminates flow-related enhancement in the blood vessel and thereby removes it from the image. In the case of renal artery MRA, a horizontal presaturation band is placed over the IVC proximal to the renal arteries, and vertical presaturation bands are placed over each kidney. Some MRI systems allow angled presaturation bands to be placed, which decreases the required number of bands from three to two. Placement of the presaturation bands requires explicit knowledge of the arterial anatomy. If the aorta is tortuous or the heart is enlarged, the band over the left kidney can diminish flow signal in the aorta and thereby decrease signal intensity in the renal arteries. If the band over the IVC is too narrow or placed too far upstream, the blood flow signal may reaccumulate and negate the effect of the presaturation band. Another disadvantage of saturation bands is that they force the TR and TE to increase. In general, we prefer a shorter TE in order to minimize intravoxel dephasing and improve image quality. A shorter TR is preferred in breath-hold techniques to minimize slice acquisition time.

The other venous flow suppression technique uses PC. By selecting a single direction of flow sensitivity, blood flow in an orthogonal direction is not detected. By selecting right-left flow direction, flow in the IVC is suppressed. Inherent to PC imaging, the direction of flow can be determined by the sign of the phase shift. If the phase shift is positive, blood flow is one direction; if the phase shift is negative, the flow is in the opposite direction. In this way the renal veins can be

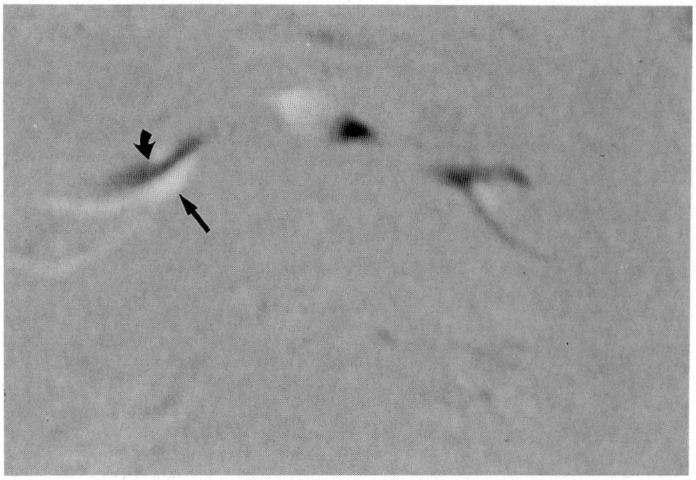

**FIGURE 8** Axial PC MRA of renal arteries. 3D PC MRA (TR/TE 24/10 ms, 20° flip-angle, 30 cm/sec VENC, right-left flow direction, 1 NEX, NP). This raw data image encodes blood flow direction. The right renal artery *(straight black arrow)* is white and the right renal vein *(curved black arrow)* is black.

A

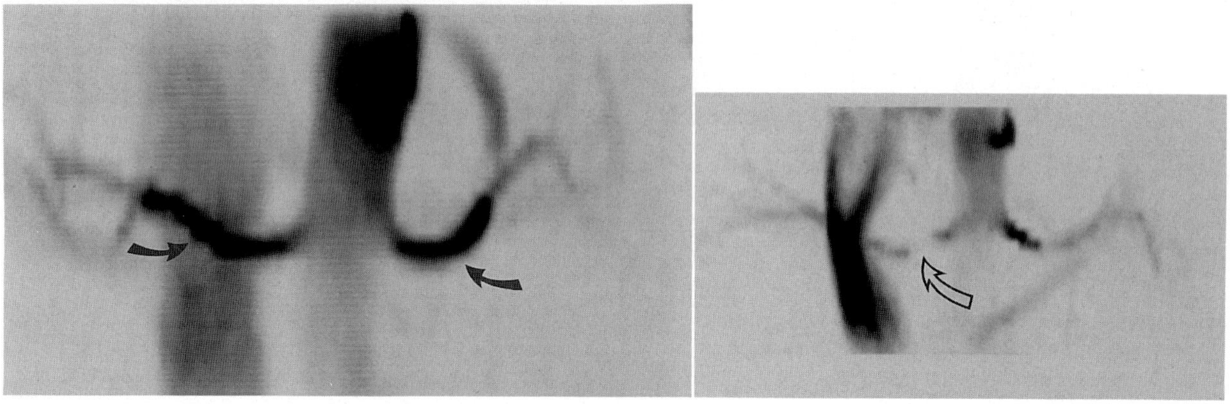

B

**FIGURE 9** Renal artery MRA. 3D PC MRA (TR/TE 24/10 ms, 20° flip-angle, 30 cm/sec VENC, all flow directions, 1 NEX, NP). *(A)* shows patent renal arteries *(curved black arrows),* while *(B)* shows a tight stenosis of the right renal artery *(curved white arrow)* that subsequently received balloon angioplasty in a patient with hypertension.

eliminated from the overlapping renal artery, since their direction of flow should be opposite to the renal artery (Fig. 8).

### Preferred MRA Technique

The technique that I have come to prefer is a two-sequence, 3D PC technique that takes advantage of the high signal-to-noise ratio and thin-slice capabilities of 3D techniques while relying on the excellent stationary tissue suppression afforded by PC. The first acquisition encodes flow only in the right-left direction and is acquired in under 3 minutes. The second acquisition is acquired only if the first acquisition is not normal and usually takes 9 minutes (Fig. 9).

## *Interpretation and Reliability*

Interpretation is based on detection of severe RAS. MRA has been particularly accurate in the diagnosis of ostial RAS. The sign of a tight stenosis is a signal dropout at the point of stenosis due to intravoxel dephasing (see Fig. 9). With the current TE and voxel size, this corresponds to approximately 75 percent diameter stenosis. If there is a narrowing in the artery, particularly at the ostia, this corresponds to a stenosis, but not an angiographically significant stenosis.

In the Cedars-Sinai series, 95 patients underwent MRA of the renal arteries from March 1990 to April 1991. Of these patients, 32 had confirmatory angiograms. Analysis of the data revealed the following: (1) in all 12 patients with a normal MRA, the angiogram was also normal; (2) angiography confirmed all 4 renal artery occlusions detected by MRA; (3) 23 tight RAS were visualized by MRA, and angiography agreed in 17 of 23 cases for a 74 percent artery specificity; (4) however, either one or both renal arteries were affected in 16 of 17 patients that had a positive MRA for a 94 percent patient specificity; and (5) the overall diagnostic accuracy of MRA was 88 percent.

## *Pitfalls and Artifacts*

MRA has been shown to be most helpful in patients with renal insufficiency and hypertension. It is most accurate for identifying ostial and proximal RAS, less accurate for distal stenoses. Some of the pitfalls for renal MRA identified were the presence of the following: accessory renal arteries, branch stenoses, and the presence of fibromuscular disease.

Artifactual sources of flow signal dropout have been observed in tortuous arteries and those arteries with sharp angulation, particularly when only a single distal branch can be observed. Mistakenly identifying the renal vein, particularly the left renal vein as the left renal artery, has been a source of false-negative evaluations. Even cases where the splenic artery and vein have been mistaken for the left renal artery have been observed.

Although angiography displays contrast displacement in arteries, MRA is sensitive to blood flow velocity. Therefore MRA cannot distinguish an occluded artery from a patent artery with minimal or absent blood flow. In patients with end-stage renal disease or congestive heart failure, MRA may show false-positive occlusions due to minimal flow in the renal arteries.

## Liver MRA

MRA has had a significant impact on vascular assessment of the liver, including pre–liver transplant evaluation. TOF MRA techniques have been used to assess the patency of the portal vein in patients with extrahepatic masses, including pancreatic head carcinomas and masses in the porta hepatis. MRA has been shown to confirm the patency of the portal vein, the splenic vein, and the superior mesenteric vein in cirrhotic patients. The role of MRA in assessing the segmental venous anatomy of the liver in presurgical liver resection planning is under investigation and may replace other imaging modalities.

### *Techniques*

Two-dimensional TOF breath-hold MRA with MIP postprocessing has become the preferred method for liver MRA at most centers. Each breath hold is 6 seconds, which allows for practically all patients to be imaged, even those patients whose respiration is compromised due to ascites. Single- or double-slice, sequential, axial and coronal images are acquired, and subvolume MIP reconstructions are created. The most relevant images are the coronal and the axial projections. Rarely the angled projections are helpful in displaying the anatomy in three dimensions.

I also have had some clinical experience with PC MRA. One pulse sequence uses 2D thick-slab PC breath-hold MRA technique that requires registration of three orthogonal views (Fig. 10); the other is a 3D acquisition (Fig. 11). We have tested axial 3D PC techniques and reviewed the component raw data; the results have been comparable to the 2D PC MRA images, but the acquisition and postprocessing times were longer.

#### Determining Direction of Blood Flow in the Portal Vein

It has been shown with conventional angiography and color duplex ultrasonography that the direction of portal vein flow correlates to the presence of portal hypertension. If bidirectional or reverse flow is present, the patient has portal hypertension.

*Presaturation.* This technique uses a wide presaturation band to eliminate reverse flow signal in the portal vein during a sagittal MRA acquisition. If the portal vein retains bright signal intensity, this verifies normal direction flow in the portal vein. This is performed in a breath hold of approximately 6 seconds. The presaturation band is then placed on the opposite side, and this can be used to detect bidirectional flow as well as distinguish slow flow from portal vein occlusion (Fig. 12).

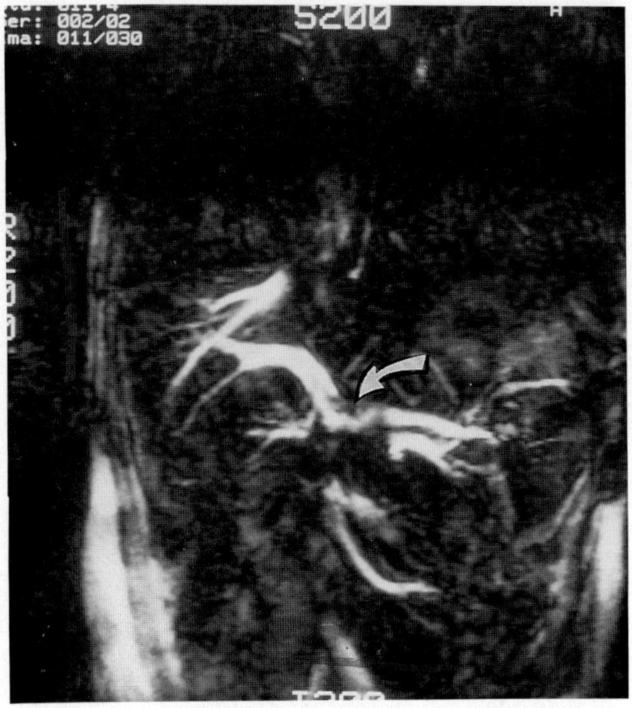


**FIGURE 10** Breath-hold 2D PC MRA of portal vein (TR/TE 24/10 ms, 20° flip-angle, 30 cm/sec VENC, right-left velocity direction, 8 cm slice thickness, SAT/s, 4 NEX). This image, encoded for flow in a single direction, was acquired in about 16 seconds of breath holding. Note the dephasing artifact at the splenoportal junction *(curved white arrow)* due to complex flow. This is an artifact and not to be confused with a thrombus.

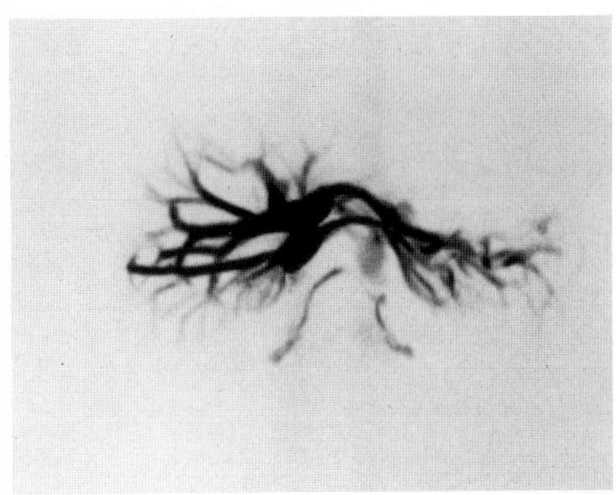

**FIGURE 11** Axial 3D PC liver MRA (TR/TE 24/10 ms, 20° flip-angle, 30 cm/sec VENC, all flow directions, 1 NEX, NP). (Courtesy of C. Dumoulin, Ph.D.)

*Phase-contrast MRA.* This method relies on a phase-weighted reconstruction where the background is gray and one direction of flow is coded white and the opposite direction is coded black (Fig. 13).

*Bolus Tracking.* Bolus tracking is a technique first described by Edelman and co-workers that relies on the use of a spatially selective presaturation pulse to turn blood flow black and measure the displacement of that black blood profile to determine the direction and velocity of blood flow.

A

B

C

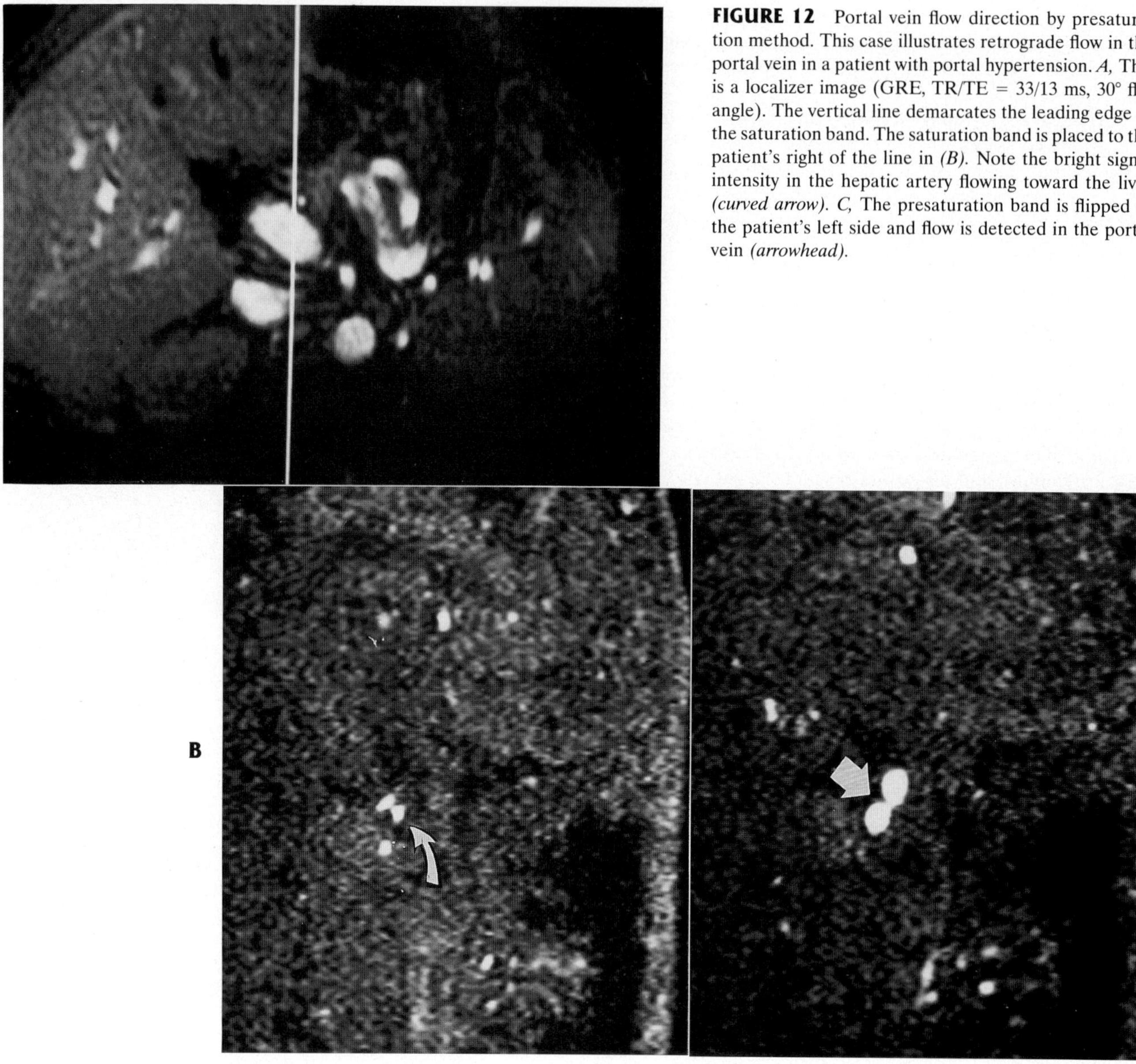

**FIGURE 12** Portal vein flow direction by presaturation method. This case illustrates retrograde flow in the portal vein in a patient with portal hypertension. *A,* This is a localizer image (GRE, TR/TE = 33/13 ms, 30° flip angle). The vertical line demarcates the leading edge of the saturation band. The saturation band is placed to the patient's right of the line in *(B).* Note the bright signal intensity in the hepatic artery flowing toward the liver *(curved arrow). C,* The presaturation band is flipped to the patient's left side and flow is detected in the portal vein *(arrowhead).*

## *Clinical Indications*

### Liver Transplantation

MRA has had a significant impact on liver transplant staging and planning. The goals of imaging before liver transplantation include assessing the patency of the portal vein and superior mesenteric vein, the status of the IVC, the presence of malignancy in the liver or other abdominal organs, and the presence of portosystemic shunts and varices. Although the identification of the arterial supply to the liver is important, this is usually performed at the time of liver transplantation and is not relevant to the donor-recipient arterial anastomosis. Although the intrahepatic portal vein may be occluded, if the extrahepatic portal vein and the splenoportal confluence is intact, the surgical plan is unchanged. If the main portal vein is occluded, the donor portal vein is anastomosed to the recipient superior mesenteric vein.

It is important to recognize the potential diagnostic problems with detection of blood flow in the portal vein. It is important to identify thrombus, even if nonoccluding, since this will likely present problems at surgery. Recanalization of the portal vein may lead to surgical problems due to postphlebitic thickening and may not provide an adequate platform for anastomosis.

### Portal Hypertension

A number of papers in the ultrasonography literature have compared the detection of various portosystemic collaterals and the direction of flow in the portal vein to the presence and severity of portal hypertension. MRA has been shown to confirm the patency of the portal vein, the splenic vein, and the superior mesenteric vein. In my experience, the cross-sectional images of TOF MRA are superior to color-flow and duplex ultrasonography for the identification of varices and portosystemic collaterals (Fig. 14). In the series of patients studied at Cedars-Sinai Medical Center, we have seen the following portosystemic collaterals: spontaneous splenorenal shunts,

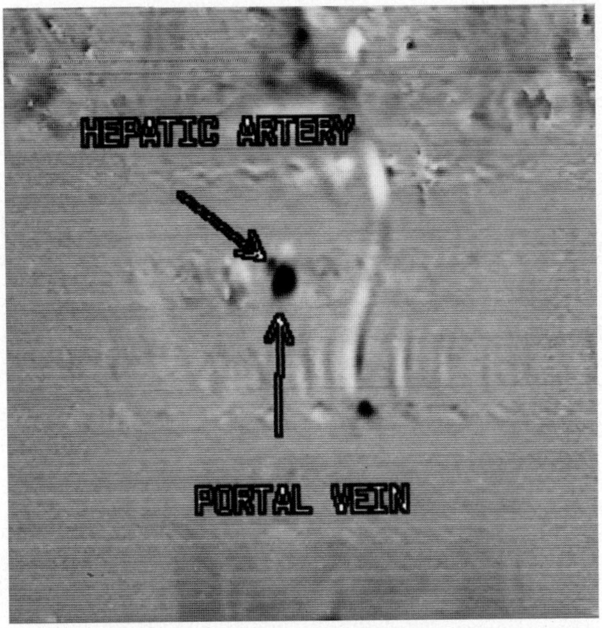


**FIGURE 13** Portal vein flow direction by phase image. Thin-slice sagittal 2D PC MRA (TR/TE 22/8 ms, 20° flip-angle, 30 cm/sec VENC, right-left velocity direction, 5 mm slice thickness, 2 NEX, NP). Note the black signal in both the portal vein and the hepatic artery, indicating the same direction of flow toward the liver.

A

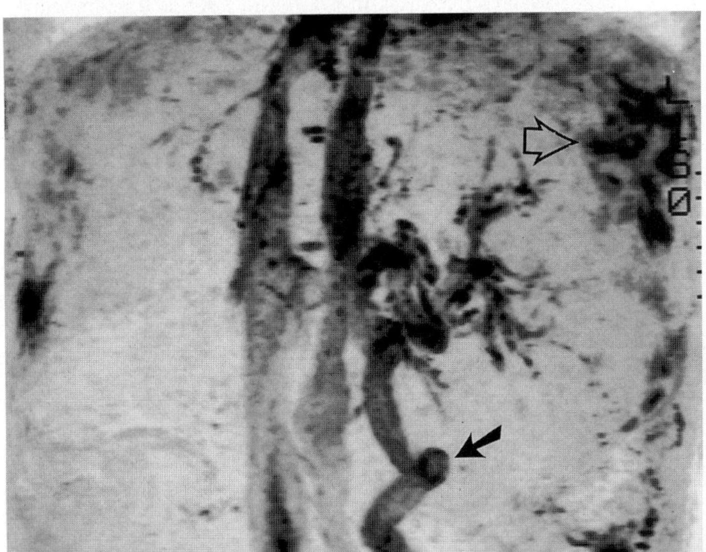

**FIGURE 14** MRA of portal hypertension. Coronal 2D TOF MRA (TR/TE 33/13 ms, 30° flip-angle, 5 mm slice thickness, 2 NEX, NP, with MIP reconstruction). *A,* Large retroperitoneal collateral *(black arrow)* drains the splenic vein as well as abdominal sidewall collaterals *(open arrowhead)* in a patient with portal vein occlusion secondary to cirrhosis. *B,* Patent portal vein *(black arrow)* and splenic vein with a dilated coronary vein and gastroesophageal varices *(open arrowhead)*. *C,* This 2-year-old patient had portal vein occlusion and cavernous transformation *(curved open arrow)* after umbilical vein catheterization. A spontaneous splenorenal shunt *(curved black arrow)*, gastroesophageal varices *(open arrowhead)*, and paraduodenal varices *(small black arrow)* are observed.

B

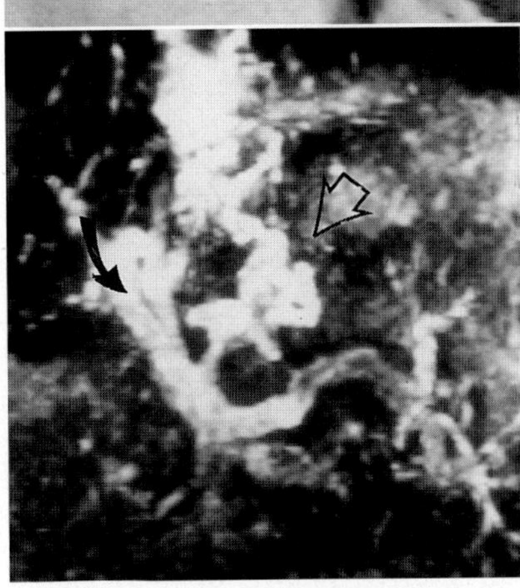

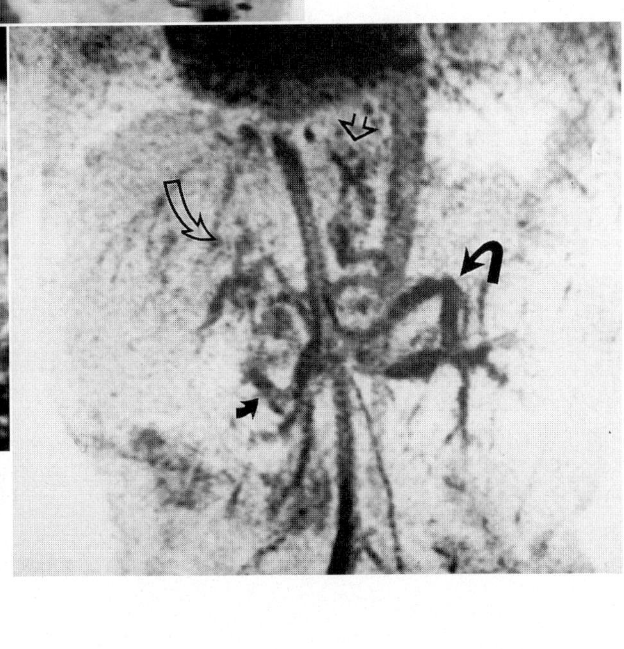

C

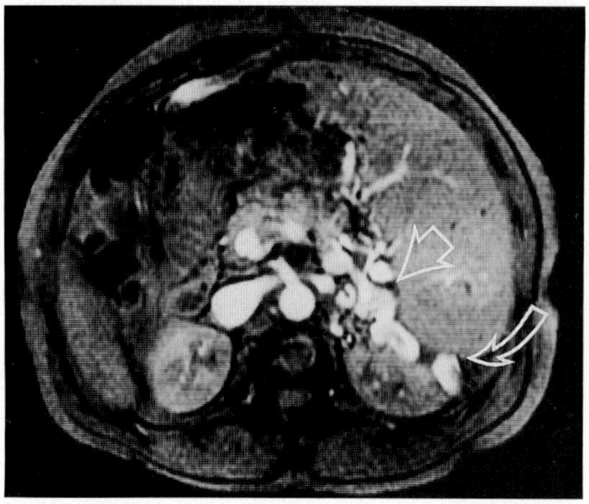

**FIGURE 15** Retroperitoneal and perisplenic varices. Breath-hold axial GRE image (TR/TE 33/13 ms, 30° flip-angle, 5 mm slice thickness, 1 NEX). Raw data image from 2D TOF MRA shows perisplenic *(straight arrow)* and retroperitoneal varices *(curved arrow)*.

gastroesophageal varices via the dilated coronary vein, retroperitoneal shunts, recanalized umbilical veins with caput medusa abdominal wall collaterals, and inferior mesenteric vein to hemorrhoidal vein and iliac vein collateral pathways. Portal vein occlusion and cavernous transformation were also more accurately detected with MRA than with color-flow ultrasonography. MRA can also be used as a noninvasive follow-up modality for portocaval and splenorenal shunts, with the limitation that shunt stenoses may be missed.

#### Hepatic Vein Occlusion

Although MRA is sensitive to flow in the large veins of the liver, segmental branches that are extrinsically compressed may not be seen. Therefore MRA can exclude large vein thromboses but may not be sensitive to smaller vein occlusions seen in Budd-Chiari syndrome.

### *Interpretation and Reliability*

The main advantage of 2D TOF MRA techniques is the detection of portosystemic collaterals. The raw data axial images afford the relevant anatomic clues to localize the locations of the varices (Fig. 15). The presence of varices probably is a better predictor of portal hypertension than the direction of portal vein blood flow.

### *Pitfalls and Artifacts*

The single greatest pitfall of all liver MRA techniques is failure to detect slow flow in the portal vein. The key factors in determining whether blood flow is present or not are the TR, slice thickness, and flip-angle. These three factors determine the minimum velocity that can be detected by TOF techniques. If the TR is set too short, this will not allow for enough flow-related enhancement. This was observed in a pediatric case using ultrashort gradient-echo techniques with the TR reduced to 6 msec. Compared with a TR of 25 msec, this technique was one-fourth as sensitive to slow flow. Another pitfall in interpretation is confusing the portal vein with either an enlarged hepatic artery or collateral vein in the porta hepatis. A key factor in determining whether the blood vessel in the porta hepatis is the portal vein is based on anatomic analysis. The vessel has to branch into the right and left intrahepatic portal vein and originate from the superior mesenteric vein and/or splenic vein. If this cannot be determined, the patency of the portal vein cannot be established with certainty. In addition, care must be taken so that intravoxel dephasing in the interior of the portal vein due to complex flow is not misinterpreted as a thrombus.

## Discussion

This chapter has attempted to include a broad range of information that is necessary to understand the technical factors responsible for the success and limitations of MRA. Currently, there is no single "push-button" technique radiologists can use in all situations. Instead, radiologists must choose from a long menu of options and create the MRA technique that can optimally image the particular clinical indication. The concept of a tailored approach to imaging is one that is familiar to most radiologists. Active research in the areas of pulse sequence design and computer postprocessing is promising to allow even greater use of MRA. However, the future of MRA in the diagnostic imaging evaluation of abdominal and peripheral vascular disease awaits further clinical and pathological correlation.

## Suggested Reading


Dumoulin CL, Yucel EK, Vock P, et al. Two and three dimensional phase contrast MR angiography of the abdomen. JCAT 1990; 145:779–784.

Edelman RR, Wentz KU, Mattle HP, et al. Projection arteriography and venography: Initial clinical results with MR. Radiology 1989; 172:351–357.

Finn JP, Edelman RR, Jenkins RL, et al. Liver transplantation: MR angiography with surgical validation. Radiology 1991; 179:265–269.

Kim D, Edelman RR, Kent KC, et al. Abdominal aorta and renal artery stenosis: Evaluation with MR angiography. Radiology 1990; 174:727–731.

Roubidoux MA, Dunnick NR, Sostman HD, Leder RA. Renal carcinoma: Detection of venous extension with gradient echo imaging. Radiology 1992; 182:269–272.

Spritzer CE, Sussman SK, Blinder RA, et al. Deep venous thrombosis evaluation with limited flip angle, gradient refocussed MR imaging: Preliminary experience. Radiology 1988; 166:371–375.

Steinberg FL, Dumoulin CL, Deutsch AL. MR angiography. In: Deutsch AL, Mink JH, Kerr R, eds. MRI of the Foot and Ankle. New York: Raven Press, 1992, 313–344.

Steinberg FL, Yucel EK, Dumoulin CL, Souza SP. Peripheral vascular and abdominal applications of MR flow imaging techniques. Magn Reson Med 1989; 14:315–320.

Yucel EK. Magnetic resonance angiography of the lower extremity and renal arteries. Semin Ultrasound CT MRI 1992; 13:291–302.

Yucel EK, Steinberg FL. Lower extremity and renal angiography. In: Potchen EJ, Haacke EM, Siebert JE, Gottshalk A, eds. Magnetic Resonance Angiography: Concepts and Applications. St. Louis: Mosby-Year Book, 1992.

# Ultrasound Diagnosis of the Peripheral Vasculature

E. KENT YUCEL, M.D.

The application of duplex Doppler and color-flow Doppler techniques to peripheral vascular imaging, in combination with the use of high-frequency transducers and new examination techniques, have dramatically extended our ability to noninvasively image peripheral venous and arterial disease.

## Lower-Extremity Venous Thrombosis

The traditional approach to noninvasive diagnosis of lower-extremity deep venous thrombosis (DVT) has relied on indirect evaluation of venous outflow using continuous-wave Doppler or impedance plethysmography. These methods, which rely on abnormalities of flow to detect DVT, have several major limitations. Sensitivity is limited by the inability to detect small, nonocclusive thrombi and calf DVT, while specificity is limited because any disorder that decreases venous outflow (e.g., extrinsic compression, right heart failure, chronic thrombophlebitis) can yield a false-positive result. Owing to these limitations, frequent recourse to venography was necessary. Compression ultrasonography (CUS) has revolutionized the noninvasive approach to DVT by rendering venography obsolete in most instances. When properly performed, CUS has been shown to have a sensitivity of 95 percent and specificity of 99 percent. Therefore venography is not required in the vast majority of instances, either to confirm a positive diagnosis or to exclude DVT above the calf.

The performance of CUS is extremely simple and easy to master. The key to its proper performance is the use of high-frequency linear transducers ($\geq$5 MHz). The femoral vein is examined with the patient in the supine position and with the leg slightly externally rotated. The common femoral vein and artery are identified in the transverse plane (vein medial). Gentle compression is applied, which causes complete obliteration of the normal vein lumen (Fig. 1). When thrombus is present in the vein, it is not possible to compress the lumen completely (Fig. 2). The examination is carried cephalad to the point where the external iliac vein dives into the pelvis and is obscured by bowel gas. The examination is then carried inferiorly to the point where the femoral vein is lost in the adductor canal. The patient is then turned into the prone or lateral decubitus position (affected side up) with the knee slightly flexed. Alternatively, the patient can remain supine while the leg is externally rotated and knee slightly flexed to allow access to the popliteal fossa. The popliteal vein and artery are then identified at their most superficial point in the popliteal fossa (vein posterior), and the vein is followed cephalad into the adductor canal and caudad to its trifurcation.

Several technical points are worthy of note. The exact degree of compression required to completely obliterate the vein lumen varies from patient to patient, depending on body habitus, presence of leg edema, depth of the vessel segment being examined, and history of thrombosis. No hard-and-fast rules can be given, and the operator's skill in this aspect of the examination improves with experience as he or she examines a wide variety of patients. It is important to remember that thrombus, especially when acute, can be partially (but never completely) compressible. The inexperienced operator must be alert to the possibility of thrombosis when firm compression causes marked but incomplete compression of the vessel. Care must be taken when examining the popliteal fossa to use minimal pressure initially lest the popliteal vein be inadvertently compressed, making the lumen difficult or impossible to identify. Slight flexion of the knee is also necessary to prevent extrinsic compression of the popliteal vein, which can also obliterate the lumen.

Despite the enthusiasm with which it has been received, CUS does have some limitations. The iliac veins are usually obscured by bowel gas and cannot be routinely imaged. Fortunately, iliac vein thrombosis is usually associated with femoral DVT. However, in cases of pelvic pathology or surgery, thrombus may be limited to the iliac vein. Normally flow in the femoral vein is spontaneous and varies with respiration.

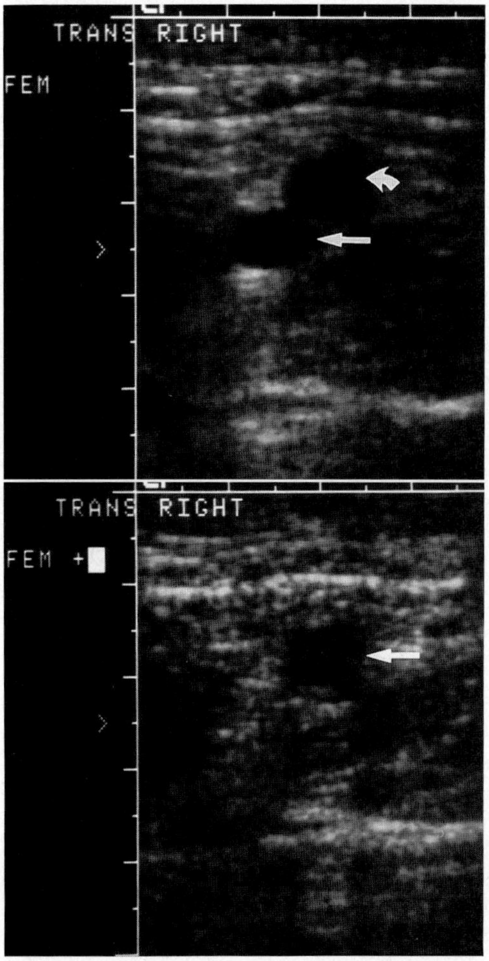


A

B

**FIGURE 1** *A,* The femoral vein *(curved arrow)* and artery *(straight arrow)* are observed in the transverse plane without compression. The vein is medial and superficial to the artery at this level. *B,* With compression, the femoral vein lumen is completely obliterated and only the femoral artery *(straight arrow)* is observed.

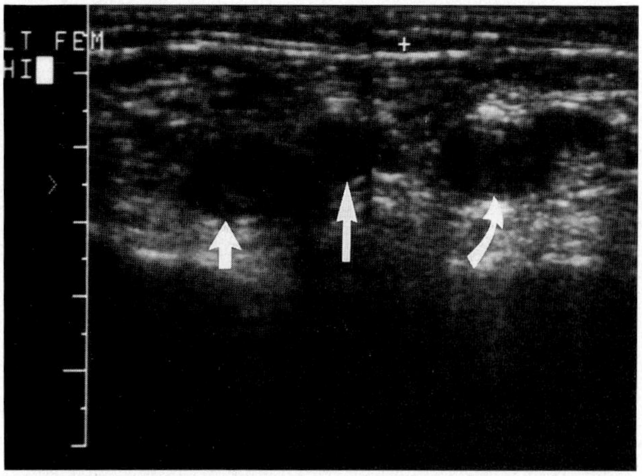


**FIGURE 2** The femoral vein *(short straight arrow)* contains echogenic material on the noncompressed image. Note the adjacent femoral artery *(long straight arrow)*. The vein lumen can still be visualized with compression *(curved arrow)*, indicating that it is filled with thrombus. Note that the adjacent artery is partially compressed, indicating that a substantial amount of force has been used.

Performance of the Valsalva maneuver causes spontaneous flow to cease, and release of the Valsalva maneuver causes marked augmentation of forward flow. Diminished spontaneous flow in the femoral vein with absence of normal respiratory variation, including response to the Valsalva maneuver, suggests iliac vein obstruction. However, as with any indirect test of venous function, extrinsic and intrinsic venous obstruction cannot be differentiated. When there is doubt as to the possibility of iliac vein thrombosis, venography is indicated.

Chronic, recurrent thrombophlebitis represents another difficult problem. After an episode of DVT, the vein may return to a normal appearance or may have residual abnormalities such as wall thickening, diminished compressibility, synechia formation, or complete occlusion. Chronic thrombophlebitis is the setting in which a false-positive CUS examination is most likely to occur. Although acute thrombus tends to be hypoechoic and to enlarge the vein, the converse is not reliable in assessing the age of thrombus. Venography is often necessary to separate acute from chronic DVT.

The calf veins have been considered a blind area for all noninvasive tests for DVT, including CUS. However, recent work has shown that calf DVT can be diagnosed by CUS. The paired posterior tibial and peroneal veins can be identified along the medial and central aspects of the calf, respectively (Fig. 3). The sural veins can be identified within the calf muscles. Criteria for diagnosis of calf DVT are the same as those used for diagnosis of femoropopliteal DVT. The use of higher-frequency transducers (e.g., 7 MHz) and distending the veins by having patients sit up and hang their legs over the edge of the stretcher are helpful in evaluating the calf veins. Preliminary results have shown a sensitivity of 88 percent and specificity of 95 percent. CUS is highly sensitive for detecting extensive calf thrombus and most likely to miss small focal thrombi. By themselves, such thrombi are unlikely to be a source of pulmonary embolism, but there is a small but definite risk of thrombus extension. Therefore, in patients with an initially negative ultrasonographic study, a follow-up sonogram or venogram is recommended in 3 to 5 days if calf symptoms persist.

Recently, color Doppler has been applied to the evaluation of DVT. Although it is not necessary for routine DVT evaluation, color Doppler has some potential applications. The color examination may be performed in either the transverse or longitudinal planes. Care must be taken to lower the color Doppler velocity scale to the minimum and to angulate the beam cephalad or caudad, either manually or electronically. Augmentation of flow by gentle, intermittent calf compression is helpful in optimizing the color signal. Color Doppler can be used to demonstrate thrombus in a manner comparable to venography. Instead of iodinated contrast material, the color-encoded flow signal is used to demonstrate the patent lumen and to outline acute thrombus as a "filling defect" (Fig. 4 and Color Plate 18). Color Doppler is especially helpful in shortening the learning curve for the beginning operator and can help speed the examination by helping to clarify problem areas. In particular, the vein in the deepest portion of the adductor canal can be difficult to compress and color Doppler can be used to document patency of this segment. Similarly, color can be helpful in patients in whom obesity or leg edema make compression of the vein difficult. Color Doppler can detect thrombus in the deep femoral vein, which is often difficult to evaluate by routine CUS as well as venography (Fig. 5 and Color Plate 19).

Color Doppler may also be helpful in the setting of chronic thrombophlebitis. Color can be used to document a patent lumen and exclude acute DVT in patients with chronically thickened vein walls and relatively incompressible veins. Color Doppler can rapidly and accurately detect the presence of venous reflux in patients with postphlebitic venous stasis ulceration (Fig. 6 and Color Plate 20). Color Doppler may be

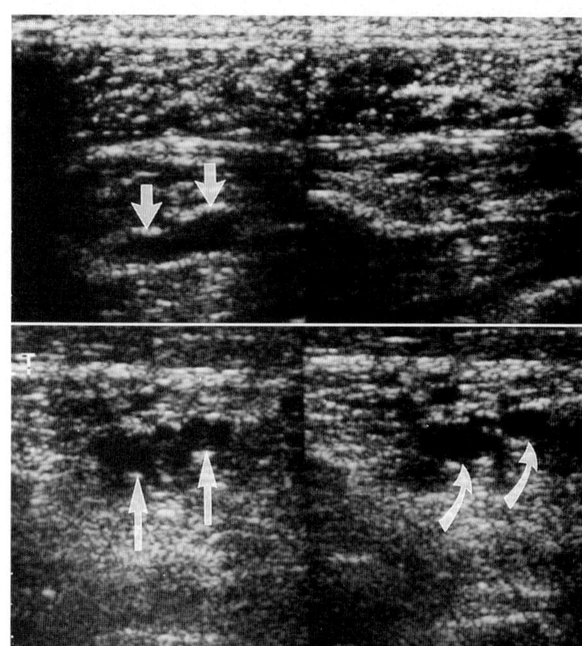

A

B

**FIGURE 3** *A,* Without compression, the paired peroneal veins are well seen *(arrows, left)* using a 7 MHz transducer and having the patient hang his legs off the side of the stretcher. With compression *(right)* the veins completely disappear. *B,* In this patient with peroneal vein thrombosis, the peroneal veins cannot be compressed (without compression, *straight arrows;* with compression, *curved arrows*). (From Yucel EK, et al. Compression ultrasound diagnosis of isolated calf vein thrombo[illegible] Radiology 1991; 179:443–446; with permission.)

A

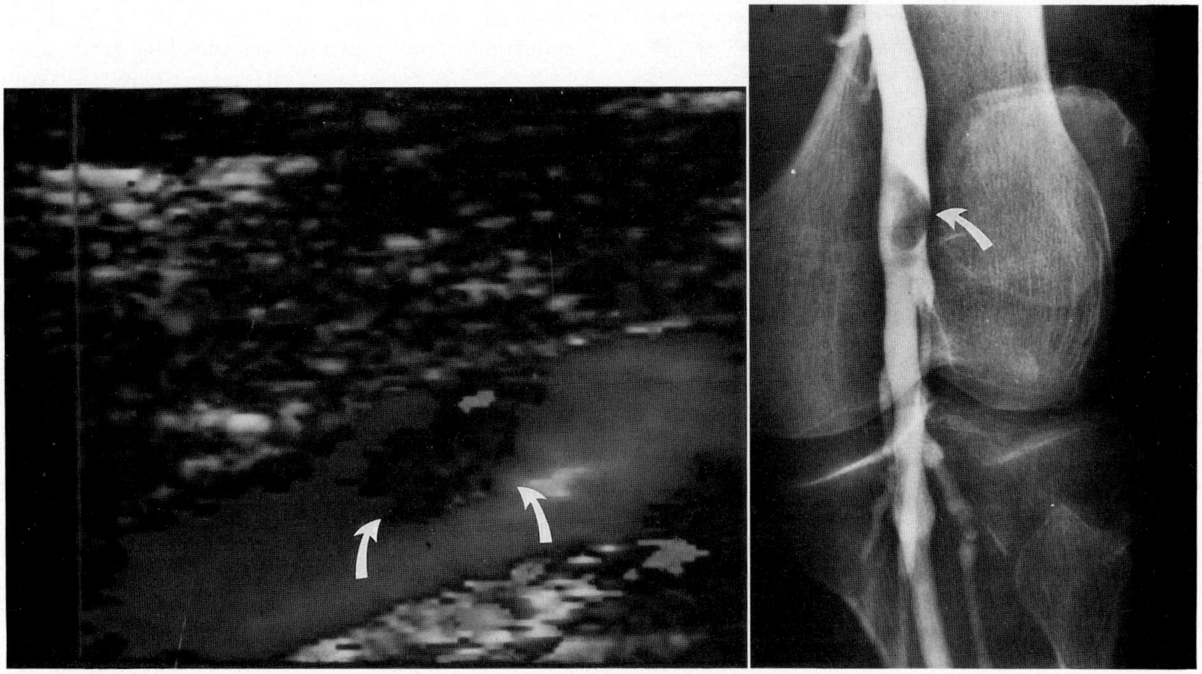

B

**FIGURE 4** *A,* Longitudinal color Doppler image of the popliteal vein *(reproduced here in black and white)* demonstrates color signal surrounding a thrombus *(curved arrows),* exactly comparable to the corresponding venographic image *(B).* See also Color Plate 18.

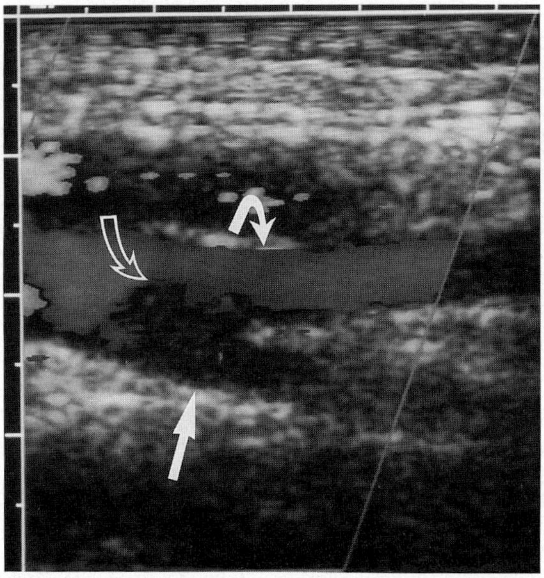

**FIGURE 5** Longitudinal color Doppler image *(reproduced here in black and white)* demonstrates normal flow in the superficial femoral vein *(curved arrow).* Thrombus fills the deep femoral vein *(straight arrow)* and extends into the lumen of the common femoral vein *(open arrow).* See also Color Plate 19.

A B C D

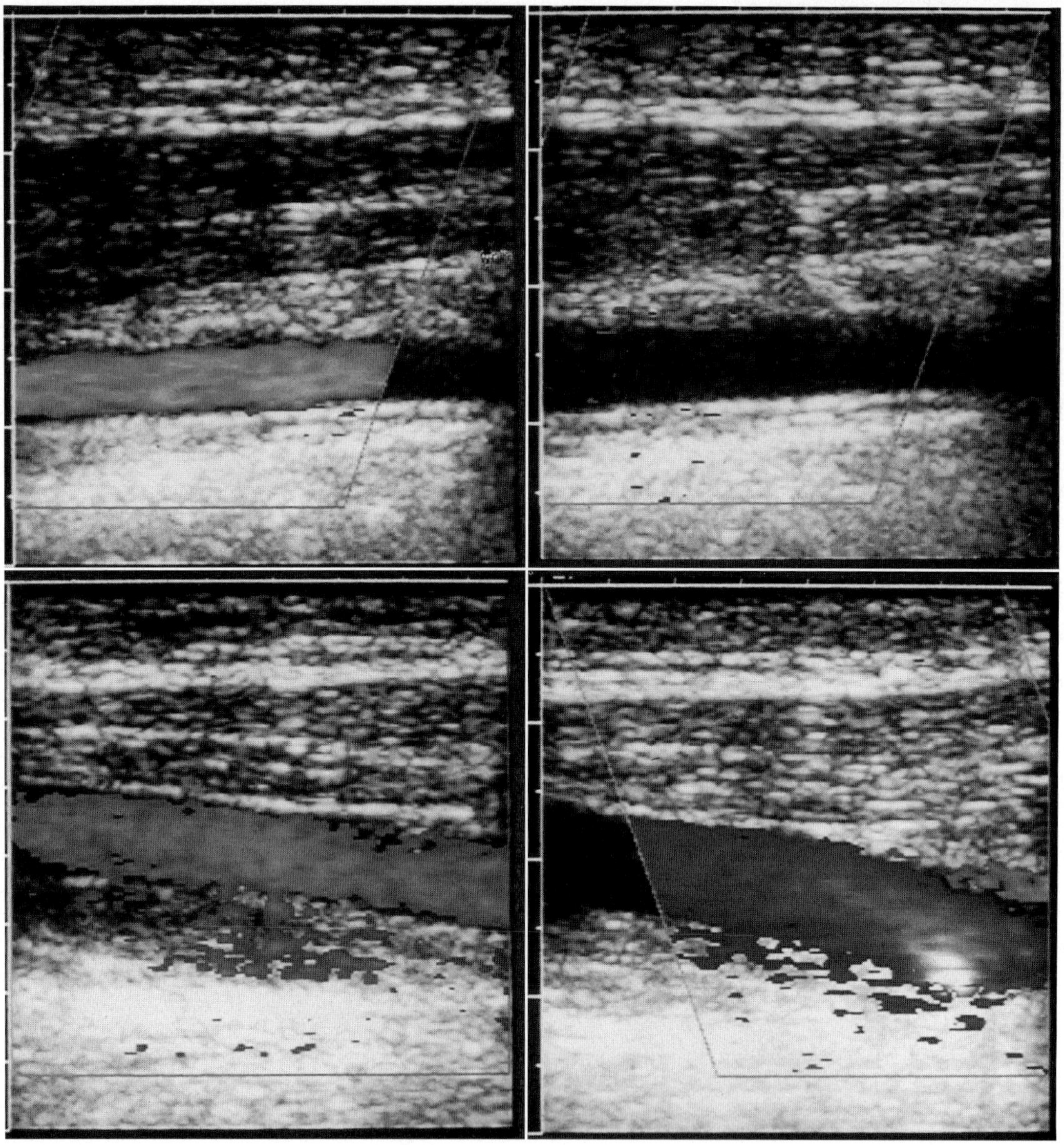

**FIGURE 6** *A,* Normal femoral vein demonstrates antegrade flow in red. *B,* With the Valsalva maneuver, flow in the normal femoral vein ceases completely. *C,* In this femoral vein in a patient with chronic venous ulceration, normal antegrade flow is red. *D,* With the Valsalva maneuver, retrograde flow in blue is detected, indicating venous valvular insufficiency. (*Note:* Colors are not visible in these black-and-white images; see Color Plate 20 for color reproduction.)

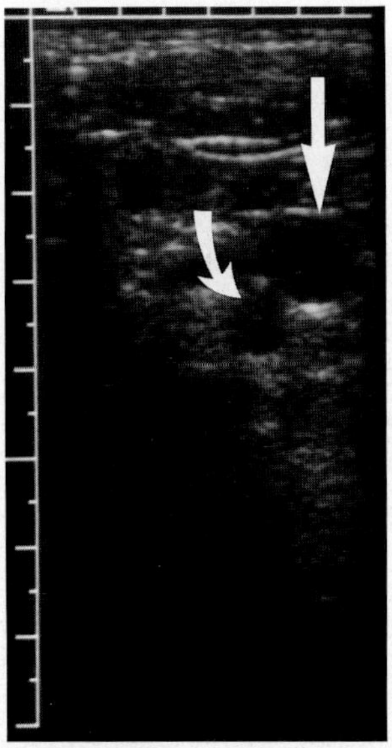

**FIGURE 7** In this sagittal gray-scale image, the larger subclavian vein *(straight arrow)* is observed in cross section, anterior and inferior to the subclavian artery *(curved arrow)*.

helpful in evaluation of the calf veins, both to identify clot within the veins and to locate the tibial veins by identifying their accompanying arteries.

## Upper-Extremity Venous Disease

Color Doppler techniques have had a major impact on evaluation of the upper-extremity veins. The subclavian vein is not readily compressible through much of its course, and Doppler techniques are essential to document venous patency. Color Doppler has the advantage over duplex Doppler of being more rapid and more accurate in the diagnosis of nonocclusive thrombus. The examination begins with the patient supine and with the arm at his or her side. Initially, the transducer is placed below the clavicle in the midclavicular line and a sagittal image is obtained. This view shows the subclavian artery and vein next to each other in cross section. The vein is typically larger and located anterior and inferior to the artery (Fig. 7). Duplex Doppler tracings may also be obtained to definitively identify the vessels. It is crucial to identify the subclavian vein in its normal location next to the artery in the sagittal plane. Otherwise, one can be easily led in cases of subclavian vein thrombosis to mistakenly follow chest wall collateral veins, which can be large and mimic the course of the subclavian vein in the axial plane. Once the subclavian vein is identified in its normal location in the sagittal plane, the transducer can be turned longitudinal to the vein in the axial oblique plane, color Doppler turned on, and the vein followed laterally to the axilla and medially to where it disappears beneath the clavicle (Fig. 8 and Color Plate 21).

Subclavian vein thrombosis is identified by lack of color signal in the vein or color surrounding a filling defect within the vein lumen (Fig. 9 and Color Plate 22). If necessary, augmentation of venous flow can be obtained by manual compression of the patient's upper arm. The transducer is then moved to the neck and the internal jugular vein imaged in the axial plane. Although color Doppler examination can also be used for the jugular vein, it is readily compressible, much like the femoral vein. This vein is then followed inferiorly in the axial plane. As one approaches the clavicle from above, the vein is followed while the transducer is rotated into the coronal plane, which gives the operator a view of the superior portion of the brachiocephalic vein where the subclavian and internal jugular veins join. At this point the veins become incompressible again and color Doppler is helpful in assessing patency. Ultrasonography is not generally capable of directly imaging the more central portions of the brachiocephalic veins or the superior vena cava (SVC). Indirect signs of central venous obstruction, such as diminished flow and decreased respiratory variation, should alert the operator to the possible presence of brachiocephalic or SVC thrombosis, which can then be pursued by venography, computed tomography, or magnetic resonance imaging.

Another application of Doppler examination to the upper extremity is in the evaluation of dialysis fistulas. Duplex Doppler is highly accurate in the identification of thrombosis (Fig. 10) and efferent (venous) limb stenosis. To identify efferent limb stenosis, it is important to follow the venous outflow from the fistula all the way to the subclavian vein, because venous stenosis can occur at any level. In one study, efferent limb stenosis was accurately identified by a maximum Doppler shift of 8 kHz, which corresponds to a velocity of about 2 m/sec with a 5 MHz transducer and 45 to 60° angle of incidence (Fig. 11). Duplex techniques were less accurate in identifying afferent limb (arterial) stenoses.

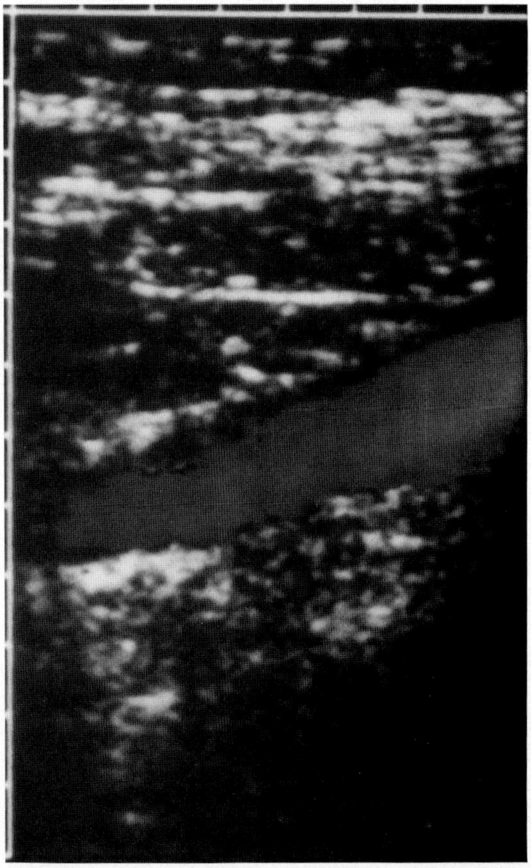

**FIGURE 8** Normal flow in the subclavian vein is displayed in blue (not visible here) in this image taken along the long axis of the vein. See also Color Plate 21.

A 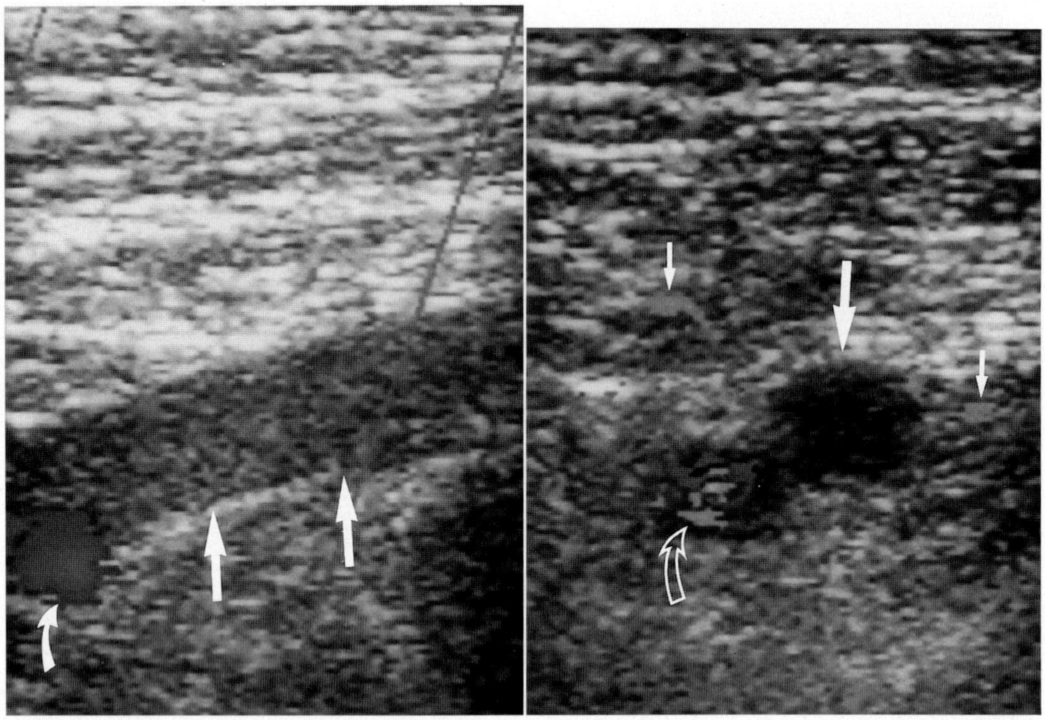 B

**FIGURE 9** *A,* Long- and *(B)* short-axis views of the subclavian vein *(straight arrows),* which is filled with hypoechoic thrombus. A small area of residual flow is displayed within the vein *(curved arrow, A).* Collateral veins *(small arrows)* and the normal subclavian artery *(open arrow)* are also displayed in *(B).* See also Color Plate 22.

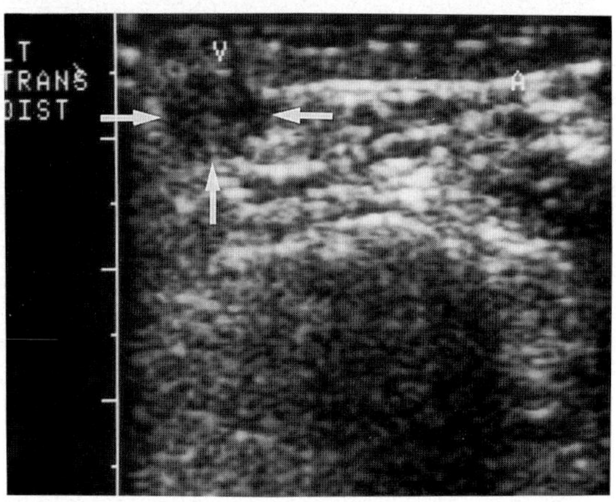


**FIGURE 10** Thrombosis of the efferent limb of a dialysis fistula is identified as echogenic thrombus filling the vein lumen *(arrows)* on this transverse gray-scale image.

## Lower-Extremity Arterial Disease

Duplex ultrasonography has been touted as a potential modality for the evaluation of native vessel atherosclerotic occlusive disease. Unfortunately this potential has not been realized for several reasons. First, it cannot replace segmental pressure measurements and plethysmography. These are the standard noninvasive studies used in the investigation of claudication and give unique hemodynamic information that the surgeon uses to complement the anatomic data on the angiogram. On the other hand, sonography cannot compete with angiography owing to difficulties in adequately visualizing the iliac and tibial arteries, the former because of overlying bowel gas and the latter because of their number, depth, and small size. Standard duplex sonographic criteria of a twofold velocity acceleration for arterial stenosis and absence of flow for arterial occlusion can be applied to the femoral and popliteal arteries. Duplex sonograms can be used to identify candidates for femoropopliteal angioplasty before arteriography by separating patients with long occlusions, who require bypass surgery, from those with short occlusions and focal stenoses, for whom angioplasty might be a suitable alternative to surgery.

Unlike its questionable role in native vessel occlusive disease, ultrasonography has several important roles to play in graft evaluation. Before bypass surgery, color Doppler sonograms can be used to identify, measure, and map on the skin the greater and lesser saphenous veins (Fig. 12). Inadequacy of the vein owing to small size, discontinuity, chronic thrombophlebitis, and varicosities can be readily identified preoperatively. This is especially helpful in patients who have had previous vein harvesting performed. After surgery, arteriovenous fistulas (AVFs) from in situ grafts can be readily identified using color Doppler and marked on the skin and anastomotic pseudoaneurysms (Fig. 13) can be evaluated. Duplex Doppler can be used to identify infrainguinal bypass graft stenosis before graft failure. Peak systolic velocities <45 cm/sec within the graft can be used to identify the presence of an obstructive lesion. Examination of the entire length of the graft for focal doubling of peak systolic velocity can accurately identify the site of stenosis (Fig. 14 and Color Plate 23). The use of duplex Doppler as part of the routine screening of infrainguinal bypass

A

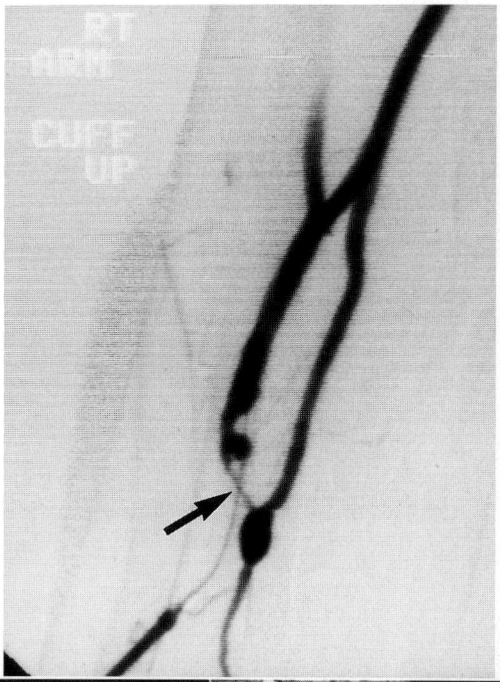


B

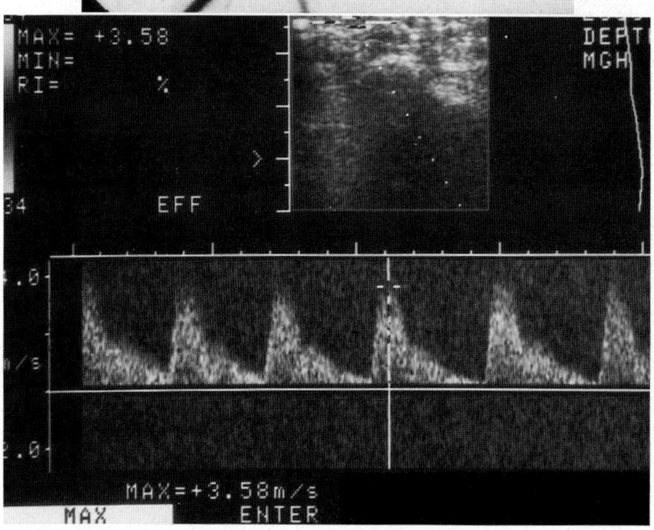


**FIGURE 11** Efferent limb stenosis *(arrow, A)* can be identified by peak systolic velocity >3.5 m/sec on Doppler tracing *(B)*.

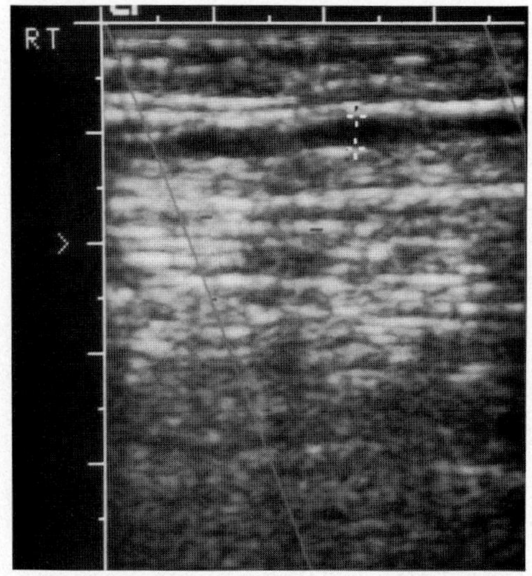


**FIGURE 12** Long-axis gray-scale image of the greater saphenous vein (between calipers).

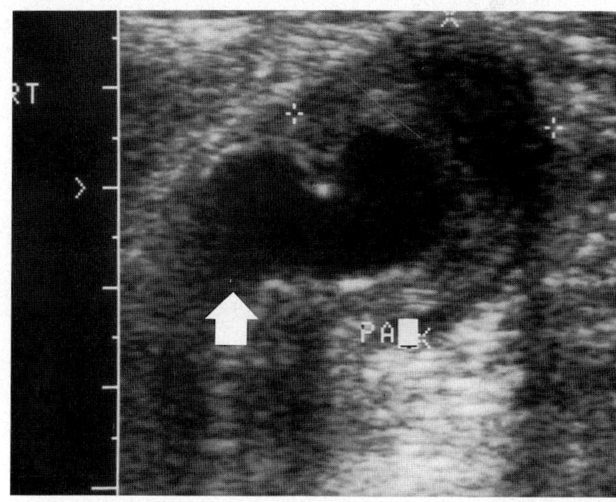

**FIGURE 13** Transverse gray-scale image demonstrates a thrombus-containing pseudoaneurysm (between calipers) arising from a graft *(arrow)* anastomosis.

grafts improves the detection rate of significant graft stenoses before graft failure in comparison to plethysmography and segmental pressure measurements alone.

Additional conditions that are amenable to color Doppler evaluation include native vessel aneurysms and postcatheterization AVFs and pseudoaneurysms. Both true aneurysms and pseudoaneurysms can be diagnosed by simple gray-scale ultrasonography. However, in the case of true aneurysms, such as aneurysms of the popliteal artery, the addition of color Doppler is helpful in identifying mural thrombus, which can be an important factor in identifying patients for surgery. In the case of pseudoaneurysms, color imaging can be used to identify the neck of the pseudoaneurysm (Fig. 15 and Color Plate 24), and sonographically guided manual compression has even been used as definitive treatment of this condition.

AVFs are rarer complications of catheterization. Duplex Doppler can be used to identify the source artery by finding low-resistance flow in the involved vessel (deep, superficial, or common femoral artery) with normal high-resistance flow elsewhere (Fig. 16). Color imaging, however, is essential in actually identifying the fistula itself, because these are usually small and difficult or impossible to observe by gray-scale imaging alone (Fig. 17 and Color Plate 25).

## Arteriovenous Malformations

Extremity and facial soft-tissue AVMs exhibit characteristic appearances on color and duplex Doppler sonograms. With color ultrasonography, numerous enlarged arterial and venous channels are observed. On duplex Doppler examination a

A

B

C

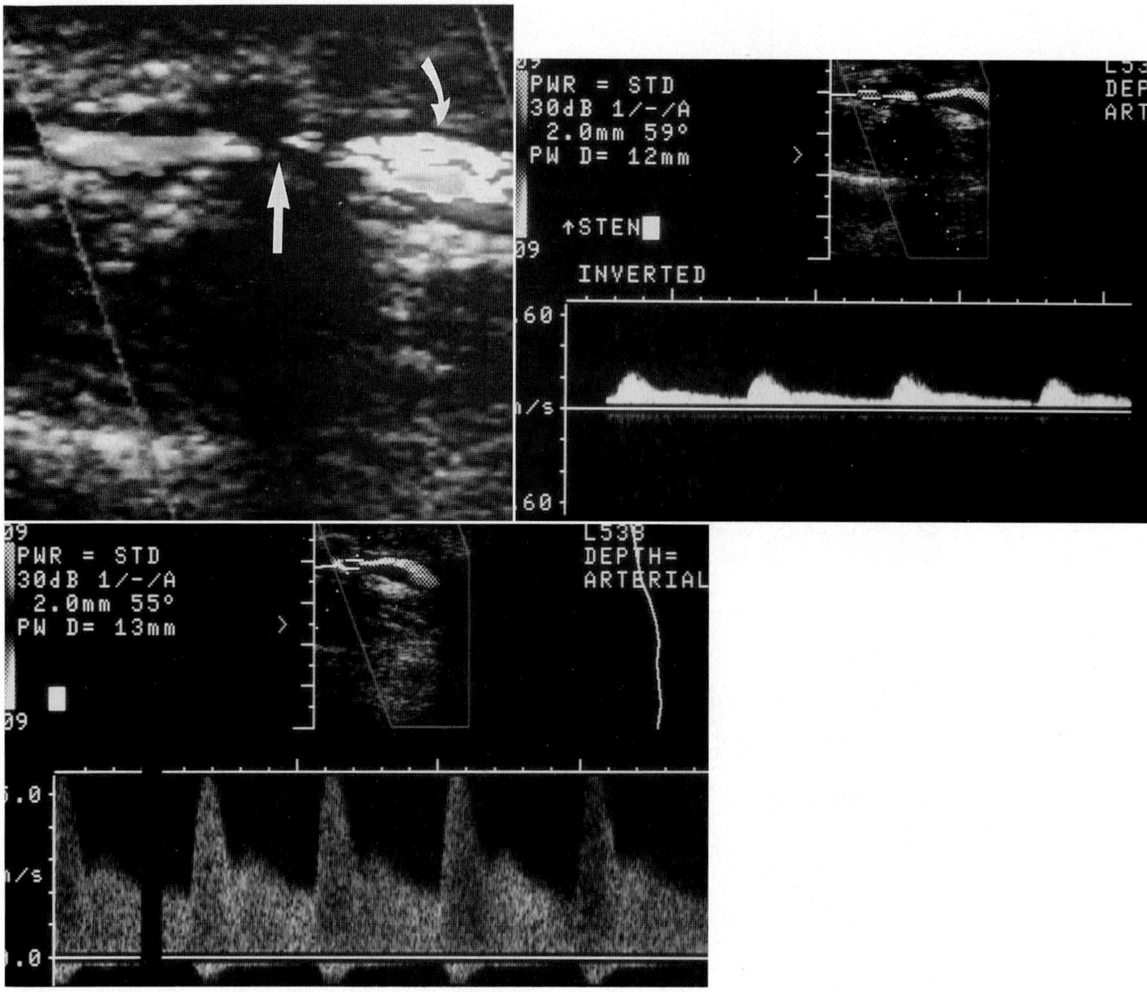


**FIGURE 14** *A,* Longitudinal color Doppler image of a bypass graft *(reproduced here in black and white)* demonstrates narrowing of the lumen *(straight arrow)* and marked velocity acceleration *(curved arrow),* indicating a significant stenosis. See also Color Plate 23. *B,* Proximal to the stenosis graft, velocities are low ( < 30 cm/sec). *C,* At the site of stenosis, peak systolic velocity is > 500 cm/sec, indicating a severe stenosis.

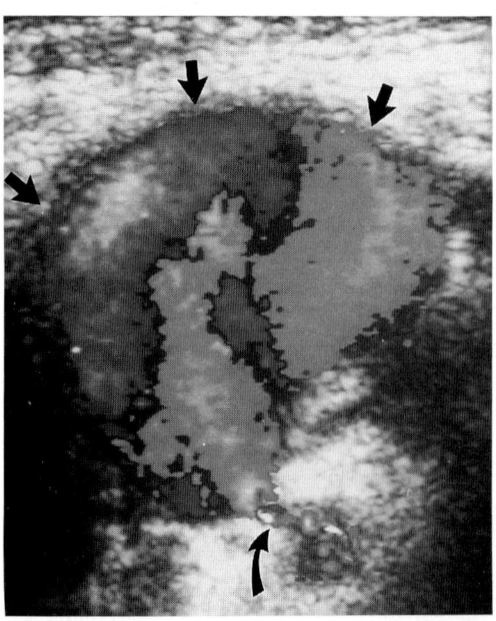

**FIGURE 15** Transverse color Doppler image *(reproduced here in black and white)* of a large postcatheterization axillary artery pseudoaneurysm *(straight arrows).* Note the neck *(curved arrow)* connecting the pseudoaneurysm to the native vessel. See also Color Plate 24.

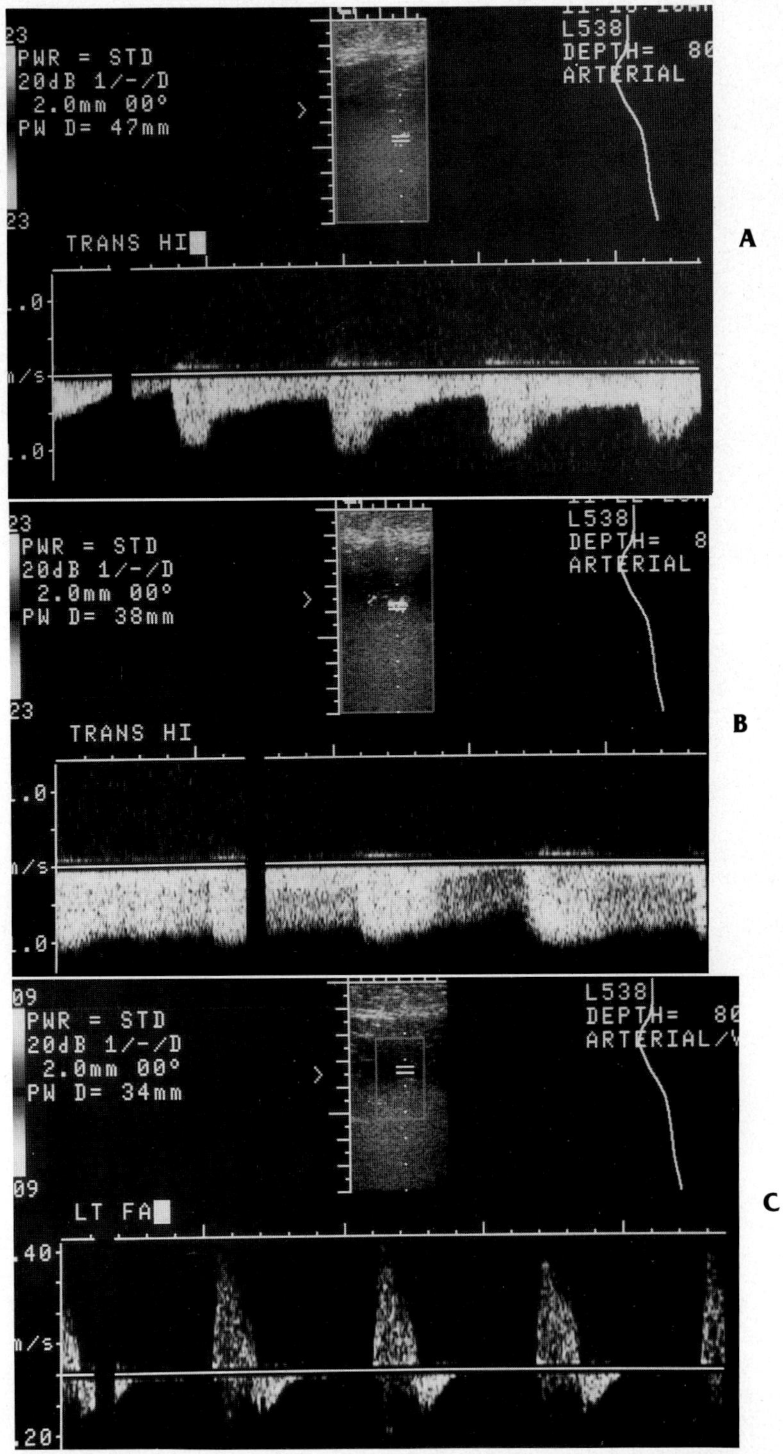


**FIGURE 16** Duplex sonogram of an iatrogenic AVF arising from the common femoral artery. *A,* Proximal to the AVF in the common femoral vein, there is abnormally high flow throughout diastole. *B,* At the site of the AVF, there is turbulent flow throughout the cardiac cycle. *C,* Beyond the AVF in the proximal superficial femoral artery, the waveform returns to the normal high-resistance type, with end-systolic flow reversal and absent flow in diastole.

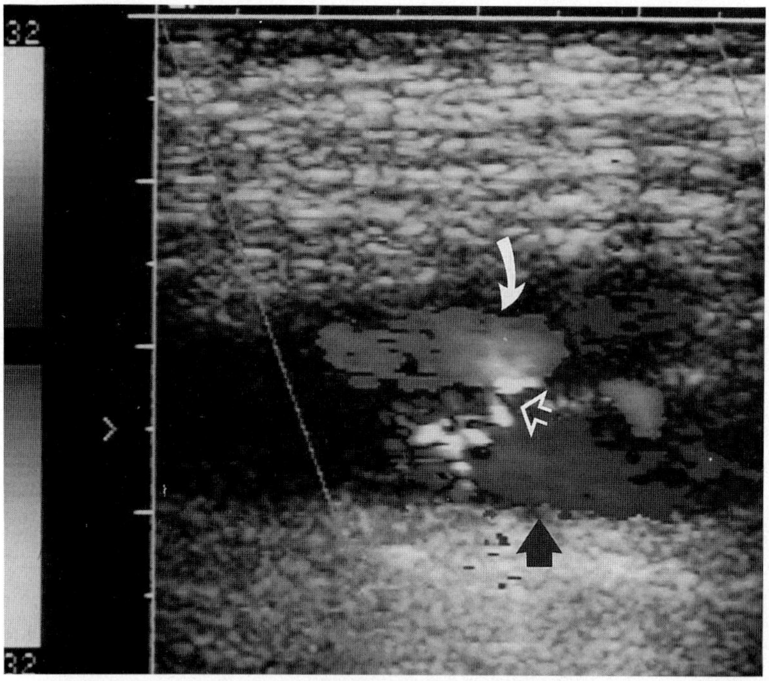

**FIGURE 17** Longitudinal color Doppler image *(reproduced here in black and white)* demonstrates high velocity through an AVF *(open white arrow)* between the superficial femoral artery *(curved white arrow)* and vein *(black arrow)*. See also Color Plate 25.

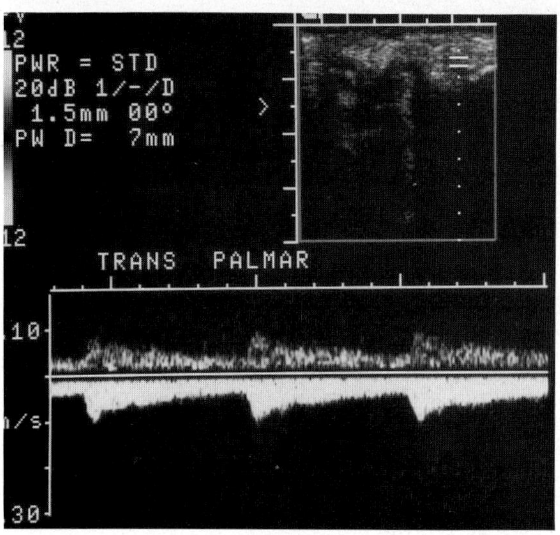


**FIGURE 18** Increased diastolic flow is observed in a palmar artery in this patient with a hand AVM.

low-resistance waveform with increased diastolic flow is observed in the arteries feeding the mass (Fig. 18). Using these techniques, AVMs can be reliably distinguished from venous malformations and hemangiomas, which do not demonstrate increased flow, and from vascular tumors, which have a discrete soft-tissue mass in association with the abnormal vascularity. In addition, soft-tissue extent, response to percutaneous interventions, and recurrence can be assessed.

## Suggested Reading

Bandyk DF, Seabrook GR, Moldenhauer RN. Hemodynamics of vein graft stenosis. J Vasc Surg 1988; 8:688–694.

Knudson GJ, Wiedmeyer DA, Erickson SJ, et al. Color Doppler sonographic imaging in the assessment of upper-extremity deep venous thrombosis. AJR 1990; 154:399–403.

Liu JBL, Merton DA, Mitchell DG, et al. Color Doppler imaging of the iliofemoral region. RadioGraphics 1990; 10:403–412.

Londrey GL, Hodgson KJ, Spadone DP, et al. Initial experience with color-flow duplex scanning of infrainguinal bypass grafts. J Vasc Surg 1990; 12:284–290.

Polak JF, Karmel MI, Meyerovitz MF. Accuracy of color Doppler flow mapping for evaluation of the severity of femoropopliteal arterial disease: A prospective study. JVIR 1991; 2:471–479.

Rose SC, Zweibel WJ, Nelson BD, et al. Symptomatic lower extremity deep venous thrombosis: Accuracy, limitations, and role of color duplex flow imaging in diagnosis. Radiology 1990; 175:639–644.

Tordoir JHM, de Bruin HG, Hoeneveld H, et al. Duplex ultrasound scanning in the assessment of arteriovenous fistulas created for hemodialysis access: Comparison with digital subtraction angiography. J Vasc Surg 1989; 10:122–128.

White RH, McGahan JP, Daschbach MM, Hartling RP. Diagnosis of deep-vein thrombosis using duplex ultrasound. Ann Intern Med 1989; 111:297–304.

Yucel EK, Fisher JS, Egglin TK, et al. Compression ultrasound diagnosis of isolated calf vein thrombosis. Radiology 1991; 179:443–446.

# Duplex Doppler and Color-Flow Imaging of the Abdomen

*EDWARD I. BLUTH, M.D.*

Since the mid-1970s, ultrasonography has been of considerable value in the evaluation of the abdomen. With the advent of Doppler and color-flow Doppler imaging (CFDI), the ability to study abdominal structures has been enhanced. Doppler and, most recently, CFDI have become vital in the evaluation of abdominal structures.

Initially, with articulated arm B-scanners, the subtle abdominal structures were difficult to visualize. With the advent of real-time sonography, the ability to obtain good diagnostic images was much improved. The field of ultrasonography has been challenged by the development of computed tomography (CT) and recently magnetic resonance imaging (MRI) since, with these modalities, reliable and reproducible examinations are easily achieved. Doppler and CFDI add a new dimension to studying the abdominal structures that is different from the other imaging modalities. Another advantage of diagnostic ultrasonography is that it is still far less expensive than CT and MRI. If answers to diagnostic questions can be obtained with these imaging methods, it is incumbent on the medical profession to use the least expensive modality.

## Examination Technique

Routinely I start an abdominal survey by scanning in the midline in the transverse plane with gray-scale only. I quickly survey the course of the abdominal aorta and retroperitoneal structures transversely. I therefore can determine the amount of bowel gas, the size and pattern of the pancreas, and the presence of nodal enlargement. I then turn the transducer 90° and evaluate in the sagittal projection the aorta and inferior vena cava. I evaluate the liver initially sagittally and then transversely. I also turn the transducer obliquely as necessary to image the common bile duct, the common hepatic duct, and the intrahepatic radicals. I quickly evaluate the gallbladder in various projections while the patient is in the supine position. I evaluate first the right kidney, sagittally and transversely. Then I reach across the abdomen to the left side and evaluate first the spleen and then the left kidney. At times, I ask the patient to turn in the right lateral decubitus position to better visualize the left kidney and the spleen. I end the examination by positioning the patient in the left lateral decubitus position to evaluate the gallbladder for subtle calculi, the common bile duct for a second evaluation, and possibly the right kidney if it has not been well seen.

Throughout the examination, I turn the color option on and off to better characterize the structures I am observing. In particular, if a lesion is identified, I always characterize it with CFDI to determine the degree of vascularity or whether vascular structures are displaced, encased, or obstructed. In my opinion, CFDI is an integral part of the routine examination rather than a separate, independent study. The amount of time spent on Doppler and CFDI depends on the questions that must be answered, the structures being studied, and the patient's ability to cooperate. For CFDI to be of added value, a more cooperative patient is usually necessary than with gray-scale alone.

Careful attention to technique is needed to ensure that the highest-frequency transducer is used that will allow the best image resolution. Frequently, transducers must be switched during the evaluation to ensure that all structures are adequately evaluated. When using CFDI, one must be careful to use the correct filter level. If a filter with a level that is too high is used, it may be impossible to detect low frequencies or low-velocity states, and structures will be falsely defined as being avascular. In general, I use either a 3.5 or 5.0 MHz transducer, depending on the patient's body habitus. I have also found a small color-field of view valuable to ensure a maximal frame rate. At times, a transducer with a frequency lower than necessary for optimal imaging is required for a better Doppler evaluation.

## Doppler Principles

An understanding of certain basic physical principles of Doppler is necessary to use CFDI successfully. The best gray-scale images are obtained when the transducer is parallel to the structure being studied, whereas the best Doppler information is obtained when the beam is parallel to the moving object. When the Doppler beam is perpendicular to a moving object, a flow void occurs. In standard duplex scanning, a compromise is made between the optimal image and the best Doppler angle. In duplex scanning the optimal scanning angle is between 45 and 60°. Angles of insonation greater than 70° produce spurious velocity data and flow patterns and should be avoided when possible. When the angle is greater than 70°, progressively smaller frequency shifts are observed, the velocity scale is compressed, and erroneously elevated velocity calculations occur. With CFDI, these frequency elevations appear as changes in color saturation (whiter). Although with CFDI these spurious changes still occur, the true course of tortuous vessels can be more easily observed than with gray-scale alone. With CFDI, a properly compensated Doppler angle that allows the operator to manipulate the velocity scale and produce accurate velocity readings can be chosen more easily than with other modalities.

Another principle is that, with CFDI, frequency shifts can be analyzed not only by using spectral analysis but also by looking carefully at the levels of color saturation. Higher-frequency shifts produce an increase in color saturation toward white. This is true whether the basic color is red or blue. The frequency shift displayed with CFDI is the mean frequency shift and not the peak frequency shift. Peak frequency shifts still must be obtained with pulsed Doppler waveform analysis. Nonmoving targets produce no phase shift and therefore no color. As in gray-scale, the echoes of nonmoving targets are assigned a shade of gray, depending on their amplitude.

The last important physical principle is that aliasing occurs with CFDI, just as it does with standard duplex imaging. In

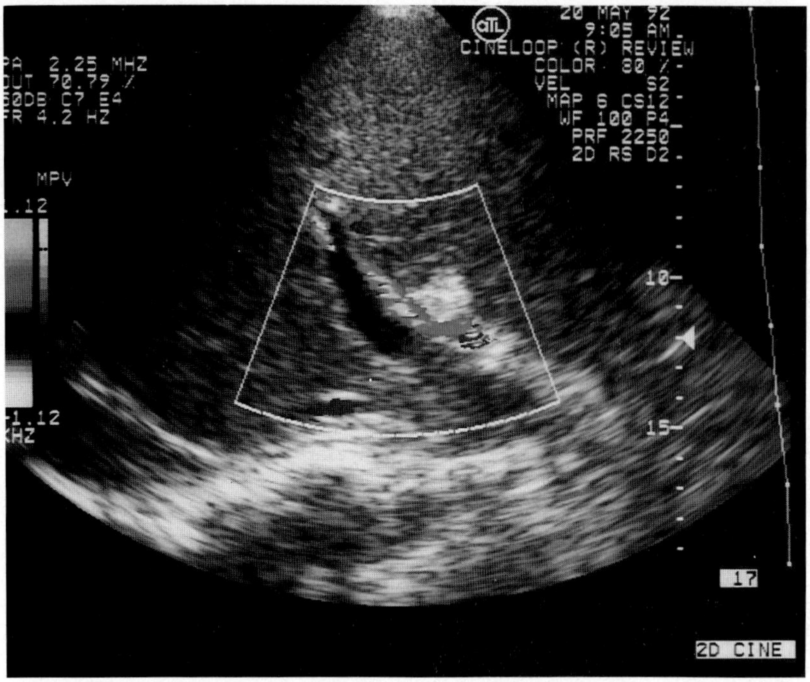


**FIGURE 1** Oblique scan demonstrates dilated obstructed portal vein and prominent hepatic artery, confirmed to represent portal vein thrombosis. See also Color Plate 26.

pulsed Doppler standard systems, when Doppler shifted frequencies exceed the Nyquist limit (one-half of the pulsed repetition frequency) aliasing occurs, resulting in spectral waveforms that appear clipped at the top. The missing spectral data are "wrapped around" and displayed in the negative portion of the frequency window. Similarly, with color systems, aliasing occurs and appears similar to the spectral waveform but appears on the color image as reversed flow or a nonlaminar flow pattern. The examiner must therefore be aware that a pattern of flow reversals or turbulence may be merely a representation of aliasing. To overcome aliasing, one can change the probe position to decrease the tissue path of the vessel, increase the Doppler incidence angle theta, or use a lower-frequency Doppler probe.

## Value of CFDI

Although CFDI is of value in studying and confirming mass lesions of the liver, it has still not significantly improved our ability to distinguish benign from malignant lesions. Cystic lesions are accurately assessed with gray-scale imaging. CFDI is of value to confirm that these are definitely cysts with no flow. Hepatocellular carcinoma has been shown by Taylor to exhibit Doppler shifts of 5 kHz or greater. However, below this frequency shift level, there is overlap among metastatic lesions, hepatocellular carcinoma, and focal nodular hypoplasia. With use of CFDI, Tanaka et al. have shown that hepatocellular carcinomas demonstrate specific characteristic flow patterns; however, others have been unable to discriminate lesions using these findings. In my experience, increased internal and peripheral flow suggests a hepatocellular carcinoma but this is not pathognomonic. Biopsy of solid lesions is still necessary to separate benign from malignant solid mass lesions.

The use of CFDI has dramatically improved our ability to evaluate vascular abnormalities. Our ability to identify vascular lesions such as portal vein thrombosis and Budd-Chiari syndrome has been made possible with CFDI (Fig. 1 and Color Plate 26). CFDI allows the examiner to more easily identify the course of the portal vein. Demonstration of flow in the portal vein rapidly excludes the diagnosis of portal vein thrombosis. The absence of flow in the portal vein, while suggestive of portal vein thrombosis, could also be the result of significantly reduced velocity, as in cases of severe portal hypertension. It can also be a result of technical problems including those caused by wall filter settings. As a result, in my experience, a definitive diagnosis of portal vein thrombosis requires arteriographic correlation. I use CFDI as a screening procedure for portal vein thrombosis because of its high negative predictive value. Similarly, I use CFDI as a screening procedure to visualize and identify as patent all of the hepatic veins and to exclude abnormalities such as Budd-Chiari syndrome. Three hepatic veins are noted to unite at the inferior vena cava. With abnormalities such as cirrhosis or hepatomegaly, the hepatic veins can be displaced or compressed. The patency of these vessels can be difficult to determine without the use of CFDI. Additionally, CFDI is valuable in the identification of venous collaterals, which adds increased confidence in the diagnosis of hepatic vein obstruction. Although these evaluations are frequently time-consuming with CFDI, they are much more difficult if not impossible with gray-scale imaging or standard Doppler alone.

On the other hand, CFDI has not added much to the differentiation of parenchymal liver patterns. The normal liver has uniform echogenicity, midway between that of the more hypoechoic renal cortex and the more echogenic pancreas. CFDI does not add to the specificity of diffuse parenchymal changes, which can be identified with gray scale alone and are observed with abnormalities such as fatty infiltration. Similarly, although sonography plays an important role in the accurate assessment of the gallbladder and bile ducts, CFDI has not added significantly to the evaluation of these structures. On occasion, I have found CFDI useful in distinguishing a dilated intrahepatic bile duct branch from a vascular structure. I have not found it helpful in identifying patients with acute cholecystitis.

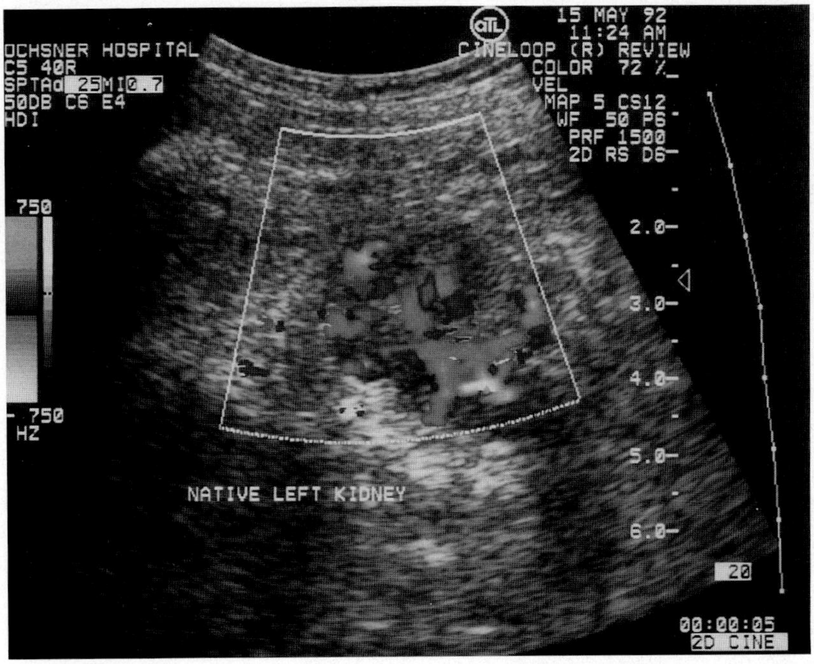


**FIGURE 2** Oblique image of left kidney demonstrates hypervascular mass lesion with increased flow, surgically proven to be a hypernephroma. See also Color Plate 27.

The identification of mass lesions in the pancreas has not been aided with the use of CFDI, since these lesions are not usually vascular. Many people consider CT to be the study of choice, because the whole organ can be visualized and extrapancreatic extension of disease more readily identified if present. Lesions of the gastrointestinal tract have long been identified with gray-scale ultrasonography. Bowel lesions throughout the gut can appear as a "pseudokidney," bull's-eye, or target sign. This occurs when bowel wall thickening occurs as a result of lesions as diverse as Crohn's disease, adenocarcinoma, or ischemia. CFDI does not aid in differentiating the types of lesions present.

In contrast to these uses, CFDI has been of considerable value in improving my diagnostic evaluation of the kidneys. When a solid mass lesion is noted, CFDI should always be used to determine whether tumor vascularity is present. Although not all hypernephromas are vascular, a significant increase in abnormal vessels makes the diagnosis more certain (Fig. 2 and Color Plate 27). Further, CFDI is useful in evaluating the renal veins and inferior vena cava to be certain there is no tumor invasion. I have found CFDI particularly helpful in distinguishing physiologic dilatation from obstructive hydronephrosis. CFDI is helpful in identifying renal vessels, which can be rapidly interrogated; as a result, vascular impedance patterns can be quantitated. In hydronephrosis, as opposed to dilatation, an increase in vascular impedance and the loss of diastolic flow are noted. The evaluation of renal artery stenosis can also be made more accurately and rapidly with CFDI. There are currently two methods: the first evaluates the origin of the renal arteries and the second evaluates the impedance pattern of segmental artery branches.

In the first method, the origin of the renal arteries is identified and velocity measurements are made and compared with the opposite side. A ratio is computed comparing the peak renal artery velocity with the velocity of the abdominal aorta. In normal patients, velocity ratios should not exceed 3.5, and generally the peak velocity is less than 100 cm/s. In the second method, which I find more rapid and easier to perform, segmental arteries are interrogated with Doppler and the waveform is analyzed. It has been my experience and the experience of others that, in cases of renal artery stenosis, there is a decreased acceleration slope as well as rounding and decrease in the peak velocity spectrum. These studies are screening tests, and arteriographic confirmation is still necessary at this time.

## Suggested Reading

Bluth EI, Merritt CRB, Sullivan MA. Ultrasonic evaluation of the stomach, small bowel, and colon. Radiology 1979; 133:677–680.

Grant EG, Tessler FN, Gomes AS, et al. Color Doppler imaging of portosystemic shunts. AJR 1990; 154:393–397.

Merritt CRB. Doppler Color Imaging. New York: Churchill Livingstone, 1992.

Mittelstaedt C. General Ultrasound. New York: Churchill Livingstone, 1992.

Rumack C, Wilson S, Charboneau W, eds. Diagnostic ultrasound. St Louis: Mosby-Year Book, 1991.

Tanaka S, Kitamura T, Fujita M, et al. Color Doppler flow imaging of liver tumors. AJR 1990; 154:509–514.

Taylor KJW, Ramos I, Morse SS, et al. Focal liver masses: Differential diagnosis with pulsed Doppler US. Radiology 1987; 164:643–647.

Tessler FN, Gehring BJ, Gomes AS, et al. Diagnosis of portal vein thrombosis: Value of color Doppler imaging. AJR 1991; 157:293–296.

# INDEX

***f* indicates figure or illustration, *t* indicates table**

**A**

**E**

**F**

## G

**I**

## J



## K



## L

## N

## O



## P

**T**